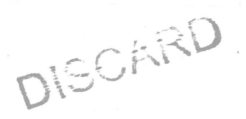

Clinical Pediatric
Urology

Clinical Pediatric Urology

Fourth edition

Edited by

A. Barry Belman, MD, MS
Professor of Urology and Pediatrics
George Washington University
Emeritus Chairman, Department of Pediatric Urology
Children's National Medical Center
Washington, DC, USA

Lowell R. King, MD
Professor of Urology (Emeritus), Duke University Medical School
Department of Surgery, Division of Urology
University of New Mexico Health Sciences Center
Albuquerque, NM, USA

Stephen A. Kramer, MD
Head, Section of Pediatric Urology
Mayo Clinic and Mayo Foundation
Professor of Urology
Mayo Medical School
Rochester, MN, USA

MARTIN DUNITZ

© 2002 Martin Dunitz Ltd, a member of the
Taylor & Francis group

First published in the USA in 1976
Second edition 1985
Third edition 1992
Fourth edition published 2002 by Martin Dunitz Ltd,
The Livery House, 7–9 Pratt Street, London NW1 0AE

Tel.: +44 (0) 20 74822202
Fax.: +44 (0) 20 72670159
E-mail: info.dunitz@tandf.co.uk
Website: http://www.dunitz.co.uk

Although every effort has been made to ensure that all owners of
copyright material have been acknowledged in this publication, we
would be glad to acknowledge in subsequent reprints or editions any
omissions brought to our attention.

The Author has asserted his right under the Copyright, Designs and
Patents Act 1988 to be identified as the Author of this Work.

Although every effort has been made to ensure that drug doses and
other information are presented accurately in this publication, the
ultimate responsibility rests with the prescribing physician. Neither
the publishers nor the authors can be held responsible for errors or
for any consequences arising from the use of information contained
herein. For detailed prescribing information or instructions on the
use of any product or procedure discussed herein, please consult
the prescribing information or instructional material issued by
the manufacturer.

A CIP record for this book is available from the British Library.

ISBN 1 901865 63 0

Produced by Gray Publishing, Tunbridge Wells

Printed and bound in China by Imago

Distributed in the USA by
Fulfilment Center
Taylor & Francis
7625 Empire Drive
Florence, KY 41042, USA
Toll Free Tel.: +1 800 634 7064
E-mail: cserve@routledge_ny.com

Distributed in Canada by
Taylor & Francis
74 Rolark Drive
Scarborough, Ontario M1R 4G2, Canada
Toll Free Tel.: +1 877 226 2237
E-mail: tal_fran@istar.ca

Distributed in the rest of the world by
ITPS Limited
Cheriton House
North Way
Andover, Hampshire SP10 5BE, UK
Tel.: +44 (0)1264 332424
E-mail: reception@itps.co.uk

Contents

Contributors

Ian A. Aaronson, MD, FAAP
Professor of Urology and Pediatrics
Director of Pediatric Urology
Medical University of South Carolina
Charleston, South Carolina

Billy S. Arant, Jr, MD, FAAP
Professor and Chairman
Department of Pediatrics
University of Tennessee
College of Medicine
Chattanooga, Tennessee

Paul F. Austin, MD
Assistant Professor in Surgery (Urology)
Washington University School of Medicine
St Louis Children's Hospital
St Louis, Missouri

Darius J. Bägli, MD, CM, FRCSC, FAAP
Assistant Professor
Department of Surgery
University of Toronto
Staff Urologist
Hospital for Sick Children
Toronto, Ontario

John M. Barry, MD
Professor of Surgery
Chairman
Division of Urology and
Renal Transplantation
Oregon Health Sciences University
Staff Surgeon
Doernbecher Children's Hospital
Portland, Oregon

Julia Spencer Barthold, MD, FAAP
Associate Professor of Urology
Associate Chief, Thomas Jefferson University
Division of Urology
du Pont Hospital
Wilmington, Delaware

Stuart B. Bauer, MD, FAAP
Professor of Surgery (Urology)
Harvard Medical School
Senior Associate in Urology
Children's Hospital
Boston, Massachusetts

A. Barry Belman, MD, MS, FAAP
Professor of Urology and Pediatrics
Emertitus Chairman, Department of Urology
The George Washington University
Children's National Medical Center
Washington, DC

David A. Bloom, MD, FAAP
Professor of Surgery
University of Michigan Medical Center
Ann Arbor, Michigan

Mark P. Cain, MD, FAAP
Assistant Professor, Pediatric Urology
Indiana University School of Medicine
James Whitcomb Riley Hospital for Children
Indianapolis, Indiana

Patrick C. Cartwright, MD, FAAP
Associate Professor of Surgery and Pediatrics
University of Utah
Primary Children's Medical Center
Salt Lake City, Utah

Anthony J. Casale, MD, FAAP
Associate Professor, Urology
Indiana University School of Medicine
James Whitcomb Riley Hospital for Children
Indianapolis, Indiana

Earl Y. Cheng, MD, FAAP
Assistant Professor of Urology
Department of Urology
University of Oklahoma Medical School
Children's Hospital of Oklahoma
Oklahoma City, Oklahoma

Allen M. Chernoff, MD
Assistant Professor of Urology
University of Illinois, Chicago, Illinois

Edith Jacobson Chernoff, MD, FAAP
Medical Genetics Fellow
National Cancer Institute
Bethesda, Maryland

Michael Erhard, MD
Assistant Professor of Urology
Mayo Medical School
Chief, Division of Urology
The Nemours Children's Clinic
Jacksonville, Florida

Fernando A. Ferrer, MD
University of Connecticut Medical School
Connecticut Children's Medical Center
Hartford, Connecticut

Israel Franco, MD, FAAP
Assistant Professor of Urology
New York Medical College
Valhalla, New York

Leo C.T. Fung, MD, FRCS(C), FAAP
Assistant Professor of Urology and Pediatrics
Chief of Pediatric Urology
Director of Pediatric Urology
Research Laboratory
University of Massachusetts Medical Center
Worcester, Massachusetts

Lawrence Gibel, MD
University of New Mexico, Health Sciences Center
Department of Surgery, Division of Urology
Albuquerque, New Mexico

Kenneth I. Glassberg, MD, FAAP
Professor of Urology
Director, Division of Pediatric Urology
State University of New York
Downstate Medical Center
Brooklyn, New York

Richard W. Grady, MD
Assistant Professor of Urology
The University of Washington Medical Center
Children's Hospital and Regional Medical Center
Seattle, Washington

Larry Greenbaum, MD, PhD, FAAP
Assistant Professor of Pediatrics
Department of Pediatrics
Medical College of Wisconsin
Milwaukee, Wisconsin

Yves L. Homsy, MD, FAAP
Children's Urology Group
Clinical Professor of Urological
Surgery and Pediatrics
Director of Pediatric Urology
University of South Florida
Tampa, Florida

Mark Horowitz, MD
Assistant Professor of Urology
Associate Director, Division of
Pediatric Urology
State University of New York
Downstate Medical Center
Brooklyn, New York

Douglas A. Husmann, MD, FAAP
Professor of Urology
Mayo Clinic and Mayo Foundation
Rochester, Minnesota

George W. Kaplan, MD, MS, FAAP
Clinical Professor of Surgery and Pediatrics
Children's Hospital of San Diego
San Diego, California

William E. Kaplan, MD, FAAP
Professor of Urology
Northwestern University
Director, Neuro-Urology
Children's Memorial Hospital
Chicago, Illinois

Evan J. Kass, MD, FAAP
Chairman, Division of Pediatric Urology
Clinical Associate
William Beaumont Hospital
Royal Oak, Michigan

Robert Kay, MD, FAAP
Section of Pediatric Urology
The Cleveland Clinic Foundation
Cleveland, Ohio

Michael A. Keating, MD, FAAP
Clinical Professor of Urology
University of South Florida and
Chairman, Department of Children's Surgery
The Arnold Palmer Hospital for
Children and Women
Orlando, Florida

William A. Kennedy II, MD
Assistant Professor, Associate Chief
of Pediatric Urology
Department of Urology
Stanford University School of Medicine
Stanford, California

Kanwal K. Kher, MD, FAAP
Chairman, Department of Nephrology
Children's National Medical Center
Associate Professor of Pediatrics
The George Washington University
Washington, DC

Antoine E. Khoury, MD, FAAP
Associate Professor
University of Toronto
Head, Division of Urology
The Hospital for Sick Children
Toronto, Ontario, Canada

Lowell R. King, MD, FAAP
Department of Surgery, Division of Urology
University of New Mexico Health Sciences Center
Albuquerque, New Mexico

Harry P. Koo, MD, FAAP
Department of Pediatric Urology
University of Michigan Medical Center
Ann Arbor, Michigan

Martin A. Koyle, MD, FAAP
Chairman, Department of Pediatric Urology
The Children's Hospital
Professor, Departments of Surgery and Pediatrics
University of Colorado School of Medicine
Denver, Colorado

Stephen A. Kramer, MD, FAAP
Professor of Urology
Mayo Medical School
Head, Section of Pediatric Urology
Mayo Clinic and Mayo Foundation
Rochester, Minnesota

Bradley P. Kropp, MD, FAAP
Associate Professor of Urology
Children's Hospital of Oklahoma
Department of Urology
University of Oklahoma Medical School
Oklahoma City, Oklahoma

Yegappan Lakshmanan, MD, FRCS (Ed)
Chief Resident of Urology
University of Massachusetts Memorial Medical Center
Worcester, Massachusetts

Steven E. Lerman, MD
Assistant Professor of Urology
Division of Pediatric Urology
UCLA School of Medicine
Los Angeles, California

Andrew J. Le Roy, MD
Associate Professor of Radiology
Mayo Clinic and Mayo Foundation
Rochester, Minnesota

Padraig S.J. Malone, MD, MCh, FRCSI, FRCS
Consultant Paediatric Urologist
Wessex Regional Centre for Paediatric Surgery
Southampton General Hospital
Southampton, UK

Jane S. Matsumoto, MD
Assistant Professor of Radiology
Mayo Clinic and Mayo Foundation
Rochester, Minnesota

Irene M. McAleer, MD, FAAP
Clinical Assistant Professor of Surgery, (Urology) and
Pediatrics, University of California
Children's Hospital of San Diego
San Diego, California

Jack W. McAninch, MD, FACS
Professor of Urology
University of California
San Francisco, California

Patrick H. McKenna, MD, FAAP
Professor of Surgery
Chairman, Division of Urology
Southern Illinois University School of Medicine
Springfield, Illinois

Gordon A. McLorie, MD, FAAP
Associate Professor, University of Toronto
Staff Urologist, The Hospital for Sick Children
Toronto, Ontario
Canada

Paul A. Merguerian, MD, FRCS(C), FAAP
Associate Clinical Professor of Pediatric Surgery
University of California
San Francisco
Fresno, California

Michael E. Mitchell, MD, FAAP
Professor of Urology
University of Washington Medical School
Director of Pediatric Urology
Children's Hospital and Regional Medical Center
Seattle, Washington

Allen F. Morey, MD, FACS
Chief, Urology Service
Brooke Army Medical Center
San Antonio, Texas

Marva Moxey-Mims, MD, FAAP
Department of Nephrology
Children's National Medical Center
Clinical Associate Professor of Pediatrics
George Washington University
Medical Center
Washington, DC

Sara M. O'Hara, MD
Department of Radiology
Children's Hospital Medical Center
Cincinnati, Ohio

Hans G. Pohl, MD
Division of Urology
Children's Hospital
Boston, Massachusetts

William G. Reiner, MD
Associate Professor
Division of Child and Adolescent Psychiatry
Division of Pediatric Urology
Johns Hopkins Medical Institutions
Baltimore, Maryland

Richard C. Rink, MD, FAAP
Robert A. Garrett Professor of
Pediatric Urologic Research
Indiana University School of Medicine
Chief, Pediatric Urology
James Whitcomb Riley Hospital for Children
Indianapolis, Indiana

Michael L. Ritchey, MD, FAAP
C. R. Bard, Inc. and Edward J. McGuire
Distinguished Chair and Director
Division of Urology
Professor of Surgery and Pediatrics
University of Texas –
Houston Medical School

Kenneth N. Rosenbaum, MD, FAAP
Associate Professor of Pediatrics
George Washington University
Director, Perinatal Genetics
Children's National Medical Center
Washington, DC

H. Gil Rushton, MD, FAAP
Professor of Urology and Pediatrics,
The George Washington University
Chairman, Department of Urology
Children's National Medical Center
Washington, DC

Joseph W. Segura, MD
Department of Urology
Mayo Clinic and Mayo Foundation
Rochester, Minnesota

Curtis A. Sheldon, MD, FAAP
Professor of Surgery
University of Cincinnati Medical Center
Director, Pediatric Urology
Children's Hospital Medical Center
Cincinnati, Ohio

Linda M. Dairiki Shortliffe, MD, FAAP
Professor and Chair
Chief of Pediatric Urology
Department of Urology
Stanford University School of Medicine
Stanford, California

Steven J. Skoog, MD, FAAP
Professor of Surgery and Pediatrics
Director of Pediatric Urology
Doernbeckers Children's Hospital
Oregon Health Science University
Portland, Oregon

Brent W. Snow, MD, FAAP
Professor of Surgery and Pediatrics
University of Utah
Primary Children's Medical Center
Salt Lake City, Utah

David F.M. Thomas, FRCP, FRCPH, FRCS
Consultant Paediatric Urologist
Honorary Reader in Paediatric Surgery
Department of Paediatric Urology
St James' University Hospital
Leeds, UK

Michael J. Wehle, MS, MD
Assistant Professor of Urology
Mayo Clinic and Mayo Foundation
Jacksonville, Florida

John S. Wiener, MD, FAAP
Associate Professor of Surgery
Assistant Professor of Pediatrics
Head, Section of Pediatric Urology
Duke University Medical Center
Durham, North Carolina

Preface to the fourth edition

Almost 10 years have elapsed since the third edition of this text. This period has seen great changes in urology and specifically in pediatric urology. General urology, aside from the treatment of cancer and advances in reconstructive procedures, has become much more office based. As a result, pediatric urology has become more important in teaching residents surgical technique. Clinical advances continue to be made at a rapid pace, as organized pediatric urology programs have greatly improved training, and the subspecialty continues to attract innovative and dedicated physicians. Additionally, much more research is being done in the laboratory by senior pediatric urologists and fellows.

For instance, although bladder augmentation and substitution is historically a relatively new endeavor, many are exploring alternatives to the use of bowel. Some, like gastrocystoplasty, use other organs with less re-absorbent capability. Other approaches involve growing replacement epithelium *ex-vivo,* implanting this product using several different methods. These concepts are explored in this edition. No area has changed as much in the past decade as hypospadias surgery. Once often frustrating, results are now good or excellent in most instances and fistulae have become relatively uncommon. The most controversial area at the moment is the way we view and treat intersex. Recommendations have changed, as many patients, especially males reared as females, are redeclaring themselves boys or men as they get older. Intersex surgery may often best be delayed in some instances. Meanwhile, the techniques of genital reconstruction are greatly improved. Laparoscopy is finding many niches, and is at least as successful as open surgery in a number of areas. The debate over how to treat obstruction in neonates discovered as a consequence of prenatal hydronephrosis continues and has stimulated important research, both in animals and babies.

All in all, this text conveys a plethora of new information. Every chapter has been revised and most completely rewritten, often by new authors. These essays are clinically oriented, and are meant to be of real help in deciding how to manage perplexing clinical problems. So, to this end, some redundances occur in order to make each chapter easily comprehensible, avoiding the need to keep refering the reader to other sections of the book. The editors have attempted to be certain that conflicting statements do not arise, except in areas in which two or three approaches are in use and a standardized technique has not yet emerged. These topics are identified, and include intersex, fetal hydronephrosis, post-natal obstruction, reflux management, and many others.

Several chapters are devoted to diagnostic evaluation, stressing the importance of making an exact diagnosis. In most instances, treatment options then become apparent. We are heavily dependent on evaluation by imaging. Of these tests, none has caused more confusion than the diuretic renogram. Pediatric urologists must understand this test, and acertain that it is properly performed if it is to be useful.

We earnestly believe that the information in this edition is the 'state of the art'. At the same time we realize that, in a text of this magnitude, omissions may occur. This work is meant to be neither an encyclopedia nor, for that matter, a compendium of rare congenital anomalies. Rather, as in the previous editions, our overriding consideration has been to present material that lives up to the title of the book – clinical in orientation and, we hope, practical in presentation. We have made an effort to include detailed and comprehensive material seldom available in one place. The multiauthor format in an area of constantly expanding knowledge permits the presentation of a complete and authoritative overview in each area; unavoidably, some areas overlap. As mentioned earlier we have generally viewed this as an advantage, realizing that this allows individual chapters to be developed in a coherent fashion. Additionally, there might be some differences in recommendations and conclusions between overlapping chapters. We hope this does not cause undue confusion and will be interpreted as honest differences in experience and opinions.

Once again, we are deeply indebted to our contributors, past and present, for their sincere efforts and cooperation despite their ever-increasing professional commitments and other responsibilities. Without them, this work would have been impossible to complete. The credit is theirs; the mistakes are ours.

We are especially indebted to Ms Lesley Gray of Gray Publishing, without whose intense efforts and perseverance this work would never have been completed.

A. Barry Belman
Lowell R. King
Stephen A. Kramer

Embryology of the genitourinary tract

Steven E. Lerman, Irene M. McAleer and George W. Kaplan

Introduction

An understanding of the significant events in the embryology of the genitourinary tract is essential to both the diagnosis of congenital anomalies and the interpretation of pathologic findings that result from disordered embryogenesis. The following synopsis is synthesized largely from standard textbooks of embryology but is amplified with newer concepts as they seem clinically pertinent. The material is arranged chronologically as well as by organ to provide a better understanding of the interrelationships between structures. A developmental 'timeline' is presented at the conclusion of the chapter for easy reference. As the authors are not embryologists, some might suggest an element of 'armchair embryology', but as this material is presented only to aid in clinical understanding this posture may be excusable.

The first events in embryology occur at the time of conception, or fertilization of the ovum by a spermatozoon. It is at this moment, or in the first few subsequent cell divisions, that the chromosomal constitution (karyotype) is established. The normal human cell contains 46 chromosomes (usually written 46,XY 46,XX), 23 of which are provided by the maternal gamete (ovum) and 23 by the paternal gamete (sperm). The future individual's genotypic sex is now established as an X chromosome is provided by the ovum and either an X or a Y chromosome by the sperm. It is mostly the presence and expression of the testis-determining factor (TDF) gene, a locus usually carried on the Y chromosome but rarely translocated to one of the other chromosomes, that results in maleness (Vilain and McCabe, 1998). In the absence of this locus, femaleness is likely to develop. Other non-Y-linked genes involved in sex determination have been found by genetic analysis of XY sex-reversed patients whose phenotype could not be explained by mutations in the TDF gene (Vilain and McCabe, 1998). It is presumably at conception, as well, that certain other genitourinary abnormalities related to the individual's karyotypic constitution are determined. For example, many of the intersex states are determined at this time, either as deletions of chromosomes (e.g. Turner syndrome, 45,XO) (Lindsten, 1963) or as extra chromosomes (e.g. Klinefelter syndrome, 47,XXY) (Jacobs and Strong, 1959). The genital abnormalities of the Aarskog–Scott syndrome are also determined at this moment as they are carried as an X-linked recessive trait (Berman et al., 1975). Many of the trisomy syndromes include abnormalities of the genitalia and of the urinary tract as part of their spectra of expression (Smith, 1982). The syndrome of Wilms' tumor and aniridia is related to a chromosomal abnormality (deletion of the short arm of the 11th chromosome) (Riccardi et al., 1978). Many other urinary abnormalities are probably also determined at this time, although the exact nature of this process is as yet unknown. Such abnormalities are those that seem to be familial in nature and include duplication anomalies (Atwell et al., 1974; Santava et al., 1990), vesicoureteral reflux (VUR) (Dwoskin, 1976; Mackintosh et al., 1989), congenital ureteropelvic junction (UPJ) obstruction (Fryns et al., 1993), renal agenesis and dysplasia (Moerman et al., 1994), and the adrenogenital syndrome (Vaughn and McKay, 1975).

In addition, in very early embryonic life teratogens such as heat, viruses, and drugs can exert an effect on the developing embryo (Table 1.1). Maternal hyperthermia can induce neural tube defects in the embryo. Hyperthermic states have also been associated with hypothalamic lesions leading to micropenis (Smith, 1982). Some viruses, when they infect the mother, may produce congenital abnormalities in the fetus. Urologic abnormalities appear more frequently than

Table 1.1 Genitourinary (GU) tract teratogens

Teratogen	Potential GU defect
Maternal hyperthermia	Micropenis
Rubella virus (congenital rubella)	Hypospadias, cryptorchidism
Progestational agents	Ambiguous genitalia
Oral contraceptives	Hypospadias
ACE inhibitors	Renal dysplasia
Ethanol (fetal alcohol syndrome)	Hypospadias, hydronephrosis
Anticonvulsants	Hypospadias, ambiguous genitalia, cryptorchidism
Cocaine	Eagle–Barrett syndrome, hypospadias, hydronephrosis
Vitamin A (excessive)	Hydronephrosis, hypospadias

ACE = angiotensin converting enzyme.

normal in the congenital rubella syndrome (Kaplan and Mclaughlin, 1973). It is well known that maternal ingestion of drugs can affect the developing fetus. Progestational agents may masculinize a female fetus (Vaugh and McKay, 1975). The maternal production of androgens by ovarian tumors can also masculinize a female fetus. Maternal use of oral contraceptive pills has been theorized to be associated with the development of hypospadias (Lopez-Camelo and Orioli, 1996). Use of angiotensin converting enzyme during pregnancy has been associated with renal dysplasia, probably due to the drug's deleterious effects on the developing renal vasculature (Mehta and Modi, 1989). The fetal alcohol syndrome, on occasion, includes urinary abnormalities (Clarren and Smith, 1978). In addition, the use of anticonvulsant medications during pregnancy has been associated with genitourinary abnormalities in the fetal hydantoin syndrome (Pinto *et al.*, 1977) and the fetal trimethadione syndrome (Zackai *et al.*, 1975). Maternal use of recreational drugs, such as cocaine and metaamphetamine, has been associated with anomalies of the genitourinary system, including Eagle–Barrett syndrome and hypospadias (Greenfield *et al.*, 1991). Excessive vitamin A ingestion during the first trimester of pregnancy has been reported to increase the risk for the development of genitourinary abnormalities (Rothman *et al.*, 1995). In addition, physical forces (e.g. compression of the fetus within the uterus secondary to oligohydramnios) can induce permanent physical changes in the fetus, even at a relatively late stage of development. These are termed 'deformation syndromes', of which Potter's syndrome is thought to be one (Thomas and Smith, 1974).

Anterior abdominal wall

During the first 3 weeks of development, the embryo is a plate of cells, the embryonic disk, whose ventral surface is a membrane called the somatopleure. The anterior abdominal wall is at first represented by the somatopleure of the overhanging head and tail folds. The somatopleure closes concentrically from the cranial, caudal, and lateral margins, centering on the future umbilical ring (Fig. 1.1).

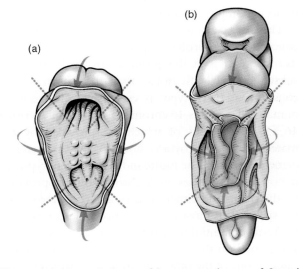

Figure 1.1 Ventral views of human embryos of 2 and 3 mm. The body stalk has been cut distal to the site of the future umbilical ring. Arrows show the direction of infolding; dotted lines indicate the arbitrary boundaries of the four infoldings. (From Gray and Skandalakis, 1972.)

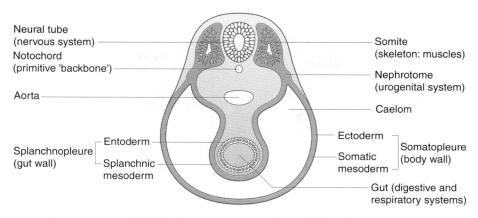

Neural tube (nervous system)
Notochord (primitive 'backbone')
Aorta
Splanchnopleure (gut wall)
Entoderm
Splanchnic mesoderm
Somite (skeleton: muscles)
Nephrotome (urogenital system)
Caelom
Ectoderm
Somatic mesoderm
Somatopleure (body wall)
Gut (digestive and respiratory systems)

Figure 1.2 Diagrammatic transverse section of a vertebrate embryo. (From Arey, 1974.)

In the 6th week of development, the midgut closes and the body stalk reduces in relative size. The somatopleure is invaded by mesoderm from myotomes on either side of the vertebral column. This mesoderm migrates laterally and ventrally as a sheet (Fig. 1.2).

The primordia of the two rectus abdominis muscles form laterally and begin to move toward the midline during the 7th week. At that time, the mesoderm laterally splits into three sheets, eventually producing the external oblique muscle, the internal oblique muscle, and the transversus abdominis muscle. These layers are all recognizable during the 7th week (Fig. 1.3). In the infraumbilical area, the formation of three muscle layers is preceded by invasion of secondary mesoderm that arises from the primitive streak just behind the cloaca. This secondary mesoderm then surrounds the cloaca and invades the body wall caudal to the body stalk, providing primary closure to the body wall between the phallus and the body stalk and forming part of the anterior bladder musculature as well (Glenister, 1958) (Fig. 1.4).

Between the 7th and 12th weeks of development, the rectus abdominis muscles meet in the midline except around the umbilicus. During this same time the secondary mesoderm forming the lower abdominal wall is reinforced externally by invading somatic mesoderm that forms the muscular layers of the lower abdominal wall.

The important urologic anomalies resulting from faulty embryogenesis of the abdominal wall are the Eagle–Barrett (prune belly) syndrome and exstrophy of the bladder or cloaca. Neither of these is an arrested stage of normal embryogenesis. The Eagle–Barrett syndrome seems most likely to be due to faulty mesodermal development during the 6th to the 12th week, as several mesodermal elements (abdominal wall, ureter, bladder, and testes) are usually involved (Spence and Allen, 1964). Another theory states that the Eagle–Barrett syndrome is a deformation of the abdominal wall produced by distended viscera or increased intra-abdominal pressure (Pagon *et al.*, 1979). A third theory attributes the urinary abnormalities to a primary abdominal wall defect resulting in decreased intra-abdominal pressure (Osler, 1901).

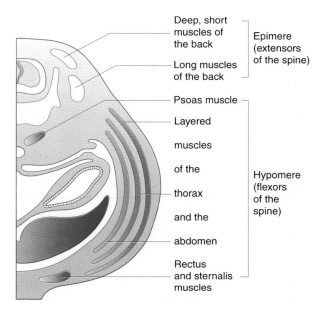

Deep, short muscles of the back
Long muscles of the back
Psoas muscle
Layered muscles of the thorax and the abdomen
Rectus and sternalis muscles
Epimere (extensors of the spine)
Hypomere (flexors of the spine)

Figure 1.3 Diagrammatic transverse hemisection through the abdomen or thorax of a 7-week human embryo. (From Arey, 1974.)

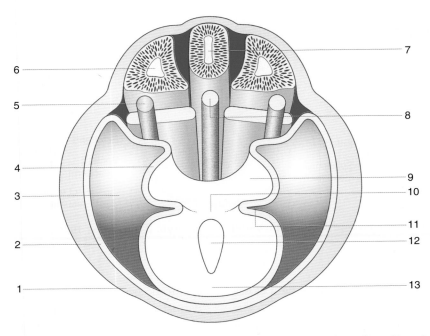

Figure 1.4 Disposition of mesoderm at the caudal end of a somite embryo as viewed working down from inside the caudal end of the embryo. 1, Surface epithelium; 2, somatic layer of the lateral plate mesoderm; 3, coelomic cavity; 4, visceral layer of the lateral plate mesoderm; 5, nephrogenic cord; 6, somite; 7, neural tube; 8, notochord; 9, unsegmented paraxial mesoderm; 10, primitive streak; 11, site of developing urorectal septum; 12, site of cloacal membrane; 13, infraumbilical abdominal wall. (From Glenister, 1958.)

Exstrophy may result from a failure of the secondary mesoderm to cover the infraumbilical abdominal wall. Rupture of the cloacal membrane prematurely could also produce such a failure. Should this occur in the 5th week, cloacal exstrophy could result (Muecke, 1964). If this does not occur until the 7th week, so that some of the secondary mesoderm is in place, classical bladder exstrophy might result. Still later (the 10th or 11th week), failure of invasion by somatic mesoderm might result in superior vesical fissure or epispadias.

Renal vasculature

The primitive vasculature is forming during the first 3 gestational weeks. Angioblasts form from cells that separate from the primary trophoblast at the same time as other mesoderm is forming. These angioblasts appear in the body stalk and form isolated vascular spaces. By growth and union of these isolated spaces plexi form, which eventually unite to form a system of closed vessels. Once this system of closed vessels is in place any new vessels that arise do so only as outgrowths of existing vessels. Mesenchyme is laid down around the endothelium of the vessels to form the intima, media, and adventitia of the vessels. By selection, enlargement, and differentiation, definitive vessels arise. The selection of the channels that result is by virtue of inherited patterns and hemodynamic factors. Research identifying specific vascular growth factors and proteases necessary for normal angiogenesis is ongoing (Gomez *et al.*, 1997; Gomez, 1998). It is during this period that paired dorsal aortae arise. In addition, paired postcardinal veins form to return blood to the heart from the caudal end of the body via a common cardinal vein. These postcardinal veins develop as vessels of the mesonephroi and run dorsal to them. The previously paired dorsal aortae fuse to form a single descending aorta in the the 4th week. Lateral branches of the dorsal aorta appear during the 5th week. They are irregularly segmental and supply structures arising from the nephrotome region, specifically the mesonephros, gonads, metanephros, and suprarenal glands. As the mesonephros involutes, the number of lateral branches is reduced, but these lateral branches eventually become the inferior phrenic, adrenal, renal, and gonadal arteries.

During the 6th week the formation of the inferior vena cava starts (Fig. 1.5). Subcardinal veins develop ventromedial to the mesonephroi and connect with each other and with the postcardinal veins. Supracardinal veins develop dorsomedial to the postcardinal veins and replace them. This process is progressing during the 6th to the 8th week of gestation, at which time the formation of the inferior vena cava is complete. Connections between the subcardinal veins persist as a common stem uniting the left renal vein,

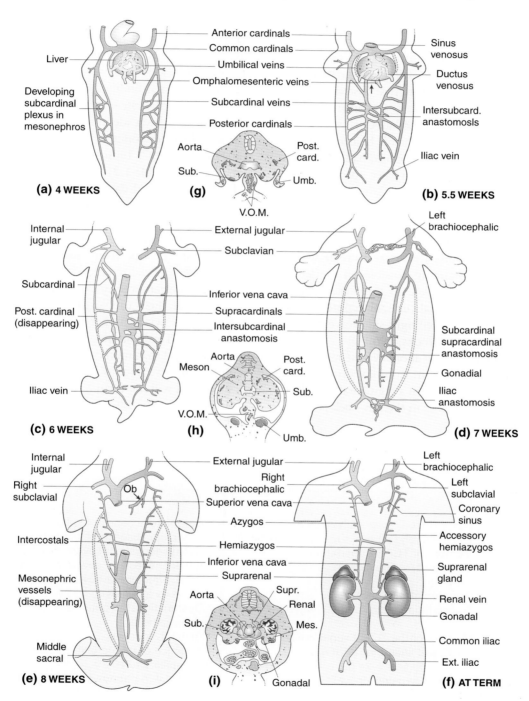

Figure 1.5 Development of the superior and inferior venae cavae. (*a–f*), anterior views; (*g–i*), cross-sectional views. Cardinal veins are black, subcardinal veins are stippled and supracardinal veins are hatched. vom = omphalomesentenc vein. (From Patten, 1976, with permission.)

the left adrenal vein, and the left gonadal vein to the vena cava. The right subcardinal vein forms the inferior vena cava at the level of the renal veins and cephalad; it is for this reason that the right adrenal vein and the right gonadal vein drain directly into the inferior vena cava. The right supracardinal vein persists as the inferior vena cava caudal to the renal veins, whereas the left supracardinal vein disappears entirely.

Although there are many normal variations in renal arterial supply they tend to fall into variations of arrangement of five segmental arteries: posterior, upper anterior, middle anterior, apical, and inferior polar (Graves, 1954). However, if the kidney is ectopic the arterial supply is from other lateral branches of the dorsal aorta that would have atrophied had the kidney ascended to its normal location. Hence, these could be considered an arrest of normal embryogenesis (Neidhart, 1972).

Should the right subcardinal vein rather than the supracardinal vein persist as the inferior vena cava caudal to the renal veins, a retrocaval ureter would result. Although theoretically possible on the left if the left subcardinal vein were to form the inferior vena cava caudal to the renal veins, all reported cases of retrocaval ureter have been right-sided except when situs inversus is present (Brooks, 1962).

Retroiliac ureter is a rare anomaly that may result if the iliac artery should form from a ventral root of the umbilical artery rather than a segmental branch of the aorta as it normally does in the 4th week (Corbus *et al.*, 1960).

Kidney and ureter

It is best to consider the development of the kidney and the ureter together as their histories are inextricably intertwined. Abnormal embryogenesis of one has a domino effect on the other. This discussion will proceed chronologically but also from cranial to caudal to cranial, as will be seen. Remarkable advances have been made in understanding the molecular basis of embryonic kidney development. The details of these experimental findings are beyond the scope of this text. Nevertheless, several genes, and their gene products, have been identified that are essential for normal kidney development (Ekbolm, 1996; Lechner and Dressler, 1997; Lipschultz, 1998; Orellana and Avner, 1998) (Table 1.2).

During the first 21 days the pronephroi arise in the cervical and thoracic region of the embryo (Fig. 1.6). The pronephros does not function in mammals but does in some animals. Seven pairs of tubules arise as dorsolateral sprouts from segmentally arranged nephrotomes (specialized areas of mesoderm). As the last tubule appears, the earliest is degenerating. The distal ends of these tubules bend dorsally, canalize, and unite one with another into a longitudinal collecting duct. This collecting duct eventually reaches the cloaca and communicates with it. If the pronephros or its duct should not develop, the mesonephros will not form.

Slightly later in this same timeframe the mesonephros arises caudal to the pronephros, again from nephrotomes; these nephrotomes, unlike those of the

Table 1.2 Genes necessary for normal kidney development

Gene	Type	Defect
WT-1	Transcription factor with zinc finger domains	Complete absence of kidney
Pax-2	Transcription factor of the paired box family	Complete absence of kidneys
GDNF	Member of TGF-B superfamily	Renal agenesis or severe dysplasia
c-ret	Receptor tyrosine kinase	Renal agenesis or severe dysplasia
α8β1	Integrin	Renal agenesis or severe dysplasia
Wnt-4	Secreted glycoprotein	Renal dysgenesis
BF-2	Transcription factor of the winged helix family	Dysfunctional stromal cells leading to renal dysgenesis
BMP-7	Member of the TGF-B superfamily	Renal dysgenesis
PDGF-B	PDGF and ligand for PFGFR-B	Absence of glomerular mesangial cells and capillary tufts
PDGFR-β	Receptor tyrosine kinase	Identical to phenotype of PDGF-B
α3β1	Integrin	Abnormal glomerular podocyte and BM; decreased branching of ureteral bud

TGF = transforming growth factor; PDGF = platelet-derived growth, factor; BM = basement membrane.

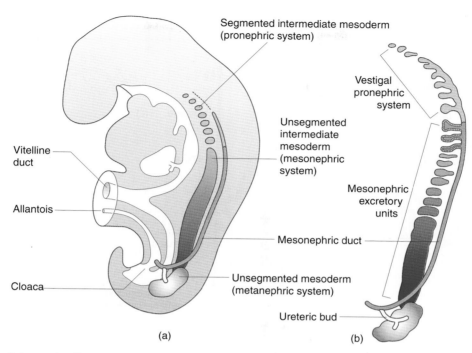

Figure 1.6 (a) Schematic diagram showing the relationship of the intermediate mesoderm of the pronephric, mesonephric, and metanephric systems. In cervical and upper thoracic regions, intermediate mesoderm is segmented; in lower thoracic, lumbar, and sacral regions, it forms a solid, unsegmented mass of tissue, the nephrogenic cord. Note the longitudinal collecting duct, formed initially by the pronephros but later by the mesonephros. (b) Schematic representation of excretory tubules of the pronephric and mesonephric systems in a 5-week-old embryo. (From Sadler, 1995.)

pronephros, are unsegmented. The mesoderm that gives rise to the mesonephros separates into a longitundinal bar that is termed the nephrogenic cord. Within this cord the mesenchyme forms into tubules. One end of the tubule becomes associated with a knot of blood vessels, while the other opens into the pronephric duct, which now is called the mesonephric duct. It is by this process that the nephrogenic cord becomes subdivided into spherical masses of cells that appear progressively from its cranial end to its caudal end. These masses tend to hollow and send out solid extensions that unite with the mesonephric duct. These solid extensions canalize and, by growth, bend into an S-shape. A knot of blood vessels (the glomerulus) indents the free end of the tubule, which now becomes Bowman's capsule (Fig. 1.7). Bowman's capsule and the glomerulus together make up the mesonephric corpuscle. Lateral branches of the aorta feed the glomerulus, while the postcardinal veins drain these tubules by sinusoids. The mesonephric tubules between the mesonephric duct and the glomerulus elongate and form a secretory segment and a collecting segment. As the tubules enlarge, the nephrogenic cord bulges into

the coelom, forming a urogenital ridge on each side of the dorsal mesentery extending roughly from the diaphragm to the cloaca (Fig. 1.8).

The pronephric tubules have completely degenerated by the 4th week but, as already stated, the pronephric duct persists as the mesonephric (wolffian) duct. The mesonephros begins to reach its stage of maximal development by the 28th day, with about 30 tubules in each mesonephros. The cranial tubules of the mesonephros are degenerating while more caudal ones are forming. The mesonephros, in contrast to the pronephros, has been shown to be functional in rabbits, cats, and pigs. The glomeruli in these animals at this stage can excrete ferrocyanide, and the tubules can secrete phenol red. At the caudal end of the nephrogenic cord, lying at the level of the sacral vertebrae deep in the plevis, the metanephros appears as a metanephrogenic mass (nephric blastema).

The mesonephric duct makes a sharp bend before it enters the cloaca (Fig. 1.9). The ureteric bud arises from the dorsal medial aspect of this bend. It hollows and grows dorsad and then cephalad. It pushes into the metanephrogenic mass, which has separated itself

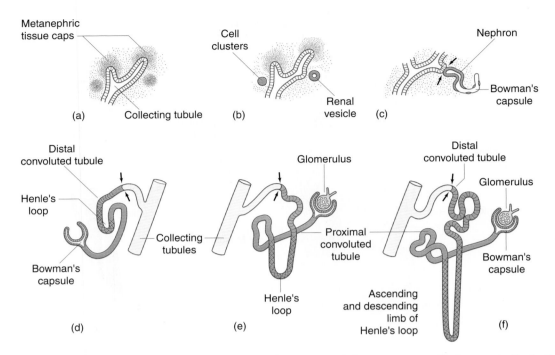

Figure 1.7 Schematic representation of development of a metanephric excretory unit. Arrows indicate the place where the excretory unit establishes an open communication with the collecting system, thus allowing the flow of urine from the glomerulus into the collecting ducts. (From Sadler, 1995.)

from the nephrogenic cord, and begins to induce nephrogenesis. The proximal end of the ureteric bud elongates to form the ureter, while the distal end (that portion pushing in to the metanephrogenic mass) becomes the renal pelvis. The metanephrogenic mass surrounds the renal pelvis like a cap.

In the 5th week the kidney is forming, having been induced by the key union of the ureteric bud with the metanephrogenic mass. The kidney is initially orient-ed in an anteroposterior direction with the ureter entering the hilum of the kidney anteriorly (Fig. 1.10). With elongation of the ureter and straighten-ing of the body, the kidney ascends from its pelvic position to its eventual normal site in the loin, but during the 5th week the kidney is still caudal to the umbilical arteries. Late in the 5th week the kidney begins to turn 90° on its vertical axis so that its dorsal border becomes its lateral border.

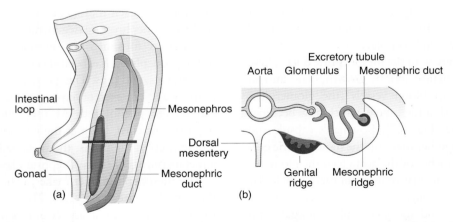

Figure 1.8 (*a*) Relationship of the genital ridge and the mesonephros. Note the location of the mesonephric duct. (*b*) Transverse section through the mesonephros and genital ridge at the level indicated in (a). (From Sadler, 1995.)

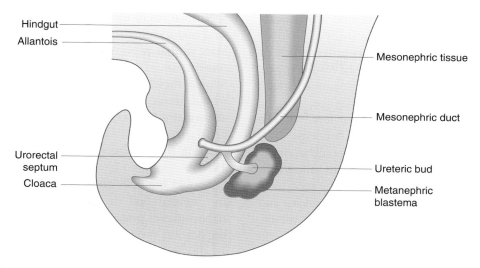

Figure 1.9 Schematic drawing showing the relationship of the hindgut and cloaca at the end of the 5th week. The ureteric bud penetrates the metanephric mesoderm (blastema). (From Sadler, 1995.)

By the 6th week, the kidney has ascended sufficiently so that it lies cephalad to the umbilical artery. The renal pelvis flattens and divides into two major calices. By the 7th week, the kidney comes into contact with the suprarenal body, shortens and widens; by the 8th week, the center of the kidney has reached its permanent level opposite the second lumbar vertebra. The caudal pole is above the iliac vessels and the cranial pole below the suprarenal gland.

From the 6th to the 20th week, the major calices progressively subdivide through 12 generations. The second, third, and fourth generations enlarge and fuse to form approximately nine minor calices. The fifth generation of branches (about 25 in number) form papillary ducts, emptying into the minor calices. The sixth to 12th generations of branches form the col-

lecting ducts in the renal medulla and project into the renal cortex as rays. All the tubules draining into a minor calyx comprise a renal pyramid, the base of which adjoins the renal cortex, while its apex (papilla) projects into a calyx. The calices, pelvis, and ureter differentiate into transitional epithelium and become invested with smooth muscle and connective tissue by specialization of the surrounding mesenchyme during the 8th week.

The cap of metanephrogenic tissue that covers the ureteral bud has two layers: an external layer, which forms the renal capsule and connective tissue, and an inner layer, which forms the nephrons. The inner layer divides as the renal pelvis branches, so that one lump of metanephrogenic tissue covers each subdivision through all 12 generations. As the renal cortex

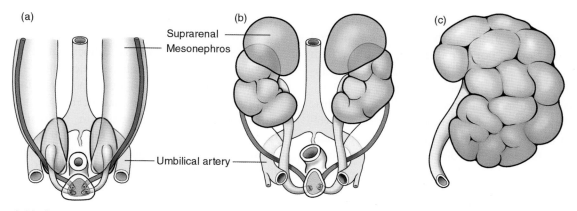

Figure 1.10 Ascent and lobation of the human kidney: (a) 6 weeks; (b) 9 weeks; (c) at birth. (From Arey, 1974.)

organizes, the region over each pyramid is demarcated from the next pyramid, so that as many as 20 lobes are formed. This lobation disappears progressively in infancy and early childhood but may be readily apparent on routine ultrasonographic examination as fetal lobulations, especially in infants.

During the 7th week, the inner layer of the metanephrogenic tissue begins to condense into spherical masses about the ends of the branches of the ureteral bud. These masses hang down into the angles between the branches. As the cortex thickens, new spheres form. The spheres change into vesicles and elongate, producing an S-shaped secretory tubule, which unites with a collecting tubule. The blind end of the secretory tubule becomes the Bowman's capsule, while the mid-portion elongates and twists. An afferent arteriole grows in, the glomerulus differentiates, and an efferent arteriole grows out. This process of nephrogenesis starts in third-generation ureteral branches in the mid-portion of the kidney and in fifth-generation branches at the poles. Nephrogenesis continues through the 36th week of gestation and then ceases, but the size of the nephron increases with age throughout somatic growth.

The fetal kidney is capable of secretion by the 10th week of gestation, and urine is produced. The bladder fills and urine is voided into the amniotic sac. The amniotic fluid is imbibed by the fetus and is an important factor in pulmonary maturation.

Multiple anomalies result from disordered embryogenesis of the ureter or kidney. Some are known to be familial, at least in some instances (e.g. ureteral duplications), whereas others are frequently associated with chromosomal abnormalities (e.g. horseshoe kidney and Turner syndrome). Most, however, seem sporadic in incidence.

If the pronephrosis fails to develop, the mesonephros will not develop; the result is renal and ureteral agenesis. Additionally, in the male, the ipsilateral genital ducts would not form. Hence, there is a high association of renal agenesis in patients with congenital absence of the vas deferens (Schlegel *et al.*, 1996). A similar situation would result if the mesohnephric duct failed; however, if the mesonephric duct developed but the mesonephros did not, the kidney would be absent, while the genital ducts, and perhaps a blind-ending ureter, could result. If both kidneys fail to develop, oligohydramnios (due to a lack of fetal urine) produces the deformation characteristic of Potter syndrome and interferes with pulmonary maturation.

Normal nephrogenesis is dependent upon the ureteral bud meeting the center of the metanephrogenic mass so that nephrogenesis is induced by the ureter (Grobstein, 1955; Mackie and Stevens, 1975). Should they not meet at all, a blind-ending ureter would result. However, should they meet in an abnormal (degenerating) part of the metanephrogenic mass, renal dysplasia would be anticipated (Mackie and Stephens, 1975; Maizels and Simpson, 1983).

Should multiple ureteral buds develop, or should the ureteral bud divide before meeting the metanephrogenic mass, complete or partial ureteral duplication (or triplication) would be the outcome. In this instance, if one bud met the center of the metanephrogenic mass and the other a pole of degenerating metanephric tissue, the former would develop normally whereas the latter might be dysplastic. This seems to explain the high association of dysplasia with ureteral ectopia (Mackie and Stephens, 1975).

Failure of renal ascent results in simple pelvic ectopia. Further ascent but failure of rotation is seen clinically as malrotation. If the two metanephrogenic masses come into contact in the pelvis they could fuse and form a pancake (lump) kidney. Fusion slightly later, perhaps secondary to delayed ascent produced by delayed straightening of the hind end of the fetus, might result in horseshoe kidney. A horseshoe kidney will be arrested in its ascent by the inferior mesenteric artery. The embryogenesis of crossed ectopia is harder to explain, but it may result from lateral bending and rotation of the tail of the embryo, thereby altering the course of ascent. In this way both ureteral buds might penetrate a single metanephrogenic mass (Cook and Stephens, 1977).

Ureteral obstructions occur primarily at the ureteropelvic and ureterovesical junctions. These obstructions are usually intrinsic in nature and the area in question is often of normal caliber but abnormally fibrous histologically, perhaps reflecting a localized vascular accident later in development. Multicystic dysplastic kidney disease has been said to result from early ureteral obstruction (Bernstein and Gardner, 1979) but seems more likely to result from disordered induction of the metanephrogenic mass by a faulty ureteral bud (Gray and Skandalakis, 1972). Involution of the cystic components of the multicystic kidney also accounts for some cases of renal agenesis.

Lower urinary tract

The development of the lower urinary tract is closely interrelated with that of the genital tract and the hindgut, but for clarity the genital tract is discussed later.

During the first 3 weeks the cloaca develops from endoderm as a blind caudal expansion of the hindgut (Fig. 1.11). The hindgut meets the ectoderm of the body wall at the cloacal membrane. This membrane extends caudally from the primitive streak and is turned under by the tailfold. It extends from the tail-bud to the body stalk. As the mesoderm grows, the extent of the cloacal membrane is decreased. The cloaca gives off a ventrally directed allantoic stalk and receives the mesonephric duct laterally and extends caudally as the tailgut.

The cloaca, during the 5th week, is divided by opposing walls of the hindgut in the allantois, meeting in a saddle-shaped notch with its apex pointing caudally. This notch fills in with mesenchyme to form the urorectal septum. This septum pushes caudally as a fold and advances, dividing the cloaca into the primitive rectum posteriorly and a urogenital sinus anteriorly (Fig. 1.12).

Various regions of the urogenital sinus are recognizable in the 6th week: the allantois, bladder, pelvic, and phallic portions of the urogenital sinus. The pelvic portion of the urogenital sinus lies cephalad to the entrance of the mesonephric duct but below the bladder, whereas the phallic portion of the urogenital sinus lies caudad to the entrance of the mesonephric duct and extends distally toward the genital tubercle.

By the 7th week the ureters empty into the bladder by a process in which nephric ducts, after the ureteral buds have appeared, are absorbed into the urogenital sinus and acquire four separate openings into the sinus (Fig. 1.13). The mesonephric ducts are shifted further caudad in the sinus and come to lie close to each other at Müller's tubercle, while the ureters shift cephalad and laterally into the bladder. It is then that the trigone is formed. The trigone is temporarily mesodermal but fills in with urogenital sinus epithelium, so that it, too, is eventually endodermal. The bladder epithelium at this time consists of a single layer.

The urorectal septum reaches the cloacal membrane and divides the cloaca into the urogenital sinus and the rectum; the cloacal membrane then ruptures (Fig. 1.12). The caudal edge of the urorectal septum, which is covered with endoderm, is exposed as the perineal body. It merges with lateral folds flanking this fissure and becomes covered with ectoderm. It is eventually marked by a median raphe and becomes the perineum. Hillocks behind the anus encircle this area and form the anal canal, which eventually becomes lined with ectoderm.

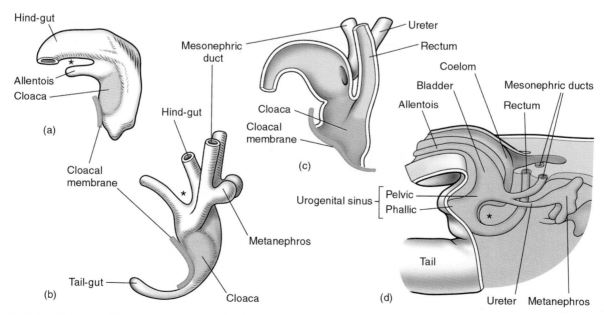

Figure 1.11 Division of the human cloaca: (*a*) 3.5 mm stage; (*b*) 4 mm stage; (*c*) 8 mm stage; (*d*) 1 mm stage. The asterisks in (*a*), (*b*) and (*d*) indicate the cloacal septum. (From Arey, 1974.)

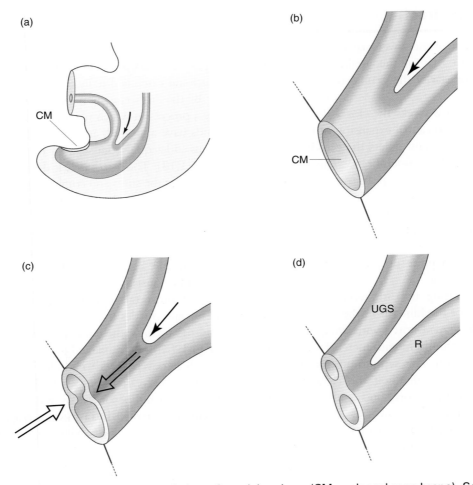

Figure 1.12 Septation of the cloaca. (a) Lateral view of caudal embryo (CM = cloacal membrane). Septation of the cloaca occurs in a coronal plane as Tourneux's fold (b) extends to the cloacal membrane from above (closed arrows), and (c) as Rathke's plicae extend towards each other from the sides (open arrows). (d) Septation establishes the primitive urogenital sinus (UGS) and rectum (R). (From Stephens and Smith, 1971.)

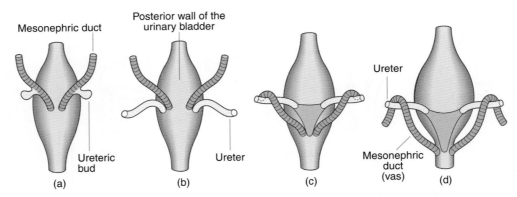

Figure 1.13 Dorsal views of the bladder to show the relationship of the ureters and mesonephric ducts during development. Initially, the ureters are formed by an outgrowth of the mesonephric duct, but with time they assume a separate entrance into the urinary bladder. Note the trigone of the bladder formed by incorporation of the mesonephric ducts. (From Sadler, 1995.)

In the 8th week the bladder muscle begins to appear as a longitudinal layer on the dorsal surface of the bladder. By the 9th week the bladder cavity begins to expand into a sac, the apex of which (the urachus) is elongated. The urachus is continuous with the allantoic stalk at the umbilicus. The bladder and urachus elongate as the infraumbilical body wall forms from the somatic mesoderm.

In the 12th week the bladder epithelium becomes transitional, and its muscular wall is formed from mesenchyme. The smooth muscle of the urinary tract is acquired in an ascending fashion from bladder to intrarenal collecting system (Baker and Gomez, 1998). The bladder epithelium over the ureteral orifice forms Chwalla's membrane, which temporarily covers and occludes the ureteral orifice. Chwalla's membrane perforates and the ureter becomes continuous with the bladder. By the 16th week the bladder is completely muscularized and the urachus is closed.

Agenesis of the bladder is a rare anomaly that may arise because the allantoic stalk fails to develop (Glenn, 1959). However, if migration of the ureters and formation of the trigone are the events that induce enlargement of the allantoic stalk, then bilateral failure of ureteral migration with resultant ureteral ectopia would result in the same anomaly.

Urachal anomalies (patent urachus, urachal cyst, urachal sinus, and urachal diverticula) may be encountered clinically (Fig. 1.14). Some result from a general mesodermal failure (the urachal diverticulum of the Eagle–Barrett syndrome); (Spence and Allen, 1964); however, most seem to result from delayed closure of the urachus. Lower urinary tract obstruction before 12

weeks of age (by virtue of bladder distension) could prevent closure (Javadpour *et al.*, 1974). There is, in addition, a definite association of patent urachus with upper tract problems, and therefore the entire urinary tract should be investigated (Rich *et al.*, 1983). Urachal cysts and sinuses presumably result from incomplete closure of the urachus.

Duplications of the bladder and urethra are usually associated with other hindgut and lower spinal cord duplications. Hence, it would appear that these result from a splitting of the hind end of the embryo at a very early stage of development.

Ureteral ectopia, VUR, and paraureteral diverticula appear to arise because the ureteral bud appears at a locus on the mesonephric duct more craniad or caudad than normal. As the ureter is incorporated into the urogenital sinus, its final site would be more craniad and lateral or caudad, respectively. The former results in VUR and diverticula, whereas the latter results in ureteral ectopia (Mackie and Stephens, 1975).

Ectopic ureteroceles probably result from abnormalities of the ureteral bud in addition to ectopia and are often associated with renal dysplasia (Mackie and Stephens, 1975). Intravesical (simple) ureteroceles are thought to be produced by persistence of Chwalla's membrane beyond the time when urine flow begins (Tanagho, 1972).

Posterior urethral valves (type 1) may result form persistence of the path of migration of the mesonephric ducts distal to Müller's tubercle so that they cross the urogenital sinus and enter anteriorly. Persistence of this portion coupled with anterior fusion

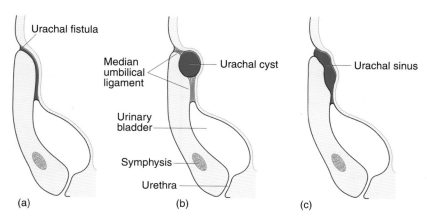

Figure 1.14 (a) Diagram of urachal fistula; (b) diagram of urachal cyst; (c) diagram of urachal sinus. The sinus may or may not be in open communication with the urinary bladder. (From Sadler, 1995.)

might then produce the diaphragm known as valves (Stephens, 1983). Another type of valves (type 3) seems to result from persistence of the cloacal membrane at the junction of the end of the phallic portion of the urogenital sinus and the bulbomembranous urethra (Field and Stephens, 1974).

Gonads, genital ducts, and genitalia

Formation of the gonads begins during the first 3 weeks. Approximately 30–50 germ cells become recognizable among the endodermal cells of the caudal portion of the yolk sac near the allantoic stalk. These begin to migrate by ameboid motion towards the genital ridge.

The gonads continue to develop during the 4th week but remain in an indifferent stage. At this time it is impossible to determine the sex of an embryo by examination. The ventral medial surface of the urogenital ridge begins to thicken and bulge into the coelom as a separate genital ridge, which lies medial and parallel to the mesonephric ridge.

The germ cells, which have been migrating dorsally in the wall of the yolk sac and gut, reach the gonadal ridge by the middle of the 5th week (Fig. 1.15). It is during this time that the genital tubercle appears on the ventral midline between the umbilical cord and the tailbud. The tubercle has a thin urogenital groove caudally, the floor of which is the cloacal membrane and the sides are the urogenital folds.

During the 6th week an indifferent gonad is recognizable in both sexes and consists of superficial germinal epithelium and an internal blastema derived from ingrowth of coelomic epithelium. The blastema forms into primary or medullary sex cords, and the germ cells and mesenchyme come to lie between these cords. The urogenital ridge is attached broadly near the root of the mesentery. In both sexes a groove appears in the urogenital ridge, located laterally on the mesonephros near the cephalic end. The cranial end of this groove remains open while caudally it

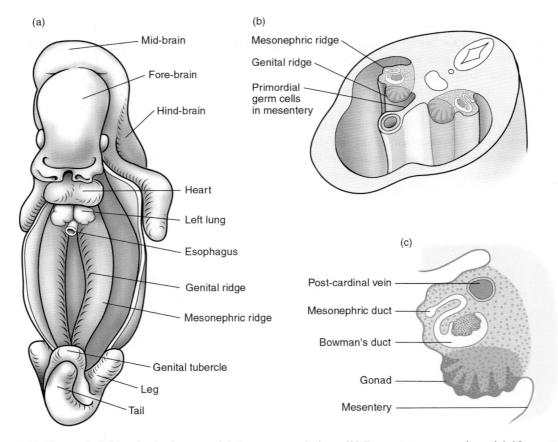

Figure 1.15 Urogenital ridge in the human: (*a*) 9 mm ventral view; (*b*) 7 mm transverse view; (*c*) 10 mm transverse view. (From Arey, 1974.)

begins to close into a tube (the müllerian duct) (Fig. 1.16). There is progressive caudal growth of the solid, blind end of the müllerian duct, guided by the mesonephros. Near the cloaca the urogenital ridges swing mesiad into the genital cord. The cranial end of the müllerian duct is forced laterally by the enlarging suprarenal glands and kidneys. Hence, each müllerian duct has two bends, a cranial one and a caudal one (Fig. 1.17).

During the 7th week in the male the attachment of the gonads to the mesonephros become the mesorchium. The medullary sex cords fuse with mesonephric tubules to form ductuli efferentes (Fig. 1.18). Some mesonephric tubules cephalad to this area persist as vestigial structures associated with the epididy-

mis and spermatic cord (the appendix epididymis, the superior and infeior vasa aberrantia, and the paradidymis). The sex cords become separated from the surface epithelium of the gonad by small cells that eventually form the tunica albuginea. The primordial germ cells become incorporated into the testis cords, and these cords become arranged radially, separated by a proliferation of mesenchyme. The cords eventually converge towards the blastemal mass, emerging as the primordia of the rete testis. In the female it is at this time that the round ligament begins to form.

The genital tubercle elongates into a phallus and its tip rounds into the glans (Fig. 1.19). Genital swellings appear lateral to the phallic base. The uro-

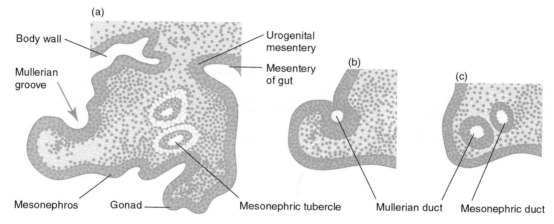

Figure 1.16 Origin of the human müllerian duct at the 12 mm stage. (*a*) Through the open groove; (*b*) Slightly lower level showing closure; (*c*) Still lower showing a tube. (From Arey, 1974.)

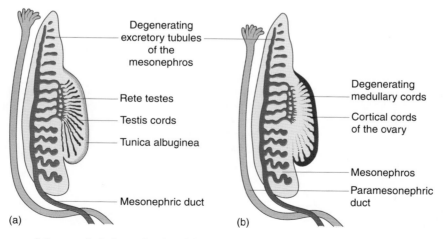

Figure 1.17 Diagram of the genital ducts in the 6th week of development in the male (*a*) and female (*b*). The mesonephric and müllerian ducts are present in both. Note the excretory tubules of the mesonephros and their relationship to the developing gonad in both sexes. (From Sadler, 1995.)

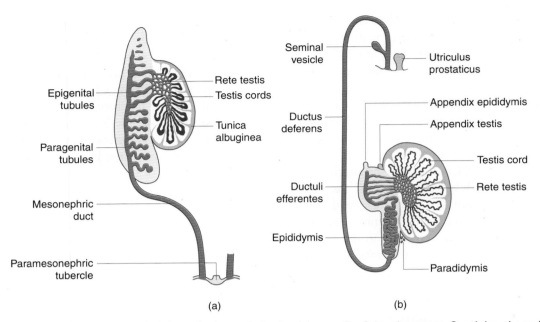

Figure 1.18 (a) Diagram of the genital ducts in the male in the 4th month of development. Cranial and caudal (para-genital tubule) segments of the mesonephric system regress. (b) Diagram of the genital ducts after descent of the testis. Note the horseshoe-shaped testis cords, rete testis, and efferent ductules entering the ductus deferens. The paradidymis is formed by remnants of the paragenital mesonephric tubules. The müllerian duct has degenerated except for the appendix testis. The prostatic utricle is an outpocketing from the urethra. (From Sadler, 1995.)

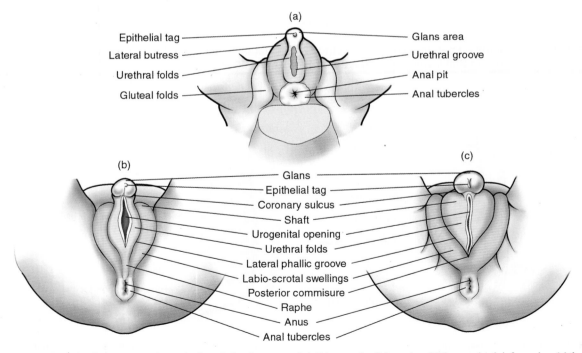

Figure 1.19 Developing external genitalia of the human: (a) 7th week; (b) male, 10th week; (c) female, 11th week (Gray and Skandalakis, 1972).

genital sinus opens at the base of the phallus by rupture of the cloacal membrane. In the male the corpora cavernosa begin to appear from mesenchymal columns in this area.

The upper five-sixths of the mesonephric ridge has been lost by the 8th week and becomes the diaphragmatic ligament of the mesonephros, which eventually will become the suspensory ligament of the gonad.

In the male, the tunica albuginea has formed a definite encapsulating layer on the gonad, and the gubernaculum begins to form. The phallus elongates, as does the urethral groove and the genital swellings rotate caudad.

In the female, clusters of indifferent cells and primordial germ cells appear. These fall into a dense primary cortex and a looser primary medulla. A mass bulges from the medulla into the mesovarium to form the rete ovarii (Fig. 1.20). The suspensory ligament of the ovary is formed from the cephalic end of the genital ridge, while the proper ligament of the ovary is formed from the terminal part of the genital ridge and unites the caudal end of the ovary to the transverse bend of the müllerian duct and eventually to the uterus.

The mesonephros consists of 34 pairs of tubules by the 9th week, but half of them are non-functional.

This is the end of the stage of maximal mesonephric development. The cranial eight to 15 pairs project against the rete testis or rete ovarii. The caudal ends of the müllerian ducts have now fused medially and end blindly at Müller's tubercle. The mesonephric ducts are now lateral to the müllerian duct caudally.

Cowper's gland in the male and Bartholin's gland in the female, which are homologs, arise as a pair of solid buds from the endodermal epithelium of the urogenital sinus distal to Müller's tubercle. In the male, they extend backwards, paralleling the urogenital sinus, and penetrate the mesenchyme of the corpus cavernosum urethrae and become glandular. They open into the bulbus urethrae. In the female, they open into the vestibule near the hymen.

By the 10th week all of the mesonephric tubules have become discontinuous. The gonads in both sexes lie at the boundary of the pelvis and the abdomen. In the male, the external genitalia are becoming visible as male structures as a result of secretion of testosterone by the fetal testis. The phallus has become the penis. The edges of the urethral folds begin to fuse progressively from posterior to anterior, forming the urethra and the median raphe. The genital swellings become scrotal swellings, which fuse forming a scrotal septum and raphe.

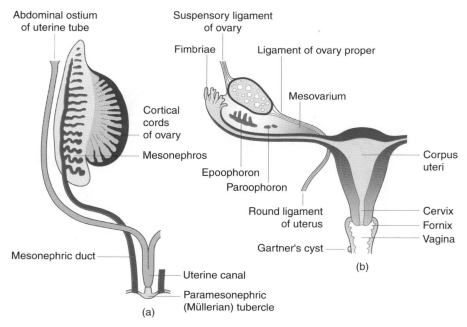

Figure 1.20 (*a*) Drawing of the genital ducts in the female at the end of the 2nd month of development. Note the müllerian tubercle and formation of the uterine canal. (*b*) Drawing of the genital ducts after descent of the ovary. The only parts remaining from the mesonephric system are the epoophoron, paroophoron, and Gartner's cyst. Note the suspensory ligament of the ovary, ligament of the ovary proper, and round ligament of the uterus. (From Sadler, 1995.)

Table 1.3 Embryologic remnants

Male	Müllerian remnants	Appendix testis Prostatic utricle
Female	Wolffian remnants	Epoophoron Paraoophoron Gartner's duct

In the 11th week the prostate arises as multiple outgrowths of endoderm both above and below the mesonephric ducts. These outgrowths arise in five different groups, each of which corresponds to a future prostatic lobe. The buds grow into the surrounding mesenchyme, which in turn provides both connective tissue and smooth muscle. In the female, the homologs of the prostate are the urethral glands, which are drained by Skene's ducts on each side.

Littre's glands bud from the male urethra in the 12th week. In the female, homologs of Littre's glands bud into the vestibule. In the male the processus vaginalis appears as an outpouching at the internal inguinal ring, and the testis lies nearby. The gubernaculum has already formed. The müllerian ducts degenerate owing to the secretion, by sertoli cells, of müllerian inhibiting factor (MIF). Müllerian remnants in the male are the appendix testis from the cranial end and the prostatic utricle from the caudal end of the müllerian duct (Table 1.3).

In the female the secondary ovarian cortex begins to form in the 12th week by division of cells of the ovarian blastema and by new growth of germinal epithelium. The early ova regress and form the medulla. The ovaries at this time lie at the pelvic brim. The round ligament is complete. Vaginal and uterine musculature appears from the mesenchyme surrounding the müllerian ducts. The distal portions of the müllerian ducts have fused below the caudal bend (Fig. 1.21).

In the 13th week, in the male, the seminal vesicles develop as lateral branches off the mesonephric duct. Branching of these seminal vesicles is evident by the 4th month of fetal life, and eventually a muscular coat is gained from the mesenchyme. In the female the mesonephric ducts begin to regress. Elongation of the fetal pelvis causes a solid epithelial cord to form between the end of the müllerian ducts and the urogenital sinus; this cord will become the upper vagina.

During the 14th week, the penile shaft continues to elongate in the male, and the urethra has fused to the base of glans penis. The penile shaft has a ventral deflection (Kaplan and Lamm, 1975). The prepuce now begins to form as a fold of skin that grows distally. By 5 months of gestational age, preputial formation is complete. The prepuce then fuses to the glans and reseparates from it under the influence of testosterone by the formation of small clefts in the preputial sac. This procedure of separation is

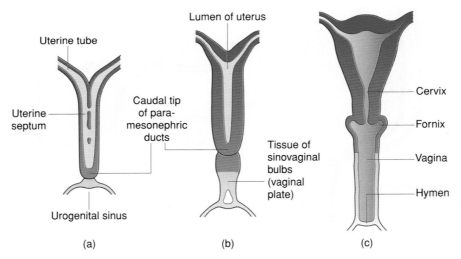

Figure 1.21 Schematic drawing showing formation of the uterus and vagina: (a) 9 weeks: note the disappearance of the uterine septum; (b) at the end of the third month: note the tissue of the sinovaginal bulbs; (c) in the newborn: the fornices and the upper portion of the vagina are formed by vacuolization of the müllerian tissue, and the lower portion of the vagina is formed by vacuolization of the sinovaginal bulbs. (From Sadler, 1995.)

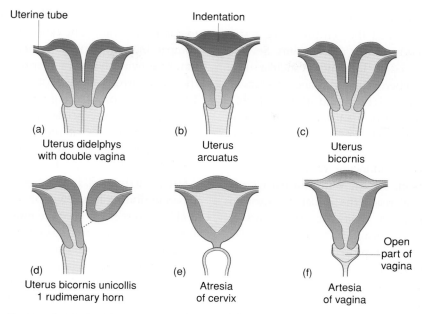

Figure 1.22 Schematic representation of the main abnormalities of the uterus and vagina, caused by persistence of the uterine septum or obliteration of the lumen of the uterine canal. (From Sadler, 1995.)

incomplete at birth and continues for several years thereafter.

By the 16th week, maximal degeneration of the mesonephric tubules has been attained. The muscles of the perineal floor are visible. The epithelium of Cowper's and Bartholin's glands is glandular in nature. In the testis, interstitial cells are very abundant. In the female, the vagina begins to form a lumen as the fornices appear as clefts in the solid epithelial cord distal to the fused müllerian ducts. The uterus forms as a fusion of müllerian ducts as they move ventrally and medially. Inappropriate fusion can result in uterine structural abnormalites such as bicornuate uterus (Fig. 1.22). During this fusion, the broad ligaments are formed. The cervix and the fallopian tubes are now evident.

The vaginal lumen and the prepuce are completely formed by the 20th week. The penile shaft is now straight (Kaplan and Lamm, 1975). Homologous structures between male and female and their embryologic origin are listed in Table 1.4.

The tunica albuginea of the ovary forms during the 24th week. In the male the lumen of the rete tubules and cranial mesonephric tubules become continuous and form the efferent ductules of the epididymis. The cranial end of the mesonephric duct convolutes, forming the body of the epididymis. The caudal end remains straight, forming the ductus deferens. The terminal end of the mesonephric duct forms the ejaculatory duct. The ampulla of the vas deferens forms from dilation of the ejaculatory duct. The processus vaginalis in the male now begins to move through the inguinal canal.

Formation of the seminal vesicles in the male is complete by the 28th week. The processus vaginalis

Table 1.4 Embryologic homologues

Embryologic Structure	Male	Female
Urogenital sinus	Prostatic urethra, prostate	Urethra, upper vagina
Genital tubercle	Glans penis	Clitoris
Genital folds	Urethra, penile shaft	Labia minora
Genital swellings	Scrotum	Labia majora

has herniated through the abdominal wall, formed the inguinal canal, and reached the scrotum. The testis then begins to descend towards the scrotum. Several factors are hypothesized to influence testicular descent. These include gubernacular guidance, increased intra-abdominal pressure (Frey and Rajfer, 1984) and, possibly, the release of a substance, descendin, from the normal testis (Levy and Husmann, 1995). In addition, the genitofemoral nerve has been studied as a potential factor in inducing testicular descent (Clarnette and Hutson, 1996). With normal factors intact, the testicle will reach the ipsilateral scrotum during the third trimester. Testis descent occurs in 60% of males by 30 weeks and 93% of males by 32 weeks (Birnholz, 1983). Cryptorchidism is a frequent anomaly whose etiology has been extensively studied but is still incompletely understood. Some instances appear to be due to intrauterine endocrine failures, whereas others seem mechanical. Intra-abdominal testes might result if the processus vaginalis did not form. Ectopic testes might result if the path of descent were obstructed or if the gubernaculum went astray,

failing to define a path for the testis to follow into the ipsilateral scrotum. The descent of the ovary is quite comparable to that of the testicle, but the gubernaculum fuses with the lateral margin of the uterus which, therefore, arrests descent of the ovary in the pelvis. Failure of fusion of the gubernaculum to the uterus may allow the ovary to descend into the labia majora.

Major anomalies of these genital organs are frequent, including intersex, hypospadias, and cryptorchidism. If the testis determining factor is present, a testis will develop. In the presence of the testis, müllerian inhibiting factor will be released by Sertoli cells and lead to regression of the müllerian ducts. In addition, elaboration of testosterone from Leydig cells will cause development of the mesonephric ducts and masculinization of the internal ducts. Masculinization of the external genitalia is dependent on the conversion of testosterone to 5-dihydrotestosterone. Failure of this conversion helps to explain some cases of ambiguous genitalia. In the absence of a testis, an ovary (or streak gonad) forms, the müllerian structures persist, and the external genitalia are feminine.

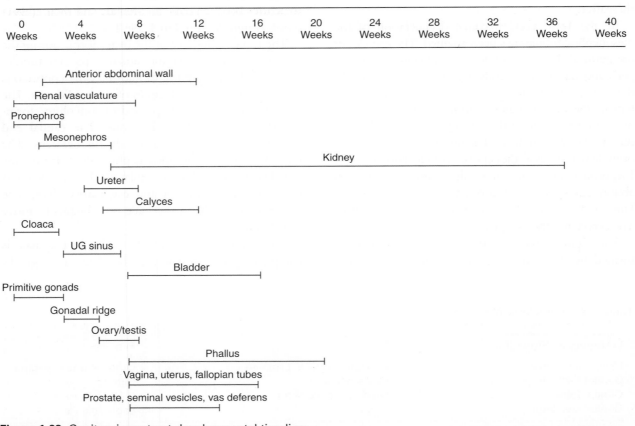

Figure 1.23 Genitourinary tract developmental timeline.

Hypospadias represents arrested formation of the phallus and phallic urethra. In many instances, the distal hypospadiac urethra is dysplastic, as is the surrounding corpus spongiosum (Avellan and Knutsscon, 1980). With severe forms of hypospadias a small müllerian remnant may persist as a diverticulum off the prostatic utricle.

Conclusions

This brief review is meant to provide a basis for understanding congenital anomalies and their relationships with one another. The mechanisms for the development of many anomalies are still incompletely understood, providing fertile ground for further investigation.

A developmental timeline of the geistourinary treat is shown in Figure 1.23.

References

Arey LB (1974) *Developmental anatomy*. 6th edition. Philadelphia, PA: WB Saunders.

Atwell JD, Cook PL, Howell CJ *et al*. (1974) Familial incidence of bifid and double ureters. *Arch Dis Child* **43**: 390.

Avellan L, Knutsson F (1980) Microscopic studies of curvature causing structures in hypospadias. *Scand J Plast Reconstr Surg* **14**: 249.

Baker LA, Gomez RA (1998) Embryonic development of the ureter and bladder: acquisition of smooth muscle. *J Urol* **160**: 545.

Berman P, Desjardins L, Fraser FC (1975) The inheritance of the Aarskog syndrome. *J Pediat* **86**: 885.

Bernstein J, Gardner KD Jr (1979) Cystic disease of the kidney and renal dysplasia. In: Harrison JH, Gittes RF, Perlmutter AD *et al*. (eds) *Campbell's urology*. 4th edition. Philadelphia, PA: WB Saunders, 1434.

Birnholz JC (1983) Determination of fetal sex. *N Engl J Med* **309**: 942.

Brooks RE Jr (1962) Left retrocaval ureter associated with situs inversus. *J Urol* **88**: 484.

Clarnette TD, Hutson JM (1996) The genitofemoral nerve may link testicular inguinoscrotal descent with congenital inguinal hernia. *Aust N Z J Surg* **9**: 612.

Clarren SK, Smith DW (1978) The fetal alcohol syndrome. A review of the world literature. *N Engl J Med* **298**: 1063.

Cook WA, Stephens FD (1977) Fused kidneys: morphologic study and theory of embryogenesis. *Birth Defects* **13**: 327.

Corbus BC, Estrem RD, Nunt W (1960) Retroiliac ureter. *J Urol* **84**: 67.

Corliss CE (1976) *Patten's human embryology*. New York: McGraw-Hill.

Dwoskin J (1976) Sibling uropathology. *J Urol* **115**: 726.

Ekbolm P (1996) Genetics of kidney development. *Curr Opin Nephrol Hypertens* **5**: 282.

Field PL, Stephens FD (1974) Congenital urethral membranes causing urethral obstruction. *J Urol* **111**: 250.

Frey HL, Rajfer J (1984) Role of gubernaculum and intraabdominal pressure in process of testicular descent. *J Urol* **131**: 574.

Fryns JP, Kleczkowska A, Moerman P *et al*. (1993) Hereditary hydronephrosis and the short arm of chromosome 6. *Hum Genet* **91**: 514.

Glenister TW (1958) A correlation of the normal development of the penile urethra and of the infraumbilical abdominal wall. *Br J Urol* **30**: 117.

Glenn JF (1959) Agenesis of the bladder. *JAMA* **169**: 2016.

Gomez RA (1998) Role of angiotensin in renal vascular development. *Kidney Int* 54 Suppl 67: S12.

Gomez RA, Norwood VF, Tufro-McReddie A (1997) Development of the kidney vasculature. *Microsc Res Tech* **39**: 254.

Graves FT (1954) The anatomy of the intrarenal arteries and their application to segmental resection of the kidneys. *Br J Surg* **72**: 132.

Gray SW, Skandalakis JE (1972) *Embryology for surgeons*. Philadelphia, PA: WB Saunders, 496.

Greenfield SP, Rutigliano E, Steinhardt G *et al*. (1991) Genitourinary tract malformations and maternal cocaine abuse. *Urology* **37**: 455.

Grobstein C (1995) Inductive interaction in the development of the mouse metanephros. *J Exp Zool* **130**: 319.

Jacobs PA, Strong JA (1959) A case of human intersexuality having a possible XXY sex-determinant mechanism. *Nature* **183**: 302.

Javadpour N, Graziano MF, Terrill R (1974) Experimental induction of patent allantoic duct by intrauterine bladder outlet obstruction. *J Surg Res* **17**: 341.

Kaplan GW, Lamm DL (1975) Embryogenesis of chordee. *J Urol* **114**: 769.

Kaplan GW, McLaughlin AP (1973) Urogenital anomalies and congenital rubella syndrome. *Urology* **2**: 148.

Lechner MS, Dressler GR (1997) The molecular basis of embryonic kidney development. *Mech Dev* **62**: 105.

Levy JB, Husmann DA (1995) The hormonal control of testicular descent. *J Androl* **16**: 459.

Lindsten J (1963) *The nature and origin of X chromosome aberrations in Turner's syndrome*. Stockholm: Almquist and Wicksell.

Lipschultz JH (1998) Molecular development of the kidney: a review of the results of gene disruption studies. *Am J Kidney Dis* **31**: 383.

Lopez-Camelo JS, Orioli IM (1996) Heterogeneous rates for birth defects in Latin America: hints on causality. *Genet Epidemiol* **13**: 469.

Mackie GC, Stephens FD (1975) Duplex kidneys:a correlation of renal dysplasia with position of the ureteral orifice. *J Urol* **114**: 274.

Mackintosh P. Almarhoos G, Heath DA (1989) HLA linkage with familial vesicoureteral reflux and familial pelvi-ureteric junction obstruction. *Tissue Antigens* **34**: 185.

Maizels M, Simpson SB Jr (1983) Primitive ducts of renal dysplasia induced by culturing ureteral buds of condensed renal mesenchyme. *Science* **219**: 509.

Mehta N, Modi N (1989) ACE inhibitors in pregnancy. *Lancet* **2**: 96.

Moerman P, Fryns JP, Sastrowijoto SH *et al.* (1994) Hereditary renal adysplasia: new observations and hypotheses. *Pediatr Pathol* **14**: 405.

Muecke EC (1964) The role of the cloacal membrane in exstrophy. *J Urol* **92**: 659.

Neidhart JH (1972) Quoted in: Gray JW, Skandalakis JF (eds) *Embryology for surgeons*. Philadelphia, PA: WB Saunders, 487.

Orellana SA, Avner ED (1998) Cell and molecular biology of kidney development. *Semin Nephrol* **18**: 233.

Osler W (1901) Congenital absence of abdominal muscles with distended and hypertrophied urinary bladder. *Bull Johns Hopkins* **12**: 311.

Pagon RA, Smith DW, Shepard TH (1979) Urethral obstruction malformation complex: a cause of abdominal muscle deficiency and the 'prune belly'. *J Pediatr* **94**: 900.

Patten (1976) *Human embryology*. New York: McGraw Hill.

Pinto W Jr, Gardner LI, Rosenbaum P (1977) Abnormal genitalia as a presenting sign in two male infants with hydantoin embryopathy syndrome. *Am J Dis Child* **131**: 452.

Riccardi JM, Sujansky E, Smith AC *et al.* (1978) Chromosomal imbalance in the aniridia–Wilms' tumor association: 11p interstitial deletion. *Pediatrics* **61**: 604.

Rich RH, Hardy BE, Filler RM (1983) Surgery for anomalies of the urachus. *J Pediatr Surg* **18**: 370.

Rothman KJ, Moore LL, Singer MR *et al.* (1995) Teratogenicity of high vitamin A intake. *N Engl J Med* **333**: 1369.

Sadler TW (1995) *Longman's medical embryology*. 7th edition. Philadelphia, PA: Williams & Wilkins.

Santava A, Utikalova A, Santavy J (1990) Hereditary and origin of duplication of the pelvicalyceal system. *Acta Univ Palacki Olomuc Fac Med* **126**: 209.

Schlegel PN, Shin D, Goldstein M (1996) Urogenital anomalies in men with congenital absence of the vas deferens. *J Urol* **155**: 1644.

Smith DW (1982) *Recognizable patterns of human malformation*. 3rd edition. Philadelphia, PA: WB Saunders.

Spence HM, Allen T (1964) Congenital absence of the abdominal musculature. *JAMA* **187**: 814.

Stephens FD (1983) *Congenital malformations of the urinary tract*. New York: Praeger, 96.

Stephens FD and Smith ED (1971) *Anorectal malformations in children*. Chicago, IL: Year Book Medical Publishers.

Tanagho EA (1972) Anatomy and management of ureteroceles. *J Urol* **107**: 729.

Thomas IT, Smith DW (1974) Oligohydramnios, cause of the non-renal features of Potter's syndrome, including pulmonary hypoplasia. *J Pediatr* **84**: 811.

Vaughn VC, McKay JR (eds) (1975) *Nelson textbook of pediatrics*. 10th edition. Philadelphia, PA: WB Saunders.

Vilain E, McCabe F. Genes controlling gonadal differentiation. *Molec Genet Metab* 1998; **65**: 74.

Zackai E, Mellman MJ, Neiderer B *et al.* (1975) The fetal trimethadione syndrome. *J Pediatrics* **87**: 280.

Renal development: fluid and electrolyte balance in neonates

2

Billy S. Arant, Jr

Introduction

The developing mammalian kidney is a remarkably complex organ. Although it has been characterized as small, immature, limited, and imbalanced and, as such, an impediment to the medical management of sick infants, this view is unwarranted. When it was first recognized that glomerular filtration rate (GFR) corrected for the body size of newborn infants was less than values measured in the adult (Barnett *et al.*, 1948), the notion of limited renal function was introduced. While the bulk of published studies on the various functions of the neonatal kidney seem to support limitation, many of these studies were misinterpreted and seemed to have conformed to the bias prevalent at the time.

It is somewhat difficult to imagine how the species survived the stress of fetal adaptation to the functional integrity of postnatal life if the neonatal kidney were indeed limited in its functional capacity. Many premature infants weighing < 1000 g at birth survived even in the 1930s to become healthy infants long before the availability of supportive measures now referred to as neonatal intensive care (Arant, 1982). Human and experimental animal studies, done more recently, provide some enlightenment and confirm the essential and unique role of the kidney at any stage of viability once the umbilical blood flow is interrupted at birth.

The kidney of the human neonate functions qualitatively like the adult kidney and is more than adequate to support functional development and growth of the infant following birth, at least within limits. These limits, however, are often exceeded by the demands imposed during the treatment of sick infants when most clinical decisions are made without concern for kidney function. Too often, perhaps, it is easier to fault the kidney because it is small rather than to understand the essence of its supporting role in health and disease. Failing to appreciate the unique responses of the neonatal kidney will, on occasion, compromise clinical decision making, especially when prescribing fluid therapy (Arant, 1982) and drugs eliminated primarily by renal excretion (Cowan *et al.*, 1980; Szefler *et al.*, 1980).

Morphologic development

The human metanephros is formed about the 5th week after conception, when the sequential branching ureteric bud contacts the caudal mesenchyma and induces glomerulogenesis. All glomeruli are contained within the cortex. The first ones formed occupy a juxtamedullary postion and have the longest loops of Henle. The ureteric bud forms the collecting duct for each nephron and continues to branch in a centrifugal pattern until 20 weeks of gestation. New glomeruli are formed until 34–36 weeks after conception when each kidney will contain approximately one million nephrons (Fig. 2.1). When birth occurs prematurely, glomerulogenesis continues. But there is speculation that the total number of glomeruli at maturity may be deficient and contribute to morbidity, mainly hypertension and renal insufficiency in later life due to glomerular hyperfiltration (Brenner and Chertow, 1994). Glomerular filtration is evident after 8 weeks' gestation, but the ureter may not be entirely patent until the 11th week. Ureteral obstruction is thought to provoke dilation of the proximal collecting system, the renal pelvis and calyces. The layers of smooth muscle and elastic fibers in the ureter are laid down after 36 weeks' gestation and continue to form for 8 weeks after birth at term. If there is an essential role of the fetal kidney, it must be to contribute the majority of amniotic fluid after the first trimester of pregnancy.

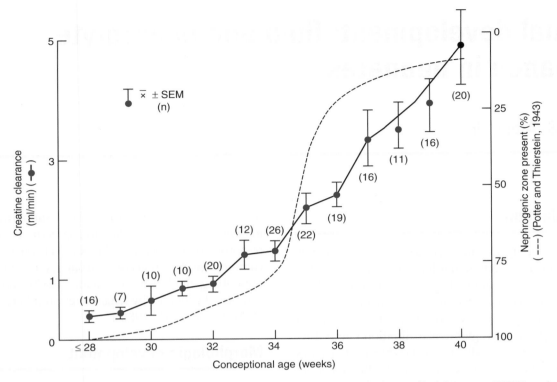

Figure 2.1 Developmental pattern of changes in creatinine clearance [glomerular filtration rate (GFR)] and the disappearance of the nephrogenic zone of the renal cortex compared with the conceptional age of human infants. (From Arant, 1992, with permission.)

Physiologic adaptation at birth

Body composition

From the moment of conception, when the composition of the fertilized ovum is 99% salt and water, there is a gradual reduction in the relative body content of water and minerals with age. While the total amounts of minerals and water provided by the placenta increase as the fetus grows, organs are formed and tissue growth occurs which incorporate these elements into cytoplasm and extracellular matrix. The higher salt and water content of the fetus assures a relative abundance of extracellular fluid which decreases from 60% of body weight at the beginning of the last trimester to 40% at birth; extracellular fluid represents only 20% of body weight in the adult (Friis-Hansen, 1961). Therefore, whether birth occurs before or at term, essentially all neonates have an expanded extracellular fluid volume that

allows them to survive naturally without intake for a few days postnatally as the volume of the mother's breast milk increases. Extracellular fluid volume expansion in the neonate influences renal function just as it does in the adult. When birth occurs at term, the total body water content has been reduced to 75% and the sodium content has decreased from 120 mmol/kg body weight at 8 weeks after conception to 85 mmol/kg (Widdowson and Dickerson, 1968). During the first week of life, there is an additional reduction in the relative body water and sodium content, mainly through urinary losses and, thus, extracellular fluid volume is reduced further. In premature infants, this abrupt reduction in total body water and sodium following birth is more pronounced and represents losses of up to 25% of body weight as water and 14 mmol/kg sodium with no change in plasma sodium concentration or blood pressure (Smith et al., 1949; Butterfield et al., 1960; Shaffer et al., 1987).

Cardiovascular hemodynamics

During fetal life, systemic vascular resistance is kept very low except in the pulmonary and renal circulations, where vascular resistance is high since neither organ contributes directly to the viability of the fetus (Arant, 1992). The explanation for the regulation of the differences in these specialized circulations may be the local formation of vasoactive substances that cause vascular smooth muscle to contract (angiotensin) or relax (prostaglandins and nitric oxide). Cardiac output in the fetus is high and varies only with heart rate since stroke volume is always at a maximum (Klopfenstein and Rudolph, 1978). Moreover, blood volume in the fetus and very preterm infant may be as high as 120 ml/kg body weight compared with 75 ml/kg in the adult (Morris *et al.*, 1974). With both cardiac output and blood volume high, how can blood pressure be so low? Normal mean arterial pressure for a preterm infant is only about 25 mmHg. The answer, therefore, must come from the balance of forces that regulate vascular resistance. There is an inverse relationship between blood volume and diastolic blood pressure in normal human adults (London *et al.*, 1977). Moreover, when fetal animals or preterm infants have their blood volumes expanded by colloid or whole blood, blood pressure does not increase and may actually decrease in some cases (Barr *et al.*, 1977; Arant, 1981). Even when the volume of blood in the placental circulation is transfused into the neonatal circulation, which could be up to 30 ml/kg, there is no sustained rise in the infant's blood pressure or right atrial pressure (Oh *et al.*, 1966). At birth, the placental circulation is interrupted, the lungs are expanded with the first breaths by the infant and pulmonary vascular resistance decreases to allow oxygen transfer across the alveolus into the blood. Then, the ductus arteriosus closes when the oxygen tension in arterial blood has increased sufficiently to cause the specialized smooth muscle in that structure to constrict. Systemic vascular resistance and blood pressure in the neonate gradually increase over the first 3 months of life to a maximum normal blood pressure of 106/63 mmHg (90th percentile for age and sex) (Task Force on Blood Pressure Control in Children, 1987).

Renal blood flow

Renal blood flow (RBF) and its intrarenal distribution have been the subject of many investigations.

Few of these studies provided results that were reproducible or explanations which were entirely satisfactory. While GFR can be measured easily by clearance methodology, the only technique for measuring RBF in human infants is still the clearance of para-aminohippurate (PAH). After concluding that RBF measured by PAH clearance was disproportionately low in newborn infants, which was part of the reason for misrepresentation of newborn kidney function, it was later learned that the extraction of PAH by the newborn kidney was less than half that of the child or adult (Calcagno and Rubin, 1963). When corrected for the PAH extraction rate, RBF and the filtration fraction or the ratio of GFR:renal plasma flow was 0.20, the same as the normal value in the adult.

RBF in the full-term infant increases from 290 ml/min per 1.73 m^2 at birth to 750 ml/min per 1.73 m^2 by 8 months of age (Rubin *et al.*, 1949; Calcagno and Rubin, 1963). This increase in RBF occurs as renal vascular resistance (RVR) decreases. No actual measurements of RVR have been reported for human infants, even though calculations made using average blood pressure for age (Fig. 2.2) provide the same pattern of developmental change as reported in the pig (Gruskin *et al.*, 1970) and dog (Seikaly and Arant, 1992).

There would appear to be a direct relationship between changes in RVR and the intracortical distribution of RBF during development. While it was once believed that there was a centrifugal redistribution of blood flow within the renal cortex, the actual pattern of blood flow distribution follows the distribution of functioning or filtering nephrons (Seikaly and Arant, 1989). Studies that fostered the former notion were conducted in anesthetized animals following acute surgical preparation, a situation known to alter total RBF and reduce outer cortical blood flow by activating the intrarenal renin–angiotensin system (Terragno *et al.*, 1977). More than half the glomeruli reside in the outer cortex at birth, and appropriately done studies have demonstrated a predominance of blood flow distribution to this area (Robillard *et al.*, 1981). Further growth of the kidney is achieved mainly by lengthening of proximal convoluted tubules which are interposed between glomeruli. At maturity, the glomeruli are evenly distributed throughout the cortex and the blood flow to each cortical region is similar.

Once it was thought that the kidney only responded to circulating hormones that affected its various

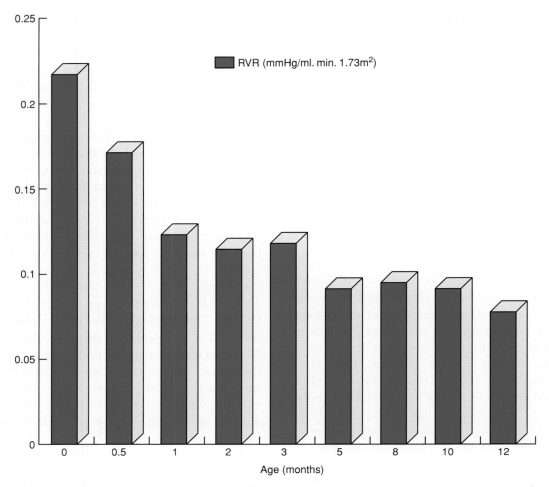

Figure 2.2 Decrease in renal vascular resistance (RVR) with the postnatal age of human infants born at term and studied during the first year of life. Renal blood flow was estimated from extraction-corrected clearances of PAH (Rubin *et al.*, 1949; Calcagno and Rubin, 1963). Age-related normal values for hematocrit and mean arterial pressure (Task Force on Blood Pressure Control in Children, 1987) were used for calculations.

functions. For instance, that renin, produced in juxta-glomerular cells and released from the kidney, acted on angiotensinogen made by the liver to synthesize angiotensin I. This, in turn, was acted on by converting enzyme in the pulmonary circulation to release the vasoconstricting hormone angiotensin II (ANGII) into the arterial circulation. However, the intrarenal production of vasoactive substances is now well known. The kidney is capable of producing large quantities of ANGII on its own, as can isolated, bloodless glomeruli (Atiyeh *et al.*, 1995). Also, molecular studies have demonstrated mRNA for renin, angiotensinogen, and angiotensin converting enzyme (ACE). In micropuncture studies of the rat kidney, ANGII concentrations were found to be 1000-fold higher in efferent arteriolar blood and proximal tubu-

lar fluid than in the systemic circulation (Seikaly *et al.*, 1990). Moreover, the kidney and glomeruli contain the enzymes for synthesizing ANGII by pathways other than ACE (Atiyeh *et al.*, 1995).

What does the kidney do with all the ANGII it produces? Both circulating levels of plasma ANGII and the urinary excretion of ANGII and its metabolites are increased in human and canine neonates (Arant and Seikaly, 1989). Moreover, the pattern of change in the urinary excretion of ANGII parallels the change in RVR following birth. In addition to effecting resistance in the renal microcirculation to regulate GFR, ANGII exerts a major influence over proximal tubular mechanisms, particularly sodium reabsorption (Schuster *et al.*, 1984). ANGII is rapidly metabolized within the kidney because the high concentrations in arteriolar blood and proximal tubular fluid are not found in either renal venous effluent or distal tubular fluid (Seikaly *et al.*, 1990). Moreover, concentrations of ANGII in tissue-free incubation medium remain constant with time but decrease in the presence of isolated glomeruli (Atiyeh *et al.*, 1995). Very little ANGII can be measured in bladder urine, but its metabolites are more abundant. Finally, ANGII is an important growth factor that, in some way, may be critical to the morphologic development of the kidney. When ACE inhibitors are given to pregnant women, both the structure and function of the fetal and neonatal kidney are altered (Pryde *et al.*, 1993). In disease states, such as diabetic nephropathy, chronic glomerulonephritis, or chronic pyelonephritis, progressive renal scarring and deterioration of renal function can be slowed dramatically by inhibiting ANGII production. This beneficial effect is mediated not only by lowering blood pressure and reducing glomerular hyperfiltration but also by the reducing the deposition of collagen in diseased renal parenchyma.

Vasoactive factors that oppose the vasoconstricting effects of ANGII include prostaglandins, particularly PGE_2 and prostacyclin, and nitric oxide. It is difficult to separate the vasodilating effects of one from the other. It may be that the prostaglandins are the mediators of nitric oxide production by the vascular endothelium, but the renal vascular and tubular responses to nitric oxide have not been studied in the developing kidney or newborn infant. Prostaglandins also mediate the effects of loop diuretics (Stokes, 1979) and reduce tubular responsiveness to arginine vasopressin (Stokes, 1981). When an inhibitor of prostaglandin synthesis is administered, therefore, the vasoconstrictor effect of ANGII is unmasked and RVR increases (Arant and Seikaly, 1990). This is clinically apparent when a non-steroidal anti-inflammatory drug is given to a patient whose endogenous ANGII synthesis is elevated, as in dehydration. If watched for, there will usually be an increase in blood pressure, a decrease in GFR, and oliguria or even anuria, which does not respond well to furosemide or fluid administration. The opposite is seen when an ACE inhibitor or AT-1 receptor blocker is given to someone whose endogenous synthesis of prostaglandins, particularly prostacyclin, is increased, as in the neonate or a patient with Bartter syndrome. This patient may become hypotensive and renal perfusion pressure reduced.

Catecholamines are produced in significant amounts in the fetus and newborn infant but their impact on renal blood flow, except in hypovolemic states, is difficult to demonstrate in clinical studies. Based on no appropriate data, the recommendation has been made for years that low doses (5 μg/kg per min) or 'renal doses' of dopamine be infused to treat infants with hypotension or hypoperfusion. The benefit of such therapy was extrapolated from studies of adults in various shock-like states (Winslow *et al.*, 1973). Studies in healthy newborn animals have not reported a consistent beneficial effect of a renal dose of dopamine (Feltes *et al.*, 1987). Although dopamine therapy may be associated with improved urine output and GFR, the effect probably is mediated through an improvement in cardiac output or blood pressure that, in turn, improves RBF, GFR, and urine volume.

Glomerular filtration rate

GFR estimated in the human fetus as early as 20 weeks gestation (Haycock, 1998) or measured at birth in minimally stressed infants from 24 weeks' gestation (Arant, 1978) has been reported to be around 0.2 ml/min, which is only about 5 ml/min per 1.73 m² and does not increase significantly above this level until a postconceptional age of 34 weeks has been reached. This pattern of change has been measured and is identical whether the fetus remains *in utero* or continues its development after a premature birth (Arant, 1978) (Fig. 2.3). In other words, the infant born after 34 weeks' gestation will exhibit a 5–7-fold increase in GFR during the first week of life, but the preterm infant born at 26 weeks' gestation will have no appreciable increase in GFR for 8 weeks. A similar developmental change in GFR has been reported to occur in every mammalian species studied. The average GFR in the normal adult is 125 ml/min, which is achieved during adolescence when the average adult body surface area is 1.73 m². After 6 months of age, however, the absolute value for GFR (ml/min) can be corrected for a body surface area of 1.73 m² in any infant or child and compared, more conveniently, to the mature value of about 125 ml/min per 1.73 m² (Barnett *et al.*, 1948).

Following some, as yet unidentified, biological signal RVR rapidly decreases and GFR increases close to the time when nephrogenesis is completed which, in the human, is at 34–36 weeks (Arant, 1978; Engle and Arant, 1983) (Fig. 2.1). This developmental

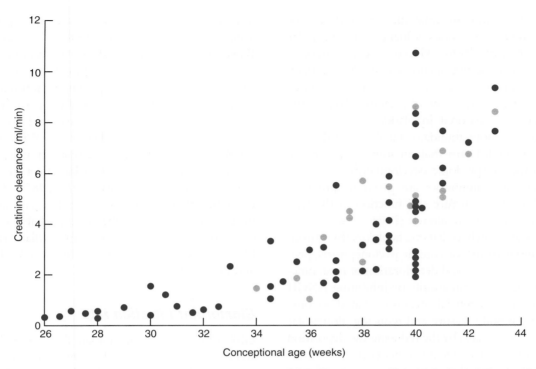

Figure 2.3 Creatinine clearance [glomerular filtration rate (GFR)] compared with conceptional age of infants from birth. Studies performed within 48 h of birth; ●: studies done at weekly intervals following birth; ● regression analysis confirmed a non-linear relationship expressed best as an exponential equation. (From Engle and Arant, 1983, with permission.)

phenomenon is mediated through changes in RVR and, probably, by changes in the intrarenal production of vasoactive substances such as ANGII, prostaglandins, and nitric oxide. Therefore, any treatment that alters the synthesis of these substances can change the developmental pattern, at least temporarily. For instance, a preterm neonate given indomethacin to effect closure of a patent ductus arteriosus will have a decreased GFR (Cifuentes *et al.*, 1979) and may have an impaired ability to increase GFR until the pharmacologic effects of the drug have diminished.

GFR in the infant can be measured directly by a clearance technique, that requires a timed urine collection and one or more blood samples, using either endogenous creatinine or an exogenous marker such as inulin or iothalomate, infused intravenously. Both timed urine collections and multiple blood samples are difficult to obtain in neonates. While many have turned to radioisotopic techniques to estimate GFR in adults, there are no normal data published for infants. Nuclear medicine studies often report the fraction of total uptake by left or right kidney and interpret the

result as a percentage of total kidney function, but this methodology provides no actual estimate of GFR.

Perhaps the most clinically useful estimate of GFR in neonates is a serial change in serum creatinine concentration compared with the pattern of change with postconceptional age expected for a normal infant. The newborn infant's serum creatinine concentration is identical to maternal values even if the infant's kidneys do not function at all (Sertel and Scopes, 1973; Arant, 1996a). GFR in infants born after 34 weeks' gestation should be expected to increase greatly and serum creatinine concentration will be reduced by 50% during the first week of life (Stuphen, 1982) (Fig. 2.4). In contrast, the infant born before 34 weeks' gestation is not expected to decrease the serum creatinine concentration until a postconceptional age of 34 weeks has been achieved because the tightly controlled GFR is sufficient only to excrete the creatinine produced each day by the infant, i.e. 8 mg/kg per day (Stuphen, 1982); the creatinine accumulated during fetal life and distributed in total body water cannot be reduced appreciably before GFR increases at around 34 weeks after conception. The normal serum creatinine concentration should be about 0.4 mg/dl by the end of the first month of life in infants born at term (Schwartz *et al.*, 1984), but preterm infants may not reach this level until 3 months of age (Arant, 1996a) (Fig. 2.4). Thereafter, a doubling of serum creatinine concentration reflects a reduction in GFR by 50%.

It may be easier to estimate GFR from serum creatinine concentration and the infant's length which,

when factored with a constant number, can provide a reasonable assessment of GFR. The formula derived by Schwartz *et al.* is:

$$\text{GFR (ml/min/1.73 m}^2) = \frac{K \times \text{length (cm)}}{\text{serum creatinine (mg/dl)}}$$

where the value for K is 0.45 for full-term infants (Schwartz *et al.*, 1984) and 0.35 for preterm infants (Brion *et al.*, 1986).

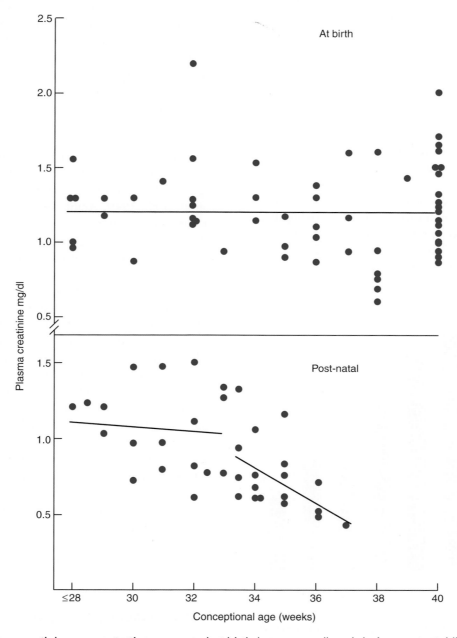

Figure 2.4 Plasma creatinine concentration measured at birth (upper panel) and during postnatal life (lower panel) compared with the conceptional age of infants. (From Arant, 1996a, with permission.)

Urinary volume

It is usual for every normal neonate, regardless of gestational age, to void some amount of urine, if not during delivery, which sometimes goes unrecognized, then, by 24 hours of age. Premature infants usually void more often and in larger volumes relative to body weight (ml/kg per h) and GFR when compared with infants born at term (Arant, 1992) (Fig. 2.5). For instance, the very small preterm infant will normally excrete about 10% of the volume of water filtered by the glomerulus when compared with 3% in the full-term infant and only 1% in the adult. One explanation for this difference is that the preterm infant has more extracellular fluid to excrete following birth than does the full-term infant, whose additional time *in utero* permitted the extracelluar fluid volume to be reduced before birth. The only way for the normal adult kidney to excrete 10% of glomerular filtrate in the urine is after massive saline expansion of the extracellular fluid volume.

The typical pattern of urinary volume in the full-term infant includes one to four voidings over the first 48 hours of life, with each subsequent voiding being somewhat smaller in volume than the last and with a higher specific gravity or osmolarity. When fed, urine production in the infant increases and the volume becomes larger and the urine less concentrated. Preterm infants, in contrast, void more frequently, with urinary flow rates usually being 3–7 ml/kg per hour during the first days of life. This urine is either isotonic or hypotonic to plasma despite a loss in body weight and reduction in extracellular fluid volume. The continued production of dilute urine depends on the volume of fluids provided to the infant and the insensible water losses experienced. Both premature and full-term infants are capable of concentrating their urines to a specific gravity >1.020 or an osmolarity of 700 mosm/kg (Smith *et al.*, 1949) once extracellular fluid volume has been reduced sufficiently to stimulate the baroreceptor-mediated release of arginine vasopressin from the hypothalamus. A marker for the end of the postnatal diuresis in a normal infant is a reduction in the frequency and volume of urine excreted, increase in urinary osmolarity, and stabilization of the infant's body weight. The extreme of this phenomenon was described in reports when premature infants were not given any fluid at all following birth for at least 72 h and, occasionally, longer (Smith *et al.*, 1949; Arant, 1982). If parenteral fluid therapy is overly aggressive, then the expanded extracellular fluid volume characteristic of the fetus will result in a continued natriuresis and diuresis in the neonate (Arant, 1992). Infants born with urologic disease, such as renal dysplasia or obstructive uropathy, may become dehydrated and hemodynamically unstable, since the ability to conserve sodium and concentrate the urine is almost certainly impaired.

In general, clinicians are comfortable when urine volume is ≥ 1 ml/kg per h, which corresponds to the urine volume of ~1500 ml/24 h in the adult. Just as one would be satisfied with slightly less urine in the adult, less urine is also acceptable in the healthy neonate. Urinary volume should never be interpreted alone, and the specific gravity or osmolarity must be considered as well. In the normal patient, neonate, or adult, there is an inverse relationship between urinary volume and urinary concentration. When urine volume changes, up or down, without a reciprocal change in concentration, an abnormal urinary tract, kidneys, or collecting system should be suspected.

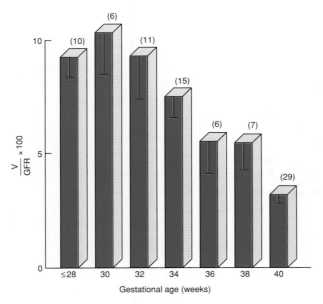

Figure 2.5 Fractional excretion of water [urine flow rate/glomerular filtration rate (GFR)] compared with gestational age of infants on the first day of life. (From Arant, 1992, with permission.)

Tubular handling of sodium

Perhaps more confusing than any other function of the neonatal kidney is its handling of sodium (Na). In the earliest reported studies, mature and premature human neonates could not excrete a NaCl load as well as an adult (Dean and McCance, 1949; Aperia *et al.*, 1974). When studies of preterm infants were performed in neonatal intensive care units, renal Na wasting was often observed even in the face of hyponatremia (Engelke *et al.*, 1978). One would think, ordinarily, that functional immaturity would be characterized first by a limited capacity of the growing renal tubule to reabsorb the Na filtered by the glomerulus. With maturation, the tubule would be able to reabsorb more. For many years, studies in both human infants and animal models held to this notion that preterm infants could not conserve sodium and full-term infants could not excrete it. The provision of Na in parenteral fluids and diet for preterm infants was decided on this basis. Then, several clinical studies were done in which the preterm infants were allowed to undergo postnatal diuresis and graduated weight loss. These infants maintained Na balance quite appropriately and very much like the adult (Lorenz *et al.*, 1982; Costarino *et al.*, 1992). In addition, preterm infants weighing <1000 g were given no Na in their fluids and only enough water to prevent the extracellular fluid from becoming hypertonic. Despite a negative Na balance from urinary losses, these very preterm infants were able to maintain a normal plasma Na concentration for the first week of life. One cannot separate the renal handling of Na from changes in effective arterial blood volume (EABV), i.e. the combined simultaneous effects of blood pressure and blood volume. When baroreceptors in the renal circulation perceive an increased EABV, whether from an increase in blood volume or blood pressure, the mature kidney responds by an increase in the renal excretion of Na and water which is facilitated by the inhibition of the release of both renin and arginine vasopressin (Arant, 1992).

One cannot completely evaluate kidney function in the newborn infant without calculating the fractional excretion of Na (FENa):

$$\text{FENa (\%)} = \frac{\text{urinary Na}^+ \text{ (mmol/l)} \times \text{serum creatinine (mg/dl)}}{\text{plasma Na}^+ \text{ (mmol/l)} \times \text{urine creatinine (mg/dl)}}$$

The result is a reliable indicator of the overall renal tubular handling of Na. FENa is <1% in the normal adult but can rise with an increase in EABV, by tubu-

lar injury as with diuretics, obstruction or renal disease, or by any maneuver that increases the fractional excretion of water (V/GFR) such as fluid overload (Arant, 1992). When the kidney is maximally conserving the circulating blood volume, as in hypovolemic shock, dehydration, or congestive heart failure, oliguria is usual, V/GFR is <1%, the urinary concentration is maximal, and the FENA is much less than 1%, often only 0.1%. This would be true even if the patient had a positive Na balance and were hypernatremic. The status of the EABV overrides any signaling from body fluid osmolarity. The renal tubular handling of Na is related directly to V/GFR rather than to the variations in the maturity of the infant or its kidney (Arant, 1988, 1992).

Acid–base balance

Unless demand becomes overwhelming the neonatal kidney is capable of reabsorbing bicarbonate filtered by the glomerulus and secreting hydrogen ions or protons in a normal or mature fashion (80 mEq/1.73 m^2 per day) (Sulyok and Heim, 1971). Most of the acidemia measured in preterm infants can be accounted for by respiratory acidosis. The relative metabolic acidosis in the neonate is implied when arterial blood gas measurement reports a significant base deficit, often calculated on the assumption that the hemoglobin is 12 g/dl, which is inappropriate in the neonate whose hemoglobin may be 18 g/dl. The normal plasma bicarbonate or serum total CO_2 in newborn infants is 13–17 mmol/l in preterm infants and 19–21 mmol/l in full-term infants (Schwartz *et al.*, 1979). If the measured or calculated bicarbonate in arterial blood is subtracted inappropriately from the 'normal' plasma bicarbonate of the adult (28–30 mmol/l), the neonate will always have a 'base deficit'. Moreover, a mild hyperchloremia (plasma chloride concentration 103–110 mmol/l) is usually observed in normal neonates. The increased EABV results in a decrease in reabsorption of nearly all substances presented to the proximal tubule: not just Na and chloride, but also bicarbonate. Once the infant's extracellular fluid excess has been reduced following birth, proximal tubular reabsorption increases, the renal threshold for bicarbonate increases, and the so-called metabolic acidosis disappears.

One should have very good basis for treating metabolic acidosis in the neonate, and more than a blood gas report. When the metabolic acidosis proves real, a reduction in renal glomerular or tubular function should be considered. Metabolic acidosis is common in urologic diseases identified in neonates. Distal tubular injury from obstruction or infection impairs the ability of that part of the nephron to secrete hydrogen ions and potassium. The metabolic acidosis and hyperkalemia in such infants suggest a tubular unresponsiveness to aldosterone or pseudohypoaldosteronism.

Renal tubular acidosis is an uncommon condition in newborn infants and should be considered only after the infant has been shown to have a metabolic acidosis, i.e. arterial blood pH < 7.35 and hyperchloremia, and the urinary anion gap is measured (urinary Na concentration + urinary potassium concentration − urinary chloride concentration). Most so-called renal tubular acidosis in infants is a complication of diarrheal disease with the intestinal loss of bicarbonate: the urine pH is always < 6.0 in these patients.

Hypertension

The incidence of hypertension in the first year of life is unknown. There is a reluctance by most healthcare providers to attempt to record blood pressure. First, there is the technical difficulty in taking the blood pressure correctly and under reproducible conditions. Most physicians do not maintain a complete assortment of cuff sizes in their offices and the size of the cuff influences the blood pressure reading significantly. The smaller the cuff, the higher the blood pressure. For the most accurate reading, the width of the cuff should cover more than 50% of the length of the humerus when the blood pressure is recorded in the upper extremity. Even if the infant is calm or sleeping, the effect of feeding and positioning has been shown to elevate the blood pressure above normal. Secondly, very few clinicians know how to interpret the blood pressure readings in infants unless very high readings are obtained (>95th percentile for age, gender, and length) (Task Force on Blood Pressure Control in Children, 1987). Consequently, it is the practice even in some tertiary pediatric facilities not to routinely record blood pressures on patients <3 years old.

If an elevated blood pressure is noted, the possible causes in the first year of life are few in number (Arar et al., 1994). The most common etiology is due to a complication of an umbilical artery catheter, either from a thrombus that forms on the tip of the catheter and embolizes into the renal artery, or from an aortic wall thrombus at or above the renal arteries that propagates to occlude one or both renal arteries. Relative renal ischemia or actual cortical necrosis will be associated with severe hypertension and heart failure. The second cause of hypertension in the first year of life is autosomal recessive polycystic kidney disease. In most cases, the cystic kidneys have been identified by fetal ultrasonography or confirmed when enlarged and irregularly shaped kidneys are detected by abdominal palpation. Neurofibromatosis is almost the only cause of renal artery stenosis in the first year of life that causes hypertension. It is unusual to find hypertension as a consequence of most other developmental abnormalities of the urinary tract. Hypertension is observed sometimes in premature infants who have suffered from barotraumas and have bronchopulmonary dysplasia, especially if they are being treated with corticosteroids. Catecholamine-producing tissues, such as pheochromocytoma and neuroblastoma, are rare causes of hypertension in infants.

Fluid therapy in the neonate

The general principle of fluid therapy in neonates is to restrict the volume of fluid given each day to less than the recommended maintenance volume (~100 ml/kg per day) until the infant has lost 5–15% of birth weight gradually, usually during the first 3–5 days of life. Premature infants will lose proportionally more weight than full-term infants. Once postnatal body weight has become constant, the urine flow rate slowed, and the urine concentration increased, the normal infant up to 10 kg body weight should receive about 100 ml/kg per day of water either by mouth, or parenterally when oral intake is not recommended. This amount represents the sum of insensible water losses (sweat, respiration, and gastrointestinal losses), which are approximately 30 ml/kg per day, and urine volume, usually about 70 ml/kg per day. Larger patients require less fluid per kilogram body weight to maintain total body water normal because of a decreasing caloric expenditure: 50 ml/kg per day for each kilogram between 11 and 20 kg and 20 ml/kg for each kilogram over 20 kg. Any condition that alters either insensible water losses or urine production must prompt a change in the volume of fluids administered; otherwise, dehydration or fluid overload is risked. After the immediate newborn period, infants will not tolerate long intervals of fluid deprivation without exhibiting signs of dehydration. Preoperatively, parenteral fluid therapy should be instituted when oral intake is discontinued.

There is only a very rare indication in pediatrics for using water or dextrose in water alone for parenteral fluid therapy. This is especially true in infants in whom water intoxication, hyponatremia, cerebral edema, and nervous system injury quickly follow the inappropriate administration of water without electrolytes. The exception will be the neonate whose insensible water losses in the first days of life only are replaced with 5–10% dextrose in water. Central diabetes insipidus is the only other clinical condition that calls for the administration of water without more electrolytes than needed to maintain the patient. To the calculated volume of water necessary for the infant or child, 1–3 mmol/kg per day of sodium, potassium, and chloride should be added (Arant, 1993). This quantity of electrolytes is required for an expanding extracellular matrix and cellular proliferation to facilitate rapid somatic growth. The faster the rate of growth, the more electrolyte is needed. Calories must be provided daily to the infant or child. One cannot rely on a 5% dextrose solution which, at best, affords only 20 kcal/kg per day when at least 65 kcal/kg per day is required to avoid catabolism in the patient. For the patient not expected to take oral feedings for more than 24 hours, consideration should be given to peripheral alimentation with up to 12.5% dextrose, essential amino acids (1 g/kg per day) and intralipid solution (1–3 g/kg per day) (Arant, 1996b).

Summary

The greatest obstacle to understanding neonatal kidney function is not knowing which reported observation is or has remained valid. Without criticism, many statements are made and referenced in review articles and textbooks that perpetuate myths of so-called clinical experience and physiologic study. When one understands the normal physiologic responses of the adult or mature kidney, then a nearly complete appreciation of the fetal and neonatal kidney is within reach. The neonatal kidney functions qualitatively like the adult kidney and its limitations come when unusual demands are made on it by stress, disease, or treatment.

References

Aperia A, Broberger O, Thodenius K *et al.* (1974) Developmental study of the renal response to an oral salt load in preterm infants. *Acta Paediatr Scand* **63**: 517–24.

Arant BS Jr (1978) Developmental patterns of renal functional maturation compared in the human neonate. *J Pediatr* **92**: 705–12.

Arant BS Jr (1981) The relationship between blood volume, prostaglandin synthesis and arterial blood pressure in neonatal puppies. In: Spitzer A (ed.) *The kidney during development. Morphology and function*. New York: Masson, 167–72.

Arant BS Jr (1982) Fluid therapy in the neonate – concepts in transition. *J Pediatr* **101**: 387–9.

Arant BS Jr (1988) Distal tubular sodium handling in human neonates: clearance studies. *Contrib Nephrol* **67**: 130–7.

Arant BS Jr (1992) Neonatal adjustments to extrauterine life. In: Edelmann CM Jr, Bernstein J, Meadow R *et al.* (eds) *Pediatric kidney disease*. Boston, MA: Little Brown, 1015–42.

Arant BS Jr (1993) Sodium, chloride, and potassium. In: Tsang RC, Lucas A, Uauy R, Zlotkin S (eds) *Nutritional needs of the preterm infant*. Baltimore, MD: Williams and Wilkins, 157–75.

Arant BS (1996a) In: Rudolph AJ (ed.) *Rudolph's Pediatrics*. 20th edition. Stamford, CT: Appleton and Lange, 1316–9.

Arant BS Jr (1996b) Pediatric fluid therapy. In: Kokko JP, Tannen RL (eds) *Fluids and electrolytes*. 3rd edition. Philadelphia, PA: WB Saunders, 819–29.

Arant BS Jr, Seikaly MG (1989) Intrarenal angiotensin II may regulate developmental changes in renal blood flow. *Pediatr Res* **25**: 334A.

Arant BS Jr, Seikaly MG (1990). Intrarenal hemodynamic effects of angiotensin II and prostaglandins are independent. *Pediatr Res* **27**: 323A.

Arar MY, Arant BS Jr, Hogg RJ, Seikaly MG (1994) Etiology of sustained hypertension in children in the Southwestern United States. *Pediatr Nephrol* **8**: 186–9.

Atiyeh BA, Arant BS Jr, Henrich WL, Seikaly MG (1995) *In vitro* production of angiotensin II by isolated glomeruli. *Am J Physiol* **268**: F266–72.

Barnett HL, Hare K, McNamara H *et al.* (1948) Measurement of glomerular filtration rate in premature infants. *J Clin Invest* **27**: 691–9.

Barr PA, Bailey PE, Sumners J *et al.* (1977) Relation between arterial blood pressure and bood volume and effect of infused albumin in sick preterm infants. *Pediatrics* **60**: 282–9.

Brenner BM, Chertow GM (1994) Congenital oligonephropathy and the etiology of adult hypertension and progressive renal injury. *Am J Kidney Dis* **23**: 171–5.

Brion LP, Fleischman AR, McCarton C *et al.* (1986) A simple estimate of glomerular filtration rate in low birth weight infants during the first year of life: noninvasive assessment of body composition and growth. *J Pediatr* **109**: 698–707.

Butterfield J, Lubchenco LO, Bergstedt J *et al.* (1960) Patterns in electrolyte and nitrogen balance in the newborn premature infant. *Pediatrics* 777–91.

Calcagno PL, Rubin MI (1963) Renal extraction of para-aminohippurate in infants and children. *J Clin Invest* **42**: 1632–9.

Cifuentes RF, Olley PM, Balfe JW *et al.* (1979) Indomethacin and renal function in premature infants with persistent patent ductus arteriosus. *J Pediatr* **95**: 583–7.

Costarino AT Jr, Gruskay JA, Corcoran L *et al.* (1992) Sodium restriction versus daily maintenance replacement in very low birth weight premature neonates: a randomized, blind therapeutic trial. *J Pediatr* **120**: 99–106.

Cowan RH, Jukkola AF, Arant BS Jr (1980) Pathophysiologic evidence of gentamicin nephrotoxicity in the neonatal puppy. *Pediatr Res* **14**: 1204–11.

Dean RFA, McCance RA (1949) The renal responses of infants and adults to the administration of hypertonic solutions of sodium chloride and urea. *J Physiol* **109**: 81–97.

Engelke SC, Shah BL, Vasan U *et al.* (1978) Sodium balance in low birth weight infants. *J Pediatr* **93**: 837–41.

Engle WD, Arant BS Jr (1983) Renal handling of beta-2-microglobulin in the human neonate. *Kidney Int* **24**: 358–63.

Feltes TF, Hansen TN, Martin CG *et al.* (1987) The effects of dopamine infusion on reional blood flow in newborn lambs. *Pediatr Res* **21**: 131–6.

Friis-Hansen B (1961) Body water compartments in children:changes during growth and related changes in body composition. *Pediatrics* **28**: 169–81.

Gruskin AB, Edelmann CM Jr, Yuan S (1970) Maturational changes in renal blood flow in piglets. *Pediatr Res* **4**: 7–13.

Haycock GB (1998) Development of glomerular filtration and tubular sodium reabsorption in the human fetus and newborn. *Br J Urol* **81** (Suppl 2): 33–8.

Klopfenstein HS, Rudolph AM (1978) Postnatal changes in the circulation and responses to volume loading in the sheep. *Circ Res* **42**: 839–45.

London GM, Safar ME, Weiss YA *et al.* (1977) Volume dependent parameters in essential hypertension. *Kidney Int* **11**: 204–8.

Lorenz JM, Kleinman LI, Kotagal UR *et al.* (1982) Water balance in very low-birth-weight-infants: relationship to water and sodium intake and effect on outcome. *J Pediatr* **101**: 423–32.

Morris JA, Hustead RF, Robinson RG *et al.* (1974) Measurement of fetoplacental blood volume in the human previable fetus. *Am J Obstet Gynecol* **118**: 927–34.

Oh W, Lind J, Gessner IH (1966) The circulatory and respiratory adaptaion to early and late cord clamping in newborn infants. *Acta Paediatr Scand* **55**: 17–25.

Pryde PG, Sedman AB, Nugent CE *et al.* (1993) Angiotensin converting enzyme inhibitor fetopathy. *J Am Soc Nephrol* **3**: 1575–82.

Robillard JE, Weismann DN, Herin P (1981) Ontogeny of single glomerular perfusion rate in fetal and newborn lambs. *Pediatr Res* **15**: 1248–55.

Rubin MI, Bruck E, Rapoport M (1949) Maturation of renal function in childhood: clearance studies. *J Clin Invest* **28**: 1144–62.

Schuster VL, Kokko JP, Jacobson HR (1984) Angiotensin II directly stimulates sodium transport in rabbit proximal convoluted tubules. *J Clin Invest* **73**: 507–15.

Schwartz GJ, Haycock GF, Edelmann CM Jr *et al.* (1979) Late metabolic acidosis: a reassessment of the definition. *J Pediatr* **95**: 102–7.

Schwartz GJ, Feld LG, Langford DJ (1984) A simple estimate of glomerular filtration rate in full-term infants during the first year of life. *J Pediatr* **104**: 849–54.

Seikaly MG, Arant BS Jr (1989) Developmental changes in renal blood flow and its intracortical distribution in conscious dogs. *Kidney Int* **35**: 473.

Seikaly MG, Arant BS Jr (1992) Development of renal hemodynamics – glomerular filtration rate and renal blood flow. *Clin Perinatol* **19**: 1–13.

Seikaly MG, Arant BS Jr, Seney FD Jr (1990) Endogenous angiotensin concentrations in specific intrarenal fluid comopartments of the rat. *J Clin Invest* **86**: 1352–7.

Sertel H, Scopes J (1973) Rates of creatinine clearance in babies less than 1 week of age. *Arch Dis Child* **48**: 717–20.

Shaffer SG, Bradt SK, Meade VM I *et al.* (1987) Extracellular fluid volume changes in very low birth weight infants during the first two postnatal months. *J Pediatr* **111**: 124–8.

Smith CA, Yudkin S, Young W *et al.* (1949) Adjustment of electrolytes and water following premature birth (with special reference to edema). *Pediatrics* **3**: 34–47.

Stokes JB (1979) Effect of prostaglandin E$_2$ on chloride transport across the rabbit thick ascending limb of Henle. *J Clin Invest* **64**: 495–502.

Stokes JB (1981) Integrated actions of renal medullary prostaglandins in the control of water excretion. *Am J Physiol* **240**: F471–80.

Stuphen JL (1982) Anthropometric determinants of creatinine excretion in preterm infants. *Pediatrics* **69**: 719–23.

Sulyok E, Heim T (1971) Assessment of maximal urinary acidification in premature infants. *Biol Neonate* **19**: 200–10.

Szefler SJ, Wynn RJ, Clarke DF *et al.* (1980) Relationship of gentamicin serum concentrations to gestational age in preterm and term neonates. *J Pediatr* **97**: 312–5.

Task Force on Blood Pressure Control in Children (1987) Report of the second task force on blood pressure control in children – 1987. *Pediatrics* **79**: 1–25.

Terragno NA, Terragno DA, McGiff JC (1977) Contribution of prostaglandins to the renal circulation in conscious, anesthetized and laporatomized dogs. *Circ Res* **40**: 590–8.

Widdowson E, Dickerson JWT (1968) Chemical composition of the body. In: Assali NS (ed.) *Biology of gestation. Volume II.* New York: Academic Press, 2–247.

Winslow EJ, Loeb HS, Rahimtoola SH *et al.* (1973) Hemodynamic studies and results of therapy in 50 patients with bacteremic shock. *Am J Med* **54**: 421–32.

Genetics and dysmorphology

Edith J. Chernoff, Allen M. Chernoff and Kenneth N. Rosenbaum

Introduction

In recent years, the field of genetics has undergone a period of extremely rapid growth with the development of clinical subspecialties, such as dysmorphology, along with dramatic advances in laboratory techniques. The urologist and geneticist share important roles in the management of the pediatric patient with a urologic abnormality. Both are frequently consulted shortly after delivery to define structural abnormalities of the genitalia, both are often placed in the position of coordinator of care for the infant with multiple malformations, yet each brings a unique but complementary approach to the clinical problem.

The purpose of this chapter is to equip the practitioner with a basic understanding of the genetic principles necessary to diagnose and formulate a management plan for the child with a dysmorphic syndrome, along with giving a brief description of common syndromes with a urologic component. Understanding common associations and their causation allows one to establish an etiology, provide accurate prognosis and to determine the need for further investigation. The patient with genetic disease may require rapid decision making. Therefore, physicians dealing with these infants should have an awareness of some of the conditions detailed in this chapter. Areas covered include the process of genetic counseling, determination of risk factors for specific urologic conditions, laboratory techniques, and prenatal diagnosis.

Significance of genetic disorders in the pediatric population

Many studies have examined the significance and cost of genetic disorders. Yoon et al. (1997) estimated the contribution of birth defects and genetic diseases to pediatric hospitalization and compared hospitalizations for these reasons with hospitalizations for other reasons. They found that 12% of pediatric hospitalizations in their population were related to birth defects and genetic diseases and that, on average, these children were 3 years younger, stayed 3 days longer, incurred 184% higher bills, and had a 4.5-fold greater in-hospital mortality than children hospitalized for other reasons. The rate of hospitalization that was related to birth defects and genetic diseases was 0.4%. Another study by Baird et al. (1988) used a database of an ongoing population-based registry to estimate the population load from genetic disease in more than 1 million consecutive livebirths. They found that 5.3% of liveborn individuals could be expected to have diseases with an important genetic component. Of these, they categorized 3.6/1000 as single-gene disorders (comprised of autosomal dominant 1.4/1000, autosomal recessive 1.7/1000, and X-linked recessive disorders 0.5/1000), 1.8/1000 as chromosomal anomalies, 46.4/1000 as multifactorial disorders, and 1.2/1000 as cases of genetic etiology for which the precise mechanism was not identified.

Dysmorphology

Credit for the foundation of modern human genetics is usually given to Gregor Mendel, an Austrian monk, whose experiments in the mid-nineteenth century demonstrated that genetic characteristics were inherited independently rather than as a result of blending of traits as was previously thought. Mendel was among the first to notice patterns of inheritance. He formulated principles, which although not strictly true have held ever since. The laws of mendelian inheritance state that genes come in pairs, that individual genes can have different alleles, which can be dominant or recessive. At meiosis, alleles segregate from each other with each gamete receiving only one allele (principle of segregation) and the segregation of different pairs of alleles is independent of one another (principle of independent assortment). Meiosis occurs once in the life cycle of a cell. It leads to the production of reproductive cells (gametes) each with half the genetic material. Mitosis, on the other hand, is the mode of cell division by which the body grows. The two daughter cells produced are identical to each other and to the parent cell.

Unfortunately, Mendel's work was poorly understood by his colleagues, and its accuracy and impact remained unknown until 1900, when three other Europeans arrived at the same conclusions (Dewald, 1977). It is not practical to list the innumerable landmarks of human genetics since that time, except to emphasize the foresight Mendel had in his observations more than 100 years ago.

Fascination with malformations and genetic disorders is not a modern phenomenon. Ancient civilizations, even prior to recorded history, fashioned idols of their malformed offspring to protect the population from recurrence of the problem, which was thought to be supernatural in origin (Warkany, 1971). Many of the examples represent varying types of conjoined twins and well-categorized conditions such as achondroplasia and other skeletal dysplasias. The Egyptians, and later the Greeks, appreciated the 'natural' origin of malformations. However, in the Middle Ages scholars viewed the birth of a malformed infant as an omen or the result of maternal impression, a concept that persists to the present.

The recognition of patterns of abnormal development, termed dysmorphology by Smith (1966), led to more objectivity in the evaluation of the malformed child. Terms such as 'FLK (funny looking kid) syndrome' have given way to the term 'dysmorphic child', which is more acceptable to families and professionals. Numerous clinical centers now exist to provide diagnosis and management of such children, and many excellent texts and journals on dysmorphology and syndromes are available (McKusiak, 1994; Buyse, 1990; Gorlin *et al.*, 1990; Jones and Smith, 1997). Classification continues to be a problem. Because the field is advancing so rapidly the dysmorphologist is faced with the unusual scenario of having to decide (often daily) whether a given patient has a previously seen syndrome or a unique complex, a situation that is infrequent in other specialties (Cohen, 1982). In addition, with improved molecular diagnostic techniques the scope of many defined syndromes has widened to include patients with subtle features; some syndromes that were previously defined separately are now recognized as being along the spectrum of the same disorder.

When evaluating the child with multiple anomalies one can consider multiple causes for the presenting phenotype. Abnormal development can be explained as malformations, disruptions, deformations, dysplasias, or syndromes. A malformation is a defect of an organ, part of an organ or larger region of the body due to an abnormal developmental process, while a disruption is a defect due to interference with an intrinsically normal developmental process. A deformation is an abnormality that results from mechanical forces, which are usually self-limiting. Dysplasia is the abnormal organization of cells into tissue. A syndrome is a recognizable pattern of malformations that are pathologically related, and an association refers to the non-random occurrence of multiple anomalies that are not necessarily part of a syndrome. Examples of these categories are shown in Table 3.1.

Two additional concepts relating to morphogenesis are field defects and sequences. A field defect is a pattern of anomalies derived from the disturbance of a single developmental field (functional embryologic unit). Examples of field defects are numerous and are seen in the facial variations of the child with a cleft lip

Table 3.1 Errors in morphogenesis

Type of error	Example	Urogenital abnormality
Malformation (syndrome)	BBB syndrome	Hypospadias
Disruption	Fetal alcohol syndrome	Renal hypoplasia
Deformation	Oligohydramnios (Potter sequence)	Renal agenesis
Dysplasia	Neurofibromatosis	Urogenital neurofibromatosis

or those frequently seen in children with underlying structural malformations of the brain. A sequence is a pattern of multiple anomalies derived from a single known anomaly or mechanical factor. Obvious clinical examples include the infant with myelomeningocele who develops limb wasting, clubfoot, and secondary renal disease.

Chromosomal disorders

Following confirmation of the chromosome number in humans as 46 and description of Down syndrome as the first clinically identified cytogenetic syndrome in 1959, there has been a proliferation of information on many new cytogenetic abnormalities. This is primarily related to the development of chromosomal banding techniques that allow for the identification of small aberrations along the length of the chromosome.

A chromosomal disorder is one in which there is a visible change in the number or structure of a chromosome. Normally, humans have 46 chromosomes, (2n). Any number which is an exact multiple of n (23) is referred to as euploid, while those which are not multiples of n are aneuploid. 3n or 4n are polyploid. A chromosome is composed of two chromatids. Each chromosome has a small arm, termed p and a long arm, termed q. A normal male is designated 46,XY. A (+) sign preceding a chromosome number signifies an entire additional chromosome, while a (−) sign signifies missing material. An individual with Down syndrome would therefore be designated 47,XY +21. A chromosome number followed by a (+) or (−) sign denotes the presence or absence of material on that particular chromosome; for example, 46 XY, 6p+ or 46 XY, 6p−. These patients are said to have a partial trisomy or partial monosomy state. The frequency of chromosomal disorders in livebirths is 6 in 1000, of which two-thirds have mental or physical disabilities.

A karyotype is a display of an individual's chromosomes. They are lined up in order from largest to smallest with the shorter arm of the chromosome pointing to the top of the page (the exception being chromosome 22, which is larger than 21). The chromosomes are further divided into groups A to G based on size and centromere position. Applying banding techniques chromosomes can be seen to be a series of light-staining and dark-staining bands (Fig. 3.1); each chromosome can be distinguished by its banding pattern. Commonly used techniques include Giemsa (G)-banding (the gold standard) and quinacrine (Q)-banding. In G-banding the dark-staining bands tend to be rich in adenosine–thymine base pairs and generally contain heterochromatin, or non-structural genetic material. Lighter-staining bands are rich in guanine–cytosine base pairs and are thought to represent areas of euchromatin, or structural gene areas. The chromosome is subdivided into regions that are numbered and then further divided into bands and subbands within regions, so that the example used above with deleted material on chromosome 6 may further be designated: 46,XY, del(6)(p23) to indicate the point at which chromosomal breakage and loss of material occurred. More sophisticated nomenclature systems have been developed to allow further subdivision of chromosomes as techniques progress and high-resolution chromosomal banding allows subdivision of the chromosomes into 850 parts, compared with 450 in standard-resolution karyotype.

Alterations in chromosomal numbers arise chiefly through non-disjunction, i.e. the failure of paired chromosomes or sister chromatids to disjoin during cell division. Aberrations in chromosomal structure may be due to loss of genetic material (deletion), gain of genetic material (duplication), inversions, translocations, or insertions. Translocations arise as a result of exchanges of blocks of chromatin between two non-homologous chromosomes. Most are 'balanced', result in no loss or gain of gene function, and so do not lead to abnormal phenotype (visible expression of heredity). However, these can lead to unbalanced offspring. A Robertsonian translocation is due to the fusion of acrocentric chromosomes at their centromeric region. (Acrosomic chromosomes are those in which the centromere is at the top of the sister chromatids so that there is only one set of arms.) The affected individual has 45 chromosomes but has a normal phenotype. However, their offspring may have an aberrant number of chromosomes. This is particularly significant in relation to the development of Down syndrome, as chromosome 21 is an acrosomic chromosome.

Gene disorders are due to mutations in one or both alleles of a gene in an autosome, a sex chromosome, or mitochondria. They are divided into autosomal recessive, autosomal dominant, sex-linked recessive, or sex-linked dominant.

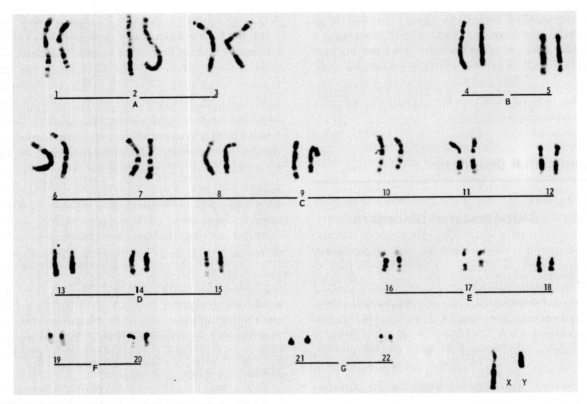

Figure 3.1 Banded karyotype from a normal male.

Multifactorial disorders are due to the interaction of one or more genes with one or more environmental factors. They account for approximately 50% of all congenital malformations, are relevant in many common chronic disorders of adulthood, and show considerable ethnic and geographic variation.

The additive effects of several mutations of different genes result in somatic cell genetic disorders. These are seen in many malignancies with the mutations confined to the tumor. Often the first step in the cascade is inherited.

More recent developments in the field of genetics include the finding of genomic imprinting. This is the modification of expression of genetic material based on the parent of origin. One may see the development of different syndromes depending on whether the genetic material is maternally or paternally derived. A clinical example of this is Angelman syndrome due to deletion of maternal 15q, and Prader–Willi syndrome due to deletion of paternal 15q. A contiguous gene syndrome is one that demonstrates a wide spectrum due to differences in the number of genes in a chromosomal sequence that are involved. The inheritance is usually sporadic, although familial associations have

been found, and examples include Wilms' tumor–aniridia association and DiGeorge sequence. Unstable triplet repeats are areas in which the genetic material contains multiple copies of a triplet of nucleotides. While these are normally found throughout the human genome with no consequences there seem to be areas where these can expand on transmission from parent to child resulting in an abnormal phenotype that worsens from generation to generation (anticipation).

Variation in gene expression

While links between genes and diseases or syndromes are rapidly being defined, there are still many unexplained phenomena. Among these are included the concepts of penetrance, expressivity, and pleiotropy. Penetrance is a gene's likelihood of being expressed. This is an all-or-none concept whereby a gene and its consequent product, be it normal or abnormal, are either on or off. Expressivity represents a phenomenon of degree. A trait may take different forms in different members of a kindred, the same gene being expressed with different severity and in different

Table 3.2 Prevalence of minor malformations and normal variations

Feature	White (%)		Black (%)	
	Male	Female	Male	Female
Epicanthal folds	1.2	1.6	0.7	1.2
Brushfield spots	7.4	7.0	0.0	0.3
Preauricular sinus (unilateral)	0.4	1.3	4.5	6.1
Diastasis recti	32.3	32.9	41.4	40.1
Umbilical hernia	0.4	1.0	3.6	8.6
Clinodactyly (fifth finger), both	5.8	4.5	5.2	8.7
Simian crease				
Unilateral	2.5	1.1	1.7	1.1
Bilateral	1.0	0.3	0.5	0.5

Adapted from Holmes (1976).

ways. Pleiotropy is the concept that one gene may lead to more than one effect. The opposite concept is the phenomenon of heterogeneity, whereby a number of differing genes may lead to the same effect; this may be seen in some of the mucopolysaccharoid storage diseases. Finally, anticipation is the apparent worsening and earlier age of onset of a disease in successive generations.

The prevalence of minor and major anomalies varies greatly between populations, while recognition varies from examiner to examiner. Major malformations are defined as those that are of medical, surgical, or cosmetic significance; 2–3% of patients with genetic syndromes have such malformations. Minor malformations are morphologic features of little or no clinical significance; these are seen in approximately 4% of the population. Table 3.2 demonstrates morphologic variation in a population.

Clinical cytogenetic syndromes

Urologic abnormalities are frequently seen in many classic cytogenetic syndromes (Table 3.3). Additions to the list include some patients who have Wilms' tumor. This includes primarily those with the aniridia–genital abnormality–retardation (WAGR) trait, who have been found to have a small deletion of 11p13 (Riccardi et al., 1978; Turleau et al., 1981). It is worth noting that this deletion has not been detected in patients with aniridia or Wilms' tumor only, without other somatic abnormalities. An increased risk for gonadoblastoma has also been noted in this group (Turleau et al., 1981).

Table 3.3 Genitourinary anomalies in selected chromosomal syndromes

Chromosomal syndrome	Malformations
Autosomes	
Trisomies (duplication)	
3q	B, E
4p	A, B, C, E
8 (mosaic)	A
9p	A, B, C, E
9 (mosaic)	A, C, E
10q	A, B, E
13	A, B, E
18	A, B, D, E
20p	A, C, E
21	A, C, E
22 (cat-eye syndrome)	E
Triploidy	A, C, E
Monosomies (deficiency)	
4p	A, B, E
5p	A, E
9p	A, C, D, E
11p	A, B, C, D
13q	A, B, E
15q (Prader–Willi syndrome)	A. C
18p	E
18q	A, C, D, E
Sex chromosomes	
XXY	A, B, C
XXXXY	A, B, C
XYY	A, B, C
X (Turner syndrome)	E

A = cryptorchidism; B = hypospadias; C = microphallus; D = ambiguous genitalia; E = renal abnormalities (including agenesis, dysplasia, horseshoe kidney, hydronephrosis, other). Adapted from Jones (1988) and Barakat and Butler (1987).

Patterns of single-gene inheritance

Autosomal dominant traits

These traits may appear in every generation, and children have a 50% risk of inheriting the trait. Unaffected members do not transmit the trait, and occurrence and transmission are not influenced by sex. In this form of inheritance, a mutation at a single locus on a given pair of chromosomes is sufficient to allow for expression (Table 3.4). An affected individual may be heterozygous for the trait, meaning that only one gene is abnormal. The molecular pathophysiology of these type of disorders includes loss of function where loss of 50% function/quantity of a gene product leads to abnormal phenotype, gain of function where a mutation alters the normal regulatory mechanism of a protein, or negative effect where production of an abnormal gene product interferes with the functioning of the product of the normal allele leading to a net decrease of more than 50%.

Autosomal recessive traits

These traits are only expressed in homozygotes; one must inherit the gene from both parents, male and females are equally affected, and there is a 25% risk with each pregnancy (Table 3.4). Spontaneous mutation is not a significant factor, and both parents are obligate carriers for the mutant gene despite a lack of findings either clinically or often biochemically. The possible causative mechanisms include loss of function or reduction in function; the basic defects include loss of enzymatic or transporter activity.

In order to calculate the frequencies of autosomal recessive disorders one must rely on the Hardy–Weinberg equilibrium equation, $p^2 + 2pq + q^2 = 1$. Here, p represents the frequency of normal genes, q represents the frequency of mutations in the general population and $2pq$ is the frequency of heterozygotes. As p approaches 1 the frequency of heterozygotes or carriers approaches $2q^2$, for example, if the frequency of cystic fibrosis in the population is 1 in 1600 births, then 1 in 20 individuals are carriers for the gene ($2\sqrt{1/1600} = 1/20$).

Another important calculation determines the risk that an unaffected child born to a family with a recessive disorder could have a child with the same condition, i.e. the risk that an unaffected family member is a carrier of the recessive disorder that runs in the family.

This is determined by multiplying the risk of carrying the mutant gene by the risk of transmitting the gene by the risk that the male is a carrier of the gene. For example, what is the risk that a couple will have a child with CF if the father has a brother with the disease and the mother is of Northern European ancestry?

The risk that the father carries the gene (A = 0.666) × risk that a carrier will pass it to a child (B = 0.5) × risk that the mother carries the gene (C = 1/2500).

Risk of child with CF

$$= A \times B \times C = 0.666 \times 0.5 \times 0.0004$$
$$= 0.00013.$$

X-linked traits

Geneticists spent years debating the mechanism of X chromosome gene action (dosage compensation) because males have only one X chromosome whereas females have two. The Lyon hypothesis accounts for this paradox by stating that, shortly after conception, one X chromosome is inactivated in all cells with two X chromosomes (Vogel and Motulsky, 1986). This process is theoretically random, with 50% of cells having the paternal X chromosome as the active one and 50% the maternal, and is usually irreversible. The inactivated X is identifiable as the Barr body in interphase cells near the nuclear membrane. Females are therefore functional mosaics for genes located on the X chromosome.

X-linked inheritance may be either recessive or, in some instances, dominant. In X-linked recessive inheritance males are hemizygotes and are affected, while females are heterozygotes or homozygotes. No male to male transmission is observed and unaffected males do not transmit the trait. All daughters of an affected male are carriers and a heterozygous female usually does not express the phenotype. For carrier females, the risk of having an affected male is 50% with every pregnancy and 50% for having a carrier female who will be clinically well. Possibly 10–15% of X-linked traits are due to spontaneous mutation (Table 3.4).

The calculation of probabilities for X-linked traits is based on Bayes' theorem, which takes into account the presence of additional historical information (such as numbers of male births) to develop a joint probability.

Table 3.4 Single-gene inheritance

Autosomal dominant
> AA = affected heterozygote
> AA = normal

Parental genotypes Aa × aa
Offspring genotypes Aa (1/2) or aa (1/2)

Autosomal recessive
> AA = normal
> Aa = heterozygote (carrier)
> Aa = homozygote (affected)

Parental genotypes Aa × Aa
Offspring genotypes AA (1/4); Aa (1/2); aa (1/4)

X-linked recessive
> XY = normal male
> X'Y = affected male (hemizygote)
> XX = normal female
> X'X = carrier female

Parental genotypes X'X × XY
Offspring genotypes X'X (1/4); X'Y (1/4); XX (1/4); XY (1/4)
Parental genotypes XX × X'Y
Offspring genotypes X'X (1/2); XY (1/2)

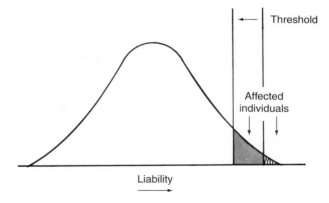

Figure 3.2 Liability curve representing model of multifactorial inheritance. (From Rosenbaum, 1978, with permission.)

X-linked dominant traits

Females who have the mutant gene are more likely to express the trait than those with X-linked recessive genes, but are more mildly affected than males owing to the phenomenon of random deactivation of the X chromosome. Numerous dysmorphic syndromes feature this mode of inheritance. The recurrence risk in male and female offspring of an affected female is 50% with each pregnancy, while all the female offspring and none of the male offspring of an affected male will be affected.

Multifactorial disorders

Multifactorial disorders are the result of the action of multiple genes with small additive effects in combination with environmental influences. Although often used interchangeably with the term polygenic inheritance, the term multifactorial allows for the role of environmental factors in the production of such traits. Multifactorial disorders are characterized by increased frequency in close relatives, and consanguinity increases the risk. Most regional malformations and other ill-defined familial disorders are thought to have a multifactorial basis.

Many measurable traits in the population, such as height, intelligence, blood pressure, and even serum cholesterol levels, reflect hereditary factors that are multifactorial and define a normal distribution or bell-shaped curve. These traits are said to be continuous, with no interruptions in the curve. At first glance, malformations appear to be discontinuous (either affected or unaffected), although it has been proposed that they also follow a gaussian curve representing liability or likelihood of developing a condition (Fig. 3.2). When the liability (genetic component) reaches a certain point (threshold), the disorder becomes manifest. Theoretically, environmental components, either extrauterine or intrauterine, may function by altering the position of the threshold, thereby increasing liability. Affected individuals have a mean liability near the tail of the curve, and first-degree relatives (siblings, parents and offspring) have a mean liability midway between the mean of the population and that of the affected group.

Calculation of recurrence risks

The multifactorial model has become the basis for the calculation of recurrence for the most isolated regional malformations, including urologic abnormalities, congenital heart disease, and neural tube defects. After exclusion of chromosomal and single-gene disorders, the theoretical risk of recurrence for a presumed multifactorial trait, as Falconer has suggested, can be expressed as:

$$\text{Risk} = \sqrt{\text{Frequency of a specific lesion.}}$$

Observed risks in populations of at-risk individuals confirm the reliability of such calculations.

Caution must be exercised in the use of theoretical figures for counseling, however, since it is based on certain assumptions. The first is that a given family is of average liability and presents with a single affected individual. Although figures are sparse for families with two affected children or an affected parent and child, the risk of recurrence then appears to increase sharply and may approach mendelian risks. It has also been observed that the more severe the defect, as in perineoscrotal versus glanular hypospadias, the greater the risk of other family members being affected.

Molecular genetic techniques for diagnosis of chromosomal abnormalities

Restriction fragment length polymorphisms

Restriction fragment length polymorphisms (RFLP) are usually non-coding regions of DNA which are unique within families or ethnic groups and are recognized by restriction endonucleases. On a particular chromosome, they are either present or not. They were initially typed by hybridizing Southern blots with radiolabeled probes (Wolfe and Hernington, 1997; Nollau and Wagener, 1997). Initial analytic methods used cloning to amplify the DNA sequences of interest. Cloning uses restriction endonucleases to cleave DNA into different sized strands that could then be incorporated into bacteria. Bacterial replication leads to amplification of the incorporated DNA. Cloning of fragments of up to one million base pairs can be accomplished in this way; however, the technology is laborious, requiring a great deal of time, money, and DNA (Strachan and Read, 1996).

Polymerase chain reaction

Developed in 1985, this technique has expanded the field of molecular genetics in a way that no other technique has been able to accomplish. Polymerase chain reaction (PCR) allows amplification of smaller fragments of DNA then cloning techniques (10–20 kilobase sequences) and does not use plasmid bacteria. Beginning with a small amount of DNA of known sequence, one can make millions of copies of a target sequence quickly, efficiently, and at a relatively low cost using DNA polymerase (Rohlfs and Highsmith, 1997).

Fluorescent in situ hybridization

In the 1990s, with the improvement of recombinant DNA technology, the technique of fluorescent *in situ* hybridization (FISH) became possible. FISH is a molecular cytogenetic technique in which a specific nucleic acid sequence (probe) is bound to its homologous segment in a fixed preparation on a glass slide. The probe used fluoreses, allowing visualization of the chromosomes and analysis. FISH is most commonly performed on metaphase (dividing) cells; however, it can be performed on interphase (non-dividing) cells as well, making it possible to use fixed cells harvested from routine tissue culture (Mark, 1994).

FISH can be used to detect marker chromosomes and mosaicism. Because it is a rapid technique it is often used when the diagnosis cannot reasonably wait for the weeks it takes for the other methods. This is particularly pertinent in prenatal diagnosis when termination of a pregnancy depends on gestational age. FISH is also commonly used in cancer cytogenetics, as malignant cells tend to yield poor chromosome spreading and suboptimal banding (Gelehrter *et al.*, 1998).

Evaluation of the dysmorphic child with urogenital abnormalities

The process of evaluating the malformed child must often, of necessity, be performed rapidly and under stressful conditions. For some isolated urologic abnormalities, such as penile agenesis or severe degrees of genital ambiguity, added pressure may be present in terms of gender identification in the delivery room. Bear in mind that one should never be pushed into making a gender assignment. It is better for the family to await the results of definitive studies than for the incorrect sex to be assigned to the newborn. The same is true for the dysmorphic child who presents with a urologic abnormality as part of a more generalized disorder. Steps that should be performed in the evaluation process are as follows.

1 *In-depth antenatal history, family history, and physical examination.* Even in the delivery room, it may be possible to elicit important information related to prenatal drug exposure, fetal activity, maternal illness, and the presence or absence of urogenital or other malformations. A rapid physical examination should then be performed looking for all abnormalities and variations.

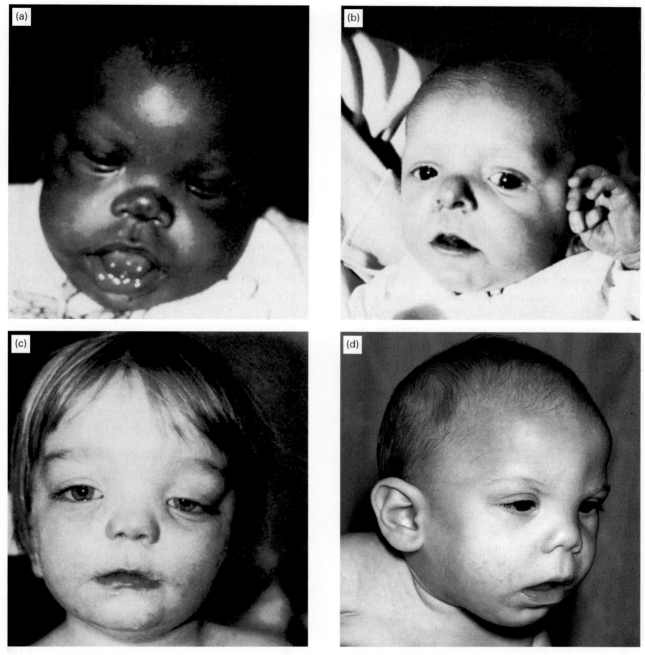

Figure 3.3 Selected dysmorphic syndromes: (*a*) hypertelorism–hypospadias syndrome; (*b*) Noonan syndrome; (*c*) Aarskog–Scott syndrome; (*d*) Smith–Lemli–Opitz syndrome.

2 *Measurements*. Objective data on facial characteristics such as interpupillary distance (to determine whether the infant has hypertelorism), ear length, and philtrum length (midline depression on upper lip), among others, are available to assist in assessment. Visual cues are often misleading; therefore, it is ideal to obtain objective measurement, if possible.

3 *Knowledge of what is normal*. As detailed in Table 3.2, many facial variations are seen so frequently in the general population that they are of little significance. Conversely, many dysmorphic syndromes are characterized by a grouping of minor variations with few, if any, major malformations. The appearance of the child with Down syndrome is an excellent example of a situation in which there

are multiple minor malformations and variations that individually are of little significance but that together allow for diagnosis.

4 *Interpretation of anomalies from the viewpoint of developmental anatomy.* A good knowledge of fetal development is essential in understanding which anomaly came first and whether it was primary or secondary. Does the patient have a true malformation, or is it explainable as a deformation or disruption?

5 *Laboratory evaluation.*

(a) Appropriate laboratory studies should be obtained in the evaluation. For the child with an isolated urologic abnormality, such as cryptorchidism or hypospadias, cytogenetic studies are not usually recommended because their yield is low. In cases of genital ambiguity, chromosomal analysis is mandatory. Buccal smears are screening tests only and decisions should not be made on the basis of their results. Falsely low percentages of Barr bodies are frequently seen in the normal newborn female, and some laboratories report low rates of false-positive Barr bodies in males. More specific is Y fluorescence, which stains the heterochromatic area of the Y chromosome intensely. Normal newborn males are 60–70% Y-chromatin positive in the authors' laboratory; again, however, this procedure remains a screening test.

(b) Preliminary chromosomal results can be obtained routinely in 72 hours; some laboratories harvest the sample as early as 48 hours if sex determination is the primary concern. High-resolution banding techniques to look for small additions or deletions usually take an additional 3–4 days. It should be stressed that the majority of children with a recognizable dysmorphic syndrome have normal chromosomes. Thus, a negative result may be falsely reassuring to physicians and parents. The greatest diagnostic yield can be anticipated from a careful physical examination by an experienced clinical geneticist or dysmorphologist.

(c) Other laboratory studies should be obtained, depending on the specific abnormality. For the genetic female with genital ambiguity, levels of serum 17-α-hydroxyprogesterone, renin, urinary 17-α-hydroxysteroids, and 17-α-ketosteroids are necessary.

6 *Radiographic studies.* Specific views of the urogenital system for the child with genital abnormalities are warranted. Depending on the clinical situation, ultrasonography, genitography, renal scanning, or voiding cystourethrography may be required.

7 *Photographs.* Documentation of physical differences is best performed with medical photographs. This is especially true of the child with life-threatening malformations or the stillborn infant, since efforts to make diagnoses often cease after death and are anticlimactic. Many geneticists routinely provide consultation through the mail on malformed infants who could not be seen personally, although this is suboptimal. Photographs also serve the purpose of reducing the mystique and fears that parents often develop about their infant's malformations.

8 *Overall diagnosis for appropriate counseling.* Without a proper diagnosis, the clinician can give little correct information about prognosis and the presence of related abnormalities. Two of the primary considerations are whether the family is at risk for recurrence of the disorder and whether prenatal diagnosis is available.

Single-gene disorders and dysmorphic syndromes with urologic anomalies

Autosomal dominant disorders

Branchio-oto-renal syndrome (Melnick–Fraser syndrome; BOR)

In 1975 Melnick *et al.* first described an association between branchial arch cysts, hearing loss, and renal anomalies. Chen *et al.* (1975) reviewed the incidence of the various anomalies in affected patients. The most frequently found abnormalities are hearing loss and periauricular pits. Branchial cleft fistulae are seen in 49% of patients, whereas renal anomalies are found at an incidence of 67%. Patients display a wide range of renal anomalies, the most common of which is renal agenesis. It has been speculated that bilateral renal agenesis results in the excess of unexplained fetal deaths in these families. Renal hypoplasia and renal dysplasia are the next most frequent renal anomalies. Anatomic abnormalities are also seen and include calyceal diverticula, ureteropelvic junction (UPJ) obstruction, hydronephrosis, pelviectasis, calyectasis and vesicoureteric reflux (VUR). All of these may be related to abnormal development of the ureteral bud.

BOR has an autosomal dominant mode of inheritance with near 100% penetrance but varied expressivity (Chen *et al.*, 1975). Its incidence is 1/40 000 births and 2% of all deaf patients are affected. Approximately 6% of patients affected will progress to renal failure (Misra and Nolph, 1998). The EYA1 gene has recently been identified as the candidate gene for BOR (Abdelhak *et al.*, 1997) and it is located on the long arm of chromosome 8 (8q13.3). Two similar syndromes, BO and BO-ureter, are likely to be different expressions of the same syndrome as BO has recently been found to be due to mutations of EYA1 as well (Vincent *et al.*, 1997).

Hypertelorism–hypospadias syndrome (Opitz G/BBB syndrome)

This syndrome was first described by Opitz *et al.* (1969a, b) as two separate disorders. Later reports of families in which findings of both BBB and G syndrome were seen suggested that they were in fact a single entity (Cordero and Holmes, 1978; Cappa *et al.*, 1987; Sedano and Gorlin, 1988). The syndrome is characterized by hypertelorism, hypospadias, and other midline anomalies (Fig. 3.3a). The common major malformations include hypospadias, cleft lip/palate, congenital heart defects (patent ductus arteriosis being most common), swallowing defects, and developmental delay (Robin *et al.*, 1996). Other common urologic anomalies are cryptorchidism (uni/bilateral), micropenis, a bifid or hypoplastic scrotum, splayed labia majora, and various renal and ureteral anomalies, most commonly VUR (Jacobson *et al.*, 1998).

Although unable to assign a specific phenotype for the different gene defects, Robin *et al.* (1995) proved that the syndrome is genetically heterogenous. There is an autosomal dominant pattern of inheritance mapped to 22q11.2 and an X-linked pattern mapped to Xp22. A broad forehead with a coarse facial appearance was suggestive of the autosomal dominant variant. Anteverted nares and classical posterior pharyngeal clefts are seen only in the X-linked group. Hypospadias and imperforate anus are more common in the X-linked families. Although Opitz (1987) reported wide clinical variability in the syndrome ranging from asymptomatic to neonatal lethality, it seems that X-linked males are the most severely affected (Robin *et al.*, 1995).

Nail–patella syndrome/hereditary osteoonychodysplasia

Nail–patella syndrome (NPS) or hereditary osteoonychodysplasia (HOOD) was first described by Sedgewick (see Little, 1987). Hawkins and Smith (1950) were the first to describe patients with NPS who also had proteinuria, cylindruria, and hematuria. It is characterized by the presence of nail dystrophy, iliac horns (pathognomonic for the syndrome), complete absence or hypoplasia of the patellae, and deformation or subluxation of the radial head (Bodziak *et al.*, 1994; Carbonara and Alpert, 1964; Miller *et al.*, 1968). Nails are thin, longitudinally ridged, hyperpigmented, or flattened. The changes are symmetrical and of decreasing severity from the thumb to the fifth digit (Carbonara and Alpert, 1964; Schmeider and Freitag, 1988). Fifty per cent of those affected will have heterochromia of the iris (Lester's sign) (Lester, 1936). Renal involvement, present in 30–50% of cases, can range from assymptomatic proteinuria or hematuria to nephrotic syndrome and renal failure (8%) (Schmeider and Freitag, 1988). Disease prevalence has been reported to be between 4.5 and 22/million (Gregory and Atkin, 1997). NPS is transmitted in an autosomal dominant pattern and has been mapped to 9q34. Severity of renal disease in the parent is no indication of the degree of involvement in the offspring (Schleutermann *et al.*, 1969; Looji *et al.*, 1988). Renal transplant is a viable option when renal failure develops (Chan *et al.*, 1988). Diagnosis may be made by ultrasound evaluation of the skeletal deformities in children and has recently been used for the prenatal diagnosis based on finding the characteristic iliac horns (Miller *et al.*, 1998; Feingold *et al.*, 1998). The diagnosis may also be made by the characteristic appearance of the glomerular basement membrane seen on renal biopsy (Morita *et al.*, 1973).

Noonan syndrome

Noonan syndrome was first described in the 1960s by Noonan and Ehmke. They reported on a group of patients with mild mental retardation, short stature, hypertelorism, low-set posteriorly rotated ears, deeply grooved philtrum, and low posterior hairlines with webbed necks (Nora *et al.*, 1974) (Fig. 3.3b). Previously, this syndrome was known as the male Turner syndrome or Turner-like syndrome. This was a misnomer as, although it phenotypically overlaps somewhat with Turner syndrome, they are unrelated. The cardinal manifestations of this syndrome, in addition to the above, include congenital heart defects (most commonly pulmonary stenosis) and chest deformities. These patients also have a higher incidence of bleeding abnormalities, generalized lymphedema and cryptorchidism that often results in inadequate secondary sexual development with deficient spermatogenesis. The incidence of Noonan syndrome is estimated to be between 1 in 1000 and 1 in 2500 births. Its inheritance is sporadic, with some evidence of direct transmission from parent to child, more commonly maternally transmitted. Diagnosis is clinical (Allanson, 1987).

Autosomal dominant polycystic kidney disease

The definition of autosomal dominant polycystic kidney disease (ADPKD) varies with the age of the patient. In an adult, diagnosis depends on documentation of bilateral renal involvement with three or more cysts, while diagnosis of children at risk is suggested by at least two unilateral or bilateral renal cysts. In addition to renal involvement, it is common for patients to have cerebral aneurysms, polycystic liver disease with hepatic cysts, cardiac valvular disease, colonic diverticula, and polycythemia (Beebe, 1996). Clinically, patients commonly present between 40 and 50 years of age with either flank or abdominal pain, gross hematuria or hypertension. Pain is believed to be due to kidney enlargement secondary to cysts. Renal complications include hypertension, hematuria, proteinuria, pain, urinary tract infections, and calculi. Ultimately, 45% will develop end-stage renal disease (ESRD) by the age of 60 years. Factors that increase the risk of developing ESRD include male gender, black race, early age at diagnosis, hypertension, gross hematuria, and proteinuria. In 1987 the causative gene for 95% of ADPKD was discovered on chromosome 16p13.11-16pter (Bear et al., 1992). More recently, a second gene has been described on chromosome 4; this mutation accounts for 4% of patients. Prenatal diagnosis is possible by amniocentesis or chorionic villae sampling and DNA analysis. Diagnosis is by renal sonography and DNA analysis. Research has been directed towards prevention of the formation of cysts in the form of chemotherapeutic agents such as taxol or methylprednisone.

Robinow syndrome (fetal face syndrome)

First described by Robinow et al. (1969), typical features of the syndrome include characteristic facies, dwarfism, and hypoplastic genitalia. The facial features include hypertelorism, depressed nasal bridge, a short upturned nose with prominent nares, and low set ears. Patients' arms are short compared with trunk length, with the forearms being most severely affected (mesomelic brachymelia). Rib and spinal abnormalities are also common (Butler and Wadlington, 1987). The urologic manifestations include cryptorchidism and hypoplastic or absent penis or clitoris (Robinow et al., 1969; Butler and Wadlington, 1987; Teebi, 1990). The penis tends to be short and broad with the base more dorsally located than normal. Wilcox's group felt the penile anomalies could be explained by their finding of an abnormal insertion of the penile crura that causes a portion of the penile shaft to be within the pelvis. They suggested that this might also be the cause of the clitoral anomalies (Wilcox et al., 1997). Other genitourinary manifestations are renal cystic disease, vaginal atresia, and cervical agenesis (Weins et al., 1990; Balci et al., 1998). In Robinow's original report the inheritance pattern was described as autosomal dominant; however, families with an autosomal recessive pattern have also been described (Teebi, 1990; Wadlington et al., 1973).

Autosomal recessive disorders

Jeune syndrome

Originally described in 1955 by Jeune and his colleagues; this syndrome is known also as asphyxiating thoracic dysplasia (ATD). It is characterized by a small thorax, short limbs more severe proximally (rhizomelic brachymelia), polydactyly, and pelvic and renal abnormalities (Chen et al., 1996). Clinically, these patients vary in phenotype from those who die hours after delivery owing to respiratory failure to those with only mild respiratory symptoms. These are classified as type I ATD, which is fatal within the first few months of life, and type II ATD. Patients with type I often have renal cysts, while those with type II sometimes develop chronic tubulointerstitial renal lesions that ultimately result in chronic renal insufficiency (Amirou et al., 1998). Jeune syndrome is a rare autosomal recessive disorder, the frequency of which is estimated at between 1 in 100 000 and 1 in 130 000 livebirths. Prenatal diagnosis is possible by a sonogram that shows a fetus with a normal head circumference, chest circumference less than fifth percentile for gestational age, short long bones, and absent breathing movements. Unfortunately, these findings are not identifiable until 18 weeks' gestation. Treatment is usually directed towards respiratory support. Should the patient develop renal insufficiency and failure, transplantation has been successful in a handful of cases.

Bardet–Biedl syndrome

First described in 1920, this syndrome's cardinal features include retinal pigmentary dystrophy that ultimately results in blindness, postaxial polydactyl, central obesity, mental retardation, short stature, renal dysplasia, and hypogonadism. Minor manifestations include hepatic fibrosis, diabetes mellitus, hearing loss, endocrinopathies, developmental delay, and speech deficits. Renal abnormalities occur in 100% of these patients, and are the major cause of morbidity and mortality; the incidence of ESRD is estimated between 14 and 55% (Devarajan, 1995). Genital abnormalities include urogenital sinus abnormalities hypoplastic uterus, ovaries and fallopian tubes, uterine duplication, septate vagina, and hemocolpos (Stoler et al., 1995). The renal and gonadal abnormalities distinguish this syndrome from Laurence–Moon. Bardet–Biedl syndrome is autosomal recessive with a heterogenous genetic basis, having at least four loci (BBS1–4) on separate chromosomes. Its highest prevalence is in the Middle East, where it occurs in 1 in 13 500, in individuals of European descent its prevalence is 1 in 160 000 and in the UK it is seen in 1 in 125 000. Diagnosis can be made clinically and confirmed using PCR and linkage analysis (Beales et al., 1997).

Fraser syndrome (cryptophthalmos syndrome)

The Fraser syndrome is an uncommon entity with variable expression of cryptophthalmos, syndactyly, craniofacial and urogenital abnormalities. For the diagnosis to be made Thomas et al. (1986) suggested that a patient needed at least two major and one minor criteria, or one major and two minor criteria. The major criteria are cryptophthalmos, syndactyly, abnormal genitalia, and an affected sibling. Minor criteria include malformations of eye, ears nose or larynx, cleft lip or palate, skeletal abnormalities, renal agenesis, and mental retardation (Sarmon et al., 1995; Comas et al., 1993). Eighty five per cent of patients have renal agenesis, which may be unilateral or bilateral, and some have suggested that it should be included among the major criteria (Lurie and

Cherstvoy, 1984). The degree of renal agenesis and laryngeal stenosis are major factors contributing to the early death of these children (Fryns et al., 1997). The most common genital abnormalities are cryptorchidism, micropenis, and hypospadias in males, and clitoral hypertrophy, bicornate uterus, and vaginal atresia in females (Sarmon et al., 1995). Fraser syndrome is most probably autosomal recessive; no gene has been found and chromosomal analysis is normal. The diagnosis can be suspected by fetal ultrasound as early as 18.5 weeks' gestation, but key to the diagnosis is a high degree of suspicion in a family with a history of an affected child (Schauer et al., 1990).

Meckel–Gruber syndrome

First described by Meckel in 1822 and subsequently by Gruber in 1936, this syndrome's cardinal features are occipital encephalocele, polydactyly, and polycystic kidneys, two of which are needed in order to make the diagnosis. Other less common features are brain malformations, cardiac anomalies, and genital ambiguity (Farag et al., 1990). It is an autosomal recessive disorder with an estimated prevalence of 1/20 000 pregnancies. The disorder is uniformly fatal, usually within minutes of birth. Although it has long been possible to make the diagnosis by prenatal ultrasound in the second and third trimester, the diagnosis has been made recently by transabdominal ultrasound as early as 11 weeks' gestation (Sepulveda et al., 1997), making issues of counseling and pregnancy termination easier.

Autosomal recessive polycystic kidney disease (ARPKD)

Affected infants characteristically have bilaterally enlarged echogenic, renoform kidneys. They often have a prenatal history of oligohydramnios developing after 20 weeks of gestation, and depending on its severity, variable degrees of 'Potter's phenotype' (Zerres et al., 1998a). Characteristic features on ultrasound are large, echogenic kidneys with poor corticomedullary differentiation, sparing of the peripheral cortex except in the most severe cases, and a radial array of ectatic tubules in the renal medulla (Jain et al., 1997). The intravenous urogram (IVU) shows a typical sunburst appearance (Glassberg, 1998). These radiographic findings are secondary to the pathologic changes of dilatation of the collecting tubules and sparing of the glomeruli. All children will have some degree of congenital hepatic fibrosis. The most critical feature in the diagnosis is its differentiation from adult polycystic kidney disease by establishing its inheritance pattern. This may be achieved by a screening renal sonography of the parents (Zerres et al., 1998b).

Zerres et al. (1998b) reported an incidence of 1/40 000. The disease can range in severity, with the earlier age at onset typically being associated with more severe renal rather than liver involvement, while the opposite is true for those diagnosed at an older age. This pattern was first described by Blyth and Ockenden (1971). Approximately 50% of patients who present at birth die within the first month of life, most often secondary to pulmonary complications (Zerres et al., 1996). In those patients who survive 1 month, the survival rate without ESRD is 86% at 1 year, 78% at 5 years, and 67% at 15 years. Hypertension develops in 39% in the first year, in 54% by 5 years, and in 60% by 15 years. Twenty three per cent of patients had variceal bleeding secondary to portal hypertension at a mean age of 12.5 years (Roy et al., 1997).

A specific gene has yet to be identified; however, ARPKD has been mapped to the short arm of chromosome 6 (6p21.1-12) and there is no evidence of genetic heterozygosity (Zerres et al., 1994). Early prenatal sonographic diagnosis is not reliable and cannot be made before 20 weeks' gestation. Zerres et al. (1998a) feel that prenatal diagnosis can reliably be made using their method of a haplotype-based approach, with multiple flanking microsatellite markers. However, they stress the importance of proper diagnosis of the first affected sibling. Further complicating genetic counseling is the disagreement over what the true degree of intrafamilial variability of severity may be (Zerres et al., 1998a; Blyth and Ockenden, 1971).

Smith–Lemli–Opitz syndrome

First described in 1964, Smith–Lemli–Opitz syndrome (SLO) is caused by a deficiency in 7-dehydrocholesterol reductase (Wassif et al., 1998). It is characterized by mental retardation and multiple congenital anomalies including holoprosencephaly (Kelley et al., 1996), microcephaly with bitemporal narrowing, eyes with downslanting palpebral fissures and ptosis, anteverted nares, low-set ears, and micrognathia.

Characteristic of the disorder is the 2/3 toe soft-tissue syndactyly, and aggressive behavior which includes self-mutilation. This is the first dysmorphic syndrome found to have a metabolic cause (Fig. 3.3d).

Ninety-one per cent of male patients with SLO have genital abnormalities (Ryan et al., 1998). Approximately one-quarter have sex reversal and one-third have ambiguous genitalia, while the remainder have hypospadias and/or cryptorchidism. All female patients with SLO have normal genitalia. In addition, approximately one-third of patients have structural renal anomalies including renal agenesis, hypoplastic kidneys, cystic kidneys, and dilatation of the renal drainage system.

The incidence of SLO is estimated to be 1 in 60 000 conceptions. The syndrome is autosomal recessive with a normal karyotype; however, investigators are currently looking at the 7q32.1 region for candidate genes. Diagnosis is made by finding low levels of cholesterol and elevated levels of 7-dehydrocholesterol. These can be determined prenatally on chorionic villus sampling (CVS) or amniocentesis in fetuses with suspicious findings by ultrasound or first-degree relatives who are affected. Studies are underway to determine the effectiveness of high cholesterol diets in the treatment of these patients.

Zellweger syndrome

Zellweger syndrome (ZS) is the paradigm of peroxisomal disorders in humans. Characteristic features include a high forehead, large anterior fontenelle, shallow orbital ridges, epicanthus, micrognathia, and external ear abnormalities. Neurologic symptoms include severe hypotonia, epileptic seizures, sensorineural hearing impairment, and eye abnormalities. Hepatomegaly is present in 80% of patients and renal cystic disease in 70% (Al-Essa et al., 1999; Fitzpatrick, 1996). ZS has an autosomal recessive inheritance pattern and patients generally have normal karyotypes. Liver biopsy will show a typical lack of peroxisomes. With simple assays that can detect high levels of very long-chain fatty acids (VLCFA), biopsy is no longer necessary for the diagnosis. VLCFA levels can be detected prenatally via chorionic villus samples (Al-Essa et al., 1999). The peroxisomal disorders are now thought to represent a spectrum of the same disease where ZS is the most severe and is uniformly fatal by the first year of life (Baumgartner et al., 1998).

X-linked disorders

Aarskog syndrome

First described by Aarskog (1970), this syndrome consists of growth impairment, a distinct facial phenotype, and genital and musculoskeletal abnormalities (Stevenson et al., 1994). The facial features include round facies with down-slanting palpebral fissures, hypertelorism, short stubby nose with anteverted nares and broad nasal bridge, and a broad upper lip with prominent philtrum (Fig. 3.3c). Musculoskeletal abnormalities described are short stature, short broad hands with mild webbing, hyperextensible interphalangeal joints, and fifth finger clinodactyly (Aarskog, 1970; Teebi et al., 1993). Patients are of normal intelligence. Genital anomalies include unilateral or bilateral undescended testes and a shawl scrotum, which is the only consistent feature. Although they undergo normal pubertal development, a high percentage is infertile and recent research suggests that this may be due to severe teratoazoospermia with defective acrosomes (Meschede et al., 1996). Inheritance of this disorder is either X-linked, with the gene mapping to Xp11.2, or autosomal dominant, with female carriers displaying a milder phenotype (Stevenson et al., 1994). Diagnosis remains clinical.

Alport's syndrome

In 1927 Alport reported deafness in a family with previously reported hereditary hematuria. In 1987 Flinter et al. proposed clinical criteria for the diagnosis of Alport's syndrome (AS) in patients with hematuria, chronic renal failure (CRF), or both. Patients must have three of the following: a family history of hematuria or CRF, characteristic electron microscopic features of the glomerular basement membrane (GBM), progressive high-tone sensorineural deafness, and characteristic ocular findings, the most common of which is anterior lenticonus (Perrin et al., 1980). Children generally present with persistent microhematuria with episodes of gross hematuria following upper respiratory tract infection. The disease progresses to renal failure by the second or third decade of life (Bodziak et al., 1994; Saborio and Scheinman, 1998). Kashtan et al. (1998) noted a correlation between age, progressive expansion of the renal interstitium, and advancing disease. Changes were not seen prior to the age of 10 years and severity correlated with creatinine clearance.

AS has a frequency of approximately 1 in 5000 in the general population, while AS cases make up 0.6–3% of patients with ESRD and 2.3% of patients undergoing renal transplant (Bodziak et al., 1994; Saborio and Scheinman, 1998; Milliner et al., 1982). AS is genetically heterogenous, with all known responsible genes affecting collagen type IV, a major component of the GBM. The COL4A5 gene on Xq22 is the gene responsible for the classic X-linked dominant type and makes up 85% of cases. COL4A3 and COL4A4, both on chromosome 2q, are thought to be responsible for the autosomal recessive variant and make up 15% of cases. The gene responsible for the rare autosomal dominant type has yet to be isolated (Smeets et al., 1996; Kashtan and Michael, 1993). Management consists of low-salt, low-phosphate, and low-protein diets (Saborio and Scheinman, 1998). Callis et al. (1999) reported that long-term treatment with cyclosporine A led to improvement and preservation of renal function in eight severely affected males. Dialysis and renal transplant are acceptable options for patients with ESRD. Post-transplant anti-GBM nephritis has been reported in as many as 7% of AS patients and should be considered with graft dysfunction. Diagnosis of anti-GBM nephritis is important as it has a high recurrence rate in subsequent transplants, and other family members may be at risk (Kashtan et al., 1998).

Oculocerebrorenal syndrome of Lowe

First described in 1952, it was not until 1965 that the oculocerebrorenal syndrome of Lowe (OCRL) was demonstrated to have X-linked recessive inheritance (Charnas and Gahl, 1991; Lavin and McKeown, 1993). This syndrome involves multiple organ systems including the eyes, the nervous system, and the kidneys. Manifestations include cataracts (100%), glaucoma (65%), miosis, corneal keloids, mental retardation, described as ranging from moderate to profound with the majority being severely limited, growth retardation, hypotonia, seizures, and Fanconi's renal syndrome (metabolic acidosis, aminoaciduria, proteinuria, and hyperphosphaturia). Patients have typical facies that become more pronounced with age; they have small, deep-set eyes, frontal bossing, and a face that becomes progressively elongated because of hypotonia (Charnas and Gahl, 1991). Carrier females have lenticular opacities in the cortex of the lens identifiable by slit-lamp exam. This examination should be performed prior to genetic counseling of a couple with an affected son and no family history. While the disorder was mapped to the Xq24-26 region, it is only recently that the gene, OCRL1, was discovered (Lin et al., 1999). The gene encodes a 105 kDa protein which is deficient in these patients. The incidence of OCRL is 1 in 200 000 live-births. While couples at risk were previously given the option of identifying the sex of the fetus and aborting males, the discovery of the gene has made prenatal diagnosis a reality. Currently, treatment revolves around control and treatment of Fanconi's syndrome using Bicitra, monitoring the patients' electrolytes with supplementation as necessary. Definitive treatment is renal transplant.

Associations and syndromes
CHARGE association

The acronym CHARGE was coined by Pagon et al. (1981) as a mnemonic for a group of associated congenital anomalies first recognized by Hall (1979). The syndrome includes colobomata, heart defects, choanal atresia, retarded growth and development, genital hypoplasia, and ear anomalies. At least four of seven anomalies are necessary for diagnosis (Pagon et al., 1981). The most common anomalies found are external ear abnormalities (88%) and ocular coloboma (86%). Various cardiac anomalies are seen in 81% of patients. Retarded growth, developmental delay or CNS abnormalities including spinal chord tethering and sacral agenesis are also commonly seen (Ragan et al., 1999).

Genitourinary abnormalities are seen in 69% of patients and vary widely (Ragan et al., 1999). The most common male genital anomalies are micropenis and cryptorchidism. Other abnormalities include penile agenesis, chordee with and without hypospadias, and bifid scrotum. Female abnormalities include hypoplasia of the labia majora, labia minora and/or clitoris, absent uterus and ovaries, and absent vagina and uterus. Ragan et al. (1999) also screened their patients with a renal ultrasound and cystourethrograms and found a 40% incidence of renal abnormalities. Abnormalities included hydronephrosis, UPJ obstruction, VUR, and neuropathic bladder. There have also been reports of renal agenesis, posterior urethral valves, and duplicated collecting systems (Pagon et al., 1981).

The incidence of CHARGE is 1 in 10 000 births. Its occurrence is generally sporadic but there have been several reports of familial cases, including autosomal recessive, autosomal dominant and X-linked inheritance patterns (Pagon et al., 1981; Arwich et al., 1982; Metlay et al., 1987; Mitchell et al., 1985). Karyotypic analyses of these patients have been normal for the most part, although a number of translocations has been reported.

Many chromosomal anomalies share common physical findings, and therefore all patients should undergo karyotypic analysis. Cardiac evaluation, renal and bladder sonography, and cystourethrograms are indicated in all patients (Ragan et al., 1999).

Goldenhar syndrome (oculo-auricular vertebral complex; OAV)

Goldenhar syndrome was originally described as a non-random association of auricular, vertebral, and ocular defects which is caused by improper development of the first two branchial arches (Zelante et al., 1997). The diagnosis requires at least two of the following: optic hypoplasia, hemifacial microsomia, lateral facial cleft, epibulbar dermoid and/or upper eyelid coloboma, and vertebral anomalies (Kumar et al., 1993). As many as 50% of patients will have other anomalies, most commonly cardiac, pulmonary, and/or urologic (Zelante et al., 1997; Ritchey et al., 1994). In a review by Ritchey et al. (1994) urologic anomalies were present in 70% of those screened, which included renal agenesis, renal ectopia, ureteral duplication, UPJ obstruction, and a multicystic dysplastic kidney. VUR was seen commonly and a left retrocaval ureter has also been described (Ishitoya et al., 1997). The incidence has been estimated at 1/3000–5000 with a slight male predominance. It is usually sporadic in nature but autosomal dominant and recessive patterns of inheritance with marked variability of expression have been described. Because of the variable expressivity, screening is suggested of family members who may have very mild findings. For the purpose of counseling, the recurrence risk has been estimated at 2–3% (Gorlin et al., 1963; Stoll et al., 1998; Schaefer et al., 1998). Once the diagnosis is made, cardiac and urologic evaluation is suggested.

MURCS association

Duncan et al. (1979) first described the association of müllerian duct aplasia, renal aplasia, and cervicothoracic somite dysplasia and coined the acronym

MURCS. The most common presenting symptom is primary amenorrhea. On physical examination, patients are found to have normal secondary sexual characteristics; however, the vagina is absent. Surgical exploration reveals normal ovaries with normal distal fallopian tubes that become rudimentary fibrous stalks with no uterus. Radiologic exam reveals characteristic fusion of cervical and upper thoracic vertebrae and occasionally abnormal scapulae and ribs, with sparing of the lower spine. Most commonly there is unilateral renal agenesis with an ectopic contralateral kidney (most often pelvic). Duncan *et al.* (1979) speculated that the association might be explained by an insult at the 4th week of embryonic development when the lower cervical, upper thoracic somites, arm buds, and pronephric ducts all share an intimate spatial relation. A male variant has been suggested where the typical renal and spinal abnormalities are associated with azoospermia (Wellesley and Slaney, 1995).

Prader–Willi syndrome

Prader–Willi syndrome (PWS) is a multisystem disorder first described in 1956 by Prader, Labhart, and Willi. Its cardinal features include infantile hypotonia of prenatal onset, hypogonadism, hyperphagia and obesity, developmental delay and mental retardation, behavioral problems, and dysmorphic facies (Cassidy, 1997; Brondum-Nielson, 1997; Gunay Aygun *et al.*, 1997). These patients classically have a narrow bifrontal diameter, a narrow nasal bridge, and a downturned mouth with a thin upper lip. Their hands and feet are small and their fingers taper. In addition, they are usually fairer in skin, hair, and eye color than other members of their family. Typical histories include decreased fetal movement, abnormal fetal position, and such profound hypotonia in infancy that they are unable to suck and often develop failure to thrive. Later (between 1 and 6 years) hyperphagia and central obesity develops, which is thought to be central in origin. Characteristic behavioral problems include temper tantrums, stubbornness, and manipulation that evolves into obsessive–compulsive disorder and occasionally (5–10%) true psychosis.

Hypogonadism and genital hypoplasia are evident at birth. In males this manifests as cryptorchidism, scrotal hypoplasia, and small penis, and in females as hypoplastic labia minora and clitoris. These patients have abnormal pubertal development, either delayed, incomplete or both. Menarche has been known to occur as late as in the 30s. In both males and females sexual activity is rare and both are infertile. Hypogonadism is hypothalamic in origin. Therefore, hormonal therapy is an effective treatment modality (Cassidy, 1997).

The prevalence of PWS is 1 in 10 000 to 1 in 15 000. This syndrome is significant for being the first identified human syndrome due to imprinting. Imprinting is a phenomenon in which there is differential expression of maternal versus paternal alleles. PWS is due to a 4–5 Mb deletion in the area of 15q11-13 of the paternal chromosome (Brondum-Nielson, 1997; Jiang *et al.*, 1998). The defect is most commonly the result of interstitial paternal deletions or maternal uniparental disomy (in which the patient has two chromosomes derived from the mother and none from the father).

The recurrence risk for PWS is based on the possibility of a paternal balanced insertion or gonadal mosaicism and is estimated at 1%. Prenatal diagnosis may be made by chorionic villae sampling or amniocentesis. Molecular diagnosis is made using PCR and FISH to identify the deleted region on chromosome 15. Treatment is symptomatic with an emphasis on weight control as obesity causes most of the morbidity and mortality in these patients.

Prune belly syndrome (PBS)

The incidence of PBS is estimated at between 1 in 30 000 and 1 in 50 000 live births. Three to five per cent of patients are females. However, Rabinowitz and Schillinger (1977), in a review of affected females, found that they either had an incomplete form or did not have PBS at all (Greskovich and Nyberg, 1988; Sutherland *et al.*, 1995). Although most cases are sporadic there have been families with multiple affected members. The possibility of an X-linked gene for PBS has been suggested. Adeyokunnu and Familusi (1982) described a family where a brother and sister as well as a male cousin were affected, and the girl had XO karyotype, strengthening the argument for an X-linked gene. Furthermore, as PBS has been described in patients with several karyotypic abnormalities, specifically trisomy 13, trisomy 18, and trisomy 21, authors have suggested that karyotypic analysis be performed on fetuses diagnosed with PBS prior to any intrauterine intervention (Frydman *et al.*, 1983; Beckman *et al.*, 1984; Amacker *et al.*, 1986). Prenatal ultrasound has been used to make the diagnosis as early as 12–14 weeks' gestation (Shimizu *et al.*, 1992).

VATER/VACTERL association

Quan and Smith (1973) first described the association of vertebral anomalies, anal atresia, T-E fistula and esophageal atresia, renal anomalies and radial malformations. The association was later expanded by Kaufman (1973) and Nora and Nora (1975) to include cardiac anomalies and limb defects (VACTERL). Although not universally accepted, at least three anomalies should be present for the diagnosis to be considered (Czeizl and Ludanyi, 1985). The most common renal anomaly is renal agenesis, but cystic renal disease, obstructive lesions, and reflux are also seen (Khoury *et al.*, 1983).

The incidence is 1.6 in 10 000 live births. There is a slightly higher incidence among whites and a male predominance has also been noted. The association is often lethal, with a 12% stillbirth rate and 48% of infants dying within the first year (Czeizl and Ludanyi, 1985; Khoury *et al.*, 1983). Most cases have been sporadic with no specific chromosomal abnormality found. A subgroup of patients who have hydrocephalus and a poorer prognosis (VACTERL-H) has been found to have an X-linked recessive mode of inheritance (Wang *et al.*, 1993; Lomas *et al.*, 1998). One theory is that VACTERL is caused by a defect in mesodermal development (Quan and Smith, 1973). Owing to the high incidence of renal involvement, renal sonography and voiding cystourography are suggested.

Genetic counseling

The process of genetic counseling is one that should be implicit in all discussions with families that include a malformed child or one with a genetic disorder. Studies show that only 15% of hospitalized patients with a genetic disorder are given genetic counseling. Physicians must keep this in mind when a child is acutely ill or the family will never receive much needed and important information (Lessick *et al.*, 1981). The purpose of such counseling is threefold: to provide useful information in an understandable fashion, to reduce the overwhelming stresses on the family, and to develop reproductive alternatives related to the risk of recurrence. Counseling is more art than science. Most genetic counselors provide nondirective counseling without making the actual decision for the family. The following steps are including in counseling a family.

1 *Rapid diagnosis.* As noted above, everything hinges on a rapid, accurate diagnosis after consideration of syndromic etiologies.
2 *Counseling parents together.* The reasons for this are obvious. During counseling, individuals hear selectively and are often unable to relay information correctly to one another. In addition, feelings of guilt are more equally divided when both members of a couple are present.
3 *Explanation of problems in biologic terms.* This step aids in reducing guilt by demonstrating that there is a scientific basis for the occurrence of a malformation or genetic disorder. Language used should be understandable, but complex terms (such as chromosomes and genes) should not be avoided.
4 *Discussion of recurrence risk.* Parents should be told what the theoretical risk of recurrence is, and it should be placed in a real-life situation. A demonstration of the mechanical basis of inheritance is reasonable at this point.
5 *Discussion of burden.* As important as risk figures may be to a family, the burden or impact of a condition on a family emotionally, financially, and medically may be what makes the decision for them. Each family views burden differently, and the counselor should not bias the information.
6 *Consideration of reproductive options.* The availability of prenatal diagnosis and other options, including donor insemination and adoption, should be introduced in an objective fashion.
7 *Written summary.* Throughout the counseling sessions, both visual and auditory cues are used. The pace of the session should be leisurely, with periodic pauses where questions would be appropriate. If possible, some written material, either informal notes of the session highlighting key points or a more formal follow-up letter, should be provided.
8 *Repetition.* Much has been written on the imperfections of counseling. Although many families may retain risk figure information, the subtleties of what occurs in a counseling session are often lost. Repetition on the part of the urologist, geneticist, and other care providers is frequently necessary to ensure a clear perception of transmitted information. Excellent reviews on the counseling process demonstrate the inherent difficulties in transmitting information to families (Leonard *et al.*, 1972; Targum, 1982).

Often it is the physician who must do the genetic counseling for prenatal testing. In many ways this is not different from obtaining informed consent for a procedure. The testing must be adequately explained, including its purpose. The risks and benefits of testing, future treatments and alternative procedures must be explained. **The patient** needs to be aware of any future decisions that may need to be made based on results of initial testing. The patient should be given ample time to ask questions and have them answered in an understandable fashion. **The patients** should understand that they may refuse testing and/or treatment. Care should be taken to ensure appropriate documentation.

Counseling for selected isolated urologic conditions

The situation that the urologist most often faces is the child with an isolated urogenital malformation and parents who desire information on the risk of recurrence. As indicated throughout much of this chapter, it is currently thought that most regional malformations are multifactorially determined, with both environmental and genetic components.

Vesicoureteral reflux

While the stimulus for the development of VUR is thought to be multifactorial there seems to be a strong genetic basis. In addition to being observed in families, the inheritance of reflux is linked to human leukocyte antigens. Segregation analysis points to VUR being inherited via a single dominant gene acting in combination with environmental factors (Chapman et al., 1985). Several studies have suggested a dominant pattern of inheritance, with one-third to one-half of the siblings of index cases having VUR and a risk of 1:2 for offspring of an affected parent (Noe et al., 1992). The gene frequency is estimated at 1 in 600 (Dillon and Goonasekera, 1998). VUR is seen in multiple conditions and syndromes, and ongoing research is attempting to identify candidate genes for VUR by analysis of these disorders. Current candidate genes include chromosome 6p, chromosome 22q11, and chromosome 10p (Devriendt et al., 1998).

Because of the high incidence of recurrence within families when the diagnosis of VUR is made in one child, younger siblings, who are at greatest risk for renal scarring, should be screened. In addition, it may be prudent to screen the offspring of parents who had VUR as children (Noe et al., 1992). While a screening ultrasound may identify hydronephrosis it is an insensitive test for identifying reflux (Blane et al., 1993). Definitive diagnosis is made by cystography.

Cryptorchidism

Undescended testis (UT) is one of the most common disorders of childhood. Although it is associated with multiple syndromes and chromosomal abnormalities, it is usually an isolated finding. UT is seen in 4% of full-term infants and 30.3% of premature infants. Birth weight is another significant risk factor in that UT occurs in 68.5% of infants less than 1800 g and 100% of infants less than 900 g (Scorer, 1964). A family history of cryptorchidism significantly increases the risk. There is a fourfold increased risk to the sibling of an affected child. There have been many reports on multiple affected siblings as well as reports of multiple affected generations, and most evidence points to a multifactorial model of inheritance (Weidner et al., 1999; Savion et al., 1984; Carragher and McLean, 1990; Corbus and O'Connor, 1922; Pardo-Mindan et al., 1975; Czeizel et al., 1981). Other risk factors include being first born and hypospadias (Weidner et al., 1999). Another interesting group at risk is the children of mothers who had late-onset menarche and short menses, raising the possibility of a hereditary hormonal abnormality (Czeizel et al., 1981).

Hypospadias

The etiology of hypospadias is unknown. Factors that have been proposed include increased maternal age, number of previous pregnancies, and drug exposure. However, none has stood up to follow-up studies and multivariate analysis. The role of fetal hormone production and the hypothalamic–pituatary–gonadal axis, although an attractive possibility, is still unclear (Zaontz and Packer, 1997; Belman, 1997). Hypospadias is one of the most common urologic anomalies, with a reported incidence of 8.2 in 1000 livebirths (Bauer et al., 1981). Although it is generally sporadic, a strong familial association exists. Bauer et al. (1981) found that the father was affected in 8% of patients with hypospadias, there was a 12% risk of a second sibling being affected, and this risk increased to 26% when both a father and sibling were affected. The recurrence risk also increases with increasing severity of the anomaly. The prevailing view is that familial clustering is polygenetic and multifactorial, although autosomal dominant, recessive, and sex-linked patterns have also been proposed (Khuri *et al.*, 1981; Harris, 1990) (Table 3.4).

Hypospadias is associated with a number of rare syndromes. In those cases that are not part of defined syndromes the most common associated anomalies are cryptorchidism and inguinal hernias, found in about 9.3% and 9.1% of patients, respectively. In one report, the incidences of both undescended testes and inguinal hernia rise dramatically, to 31.6% and 17%, respectively, in boys with severe forms of hypospadias (Khuri *et al.*, 1981). Most authors agree that in patients with milder forms of hypospadias and palpable gonads no further evaluation is necessary. However, with penoscrotal or perineal hypospadias and/or the presence of a non-palpable gonad an evaluation for intersex should be performed (Zaontz and Packer, 1997; Belman, 1997; Smith and Wacksman, 1997). The diagnosis of hypospadias has been made by prenatal ultrasound as early as the second trimester based on a typical anomalous distal penile morphology and an anomalous urinary stream (Devesa *et al.*, 1998).

Posterior urethral valves

Posterior urethral valves (PUV) are the most common cause of congenital lower urinary tract obstruction. Theories of its etiology include an anomalous development of the mesonephric duct or origination from the urogenital sinus. One-third of patients will eventually develop some degree of impaired renal function (Dineen and Duffy, 1996). The incidence of PUV has been estimated at between 1 in 5000 and 1 in 12 500 livebirths (Rajab *et al.*, 1996). A genetic basis for the disease is suggested by multiple reports of affected siblings including monozygotic twins. Recently, a single family with male-to-male transmission has been reported, suggesting an autosomal dominant mode of transmission (Hanlon-Lundberg *et al.*, 1994). Further strengthening the argument for a genetic basis of the disease is the report by Rajab *et al.* (1996) who found a nearly fourfold increased incidence of PUV in Oman. In those families affected there was a higher incidence of consanguinity and there was also a higher incidence in specific tribes. No gene has been identified and most investigators suggest a polygenic or multifactorial model of inheritance (Hanlon-Lundberg *et al.*, 1994; Livne *et al.*, 1983; Thomalla *et al.*, 1989). Antenatal diagnosis is possible

via ultrasound and some have suggested that earlier diagnosis portends a poorer prognosis (Dineen and Duffy, 1996; Hutton *et al.*, 1994).

Exstrophy and epispadias

The exstrophy/epispadias complex describes a spectrum of disease ranging from mild forms of distal epispadias to the most severe form, that of cloacal exstrophy. The prevailing causal theory is that of Marshall and Muecke (1962), who proposed that the medial migration of the lateral mesenchyme is prevented by the abnormal growth of a cloacal membrane that is prone to rupture. Severity is determined by the timing of the rupture of the cloacal membrane: the earlier the rupture the more severe the result (Gearhart and Jeffs, 1998). The incidence of classic bladder exstrophy is between 1 in 25 000 and 1 in 40 000 live births, although one multicenter study found an incidence as low as 3.3 in 100 000 live births. Cloacal exstrophy is even rarer, with an approximate incidence of 1 in 400 000, and is associated with anomalies of multiple organ systems (Zaontz and Packer, 1997; Cacciari *et al.*, 1999; Messelink *et al.*, 1994). Males predominate, with a 2.3:1 male to female ratio (Cacciari *et al.*, 1999). Shapiro *et al.* (1984) reported the incidence of bladder exstrophy in siblings to be less than 1%. Messilink *et al.* (1994) reported two families with an apparent familial occurrence of exstrophy, one with a mother to son mode of inheritance, bringing the number of familial cases reported to 20. For the purpose of counseling, the risk of having an affected sibling is 1%, while the risk of having an affected offspring to an affected parent is 1 in 70. The genetics is believed to be multifactorial. Prenatal diagnosis can be made with ultrasound as early as 14 weeks, and diagnostic criteria include a non-visualized bladder (the study should be repeated to ensure that this is the case), a lower abdominal mass, and low insertion of the umbilical cord (Cacciari *et al.*, 1999; Austin *et al.*, 1998).

Wilms' tumor syndromes

Several syndromes include an increased susceptibility to Wilms' tumor (WT) formation as a common denominator. These include WAGR (**W**ilms' tumor, **a**niridia, **g**enital abnormalities, and mental **r**etardation), Beckwith–Wiederman syndrome (BWS) and the Denys–Drash syndrome. The genital abnormalities of the WAGR and Denys–Drash syndromes are similar and include genital ambiguity, male pseudo- and true hermaphroditism, and streak gonads (Mueller, 1994). Both the WAGR and Denys–Drash syndromes also share a common gene, although the defects are different. WAGR is caused by deletion of the WT1 gene on 11p13 that follows the Knudson hypothesis of tumor suppressor genes. The genetics of Denys–Drash is more complex. This syndrome is due to mutations of the zinc finger domain of the WT1 gene leading to a dominant negative mutation (Grundy et al., 1995; Devriendt et al., 1996). The distinguishing feature of the Denys–Drash syndrome is the progressive nephropathy leading to early renal failure caused by mesangial sclerosis. Because of the risk of gonadoblastoma, gonadal excision is recommended for those patients with hermaphroditism (Rudin et al., 1998). BWS is the most common overgrowth syndrome, with an incidence of 1 in 13 000. Diagnostic criteria include omphalocele, macroglossia and macrosomia, neonatal hypoglycemia, generalized or regional overgrowth, and visceromegaly. Children are at increased risk for tumor development in the first 5 years of life, most commonly Wilms' tumor. A mutated paternal WT2 gene found on 11p15 is responsible and the mechanism is that of genetic imprinting (Grundy et al., 1995; Li et al., 1997). For the most part these syndromes are sporadic but familial cases have been reported. From linkage studies of four large families with a hereditary predisposition for WT, a third gene has been predicted (Grundy et al., 1995). Many of the anomalies are detectable with prenatal ultrasound.

Turner syndrome

Turner first described this syndrome in 1938 when he noted that a group of adolescent girls with failure to enter puberty had other findings in common. In addition to streak ovaries, these girls have congenital lymphedema, short stature, webbed neck, cubitus valgus (increased carrying angle), shield chest, and coarctation of the aorta (Saenger, 1996; Persky and Owens, 1971). They are at increased risk for otitis media due to distortion of the eustachian tube, scoliosis, glucose intolerance, hypothyroidism, gastrointestinal bleeding, and renal dysgenesis (Saenger, 1996). Persky and Owens (1971) found that approximately two-thirds of patients with Turner syndrome have significant anatomical aberration of the urogenital tract. Major

disorders noted include malrotation and duplications, non-functioning kidneys, hydronephrosis, and ectopia; horseshoe kidney is the most common anomaly (Persky and Owens, 1971; Litvak et al., 1978). Turner syndrome is the most common sex chromosome abnormality in females. Its frequency among liveborn female infants is estimated to be between 1/1500 and 1/2500. Although the first patients diagnosed with this disorder had a karyotype of 45,X, more than half are mosaics with 45,X/46,XX. Flynn et al. (1996) found a greater association of renal malformations in patients with monsomy 45,X than those with mosaicism. Patients with Turner syndrome require renal ultrasound upon diagnosis with further studies, if indicated.

Prenatal diagnosis

Since the 1960s, several tools have been developed to allow assessment of the genetic make-up of the fetus. With improved techniques and the beginnings of the field of interventional perinatal medicine, more aggressive diagnosis is being sought by many practitioners and patients.

Indications

The leading indication for prenatal diagnosis is advanced maternal age, generally accepted as 35 years or older at the time of delivery. With increasing age of the mother, there is a corresponding increase in the risk of having a child with a chromosomal abnormality. Primarily, this is the result of non-disjunctional events such as trisomy 21, trisomy 13, trisomy 18, and Klinefelter syndrome. The risk for structural chromosomal abnormalities such as unbalanced translocations and for conditions such as Turner syndrome is not increased. The risk for Down syndrome at selected maternal ages is shown in Table 3.5 (Hook and Lindsje, 1978).

Other indications for seeking prenatal diagnosis include the following.

1 *Positive family history.* The presence of a genetic disorder or birth defect in a close relative may warrant prenatal diagnosis. For families that have had a child with a single gene disorder (dominant, recessive, or X-linked), prenatal diagnosis may exist for the condition. For certain X-linked traits, sex determination may be offered if a more exact diagnosis cannot be obtained.

Table 3.5 Risk of giving birth to a child with Down syndrome at selected maternal ages

Maternal age (years)	Risk at birth
30	1/885
33	1/592
35	1/365
37	1/225
40	1/109
45	1/32

Adapted from Hook and Lindsje (1978), courtesy of the University of Chicago Press.

2 *Previously affected child with chromosomal abnormality*. The risk of having a second liveborn child with a chromosomal abnormality (e.g. Down syndrome) increases to approximately 1% plus the age-related risk. This is equally true for less common conditions where the risk seems more related to chromosomal non-disjunction in general. For families in which a parent has been identified as having a balanced translocation, with no net loss or gain of genetic material, the risk for unbalanced offspring may rise dramatically.

3 *Recurrent miscarriages or infant loss*. Approximately 5% of couples experiencing more than two unexplained spontaneous abortions carry a balanced translocation in one member of the couple.

4 *Abnormal α-fetoprotein result*. Screening for malformations of the neural tube in 'low-risk' families has been accomplished by measurement of maternal serum α-fetoprotein (MSAFP) levels (Burton, 1986; Main and Mennuti, 1986). Elevations of this protein correlate well with an increased risk for myelomeningocele and anencephaly as well as other neural tube defects. Awareness of low MSAFP levels in fetuses with Down syndrome may allow for more accurate determination of risk. Using a cutoff value of 1/270 (comparable with the risk of having a child with Down syndrome at the age of 35), DiMaio *et al*. (1988) found that one-quarter to one-third of pregnancies in which the fetus had Down syndrome could be detected using MSAFP screening. Most centers would view an MSAFP level below 0.5 multiples of the median as significant. Tables exist from a variety of sources to allow for more accurate calculations of exact risk in such a family.

5 *Abnormal fetal sonogram*.

6 *Drug exposure*. The exposure of the fetus to certain substances during pregnancy can substantially increase the risk of birth defects. Level II ultrasonography should be offered to these families for reassurance and management.

7 *Maternal illness*. The risk for malformations is increased for specific maternal illnesses, with diabetes being the most prevalent. In this situation, the risk for malformation is at least two to three times greater than the general population. In a large collaborative study, Mills *et al*. (1988) have demonstrated that improved diabetic control can reduce, but not eliminate, the risk of malformation.

Methods and techniques

Maternal α-fetoprotein (triple screen)

α-Fetoprotein is produced by the fetus in increasing concentrations in early fetal life, peaking at 12–14 weeks (Willner, 1998). It can be detected in maternal serum and in amniotic fluid. MSAFP is elevated in open body defects, most notably neural tube defects. It is also elevated in the presence of open ventral wall defects, with sensitivity estimated between 75 and 90% (Palomaki *et al*., 1988; Wald and Cuckle, 1977) providing an effective screen. In addition, MSAFP will be low in aneuploidy fetuses, for example Down syndrome. In women under the age of 35 years, measuring MSAFP, human chorionic gonadotropin (hCG), and unconjugated estriol (uE3) is an effective screen for neural tube defects and triploidies (with a sensitivity of 60–65% for detecting Down syndrome). However, in women over 35 years of age, as their risk of aneuploidy fetuses is greater, the triple screen is not a substitute for amniocentesis (Ormond, 1997). It is currently the recommendation of the American College of Obstetrics and Gynecology (ACOG) and the American College of Medical Genetics (ACMG) that all pregnant women be offered serum screening. However, which markers should be used is not specified (ACOG, 1992; ACMG, 1996).

The best time to draw a triple screen is between 16 and 18 weeks' gestation (Wald and Cuckle, 1977). MSAFP values are converted into multiples of the median, which takes into account maternal weight, insulin-dependent diabetes mellitus, the presence of multiple gestations, and maternal race. Abnormalities in values warrant sonographic follow-up to evaluate the fetus, check the accuracy of dates, and determine whether there are multiple fetuses. The majority of abnormal results is due to inaccurate dating. An abnormal sonogram warrants further investigation based on the findings, but most commonly an amniocentesis and karyotyping are done when screening results are confirmed to be abnormal.

Sonography

Sonography is a non-invasive radiologic imaging technique. It is safe for use during pregnancy at any stage of fetal development. Indications for ultrasonic examination include discrepancy in fundal height for gestational age, increased maternal α-fetoprotein, and history of a previous pregnancy with an associated congenital abnormality (Mandell *et al.*, 1991). However, many centers are now offering ultrasound exams routinely to all pregnant women (Garmel and C'Alton, 1994). Initial studies are performed between 16 and 20 weeks' gestation and include evaluation of head, spine, heart, and lungs, and measurements of the limbs and abdomen.

The number of fetal urogenital abnormalities detected has risen as a result of the performance of routine fetal sonograms. Urinary tract abnormalities can be identified *in utero* by ultrasound as early as 12–14 weeks' gestation, with an accuracy of 84.4–97% (Corteville *et al.*, 1991). To improve the yield with respect to genitourinary abnormalities there needs to be a systematic approach to assessment. Aside from localization and characterization of the genitourinary abnormality, these include determining fetal size and maturity, amniotic fluid volume, gender (if possible), and identification of other associated anomalies (Reddy and Mandell, 1998). Once identified, lesions should be monitored and their impact on fetal health assessed. Management should include a level II sonogram to look for additional malformations, consideration of a fetal echocardiogram, if not included in the original sonogram, a rapid karyotype through amniocentesis, placental biopsy, or umbilical cord blood sampling, genetic counseling, and appropriate subspecialty visits as indicated.

The presence of an apparently isolated malformation on ultrasonography should routinely raise the question as to whether the malformation is truly isolated or is part of a broader malformation syndrome. Similarly, the frequency of chromosomal syndromes in this 'isolated' group is significant. In many centers, families are routinely offered amniocentesis or rapid fetal karyotyping in this situation. An abnormal karyotype has the potential for making profound changes in prenatal and postnatal management even if the abnormality is detected beyond 25 weeks' gestation. The frequency of chromosomal abnormalities in fetuses with any ultrasonographically detected malformations ranges from 13 to 35% (Donnefeld and Mennuti, 1988; Eydoux *et al.*, 1989; Nicolaides *et al.*, 1986; Williamson *et al.*, 1987).

Amniocentesis

Amniocentesis was first performed for genetic studies in the 1950s and for prenatal diagnosis in the late 1960s (Reece, 1997). This procedure involves transabdominal needle extraction of a small amount of amniotic fluid from the uterine cavity under ultrasonic guidance. It is generally performed between 15 and 17 weeks' gestation, as at this time there is sufficient amniotic fluid and the ratio of viable to nonviable cells is greatest (Emery, 1970). Complications from this procedure include transplacental hemorrhage and maternal isoimmunization in Rh-negative women. Fluid leakage, vaginal spotting, and contractions almost always resolve on their own (Lynch and Berkowitz, 1992). Multicenter studies in both the USA and Canada have shown that the number of stillbirths, neonatal deaths, and spontaneous abortion attributable to second trimester amniocentesis are not significantly different from controls, and the risk of loss of pregnancy is estimated at between 0.5 and 1% (Canadian Collaborative Chorionic Villae Sampling—Amniocentesis Clinical Trial Group, 1989; NICD National Registry for Amniocentesis Study Group, 1976).

Early amniocentesis can be done between 10 and 14 weeks of gestation. The safety of the procedure at that time has not been as well documented. Comparisons of early amniocentesis with CVS seem to show comparable risk of culture failure; however, early amniocentesis had a higher risk of spontaneous abortion, with an estimated risk between 3.5 and 4.7%. There has also been a higher incidence of talipes equinovarus associated with early amniocentesis than with CVS (Hanson *et al.*, 1987). The advantage of early amniocentesis over CVS is that the former is more cytogenetically accurate and allows analysis of α-fetoprotein and acetylcholinesterase levels.

Chorionic villae sampling

This technique was first used by the Chinese in the early 1970s. Subsequently, the method has been refined and is currently considered a safe technique for first trimester prenatal diagnosis. CVS is performed between 9 and 12 weeks of gestation. At this time, the developing sac does not fill the uterus and it is possible, under ultrasonic guidance, to take a sampling of the chorionic frondosum, the area where the villae are mitotically active. The villae are made up of both syncytiotrophoblasts that may be cultured and cytotrophoblasts that can be used for direct karyotyping. In addition, this timing avoids the high background spontaneous miscarriage rate normally present early in pregnancy, but allows sufficient time to obtain results within the first trimester (Wapner, 1997).

CVS may be performed transcervically or transabdominally; both techniques are equally safe and efficacious (Wapner, 1997; Jackson et al., 1991). The rate of miscarriage from the time of CVS until 28 weeks' gestation is approximately 2–3% (Jackson et al., 1992). Investigators who have compared the risk of spontaneous abortion after amniocentesis to that after CVS have found no difference between the two (Canadian Collaborative Chorionic Villae Sampling—Amniocentesis Clinical Trial Group, 1989; Rhoads et al., 1989). However, CVS may be associated with the occurrence of severe limb abnormalities. Oromandibular–limb hypogenesis syndrome was seen in infants whose mothers had CVS performed between 55 and 66 days' gestation at a rate of >1% (Wapner, 1997; Foster-Iskenius and Baird, 1989), while those whose CVS was performed after day 70 of gestation did not demonstrate a risk of limb abnormalities greater than that of the general population.

Complications of CVS include vaginal bleeding in 7–10% of women after transabdominal CVS and up to one-third of women when done transcervically CVS (Rhoads et al., 1989). The bleeding is usually self-limited and does not affect the outcome of the pregnancy. Infection is a concern; however, the incidence of post-CVS infection is only 0.3%. Rare complications include acute rupture of the membranes and Rh sensitization in Rh-negative women with vaginal bleeding. It must be noted that women tested for α-fetoprotein after CVS will have an elevated value. The levels take a few weeks to drop to normal and should be within a normal range by 16–18 weeks' gestation, allowing the usual prenatal screening to be done.

Percutaneous umbilical blood sampling

Percutaneous umbilical blood sampling (PUBS) is a procedure in which the umbilical cord is used to draw blood from the fetus or for transfusion of blood products into the fetus. Initially, PUBS was used therapeutically in anemic fetuses (erythroblastosis fetalis) and those with thrombocytopenia, as well as for diagnosis of congenital infectious disease or hematologic disorders (Willner, 1998). More recently, the procedure has been used increasingly for molecular diagnostic purposes. As its indications have changed so has its timing, with PUBS being performed later in gestation. PUBS is rarely the first line of testing, rather it is performed after an abnormal result is detected by another method. It is never used as a screening procedure. The most common indication for PUBS is ultrasonic detection of a fetal anomaly; PUBS is used for rapid karyotyping in the second and third trimesters (Buscaglia et al., 1996). Other indications include mosaicism on CVS or amniocentesis, and fetal evaluation for metabolic disease in fetuses with growth retardation. Complications include umbilical hematoma, fetal bradycardia, and miscarriage. Maternal complications include hematoma of the uterine wall, chorioamnionitis, and placental rupture (Duchatel et al., 1993). These complications decrease with increasing gestational age. The rate of fetal demise is estimated at between 2.4 and 5% dependent on the experience of the physician performing the procedure, gestational age of the fetus, number of needle insertions, and duration of the procedure. Duration greater than 10 min, more than three needle insertions, and decreased gestational age lead to increased risk of pregnancy loss (Buscaglia et al., 1996; Duchatel et al., 1993). Approximately 80% of PUBS can be done within these boundaries. There seems to be a higher risk of loss in fetuses who were referred for the procedure because of structural or chromosomal abnormality than those referred for therapeutic reasons.

Magnetic resonance imaging

Although sonography is the modality of choice for routine antenatal imaging, it is not always possible to detect abnormalities using ultrasound. Magnetic resonance imaging (MRI) is being used increasingly in cases where clear sonographic images cannot be obtained. MRI, like ultrasound, is non-invasive and provides multiplanar imaging. However, MRI tends to provide better soft-tissue contrast and cerebral images than does sonography. Indications for its use include visualization of lesions not seen well sonographically or clarification of sonographic findings (Garel *et al.*, 1998). At present, fetal MRI is being used almost exclusively for evaluation of the fetal brain, but its use in fetal cardiac imaging is being evaluated.

The risk to the fetus from fetal MRI is unclear. Animal studies found a correlation between prolonged high-level exposure to electromagnetic radiation and fetal anomalies, including chromosomal mutations. To date there is no evidence of this in human fetuses; however, fetal MRI is not recommended in the first trimester to avoid these potential risks (Beers, 1989). This method of fetal evaluation is currently used in a limited number of cases.

References

Aarskog D (1970) A familial syndrome of short stature associated with facial dysplasia and genital anomalies. *J Pediatr* 77: 856–61.

Abdelhak S, Kalatzis V, Heilig R *et al.* (1997) A human homologue of the Drosophila eyes absent gene underlies branchio-oto-renal (BOR) syndrome and identifies a novel gene family. *Nature Genet* 15: 157–64.

ACOG (1992) Technical Bulletin No. 154, April 1991 Alpha-fetoprotein. *Int J Gynecol Obstet* 38: 241–7.

Adeyokunnu AA, Familusi JB (1982) Prune belly syndrome in two siblings and a first cousin. Possible genetic implications. *Am J Dis Child* 136: 23–5.

Al-Essa M, Dhaunsi GS, Rashed M *et al.* (1999) Zellweger syndrome in Saudi Arabia and its distinct features. *Clin Pediatr* 38: 77–86.

Allanson JE (1987) Noonan syndrome. *J Med Genet* 24: 9–13.

Alport AC (1927) Hereditary familial congenital haemorrhagic nephritis. *BMJ* 1: 504–6.

Amacker EA, Grass FS, Hickey DE, Hisley JC (1986) Brief clinical report: an association of prune belly syndrome with trisomy 21. *Am J Med Genet* 23: 919–23.

American College of Medical Genetics (ACMG) (1996) ACMG position statement on multiple marker screening in women 35 and older.

Amirou M, Bourdat M, Huet G *et al.* (1998) Successful renal transplantation in Jeune syndrome type 2. *Pediatr Nephrol* 12: 293–4.

Arwich PD, Flannery DB, Robertson L, Mamunes P (1982) CHARGE association anomalies in siblings. *Am J Hum Genet* 34: 80A.

Austin PF, Homsy YL, Gearhart JP *et al.* (1998) The prenatal diagnosis of cloacal exstrophy. *J Urol* 160: 1179–81.

Baird PA, Anderson TW, Newcombe HB, Lowry RB (1988) Genetic disorders in children and young adults: a population study. *Am J Hum Genet* 42: 677–93.

Balci S, Beksac S, Haliloglu M *et al.* (1998) Robinow syndrome, vaginal atresia, hematocolpos, and extra middle finger. *Am J Med Genet* 79: 27–9.

Barakat AY, Butler MG (1987) Renal and urinary tract abnormalities associated with chromosome aberrations. *Int J Pediatr Nephrol* 8: 215–26.

Bauer SB, Retik AB, Colodny AH (1981) Genetic aspects of hypospadias. *Urol Clin N Am* 8: 559–64.

Baumgartner MR, Poll-The BT, Verhoeven NM *et al.* (1998) Saudubray JM. Clinical approach to inherited peroxisomal disorders: a series of 27 patients. *Ann Neurol* 44: 720–30.

Beales PL, Warner GA, Thakker R, Flinter FA (1997) Bardet–Biedl syndrome: a molecular and phenotypic study of 18 families. *J Med Genet* 34: 92–8.

Bear JC, Parfrey PS, Morgan JM *et al.* (1992) Autosomal dominant polycystic kidney disease: new information for genetic counselling. *Am J Med Genet* 43: 548–53.

Beckman H, Rehder H, Rauskolb R (1984) Prune belly sequence associated with trisomy 13. *Am J Med Genet* 19: 603–4.

Beebe DK (1996) Autosomal dominant polycystic kidney disease. *Am Fam Physician* 15: 925–31.

Beers GJ (1989) Biological effects of weak electromagnetic fields from 0 Hz to 200 MHz: a survey of the literature with special emphasis on possible magnetic resonance effects. *Magn Reson Imaging* 7: 309–31.

Belman AB (1997) Hypospadias update. *Urology* 49: 166–72.

Blane HH, Di Pietro, Zeim JM (1993) Renal is not a reliable screening exam for vesicoureteral reflux. *J Urol* 150: 752–5.

Blyth H, Ockenden BG (1971) Polycystic disease of kidneys and liver presenting in childhood. *J Med Genet* 8: 257–84.

Bodziak KA, Hammond WS, Molitoris BA (1994) Inherited diseases of the glomerular basement membrane. *Am J Kidney Dis* 23: 605–18.

Brondum-Nielson K (1997) The genetic basis for Prade–Willi syndrome: the importance of imprinted genes. *Acta Pediatr* 423 (suppl): 55–7.

Burton BK (1986) Alpha-fetoprotein screening. *Adv Pediatr* 33: 181–96.

Buscaglia M, Ghisoni L, Belloti M *et al.* (1996) Percutaneous umbilical blood sampling: indication changes and procedure loss rate in a nine years' experience. *Fetal Diagn Ther* 11: 106–13.

Butler MG, Wadlington WB (1987) Robinow syndrome: report of two patients and review of the literature. *Clin Genet* 31: 77–85.

Buyse ML (1990) *Birth defects encyclopedia: the comprehensive systematic, illustrated reference for diagnosis, delineation, etiology, biodynamics, occurrence, prevention and treatment of human anomalies of clinical relevance.* Dover, MA: Center for Birth Defects Information Services; Cambridge, MA: Blackwell Scientific Publications.

Cacciari A, Pilu GL, Mordenti M *et al.* (1999) Prenatal diagnosis of bladder exstrophy: what counseling? *J Urol* 161: 259–62.

Callis L, Vila A, Carrera M, Nieto J (1999) Long-term effects of cyclosporine A in Alport's syndrome. *Kidney Int* 55: 1051–6.

Canadian Collaborative Chorionic Villae Sampling — Amniocentesis Clinical Trial Group (1989) Multicentre randomized clinical trial of chorionic villae sampling and amniocentesis. *Lancet* i: 1.

Cappa M, Borrelli P, Marini R, Neri G (1987) The Opitz syndrome: a new designation for the clinically indistinguishable BBB and G syndromes. *Am J Med Genet* **28**: 303–9.

Carbonara P, Alpert M (1964) Hereditary osteo-onychodysplasia (HOOD). *Am J Med Sci* **248**: 139–51.

Carragher AM, McLean RDW (1990) Familial bilateral cryptorchidism. *Br J Clin Pract* **44**: 688–9.

Cassidy SB (1997) Prader–Willi syndrome. *J Med Genet* **34**: 917–23.

Chan PCK, Chan KW, Cheng IKP, Chan MK (1988) Living-related renal transplantation in a patient with nail-patella syndrome. *Nephron* **50**: 164–6.

Chapman CJ, Bailey RR, Janus ED et al. (1985) Vesicoureteral reflux: segregation analysis. *Am J Med Genet* **20**: 577–84.

Charnas LR, Gahl WA (1991) The oculocerebrorenal syndrome of Lowe. *Adv Pediatr* **38**: 75–107.

Chen A, Francis M, Ni L et al. (1975) Phenotypic manifestations of branchiootorenal syndrome. *Am J Med Genet* **58**: 365–70.

Chen CP, Lin SP, Jan SW et al. (1996) Prenatal diagnosis of asphyxiating thoracic dysplasia (Jeune syndrome). *Am J Perinatol* **13**: 495–8.

Cohen MM (1982) *The child with multiple birth defects.* New York: Raven Press.

Comas C, Martinez Crespo JM, Puerto B et al. (1993) Bilateral renal agenesis and cytomegalovirus infection in a case of Fraser syndrome. *Fetal Diagn Ther* **8**: 285–90.

Corbus BC, O'Connor VJ (1922) The familial occurrence of undescended testes. *Surg Gynecol Obstet* **34**: 237–40.

Cordero JF, Holmes LB (1978) Phenotypic overlap of the BBB and G syndromes. *Am J Med Genet* **2**: 145–52.

Corteville JE, Gray DL, Crane JP (1991) Congenital hydronephrosis: correlation of fetal ultrasonographic findings with infant outcome. *J Pediatr Surg* **165**: 384–8.

Czeizel A, Erodi E, Toth J (1981) Genetics of undescended testis. *J Urol* **126**: 528–9.

Czeizel A, Ludanyi I (1985) An aetiological study of the VACTERL-association. *Pediatrics* **144**: 331–7.

Devarajan P (1995) Letter to the Editors: Obesity and genitourinary anomalies in Bardet–Biedl syndrome after renal transplantation. *Pediatr Nephrol* **9**: 397–402.

Devesa R, Munoz A, Torrents M et al. (1998) Prenatal diagnosis of isolated hypospadias. *Prenat Diagn* **18**: 779–88.

Devriendt K, Groenen P, Van Esch H et al. (1998) Vesicoureteral reflux — a genetic condition? *Eur J Pediatr* Apr. **157**: 265–71.

Devriendt K, van den Berghe K, Moerman P, Fryns JP (1996) Elevated maternal serum and amniotic fluid alpha fetoprotien levels in Denys-Drash syndrome. *Prenat Diagn* **16**: 455–7.

Dewald GW (1977) Gregor Johann Mendel and the beginning of genetics. *Mayo Clin Proc* **52**: 513–18.

Dillon MJ, Goonasekera CD (1998) Reflux nephropathy. *J Am Soc Nephrol* **9**: 2377–88.

DiMaio MJ, Baumgarten A, Greenstein RM (1988) Screening for fetal Down's syndrome in pregnancy by measuring maternal alpha-fetoprotein levels. *N Engl J Med* **317**: 342–6.

Dineen MD, Duffy PG (1996) Posterior urethral valves. *Br J Urol* **78**: 275–81.

Donnefeld AE, Mennuti MT (1988) Sonographic findings in fetuses with comon chromosome abnormalities. *Clin Obstet Gynecol* **31**: 80–96.

Duchatel F, Oury JF, Menneson B, Murray JM (1993) Complications of diagnostic ultrasound guided percutaneous umbilical blood sampling: analysis of a series of 341 cases and review of the literature. *Eur J Obstet Gynecol Reprod Biol* **53**: 95–104.

Duncan PA, Shapiro LR, Stangel JJ et al. (1979) The MURCS association: mullerian duct aplasia, renal aplasi, and cervicothoracic somite dysplasia. *J Pediatr* **95**: 399–402.

Emery EAH (1970) Antenatal diagnosis of genetic disease. *Mod Trends Hum Genet* **1**: 267.

Eydoux P, Choiset A, Le Porrier N (1989) Chromosomal prenatal diagnosis: study of 936 cases of intrauterine abnormalities after ultrasound assessment. *Prenat Diagn* **9**: 255–69.

Farag TI, Usha R, Uma R et al. (1990) Phenotypic variability in Meckel–Gruber syndrome. *Clin Genet* **38**: 176–9.

Feingold M, Itzchak Y, Goodman RM (1998) Ultrasound prenatal diagnosis of the nail-patella syndrome. *Prenat Diagn* **18**: 854–6.

Fitzpatrick DR (1996) Zellweger syndrome and associated phenotypes. *J Med Genet* **33**: 863–8.

Flinter FA, Bobrow M, Chantler C (1987) Alport's syndrome of hereditary nephritis. *Pediatr Nephrol* **1**: 438–40.

Flynn MT, Ekstrom L, Miguel de Arce et al. (1996) Prevalence of renal malformation in Turner's syndrome. *Pediatr Nephrol* **10**: 498–500.

Foster-Iskenius U, Baird P (1989) Limb reduction defects in over 1,000,000 consecutive live births. *Teratology* **39**: 127–35.

Frydman M, Megenis RE, Mohandas TK, Kaback MM (1983) Chromosome abnormalities in infants with prune belly anomaly: association with trisomy 18. *Am J Med Genet* **35**: 145–8.

Fryns JP, van Schoubroeck D, Vandenberghe K et al. (1997) Diagnostic echocardiographic findings in cryptopthalmos syndrome (Fraser syndrome). *Prenat Diagn* **17**: 582–4.

Garel C, Brisse H, Sebag G et al. (1998) Magnetic resonance imaging of the fetus. *Pediatr Radiol* **28**: 201–11.

Garmel SH, C'Alton ME (1994) Diagnostic ultrasound in pregnancy: an overview. *Semin Perinatol* **18**: 117–32.

Gearhart JP, Jeffs RD (1998) Exstrophy–epispadias complex and bladder anomalies. In: Walsh PC, Retik AB, Vaughan ED, Wein AJ (eds) *Campbell's urology.* 7th edition. Philadelphia, PA: WB Saunders, 1939–90.

Gelehrter TD, Collins FS, Ginsburg D (1998) *Principles of medical genetics.* 2nd edition. Baltimore, MD: Williams and Wilkins.

Glassberg KI (1998) Renal dysplasia and cystic renal disease of the kidney. In: Walsh PC, Retik AB, Vaughn ED, Wein AJ (eds) *Campbell's urology*. 7th edition. Philadelphia, PA: WB Saunders, 1757–813.

Gorlin RJ, Cohen MM, Levin LS (1990) *Syndromes of the head and neck*. 3rd edition. New York: Oxford University Press.

Gorlin RJ, Jue KL, Jacobsen U, Goldschmidt E (1963) Oculoauriculovertebral dysplasia. *J Pediatr* **63**: 991–9.

Gregory MC, Atkin CL (1997) Alport's syndrome, Fabry's disease and nail-patella syndrome. In: Schrier RW, Gottschalk CW (eds) *Diseases of the kidney*. 6th edition. Boston, MA: Little, Brown & Co., 561–90.

Greskovich FJ, Nyberg L (1988) The prune belly syndrome: a review of its etiology, defects, treatment and prognosis. *J Urol* **140**: 707–12.

Grundy P, Coppes MJ, Haber D (1995) Molecular genetics of Wilms tumor. *Hematol Oncol Clin North Am* **9**: 1201–15.

Gunay Aygun M, Cassidy SB, Nicholls RD (1997) Prader–Willi and other syndromes associated with obesity and mental retardation. *Behav Genet* **27**: 307–24.

Hall BD (1979) Choanal atresia and associated multiple anomalies. *J Pediatr* **95**: 395–8.

Hanlon-Lundberg KM, Verp MS, Loy G (1994) Posterior urethral valves in successive generations. *Am J Perinatol* **11**: 37–9.

Hanson FW, Zorn EM, Tennant FR (1987) Amniocentesis before 15 weeks gestation. Outcomes, risks and technical problems. *Am J Obstet Gynecol* **156**: 1524–131.

Harris EL (1990) Genetic epidemiology of hypospadias. *Epidemiol Rev* **12**: 29–40.

Hawkins CF, Smith OE (1950) Renal dysplasia in a family with multiple hereditary abnormalities including iliac horns. *Lancet* **1**: 803–8.

Holmes LB (1976) The malformed newborn: practical perspectives (unpubl).

Hook EJ, Lindsje A (1978) Down syndrome in live births by single year maternal age interval in Swedish study: comparison with results from a New York State study. *Am J Hum Genet* **30**: 19–27.

Hutton KAR, Thomas FFM, Arthur RJ *et al.* (1994) Prenatally detected posterior urethral valves: is gestational age at detection a predictor of outcome? *J Urol* **152**: 698–701.

Ishitoya S, Arai Yoichi, Waki K *et al.* (1997) Left retrocaval ureter associated with the Goldenhar syndrome (branchial arch syndrome). *J Urol* **158**: 572.

Jackson LG, Wapne RJ, Brambati B (1991) Limb abnormalities and chorionic villae sampling. *Lancet* **337**: 1422–4.

Jackson LG, Zachary ZM, Fowler SS (1992) Randomized comparison of transcervical and transabdominal chorionic villae sampling. *N Engl J Med* **327**: 594–8.

Jacobson Z, Glickstein J, Hensle T, Marion RW (1998) Further delineation of the Opitz G/BBB syndrome: report of an infant with complex congenital heart disease and bladder exstrophy, and review of the literature. *Am J Med Genet* **78**: 294–9.

Jain M, LeQuesne GW, Bourne AJ, Henning P (1997) High-resolution ultrasonography in the differential diagnosis of cystic diseases of the kidney in infancy and childhood: preliminary experience. *J Ultrasound Med* **16**: 235–40.

Jiang YH, Tsai TF, Bressler J, Beaudet AL (1998) Imprinting in Angelman and Prader–Willi syndromes. *Curr Opin Genet Dev* **8**: 334–42.

Jones KL (1988) *Smith's recognizable patterns of human malformation*. 4th edition. Philadelphia, PA: WB Saunders.

Jones KL, Smith DW (1997) *Smith's recognizable patterns of human malformation* 5th edition. Philadelphia, PA: WB Saunders.

Kashtan CE, Gubler MC, Sisson-Ross S, Mauer M (1998) Chronology of renal scarring in males with Alport syndrome. *Pediatr Nephrol* **12**: 269–74.

Kashtan CE, Michael AF (1993) Alport syndrome: from bedside to genome to bedside. *Am J Kidney Dis* **22**: 627–40.

Kaufman RL (1973) Birth defects and oral contraceptives. *Lancet* **i**: 1396.

Kelley RL, Roessster E, Hennekam RC *et al.* (1996) Holoprosencephaly in RSH/Smith–Lemli–Opitz syndrome: does abnormal cholesterol metabolism affect the function of sonic hedgehog. *Am J Med Genet* **66**: 478–84.

Khoury MJ, Cordero JF, Greenberg F *et al.* (1983) A population study of the VACTERL association: evidence for its etiologic heterogeneity. *Pediatrics* **71**: 815–20.

Khuri FJ, Hardy BE, Churchill BM (1981) Urologic anomalies associated with hypospadias. *Urol Clin North Am* **8**: 565–71.

Kumar A, Friedman JM, Taylor GP, Patterson MWH (1993) Pattern of cardiac malformation in oculoauriculovertebral spectrum. *Am J Med Genet* **46**: 423–6.

Lavin CW, McKeown CA (1993) The oculocerebrorenal syndrome of Lowe. *Int Ophthal Clin* **33**: 179–91.

Leonard CO, Chase GA, Childs B (1972) Genetic counseling: a consumer's view. *N Engl J Med* **287**: 433–9.

Lessick ML, VanPutte AW, Rowley PT (1981) Assessment of evaluation of hospitalized pediatric patients with genetic disorders. *Clin Pediatr* **20**:178–83.

Lester AM (1936) Familial dyschondroplasia associated with anonychia and other deformities. *Lancet* **ii**: 1519.

Li M, Squire, JA, Weksberg R (1997) Molecular genetics of Beckwith–Wiedermann syndrome. *Curr Opin Pediatr* **9**: 623–9.

Lin T, Lewis RA, Nussbaum RL (1999) Molecular confirmation of carriers for Lowe syndrome. *Opthalmology* **106**: 119–22.

Little EM (1987) Congenital absence or delayed development of the patella. *Lancet* **2**: 781–4.

Litvak AS, Rousseau TG, Wrede LD *et al.* (1978) The association of significant renal anomalies with Turner's syndrome. *J Urol* **120**: 671–2.

Livne PM, Delaune J, Gonzales ET (1983) Genetic etiology of posterior urethral valves. *J Urol* **130**: 781–4.

Lomas FE, Dahlstrom JE, Ford JH (1998) VACTERL with hydrocephalus: family with X-linked VACTERL-H. *Am J Med Genet* **76**: 74–8.

Looji BJ, TeSlaa RL, Hogewind BL, van de Kamp JJP (1988) Genetic counseling in the hereditary osteo-onychodysplasia (HOOD, nail-patella syndrome) with nephropathy. *J Med Genet* **25**: 682–6.

Lurie IW, Cherstvoy ED (1984) Renal agenesis as a diagnostic feature of the cryptopthalmos-syndactyly syndrome. *Clin Genet* **25**: 528–32.

Lynch L, Berkowitz RL (1992) Amniocentesis, skin biopsy and umbilical cord blood sampling in the prenatal diagnosis of genetic disorders. In: Reece EA, Hobbins JG, Mahoney MJ (eds) *Medicine of the fetus and mother*. Philadelphia, PA: JB Lippincott, 641–52.

Main DM, Mennuti MT (1986) Neural tube defects: issues in prenatal diagnosis and counseling. *Obstet Gynecol* **67**: 1–16.

Mandell J, Blyth BR, Peters CA *et al.* (1991) Structural genitourinary defects detected *in utero*. *Radiology* **178**: 193–6.

Mark HFL (1994) Fluorescent *in situ* hybridization as an adjunct to conventional cytogenetics. *Ann Clin Lab Sci* **24**: 153–63.

Marshall VF, Mueke EC (1962) Variations of exstrophy of the bladder. *J Urol* **88**: 766.

McKusick VA (1994) *Mendelian inheritance in man: catalogue of autosomal dominant, autosomal recessive and X-linked phenotypes*. 9th edition. Baltimore, MD: Johns Hopkins University Press.

Melnick M, Bixler D, Silk K *et al.* (1975) Autosomal dominant branchiotorenal dysplasia. *For the National Foundation – March of DIMES*. BD: OAS XI, **5**: 1212–28.

Meschede D, Rolf C, Neugebauer D *et al.* (1996) Sperm acrosome defects in a patient with Aarskog–Scott syndrome. *Am J Med Genet* **66**: 340–2.

Messelink EJ, Aronson DC, Knuist M *et al.* (1994) Four cases of bladder exstrophy in two families. *J Med Genet* **31**: 490–2.

Metlay LA, Smythe PS, Miller ME (1987) Familial CHARGE syndrome: clinical report with autopsy findings. *Am J Med Genet* **26**: 577–81.

Miller EI, Dorsey TJ, Moran ET, Rowen M (1968) Hereditary osteo-onycho-dysplasia — the nail patella syndrome. *Calif Med* **108**: 377–80.

Miller TT, Shapiro MA, Schultz E *et al.* (1998) Sonography of patellar abnormalities in children. *AJR* **171**: 739–42.

Milliner DS, Pierides AM, Holley KE (1982) Renal transplantation in Alport's syndrome. Anti-glomerular basement membrane glomerulonephritis in the allograft. *Mayo Clin Proc* **57**: 35–43.

Mills JL, Knopp RH, Simpson JL *et al.* (1988) Lack of relation of increased malformation rates in infants of diabetic mothers to glycemic control during organogenesis. *N Engl J Med* **318**: 671–6.

Misra M, Nolph K (1998) Renal failure and deafness: branchio-oto-renal syndrome. *Am J Kidney Dis* **32**: 334–7.

Mitchell JA, Giangiacomo J, Hefner MA *et al.* (1985) Dominant CHARGE association. *Opthal Pediatr Genet* **6**: 31.

Morita T, Laughlin LO, Kawano K *et al.* (1973) Nail-patella syndrome. Light and electron microscopic studies of the kidney. *Arch Intern Med* **31**: 271–7.

Mueller RF (1994) The Denys–Drash syndrome. *J Med Genet* **31**: 471–7.

NICD National Registry for Amniocentesis Study Group (1976) Midtrimester amniocentesis for prenatal diagnosis; safety and accuracy. *JAMA* **236**: 1471–6.

Nicolaides KH, Rodeck GH, Gosden CM (1986) Rapid karyotyping in nonlethal fetal malformations. *Lancet* **i**: 283–7.

Noe HN, Wyatt RJ, Peeden JN, Rivas ML (1992) The transmission of vesicoureteral reflux from parent to child. *J Urol* **148**: 1869–71.

Nollau P, Wagener C (1997) Methods for detection of point mutations: performance and quality assessment. *Clin Chem* **43**: 1114–28.

Nora AH, Nora JJ (1975) A syndrome of multiple congenital anomalies associated with teratogenic exposure. *Arch Environ Health* **30**: 17–22.

Nora JJ, Nora AH, Sinha AK *et al.* (1974) The Ullrich–Noonan syndrome (Turner phenotype). *Am J Dis Child* **127**: 48–55.

Opitz JM (1987) G syndrome (hypertelorism with esophageal abnormality and hypospadias, or hypospadias–dysphagia, or 'Opitz–Frias' or 'Opitz G' syndrome) — perspective in 1987 and bibliography. *Am J Med Genet* **28**: 275–85.

Opitz JM, Summitt RL, Smith DW (1969a) The BBB syndrome: familial telecanthus with associated congenital anomalies. *Birth Defects* **V(2)**: 86–94.

Opitz JM, Frias JL, Gutenberger JE, Pellet JR (1969b) The G syndrome of multiple congenital anomalies. *Birth Defects* **V(2)**: 95–101.

Ormond KE (1997) Update and review: maternal serum screening. *J Genet Counsel* **6**: 395–417.

Pagon RA, Graham JM, Zonana J, Yong S (1981) Coloboma, congenital heart disease and choanal atresia with multiple anomalies: CHARGE association. *J Pediatr* **99**: 223–7.

Palomaki GE, Hill LE, Knight GJ *et al.* (1988) Second trimester maternal alpha-fetoprotein levels in pregnancies associated with gastroschisis and omphalocele. *Obstet Gynecol* **71**: 906–9.

Pardo-Mindan FJ, Vargas TF, Garcia JG, Virto RMT (1975) Familial cryptorchidism. *Pediatrics* **56**: 616.

Perrin D, Junger P, Grunfeld JG *et al.* (1980) Perimacular changes in Alport syndrome. *Clin Nephrol* **13**: 163–7.

Quan L, Smith DW (1973) The VATER association. *J Pediatr* **82**: 104–7.

Rabinowitz R, Schillinger JF (1977) Prune belly syndrome in the female patient subject. *J Urol* **118**: 454–6.

Ragan DC, Casale AJ, Rink R *et al.* (1999) Genitourinary anomalies in the CHARGE Association. *J Urol* **161**: 622–5.

Rajab A, Freeman NV, Patton M (1996) The frequency of posterior urethral valves in Oman. *Br J Urol* **77**: 900–4.

Reddy PR, Mandell J (1998) Prenatal diagnosis: therapeutic implications. *Urol Clin North Am* **25**: 171–80.

Reece EA (1997) Early and midtrimester genetic amniocentesis. *Obstet Gynecol Clin North Am* **24**: 71–81.

Rhoads GE, Jackson LG, Schlesselman SE (1989) The safety and efficacy of chorionic villae sampling for early prenatal diagnosis of cytogenetics abnormalities. *N Engl J Med* **320**: 609–17.

Riccardi VM, Sujansky E, Smith AC *et al.* (1978) Chromosomal imbalance in the aniridia Wilms' tumor association: 11p interstitial deletion. *Pediatrics* **61**: 604–16.

Ritchey ML, Norbeck J, Huang C *et al.* (1994) Urologic manifestations of Goldenhar syndrome. *Urology* **43**: 88–91.

Robin NH, Opitz JM, Muenke M (1996) Opitz G/BBB syndrome: clinical comparisons of families linked to Xp22 and 22q, and a review of the literature. *Am J Med Genet* **62**: 305–17.

Robinow M, Silverman FN, Smith HO (1969) A newly recognized dwarfing syndrome. *Am J Dis Child* **117**: 645–51.

Rohlfs E, Highsmith WE Jr (1997) PCR-based methods for mutation detection. In: Coleman WB, Tsongalis GJ (eds) *Molecular diagnostic: for clinical laboratorian. Pathology and Laboratory Medicine*. Volume 1. New Jersey: Humana Press.

Roy S, Dillon MJ, Trompeter RS, Barratt TM (1997) Autosomal recessive polycystic kidney disease: long-term outcome of neonatal survivors. *Pediatr Nephrol* **11**: 302–6.

Rudin C, Pritchard J, Fernando ON *et al.* (1998) Renal transplantation in the management of bilateral Wilms' tumor (BWT) and of Denys–Drash syndrome (DDS). *Nephrol Dial Transplant* **13**: 1506–10.

Ryan AK, Bartlett K, Clayton P *et al.* (1998) Opitz syndrome: a variable clinical and biochemical phenotype. *J Med Genet* **35**: 558–65.

Saborio P, Scheinman J (1998) Genetic renal disease. *Curr Opin Pediatr* **10**: 174–83.

Saenger P (1996) Turner's syndrome. *N Engl J Med* **335**: 1749–54.

Sarmon G, Speer M, Rudolph AJ (1995) Fraser syndrome (cryptopthalmos [hidden eye]-syndactyly syndrome). *J Perinatol* **15**: 503–6.

Savion M, Nissenkorn I, Servadio C, Dickerman Z (1984) Familial occurrence of undescended testes. *Urology* **23**: 355–8.

Schaefer GB, Olney AH, Kolodziej P (1998) Oculo–auricular–vertebral spectrum. *ENT* **77**: 17–18.

Schauer GM, Dunn LK, Godmilow L *et al.* (1990) Prenatal diagnosis of Fraser syndrome at 18.5 weeks gestation, with autopsy findings at 19 weeks. *Am J Med Genet* **37**: 583–91.

Schleutermann DA, Bias WB, Murdoch JL, McKusizk VA (1969) Linkage of the loci for the nail-patella syndrome and adenylate kinase. *Am J Hum Genet* **21**: 606–13.

Schmeider G, Freitag DS (1988) The nail-patella syndrome. *Am Fam Physician* **38**: 193–4.

Scorer CG (1964) The descent of the testis. *Arch Dis Child* **39**: 605–9.

Sedano HO, Gorlin RJ (1988) Opitz oculo-genital-laryngeal syndrome (Opitz BBB/G compound syndrome). *Am J Med Genet* **30**: 847–19.

Sepulveda W, Sebire NJ, Souka A *et al.* (1997) Diagnosis of the Meckel–Gruber syndrome at eleven to fourteen weeks gestation. *Am J Obstet Gynecol* **176**: 316–19.

Shapiro E, Lepor H, Jeffs RD (1984) The inheritance of classical bladder exstrophy. *J Urol* **132**: 308–10.

Shimizu T, Ihara Y, Yomura W *et al.* (1992) Antenatal diagnosis of prune belly syndrome. *Arch Gynecol Obstet* **251**: 211–14.

Smeets HJ, Knoers VV, Van de Heuvel LP *et al.* (1996) Hereditary disorders of the glomerular basement membrane. *Pediatr Nephrol* **10**: 779–88.

Smith DW (1966) Dysmorphology (teratology). *J Pediatr* **69**: 1150–169.

Smith EP, Wacksman J (1997) Evaluation of severe hypospadias. *J Pediatr* **131**: 344–6.

Stevenson RJ, May M, Arena JF *et al.* (1994) Aarskog–Scott syndrome: confirmation of linkage to the pericentromeric region of the X chromosome. *Am J Med Genet* **52**: 339–45.

Stoler JM, Herrin JT, Holmes LB (1995) Genital abnormalities in females with Bardet–Biedl syndrome. *Am J Med Genet* **55**: 276–8.

Stoll C, Viville B, Treisser A, Gasser B (1998) A family with dominant oculovertebral spectrum. *Am J Med Genet* **78**: 345–9.

Strachan T, Read AP (1996) *Human molecular genetics*. New York: Bios Scientific Publishers Wiley-Liss.

Sutherland RS, Mevorach RA, Kogan BA (1995) The prune belly syndrome: current insights. *Pediatr Nephrol* **9**: 770–8.

Targum SD (1982) Psychotherapeutic considerations in genetic counseling. *Am J Med Genet* **8**: 281–9.

Teebi AS (1990) Autosomal recessive Robinow syndrome. *Am J Med Genet* **35**: 64–8.

Teebi AS, Rucquoi JK, Meyn MS (1993) Aarskog syndrome: report of a family with review and discussion of nosology. *Am J Med Genet* **46**: 501–9.

Thomalla JV, Mitchell ME, Garett RA (1989) Posterior urethral valves in siblings. *Urology* **33**: 291–4.

Thomas IT, Frias JL, Felix V *et al.* (1986) Isolated and syndromic cryptopthalmos. *Am J Med Genet* **25**: 85–98.

Turleau C, de Grouchy J, Dufier JL *et al.* (1981) Aniridia, male pseudo-hermaphroditism, gonadoblastoma, mental retardation, and del11p13. *Hum Genet* **57**: 300–6.

Vincent C, Kalatzis V, Abdelhak S *et al.* (1997) BOR and BO syndromes are allelic defects of EYA1. *Eur J Hum Genet* **5**: 242–6.

Vogel F, Motulsky AG (1986) Human chromosomes; dosage compensation for mammalian X chromosome. In: *Human genetics: problems and approaches*, 2nd edition. Berlin: Springer.

Wald NJ, Cuckle HS (1977) Maternal serum AFP measurement in antenatal screening for anencephaly and spina bifida in early pregnancy: report of UK collaborative study on alpha-fetoprotein in relation to neural tube defects. *Lancet* **ii**: 1323–32.

Wang H, Hunter AGW, Clifford B *et al.* (1993) VACTERL with hydrocephalus: spontaneous chromosome breakage and rearrangement in a family showing apparent sex-linked recessive inheritance. *Am J Med Genet* **47**: 114–17.

Wapner RJ (1997) Chorionic villae sampling. *Obstet Gynecol Clin North Am* **24**: 83–110.

Warkany J (1971) Teratology of the past. In: Warkany J (ed.) *Congenital malformations: notes and comment*. Chicago, FL: Year Book Medical Publishers.

Wassif CA, Maslen C, Kachelili-Linjewile S *et al.* (1998) Mutations in human sterol delta 7–reductase gene at 11q12–13 cause Smith–Lemli–Opitz syndrome. *Am J Hum Genet* **63**: 55–62.

Weidner IS, Moller H, Jensen TK, Skakkebaek NE (1999) Risk factors for cryptorchidism and hypospadias. *J Urol* **161**: 1606–9.

Weins L, Strickland DK, Sniffen B, Warady BA (1990) Robinow syndrome: report of two patients with cystic kidney disease. *Clin Genet* **37**: 481–4.

Wellesley DG, Slaney SF (1995) MURCS in a male. *J Med Genet* **32**: 314–15.

Wilcox DT, Quinn FMJ, Ng CS *et al.* (1997) Redefining the genital abnormality in the robinow syndrome. *J Urol* **157**: 2312–14.

Williamson RA, Weiner CP, Patil S (1987) Abnormal pregnancy sonogram: selective indication for fetal karyotype. *Obstet Gynecol* **59**: 15–20.

Willner JP (1998) Reproductive genetics and today's patient options: prenatal diagnosis. *Mount Sinai J Med* **65**: 173–7.

Wolfe KQ, Herrington CS (1997) Interphase cytogenetics and pathology: a tool for diagnosis and research. *J Pathol* **181**: 359–61.

Yoon PW, Olney RS, Khoury MJ *et al.* (1997) Contribution of birth defects and genetic diseases to pediatric hospitalizations. A population-based study. *Arch Pediatr Adolesc Med* **151**: 1096–103.

Zaontz MR, Packer MG (1997) Abnormalities of the external genitalia. *Pediatr Clin North Am* **44**: 1267–97.

Zelante L, Gasparini P, Scanderbag AC *et al.* (1997) Goldenhar complex: a further case with uncommon associated anomalies. *Am J Med Genet* **69**: 418–21.

Zerres K, Mucher G, Bachner L *et al.* (1994) Mapping of the gene for autosomal recessive polycystic kidney disease (ARPKD) to chromosome 6p21–cen. *Nature Genet* **7**: 429–32.

Zerres K, Mucher G, Becker J *et al.* (1998a) Prenatal diagnosis of autosomal recessive polycystic kidney disease (ARPKD): molecular genetics, clinical experience, and fetal morphology. *Am J Med Genet* **76**: 137–44.

Zerres K, Rudnik-Schoneborn S, Deget F *et al.* (1996) Clinical course of 115 children with autosomal recessive polycystic kidney disease. *Acta Paediatr* **85**: 437–45.

Zerres K, Rudnik-Schoneborn S, Steinkamm C *et al.* (1998b) Autosomal recessive polycystic kidney disease. *J Mol Med* **76**: 303–9.

Fetal urology and prenatal diagnosis

4

David F.M. Thomas

Introduction

Two decades have elapsed since the first reports on the ultrasonographic detection of fetal urinary tract anomalies began to appear in the literature. In the intervening years sonography has been widely adopted within routine obstetric practice throughout the developed world. The impact on pediatric urology has been profound, although it must be acknowledged that in some areas the clinical benefits to children and parents remain unproven. In one respect, however, prenatal diagnosis has been of unqualified benefit, by stimulating clinical and experimental research into the functional development of the urinary tract and pathophysiology of congenital uropathy. Advances in developmental biology are also shedding valuable new light on the genetic mechanisms regulating the embryologic development of the urogenital tract and on the molecular pathogenesis of genitourinary malformations.

Although this chapter is concerned primarily with the clinical aspects of prenatal diagnosis it will also consider the contribution being made by prenatal diagnosis to the scientific foundations of pediatric urology.

Functional development of the normal urinary tract

For a detailed account of the embryology of the genitourinary tract the reader is referred to Chapter 1. The pivotal event in functional development occurs at around 32 days when the ureteric bud fuses with the metanephric mesenchyme to initiate the formation of excretory nephrons. Without the inductive influence of the ureteric bud the metanephric mesenchyme is 'programmed' to regress by undergoing cellular apoptosis. Normal nephrogenesis proceeds by a process of reciprocal induction whereby the metanephros contributes the glomeruli, proximal tubules, and loops of Henle to the embryonic kidney, whereas the collecting ducts, calyces, and renal pelvis arise by serial branching of the ureteric bud. Branching of the ureteric bud derivatives ceases between 15 and 20 weeks but nephrogenesis continues until around 36 weeks with the formation of an estimated 11 generations of new glomeruli. Thereafter, the total number of nephrons remains fixed at approximately 0.7–1 million per kidney.

Fetal urine production and renal function

Urine production by the primitive nephrons commences at around the 9th week of gestation. Initially, the composition of urine reflects its origin as an ultrafiltrate of plasma, but as gestation progresses and tubular function matures, fetal urine begins to acquire the low-electrolyte, high-creatinine composition that characterizes normal urine in postnatal life (Glick *et al.*, 1985).

Fetal urinary flow rate at different stages in gestation has been studied by ultrasonography of the fetal bladder in healthy fetuses (Rabinowitz *et al.*, 1989) (Fig. 4.1). In the third trimester, hourly fetal urine production is as high as 30–40 ml/h and fetal urine comprises up to 90% of amniotic fluid volume. The role of the fetal kidney lies principally in fluid excretion, whereas homeostatic regulation of extracellular fluid composition is undertaken by the placenta. Thus, the plasma concentrations of electrolytes, urea, and creatinine of an anephric infant surviving to term mirror those in the maternal circulation. For this reason creatinine clearance is not a meaningful measure of fetal renal function. However, extrapolation of values derived from iothalamate clearance studies in the fetal lamb suggests that at 36 weeks of

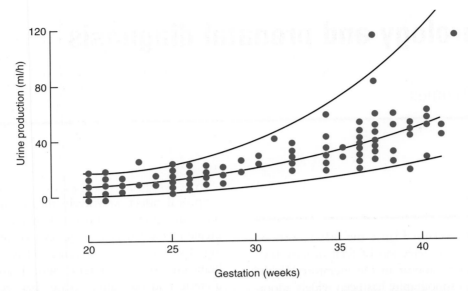

Figure 4.1 Fetal production at difference stages in normal pregnancy (Adapted from Rabinowitz *et al.*, 1989).

gestation the fetal glomular filtration rate (GFR) probably approximates 5% of the surface-corrected adult value (Haycock, 1998).

The kidney lung loop

Amniotic fluid, of which fetal urine is the major constituent, has long been known to fulfill a key role in lung development. Oligohydramnios is associated with varying degrees of pulmonary hypoplasia depending on the timing and severity of the impairment of fetal urinary output and the consequent reduction in amniotic fluid volume. The contribution of amniotic fluid to lung development extends beyond simple mechanical stenting of the airways (DeMello and Reid, 1997). Proline of renal origin has been shown to contribute to collagen formation in the fetal lung, and other renal-derived growth factors are almost certainly involved at different stages of lung development. The intriguing observation that renal mass is increased in infants with lethal congenital diaphragmatic hernias points to the existence of a reciprocal lung–kidney loop, possibly mediated by lung-derived growth factors such as hepatocyte growth factor (HGF) (Yanagita *et al.*, 1992).

Changes at the time of birth

In the latter stages of pregnancy the fetus is in a physiological state of volume expansion. A high fluid intake maintained by swallowing of amniotic fluid is matched by a high obligatory urine output. In effect, the fetus is recycling water and electrolytes. If a comparable level of diuresis were maintained after birth, dehydration and volume depletion would rapidly ensue; however, at the time of birth renal physiology rapidly switches to a fluid restrictive pattern prompted, in part, by high circulating levels of aldosterone, vasopressin, and catecholamines. More importantly, parenchymal perfusion and GFR increase dramatically in response to a fall in peripheral renovascular resistance and dramatically increased renal blood flow. While these physiological mechanisms equip the fetus to survive the transition to postnatal life renal function nevertheless remains relatively marginal, with a corrected GFR at birth averaging only 30 ml/min per 1.73 m². The normal surface-corrected value of approximately 127 ml/min per 1.73 m² is not achieved until 5 years of age (Brocklebank, 1997).

Pathophysiology of fetal uropathy

Failed induction of nephrogenesis

The pivotal role of the ureteric bud has been considered briefly above. Experimental ablation of the mesonephric ducts (the origin of the ureteric bud) has been shown to result in failure of metanephric development. A comparable etiology can be invoked in girls in whom unilateral agenesis of the paramesonephric duct derivative is associated with ipsilateral renal agenesis. At a molecular level, ablation of the *HOXa*, *PAX2*, and *WT1* genes in null mutant mice results in failed induction of the renal mesenchyme and consequent renal agenesis (Woolf, 1998).

Obstructive uropathy

Upper tract

Beck's early experimental studies in the fetal lamb (which have subsequently been reproduced by others) demonstrated that complete ureteric obstruction results in differing patterns of congenital damage depending on the timing of the obstructive insult (Beck, 1971). In these experiments unilateral ureteric ligation in the first half of gestation resulted in the morphological and some of the histological characteristics of renal dysplasia but in later gestation the same obstructive insult resulted in a hydronephrotic but otherwise recognizable kidney.

At a cellular level even brief periods of obstruction during nephrogenesis have been shown to induce apoptosis, aberrations of cell proliferation, and trans-differentiation of mesenchyme into smooth muscle phenotype, a characteristic histological feature of renal dysplasia. Mechanisms of obstructive injury in later gestation are also being studied at a molecular level. For example, Peters and associates have recently documented important alterations in gene expression of critical components of the renal renin–angiotensin system in the obstructed fetal lamb model (Gobet *et al.*, 1999b).

Partial upper tract obstruction of the type more commonly encountered in clinical practice is difficult to reproduce in experimental models such as the fetal lamb. In an attempt to overcome this problem incomplete obstruction has been reproduced in neonatal animals of species such as rats and guinea-pigs in which nephrogenesis continues after birth (corresponding to the second half of gestation in humans). In these experimental models renal blood flow and glomerular perfusion are reduced and histologic changes of progressive glomerular sclerosis, tubular atrophy, and fibrosis ensue (Nguyen and Kogan, 1998).

Lower urinary tract: bladder outlet obstruction

Models of partial and complete infravesical obstruction have been studied extensively by Harrison and his colleagues in San Francisco. In one such published study experimental obstruction was induced by positioning an ameroid constrictor around the urethra and ligating the urachus in fetal lambs at 93–107 days' gestation (Harrison *et al.*, 1982b). Fetal lambs which did not undergo any further intervention developed hydronephrosis, urinary ascites, and fatal pulmonary hypoplasia. However, in those lambs in which the obstructed bladder was subsequently decompressed *in utero* by cutaneous cystostomy at a median of 120 days, significant resolution of urinary tract dilatation occurred. Following delivery at 136–146 days the majority of lambs in the treated group survived and lung weights were higher than in the untreated group.

The detailed experimental studies conducted by the San Francisco group in the early to mid-1980s provided the scientific rationale for introducing intrauterine drainage procedures into clinical practice. Unfortunately, conclusions derived from animal studies have not translated into clinical practice. Experience with fetal intervention coupled with the evidence of second trimester ultrasonography and fetal autopsy findings has raised serious doubts about the validity of extrapolating the results obtained in the fetal lamb studies to the pathogenesis and timescale of renal dysplasia in humans. The current status of fetal intervention is considered in more detail below.

Vesicoureteric reflux

Severe renal functional impairment of the type encountered predominantly in conjunction with grade V reflux is best explained by the ureteric bud hypothesis of Mackie and Stephens (1996). In contrast; kidneys that have been exposed to mild or moderate reflux *in utero* either appear normal on dimercaptosuccinic acid (DMSA) or demonstrate symmetrical global reduction in size. Focal scarring appears to be a feature of postnatal infection (Crabbe *et al.*, 1992; Elder, 1998).

While the mechanical 'water hammer' effect of sterile reflux is not thought to be implicated in the etiology of renal damage (reflux nephropathy) in postnatal life, very little is known of the impact of sterile reflux on the developing fetal kidney. Similarly, we have very little insight into normal and abnormal voiding dynamics in the fetus. The relationship between fetal reflux and renal development is now being studied in models of experimentally induced vesicoureteric reflux (VUR) in the fetal lamb. Studies undertaken jointly at the Children's Hospitals of Zurich and Boston have revealed significant changes in tubular function and DMSA appearances in kidneys exposed to reflux created experimentally at 95 days' gestation.

Prenatal diagnosis: clinical considerations

In the UK, as in other countries with universal access to national healthcare systems, virtually ever mother is routinely scanned at least once in pregnancy. Seventeen to 20 weeks of gestation have been favored by UK obstetricians as the optimum time for the routine 'fetal anomaly' scan. More recently, ultrasonographic assessment of nuchal pad thickness at around 10 weeks has also been introduced in some centers to facilitate the early diagnosis of Down syndrome. Certain gross central nervous system (CNS) malformations such as anenecephaly can also be identified at this early stage in gestation, but major renal and cardiac anomalies cannot be detected with an acceptable level of sensitivity at 10 weeks. For this reason, the 10-week 'nuchal pad thickness' scan is unlikely to replace the second trimester fetal anomaly scan as the mainstay of fetal anomaly screening. Ultrasonographic evaluation of urinary tract anomalies should routinely include an assessment of amniotic fluid volume and a systematic search for coexisting anomalies in other systems.

Limitations of prenatal ultrasonography

Technical factors

The diagnostic sensitivity and specificity of ultrasonography is subject to certain limitations, which include:

- image resolution of the equipment used;
- experience of the sonographer or radiologist performing and/or interpreting the study;
- maternal size and obesity.

It is evident from the above that uropathies that might otherwise have been detected may be missed because of faulty or outdated equipment, operator error, or maternal obesity. Most renal anomalies are detected by virtue of dilatation, but anomalies such as renal ectopia that are not accompanied by dilatation are more readily missed. Similarly, unilateral renal agenesis may be particularly difficult to diagnose on second trimester scanning.

Natural history of uropathy

Even potentially serious anomalies, such as posterior urethral valves, with embryological origins presumed to date from the first trimester, do not necessarily give rise to detectable dilatation at 17–19 weeks. Similarly, 20% of prenatally detected multicystic dysplastic kidneys are not apparent on sonography before 24 weeks (Liebeschuetz, 1997). In the majority of cases of pelviureteric junction obstruction and VUR the urinary tract appears normal in the second trimester and dilatation only develops later in the pregnancy. Failure to appreciate the natural history of fetal uropathy and the timescale of dilatation may prompt misguided accusations of negligence for missed diagnosis.

Rationale for prenatal sonographic diagnosis

It is important to recognize that prenatal urological diagnosis has emerged as a 'by product' of obstetric practice rather than a goal specifically sought by urologists. Routine second trimester sonography for fetal anomalies constitutes a formal systematic screening program of the general, low-risk fetal population, whereas additional studies at different gestational ages represent *ad hoc* forms of screening which reflect local obstetric policy and the practice of individual obstetricians.

Abnormalities of the fetal urinary tract revealed by ultrasonography span a very broad pathological spectrum and are best considered according to severity. They include lethal uropathy, severe non-lethal uropathy resulting in early-onset renal failure, non-lethal uropathy with a low risk of renal failure, and mild dilatation.

Lethal uropathy

In a 3-year prospective study covering approximately 175 000 pregnancies in the Yorkshire Region of the UK (Brand et al., 1994), 2261 anomalies were detected, of which 369 (16%) resulted in termination of pregnancy. Autopsy was performed in 97% of aborted fetuses. Urinary tract malformations accounted for 35 terminations (approximately 10% of the total), of which renal agenesis and multicystic dysplasia, individually or in combination, accounted for 63%. Severe infravesical obstruction in male fetuses (urethral atresia or urethral valves) constituted the other main

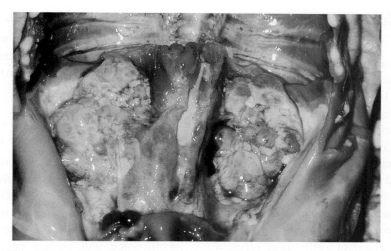

Figure 4.2 Bilateral multicystic renal dysplasia: autopsy findings following termination of pregnancy.

group of lethal uropathies. These and similar findings mirror those of previous autopsy studies which documented the importance of bilateral renal agenesis as a cause of stillbirth or neonatal death of renal origin.

Some lethal renal malformations have an inherited basis. Bilateral renal agenesis has a quoted empirical recurrence risk of 3.5% for further pregnancies (Carter and Pescia, 1979), and other urinary tract malformations have been identified in 7.4% of parents of children with bilateral renal agenesis (Roodhoft *et al.*, 1984). Bilateral multicystic dysplastic kidney occurs in approximately 1 in 20 000 pregnancies but possible patterns of inheritance have yet to be systematically studied (Fig. 4.2).

Non-lethal uropathy: early onset of renal failure

Posterior urethral valves (PUV) (Figs. 4.3, 4.4) account for only 10% of significant prenatally detected uropathies in liveborn infants (Peters, 1998), yet generate the greatest burden of serious renal morbidity in infancy and early childhood. The scale of this morbidity is evident from the observation that males account for 90% of children in renal failure in the first 4 years of life (Minoja *et al.*, 1995). North American Transplant Registry data, derived from 3223 children over a 6-year period, identified obstructive uropathy (predominantly PUV) and dysplasia as the indication for 69% of transplants in children under 1 year of age and 66% of those aged 2–5 years (Arner *et al.*, 1995).

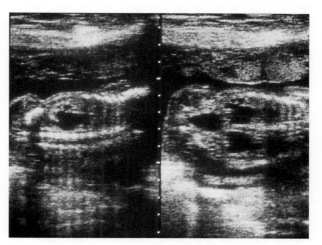

Figure 4.3 Posterior urethral valves: the fetal spine and thoracic cage are clearly visualized. Bilateral hydronephrosis and bladder distension can be seen.

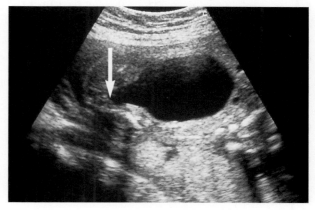

Figure 4.4 'Keyhole' sign. Dilatation of fetal bladder accompanied by distinctive dilatation of posterior urethra (*arrow*) and posterior urethral valves.

Sonographic predictors of functional outcome

Dineen and associates at Great Ormond Street Hospital reported that dilatation had only been apparent in 3 out of 19 boys (16%) with prenatally detected posterior urethral valves who had sonograms before the 24th week of gestation (Dineen *et al.*, 1992). The present author's experience was somewhat different: in 31 boys with prenatally detected posterior urethral valves, 17 (55%) had dilatation before 24 weeks, whereas in 14 boys (45%) the urinary tract had appeared normal in the second trimester and dilatation only became apparent later in the pregnancy (Hutton *et al.*, 1994). The data furthermore revealed a statistically significant correlation between the onset of dilatation and functional outcome. When dilatation had been evident on sonography before 24 weeks, 24% of infants subsequently died from pulmonary and/or renal failure and a further 35% developed significant renal impairment. In contrast, all infants with posterior urethral valves whose second trimester scans had been normal and in whom dilatation only became apparent later in the pregnancy survived and 93% had normal renal function at the time of follow-up. Assessment of qualitative parameters of the second trimester sonographic appearances enabled the poor prognosis group to be identified with even greater sensitivity (Hutton *et al.*, 1997).

Quinn *et al.* (1996) documented the prognosis of 26 male and two female fetuses with ultrasonic enlargement of the fetal bladder. Regardless of underlying etiology, the sonographic finding of an enlarged fetal bladder before 28 weeks of gestation predicted unfavorable functional outcome for those fetuses surviving to term. The value of fetal bladder distension (particularly in conjunction with bladder wall thickening, oligohydramnios, and increased renal echogenicity) as a predictor of obstructive etiology and functional outcome has also been highlighted by Kaefer *et al.* (1997) in Boston.

In summary, sonographic criteria have now been defined which make it possible to identify with considerable accuracy those fetuses with obstructive uropathy at the greatest risk of pulmonary hypoplasia and renal dysplasia:

- male fetus;
- dilated bladder;
- hydroureteronephrosis;
- dilated posterior urethra (keyhole sign).

Predictors of poor functional prognosis include:

- dilatation present before 24 weeks' gestation;
- moderate/severe hydroureteronephrosis (renal pelvis AP diameter ≥ 10 mm);
- thick-walled bladder;
- oligohydramnios;
- sonographic evidence of renal dysplasia, i.e. echogenic cortex, microcystic renal changes.

On the basis of this information a number of options exist for parents and their medical advisers. Without intervention, spontaneous abortion or intrauterine death will ensue in some cases. Those liveborn infants who do not succumb to respiratory insufficiency will mostly progress to early-onset renal failure and the requirement for renal replacement therapy in the first few months or years of life.

Fetal intervention

Historical aspects

In the 1980s the concept of fetal intervention ('fetal surgery') was adopted enthusiastically, if uncritically, by obstetricians in many centers. Where results have been published they have been uniformly disappointing and the initial promise has been largely unfulfilled. Early results from the Fetal Surgery Registry in 1986 identified an overall mortality rate of 59% in a series of 73 cases (Manning *et al.*, 1986). In many instances, however, the underlying diagnosis and indications for intervention were unclear. Reviewing a further 57 published cases, Elder *et al.* (1987) noted a 45% incidence of significant procedure-related complications, including premature labor. By the close of the 1980s, enthusiasm for fetal intervention was already waning. Mandell *et al.* (1990) identified 24 related publications between 1982 and 1985 but only seven publications between 1985 and 1989, of which two were single case reports. Throughout the 1990s fetal intervention has been undertaken in fewer centers and on a largely unreported basis. However, the Detroit group have not only persisted with intervention but adopted a commendably rigorous approach to analysing and publishing their results (Freedman *et al.*, 1999). In the period 1987–1996, 34 fetuses were treated by vesicoamniotic shunting. Thirteen died either *in utero* or postnatally and 17 survived. Fourteen infants were reassessed after 2 years of age.

Six (43%) had normal renal function and eight (57%) had renal insufficiency, of whom five had already required renal transplantation.

Selection for fetal intervention

Once the futility of treating severely affected fetuses with irreversible renal dysplasia had been recognized, efforts were directed towards selecting those fetuses with deteriorating, but potentially recoverable, function. Criteria for selective intervention have been based on sonographic appearances coupled with information derived from serial measurement of fetal urinary markers, notably urinary electrolytes. From a retrospective analysis of 40 fetuses the San Francisco group concluded that values for urinary sodium of < 100 mEq/l, chloride < 90 mEq/l and osmolality < 210 osm/l served to identify fetuses with a better prognosis who were more likely to benefit from intervention (Crombleholme *et al.*, 1990).

Other urinary constituents have been investigated as potential prognostic indicators, of which β_2-microglobulin is perhaps the most promising. This low molecular weight protein does not cross the placental barrier but is filtered by the glomerulus and is normally reabsorbed in the proximal tubule. Tubular damage results in elevated concentrations of β_2-microglobulinin in fetal urine and amniotic fluid, whereas plasma levels are reduced. Conversely, in the presence of total fetal anuria, plasma levels are increased. Unfortunately, β_2-microglobulin and urinary calcium, which have also been studied in this context, are subject to similar limitations as urinary electrolytes. There are scatter and overlap of pathological and normal values, and lack of normal reference range data at different gestational ages. Selection for fetal intervention remains, at best, an inexact exercise.

Techniques of fetal intervention

Open fetal surgery

The first case, reported by Harrison *et al.* (1982a), was a fetus with urethral obstruction delivered via hysterotomy at 21 weeks and treated by bilateral cutaneous ureterostomies before being returned to the uterus. Despite technically successful upper tract decompression, death from pulmonary insufficiency supervened within hours of subsequent delivery at 35 weeks. Although the San Francisco group persisted with further cases managed by hysterotomy and open

fetal surgery, this approach was soon superseded by the advent of percutaneously inserted vesicoamniotic shunt catheters.

Vesicoamniotic shunting

Under sonographic guidance the fetal bladder is punctured with a trochar and cannula introduced via the maternal abdominal wall and a JJ or pigtail type vesicoamniotic catheter inserted into the fetal bladder. Modifications in catheter design have not entirely eliminated the problems of occlusion and catheter displacement, with the result that further, possibly repeated, shunt insertion may be required. Other procedure-related complications include chorioamnionitis, damage to adjacent anatomical structures, and premature labor (Bewley and Rodeck, 1997) (Fig. 4.5).

Fetoscopy

Minimally invasive fetal laparoendoscopic technology is now being developed in some centers with the aim of creating a vesicostomy under direct vision or directly treating the underlying urethral obstruction *in utero*. Using a semirigid fetal cystoscope 1.3 mm in diameter, introduced via a trochar and cannula, Agarwal *et al.* (1999) treated five fetuses with posterior urethral valves at a mean gestational age of 19

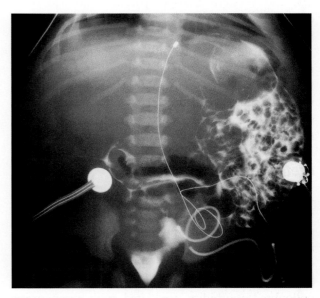

Figure 4.5 Complication of vesicoamniotic shunting. A postnatal contrast study reveals intraperitoneal placement of shunt with extravasation of contrast and urinary ascites. Despite shunting, this neonate succumbed to pulmonary hypoplasia.

weeks without fetal loss or maternal complications. It is too early to judge whether such techniques represent a genuine therapeutic advance or 'technology in search of an application'. In any event, the more fundamental problem of selection remains unresolved. Unless laparoendoscopic techniques can be safely extended into earlier gestation, i.e. before the onset of irreversible renal dysplasia, it seems unlikely that they will lead to an improved prognosis for renal function in affected infants.

Status of fetal intervention

Ransley (1996) has advocated a reappraisal of fetal intervention, arguing that our thinking has been unduly colored by poor outcomes in high-risk, poor prognosis cases. Perhaps the potential benefits of fetal intervention would only be fully realized by expanding the indications for intervention to encompass virtually every fetus with evidence of outflow obstruction. Unfortunately, Ransley's provocative hypothesis would prove difficult to test to an acceptable level of scientific credibility. Too many variables are involved, controls would be difficult to match to treated fetuses and the comparative results would take many years to assess in view of the protracted timescale of renal insufficiency in boys with PUV. At a practical level one could also anticipate that (in the UK and Western Europe) parents who had been counseled on the risks of renal failure would increasingly opt for termination.

The possible benefit from intervention in individual cases cannot be discounted but, paradoxically, fetal intervention may ultimately add to the burden of morbidity and renal failure by permitting survival of some infants who might otherwise have succumbed to lethal pulmonary hypoplasia.

Preterm delivery

Anecdotally, there is an impression that some infants with posterior urethral valves who have been born prematurely and treated promptly *ex utero* have experienced a better functional outcome than might otherwise have been anticipated. However, any perceived benefit for renal function must be offset against the undoubted morbidity associated with prematurity and the potential risks to the mother. At the present there seems insufficient evidence to justify elective preterm delivery. But when premature labor occurs spontaneously after 34 weeks, it would seem reason-

able to allow it to proceed providing there is evidence of adequate lung maturity.

Termination of pregnancy

Attitudes towards the termination of pregnancy for fetal anomalies vary in different countries, reflecting legal considerations and differing moral and religious climates. In most Western European countries, including those that espouse Roman Catholicism, termination of pregnancy for fetal anomalies is legal (subject to gestational age and obstetric criteria) and is widely practiced. The situation is somewhat different in the USA, where access to antenatal care (including second trimester sonography) is more limited in certain socioeconomic groups and where abortion is a more divisive political issue.

In the UK, termination is not confined to severe renal anomalies but is also undertaken for prenatally diagnosed cloacal and uncomplicated bladder exstrophy (Fig. 4.6). Many pediatric urologists view this with concern, pointing to the availability of newer reconstructive procedures and the achievements of some of their exstrophy patients. However, for the parents of a fetus with prenatally diagnosed exstrophy

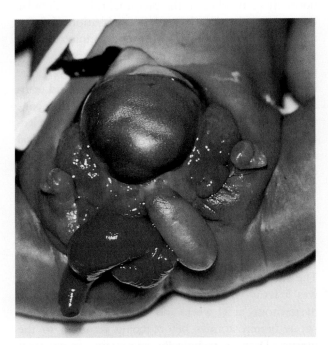

Figure 4.6 Cloacal exstrophy. Although cloacal and uncomplicated forms of bladder exstrophy are not generally associated with a significant risk of renal failure, prenatal diagnosis and possible termination of pregnancy raise serious ethical issues relating to quality of life.

these may prove unconvincing arguments when compared with the requirement for major surgery, entailing prolonged or repeated hospitalization and the prospect that continence may ultimately be dependent on lifelong self-catheterization. Pediatric urologists can play a valuable role in counseling parents to ensure that difficult decisions are made with the benefit of all the relevant information. At the Hospital for Sick Children in London four out of five sets of parents receiving expert pediatric urological counseling on exstrophy nevertheless opted to terminate the pregnancy.

Non-lethal uropathy with a low risk of renal failure

This category accounts for the largest number of infants with prenatally detected uropathy referred to pediatric urologists. Pyelocaliectasis is the single most common diagnosis. In one study, the contribution made by prenatal diagnosis to the management of 258 children was judged to have been of 'definite' value, defined as revealing clinically unsuspected obstruction or high-grade reflux affecting both kidneys or a solitary kidney, in 17%, of 'probable' value [unilateral pathology such as ureteropelvic junction (UPJ) obstruction in infants with a normal contralateral kidney] in 37%, and of 'doubtful' value (mild dilatation of questionable clinical significance) in 46% (Thomas DFM, unpublished data).

Gestational age is an important determinant of diagnostic sensitivity. Hydronephrosis of mild to moderate severity and VUR do not generally give rise to detectable dilatation by the time routine 'dating' or 'fetal anomaly' sonograms are performed in the second trimester.

One study analysed the reasons why children with urological abnormalities continue to present with symptomatic urinary infection despite having sonograms in pregnancy (Lakhoo et al., 1996). The most frequent explanation (accounting for 56% of cases) was that the fetal urinary tract had appeared normal (i.e. the uropathy in question had yet not given rise to detectable dilatation) at the time of a single study performed in the second trimester.

Postnatal evaluation: general considerations

Physical examination should always precede diagnostic imaging since it may provide confirmatory evidence of the underlying uropathy (renal mass, palpable bladder, etc.) or reveal a relevant coexisting abnormality or syndrome.

Ultrasonography

Newborn infants, particularly when breastfed, experience a short period of relative dehydration. For this reason it has been generally recommended that the initial postnatal sonogram should be deferred for 24–48 hours when the urinary tract is subjected to a more representative diuretic load. While this remains the ideal, the risk of missing significant pathology, as opposed to mild dilatation or reflux, has probably been overstated. Moreover, it may prove difficult to defer the initial study for 24–48 hours since many mothers opt for early discharge. Practice may be guided by the prenatal findings. When the possibility of a significant uropathy has been raised by prenatal findings such as bilateral dilatation, thick-walled bladder, or ureteric dilatation, the affected infant remains in hospital to be screened at 24–48 hours of age. Further investigations, notably voiding cystourethrography (VCU), are performed where indicated. Conversely, healthy infants whose prenatal sonograms have revealed only mild or equivocal dilatation are discharged, with arrangements to return for a scheduled postnatal sonogram at around 2 weeks of age. These children should be discharged on low-dose antibacterial prophylaxis.

Quantifying severity of dilatation

Measurement of the anteroposterior diameter of the renal pelvis is now routinely performed in most major centers. Although subject to operator variability and the state of hydration, measurement of renal pelvic AP diameter is greatly preferable to subjective descriptors such as 'mild' or 'moderate' dilatation, 'full' or 'baggy' renal pelvis, etc. The grading system advocated by the Society for Fetal Urology (SFU) (Maizels et al., 1992) encompasses the appearances of the collecting system 'central renal complex' and renal parenchymal thickness (Fig. 4.7, Table 4.1). These aspects of sonographic appearances should be documented, even if the formal SFU protocol is not adopted.

Voiding cystourethrography (VCU)

Centers vary considerably in the extent to which VCU is routinely employed for the postnatal evaluation of

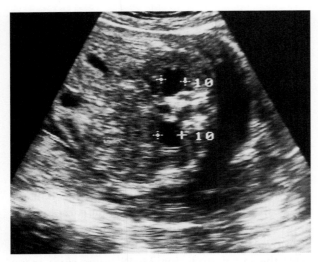

Figure 4.7 Bilateral renal pelvic dilatation. Anteroposterior diameters = 1.0 cm at 26 weeks' gestation. No underlying pathology was identified on postnatal investigation.

- ureteric dilatation demonstrated on ultrasonography, either prenatally or postnatally;
- thick-walled bladder or other evidence of outflow obstruction;
- bilateral upper tract dilatation in a male fetus or infant;
- caliceal dilatation (usually in conjunction with pelvic dilatation): this is a relative indication for VCU since it may be a sonographic feature of high-grade VUR as well as obstruction.

VCU in this age group should always be undertaken under antibiotic cover and a catheter or feeding tube should be left in the bladder when urethral obstruction is demonstrated. Where there is already strong presumptive evidence of a posterior urethral valve there may be an advantage to performing the VCU through a percutaneously inserted neonatal suprapubic catheter rather than via the urethral route, particularly if catheterization is difficult.

Isotope imaging

The choice of modality is determined by the nature of the anomaly. [Technetium-99m]dimercaptosuccinic acid ([^{99m}Tc]DMSA) is most suitable for confirming

infants with prenatally detected dilatation. To avoid subjecting large numbers of healthy infants to an invasive investigation, a more selective approach can be used, based on:

Table 4.1 Classification of prenatal hydronephrosis (Society for Fetal Urology)

Renal image		
Grade of hydronephrosis	Central renal complex (intrarenal pelvis, calyces)	Renal parenchymal thickness
0	Intact	Normal
1	Slight splitting	Normal
2	Evident splitting, complex confined within renal border	Normal
3[a]	Wide splitting, pelvis dilated outside renal border, *and* calices *uniformly* dilated.	Normal
4	Further dilatation of pelvis and calices (calices may appear convex)	Thin

Grade of ureteral dilatation (UD Gr)	
UD Gr	Diameter of ureter (mm)
1	< 7
2	7–10
3	> 10

[a]An extrarenal pelvis extending outside the renal border which is not accompanied by calyceal dilatation corresponds to grade 2 hydronephrosis.
The grading system was devised as a guide to postnatal assessment but can also be used in the third trimester to counsel parents on the clinical significance, or otherwise, of prenatal sonogram findings.
From Maizels *et al*. (1992).

total absence of function in a multicystic dysplastic kidney or for documenting differential function and patterns of parenchymal damage associated with VUR. Dynamic renography with [^{99m}Tc]mercapto-acetyltriglycine (MAG-3) is used primarily in the diagnosis of obstruction. Furosemide washout is an essential component of the study and it is important to obtain postvoiding images of the upper tracts. The interpretation of drainage curves is particularly problematic in young infants during the period of 'transitional renal function'. A normal drainage washout response to furosemide can reasonably be interpreted as excluding obstruction. However, the converse may not be true, and an abnormal drainage curve cannot necessarily be construed as definite evidence of obstruction particularly where function in the relevant kidney is significantly impaired or dilatation is severe. Fortunately, the information derived from diuretic renography is rarely crucial to management in the first few weeks or months of life and this investigation can generally be deferred for 2–4 weeks, when the results can be interpreted more reliably.

Postnatal investigation: general considerations

The risk of urinary infection merits antibiotic prophylaxis until a urologic diagnosis has been established. In contrast, the requirement for early postnatal surgical intervention is virtually confined to relieving outflow obstruction (usually boys with posterior urethral valves) and draining gross hydronephrosis. Most infants with prenatally detected anomalies are asymptomatic and their overall renal function is not at immediate risk. Thus, the timing and pattern of further imaging can be guided largely by the initial ultrasound findings and an assessment of differential diagnosis. Investigative protocols vary considerably but the one that has evolved in Leeds, UK, is illustrated in Figure 4.8.

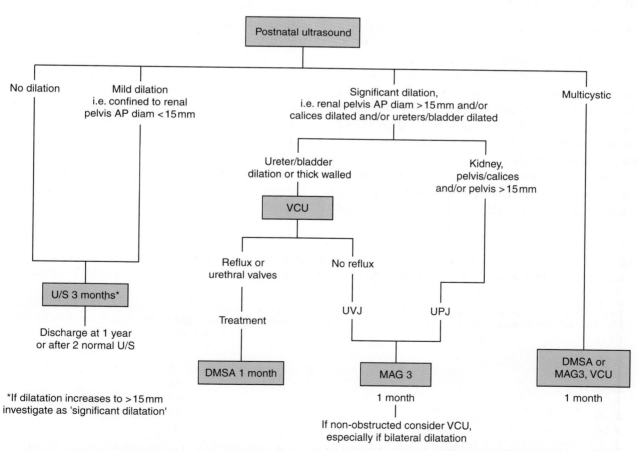

Figure 4.8 Protocol for the early postnatal investigation of prenatally detected dilatation. (VCU = voiding cysto-urethrography; UVJ = ureterovesical junction; UPJ = ureteropelvic junction.)

Ureteropelvic junction obstruction

Clinically significant hydronephrosis (as opposed to mild pelvic or pelvicaliceal dilatation) has an estimated incidence of 1 in 600 to 1 in 800 fetuses. The most common final diagnosis is UPJ obstruction, which accounts for 35–50% of all prenatally detected uropathies (Thomas and Barker, 1997; Nguyen and Kogan, 1998).

Differential diagnosis

In addition to UPJ obstruction, ureterovesical junction obstruction (megaureter), vesicoureteral reflux, dilatation of one moeity of a duplex kidney, and multicystic dysplastic kidney may all give rise to diagnostic uncertainty on prenatal sonography. But in a male infant the possibility of outflow obstruction should always be considered first as the explanation for bilateral upper tract dilatation.

Management: prenatal

Fetal intervention (nephrostomy) was performed on a very limited and largely anecdotal basis in the 1980s, but it is highly doubtful whether UPJ obstruction could ever be regarded as a legitimate indication for intervention *in utero*. The main benefits of prenatal diagnosis lie in counseling parents on the likely requirement for postnatal pyeloplasty and providing an opportunity to avert urinary infection or postnatal functional deterioration.

A broad correlation can be demonstrated between the duration and severity of fetal dilatation and the postnatal outcome for differential renal function, and thus the predicted requirement for pyeloplasty. However, the predictive sensitivity of the prenatal findings is weak and in one study statistical significance was only reached in those obstructed kidneys showing evidence of severe dilatation (i.e. renal pelvis diameter > 15 mm) in the second trimester (Thomas and Barker, 1997). The data of Dhillon and associates indicate that a maximal renal pelvic anteroposterior (AP) diameter of > 30 mm recorded either *in utero* or postnatally is associated with a 60–100% risk of functional impairment, depending on the severity of dilatation (Dhillon, 1998a) (Table 4.2).

During the 1990s a non-surgical approach has evolved with respect to obstructed kidneys that maintain normal levels of differential function (defined by Ransley and Manzoni, 1985, as a figure of >40% in the affected kidney). This approach has been endorsed by Koff and Campbell (1994), who have documented spontaneous maturation of individual kidney GFR to normal levels despite the presence of severe UPJ obstruction on diuretic renography.

The natural history of prenatally detected UPJ obstruction has been studied in a randomized controlled trial of surgical versus non-surgical treatment undertaken at the Hospital for Sick Children, London. Forty-eight children underwent pyeloplasty and 52 were managed non-operatively. Nine (17%) of those in the observation group came to pyeloplasty because of functional deterioration, which in most instances recovered postoperatively. Fourteen kidneys (27%) showed evidence of resolving obstruction, whereas 29 (56%) remained obstructed but with stable function over the duration of the study (Dhillon, 1998b).

Table 4.2 Prenatally detected ureteropelvic junction obstruction: correlation between maximum recorded anteroposterior (AP) diameter of renal pelvis and likelihood of impaired differential function on initial postnatal evaluation or during follow-up

Maximal AP diameter of renal pelvis (mm)	Requirement for surgical intervention (based on functional criteria) (%)
< 15	2
15–20	7
20–30	29
30–40	61
40–50	67
> 50	100

Findings derived from prospective studies undertaken at the Hospital for Sick Children Great Ormond Street, London (Dhillon, 1998a).

Legitimate concerns have been voiced regarding the potential for recovery of function in those kidneys that come to pyeloplasty because of functional deterioration during 'conservative' follow-up. Subramaniam *et al.* (1999) reported that postoperative functional recovery was significantly less after delayed pyeloplasty at a mean age of 2.2 years than early pyeloplasty at a mean age of 4.8 months. However, their study also revealed a correlation between the AP diameter of the renal pelvis and functional deterioration in the delayed pyeloplasty group. This observation is consistent with data from Great Ormond Street Hospital, Leeds, and other centers confirming the correlation between the severity of dilatation and the requirement for surgery, based on functional criteria at the time of initial assessment or deteriorating function on follow-up. Thus, it is seems clear that the development of increasing dilatation represents an indication to abandon non-operative management without waiting for functional deterioration to become apparent. In this way it may be possible to minimize the risk of long-term functional impairment associated with observation.

The author's current protocol for the management of prenatally detected UPJ obstruction can be broadly summarized as follows.

Pyeloplasty is advised if there is evidence of significant functional impairment (< 40% on renography at 3–6 months) or gross hydronephrosis (AP diameter > 30 mm). The Great Ormond Street long-term data indicate that deteriorating renal function rarely occurs when the initial AP diameter is less than 20 mm.

Non-operative management is chosen when differential function in the affected kidney exceeds 40% and the maximum recorded AP diameter of the renal pelvis is less than 30 mm. Indications for surgery include:

- deteriorating function (falling below 35–40% on follow-up);
- increasing dilatation, which often precedes a drop in function (see above);
- persisting obstruction with stable function but no evidence of improving drainage after 4–5 years of observation.

In bilateral UPJ obstruction, management is more problematic in view of the difficulties inherent in interpreting differential function in the presence of bilateral pathology. Bilateral pyeloplasty is justified where the dilatation is severe but in other cases it is reasonable to operate on the more severely affected kidney and monitor the contralateral kidney.

Vesicoureteral reflux

Ultrasonography is an unreliable modality for the detection of VUR, both prenatally and postnatally. Nevertheless, clues to the presence of VUR can be inferred from certain sonographic findings, namely ureteral dilatation, caliceal dilatation, 'bright' renal parenchyma, and other features of renal dysplasia.

Primary VUR accounts for 15–20% of prenatally detected uropathies. Low-grade, non-dilating VUR may also be identified as an incidental finding on a VCU included as part of the routine evaluation of co-existing prenatally detected abnormalities. For example, multicystic dysplastic kidney is associated with a 20–40% incidence of contralateral VUR which is generally low grade and undetectable sonographically.

Prenatally detected primary VUR is predominantly a disorder of male infants, who outnumber females by a ratio of approximately 5:1 (Thomas, 1997). High intravesical pressures, i.e. 100–230 cmH_2O have been documented in urodynamic studies of male infants with high-grade primary VUR in studies reported by Sillen (1998) and Chandra *et al.* (1996). Similar findings were published by Yeung *et al.* (1997), who also noted that early resolution of VUR occurred more frequently in those boys whose voiding dynamics reverted to normal during the period of follow-up.

Some caution is needed when interpreting the significance of these urodynamic findings in very young infants in view of the paucity of control data. Nevertheless, when viewed together the evidence implicates bladder dysfunction in the etiology of 'Primary' VUR in male infants. The underlying cause remains unclear, although the legacy of transient urethral obstruction *in utero* by Cowper's duct cysts has been invoked as the explanation in some cases. Homsy and Kokoua (1998) studied the embryological development of the external sphincter complex and speculated that delayed or abnormal sphincter maturation could result in a period of functional obstruction.

Experimental fetal models of VUR and incomplete urethral obstruction are now being developed which may provide much needed information on the interrelationship between bladder dysfunction and reflux *in utero* (Gobet *et al.*, 1999a).

Postnatal investigation and management

Antibiotic prophylaxis should be instituted from the first day of life in all infants in whom VUR figures in the differential diagnosis. In addition, an early VCU is advisable because of the difficulty in distinguishing between primary VUR and less severe forms of PUV. For reasons already considered, DMSA renography may be best deferred until 4–6 weeks of age. Some surgeons have advocated early surgical correction of prenatally detected VUR but the informed consensus favors a more selective approach to surgical correction, particularly in view of the well-documented potential for even moderately high grades of VUR to resolve spontaneously in male infants.

Reviewing the results of seven series published between 1991 and 1997 (totaling 413 refluxing units detected prenatally), Elder (1998) found that the reported resolution rates for different grades of VUR by 1–2 years were: 91% for grade I, 84% for grade II, 71% for grade III, 40% for grade IV, and 14% for grade V. For grades I–III the overall figure was 78%, and for grades IV–V 36%. During 1–2 years of follow-up 13% of males developed urinary infection.

Where break-through urinary infection prompts surgical intervention in the first 9 months the author's preference is usually for cutaneous vesicostomy, particularly for those with high-grade reflux. Thereafter, ureteral reimplantation is performed after the marked ureterectasis resolves.

Multicystic dysplastic kidney

The advent of prenatal sonography has revealed that the true prevalence of multicystic dysplastic kidney (MDK) is far higher than was previously suspected. Data collected in Leeds, UK (Gordon *et al.*, 1988), indicated that unilateral MDK was present in 1 in 4300 livebirths. More recently, data derived with more sensitive, modern equipment over a 10-year period at Northwick Park Hosptial, London (Liebeschuetz and Thomas, 1997), put the figure at 1 in 2400 livebirths.

Etiology

Experimental ureteric ligation in the fetal lamb during the first half of gestation results in some cystic dysplastic changes, but the characteristic features of MDK have not been convincingly reproduced in an experimental model. The high incidence of coexisting ipsilateral and contralateral VUR and the well-documented association with renal agenesis raise the possibility that MDK may reflect the outcome of an underlying ureteric bud anomaly, rather than ischemic atresia or ureteric obstruction that has been previously suggested. Although MDK generally behaves as a sporadic anomaly, affected families have been described in whom the probable mode of inheritance is an autosomal dominant trait with variable penetrance (Belk *et al.*, 1997). Additionally, the high incidence of contralateral reflux supports this theory.

Diagnosis

MDK may sometimes be difficult to distinguish sonographically from hydronephrosis, and, indeed, intermediate forms have been described (Carey and Howards, 1993). Although the majority of unilateral MDKs are now detected in otherwise healthy infants, MDK also appears frequently in association with esophageal atresia and verterbral and limb anomalies.

Postnatal evaluation comprises sonography and DMSA renal scan. Opinion is divided on the need for a routine VCU since, in the absence of dilatation, any coexisting VUR is generally low grade and rarely of clinical significance.

The predilection for MDKs to involute is well documented postnatally. This phenomenon can also occur *in utero*, mimicking renal agenesis (Mesrobian *et al.*, 1993). The natural history of MDK, the controversy surrounding its management, and the perceived risks of hypertension and malignancy are detailed elsewhere.

Mild dilatation (pelviectasis)

Mild dilatation of one or both fetal kidneys is a feature of 1 in 100 to 1 in 200 pregnancies (Chitty *et al.*, 1990). This common sonographic finding may reflect a simple anatomical variant, a prominent extrarenal pelvis, or low-grade or 'burnt-out' UPJ obstruction or VUR. For the clinician, the challenge lies in distinguishing potentially pathologic causes of mild dilatation, notably VUR and UPJ obstruction, from simple anatomical variants and physiological dilatation of little clinical significance.

Anteroposterior pelvic diameter

In an attempt to differentiate between 'pathological' and 'physiological' dilatation, and thus to identify infants meriting further investigation, greatest emphasis has been placed on the severity of dilatation, as measured by renal pelvic diameter. Taking an AP pelvic diameter of 5 mm as the normal upper limit, Arger *et al.* (1985) reported a surprisingly low false-positive rate of only 18%. Since the 1980s, 10 mm has been widely regarded as the upper limit of the 'normal' renal pelvic diameter. However, this arbitrary figure has never been convincingly validated as a predictor of pathology. In a prospective study of 6292 pregnancies screened at 28 weeks' gestation, Livera *et al.* (1989) reported a false-positive rate (no abnormality found on postnatal investigation) of 56% based on an AP pelvic diameter of 10 mm. Other authors have reported 'false-positive' rates ranging from 9 to 50% for an AP diameter of 10 mm and less.

Above 15 mm AP diameter, Grignon *et al.* (1986) reported a false-positive rate of only 6%. In the context of UPJ obstruction the predictive value of the 15 mm figure has been largely validated by the findings of Dhillon (1998a), who concluded that, when the AP diameter was 15 mm or less, the risk of functional impairment or deterioration resulting in a requirement for pyeloplasty was only 2%. Even in the 15–20 mm range, the overall requirement for pyeloplasty, based on functional criteria, was only 7%.

In summary, active obstruction of sufficient severity to pose an ongoing threat of renal impairment is most unlikely when dilatation is confined to the renal pelvis or where pelvicaliceal dilatation is associated with a pelvic AP diameter of less than 15 mm. Since the results of isotope renography rarely contribute to the practical management of mild dilatation there is little justification in submitting such infants to this invasive investigation. However, a repeat sonogram should be done within 12 months.

Mild dilatation and vesicoureteric reflux

In contrast to the understanding of obstruction the significance of mild pelvic and/or pelvicaliceal dilatation as a marker of VUR is still poorly validated, not least because of the unreliability of sonography for the detection of VUR at any age. The simplistic solution consists of routinely investigating every infant with any degree of prenatally detected dilatation by VCU. However, this approach inevitably entails submitting large numbers of healthy infants to an invasive inves-

tigation, which in the majority of instances is destined to yield negative or clinically irrelevant findings. In a study of 29 infants with mild dilatation followed to a mean age of 4.2 years, representing a total of 122 child-years of follow-up, only two episodes of urological morbidity were documented, neither of which was related to reflux (Thomas *et al.*, 1994). In the author's clinic, VCU is generally limited to those infants whose 'mild' pelvic dilatation is accompanied by ureteric and/or caliceal dilatation on sonography. Some cases of predominantly low-grade VUR will be missed by adopting a selective approach but experience and the limited available evidence indicate that this risk is outweighed by the benefit of reducing the burden of unnecessary invasive investigation in healthy infants. Unfortunately, this belief may not be shared by the lawyers. In the prevailing climate of litigation the investigation of mild dilatation may be increasingly determined by defensive medicine rather

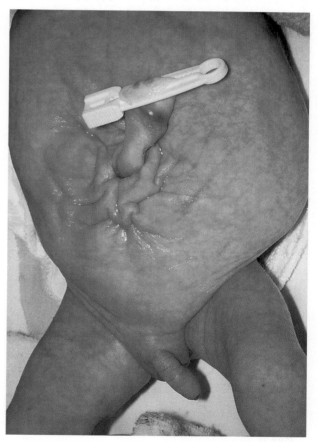

Figure 4.9 Newborn infant with characteristic features of prune belly syndrome, which is a disappearing disorder. Most major centers report a dramatic decline in incidence following the advent of prenatal diagnosis and termination of pregnancy.

than evidence-based medicine. An authoritative prospective study is needed to put the risks in context. Until then, parents should be informed of the risks and, ideally, should be party to any decision on whether or not to proceed to VCU.

Conclusions

Ultrasonography is now so firmly rooted in obstetric practice that it would be unthinkable for pediatric urology to return to the preultrasonography era. The impact of termination of pregnancy is already evident in the dramatic fall in new cases of prune belly syndrome (Fig. 4.9). As termination of pregnancy extends to include other severe, non-lethal fetal uropathies the number of infants and young children requiring renal replacement therapy and transplantation (predominantly males with urethral obstruction and renal dysplasia) will probably also diminish. For reasons already considered the incidence of cloacal and uncomplicated bladder exstrophy is also destined to decline in countries where termination is offered. Few changes are envisaged in the management of most other non-lethal uropathies, although the next few years will probably witness a moderate swing of the surgical pendulum back in favor of pyeloplasty for a higher proportion of prenatally detected UPJ obstructions.

In the longer term the rapidly advancing science of developmental biology is destined to yield discoveries of fundamental importance to pediatric urology.

References

Agarwal S, Mlouf D, Welsh A, Fisk N (1999) Endoscopic management of foetal obstructive uropathy. *Br J Urol Int* **83**(4): Abstract 98,46.

Arger PH, Coleman BG, Mintz MC *et al.* (1985) Routine fetal genitourinary tract screening. *Radiology* **156**: 485–9.

Avner ED, Chavers B, Sullivan EK *et al.* (1995) Renal transplantation and chronic dialysis in children and adolescents: the 1993 annual report of the North American Paediatric Renal Transplant Cooperative Study. *Pediatr Nephrol* **9**: 61–73.

Beck AD (1971) The effect in intra-uterine urinary obstruction upon the development of the fetal kidney. *J Urol* **105**: 784–9.

Belk RA, Thomas DFM, Mueller RF *et al.* (1997) Multicystic dysplastic kidney: an inherited anomaly? Presentation to Section of Urology, American Academy of Paediatrics, New Orleans, Louisiana, November 1–3, Abstract **128**: 210.

Bewley S, Rodeck CH (1997) Fetal intervention. In: Thomas DFM (ed.) *Urological disease in the fetus and infant*. Oxford: Butterworth-Heinemann, 96–114.

Brand IR, Kaminopetros P, Cave M *et al.* (1994) Specificity of antenatal ultrasound in the Yorkshire region: a prospective study of 2261 ultrasound detected anomalies. *Br J Obstet Gynaecol* **101**: 392–7.

Brocklebank JT (1997) Renal function in the infant and management of renal failure. In: Thomas DFM (ed.) *Urological disease in the fetus and infant*. Oxford: Butterworth-Heinemann, 124–49.

Carey PO, Howards SS (1993) Multicystic dysplastic kidneys and diagnostic confusion on renal scan. *J Urol* **139**: 83–4.

Carter CO, Pescia G (1979) A family study of renal agenesis. *J Med Genet* **16**: 176–88.

Chandra M, Maddix H, McVicar M (1996) Transient urodynamic dysfunction of infancy: relationship to urinary tract infections and vesicoureteral reflux. *J Urol* **155**: 673–7.

Chitty LS, Pembrey E, Chudleigh PM, Campbell S (1990) Multicentre study of antenatal calyceal dilation detected by ultrasound. *Lancet* **336**: 875.

Crabbe DCG, Thomas DFM, Gordon AC *et al.* (1992) Use of ^{99m}technetiumdimercaptosuccinic acid to study patterns of renal damage associated with prenatally detected vesicoureteral reflux. *J Urol* **148**: 1229–31.

Crombleholme TM, Harrison MR, Golbus MS *et al.* (1990) Fetal intervention in obstruction uropathy: prognostic indicators and efficacy of intervention. *Am J Obstet Gynecol* **162**: 1239–44.

De Mello D, Reid LM (1997) The kidney/lung loop. In: Thomas DFM (ed.) *Urological disease in the fetus and infant*. Oxford: Butterworth-Heinemann, 62–77.

Dhillon HK (1998a) Data presented to the 9th Annual Meeting European Society of Paediatric Urology, Salzburg.

Dhillon HK (1998b) Prenatally diagnosed hydronephrosis: the Great Ormond Street Experience. *Br J Urol* **81**(2): 39–44.

Dineen MD, Dhillon HK, Ward HC *et al.* (1992) Antenatal diagnosis of posterior urethral valves. *Br J Urol* **72**: 364–9.

Elder J (1998) Prenatally diagnosed reflux: current guidelines. *Dialog Paediatr Urol* **21**(4): 5.

Elder JS, Duckett JW, Snyder HM (1987) Intervention for fetal obstructive uropathy: has it been effective? *Lancet* **ii**: 1007–10.

Freedman AL, Johnson MP, Smith CA *et al.* (1999) Long-term outcome in children after antenatal intervention for obstructive uropathies. *Lancet* **354**: 374–7.

Glick PL, Harrison MR, Golbus MS *et al.* (1985) Management of the fetus with congenital hydronephrosis II. Prognostic criteria and selection for treatment. *J Pediatr Surg* **20**: 376–87.

Gobet R, Cisek LR, Chang B *et al.* (1999a) Experimental fetal vesicoureteral reflux induces renal tubular and glomerular damage, and is associated with persistent bladder instability. *J Urol* **162**: 1090–5.

Gobet R, Park B, Chang H *et al.* (1999b) Dysregulation of the renal renin/angiotensin system caused by partial bladder outlet obstruction in foetal sheep. *Brit J Urol* **83**(3): 79.

Gordon AC, Thomas DFM, Arthur R *et al.* (1988) Multicystic dysplastic kidney: is nephrectomy still appropriate? *J Urol* **140**: 1231–4.

Grignon A, Filiatrault D, Homsy Y *et al.* (1986) Ureteropelvic junction stenosis: antenatal ultrasonographic diagnosis, postnatal investigation, and follow up. *Radiology* **160**: 649–51.

Harrison MR, Golbus MS, Filly RA *et al.* (1982a) Fetal surgery for congenital hydronephrosis. *N Engl J Med* **306**: 591–3.

Harrison MR, Nakayam DK, Noall R *et al.* (1982b) Correction of congential hydronephrosis *in utero* II. Decompression reverses the effects of obstruction on the fetal lung and urinary tract. *J Pediatr Surg* **17**: 965–74.

Haycock GB (1998) Development of glomerular filtration and tubular sodium reabsorption in the human fetus and newborn. *Br J Urol* **81**: 33–8.

Homsy YI, Kokoua A (1998) Maturation of the human external urinary sphincter. *Dialog Paediatr Urol* **21(4)**: 6–8.

Hutton KAR, Thomas DFM, Arthur RJ *et al.* (1994) Prenatally detected posterior urethral valves: is gestational age at detection a predictor of outcome? *J Urol* **152**: 698–701.

Hutton KAR, Thomas DFM, Davies BW (1997) Prenatally detected posterior urethral valves: qualitative assessment of second trimester scans and prediction of outcome. *J Urol* **158**: 1022–5.

Kaefer M, Peters CA, Retik AB, Benacerraf BR (1997) Increased renal echogenicity: a sonographic sign for differentiating between obstruction and nonobstructive etiologies of *in utero* bladder distension. *J Urol* **158**: 1026–9.

Koff SA, Campbell KD (1994) The non-operative management of unilateral neonatal hydronephrosis. Natural history of poorly functioning kidneys. *J Urol* **152**: 593–5.

Lakhoo K, Thomas DFM, Fuenfer M, D'Cruz AJ (1996) Failure of prenatal ultrasonography to prevent urinary infection associated with underlying urological abnormalities. *Br J Urol* **77**: 905–8.

Liebeschuetz S, Thomas R (1997) Letter to the Editor: Unilateral multicystic dysplastic kidney. *Arch Dis Child* **77**: 369.

Livera LN, Brookfield DS, Egginton JA, Hawnaur JM (1989) Antenatal ultrasonography to detect fetal renal abnormalities: a prospective screening programme. *BMJ* **298**: 1421–3.

Mackie GG, Stephens FD (1996) Duplex kidneys: a correlation of renal dysplasia with position of the urethral orifice. In: Stephens FD, Smith ED, Hutson JM (eds) *Congenital anomalies of the urinary and genital tract*. Oxford: Isis, 307–16.

Maizels M, Reisman EM, Flom LS *et al.* (1992) Grading nephrouretral dilatation detected in the first year of life – correlation with obstruction. *J Urol* **148**: 609–14.

Mandell J, Peters CA, Retik AB (1990) Current concepts in the perinatal diagnosis and management of hydronephrosis. *Urol Clin North Am* **17**: 247–61.

Manning FA, Harrison MR, Rodeck C *et al.* (1986) Catheter shunts for fetal hydronephrosis and hydrocephalus. *N Engl J Med* **315**: 336.

Mesrobian HGJ, Rushton HG, Bulas D (1993) Unilateral renal agenesis may result from utero regression of multicystic renal dysplasia. *J Urol* **150**: 793–4.

Minoja M, Hirschman G, Jones C *et al.* (1995) Incidence and causes of ESRD in children in the USA. *J Am Soc Nephrol* **6**: 396.

Nguyen HT, Kogan BA (1998) Upper urinary tract obstruction: experimental and clinical aspects. *Br J Urol* **81(2)**: 13–21.

Peters CA (1998) Lower urinary tract obstruction clinical and experimental aspects. *Br J Urol* **81(2)**: 22–32.

Quinn FMJ, Deans A, Dhillon HK *et al.* (1996) The dilated fetal bladder on antenatal ultrasound: diagnosis and outcome. *Pediatrics* **98**: 622.

Rabinowitz R, Peters MT, Vyas S *et al.* (1989) Measurement of fetal urine production in normal pregnancy by real-time ultrasonograhpy. *Am J Obstet Gynecol* **161**: 1264–6.

Ransley PG (1996) Impact of prenatal diagnosis on paediatric urology. Read at Annual Meeting of the American Urological Association, Orlando, FL, May 4–9.

Ransley PG, Manzoni GA (1985) 'Extended' role of DTPA scan in assessing function and PUJ obstruction in neonates. *Dialog Paediatr Urol* **8**: 3.

Roodhoft AM, Birnholz J, Holmes L (1984) Familial nature of congenital absence and severe dysgenesis of both kidneys. *N Engl J Med* **310**: 1341–5.

Sillen U (1998) Neonatal urodynamic. *Dialog Paediatr Urol* **21(4)**: 5.

Subramaniam R, Kouriefs C, Dickson AP (1999) Antenatally detected pelvi-ureteric junction obstruction: concerns about conservative management. *Br J Urol Int* **84**: 335–8.

Thomas DFM (1997) Veiscoureteric reflux. In: Thomas DFM (ed.) *Urological disease in the fetus and infant*. Oxford: Butterworth-Heinemann, 209–21.

Thomas DFM, Madden NP, Irving HC *et al.* (1994) Mild dilation of the fetal kidney: a follow up study. *Br J Urol* **74**: 236–9.

Woolf AS (1998) Molecular control of nephrogenesis and the pathogenesis of kidney malformation. *Br J Urol* **81**: 1–7.

Yanagita K, Nagaike M, Ishibashi H *et al.* (1992) Lung may have an endocrine function producing hepatocyte growth factor in response the injury of distal organs. *Biochem Biophys Res Commun* **182**: 802–9.

Yeung CK, Godley ML, Dhillion HK *et al.* (1997) The characteristics of primary veisco-ureteric reflux in male and female infants with pre-natal hydronephrosis. *Br J Urol* **80**: 319–27.

Pediatric imaging

5

Jane S. Matsumoto and A.J. Le Roy

Introduction

The radiological evaluation of children with urological disease can be a complex process. It is often not limited to one imaging test or one imaging modality. A number of tests may be performed to provide the best diagnostic evaluation of the child's urologic tract (Fernbach, 1998). The continually evolving modalities such as ultrasound, computed tomography (CT), magnetic resonance imaging (MRI) and nuclear medicine offer ever more complex evaluations. The standard voiding cystourethrogram (VCUG) is irreplaceable in the evaluation of the lower urinary tract. Excretory urography and plain film, which are often overlooked, should be part of the uroradiologic armamentarium. There are many factors to consider when choosing imaging tests. It is important to know the strengths and weaknesses of each modality. Considerations also include cost, radiation exposure (Table 5.1), contrast allergy, and the need for sedation. There is no gold standard in imaging of the urologic system. The urology imaging tests are comple-

mentary and each offers its own unique piece of information. The uroradiologic evaluation is best and most efficiently performed when there is good communication and consultation between the radiologist and the pediatric urologist. The work-up is likely to be more successful and less stressful when there are radiology personnel who are skilled in working with children and families and are sensitive to their varying needs and concerns. It is also helpful to have child-friendly facilities.

Modalities

Plain film

The abdominal plain film is the most basic imaging evaluation. It is valuable for evaluation of bowel pattern, stones, and bony abnormalities. It can often guide the next choice of tests. Renal or bladder stones may be readily apparent. Plain film can demonstrate changes in skeletal dysplasias, which may be associated with renal abnormalities. Spinal dysraphism may be obvious in children with suspected bladder abnormalities.

Excretory urography

The excretory urogram was the standard for renal evaluation before the advent of ultrasound and CT. CT is basically an excretory urogram with axial tomographic reconstruction. Ultrasound and CT, with its finer detail and added dimension, have largely replaced excretory urography in evaluation of the renal parenchyma. Because of their orientation and course, there are aspects of the renal collecting systems that are often best evaluated in the coronal plane. Plain film after contrast or excretory urography best accomplishes this. This type of imaging can also be done in conjunction with a CT without oral contrast,

Table 5.1 Radiation exposure

Examination	Entrance skin exposure (R)	
	Infant (0–1 year old)	Child (5–7 years old)
Lumbar projection, AP	0.03	0.05
Kidney tomogram	0.25	0.5
Voiding cystourethrogram	0.25	0.5
Spiral CT abdomen	3.1	3.1
Electron beam CT abdomen	1.6	3.2

AP = anteroposterior;
CT = computed tomography.

to obtain an excellent overall evaluation of the renal parenchyma, the collecting system, and bladder.

Excretory urography typically consists of a scout film before administration of intravenous contrast. This allows for evaluation of possible stones or other radiopacities before they may be obscured by intravenous contrast. Intravenous contrast material is administered and a film over the kidneys is obtained at 2–3 min followed by tomographic images of the kidneys. Prone films of the whole abdomen are obtained at 10 min and potentially at 20 min. The prone position optimizes visualization of the collecting systems. The bladder should be catheterized during the study if the child is known to have vesicoureteral reflux (VUR). This prevents the false impression of function within a non-functioning or poorly functioning refluxing kidney. With an obstructive picture, delayed films are obtained and intravenous Lasix may be given to assess clearing of the contrast within the collecting systems.

Sonography

For many, sonography is the initial study for evaluation of children's kidneys. The advantages include good visualization of the renal parenchyma and collecting system, lack of radiation, little if any need for sedation, portability, and relatively low costs. Sonography is the best screening modality for possible renal obstructive processes. It also offers exquisite visualization of the renal parenchyma of the neonate and infant.

The sonographic examination is very operator dependent. It is important to have skilled, experienced sonographers and routine protocols, so that the studies are reproducible and comparable over time. Renal sonograms should include both supine and prone views with images in both transverse and longitudinal projections, as well as additional concentrated views of the upper and lower poles.

Sonography offers an accurate evaluation of renal length and growth. Nomographic charts are available for renal size for age and body size, and for the child with a single kidney (Shan et al., 1992; Zerin and Blane, 1994; Rottenberg et al., 1996; De Sanctis et al., 1998) (Figure 5.1).

Although sonography offers a good evaluation of the appearance of the renal parenchyma, dilatation of the collecting system and renal length, it is not as sensitive as a dimercaptosuccinic acid (DMSA) renal

scan in detecting renal scarring or pyelonephritis (Bjorgvinsson et al., 1991; Conway and Cohn, 1994).

Bladder views may offer important information and must be included in every examination. The bladder should be well distended. These views may be difficult to obtain in infants and the bladder should be checked early in the examination. If it is full, images should be obtained before the infant voids. If the bladder is empty, the child should be given oral fluids and the bladder checked at intervals, until it can be well evaluated. Bladder views may reveal dilated distal ureters, filling defects such as ureteroceles, or polyps, diverticula, thickened bladder wall and stones.

Doppler evaluation is a unique sonographic tool and is used in the evaluation of the vasculature of the kidneys, ovaries, and testes. It offers invaluable information in cases such as renal vein thrombosis, testicular or ovarian torsion, and renal artery stenosis. The opportunity to evaluate blood flow in children, without necessarily using intravenous contrast or angiography, is a wonderful advance in imaging.

Computed tomography

Technological advances have been made in CT imaging during the 1990s, with the development of spiral CT and electron beam CT, resulting in improved evaluation of the kidneys, the collecting systems, and the renal vasculature. CT has developed remarkably fast image acquisition. State-of-the-art CT can acquire 40 images or more in less than 1 min. The whole abdomen and pelvis can be imaged in less than 1 min with a few breathholds. Images are acquired in an axial mode with sagittal and coronal reformatting capabilities.

This fast acquisition time allows multiple stages of enhancement to be potentially captured in the first few minutes. The contrast bolus and scan time can be planned to obtain the arterial, parenchymal, and/or venous phases. After the initial bolus of intravenous contrast, single or multiphasic images are acquired. Delayed images after 3–5 min can be obtained to identify contrast filling the collecting systems and bladder.

Early contrast bolus ultrathin 1 mm images potentially allow an evaluation of the renal arteries. Imaging during the early contrast bolus will also offer a cortical nephrographic phase. While this allows optimal evaluation of the cortex, the medullary

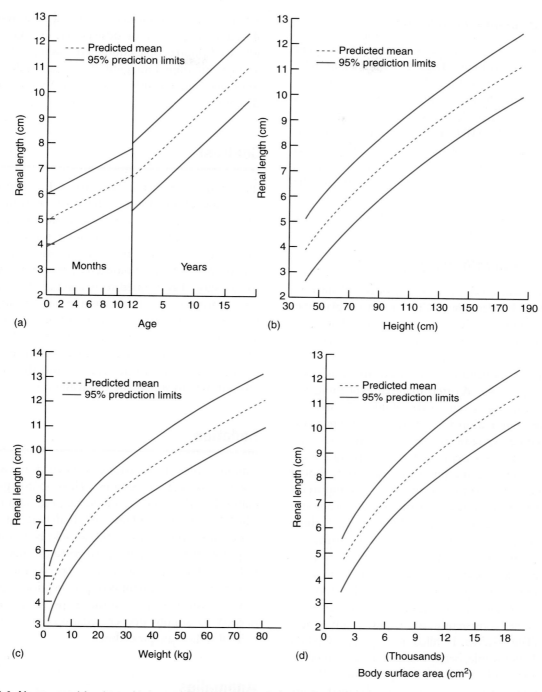

Figure 5.1 Nomographic chart. (Adapted from Han and Babcock, 1986.)

pyramids are not yet filled with contrast and are low density. Abnormalities in the medullary pyramids may be masked at this time. The medullary pyramids will normally fill with contrast within 1–2 min. The renal veins and inferior vena cava (IVC) are also usu-ally opacified at this time. Non-contrast single breath-hold thin-section CT is increasingly used in the eval-uation of renal stones. CT offers the additional advan-tage of imaging the remaining organs of the abdomen.

Magnetic resonance imaging

MRI is not used in children as often as in the adult population for urologic imaging, owing to its relatively long acquisition time, frequent need for sedation, and relatively high cost. In children under 5 years, sedation is usually necessary in order to obtain a diagnostic study. MRI may offer valuable information in the evaluation of renal masses and potential invasion of the renal vein and IVC. It has also shown efficacy in the evaluation of renal artery stenosis. The role of MRI in the evaluation of acute infections and obstruction has shown promise and will no doubt be developed in the future (Pennington et al., 1996).

Voiding cystourethrography

Although it can be difficult to perform and uncomfortable for children, the VCUG is an irreplaceable urologic imaging study. It is important to have personnel who are skilled in this study and can work with the child and family to decrease their apprehension, increase their cooperation, and make them as comfortable as possible. Written material explaining the procedure may be given to the child and caregiver before the examination to help them to prepare for the procedure. Questions are answered when the child and family or caregivers arrive at the radiology department. During the procedure each step should be explained again to the aware child. It is important to be sensitive to the needs of the preadolescent and adolescent child. Even in a teaching hospital, there should not be excessive staff in the room during the study. It is often less intimidating and easier to initiate voiding when medical personnel of the same sex as the patient are staffing the room during the study.

There is skill and a large degree of patience involved in being able consistently to acquire high-quality VCUGs. The bladder is filled to capacity. Cyclical studies, when possible, better evaluate the possibility of reflux (Paltiel et al., 1992). Anteroposterior (AP) and oblique images of the full bladder are obtained, as are images of the urethra during voiding in males. Intermittent fluoroscopic examination of the bladder is performed during voiding. Postvoid images of the bladder and the renal fossa are obtained.

The VCUG is most commonly employed to evaluate for possible VUR. It is also used to rule out urethral and bladder abnormalities. It offers the best evaluation of the bladder and urethra, not only anatomically, but also the physiological appearance during voiding. Radionuclide cystography traditionally has a lower radiation dose than a VCUG but with advanced fluoroscopic equipment, using pulsed fluoroscopy and digital imaging, the radiation dosage can be reduced significantly on standard VCUG (Klein et al., 1994).

Contrast

Intravenous contrast is used for CT and excretory urography examinations. The dose of contrast for children is 2 ml/kg. There is a small risk of allergic reaction with intravenous contrast for children, as well as adults (Cohen, 1994). In facilities where intravenous contrast is administered, the radiology personnel should be trained to recognize and treat contrast reactions. Resuscitation equipment, including pediatric-sized airway equipment and emergency medication, should be readily available. Non-ionic contrast is recommended for children because of the decreased risk of allergic reaction and the decreased morbidity with soft-tissue extravasation.

Sedation

Children may need to be sedated for radiologic evaluations and procedures. This occurs predominantly in MRI, nuclear medicine, and angiography. The American Academy of Pediatric guidelines (Committee on Drugs, 1992) should be followed for all procedures and studies performed on children with sedation. The guidelines include criteria for sedation, monitoring, documentation, education, and discharge instructions. Anesthesia personnel may be needed to supply deeper sedation in children for painful radiologic procedures.

Anomalies

Anomalies of the genitourinary tract are fairly common. Anomalies include renal agenesis, renal ectopia, horseshoe kidney, renal duplication, and crossed fused ectopia. The kidneys may not be in their expected locations. This development occurs in early embryonic stages with lack of normal movement of the kidneys in relationship to other abdominal organs. The kidney may be located anywhere from the pelvis to the thoracic cage. During initial sonographic evaluation, if there is no kidney identified in the renal fossa, the paraspinal region and pelvis should be evaluated. Ectopic kidneys may be very small and dysplastic, or may have other anomalies such as obstruction or fusion, or be multicystic dysplastic (Figure 5.2). This

may make it difficult to identify the tissue as being renal in origin, and a renal scan or CT scan may offer the next step in radiologic evaluation.

Horseshoe kidneys are fused across the midline by their medial lower poles (Figure 5.3). The fused portion may consist of fibrous tissue or normal renal parenchyma. The kidney is supplied by multiple renal arteries arising from the lower abdominal aorta. These kidneys are at higher risk for reflux, infection, and stones. Horseshoe kidneys are associated with Turner syndrome.

Renal duplication is a common anomaly. The collecting system is duplicated with two renal pelves and two ureters. The ureters may join into one ureter anywhere along their course or may enter the bladder through two separate orifices. Most renal duplications are uncomplicated and asymptomatic. They may, however, be associated with both obstruction and VUR. The upper pole ureter may be associated with an ectopic ureterocele. The ureterocele can be large enough to obstruct not only the lower pole ureteral orifice but also the ureter of the opposite kidney.

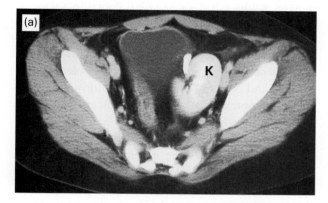

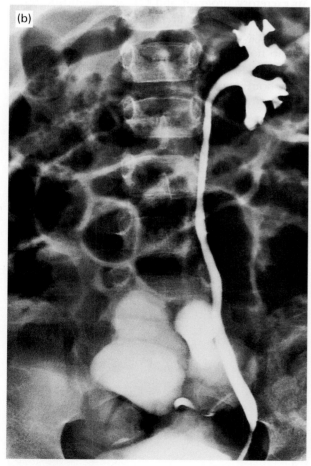

Figure 5.2 (*a*) CT of the left pelvic kidney (K); (*b*) bilateral retrograde ureterogram. Right pelvic kidney with a ureteropelvic junction obstruction.

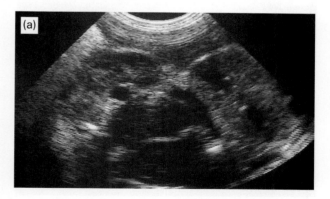

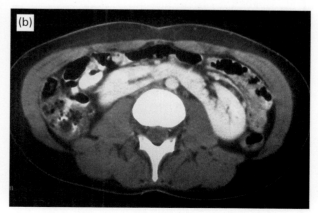

Figure 5.3 (*a*) Sonogram; and (*b*) CT of horseshoe kidney.

These children may present with bilateral hydroureteronephrosis. The ureterocele may extend into the bladder outlet and cause bladder outlet obstruction (Figure 5.4). Conversely, the ureter may not enter the bladder at all but may insert ectopically into other tissue within the pelvis, such as the vagina or urethra. This may be associated with obstruction at the ectopic

insertion site or it may result in incontinence in girls, because it inserts into either the urethra, vagina, or perineum. The lower pole ureter may insert abnormally and is at increased risk for reflux.

With a complete renal duplication a VCUG may demonstrate reflux into a lower pole moiety, with a 'drooping lily' appearance (Figure 5.5). There will be contrast within fewer calyces than would be expected for a single collecting system. This may be the first indication that a duplication is present. The ureter and lower pole moiety may be displaced laterally by an obstructed hydronephrotic upper pole system. Voiding and postvoid images may demonstrate reflux into an ectopic ureter, arising from near the bladder neck or the urethra (Figure 5.6).

Crossed fused ectopia is an uncommon entity. One of the kidneys crosses the midline and fuses to the lower pole of the other. This entity may be difficult to differentiate from a solitary kidney on sonography. An excretory urogram and CT are diagnostic tests. They demonstrate the ureter from the crossed kidney to extend across the midline and insert in the bladder on the normal side. Variations of this include the 'pancake' kidney, which is a rounded, sometimes amorphous mass of renal parenchyma, not in the

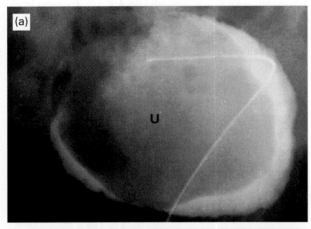

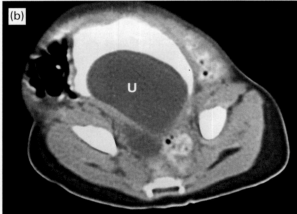

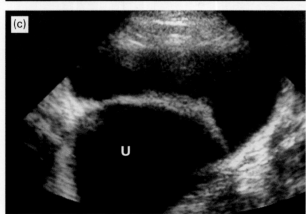

Figure 5.4 (*a*) VCUG; (*b*) CT; and (*c*) sonogram of large ureteroceles (U).

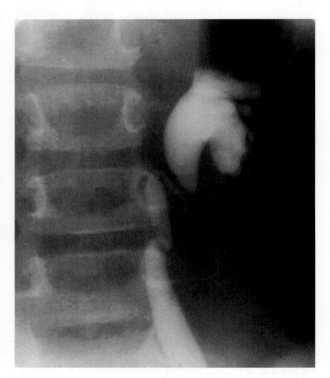

Figure 5.5 VCUG of refluxing 'drooping lily' of duplicated left kidney.

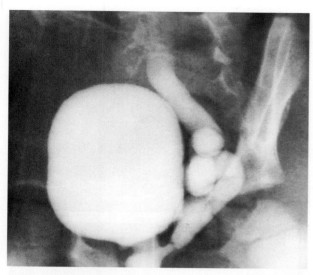

Figure 5.6 VCUG of reflux in ectopic ureter, inserting in posterior urethra.

normal reniform shape, commonly in the pelvis with ureters arising from it. This can be associated with other congenital organ malformations.

Obstruction

Congenitally obstructed kidneys are increasingly detected during routine prenatal ultrasound evaluations (Mandell *et al.*, 1991). The *in utero* diagnosis of hydronephrosis was initially made on the basis of dilatation of the renal pelvis. A scoring system has been developed which gives a more detailed evaluation of dilatation of specific renal segments and the presence of renal parenchymal thinning (Fernbach *et al.*, 1993). Although sonograms are most often obtained in the first few days of life, accurate postnatal evaluation of the kidneys for hydronephrosis should be repeated 3–4 weeks after birth for the best evaluation of possible obstructive processes. Before this time, renal function and urine output are not optimal and obstructive processes may not yet be apparent (Clautic-Engle *et al.*, 1995; Dremsek *et al.*, 1997). Patients who may need more immediate attention include infants with bladder outlet obstruction from entities such as posterior urethral valves or obstructing ureteroceles.

Postnatal sonography may not confirm the prenatal diagnosis of hydronephrosis (Kletcher *et al.*, 1991). There may be a prominent extrarenal pelvis with no true dilatation of the calyces to suggest obstruction. The dilatation may have been due to reflux (Zerin *et al.*, 1993). The question of obstructed or non-obstructed dilatation is the focus of much of the radiographic evaluation of hydronephrosis in the newborn. Non-obstructed systems include reflux, megaureter, megacalycosis, and Eagle–Barrett or prune belly syndrome. Obstructed causes include ureteropelvic junction (UPJ), ureterovesical junction (UVJ), complex duplication with obstructed ureters, and bladder outlet obstruction such as posterior urethral valves (PUV).

Sonography is an ideal imaging modality for initial evaluation of a dilated collecting system in infants and children. The whole drainage system, including the ureters and bladder, are included in the evaluation to look for a level of transition from a dilated to a normal caliber. If hydronephrosis is present, a VCUG should be performed to determine whether this represents reflux. If no reflux is present, diuretic renography is the next step to differentiate between obstructed and non-obstructed dilatation. Radionuclide studies are usually the preferred test because of their ability to quantify digitally both renal function and collecting system washout. However, excretory urography, with Lasix, may also give valuable anatomic information about the kidneys, ureters, and bladder. It may give qualitative information about renal function and contrast excretion, including the general degree of obstruction, if present. Because of its coronal plane and highly detailed images, it is a good imaging modality for evaluation of the collecting system of a renal duplication (Figure 5.7).

A UPJ obstruction is the most common congenital obstruction. The calyces and renal pelvis are dilated to a varying degree with no ureteral dilatation (Figure 5.8). The renal pelvis may often be disproportionately more dilated than the calyces. A prominent or large renal pelvis does not necessarily mean that there is hydronephrosis or an obstruction. There can be a prominent renal pelvis without calyceal dilatation. If the calyces are not dilated, then there is not likely to be obstruction. The renal parenchyma may be thinned to a varying degree. In severe obstruction, the parenchyma may be pencil thin, measuring only a few millimeters. The renal parenchyma may also appear echogenic and even contain tiny, non-communicating cysts. This may indicate an element of dysplasia due to long-standing severe obstruction (Figure 5.9). In UPJ obstruction the ureter is not dilated and usually not visualized. The renal pelvis may have a funnel appearance and extend inferiorly towards the bladder.

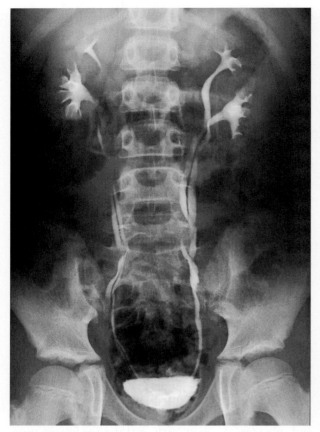

Figure 5.7 Excretory urogram of bilateral renal duplication.

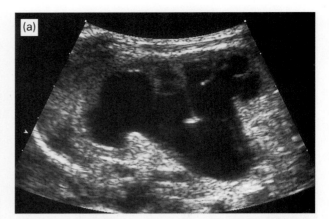

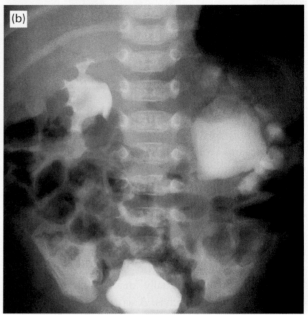

Figure 5.8 (*a*) Sonogram; and (*b*) excretory urogram of ureteropelvic junction obstruction.

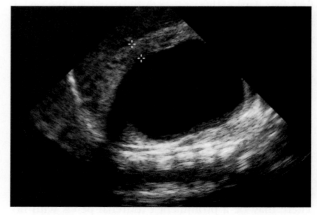

Figure 5.9 Neonatal sonogram of obstructed kidney with hyperechoic renal parenchyma.

This can be mistaken for dilatation of the proximal ureter on sonographic and renal scan evaluation. It is delineated more clearly as part of the renal pelvis and not the ureter on excretory urography. UPJ obstructions can be due to intrinsic stenosis, scarring, polyps, or extrinsic causes such as crossing vessels.

Obstruction of the UVJ is much less common than a UPJ obstruction. There is hydroureteronephrosis down to the level of the bladder with varying degrees of dilatation. The calyces may be mildly dilated with more marked dilatation of the distal ureter. Primary megaureter, an entity caused by an adynamic segment of distal ureter, may be part of an obstructed or non-obstructed system. These two entities are not always easily separated. Lasix washout studies can be invaluable in differentiating obstructed from non-obstructed ureters. The ureter, though, has the potential to act as a reservoir, resulting in apparent clearing of contrast of the upper collecting system, into what is actually an obstructed distal system (Figure

5.10). UVJ obstruction may be due to intrinsic causes such as distal ureteral stenosis, stones, or scarring, or extrinsic causes such as pelvic masses. High-grade reflux can give the appearance of a UVJ obstruction if post-void films are not taken to demonstrate drainage.

Hydroureteronephrosis may be associated with obstruction of an upper pole renal duplication. This is caused either by an ectopic ureterocele or ectopic insertion of the distal ureter of the upper pole moiety (Figure 5.11). The upper pole moiety may be small with a dilated pelvis and a varying amount of renal parenchymal thinning. Sometimes an upper pole moiety is not identified at all. There is just a dilated ureter extending medially, which appears to end just above the lower pole (Figure 5.12). There may be parenchymal dyplasia of the upper pole moiety.

PUV is a common cause of bilateral hydroureteronephrosis in boys. It is commonly diagnosed on routine prenatal sonography. Characteristically, there is fairly symmetric high-grade bilateral hydroureteronephrosis. The ureters may be very tortuous and difficult to follow and even resemble fluid-filled small bowel loops on sonography. Uncommonly, there may be only unilateral hydroureteronephrosis with high-grade reflux into the affected kidney. The opposite kidney may be normal in appearance or may

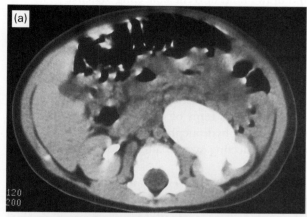

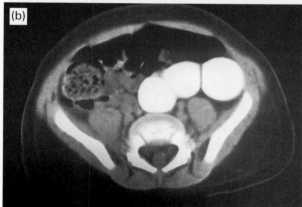

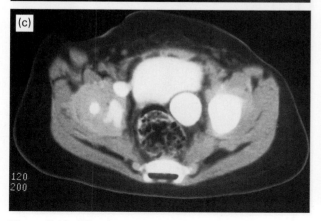

Figure 5.10 CTs of ureterovesical junction, with the ureter acting as a reservoir.

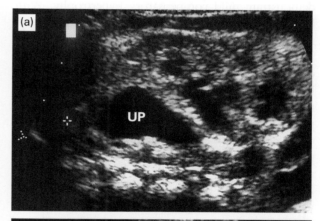

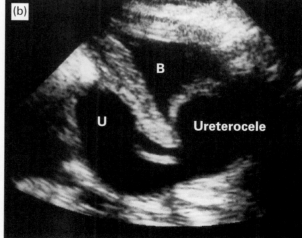

Figure 5.11 (*a*) Sonogram of obstructed upper pole segment (UP); (*b*) pelvic image demonstrating bladder (B), dilated upper pole ureter (U) and ureterocele.

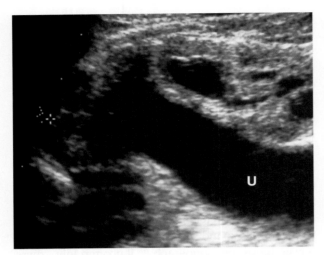

Figure 5.12 Sonogram massive dilated ureter and atrophic upper pole parenchyma (U = ureter).

demonstrate mild compensatory hypertrophy. With bilateral hydroureteronephrosis, the renal parenchyma is variably thinned. There may be renal dysplasia with echogenic renal parenchyma and small renal cysts (Slovis *et al.*, 1993; Kaefer *et al.*, 1997). The bladder wall is thickened and trabeculated owing to the chronic high pressure needed to generate flow past the obstructing valves. There is focal narrowing or a change in caliber at the level of the valves in the posterior urethra during voiding (Figure 5.13). This narrowing can be masked by an indwelling catheter. It is important to evaluate the urethra during voiding without an indwelling catheter. PUV are very thin and may not be visualized, but the secondary effect of the valves is demonstrated. The posterior urethra is widened and elongated. The anterior urethra is normal in contour but is not well filled out with voiding and may appear small in caliber.

Bilateral hydroureteronephrosis can be due to non-obstructed dilatation such as non-obstructed and non-refluxing megaureters or to reflux. The VCUG is an important diagnostic test to distinguish between these entities. The VCUG will evaluate the presence of reflux, a neuropathic bladder, bladder outlet obstructing lesions, such as a polyp or ureterocele, or urethral abnormalities such as valves, strictures, or diverticula.

Acquired obstructions of the collecting system may be intrinsic or extrinsic. Intrinsic causes include stones, hemorrhage, polyps, tumors, and scarring from previous surgery, trauma, or radiation therapy.

Extrinsic lesions include malignancy and inflammatory processes.

The child should be well hydrated for the best radiographic evaluation of the collecting system. If the child is fasting for sonography, the amount of collecting system dilatation can be underappreciated. Although children are fasting for CT or excretory urography before intravenous contrast material is administered, the contrast tends to serve as a diuretic and draws fluid into the collecting systems.

The renal parenchyma is best appreciated on the early images from CT or excretory urography. If there is a significant obstructive process, a delayed nephrogram is present. Contrast is normally excreted into the collecting system after 2–3 min, with contrast throughout the collecting system, including the bladder, on delayed films of 10 min. A full bladder may result in mild hydronephrosis. It is worthwhile imaging the collecting system after voiding, to determine

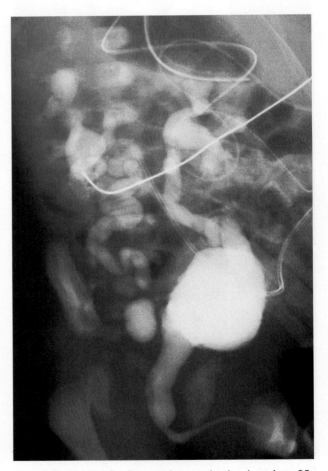

Figure 5.13 VCUG of posterior urethral valves in a 28-week gestation neonate with urinary ascites.

whether the hydronephrosis resolves. If there appears to be dilatation of the collecting system, intravenous Lasix may be given to evaluate how well the contrast washes out. This does not quantify the amount of washout or excretion, as does the radionuclide scan, but gives a visual or analog-type picture, which can yield useful information.

Infection

Urinary tract infection (UTI) is one of the most common reasons for imaging the urinary tract in children. In order to maintain renal function and prevent renal scarring and possible hypertension and renal failure later in life, most UTIs are actively worked up. Imaging of both the upper and lower urinary tracts is an essential part of the evaluation of UTI (Slovis, 1992).

The upper tracts are evaluated not only for detection of pyelonephritis, pyonephrosis, or abscess, but also for possible underlying causes of infection such as obstruction, stones, or tumor. Renal sonography is often the initial study of choice for the upper tracts. It is a non-invasive study with no ionizing radiation and relatively low cost. The sonogram is valuable in being able to rule out obstructive processes and tumors. If performed with diligence and attention to detail, it

offers an accurate indication of renal length and growth (Zerin and Blane, 1994; De Sanctis *et al.*, 1998). It is not as accurate as renal DMSA or excretory urography in the evaluation of renal scarring (Majd and Rushton, 1992; Shan *et al.*, 1992).

Sonography of pyelonephritis may demonstrate an asymmetric enlargement of the affected kidney with compression of the collecting system due to edema. Although sonography is not sensitive in detecting VUR, it may offer indirect evidence of reflux. The wall of the renal pelvis may be thickened, owing to intermittent distention from reflux (Figure 5.14) (Babcock, 1997). With a full bladder, there may be mild intermittent hydroureteronephrosis from ongoing reflux. In an active infection, echogenic debris may be floating within the bladder, ureter, and renal pelvis.

An area of pyonephrosis may appear as a small renal mass on sonography. In the appropriate clinical setting, this should be suspected to be an infectious process. Color flow Doppler can demonstrate decreased perfusion within areas of significant parenchymal inflammation (Dacher *et al.*, 1996). Both CT and DMSA are exquisitely sensitive in demonstrating perfusion defects (Figure 5.15). Radionuclide studies are discussed in detail in Chapter 6. On contrast-enhanced CT there will be multifocal, often streaky, peripheral areas of decreased density due to diminished perfusion from

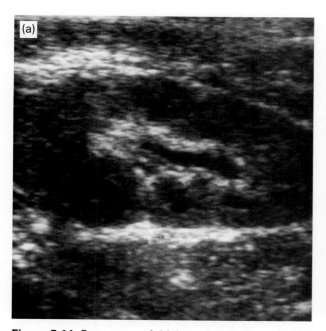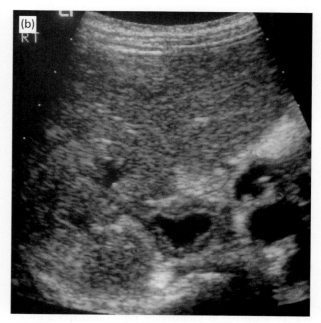

Figure 5.14 Sonogram of thickened wall of renal pelvis secondary to reflux.

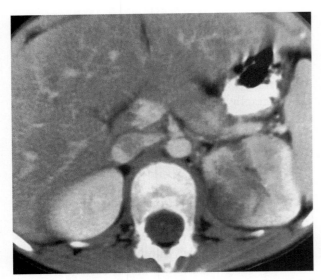

Figure 5.15 CT of pyelonephritis with decreased renal parenchymal enhancement.

edema and infection. Perinephric abscesses appear as low-density material within the perinephric space. These fluid collections may have thin enhancing walls and may extend into the adjacent psoas muscle.

Stones may predispose to renal infection. They may obstruct portions of the collecting system, form within areas of chronic obstruction from stasis, or act as foci of chronic infection. CT offers the best evaluation of renal stones, both intrarenal and extrarenal.

Uncommonly, renal tumors may present with signs and symptoms of a UTI. Therefore, it is always important to evaluate not only the lower tract but also the upper tract in cases of UTI.

The lower urinary tract is evaluated for reflux and urethral or bladder abnormalities, which would predispose to infection. Pyelonephritis is often secondary to VUR.

The lower urinary tract can be evaluated with a radionuclide or radiographic VCUG. The radiographic VCUG offers the best anatomical evaluation of the bladder and urethra in males and is usually done as the initial VCUG. It can demonstrate diverticula and trabeculations of the bladder wall, as well as filling defects and abnormalities of the urethra. Radionuclide cystography, although it does not have the anatomic resolution of the standard X-ray study, is very sensitive in identifying reflux and has a lower radiation exposure. After the VCUG has delineated

the anatomy on the initial study, reflux may be followed with radionuclide studies. Radionuclide may also be the study of first choice in asymptomatic siblings of children with reflux. Reflux occurs in up to one-third of these siblings (Tannous *et al.*, 1989). Reflux, which predisposes to the development of upper UTI, is present in 35% of white children with a UTI (Strife *et al.*, 1989). Children with an abnormal insertion of the distal ureter, or with structural abnormalities of the bladder such as Hutch diverticulum, bladder outlet obstruction, or neuropathic bladders are predisposed to reflux.

Acute pyelonephritis and subsequent renal scarring can occur in the absence of reflux. Imaging of the kidneys, in the absence of reflux, may reveal areas of infection and subsequent scarring. This may best be demonstrated on renal scintigraphy or CT.

The VCUG includes both filling and voiding phases. If the bladder is not filled to capacity, reflux may not be demonstrated. Reflux may only be present with a full bladder and during the higher pressure stages of voiding. Cyclical VCUG will detect reflux an additional 10% of the time (Paltiel *et al.*, 1992), although it is not always feasible to perform more than one cycle. Two cycles allow a more reliable evaluation of bladder capacity and the reproducibility of reflux during voiding. Reflux is graded according to the International Classification of grade I–V (Figure 5.16) (Leibowitz *et al.*, 1985). The appearance of the ureters, renal pelvis, and calyces during reflux may offer additional information beyond the grade of reflux. There may be reflux into the lower pole of a duplicated system, into scarred and deformed calyces from reflux nephropathy (Figure 5.17), intrarenal reflux, or high-grade reflux into a secondary UPJ obstruction. The ureters can be significantly wider and more patulous during a dynamic voiding study than during static upper tract imaging, such as an excretory urogram or CT. Fluoroscopy offers a physiological, as well as an anatomic, evaluation. There may be reflux only with voiding or throughout both filling and voiding stages. The child may void intermittently without a continuous contraction. Diverticula may enlarge during voiding and only be visualized at the end of the voiding cycle. The dynamic evaluation of the bladder during voiding offers useful information in the care of the child with an abnormal bladder or one who is a dysfunctional voider.

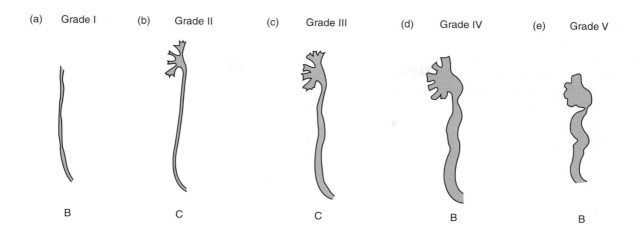

(a)   Grade I   (b)   Grade II   (c)   Grade III   (d)   Grade IV   (e)   Grade V

B   C   C   B   B

Figure 5.16 International classification of grade I–V vesicoureteral reflux. (Adapted from Leibowitz *et al.*, 1985.)

Stones

There are several predisposing factors to stone forma-tion in children. Nephrocalcinosis is the abnormal deposition of calcium in the renal parenchyma. This may be limited to the medullary pyramids, which is more common, or may be diffuse.

Very low birth weight premature infants are at risk of developing medullary nephrocalcinosis (Short and Cooke, 1991; Adam and Rowe, 1992). Nephro-calcinosis may occur on the basis of hypercalciuria owing to a combination of factors including diuretics, relative immobility, immature gastrointestinal tracts, and familial predisposition to stone formation (Karlo-wicz *et al.*, 1994). Children with nephrocalcinosis from other causes of hypercalciuria include those with underlying hypervitaminosis D, milk-alkali syndrome, sarcoidosis, hyperparathyroidism, hypercalcemia, hypophosphatemia, Bartter syndrome, Williams syn-drome, renal tubular acidosis, hyperoxaluria, and hyperuricemia.

Sonography is very sensitive in the evaluation of nephrocalcinosis. The deposition of minerals within the tubules of the medullary pyramids causes increas-ed interfaces for the ultrasound beam, which results in increased echogenicity. The ultrasound examination also has the advantage of being portable for the infant in the neonatal intensive care unit (NICU). Higher power linear transducers, such as a 7 MHz machine, offer superb resolution of the renal parenchyma and the cortical medullary echotecture. In medullary

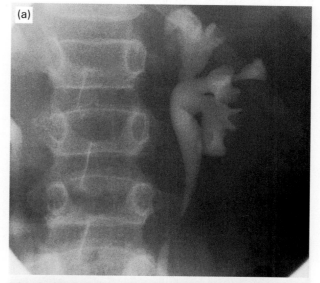

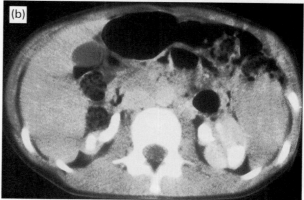

Figure 5.17 (*a*) VCUG and (*b*) CT of reflux nephropathy with renal scarring.

nephrocalcinosis, there is increased echogenicity of the medullary pyramids (Figure 5.18) (Myracle *et al.*, 1986). This tends to affect both kidneys symmetrically. If one of the kidneys has an underlying obstructive process, the nephrocalcinosis may be more prominent owing to the increased stasis within the tubules. Causes of echogenic medullary pyramids, other than nephrocalcinosis, include Tamm–Horsfall proteinuria, vascular congestion, infection, and autosomal recessive polycystic disease (Hernanz-Schulman, 1991). The calcium aggregates in the medulla and may form plaques and extend into the caliceal tips, serving as a nidus for the formation of well-defined stones (Gearhard *et al.*, 1991). There is a range in the appearance of medullary nephrocalcinosis. Mild nephrocalcinosis may demonstrate a peripheral rim of increased echogenicity. As the mineral content increases, the medullary pyramids fill in and become diffusely echogenic (Patriquin and Robitaille, 1988). The nephrocalcinosis may or may not cause shadowing. If stones form, they may cause urinary tract obstruction.

The incidence of urolithiasis, or discrete stones within the collecting system, in children is less than 0.1% (Gearhard *et al.*, 1991). Children may develop stones due to infection, obstruction, or hypercalcuria from diuretic therapy, to metabolic abnormalities such as hypercalcemia, hypercalciuria, hyperoxaluria, cystinuria, uricosuria, or xanthinuria, and to enzymatic abnormalities such as renal tubular acidosis. These children come to medical attention either in a genetic screening work-up or acutely in pain from a stone obstructing the collecting system. Most typically, children with obstructing stones present with pain and hematuria and possibly with proteinuria and leukocytosis. Like appendicitis, the renal stone presentation in children is often not classic and is worked up within a broad differential. For this reason, the plain abdominal film is the initial study of choice. It may confirm renal stones or suggest a separate disease process causing the abdominal pain. Stones are calcified 85% of the time.

If renal stones are strongly suspected clinically or by plain film, sonography may help to localize the site of the stone and the level of obstruction (Figure 5.19). The sensitivity of sonography for renal stones is 96% (Middleton *et al.*, 1988). Stones within the ureters may be obscured on sonography by overlying bowel gas. In some early cases of acute obstruction, there may not be hydronephrosis and the sonogram may offer a false-negative result. CT without contrast is the most sensitive modality for the detection of renal stones within either the kidney or the collecting system (Perlman *et al.*, 1996). Thin 3–6 mm section images are obtained continuously in a single breathhold, if possible for the child. This minimizes any 'skip' areas where stones may not be imaged because they are between slices. Stones are fairly easily detected on CT because of their inherent high density. Some obstructing stones may be only millimeters in size, however, and identified on only a single image. There is pre-

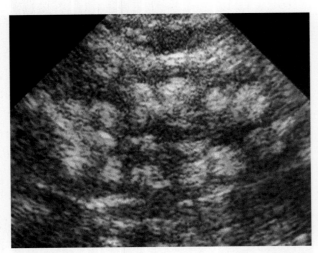

Figure 5.18 Sonogram of nephrocalcinosis, with increased echogenicity throughout the medullary pyramids.

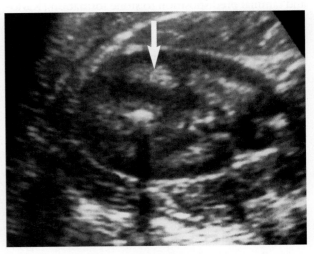

Figure 5.19 Sonogram of single renal stone with sharp focal area of increased echogenicity and posterior shadowing.

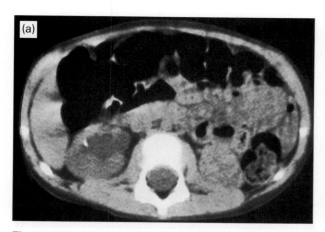

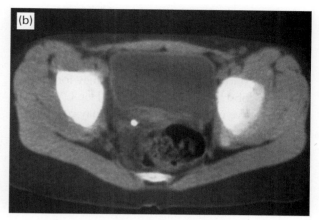

Figure 5.20 Non-contrast CT of right hydronephrosis, with distal obstructing right ureteral stone.

sumptive evidence of an obstructing stone when there is associated dilatation of the affected collecting system. There may be thickening of the wall of the collecting system and inflammatory stranding and edema in the soft tissue surrounding the renal pelvis and ureter. The CT study not only includes the kidneys but extends through the lower abdomen and pelvis to evaluate for possible ureteral or bladder stones (Figure 5.20). It is usually not necessary to administer intravenous contrast material to make the diagnosis of obstructing urolithiasis. If intravenous contrast is given, there may be delayed enhancement of the obstructed kidney. Excretory urography will often demonstrate evidence of renal obstruction with a delayed nephrogram and dilated collecting system. However, subtle cases may be difficult to diagnose with certainty, and thin section non-contrast CT has proven more reliable in making the diagnosis than excretory urography (Perlman *et al.*, 1996).

Sonography is not as reproducible or specific as CT in the staging of non-obstructing renal stones. CT is more accurate in following the number, size, and location of stones. Sonography is useful in detecting medium to large stones but if the stones are numerous it may be difficult to track their number and size accurately. Tiny stones may not be visualized on sonography. There can be small focal echogenic material in the renal parenchyma such as fat, prominent vessels, or gas, which may be difficult to differentiate from tiny stones. Air within the collecting system, following a VCUG, is a classic mimic of stones (Figure 5.21). MRI is not sensitive in the detection of stone material.

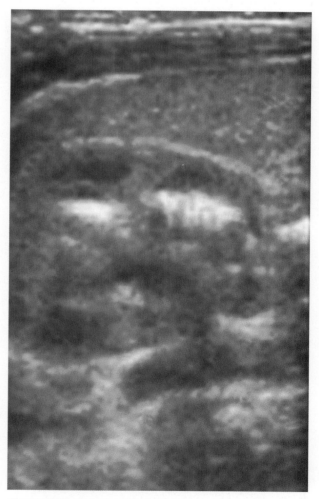

Figure 5.21 Sonogram of air within the calyces that is echogenic and mimics stones. The air within the collecting system was due to VCUG prior to the sonogram in a child with reflux.

Stones may be associated with infection. They may represent a chronic focus of infection that prevents a UTI from clearing. They may also form as a secondary reaction to chronic infection because of an altered pH status of the urine. Stones may form proximal to an obstruction, such as a UPJ or UVJ, in an area of relative urinary stasis. Stones may continue to form after the obstruction is relieved by surgery.

Tumors

Wilms' tumor

This is the most common malignant renal tumor of childhood. Wilms' tumor develops from primitive metanephric blastema and is known for its histologic diversity. It represents 6% of childhood cancers. The mean age at diagnosis is 3–4 years for unilateral disease and 2–3 years for bilateral disease. It is associated with anomalies such as aniridia, hemihypertrophy, hypospadias, and cryptorchidism (Green *et al.*, 1997).

Wilms' tumor typically presents as an abdominal mass. Clinical findings may include hematuria, pain, fever, and hypertension. Radiographically, Wilms' tumor typically appears as a large, well-defined mass arising out of the kidney with compression of adjacent renal parenchyma and distortion and/or obstruction of the adjacent renal pelvis and calyces. A thin rim of normal appearing renal parenchyma can usually be identified extending along the periphery of the mass. It uncommonly invades the collecting system. While the masses are typically very large and often cross the midline, they do not often encase vessels and invade adjacent organs, unlike a neuroblastoma, which is the main differential in this age group. Neuroblastoma tends to encase adjacent structures early in its course, has a characteristic speckled calcification in 90% of cases and commonly contains large areas of necrosis and hemorrhage (Figure 5.22). These features and its younger age at presentation, with a median age of 18 months, helps to differentiate neuroblastoma from Wilms' tumor. Wilms' tumor tends to displace and compress but does not invade or infiltrate until late stages. Favorable histology Wilms' tumors, despite their large size, are often totally surgically resectable at presentation, owing to relatively late extension and late metastatic disease. Stage 1 favorable histology Wilms' has a prognosis of 90% survival, regardless of its size (Cohen, 1996).

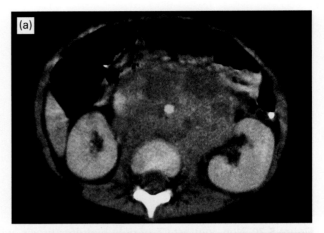

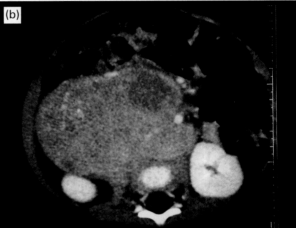

Figure 5.22 CT of neuroblastoma, with a large, partially necrotic calcified retroperitoneal mass encasing vessels.

On sonography, Wilms' tumor may have a relatively homogeneous echotecture or may be inhomogeneously echogenic with scattered internal cystic areas representing hemorrhage or necrosis (Figure 5.23). Fat or calcification may appear as focal areas of markedly increased echogenicity. Normal compressed renal parenchyma can be identified at the periphery of the mass. Smaller hypoechoic solid masses in the same or opposite kidney may indicate second tumors, bilateral disease, or areas of nephroblastomatosis (Figure 5.24).

Color-flow Doppler evaluation of the renal vein and IVC for extension of tumor thrombus, which occurs in 5–10% of cases, is an important part of the sonographic examination. Demonstrating patency of the renal vein by color-flow Doppler does not exclude

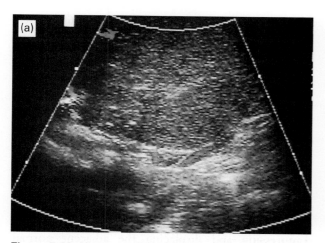
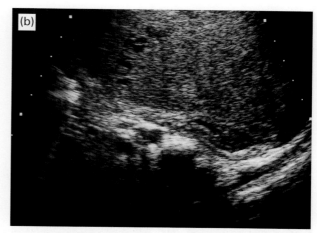

Figure 5.23 Ultrasound scans of large Wilms' tumors replacing and compressing much of the kidneys.

extension of non-occlusive tumor thrombus in the renal veins or IVC. Gray-scale evaluation of the renal vein and IVC is necessary to exclude tumor involvement, which appears as a fairly well-defined intraluminal echogenic mass, surrounded by anechoic flowing blood. Extensive thrombus tends to enlarge the renal vein and/or IVC, often making it easier to visualize (Figure 5.25). The renal vein may be difficult to visualize owing to the distortion of the normal renal parenchyma and hilum by the tumor. Collateral veins may develop at the renal hilum that may be indistinguishable from the renal vein.

CT is valuable, not only in evaluation of the primary renal mass, but also in staging of the entire abdomen. Calcifications can be demonstrated on non-contrast CT in 10% of Wilms' tumors (Kaufman *et al.*, 1978). Non-contrast CT may demonstrate focal areas of internal hemorrhage, which will be slightly higher in density than the adjacent parenchyma. Contrast-enhanced CT demonstrates inhomogeneous enhancement of the mass, with some central areas of low density representing necrosis. There will be a variable rim of enhancing, normal renal parenchyma stretched along the edge of the mass, known as the

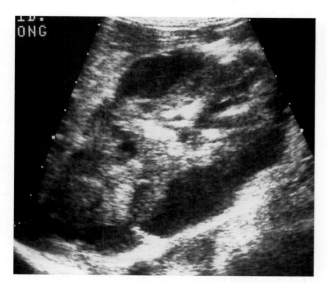

Figure 5.24 Sonogram of nephroblastomatosis with multiple hypoechoic peripheral renal masses.

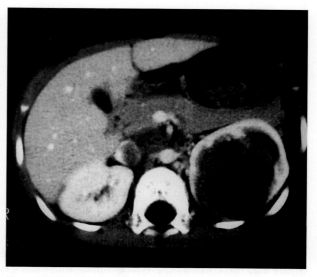

Figure 5.25 CT of a left renal Wilms' tumor, with extension into the renal vein and inferior vena cava.

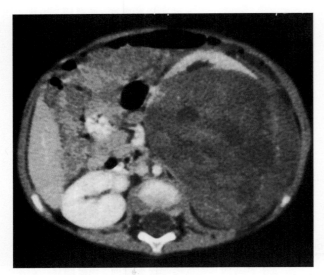

Figure 5.26 CT of left Wilms' tumor, with a thin rim or claw sign or normal parenchyma stretched around the tumor.

claw sign. This helps to identify the kidney as the origin of the mass. The large tumor often creates an obstructive process with delay of contrast filling the collecting system of the involved kidney (Figure 5.26). Delayed images may be needed to delineate further the location and possible involvement of the renal pelvis and ureter. Extension of tumor into the collecting system may be visualized as a filling defect on these delayed images (Mitchell and Yeo, 1997). Involvement of the lymph nodes at the renal hilum

and in the retroperitoneum occurs in 20% of cases. Enlarged lymph nodes are not specific for malignant involvement and may be due to a reactive process or lymphatic engorgement secondary to venous or lymphatic obstruction. Extension of tumor beyond the renal capsule may be suggested by irregularity and loss of the sharp margin or contour of the tumor capsule with ill-defined tissue extending into the perirenal space. Adjacent organs, such as the liver, spleen, and pancreas, are usually compressed and displaced by the Wilms' tumor. It may be difficult on CT to exclude tumor extension into the adjacent liver, due to the appearance on axial imaging of tumor compressing and displacing the adjacent normal hepatic tissue. MRI and ultrasound may offer a better evaluation of the margins of the tumor because of their ability to image in the coronal and sagittal planes.

Extension of tumor into the renal veins and IVC may be identified as well on CT as on ultrasound, depending on the staging of intravenous contrast enhancement. With fast CT technology, a biphasic CT examination can highlight both the arterial and venous phase of intravenous contrast enhancement. Uncommonly, tumor may extend into the distal intrahepatic IVC, with resulting obstruction of the hepatic veins. This creates hepatic congestion and a Budd–Chiari type of picture (Figure 5.27). Rarely, there may be intracardiac extension of tumor, which can impede right heart cardiac output (Figure 5.28) (Ritchey et al., 1988).

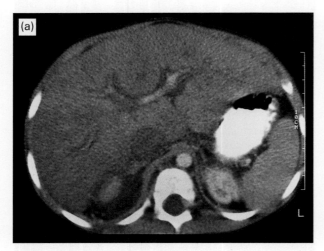
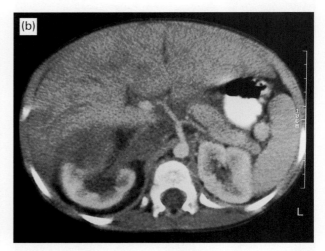

Figure 5.27 (a) CT of a right Wilms' tumor with extension into the right renal vein and inferior vena cava; and (b) CT showing that the thrombus obstructs the hepatic veins, resulting in hepatic congestion, delayed hepatic enhancement, and a Budd–Chiari type of appearance.

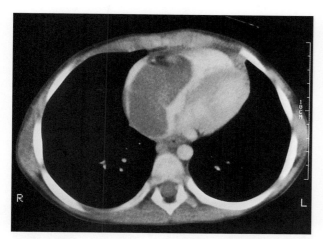

Figure 5.28 CT of intracardiac extension of Wilms' tumor.

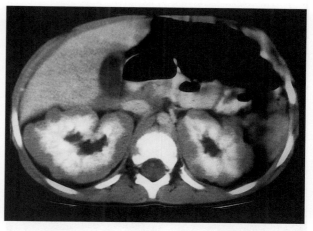

Figure 5.30 CT of nephroblastomatosis, with multiple small, low-density masses in the periphery of both kidneys (see also Figure 5.24).

MRI is ideal for evaluation of possible tumor extension into the renal veins, IVC, hepatic veins, and heart. It also offers an excellent evaluation of the primary renal mass and involvement of the opposite kidney, liver, and renal hilar adenopathy (Belt *et al.*, 1986; Gylys-Morin *et al.*, 1993). There is little role for invasive angiography, except for presurgical evaluation of anomalous vasculature or complex vascular involvement.

There is bilateral renal involvement in 5% of cases (Figure 5.29). This is most commonly synchronous but can be metachronous. Bilateral involvement is more common with associated congenital anomalies, younger age, and nephroblastomatosis. Multifocal disease in the same kidney is also associated with nephroblastomatosis. Nephroblastomatosis is charac-

terized by multifocal involvement of the kidneys with embryonic nephrogenic rests, which are precursors of malignant Wilms' tumors (Figure 5.30). Nephroblastomatosis rests are found in 30% of Wilms' tumor cases. These children are at higher risk of developing recurrent Wilms' tumor. The recurrence can occur many years after apparently successful treatment and thus mandates long-term imaging follow-up. The child may present with any number of masses of varying size within each or both kidneys. Nephroblastomatosis classically occurs in the subcapsular region of the renal cortex. It may be single or multiple. They may be so numerous that they create a lobular scalloped ring around the periphery of the kidney. They are classically hypoechoic on sonography (Figure 5.24) and display minimal enhancement on CT (Figure 5.30). A biopsy specimen and an experienced renal pathologist is needed to differentiate Wilms' tumor from nephroblastomatosis.

The staging of Wilms' depends on tumor extension and metastatic disease. The prognosis depends more on histology than on stage. Favorable histology Wilms' tumor make up 90% of the cases. The unfavorable histology Wilms' has a worse prognosis than favorable histology. Rhabdoid and clear cell sarcoma are two types of malignant renal tumors in children that are not classified as Wilms' variants. Both of these tumors have a much less favorable prognosis than Wilms', with a higher rate of relapse and death. They metastasize to lung, bone, and brain. Rhabdoid tumor should be considered in an infant of less than 6 months who presents with a solid renal tumor.

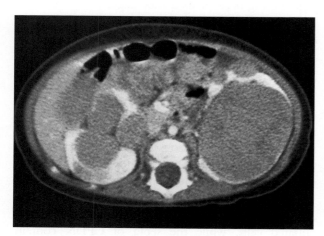

Figure 5.29 CT of bilateral Wilms' tumor.

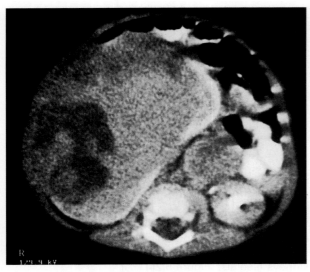

Figure 5.31 CT of rhabdoid tumor of right kidney in a 4-month-old child. There is extension outside of the renal capsule and malignant adenopathy on the left para-aortic region.

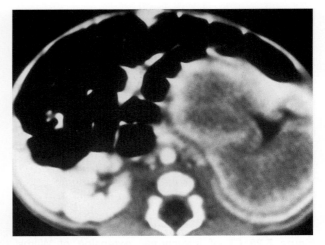

Figure 5.32 CT of mesoblastic nephroma.

Radiologically, it is difficult to differentiate Wilms' from a rhabdoid or a clear cell sarcoma. The latter two malignancies may present with a more aggressive malignant picture than favorable histology Wilms', which tends to stay encapsulated and localized until late in its course (Figure 5.31).

Staging of a Wilms' tumor should include close evaluation of the opposite kidney for a mass with CT or MRI. Chest radiography is not adequate in detecting and quantifying metastatic lung nodules. Chest CT offers the best evaluation of the lungs for possible metastatic disease (Owens *et al.*, 1993). The renal vein and IVC should be evaluated with CT, ultrasound or MRI for extension of tumor. Extension of tumor into the IVC is of paramount importance for the surgeon to know before attempting resection. With bilateral renal tumors or IVC extension, the child may be placed on a course of chemotherapy before surgical resection is attempted.

Congenital mesoblastic nephroma

Although unusual, this is the most common solid renal tumor of infancy. The median age at presentation is 2 months and it has even been identified on fetal sonography (Bolande *et al.*, 1967; Matsumura *et al.*, 1993). There is a male predominance. Pathologically, it is characterized by spindle cells infiltrating into the renal parenchyma and the perinephric spaces.

There is variable opinion by pathologists on the malignant potential of mesoblastic nephroma. The more cellular mesoblastic nephroma, presenting over 3 months of age, may have potential for malignant behavior. Overall, it is associated with good outcomes and is usually treated only by nephrectomy. Wide margins of surgical resection and close follow-up are recommended.

Radiographically, mesoblastic nephroma presents as a large, solid, renal mass. It may have ill-defined margins because of its infiltration into perirenal soft tissue. It may not be able to be differentiated from a Wilms' tumor, except for the young age at presentation. On sonography it is relatively hypoechoic and on CT it has a low density with little enhancement (Hartman *et al.*, 1981; Kirks and Kaufman, 1989) (Figure 5.32). It may have internal cystic regions representing necrosis or hemorrhage.

Multilocular cystic nephroma

This uncommon cystic renal tumor affects mainly young boys and older women (Agrons *et al.*, 1995). It appears as a large, complex, cystic mass arising out of the kidney. The tumor is a well-encapsulated, multiloculated cystic renal mass with multiple internal septations. There are no solid components of this tumor other than the septa. Pathologically it is divided into two types: cystic nephroma (CN) and cystic poorly differentiated nephroblastoma (CPDN). Microscopically the septa of CN contain well-differentiated cells, while the septa of CPDN contain blastemal elements. Histologically they are benign.

Some regard CPDN as a transition between the benign CN and the malignant Wilms' tumor (Joshi and Beckwith, 1989). Nephrectomy with total tumor resection is usually curative. There is potential for CPDN to recur and close radiographic follow-up is warranted.

Radiographically, CN and CPDN are similar in appearance. On ultrasound, CT and MRI they appear as an encapsulated multilocular cystic mass. There may be fine calcifications within the septa. The septations are thin, with no solid nodular components. If a solid component is identified, other renal masses such as a necrotic Wilms' should be considered. On sonography the multiple cysts may be so small as not to be discretely identifiable and the mass may appear echogenically solid (Banner *et al.*, 1981). On CT the septa may enhance after intravenous contrast, but the cystic spaces remain low in density (Parienty *et al.*, 1981). If the cysts are very small, the mass may appear solid. Limited MRI experience with cystic nephroma demonstrates the capsule and septa to be low signal on T1-weighted images. The septa may enhance after gadolinium. The cysts themselves are of variable signal intensity, depending on the proteinaceous or hemorrhagic content of the fluid. The cysts do not enhance after gadolinium (Dikengil *et al.*, 1988). The differential diagnosis of multilocular cystic nephroma includes multicystic dysplastic kidney, which is usually smaller and does not have a normal appearing renal parenchyma. A very necrotic or hemorrhagic Wilms' tumor, clear cell sarcoma, or a cystic variant of mesoblastic nephroma may be suggestive of a cystic nephroma but have solid components that a multicystic nephroma does not (Madewell *et al.*, 1983).

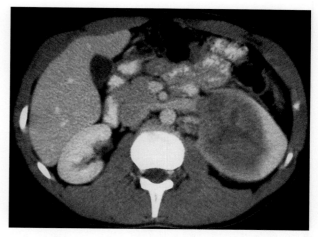

Figure 5.33 CT of renal cell cancer with a single left renal mass in a 15-year-old adolescent.

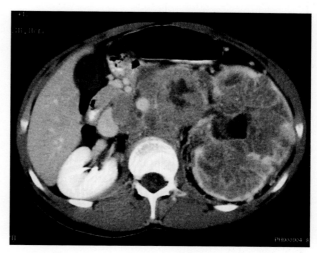

Figure 5.34 CT of a left renal cell cancer in a 14-year-old with extensive retroperitoneal metastasis.

Renal cell carcinoma

This is rare in children. It presents with a flank mass, pain, and or hematuria. The incidence of renal cell carcinoma approaches that of Wilms' in the adolescent age group (Douglas and Pratt, 1997). The median age at presentation for children is 11 years. It presents as a solid renal mass, usually smaller than Wilms' tumor. On CT it appears as a solid mass with some degree of enhancement (Figure 5.33). It is usually encapsulated but may be infiltrating with poorly defined margins. There are focal calcifications in 25% of cases. Sonography demonstrates a solid mass of variable echogenicity. MRI demonstrates a solid

mass, which may have areas of hemorrhage or necrosis. Doppler ultrasound is used to evaluate the renal vein and IVC. Renal cell carcinoma spreads to nodes at the renal hilum and metastasizes to the lung, bone, and liver (Figure 5.34). The prognosis depends on stage at presentation. If resectable, it may be curable by surgery. Renal cell carcinoma is poorly amenable to chemotherapy.

Lymphoma and leukemia

These may both secondarily involve the kidneys. They may both present as diffuse infiltrative enlargement of

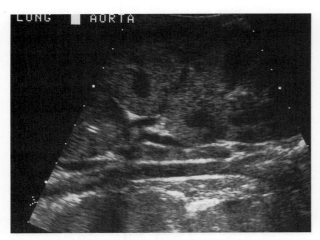

Figure 5.35 Sonogram of massive bilateral renal enlargement secondary to acute lymphoblastic leukemia in a 2-year-old child.

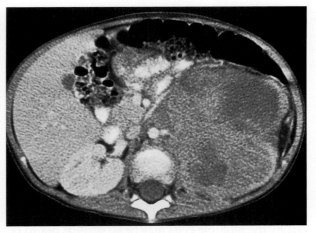

Figure 5.37 CT of neuroblastoma, with extension into the upper pole of the left kidney.

the kidneys without evidence of a focal mass (Figure 5.35). Lymphoma most commonly involves the kidney as multiple solid renal masses of varying sizes. These masses are commonly hypoechoic on sonography and low density with mild enhancement on CT (Figure 5.36). It can present as a single mass, multiple bilateral renal masses, or with extension into adjacent retroperitoneal lymph nodes. Hydronephrosis may develop from obstructing retroperitoneal or pelvic adenopathy (Hartman *et al.*, 1982; Weinberger *et al.*, 1990).

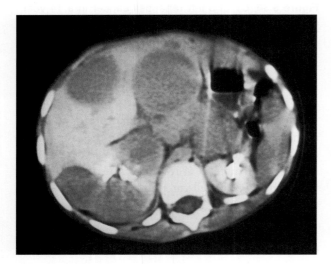

Figure 5.36 CT of hepatic and renal masses from Burkitt's lymphoma.

Neuroblastoma

Uncommonly, this may invade the kidney by extension from a suprarenal retroperitoneal origin. If this invasion is extensive, it may make it difficult to differentiate a neuroblastoma from a primary renal malignancy (Figure 5.37). Features such as encasement of vessels and internal calcification help to characterize it as a neuroblastoma.

Angiomyolipoma

This type of hamartoma is a benign solid renal tumor, associated with tuberous sclerosis. It may present as a solitary mass or multiple renal masses of variable size. Sonography typically demonstrates well-defined echogenic masses. The amount of increased echogenicity depends on the fat content. The angiomyolipomas may diffusely involve the kidney replacing much of the normal renal parenchyma (Figure 5.38). Fat within an angiomyolipoma commonly demonstrates characteristic low density on non-contrast CT; if the fat content is minimal, the angiomyolipoma may have a non-specific appearance. Patients with tuberous sclerosis may also have lymphangiomatous involvement of the kidneys and perinephric space.

Lymphangiomas

These may affect the kidneys. Lymphangiomas may be sporadic or associated with tuberous sclerosis or Klippel Trenaunay syndrome. Lymphangiomas pre-

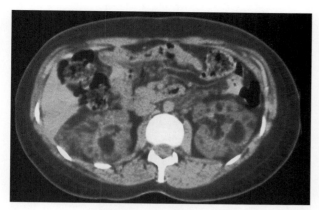

Figure 5.38 CT of diffuse angiomyolipomas with multiple fatty density renal masses.

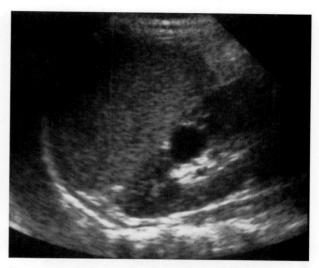

Figure 5.40 Sonogram of a simple cyst in a 5-year-old child.

sent less as a well-defined mass than as an infiltrative process. On sonography, they are inhomogeneously echogenic with ill-defined margins. On CT, there are low-density areas interspersed within more normal appearing tissue (Figure 5.39). If there is a hemangiomatous component, there may be areas of hazy enhancement after administration of intravenous contrast.

Cystic kidney disease

While not as commonly as in the adult population, children may have benign, simple renal cysts. These cysts are variable in size but may be large enough to compress adjacent renal parenchyma (Figure 5.40).

Cysts demonstrated by ultrasound appear as well-defined anechoic masses with thin walls. There are cystic appearing structures on ultrasound that may not represent the cysts. For example, it may be difficult to differentiate a calyceal diverticulum from a renal cyst. In newborns, the medullary pyramids may be so hypoechoic and rounded in configuration that, depending on the sonographic technique, they may be mistaken for multiple renal cysts (Figure 5.41). Marked dilatation of the calyces, if they are not visually connectable to the renal pelvis on sonography, may be mistaken for cystic kidney disease.

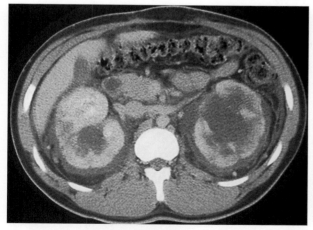

Figure 5.39 CT of a lymphangioma with involvement of both kidneys with low-density material in the perinephric space and extending into the renal parenchyma.

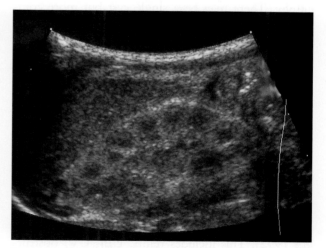

Figure 5.41 Sonogram of prominent hypoechoic normal renal pyramids in a newborn.

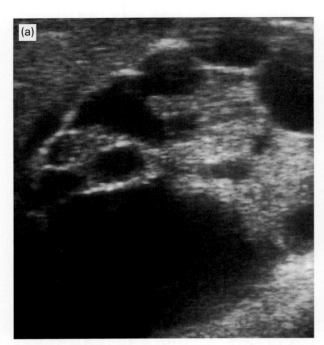

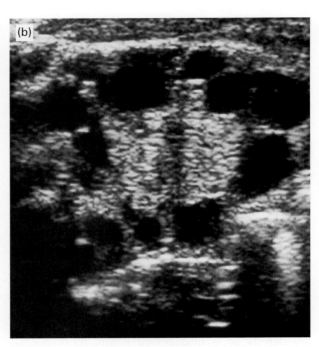

Figure 5.42 Sonograms of multicystic dysplastic kidneys with multiple cysts of varying sizes that do not communicate.

Numerous renal cysts of various sizes and configurations may be present in a spectrum of underlying cystic renal diseases. These would include autosomal dominant and recessive polycystic kidney disease (ADPKD and ARPKD), cystic disease of tuberous sclerosis, glomerulocystic disease, and MCDK.

Multicystic dysplastic kidney

MCDK has a characteristic appearance on sonography. There may be a single cyst but more commonly there are multiple, thin-walled cysts of varying sizes, which do not communicate. No definite renal pelvis is identified. Little, if any, solid renal parenchymal tissue is identified (Figure 5.42). If present, it does not have the expected appearance of renal tissue. There is absent or only a minimal amount of blood flow detected by Doppler ultrasound. The cysts commonly regress over time and may disappear altogether (Gordon *et al.*, 1988; Vinocur *et al.*, 1988; Strife *et al.*, 1993). Conversely, the cysts may grow or remain stable in appearance over time. There is an abnormality of the opposite kidney, besides compensatory hypertrophy, in 30% of patients (Atiyehm *et al.*, 1992). This includes reflux, UPJ, UVJ obstruction, and duplication. A MCDK may demonstrate other anomalies, such as an ectopic location, or be part of a duplicated kidney (Figure 5.43). In a child with a MCDK it is worthwhile to perform a VCUG to rule out reflux and closely evaluate the opposite solitary kidney. It is not uncommon to detect reflux into the distal remnant ureter of a MCDK. This suggests early development of a renal collecting system, which has become discontinuous and atretic at some time during embryonic life. A MCDK may represent extreme obstruction early in embryonic life of the collecting system (Avni *et al.*, 1986). The renal pelvis

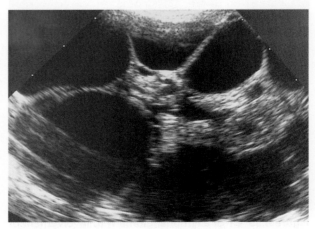

Figure 5.43 Sonogram of multicyctic dysplastic kidney in the upper pole of a renal duplication.

and calyces become discontinuous, forming multiple cystic structures in the renal fossa (Fig. 5.44). There may be cases in which it is difficult to differentiate with certainty a MCDK from a severe UPJ obstruction by sonography. Definitive diagnosis of MCDK is made when non-function on the renal scan is found in conjunction with the typical cystic appearance on sonogram.

Autosomal recessive polycystic kidney disease

This inherited disorder of the renal tubules also affects the hepatic parenchyma at later stages in life. Sonography offers a fairly characteristic appearance of ARPKD. The kidneys are symmetrically enlarged and inhomogeneously echogenic. The increased echogenicity is due to the ectasia of the tubules. This myriad of mildly dilated tubules, or microscopic cysts, results in multiple interfaces and an echogenic appearance (Figure 5.45). There may be an occasional macroscopic cyst, but these are not the dominant picture as they are in ADPKD. There may be little or no cortical medullary differentiation or the medullary pyramids may have an increased speckled echotecture in relationship to the renal cortex. The renal pelvis and calyces tend to be patulous rather than hydronephrotic. Evaluation of the liver may demonstrate a few small cysts. Over time, the liver demonstrates slightly increased echotecture and the spleen becomes enlarged owing to portal hypertension. If the renal involvement is minimal, the child may present in the second decade of life with hepatic involvement and gastrointestinal bleeding due to varices.

Contrast-enhanced CT and excretory urography demonstrate a unique and characteristic appearance of ARPKD. They may not be able to be performed if the child's creatinine is elevated. There is a striated appearance of the nephrogram, with delayed filling of the tubules. Streaky, linear, low-density areas are interspersed with more normally enhancing parenchyma. There is no distinct separation between the cortical and medullary enhancement (Figure 5.46).

Autosomal dominant polycystic kidney disease

This can present in late childhood or adolescence with multiple cysts, which are relatively small in size, initially. The cysts grow in size and number over time.

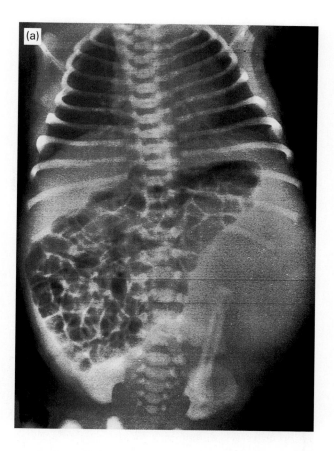

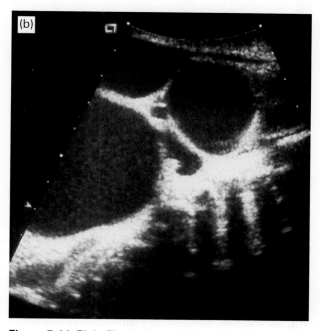

Figure 5.44 Plain film and sonogram of large left multicystic dysplasia kidney in a newborn.

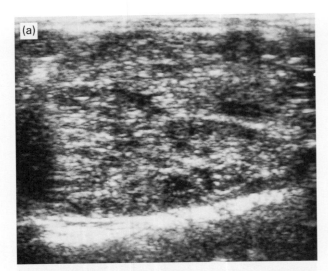

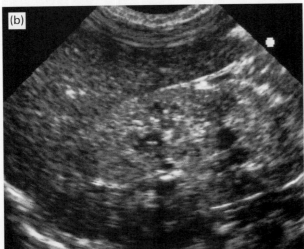

Figure 5.45 Sonograms of two infants with autosomal recessive polycystic kidney disease. The kidneys are enlarged and inhomogeneous.

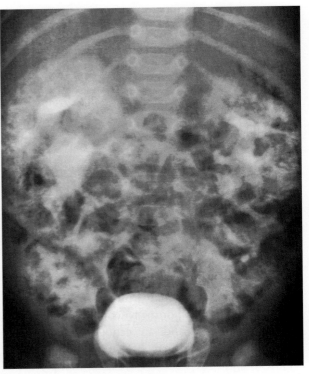

Figure 5.46 Excretory urography of autosomal recessive polycystic kidney disease, with bilaterally enlarged kidneys with inhomogeneous enhancement and patulous renal calyces and pelves.

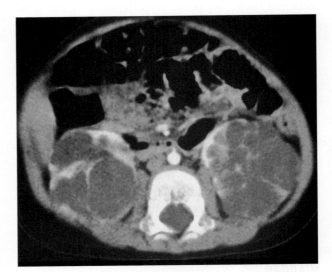

Figure 5.47 CT of autosomal dominant polycystic kidney disease with multiple cysts of varying sizes within bilaterally enlarged kidneys with distorted but otherwise normal appearing parenchyma.

The renal parenchyma is normal in echotecture early on. With time, the parenchyma becomes compressed by the multiple cysts. The collecting system also becomes distorted, compressed and obstructed by the cysts. CT, ultrasound, and MRI all demonstrate the characteristic appearance of ADPKD. CT and MRI offer the most global view of the massively enlarged kidneys (Figure 5.47). It may be difficult on sonography to reliably reproduce findings between examinations and to evaluate totally both kidneys in fine detail. While most of the cysts are low density on CT and anechoic on sonography, some may be higher in density if they contain elements of hemorrhage. These higher density cysts should not enhance after intravenous contrast administration and should demonstrate through transmission on sonography. Calcification in the wall of the cysts is a common finding. Patients with ADPKD are at slightly greater risk of developing renal cell carcinoma later in life.

Uncommonly, there may be overlap between the appearance of ADPKD and ARPKD. Children with ADPKD may present in infancy with enlarged hyperechoic kidneys resembling ARPKD. Some children with ARPKD may have multiple macroscopic cysts within enlarged kidneys that resemble ADPKD. Both groups of patients may develop multiple hepatic cysts. Inheritance patterns and screening of parents and siblings can help to differentiate these two entities.

Tuberous sclerosis

Children with tuberous sclerosis may develop polycystic renal disease that mimics ADPKD. There may be multiple cysts of varying sizes throughout both kidneys. There are cases of children with tuberous sclerosis who also have ADPKD.

Glomerulocystic renal disease

This is associated with multiple congenital anomalies. The kidneys are mildly enlarged and contain multiple relatively smaller cysts. The cysts do not enlarge as much as in ADPKD. The renal echotecture is homogeneously increased, in comparison with ARPKD, in which the parenchyma is inhomogeneously increased in echotexture.

Glomerulocystic renal disease is a non-specific term. It is used to describe kidneys that on ultrasound may be small in size and diffusely increased in echotecture, and contain any number of small, scattered cysts. These kidneys may have suffered a significant insult, such as severe reflux or obstruction, during development, so that the parenchyma never developed normally. They may also represent congenitally dysplastic renal mesenchyma, which was abnormal in the initial stages of development. In either case, when these kidneys are identified, it is difficult to tell how well and for how long they will function.

Renal parenchymal disease

There are numerous causes of acute inflammatory conditions of the kidneys. Some of these are due to infectious causes such as pyelonephritis, poststrepto-coccal glomerulonephritis, and hemolytic uremic syndrome. Others causes of acute inflammation include non-infectious glomerulonephritis, nephrotic syndrome, or vasculitides such as Henoch Schönlein purpura and polyarteritis nodosa. On sonography, the kidneys may appear normal in size or may be enlarged. The renal parenchyma may be normal in echotecture or there may be increased cortical echogenicity, with preservation of cortical medullary differentiation (Figure 5.48) (Hricak *et al.*, 1982). The enlargement and increased echotecture may be due to edema and infiltration from the inflammatory/vasculitic process.

These children may be unable to tolerate CT with intravenous contrast material due to poor renal funtion. Non-contrast CT may demonstrate symmetrically enlarged kidneys, which are slightly lower in density than expected. If intravenous contrast is able to be given, the kidneys may appear enlarged with diminished enhancement. Ascites may be present.

Some of these entities may ultimately result in chronic renal disease. The appearance of the kidneys in chronic end-stage renal disease (ESRD) is non-specific for etiology. On sonographic evaluation, the kidneys are small in size and diffusely increased in echotecture with loss of cortical medullary echogenicity (Rosenfield and Siegel, 1981).

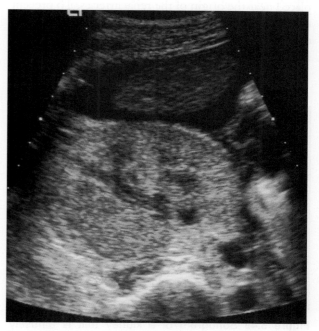

Figure 5.48 Sonogram of renal parenchymal disease with enlarged kidneys.

Vascular disease

Renal vein thrombosis during infancy and childhood is associated with dehydration, infants of diabetic mothers, nephrotic syndrome, coagulopathies, sepsis, and malignancies such as Wilms' tumor. Hematuria, proteinuria, and hypertension are the non-specific presenting symptoms. On sonography, the affected kidney is diffusely enlarged and inhomogeneously increased in echotecture due to edema and hemorrhage (Figure 5.49) (Rosenfield *et al.*, 1980). There is loss of the normal renal architecture with little or no corticomedullary differentiation. Clot may be identified within the renal vein and/or the IVC. Doppler evaluation may show little or no flow in the renal vein. There may be high-resistance flow in the renal artery with diminished diastolic arterial flow. This is due to vascular congestion from obstructed venous outflow. Venous flow is re-established by the development of venous collaterals and recanalization of the thrombosed veins. The extent and length of venous occlusion will affect the degree of renal recovery. If the renal vein thrombosis is highly occlusive, there will be long-term atrophy of the kidney with persistent increased echotecture of the renal parenchyma (Laplante *et al.*, 1992) (Figure 5.50).

Renal artery thrombosis may occur during the neonatal period from an umbilical artery catheter placed near the origin of the renal arteries. To prevent this problem, most such catheters are placed below L_2 or above T_{10}. Other causes of renal artery thrombosis include dehydration, sepsis, and emboli. The kidney

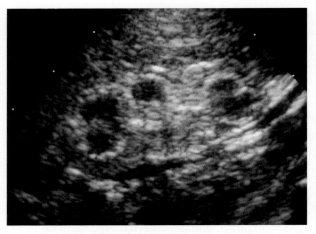

Figure 5.50 Follow-up sonogram of a small atrophic kidney due to renal vein thrombosis 3 months earlier (same patient as Figure 5.49).

may be normal in size and increased in echotecture from edema. Doppler evaluation will be unable to detect arterial flow at the renal hilum and thrombus may be detected within the renal artery lumen. Over time, collateral arteries will develop at the periphery of the kidney. Similarly to renal vein thrombosis, kidney atrophy depends on the length and degree of arterial compromise.

Renal artery occlusion may also occur following trauma. Hematuria may or may not be present. CT, which is the imaging modality of choice following

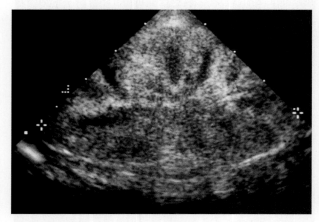

Figure 5.49 Sonogram of a kidney that is diffusely enlarged and echogenic due to renal vein thrombosis in a newborn with hypertension.

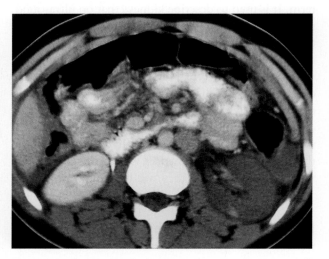

Figure 5.51 CT demonstrating non-enhancement of the left kidney, due to renal artery dissection in a child kicked by a horse.

significant trauma, will demonstrate lack of enhancement of the affected kidney in comparison with the opposite kidney (Figure 5.51). Occlusion or dissection of a segmental renal branch will result in lack of enhancement of a sharply demarcated portion of the kidney in a wedge-shaped distribution. Delayed images of complete renal artery occlusion will fail to demonstrate contrast within the collecting system. Angiography will offer the best anatomic resolution of renal artery damage.

Renal artery narrowing in children may be due to fibromuscular dysplasia, radiation arteritis, congenital stenosis, neurofibromatosis, and arteritides such as Takayasu's. Other causes of hypertension include reflux nephropathy with significant scarring, and tumors. The radiographic work-up of hypertension includes Doppler sonography, CT and MRI, captopril-enhanced renal scan, or radiographic angiography of the renal arteries. Angiography is considered the gold standard for evaluation of vascular stenosis but represents an invasive procedure with some risks involved for the child.

Doppler evaluation is the initial study of choice. The entire length of both renal arteries is evaluated to identify an area of increased velocity that would indicate a focal area of stenosis. Classically, there will be a significant elevation of the peak systolic velocity, >180 cm/s, and a ratio of renal artery to abdominal aortic velocity of >3.5:1. There is turbulence distal to the site of stenosis and increased resistance proximally (Babcock and Patriquin, 1998) (Figure 5.52). Evaluation of intrarenal branch vessels can suggest significant renal artery stenosis. Indirect evidence of stenosis including a dampened systolic waveform, decreased flow velocity, and slowed acceleration of the systolic upstroke (Patriquin et al., 1992; Postma et al., 1992; Stavros et al., 1992).

Carefully performed Doppler evaluation is sensitive in detecting significant stenosis in 60–100% of cases (Rosendahl et al., 1994; Ellis et al., 1995;

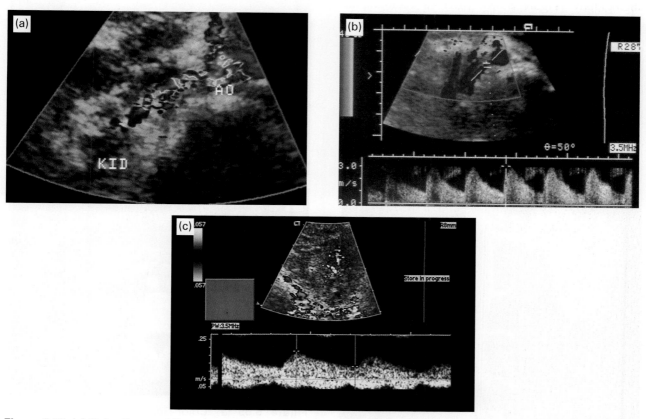

Figure 5.52 (a) Color-flow and Doppler sonography with significant right renal artery stenosis. (b) There is increased peak systolic velocity in the proximal renal artery at the site of the stenosis. (c) There is blunted systolic peak in the arcuate arteries.

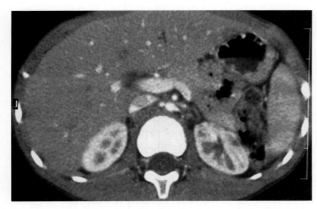

Figure 5.53 CT of aortic coarctatian with renal artery stenosis.

Brun *et al.*, 1997). If renal artery stenosis is suspected but Doppler sonography is not diagnostic, it is worthwhile pursuing further radiographic evaluation. Ultrathin-section CT with bolus contrast may offer an angiographic quality image of the renal arteries without resorting to the more invasive angiography (Figure 5.53). MRI or radiographic angiography (Figure 5.54) would be the next step in evaluation.

Vascular malformations, including hemangiomas, aneurysms, and arteriovenous fistulae, are uncommon. Aneurysms and AV fistulae may occur after trauma, surgery, or biopsy. If the malformation is large, sonography with color-flow Doppler may reveal abnormal vessels and waveforms (Figure 5.55a). A negative ultrasound study does not exclude a vascular malformation. On CT with multiphase contrast, vascular malformations may demonstrate a prominent focal area of enhancement (Figure 5.55b). AV fistulae and aneurysms will have rapid washout of contrast during the venous phase. Hemangiomas may have persistent contrast enhancement with a slower washout.

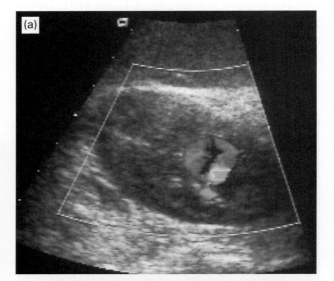

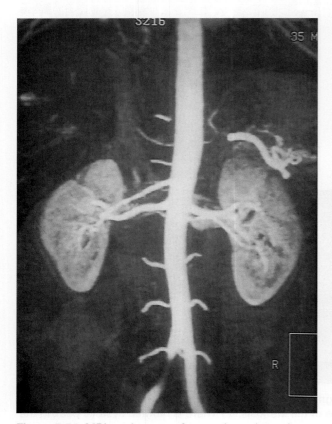

Figure 5.54 MRI angiogram of normal renal arteries.

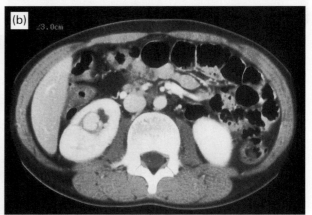

Figure 5.55 (*a*) Color-Doppler sonography of an arteriovascular malformation due to previous biopsy; (*b*) CT of an arteriovascular malformation due to a previous biopsy.

Renal transplantation

Renal transplantation for children with ESRD has a high success rate. Causes of ESRD in children include severe bilateral VUR with resulting nephropathy, bilateral obstructive processes such as PUV, or chronic inflammatory conditions such as glomerulonephritis. Many children receive a donor kidney from a parent.

The transplant may develop hydronephrosis from obstruction by perinephric fluid collections such as lymphoceles, ureteral stricture, stenosis, kinking, stones or bladder dysfunction. Stones or mineralizing sludge may develop within the transplant due to stasis from delayed drainage, even in children who were not previously stone formers. Due to underlying bladder pathology some transplant ureters may drain into an augmented or neobladder or an ileal conduit. These all have an increased risk of stone formation secondary to mucous secretion, changed urine pH and stasis.

Routine ultrasound studies include Doppler evaluations of the renal artery and vein, the arcuate arteries, and the iliac artery and vein if they are the sites of the venous and arterial anastomosis. Renal artery stenosis characteristically demonstrates a focally elevated peak systolic velocity, dampened intrarenal arterial flow, and turbulence. Renal arterial stenosis is most common at the anastomotic site but can occur at other sites along the course of the artery. It can occur at vascular clamp sites. Renal arterial and venous thrombosis are also complications of trans-

plantation (Solvis *et al.*, 1984; Dodd *et al.*, 1991) (Figure 5.56). In renal vein thrombosis, echogenic material within the lumen may be demonstrated. The transplant parenchyma may be enlarged and hypoechoic or hyperechoic. There may be reversal of diastolic flow and a sharp, narrow systolic peak (Reuther *et al.*, 1989). Resistive indices of the arcuate arteries normally range between 40 and 80% (Siegal, 1995). Elevated resistive indices indicate increased resistance to arterial flow and diminished diastolic flow. Elevated resistive indices are not specific but can be abnormal in various phases of rejection, infection, or venous outflow obstruction. AV fistulae and pseudoaneurysms are potential complications of percutaneous needle biopsy, which may be detected on Doppler sonography.

In allograft rejection the renal transplant may be normal, increased, or decreased in echogenicity (Slovis *et al.*, 1984). The transplant may be enlarged owing to edema and/or infiltration. Fluid collections that develop around renal transplants can represent lymphoceles, seromas, or urinomas. These fluid collections are easily imaged on sonography. Their exact relationship to the kidney, ureter, and bladder are best appreciated on CT. Enlarged lymphoceles may require draining if they interfere with urine flow. Urine may collect because of perforation within the pelvis, ureter, or bladder. These perforations can result from ischemic changes, suture breakdown, or other postsurgical or postprocedural complications.

Bladder abnormalities

The bladder is a unique part of the urinary tract. It acts as a reservoir for urine excreted from the kidneys. The function of the bladder and urethra may significantly impact the status of the upper urinary tract collecting system and the renal parenchyma. Evaluation of the bladder is an important component of the radiological work-up of renal disease in children.

Bladder exstrophy is an abdominal wall defect, apparent at birth. Initial imaging of these infants includes evaluation of the kidneys to identify any associated renal anomalies or hydronephrosis. At birth the kidneys are usually normal. After closure of the bladder, interval VCUGs are needed to evaluate the size and function of the bladder and to check for development of reflux. If the bladder size is small, it may predispose to reflux or hydronephrosis.

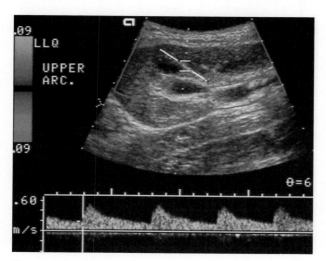

Figure 5.56 Doppler sonography of a renal transplant-demonstrates a normal arterial waveform.

Cloacal abnormalities, such as cloacal exstrophy, are caused by a defect in the inferior anterior abdominal wall. There is maldevelopment of the urorectal septum. There is an increased incidence of associated spinal cord abnormalities in children with cloacal abnormalities.

Megacystis, microcolon with hypoperistalsis syndrome usually presents in the neonatal period. The bladder is massively enlarged, extending above the umbilicus. Hydroureteronephrosis may or may not be present initially, although it may develop over time. There is no mechanical evidence of obstruction, although the bladder may act as a functional obstruction because of its poor emptying. The urethra is normal in appearance. There is microcolon and markedly delayed small bowel peristalsis. There is no evidence of anatomic bowel obstruction but upper gastrointestinal imaging (UGI) may demonstrate a delayed transit time through the small bowel of over 24 hours. These children may become candidates for small bowel transplantation.

The bladder during embryonic development is connected to the umbilicus through the urachus. The urachus should regress and disappear during gestation. Persistent urachal remnants may be connected to or separate from the bladder. There may be a patent urachus with an open communication from the bladder to the umbilicus. There may be a urachal sinus with a blind-ending tract extending to the umbilicus, a closed ending urachal diverticulum extending off the bladder, and a non-communicating urachal cyst. Urachal cysts are at risk of becoming infected. Urachal remnants are located immediately beneath the umbilicus and may be easily identified by sonography.

Bladder diverticula may be congenital but more commonly develop over time secondary to obstruction, reflux, or a neuropathic bladder. Bladder diverticula at the UVJ may predispose to reflux and are referred to as paraureteral diverticula (Figure 5.57). Bladder diverticula are radiologically diagnosed by VCUG or on sonography. The advantage of fluoroscopy is that diverticula may only become apparent as they enlarge during voiding and dynamic imaging is needed to confirm the diagnosis. On sonography they appear as anechoic outpouchings of the bladder wall. They are usually at the base of the bladder.

Thickening of the bladder wall may develop from chronic inflammation, chronic bladder outlet obstruction, radiation or hemorrhagic cystitis, or neurogenic causes. Bladder wall thickening may be the only

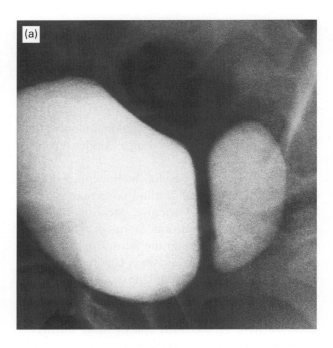

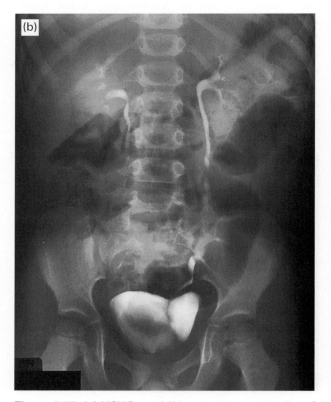

Figure 5.57 (*a*) VCUG; and (*b*) excretory urography of a left paraureteral diverticulum.

evidence of chronic UTI in children. Bladder wall thickening is well evaluated on sonography. A well-distended bladder with a wall that measures more than 3 mm in thickness is abnormal (Jequier and Rosseau, 1987). A bladder that is not well distended may appear to be thick walled.

With a UTI there may be echogenic material within the bladder from debris, hemorrhage, and inflammatory cells. Clumps of clot or aging thrombus within the bladder can be identified with hemorrhagic cystitis. Neuropathic bladders and bladders with chronic outlet obstruction may not only be thick walled but also have multiple diverticula or cellules of varying sizes.

VCUG may demonstrate a 'Christmas tree' appearance of a neuropathic or high-pressure bladder. The bladder is pear shaped with a vertical orientation and contains multiple diverticula, which have the appearance of bulbs on a Christmas tree (Figure 5.58). There may or may not be associated reflux with neuropathic bladders. Some are not thick walled but are large in volume or high capacity for age. These children may not be capable of voiding and may have overflow incontinence when the bladder capacity reaches a certain volume. If a child has what appears to be a neuropathic bladder, a work-up of the spine, including plain films and MRI, is warranted.

Ureteroceles present as round cystic masses of varying sizes within the base of the bladder. They may be bilateral, associated with a single system or with the upper pole ureter from a renal duplication. They are variable in size; some may be so large that they obstruct the upper pole ureter, the opposite ureter, and even the bladder outlet (Figure 5.59). Uretero-celes have a unique appearance on sonography. They appear as a thin-walled simple cystic mass at the bladder base. The ureterocele lies in continuity with an often dilated distal ureter coursing along the posterior wall of the bladder. Excretory urography offers a classic 'cobra head' appearance of the small, intravesical ureterocele. At times a ureterocele can be so massive that it fills the bladder and is mistaken for the bladder itself on ultrasonography instead of a large cystic mass within the bladder (Figure 5.60).

Bladder stones may be due to stones passed from the kidneys or the result of urine stasis, calcified foreign body, and bladder augmented with mucus-producing bowel. Because stones are high density, they have unique imaging characteristics and may be identified by ultrasound, non-contrast CT or plain film. Plain film is easily performed and can be the first step in identifying moderate- or large-sized stones within

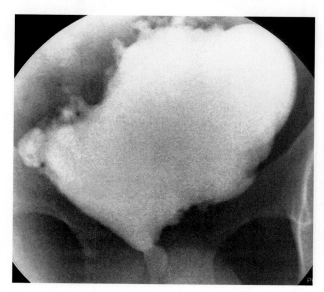

Figure 5.58 VCUG of a 'Christmas tree' or neuropathic bladder due to a tethered cord.

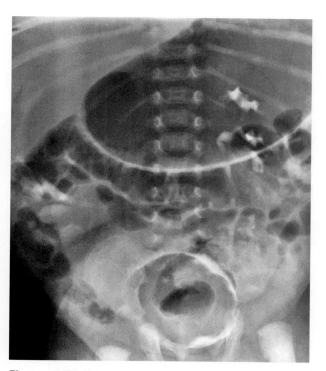

Figure 5.59 Excretory urography of a right renal duplication with an obstructed upper pole due to a ureterocele, causing the lower pole system to be deflected inferiolaterally.

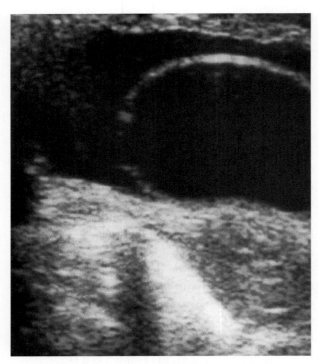

Figure 5.60 Sonogram of a large ureterocele.

the bladder. On sonography, stones appear as well-defined, highly echoic homogenous foci, that shadow sharply. On CT, stones appear as foci of high density. It is important to perform the CT without oral or intravenous contrast, which may mask stones or make them difficult to identify. If the bladder has been augmented or there is an ileal conduit, both of which predispose the patient to stones, they may be more difficult to identify because of the altered anatomy and redundant mucosal folds. A CT scan may offer the best evaluation in these cases. It is important to identify the staple lines and sutures from previous surgery. Comparison with previous studies is invaluable in these cases.

Solid masses that appear in the bladder include polyps, adenomas, and malignancies. Urethral polyps may present as solid, small, lobular, soft-tissue masses at the bladder neck (Figure 5.61).

Rhabdomyosarcoma is the most common malignancy affecting the bladder in children. It typically presents between 3 and 4 years of age (Wexler and Helman, 1997). It may arise from the bladder itself or from tissue adjacent to the bladder. Rhabdomyosarcoma may arise from the prostate in males and the vagina in females, and invade the bladder base with

potential obstruction of not only the bladder outlet but also the distal ureters (Figure 5.62). Children may present with bladder outlet obstruction, hematuria, or a lower abdominal mass. MRI offers the best detail in the relationship of the mass to adjacent pelvic organs such as the bladder, prostate, uterus, urethra, and rectum. It is the study of choice in staging pelvic tumors. Rhabdomyosarcomas are typically large, solid, and lobular in contour. Although commonly midline, they can arise from tissue on either side of the midline. The bladder wall may be thickened as a result of the high pressure needed to overcome the partially obstructing mass at the outlet. If large, they may contain areas of necrosis or hemorrhage. CT or MRI is used in staging the remainder of the abdomen for liver metastasis or retroperitoneal adenopathy. Chest CT is needed to evaluate the lungs for metastatic disease.

Transitional cell carcinoma of the bladder, while common in the adult population, is extremely rare in children (Lalmand *et al.*, 1987).

Pelvic masses, which may secondarily affect the bladder by external compression and cause displacement of distal ureteral obstruction, include malignant, inflammatory, or hemorrhagic processes. Malignancies which may involve the pelvis include lymphoma, neuroblastoma, and sacrococcygeal teratoma. Pelvic abscesses, most commonly from perforated appendices in children, or hematoma from trauma

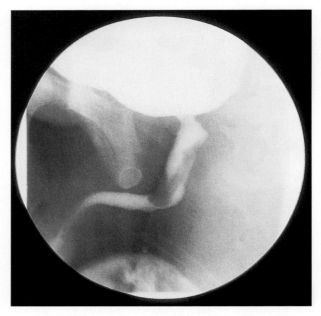

Figure 5.61 VCUG of a urethral polyp with long, tubular filling defect in the posterior urethra.

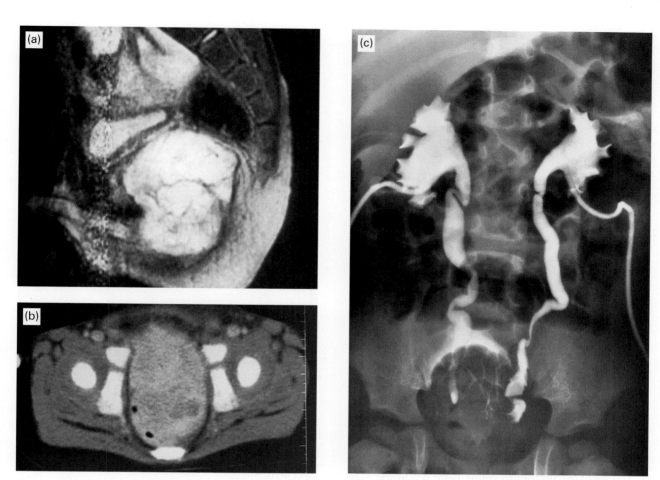

Figure 5.62 CT and nephrostogram of prostatic rhabdomyosarcoma causing bladder outlet obstruction.

may similarly affect the bladder by compression and displacement. CT offers the best evaluation of these processes.

Urethral abnormalities

There are few urethral abnormalities in females. In the adrenogenital syndrome, a male type urethra develops (Figure 5.63). The vagina may connect to or extend off the urethra and have the appearance of a large utricle. The urethra may also be maldeveloped in association with cloacal abnormalities.

The normal male urethra has multiple components: the bladder neck, the posterior urethra with the prostatic component, the veru montanum, the external sphincter, the anterior urethra with its bulbous and penile components, and the meatus (Figure 5.64).

Urethral abnormalities in males that result in obstruction to urine outflow from the bladder include anterior and posterior urethral valves, polyps, diverticula, stricture, stones, and dissection or disruption from trauma.

PUV is the most common urethral obstructing lesion in infancy. It is characterized by a dilated and elongated posterior urethra, a focal change in caliber at the expected level of the valve, a normal appearing but not well-distended anterior urethra and a thick-walled enlarged bladder (Figure 5.65). Anterior urethral valves are much less common. They obstruct in the same fashion as PUV. Strictures occur from previous trauma or instrumentation. When the child is voiding with a full stream the urethra should be well distended. A focal caliber change of the urethra with dilatation proximally should be suspect for an obstructing lesion.

Flow is disrupted but not necessarily obstructed by diverticula and fistulae. Diverticula may cause pooling

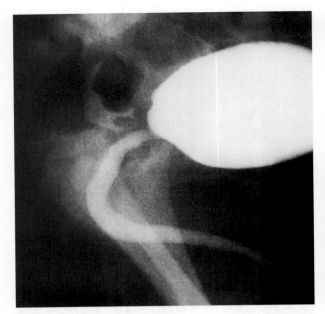

Figure 5.63 VCUG of male type urethra in adreno-genital syndrome.

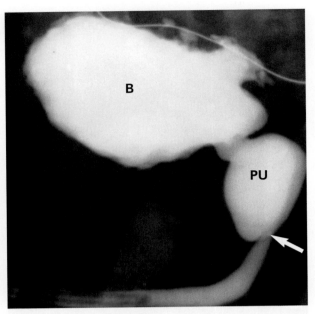

Figure 5.65 VCUG of posterior urethral valve (*arrow*). (B = bladder; PU = prostatic urethra.).

of urine with loss of the normal evacuation of urine from the urethra. This may result in a partially obs-tructive process with poor bladder emptying. Stones may develop in the diverticulum as a result of stasis.

The prostatic urethra in prune belly syndrome may be quite dilated and appear similar to that with PUV. Congenital abnormalities of the urethra include epis-padias and hypospadias. Rarely there may be a urethral duplication. Mixed gonadal dysgenesis patients may have a normal appearing male genitalia with an enlarged utricle, representing the remnant müllerian duct structure.

The urethra is best evaluated radiographically by standard VCUG or retrograde urethrogram. The ure-

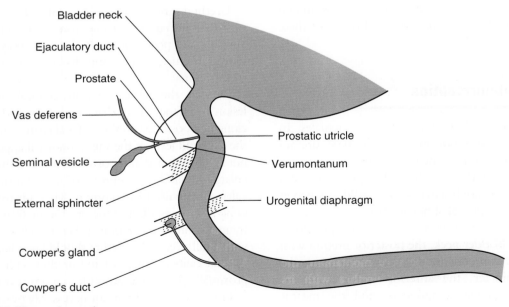

Figure 5.64 The male urethra.

thra should be evaluated in its entirety because abnormalities can occur anywhere along its course. In most circumstances, the male urethra is best evaluated during voiding without an indwelling catheter on VCUG. In cases of trauma a retrograde urethrogram is needed initially before the VCUG to rule out urethral disruption.

Gynecological abnormalities

The uterus is prominent in newborn females owing to maternal hormonal stimulation during pregnancy. It is easily identifiable on sonography as a lobular soft-tissue mass posterior to the bladder (Nussbaum *et al.*, 1986). An endometrial echo strip may be identifiable. After early infancy, the uterus becomes small in size and the endometrial echostripe cannot be identified. The uterus remains a small, tubular structure until hormonal stimulation begins in early puberty. The uterus then becomes longer and thicker and the endometrial canal can be identified (Orsini *et al.*, 1989). Ultrasound is the study of first choice in evaluating the uterus and ovaries at any age. It is especially advantageous in infants and children because there is no radiation, no need for sedation, and good resolution because of the child's relatively small size.

Hydrometrocolpos or hematometrocolpos may develop in the newborn period or early adolescence secondary to vaginal obstruction. The obstruction is most commonly due to an imperforate hymen or membrane, vaginal atresia or stenosis, or cloacal abnormalities (Rosenberg *et al.*, 1982; Blask *et al.*, 1991a, b). Hemorrhage or secretions may greatly distend the vagina so that it has the appearance of a large, rounded, tubular shaped mass. On sonography there is a large elongated mass with a thin uniform wall and low-level internal echoes lying directly posterior to the bladder (Figure 5.66). The echoes may move with change in position of the patient, confirming their fluid nature. The uterus contains a smaller amount of echogenic material and is small in comparison with the vagina. The vagina may be so large as to obstruct the distal ureters and cause hydronephrosis.

Hematometrocolpos may develop in one horn of a duplicated uterus and a septated vagina. A normal appearing uterine horn may be identified in addition to the expected findings of hematometrocolpos on the obstructed side. This can be associated with renal

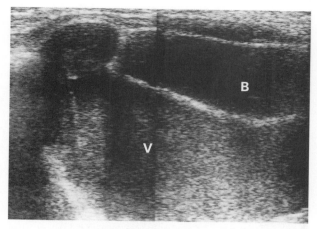

Figure 5.66 Sonogram of hematometrocolpos with hypoechoic material throughout a massively dilated vagina and a small amount in the uterus in a 14-year-old girl. (B = bladder; V = vagina.)

agenesis on the side of the obstructed uterine horn (Figure 5.67).

Other uterine abnormalities include septated uterus and unicornuate uterus. These anomalies are difficult to identify in the prepubertal child and typically present in adolescence or later in adult life.

Uterine agenesis is the hallmark of Rokitansky–Meyer syndrome. It presents in adolescence with amenorrhea. The lower third of the vagina, which develops from the urogenital sinus, is present. The upper two-thirds of the vagina and the uterus, which develop from the müllerian ducts, are absent. These children have XX chromosomes. The ovaries develop normally and separately from the uterus and the girls have normal secondary sexual characteristics. There may be a tiny remnant uterus.

There may be a hypoplastic or absent uterus with various chromosomal anomalies, including mixed gonadal dysgenesis and Turner syndrome. MRI is the most sensitive modality for evaluation of uterine anomalies and would be the second study of choice if the initial sonogram suggests uterine anomalies or absence.

Rhabdomyosarcoma is the most common uterine malignancy in childhood, although it is uncommon. It presents most often in children younger than 5 years, but can occur later in childhood and adolescence. The child may have uterine bleeding or an abdominal mass. Rhabdomyosarcoma appears on sonography as a solid, inhomogeneously echogenic mass of varying size. It may be localized to the vagina

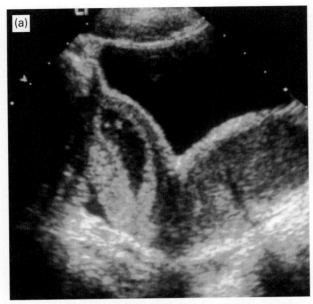

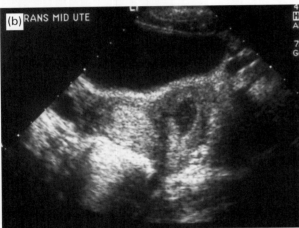

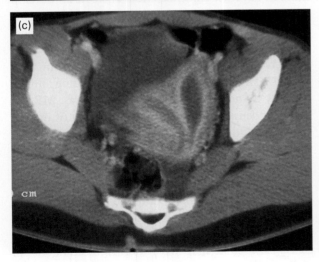

Figure 5.67 Ultrasound and CT of hematometrocolpos from obstruction of one horn of uterine didelphys in a 14-year-old girl.

or uterus if it is detected early (Figure 5.68). Later in its course, it may present as a huge bulky pelvic mass that obscures adjacent organs, making it difficult to determine the site of origin. It may involve the vagina and uterus and compress, obstruct, or invade the bladder and distal ureters. Sarcoma botryoides is the term used for rhabdomyosarcomas having the appearance of a cluster of grape-like, small, rounded masses.

The ovaries, like the uterus, may be prominent at birth owing to hormonal stimulation during pregnancy. Ovarian cysts are not uncommon in the newborn and those larger than 3 cm are at risk for torsion. Internal echoes within large ovarian cysts may be due to hemorrhage from torsion. Ovarian cysts will appear as a cystic mass, separate from any solid abdominal organ, such as the liver or kidneys. They are the most common abdominal cystic mass of newborn girls. On sonography, an ovarian cyst has a thin, single wall, as distinct from the thicker wall of a duplication cyst of the bowel (Figure 5.69).

Ovaries of preadolescent girls are often identified on sonography. They may contain small cysts and follicles due to low levels of hormonal stimulation (Stanhope *et al.*, 1985; Cohen *et al.*, 1993). Ovarian volume is used for the most consistent and comparable measurement of ovarian size (Cohen *et al.*, 1990). It is a helpful tool in the evaluation of girls with precocious puberty.

Ovarian tumors are uncommon in children. They are classified as germ cell or non-germ cell. Germ cell tumors are the most common and make up 60% of ovarian masses (Castleberry *et al.*, 1991). Germ cell tumors include teratomas, dysgerminomas, endoder-

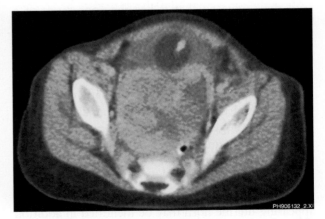

Figure 5.68 CT of vaginal rhabdomyosarcoma in a 10-month-old girl.

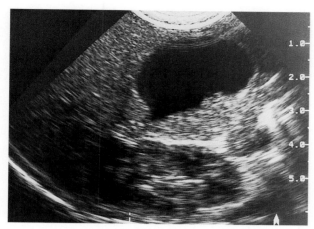

Figure 5.69 Sonogram of a right ovarian cyst in a newborn girl. The ovarian cyst has dependent internal debris, which may be due to torsion.

mal sinus tumors, embryonal carcinoma, choriocarcinoma, mixed germ cell tumors, and gonadoblastoma. Non-germ cell tumors include sex cord–stromal tumors such as granulosa-theca cell, and epithelial tumors such as serous and mucinous cystadenomas. Tumors within the ovary may place the ovary at increased risk for torsion.

Teratomas are the most common germ cell tumor of the ovary. They are benign in 90% of cases. Teratomas have a variable appearance on sonography. They may appear as a cystic, complex cystic, or solid inhomogeneous mass. They may have focal areas of increased echogenicity with shadowing if calcification is present. Fatty tissue within the tumors will also appear echogenic (Figure 5.70). The characteristic CT appearance of calcification and fat within an ovarian mass is diagnostic of teratomas (Figure 5.71).

Malignant tumors make up 35% of ovarian masses and 1–2% of all childhood malignancies (Castleberry *et al.*, 1991). Germ cell tumors are the most common ovarian malignancy, with dysgerminoma being the most common of these tumors. Stromal sex cord tumors are the second most common ovarian malignancies.

Cystadenomas account for 10% of ovarian masses. They may present as large, complex cystic masses with thin walls and internal septations (Figure 5.72). Doppler evaluation may demonstrate flow within the wall and internal septations of the mass. They may be massive, involving so much of the abdomen and pelvis that it is difficult to tell their origin. Rarely, these may be cystadenocarcinomas.

Paraovarian cysts present as adnexal cystic masses. They are variable in size and originate within the uterine ligaments. The normal ovary may or may not be identified separately from the paraovarian cyst. They do not fluctuate in size with the menstrual cycle.

Hemorrhagic ovarian cysts are the most common complex cystic ovarian mass. They may appear as large inhomogeneous, partially cystic complex ovarian masses (Figure 5.73). Normal ovarian tissue can usually be identified along the margins of the mass. Follow-up sonography within 2–4 weeks will demonstrate aging of the hemorrhagic component and a decrease in size, or possibly even complete resolution of the cystic mass.

Endometriosis is uncommon in adolescents. Sonography is not sensitive in identifying small areas of endometriosis. If large enough, it can present as an ovarian mass and is indistinguishable from other solid ovarian masses on sonography. MRI is the sensitive and specific modality for detection of endo-

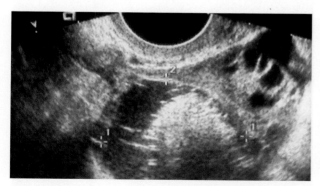

Figure 5.70 Sonogram of a right ovarian teratoma with an inhomogeneous echogenic mass due to internal fat.

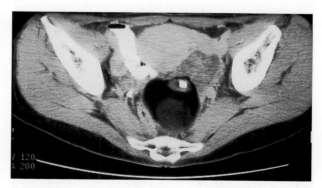

Figure 5.71 CT of a left ovarian teratoma demonstrating internal calcification and fat.

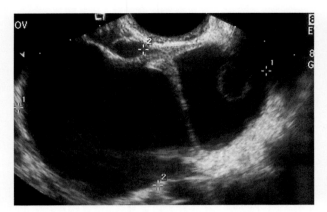

Figure 5.72 Sonogram of ovarian cystadenoma with a large, complex cystic mass with internal septations.

Figure 5.73 Sonogram of a hemorrhagic ovarian cyst with internal echoes and septations.

metriosis. Endometriomas will demonstrate signals characteristic of hemorrhage.

Ectopic pregnancies are in the differential of adnexal masses in any sexually active adolescents. If the pregnancy test is positive and a fetal pole or yolk sac is not yet identified within the endometrial canal, any ovarian mass must be viewed as a potential ectopic pregnancy. Endovaginal sonography affords the opportunity to visualize a fetal pole or yolk sac 1–2 weeks earlier than transabdominal ultrasound.

Ovarian torsion can present in infancy or more commonly in adolescence. The ovary is quite enlarged and inhomogeneous with loss of the normal ovarian echotecture due to edema from ischemia. Multiple, small, peripheral cysts have been described as a common finding in torsion (Graif and Itzhak, 1988; Rosado et al., 1992). Doppler evaluation may show either no flow,

flow in the paraovarian soft tissue, or, uncommonly, a small amount of intraovarian flow (Figure 5.74). An ovarian mass may predispose to torsion. It is usually quite painful and the differential includes appendicitis, ectopic pregnancy, and endometriomas. There is commonly free fluid within the pelvis.

Other cystic masses within the pelvis, which are not ovarian in origin, are cystic sacrococcygeal teratoma, anterior meningoceles, and rectal duplication cysts.

Scrotal abnormalities

Sonography ideally visualizes most scrotal abnormalities and has the added benefit of vascular interrogation by Doppler ultrasound (Finkelstein et al., 1986; McAlister and Sisler, 1990; Castleberry et al., 1991).

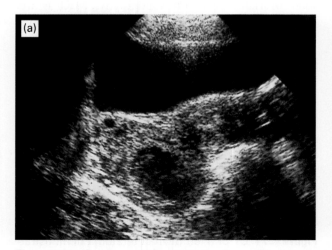

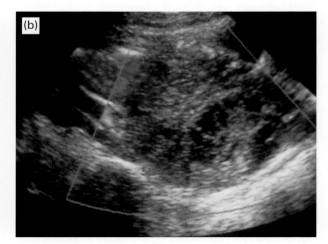

Figure 5.74 Sonogram of ovarian torsion, with an enlarged inhomogeneous ovary.

Undescended testes are one of the most common scrotal abnormalities in infant boys. The testes can be quite mobile in infants and move between the inguinal canal and the scrotum. The testes are round, well defined and homogeneous, and are readily identified within the inguinal canal or scrotum by sonography. If the testis cannot be identified, it may not have descended and may lie within the abdomen. MRI of the pelvis has limited benefit, since failure to visualize testicular tissue does not assure absence. Gonads have bright signal characteristics on MRI with T_2-weighted sequencing.

Testicular torsion may occur at any time but is most common perinatally and during adolescence. Torsion may even occur *in utero* and the only evidence of it at birth may be a small remnant of partially calcified testis (Brown *et al.*, 1990). Acute testicular torsion presents as a swollen, reddened painful hemi-scrotum. Testicular torsion is an emergent situation, with testicular salvage highest within the first 6 hours of onset. In cases where the clinical history and examination are strongly suggestive of torsion, the child may be taken immediately to surgery. If they are immediately available, either sonography with Doppler imaging or nuclear scintigraphy are the imaging studies of choice. Both methods can offer valuable information about the status of flow to the testis. The clinical situation, availability of the imaging test, and the radiology expertise of the particular medical institute often dictate what approach is best taken. Sonography with Doppler has made immense technological advances, so that it is often the imaging study of first choice for patients with a painful, red, swollen testis (McCartney, 1992; Patrquin *et al.*, 1993; Luk and Siegel, 1994; Lewis *et al.*, 1995).

The main differential for the painful, red, swollen testis is torsion, epididymitis/orchitis, and trauma. Trauma should have an antecedent history suggesting that as the etiology.

An intratesticular hematoma may appear as a poorly defined hypoechoic region. Close follow-up with sonography should be obtained to ensure resolution of the hematoma and that the mass does not represent tumor, unrelated to the traumatic episode. With testicular rupture, the normal egg shape of the testis is lost and the contour is disrupted. The testicular parenchyma loses its normal homogeneous echotecture and becomes inhomogeneous (Figure 5.75). These children are taken to surgery for repair and salvage.

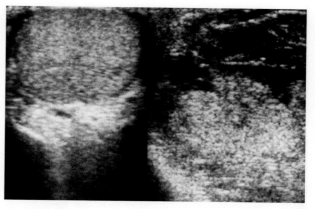

Figure 5.75 Sonogram of left testicular rupture, with normal right testis for comparison. There is loss of the normal testicular contour and shape and the testicular parenchyma is diffusely inhomogeneous.

There is prominent increased flow within the testis and epididymis with orchitis/epididymitis. The affected testes is asymmetrically enlarged and mildly inhomogeneous in echotecture (Figure 5.76).

With testicular torsion, sonography demonstrates a high-lying, echogenic, inhomogeneously enlarged testis with no intratesticular flow identifiable by Doppler (Figure 5.77). It is important to evaluate flow with both Doppler interrogation and color-flow. A slight movement of the child or transducer may create an artificial color signal. An arterial waveform is definite evidence of vascular flow (Meza *et al.*, 1992). Doppler ultrasound has made significant

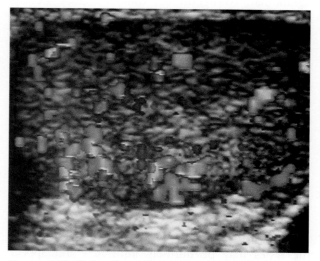

Figure 5.76 Color-flow ultrasound of orchitis, with diffusely increased testicular flow.

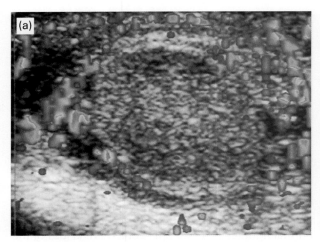
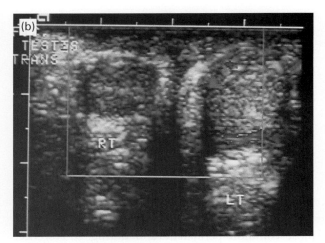

Figure 5.77 (*a*) Color-flow ultrasound of left testicular torsion, within enlarged left testis and paratesticular flow with no internal flow. (*b*) Normal right testis.

technological advances in its ability to detect low vascular flow. Testicular flow can often be demonstrated in the preadolescent male. The opposite, normal testis, is valuable in offering a baseline comparison of flow and echotecture. If the torsion is late, there may be paratesticular flow, which corresponds to the 'ring' or 'halo' sign present on nuclear medicine scans.

Testicular tumors may be benign or malignant. Testicular tumors can be divided into germ cell and non-germ cell types (Castleberry *et al.*, 1991). Germ cell tumors are the most common, accounting for 90% of cases. Germ cell tumors include yolk sac tumors, teratomas, embryonal carcinomas, teratocarcinomas, mixed germ cell, choriocarcinomas, and seminomas. Non-germ cell tumors include Leydig cell and Sertoli cell. Yolk sac tumors are the most common germ cell tumor of the testes in infants and young boys. Seminomas are rare in infants and young boys and uncommon in adolescence. Choriocarcinoma and embryonal carcinoma usually occur as part of a mixed malignant germ cell tumor. Testicular tumors are well evaluated on sonography (Schwerk *et al.*, 1987). They may appear hypoechoic or be inhomogeneous with areas of increased echogenicity, even with calcification, in the germ cell tumors (Figure 5.78). There may be evidence of extensive metastatic disease, in spite of the primary testicular tumor remaining relatively small. Testes may be secondarily involved with leukemia and lymphoma. In these cases the testes may be diffusely infiltrated and appear enlarged, or there may be a discrete testicular mass or masses.

Although extratesticular scrotal massses are generally considered benign in the adult, in children and adolescents malignancy should also be considered. Malignancies that may involve the paratesticular soft tissue include rhabdomyosarcoma, neuroblastoma, lymphoma, and other soft-tissue sarcomas (Figure 5.79). These are best evaluated initially with ultrasound. MRI or CT is needed for further staging of possible extension of the malignancy.

Testicular tumors are usually well-defined masses on sonography. Teratomas may contain calcification, fat, or fluid. On sonography there may be inhomogeneous masses with anechoic areas representing necrosis and focal areas of increased echogenicity that may

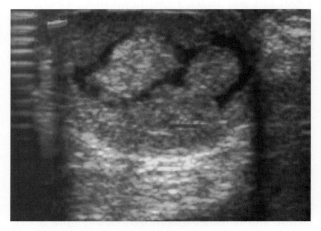

Figure 5.78 Sonogram of a germ cell tumor of the testis.

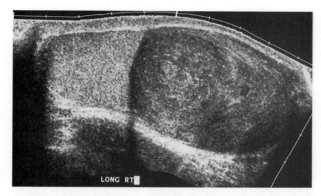

Figure 5.79 Sonogram of a large paratesticular rhabdomyosarcoma in a 17-year-old. The mass compresses the adjacent normal testis.

represent fat or, if there is shadowing, calcification. Seminomas tend to appear as homogeneously hypoechoic solid masses. Epidermoid tumors are one of the few benign testicular tumors.

Although not as common as in the adult population, children may develop epididymitis and orchitis. They present with a red, swollen, painful scrotum, similar to testicular torsion. Sonography is useful in differentiating these two entities. With epididymitis and orchitis there will be increased flow throughout the testis and epididymis consistent with inflammation. It is important to differentiate paratesticular flow, which may be present in torsion, from internal testicular flow, which will be increased in orchitis. Scrotal abscesses are uncommon in children. There would be echogenic fluid and an inhomogeneous enlarged testis from inflammation.

Testicular microlithiasis (Figure 5.80) is a unique entity with a characteristic appearance on sonography. The testes are usually normal in size. They contain multiple, small, bright foci of increased echotecture, which may shadow. These represent tiny calcifications within the tubules of the testes. These are of uncertain etiology but there may be an increased association with future malignancy.

Hydroceles are common in infancy and most resolve spontaneously. Premature infants commonly have inguinal hernias. They can often be differentiated from large hydroceles by visualizing bowel with the sac on sonogram.

In utero bowel perforation may result in meconium within the scrotum through a patent process vaginalis in the inguinal canal. The meconium usually calcifies. The process vaginalis may close over time and the only evidence of the perforation will be speckles of calcified meconium within the scrotum at birth (Figure 5.81).

Renal trauma

CT with intravenous contrast offers a fast and relatively all-inclusive evaluation of the abdomen in cases of trauma. CT is sensitive for the detection of abdominal organ injury. With the advent of rapid image acquisition, high-quality images of the abdominal organs and much of the abdominal vasculature can be obtained during bolus contrast enhancement. CT without intravenous contrast is not usually indicated in cases of trauma. Non-contrast CT is most advantageous when looking for evidence of stones or calcifi-

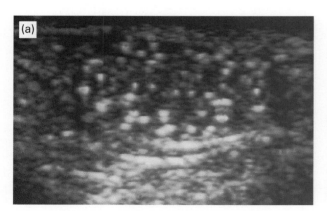
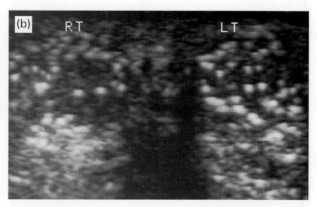

Figure 5.80 Sonogram of testicular microlithiasis with speckled punctate areas of calcification through both testes.

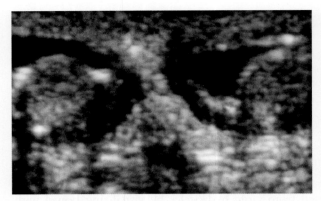

Figure 5.81 Sonogram of calcified meconium in the scrotum, with small focal areas of increased echotexture within the scrotum.

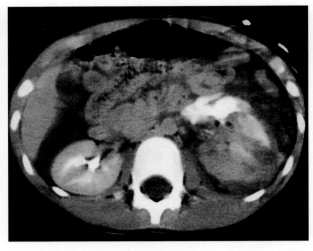

Figure 5.83 Delayed CT of left renal injury, with extravasation of contrast into the left perinephric space (same patient as Figure 5.82).

cation. It can be useful if there is a question of whether or not a fluid collection represents hemorrhage. Acute hemorrhage will be relatively high in density on non-contrast images.

CT imaging during bolus intravenous contrast injection will demonstrate enhancement of the aorta, renal arteries, and renal parenchyma. If there is renal injury there will be focal areas that are not enhancing, suggesting non-perfusion due to contusion or laceration (Figure 5.82). The renal contour may be disrupted and there may be blood within the perinephric space. The hematoma can extend inferiorly, surrounding the ureter. It is helpful to investigate the opposite, hopefully, normal kidney for comparison. If there is a main renal artery occlusion or dissection, the whole kidney may not enhance. Renal vein thrombosis or occlusion may result in a very prolonged

nephrogram. Delayed images are needed to evaluate excretion of contrast into the collecting system. If there is extravasation of contrast due to disruption of the collecting system, this may not be evident on the early images before contrast fills the renal pelves, ureters, and bladder (Figure 5.83).

Bladder disruption may be intraperitoneal or extraperitoneal. Delayed images with a contrast-filled bladder are needed to identify extravasation of contrast from the bladder into the pelvis (Figure 5.84). Pelvic fractures will result in hematomas, which may displace and compress the bladder. CT is not an adequate evaluation of the integrity of the urethra and a retrograde urethrogram (RUG) is warranted if there is a question of urethral disruption (Figure

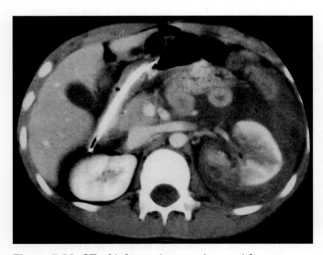

Figure 5.82 CT of left renal contusion and fracture.

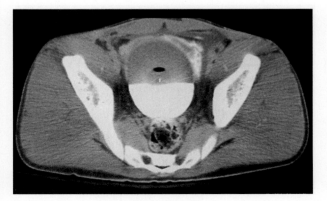

Figure 5.84 Delayed CT of bladder perforation of with extravasation of contrast around the bladder.

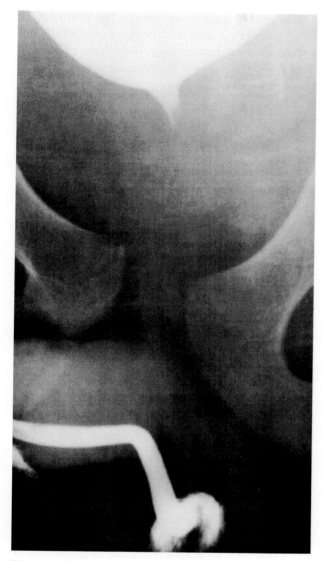

Figure 5.85 RUG of urethral disruption.

ously, the widespread use of ultrasound and CT imaging has enhanced both the performance and the range of application of percutaneous needle and catheter techniques for both diagnosis and therapeutic interventions in this group of patients. A wide variety of complex endourologic techniques has evolved, based on the initial creation of safe and reliable percutaneous access into the urinary tracts (Ball *et al.*, 1986). The optimal clinical applications of these procedures have resulted from the continuing frequent consultation and interaction between pediatric radiologists and pediatric urologists.

Antegrade pyelography is a minimally invasive technique best used to define collecting system anatomy (Riedy and Lebowitz, 1986). In older children, only mild sedation is needed to limit anxiety, but in infants and young children, deeper levels of anesthesia are frequently needed for patient comfort. Real-time ultrasound guidance is used for initial renal localization and subsequent needle insertion. After the injection of a local anesthetic at the puncture site, the operator percutaneously inserts a 21- or 22-gauge needle into the renal collecting system, preferably choosing a posterolateral calyx. With markedly dilated collecting systems, fluoroscopic-guided needle insertion can be equally effective. Following initial aspiration of urine for bacterial cultures, contrast material is injected into the collecting system under fluoroscopic observation. Precise preoperative definitions of collecting system abnormalities and postoperative anastomoses are often best defined with fluoroscopy (Figure 5.86). Minimal complications are encountered with this technique because of the small needles used, permitting outpatient evaluation.

Percutaneous nephrostomy placement is a direct extension of antegrade pyelography. Following percutaneous needle placement into a selected calyx, a guidewire is advanced through the needle into the collecting system and coiled in the renal pelvis. The percutaneous tract is then dilated and a nephrostomy tube is inserted. While infants' kidneys are adequately drained by a 6 Fr catheter, in larger children, an 8 or 10 Fr catheter provides better drainage. The widely used, self-retaining loop drainage catheters greatly reduce the incidence of catheter dislodgement and aid in maintaining catheter stability, particularly in acutely ill, uncooperative children.

The acute complications of antegrade pyelography and percutaneous nephrostomy placement are minimal. Postprocedural hematuria develops in all patients

5.85). A catheter should not be passed into the bladder without verifying, through a retrograde injection, that it is completely intact. A false urethral passage may be created by a catheter passed blindly into a partially or fully disrupted urethra.

Percutaneous interventional procedures

The extensive application of non-invasive imaging techniques to the evaluation of the urinary tracts in pediatric patients during the 1980s and 1990s has greatly improved the anatomic delineation of abnormalities and augmented surgical planning. Simultane-

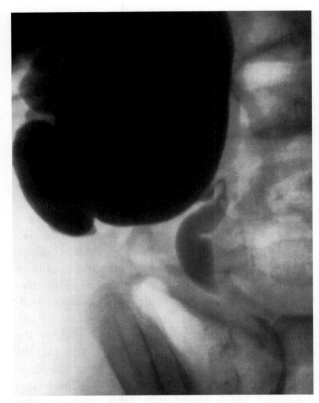

Figure 5.86 Left antegrade pyelogram with the infant prone showed marked dilatation of the left renal pelvis despite previous pyeloplasty. The focal obstruction of the left upper ureter was due to a combination of a small anomalous crossing renal artery and postoperative scar tissue and required dismembered pyeloplasty.

and usually clears within 24 hours, except in profoundly uremic patients. Repeated, postprocedural gross hemorrhage into the collecting systems occurs in fewer than 1% of patients undergoing these percutaneous manipulations, and their small, intrarenal arterial injuries are best diagnosed and treated with transcatheter angiographic embolization. Percutaneous catheter placement into a collecting system containing infected urine may lead to clinical signs of sepsis. This complication is best limited by adequate pre-instrumentation antibiotic coverage, minimizing the manipulations required for tube placement in the acute setting, and delaying comprehensive pyelography for 48 hours after initial tube insertion. Flank pain related to acute nephrostomy insertion usually becomes minimal after 48 hours and prolonged nephrostomy drainage can be maintained with minimal discomfort.

The clinical indications for the performance of antegrade pyelography and nephrostomy placement in the pediatric patient have been lessened by the application of extensive cross-sectional imaging and the development of improved retrograde transurethral access techniques. The wide variety of percutaneous endourologic techniques that can be performed through the percutaneous tract has supported the continued expansion of clinical applications of basic collecting system access techniques. Nephrostomy tube insertion for collecting system obstruction provides urinary drainage, which allows healing of obstructive postoperative edema, direct assessment of renal function, or drainage of infected urine to improve overall clinical status (Towbin and Ball, 1988). Complex postoperative collecting system leaks or anastomotic dysfunction often require initial drainage, repeated nephrostograms, and subsequent catheter manipulations. During the 1990s, equipment manufacturers have effectively miniaturized the stents and endourologic tools that were initially developed for adult patient applications. Working through small sheaths inserted through the percutaneous nephrostomy tract, a wide variety of balloon dilation catheters, baskets, and ureteral stents can be efficiently used in pediatric patients. Even in neonates, 3–4 Fr ureteral stents provide adequate flow rates to permit internalization of these urinary catheters, thus eliminating the risk of external nephrostomy catheter dislodgement or a secondary collecting system infection along the percutaneous tract.

Contraindications to percutaneous intervention are few. Correction of an underlying bleeding diathesis or reversal of systemic anticoagulation is necessary prior to needle/catheter placement to prevent hemorrhagic complications. In acute renal failure, rapid elevation of the serum potassium levels may require transvenous hemodialysis to normalize the potassium level prior to percutaneous nephrostomy placement. Body habitus abnormalities, such as severe scolioses, may alter the usual internal anatomic relationships of the abdominal contents and preclude the creations of safe, percutaneous access. This situation is best addressed by preprocedural CT scanning.

The clinical implications of persistent postoperative collecting system dilatation are often difficult to assess, even with comprehensive cross-sectional imaging. Pressure–flow evaluation (the Whitaker test) of these dilated collecting systems is an important application of percutaneous techniques (Whitaker, 1973).

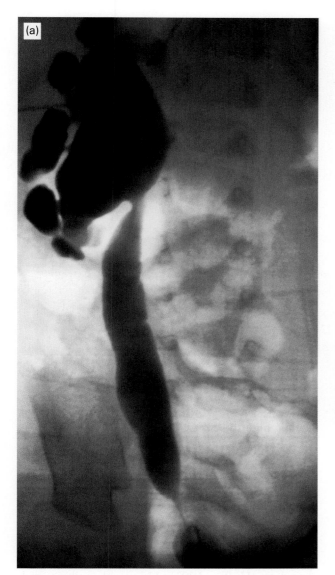

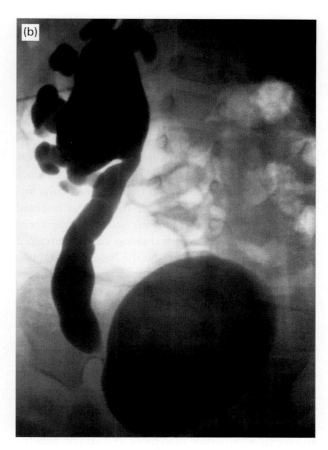

Figure 5.87 Left Whitaker test was performed through a 4 Fr percutaneous catheter in the renal pelvis, with the patient prone. (*a*) Intrarenal injection showed a widely patent ureterovesical junction after ureteroneocystotomy with no obstruction when the urinary bladder was empty. (*b*) Antegrade Whitaker test shows ureterovesical junction obstruction with the urinary bladder full. Renal function stabilized with a frequent timed voiding schedule to keep the bladder at minimal volume.

Through small needles, or more reliably through small nephrostomy tubes, infusion of fluid into the collecting system at a defined rate is accompanied by monitoring of pressure within the renal pelvis and urinary bladder. After the infusion of 10 ml/min, an increase of more than 10 cmH$_2$O above the baseline pressure differential between the renal pelvis and the bladder is considered abnormal. Monitoring of urinary bladder pressures and control of urinary bladder volume are important components of the Whitaker test

because bladder dynamics may affect antegrade urine flow in the postoperative patient (Figure 5.87) (see Chapter 20).

The creation of an appropriate percutaneous nephrostomy tract is the initial technique in the performance of complex endourologic therapy within the urinary tract. Similar to the experience in adult patients, percutaneous renal and ureteral stone removal techniques are widely adaptable to manage successfully nearly all presentations of stone disease

(Woodside *et al.*, 1985; Mor *et al.*, 1997). In the pediatric patient population, comprehensive percutaneous stone removal therapy additionally often includes endourologic surgical repair of an underlying collecting system abnormality such as endopyelotomy for UPJ obstruction or incision of an infundibular stenosis (Douenias *et al.*, 1990; Wilkinson and Azmy, 1996). Percutaneous obliteration of collecting system diverticula usually requires direct percutaneous access into the diverticulum, followed by removal of stones if present, and then elimination of the diverticular lining with electrocautery or laser energy. An essential component of all percutaneous stone management techniques is laboratory evaluation of the extracted stone material, complementing the baseline metabolic evaluation. This is particularly important in pediatric patients with medical conditions presenting with frequent and recurrent stone formation, such as hyperoxaluria and cystinuria. Complex endourologic procedures often require additional equipment and expertise, optimally provided through the cooperative efforts of radiologists and pediatric urologists. General anesthesia is usually needed for these complex endoscopic procedures.

The use of percutaneous antegrade pyelography and nephrostomy tube placement in pediatric patients with renal transplants closely parallels the use of these techniques in native kidneys. The complete range of percutaneous interventional techniques can be used in renal transplants, ranging from simple urinary drainage to stricture dilation and stenting or removing stones or foreign bodies (Figure 5.88). Percutaneous drainage of pelvic fluid collections, such as lymphoceles causing ureteral obstruction, may preclude the need for renal puncture and intubation.

Percutaneous drainage of renal, perinephric, and retroperitoneal abscesses has been shown to be an effective means of obtaining material for bacterial culture, as well as an alternative to surgical intervention in selected cases (Zerin, 1997). However, renal abscesses resulting from pyelonephritis usually resolve without drainage, once proper therapy has been initiated. In those patients with an underlying anatomic abnormality, percutaneous abscess drainage improves the patient's physical condition and often permits a delayed single-stage surgical reconstruction, rather than requiring complex staged surgical procedures (Towbin *et al.*, 1994). Frequent tube injection and catheter manipulations may be needed to treat multiloculated collections, but the rapid healing ability of

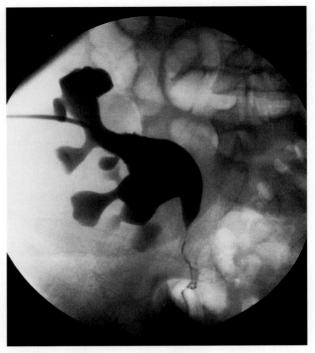

Figure 5.88 Right pelvic renal transplant kidney nephrostogram showed a stricture of the ureter secondary to ureteral ischemia. Percutaneous nephrostomy was inserted to improve urine flow and renal function prior to surgical repair.

most children complements this minimally invasive percutaneous therapy of complex processes.

Percutaneous biopsy of renal and abdominal masses in the pediatric population has been included in earlier sections of this chapter as a safe and effective procedure (Hoffer, 1991). Using either ultrasound, CT, or fluoroscopic guidance, nearly all intra-abdominal lesions can be biopsied percutaneously. In the pediatric population, the use of adequate intravenous sedation and small percutaneous biopsy needles allows outpatient intervention.

Angiography

Transfemoral catheter angiography is a valuable technique in pediatric patients in evaluating the abdominal aorta and renal arteries in those patients with intrinsic vascular diseases. The introduction of ultrasound and CT has eliminated the clinical use of angiographic evaluation of renal parenchymal disease or mass lesions. Similarly, direct injection of the inferior vena cava for the evaluation of tumor thrombus extent has been replaced with less invasive ultrasonic or MRI examinations. Screening renal artery evaluation with ultrasound including Doppler evaluation is performed initially in patients with suspected vascular disease (Gordon, 1994), as described earlier in this chapter. Progressive improvements in CT angiography and MR angiography accurately allow the identification of major renal arteries and veins, but catheter angiography still produces the best images of large and small vessel pathology, particularly of abnormalities within intrarenal parenchymal arterial branches.

The standard technique of percutaneous transfemoral angiography by the Seldinger technique provides safe, accurate diagnostic examinations by skilled operators. Because of the more invasive nature of arterial catheter placement, the greater risk of this technique must be balanced against the clinical necessity. Localized hematoma formation at the site of the arterial puncture can be avoided by applying continuous localized pressure for at least 10 min. Distal arterial occlusion from clot formation on the intraarterial catheter and excessive pressure at the puncture site are technical complications that can be avoided with operator awareness. Segmental renal parenchymal infarction from guidewire–catheter manipulations is also an avoidable technical complication.

Preprocedural discussion of angiographic indications allows the performance of initial diagnostic and subsequent therapeutic procedures in one setting. Transcatheter embolization of arteriovenous fistulae created by renal parenchymal biopsy or percutaneous intervention is an important clinical technique in both native and transplant kidneys. Percutaneous transluminal angioplasty is useful for treating renal artery-induced systemic hypertension secondary to fibromuscular dysplasia or non-specific aortoarteritis (Stanley *et al.*, 1984; Sharma *et al.*, 1996). Thrombolysis techniques may also be needed for acute renal venous thrombosis or aortic emboli. Transcatheter renal parenchymal obliteration with ethanol injection into the renal artery is occasionally used to reduce systemic hypertension caused by end-stage renal parenchymal dysfunction (Nanni *et al.*, 1983; Garel *et al.*, 1986). Debilitating massive proteinuria in children on hemodialysis for chronic renal failure may be greatly decreased with transarterial ethanol ablation of the renal parenchyma.

References

Adams ND, Rowe JC (1992) Nephrocalcinosis. *Clin Perinatal* **19**: 179–95.

Agrons GA, Wagner BJ, Davidson AJ *et al.* (1995) Multilocular cystic renal tumor in children: radiologic–pathologic correlation. *Radiographics* **15**: 653–69.

Atiyehm B, Husmann D, Maum M 1992 Contralateral renal abnormalities in multicystic–dysplastic kidney disease. *J Pediatr* **121**: 65–7.

Avni EF, Thoua Y, Lalmand B *et al.* 1986 Multicystic dysplastic kidney: evolving concepts – *in utero* diagnosis and post-natal follow-up by ultrasound. *Ann Radiol* **29**: 663–8.

Babcock DS (1997) Sonography of wall thickening of the renal collecting system: a nonspecific finding. *J Ultrasound Med* **6**: 29–32.

Babcock DS, Patriquin HB (1998) The pediatric kidney and adrenal glands. In: Rumack CM, Wilson SR, Charboneau JW (eds) *Diagnostic ultrasound*. 2nd edition. St Louis: Mosby, 1704–9.

Ball WS Jr, Towbin R, Strife JL, Spencer R (1986) Interventional genitourinary radiology in children: a review of 61 procedures. *AJR Am J Roentgenol* **147**: 791.

Banner MP, Pollack HM, Chatten J *et al.* (1981) Multilocular renal cysts: radiologic–pathologic correlation. *AJR Am J Roentgenol* **136**: 239–47.

Belt TG, Cohen MD, Smith JA *et al.* (1986) MRI of Wilms' tumor: promise as the primary imaging modality. *AJR Am J Roentgenol* **146**: 955–61.

Bjorgvinsson E, Majd M, Effli KD (1991) Diagnosis of acute pyelonephritis in children: Comparison of sonography and ^{99}mTc DMSA scintigraphy. *AJR Am J Roentgenol* **157**: 539–43.

Blask ARN, Sanders RC, Gearhart JP (1991a) Obstructed uterovaginal anomalies: demonstration with sonography. Part I: neonates and infants. *Radiology* **179**: 79–93.

Blask ARN, Sanders RC, Rock JA (1991b) Obstructed uterovaginal anomalies: demonstration with sonography. Part II: teenagers. *Radiology* **179**: 84–8.

Bolande RP, Brough AJ, Azant RJ Jr (1967) Congenital mesoblastic nephroma of infant: a report of eight cases and the relationship to Wilms' tumor. *Pediatrics* **40**: 272–8.

Brown SM, Casillas VJ, Montalvo BM *et al.* (1990) Intrauterine spermatic cord torsion in the newborn: sonographic and pathologic correlation. *Radiology* **177**: 755.

Brun P, Kchouk H, Mouchet B *et al.* (1997) Value of Doppler ultrasound for the diagnosis of renal artery stenosis in children. *Pediatr Nephrol* **11**: 27–30.

Castleberry RP, Kelly DR, Joseph DB, Cain WS (1991) Gonadal and extragonadal germ cell tumors. In: Fernbach DJ, Vietti TJ (eds) *Clinical pediatric oncology*. St Louis: Mosby Year Book, 577–94.

Clautic-Engle T, Anderson NG, Allan RB (1995) Diagnosis of obstructive hydronephrosis in infants: comparison sonograms performed 6 days and 6 weeks after birth. *Am J Roentgenol* **199**: 441.

Cohen MD (1994) Intravenous use of ionic and nonionic contrast agents in children. *Radiology* **191**: 793–4.

Cohen MD (1996) Commentary: imaging and staging of Wilms' tumors: problems and controversies. *Pediatr Radiol* **26**: 307–11.

Cohen HL, Tice HM, Mandel FS (1990) Ovarian volumes measures by US: bigger than we think. *Radiology* **177**: 189–92.

Cohen HL, Shapiro MA, Mandel FS, Shapiro ML (1993) Normal ovaries in neonates and infants: a sonographic study of 77 patients 1 day to 24 months old. *Am J Roentgenol* **160**: 583–6.

Committee on Drugs (1992) Guidelines for monitoring and management of pediatric patients during and after sedation for diagnostic and therapeutic procedures. *Pediatrics* **89**: 1110–15.

Conway J, Cohn R (1994) Evolving role of nuclear medicine for the diagnosis and management of urinary tract injection. *J Pediatr* **124**: 87–90.

Dacher J-M, Pfister C, Monroc M *et al.* (1996) Power Doppler sonographic pattern of acute pyelonephritis in children: comparison with CT. *Am J Roentgenol* **166**: 1451.

De Sanctis JT, Connolly SA, Bramson RT (1998) Effect of patient position on sonographically measured renal length in neonates, infants, and children. *Am J Roentgenol* 170.

Dikengil A, Benson M, Sanders L *et al.* (1988) MRI of multilocular cystic nephroma. *Urol Radiol* **10**: 95–9.

Dodd GD III, Tublin ME, Shah A, Zajko AB (1991) Imaging of vascular complications associated with renal transplants. *AJR Am J Roentgenol* **157**: 449–59.

Douenias R, Smith AD, Brock WA (1990) Advances in the percutaneous management of the ureteropelvic junction and other obstructions of the urinary tract in children. *Urol Clin North Am* **17**: 419.

Douglas EC, Pratt CB (1997) Management of Infrequent Cancers of Childhood. In: Pizzo PA, Poplack DG (eds) *Principles and practice of pediatric oncology*. 3rd edition. Philadelphia, PA: Lippincott-Raven, 985–7.

Dremsek PA, Gindl K, Voitl P *et al.* (1997) Renal pyelectasis in fetus and neonates: diagnostic value of renal pelvis diameter in pre and postnatal sonographic screening. *Am J Roentgenol* **168**: 1017–19.

Ellis D, Shapiro R, Scantlebury VP *et al.* (1995) Evaluation and management of bilateral renal artery stenosis in children: a case series and review. *Pediatr Nephrol* **9**: 259–67.

Fernbach SK (1998) Pediatric uroradiology – 1997. *World J Urol* **16**: 46–51.

Fernbach SK, Maizels M, Conway JJ (1993) Ultrasound grading of hydronephrosis: introduction to the system used by the Society for Fetal Urology. *Pediatr Radiol* **23**: 478–80.

Finkelstein MS, Rosenberg HK, Snyder HM, Duckett JW (1986) Ultrasound evaluation of scrotum in pediatrics. *Urology* **27**: 1–9.

Garel L, Mareschal J, Gagnadouz M *et al.* (1986) Fatal outcome after ethanol renal ablation with child with end stage kidneys. *Am J Roentgenol* **146**: 593.

Gearhard JP, Hertzberg GZ, Jeffs RD (1991) Childhood urolithiasis: experience and advances. *Pediatrics* **87**: 445.

Gordon AC, Thomas DFM, Arthur RJ, Irving HC 1988 MCDK: is nephrectomy still appropriate? *J Urol* **140**: 1231–4.

Gordon I (1994) Imaging in systemic hypertension in pediatrics. *J Hum Hypertens* **8**: 377–9.

Graif M, Itzhak Y (1988) Sonographic evaluation of ovarian torsion in childhood and adolescence. *AJR Am J Roentgenol* **150**: 647–9.

Green DM, Coppes MJ, Breslow NE *et al.* (1997) Wilms' tumor. In: Pizzo PA, Poplack DG (eds) *Principles and practice of pediatric oncology*. 3rd edition. Philadelphia, PA: Lippincott-Raven, 713–37.

Gylys-Morin V, Hoffer FA, Kozakewich H *et al.* (1993) Wilms' tumor and nephroblastomatosis: imaging characteristics at gadolinium-enhanced MR imaging. *Radiology* **188**: 517–21.

Han BK, Babcock DS (1986) Sonographic measurement and appearance of normal kidneys in children. *Am J Roentgenol* **145**: 613.

Hartman DS, Lesar MSL, Madewell JE *et al.* (1981) Mesoblastic nephroma: radiologi–pathologic correlation of 20 cases. *Am J Roentgenol* **136**: 69–74.

Hartman DS, Davis CJ Jr, Goldman SM *et al.* (1982) Renal lymphoma: radiologic–pathologic correlation of 21 cases. *Radiology* **144**: 759–66.

Hernanz-Schulman M (1991) Hyperechoic renal medullary pyramids in infants and children. *Radiology* **186**: 9–11.

Hoffer F (1991) Imaging guided aspiration and biopsy in children. *Semin Intervent Radiol* **8**: 188–94.

Hricak H, Cruz C, Romanski R *et al.* (1982) Renal parenchymal disease: sonographic–histologic correlation. *Radiology* **144**: 141–7.

Jequier S, Rosseau O (1987) Sonographic measurements of the normal bladder wall in children. *Am J Roentgenol* **149**: 563–6.

Joshi VV, Beckwith JB (1989) Multilocular cyst of the kidney (cystic nephroma) and cystic, partially differentiated nephroblastoma: terminology and criteria for diagnosis. *Cancer* **64**: 466–79.

Kaefer M, Peters CA, Retik AB *et al.* (1997) Increased renal echogenicity: a sonographic sign for differentiating between obstructive and nonobstructive etiologies of in uretero bladder distension. *J Urol* **158**: 1026–9.

Karlowicz MG, Katz ME, Adelman RD *et al.* (1994) Nephrocalcinosis in very low birth weight neonates: family history of kidney stones and ethnicity as independent risk factors. *J Pediatr* **122**.

Kaufman RA, Holt JF, Heidelberger KP (1978) Calcification in primary and metastatic Wilms' tumor. *Am J Roentgenol* **130**: 783–5.

Kirks DR, Kaufman RA (1989) Function within mesoblastic nephroma: imaging pathologic correlation. *Pediatr Radiol* **19**: 136–9.

Klein PK, Diamond DA, Karellas A *et al.* (1994) Tailored low-dose fluoroscopic voiding cystourethrography for the reevaluation of vesicoureteral reflux in girls. *Am J Roentgenol* **162**: 1151–4.

Kletcher B, Badiola F de, Gonzalez R (1991) Outcome of hydronephrosis diagnosed antenatally. *J Pediatr Surg* **26**: 455–60.

Lalmand B, Avni EF, Simon J *et al.* (1987) Transitional cell papillary carcinoma of the bladder in a child. *Pediatr Radiol* **17**: 77–9.

Laplante S, Patriquin HB, Robitaille P *et al*. (1992) Renal vein thrombosis in children: evidence of early flow recovery with Doppler US. *Radiology* **184**: 479–85.

Leibowitz RL, Olbing H, Parkkulainen KV *et al*. (1985) International system of radiographic grading of vesicoureteral reflux. *Pediatr Rad* **15**: 105.

Lewis AG, Bukoshi TP, Jarvis PD *et al*. (1995) Evaluation of acute scrotum in the emergency department. *J Pediatr Surg* **30**: 277.

Luk GD, Siegel MJ (1994) Color Doppler sonography of he scrotum in children. *Am J Roentgenol* **163**: 649.

McAlister WH, Sisler CL (1990) Scrotal sonography in infants and children. *Curr Prob Radiol* **6**: 201–51.

McCartney WH (1992) Radionuclide genital imaging. *Urol Radiol* **14**: 96.

Madewell J, Goldman S, Davis C *et al*. (1983) Multilocular cystic nephroma: a radiographic–pathologic correlation of 58 patients. *Radiology* **146**: 309–21.

Majd M, Rushton HG (1992) Renal cortical scintigraphy in the diagnosis of acute pyelonephritis. *Semin Nucl Med* **22**: 98.

Mandell J, Blyth BR, Peters CA *et al*. (1991) Structural genitourinary tract defects detected *in utero*. *Radiology* **178**: 193.

Matsumura M, Nishi T, Sasaki Y *et al*. (1993) Prenatal diagnosis of treatment strategy for congenital mesoblastic nephroma. *J Pediatr Surg* **28**: 1607–9.

Meza MP, Amundson GM, Aquilina JW, Reitelman C (1992) Color flow imaging in children with clinically suspected testicular torsion. *Pediatr Radiol* **22**: 370–3.

Middleton WD, Dodd WJ, Lawson TL, Foley WD (1988) Renal calculi: sensitivity for detection with US. *Radiology* **167**: 239–44.

Mitchell CS, Yeo TA (1997) Noninvasive botryoid extension of Wilms' tumor into the bladder. *Pediatr Radiol* **27**: 818–20.

Mor Y, Elmasry YE, Kellett MH, Duffy PG (1997) The role of percutaneous nephrolithotomy in the management of pediatric renal calculi. *J Urol* **158**: 1319–21.

Myracle MR, McGahan JP, Goetzman BW *et al* (1986) Ultrasound diagnosis of renal calcifications in infants of chronic furosemide therapy. *J Clin Ultrasound* **14**: 281–7.

Nanni G, Hawkins IJ, Orak J (1983) Control of hypertension of ethanol renal ablation. *Radiology* **148**: 51.

Nussbaum AR, Sanders RC, Jones MD (1986) Neonatal uterine morphology as seen on real-time US. *Radiology* **160**: 641–3.

Orsini LF, Salardi S, Pilu G *et al*. (1989) Pelvic organs in premenarcheal girls: real-time ultrasonography. *Radiology* **170**: 557–8.

Owens CM, Burnett SJ, Veys PA *et al*. (1993) Role of pulmonary CT in staging and management of Wilms' tumor. Presented at the annual meeting of the Radiologic Societey of North America, Chicago, IL November 28–December 3, 1993.

Paltiel HJ, Rupich RC, Kirulata HG (1992) Enhanced detection of vesicouretral reflux in infants and children with use of cyclic voiding cystourethrography. *Radiology* **184**: 753–5.

Parienty RA, Pradel J, Imbert MC *et al*. (1981) Computed tomography of multilocular cystic nephroma. *Radiology* **140**: 135–9.

Patriquin H, Robitaille P (1988) Renal calcium deposition in children: sonographic demonstration of the Anderson–Carr progression. *Am J Roentgenol* **146**: 1253–6.

Patriquin H, Lafortune M. Jequier JC *et al*. (1992) Stenosis of the renal artery: assessment of slowed systole in the downstream circulation with Doppler sonography. *Radiology* **184**: 479–85.

Patrquin HB, Yazbeck S, Trinh B *et al*. (1993) Testicular torsion in infants and children: diagnosis with Doppler sonography. *Radiology* **188**: 781.

Pennington DJ, Lonergan GJ, Flack CE *et al*. (1996) Experimental pyelonephritis in piglets: diagnosis with MR imaging. *Radiology* **201**: 199.

Perlman ES, Rosenfield AT, Wexler JS *et al*. (1996) CT urography in the evaluation of urinary tract disease. *J Comput Assist Tomog* **20**: 620.

Postma CT, Van Aalen J, De Boo T *et al*. (1992) Doppler ultrasound scanning in the detection of renal artery stenosis in hypertensive patients. *Br J Radiol* **65**: 857–60.

Reuther G, Wanjura D, Bauer H (1989) Acute renal vein thrombosis in renal allografts: detection with duplex Doppler US. *Radiology* **170**: 557–8.

Riedy MJ, Lebowitz RL (1986) Percutaneous studies of the upper urinary tract in children with special emphasis on infants. *Radiology* **160**: 231.

Ritchey ML, Kelalis PP, Breslow N *et al*. (1988) Intracaval and atrial involvement with nephroblastoma: review of National Wilms' Tumor Study 3. *J Urol* **140**: 1113–18.

Rosado WM Jr, Trambert MA, Gosink BB, Pretorius DH (1992) Adnexal torsion: diagnosis by using Doppler sonography. *AJR Am J Roentgenol* **159**: 1251–3.

Rosenberg HK, Udassin R, Howell C *et al*. (1982) Duplication of the uterus and vagina, unilateral hydrometrocolpos, and episilateral renal agenesis: sonography aid to diagnosis. *J Ultrasound Med* **1**: 289–91.

Rosendahl W, Grunert D, Schoning M (1994) Duplex sonography of renal arteries as a diagnostic tool in hypertensive children. *Eur J Pediatr* **153**: 588–93.

Rosenfield AT, Siegel NG (1981) Renal parenchymal disease: histopathologic sonographic correlation. *Am J Roentgenol* **137**: 793–8.

Rosenfield AT, Zeman RK, Cronan JJ *et al*. (1980) Ultrasound in experimental and clinical renal vein thrombosis. *Radiology* **137**: 735–41.

Rottenberg GT, De Bruyn R, Gordon I (1996) Sonographic standards for a single functioning kidney in children. *Am J Roentgenol* **167**: 1255–9.

Schwerk WB, Schwerk WN, Rodeck G (1987) Testicular tumors: prospective analysis of real-time US findings and abdominal staging. *Radiology* **164**: 369–74.

Shan A, Feldman W, McDonald P *et al*. (1992) Evaluation of renal scars by technetium-labeled dimercaptosuccinic acid scan, intravenous urography, and sonography: a comparative study. *J Pediatr* **129**: 399–403.

Sharma S, Thatai D, Saxena A *et al*. (1996) Renovascular hypertension resulting from nonspecific aortoarteritis in children: midterm results of percutaneous transluminal angioplasty and predictors of restenosis. *Am J Roentgenol* **166**: 157–62.

Short C, Cooke RWI (1991) The incidence of renal calcification in preterm infants. *Arch Dis Child* **66**: 412–17.

Siegal M (1995) Urinary tract. In: Siegel M (ed.) *Pediatric sonography*, 2nd edition. New York: Raven Press, 411–22.

Slovis TL (1992) Is there a single most appropriate imaging workup of a child with an acute febrile urinary tract infection? *J Pediatr* **129**: 399–403.

Slovis TL, Babcock DS, Hricak H *et al*. (1984) Renal transplant rejection: sonographic evaluation in children. *Radiology* **153**: 659–65.

Slovis TL, Bernstein J, Gruskin A (1993) Hyperechoic kidneys in the newborn and young infants. *Pediatr Nephrol* **7**: 294–302.

Stanhope R, Adams J, Jacobs HS, Brook CGD (1985) Ovarian ultrasound assessment in normal chilren, idiopathic precocious puberty, and during low dose pulsatile gonadotropin releasing hormone treatment of hypogonadotropic hypogonadism. *Arch Dis Child* **60**: 116–19.

Stanley P, Hieshima G, Mehringr M (1984) Percutaneous transluminal angioplasty for pediatric renal vascular hypertension. *Radiology* **153**: 101.

Stavros AT, Parker SH, Yakes WF *et al*. (1992) Segmental stenosis of the renl artery: pattern recognition of tardus and parvus abnormalities with duplex sonography. *Radiology* **184**: 487.

Strife JL, Bisset GS, Kirks DR *et al*. (1989) Nuclear cystography and renal sonography: findings in girls with urinary tract infection. *Am J Roentgenol* **148**: 479.

Strife JL, Souza AS, Kirks DR *et al*. (1993) Multicystic dysplastic kidney in children: US follow-up. *Radiology* **186**: 785–8.

Tannous WN, Azou EM, Homsy YL *et al*. (1989) Computed tomography and ultrasound imaging of pelvic rhabdomyosarcomas in children: a review of 56 patients. *Pediatr Radiol* **19**: 530.

Towbin RB, Ball WS JR (1988) Pediatric interventional radiology. *Radiat Clin North Am* **26**: 419–40.

Towbin R, Kaye R, Bron K (1994) Intervention in the critically ill patient. *Crit Care Clin* **10**: 437–54.

Vinocur L, Slovis TL, Perlmutter AD *et al*. (1988) Follow-up studies of multicystic dysplastic kidneys. *Radiology* **167**: 311–15.

Weinberger E, Rosenbaum DM, Pendergrass TW (1990) Renal involvement in children with lymphoma: comparison of CT with sonography. *Am J Roentgenol* **155**: 347–9.

Wexler LH, Helman LJ *et al*. (1997) Rhabdomyosarcoma and the undifferentiated sarcomas. In: Pizzo PA, Poplack DG (eds) *Principles and practice of pediatric oncology*, 3rd edition. Philadelphia, PA: Lippincott-Raven, 799–824.

Whitaker RH (1973) Diagnosis of obstruction in dilated ureters. *Ann R Coll Surg Engl* **53**: 153–66.

Wilkinson AG, Azmy A (1996) Balloon dilatation of the pelviureteric junction in children: early experience and pitfalls. *Pediatr Radiol* **26**: 882.

Woodside JR, Stevens GF, Stark GL *et al*. (1985) Percutaneous stone removal in children. *U Urol* **134**: 1166.

Zerin JM (1997) Uroradiologic emergencies in infants and children. *Radiat Clin Am* **35**: 897–919.

Zerin JM, Blane CE (1994) Sonographic assessment of renal length in children: a reappraisal. *Pediatr Radiol* **24**: 101–6.

Zerin JM, Ritchey ML, Change AC (1993) Incidental vesicoureteral reflux in neonates with antenatally detected hydronephrosis and other renal abnormalities. *Radiology* **187**: 157.

Nuclear medicine

6

Sara M. O'Hara

Introduction

Nuclear medicine and sonography have become the current mainstays in the diagnosis and management of urologic problems in infants and children. The combined physiologic and anatomic information provided by these two imaging modalities helps to determine the necessity and timing of intervention, and assess response to therapy. The introduction of better radiopharmaceuticals, the improvement in imaging devices (gamma cameras), and the use of computers in analysis of the functional parameters of the genitourinary system have all contributed to increased utilization of nuclear imaging in pediatric urology. Sonography and nuclear medicine studies have virtually replaced excretory urography in the pediatric population today.

Nuclear medicine procedures are generally minimally invasive, requiring at most intravenous access and a bladder catheter. Sedation is seldom necessary when those performing the examination pay sufficient attention to patient comfort, immobilization, and parental/caregiver participation. Children do not need to fast, follow bowel preparation regimens, or be hospitalized for these examinations. The radiopharmaceuticals used in urologic imaging have no systemic pharmacologic effects and do not cause any allergic reaction. Absorbed radiation doses from the radionuclide studies do not reach a harmful range and, in some instances, are much lower than the doses from comparable radiographic tests. Most importantly, radionuclide studies offer quantitative functional information currently not available with other imaging modalities. Furthermore, they lend themselves to a variety of physiologic and pharmacologic interventions that can enhance their diagnostic accuracy. Notable examples of the use of pharmacologic intervention in renal studies are diuretic renography and captopril-enhanced renal scintigraphy. Many disorders of the genitourinary system in children are part of a dynamic process that necessitates serial assessment. Nuclear imaging studies provide optimal means of evaluating and following the course of such disorders (Taylor *et al.*, 1989).

Renal imaging and functional analysis

Radiopharmaceuticals

Radionuclide renal studies are used to assess renal perfusion and various aspects of renal function and structure. The radiopharmaceuticals are cleared by glomerular filtration, tubular secretion, and tubular binding in varying proportions. The information gained depends on which radiopharmaceutical is used. Currently, the following radiopharmaceuticals are used for the evaluation of the kidneys.

Technetium-99m-mercaptoacetyltriglycine

Technetium-99m-mercaptoacetyltriglycine ($[^{99m}Tc]$ MAG-3) is a relatively new renal radiopharmaceutical that combines the desirable biologic properties of an older agent, Hippuran [orthoiodohippurate(OIH)], and the imaging properties of technetium-99m. This agent is rapidly cleared by tubular secretion and is not retained in the parenchyma of normal kidneys. Although extraction of MAG-3 from blood in each passage through the kidney is less than that of OIH, the rates at which the two tracers appear in the urine are almost identical. This is primarily due to the fact that MAG-3 is more highly protein bound than OIH and a greater percentage of the injection dose remains in the intravascular compartment. Furthermore, in contrast to OIH, very little, if any, MAG-3 enters the red blood cells. Therefore, a higher percentage of the injected dose of MAG-3 is available for renal clearance (Taylor *et al.*, 1989).

Owing to its superior imaging qualities and lower radiation doses, [^{99m}Tc]MAG-3 is rapidly gaining acceptance as the first choice in renal perfusion and drainage studies. The quality of MAG-3 images is also superior to the quality of diethylenetriaminepentaacetic acid (DTPA) images. This is due to a much smaller volume of distribution and faster clearance, resulting in higher target-to-background ratio, even in premature infants with low glomerular filtration rates (GFR). Therefore, MAG-3 appears to be a good replacement for DTPA in certain applications, such as diuretic renography. These favorable qualities of [^{99m}Tc]MAG-3 make it particularly appealing for use in the pediatric age group.

Technetium-99m-diethylenetriamine pentaacetic acid

[^{99m}Tc]DTPA is commonly used for quantitative GFR and other renal studies. Renal clearance of DTPA is almost exclusively by glomerular filtration, with no significant tubular secretion or cortical retention. Therefore, its rate of clearance provides an accurate measurement of the GFR. Its initial transit through the kidney reflects renal perfusion. Accumulation of the tracer in each kidney between 1 and 3 min after injection is proportional to its GFR. Because of rapid clearance, the high concentration of [^{99m}Tc]DTPA in the urine provides excellent visualization of the pelvicalyceal systems, ureter, and bladder. Because of its low retention in the renal cortex, however, this agent may fail to demonstrate small cortical lesions.

Technetium-99m-glucoheptonate

[^{99m}Tc]glucoheptonate (GHA) is cleared by a combination of glomerular filtration and tubular extraction. Most of the agent is rapidly excreted in the urine, allowing moderately good visualization of the pelvicalyceal systems, ureters, and bladder. Approximately 20% of the administered dose of glucoheptonate, however, remains in the renal cortex, firmly bound to the tubular cells. Therefore, delayed imaging at 2–4 hours provides visualization of the renal cortex. GHA, owing to its complex mode of clearance, is not a suitable agent for measuring GFR. However, its accumulation in each kidney between 1 and 3 min after injection can be used as a measure of relative renal function.

Cortical uptake of glucoheptonate in each kidney on the delayed images can also be used for calculation of differential renal function, provided that there is no retention of the tracer in the pelvicalyceal system. In patients with impaired renal function, hepatobiliary excretion of glucoheptonate increases and may show tracer activity in the gallbladder or bowel. Because this agent lies between the filtration/drainage agents and the purely cortical agents, it provides a good overall assessment of differential renal function, pelviureteral washout, and cortical pathology.

Technetium-99m-dimercaptosuccinic acid

[^{99m}Tc]dimercaptosuccinic acid (DMSA) is presently the best cortical imaging agent available. The majority is tightly bound to the renal tubular cells, and only a small amount is excreted in the urine. Approximately 50% of the injected dose is bound to the tubules in the renal cortex after 1 hour (Enlander *et al.*, 1974). DMSA allows excellent visualization of the renal parenchyma without interference from pelvicalyceal activity and is therefore recommended for detection of cortical lesions such as acute pyelonephritis, cortical scars, or infarcts. The uptake of [^{99m}Tc]DMSA by each kidney is an accurate measure of relative functioning tubular mass and in most situations correlates well with the relative GFR and other parameters of renal function (Taylor, 1982).

Iodine-131-orthoiodohippurate

[^{131}I]OIH, (Hippuran) is primarily a tubular agent. Approximately 80% of OIH entering the kidney is extracted with each pass, of which 85–90% is removed by tubular secretion and the remaining 10–15% by passive glomerular filtration. Despite these excellent biologic properties, which mimic paraaminohippurate clearance, and its past popularity, [^{131}I]OIH currently has little place in pediatric nuclear medicine. The major disadvantages of this agent are poor characteristics of its gamma radiation for imaging and high radiation dose resulting from its emission of beta particles. This necessitates the use of a low dose of the tracer, leading to a poor-resolution image.

Iodine-123-orthoiodohippurate

[^{123}I]labeled OIH, in contrast, is an excellent renal imaging agent. ^{123}I is a pure gamma emitter with an energy level suitable for imaging with the scintillation camera. It can be used in millicurie doses with a significantly lower radiation dose than would be received from microcuries of [^{131}I]OIH. Cyclotron produced, radiochemically pure [^{123}I]OIH, however, is not readily available, is costly, and has a short half-life. Thus, this agent is seldom used.

Procedures

Renal scintigraphy

The conventional renal scan should consist of a radionuclide angiogram followed by sequential functional images of the kidneys, ureters, and bladder. The techniques used in different institutions vary greatly. The following technique, modified from the Society of Nuclear Medicine Guidelines (Mandell *et al.*, 1997) is currently used in this author's laboratory.

After establishing intravenous access, the patient is hydrated and comfortably immobilized. If diuretic scintigraphy is being performed, a bladder catheter is also inserted. After a rapid intravenous injection of an appropriate amount of the tracer (MAG-3, DTPA, or GHA), a series of 2-second dynamic posterior images of the kidneys is obtained during the first minute, angiographic phase (Fig. 6.1). This is followed by a series of 1-min images of the kidney, ureters, and bladder for 20 min for the evaluation of renal excretion and drainage of the tracer. In cases of known hydronephrosis or suspected obstruction, furosemide (Lasix) is given at this point and imaging continues for an additional 20 min. Further delayed images, and images after standing upright, are obtained if necessary.

Digital images are also acquired on a computer at the rate of one image per second for 60 seconds (angiographic phase) followed by a series of 15-second images for 20 min. The early digital images, after the angiographic phase and before accumulation of the tracer in the collecting systems, are used to generate time–activity curves for assessment of relative renal function.

Although analog images allow for a rough visual assessment of renal vascular perfusion, computer

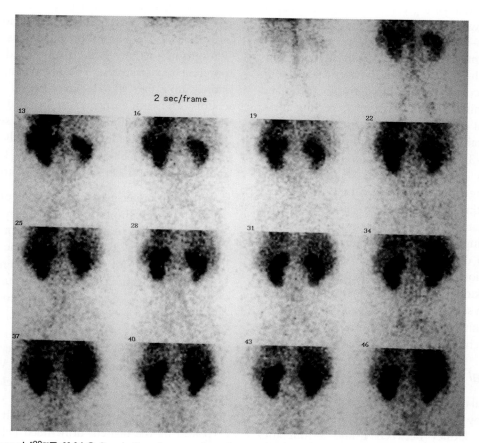

Figure 6.1 Normal [^{99m}Tc]MAG-3 scintiangiogram in a 1 month-old infant. Images taken at 2 seconds/frame show renal perfusion simultaneously, within 2 seconds of radiotracer appearance in the mid-aorta.

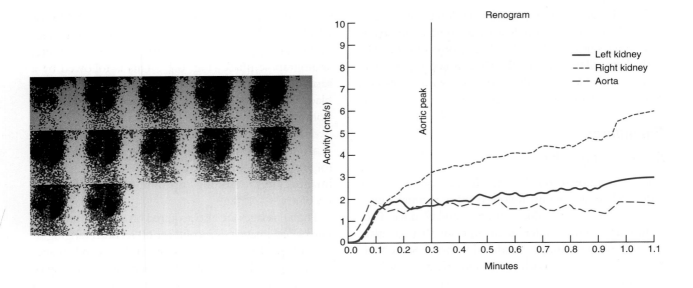

Figure 6.2 Normal time–activity curves in the same infant, showing aortic peak occurring just prior to renal upslope. Note the flattening of the aortic curve with time while the renal curves continue to rise.

analysis is essential for a precise assessment. Areas of interest are drawn over the abdominal aorta and the kidneys. Time–activity curves are generated from these areas of interest. The renal slopes are then compared with each other and with the aortic slope (Fig. 6.2). Normal curves show a rapid rise in aortic and renal activity initially, then stable or decreasing aortic activity as renal counts continue to rise.

Renal cortical imaging is accomplished by delayed imaging 1.5–3 hours after injection of either [^{99m}Tc]DMSA or [^{99m}Tc]GHA. Magnified, high-resolution images of each kidney, in posterior and posterior oblique projections, are obtained using a pinhole collimator. In addition, a posterior image of the kidneys using a parallel hole collimator is obtained for calculation of differential renal function. Single-photon emission computed tomography (SPECT) images of the kidneys are used routinely in some institutions, and in selected cases at the author's center.

Captopril-enhanced renal scintigraphy, a variation on the above scheme, is discussed later in this chapter.

Relative renal function

The differential or relative function of each kidney can be calculated by determining the accumulation of the tracer in each kidney between 1 and 3 min after injection. During this period, all of the radioactivity within the kidney is confined to the blood pool and

functioning renal parenchyma, as the tracer has not yet reached the collecting system. Regions of interest are selected for each kidney and its background. Background activity is then subtracted from corresponding renal activity. The net counts within each kidney are expressed as a percentage of the total renal counts. The same principle can be used in calculating the relative contribution of different segments of a kidney to its total function. The pitfalls of the differential function analysis, based on the 1–3 min accumulation of the tracer in the kidneys, are as follows.

1   While computer-generated regions of interest suffice in cases without unusual anatomy or significant dysfunction, the technique is operator dependent in abnormal cases. The selection of the time interval and the regions of interest affect the results. This is particularly critical for the background regions of interest, which may include a portion of the liver and spleen, areas containing a high concentration of the tracer.

2   The results may be invalid in the presence of extreme hydronephrosis or delayed function. When the cortex is thin and poorly functioning, selecting an area of interest is difficult. Attenuation of the counts from the anterior parenchyma, which is widely displaced by the dilated, urine-filled pelvicalyceal system, results in inaccurate calculation of the total activity contained in the entire renal parenchyma.

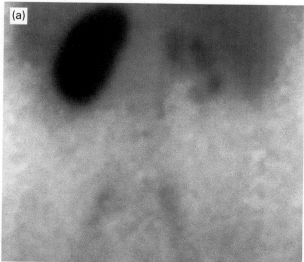

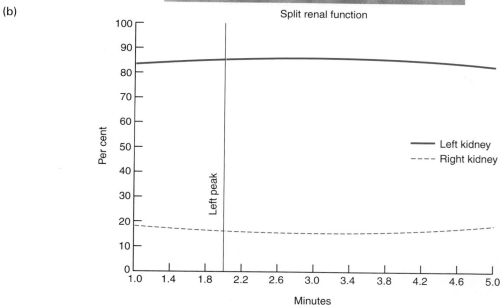

Figure 6.3 (*a*) Posterior image at 1–3 min after injection of [99mTc]MAG-3 shows a poorly functioning right kidney with central photopenia, probably related to hydronephrosis. (*b*) The split function curve in the same patient shows that the right kidney contributes less than 20% of total renal function. Function on this side did not improve with time, reflecting parenchymal damage in this chronically obstructed and atrophic kidney.

3 In cases of delayed function, graphic display of split renal function over the first several minutes of the examination can demonstrate increasing function with time. One should be careful to take into account activity that may appear early in the collecting system of a normal contralateral kidney (Fig. 6.3a, b).

The relative renal function can also be calculated on delayed images (1.5–3 hours) using [99mTc]DMSA (Fig. 6.4) or [99mTc]glucoheptonate. The advantages to this method are as follows.

1 The background activity is negligible by that time, and thus one source of potential error is eliminated.
2 Both anterior and posterior images can be obtained from which a geometric mean value can be calculated. The geometric mean may be more reliable than the count ratios from posterior images alone as routinely obtained when MAG-3 or DTPA is used, particularly when the kidneys are at different depths.

Several investigations have confirmed the validity of these methods of calculating differential renal function by comparing results from DMSA, DTPA, and ureteral catheterization studies with split creatinine clearances (Daly *et al.*, 1979; Powers *et al.*, 1981). The percentages calculated using DTPA and glucoheptonate are the same, in spite of their different modes of renal excretion. Furthermore, the glucoheptonate ratios calculated on the basis of early and delayed images are similar.

The differential renal functional analysis is an index only of relative function of the kidneys and does not provide information about absolute function of each kidney. Reliable quantitation of absolute renal function in pediatric patients requires blood or urine sampling and is merely estimated by imaging methods alone.

Total and separate glomerular filtration rates

Since [^{99m}Tc]DTPA is excreted almost exclusively by glomerular filtration, its rate of clearance from blood is an accurate measure of GFR. A variety of methods may be used to calculate GFR using [^{99m}Tc]DTPA (Russell *et al.*, 1985; Mulligan *et al.*, 1990; Blaufox *et al.*, 1996). The simplest method, which employs two blood samples drawn at 1 and 3 hours after injection, is based on single compartmental analysis of the DTPA clearance (Fig. 6.5). There is excellent correlation between this technique and 24-hour urinary creatinine clearance (Braren *et al.*, 1979). Absolute GFR

of each kidney can then be calculated by multiplying the total calculated GFR in milliliters per minute by the percentages obtained from the imaging assessment of differential renal function. This method of GFR calculation is relatively non-invasive and obviates the need for 24-hour urine collection. Because of the need for multiple venous punctures, however, the test is unpleasant for children and their parents. Because of uncertainty about the effect of diuretics on the GFR in different pathologic states, the test cannot be reliably performed in conjunction with diuretic renography. Some antihypertensive medications, namely angiotensin converting enzyme (ACE) inhibitors, can also alter GFR results.

Other methods of calculating GFR based on external counting without blood samples or with a single blood sample have been developed (Gates, 1982; Shore *et al.*, 1984). These methods have become popular in adult nuclear medicine, but their reliability for use in children has not been proven.

Clinical applications

What the radionuclide renal scan lacks in anatomic resolution is far surpassed in physiologic assessment. Renal scans provide quantitative measures of renal function, despite overlying bowel contents and bony structures, and enable easy identification of ectopic parenchyma and renal tissue with a very low level of

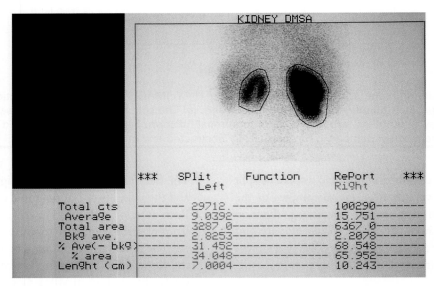

Figure 6.4 Differential function as calculated from delayed posterior image of [^{99m}Tc]DMSA exam. The patient has a history of high-grade reflux on the left. The left kidney is globally scarred and has virtually no function in the lower pole. Note the small scar in the right kidney laterally. From the regions of interest drawn, differential function is 31% left and 69% right.

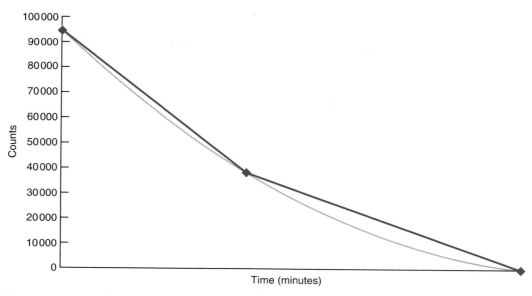

Figure 6.5 Graphic display of serum sample counts of [99mTc]DTPA, drawn 1 and 3 hours after radiopharmaceutical bolus. From the slope of the curve and the child's body surface area, GFR was calculated to be 88 ml/min per 1.73 m². This value is below normal, but stable in this teenage patient with glomerulonephritis.

function. These advantages are particularly important in neonates. At birth, the GFR is about 21% of the corrected adult value and reaches only 44% by 2 weeks of age (McCrory, 1972). The low GFR, together with overlying bowel gas, generally results in poor visualization of kidneys on the excretory urogram. The radiation exposure from multiple radiographs and, occasionally, tomography far exceeds the radiation exposure from nuclear imaging techniques. Thus, excretory urography may expose the child to an unacceptably high radiation dose. In addition, the iodinated contrast media may produce osmotic side-effects (Wood and Smith, 1981) and allergic reactions not seen with radiopharmaceuticals discussed in this chapter. Radionuclide scanning, which is limited only by renal function, is superior to excretory urography for localization and functional analysis of the kidneys in all ages, including the newborn.

Congenital anomalies

Any functioning renal tissue, irrespective of its location, can be visualized on renal scan. Ectopic kidneys, that are often superimposed on bones and may remain obscure on an excretory urogram, can be easily demonstrated and differentiated from renal agenesis. The horseshoe kidney and other variants of fused kidneys are also often more apparent on a renal scan than on sonograms or excretory urograms (Fig. 6.6).

The renal scan is frequently useful to confirm renal duplication suspected on the excretory urogram or sonogram or even to diagnose unsuspected cases. The function of each moiety of a duplicated kidney relative to the other and to the opposite kidney can be assessed. This may be important in deciding whether there is enough function to salvage a hydronephrotic, poorly functioning moiety.

The two most common flank masses in the neonatal period are multicystic dysplastic kidney (MCDK)

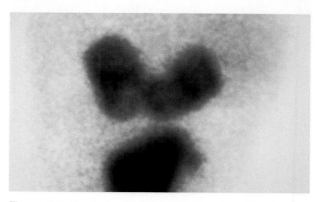

Figure 6.6 Posterior image approximately 30 min after administration of [99mTc]GHA shows abnormal orientation of the kidneys, horseshoe variant. Note the full bladder in this toddler.

and hydronephrosis caused by congenital uretero-pelvic junction (UPJ) obstruction. The multicystic dysplastic kidney is postulated to be caused by atresia of the ureter, renal pelvis, or both during the metanephric stage of renal development and is probably the end of the spectrum of ureteral obstruction (Felson and Cusson, 1975; Griscom *et al.*, 1975). The continuing function of a few glomeruli and tubules creates hydronephrosis proximal to the obstruction. With time, the altered excretory function inhibits cellular development and the kidney becomes dysplastic. Depending on the number of functioning glomeruli remaining, the kidney may show minimal or no function. In contrast, a kidney with congenital UPJ obstruction without dysplasia of the renal parenchyma usually retains significant function, unless prolonged obstruction has existed or infection has supervened. Therefore, the presence or absence of functioning renal tissue dictates management. The additional association of MCDK with contralateral abnormalities necessitates early work-up and intervention (Fig. 6.7).

Sonography is the ideal initial imaging procedure in the evaluation of neonatal abdominal masses. It shows whether the mass is of renal or extrarenal origin and establishes the tissue character of the mass (solid, cystic, or mixed). The next step in the evaluation of proven renal pathology is often renal scinti-graphy to evaluate renal function. Both multicystic kidney and severe hydronephrosis appear as a relatively avascular mass on the angiographic phase of the examination. Because the dysplastic tissue of a MCDK is still perfused, transient radiotracer accumulation is often seen. The delayed functional images in multicystic kidney show either no evidence of functioning renal tissue or only very minimal function without excretion into the collecting system. In contrast, the salvageable hydronephrotic kidney demonstrates a rind of functioning cortex of varying thickness at the periphery on the early static images, while the delayed images show significant accumulation of the tracer in the dilated pelvicalyceal system.

Hydronephrosis

With the increasing use of antenatal sonography, renal anomalies, including hydronephrosis, are being diagnosed much earlier and with greater frequency. In fact, hydronephrosis is the most common abnormality found on prenatal sonograms. Patients with hydronephrosis or hydroureteronephrosis may also present with urinary tract infection (UTI) or an abdominal mass. Assessment of renal function and differentiation between obstructive and non-obstructive hydronephrosis are essential in the management of these patients. The diagnostic procedures used in the evaluation of hydronephrosis include cysto-

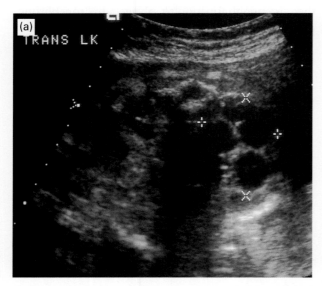 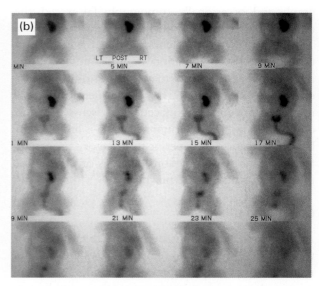

Figure 6.7 (*a*) *In utero* axial sonogram shows multiple cysts in the left renal fossa adjacent to the dark shadow created by the spine. Differential considerations are hydronephrotic kidney and MCDK. (*b*) [99mTc]MAG-3 study performed shortly after delivery shows no function in the left kidney and normal uptake and drainage on the right. Note the bladder catheter draining activity. The baby had MCDK.

graphy, renal sonography, renal scintigraphy with or without diuretic enhancement, and increasingly, magnetic resonance imaging (MRI). Pressure perfusion studies (the Whitaker test), excretory urography, retrograde pyelography and computed tomography (CT) are seldom used in the current work-up of these pediatric patients.

Vesicoureteral reflux (VUR) as the cause of hydronephrosis is readily diagnosed by radiographic or radionuclide cystography. It should be noted, however, that reflux and obstruction may coexist (Lebowitz and Blickman, 1983). The conventional excretory urogram is occasionally diagnostic of obstruction but frequently does not differentiate between obstructive and non-obstructive hydronephrosis. A retrograde pyelogram may define the site of the change in ureteral caliber, but does not provide functional information about the renal parenchyma that it subtends and is rarely indicated.

The pressure perfusion study (the Whitaker test) is based on the hypothesis that the dilated upper urinary tract can transport 10 ml/min without an inordinate increase in pressure. The hydrostatic pressure in the system is then thought to be within physiologically normal levels and should not cause deterioration of renal function, and the degree of obstruction, if any, is insignificant. The Whitaker test is generally accepted as the standard for distinguishing obstructive from non-obstructive hydronephrosis. Its invasive nature, however, makes it undesirable for screening purposes and particularly for serial assessments. Furthermore, it does not provide any information about renal function.

The conventional renal nuclear scan demonstrates the presence, extent, and severity of hydronephrosis, and allows quantitative assessment of residual renal function. The addition of Lasix (furosemide) is needed to differentiate obstructive from non-obstructive hydronephrosis. Diuretic excretory urography was based on the principle that, in the presence of significant obstruction, the urinary tract is unable to transport fluid over the physiologic range of flow rate and diuresis produces a significant increase in the dimensions of the pelvicalyceal system. A 20–22% increase in the area of the pelvicalyceal system after furosemide-induced diuresis has been reported to indicate significant obstruction (Whitfield et al., 1977). Quantification by planimetry of the changes in the size of the pelvicalyceal system, however, is imprecise, and the test is not reliable. The following modifications of radionuclide renography offer more objective means of differentiating obstructed from non-obstructive dilatation.

Diuretic-augmented radionuclide renography

This provocative test is based on the hypothesis that prolonged retention of the radiotracer in the non-obstructed, dilated upper urinary tract is due to a reservoir effect and that increased urine flow following diuretic administration should result in prompt washout of the tracer. Conversely, in obstructive hydronephrosis there should not be any significant washout following diuretic challenge. In cases of partial obstruction, increased urine flow may potentiate flank pain and unmask flow-dependent obstruction. The techniques and analytical methods used by different investigators vary widely. Diuretic renography is dependent on several physiologic, mechanical, and technical factors. Understanding the principles of the test, its limitations, and sources of error is essential in the interpretation of the results and effective use of the test. Figure 6.8 is an example of a normal pediatric diuretic renogram using MAG-3.

Factors affecting the renogram

The factors that affect the rate of the washout of the tracer and the shape of the renogram curve include the following.

State of hydration

Adequate hydration is essential for diuresis. In addition to prescribing oral intake of fluid before the test, the patient may be hydrated with intravenous 5% dextrose in one-half normal saline. This improves excretion of the tracer, enhances the response to furosemide, and prevents dehydration.

Fullness of the bladder

Increased intravesical pressure associated with a full bladder may significantly affect the drainage from the upper urinary tract. An indwelling catheter should be inserted for continuous drainage of urine unless the patient can void independently on command as the bladder fills. This has the following advantages.

- It eliminates the effect of a full bladder on the washout.
- It allows measurement of the urine output at any chosen interval before and after injection of furosemide.

It eliminates the discomfort of a full bladder, which can cause the patient to move during acquisition of computer data.

It decreases radiation dose to the gonads by rapidly draining the radioactive urine.

It eliminates the effect of vesicoureteral reflux should reflux exist (Fig. 6.9a, b).

Variable degrees of obstruction

Practically all cases of obstruction are partial with varying degrees of severity. It is often difficult to predict what degree of obstructions will lead to deterioration of renal function. Some cases of obstruction are intermittent. Furthermore, the obstructive process, particularly in a young infant,

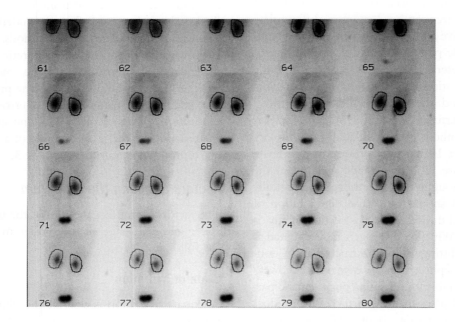

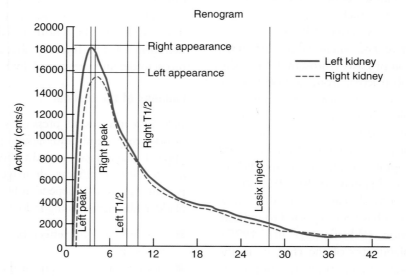

Figure 6.8 Normal [^{99m}Tc]MAG-3 renogram demonstrating good uptake of radiotracer and prompt excretion bilaterally. The time–activity curves show a sharp rise to peak activity and steep washout curve.

Renogram

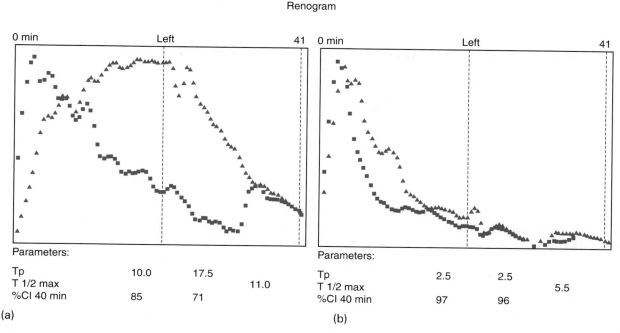

Parameters:

Tp	10.0	17.5	
T 1/2 max			11.0
%Cl 40 min	85	71	

(a)

Parameters:

Tp	2.5	2.5	
T 1/2 max			5.5
%Cl 40 min	97	96	

(b)

Figure 6.9 (*a*) [⁹⁹ᵐTc]MAG-3 study in a child with known right reflux. This study was performed without a bladder catheter and the patient was unable to void voluntarily. The left kidney appears to have an equivocal curve, while the right kidney appears obstructed. Note the change in the time–activity curves, reflecting reflux on the right and back pressure on the left. (*b*) The study was repeated 1 week later with a Foley catheter in the bladder. Neither kidney is obstructed. ▲ = right; ■ = left.

may be progressive. Therefore, the definition of significant obstruction remains imprecise.

Variable impairment of renal function

The rate of accumulation of radionuclide in the dilated collecting system, as well as the response to diuretic, is dependent on renal function. Therefore, in the presence of poor renal function the test is unreliable. Unfortunately, the level of renal function below which the diuretic renogram becomes unreliable is not clearly defined. The author's experience suggests that when the collecting system does not completely fill within 1 hour after injection of the tracer, or if the affected kidney has less than 20% of the total renal function, a prolonged washout may not be absolutely indicative of obstruction.

Age of patient

It is commonly suggested that, because of renal immaturity, the child under 1 month of age is not a candidate for diuretic renography. The concern is that younger kidneys cannot concentrate the radioisotope

or respond properly to the diuretic agent. Chung *et al.* (1993) reviewed the results of diuretic renograms of 17 consecutively studied neonates (<28 days of age). The youngest child was 3 days with nine under 2 weeks. All had follow-up scans and the results compared with the initial study. There was no statistically significant difference between initial and follow-up renal function nor reponse to diuresis. The conclusion was that when properly performed, the Lasix renal scan is applicable to all age groups.

Capacity and compliance of the dilated system

In the presence of massive hydroureteronephrosis, even a very good response to furosemide may have little effect on the washout of tracer from the huge pool of retained tracer and may cause false-positive results. Distensibility or compliance of the dilated collecting system also plays a role.

Dose of diuretic

The response to furosemide is dose dependent. A dose of 1 mg/kg (maximum 40 mg) has been found to be very effective and safe. Lower doses of furosemide do not yield reliable washout curves (Gordon *et al.*, 1991).

Time of diuretic injection

Some have advocated injection of the diuretic shortly (2–3 min) after injection of the tracer (Sfakianakis and Sfakianakis, 1988). This may not adversely affect the washout curves of the mildly dilated, non-obstructed systems. But, more severely dilated systems will probably remain incompletely filled during the acquisition of the computer data and the washout will appear falsely prolonged. Others have advocated injection of furosemide 15 min before or coincident with injection of the tracer (English *et al.*, 1987; Sfakianakis *et al.*, 1999). This is based on the assumption that the peak effect of furosemide is at about 30 min after injection. In the experience of several large pediatric nuclear imaging departments, based on routine measurement of urine output at 10-min intervals, maximal diuresis usually occurs within a few minutes of furosemide in the hydrated child. Therefore, it seems logical to administer furosemide after most of the injected tracer has cleared from the blood, at which time concentration of the tracer in the retained urine is at its maximum and in the incoming urine at its minimum. In well-hydrated patients with normal real function, this occurs at about 20–30 min after injection of the tracer. Alternatively, the accumulation of tracer can be continuously monitored and when the dilated collecting system is maximally filled, the furosemide injected (Majd, 1992).

Patient position

Washout of the retained tracer is occasionally affected by the position of the patient. The easiest and most practical position for immobilization and observation of the patient and for performance of diuretic renography in the pediatric age group is supine, with the camera positioned underneath the patient. However, if drainage is markedly delayed during the first 30 min after diuretic injection, the patient can be placed in the prone or upright seated position and additional images obtained for 10–15 minutes. Markedly improved drainage with alteration in patient position makes high-grade obstruction less likely and is usually associated with preservation of renal function.

Radiopharmaceutical

The ideal radiopharmaceutical for diuretic renography should have rapid blood clearance, a short physical half-life, and radiation characteristics suitable for imaging. And, it should be readily available. At present, [^{99m}Tc]MAG-3 is clearly the radiopharmaceutical of choice for diuretic renography.

Region of interest

Appropriate regions of interest should be chosen for generation of the curves. The changes in the amount of tracer in a portion of dilated system may not be representative of the drainage from the entire system. In the presence of both pelvic and ureteral dilatation, the ureter can function as a reservoir for the tracer drained from the renal pelvis. Therefore, time–activity curves using a region of interest including the entire dilated collecting system are sometimes helpful (Fig. 6.10).

Technique of diuretic renography

It is desirable to adopt a standard technique that eliminates or reduces the effect of as many of the aforementioned variables as possible. The following technique has evolved from personal experience at several institutions and is in accordance with the Society of Nuclear Medicine Guidelines (Mandell *et al.*, 1997).

The patient is positioned supine on the scanning table with the gamma camera underneath. An intravenous line is established and an indwelling bladder catheter is inserted. The patient is hydrated by intravenous administration of 5% dextrose in one-half normal saline during the test (total 15 ml/kg, starting before the injection of the tracer) and with oral fluids *ad libitum*. A conventional renal scan using either [^{99m}Tc]MAG-3 (100 μCi/kg, minimum 500 mCi) or [^{99m}Tc]DTPA (100 μCi/kg, minimum 1 mCi) is obtained. Accumulation of the tracer is continuously monitored, and when the dilated system is filled with tracer, typically at 20 min, furosemide is injected intravenously in a dose of 1 mg/kg, up to 40 mg. Digital images are stored on a computer from the time of injection of the tracer until 20–25 min after injection of furosemide. Urine output is measured during the period before injection of furosemide and afterward at 10-min intervals. The computer data are then processed to generate the renogram time–activity curve and calculate the clearance half-time of the tracer from the dilated upper urinary tract (Fig. 6.11).

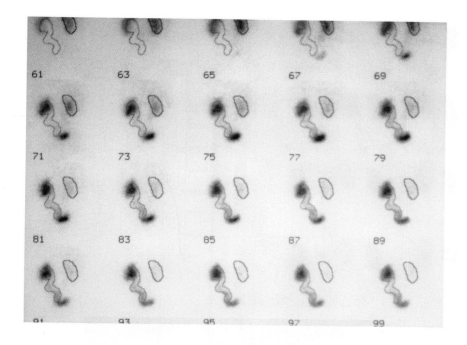

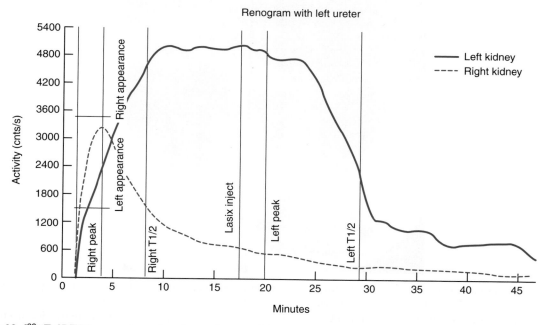

Renogram with left ureter

Figure 6.10 [^{99m}Tc]DTPA renogram showing a time–activity curve that includes a dilated left ureter. The washout on the left is delayed, but responds to Lasix in this patient with non-obstructive megaureter.

Analysis and interpretation of diuretic renography

There are basically two methods for analysing a diuretic renogram curve: pattern recognition and quantitative analysis.

The pattern recognition method is based in the subjective analysis of the shape of the curve (O'Reily

et al., 1979; Thrall *et al.*, 1981). There is a spectrum of responses ranging from very rapid drainage to no drainage at all. Characteristic patterns are seen at the ends of the spectrum for non-obstructed hydronephrosis and for high-grade obstruction that are easily recognizable. However, many curves demonstrate an intermediate response, which may indicate mild to

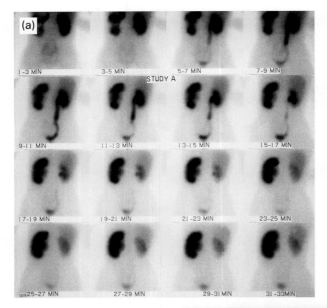

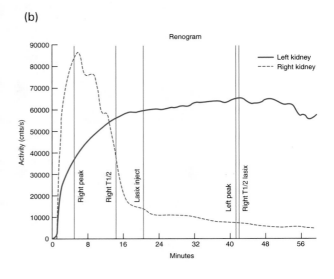

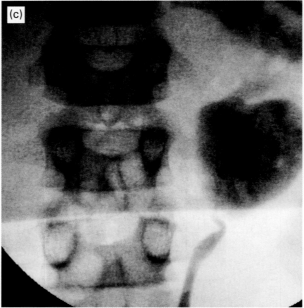

Figure 6.11 (*a*) Serial images during a [^{99m}Tc]MAG-3 study show marked hydronephrosis on the left. The left ureter is never visualized. (*b*) Time–activity curve shows normal drainage on the right and no washout following Lasix on the left. The $t_{1/2}$ cannot be calculated on the left (> 20 min). (c) Retrograde injection of the patient's left ureter in the operating room confirms the tight UPJ obstruction.

moderate obstruction (Fig. 6.12). Determination of the significance of obstruction, if any, based on the subjective interpretation of the shape of the intermediate curves is often difficult.

Quantitative analysis methods based on the washout half-time or some other measure of the washout rate help to reduce subjectivity in the interpretation of the curve and decrease the number of indeterminate

results. This is particularly helpful when serial examinations are compared. Based on extensive pediatric clinical experience, including surgical findings, comparative studies with Whitaker test, and long-term follow-up studies, it has been shown that a drainage half-time of ≥20 min is almost always associated with significant obstruction, whereas a washout half-time of ≤ 10 min usually represents no significant obstruction. Washout

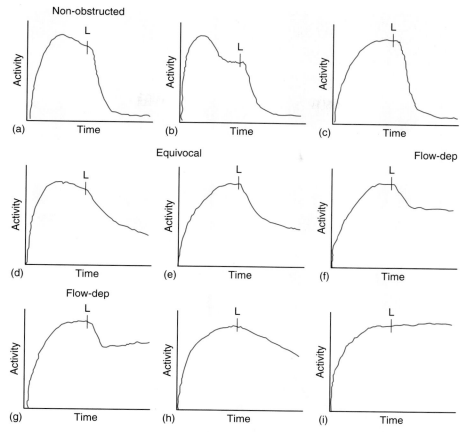

Figure 6.12 Examples of time–activity curves of hydronephrotic kidneys with diuretic injection (L) at the midpoint of a 60-min acquisition. Patterns (*a*), (*b*), and (*c*) are seen with unobstructed systems. Patterns (*d*) and (*e*) are equivocal. Patterns (*f*), (*g*), (*h*), and (*i*) indicate significant obstruction. Patterns (*f*) and (*g*) are examples of flow-dependent obstruction.

half-times between 10 and 20 min, particularly on a single study, are considered indeterminate and warrant close observation and follow-up. It is always wise to remember when considering any computed result that the quantitative data should corroborate the trends visible in the original data, as in this case the drainage images. In addition, the washout half-time ($t_{1/2}$) may be calculated from peak activity or from Lasix injection. The report should specify which method was used.

In addition to the washout half-time, the shape of the curve should be considered in the analysis of the diuretic renogram. The curve may show an initial rapid drop with a short calculated washout half-time, but instead of continuing to drop exponentially to a low level of residual activity, it may plateau at a high level of activity or it may even rise. These biphasic curves are almost always due to flow-dependent obstruction. This information may be lost when furosemide is given prior to 20 min or if the collecting system has not completely filled with marker.

Improvement in the washout of the tracer after pyeloplasty varies greatly. In some, the half-time returns to the non-obstructed range in a short period, whereas in others this may take significantly longer. In many instances, the washout half-time remains in the obstructed or equivocal range for at least 6 months. Similar results have been reported with sonographic follow-up following pyeloplasty (Amling *et al.*, 1996). Specifically, it takes 6–24 months to see improvement in the degree of pelvicaliectasis following pyeloplasty in the majority of patients. The dilated collecting system does not shrink immediately. If function remains stable in the perioperative period, there is no need for concern.

In summary, diuretic-augmented radionuclide renography is a safe and valuable tool for the evaluation and management of hydronephrosis in infants and children. Its effectiveness is dependent on the technique of the examination, meticulous analysis of the results, and recognition of its pitfalls and limitations (Fig. 6.13).

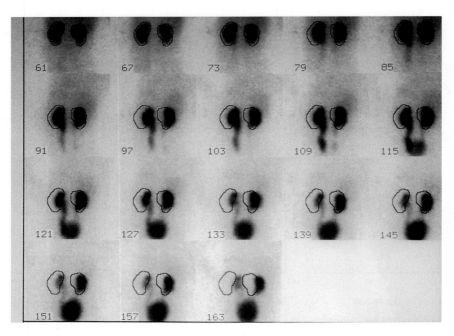

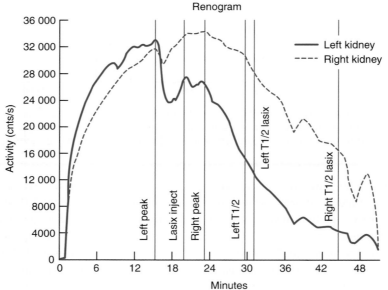

Figure 6.13 Example of a pitfall during acquisition and processing of a [^{99m}Tc]MAG-3 study. The patient was moving on the examination table and his kidneys have migrated out of the region of interest (ROI) chosen for the curves. This can cause a dilated collecting system to move out of the ROI and seem to plummet on the curve, when no drainage has actually occurred.

Urinary tract infections

UTI may be limited to the bladder (cystitis) or upper collecting systems (ureteritis, pyelitis), or it may involve the renal parenchyma (pyelonephritis). Acute pyelonephritis is a major cause of morbidity in children with UTI and can result in irreversible renal scarring. Well-recognized late sequelae of pyelonephritic scarring include hypertension and chronic renal failure. Clinical and experimental studies have demonstrated that renal scarring can be prevented or diminished by early diagnosis and aggressive treatment of acute pyelonephritis. Therefore, accurate diagnosis of pyelonephritis has significant clinical relevance.

Acute pyelonephritis in adults is usually diagnosed on the basis of clinical signs and symptoms. In infants and children, however, differentiation of acute pyelonephritis from lower UTI based on clinical and laboratory findings is often difficult and the use of diagnostic imaging becomes necessary. Excretory urography has a very low sensitivity for the diagnosis of pyelonephritis. Sonography is more sensitive than urography, especially when power Doppler is added, but still only detects roughly one-half of the cases. Renal sonography is also useful in detection of renal or perirenal abscesses. CT is a more sensitive and effective technique than sonography for the diagnosis of pyelonephritis, but its routine use in the evaluation of children with UTI is not practical, owing to cost and radiation exposure. Although MRI is very accurate in the diagnosis of acute pyelonephritis, it is also costly and less readily available. Radionuclide imaging procedures using gallium-67 citrate or [99mTc]-labeled leukocytes may be very reliable in the diagnosis of acute pyelonephritis. These imaging procedures, however, result in high radiation absorbed doses, require 24–48 hours to perform and, more importantly, do not provide any information about the function or morphology of the kidneys.

Clinical studies have shown renal cortical scintigraphy using [99mTc]DMSA or GHA to be significantly more sensitive than intravenous pyelography (IVP) and renal sonography in the detection of acute pyelonephritis. [99mTc]DMSA renal cortical scintigraphy has also been evaluated in experimentally induced acute pyelonephritis in piglets. In that study, unilateral VUR of infected urine was surgically induced in 22 piglets. DMSA and histopathologic examinations were compared in a blinded fashion. DMSA scans showed scintigraphic evidence of acute pyelonephritis with a sensitivity of 87% and specificity of 100%. There was an overall 94% agreement between the DMSA scan and histopathologic findings for the detection of individual segmental lesions (Majd and Rushton, 1992). Others have reported similar results. Therefore, DMSA renal cortical scintigraphy is a highly sensitive and reliable technique for the detection and localization of acute pyelonephritis (Fig. 6.14).

Renal cortical imaging has also proved to be more accurate than excretory urography in detection of

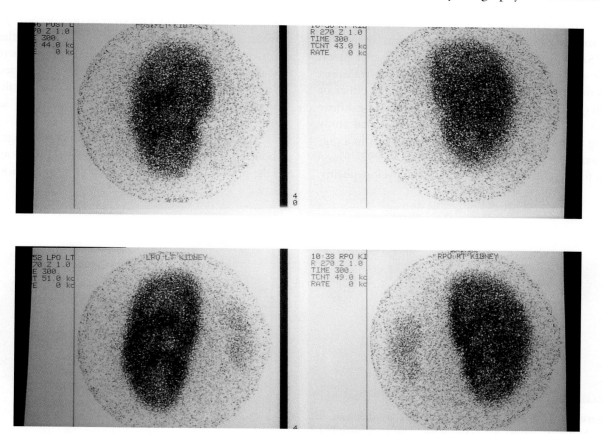

Figure 6.14 Pinhole views of normal kidneys 2 hours after [99mTc]DMSA injection. The cortical margins are smooth with mildly decreased counts in the thinner polar regions of the kidneys.

pyelonephritic scarring (Fig. 6.15). Merrick *et al.* (1980) compared renal cortical imaging and excretory urography in 79 children with proven UTI followed for a period of 1–4 years. Both techniques were in agreement as to the presence or absence of scarring as well as to the extent of abnormality in 93.5% of the kidney studies. There was, however, discrepancy in ten kidneys. Excretory urography had a sensitivity of 86% and a specificity of 92% in the detection of pyelonephritic scarring, whereas renal cortical imaging had a sensitivity of 96% and a specificity of 98%. Detection of focal scarring with sonography is also limited by the dedication of the sonographer.

The scintigraphic pattern of acute pyelonephritis is one of decreased cortical uptake of the tracer without any volume loss (Fig. 6.16). This can be focal, multifocal, or diffuse. Cortical scars are usually associated with loss of volume and present as a crescent-shaped defect or thinning and flattening of the cortex (Fig. 6.17). Cortical imaging also offers the quantitative evaluation of relative renal function and a non-invasive method of assessing response to treatment.

The pathophysiologic mechanisms that account for the decreased uptake of DMSA in acute pyelonephritis are probably multifactorial. Cortical uptake of DMSA is determined primarily by intrarenal blood flow and proximal tubular cell membrane transport function. Any pathologic process that alters either or both of these parameters may result in focal or diffuse areas of decreased uptake. In an experimental study using sodium chromate (^{51}Cr) microspheres in a piglet model of pyelonephritis, Majd *et al.* (1992) found that focal ischemia does occur in acute pyelonephritis.

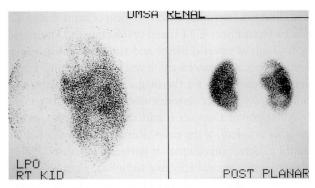

Figure 6.16 Pinhole and planar images in a 2-year-old child with fever of unknown origin and negative urine culture following antibiotics for otitis media. Large wedge-shaped areas of decreased radiotracer accumulation are seen in both the upper and lower pole of the right kidney, consistent with acute pyelonephritis.

In some lesions the decrease in uptake of DMSA is proportional to focally decreased blood flow, whereas in other lesions DMSA uptake is more severely decreased than regional blood flow. This suggests that focal ischemia is an early event that precedes tubular damage. Therefore, the DMSA scan may become positive in a very early stage of the parenchymal inflammatory response to the invasion by bacteria. It is reasonable to assume that adequate treatment of acute pyelonephritis in this very early stage should result in complete resolution without progression to scar formation.

[^{99m}Tc]DMSA is an excellent renal cortical agent. About 60% of the administered dose is tightly bound to the proximal tubular cells, and only a small amount

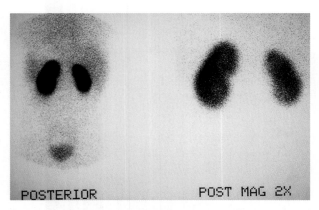

Figure 6.15 Posterior planar and magnified views of the kidneys using [^{99m}Tc]DMSA show a smaller, scarred right kidney compared to the left. However, there is no evidence of recent pyelonephritis.

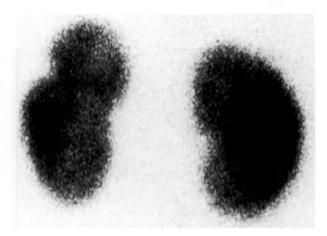

Figure 6.17 Cortical scar in the lateral aspect of the upper pole of the left kidney.

is slowly excreted in the urine. DMSA allows visualization of renal parenchyma without interference from retained tracer in the collecting systems.

Concerns regarding higher radiation absorbed dose with DMSA have been expressed. It is true that radiation to the cortex of the kidneys per millicurie administered dose is about three times higher with DMSA than with GHA. This is due to cortical fixation of a larger fraction of DMSA. Therefore, the administered dose of DMSA can be one-third that of GHA. With this adjustment in the administered dose, total DMSA retained in the kidney and resultant renal radiation doses are equal to those of GHA; however, owing to the accumulation of a smaller amount of DMSA in the bladder, the gonadal radiation dose is significantly lower. Therefore, DMSA is a preferred renal cortical imaging agent, particularly in infants.

[99mTc]glucoheptonate is cleared from circulation by both glomerular filtration and cortical fixation. About 20% of the administered dose is firmly bound to the tubular cells. Therefore, delayed imaging provides visualization of the cortex similar to DMSA images (Fig. 6.18b). Most of the administered dose is excreted in the urine, allowing moderately good visualization of the renal collecting systems (Fig. 6.18a). This additional information provided by GHA makes it the agent preferred by some. However, the anatomic state of the collecting systems is best evaluated

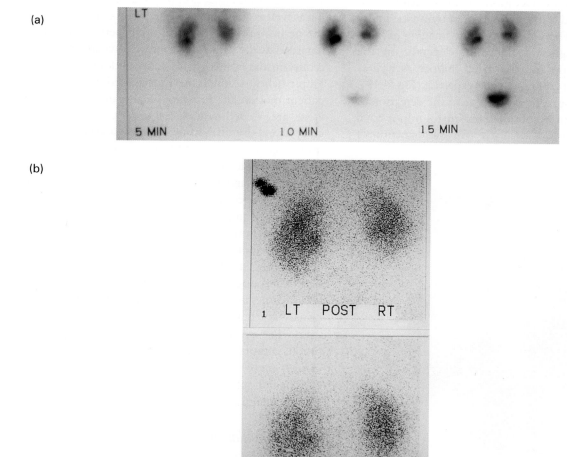

Figure 6.18 (a) Early phase of [99mTc]GHA scan showing excretion into the collecting system. Renal function is symmetric. (b) Normal late phase of same patient examination showing pinhole views of the kidneys obtained for cortical detail. The count statistics are much lower with GHA than with DMSA, reflected in the image resolution of these two studies.

by renal sonography, which is usually obtained in conjunction with the renal scan. There is often some hepatobiliary excretion of GHA, particularly in infants. Tracer in the gallbladder or small bowel may superimpose on the right kidney and cause confusion.

Trauma

Renal injuries are typically due to blunt abdominal trauma or, less commonly, to penetrating injuries. Iatrogenic injuries may also occur as a result of surgical intervention, renal biopsy, retrograde pyelography, or interventional radiographic procedures. Diagnostic imaging procedures used in the evaluation of renal trauma include CT, sonography, angiography, and excretory urography. Occasionally, radionuclide studies are well suited to the evaluation of traumatic injury to the kidneys. The position of these imaging modalities in the diagnostic algorithm depends on the patient's condition and associated injuries as well as the availability of equipment and expertise (Fig. 6.19).

Excretory urography is sensitive in the detection of renal pedicle injuries, but underestimates minor renal injuries. It has a low sensitivity for the detection of

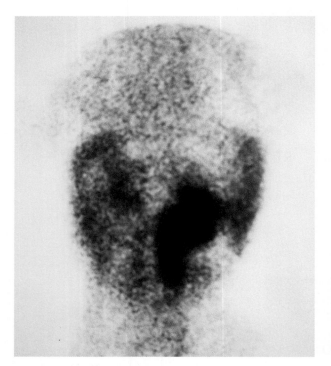

Figure 6.19 [^{99m}Tc]DTPA scan after a nephrostomy tube was inadvertently removed from this infant shows urine leakage into the peritoneum and marked hydronephrosis on the right.

urinary leakage and does not provide information about injury to the other organs.

Angiography is the best method for demonstrating vascular injury directly and also offers an opportunity to control active hemorrhage by selective arterial embolization. It is, however, invasive and not suitable for screening or serial evaluation.

Renal sonography is useful in the detection of subcapsular and perirenal hematomas, lacerations, blood clots in the renal pelvis, and urinary tract obstruction. The use of Doppler studies allows evaluation of renal blood flow. Renal sonography, however, does not provide any information about renal function.

CT of the abdomen with intravenous contrast enhancement provides superior anatomic detail that allows accurate evaluation of the extent of renal trauma as well as simultaneous evaluation of other organs, the peritoneal cavity, and the retroperitoneum. It is regarded as the single most informative imaging procedure in the evaluation of acute abdominal trauma. Faster helical scanners have decreased artifacts from patient motion and improved image quality. Delayed views are needed to look for urine extravasation, as complete abdominal scans are now accomplished in several seconds, well in advance of contrast excretion.

Radionuclide renal imaging provides information about global and regional perfusion and function of the kidneys. Despite its extreme sensitivity in detecting renal pedicle injuries, segmental infarctions, contusions, lacerations, and urine extravasation, renal scintigraphy is seldom chosen over CT or sonography in the acute setting. Radionuclide renal studies, in conjunction with sonography, are particularly useful in follow-up assessments of healing of traumatic injuries to the urinary tract and detection of secondary complications. Pre-existing congenital anomalies, such as fusion, ectopia, and hydronephrosis, which make the kidneys more susceptible to trauma, are easily detected. The radiopharmaceuticals of choice for the evaluation of renal trauma are [^{99m}Tc]MAG-3 and GHA.

Renal vascular abnormalities

Renovascular hypertension

Hypertension in children is often of renal origin. Some of the renal causes of hypertension, such as infarction, postpyelonephritic cortical scarring, and post-traumatic injuries, are easily diagnosed by renal sonography, CT, or scintigraphy. These methods, however, are less reliable in the diagnosis of renovascular hypertension. Renal artery stenosis is the cause of approximately 5% of all cases of childhood hypertension. The prevalence is considerably higher when the hypertension occurs in association with neurofibromatosis or aortic anomalies. In half of all hypertensive children younger than 10 years of age, there is a vascular cause for the disease.

Renal arteriography and renal vein renin measurements are needed for definitive diagnosis and management of the renal vascular causes of hypertension. Renal arteriography, however, is an invasive procedure and is not suitable for screening. The role of less invasive CT angiography for this purpose is promising, but unproven in large series. Doppler sonography for the diagnosis of renal artery stenosis is highly sensitive, but challenging in pediatric patients. Up to 20% of these examinations are technically unsatisfactory (Dillon, 1997).

Conventional radionuclide renography in the presence of unilateral renal artery stenosis can show evidence of decreased renal perfusion and function on the affected side. In the presence of hypertension, however, the kidney with a stenotic artery may remain adequately perfused and, owing to the autoregulation mechanism, the renal scan and renogram may remain normal. Arlat *et al.* (1979), reporting on a group of 105 patients with angiographically proven unilateral renal artery stenosis and 45 patients with essential hypertension, found 18% false-negative and 13% false-positive renal scans for renal artery stenosis. The percentages for Hippuran renography were 17% and 26%, respectively. Radionuclide studies are even less efficacious in the diagnosis of bilateral or segmental renal artery stenosis.

Captopril-enhanced scintigraphy

The observation that captopril therapy in hypertensive children with renal artery stenosis caused dramatic but reversible deterioration of renal function prompted Majd *et al.* (1983) to investigate ACE inhibitor renography. Captopril is the drug most commonly used as a provocative test to increase the efficacy of renal scanning in the detection of renal artery stenosis. Since the early 1980s, extensive experimental and clinical studies have substantiated the usefulness of this pharmacologic intervention in the diagnosis of renovascular hypertension.

In the presence of renal artery stenosis, the intrarenal perfusion pressure is decreased and there is a tendency for GFR to fall. However, within a wide range of perfusion pressure GFR is maintained at normal levels by an autoregulation mechanism mediated by the renin–angiotensin system. A major factor in maintaining GFR is the transcapillary pressure gradient across the glomerulus related to the difference in resistance at the level of the afferent and efferent arterioles. This is regulated by angiotensin II-induced selective constriction of the efferent arteriole of the glomerulus. Captopril, an angiotensin-converting enzyme inhibitor, blocks the formation of angiotensin II, causing dilatation of efferent arterioles and a decrease in the transcapillary pressure gradient. This leads to a significant, but reversible, decrease in renal function.

The choice of radiopharmacutical, ACE inhibitor, and technique of examination varies among institutions. Either glomerular or tubular agents can be used. The original work in pediatric patients was done with the use of DTPA and captopril. Subsequent experience has shown this to be a reliable method. Currently, MAG-3, which has replaced OIH for clinical use, is being evaluated for captopril renography and appears to be promising, particularly in cases of segmental renal artery stenosis. Either captopril or enalapril maleate can be used as a choice of ACE inhibitor. Their mechanisms of action are similar, but the advantage of enalaprilat is that it is administered intravenously and, unlike oral captopril, its effect is not dependent on variable absorption through the gastrointestinal tract. Most centers routinely obtain a baseline renal scan, followed by a second study either 1 hour after oral administration of captopril or 10 min after intravenous administration of enalaprilat.

The scintigraphic manifestation of decreased renal function after administration of the ACE inhibitor depends on which radiopharmaceutical is used. With DTPA, there is decreased extraction and delayed appearance of the tracer in the collecting systems; with MAG-3, there is prolonged parenchymal retention of the tracer (Fig. 6.20).

Other vascular abnormalities

Other vascular abnormalities of the kidney, such as thrombosis of the main or segmental renal veins or arteries, can often be diagnosed on the radionuclide studies. Renal vein thrombosis occurs most often in neonates and is usually secondary to hemoconcentration. The renal scan generally shows both decreased perfusion and function in an enlarged kidney. Renal artery thrombosis in the neonate occurs most

(a)

(b)

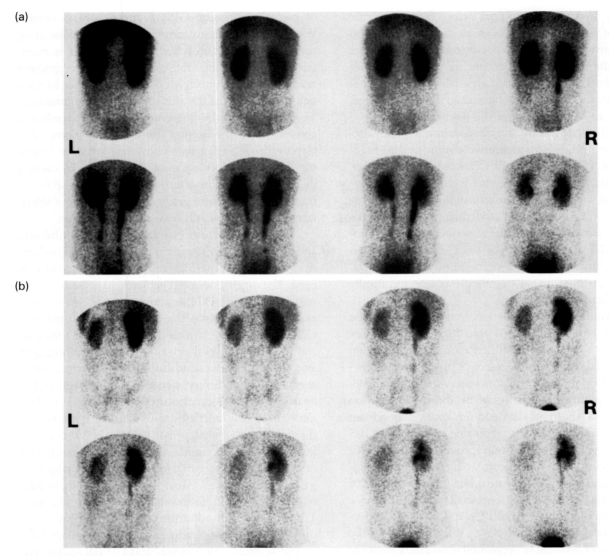

L   R

Figure 6.20 Effect of captopril on renal function in the presence of renal artery stenosis. (*a*) The renal scan obtained as a part of the initial hypertensive work-up was normal. (*b*) The repeat study after 2 months of captopril therapy showed marked deterioration of the left renal function. (*c*) and (*d*) Shown opposite.

commonly as a complication of an indwelling aortic catheter. Renal artery thrombosis also causes decreased perfusion and function of the kidney but, unlike renal vein thrombosis, usually does not cause enlargement of the kidney. Scintigraphic findings of renal vascular occlusion are non-specific and should be interpreted in the clinical context.

Renal masses

Most renal masses are adequately localized and characterized by sonography or CT. Radionuclide renal cortical imaging, however, may be of value in differentiating functioning pseudotumors (such as promi-

nent columns of Bertin), fetal lobulation, and dromedary humps from true nonfunctioning pathology, such as tumor, infarct, or hemorrhage.

The relative sensitivity of different diagnostic imaging modalities in early detection of Wilms' tumor in children with aniridia or hemihypertrophy has not been defined.

Renal transplantation
Evaluation of donor

Renal scanning (including total and separate GFR determination) is often used in the evaluation of the living donor to ensure that he or she has two kidneys with normal function. This is usually followed by selective renal arteriography. When the use of the kidney from a 'brain-dead' patient is contemplated, a cerebral flow study may be performed as part of [99mTc]DTPA renal scan both to confirm brain death and to evaluate renal function.

Evaluation of the transplanted kidney

A variety of radionuclide studies has been used to evaluate perfusion and function of a transplanted kidney. The most common procedure in children is [99mTc]DTPA renal scintigraphy, including evaluation of the first transit of tracer from the aorta and iliac artery to the transplanted kidney. The renal time–activity curve of the first transit is compared with that of the aorta or iliac artery. A normally perfused transplanted kidney shows a sharp rise and fall in the renal time–activity curve, which closely parallels the aortic curve. Qualitatively, the images should show prompt perfusion of the transplant simultaneous with the radionuclide reaching the iliac vessels (Fig. 6.21).

Complications

Possible complications following renal transplantation can be classified into two general categories: (1) those due to parenchymal failure, such as acute tubular necrosis (ATN), rejection, cyclosporine toxicity, and infection; and (2) those due to mechanical injuries, including complete or partial obstruction of

(c)

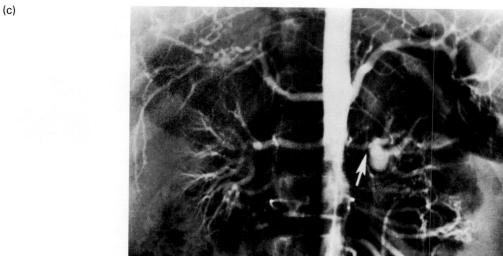

(d)

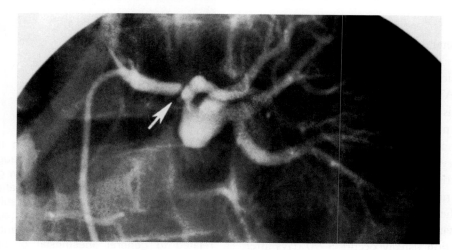

Figure 6.20 *Continued.* (*c*) An abdominal aortogram and (*d*) a selective left renal arteriogram showed stenosis of the left renal artery (*arrow*) with poststenotic aneurysmal dilatation.

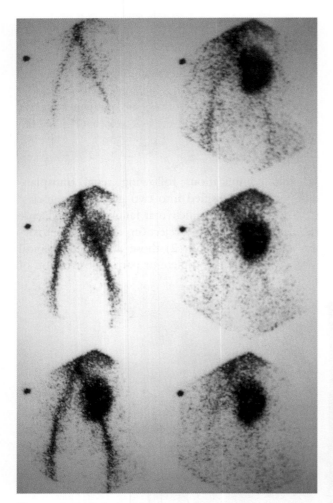

Figure 6.21 Scintiangiogram of left lower quadrant transplant kidney. These anterior images show excellent perfusion of transplant and rapid clearance of blood pool activity.

blood vessels, ureteral obstruction, urinary leak, and lymphocele.

Certain complications occur at specific times after transplantation. ATN secondary to ischemic damage prior to grafting is present in the majority of cadaveric transplants. It may rarely occur in a living, related donor transplant as a result of technical problems at the time of surgery, severe hypotension, or reaction to radiographic contrast medium. Cyclosporine toxicity can occur at any time, but is less common during the first month of therapy. Hyperacute rejection occurs immediately or within the first 24 h after transplantation. Acute rejection usually occurs 5–90 days after transplant. Chronic rejection is a slow process and is usually manifested months to years later.

Radionuclide studies are very useful in the diagnosis of acute renal vessel occlusion, poor parenchymal function, renal infarction, ureteral obstruction, and extravasation of urine. However, the scintigraphic patterns of parenchymal dysfunction are usually nonspecific and do not allow differentiation among ATN, rejection, cyclosporine toxicity, and complete obstruction (Fig. 6.22).

In ATN, renal function decreases, whereas renal perfusion usually remains relatively normal; in rejection, both perfusion and function decrease proportionally. Differentiation of rejection from ATN on the basis of a single study, however, is often difficult, and serial studies over several days or weeks may be necessary. A kidney injured by ATN generally displays its lowest level of perfusion and function by 24–48 hours after transplantation. Therefore, on serial examinations the perfusion and function should improve or remain unchanged. By contrast, deterioration of renal

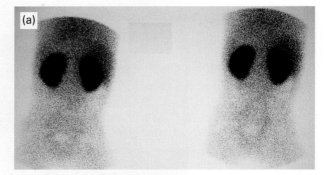

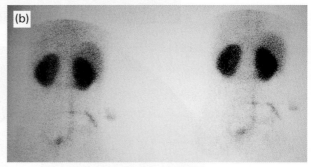

Figure 6.22 (a) Early images from a [99mTc]MAG-3 study following complex bladder augmentation and bilateral reimplantation surgery show good uptake but no excretion of radiotracer. The patient was anuric. (b) On delayed images there is still no excretion, although faint activity is seen in a surgical drainage tube. These findings could represent ATN (possibly related to general anesthesia) or obstruction. The patient passed clots within hours of the study and relieved the obstruction.

perfusion and function due to rejection, if untreated, is generally progressive.

It is important to obtain a baseline renal scan shortly after surgery, preferably within the first 24 h. The same protocol and technical parameters should be used in all follow-up examinations to facilitate comparison. The patient should be well hydrated and the bladder emptied before the examination.

Complete renal arterial or venous occlusion as well as hyperacute rejection result in non-perfusion of the transplant and cannot be differentiated by radionuclide angiography alone. The scintigraphic findings of a 'photon-deficient' zone (renal activity distinctly less than surrounding background activity) indicate a non-salvageable transplant.

Hypertension may be due to stenosis of the vascular graft or vascular disease of the native kidney. Captopril-enhanced renal scintigraphy is helpful in the detection of renal artery stenosis.

Obstructive uropathy and urinary extravasation are readily detected on the renal scan, provided that renal function is adequate. A photon-deficient zone adjacent to the kidney on the early images may be due to urinary extravasation or lymphocele. In the case of urinary extravasation, delayed images demonstrate accumulation of tracer in the area, whereas a lymphocele remains photon deficient (Fig. 6.23). Sonography is complementary to scintigraphy in the detection of the urologic complications of renal transplantation.

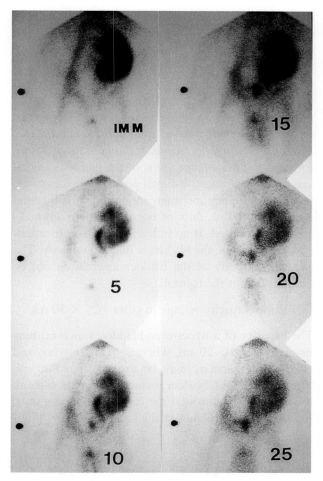

Figure 6.23 [^{123}I]OIH study in a 14-year-old patient with recent transplant showing a photopenic area medial to the transplant, which was a lymphocele.

Radionuclide cystography

The use of radionuclides for the detection of VUR dates back to 1959, when Winter reported the appearance of radioactivity in the area of the kidneys after [^{131}I]iodopyracet (Diodrast) or [^{131}I]Rose Bengal had been instilled into the bladder. For these studies, scintillation probes were positioned over the kidneys. In 1964 others reported the use of colloidal gold-198 for cystography and emphasized the advantage of its low radiation dose compared with that of retrograde X-ray cystography. With the advent of the gamma camera and ^{99m}Tc compounds, retrograde radionuclide cystography with isotope directly instilled in the bladder was modified by several researchers and was popularized by Conway *et al.* (1972). This technique is also known as direct radionuclide cystography.

Dodge (1963) reported his observation that a brisk rise in activity occurred in some patients with known

reflux upon voiding at the end of a radionuclide renogram. This suggested a new technique for the detection of VUR using intravenous injection of [^{131}I]Hippuran and external scintillation counting over the renal area. This technique of indirect (intravenous) cystography was later modified.

Direct (retrograde) radionuclide cystography

No preparation or sedation is needed. The patient is positioned supine with the gamma camera underneath the examination table. Using aseptic technique, the urethra is catheterized with an 8 Fr Foley catheter or an infant feeding tube. The bladder is emptied and a urine sample is collected in a sterile container for culture. The catheter is connected to a bag of normal saline by a regular intravenous infusion tubing set. The bag of saline is placed 100 cm above the table top. After the flow of normal saline is established, 1mCi of [^{99m}Tc]pertechnetate or sulfur colloid (0.5 mCi in neonates) is injected into the stream of saline through the rubber injection site of the infusion tube. The patient is positioned with the bladder on the lower edge of the field of view of the gamma camera (Fig. 6.24).

While the bladder is filling, it is continuously monitored on the persistence scope of the gamma camera, and multiple analog and digital posterior images of the bladder and upper abdomen are obtained. If bilateral reflux is observed, flow of normal saline is immediately discontinued. If no reflux is seen or only unilateral reflux occurs, the bladder is filled to capacity. The expected capacity of the bladder in children can be estimated from the formula:

Bladder capacity = (age in years +2) $\times$ 30 ml.

The capacity of a hypertonic bladder, however, may be as low as 10–20 ml, whereas in those who void infrequently capacity may be greater than 500 ml. The signs of a full bladder include backup of saline in the tube, leakage around the catheter, upgoing toes, irritability, and crossing of the legs.

When reflux is seen, the volume of instilled saline is recorded. After adequate filling, the older patient is seated on a bedpan in front of a gamma camera, that has been reoriented in a vertical position. The catheter is untaped or the Foley balloon deflated, and the patient is encouraged to void. Analog and digital images are obtained before, during, and after voiding. The total volume of instilled saline and the volume of voided fluid are recorded. These values, together with the volume at the time of reflux, are used to calculate residual postvoid bladder volume. The volume of reflux and the rate of its drainage back into the bladder can also be assessed (Fig. 6.25a, b). In infants, the voiding phase of the examination is carried out with the child in the supine position without measuring the voided urine volume. The volume of instilled saline at the time of reflux is accepted as the total bladder volume at that time.

Advantages

Low radiation dose

The most important advantage of direct radionuclide cystography is its extremely low radiation dose. With 1 mCi of [^{99m}Tc]pertechnetate or ^{99m}Tc sulfur colloid

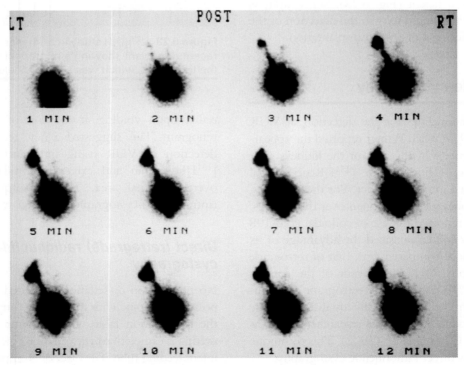

Figure 6.24 Posterior images during a radiocystogram demonstrate bilateral reflux, much greater on the left than on the right.

(a)

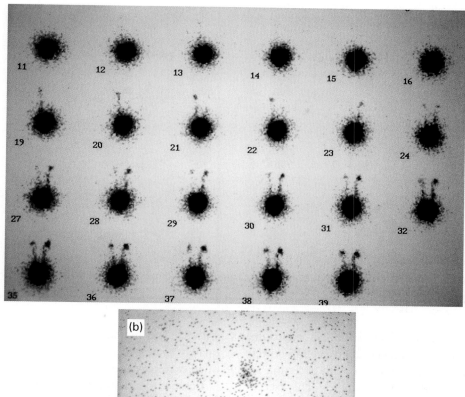

(b)

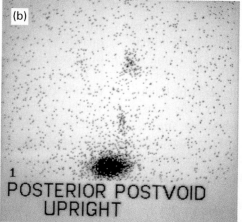

1
POSTERIOR POSTVOID
UPRIGHT

Figure 6.25 (*a*) Posterior images obtained at 10 s/frame show transient vesicoureteral reflux initially that becomes constant at higher bladder volume. (*b*) A final image obtained after upright positioning, documenting good drainage from the upper tract collecting system.

in 200 ml of saline, the dose to the bladder wall during direct radionuclide cystography is about 1 mrad per minute of contact. In the author's experience, the average length of bladder exposure is only about 15 minutes, resulting in a radiation dose of about 15 mrad to the bladder wall. The dose to the gonads, which in boys are at a considerable distance from the bladder wall, is probably less than 5 mrad. In contrast, gonadal dose with standard X-ray voiding cystourethrography ranges from 75 mrad to several rads, depending on the fluoroscopy time and the number of films taken. Therefore, the gonadal dose is less than one-tenth that of standard X-ray studies. The total body radiation that may result from possible absorption of a minimal amount of [^{99m}Tc]pertechnetate is negligible.

Sensitivity

Reflux is a dynamic, intermittent phenomenon. A considerable amount of reflux may vanish within a matter of seconds. With standard X-ray voiding cystourethrography, continuous extended observation under fluoroscopy is unacceptable because of excessive radiation. With direct radionuclide cystography, the urinary tract is monitored continuously during filling, during voiding, and after voiding with no

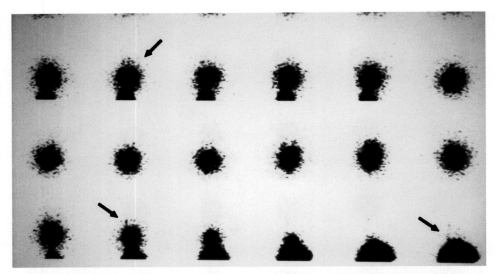

Figure 6.26 Images from a radiocystogram at near maximal bladder capacity, showing faint grade I vesicoureteral reflux transiently bilaterally (*arrows*).

increase in the amount of radiation. In addition, reflux is more easily detected because overlying bowel contents and bones do not interfere with detection as they may during standard X-ray studies. The exception is minimal reflux to the distal ureter, which may be obscured by the isotope-filled bladder (Fig. 6.26). This pitfall can be minimized by obtaining shallow oblique views of the pelvis at maximal bladder capacity. Direct radionuclide cystography is more sensitive than X-ray cystography in detecting VUR.

Quantitative analysis

Parameters such as residual urine volume, bladder volume at the time of reflux, volume, and rate of clearance of reflux can be calculated. The clinical significance of these functional parameters is not clear. Bladder volume at the time of reflux appears to have a prognostic significance. If the bladder volume at the time of demonstration of reflux increases on annual serial examinations, it may indicate a better prognosis for spontaneous cessation of reflux. Maizels *et al.* (1979) recorded intravesical pressures during nuclear cystography and reported that this combined information facilitates the management of children with VUR and voiding abnormalities.

Disadvantages

The major disadvantage of direct radionuclide cystography is its unsuitability for evaluation of the male urethra. Therefore, its use for the initial study in boys

with UTI is not advised unless the urethra is adequately evaluated on a voiding film obtained as part of an excretory urogram.

Because the anatomic resolution of direct radionuclide cystography is not as good as that of X-ray voiding cystourethrography, reflux cannot be graded accurately. The extremes of the spectrum (grades I, II, and V) can be differentiated, but grades III and IV cannot be accurately separated. Major abnormalities, such as large filling defects in the bladder (ureterocele), distortion and displacement of the bladder, and most duplications associated with reflux, can be appreciated, but minor abnormalities of the bladder wall, such as diverticula, will be missed.

Indirect (intravenous) radionuclide cystography

Indirect radionuclide cystography is now primarily of historical interest. The examination is a means of identifying reflux without bladder catheterization. It is based on the ideal condition of rapid and complete renal clearance of an intravenously injected radiopharmaceutical. The well-hydrated patient is injected with [^{99m}Tc]DTPA or [^{99m}Tc]MAG-3, and a conventional renal scan is obtained. The patient is instructed not to void and is monitored intermittently. When the upper urinary tract has drained and most of the tracer is contained in the bladder, the child is placed before the gamma camera in a sitting or standing position and images are obtained before, during and after voiding. A sudden increase in radioactivity over a kidney or ureter indicates VUR.

Advantages

The theoretical advantages of indirect radionuclide cystography are that unpleasant catheterization is avoided, voiding may be more normal because the urethra is not irritated, and the study is performed without overdistending the bladder. A final advantage is that renal function and morphology as well as reflux may be evaluated simultaneously.

Disadvantages

Although some reports indicated good correlation between indirect radionuclide cystography and X-ray voiding cystourethrography, other studies (Majd *et al.*, 1985) had a low sensitivity with an overall false-negative rate of 41%. A positive study is reliable, but the negative studies should be confirmed by direct cystography.

Other disadvantages of the indirect method include its dependence on renal function and adequate drainage as well as cooperation by the patient, who must be able to void on request. The study is not practical in children who have a neuropathic bladder and in those who are not toilet trained. The radiation dose is higher than that used for the direct cystogram and may become considerable if the child withholds urine for a protracted interval.

Clinical applications of (direct) nuclear cystography

Direct radionuclide cystography, because of its superior sensitivity and minimal radiation dose, is the method of choice in the following situations:

- all follow-up examinations in patients with known reflux or who have had antireflux surgery;
- as a screening test to detect familial reflux;
- for serial evaluation of children with neuropathic bladders who are at risk for reflux to develop;
- as the initial screening test for detection of reflux in girls with UTI.

Scrotal scintigraphy

Diagnostic testicular scanning was first proposed by Nadel *et al.* (1973). Since then, radionuclide scrotal imaging has been refined and has proved a useful adjunct in differentiating 'surgical' from 'non-surgical' disorders of the scrotal contents. This study, if done properly in patients presenting with an acutely enlarged and painful hemiscrotum, may drastically decrease the number of negative surgical explorations. Scrotal scintigraphy and sonography are close competitors in both speed and sensitivity when evaluating the acute scrotum.

Technical considerations

Thyroid uptake of [^{99m}Tc]pertechnetate can be blocked by oral administration of potassium perchlorate in a dose of 5 mg/kg immediately prior to the test. The child is positioned supine on the imaging table. The penis is taped up over the pubis. The scrotum is supported by towels positioned between the thighs or by a tape sling. Lead shielding under the scrotum is not recommended for the angiographic phases of the examination, but is used for the static images, particularly in younger children. A lead shield under the scrotum facilitates detection of areas of decreased blood flow. The scrotum is positioned under the center of a gamma camera that is equipped with converging collimator or electronic magnification capability.

After rapid intravenous injection of [^{99m}Tc]pertechnetate in a dose of 200 µCi/kg, multiple 3-second dynamic images (radionuclide angiogram) are obtained. Immediately after the angiographic phase, early static images ('blood pool' or 'tissue phase') are obtained. This is usually followed by the use of a pinhole collimator to obtain high-resolution magnified static images.

Physical examination of the scrotum and accurate localization of the testicles by the nuclear physician are crucial in correct interpretation of the scintigraphic findings.

Scintigraphic patterns

Basic knowledge of the vascular anatomy of the scrotum and its contents is essential for understanding the scintigraphic findings. A dual blood supply exists. The main blood supply includes the spermatic and defferential arteries, supplying the testis and epididymis, and cremasteric vessels from the inferior epigastric vessels. These vessels enter at different levels and usually anastomose in and around the testicular mediastinum. The cremasteric artery forms a network over the tunica vaginalis and also participates in anastomoses with vessels supplying the scrotal wall. The second pathway is composed of the vessels that do not enter the spermatic cord. These include the internal pudendal artery and the superficial and deep external pudendal arteries. These arteries supply the scrotum and penis.

Normal scrotal scintigram

In a normal scrotal scintigram, the iliac arteries are well visualized. However, owing to their size and the relatively small amount of blood flow, the vessels supplying the scrotal contents are ill defined and the scrotum and its contents blur into a homogeneous area of tracer accumulation similar in intensity to that in the image of the thigh. Dartos activity cannot be separated from testicular or epididymal activity.

Testicular torsion

The scintigraphic pattern in testicular torsion depends on the duration of torsion.

Early phase (acute torsion)

In the early phase (probably within the first 6 hours), the radionuclide angiogram may show decreased blood flow to the hemiscrotum or may appear normal. Blood flow to the hemiscrotum is not increased at this stage. The static images ('tissue phase') show decreased accumulation of the tracer in the testicle without the reactive surrounding halo of increased activity seen in the later phases.

Midphase

After a few more hours, there is reactive hyperemia in the region supplied by the pudendal arteries. The radionuclide angiogram shows increased blood flow to the dartos, and the early static images show a halo of mildly increased activity around a cold center. The halo of increased activity gradually disappears on the subsequent images. This pattern is usually seen in patients who have been symptomatic for 6–18 hours.

Late phase

If the patient with torsion does not seek immediate medical attention or is erroneously diagnosed, irreversible testicular infarction occurs. The pain and swelling resolve in a few days to weeks with subsequent atrophy of the testicle. It is important to diagnose late-phase testicular torsion in order to perform orchiopexy on the contralateral side.

Late-phase torsion reveals a characteristic scintigraphic pattern. The angiographic phase shows marked increased blood flow to the dartos, and static images reveal a complete rim or halo of increased activity around a cold center. The halo persists throughout the examination, which usually takes about 15–20 min (Fig. 6.27).

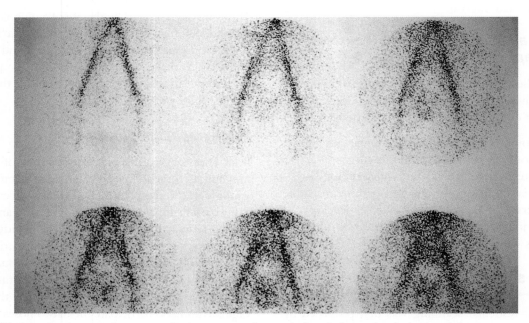

Figure 6.27 Anterior images from a testicular scan performed after 3 days of pain in the right scrotum, showing a rim of activity around a late phase torsion.

Spontaneous detorsion

A spontaneously detorsed testicle may appear normal on the scans or may show slight, diffuse increased scrotal vascularity if the scan is obtained shortly after detorsion. The diagnosis is best made on the basis of clinical history if the examination has not been carried out prior to the detorsion. Demonstration of an intact blood supply to the testicle obviates only the need for emergency surgery. If the history is typical, but physical examination shows the testis to be normally positioned and the scrotal scan demonstrates intact perfusion and slightly increased activity, intermittant torsion should be considered

Acute epididymitis

In acute epididymitis, the radionuclide angiogram and the static images show markedly increased blood flow and blood pool activity to the area corresponding to the epididymis. The entire hemiscrotum may be inflamed, if epididymoorchitis is present (Fig. 6.28). Intense, increased activity in the epididymis may occasionally resemble the halo of late-phase torsion. But, unlike the halo of late-phase torsion, the rim is incomplete and asymmetric. Epididymitis in infants and young children may be secondary to an underlying anatomic abnormality, such as an ectopic ureter or vas, and warrants complete investigation of the genitourinary system.

Torsion of the testicular appendages

Torsion of the appendix testis or epididymis may be visualized as a focal area of increased blood flow and blood pool activity, probably secondary to reactive hyperemia around the torsed appendix. The ischemic appendix itself is too small to be resolved on the images. A more common scintigraphic pattern is that of mild generalized increased blood flow and blood pool activity indistinguishable from that seen with epididymitis. This differentiation is of no surgical significance because both epididymitis and torsion of the appendix testis are generally considered to be nonsurgical problems. Radionuclide studies in the early phase of torsion of the appendix testis, prior to a significant inflammatory response, may be normal.

Scrotal trauma

The scintigraphic pattern following scrotal trauma depends on the extent of injury as well as the time

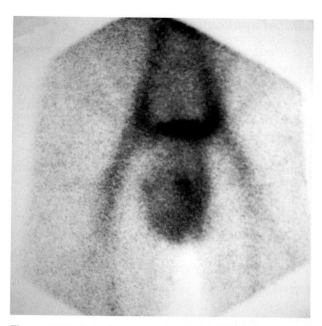

Figure 6.28 Anterior image from a testicular scan performed after several hours of left-sided scrotal pain and swelling, revealing hyperemia and increased radiotracer accumulation, most consistent with epididymitis.

elapsed between the trauma and the scan. Mild, traumatic changes may appear as slightly to moderately diffuse increased tracer accumulation. Intratesticular or intrascrotal hematoma may appear as a cold lesion with or without a surrounding halo of increased activity similar to testicular torsion. Testicular rupture is also a surgical problem. Ultrasonography may be a useful adjunct in localizing a hematoma in relation to the testicle.

Hydrocele

The diagnosis of a simple hydrocele is made by physical examination and transillumination. In secondary hydrocele, which is seen in association with torsion, epididymitis, trauma, or following herniorrhaphy, scintigraphic findings reflect the underlying condition. Hydroceles often appear as a horseshoe or a half-moon-shaped photon deficiency surrounding the testicle.

Abscess

Scans of testicular or intrascrotal abscesses demonstrate a cold center surrounded by a rim of increased activity similar to that of late-phase torsion. The diagnosis is usually made in the context of the clinical history.

Clinical applications

The scintigraphic patterns in the acute hemiscrotum can be divided into two groups:

1 diffuse or focal increased blood flow and blood pool activity without any cold component. This pattern is seen in patients with epididymitis, torsion of the appendix testis, and minor posttraumatic abnormalities, all of which are non-surgical conditions. The problem of differentiation between these conditions and spontaneous detorsion is usually resolved on the basis of clinical history;

2 cold lesions with or without a surrounding rim of increased activity (excluding typical hydrocele). This pattern is seen in patients with testicular torsion, hematoma, and abscess, all of which are surgical conditions.

Acute hemiscrotum

When the clinical presentation and physical findings are typical of the early phase of acute testicular torsion, surgery should be performed immediately without delaying for any imaging.

When the history suggests inflammatory disease or conditions other than acute torsion, or when the patient cannot be properly examined because of extreme swelling and tenderness, testicular scanning is indicated and can reliably differentiate 'surgical' from 'non-surgical' conditions.

Non-acute indications

Testicular scanning may also be helpful (1) if there is any clinical doubt as to testicular viability after corrective detorsion and orchiopexy, and (2) in the occasional patient with suspected incompletely treated epididymoorchitis when the question of abscess arises.

Positron emission tomography in oncology

The most recent development in functional imaging in nuclear medicine is positron emission tomography (PET). The technique uses short-lived radiopharmaceuticals produced in a cyclotron that decay by positron emission. When the positron reacts with nearby electrons, two 511-keV photons are emitted in an annihilation reaction. The specially designed gamma camera for PET senses these photon pairs, and com-

puter analysis of these coincident detections generates an image of their source. The most commonly used radiopharmaceutical is [^{18}F]fluordeoxyglucose (FDG). FDG is accumulated in malignant tissues to a greater extent than normal tissues both because of increased metabolic activity and because of greater numbers of active transport sites on cell membranes. Once in the cancer cell, FDG enters the glycolytic pathway, but is trapped after the first phosphorylation and cannot be processed further. These factors cause disproportionate accumulation of FDG in tumor cells, making them apparent on PET images. The majority of FDG is excreted via the urinary system.

FDG PET has already gained acceptance in evaluating cancers of the lung, colon, rectum, brain, and melanoma. Its use is rapidly expanding to lymphoma, bone, soft-tissue, and gynecologic malignancies. In terms of pediatric urologic applications, it may prove helpful in initial staging and in determining the response to therapy for renal, retroperitoneal, and pelvic tumors. At this time, it has been most useful in evaluating the nature of tissue remaining in surgical beds (O'Hara et al., 1999). Scar tissue and inflammation do not accumulate FDG to the extent that residual or recurrent tumor does.

Acknowledgements

The author thanks Dr Massoud Majd, who authored this chapter in previous editions of this book, for his assistance in this current edition, his patient, concise manner of teaching, and the example he sets through his care of pediatric patients.

References

Amling CL, O'Hara SM, Wiener JS et al. (1996) Ultrasound changes after pyeloplasty in children with ureteropelvic junction obstruction: long-term outcome in 47 renal units. J Urol 156: 2020–24.

Arlart I, Rosenthal J, Adam WE et al. (1979) Predictive value of radionuclide methods in the diagnosis of unilateral renovascular hypertension. Cardiovasc Radiol 2: 115–25.

Blaufox MD, Aurell M, Bubeck B et al. (1996) Report of the radionuclides in nephrourology Committee on Renal Clearance. J Nucl Med 37: 1883–90.

Braren V, Versage PN, Touya JJ et al. (1979) Radioisotopic determination of glomerular filtration rate. J Urol 121: 145–7.

Chung S, Majd M, Rushton HG et al. (1993) Diuretic renography in the evaluation of neonatal hydronephrosis: Is it reliable? *J Urol* **150**: 765–8.

Conway JJ, King LR, Belman AB *et al.* (1972) Detection of vesicoureteral reflux with radionuclide cystography. *Am J Roentgenol Radium Ther Nucl Med* **115**: 720–7.

Daly MJ, Jones W, Rudd TG *et al.* (1979) Differential renal function using technetium-99m dimercaptosuccinic acid (DMSA): *in vitro* correlation. *J Nucl Med* **20**: 63–6.

Dillon MJ (1997) The diagnosis of renovascular disease. *Pediatr Nephrol* **11**: 366–72.

Dodge EA (1963) Vesicoureteral reflux: diagnosis with iodine-131 sodium ortho-iodohippurate. *Lancet* **i**: 303–6.

English PJ, Testa HJ, Lawson RS *et al.* (1978) Modified method of diuresis renography for the assessment of equivocal pelviureteric junction obstruciton. *Br J Urol* **59**: 10–14.

Enlander D, Weber PM, dosRemedios LV (1974) Renal cortical imaging in 35 patients: superior quality with ^99mTc^-DMSA. *J Nucl Med* **15**: 743–9.

Felson B, Cussen LJ (1975) The hydronephrotic type of unilateral congenital multicystic disease of the kidney. *Semin Roentgenol* **10**: 113–23.

Gates GF (1982) Glomerular filtration rate: estimation from fractional renal accumulation of 99m Tc-DTPA (stannous). *AJR AM J Roentgenol* **138**: 565–70.

Gordon I, Dhillon HK, Gatanash H (1991) Antenatal diagnosis of pelvic hydronephrosis: assessment of renal function and drainage as a guide to management. *J Nucl Med* **32**: 1649–54.

Griscom NT, Wawter GF, Fellers FX (1975) Pelvoinfundibular atresia: the usual form of multicystic kidney: 44 unilateral and two bilateral cases. *Semin Roentgenol* **10**: 125–31.

Lebowitz RL, Blickman JG (1983) The coexistence of ureteropelvic junction obstruction and reflux. *AJR AM J Roentgenol* **140**: 231–8.

McCrory WW (1972) *Developmental nephrology*. Cambridge, MA: Harvard University Press, 96.

Maizels M, Weiss S, Conway JJ *et al.* (1979) The cystometric nuclear cystogram. *J Urol* **121**: 203–5.

Majd M (1992) Nuclear medicine in pediatric urology. *Clinical pediatric urology*, 3rd edition, LR King, PP Kelalis and AB Belman (eds), WB Saunders, Philadelphia.

Majd M, Rushton HG (1992) Renal cortical scanning in the diagnosis of acute pyelonephritis. *Semin Nucl Med* **22**: 98–111.

Majd M, Potter BN, Guzzeta PC, Ruley EJ (1983) Effect of Captopril on efficacy of renal scintigraphy in detection of renal artery stenosis (abstract). *J Nucl Med* **24**: 23.

Majd M, Kass EJ, Belman AB (1985) Radionuclide cystography in children: comparison of direct (retrograde) and indirect (intravenous) techniques. *Ann Radiol* **28**: 322–8.

Mandell GA, Cooper JA, Leonard JC *et al.* (1997) Procedure guideline for diuretic renography in children. *J Nucl Med* **38**: 1647–50.

Merrick MV, Uttley WS, Wild SR (1980) The detection of pyelonephritic scarring in children by radioisotope imaging. *Br J Radiol* **53**: 544–56.

Mulligan JS, Blue PW, Hasbargen JA (1990) Methods of measuring GFR with technetium 99m-DTPA: an analysis of several common methods. *J Nucl Med* **31**: 1211–19.

Nadel NS, Gitter MH, Hahn LC *et al.* (1973) Pre-operative diagnosis of testicular torsion. *Urology* **1**: 478–9.

O'Hara SM, Donnelly LF, Coleman RE (1999) Pediatric body applications of FDG PET. *AJR Am J Roentgenol* **172**: 1019–24.

O'Reily PH, Lawson RS, Shields RA *et al.* (1979) Idiopathic hydronephrosis — the diuresis renogram: a new noninvasive method of assessing equivocal pelviureteral junction obstruction. *J Urol* **121**: 153–5.

Powers TA, Stone WJ, Grove RB *et al.* (1981) Radionuclide measurement of differential glomerular filtration rate. *Invest Radiol* **16**: 59–64.

Russell CD, Bischoff PG, Kontzen FN *et al.* (1985) Measurement of glomerular filtration rate: single injection plasma clearance method without urine collection. *J Nucl Med* **26**: 1243–7.

Sfakianakis GN, Sfakianakis ED (1988) Nuclear medicine in pediatric urology and nephrology. *J Nucl Med* **29**: 1287–93.

Sfakianakis GN, Cole C, Georgiou MF *et al.* (1999) Optimal timing of diuretic administration in diuretic renography (Abstract). *J Nucl Med* **40** Suppl: 51.

Shore RM, Koff SA, Mentser M *et al.* (1984) Glomerular filtration rate in children: determination form the Tc-99m DTPA renogram. *Radiology* **151**: 627–33.

Taylor A Jr (1982) Quantitation of renal function with static imaging agents. *Semin Nucl Med* **12**: 330–44.

Taylor A Jr, Ziffer JA, Steves A *et al.* (1989) Clinical comparison of I-131 orthoiodohippurate and the kit formulation of Tc-99m mercaptoacetyltriglycine. *Radiology* **170**: 721–5.

Thrall JH, Koff SA, Keyes JW Jr (1981) Diuretic radionuclide urography and scintigraphy in the differential diagnosis of hydronephrosis. *Semin Nucl Med* **11**: 89–104.

Whitfield HN, Britton KE, Fry IK *et al.* (1977) The obstructed kidney: correlation between renal function and urodynamic assessment. *Br J Urol* **49**: 615–18.

Winter CC (1959) A new test for vesicoureteral reflux: an external technique using radioisotopes. *J Urol* **81**: 105–11.

Wood BP, Smith WL (1981) Pulmonary edema in infants following injection of contrast media for urography. *Radiology* **139**: 377–9.

Prenatal and postnatal urologic emergencies

7

Patrick H. McKenna and Fernando A. Ferrer

Introduction

There are few true urologic emergencies. The object of this chapter is to cover the practical management of urgent consultations from the antenatal period through childhood. This includes a discussion of abdominal masses and intraoperative consultations. Several factors have impacted on the identification and management of fetuses and children with many urologically related anomalies. One of the most important factors has been the ability to identify many urologic problems during fetal development. This has occurred because of increasingly accurate imaging, genetic screening, and the active participation of pediatric urologists in a multidisciplinary approach to urologic problems. As technology and genetic understanding of diseases continue to advance, the frequency with which diseases are identified in the prenatal period will continue to increase.

Antenatal period

Intervention during the antenatal period takes many forms, including medical treatment, termination of pregnancy, early delivery induction, and surgical intervention. The incidence of intervention is gradually increasing but remains rare. There are ethical, technical, and medical issues surrounding fetal surgery (Nichols and Bianchi, 1996).

Pertinent ethical issues also surround the decision to terminate a pregnancy. Discussion of the ethics concerning termination is beyond the scope of this chapter and is societal in nature. The pertinent ethical issues facing maternal fetal obstetricians and pediatric urologists that are germane to this discussion are the accuracy of the antenatal diagnosis and correct explanation of the long-term outcome of antenatally detected problems to the expecting parents. These issues are especially important in countries such as the USA where there is a time limit on the developmental date when elective termination can be performed.

Most initial screening antenatal sonograms are performed in an obstetric office. When significant abnormalities are identified, patients should be referred to centers with experience with these abnormalities to confirm the diagnosis and provide an accurate explanation of the consequences and long-term outcome. The difficult task is providing an accurate assessment of the quality of life for patients with severe congenital abnormalities so that parents can make an educated decision about intervention or pregnancy termination. Currently, severe urinary tract obstruction and congenital abnormalities, complications of intervention, and intersex disorders are the most commonly encountered antenatal problems that may involve an urgent antenatal consultation.

Urinary tract obstruction with oligohydraminous

It is estimated that only one in 30 000 pregnancies may be a candidate for antenatal intervention because of an obstructive lesion (Housley and Harnison, 1998 and Herndon et al., 2000). The most common form of intervention is the induction of an early delivery after lung maturity is established. Treating the mother with steroids may accelerate lung maturity in the fetus (Leviton et al., 1999). Since this is such a rare event, much of the effort of pediatric urologists has been spent in preventing unindicated antenatal intervention. There are few scientific data to support the efficacy of early intervention (Elder et al., 1987; Crombleholme et al., 1990; Johnson et al., 1994, 1995; Freedman et al., 1996, 1999). Published reports concerning results of intervention are mostly retrospective in nature and none has long-term fol-low-up (McCurdy and Seeds, 1993). In addition, the natural history of these lesions differs in the timing of presentation and their severity, even during the ante-natal period, making case comparisons difficult (Hutton *et al.*, 1994). Early severe obstruction impacts on lung development, leading to pulmonary hypoplasia (Harrison *et al.*,1982; Peters *et al.*, 1991a, b; Chevalier and Klahr, 1998).

Urethral atresia is the most common cause of early severe hydroureteronephrosis. Posterior urethral valves (PUV) (Fig. 7.1) may present either early or late in the pregnancy with varying degrees of renal injury. A ball valving urterocele blocking the bladder neck is another rare form of bladder neck obstruction. These issues may be approached by working with maternal–fetal obstetricians to educate the general obstetricians on the correct differential diagnosis of antenatal urologic abnormalities. The flow diagram in Figure 7.2 is designed to focus the obstetrician on the importance of oligohydramnios when considering intervention. Education of obstetricians is important because ultimately they make the decision about inter-vention and also determine the timing of intervention. If the flow diagram is followed, only patients with oligohydramnios are even considered intervention candidates. Good prenatal sonography is accurate in making the diagnosis of PUV (Cohen *et al.*, 1998). The correct management of these problems should involve a multidisciplinary approach since the bulk of the care resulting from the early intervention will fall to the pediatrician and pediatric urologist.

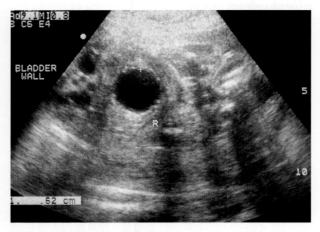

Figure 7.1 Prenatal posterior urethral valves: prenatal sonogram showing bilateral dilated renal pelvises and bladder with oligohydramnios.

In the rare instance where intervention is consid-ered, oligohydramnios should be present, other severe congenital abnormalities should be ruled out and evi-dence of recoverable renal function should be estab-lished (Golan *et al.*, 1994) (Fig. 7.3). Infusion of fluid into the amniotic space may be required to conduct an accurate sonographic survey for other severe con-genital abnormalities incompatible with survival. In addition, chromosome analysis should be obtained. Assessment of viable renal function is more difficult. It has been suggested that serial urine samples from the fetus be obtained to confirm renal function. Normal values (Table 7.1) may predict a better prog-nosis, as does the rate with which the bladder refills after tapping off the urine (Glick *et al.*, 1985; Evans *et al.*, 1991; Lipitz *et al.*, 1993; Johnson *et al.*, 1994, 1995). The reliability of these tests needs to be further documented (Wilkins *et al.*, 1987; Guez *et al.*, 1996). No assessment was done concerning quality of life issues in these patients. In cases of significant obstruc-tion the picture of increasing dilatation of the renal pelvic correlates with a greater likelihood of obstruc-tion (Anderson *et al.*, 1995). The *in utero* progression of mild hydronephrosis is usually less than 15% (Bobrowski *et al.*, 1997). No prospective studies have been performed comparing intervention to observa-tion. Since these abnormalities are so rare, single-cen-ter experiences are always small. A multicenter reg-istry has been attempted in the past but only a small number of patients was entered and long-term follow-up was not obtained (Manning *et al.*, 1986). The sin-gle-center review by Freedman *et al.*, (1999) of 14 patients with follow-up greater than 2 years revealed that five patients required renal transplantation, three had renal insufficiency, and six had normal renal func-tion. Ultimately, multicenter studies will be required to answer many of the questions concerning appro-priateness of intervention. A recent survey of practic-ing pediatric urologists confirmed that few recom-mend antenatal intervention. When it is considered, the strict criteria outlined above should be followed (Herndon *et al.*, 1999).

Complications of antenatal intervention

Intervention in the antenatal period can take various forms, from medical treatment to actual surgical intervention. The consequences of antenatal medical treatment for congenital adrenal hyperplasia (CAH) exemplify some of the ethical and practical problems

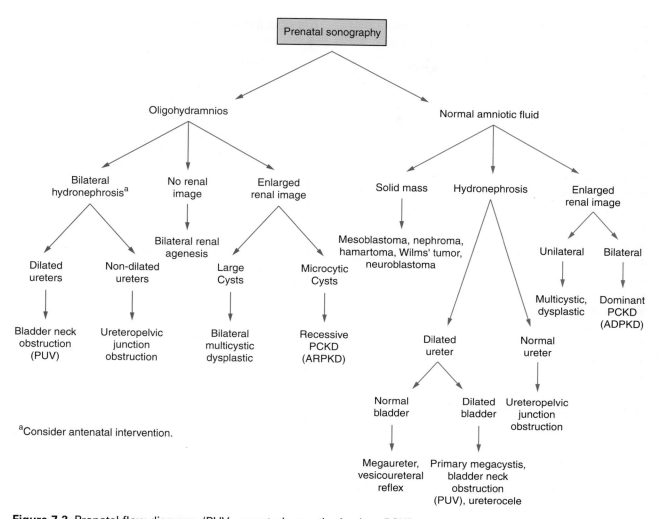

Figure 7.2 Prenatal flow diagram. (PUV = posterior urethral value; PCKD = polycystic kidney disease.)

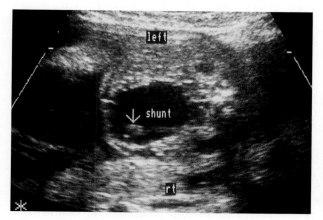

Figure 7.3 Antenatally detected posterior urethral valves with percutaneously placed vesicoamniotic shunt.

Table 7.1 Fetal urine electrolytes suggesting good renal function (bladder aspirates)

	Value
Sodium	< 100 mEq/l
Chloride	< 90 mEq/l
Osmolarity	< 210 mOSM/l
Urine output	> 2 ml/h
β_2-Microglobulin	< 6 mg/l

with prenatal treatment of the fetus with medication. The risks to the fetus escalate the more invasive the form of antenatal intervention. Amniocentesis during the second trimester has become almost a routine procedure. When it is done with ultrasound guidance there is a 1% incidence of spontaneous abortion (Tabor *et al.*, 1986; Hsieh *et al.*, 1989). Fetal hemorrhage, cord laceration, direct fetal injury, uterine injury, and chorioamnionitis have been reported after amniocentesis. But, when amniocentesis is performed using specific guidelines by experienced teams, these risks are minimal (Bahado-Singh, 1992). Chorionic villae sampling has a fetal loss rate of approximately 3.5% (Rhoads *et al.*, 1989) and infection rates of 0.25–0.5% (Kuliev *et al.*, 1996). The complications for this procedure are also decreasing and in some centers are not statistically different from those of amniocentesis (Donner *et al.*, 1995).

More invasive intervention, including percutaneous procedures and open surgery, are associated with more significant problems. The main abnormalities currently considered for intervention include fetal urinary tract obstruction, myelomeningocele, fetal diaphragmatic hernia, fetal cystic adenomatoid malformation, and fetal sacrococcygeal teratoma (Farmer, 1998). Even the most invasive procedures have minimal maternal risks or effect on future fertility (Farrell *et al.*, 1999).

The main risk of intervention with hysterotomy is subsequent uncontrolled uterine contractions with spontaneous delivery (Longaker *et al.*, 1991; Harrison, 1996). Development of better tocolytic agents and other methods to prevent uterine contraction is crucial to successful prenatal surgery. The increased use of percutaneous laparoscopic surgery may decrease the problems of uncontrolled uterine contractions. However, laparoscopy is associated with an increased risk of percutaneous access wounds. Risks include injury to other fetal organs and to the abdominal wall (Robichaux *et al.*, 1991; Estes *et al.*, 1992; Quintera *et al.*, 1995; Coplen *et al.*, 1996; Coplen *et al.*, 1997; Herndon and McKenna, 1998; Lewis *et al.*, 1998; Oberg *et al.*, 1999). Once intervention is anticipated, the pediatric team, including the maternal-fetal obstetrician, pediatric urologist, and neonatologist, should be available because complications such as uncontrolled uterine contraction or serious fetal injury may require immediate delivery, infant resuscitation, or surgical intervention (Herndon and McKenna, 1998).

Classic bladder exstrophy

The antenatal identification of exstrophy is relatively straightforward. A combination of characteristics can be identified on a screening sonogram. The five most commonly identified findings are: (1) no visualization of the bladder; (2) a lower abdominal bulge; (3) small penis and anteriorly placed scrotum; (4) a low-set umbilicus; and (5) abnormal widening of the iliac crests (Gearhart *et al.*, 1995). Omphaloceles are usually associated with a midline defect at the umbilical insertion, gastroschisis most frequently consists of a small, right-sided paraumbilical defect, and large lateral defects usually occur in the limb–body wall complex. In addition, specific organ evisceration and other associated abnormalities assist in the differential diagnosis (Emanuel *et al.*, 1995; Dykes, 1996).

The challenge in the antenatal identification of these abnormalities is to provide correct counseling to the parents at the time when the abnormalities are identified (Cacciari *et al.*, 1999). The correct approach is to involve a physician familiar with the long-term outcome of patients with these complex reconstructive problems. Initial work on the psychosocial and physical outcome of patients treated with various surgical approaches has begun but the outcome is known in a small number of patients (Woodhouse *et al.*, 1983; Feitz *et al.*, 1994; Ben-Chaim *et al.*, 1996). Although some broad generalizations can be made, more outcome data will be required to confirm early results. In the initial reviews, concerns centered primarily on worries about sexual function and sexual disfigurement, while education, family life, and employment appear to be less prominent. The males were concerned about the appearance of their external genitalia, even though their sexual function was preserved. The female patients were less concerned about disfigurement and had normal sexual function, sexuality, and fertility. A complete understanding of the underlying anatomical abnormalities and the approach in the surgical reconstruction are requirements to the appropriate counseling of these patients.

Neural tube defects

Although not primarily a urologic abnormality, neural tube defects result in significant urologic morbidity. The accurate diagnosis of neural tube defects during the antenatal period can result from a combination of routine screening of maternal serum α-fetoprotein and targeted sonography (Vintzileos *et al.*, 1999). Neuropathic bladder effects have been detected before birth (Kopp and Greenfield, 1993). The decreasing incidence of neural tube defects in the newborn period is secondary to the increased use of folic acid by childbearing women (Christensen and Rosenblatt, 1995; Neuhouser *et al.*, 1998) and the increase in termination of affected fetuses during pregnancy (Cromie *et al.*, 1998). The Public Health Service of the USA currently recommends that all women capable of childbearing consume 0.4 mg folic acid per day to decrease the risk of neural tube defects and anencephaly. Recently, it has been determined that the neurologic abnormalities associated with neural tube defects may results primarily from prolonged exposure of the neural tube to the amniotic fluid. Early antenatal intervention to close these defects has gained increased acceptance. The level of the defect, timing of repair and type of repair all effect the outcome. Long-term follow-up of antenatally treated patients is not available and urologic participation in the postnatal evaluation and follow-up will be crucial to determine the possible benefits of the antenatal surgical approach.

Solid masses

The antenatal identification of a solid mass seldom requires early intervention but often generates an urgent consultation. The commonly detected antenatal masses include:

- adrenal hemorrhage
- neuroblastoma
- congenital mesoblastic nephroma
- Wilms' tumor
- pulmonary sequestration
- teratoma
- sacrococcygeal teratoma
- hepatic lesions
- rhabdomyosarcoma.

Since hydronephrotic and cystic lesions are easily distinguished by sonography the list is predominantly made up of rare but reported lesions. The recommendation should be to evaluate these patients with a complete work-up after delivery.

Intersex disorders

The identification of intersex disorders in the antenatal period is the result of better screening techniques and advances in the understanding of the genetic inheritance of these diseases. Unlike the postnatal period, where ambiguous genitalia is the initiating factor, amniocentesis, chorionic villae sampling, and better sonographic techniques allow early identification of many intersex disorders in the antenatal period (Elejalde *et al.*, 1985; Doran, 1990; Mandell *et al.*, 1995; Herndon and McKenna, 1999). The prenatal identification of these problems results in the need to provide adequate prenatal counseling (Kemp *et al.*, 1998). Identifying CAH before birth provides the opportunity to treat the fetus in the hope of preventing androgen effects on fetal development (David and Forest, 1984; Evans *et al.*, 1985; Speiser *et al.*, 1990; Forest *et al.*, 1993; Mercado *et al.*, 1995; Lajic *et al.*, 1998).

Most intersex disorders other than CAH are identified inadvertently (Ross and Elias, 1997). In some cases this is the result of an amniocentesis because of a simple parental request to know the sex of the fetus. In other cases, there can be an issue of other known inheritable diseases such as determining the likelihood of an X-linked disorder (e.g. hemophilia). Knowing the sex may be helpful in confirming the cause of a structural disorder (e.g. PUV) that does not occur in girls. In cases with a family history of CAH genetic sampling can identify the inherited genetic disorder. The identification of an intersex disorder may also result from routine screening of an older mother. In situations where the genetic sex is known, but the genital screening by ultrasound does not appear to match the genotype, clinicians should consider the possibility of an intersex disorder. In the case of a 46,XY karyotype with female-appearing genitalia, the differential diagnosis should include gonadal dysgenesis or androgen insensitivity. In severely androgenized females with CAH, a 46,XX karyotype may be associated with ultrasound findings suggesting male genitalia. Table 7.2 lists the chromosomal analyses and possible intersex disorders.

The ability to identify and medically treat a disease in the antenatal period will probably become the norm in the future; however, the consequences of prenatal treatment need to be completely understood before it is openly embraced. Accuracy of the antenatal diagnosis and the effect of the medical treatment on other aspects of the fetus' development must be understood before treatment becomes routine. There is no better example of this controversy than the current debate over prenatal treatment of CAH (Speiser,

Table 7.2 Chromosomal analyses and possible intersex disorder

46,XX	Female pseudohermaphrodite (usually CAH)
	Male pseudohermaphrodite (i.e. SRY positive)
	True hermaphrodite
	Gonadal dysgenesis
46,XY	Male pseudohermaphrodite
	True hermaphrodite
46,XX/XY	True hermaphrodite
45,X, 45,X/46,XX,	Gonadal dysgenesis
45,X/46,XY,	Mixed gonadal dysgenesis
others	Male pseudohermaphrodite
	True hermaphrodite

1999; Miller, 1999). Prenatal treatment of CAH needs to start before 6 weeks' gestation to completely prevent androgenic effects. Chorionic villae sampling to obtain fetal DNA cannot be done until 10–12 weeks' gestation.

The most common cause of CAH is 21-hydroxylase deficiency. This deficiency results in the inability to synthesize cortisol. The pituitary and hypothalamus overstimulate the adrenal gland, causing the overproduction of androstenedione. The androstenedione is further metabolized, predominantly to testosterone and dihydrotestosterone, resulting in the prenatal virilization of the female fetus. Early treatment with dexamethasone can prevent or minimize severe genital abnormalities in some patients (Pang *et al.*,1990; Forest *et al.*,1993; Speiser and New, 1994; New and White, 1995). The risk of having an infant with CAH for a mother with classic 21-hydroxylase deficiency is 1 in 8. The complications of prenatal treatment to the fetus, maternal risks, and long-term effects to the child are incompletely understood. Since antenatal treatment with dexamethasone needs to begin at 6 weeks' gestation, seven fetuses are treated unnecessarily to affect the external genital development of one fetus. This has significant ethical implications. The fetal metabolism of dexamethasone is not understood, and the doses recommended for treatment are greater then required to surpress the adrenal in the adult (Miller, 1999). The effect on normal fetuses is not completely known. Despite these concerns, the possibility of preventing androgen imprinting of the brain in the affected female fetuses justifies a controlled long-term study.

Postnatal period

In the past, urologic problems identified at birth were primarily obvious congenital abnormalities such as exstrophy. Now, the majority of urologic problems seen by urologists in the immediate postnatal period are identified by prenatal sonography. In the evaluation and treatment of these problems physicians need to consider the unique aspects of bonding between the infant and the parents (Klaus and Kennell, 1982; Crouch and Manderson, 1995). Bonding can be affected by separation of the infant from the parents and by severely disfiguring congenital anomalies (Riski, 1991; Bradbury and Hewison, 1994). These considerations should impact the treatment of infants with and without obvious congenital abnormalities. The support needs go beyond helping the family to come to grips with the congenital anomaly, and should include dealing with parental fears concerning job loss, financial difficulties, and effects on other family members (Riski, 1991). One should encourage early discharge of infants who can be adequately managed as outpatients. When prolonged hospitalization is required, parental rooming-in with the infant is encouraged. A psychiatrist and staff educated on bonding issues should be actively involved in patient and parental management (Drotar *et al.*, 1975; Quine and Pahl, 1987; Varni and Setoguchi, 1993).

Congenital anomalies noted at birth
Anorectal malformations

Anorectal malformations (imperforate anus) are congenital lesions of the cloaca (Fig. 7.4). It is important for urologists to be familiar with these malformations because they are often associated with urologic abnormalities. There is also a high incidence of other congenital abnormalities associated with such malformations. There are multiple classification systems but none has gained wide acceptance. From a urologic perspective the simple distinction of 'high', 'intermediate', or 'low' anorectal lesions is probably sufficient: low lesions are those that occur inferior to the levator muscles, high lesions occur above the levator muscles, and intermediate ones in between (Fig. 7.5) (Belman and King, 1972b). From a clinical point of view most intermediate lesions are treated as high lesions. The surgical correction of these malformations is most often by a technique popularized by de Vries and Pena (1982) using the posterior

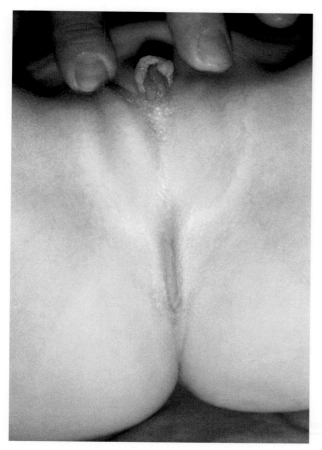

Figure 7.4 Patient with imperforate anus. (From Dr Donald W. Hight, Connecticut Children's Medical Center, with permission.)

sagittal approach. Associated urologic abnormalities occur in up to 20% of patients with low lesions and up to 60% of those with high lesions (McLorie *et al.*, 1987; Levitt *et al.*, 1997). The most common findings are vesicoureteral reflux (VUR), neuropathic bladder, renal agenesis, renal dysplasia, and cryptorchidism. It is not surprising that there is a high incidence of neuropathic bladder because of the likely association of vertebral abnormalities with anorectal malformations, especially with high lesions. Neuropathic bladder may occur in as many as 50% of patients (McLorie *et al.*, 1987). The most common anatomic abnormality in patients with vertebral abnormalities is a tethered cord. Only recently has this association been identified and linked to the high incidence of neuropathic bladders and dysfunctional pelvic floors. Patients with anorectal malformations should be studied urodynamically, especially if they have high lesions and/or spinal abnormalities.

Exstrophy

Classic bladder exstrophy still most commonly presents at the time of birth despite the known specific antenatal sonographic findings (Gearhart *et al.*, 1995) (Fig. 7.6). The typical infant is male and is otherwise healthy. An exstrophic bladder, abdominal wall defect, epispadias, pelvic diastasis, VUR after bladder closure, and bilateral inguinal hernias characterize the anomaly. Initially, much time is spent with the family explaining the disease and planning the bladder closure. Patients should be managed in a center with exstrophy closure experience. The initial treatment is to protect the exposed bladder mucosa. If a plastic umbilical clamp was placed in the delivery suit it should be removed and replaced with a suture. If possible, nothing should come into contact with the bladder mucosa. A modified humidifier tent can be placed over the bladder, but for transport a cellophane non-adherent dressing may be utilized.

The methods of reconstruction used by the present authors are based on a staged strategy (Jeffs *et al.*, 1982; Gearhart and Rock, 1989), the first stage involving bladder and abdominal wall closure with pelvic osteotomy in most cases (Fig. 7.7). The epispadias is reconstructed in the next stage, and finally the incontinence and reflux. Recently, Mitchell has advocated combining the first stages into one operation soon after birth (see Chapter 27). Initial reports are encouraging but relatively few patients have been treated in this way and little long-term follow-up is yet available (Grady and Mitchell, 1999).

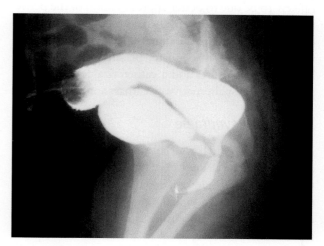

Figure 7.5 Radiographic picture of high bowel–urethral fistula. (From Dr Donald W. Hight, Connecticut Children's Medical Center, with permission.)

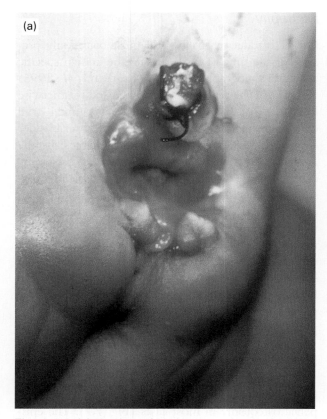
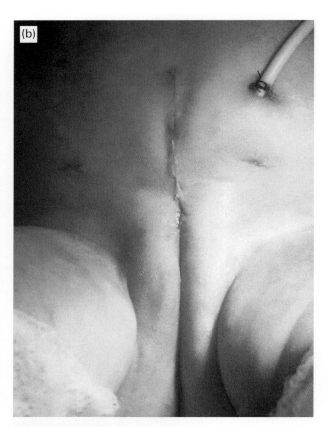

Figure 7.6 (*a*) Newborn female exstrophy patient; (*b*) 4 weeks after initial closure.

Exstrophy reconstruction has led to a greater understanding of sphincter and pelvic floor anatomy and function. Patients have improved pelvic floor reconstruction and better continence rates after osteotomy (McKenna, 1993; McKenna *et al.*, 1993, 1994). This is likely to be due to better approximation of the pelvic floor muscle. In addition, there is a close relationship between bladder size and continence. In situations where capacity is inadequate, bladder augmentation, bladder neck closure, and a catheterizable stoma may provide the best alternative (Gearhart and Jeffs, 1988).

Prune belly syndrome

Deficient abdominal wall musculature, cryptorchism, and urinary tract dilatation characterize this syndrome. Other names include: triad syndrome, Eagle–Barrett syndrome, and abdominal muscular deficiency syndrome. The spectrum of this disease is wide. It ranges from *in utero* demise, renal dysplasia and subsequent renal failure, to normal renal function. The pathogenesis is not completely understood (Wheately *et al.*, 1996). The presumptive prenatal diagnosis has been

made as early as 12 weeks' gestation (Hoshino *et al.*, 1998). In the most severe forms, identified antenatally, there is complete urethral obstruction. In the antenatal period these patients are often confused with patients who have severe PUV and may be inadvertently combined in retrospective reviews (Johnson *et al.*, 1994). One terminated fetus had urethral atresia

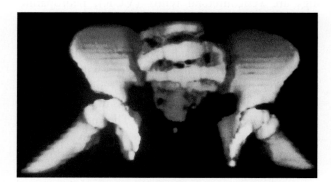

Figure 7.7 Three-dimensional CT reconstruction of a 5-year-old male with uncorrected classic bladder exstrophy showing a wide separation of the pubic bones and flattening of the ilial bones.

with histologically normal kidneys, which may mean that there is a role for intervention in cases identified very early (Shigeta *et al.*, 1999). The postnatal evaluation should include sonography, voiding cysto-urathrography (VCUG), and renal scan when indicated. Although predominatly affecting males, a female variety has been described (Hirose *et al.*, 1995). Initially, medical treatment (i.e. antibacterial prophylaxis and prehaps circumcision in babies with reflux) and close surveillance is indicated in all but the most severe cases where vesicostomy or upper tract diversion may be needed (Burbige *et al.*, 1987; Woodard and Zucker, 1990; Druschel, 1995). In the long term, a combination of continuous antibacterial prophylaxis, well-planned surgery, and close surveillance is the best means to ensure an optimal outcome (Reinberg *et al.*, 1989, 1991; Woodard and Zucker, 1990; Bukowski and Perlmutter, 1994; Noh *et al.*, 1999). Severity of the congenital renal dysplasia, nadir creatinine greater than 0.7 mg/dl, recurrent pyelonephritis, and renal obstruction all correlate with eventual development of renal failure (Reinberg *et al.*, 1991; Noh *et al.*, 1999). Treatment of the undescended testes should be similar to that recommended for other patients with abdominal testes. Early orchidopexy should be accomplished and may be facilitated by laparoscopy (Docimo *et al.*, 1995). No prune belly patient has been known to father a child; however, early testis biopsy has identified spermatogonia so fertility is possible using *in vitro* fertilization (Woodhouse and Snyder, 1985; Orvis *et al.*, 1988). The histologic findings of significantly reduced spermatogonia and marked Leydig cell hyperplasia suggest that the pathology of the testis in prune belly syndrome is secondary to more than just its abdominal location. Testis tumors have developed in these patients (Woodhouse and Ransley, 1983; Parra *et al.*, 1991; Massad *et al.*, 1991).

Myelodysplasia

In the past this was the most common cause of neurogenic bladder dysfunction in children. Its incidence has been steadily decreasing because of early detection in the antenatal period resulting in termination of the pregnancy (Cromie *et al.*, 1998), and maternal folic acid treatment which markedly decreases the likelihood of developing spinal defects (Stein *et al.*, 1982; Anon. 1991; Lewis DP *et al.*, 1998). There is a slight increase in the incidence of myelodysplasia if other

family members also have the condition (Scarff and Fronczak, 1981).

Open myelomeningoceles (Fig. 7.8) are readily identifiable at birth. The level of the lesion does not determine the neurologic effect because some nerve roots may be left intact. An Arnold–Chiari malformation can affect the brainstem and pontine center. Tethering of the spinal cord and different growth rates in the distorted vertebral bodies can affect the final neurologic deficit (Lais *et al.*, 1993). Likewise, immediately after birth and during infancy and early childhood, a changing pattern is often seen in the urodynamics of these patients (Bauer, 1984; Roach *et al.*, 1993; Sillén *et al.*, 1996). It is impossible to make broad generalizations but in children with high thoracic lesions, patients may have an intact sacral reflex arc. Those with lesions at S1 and below can have normal bladder function but upper or lower motor lesions involving the bladder and or pelvic floor are also seen. Complete urologic evaluation after closure of the defects including renal sonography, VCUG, and full urodynamic assessment is advisable because sphincter dyssynergia and uninhibited

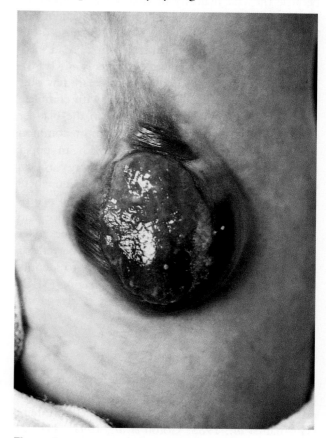

Figure 7.8 Newborn with myelomeningocele.

bladder contractions may be predictive of future upper tract deterioration (McGuire *et al.*, 1981; van Gool *et al.*, 1982; Bauer, 1984; Dator *et al.*, 1992; Andros *et al.*, 1998). Clear evidence exists that starting prophylactic treatment in situations where there is high risk for deterioration (uninhibited bladder contraction and elevated storage pressure in association with sphincter dyssynergy) is beneficial in decreasing the likelihood of upper tract and bladder deterioration (Perez *et al.*, 1992; Wu *et al.*, 1997; Bauer, 1998). Management usually involves initiation of clean intermittent catheterization (CIC) and anticholinergic medication. The dynamic nature of this disease requires routine surveillance throughout the patient's life, but particularly during periods of rapid linear growth, when spinal cord tethering may occur (Bauer *et al.*, 1992; Bauer, 1998).

Lipomeningocele

This abnormality is difficult to identify on physical examination. It is important to have a high level of suspicion and to examine the lower spine carefully because the vast majority of children with lipomeningocele have an identifiable superficial or cutaneous lesion. The neurologic changes occur because of an intradural lipoma. This lesion results in a broad spectrum of disease and presentation (Foster *et al.*, 1990). Typically, during early childhood, there are few outward physical abnormalities and only with complete urodynamic assessment is the effect on the bladder identified (Atala *et al.*, 1992). The most common urodynamic findings are consistent with an upper motor neuron lesion. Sphincter dyssynergy is less often identified in this group. In older children where the diagnosis has been delayed there are often neurologic changes in the lower extremity (Bruce and Schut, 1979). The bladder changes in the older group are mixed between detrusor hyperreflexia and detrusor areflexia. The best methods to identify these lesions are magnetic resonance imaging (MRI) and complete urodynamic assessment (Colak *et al.*, 1998).

Sacral agenesis

This lesion is even more difficult to identify on physical examination and often the patient presents at an older age with failure to become continent (Guzman *et al.*, 1983; Gotoh *et al.*, 1991). Loss of the lower vertebral bodies can be easily seen on a lateral lower plain film of the spine or on an MRI study. White and Klauber (1976) suggested that palpation of the coccyx could identify absent vertebral bodies, but radiographic confirmation is the best method. These patients have a stable neurologic lesion that does not progress with growth. However, the results of urodynamic studies are variable (Koff and DeRidder, 1977). Patients may have no sign of denervation or hyperreflexia, areflexia, intact sphincter function, or sphincter dyssynergy, and some have absent control over the sphincter (Borrelli *et al.*, 1985). A high level of suspicion and complete urodynamics help to guide treatment (Guzman *et al.*, 1983). Specific intervention is based on the identified findings (Gotoh *et al.*, 1991).

Scrotal masses

Palpation of a scrotal mass commonly results in an urgent consultation. When it is of an acute nature with pain, testicular torsion is the most important diagnosis to consider. This represents a true surgical emergency. It is best managed by early exploration, detorsion and, when the testis is salvageable, fixation. If the testis is not salvageable it should be removed. In either instance, the contralateral testis should also be sutured to the scrotal wall.

The history should focus on the age of the patient, whether there is associated pain, and whether there is a history of trauma. The onset and severity of pain may be helpful in the differential diagnosis of torsion versus epididymitis. The physical examination should focus on identifying the location of the mass in relation to the testis. The orientation of the testis should be evaluated. Normally, the epididymis is posterior and lateral to the testis. Careful palpation will identify torsion of appendices such as the appendix testis, both anterior and superior appendices of the epididymis, and the hydatid of Morgagni that is located in the posterior inferior epididymal testicular ridge (Noske *et al.*, 1998). In non-acute masses sonography is important to confirm the location and architecture of the mass. Possible scrotal masses are:

- hydrocele
- incarcerated hernia
- torsion of the testis
- appendage torsion
- testis tumor
- epididymitis

- epididymal cyst
- epididymal tumor
- paratesticular tumor
- varicocele
- Henoch–Schönlein purpura
- idiopathic edema
- cavernous hemangioma
- funiculitis
- lesions that result from a patent process vaginalis.

Neonatal scrotal masses

History plays very little role in the diagnosis in neonates (Siegel and Herman, 1994). The specific diferential diagnosis of such masses includes:

- hydrocele
- incarcerated hernia
- torsion
- lesion secondary to patent processus vaginalis
    meconium
    intraperitoneal bleeding
- testis tumors
- trauma.

The initial evaluation of these infants involves a complete physical examination. Perinatally firm enlarged scrotal masses may be hydroceles but the diagnosis of bilateral torsion should be considered (Gross et al., 1993). Positive transillumination can often aid the differential diagnosis. Occasionally a plain abdominal film may be helpful in identifying bowel gas in the scrotal mass that would indicate a communicating hydrocele with bowel in the scrotum. If the mass is associated with thickened cord structures or if it can be reduced, a hernia is likely. Ultrasound examination can differentiate solid and cystic masses. Doppler ultrasound can often confirm blood flow, but is often misleading in the small child.

Prenatal testis torsion is also referred to as neonatal torsion, intrauterine torsion, antenatal torsion, perinatal torsion, and newborn torsion. There is controversy over the mechanism of the torsion, risk of bilaterality, and need for and timing of contralateral fixation (Baptist and Amin, 1996; Pinto et al., 1997; Driver and Losty, 1998). When torsion occurs before delivery it has been thought to occur extravaginally, involving the entire spermatic cord and its tunics. Some physicians believe that this process can occur very early in the pregnancy and that it is responsible for most instances of testicular agenesis (Huff et al., 1991; Cilento et al., 1993; Gong et al., 1996). It is

impossible to determine whether all cases are extravaginal and at least some are probably intravaginal torsion, as seen in older boys. When torsion occurs prior to delivery the presentation is one of a non-tender, discolored, solid scrotal mass. Doppler ultrasound is generally accurate in confirming the diagnosis (Cartwright et al., 1995; Stone et al., 1995; Groisman et al., 1996; Hernanz-Schulman et al., 1997; Zinn et al., 1998). The torsion is most often unilateral but over 30 bilateral cases have been reported (Tripp and Homsy, 1995; Groisman et al., 1996; Cooper et al., 1997). A strong case has been made for early exploration, with orchiectomy when the testis is necrotic, and contralateral fixation, as many examples of subsequent contralateral torsion have now been reported (LaQuaglia et al., 1987; Das and Singer, 1990; Calleja and Archer, 1996). The arguments in favor of early exploration include: relative safety of anesthesia in the neonatal period, possibility of testicular salvage (10%), particularly the hormonal function, ability to fix the contralateral testis to prevent dyssynchronous torsion in the future, and to confirm the diagnosis.

Lesions that result from a patent processus vaginalis include meconium mass, hemoscrotum from intra-abdominal hemorrhage, and tumor seeding from renal or adrenal tumors (Putnam, 1989; Ring et al., 1989; McAlister and Sisler, 1990; Stokes and Flom, 1997; Han et al., 1998). Spontaneous rupture of the bowel can occur during fetal development resulting in meconium peritonitis. If the processus vaginalis is still open at that time the meconium can fall into the scrotum and present as a solid mass at birth. Stippled calcification is usually present. Likewise, other anomalies such as adrenal hematomas, neuroblastoma, and Wilms' tumor can also seed the scrotum through a patent canal and should be considered in the differential diagnosis of neonatal scrotal masses.

Testis tumors are also seen in the neonatal period but are rare (Table 7.3) (Levy et al., 1994). Yolk sac tumors, teratomas, gonadal stromal tumors and juvenile granulosa cell tumors are the most common. Early radical surgical removal is the recommended treatment for those with malignant potential, with chemotherapy in selected cases.

Pediatric scrotal masses

In older patients history plays a greater role in the differential diagnosis. Torsion has a bimodal distribution:

Table 7.3 Neonatal testicular tumors

Tumor	Frequency (%)
Yolk sac	27
Gonadal stromal tumors	27
Juvenile granulosa cell tumors	27
Gonadal blastoma	9
Teratoma	5
Harmartoma	5
Adapted from Levy *et al*. (1994).	

in the perinatal period and at or before puberty (Melekos, 1988). When there is sudden onset of severe pain associated with nausea and scrotal swelling, torsion should be suspected and represents a true surgical emergency. On examination of the scrotum there is no spermatic cord swelling. The cremasteric reflex is generally absent (Caldamone *et al*., 1984) and the testis is tense to palpation and rides high in the scrotum. The epididymis will either not be palpable or is palpable in an abnormal location. Urinalysis is usually normal. Torsion is usually confirmed by surgical exploration; however, in centers with rapid access to color Doppler ultrasound the diagnosis can be confirmed before intervention (Patriquin *et al*., 1993; Kass *et al*., 1993; Yazbeck and Patriquin, 1994). In most cases history and physical examination are sufficient for diagnosis, and radiologic evaluation is only performed in those in whom the diagnosis is unlikely. Detorsion can take place prior to exploration by manually untwisting the involved testis. The most common direction of torsion is from lateral to medial (when viewing the scrotum from the patient's feet), so detorsion manually should be from medial to lateral (again viewing the scrotum from the patient's feet). If detorsion is unsuccessful attempts in the other direction can be tried. Once the direction is determined the testis will spin rapidly and complete resolution of pain confirms detorsion. The testis should still be fixed in place by suture to prevent recurrent torsion. Torsion in the pediatric period is usually intravaginal and secondary to a bell-clapper deformity. Torsion should be relieved within 4 hours to be certain of testis viability, but detorsion after 12 hours has resulted in viable testis tissue in some cases; by 24 hours there is almost uniform atrophy (Brandell and Brock, 1993; Tryfonas *et al*., 1994; Rampaul and Hosking, 1998). Cases where there has been testicular salvage after longer periods probably represent intermittent torsion. Spermatogonia appear to be more sensitive to ischemia then the Sertoli and Leydig cells (Mikuz, 1985). Since the bell-clapper deformity affects both testes the contralateral testis should be pexed at the time that the involved testis is explored. In a typical pediatric emergency room 16% of the patients who present with an acute scrotum will have testis torsion, 46% of whom will have torsion of an appendix of the testis, 35% will have epididymitis, and the remainder are other lesions (Lewis *et al*., 1995). It appears that treatment with human chorionic gonadotropin (hCG) may occasionally induce torsion in the unde-

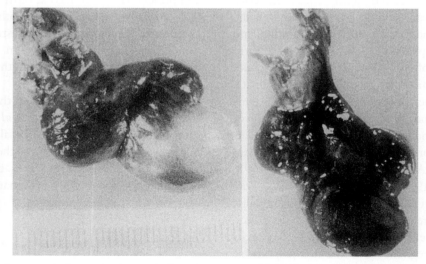

Figure 7.9 Infarcted testes and spermatic cord after treatment with hCG: (*a*) external appearance; (*b*) longitudinal sections. (From Sawchuk *et. al.*, 1993, with permission.)

scended testes (Sawchuk *et al.*, 1993) (Fig. 7.9).

Epididymitis should also be considered in boys with acute scrotal pain. It usually presents as scrotal swelling with gradually increasing pain. Physical examination isolates pain to the epididymis. The cremasteric reflex is often intact (Kadish and Bolte, 1998). Elevation of the testis may improve the pain (Prehn's sign). When pyuria is present this supports the diagnosis but in children it is often not present. Sonography shows a hyperemic swollen epididymis (Hamm, 1997). The causes of epididymitis include trauma, infection, or reflux of sterile urine. Since the cause may not be identified at diagnosis, treatment should include scrotal elevation, bed rest, antibiotics, and an anti-inflammatory medication. In sexually active teenagers possible *Chlamydia trachomatis* infection should be treated, and in non-sexually active children treatment should be directed toward *Escherichia coli*. In boys with proven bacterial epididymitis there is a high probability of an anatomic abnormality. After treatment full examination of the upper and lower urinary tract should be accomplished with ultrasound and a VCUG (Lewis *et al.*, 1995).

Pediatric scrotal tumors are rare and include primary testis lesions, paratesticular tumors, and metastatic or lymphatic tumors (Sugita *et al.*, 1999):

- mature teratoma
- teratocarcinoma
- yolk sac tumor
- paratesticular rhabdomyosarcoma
- gonadal stromal tumors
- granulosa cell tumors

- cavernous hemangioma
- gonadoblastoma
- metastatic tumors.

Ultrasound is helpful in locating the origin of these lesions but the diagnosis is made by surgical exploration through a groin incision. It is inadvisable to explore tumors through a scrotal lesion because such intervention can change the direction of lymphatic spread of the tumor. Once the tumor is removed pathologic evaluation determines the diagnosis. A combination of surgery, chemotherapy, and radiation has resulted in a high cure rate (Levy *et al.*, 1994; Sugita *et al.*, 1999).

Another scrotal lesion that may present as a scrotal mass is a varicocele. It is usually left sided and disappears when the patient lies flat. Intervention is indicated if it is associated with ipsilateral testicular growth failure. Other intrascrotal lesions are extremely rare, usually benign and identified by history, physical, ultrasound, and biopsy (Ferrer and McKenna, 1995; Aragona *et al.*, 1996; Sugita *et al.*, 1999) (Fig.

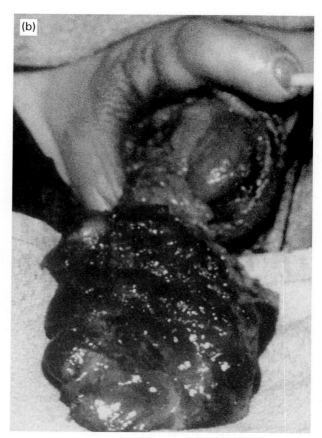

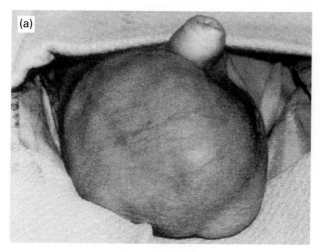

Figure 7.10 (*a*) Preoperative picture of scrotal cavernous hemangioma; (*b*) intraoperative picture of a cavernous hemangioma.

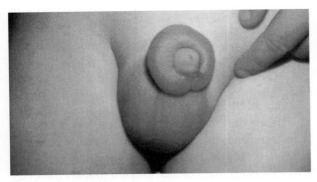

Figure 7.11 Idiopathic edema.

7.10). The more common superficial lesions such as funiculitis and idiopathic edema should be considered when the scrotal contents are normal (Fig. 7.11).

Intersex disorders

A consultation for ambiguous genitalia is one of the urgent problems that a urologist must face. The initial approach to managing intersex patients is to identify and treat possible life-threatening abnormalities (Donahoe *et al.*, 1991; Lee, 1991; Donahoe and Schnitzer,

1996; Lee and Donahoe, 1997). In most instances sexual assignment is straightforward and where it is not, consideration should be given to delaying the decision to intervene surgically until the infant is older (Donahoe and Schnitzer, 1996; Meyer-Bahlburg 1999) (see Chapter 29).

CAH is the most common form of ambiguous genitalia at birth. It is the only form of intersex that can be life threatening. The possible enzyme deficiencies include: 21-hydroxalase, 11-betahydroxalase, 20,22-desmolase, and 3B-hydroxysteroid dehydrogenase. In 21-hydroxalase deficiency lack of mineralocorticoid and glucocorticoid cause an electrolyte imbalance resulting in elevated serum potassium and low sodium that lead to dehydration or potentially lethal cardiac arrhythmias. The excess androstenedione that builds up behind the enzymatic block metabolizes to testosterone and dihydrotestosterone causing virilization of the female infant (Fig. 7.12). Physical examination and screening laboratory studies facilitate the differential diagnosis relatively rapidly. The infant will have varying degrees of virilization, from hypertrophy of the clitoris and mild labioscrotal development to a normal appearing male phallus and scrotum. The

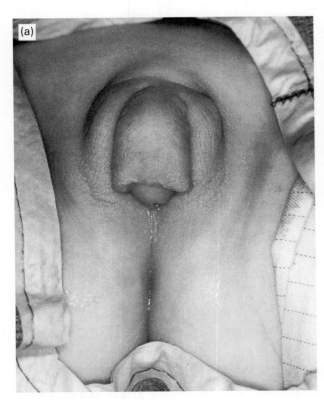
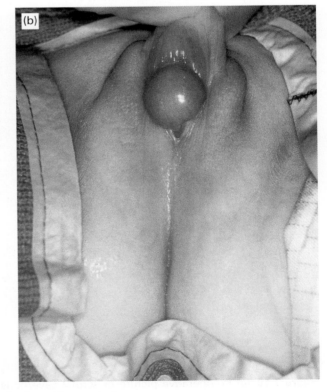

Figure 7.12 Severely androgenized patient with congenital adrenal hyperplasia.

gonads are symmetrical and typically non-palpable. The Barr body is positive, and pelvic sonography identifies a uterus and ovaries. Müllerian inhibiting substance is undetectable, and the chromosome evaluation is 46,XX. Serum studies should include electrolytes, glucose, gonodotropin, dihydrotestosterone, testosterone, and adrenal steriod levels. Initial treatment involves glucocorticoid and mineralocorticoid replacement. It is strongly recommended that these patients be reared as female because of the chromo-

somal sex and potential fertility, but in the most virilized form questions have arisen as to the best sex of rearing (Colapinto, 1997; Meyer-Bahlburg, 1999).

Although CAH is the most common intersex disorder, it is important to have a diagnostic plan for evaluating all intersex patients. The differential diagnosis method used by the authors is based on history, chromosome determination, serum tests, screening radiological studies, and pathology (Fig. 7.13).

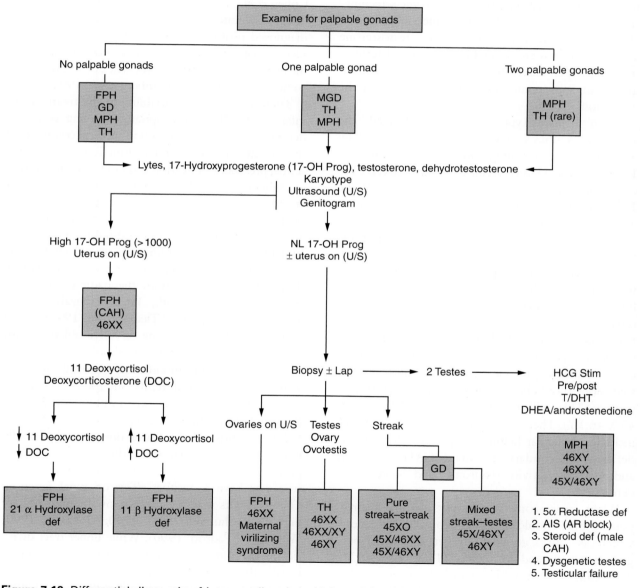

Figure 7.13 Differential diagnosis of intersex disorders. (Adapted from flow diagram presented to the Society for Fetal Urology in 1999 by Thomas Kolon, MD.) (FPH = female pseudohermaphroditism; GD = gonal dysgenesis; MPH = male pseudohermaphroditism; TH = true hermaphroditism; MGD = mixed gonadal dysgenesis; CAH = congenital adrenal hyperplasia.)

The initial history should focus on pedigree and drug ingestion history. Physical examination should concentrate on palpating the gonads. If no gonads can be palpated in the masculinized baby, one should consider female pseudohermaphroditism (FPH), gonadal dysgenesis (GD), male pseudohermaphroditism (MPH), and true hermaphroditism (TH). When only one gonad is palpable one should consider mixed gonadal dysgenesis (MGD), TH and MPH. When both gonads are palpated one should consider MPH and rarely TH. The next step involves targeted laboratory and radiologic screening. Initial evaluation should include measuring serum electrolyte, 17-hydroxyprogesterone, testosterone and dihydrotestosterone (DHT) levels, and determining karyotype. Screening sonography and genitography in appropriate situations are helpful in the evaluation.

When 17-hydroxyprogesterone is elevated, the karyotype is 46,XX, and a uterus is identified by ultrasound, one is dealing with CAH. Checking the 11-deoxycortisol levels can differentiate between 21α-hydroxylase and 11β-hydroxylase deficiency. If the 17-hydroxyprogesterone levels are normal and a uterus and ovaries are identified in a child with a 46,XX karyotype a maternal virilizing syndrome should be considered.

In the remainder of cases, 17-hydroxyprogesterone will not be elevated. A combination of ultrasound findings and laparoscopy with or without biopsy is often required to make a definitive diagnosis. If two testes are identified an hCG stimulation test should be performed. Serum testosterone, DHT, dehydroepiandrosterone (DHEA) and androstenedione should be measured before and after stimulation. This will identify MPH (46,XY, 46,XX, 45,X/46,XY). There are a number of causes of MPH, including testicular failure, dysgenetic testes, steroid deficiency secondary to male CAH, complete androgen insensitivity syndrome, and 5α-reductase deficiency.

When laparoscopy and biopsy identify a streak gonad, one should consider gonadal dysgenesis, which is pure gonadal dysgenesis with both gonads represented as streaks (45,X, 45,X/46,XX, 45,X/46,XY), or mixed gonadal dysgenesis with a streak gonad and testis (45,X/46,XY, 46,XY). In cases with both a testis and ovary or ovotestes, one should consider true hermaphroditism (46,XX, 46,XX/XY, 46,XY).

Posterior urethral valves and lower urinary tract abnormalities

This cause of lower urinary tract obstruction is now commonly diagnosed presumptively in the antenatal period. Previously, infants presented with failure to thrive, an abdominal mass, or urosepsis (Dinneen et al., 1993). Common antenatal ultrasound findings include a distended thick-walled bladder, bilateral hydronephrosis, and oligohydramnios in some cases (Dinneen et al., 1993; Dewan and Goh, 1995; Cohen et al., 1998). While the outcomess of patients diagnosed antenatally may be worse than those diagnosed postnatally, this is indicative of a greater severity of disease and should not be taken to mean that antenatal diagnoses will not improve outcome in these patients (Reinberg et al., 1992).

There is significant variability in the treatment of infants with PUV. Appropriate treatment is usually determined based on the overall medical condition of the infant, including renal function, hydrational status, presence of infection and lung maturity, as well as caliber of the urethra. In general, some basic tenets are applicable to most cases. Catheter drainage of the bladder will allow decompression of the urinary tract and prophylactic antibiotics should be initiated. Initial measures of renal function are reflective of the mother's kidney function; therefore, catheter drainage should be maintained until the nadir creatinine is reached (Churchill et al., 1990; Gonzales, 1990; Merguerian et al., 1992; Tietjen et al., 1997). If the creatinine falls below 1 mg/dl, valve ablation with pediatric endoscopic equipment should be performed, after which careful monitoring of renal function, bladder function, and reflux should be continued while the child remains on antibiotic prophylaxis (Smith et al., 1996; Close et al., 1997).

Infants whose renal function does not substantially improve pose a much more difficult management problem. In these patients minimizing intrarenal pressure *may* have a positive effect on renal function. These patients may have either low or high urinary diversion (Churchill et al., 1990; Gonzales, 1990; Walker and Padron, 1990). While upper tract diversion was commonly used in the past, vesicostomy is usually the initial step to decompress these kidneys. Consideration to upper tract diversion may be given in severe cases in order to minimize intrapelvic pressures and in those with urinary infection, as this optimizes renal drainage. However, little evidence exists that upper tract diversion really helps, unless infection has been present. Long-term outcome in these patients depends essentially on the degree of renal damage and on bladder function (Parkhouse and Woodhouse, 1990; Reinberg *et al.*, 1992). Older children may require anticholinergics and/or bladder augmentation for the 'valve bladder' with high storage pressures. Reimplantation to correct reflux may be necessary: The worst cases come to dialysis and eventual transplantation.

An ectopic ureterocele can present as an obstructing lesion at the bladder neck. This condition occurs with a female prevalence of approximately 3–4:1 (Mor *et al.*, 1992; Sherer and Hulbert, 1995; Gloor *et al.*, 1996). Cases in which the ureterocele creates a ball-valve obstructive mechanism have been reported and these have been detected antenatally (Gloor *et al.*, 1996). Bilateral ureteroceles have also been diagnosed by ultrasound prior to birth. In general, these patients are managed initially by transurethral incision (Blyth *et al.*, 1993; Smith *et al.*, 1994; Di Benedetto *et al.*, 1997; Coplen, 1998; Pfister *et al.*, 1998) (Fig. 7.14). Once stabilized they undergo final management, which may include treatment of reflux, excision of the ureterocele and in some cases upper pole nephrectomy and ureterectomy (Mor *et al.*, 1992). As in all cases of lower urinary tract obstruction, treatment of long-term bladder dysfunction may be required. Infection is another indication for ureterocele incision.

VUR can be the cause of the upper tract dilatation in as many as 35% of children with antenatal hydronephrosis (Herndon *et al.*, 1999). Recent reviews suggest that this is a rare occurrence in African–Americans and more common in males than females (Avni and Schulman, 1996; Yeung *et al.*, 1997). Children with dilated upper tracts should have a VCUG to rule out reflux prior to treatment for other urinary tract abnormalities (Tibballs and De Bruyn, 1996).

Circumcision injuries

Circumcision is of the most common surgical procedures performed in the USA, with approximately 600 000–700 000 operations performed annually (Poland, 1990). The indications for neonatal circumcisions are few (Gordon and Collin, 1993; Wiswell *et al.*, 1993). In neonates with prenatally detected hydronephrosis, especially when reflux is identified, circumcision may be recommended because it decreases the likelihood of an early urinary tract infection (UTI) (Barnhouse *et al.*, 1992; Spach *et al.*, 1992; Herndon *et al.*, 1999). Indications in older children include persistent phimosis, paraphimosis, and recurrent balanitis. Paraphimosis is best treated by pressure on the edematous preputial skin and reduction of the paraphimotic skin. If the glans cannot be replaced a dorsal slit incision in the phimotic skin allows reduction. Circumcision in infants with known bleeding disorders, hypospadias, and congenital anomalies of the penis, buried penis, or prematurity should be delayed to a later date (Alter *et al.*, 1994).

Complications of circumcisions occur in 0.2–10%:

1 Early acute complications:
- bleeding
- infection
- amputation, usually partial
- urinary retention
- skin loss
- necrosis, sometimes due to overuse of cautery.
2 Non-acute complications:
- skin excess
- skin asymmetry
- skin bridges
- skin chordee
- epidermal inclusion cysts
- concealed (buried) penis
- phimosis
- meatal stenosis
- urethrocutaneous fistula
- circumcision despite hypospadias, removing skin needed for repair
- plastibell specific
- lymphedema.

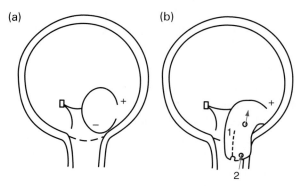

(a)   (b)

Figure 7.14 Technique for incision of ureteroceles: (*a*) incision for an intravesical ureterocele; (*b*) techniques for an ectopic ureterocele: (1) incising proximally, (2) puncturing urethal and intravesical segments separately. (From Blyth *et al.*, 1993, with permission.)

The majority are minor (Willams and Kapila, 1993; Eason *et al.*, 1994; Smith *et al.*, 1994; Persad *et al.*, 1995; Bliss *et al.*, 1996; Neulander *et al.*, 1996; Stirimling, 1996; Ozdemir, 1997). The incidence of complications is probably higher than reported in the urologic literature since many are treated without referral and some do not present until the patient is much older. Complications are best prevented by strict attention to the details of the procedure, which include sterile technique, hemostasis, protection of the glans, and removing the appropriate amount of inner and outer preputial skin (Kaplan, 1983; Niku *et al.*, 1995; Davenport, 1996). When complications occur, immediate attention and treatment is the best management (Gearhart and Rock, 1989; Gluckman *et al.*, 1995; Sherman *et al.*, 1996; Baskin *et al.*, 1997; Ozkan and Gurpinar, 1997). Bleeding is best managed by pressure, placing an absorbable stitch, or with electrocautery. Most of the cases that require immediate repair involve amputation of a portion of the glans (Fig. 7.15). Commonly, these result from a circumcision done using a Mogen clamp placed at an angle incorporating the frenulum which draws up the glans into the clamp (Sherman *et al.*, 1996). When amputation occurs the amputated portion of the glans should be wrapped sterilely and kept cool on ice, but not submerged in saline. In most instances it can be reattached (Sotolongo *et al.*, 1985; Gluckman *et al.*, 1995; Sherman *et al.*, 1996; Ozkan and Gurpinar, 1997). Most urethral injuries should have a staged reconstruction, although fistulae can be closed immediately if recognized (Baskin *et al.*, 1997). Sometimes an apparently normal penis with a complete circumferential prepuce is found to have a hypospadiac meatus when the skin is incised or retracted. This rare form of hypospadias is called megameatus with intact prepuce. The circumcision should be discontinued and any remaining skin left attached for possible later use in hypospadias repair. Plastibell circumcisions have there own specific complications, including a higher incidence of delayed wound infections and retained plastic cuff. Concealed or buried penis can result when the glans penis recedes below the circumcision scar and the scar then contracts (Kon, 1983).

Recently, much emphasis has been placed on using local anesthesia. The best method of providing a penile block is with a ring block using lidocaine (Stang *et al.*, 1988; Snellman and Stand, 1995; Hardwik-Smith *et al.*, 1998; Horger *et al.*, 1998; Howard *et al.*, 1998). Single injection on the dorsum is the next best approach. EMLA® cream requires a prolonged exposure to provide deep superficial analgesia (Benini *et al.*, 1993) and often results in moderate preputial edema, so it is not the method of choice (Lander *et al.*, 1997).

Abdominal masses in the infant

The neonate presenting with an abdominal mass is of particular importance to the pediatric urologist because the majority of such lesions arises in the retroperitoneum in general and the kidney specifically (Caty and Shamberger, 1993; Xue *et al.*, 1995). Traditionally, they presented with a palpable mass. Although some still present this way, masses are far more likely to be detected by prenatal sonography. At the time of presentation to the urologist most have already been categorized as solid, cystic, or hydronephrotic. The urologist must be familiar with the masses that originate from the genitourinary tract as well as the following broad spectrum of other potential etiologies:

1 Hydronephrotic and cystic lesions:
 ■ hydronephrosis
 ■ multicystic dysplastic kidney
 ■ cystic nephroma
 ■ autosomal recessive polycystic kidney disease
 ■ autosomal dominant polycystic kidney disease.
2 Midline cystic lesions:
 ■ hydrometrocolpos
 ■ ovarian cyst
 ■ distended bladder
 ■ urinary ascites

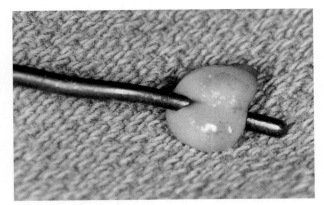

Figure 7.15 Amputation of the distal portion of the glans shown with urethra intubated. This was successfully reattached.

3 Solid lesions:
- neuroblastoma
- congenital mesoblastic nephroma
- Wilms' tumor
- renal vein thrombosis
- renal artery thrombosis
- adrenal hemorrhage.

4 Non-genitourinary lesions:
- pulmonary sequestration
- hepatic lesions
- gastrointestinal lesions
- germ cell tumors
- sarcoma
- sacrococcygeal teratoma.

Figure 7.16 provides a flow diagram that outlines the general framework used to evaluate the lesions identified antenatally. The evaluation of an infant with a mass often becomes a continuum of the evaluation that began prenatally. It is important to note that neonates with masses represent a diagnostic emergency for both parent and referring physician, but rarely do they require emergency surgery and prenatal intervention is almost never indicated.

Hydronephrotic lesions

Ureteropelvic junction (UPJ) obstruction and pyelo-calycetasis causing hydronephrosis remain the most common causes of an abdominal mass in the neonate (Griscom *et al.*, 1977) Currently, this diagnosis is almost always made by prenatal ultrasound (Dhillon, 1998). Barring the development of oligodramnios or anhydramnios, most fetuses are observed until term

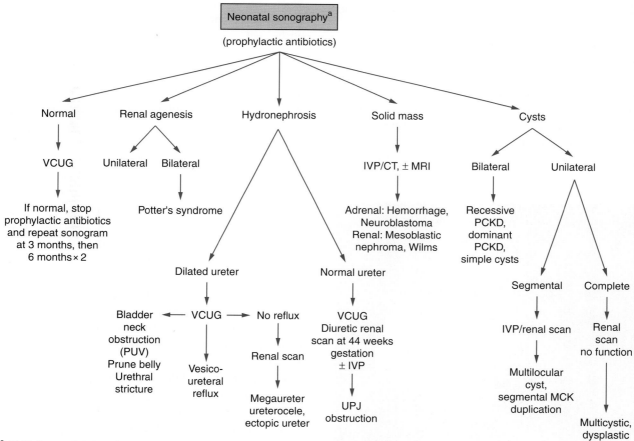

[a] (1) Unilateral hydronephrotic and cystic lesions can be evaluated as an outpatient.
(2) Bilateral lesions should be evaluated prior to discharge.
(3) Masses should be evaluated prior to discharge.

Figure 7.16 Postnatal flow diagram. (VCUG = voiding cystourethrography; IVP = intravenous pyelogram; CT = computed tomography; MRI = magnetic resonance imaging; PCKD = polycystic kidney disease; PUV = posterior urethal valves; UPJ = ureteropelvic obstruction.)

delivery. The UPJ obstruction is usually unilateral but can be bilateral in up to 20–40% of cases. (Murphy *et al.*, 1984). The incidence of bilaterality is higher than seen in older children.

At birth, prophylactic antibiotics are begun and postnatal sonography is performed. If hydronephrosis is detected and no ureter is visualized the presumed diagnosis of UPJ is pursued. Confirmation of the diagnosis of UPJ and differentiation from other potential diagnoses is also done radiographically. A VCUG will exclude the possibility of ipsilateral or contralateral reflux. This test should be performed before any intervention is considered. To establish the diagnosis, a well-tempered renogram is performed. When performing Lasix renograms it is important to optimize the study by following an accepted protocol and ensuring that the infant is well hydrated (Conway and Maizels, 1992; O'Reilly *et al.*, 1996). Prophylactic antibiotics are discontinued when reflux and obstruction are excluded.

In cases where it is believed that the obstructed kidney may have minimal function, proceeding with further evaluation and treatment earlier is often indicated because the neonatal kidney has significant ability to recoup function. A biopsy at the time of surgical correction has the best predictive value with regard to future renal function (Fig. 7.17). If no function is present on the renal scan the diagnosis of multicystic

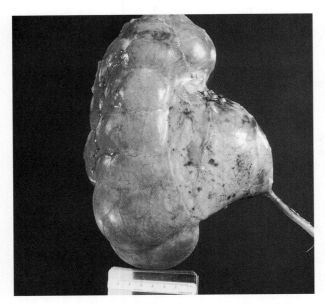

Figure 7.17 End-stage-ureteropelvic junction obstruction showing how the dilated calyces can mimic cystic structures.

dysplastic kidney (MCDK) becomes much more likely.

Treatment of the UPJ is dependent on the degree of obstruction and whether the lesion is unilateral or bilateral (Palmer *et al.*, 1998). Clearly, children with significant bilateral obstruction require early intervention. Since surgical repair of UPJ in infants does not have a higher complication rate than in larger children, age does not affect the decision to intervene surgically (King *et al.*, 1984).

Cystic lesions

Increasingly, cystic mass lesions in the neonatal period are detected antenatally by sonography. In evaluating these lesions it is useful to divide them into unilateral and bilateral categories. This allows a natural division of diagnostic possibilities (McVicar, 1991). Most lesions are detected antenatally but do not require intervention or further evaluation until after birth.

Unilateral lesions

MCDK is the second most common cause of an abdominal mass in infants (Pathak and Williams, 1964). Usually the mass is unilateral and may be palpable as a multilobular 'cluster of grapes' that readily transilluminates. These lesions may be quite large and can impede normal feeding because of compression of the stomach; alternatively, they may impinge on the diaphragm and affect respiration. Importantly, this lesion has a high incidence of associated contralateral renal abnormalities that should be aggressively sought. Contralateral lesions are seen in upwards of 25% of these children (Glassberg, 1987; Al-Khaldi *et al.*, 1994). The two most common kidney lesions are UPJ obstruction and MCDK. There is also a high incidence of contralateral VUR. For this reason patients with suspected MCDK should have a VCUG.

Diagnosis of MCDK is usually made postnatally with a songram, which shows a multiloculated mass with little parenchyma (Fig. 7.18). The cysts are generally non-connected. When the cysts appear to be connected the diagnosis of severe UPJ obstruction should be entertained. The diagnosis is confirmed with a dimercaptosuccinic acid (DMSA) scan that demonstrates no function of the affected side. Contralateral imaging with sonography to rule out obstruction or bilateral MCDK is mandatory. Ureteral atresia is asso-

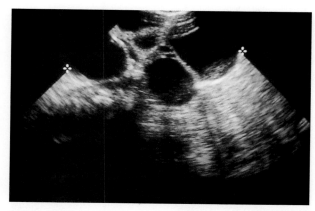

Figure 7.18 Sonogram of multicystic dysplastic kidney. (From Anthony Balcom, Milwaukee, WI, with permission.)

ciated with a higher incidence of contralateral abnormalities then is renal pelvic atresia (de Klerk *et al.*, 1977).

Treatment previously consisted of nephrectomy; however, with the advent of advanced sonographic imaging the lesion is usually followed. Multicystic kidneys typically regress (Kessler *et al.*, 1998; Perez *et al.*, 1998). Rare reports of malignancy have led some to suggest that these lesions should be removed if they persist, and only lesions that involute be managed non-operatively (Birken *et al.*, 1985; Dimmick *et al.*, 1989). In addition, lesions that compromise respiration or feeding, and the rare MCDK associated with hypertension, should also be excised (Susskind *et al.*, 1989).

Bilateral lesions

Autosomal recessive polycystic kidney disease (ARPKD) is a rare congenital renal disorder with an overall incidence of approximately 1: in 40 000 and presents with varying degrees of severity (Zerres *et al.*, 1998). Children are born with massively enlarged kidneys that are typically seen on antenatal or postnatal sonograms as homogeneously hyperechogenic. In severe cases oligohydramnios and Potter's facies may be present. The sonographic pattern is sufficiently different from that of MCDK and autosomal dominant polycystic kidney disease (ADPKD) to distinguish reliably between these. Associated conditions include pulmonary hypoplasia and hepatic fibrosis, which both contribute significantly to morbidity. Prognosis for these children is dependent

on the spectrum of their disease, but is generally poor, with those surviving the neonatal period requiring hemodyalisis and transplantation (Cole *et al.*, 1987).

ADPKD has an incidence of 1 in 500 to 1 in 1000 births, and two gene sequences on chromosomes 4 and 16 have been associated with this disorder (Reeders and Germino, 1989; Peters *et al.*, 1993). While formally called 'adult' polycystic kidney disease, this name is inaccurate as the condition has been identified in children. Children with this disease are typically diagnosed by prenatal sonogram. Sonography is also the primary modality used to screen potentially affected siblings (Papadopoulou *et al.*, 1999). Infants born with this disorder often have massive renomegaly and severely affected infants have poor survival. Children who do not present in the initial neonatal period often come to attention later in life with hypertension, impaired renal function, proteinuria, or hematuria. Associated conditions include hepatic and pancreatic cysts as well as cerebral aneurysms. Although the outlook for these patients is improving a significant number eventually develop renal failure (Glassberg, 1999).

Other midline cystic abdominal lesions

As with UPJ and MCDK, modern ultrasonography has greatly facilitated the diagnosis of other less common cystic abdominal masses in infants. Previously, children would often undergo laparotomy to establish such a diagnosis.

Hydrocolpos refers to the distension of the vagina generally with mucus derived from the cervix. It results from vaginal obstruction secondary to imperforate hymen or other obstructive vaginal anomalies. Maternal estrogens stimulate these secretions (Hahn-Pedersen *et al.*, 1984). It most commonly presents as a midline abdominal mass and/or a protruding mass in the perineum, which is the bulging imperforate hymen. However, the diagnosis has also been made antenatally sonographically (Hill and Hirsch, 1985; Banerjee *et al.*, 1992). Careful physical examination will show that the mass is anterior to the rectum. Sonography will indicate that the lesion is behind the bladder. A common finding in these patients is lower urinary tract obstruction and hydronephrosis (Turner and Leonard, 1997). Once the diagnosis is made, incision of the hymen and drainage result in resolution of the mass. Hydronephrosis then usually resolves with time. Care must be taken because simple percutaneous drainage may result in reaccumulation of secretions within the vagina. Serial ultrasonography should be performed to ensure that the hydronephrosis resolves.

Ovarian cysts are another cause of an abdominal mass in an infant. This diagnosis has been made prenatally by ultrasound as well as postnatally (Armentano *et al.*, 1998). Adnexal torsion in females followed by cystic degeneration of the ovary may occur. This situation is typically managed by excision of the cystic mass (Fig. 7.19). This can be accomplished by open surgery or may be achieved laparoscopically, even in infants (Decker *et al.*, 1999) (Fig. 7.20).

Sacrococcygeal teratoma represents the most common fetal neoplasm, with an estimated incidence of 1 in 40 000 births (Flake, 1993). The majority occurs in females. Intrapelvic lesions may be difficult to diagnose. The presumptive *in utero* diagnosis has been made by ultrasound. When this lesion is suspected in the postnatal period it is best evaluated by computed tomography (CT) or magnetic resonance imaging (MRI) (Chisholm *et al.*, 1999). The tumor may cause obstruction of the urinary tract with resultant hydronephrosis. Treatment typically consists of surgical excision.

Neonatal urinary ascites previously presented as an enlarged abdomen in newborns; however, today the diagnosis is frequently made *in utero* by antenatal sonography (Blessed *et al.*, 1993; Adams *et al.*, 1998). Ascites in the fetus or newborn can be from

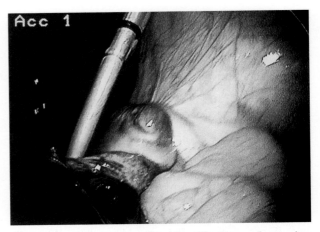

Figure 7.20 Laparoscopic identification of ovarian torsion.

urologic and non-urologic causes. Among urologic causes, lower urinary tract obstruction and trauma are the most common. Specifically, PUV, urethral stenosis, distal ureteral stenosis, and obstructing ureteroceles have all been associated with neonatal urinary ascites (Mann *et al.*, 1974; Forrest *et al.*, 1980; Kay *et al.*, 1980; Cass *et al.*, 1981; Greenfield *et al.*, 1982) (Fig. 7.21). Less frequently, obstructed and hydronephrotic kidneys may also be the cause. Some believe that this serves as a protective mechanism allowing the kidney to decompress, minimizing damage from obstruction (Parker, 1974; Wasnick, 1987; Reha and Gibbons, 1989). In these cases extravasation of urine occurs either from the bladder or, more commonly, from a forniceal rupture in the kidney (Sahdev *et al.*, 1997). Ascites from unilateral obstructive lesions have been reported, although far less commonly than in cases of bilateral obstruction (Chun and Ferguson, 1997). Alternatively, perinatal trauma to the urinary tract may also cause neonatal ascites (Smith, 1998). In particular, umbilical artery catheterization with inadvertent bladder perforation is an important cause of neonatal urinary ascites (Mata *et al.*, 1987; Diamond and Ford, 1989).

Sonography and VCUG can usually determine the urologic abnormality and site of extravasation in those with neonatal urinary ascites. Historically, plain film X-ray findings of a ground-glass appearance of the abdomen with floating loops of bowel have been described in patients with ascites. Neonatal urinoma, which may or may not be associated with ascites, can

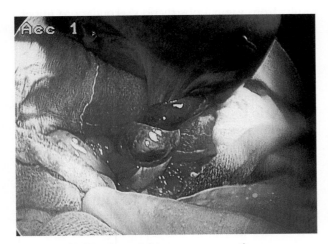

Figure 7.19 Torsion of the ovary presenting as a complex cyst.

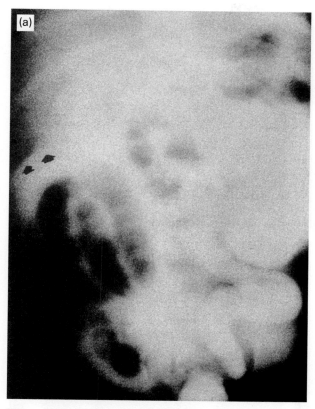

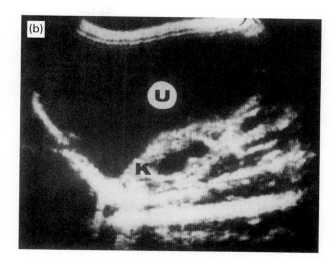

Figure 7.21 (*a*) Voiding cystourethrogram of urinary ascites: the black arrows point to the liver edge; (*b*) ultrasound study showing a retroperitoneal urinoma. K, kidney; U, urine collection. (From Rittenberg *et al.*, 1988, with permission.)

be identified by a 'c' sign, a rim of opacified contrast around the kidney on intravenous pyelography (IVP) (Barry *et al.*, 1974). Clinically, these patients can be quite ill. The primary metabolic abnormality is hyponatremia (Clarke *et al.*, 1993). Other abnormalities, such as an increase in the blood urea nitrogen/creatinine ratio, because of peritoneal absorption of urea, are seen less frequently than hyponatremia but may also be present. Treatment is individualized, but urinary drainage with a urethral catheter allowing the intraperitoneal urine to be reabsorbed, along with urinary antibiotic prophylaxis, is often sufficient. Open drainage may be required in instances where infection of the urine occurs or when respiratory embarrassment is due to the mass effect. The outlook for these patients has improved substantially. Previous reports of 70% mortality have improved to less than 15% in more recent series (Scott, 1976; Tank *et al.*, 1980; Greenfield *et al.*, 1982). Non-urologic causes of neonatal ascites include

erythroblastosis fetalis, cardiac or hepatic abnormalities, sepsis, and gastrointestinal perforation (Griscom *et al.*, 1977).

Solid lesions

As with cystic lesions, solid lesions in children are being detected prenatally with increasing frequency. One of the best examples is neuroblastoma (Fowlie *et al.*, 1986; Giulian *et al.*, 1986). While early detection of neuroblastoma does not necessarily change initial management, it results in the child receiving treatment sooner. In addition, patients with neuroblastomas detected early in life have a better outlook. Thus, early diagnosis probably improves the prognosis (Fowlie *et al.*, 1986). As a rule, solid lesions detected antenatally are followed before delivery, and then after birth are imaged by CT scan or MRI. Ocassionally, a postcontrast CT kidney, ureter, and bladder (KUB) scan may clarify the diagnosis. No indications for antenatal intervention exist for solid lesions.

Neuroblastoma remains the most common solid malignant tumor in neonates and is characterized by its variability in presentation (Lukens, 1999). It is often identified prenatally (Liyanage and Katoch, 1992; Jennings *et al.*, 1993; Ho *et al.*, 1993; Toma *et al.*, 1994). Many factors, including age at detection and location, affect overall outcome. Early diagnosis and treatment may be critical in some cases (Haase *et al.*, 1999). However, information derived from countries with mandatory postnatal screening for neuroblastoma suggest that many tumors detected in the perinatal period regress. Therefore, some infants diagnosed very early may have unnecessary interventions (McWilliams, 1987; Woods and Tuchman, 1997; Erttman *et al.*, 1998).

On physical examination, neuroblastoma has classically been described as a firm, fixed lesion that may cross the midline. Children may also present with bulky metastatic disease that includes a palpable liver and subcutaneous nodules that characterize stage IV-S disease. This form usually undergoes spontaneous regression. (van Noessel *et al.*, 1997). Imaging by ultrasound can usually suggest the diagnosis. Confirmation is made by CT scan or MRI. These studies show a lesion that displaces the kidney but does not arise from the kidney (Fig. 7.22). The appearance of a tumor arising from the kidney will cause a beaking effect of the renal tissue (Fig. 7.23). Despite modern imaging techniques the diagnosis of neuroblastoma may be confused with other less common conditions, such as pulmonary sequestration (Matzinger *et al.*, 1992). Cystic neuroblastomas detected prenatally have also been reported, so the diagnosis should not be excluded on the basis of a cystic component (Eklof *et al.*, 1986; Croitoru *et al.*, 1992; Richard *et al.*, 1995; Acharya *et al.*, 1997; Hamada *et al.*, 1999). Most patients present with elevations of urinary catecholamines, which should be checked in all such patients.

Treatment generally consists of surgery for those patients with early-stage localized disease. Multimodal therapy, including chemotherapy and radiotherapy, is indicated in patients with advanced disease. Outcome is variable but patients with advanced disease tend to do poorly despite aggressive treatment (Hosoda *et al.*, 1992; Haase *et al.*, 1999).

Congenital mesoblastic nephroma is a rare renal tumor that is the most common solid renal mass in children less than 6 months of age (50%). Eighty per

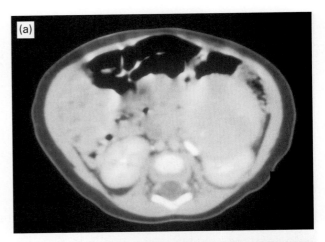

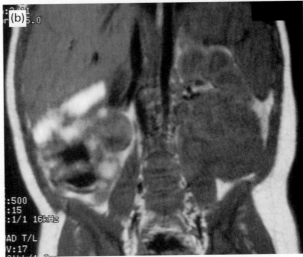

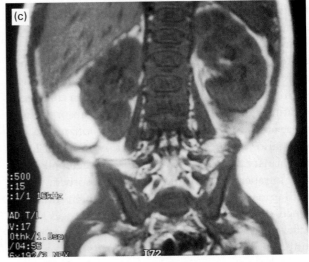

Figure 7.22 (*a*) CT scan showing displacement of the kidney by neuroblastoma (note no beaking of the renal tissue); (*b*) MRI showing neuroblastoma in relation to the kidney; (*c*) MRI showing normal renal contour confirming that the tumor is separate from the kidney.

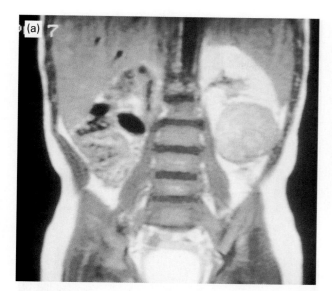

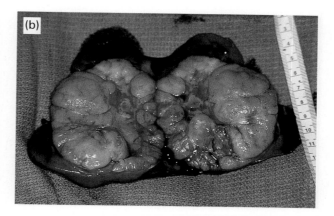

Figure 7.23 (a) Wilms' tumor showing beaking of the renal tissue, confirming its intrarenal location; (b) bivalved tumor showing the beaking effect of the normal renal tissue around the mass.

cent of these lesions are discovered in the first month of life (Campagnola *et al.*, 1998). Congenital mesoblastic nephroma has been detected prenatally, where it is most commonly associated with polyhydramnios and subsequent prematurity (Haddad *et al.*, 1996). Typically, the lesion is noted as a solid intrarenal mass on sonogram that appears fibroid when removed (Chan *et al.*, 1987) (Fig. 7.24). A cystic form can also occur (Campagnola *et al.*, 1998) (Fig. 7.25). *In utero* treatment usually consists of observation and management of polyhydramnios with its attendant complications. While this lesion almost never metastasizes, it can be locally invasive. Therefore, elective nephrectomy is recommended (Heidelberger *et al.*, 1993). Cases requiring urgent surgery following

tumor rupture and hemorrhage have been reported. (Arensman and Belman, 1980; Matsumura *et al.*, 1993).

Wilms' tumor, which is more common in older children, is seldom the cause of a renal mass in the newborn (Brove, 1999). Even less common is confirmation of prenatal detection of a Wilms' tumor, as these masses are usually found to be mesoblastic nephromas on postnatal examination (Beckwith, 1999). Current evidence clearly supports genetic mutation on chromosome 11p13 in the etiology of Wilms' tumor. Bilateral nephroblastomatosis, aniridia, and 11p13 deletion result in the development of Wilms' tumor in close to 100% of affected individuals (Fig. 7.26). These patients may develop bilateral Wilms' tumor, requiring

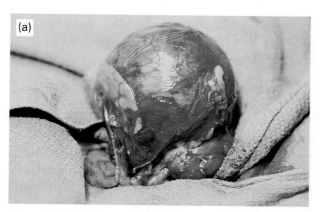

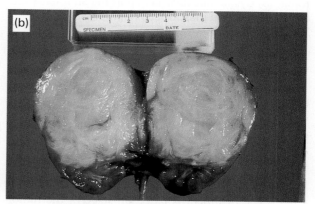

Figure 7.24 Solid mesoblastic nephroma in a 3-day-old patient: (a) surgical picture; (b) bivalved lesion showing a typical fibroid appearance.

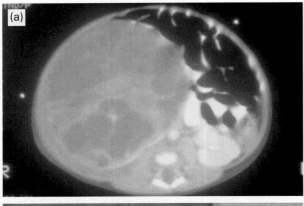

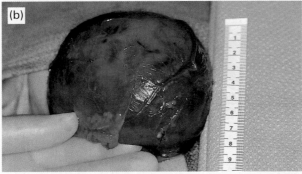

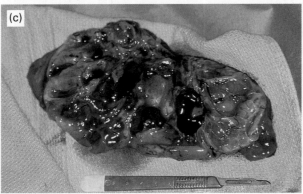

Figure 7.25 (*a*) CT scan of cystic mesoblastic nephroma; (*b*) Cystic mesoblastis nephroma after excision; (*c*) Bivalved cystic mesoblastic nephroma.

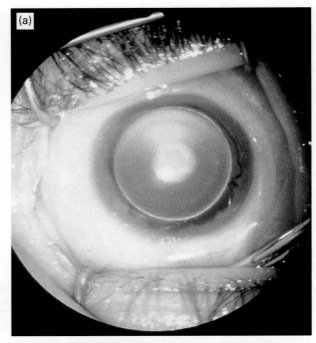

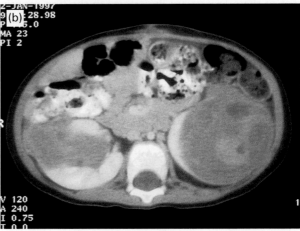

Figure 7.26 (*a*) Aniridia with red reflex; (*b*) bilateral Wilms' tumor in a patient with aniridia.

nephron-sparing surgical techniques. Evaluation of the vascular anatomy is best performed with MR angiography (Ferrer *et al.*, 1994) (Fig. 7.27). Multiple congenital disorders associated with this disease include WAGR syndrome, hemihypertrophy, Beckwith–Wiedemann syndrome, and neurofibromatosis (Bove, 1999). The treatment is based on stage of the tumor and involves surgery, chemotherapy, and sometimes radiation therapy.

Renal vein thrombosis (RVT) may be the cause of a mass in a neonate. The characteristic clinical presentation has been one of an enlarged kidney, hematuria and proteinuria in an ill infant (Fig. 7.28). Proteinuria is less prominent than in cases seen in adults. Low platelet counts due to consumption by the developing thrombus help to confirm the diagnosis. Infants appear to be predisposed to this condition because of lower renal arterial and venous flow rates. Recently, reports of prenatal diagnoses of RVT have

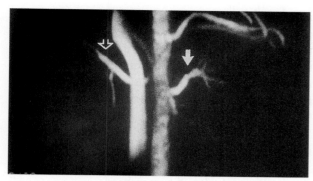

Figure 7.27 Phase-contrast magnetic resonance angiography. The open arrow indicates the superiorly displaced right renal artery from a Wilms' tumor. The solid arrow indicates the single left renal artery. (From Ferrer *et al.*, 1994, with permission.)

genic, with loss of corticomedullary differentiation (Hibbert *et al.*, 1997). Treatment of unilateral RVT is supportive, with hydration and correction of any predisposing abnormalities (Belman and King, 1972a). Bilateral thrombosis requires more aggressive treatment and has a worse prognosis, but thrombus removal has not proven helpful. These patients warrant treatment with either heparin or systemic thrombolytic therapy in order to minimize morbidity (Duncan *et al.*, 1991; Nuss *et al.*, 1994). Patients with unilateral thrombosis usually do well, while those with bilateral thrombosis have a higher rate of complications such as renal failure (Keidan *et al.*, 1994). All patients must have long-term monitoring of renal function and evaluation for hypertension (Jobin *et al.*, 1982; Laplante *et al.*, 1993).

Renal artery thrombosis does not commonly present as a neonatal mass (Durante *et al.*, 1976). The occurrence of this disorder has increased significantly in relation to the increased use of umbilical artery catheters, despite the fact that a causal relationship was made some time ago (Bauer *et al.*, 1975). The diagnosis is commonly made with Doppler ultrasound, which demonstrates the absence of flow in the renal artery. Treatment varies from supportive to surgical depending on the extent of thrombosis and whether or not aortic involvement exists (Kavaler, 1997; Greenberg *et al.*, 1998).

appeared (Cozzolino and Cendron, 1997). RVT is most commonly associated with risk factors that include dehydration, sepsis, birth asphyxia, maternal diabetes, polycythemia, and an umbilical catheter. The thrombosis starts in the venules within the kidney and progressively extends to the major renal vein or veins. The diagnosis is most commonly made by ultrasound (Fig. 7.29). Initially, the lesion appears as highly echogenic streaks within the kidney. Subsequently, the kidney becomes enlarged and echo-

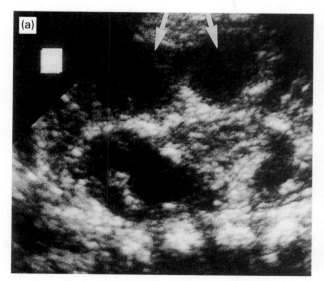

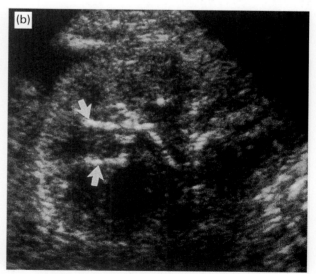

Figure 7.28 Renal vein thrombosis; (*a*) enlarged left kidney with echogenic intermedullary streaks and echopoor medullary pyramids (*arrows*); (*b*) same patient's right kidney showing swelling of the upper pole and focal echogenic intermedullary streaks. (From Hibbert, 1997, with permission.)

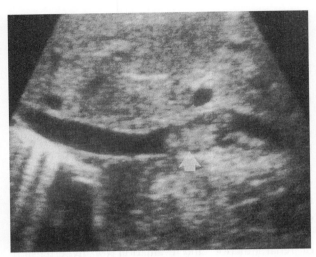

Figure 7.29 Renal vein thrombosis. Ultrasound through the IVC showing thrombus within the IVC at the level of the renal vein. (From Hibbert, 1997, with permission.)

Neonatal adrenal hemorrhage is associated with traumatic or difficult labor, neonatal hypoxia, septicemia, or coagulopathy. Traditionally, it is believed that the relatively large size and vascularity of the newborn gland predisposes it to bleeding. A recent study using ultrasound to screen newborns for adrenal hemorrhage in 8374 pregnancies reported an incidence of 1.9 per 1000 births (Felc, 1995). In this report, 13 cases were on the right, two on the left and one was bilateral. These findings corroborate previous reports

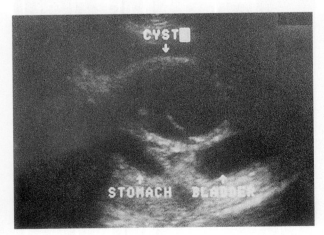

Figure 7.30 Prenatal adrenal hemorrhage identified as a complex cyst on sonogram. (From Burbige, 1993, with permission.)

indicating a right-sided predominance and 10% bilaterality. Diagnosis is made by ultrasound, and antenatal diagnosis has been made in the second and third trimesters (Fig. 7.30). Identification by ultrasound is usually reliable, but in some cases it is difficult to differentiate from an adrenal neuroblastoma (Burbige, 1993; Chen *et al.*, 1998; Fang *et al.*, 1999) (Fig. 7.31). In difficult cases CT and MRI may be helpful in the diagnosis (Willemse *et al.*, 1989; Hoeffel *et al.*, 1995). Negative urine catecholamines also support the diagnosis of adrenal hemorrhage.

Experience has confirmed the initial belief that the majority with adrenal hemorrhage require no treatment except for occasional phototherapy and, rarely, transfusion (Khuri *et al.*, 1980; Sherer *et al.*, 1994). Even less common are instances of adrenal insufficiency related to adrenal hemorrhage. Observation for resolution and monitoring of hematocrit and bilirubin should be routine. Occasionally, steroid replacement for adrenal insufficiency is required.

Cystic nephroma is a rare benign renal neoplasm. Lesions may be unilateral or bilateral, and bilateral metachronous lesions have been reported (Ferrer and McKenna, 1994). Partial nephrectomy is appropriate when possible to preserve renal parenchyma (Fig. 7.32).

Rhabdomyosarcoma is an uncommon neoplasm of the lower urinary tract in children. Lesions may occur in the bladder, prostate, vagina, or uterus (Fig. 7.33). Presentation in infancy depends on the organ of origin and may include hematuria, vaginal bleeding, or obstruction of the urinary tract. Treatment is multimodal, including chemotherapy, radiation therapy, and exenteration followed by reconstructive surgery (Duel *et al.*, 1996; Merguerian *et al.*, 1998). As a result of collaborative efforts by the Intergroup Rhabdomyosarcoma Study, treatment results for these patients are improving. Current efforts are focused on bladder preservation (Hays *et al.*, 1995). Dysfunctional bladders may result, however, from high does of chemotherapy and radiation.

Germ cell tumors are rare in children and their presentation as a lower abdominal mass is extremely uncommon. They may occur as an ovarian mass (Laza and Stolar, 1998) or as a mass in an undescended testis (Mukai *et al.*, 1998). Treatment for these tumors is dependent on stage at diagnosis but is usually multimodal including surgery and platinum-based chemotherapy, depending on histology.

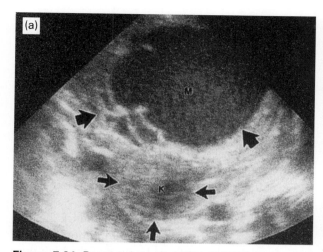
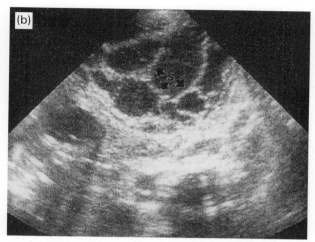

Figure 7.31 Postnatal confirmation of a complex cystic lesion superior to the kidney. Surgical exploration later confirms adrenal hemorrhage. (From Burbige, 1993, with permission.)

Enterocystoplasty and the acute abdomen

Bladder augmentation with bowel segments is commonly performed in children with neuropathic bladders, bladder tumors, and exstrophy. Most of these patients require clean intermittent catheterization after bladder augmentation and have poor bladder sensation. A combination of poor sensation and over distension can lead to a spontaneous augmentation rupture, an acute abdomen, and life-threat-

ening sepsis. The presentation can be confusing because most patients have altered abdominal sensation, so identifying the source of sepsis can be difficult. A cystogram may not reveal extravasation and the best screening study is a sonogram that shows floating loops of bowel. Early surgical exploration is indicated. The rupture is usually located at the posterior suture line between the bladder and augmented bowel. Whenever a patient with a bladder augmentation presents with sepsis this diagnosis should be considered.

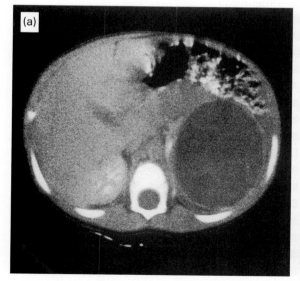
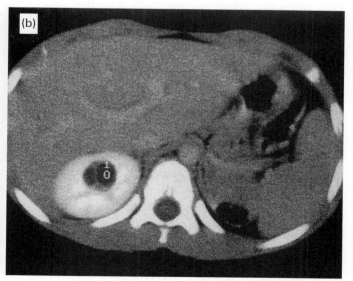

Figure 7.32 Multilocular cyst of the kidney (cystic nephroma). (a) CT scan of cystic nephroma in the left kidney with a normal right kidney; (b) CT scan of the same patient 2 years later with a solitary right kidney and metachronous cystic nephroma. (From Ferrer and McKenna, 1994, with permission.)

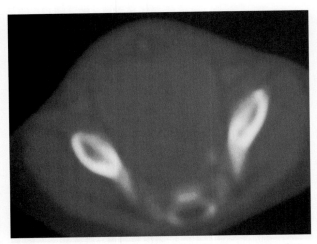

Figure 7.33 Pelvic sarcoma with displacement of the bladder superiorly. Note Foley balloon in the bladder.

Intraoperative consultations

The best approach to intraoperative consultations is to take the time to obtain a complete history. This usually is chart based but may include talking to the parents prior to making a quick decision about a complex question. This is also the case when one is asked about a surgical finding or called to address a surgical complication. After the chart review and appropriate history, it is best to scrub into the case and review the exact location of the lesion from the skin to the region of question. One must take a fresh look at the situation and not rely totally on the primary physician. When any questions arise that deal with surgical excision of a mass, multiple radiologic modalities can be used intraoperatively, and frozen section sampling is available. There is little to be lost in closing the patient who needs further evaluation which cannot be undetaken in the operating room, and reoperating when the problem is better understood.

Many unusual structures may be found during a pediatric hernia repair. Among these is the finding of reproductive organs appropriate to the opposite sex. Although rare, this will usually generate an intraoperative consultation. In males, the finding of female organs, such as a fallopian tube or uterus, is termed persistent müllerian duct syndrome (Sloan and Walsh, 1976) or hernia uterine inguinale. The cause of this anomaly is a failure of Sertoli cell production of Müllerian inhibiting substance (MIS), leading to feminization of pelvic structures. The testis should be undescended, but otherwise the patient is phenotypi-cally male. Intraoperative biopsy confirms the presence of a normal testis. Excision of the female structures should be performed with care, avoiding injury to the adjacent functioning wolffian duct structures. Excision is important because of the risk of future malignancy arising in these tissues (Allen, 1976). Others have recommended that they be left in place to avoid potential injury (Rajfer and Walsh, 1978). In phenotypic females, the finding of male reproductive structures during hernia repair suggests testicular feminization. Here, the timing of excision of the male gonads is controversial: if removed early, exogenous estrogens must be administered to induce normal maturation at puberty; if left *in situ* until puberty the testis must then be removed because of the high possibility of developing gonadoblastoma (Verp and Simpson, 1987). Laparoscopic removal of the testis allows for a minimally invasive approach yet permits direct molecular analysis of the specimen (Kanayama *et al.*, 1999). Over 40 other tissues have been identified in and around the hernia sac. They include normal structures drawn into the sac, organ duplications as 'rests', inflammatory lesions, tumors, and drainage from the abdomen into a patent processus vaginalis (Bloom *et al.*, 1992):

1 Organs drawn into the hernia sac:
   - appendix
   - bladder
   - gonad
   - Meckle's diverticulum
   - omentum
   - bowel
   - pelvic kidney
   - ureter
   - uterus.
2 Aberrant rests:
   - adrenal
   - ectopic renal tissue
   - accessory spleen.
3 Inflammatory lesions:
   - abscess
   - funniculitis
   - granulomas
   - sarcoidosis
   - meconium granuloma
   - parasitic disease
   - peritonitis
   - polyarteritis nodosa
   - vasitis nodosa
   - xanthrogranuloma.

4 Tumors and benign lesions:
- adrenal tumor
- dermoid cyst
- epidermoid cyst
- epididymal cysts and nodules
- calculi
- hemangioma
- lymphangioma
- mesenchymoma
- neuroblastoma
- paratesticular cyst/rhabdomyosarcoma
- spermatic cord tumors
- spermatocele
- tunica albuginea cyst
- tunica vaginalis cyst
- venous thrombosis
- Wilms' tumor.

5 Lesions that appear because of patent processus vaginalis:
- adrenal hemorrhage
- endometriosis
- meconium
- blood.

Unusual findings in the spermatic cord of which the urologist should be aware include those listed above, particularly ectopic adrenal tissue and accessory spleens (Mares *et al.*, 1980; Paul *et al.*, 1997). In cases of ectopic adrenal tissue the yellow color and an appearance similar to the normal gland usually help to identify adrenal tissue. Neuroblastoma has also been reported to present as a mass in the spermatic cord (Knoedler *et al.*, 1989). In addition to the more common scrotal masses, heterotopic Wilms' tumor and neuroblastoma have been reported (Kay, 1985). Both adrenal and splenic tissue have also been found in the sctotum and splenogonadal fusion is not uncommon with an undescended left testis. Excision of these masses is usually best, with careful pathologic evaluation to confirm the diagnosis.

Although vasal injuries are most commonly diagnosed later in life during the work-up of infertility, vasal injury during pediatric hernia repair mandates intraoperative pediatric urologic consultation. Previous studies have documented the ease with which vasal trauma may occur secondary to intraoperative manipulation (Schandling and Jank, 1981). In cases of transection immediate microvascular repair is indicated. Crush injuries may result in future obstruction. In these situations the decision regarding treatment must be individualized. In most instances observation is indicated. However, when a severe crush injury has occurred, as when a clamp is applied and closed with obvious injury, excision and primary reanastomosis is indicated.

Intraoperative consultations relating to the bladder are usually a result of trauma or iatrogenic injury during surgery. Intraoperative injury to the bladder is rare but may occur secondary to percutaneous laparoscopic procedures or during inguinal hernia repair. When it happens it is best managed by primary closure, and bladder drainage in the postoperative period via a urethral catheter and or suprapubic tube. Perivesical drainage is also appropriate in the immediate postoperative period. A cystogram to confirm the absence of extravasation should be performed prior to removal of drainage catheters. Rarely, during umbilical hernia repair, a urachal abnormality is discovered. In these cases the urachus should be traced to the dome of the bladder and excised with primary closure of the bladder (Kay, 1985). If the diagnosis is uncertain an intraoperative cystogram may clarify the picture.

Most consultations related to the kidney and ureter are in patients with renal trauma. The basic recommendation is not to explore the flank even when an expanding mass is present until normal function of the contralateral kidney has been assured. When an expanding retroperitoneal mass is explored after trauma, early renal vascular control should be the main objective. Traumatic separation of the ureter and pelvis occasionally occurs in children. Unlike many injuries where drainage and observation is indicated, complete avulsion of the ureter should be surgically repaired as quickly as possible. It is a more complex procedure that a standard UPJ repair because the pelvis is almost always intrarenal and mobilization of the kidney and ureter to prevent tension on the anastomosis can be difficult. The procedure is much more difficult if the correction is delayed because of edema with subsequent scar formation.

As a result of advancements in imaging and thorough preoperative evaluations, consultations because of a previously undiagnosed renal mass, formerly common, are now unusual. Despite this, the urologic surgeon should bear in mind that occasionally an ectopic or a pelvic kidney may be confused with a pelvic mass and indicate intraoperative consultation. Reports of inadvertent nephrectomy in patients with solitary ectopic kidneys are found in the literature

(Kay, 1985). When it is unclear whether the mass in question is a solitary kidney, intraoperative imaging may be necessary to clarity the situation. This is critical as reports indicate that up to 10% of all pelvic kidneys are solitary (Zabbo, 1985). Intraoperatively, it is important to remember that ectopic kidneys may not be reniform in shape and have an anomalous blood supply derived from the aorta and iliac vessels, or the superior mesenteric artery (Zabbo, 1985). Simple needle aspiration to confirm the presence of urine may also be useful in identifying a kidney. Fusion anomalies and horseshoe kidneys may also be a source of confusion and prompt urologic consultation.

Occasionally, the urologist will be called to evaluate an infant for difficulty in placing an urethral catheter. Initially, properly lubricating the urethra by injecting 2% lidocaine jelly facilitates catheter insertion. Most commonly, these will be male neonates who have had multiple attempts at catheterization before urologic consutation. In these cases a good option may be to use a curved-tip 'coude' catheter, which have recently become available in pediatric sizes. When these are not available, or will not pass, a small catheter guide may be placed within a pediatric feeding tube and manipulated into the bladder. If no guides are available bending a heavy wire suture for use as a catheter guide may be successful (Gerber, 1982; Redman, 1994). Lubricating jelly must be placed on the guide to facilitate its removal. In cases where this fails proceeding directly to cystoscopy to evaluate the possibility of a false passage, and the use of a guide wire placed under direct vision followed by catheter placement over the wire ensures proper catheter placement. When the bladder is palpable, a percutaneous cystotomy may be performed under local anesthesia or in the operating room. Alternatively, a large-gauge needle placed into the distended bladder will permit insertion of a guidewire, dilation of the tract, and placement of a suprapubic catheter.

References

Acharya S, Jayabose S, Kogan SJ et al. (1997) Prenatally diagnosed neuroblastoma. Cancer 80: 304–10.

Adams MC, Ludlow J, Brock JW III, Rink RC (1998) Prenatal urinary ascites and persistent cloaca: risk factors for poor drainage of urine or meconium. J Urol 160: 2179–81.

Al-Khaldi N, Watson AR, Zuccollo J et al. (1994) Outcome of antenatally detected cystic dysplastic kidney disease. Arch Dis Child 70: 520–2.

Allen TD (1976) Disorders of sexual differentiation. Urology 7(Suppl 4): 1–32.

Alter GJ, Horton CE Jr, Horton CE Jr (1994) Buried penis as a contraindication for circumcision. J Am Coll Surg 178: 487–9.

Anderson N, Clautice-Engle T, Allan R et al. (1995). Detection of obstructive uropathy in the fetus. Am J Roentgenol 164: 719–23.

Andros GJ, Hatch DA, Walter JS et al. (1998). Home bladder pressure monitoring in children with myelomeningocele. J Urol 160: 518–21.

Anon. (1991) Use of folic acid for prevention of spina bfida and other neural tube defects. Morb Mort Weekly Rep 40: 513–16.

Aragona F, Pescatori E, Talenti E et al. (1996) Painless scrotal masses in the pediatric population: prevalence and age distribution of different pathological conditions – a 10 year retrospective multicenter study. J Urol 155: 1424–26.

Arensman RM, Belman AB (1980) Ruptured congenital mesoblastic nephroma: chemotherapy and irradiation as adjuvants to nephrectomy. Urology XV: 394–6.

Armentano G, Dodero P, Natta A et al. (1998) Fetal ovarian cysts: prenatal diagnosis and management. Report of two cases and review of literature. Clin Exp Obstet Gynecol 25: 88–91.

Atala A, Bauer SB, Dyro FM et al. (1992) Bladder functional changes resulting from lipomeningocele repair. J Urol 148: 592–4.

Avni EF, Schulman CC (1996) The origin of vesico-ureteric reflux in male newborns: further evidence in favour of a transient fetal urethral obstruction. Br J Urol 78: 454–9.

Bahado-Singh R, Schmitt R, Hobbins JC (1992) New technique for genetic amniocentesis in twins. Obstet Gynecol 79: 304–7.

Banerjee AR, Clarke O, MacDonald LM (1992) Sonographic detection of neonatal hydrometrocolpos. Br J Radiol 65: 268–71.

Baptist EC, Amin PV (1996) Perinatal testicular torsion and hard testicle. J Perinatol 16: 67–8.

Barnhouse DH, Chin DL, Lewis DD et al. (1992) Circumcision and urinary tract infection. JAMA 268: 54–5.

Barry JM, Anderson JM, Hodges CV (1974) The subcapsular C sign: a rare radiographic finding associated with neonatal urinary ascites. J Urol 112: 836–9.

Baskin LS, Canning DA, Snyder HM III, Duckett JW Jr (1997) Surgical repair of urethal circumcision injuries. J Urol 158: 2269–71.

Bauer SB (1984) Management of neurogenic bladder dysfunction in children. J Urol 132: 544–5.

Bauer SB (1998) Editorial: the challenge of the expanding role of urodynamic studies in the treatment of children with neurological and functional disabilities. J Urol 160: 527–8.

Bauer SB, Feldman SM, Gellis SS, Retik AB (1975) Neonatal hypertension. A complication of umbilical-artery catheterization. N Engl J Med 293: 1032–3.

Bauer SB, Lais A, Scott RM (1992) Continuous urodynamic surveillance of babies with myelodysplasia: implications for further neurosurgery. *Eur J Pediatr Surg* **1** (Suppl 2): 35–6.

Beckwith JB (1999) Pernatal detection of a Wilms' tumor. *Pediatr Radiol* **29**: 64–5.

Belman AB, King LR (1972a) The pathology and treatment of renal vein thrombosis in the newborn. *J Urol* **107**: 852–5.

Belman AB, King LR (1972b) Urinary tract abnormalities associated with imperforate anus. *J Urol* **108**: 823–4.

Ben-Chaim J, Jeffs RD, Reiner WG, Gearhart JP (1996) The outcome of patients with classic bladder exstrophy in adult life. *J Urol* **155**: 1251–2.

Benini F, Johnston CC, Faucher D, Aranda JV (1993) Topical anesthesia during circumcision in newborn infants. *JAMA* **270**: 850–3.

Birken G, King D, Vane D, Lloyd T (1985) Renal cell carcinoma arising in a multicystic dysplastic kidney. *Pediatr Surg* **20**: 619–21.

Blessed WB, Sepulveda W, Romero R *et al.* (1993) Prenatal diagnosis of spontaneous rupture of the fetal bladder with color Doppler ultrasonography. *Am J Obstet Gynecol* **169**: 1629–31.

Bliss DP Jr, Healey PJ, Waldhausen JHT (1996) Necrotizing fasciitis after plastibell circumcision. *J Pediatr* **131**: 459–62.

Bloom DA, Wan J, Key D (1992) Disorders of the male external genitalia and inguinal canal. *Clin Pediatr Urol* **2**: 1015–49.

Blyth B, Passerini-Glazel G, Camuffo C *et al.* (1993) Endoscopic incision of ureteroceles: intravesical versus ectopic. *J Urol* **149**: 556–60.

Bobrowski RA, Levin RB, Lauria MR *et al.* (1997) *In utero* progression of isolated renal pelvis dilation. *Am J Perinatol* **14**: 423–6.

Borrelli M, Bruschini H, Nahas WC *et al.* (1985). Sacral agenesis: why is it so frequently misdiagnosed? *Urology* **26**: 351–5.

Bove KE (1999) Wilms' tumor and related abnormalities in the fetus and newborn. *Semin Perinatol* **23**: 310–8.

Bradbury ET, Hewison J (1994) Early parental adjustment to visible congenital disfigurement. *Child Care Health Dev* **20**: 251–66.

Brandell RA, Brock JW III (1993) Common problems in pediatric urology. *Comprehens Therapy* **19**: 11–6.

Bruce DA, Schut L (1979) Spinal lipomas in infancy and childhood. *Brain* **5**: 192–203.

Bukowski TP, Perlmutter AD (1994) Reduction cystoplasty in the prune belly syndrome: a long-term followup. *J Urol* **152**: 2113–6.

Burbige KA (1993) Prenatal adrenal hemorrhage confirmed by postnatal surgery. *J Urol* **150**: 1867–9.

Burbige KA, Amodio J, Berdon WE *et al.* (1987) Prune belly syndrome: 35 years of experience. *J Urol* **137**: 86–90.

Cacciari A, Pilu GL, Mordenti M *et al.* (1999) Prenatal diagnosis of bladder exstrophy: what counseling? *J Urol* **161**: 259–61.

Caldamone AA, Valvo JR, Altebarmakian VK, Rabinowitz R (1984) Acute scrotal swelling in children. *J Pediatr Surg* **19**: 581–4.

Calleja R, Archer TJ (1996) Bilateral testicular torsion in a neonate. *Br J Urol* **78**: 793–804.

Campagnola S, Fasoli L, Flessati P *et al.* (1998) Congenital cystic mesoblastic nephroma. *Urol Int* **61**: 254–6.

Cartwright PC, Snow BW, Reid BS, Shultz PK (1995) Color Doppler ultrasound in newborn testis torsion. *Urology* **45**: 667–70.

Cass AS, Khan AU, Smith S, Godec C (1981) Neonatal perirenal urinary extravasation with posterior urethral valves. *Urology* **18**: 258–61.

Caty MG, Shamberger RC (1993) Abdominal tumors in infancy and childhood. *Pediatr Clin North Am* **40**: 1253–71.

Chan HSL, Cheng M, Mancer K *et al.* (1987) Congenital mesoblastic nephroma: a clinicoradiologic study of 17 cases representing the pathologic spectrum of the disease. *J Pediatr* **III**: 64–70.

Chen C, Shih S, Chuang C *et al.* (1998) *In utero* adrenal hemorrhage: clinical and imaging findings. *Acta Obstet Gynecol Scand* **77**: 239–41.

Chevalier RL, Klahr S (1998) Therapeutic approaches in obstructive uropathy. *Semin Nephrol* **18**: 652–8.

Chisholm CA, Heider AL, Kuller JA *et al.* (1999) Prenatal diagnosis and perinatal management of fetal sacrococcygeal teratoma. *Am J Perinatol* **16**: 47–50.

Christensen B, Rosenblatt DS (1995) Effects of folate deficiency on embryonic development. *Baillieres Clin Haematol* **8**: 617–37.

Chun KE, Ferguson RS (1997) Neonatal urinary ascites due to unilateral vesicourerteric junction obstruction. *Pediatr Surg Int* **12**: 455–7.

Churchill BM, McLorie GA, Khoury AE *et al.* (1990) Emergency treatment and long-term followup of posterior urethral valves. *Urol Clin North Am* **17**: 343–60.

Cilento BG, Najjar SS, Atala A (1993) Cryptorchidism and testicular torsion. *Pediatr Clin North Am* **40**: 1133–49.

Clarke HS Jr, Mills ME, Parres JA, Kropp KA (1993) The hyponatremia of neonatal urinary ascites: clinical observations, experimental confirmation and proposed mechanism. *Urology* **150**: 778–81.

Close CE, Carr MC, Burns MW, Mitchell ME (1997) Lower urinary tract changes after early valve ablation in neonates and infants: is early diversion warranted? *J Urol* **157**: 984–8.

Cohen HL, Zinn HL, Patel A *et al.* (1998) Prenatal sonographic diagnosis of posterior urethral valves: identification of valves and thickening of the posterior urethral wall. *J Clin Ultrasound* **26**: 366–70.

Colak A, Pollack IF, Albright AL (1998) Recurrent tethering: a common long-term problem after lipomyelomeningocele repair. *Pediatr Neurosurg* **29**: 184–90.

Colapinto J (1997) The true story of John/Joan. *Rolling Stone*, February, 55–96.

Cole BR, Conley SB, Stapleton FB (1987) Polycystic kidney disease in the first year of life. *Pediatrics* **III**: 693–9.

Conway JJ, Maizels MJ (1992) The 'well tempered' diuretic renogram: a standard method to examine the asymptomatic neonate with hydronephrosis or hydroureteronephrosis. A report from combined meetings of The

Society for Fetal Urology and members of The Pediatric Nuclear Medicine Council–The Society of Nuclear Medicine. *Nucl Med* **33**: 2047–51.

Cooper CS, Snyder OB, Hawtrey CE (1997) Bilateral neonatal testicular torsion. *Clin Pediatr* **36**: 653–6.

Coplen DE (1997) Prenatal intervention of hydronephrosis. *J Urol* **157**: 2270–7.

Coplen DE (1998) Editorial: neonatal ureterocele incision. *J Urol* **159**: 1010.

Coplen DE, Hare JY, Zderic SA *et al.* (1996) 10-year experience with prenatal intervention for hydronephrosis. *J Urol* **156**: 1142–5.

Cozzolino DJ, Cendron M (1997) Bilateral renal vein thrombosis in a newborn: a case of prenatal renal vein thrombosis. *Urology* **50**: 128–31.

Croitoru DP, Sinsky AB, Laberge J (1992) Cystic neuroblastoma. *J Pediatr Surg* **27**: 1320–1.

Crombleholme TM, Harrison MR, Golbus MS *et al.* (1990) Fetal intervention in obstructive uropathy: prognostic indicators and efficacy of intervention. *Am J Obstet Gynecol* **162**: 1239–44.

Cromie WJ, Lee K, Houde K, Holmes L (1998) Implications of the decrease in major genitourinary malformations in the United States, 1972–1974. *American Academy of Pediatrics, Annual Meeting*, San Francisco, CA; Abstract **106**.

Crouch M, Manderson L (1995) The social life of bonding theory. *Soc Sci Med* **41**: 837–44.

Das S, Singer A (1990) Controversies of perinatal torsion of the spermatic cord: a review, survey and recommendations. *J Urol* **143**: 231–3.

Dator DP, Hatchett L, Dyro FM *et al.* (1992) Urodynamic dysfunction in walking myelodysplastic children. *J Urol* **148**: 362–5.

Davenport M (1996) Problems with the penis and prepuce. (ABC of general surgery in children) *BMJ* **312**: 299–301.

David M, Forest MG (1984) Prenatal treatment of congenital adrenal hyperplasia resulting from 21-hydroxylase deficiency. *J Pediatr* **105**: 799–803.

Decker PA, Chammas J, Sato TT (1999) Laparoscopic diagnosis and management of ovarian torsion in the newborn. *JSLS* **3**: 141–3.

De Klerk DP, Marshall FF, Jeffs RD (1977) Multicystic dysplastic kidney. *J Urol* **118**: 306–8.

deVries PA, Pena A (1982) Posterior sagittal anorectoplasty. *J Pediatr Surg* **17**: 638–43.

Dewan PA, Goh DG (1995) Variable expression of the congenital obstructive posterior urethral membrane. *Urology* **45**: 507–9.

Dhillon HK (1998) Prenatally diagnosed hydronephrosis: the great Ormond Street experience. *Br J Urol* **81**: 39–44.

(1990) Diagnostic and therapeutic technology assessment. Chorionic villus sampling: a reassessment. *JAMA* **263**: 305–6.

Diamond DA, Ford C (1989) Neonatal bladder rupture: a complication of umbilical artery catheterization. *J Urol* **142**: 1543–4.

Di Benedetto V, Morrison-Lacombe G, Bagnara V, Monfort G (1997) Transurethral puncture of ureterocele associated with single collecting system in neonates. *J Pediatr Surg* **32**: 1325–27.

Dimmick JE, Johnson HW, Coleman GU, Carter M (1989) Discussion 489 Wilms tumorlet, nodular renal blastema and multicystic renal dysplasia. *Urology* **142**: 484–5.

Dinneen MD, Dhillon HK, Ward HC *et al.* (1993) Antenatal diagnosis of posterior urethral valves. *Br J Urol* **72**: 364–9.

Docimo SG, Moore RG, Kavoussi LR (1995) Laparoscopic orchidopexy in the prune belly syndrome: a case report and review of the literature. *Urology* **45**: 679–81.

Donahoe PK, Schnitzer JJ (1996) Evaluation of the infant who has ambiguous genitalia, and principles of operative management. *Semin Pediatr Surg* **5**: 30–40.

Donahoe PK, Powell DM, Lee MM (1991) Clinical management of intersex abnormalities. *Curr Probl Surg* **28**: 513–79.

Donner C, Simon P, Karioun A *et al.* (1995) Experience with ^{125}I transcervical chorionic villus samplings performed in the first trimester by a single team of operators. *Eur J Obstet Gynecol Reprod Biol* **60**: 45–51.

Doran TA (1990) Chorionic villus sampling as the primary diagnostic tool in prenatal diagnosis. Should it replace genetic amniocentesis? *J Reprod Med* **35**: 935–40.

Driver CP, Losty PD (1998) Neonatal testicular torsion. *Br J Urol* **82**: 855–8.

Drotar D, Baskiewicz A, Irvin N *et al.* (1975) The adaptation of parents to the birth of an infant with a congenital malformation: a hypothetical model. *Pediatrics* **56**: 710–7.

Druschel CM (1995) A descriptive study of prune belly in New York state, 1983 to 1989. *Arch Pediatr Adolesc Med* **149**: 70–6.

Duel BP, Hendren WH, Bauer SB *et al.* (1996) Reconstructive options in genitourinary rhabdomyosarcoma. *J Urol* **156**: 1798–804.

Duncan BW, Adzick NS, Longaker MT *et al.* (1991) *In utero* arterial embolism from renal vein thrombosis with successful postnatal thrombolytic therapy. *Pediatr Surg* **26**: 741–3.

Durante D, Jones D, Spitzer R (1976) Neonatal renal arterial embolism syndrome. *Pediatrics* **89**: 978–81.

Dykes EH (1996) Prenatal diagnosis and management of abdominal wall defects. *Semin Pediatr Surg* **5**: 90–4.

Eason JD, McDonnell M, Clark G (1994) Male ritual circumcision resulting in acute renal failure. *BMJ* **309**: 660–1.

Eklof O, Mortensson W, Sandstedt B (1986) Suprarenal haematoma versus neuroblastoma complicated by haemorrhage. *Acta Radiol Diag* **27**: 3–10.

Elder JS, Duckett JW Jr, Snyder HM (1987) Intervention for fetal obstructive uropathy: has it been effective? *Lancet* **2**: 1007–10.

Elejalde BR, de Elejalde MM, Heitman T (1985) Visualization of the fetal genitalia by ultrasonography: a review of the literature and analysis of its accuracy and ethical implications. *J Ultrasound Med* **4**: 633–9.

Emanuel PG, Garcia GI, Angtuaco TL (1995) Prenatal detection of anterior abdominal wall defects with US. *Radiographics* **15**: 517–30.

Erttman R, Tafese T, Berthold F *et al.* (1998) 10 years' neuroblastoma screening in Europe: preliminary results of a clinical and biological review from the Study Group for Evaluation of Neuroblastoma Screening in Europe (SENSE). *Eur J Cancer* **34**: 1391–7.

Estes JM, MacGillivray TE, Hedrick MH *et al.* (1992) Fetoscopic surgery for the treatment of congenital anomalies. *J Pediatr Surg* **27**: 950–4.

Evans MI, Chrousos, Mann GP *et al.* (1985) Pharmacologic suppression of the fetal adrenal gland *in utero*. Attempted prevention of abnormal external genital masculinization in suspected congenital adrenal hyperplasia. *JAMA* **253**: 1015–20.

Evans MI, Sacks AJ, Johnson MP *et al.* (1991) Sequential invasive assessment of fetal renal function and the intrauterine treatment of fetal obstructive uropathies. *Obstet Gynecol* **77**: 545–50.

Fang SB, Lee HC, Sheu JC *et al.* (1999) Prenatal sonographic detection of adrenal hemorrhage confirmed by postnatal surgery. *J Clin Ultrasound* **27**: 206–9.

Farmer DL (1998) Fetal surgery: a brief review. *Pediatr Radiol* **28**: 409–13.

Farrell JA, Albanese CT, Jennings RW *et al.* (1999) Maternal fertility is not affected by fetal surgery. *Fetal Diagn Ther* **14**: 190–2.

Feitz WF, Van Gruns-Venn EJ, Froeling FM, de Vries JD (1994) Outcome analysis of psychosexual and socioeconomic development of adult patients born with bladder exstrophy. *J Urol* **152**: 1417–19.

Felc A (1995) Ultrasound in screening for neonatal adrenal hemorrhage. *Am J Perinatol* **12**: 363–6.

Ferrer FA, McKenna PH, Donnal JF (1994) Noninvasive angiography in preoperative evaluation of complicated pediatric renal masses using phase contrast magnetic resonance angiography. *Urology* **44**: 254–9.

Ferrer FA, McKenna PH (1994) Partial nephrectomy in a metachronous multilocular cyst of the kidney (cystic nephroma). *J Urol* **151**: 1358–60.

Ferrer FA, McKenna PH (1995) Cavernous hemangioma of the scrotum: a rare benign genital tumor of childhood. *J Urol* **153**: 1262–4.

Flake AW (1993) Fetal sacrococcygeal teratoma. *Semin Pediatr Surg* **2**: 113–20.

Forest MG, David M, Morel Y (1993) Prenatal diagnosis and treatment of 21-hydroxylase deficiency. *J Steroid Biochem Mol Biol* **45**: 75–82.

Forrest JR, Buschi AJ, Howards SS (1980) Neonatal urinary ascites sedcondary to distal ureteral stenosis. *J Urol* **124**: 919–20.

Foster LS, Kogan BA, Cogan PH, Edwards MSB (1990) Bladder function in patients with lipomyelomeningocele. *J Urol* **143**: 984–6.

Fowlie F, Giacomantonio M, McKenzie E *et al.* (1986) Antenatal sonographic diagnosis of adrenal neuroblastoma. *Can Assoc Radiol J* **37**: 50–1.

Freedman AL, Bukowski TP, Smith CA *et al.* (1996) Fetal therapy for obstructive uropathy: specific outcomes diagnosis. *J Urol* **156**: 720–4.

Freedman AL, Johnson MP, Smith CA *et al.* (1999) Long-term outcome in children after antenatal intervention for obstructive uropathies. *Lancet* **354**: 374–7.

Gearhart JP, Jeffs RD (1988) Augmentation cystoplasty in the failed exstrophy reconstruction. *J Urol* **139**: 790–3.

Gearhart JP, Rock JA (1989) Total ablation of the penis after curc with electrocautery: a method of management and long-term followup. *J Urol* **142**: 799–801.

Gearhart JP, Ben-Chaim J, Jeffs RD, Sanders RC (1995) Criteria for the prenatal diagnosis of classic bladder exstrophy. *Obstet Gynecol* **85**: 961–4.

Gerber WL (1982) Catheter guide for neonates. *Urology* **20**: 87.

Giulian BB, Chang CCN, Yoss BS (1986) Prenatal ultrasonographic diagnosis of fetal adrenal neuroblastoma. *J Clin Ultrasound* **14**: 225–7.

Glassberg KI (1999) Unilateral renal cystic disease. *Urology* **53**: 1227–8.

Glassberg KI, Stephens FD, Lebowitz RL *et al.* (1987) Renal dysgenesis and cystic disease of the kidney: a report of the Committee on Terminology, Nomenclature and Classification, Section on Urology. American Academy of Pediatrics. *J Urol* **138**: 1085–92.

Glick PL, Harrison MR, Globus MS *et al.* (1985) Management of the fetus with congenital hydronephrosis II: prognostic criteria and selection for treatment. *J Pediatr Surg* **20**: 376–87.

Gloor JM, Ogburn P, Matsumoto J (1996) Prenatally diagnosed ureterocele presenting as fetal bladder outlet obstruction. *J Perinatol* **16**: 285–7.

Gluckman GR, Stoller ML, Jacobs MM, Kogan BA (1995) Newborn penile glans amputation during circumcision and successful reattachment. *J Urol* **153**: 778–9.

Golan A, Lin G, Evron S *et al.* (1994) Oligohydramnios: maternal complications and fetal outcome in 145 cases. *Gynecol Obstet Invest* **37**: 91–5.

Gong M, Geary ES, Shortliffe LMD (1996) Testicular torsion with contralateral vanishing testis. *Urology* **48**: 306–7.

Gonzales ET (1990) Alternatives in the management of posterior urethral valves. *Urol Clin North Am* **17**: 335–42.

Gordon A, Collin J (1993) Save the normal foreskin: widespread confusion over what the medical indications for circumcision are. *BMJ* **306**: 1–2.

Gotoh T, Shinno Y, Kobayashi S *et al.* (1991) Diagnosis and management of sacral agenesis. *Eur Urol* **20**: 287–92.

Grady RW, Mitchell ME (1999) Complete primary repair of exstrophy. *J Urol* **162**: 1415–20.

Greenberg R, Waldman D, Brooks C *et al.* (1998) Endovascular treatment of renal artery thrombosis can be caused by umbilical artery catheterization. *J Vasc Surg* **28**: 949–53.

Greenfield SP, Hensle TW, Berdon WE, Geringer AM (1982) Urinary extravasation in the newborn male with posterior urethral valves. *Pediatr Surg* **17**: 751–6.

Griscom NT, Colodny AH, Rosenberg HK *et al.* (1977) Diagnostic aspects of neonatal ascites: report of 27 cases. *AJR Am J Roentgenol* **128**: 961–70.

Groisman GM, Nassrallah M, Bar-maor JA (1996) Bilateral intra-uterine testicular torsion in a newborn. *Br J Urol* **78**: 800–1.

Gross BR, Cohen HL, Schlessel JS (1993) Perinatal diagnosis of bilateral testicular torsion: beware of torsions simulating hydroceles. *J Ultrasound Med* **12**: 479–81.

Guez S, Assael BM, Melzi ML *et al*. (1996) Shortcomings in predicting postnatal renal function using prenatal urine biochemistry in fetuses with congenital hydronephrosis. *J Pediatr Surg* **31**: 1401–4.

Guzman L, Bauer SB, Hallet M *et al*. (1983) The evaluation and management of children with sacral agenesis. *Urology* **23**: 506–9.

Haase GM, Perez C, Atkinson JB (1999) Current aspects of biology, risk assessment, and treatment of neuroblastoma. *Semin Surg Oncol* **16**: 91–104.

Haddad B, Haziza J, Touboul C *et al*. (1996) The congenital mesoblastic nephroma: a case report of prenatal diagnosis. *Fetal Diagn Ther* **11**: 61–6.

Hahn-Pedersen J, Kvist N, Nielsen OH (1984) Hydrometrocolpos: current views on pathogenesis and management. *J Urol* **132**: 537–40.

Hamada Y, Ikebukuro K, Sato M *et al*. (1999) Prenatally diagnosed cystic neuroblastoma. *Pediatr Surg Int* **15**: 71–4.

Hamm B (1997) Differential diagnosis of scrotal masses by ultrasound. *Eur Radiol* **7**: 668–9.

Han K, Mata J, Zaontz MR (1998) Meconium masquerading as a scrotal mass. *Br J Urol* **82**: 765–7.

Hardwick-Smith S, Mastrobattista JM, Wallace PA, Ritchey ML (1998) Ring block for neonatal circumcision. *Obstet Gynecol* **91**: 930–4.

Harrison MR (1996) Fetal surgery. *Am J Obstet Gynecol* **174**: 1255–64.

Harrison MR, Nakayama DK, Noall R, deLorimier AA (1982) Correction of congenital hydronephrosis in utero II: decompression reverses the effects of obstruction on the fetal lung and urinary tract. *J Pediatr Surg* **17**: 965–74.

Hays DM, Raney RB, Wharam MD *et al*. (1995) Children with vesical rhabdomyosarcoma (RMS) treated by partial cystectomy with neoadjuvant or adjuvant chemotherapy, with or without radiotherapy. A report from the Intergroup Rhabdomyosarcoma Study (IRS) Committee. *J Pediatr Hematol Oncol* **17**: 46–52.

Heidelberger KP, Ritchey ML, Dauser RC *et al*. (1993) Congenital mesoblastic nephroma metastatic to the brain. *Cancer* **72**: 2499–502.

Hernanz-Schulman M, Yenicesu F, Heller RM, Brock JW III (1997) Sonographic identification of perinatal testicular torsion. *J Ultrasound Med* **16**: 65–7.

Herndon CDA, McKenna PH (1998) Survival after vascular injury with prenatal intervention: review of the complications. *Soc Fetal Urol* **5**(2): 4.

Herndon CDA, McKenna PH (1999) The antenatal detection of a 45X male. *Urology* **53**: 1033.

Herndon CDA, McKenna PH, Kolon TF *et al*. (1999) A multicenter outcomes analysis of patients with neonatal reflux presenting with prenatal hydronephrosis. *J Urol* **162**: 1203–8.

Herndon CDA, McKenna PH, Freedman AL (2000) Consensus on antenatal intervention. *J Urol* **164**: 1052–6.

Hibbert J, Howlett DC, Greenwood KL *et al*. (1997) The ultrasound appearances of neonatal renal vein thrombosis. *Br J Radiol* **70**: 1191–4.

Hill SJ, Hirsch JHA (1985) Sonographic detection of fetal hydrometrocolpos. *Ultrasound Med* **4**: 323–5.

Hirose R, Suita S, Taguchi T *et al*. (1995) Prune-belly syndrome in a female, complicated by intestinal malrotation after successful antenatal treatment of hydrops fetalis. *J Pediatr Surg* **30**: 1373–5.

Ho PTC, Estroff JA, Kozakewich H *et al*. (1993) Prenatal detection of neuroblastoma: a 10 year experience from the Dana-Farber Cancer Institute and Children's Hospital. *Pediatrics* **92**: 358–64.

Hoeffel C, Legmann P, Luton JP *et al*. (1995) Spontaneous unilateral adrenal hemorrhage: computerized tomography and magnetic resonance imaging findings in 8 cases. *J Urol* **154**: 1647–51.

Horger EO III, Arnett RM, Jones JS *et al*. (1998) Local anesthesia for infants undergoing circumcision. (Letter to the Editor). *JAMA* **279**: 1169.

Hoshino T, Ihara Y, Shirane H, Ota T (1998) Prenatal diagnosis of prune belly syndrome at 12 weeks of pregnancy: case report and review of the literature. *Ultrasound Obstet Gynecol* **12**: 362–6.

Hosoda Y, Miyano T, Kimura K *et al*. (1992) Characteristics and management of patients with neuroblastoma. *J Pediatr Surg* **27**: 623–5.

Housley HT, Harrison MR (1998) Fetal urinary tract abnormalities. *Urol Clin* **1**: 63–73.

Howard CR, Howard FM, Garfunkel LC *et al*. (1998) Neonatal circumcision and pain relief: current training practices. *Pediatrics* **101**: 423–8.

Hsieh TT, Lee JD, Kuo DM *et al*. (1989) Perinatal outcome of chorionic villus sampling versus amniocentesis. *Taiwan I Hsueh Hui Tsa Chih* **88**: 894–9.

Huff DS, Wu H, Snyder HM III *et al*. (1991) Evidence in favor of the mechanical (intrauterine torsion) theory over the endocrinopathy (cryptorchidism) theory in the pathogenesis of testicular agenesis. *J Urol* **146**: 630–1.

Hutton KAR, Thomas DFM, Arthur RJ *et al*. (1994) Prenatally detected posterior urethral valves: is gestational age at detection a predictor of outcome? *J Urol* **152**: 698–701.

Jeffs RD, Guice SL, Oesch I (1982) The factors in successful exstrophy closure. *J Urol* **127**: 974–7.

Jennings RW, LaQuaglia MP, Leong K *et al*. (1993) Fetal neuroblastoma: prenatal diagnosis and natural history. *J Pediatr Surg* **28**: 1168–74.

Jobin J, O'Regan S, Demay G *et al*. (1982) Neonatal renal vein thrombosis – long-term follow-up after conservative management. *Clin Nephrol* **17**: 36–40.

Johnson MP, Bukowski TP, Reitleman C *et al*. (1994) *In utero* surgical treatment of fetal obstructive uropathy: a new comprehensive approach to identify appropriate candidates for vesicoamniotic shunt therapy. *Am J Obstet Gynecol* **170**: 1770–6.

Johnson MP, Corsi P, Bradfield W *et al*. (1995) Sequential fetal urine analysis provides greater precision in the evaluation of fetal obstructive uropathy. *Am J Obstet Gynecol* **173**: 59–65.

Kadish HA, Bolte RG (1998) A retrospective review of pediatric patients with epididymitis, testicular torsion, and torsion of testicular appendages. *Pediatrics* **102**: 73–6.

Kanayama H, Naroda T, Inoue Y *et al.* (1999) A case of complete testicular feminization: laparoscopic orchietomy and analysis of androgen receptor gene mutation. *Int J Urol* **6**: 327–30.

Kaplan GW (1983) Complications of circumcision. *Urol Clin North Am* **10**: 543–9.

Kass EJ, Stone KT, Cacciarelli AA, Mitchell B (1993) Do all children with an acute scrotum require exploration? *J Urol* **150**: 667–9.

Kavaler E, Hensle TW (1997) Renal artery thrombosis in the newborn infant. *Urology* **50**: 282–4.

Kay R (1985) Pediatric urologic intraoperative consultation. *Urol Clin North Am* **12**: 461–8.

Kay R, Brereton RJ, Johnson JH (1980) Urinary ascites in the newborn. *Br J Urol* **52**: 451–4.

Keidan I, Lotan D, Gazit G *et al.* (1994) Early neonatal renal venous thrombosis: long-term outcome. *Acta Paediatr* **83**: 1225–7.

Kemp J, Davenport M, Pernet A (1998) Antenatally diagnosed surgical anomalies: the psychological effect of parental antenatal counseling. *J Pediatr Surg* **33**: 1376–9.

Kessler OJ, Ziv N, Livne PM *et al.* (1998) Involution rate of multicystic renal dysplasia. *Pediatrics* **102**: E73.

Khuri FJ, Alton DJ, Hardy BE *et al.* (1980) Adrenal hemorrhage in neonates: report of 5 cases and review of the literature. *J Urol* **124**: 684–7.

King LR, Coughlin PW, Bloch EC *et al.* (1984) The case for immediate pyeloplasty in the neonate with ureteropelvic junction obstruction. *J Urol* **132**: 725–8.

Klaus M, Kennell J (1982) Interventions in the premature nursery: impact on development. *Pediatr Clin North Am* **29**: 1263–73.

Knoedler CJ, Kay R, Knoedler JP Sr, Wiig Th (1989) Pelvic neuroblastoma. *J Urol* **141**: 905–7.

Koff SA, DeRidder PA (1977) Patterns of neurogenic bladder dysfunction in sacral agenesis. *J Urol* **118**: 87–9.

Kon M (1983) A rare complication following circumcision: the concealed penis. *J Urol* **130**: 573–4.

Kopp C, Greenfield SP (1993) Effects of neurogenic bladder dysfunction in utero seen in neonates with myleodysplasia. *Br J Urol* **71**: 739–42.

Kuliev A, Jackson L, Froster U *et al.* (1996) Chorionic villus sampling safety. Report of World Health Organization/ EURO meeting in association with the Seventh International Conference on Early Prenatal Diagnosis of Genetic Diseases, Tel-Aviv, Israel, May 21, 1994. *Am J Obstet Gynecol* **174**: 807–11.

Lais A, Kasbian NG, Dyro FM *et al.* (1993) The neurosurgical implications of continuous neurourologocial surveillance of children with myelodysplasia. *J Urol* **150**: 1879–83.

Lajic S, Wedell A, Bui T-H *et al.* (1998) Long-term somatic follow-up of prenatally treated children with congenital adrenal hyperplasia. *J Clin Endocrinol Metab* **83**: 3872–80.

Lander J, Brady-Fryer B, Metcalfe JB *et al.* (1997) Comparison of ring block, dorsal penile nerve block, and topical anesthesia for neonatal circumcision: a randomized controlled trial. *JAMA* **278**: 2157.

Laplante S, Patriquin HB, Robitaille P *et al.* (1993) Renal vein thrombosis in children: evidence of early flow recovery with Doppler US. *Radiology* **189**: 37–42.

LaQuaglia MP, Bauer SB, Eraklis A *et al.* (1987) Bilateral neonatal torsion. *J Urol* **138**: 1051–4.

Lazar EL, Stolar CJ (1998) Evaluation and management of pediatric solid ovarian tumors. *Semin Pediatr Surg* **7**: 29–34.

Lee MM (1991) Clinical management of intersex abnormalities. *Curr Probl Surg* **8**: 519–79.

Lee MM, Donahoe PK (1997) The infant with ambiguous genitalia. *Curr Ther Endocrinol Metab* **6**: 216–23.

Leviton LC, Goldenberg RL, Baker CS *et al.* (1999) Methods to encourage the use of antenatal corticosteroid therapy for fetal maturation: a randomized controlled trial. *JAMA* **281**: 46–52.

Levitt MA, Rodriguez G, Gaylin DS, Pena A (1997) The tethered spinal cord in patients with anorectal malformations. *J Pediatr Surg* **32**: 462–8.

Levy DA, Kay R, Elder JS (1994) Neonatal testis tumors: a review of the Prepubertal Testis Tumor Registry. *J Urol* **151**: 715–17.

Lewis AG, Bukowski TP, Jarvis PD *et al.* (1995) Evaluation of acute scrotum in the emergency department. *J Pediatr Surg* **30**: 277–82.

Lewis DP, Van Dyke DC, Stumbo PJ, Berg MJ (1998) Drug and environmental factors associated with adverse pregnancy outcomes. Part II: improvement with folic acid. *Ann Pharmacother* **32**: 947–61.

Lewis KM, Pinckert TL, Cain MP, Ghidini A (1998) Complications of intrauterine placement of a vesicoamniotic shunt. *Obstet Gynecol* **91**: 825–7.

Lipitz S, Ryan G, Samuell C *et al.* (1993) Fetal urine analysis for the assessment of renal function in obstructive uropathy. *Am J Obstet Gynecol* **168**: 174–9.

Liyanage IS, Katoch D (1992) Ultrasonic prenatal diagnosis of liver metastases from adrenal neuroblastoma. *J Clin Ultrasound* **20**: 401–3.

Longaker MT, Golbus MS, Filly RA *et al.* (1991) Maternal outcome after open fetal surgery. A review of the first 17 human cases. *JAMA* **265**: 737–41.

Lukens JN (1999) Neuroblastoma in the neonate. *Semin Perinatol* **23**: 263–73.

McAlister WH, Sisler CL (1990) Scrotal sonography in infants and children. *Curr Probl Diagn Radiol* **19**: 201–42.

McCurdy CM Jr, Seeds JW (1993) Oligohydramnios: problems and treatment. *Semin Perinatol* **17**: 183–96.

McGuire EJ, Woodside JR, Borden TA *et al.* (1981) Prognostic value of urodynamic testing in myelodysplasia patients. *J Urol* **126**: 205–9.

McKenna PH (1993) A functional classification of ectopic ureteroceles based on renal unit jeopardy. *Dialog Pediatr Urol* **16**: 9.

McKenna PH, Khoury AE, McLorie GA *et al.* (1993) Anterior diagonal mid-innominate osteotomy. *Dialog Pediatr Urol* **16**: 1.

McKenna PH, Khoury AE, McLorie GA *et al.* (1994) Iliac osteotomy: model to compare options in bladder and cloacal exstrophy reconstruction. *J Urol* **151**: 182–6, Discussion 186–7.

McLorie GA, Sheldon CA, Fleisher M, Churchill BM (1987) The genitorurinary system in patients with imperforate anus. *J Pediatr Surg* **22**: 1100–4.

McVicar M, Margouleff D, Chandra M (1991) Diagnosis and imaging of the fetal and neonatal abdominal mass: an antegrated approach. *Advan Pediatr* **38**: 135–49.

McWilliams NB (1987) Screening infants for neuroblastoma in North America. *Pediatrics* **79**: 1048–9.

Mandell J, Bromley B, Peters CA, Benacerraf BR (1995) Prenatal sonographic detection of genital malformations. *J Urol* **153**: 242–6.

Mann CM, Leape LL, Holder TM (1974) Neonatal urinary ascites: a report of 2 cases of unusual etiology and a review of the literature. *J Urol* **111**: 124–8.

Manning FA, Harrison MR, Rodeck C (1986) Catheter shunts for fetal hydronephrosis and hydrocephalus. Report of the international fetal surgery registry. *N Engl J Med* **315**: 336–40.

Mares AJ, Shkolnik A, Sacks M, Feuchtwanger MM (1980) Aberrant (ectopic) adrenocortical tissue along the spermatic cord. *Pediatr Surg* **15**: 289–92.

Massad CA, Cohen MB, Kogan BA, Beckstead JH (1991) Morphology and histochemistry of infant testes in the prune belly syndrome. *J Urol* **146**: 1598–600.

Mata JA, Livne PM, Gibbons MD (1987) Urinary ascites: complication of umbilical artery catheterization. *Urology* **30**: 375–7.

Matsumura M, Nishi T, Sasaki Y *et al.* (1993) Prenatal diagnosis and treatment strategy for congenital mesoblastic nephroma. *J Pediatr Surg* **28**: 1607–9.

Matzinger MA, Matzinger FR, Matzinger KE, Black MD (1992) Antenatal and postnatal findings in intra-abdominal pulmonary sequestration. *Can Assoc Radiol J* **43**: 212–4.

Melekos MD (1988) Re: Testicular torsion in a 62-year-old man. *J Urol* **140**: 387–9.

Mercado AB, Wilson RC, Cheng KC *et al.* (1995) Prenatal treatment and diagnosis of congenital adrenal hyperplasia owing to steroid 21-hydroxylase deficiency. *J Clin Endocrinol Metab* **80**: 2014.

Merguerian PA, McLorie GA, Churchill BM *et al.* (1992) Radiographic and serologic correlates of azotemia in patients with posterior urethral valves. *J Urol* **148**: 1499–503.

Merguerian PA, Agarwal S, Greenberg M *et al.* (1998) Outcome analysis of rhabdomyosarcoma of the lower urinary tract. *J Urol* **160**: 1191–4, Discussion **1216.**

Meyer-Bahlburg HF (1999) Gender assignment and reassignment in 46,XY pseudohermaphroditism and related conditions. *J Clin Endocrinol Metab* **84**: 3455–8.

Meyer-Bahlburg HF, Heino FL (1999) New York State Psychiatric Institute, Dept of Psychiatry, Columbia University, New York, NY. Gender assignment and reassignment in intersexuality: controversies, data, and guidelines for research. In: Zderic SA, Canning DA, Snyder HM III, Carr MC (eds) *Pediatric gender reassignment: a critical reappraisal*. New York: Plenum, 12–24.

Mikuz G (1985) Testicular torsion: simple grading for histological evaluation of tissue damage. *Appl Pathol* **3**: 134–9.

Miller WL (1999) Dexamethasone treatment of congenital adrenal hyperplasia *in utero*: an experimental therapy of unproven safety. *J Urol* **162**: 537–40.

(1991) Use of folic acid for prevention of spina bifida and other neural tube defects–1983–1991. *MMWR Morb Mortal Wkly Rep* **40**: 513–6.

Mor Y, Ramon J, Raviv G *et al.* (1992) A 20-year experience with treatment of ectopic ureteroceles. *J Urol* **147**: 1592–4.

Mukai M, Takamatsu H, Noguchi H, Tahara H (1998) Intra-abdominal testis with mature teratoma. *Pediatr Surg Int* **13**: 204–5.

Murphy JP, Holder TM, Ashcraft KW *et al.* (1984) Ureteropelvic junction obstruction in the newborn. *Pediatr Surg* **19**: 642–8.

Neuhouser ML, Beresford SA, Hickok DE, Monsen ER (1998) Absorption of dietary and supplemental folate in women with prior pregnancies with neural tube defects and controls. *J Am Coll Nutr* **17**: 625–30.

Neulander E, Walfisch S, Kaneti J (1996) Amputation of distal penile glans during neonatal ritual circumcision – a rare complication. *Br J Urol* **77**: 924–5.

New M, White P (1995) Genetic disorders of steroid hormone synthesis and metabolism. *Baillieres Clin Endocrinol Metab* **9**: 525–54.

Nichols VG, Bianchi DW (1996) Prenatal pediatrics: traditional specialty definitions no longer apply. *Pediatrics* **97**: 729–32.

Niku SD, Stock JA, Kaplan GW (1995) Neonatal circumcision. *Urol Clin North Am* **22**: 57–65.

Noh PH, Cooper CS, Winkler AC *et al.* (1999) Prognostic factors for long-term renal function in boys with the prune belly syndrome. *J Urol* **162**: 1399–401.

Noske HD, Kraus SW, Altinkilic BM, Weidner W (1998) Historical milestones regarding torsion of the scrotal organs. *J Urol* **159**: 13–16.

Nuss R, Hays T, Manco-Johnson M (1994) Efficacy and safety of heparin anticoagulation for neonatal renal vein thrombosis. *Am J Pediatr Hematol Oncol* **16**: 127–31.

Oberg KC, Robles AE, Ducsay CA *et al.* (1999) Endoscopic intrauterine surgery in primates: overcoming technical obstacles. *Surg Endosc* **13**: 420–6.

O'Reilly P, Aurell M, Britton K *et al.* (1996) Consensus on diuresis renography for investigating the dilated upper urinary tract. *J Nucl Med* **37**: 1872–76.

Orvis Br, Bottles K, Kogan BA (1988) Testicular histology in fetuses with the prune belly syndrome and posterior urethral valves. *J Urol* **139**: 335–7.

Ozdemir E (1997) Significantly increased complication risks with mass circumcisions. *Br J Urol* **80**: 136–9.

Ozkan S, Gurpinar T (1997) A serious circumcision complication: penile shaft amputation and a new reattachment technique with a successful outcome. *J Urol* **158**: 1946–7.

Palmer LS, Maizels M, Cartwright PC *et al.* (1998) Surgery versus observation for managing obstructive grade 3 to 4 unilateral hydronephrosis: a report from the Society for Fetal Urology. *J Urol* **159**: 222–8.

Pang SY, Pollack MS, Marshall RN, Immken L (1990) Prenatal treatment of congenital adrenal hyperplasia due to 21-hydroxylase deficiency. *N Engl J Med* **322**: 111–15.

Papadopoulou D, Tsakiris D, Papadimitriou M (1999) The use of ultrasonography and linkage studies for early diagnosis of autosomal dominant polycystic kidney disease (ADPKD). *Ren Fail* **21**: 67–84.

Parker RM (1974) Neonatal urinary ascites. A potentially favorable sign in bladder outlet obstruction. *Urology* **III**: 589–94.

Parkhouse HF, Woodhouse CRJ (1990) Long-term status of patients with posterior urethral valves. *Urol Clin North Am* **17**: 373–8.

Parra RO, Cummings JM, Palmer DC (1991) Testicular seminoma in a long-term survivor of the prune belly syndrome. *Eur Urol* **19**: 79–80.

Pathak IG, Williams DI (1964) Multicystic and cystic dysplastic kidneys. *Br J Urol* **36**: 318–31.

Patriquin HB, Yazbeck S, Trinh B *et al.* (1993) Testicular torsion in infants and children: diagnosis with Doppler sonography. *Radiology* **188**: 781–5.

Paul R, Bielmeier J, Breul J *et al.* (1997) Accessory spleen of the spermatic cord. *Urologe A* **36**: 262–4.

Perez LM, Khoury J, Webster GD (1992) The value of urodynamic studies in infants less than one year old with congenital spinal dysraphism. *J Urol* **148**: 584.

Perez LM, Naidu SI, Joseph DB (1998) Outcome and cost analysis of operative versus nonoperative management of neonatal multicystic dysplastic kidneys. *J Urol* **160**: 1207–11.

Persad R, Sharma S, McTavish J *et al.* (1995) Clinical presentation and pathophysiology of meatal stenosis following circumcision. *Br J Urol* **75**: 91–3.

Peters CA, Docimo SG, Luetic T *et al.* (1991a) Effect of *in utero* vesicostomy on pulmonary hypoplasia in the fetal lamb with bladder outlet obstruction and oligohydramnios: a morphometric analysis. *J Urol* **146**: 1178–83.

Peters CA, Reid LM, Docimo S *et al.* (1991b) The role of the kidney in lung growth and maturation in the setting obstructive uropathy and oligohydramnios. *J Urol* **146**: 597–600.

Peters DJ, Spruit L, Saris JJ *et al.* (1993) Chromosome 4 localization of a second gene for autosomal dominant polycystic kidney disease. *Nat Genet* **5**: 359–62.

Pfister C, Ravasse P, Barret E *et al.* (1998) The value of endoscopic treatment for ureteroceles during the neonatal period. *J Urol* **159**: 1006–9.

Pinto KJ, Noe HN, Jerkins GR (1997) Management of neonatal testicular torsion. *J Urol* **158**: 1196–7.

Poland RL (1990) The question of routine neonatal circumcision. *N Engl J Med* **322**: 1312–15.

Putnam MH (1989) Neonatal adrenal hemorrhage presenting as a right scrotal mass. *JAMA* **261**: 2958.

Quine L, Pahl J (1987) First diagnosis of severe handicap: a study of parental reactions. *Dev Med Child Neurol* **29**: 232–42.

Quintera RA, Johnson MP, Romero R *et al.* (1995) In-utero percutaneous cystoscopy in the management of fetal lower obstructive uropathy. *Lancet* **346**: 537–40.

Rajfer J, Walsh PC (1978) Testicular descent. Normal and abnormal. *Urol Clin North Am* **5**: 223–35.

Rampaul MS, Hosking SW (1998) Testicular torsion: most delay occurs outside hospital. *Ann R Coll Surg Engl* **80**: 169–72.

Redman JF (1994) A catheter guide to obviate difficult urethral catheterization in male infants and boys. *J Urol* **151**: 1051–2.

Reeders ST, Germino GG (1989) The molecular genetics of autosomal dominant polycystic kidney disease. *Semin Nephrol* **9**: 122–34.

Reha WC, Gibbons MD (1989) Neonatal ascites and ureteral valves. *Urology* **33**: 468–71.

Reinberg Y, Manivel JC, Fryd D *et al.* (1989) The outcome of renal transplantation in children with the prune belly syndrome. *J Urol* **142**: 1541–2.

Reinberg Y, Manivel JC, Pettinato G, Gonzalez R (1991) Development of renal failure in children with the prune belly syndrome. *J Urol* **145**: 1017–9.

Reinberg Y, De Castano I, Gonzalez R (1992) Prognosis for patients with prenatally diagnosed posterior urethral valves. *J Urol* **148**: 125–6.

Rhoads GG, Jackson LG, Schlesselman SE *et al.* (1989) The safety and efficacy of chorionic villus sampling for early prenatal diagnosis of cytogenetic abnormalities. *N Engl J Med* **320**: 609–17.

Richard ML, Gundersen AE, Williams MS (1995) Cystic neuroblastoma of infancy. *J Pediatr Surg* **30**: 1354–7.

Ring KS, Axelrod SL, Burbige KA, Hensle TW (1989) Meconium hydrocele: an unusual etiology of a scrotal mass in the newborn. *J Urol* **141**: 1172–3.

Riski JE (1991) Parents of children with cleft lip and plate. *Clin Commun Disord* **1** (3): 42–7.

Rittenberg M, Hulbert WC, Snyder HM 3rd *et al.* (1988) Protective factors in posterior urethal valves. *J Urol* **140**: 993–6.

Roach MB, Switters DM, Stone AR (1993) The changing urodynamic pattern in infants with myelomeningocele. *J Urol* **150**: 944–7.

Robichaux AG III, Greene MJ, Greene MF *et al.* (1991) Fetal abdominal wall defect: a new complication of vesicoamniotic shunting. *Fetal Diagn Ther* **6**: 11–3.

Ross HL, Elias S (1997) Maternal serum screening for fetal genetic disorders. *Obstet Gynecol Clin North Am* **24**: 33–47.

Sahdev S, Jhaveri RC, Vohra K, Khan AJ (1997) Congenital bladder perforation and urinary ascites caused by posterior urethral valves: a case report. *J Perinatol* **17**: 164–5.

Sawchuk, T, Costabile RA, Howards SS, Rodgers BM (1993) Spermatic cord torsion in an infant receiving human chorionic gonadotropin. *J Urol* **150**: 1212–3.

Scarff TB, Fronczak S (1981) Myelomeningocele: a review and update. *Rehab Lit* **42**: 143–6.

Scott TW (1976) Urinary ascites secondary to posterior urethral valves. *Urology* **116**: 87–91.

Shandling B, Jank JJ (1981) The vunerability of the vas deferens. *J Pediatr Surg* **16**: 461–4.

Sherer DM, Hulbert WC (1995) Prenatal sonographic diagnosis and subsequent conservative surgical management of bilateral ureteroceles. *Am J Perinatol* **12**: 174–7.

Sherer DM, Kendig JW, Sickel JZ *et al.* (1994) *In utero* adrenal hemorrhage associated with fetal distress, subsequent transient neonatal hypertension, and a nonfunctioning ipsilateral kidney. *Am J Perinatol* **11**: 302–4.

Sherman J, Borer JG, Horowitz M, Glassberg KI (1996) Circumcision: successful glanular reconstruction and survival following traumatic amputation. *J Urol* **156**: 842–4.

Shigeta M, Nagata M, Shimoyamada H *et al.* (1999) Prune belly syndrome diagnosed at 14 weeks' gestation with severe urethral obstruction but normal kidneys. *Pediatr Nephrol* **13**: 135–7.

Siegel MJ, Herman TE (1994) Neonatal spermatic cord torsion and testicular infarction. *J Perinatol* **14**: 431–2.

Sillén U, Hansson E, Hermansson G *et al.* (1996) Development of the urodynamic pattern in infants with myelomeningocele. *Br J Urol* **78**: 596–601.

Sloan WR, Walsh PC (1976) Familial persistent Mullerian duct syndrome. *J Urol* **115**: 459–61.

Smith C, Gosalbez R, Parrott TS *et al.* (1994) Transurethral puncture of ectopic ureteroceles in neonates and infants. *J Urol* **152**: 2110–2.

Smith DJ, Hamdy FC, Chapple CR (1994) An uncommon complication of circumcision. *Br J Urol* **73**: 459–60.

Smith DP (1998) Can perinatal events cause neonatal urinary ascites? *Urology* **159**: 1652–3.

Smith GHH, Canning DA, Schulman SL *et al.* (1996) The long-term outcome of posterior urethral valves treated with primary valve ablation and observation. *J Urol* **155**: 1730–4.

Snellman LW, Stand HJ (1995) Prospective evaluation of complications of dorsal penile nerve block for neonatal circumcision. *Pediatrics* **95**: 705–9.

Sotolongo JR Jr, Hoffman S, Gribetz ME (1985) Penile denudation injuries after circumcision. *J Urol* **133**: 102–3.

Spach DH, Stapleton AE, Stamm WE (1992) Lack of circumcision increases the risk of urinary tract infection in young men. *JAMA* **267**: 679–82.

Speiser PW (1999) Prenatal treatment of congenital adrenal hyperplasia. *J Urol* **162**: 534–6.

Speiser PW, New MI (1994) Prenatal diagnosis and management of congenital adrenal hyperplasis. *Clin Perinatol* **21**: 631–8.

Speiser PW, Laforgia N, Kato K *et al.* (1990) First trimester prenatal treatment and molecular genetic diagnosis of congenital adrenal hyperplasia (21-hydroxylase deficiency). *J Clin Endocrinol Metab* **70**: 838–48.

Stang HJ, Gunnar MR, Snellman L *et al.* (1988) Local anesthesia for neonatal circumcision: effects on distress and cortisol response. *JAMA* **259**: 1507–9.

Stein SC, Feldman JG, Freidlander M, *et al.* (1982) Is myelomeningocele a disappearing disease? *Pediatrics* **69**: 511–13.

Stirimling BS (1996) Partial amputation of glans penis during Mogen clamp circumcision. *Pediatrics* **97**: 906–8.

Stokes S III, Flom S (1997) Meconium filled hydrocele sacs as a cause of acute scrotum in a newborn. *J Urol* **158**: 1960–1.

Stone KT, Kass EJ, Cacciarelli AA, Gibson DP (1995) Management of suspected antenatal torsion: what is the best strategy? *J Urol* **153**: 782–4.

Sugita Y, Clarnette TD, Cooke-Yarborough C *et al.* (1999) Testicular and paratesticular tumours in children: 30 years' experience. *Aust NZ J Surg* **69**: 505–8.

Susskind MR, Kim KS, King LR (1989) Hypertension and multicystic kidney. *Urology* **34**: 362–6.

Tabor A, Philip J, Madsen M *et al.* (1986) Randomised controlled trial of genetic amniocentesis in 4606 low-risk women. *Lancet* i: 1287–93.

Tank ES, Carey TC, Seifert AL (1980) Management of neonatal urinary ascites. *Urology* **XVI**: 270–3.

Tibballs JM, De Bruyn R (1996) Primary vesicoureteral reflux – how useful is postnatal ultrasound? *Arch Dis Child* **75**: 444–7.

Tietjen DN, Gloor JM, Husmann DA (1997) Proximal urinary diversion in the management of posterior urethral valves: is it necessary? *J Urol* **158**: 1008–10.

Toma P, Lucigrai G, Marzoli, Lituania M (1994) Prenatal diagnosis of metastatis adrenal neuroblastoma with sonography and MR imaging. *Am J Roentgenol* **162**: 1183–4.

Tripp BM, Homsy YL (1995) Prenatal diagnosis of bilateral neonatal torsion: a case report. *J Urol* **153**: 1990–1.

Tryfonas G, Violaki A, Tsikopoulos G *et al.* (1994) Late postoperative results in males treated for testicular torsion during childhood. *J Pediatr Surg* **29**: 553–6.

Turner JH, Leonard JC (1997) Renal scintigraphic findings in a patient with hydrometrocolpos. *Clin Nucl Med* **22**: 394–6.

van Gool JD, Kuijten RH, Donckerwolcke RA, Kramer PP (1982) Detrusor-sphincter dyssynergia in children with myelomeningocele: a prospective study. *Z Kinderchir* **37**: 148–54.

van Noesel MM, Hahlen K, Hakvoort-Cammel FG, Egeler RM (1997) Neuroblastoma 4S: a heterogeneous disease with variable risk factors and treatment strategies. *Cancer* **80**: 834–43.

Varni JW, Setoguchi Y (1993) Effects of parental adjustment on the adaptation of children with congenital or acquired limb deficiencies. *J Dev Behav Pediatr* **14**: 13–20.

Verp MS, Simpson JL (1987) Abnormal sexual differentiation and neoplasia. *Cancer Genet Cytogenet* **25**: 191–218.

Vintzileos AM, Ananth CV, Fisher AJ *et al.* (1999) Cost–benefit analysis of targeted ultrasonography for prenatal detection of spina bifida in patients with an elevated concentration of second-trimester maternal serum alpha-fetoprotein. *Am J Obstet Gynecol* **180**: 1227–33.

Walker RD, Padron M (1990) The management of posterior urethral valves by initial vesicostomy and delayed valve ablation. *J Urol* **144**: 1212–4.

Wasnick RJ (1987) Neonatal urinary ascites secondary to ureteropelvic junction obstruction. *Urology* **30**: 470–1.

Wheatley JM, Stephens FD, Hutson JM (1996) Prune belly syndrome: ongoing controversies regarding pathogenesis and management. *Semin Pediatr Surg* **5**: 95–106.

White RI, Klauber GT (1976) Sacral agenesis. Analysis of 22 cases. *Urology* **8**: 521–5.

Wilkins IA, Chitkara U, Lynch L *et al.* (1987) The non-predictive value of fetal urinary electrolytes: preliminary report of outcomes and correlations with pathologic diagnosis. *Am J Obstet Gynecol* **157**: 694–8.

Willemse AP, Coppes MJ, Feldberg MA *et al.* (1989) Magnetic resonance appearance of adrenal hemorrhage in a neonate. *Pediatr Radiol* **19**: 210–1.

Williams N, Kapila L (1993) Complications of circumcision. *Br J Surg* **80**: 1231–6.

Wiswell TE, Tencer HL, Welch CA, Chamberlain JL (1993) Circumcision in children beyond the neonatal period. *Pediatrics* **92**: 791–4.

Woodard JR, Zucker I (1990) Current management of the dilated urinary tract in prune belly syndrome. *Urol Clin North Am* **17**: 407–18.

Woodhouse CR, Ransley PG (1983) Teratoma of the testis in the prune belly syndrome. *Br J Urol* **55**: 580–1.

Woodhouse CR, Snyder HM III (1985) Testicular and sexual function in adults with prune belly syndrome. *J Urol* **133**: 607–9.

Woodhouse CRJ, Ransley PC, Williams DI (1983b) The exstrophy patient in adult life. *Br J Urol* **55**: 632–42.

Woods WG, Tuchman M (1997) Neuroblastoma: the case for screening infants in North America **79**: 869–73.

Wu HY, Baskin LS, Kogan BA (1997) Neurogenic bladder dysfunction due to myelomeningocele: neonatal versus childhood treatment. *J Urol* **157**: 2295–7.

Xue H, Horwitz JR, Smith MB *et al.* (1995) Malignant solid tumors in neonates: a 40-year review. *J Pediatr Surg* **30**: 543–5.

Yazbeck S, Patriquin HB (1994) Accuracy of Doppler sonography in the evaluation of acute conditions of the scrotum in children. *J Pediatr Surg* **29**: 1270–2.

Yeung CK, Godley ML, Dhillon HK *et al.* (1997) The characteristics of primary vesico-ureteric reflux in male and female infants with pre-natal hydronephrosis. *Br J Urol* **80**: 319–27.

Zabbo A, Montie JE (1985) Intraoperative consultation for the kidney. *Urol Clin North Am* **12**: 405–10.

Zerres K, Rudnik-Schoneborn S, Steinkamm C *et al.* (1998) Autosomal recessive polycystic kidney disease. *J Mol Med* **76**: 303–9.

Zinn HL, Cohen HL, Horowitz M (1998) Testicular torsion in neonates: importance of power Doppler imaging. *J Ultrasound Med* **17**: 385–8.

Office pediatric urology

8

Patrick C. Cartwright and Brent Snow

Introduction

The environment of a medical office can play a pivotal role in making pediatric patients and their families comfortable. Engaging decorations, bright colors, toys, and play areas often help to calm nervous children. A bulletin board with patient photos and cards often softens the feel of the office as well. Every effort should be made to allow parents to be with their child at all times to provide reassurance. Each physician's style and personality is different, but often those who deal with children usually forego the formality of a white coat so that the encounter might be more familiar to the patient. It is important upon entering the examination room first to engage the patient in gentle conversation, when possible, to develop rapport and place the child at ease even before talking to the parent. If the child is old enough, history taking generally begins with the child and is supplemented by parental input.

The physical examination is generally performed on the examining table with a parent standing beside the physician at the head of the bed. It is important to let the child know that they will not be poked or hurt but 'gently checked'. As children approach puberty, they may be relieved to have one or both of their parents leave for the examination if given this opportunity by the physician. After the examination is completed it is important to let the patient know that they are finished so they will no longer be ill at ease. Upon leaving the office, children are often rewarded with a treat for their good behavior so that they will look forward to return visits.

Most physicians find that dealing with children in an honest, straightforward manner is best. It is appropriate to tell the child before any uncomfortable or painful procedures are undertaken so that they will not be fearful the entire time, but only for the first few moments that it occurs. Surprising a child with an unpleasant examination or injection results in a loss of trust and faith in the physician which is difficult to regain. Parents are encouraged to tell their children honestly about diagnostic X-ray examinations and office visits so that the children can be appropriately prepared. Under these circumstances, the examination and history may be completed accurately with little threat to the child.

The penis

Foreskin and phimosis

The appropriate management of penile problems in childhood is based on a reasonable understanding of genital embryology and postnatal penile development. Genital differentiation takes place between the 9th and 13th weeks of gestation. The glans penis forms from the genital tubercle and is covered with a prepuce that is adherent to its surface. The preputial attachments persist throughout gestation and the epithelial layer of the inner prepuce and the glans penis are fused at birth. The newborn foreskin cannot be retracted without disrupting this natural adherence. Subsequently, glanular secretions and desquamated epithelial debris, collectively called smegma, collect between the inner prepuce and the glans penis, gradually separating these two layers. The build-up of this material can be impressive and patients may present with a mass that can be seen through the thin foreskin. This has been referred to as a 'foreskin pearl'. Treatment is not required as the pearl eventually erupts at the foreskin meatus, disrupting the adherence and resulting in partial separation of the foreskin (Caldamone *et al.*, 1996). This sequence is often misdiagnosed as a penile infection, the smegma presumed

Table 8.1 Incidence of phimosis in children

Age (years)	Phimosis (%)	Tight prepuce (%)
6–7	8	1
8–9	6	2
10–11	6	2
12–13	3	3
14–15	1	1
16–17	1	1

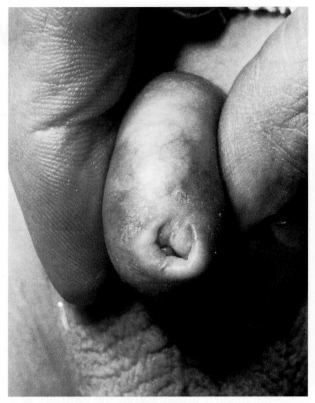

Figure 8.1 This prepuce displays a true 'phimotic ring' laterally and inferiorly with thickened skin, while superiorly the skin shows a more normal, effaced (thin) appearance when the foreskin is pushed gently toward the base of the penis.

to be 'pus'. Hopefully, physicians easily recognize that this is not an infection but the physiologic appearance of smegma. Reassurance usually quiets parental concerns.

The physiologic adherence (physiologic phimosis) resolves spontaneously, but may remain present for several years. Texts suggest that most physiologic phimosis resolves by age of 3–5 years, such that the glans penis can be fully exposed (Walker, 1992). In the authors' experience, limited adherence of little significance may remain for years longer. In a longitudinal study, Oster (1968) reported that physiologic phimosis in school-aged boys resolved over time (Table 8.1).

Physiological phimosis should be distinguished from pathologic or true phimosis. Physiologic phimosis exists when the adherence between the inner prepuce and glans penis persists as filmy attachments. True phimosis occurs when the foreskin cannot be retracted after it has been previously retractable, if there is a densely thickened prepuce that will not retract, or one that remains non-retractile after a patient has completed pubertal development.

The easiest way to differentiate physiologic phimosis from pathologic phimosis is careful examination. Forceful separation of foreskin adherence is not recommended because of pain and trauma to the patient, but gentle proximal traction of the foreskin may enable one to differentiate between normal and abnormal. If the foreskin retracts part way and then lays flat against the glans penis and effaces or thins, the remaining attachments are likely to be physiologic and more time is required for natural separation to occur. If, when the foreskin is retracted to the point of attachment, and there is a thickened, rolled edge this is likely to be pathologic phimosis due to scarring and inflammation (Fig. 8.1). This is unlikely to resolve on its own and may require circumcision.

Ballooning of the foreskin during voiding is often associated with true phimosis as well. There have been recent studies suggesting that steroids applied to the prepuce and glans penis will help to separate physiologic adhesions, aiding in the resolution of this diagnostic dilemma (Chu *et al.*, 1999).

Questions often arise about the care of the uncircumcised penis. The genital area should be cleaned as any other skin area and the foreskin may gently be retracted to the extent allowable without discomfort for cleaning. Forcible retraction may result in tearing of the foreskin meatus, inflammation, and secondary scarring leading to true phimosis.

Post-circumcision phimosis (entrapped penis)

Following routine neonatal circumcision with any standard circumcision clamp, an unusual type of secondary phimosis can develop. Since the circumcision scar is circumferential, and the process of wound healing involves contracture, this may cause narrowing of the shaft skin at the circumcision site. If the circumcision site is mobile and sufficient inner foreskin remains, the circumcision site can migrate distally over the glans and begin to contract in this position (Fig. 8.2). This contraction and scarring may be tight enough that the glans penis can no longer be seen and occasionally urinary flow may be restricted. This type of phimosis (penile entrapment, secondary phimosis) can often be avoided by firmly seating the bell of the newborn clamp at the coronal margin so that there is not redundant inner prepuce remaining which might let the circumcision scar ride distally over the coronal margin. This seems to be a more common problem in young boys with an abundant pubic fat pad who may not be candidates for circumcision in the first place (Fig. 8.3). If secondary phimosis is discovered early after circumcision, aggressive foreskin retraction by stretching the ring with a hemostat dilates the scar

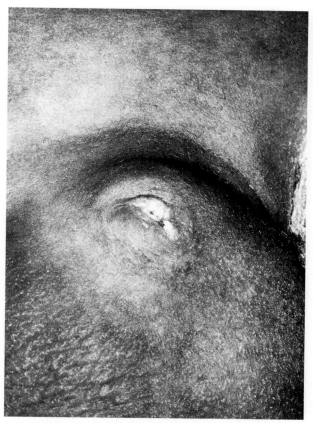

Figure 8.3 Severe penile entrapment. This required incision of the phimotic ring in two locations followed by horizontal closure of the vertical incision lines.

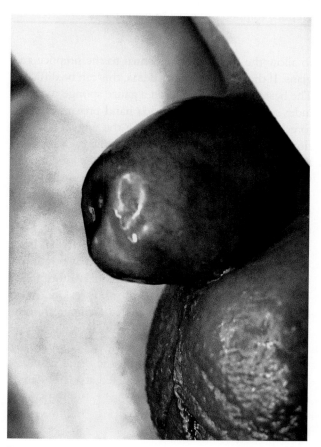

Figure 8.2 Entrapped penis following circumcision (secondary phimosis).

and the need for later revision of the circumcision is avoided. In other cases, the phimotic ring may be anaesthetized and snipped in the office, incising vertically and closing horizontally to create a wider circumference. This may not resolve the problem in all patients and formal circumcision revision may be necessary in some, tailoring the inner foreskin length so that the circumcision scar cannot migrate past the coronal margin; occasionally, removal of more shaft skin becomes necessary.

Penile glanular adhesions (skin bridges)

After newborn circumcision, the glans epithelium is denuded owing to separation of the physiologic adherence with the foreskin. The circumcision site is also a raw surface and if the glans epithelium and the circumcision site rest together for a prolonged period a postsurgical adhesion may form (Fig. 8.4). These are dense adhesions that cannot be teased apart in the

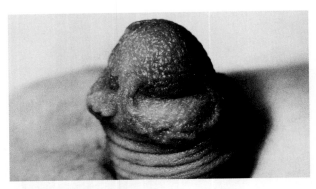

Figure 8.4 Postcircumcision skin bridges.

office. These adhesions usually occur as 'skin bridges' so that an instrument tip can be passed underneath them, and their blood supply comes from both the shaft skin and the glans. Surgical division of such skin bridges is required.

This usually requires some sort of analgesic agent, which may be EMLA® cream, or a local injection in the office, or if more extensive, general anesthesia. After appropriate analgesia, a hemostat is used to crush the bridge near the glans and the adhesion is divided with scissors, rotating the blade and cutting the skin bridge nearly flush with the glans epithelium. Sometimes a second cut flush with the shaft skin is necessary for good cosmesis. It is important not to cut the skin bridge in the middle because this often leaves a skin tag of shaft skin on the glans penis which is a noticeable cosmetic problem. Suturing may or may not be required. Ointment is then placed on the penis twice daily for 7–10 days; gently retracting the shaft skin prevents the two edges from coming into contact to re-form the adhesion.

Paraphimosis

Paraphimosis is the term applied when the foreskin has been retracted and cannot then be brought back over the glans penis (Fig. 8.5). This may happen after the foreskin has been forcefully separated for the first time, disrupting the preputial adherence to the glans. In the hospital this often occurs when the foreskin is retracted for the placement of an indwelling catheter. Once the catheter has been secured, medical personnel neglect to replace the foreskin over the glans penis. With the tight foreskin proximal to the glans penis, venous congestion leads to progressive swelling. When paraphimosis is recognized it is imperative that the foreskin be immediately placed back over the glans

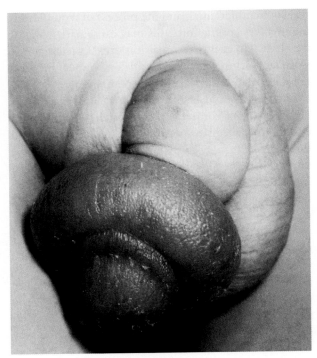

Figure 8.5 Paraphimosis with edematous, discolored prepuce trapped proximal to glans penis.

to allow the blood flow to return to the prepuce and glans. If there is significant edema, this can be difficult. The best technique is to hold a gauze sponge with the index and third fingers of each hand proximal to the foreskin, with the gauze covering the fingers for traction. The thumbs push the glans penis back through the paraphimotic ring between the other four fingers that are supporting it. A minute or two of steady pressure may be required to decompress the glans and force the foreskin edema proximally to allow the glans to suddenly slip through to the paraphimotic ring. Placing ice on the penis before this procedure has been advocated and a penile anesthetic block may be administered before the manual reduction. Additionally, infiltration of the edematous foreskin with hyaluronidase has been reported to facilitate decompression (DeVries, 1996). If manual reduction is unsuccessful, a dorsal slit of the tight preputial ring will restore venous drainage from the distal tissue. A formal circumcision can be completed at a later date if necessary.

Meatal stenosis

Stenosis of the urethral meatus may occasionally be associated with hypospadias, but seems to be largely an acquired problem of circumcised boys. Recurrent meatitis or meatal inflammation secondary to prolonged exposure of the meatus to the moist and irritating environment of the diaper (ammoniacal dermatitis) or other inflammatory skin diseases can induce this problem. In the former, the delicate meatal skin edges lose their superficial epithelial lining when inflamed, and, as a result, become adherent in a side-to-side fashion. This almost always occurs ventrally and progresses dorsally, and boys are left with a small or even pinpoint meatus at the apex of the glans. Some authors have suggested that the advent of disposable diapers has led to an increasing prevalence of this problem since the 1980s. The occurrence of meatal stenosis is distinctly unusual in an uncircumcised boy and therefore is best considered a potential side-effect of circumcision.

Causes beyond simple irritation that can induce strictures of the meatus include: prior hypospadias repair or other penile surgery, prolonged urethral catheterization, trauma, or balanitis xerotica obliterans (BXO). These diagnoses are often apparent on examination or when reviewing the child's history. BXO induces a characteristic whitish circumferential discoloration of much of the glans and may induce a narrowing of the urethra extending more proximal than simple irritative meatal stenosis. BXO is also more difficult to treat.

Normal meatal caliber based on age has been reported in boys. In general, a boy under the age of 1 year should have a meatus that easily accepts a 5 Fr feeding tube. Between the ages of 1 and 6 years this increases to at least an 8 Fr size. It can be difficult to estimate meatal size accurately when inspecting this visually. However, gentle lateral traction on the meatal edges to open the meatus side to side reveals the typical fused appearance of the ventral edges, confirming some degree of stenosis. On the other hand, if normal urethral mucosa can be everted, meatal size is probably adequate. Final confirmation is obtained by observing voiding. There is a characteristic dorsal deflection of the stream due to a ventral lip of scar tissue as a result of fusion of the meatal edges. The patient also demonstrates a very fine-caliber, forceful stream with a long voiding distance. This is due to the acute decrease in the size of the lumen of the urethra distally and the secondary accelerated velocity of the urine. Some patients will learn to direct their penis towards their feet during voiding so that the stream will enter the toilet bowl, while others seem not to catch on and miss the bowl entirely.

Meatal stenosis is uncommonly diagnosed prior to a boy becoming toilet trained. There may be intermittent dysuria with discomfort at the tip of the glans and occasional blood spotting in the underwear due to recurrent inflammation at the meatus. Patients with meatal stenosis demonstrate a prolonged voiding time and some boys decide that it is simpler to sit during voiding rather than try to direct their streams while standing. It should be noted that meatal stenosis is an unlikely cause of recurring urinary tract infection (UTI) or true obstruction to the lower urinary tract. When the history, penile examination, and observation of the urinary stream suggest meatal stenosis no further diagnostic evaluation is required.

When any of the above symptoms are present, and voiding is characteristic, treatment of meatal stenosis is generally warranted. Simple dilation of the urethral meatus will often result in tearing of the skin edges and a high rate of recurrent stenosis. Urethral meatotomy is, therefore, the preferred method of treatment. Meatotomy is a very simple procedure in which one prong of a hemostat is inserted within the urethral meatus and directed toward the ventrum and midline of the glans a few millimeters proximal to the stenotic pinpoint meatus. The glans is engaged and the skin edges crushed together for 1–2 min. Once the clamp is removed, fine scissors are used to incise the ventral midline, thus reopening the meatus (Fig. 8.6). The

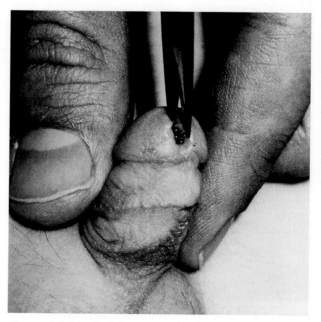

Figure 8.6 Vertical incision for meatotomy following 60 s of clamping with a hemostat.

crushed skin remains together, generating appropriate hemostasis.

Options exist in terms of analgesic techniques for meatotomy. The procedure may be performed under a general anesthetic in the operating room as a quick and simple outpatient procedure; however, this is generally not necessary. Some urologists have performed this procedure in an office setting by injecting a small amount of lidocaine with epinephrine directly into the ventral meatal skin using a small-caliber needle. This provides analgesia and hemostasis. However, most boys will not tolerate this since the injection is distinctly uncomfortable.

More recently, the authors have reported using topical EMLA cream (eutectic mixture of local anesthetics) applied over the entire glans to anesthetize the meatus and perimeatal skin for urethral meatotomy (Cartwright *et al.*, 1996; Brown *et al.*, 1997). Others have recently reported a similar use for EMLA cream (Hoebeke *et al.*, 1997). At the time of writing, the authors have performed urethral meatotomy in the office using EMLA cream in 226 patients. The EMLA cream is applied liberally over the entire glans, especially on the ventrum. It is secured in place with an occlusive dressing and left in contact with the glans skin for 1–1.5 h before the procedure (Fig. 8.7).

The cream is removed and the meatotomy is completed. The vast majority of patients will experience no discomfort when EMLA cream is used with this technique. Occasionally, there will be a sensation of 'pressure' when the hemostat is clamped. In an occasional patient the EMLA cream may be supplemented with a small amount of injected lidocaine with epinephrine, which seems to be minimally uncomfortable when given following EMLA. One patient required a suture on each side of the meatotomy for oozing from the meatal edges following the procedure.

Patient tolerance of the procedure overall is quite good as long as a caring and patient approach is taken to reassure boys before and during the procedure. The room is quiet with minimal lighting and parents bring some of the child's books and hand-held toys for the waiting period after the EMLA is applied. Parents stay in the room during the procedure and this further reassures the child. The authors have chosen, based on parental preference and patient personality, to use midazolam hydrochoride as an anxiolytic with good results in 23 patients. However, the general observation has been that midazolam is unnecessary for the majority of patients.

Following meatotomy, it is crucial to keep the edges of the meatus separated so that restenosis does not occur. Immediately following meatotomy, while still in the office, the parent is shown how to apply antibiotic ointment within the meatus. The parent then continues this at home, using one hand to separate the meatus while the other index finger is used to place a small amount of ointment directly into the meatus. This is performed twice daily for the first 2 weeks and then once daily for another 4 weeks. Alternatively, a small tube of ophthalmic ointment (Lacrilube) may be used as a meatal dilator. A small amount of the ointment is extruded from the metal tip for lubrication and the tip is then passed within the meatus. It is of appropriate size to serve as a dilator for most boys undergoing meatotomy. The use of meatal dilation may be helpful in certain cases if readherence of meatal edges is problematic, but the authors do not feel that it is routinely required.

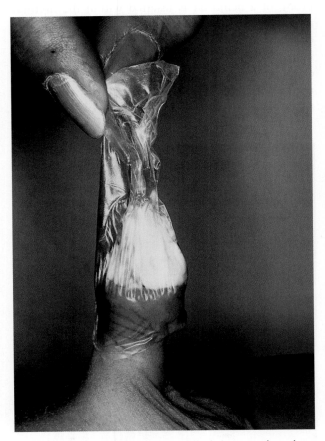

Figure 8.7 EMLA cream is applied over entire glans prior to meatotomy. This remains for at least 60 min before the procedure.

Patients may be expected to experience mild dysuria for the first 1–2 days postoperatively. It has generally been helpful to have them take ibuprofen or acetaminophen 2 hours prior to the procedure to decrease discomfort. Boys at the age of 3 or 4 years may respond to meatotomy by holding their urine for prolonged periods. Placing them in a warm tub often stimulates voiding in this circumstance. One value of keeping ointment over the meatal edges is that it functions as a barrier to shield the surface from the passage of urine and the resulting discomfort. It should also be noted that increasing the fluid intake for the first day or two following the procedure dilutes the urine and leads to less dysuria. Minor blood spotting in the underwear following meatotomy is common for 1–2 days. Printed handouts are given to parents with these recommendations and they are warned of the risk for restenosis when the instructions are not followed. In addition, boys who remain wet following meatotomy, from either still being in a diaper or having problems with persistent incontinence, are at risk for redeveloping stenosis based on recurrent inflammation of the meatus. This group may not be candidates for treatment until dryness is achieved. Two out of 226 patients seen by the authors required a second meatotomy. Over the same period that they have used EMLA cream for analgesia, the authors have chosen to perform meatotomy in the operating room in three boys because of patient behavioral issues including extreme attention deficient disorder. As experience has been gained it has become apparent that midazolam works well in the moderately, overactive, anxious, or difficult young boy, and meatotomy in the operating room should be reserved for the patient with BXO or posthypospadias meatal stenosis.

Non-neonatal circumcision

The pros and cons of newborn circumcision have been and will continue to be debated. Less discussion surrounds circumcision after the newborn period, when it is estimated that 1 in 100 uncircumcised boys will require circumcision (Bloom *et al.*, 1992). During childhood the most common indication for circumcision is phimosis. This develops because of preputial irritation leading to inflammation, scarring, and thickening of the preputial opening so that the foreskin cannot retract. Hygiene then becomes a problem and, occasionally, this process is so severe

that urine flow is affected and the preputial sac dilates with urine dribbling out after voiding. In some patients with chronic skin irritation and inflammation, fissures of the prepuce develop. This makes spontaneous erections and retraction of the foreskin painful and discomfort occasionally awakens the patient during sleep. Steroid ointments may reduce inflammation, but circumcision is indicated if fissures persist.

Balanoposthitis is an infection of the glans and preputial sac. This infection occurs uncommonly, but can be painful. Skin flora are usually the predominant organisms found on culture. If the balanoposthitis is mild, sitz baths and topical antibiotic ointment (bacitracin) may be sufficient. If cellulitis and fever are present, then a systemic antibiotic (cephalexin) is added. The first episode of balanoposthitis is not a mandatory indication for circumcision. Recurrent episodes strengthen the argument for circumcision. Penile hygiene should be reviewed with the parents and patient.

UTIs are more common in uncircumcised boys, especially during the first 6 months of life. Some consider a UTI in a boy an indication for circumcision. After 1 year of age the increased risk for UTI in the uncircumcised male diminishes.

Penile cancer is known to be prevented by newborn circumcision. It is thought that the development of penile cancer closely correlates with penile hygiene, and in developed countries, where hygiene is good, the rate of penile cancer is very low regardless of circumcision status. Since penile cancer is very uncommon, the likelihood of a serious circumcision complication may be higher than the eventual possibility of penile cancer.

Occasionally, trauma to the prepuce leads to circumcision. Zipper trauma is the most common occurrence. Usually, with local anesthesia, the zipper can be dislodged by simple advancement or at times by cutting the median bar of the zipper, thereby allowing the teeth to separate. Occasionally, circumcision may be warranted acutely.

After the newborn period the indications for circumcision are relatively few. Circumcision is performed under general anesthesia after the newborn period, although a recent report documents the use of local blocks and circumcision in boys beyond this period (Jayanthi *et al.*, 1999). Depending on the age of the patient and the size of the penis, surgical excision and suturing or newborn clamps may be used. The procedure is usually successful with low complication rates and is performed on an outpatient basis. Recovery is generally prompt, with the older patients experiencing more discomfort and having a longer recovery period.

Genital holding

Children who hold or clutch their genitalia are often of concern to their parents. This behavior begins shortly after toilet training and may last through the prepubertal years. It is more common in boys than girls. In boys, some degree of genital holding is almost universal. This behavior is thought to have no significant sexual or psychological implications, (Caldamone *et al.*, 1996) is thought to be normal and does not warrant any diagnostic studies. Seldom is there any underlying physical cause and evaluation beyond physical examination and urinalysis is not warranted. The best advice for parents is to have them redirect the child's attention without placing great emphasis on this behavior. Generally, over time, children learn more acceptable public behavior without the apparent preoccupation for genital holding. Occasionally, very persistent holders may be told that the behavior may make others uncomfortable, and that for this reason, if they must hold themselves, they should do this in private. Parental education and reassurance is the best course of management.

Female-specific problems

Urethral prolapse

The circumferential eversion of urethral mucosa through the urethral meatus in girls is termed urethral prolapse. It is associated with vascular congestion and possible strangulation of the prolapsed tissue. It is possible to have a partial or incomplete prolapse, but complete urethral prolapse is more common (Shah and Tunnesen, 1995). The etiology of urethral prolapse is unclear. Suggested causes include: poor attachment between the inner longitudinal and outer circular and oblique smooth muscle layers of the urethra associated with antecedent episodes of increased abdominal pressure, mucosal redundancy and vaginal mucosal atrophy, estrogen deficiency leading to lax periurethral fascia, neuromuscular disorders, urethral malposition, increased width of the urethra, poor bladder support, and deficient elastic tissues (Kleinjan and Vos, 1996). Predisposing valsalva maneuvers

such as chronic coughing, asthma, and constipation, as well as UTI and trauma have been reported (Kamat *et al.*, 1969; Jerkins *et al.*, 1984; Lowe *et al.*, 1986; Fernandes *et al.*, 1993).

Urethral prolapse is often misdiagnosed as the cause of urogenital bleeding in girls. The correct diagnosis at presentation has been reported at only 21% (Anveden-Hertzberg *et al.*, 1995). It is important to recognize that prolapse appears as a doughnut-shaped mass protruding at the vulva (Fig. 8.8). The mucosa is edematous, friable, bright red, or blue–black. As time goes on it may become infected, ulcerated, necrotic, or gangrenous (Shah and Tunnessen, 1995). The differential diagnosis of urethral prolapse includes: a prolapsing ectopic ureterocele, prolapsed urethral polyp, ectopic ureter, prolapsed bladder, urethral cyst, hydrometrocolpos, condyloma acuminatum, sarcoma botryoides, and periurethral abscess. The diagnosis of urethral prolapse is visual and based on the typical circumferential appearance of the lesion around the meatus. None of

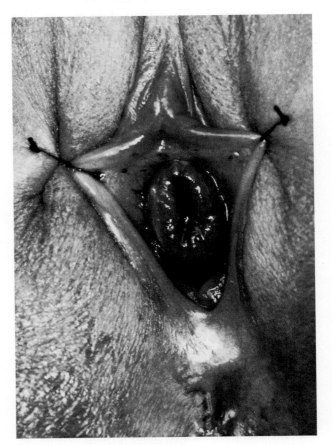

Figure 8.8 Urethral prolapse: note the doughnut appearance with urethral meatus centrally.

the other stated conditions has a similar appearance. At times, diagnostic confirmation is made by placing a catheter or an instrument tip demonstrating that the urethra is actually in the center of the edematous tissue. Imaging studies are not necessary, but a VCUG can show a narrow, distal urethra (Potter, 1971). The age range at diagnosis in pediatric series is from 5 days to 11 years, with a mean of 4.5–6 years (Richardson *et al.*, 1982; Bullock, 1983; Jerkins *et al.*, 1984; Anveden-Hertzberg *et al.*, 1995; Fernandes *et al.*, 1993). Urethral prolapse has been reported in identical twins (Mitre *et al.*, 1987). There is a significant preponderance of urethral prolapse in patients of African descent, with reports being 90% or greater (Jerkins *et al.*, 1984; Rock and Azziz, 1987; Anveden-Hertzberg *et al.*, 1995).

In addition to bleeding, symptoms include dysuria or frequency in 25% (Richardson *et al.*, 1982; Jerkins *et al.*, 1984; Fernandis *et al.*, 1993; Anveden-Hertzberg *et al.*, 1995). Nine per cent of the patients are asymptomatic, with the urethral mucosa showing no tenderness (Fernandes *et al.*, 1993; Shah and Tunnessen, 1995). Urogenital bleeding due to urethral prolapse may be mistaken for a vaginal source (Richardson *et al.*, 1982; Jerkins *et al.*, 1984; Fernandes *et al.*, 1993; Trotman and Brewster, 1993; Anveden-Hertzberg *et al.*, 1995).

Treatment options vary for urethral prolapse. Simple options may be tried first, including observation alone, topical antibiotic ointment, topical estrogen cream, and sitz baths. Surgical treatments include primary excision, reduction and catheterization, and suture ligation of the prolapsed tissue over a catheter, and in adult women cryoablation has been reported (Friedrich, 1977). Most published series recommend conservative therapy (Redman, 1982; Richardson *et al.*, 1982; Jerkins *et al.*, 1984; Carlson *et al.*, 1987; Trotman and Breuster, 1993; Anveden-Hertzberg *et al.*, 1995). Surgical treatment should be reserved for those rare instances of recurrence or persistent, symptomatic prolapse (Richardson *et al.*, 1982; Jerkins *et al.*, 1984; Trotman and Brewster, 1993; Anveden-Hertzberg *et al.*, 1995; Kleinjan and Vos, 1996).

Labial adherence

Labial adherence, midline fusion of the labia minora, is a common acquired lesion in young girls. Before puberty the labia minora are covered with a thin hypoestrogenized epithelium (Rock and Azziz, 1987; Starr, 1996). An irritating event, such as infection,

trauma, or inflammation, causes the area to become denuded and inflamed, and the medial labial surfaces adhere with a fibrinous exudate over their surfaces (Rock and Azziz, 1987). Perhaps the most common inciting event is ammoniacal irritation. Adherence generally begins posteriorly and progresses anteriorly, leaving a small opening for the urine just inferior to the glans clitoris (Clair and Caldamone, 1988) (Fig. 8.9). Occasionally the process begins near the clitoris, forming a 'preputial fusion' (Rock and Azziz, 1987). Labial adherence is also known as labial adhesions, labial agglutination, gynatresia, vulvar fusion, coalescence of the labia minora, vulvar synechiae, labial fusion, and occlusion of the vaginal vestibule. Differential diagnosis includes scarring of the labia minora, imperforate hymen, vaginal agenesis, clitoral hypertrophy, and intersex disorders (Starr, 1996).

Labial adherence is fairly common and accounts for a large number of the genital abnormalities seen in

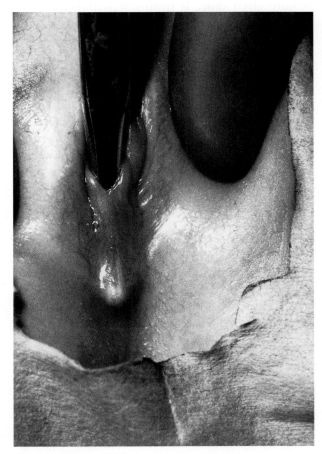

Figure 8.9 Labial adhesions characterized by fusion of the labia minora. There is generally a small opening anteriorly.

girls. The peak incidence is between birth and 2 years old and again around the age of 6–7 years, although fusion can be seen until puberty (Clair and Caldamone, 1988; Starr, 1996). Most girls with fused labia are asymptomatic but some have a deflected urinary stream or vaginal pooling of urine. Dysuria, generally secondary to the underlying inflammatory process, may be a persistent complaint. Patients may present with the diagnosis of UTI (Clair and Caldamone, 1988); however, the suspected infection may simply be a contaminated specimen, as urine pools beneath the fused labia before exiting. True adhesion of the labia can occur in sexually abused girls with an incidence of approximately 3% (Muram, 1988; Starr, 1996). This scarring is often thick and irregular in texture, and involves deeper layers (McCann *et al.*, 1988).

Treatment of adherent labia minora is not routinely required. Parents and referring primary-care physicians should be reassured that they will lyse spontaneously given time. If treatment is thought to be necessary, estrogen cream can be applied daily, with successful separation reported to be as high as 90% at 8 weeks (Starr, 1996). The side-effects of the estrogen cream will include vulvar pigmentation in all patients and breast tenderness in 6% that resolves after the estrogen therapy is discontinued (Clair and Caldamone, 1988). However, the long-term effects of estrogen given to prepubertal girls are unknown and treatment beyond 2 weeks is probably unwarranted. Persisting adherence can be separated in the office using topical anesthetic (EMLA) and gentle, blunt separation (Rock and Azziz, 1987; Clair and Caldamone, 1988; Starr, 1996). An oral anxiolytic should be considered in such girls for this procedure. Following separation, daily separation of the labia with application of a water soluble ointment should be continued indefinitely to prevent recurrence (Clair and Caldamone, 1988; Starr, 1996). Forceful separation without analgesia not recommended.

Vaginal cysts

Introital cysts are uncommon but may be found in the newborn period, possibly as a consequence of stimulation by maternal estrogens. They are usually single and between 1 and 3 cm in diameter. When recognized in newborns, evaluation should include passage of a catheter or instrument into the vaginal introitus to assure patency. Rarely, ultrasonography may be necessary to ensure that the vagina is normal and

not obstructed. These cysts almost always rupture spontaneously or resolve over a few weeks and need no further treatment.

Gartner's duct cyst

Gartner's duct is the distal rudimentary portion of the wolffian (mesonephric) duct in girls. These ducts in girls usually regress and almost completely disappear. If remnants persist they are found along the anterolateral walls of the vagina. Flat, cuboidal cells line the cyst (Klein *et al.*, 1986). Gartner's duct cysts present as a perivaginal mass and usually appear in infants (Muram and Jerkins, 1988). These cysts can be large enough to protrude from the vaginal introitus or fill the vagina and block its opening (Gallup and Talledo, 1987; Muram and Jerkins, 1988). The cyst membrane is usually very thin and lined with epithelium. They are generally asymptomatic, although they may become infected if they persist into the sexually active years. Treatment consists of marsupialization within the vaginal vault (Muram and Jerkins, 1988).

Müllerian duct cyst

Müllerian duct cysts are remnants of non-fused portions of the Müllerian ducts. They are generally asymptomatic and do not usually cause problems until menarche. After menarche they may fill with fluid or menstrual discharge and cause symptoms such as a visible or palpable introital or abdominal mass, dyspareunia, voiding disturbances, vaginal discharge, or pain. Ultrasound shows a fluid-filled structure between the uterus and bladder. Treatment consists of drainage into the vagina to prevent reaccumulation (Gallup and Talledo, 1987). A blind-ending sac filled with mucinous fluid or blood that has the same lining as the vagina is found at surgery.

Epithelial inclusion cyst

Most epithelial inclusion cysts are remnants of the urogenital sinus. Following trauma or surgery, buried vulvar or vaginal epithelium may also cause epithelial inclusion cysts. These are rare in children, although not uncommon in older women (Klein *et al.*, 1986). They usually occur posteriorly and in the midline of the vagina (Beazley, 1977). The cysts contain thick, caseous material with a squamous epithelium lining their inner surface (Klein *et al.*, 1986). Surgical excision is the treatment of choice (Gallup and Talledo, 1987).

Hydrocolpos

Distension of the vagina with fluid or mucous secretions is called hydrocolpos. If the uterus is involved the term is hydrometrocolpos. In newborns the secretions are due to maternal estrogen stimulation of the uterus and cervical glands. The vagina can be obstructed from an imperforate hymen, transverse vaginal septum, or atretic vaginal introitus (Nussbaum and Lebowitz, 1983). This produces a bulging, shiny, pearly gray protuberance observed over the vaginal introitus (Nussbaum and Lebowitz, 1983; Muram and Jerkins, 1988). The urethral meatus can be noted anterior to the mass (Fig. 8.10). Large abdominal masses can be palpable or identified on ultrasonography. Occasionally, urinary retention can be due to the mass effect. Ultrasonography shows a retrovesical oval cystic mass occasionally causing hydroureteronephrosis (Patel *et al.*, 1992). Treatment consists of drainage of the obstructed vagina perineally, but occasionally temporary abdominal vaginostomy may be necessary.

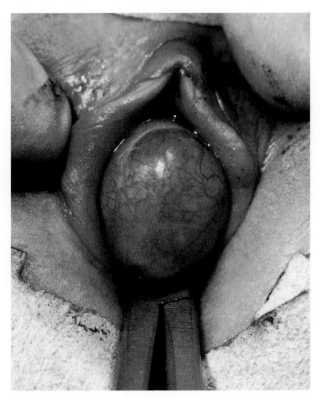

Figure 8.10 Hydrocolpos with duplicated vagina. The urethral meatus is seen splayed above the bulging mass while the hemostat is placed in the patent (second) vaginal opening.

Other interlabial masses

Paraurethral cysts are known to occur along the distal one-third of the urethrovaginal wall (Klein *et al.*, 1986). The urethral meatus can be displaced causing compression and a deflected urinary stream or dysuria. These cysts are lined with transitional epithelial cells and usually rupture spontaneously (Nussbaum and Lebowitz, 1983; Emans and Goldstein, 1990).

Rhabdomyosarcoma of the vagina (sarcoma botryoides) is the most common primary malignancy involving the vagina, uterus, and bladder in children. It has an appearance of a cluster of grapes extruding through the introitus. Radiographic imaging is necessary to evaluate tumor size, location, and metastatic disease status (Nussbaum and Lebowitz, 1983). Other interlabial masses can include prolapsing ectopic ureteroceles, condyloma acuminatum, and benign urethral polyps (Duckman *et al.*, 1984; Gallup and Talledo, 1987; Klee *et al.*, 1993).

Vaginal disorders

It is helpful to understand the changes in the vagina from birth to puberty. The neonatal vagina is sterile with an alkaline pH (Danesh *et al.*, 1995). During the first several weeks of life the vagina is under maternal estrogen stimulation which causes the pH to decrease to around 4.8 and colonize with Döderlein's bacilli (Jenny, 1992; Danesh *et al.*, 1995). During the maternal estrogen stimulation period the vagina is lined by stratified squamous epithelial cells (Judson and Ehret, 1994). After approximately 3–6 weeks of life, estrogen stimulation diminishes until menarche. The vaginal pH returns to neutral and bacterial colonization diminishes (Jenny, 1992; Danesh *et al.*, 1995). The vaginal lining changes to cuboidal epithelial cells which then return to squamous epithelial cells at puberty (Judson and Ehret, 1994).

Vaginitis

Vulvovaginitis is the most common cause of vaginal bleeding in the pediatric age group (Fishman and Paldi, 1991). Vulvitis is vulvar irritation secondary to trauma, topical allergens, mechanical irritation, chemical irritation, or poor hygiene (Jenny, 1992). Vaginitis is erythema and inflammation of the vaginal mucosa generally associated with discharge. Vulvovaginitis is very often a self-limiting problem and immediate work-up is not necessary. As the symptoms persist or become more annoying, work-up should include sampling of the vaginal pool for pH, wet mount, potassium hydroxide swab, and examination for chlamydia and gonorrhea. A urinalysis with culture may be diagnostic. If specific treatment is desired a definitive diagnosis must be made (Fishman and Paldi, 1991). Vaginal cultures may be helpful and are more reliable if two confirmatory tests are completed (Judson and Ehret, 1994). Non-infectious causes in infants and children should be investigated, including ruling out the presence of a vaginal foreign body. Foreign body vaginitis symptoms are similar to other types of vaginitis. Toilet paper remnants are the most common objects found in the vagina. Vaginal symptoms can arise from psychosomatic illnesses such as school phobia, guilt about sexual activity, or fear of sterility (Brown, 1989; Rosenfeld and Clark, 1989; Emans and Godstein, 1990; Strasburger, 1990; Sparks, 1991).

Non-specific vulvovaginitis

Non-specific vulvovaginitis refers to a non-purulent, non-odorous discharge with a neutral pH and normal flora on wet mount. It accounts for 25–75% of all vulvovaginitis seen in premenarchal girls (Emans and Goldstein, 1990). The etiology includes poor hygiene, urinary soiling, tight clothing, or chemical irritants such as harsh soaps. When testing is normal, treatment consists of reassurance and encouragement of good hygiene and appropriate clothing.

Newborn physiologic leukorrhea

It is normal for newborn girls under maternal estrogen stimulation to have a vaginal discharge. It is usually clear with white–gray mucus not associated with odor or irritation. Wet mount shows numerous epithelial cells without pathogenic bacteria or leukocytes. The discharge diminishes once maternal estrogen stimulation subsides. The tendency towards treatment with vaginal creams and antibiotics should be discouraged.

Genital infections in the young

Chlamydia trachomatis

A chlamydia infection is caused by *Chlamydia trachomatis*, which is an obligate intracellular Gram-negative organism capable of infecting the atrophic cuboidal epithelium of the prepubertal, non-estrogenized vagina (Jenny, 1992). Chlamydia is a common sexually transmitted disease in sexually active adoles-

cents and adults. Young children may acquire chlamydia by passing through an infected birth canal or by sexual abuse. In newborns, chlamydia may infect the conjunctiva, pharynx, vagina, or anus. It is estimated that 50–75% of newborns become infected if their mothers were infected with chlamydia (Hammerschlag, 1994). The organism may persist for as long as 3 years, making positive cultures in young children difficult to interpret (Jenny, 1992; Hammerschlag, 1994). It is estimated that 2–13% of sexually abused children have rectogenital chlamydia infections (Ingram *et al.*, 1984; Hammerschlag, 1994). Chlamydial infections may be asymptomatic or present with a mucopurulent vaginal discharge or urethritis. When suspected, the diagnosis should be confirmed by culture inoculation on 0.2 M sucrose–phosphate-buffered transport medium and either cultured immediately or stored at –80°C until cultured. Non-culture tests used in adults, such as enzymes immunoassay, direct fluorescent antibody tests, or DNA probes should not be used for rectal or vaginal sites in children owing to poor test sensitivity and specificity (Jenny, 1992; Hammerschlag, 1994). Treatment of chlamydia consists of erythromycin or tetracycline. Tetracycline is generally not used in children younger than 8 years or until their permanent teeth are established. Single-dose azithromycin may be used in boys and non-pregnant girls.

Gonorrhea

Gonorrhea is the most common sexually transmitted disease in abused children and is unlikely in children who are not sexually abused (Jenny, 1992; Judson and Ehret, 1994). It is important to recognize gonorrhea to prevent sequelae and to identify the child who is sexually abused. Infants can be contaminated through vaginal secretions in the birth canal colonizing their oropharynx, vagina, and rectum. The infection may remain asymptomatic. However, a white, yellow, or greenish, thick vaginal discharge with odor may be present. Labial erythema, urethral irritation, proctitis, or dysuria may be present. The discharge may not persist even though the gonorrhea does. The gonococcal infection may become symptomatic if a child contracts measles, chicken pox, or scarlet fever (Ingram, 1994). The diagnosis is suspected when Gram-negative, oxidase-positive diplococci are observed. Appropriate culture is mandatory because of the implications of the diagnosis in children. If abuse is suspected, a culture should be obtained from hymenal tissues and the distal vagina even in the absence of symptoms or discharge (Ingram, 1994). Selective media such as Thayer–Martin should be used in incubated temperatures of 34–36°C in 3–10% CO_2 and 70% humidity. If there is doubt, the organism should be sent to a reference laboratory for confirmation. Treatment of asymptomatic individuals is ceftriaxone (25–50 mg/kg i.v./i.m.) in a single dose, not to exceed 125 mg.

Candida

Other than the cutaneous variety associated with diaper rash, yeast infections are more common in adult females than in prepubertal girls. The alkaline vaginal pH of childhood is hostile to yeast (Jenny, 1992). Most yeast vaginitis is caused by *Candida albicans*. Other yeast can cause vaginal infections, including non-albicans *Candida* species, *Torulopsis glabrata*, *Cryptococcus*, and *Saccharomyces*. Candida infections in girls may be due to poor hygiene with transfer of the organisms from the gastrointestinal tract to the vagina (Strasburger, 1990). However, most often they are secondary to such predisposing host factors as depressed cellular immunity or antibiotic use, especially broad-spectrum antibiotics effective against lactobacillus, such as cephalosporins, ampicillin, and tetracycline. Usually there is vulvar erythema and edema, minimal vaginal soreness, non-odorous discharge, pruritus, dysuria, and epithelial fissures. Sometimes there is a whitish discharge adherent to the erythematous mucosa of the introitus. Few young patients exhibit the classic thick 'cottage-cheese' discharge seen in adult women. In infants and young girls a perineal rash with classic satellite lesions is common. The vaginal pH is less than 4.5 and 10% KOH preparation identifies budding yeast and hyphae. Treatment includes imidazole, miconazole, or clotrimazole applied topically.

Bacterial vaginosis

Less commonly, vaginal infections can be due to bacteria and are often listed as non-specific or *Gardnerella* vaginitis. This is now recognized to be caused by a mixed flora including anaerobic bacteria such as the *Gardnerella* species and other organisms including *Mycoplasma*, *Bacteroides*, *Peptostreptococcus*, *Peptococcus*, *Eubacterium*, *Prevotella*, and *Mobiluncus* species. Prior to infection, the normal lactobacillus is replaced by increased numbers of *Gardnerellae*. Bacterial vaginosis generally affects adult women. However, it can rarely be found in prepubertal girls and has been noted in increased prevalence in girls who have been sexually abused (Hammerschlag *et al.*, 1985). Physical signs include a thin, homogeneous, malodorous discharge. Laboratory investigations demonstrate a pH of greater than 4.5, clue cells (vaginal epithelial cells with ill-defined margins caused by bacteria on the surface), and positive whiff test (a fishy odor with 10% KOH). Culture is seldom helpful because of the mixed flora origin (Rosenfeld and Clark, 1989). Treatment is metronidazole and clindamycin, ampicillin, or amoxicillin. For older adolescents intervaginal therapies include chlorhexidine suppositories, vaginal metronidazole, or clindamycin for treatment failures (Faro, 1991; Biswas, 1993).

Trichomonas

Trichomonas is a common cause of vaginitis in sexually active women and rarely a cause of neonatal infection (Danesh *et al.*, 1995). Prevalence increases with numbers of sexual partners and level of sexual activity (Rosenfeld and Clark, 1989; Heine and McGregor, 1993). Premenarchal girls are unlikely to become infected because of their alkaline vaginal pH (Danesh *et al.*, 1995). Vaginal secretions in the birth canal can contaminate the nasopharynx and vagina of newborns (Jenny, 1992; Danesh *et al.*, 1995). Vaginitis caused by *Trichomonas vaginalis* leads to a malodorous, frothy, yellow–green discharge with pruritus. Only one-third to one-half of infected patients have the classic findings (Rosenfeld and Clark, 1989; Heine and McGregor, 1993). Other symptoms include dysuria, lower abdominal pain, and vaginal erythema and dyspareunia in sexually active adolescents. Vaginal pH is greater than 4.5 with a positive whiff test with 10% KOH. Metronidazole is the treatment of choice, with clotrimazole intravaginal cream as an alternative treatment for adolescents (Heine and McGregor, 1993).

References

Anveden-Hertzberg L, Gauderer WL, Elder JS (1995) Urethral prolapse: an often misdiagnosed cause of urogenital bleeding in girls. *Pediatr Emerg Care* 11: 212.

Beazley JM (1979) Congenital anomalies of the female genital tract excluding intersex. *Clin Obstet Gynecol* 20: 533.

Biswas MK (1993) Bacterial vaginosis. *Clin Obstet Gynecol* 36: 166.

Bloom DA, Wan J, Key D (1992) Disorders of the male external genitalia and inguinal canal. In: Kelalis PP, King LR, Belman AB (eds) *Clinical pediatric urology*. Philadelphia, PA: WB Saunders, 1015–18.

Brown JL (1989) Hair shampooing technique and pediatric vulvovaginitis. *Pediatrics* **83**: 146.

Brown MR, Cartwright PC, Snow BW (1997) Common office problems in pediatric urology and gynecology. *Pediatr Clin North Am* **44**: 1091–115.

Bullock KN (1983) Strangulated prolapse of female urethra. *Urology* **21**: 46.

Caldamone AA, Schulman S, Rabinowitz R (1996) Outpatient pediatric urology. In: Gillenwater JY, Grayhack JT, Howards SS *et al*. (eds): *Adult and pediatric urology*. St Louis: Mosby-Year Book, 2730–1.

Carlson NJ, Mercer LJ, Hajj SN (1987) Urethral prolapse in the premenarchal female. *Int J Gynecol Obstet* **25**: 69.

Cartwright PC, Snow BW, McNees DC (1996) Office meatotomy utilizing EMLA® cream as the anesthetic. *J Urol* **156**: 857.

Chu C, Chen K, Diau G (1999) Topical steroid treatment of phimosis in boys. *J Urol* **162**: 861.

Clair DL, Caldamone AA (1988) Pediatric office procedures. *Urol Clin North Am* **15**: 715.

Danesh JS, Stephen JM, Gorbach J (1995) Neonatal trichomonas vaginalis infection. *J Emerg Med* **13**: 51.

DeVries C, Miller AK, Packer MG (1996) Reduction of paraphimosis with hyaluronidase. *Urology* **48**: 464–5.

Duckman S, Suarez J, Spitaleri J (1984) Vaginal pregnancy presenting as a suburethral cyst. *Am J Obstet Gynecol* **149**: 572.

Emans SJH, Goldstein DP (1990) *Pediatric and adolescent gynecology*, 3rd edition. Boston, MA: Little, Brown and Co.

Faro S (1991) Bacterial vaginitis. *Clin Obstet Gynecol* **34**: 582.

Fernandes ET, Dekermacher S, Sabadin MA *et al*. (1993) Urethral prolapse in children. *Urology* **41**: 240.

Fishman A, Paldi E (1991) Vaginal bleeding in premenarchal girls: a review. *Obstet Gynecol Survey* **46**: 457.

Friedrich EG (1977) Cryosurgery for urethral prolapse. *Obstet Gynecol* **50**: 359.

Gallup DG, Talledo OE (1987) Benign and malignant tumors. *Clin Obstet Gynecol* **30**: 662.

Hammerschlag MR (1994) *Chlamydia trachomatis* in children. *Pediatr Ann* **23**: 349.

Hammerschlag MR, Cummings M, Doraiswamy B *et al*. (1985) Nonspecific vaginitis following sexual abuse in children. *Pediatrics* **75**: 1028.

Heine P, McGregor JA (1993) Trichomonas vaginalis: a reemerging pathogen. *Clin Obstet Gynecol* **36**: 137.

Hoebeke P, Dupawn P, Van Laecke E *et al*. (1997) The use of EMLA® cream as anaesthetic for minor urological surgery in children. *Acta Urol Belg* **65**: 25–8.

Ingram DL (1994) *Neisseria gonorrhoeae* in children. *Pediatr Ann* **23**: 341.

Ingram DL, Runyan DK, Collins AD *et al*. (1984) Vaginal *Chlamydia trachomatis* infection in children with sexual contact. *Pediatr Infect Dis J* **3**: 97.

Jayanthi VR, Burns JE, Koff SA (1999) Post neonatal circumcision with local anesthesia: a cost-effective alternative. *J Urol* **161**: 1301.

Jenny C (1992) Sexually transmitted diseases and child abuse. *Pediatr Ann* **21**: 497.

Jerkins GR, Verheeck K, Noe HN (1984) Treatment of girls with urethral prolapse. *J Urol* **132**: 732.

Judson FN, Ehret J (1994) Laboratory diagnosis of sexually transmitted infections. *Pediatr Ann* **23**: 361.

Kamat MH, DelGaizo A, Seebode JJ (1969) Urethral prolapse in female children. *Am J Dis Child* **118**: 691.

Klee LW, Rink RC, Gleason PE *et al*. (1993) Urethral polyp presenting as interlabial mass in young girls. *Urology* **41**: 132.

Klein FA, Vick CW, Broecker BH (1986) Neonatal vaginal cysts: diagnosis and management. *J Urol* **135**: 371.

Kleinjan JH, Vos P (1996) Strangulated urethral prolapse. *Urology* **47**: 599.

Lowe FC, Hill GS, Jeffs RD *et al*. (1986) Urethral prolapse in children: Insights into etiology and management. *J Urol* **135**: 100.

McCann J, Voris J, Simon M (1988) Labial adhesions and posterior fourchette injuries in childhood sexual abuse. *Am J Dis Child* **142**: 663.

Mitre A, Nahas W, Gilbert A *et al*. (1987) Urethral prolapse in girls: familial case. *J Urol* **137**: 115.

Muram D (1988) Labial adhesions in sexually abused children. *JAMA* **259**: 352.

Muram D, Jerkins GR (1988) Urinary retention secondary to a Gartner's duct cyst. *Obstet Gynecol* **72**: 510.

Nussbaum AR, Lebowitz RL (1983) Interlabial masses in little girls: review and imaging recommendations. *AJR Am J Roentgenol* **141**: 65.

Oster J (1968) Further fate of the foreskin: incidence of preputial adhesions, phimosis and smegma among Danish schoolboys. *Arch Dis Child* **43**: 200.

Patel VH, Merchant SA, Kedar RP *et al*. (1992) Isolated hydrocolpos: ultrasound findings and the importance of confident preoperative diagnosis. *J Clin Ultrasound* **20**: 85.

Potter BM (1971) Urethral prolapse in girls. *Radiology* **98**: 287.

Redman JF (1982) Conservative management of urethral prolapse in female children. *Urology* **19**: 505.

Richardson DA, Hajj SN, Herbst AL (1982) Medical treatment of urethral prolapse in children. *Obstet Gynecol* **59**: 69.

Rock JA, Azziz R (1987) Genital anomalies in childhood. *Clin Obstet Gynecol* **30**: 682–96.

Rosenfeld WD, Clark J (1989) Vulvovaginitis and cervicitis. *Pediatr Clin North Am* **36**: 489.

Shah BR, Tunnessen WW (1995) Picture of the month. *Arch Pediatr Adolesc Med* **149**: 462.

Sparks JM (1991) Vaginitis. *J Reprod Med* **36**: 745.

Starr NB (1996) Labial adhesions in childhood. *J Pediatr Health Care* **10**: 26.

Strasburger VC (1990) *Basic adolescent gynecology*. Baltimore, MD: Urban and Schwarzenberg.

Trotman MDW, Brewster EM (1993) Prolapse of the urethral mucosa in prepubertal West Indian girls. *Br J Urol* **72**: 503.

Walker RD (1992) Presentation of genitourinary disease and abdominal masses. In: Kelalis PP, King LR, Belman AB (eds) *Clinical pediatric urology*. Philadelphia, PA: WB Saunders, 231.

Pediatric endourology

9

Michael Erhard

Introduction

The field of pediatric endourology, i.e. the endoscopic or percutaneous treatment of pediatric conditions, has expanded as technology has evolved. Many techniques are based on experience gained in the adult population; however, several of these procedures do not have clear-cut advantages when they are adapted to children. Endourology has well-documented beginnings and urologic surgeons have long been innovators. Hopefully, this energy will help to define improved treatment alternatives for the pediatric population. As with anything new, techniques, outcomes, and treatment criteria need to be established before there is widespread acceptance.

The history of cystoscopy began with Nitze who, in 1891, introduced the refined operative cystoscope (Nitze, 1891). His contribution was clearly based on Bozzini who, in 1806, published his ideas on endoscopy for examination of natural openings and cavities. Bozzini's device, called the 'lichtleiter' or light conductor, was to be used in the vagina, nasopharynx, urethra, and rectum, but it lacked optical magnification and had a poorly controllable light source (Bozzini and Lichtleiter, 1806). It is de'Sormeaux who was credited with the first endourologic operation in 1853, when he removed a tumor from the urethra (de'Sormeaux, 1865). Many improvements developed as technology and ideas matured. Arguably, the individual most responsible for the advancement of endourology in the twentieth century is Harold Hopkins. In 1954, Dr Kapany and he published an article reporting the transmission of images along tiny fibers of glass. This was similarly reported by VanHeel, but it was Hopkins and Kapany who refined the technology (Gow, 1998).

Optics: rigid versus fiberoptic

Current rigid optical systems are based on the revolutionary design of the rod lens system in 1959 by

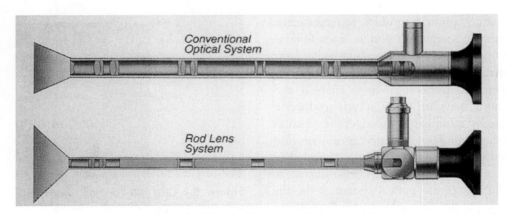

Figure 9.1 Hopkins' rod lens system (*bottom*). This revolutionary design greatly improved endoscopic visualization.

Hopkins (Fig. 9.1). Before this, endoscopic telescopes consisted of a hollow tube with a distal objective lens, an ocular lens, and a series of relay lenses throughout the length of the tube. This particular design resulted in poor image transmission and inadequate transmission of light. Hopkins' rod lens system replaced the hollow air spaces with glass rods. Glass lenses allowed for a much higher refractive index, which enabled more efficient transmission of both light and operative images.

Objective lenses for rigid optic systems are available with angles of view varying from 0° to 120° which allow for complete endoscopic visualization of the urinary tract. After the challenge of the rod lens system was met, the next hurdle was to improve the delivery of light to the endoscopic surgical field. Dr Hopkins devised a fiberoptic bundle to deliver light from the proximal to the distal tip of the endoscope. This is termed an incoherent bundle, in that there is no need for the fibers to correspond in position with one another at both the proximal and distal end. This is in contrast to the organized fibers of a coherent bundle, which is necessary for the precise transmission of the operative image back to the lens. Fortunately, the magnitude of Hopkins' findings was recognized by Storz, who mass produced this technology.

Fiberoptics

Tyndall defined the principle of internal reflection within glass fibers in 1854 (Barlow, 1990). This principle is responsible for the transmission of images along glass fibers, and involves the functional bending of light within flexible glass. The conveyance of light from the proximal to distal end of any fiberoptic endoscope is accomplished through an incoherent bundle of fibers. In a coherent bundle, each fiber is positioned in order, which corresponds to its position at the proximal as well as the distal end. Improvements in fiberoptic technology have enabled the bundling of more individual fibers, which produces a sharper image. By minimizing the cladding (insulation) around these bundles, the diameter of fiberoptic endoscopes has gradually decreased.

The angle of view for fiberoptic instruments is dictated by the axis of the optical system at the tip of the scope. Typically, this angle varies from 0° to approximately 10°. Although clarity of the image may be less for fiberoptic endoscopes than for rigid lens systems, image enhancement can be improved through the use of endoscopic filters (Aslan *et al.*, 1999).

The magnification of any image is dependent on the diameter of the view lens; therefore, the size of a magnified image will always be smaller in a smaller diameter lens. An advantage of the rod lens system over fiberoptics is excellent clarity of vision and sharper resolution; however, any distortion of the shaft may produce a 'half-moon' image. The smaller diameter lenses are more prone to damage and need to be handled with care.

Endourology set-up

One advantage of endoscopic surgery is the ability to transmit a clear, magnified operative field image on a video system. Two significant advancements have been the development of the charged-coupled device (CCD) chip camera and digital video imaging (Preminger, 1996) (Fig. 9.2). The CCD chip cameras contain either a single- or three-chip microprocessor. The main advantage of a three-chip over a single-chip camera is a clearer, more precise image. The cameras may be cleaned in a cold disinfectant solution, making them readily available for multiple procedures. Most cameras have the ability to adjust automatically to the varying light conditions frequently encountered during endoscopic procedures. An important addition is

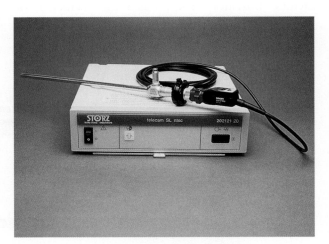

Figure 9.2 Charged-coupled device (CCD) cameras provide excellent image enhancement as well as magnification.

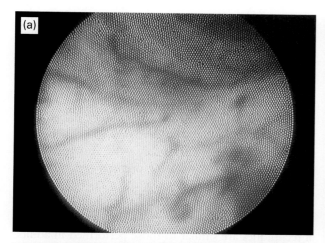

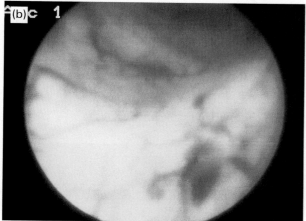

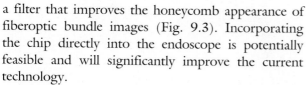

Figure 9.3 Endoscopic camera filter: (*a*) typical honey-comb appearance of fiberoptic bundles; (*b*) endo-scopic filters built into camera systems can remove bundle image distortion.

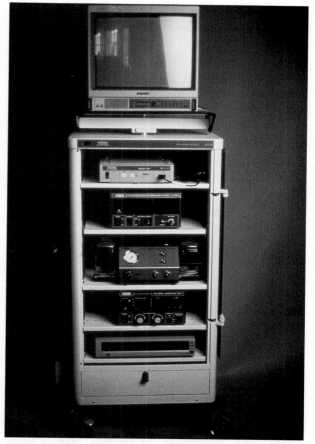

Figure 9.4 Endourology video cart. This allows for a self-contained system which is easily stored and transported.

a filter that improves the honeycomb appearance of fiberoptic bundle images (Fig. 9.3). Incorporating the chip directly into the endoscope is potentially feasible and will significantly improve the current technology.

A high-intensity light source is needed for proper illumination. Halogen and xenon are the most common. Care should be taken not to allow the cable end to come in contact with either the patient or surgical drapes because of the intense heat generated. Some light systems can automatically adjust to the variation in lighting encountered during a procedure.

Documentation capabilities are also an important part of any endourology system. This should include hard-copy photography, as well as video tape-record-

ing capability, to permit accurate depiction of a procedure and expedite chart documentation. Digital still-image recording produces high-resolution files, which can then be placed into electronic medical records, incorporated into slide presentations, and stored for easy accessibility (Kuo *et al.*, 1999).

In summary, the basic endourology video cart should contain image electronics (video camera and video screen), a halogen or xenon light source, a hard-copy printer, and a video recorder (Fig. 9.4). In addition, laparoscopic procedures require insufflation equipment. All equipment should be housed on a portable cart to allow for streamlined storage and easy transportability between surgical suites. In the future, fiberoptic or satellite transmission will allow for intraoperative linkage between distant sites for virtual consultation services.

Cystourethroscopes

Traditional rod lens pediatric cystoscopes range in size from 7 to 13 Fr. The smallest endoscopes do not have a working channel and can be used for observation only. The 10 Fr size accommodates a 3 Fr working instrument, while the 13 Fr cystoscope has a working channel of 5 Fr.

With fiberoptic technology has come the development of small-caliber pediatric endoscopes, with larger working channels. The size of these various instruments ranges from approximately 6 to 10 Fr (Fig. 9.5). Irrigating and working channels also vary in size. Some contain straight channels, which allow for the use of reusable rigid instruments. A summary of semirigid fiberoptic pediatric endoscopes is shown in Table 9.1. There are several advantages to fiberoptic endoscopes. They can accommodate significant bending without producing a diminished visual field. They are also a self-contained system in that there are no lens telescopes and, therefore, they are less fragile. The small-caliber fiberoptic endoscopes allow for safe diagnostic and therapeutic procedures in newborn premature infants.

Neonatal and pediatric resectoscopes have an outside diameter of approximately 8.5 Fr (Fig. 9.6a). A variety of electrodes can be fitted to these instruments for both cutting and coagulative procedures. Pediatric urethrotomes of approximately 9 Fr also permit the use of cold knife cutting of urethral strictures and valves (Fig. 9.6b).

Caution must be exercised during cystourethroscopy in the pediatric patient. Although the procedural techniques are similar to those performed in adults, certain anatomic considerations need to be kept in mind. The normal male neonatal urethra can usually accommodate an 8 Fr instrument (Allen *et al.*, 1972). The size is often dictated by the caliber of the urethral meatus, which is the narrowest portion of the male urethra (Litvak *et al.*, 1976). The urethra is more

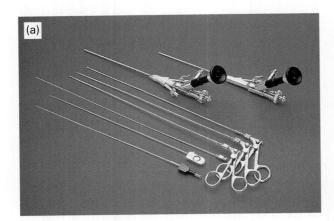

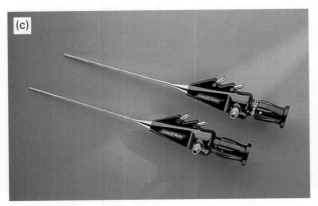

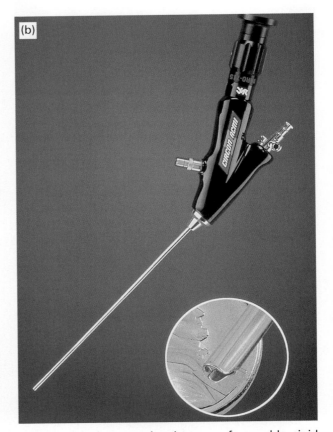

Figure 9.5 Minirigid fiberoptic endoscopes: (*a, b*) offset eyepiece design permits the use of reusable rigid equipment because of a straight working channel; (*c*) dual channels allow for use of flexible instruments while maintaining a separate irrigating port.

Table 9.1 Fiberoptic pediatric cystourethroscopes

	Shaft (Fr) Tip/Proximal	Angle of view (degrees)	Length (cm)	Irrigating/working channels (Fr)
Circon/Acmi				
MR-PC	6.9/10.2	5°	15.5	2.3, 3.4
MR-915	9.4/12.4	5°	15.5	2.1, 5.4
MRO-715	7.7/10.8	5°	15.5	5.4, straight
Olympus				
S-1234/1[a]	6.4/7.8	7°	13.0	4.2, straight
S-1234/2[a]	8.6/9.8	7°	14.0	6.6, straight
Storz				
27030K[a]	7.5/8.5	0°	11.0	2.4, 3.5, straight
27030K[a]	10.0/10.5	0°	11.0	5.5, straight
Wolf				
4615.401	4.5/6.0	0°	11.0	2.4
8616.411[a]	6.0/7.5	0°	14.0	4.0
8626.431[a]	9.5	5°	11.6	5.0, straight

[a]Autoclavable for sterilization.

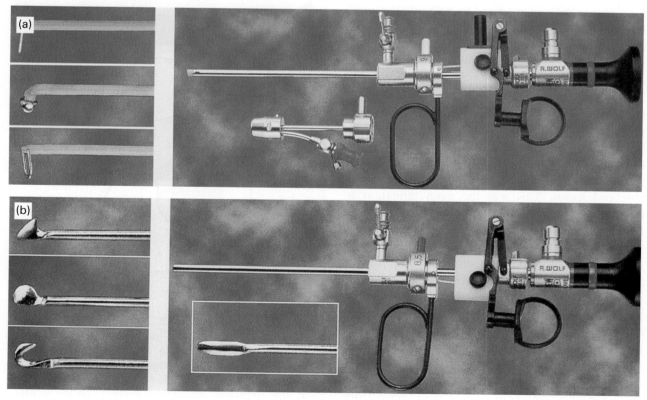

Figure 9.6 Pediatric/neonatal (*a*) resectoscope; (*b*) urethrotome.

fragile and delicate in the child than in the adult; therefore, any degree of trauma may result in stricture formation. Overdistension of the pediatric bladder can occur quickly and must be recognized to prevent overstimulation under light anesthesia, as well as bladder rupture.

Ureteroscopes

Pediatric cystoscopes were the first rigid rod lens instruments to be used as ureteroscopes. Hampton Young performed the first documented ureteroscopic procedure in 1912 in a 2-month-old child with massively dilated ureters secondary to a posterior urethral valve (PUV). The ureteral dilation allowed the placement of a 9.5 Fr pediatric cystoscope into the renal pelvis with visualization of the intrarenal collecting system. This was not reported until 1929 (Young and McKay, 1929). The next reported use of rigid ureteroscopy was in the late 1970s when Goodman and Lyons independently reported the use of an 11 Fr pediatric cystoscope for ureteroscopy (Goodman, 1977; Lyons et al., 1978).

The first endoscope which was designed specifically for ureteroscopy was produced by Richard Wolf medical instruments (Vernon Hills, IL, USA) and was first reported by Lyons et al. (1979). Its working length was 23 cm and its design was similar to the pediatric cystoscope. It was available in sizes varying from 13 to 16 Fr. This made available the use of endoscopic equipment for the manipulation and removal of ureteral stones. Subsequent changes in both diameter and length allowed for more ready access to the upper urinary tract, including the renal pelvis.

The early rigid ureteroscopes all used interchangeable rod lenses. This was the main limitation to downsizing their diameter. An offset lens semirigid fiberoptic endoscope has a straight working channel, which will accept rigid reusable instruments. By shortening the length, these semirigid ureteroscopes have become useful cystourethroscopes for children.

Through the use of fiberoptic bundle imaging there has been significant miniaturization. Fiberoptics allows bending of the endoscope without distortion of the image and enables a large-diameter working channel.

Even though rigid ureteroscopy was reported much earlier, the clinical use of flexible ureteroscopes predates published reports of routine rigid ureteroscopy (Marshall, 1964; Brush et al., 1970; Takagi et al.,

1971). Early urologic endoscopy involved the use of modified bronchoscopes, as well as gastroscopes. The first flexible ureteroscope was cumbersome because of problems with irrigation and deflection. It was difficult to pass the instrument through the intramural ureter. It was not until the 1980s that a renewed interest in flexible endoscopy occurred, brought about by improvements in miniaturization as well as the

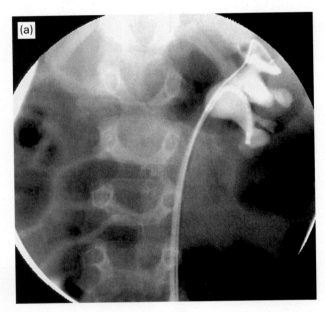

(a)

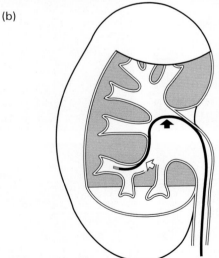

(b)

Figure 9.7 (a) Active tip deflection usually enables access to the lower pole calyces; (b) occasionally active (*open arrow*) combined with secondary passive (*closed arrow*) deflection is required to reach all areas of the intrarenal collecting system. (After Grasso, 1996b.)

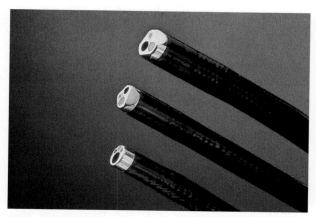

Figure 9.8 Tip design of various flexible uretero-scopes.

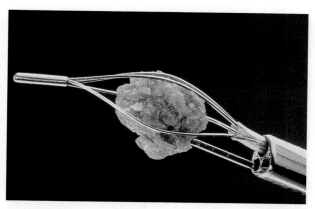

Figure 9.9 A triangular sheath design maximizes the size of independent working/irrigating channels.

addition of active deflection, adequate working channels, and small-diameter working instruments. Improvements in the ability to bundle more individual fibers resulted in sharper images (Barlow, 1990). Current flexible ureteroscopes are designed with active tip deflection as well as secondary passive deflection which effectively lengthens the deflected segment permitting inspection of the entire intrarenal collecting system (Bagley, 1993) (Fig. 9.7).

The working channel of a flexible ureteroscope consists of a smooth, cylindrical plastic tube located eccentrically at the tip (Fig. 9.8). Most flexible ureteroscopes have a working channel of 3.6 Fr, which is adequate for working instruments while still maintaining irrigation capabilities. Unfortunately, the placement of instruments through the working channel decreases the amount of active tip deflection (Grasso and Bagley, 1994a; Poon *et al.*, 1997). It is recommended that the tip of the ureteroscope be straight prior to the passage of any working instrument. A silicone lubricant may aid in decreasing resistance during deployment.

Because of their flexible design, ureteroscopes are delicate instruments and need to be handled with care. The fiberoptic fibers can be damaged, and if enough fibers become broken, the image becomes distorted and the endoscope needs to be repaired. Flexible endoscopes cannot be autoclaved but can be safely soaked in cold sterilization solution (Gregory *et al.*, 1988).

In contrast, rigid ureteroscopes use one or more working channels. The advantage of two separate channels is that one can be used for irrigation while the other permits passage of working instruments. The metal sheath of these scopes is usually triangular or oval in shape, which increases the size of the working channels (Fig. 9.9). It also protects the delicate fiberoptic bundles, making the minirigid endoscopes quite durable. Most minirigid endoscopes can be safely autoclaved for sterilization.

Ureteroscopy technique

Ureteroscopy is accomplished using general anesthesia. The patient is placed in the dorsal lithotomy position in either stirrups or a frog-legged position. The child should be well padded in order to prevent any excessive limb abduction or pressure on nerves and limbs.

A small-diameter, semirigid cystourethroscope with an offset lens and a large-caliber working channel is passed under vision. The author uses an endoscope with a distal tip of approximately 7 Fr. A straight working channel of greater than 5 Fr allows for the placement of a 5 Fr open-ended ureteral catheter. After the bladder has been inspected the ureteral orifice is visualized and an attempt is made at direct intubation using the open-ended catheter. There are clear anatomic differences between adults and children, especially in the diameter and size of the ureter. These parameters are age dependent and are based on work by Cussen (1971). If the orifice

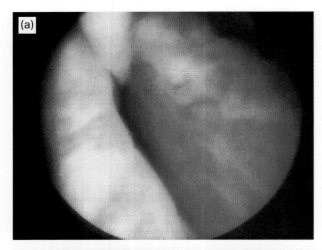

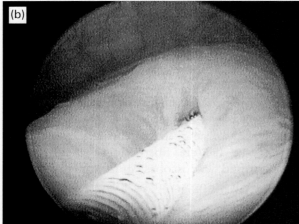

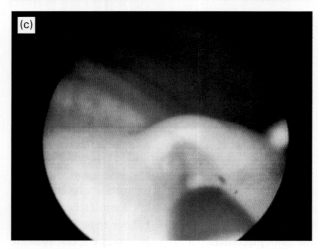

Figure 9.10 Various ureteral orifice configurations: (*a*) tenting up the mucosa makes placement of a uretero-scope much easier; (*b*) a 0.035 inch (0.9 mm) guidewire is used to gauge accessibility. A minirigid ureteroscope should be able to be passed over this wire into the ureter under direct vision; (*c*) a ureteral orifice that barely accepts a 3 Fr catheter will require active dilation.

accepts a 5 Fr catheter, then a small-diameter mini-rigid ureteroscope can be safely placed across the intramural ureter under direct vision. If the orifice accepts a 3 Fr open-ended catheter for a retrograde ureteropyelogram, then active dilation of the ureteral orifice is undertaken (Fig. 9.10). Previously published reports have demonstrated the effectiveness and safe-ty of balloon dilation in children (Shepherd *et al.*, 1988; Thomas *et al.*, 1993b), but this may be more extensive dilatation than is necessary for placement of small-diameter ureteroscopes. Therefore, graduated dilation from 3 to 8 Fr may be used, with a single graduated catheter of 4–8 Fr. Performing this through a cystoscopic sheath decreases the chance of buckling within the bladder, and is best performed over a stiff guidewire.

If therapeutic maneuvers are anticipated, a 0.035 inch (0.9 mm) guidewire is left in place as a safety wire. If an electrosurgical procedure is planned, the wire should be hydrophilic coated, or insulated with an open-ended catheter, in order to prevent energy transmission along the wire. A semirigid ureteroscope can be inserted alongside the guidewire, using the wire to tent-up the wall of the ureteral orifice (Fig. 9.10a), or placed between two guidewires after one is placed through the working channel of the uretero-scope. If therapeutic flexible ureteropyeloscopy is to be performed, a second guidewire is placed as a work-ing wire to allow for advancement of the flexible ureteroscope into the proximal collecting system in a monorail fashion (i.e. over the wire) (Fig. 9.11). The ureteroscope is guided into the ureter using fluoro-scopic visualization. If difficulty is encountered, the ureteroscope should be repositioned sequentially in 90° clockwise rotations, and attempts made to pass the instrument once again (Fig. 9.12). If there is con-tinued difficulty, a larger graduated ureteral dilator of 5–10 Fr may be helpful in gaining access.

The ureter has three physiologic areas of narrow-ing. The first is at the ureterovesical intramural portion, the next is over the area of the iliac vessels, and the third is at the ureteropelvic junction (UPJ). During any endourologic procedure, it is important to maintain a three-dimensional image of the position within the collecting system. It is impor-tant to keep in mind surrounding structures such as the iliac and gonadal vessels, and the vas deferens in males.

As the ureteroscope is advanced proximally, changes are appreciated in the configuration as well as

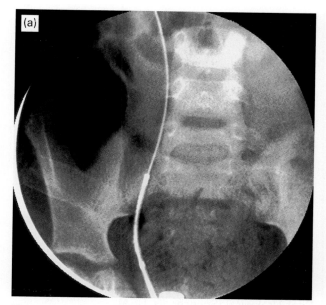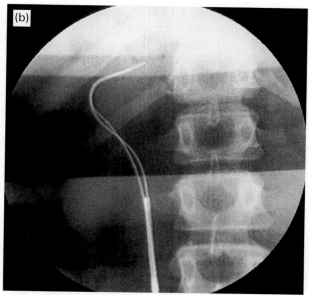

Figure 9.11 Flexible ureteroscopes can be passed over a guidewire in a 'monorail' fashion: (*a*) one wire is sufficient for diagnostic procedures; (*b*) a second safety wire should be used when performing therapeutic maneuvers in the proximal collecting system.

movement of the ureter. In the proximal ureter, one can see caudal movement of the renal pelvis and upper ureter with inspiration and cephalad movement with expiration. The intrarenal collecting system consists of many infundibula with compound upper and lower pole calyces. Radiographic contrast should be used to confirm complete inspection of the entire renal collecting system.

Although in the majority of cases safe access can be accomplished into the upper urinary tract using minimal dilation, there are instances when the need arises for more extensive ureteral dilation. If difficulty is encountered while passing a flexible instrument proximally, then direct visualization should be used to see whether the endoscope can be visually directed around any obstruction. If, after repeated attempts,

advancement is still unsuccessful, then the placement of a temporary indwelling ureteral stent will allow for passive dilation of the ureter and possibly make subsequent ureteroscopy more successful at a later date. It is prudent to approach these situations conservatively. The routine use of preoperative stenting of the pediatric ureter is not necessary.

Percutaneous endourology

The most basic form of percutaneous endourology involves the placement of a percutaneous nephrostomy tube for either diagnostic or therapeutic reasons. Hillier can be credited with the description of the first therapeutic percutaneous renal drainage of what

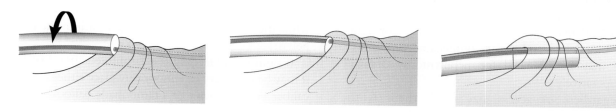

Figure 9.12 Sequential rotation of the ureteroscope may allow for subsequent successful intubation. (After Huffman *et al.*, 1988.)

probably represented UPJ obstruction (Bloom *et al.*, 1989). The first procedure was performed in 1864. In 1865 he had described the percutaneous tapping of giant hydronephrosis due to UPJ obstruction in a 4-year-old boy, but unfortunately in 1868 the boy succumbed to septicemia after one of the procedures.

In 1941 Rupel removed renal calculus debris through a nephrostomy tract using endoscopic equipment (Rubel and Brown, 1955). Goodwin *et al.* (1955) reported on percutaneous trocar nephrostomy for hydronephrosis in 16 patients. Despite these reports, it was several more decades before the technique of percutaneous access for both diagnostic and therapeutic intervention became a routine part of the urologist's armamentarium (Fernstrom and Johansson, 1976).

Initial recommendations for percutaneous endourologic procedures in children suggested that they be limited to those older than 8 years of age (Hulbert *et al.*, 1985). This recommendation was based on the observation that large-caliber tract dilation (i.e. ≥ 24 Fr) in young children resulted in an increased risk of blood loss. Subsequent reports have demonstrated that this procedure is technically feasible and efficacious in children less than 8 years of age (Woodside *et al.*, 1985; Boddy *et al.*, 1987; Callaway *et al.*, 1991; Burns and Joseph 1993; Dushinski *et al.*, 1997b; Jackman *et al.*, 1998; Desai *et al.*, 1999). Because of concerns about blood loss, the technique of smaller access, percutaneous procedures has been developed in the pediatric population. Desai *et al.* (1999) demonstrated a significant difference in blood loss between a single percutaneous tract dilated to less than 21 Fr and tracts dilated to greater than 21 Fr. These same concerns prompted Helal *et al.* (1997) to present their experience using a 15 Fr peel-away sheath in a 2-year-old child for percutaneous stone removal. More recently, the 11 Fr ('mini-perc') technique has been reported (Jackman *et al.*, 1998). After percutaneous access is obtained, single-step dilation with sheath placement reduces trauma to the renal tissue (Fig. 9.13). There have been no reports of significant blood loss and, in uncomplicated procedures, there may be no need for nephrostomy drainage postoperatively.

Regardless of access size used, there is the need for dilation of the tract. Once needle placement has been accomplished, a wire is passed down the ureter into the bladder to help with tract dilation

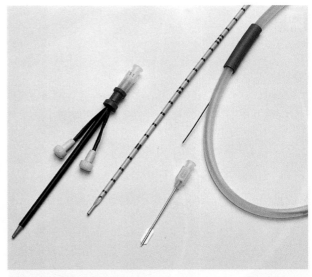

Figure 9.13 The 'mini-perc' system prepackaged from Cook Urological (Spencer, IN, USA).

and prevent accidental loss of access to the collecting system. If ureteral placement is not possible, the wire should be coiled within the collecting system.

Once safe access has been confirmed, there are two techniques for tract dilation. One involves using graduated dilators (Amplatz), while the other involves active balloon dilation. Because of its potential shearing effect, there may be increased risk for bleeding, as well as an increased risk for renal pelvic disruption, if the sequential dilating system is advanced too far medially.

For balloon dilation of the tract, the distal radiographic marker is placed into the renal pelvis while the proximal portion of the balloon is located externally. The balloon is then inflated to its maximum pressure and left fully inflated until there is no longer evidence of waisting at the level of the fascia. It should be left inflated for several minutes to aid in hemostasis. The balloon is then partially deflated, while the access sheath is guided over it into the renal pelvis.

If significant bleeding is encountered after dilation, it may be necessary to temporarily place either a large-caliber Foley catheter or a tamponade balloon. If this simple technique does not result in satisfactory hemostasis, the catheter may be left in place and the procedure performed at another time.

After the working sheath has been placed, the planned procedure is undertaken. This may require the use of both rigid and flexible instruments. Endourologic instrumentation is similar to that used for other procedures.

One unique anatomic consideration for young patients is the relative paucity of retroperitoneal fat surrounding the kidney. This makes the kidney a more freely mobile target for both initial access and subsequent dilation. Another important technical consideration in children is to avoid injury to the infundibulum and renal parenchyma during leverage of the nephroscope. The use of warmed saline irrigant during the procedure is encouraged. This may be switched to water or glycine if an electrosurgical procedure is planned. It is extremely important to maintain safety wire access in case of dislodgment of the operating access sheath.

Working instruments

Guidewires

Concurrent with the development of smaller rigid and flexible endoscopes came the availability of small-diameter working instruments to perform diagnostic and therapeutic procedures. Guidewires are the most commonly used instrument in endourology. Not only do they provide initial access to the ureter, they also ensure access as safety wires in the event of intraoperative complications during ureteroscopy. Their basic design revolves around a solid core wire, which has wrapped around it a tightly coiled spring wire. There are different diameters, ranging from 0.018 to 0.038 inches (0.64–0.97 mm). Their distal tip may be straight or angled and the floppy flexible tip varies in size from 1 to 15 cm. Some have a moveable core wire, which offers varying lengths of distal flexibility. Overall length ranges from 80 to 260 cm. Wires with a proximal flexible tip may decrease the chance of damage to the working channel of a flexible instrument when passed over the guidewire in the monorail fashion. There are several types of coating, the most common being Teflon. Hydrophilic polymer coatings decrease the friction of wires, making them useful for negotiating tortuous or narrowed ureters and for placement of a wire proximal to an impacted ureteral calculus. Although hydrophilic guidewires are helpful in negotiating the ureter, they can be difficult to handle and may become dislodged easily because of their slippery coating. For this reason, they should not be used routinely as a safety wire. A moistened gauze sponge or locking torque device significantly improves handling.

The stiffness of the wire can be varied by increasing the diameter of the core wire. The stiffer Amplatz wires are helpful for straightening significant kinks when using graduated dilators. They should not be used as working wires for flexible endoscopes owing to an increased risk of damage to the delicate working channel.

Electrosurgical probes

Several cutting and fulgurating electrodes are available, ranging in size from 2 to 5 Fr. Multiple designs enable them to be used in a variety of situations (Fig. 9.14). Straight-tip electrodes for cutting are available as small as 2 Fr. Most angled tips are 3 Fr. Some are reusable, but most are disposable. Conduction of electrical current is possible over uncoated guidewires; therefore, it is imperative either to insulate the guidewire with a catheter, or to use a wire with a non-conductive coating (i.e. hydrophilic). Direct contact with the wire should always be avoided, but in small working areas this is not always possible.

Baskets and graspers

A number of designs exist for the baskets and graspers used for endoscopic procedures. Diameters vary from 1.9 to 4.5 Fr. The basic design is similar for both baskets and graspers. There is a working handle, which allows for advancement and retraction of the basket or grasper. They are contained within a hydrophilic sheath to facilitate passage through endoscopes.

Baskets come as either a flat wire (Segura) or a helical design (Fig. 9.15). The helical baskets range in size from 1.9 to 4.5 Fr. They are usually made of either three or four wires, and some contain double wires to help with radial expansion of the ureter. The helical basket is passed proximal to the stone and then drawn back while deployed to engage the calculus. A design advantage to the helical basket is the ability to rotate and engage a stone.

Flat wire non-helical baskets vary in design with either four or six wires and diameters of 2.4–4.5 Fr. There is a larger space between wires, which allows for easier stone entrapment. Unlike the helical basket,

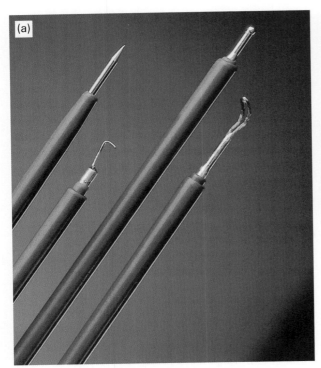

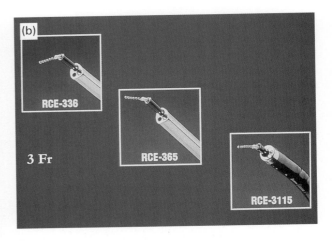

Figure 9.14 3 Fr electrosurgical probes come in various shapes and lengths; (*a*) the Hulbert set (Cook Urological, Spencer, Indiana); (*b*) the Ritecut from Circon, ACMI (Stamford, Connecticut).

a flat wire basket should be positioned alongside a stone in order for proper engagement. A flat wire basket can be helpful for biopsy and removal of pedunculated lesions of the collecting system.

A significant improvement in design is the tipless nitinol (nickel–titanium; Cook Urological, Spencer, IN, USA) basket (Fig. 9.16). It is particularly helpful in accessing calculi contained within the lower pole collecting system because it does not significantly effect active deflection of flexible ureteroscopes.

Because of the tipless design and increased flexibility of the individual wires, it is particularly safe and useful for the extraction of calculi contained within calyces (Honey, 1998). It does not have significant radial expansive pressure, which can make it difficult to engage impacted ureteral calculi. Some baskets have an inner central channel, which allows the simultaneous placement of an electrohydraulic or laser lithotripsy device. This may be necessary if a basketed stone becomes trapped within the ureter.

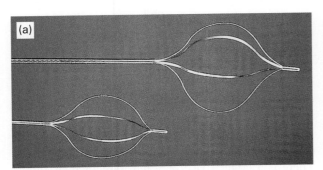

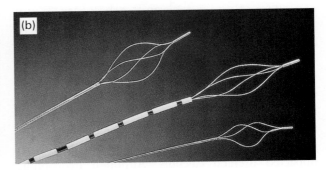

Figure 9.15 Basic basket design: (*a*) flat wire (Segura); (*b*) helical.

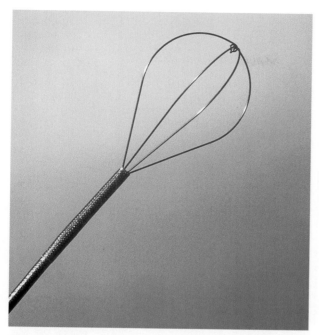

Figure 9.16 A nitinol (nickle titanium) wire basket (Cook Urological, Spencer, IN, USA). The tipless design minimizes calyceal trauma and its flexibility maintains active deflection.

Graspers

Grasping forceps have proven to be useful during endoscopic stone extraction (Bagley, 1992). A small-diameter flexible ureteroscope is excellent for removal of calculi located in the mid- and upper ureter, as well as the intrarenal collecting system. Grasping forceps aid in stone removal. They are made with two, three,

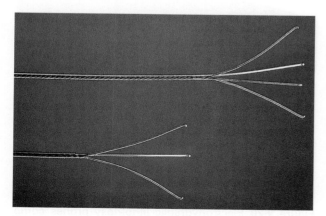

Figure 9.17 Standard design of three and four-pronged grasping forceps.

and four wires and are available in sizes from 1.9 to 4.5 Fr (Fig. 9.17). One advantage of forceps over baskets is that they will disengage from a stone when it becomes lodged in a relatively narrow ureteral segment. This helps to prevent trauma to the ureteral wall and eliminates basket entrapment during stone removal. Stone engagement with forceps involves a different technique from that used for helical and flatwire baskets (Fig. 9.18). Upon opening a grasping forceps, the individual wires are advanced away from the operator. Because the forcep advances towards the stone, slight retraction is necessary during deployment in order to avoid pushing the stone proximally. The forceps should be opened only as wide as needed to engage the calculus. Once opened to the appropriate size, they are advanced while simultaneously closing the graspers. This ensures that contact is maintained with the calculus.

Intracorporeal lithotripsy

Four techniques of intracorporeal lithotripsy are available: electrohydrolic, ultrasonic, ballistic, and laser. All four modes of lithotripsy have been extensively studied and evaluated, and the pros and cons for each of these will be discussed.

Electrohydraulic lithotripsy

Yutkin (1955) is credited with the discovery of electrohydraulic lithotripsy (EHL) while working as an engineer at the University of Kiev. The principle of EHL involves the generation of an electrical spark that produces two different effects. The first effect is a shock wave from the spark itself, which produces a cavitation bubble from superheated steam generated by its energy. This cavitation bubble produces energy sufficient enough for the fragmentation of calculi. There is an initial expansion phase followed by collapse, which produces the energy for lithotripsy. The energy of the shockwave decreases by the square root of the distance from the tip of the probe to the stone. This energy is maximized at a range of approximately 1 mm (Fig. 9.19). It is important, therefore, that the probe is not held directly in contact with the stone because this inhibits adequate generation of this cavitation bubble.

Probes vary in size and are available as small as 1.6 Fr (Fig. 9.20). As they have decreased in size so

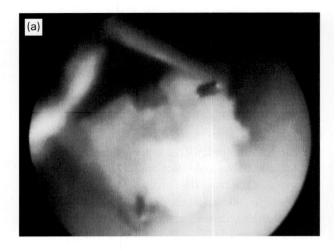

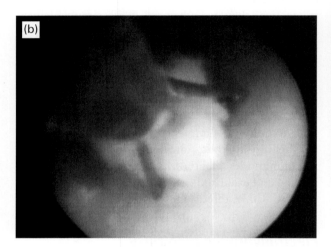

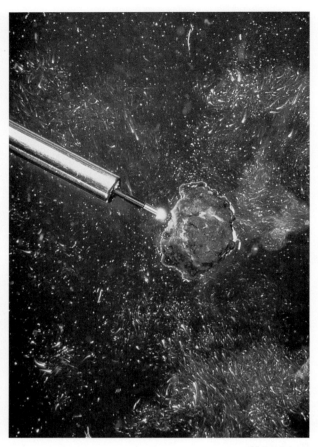

Figure 9.19 The electrohydraulic probe should be at least 1 mm from the surface of the stone in order to maximize lithotripsy potential.

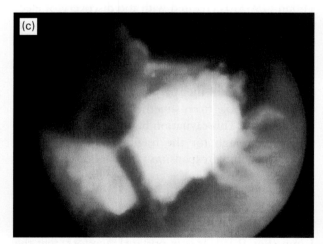

Figure 9.18 The technique for using forceps for stone removal involves (*a*) opening of wires only as large as needed to engage the stone while slowly retracting to prevent migration. Once the stone has been entrapped (*b*) it should be pulled closer to the endoscope tip (*c*) prior to removal of the entire system.

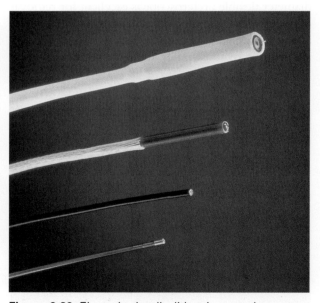

Figure 9.20 Electrohydraulic lithotripsy probes come in various sizes for use in the bladder, ureter, and kidney.

have the overall complications associated with their use. One particular advantage is that they restrict the deflection of flexible ureteroscopes to a lesser degree than other intracorporeal devices. Improvements in tip design have helped to reduce the amount of lateral disbursement of energy, thereby decreasing the risk of injury to surrounding tissues.

Ultrasonic lithotripsy

Mulvaney (1953) is credited with the first description of ultrasound energy for the disintegration of urinary calculi. The ultrasound probe is made of metal, which transmits vibrational energy to the tip. When in contact with the stone this causes resonation at high frequency with subsequent disintegration due to cleavage of the crystal matrix. There is associated high heat energy that is dissipated along the ultrasound probe; therefore, it is important to have a constant flow of irrigation fluid to help cool the system. The metal probe should not be touched during use to prevent thermal injury.

Solid probes as small as 2.5 Fr have been used for stone fracture; however, larger fragments require removal using an endoscopic forcep or basket (Chaussy et al., 1987). Hollow probes as small as 4.5 Fr are useful during percutaneous procedures to allow simultaneous suction extraction of stone debris (Fig. 9.21). One disadvantage to its use in the ureter is that the stone may move proximally as a result of vibration; therefore, stone immobilization through the use of a basket is often necessary. It is also necessary to apply pressure directly to the stone in order to achieve maximal success; therefore, it is important not to push the stone through the ureter or into the renal parenchyma. A benefit of this form of lithotripsy, owing to the non-transmission of vibrational energy, is the minimal tissue damage when it comes in contact with the ureter or bladder (Piergiovanni et al., 1994). The ultrasonic probe is reusable and relatively inexpensive to maintain. Ultrasonic lithotripsy is particularly useful for the percutaneous removal of large stone burdens.

Ballistic lithotripsy

This type of lithotripsy involves the mechanical impaction of stones by probes (Ten et al., 1998). There are two different mechanical design principles. The first works using a metal rod, which is struck at its proximal end by a metallic bullet. This drives the probe forward, mechanically impacting the stone. There are both rigid probes for use within semirigid miniscopes and a more flexible version for use within flexible endoscopes. The technique is quite effective in fragmenting all types of stone (Schulze et al., 1993; Haupt et al., 1995). One disadvantage of this device is that the probe needs to be relatively straight, since there is a substantial loss of power if bowing of more than 10° occurs. Another shortcoming of this technology is retrograde migration of the stone due to the mechanical impaction.

The second design uses a nitinol probe to impact the stones mechanically (Loisides et al., 1995). It has been used experimentally through flexible ureteroscopes and has been shown to be effective for lithotripsy even at a deflection of 90°. Once again, because of the pneumatic impaction there may be problems with retrograde stone migration.

Laser lithotripsy

The first laser to be developed was the ruby laser at a wavelength of 690 nm. It was able to generate enough energy to produce fragmentation of calculi (Mulvaney and Beck, 1968). Although this laser is not used routinely today, it cleared the way for the development of laser lithotripsy. There continues to be significant refinement to this technology.

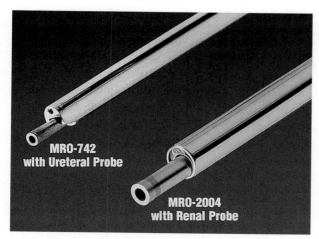

Figure 9.21 Hollow ultrasonic lithotripsy metal probes come as small as 4.5 Fr (*left*) for use with small-diameter fiberoptic minirigid endoscopes. Larger hollow probes (*right*) require a 4 or 5 mm working channel and are good for removing large stone burdens.

Tunable dye laser

The coumarian green dye laser at 504 nm was the first laser to be studied extensively for its fragmentation ability (Watson et al., 1987). Delivery through a fiber of 250 or 320 μm allowed enough energy to be transmitted for adequate lithotripsy. This type of laser worked well on most stones, although it had difficulty in the fragmentation of cystine and calcium oxalate monohydrate stones (Dretler and Bhatta 1991; Grasso and Bagley 1994b). As with any laser energy, the probe needs to be maintained in contact with the stone in order to prevent energy disbursion with local tissue damage. Although it proved to be quite effective, it was very expensive to purchase and maintain.

Alexandrite

Unlike coumarian dye, the alexandrite laser is a solid medium laser with a wavelength of 775 nm. It was first introduced in 1991 as a laser lithotriptor (Weber et al., 1991). This particular laser was an improvement over the pulsed dye lasers, but unfortunately it is unable to fragment all calculi, and therefore is not used routinely (Pearle et al., 1998).

Holmium: yttrium aluminum garnet (YAG)

The holmium lithotriptor is a 2100 nm laser delivered through 200, 365, 500, and 1000 μm fibers (Fig.

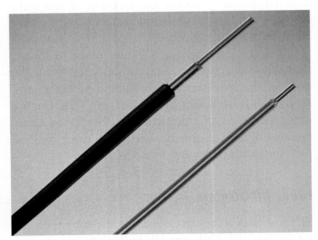

Figure 9.22 The holmium laser fibers are reusable and are usually made of low water content quartz. Not only is this wavelength able to fragment all calculi, but it also incises and ablates tissue at higher energy levels. Fibers are small enough to be used in most flexible and rigid fiberoptic endoscopes.

9.22). It has been effective in fragmenting all types of stones (Grasso, 1996a). Unlike other lasers that rely on shockwave energy, the mechanism of holmium lithotripsy involves direct stone absorption of laser energy with subsequent disintegration (Vassar et al., 1999). A particular advantage of this type of laser is its ability to ablate tissue and, therefore, act as a cutting instrument. It has also been shown to be safe for use in all areas of the urinary system (Erhard and Bagley, 1995). Because of its ability to fragment all types of calculi, as well as to incise and ablate tissue, it is particularly well suited for use within the genitourinary system. Energy settings required for stone fragmentation are usually less than 1 J, with a frequency of less than 10 pulses/sec. These settings need to be increased for tissue ablative effects.

Erbium laser

The erbium laser at 2900 nm is a wave length that has been clinically shown to be a more effective energy source for lithotripsy. Currently, this wavelength is used for other medical indications and is not yet suited for endourologic use. Hopefully, in the future this may provide a less expensive, more efficient method of laser lithotripsy.

Endourologic clinical applications

Ureteroceles

A ureterocele is a congenital cystic dilation of the submucosal portion of the intravesical ureter. The American Academy of Pediatrics Section on Urology has come to a consensus as to the nomenclature of this condition. An intravesical ureterocele is one located entirely within the bladder, and an ectopic ureterocele is defined as one in which any portion of the ureterocele is located permanently at either the bladder neck or within the urethra. Approximately 60% of ureteroceles are ectopic in nature, and are more prevalent in females. Approximately 80–90% of ureteroceles are associated with the upper pole segment of a duplex collecting system. Ureteroceles occur bilaterally in 10% of cases.

The treatment of asymptomatic ureteroceles remains controversial. Initial reports of the endo-

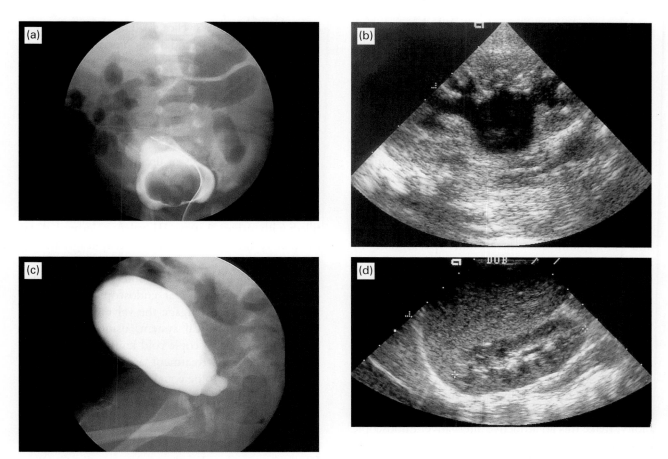

Figure 9.23 (*a*) Voiding cystourethrogram (VCUG) reveals a large intravesicle single system ureterocele of a solitary right kidney; (*b*) preoperative sonogram (U/S) reveals significant hydronephrosis; (*c*) postoperative VCUG after limited puncture shows decompression without reflux; (*d*) postoperative U/S confirms resolution of hydronephrosis.

scopic decompression of ureteroceles often resulted in secondary reflux (Monfort *et al.*, 1985; Tank, 1986). Interest has been regenerated by observations that a limited puncture may decrease the risk of secondary vesicoureteral reflux (VUR) in intravesical ureteroceles (Fig. 9.23). However, endoscopic decompression of ectopic ureteroceles rarely constitutes definitive therapy, but helps to correct associated conditions of urosepsis and azotemia (Blyth *et al.*, 1993; Smith *et al.*, 1994; Pfister *et al.*, 1998).

Once the decision has been made for endoscopic treatment, the procedure is tailored to findings at the time of surgery. After induction of general anesthesia, the patient is put in the dorsal lithotomy position. Intraoperative antibiotic prophylaxis is suggested. The most common cutting device used is a 3 Fr electrode which allows simultaneous

ablation and coagulation. Laser energy may also be used.

The surgical principle is similar regardless of the type of ureterocele present or the energy source used for treatment. A small limited incision or puncture is used (Rich *et al.*, 1990; Blyth *et al.*, 1993). In instances of urosepsis with associated VUR into the lower pole moiety, a larger transverse incision is appropriate to insure decompression. The intravesical ureterocele is punctured on the anterior wall close to the level of the bladder neck. It is important to make certain that the opening is within the bladder, so that upon bladder neck closure, there will be no obstruction to the drainage of the ureterocele. When incising an ectopic ureterocele, it is also important that the portion extending into the urethra is adequately drained. In order to accomplish this, it may be necessary to perform a longitudinal incision from the base of the ureterocele cephalad. An alternative is to perform a through-and-through puncture by guiding the electrode from the initial puncture site within the urethra through to the anterior wall of the intravesical portion. Adequate decompression should be confirmed in all cases before completion of the procedure.

Postoperatively, a catheter is not routinely needed, and the procedure can be performed as an outpatient. Morbidity related directly to the incisional portion of the procedure is minimal and includes localized bleeding and urinary tract infection. Radiographic imaging should include a voiding cystourethrogram and sonogram. An intravenous pyelogram or radionuclide renal scan is indicated to document excretion and function.

When deciding on appropriate therapy for children with ureteroceles, each case should be individualized (Spencer-Barthold, 1998). Puncture should be considered for definitive treatment of intravesical ureteroceles, whether associated with a duplex or single collecting system. The relatively low incidence of secondary VUR, as well as the high likelihood of surgical decompression with minimal overall morbidity, make this an attractive alternative. Endoscopic decompression of ectopic ureteroceles may rarely constitute definitive therapy and therefore should be used infrequently as primary therapy. It can be considered appropriate acute treatment for patients with urosepsis and bladder outlet obstruction with azotemia.

Urethral valves

Posterior urethral valves

Posterior urethral valves are the most common congenital urethral obstruction in newborn males. Prenatal ultrasonography has enabled most cases to be diagnosed in the neonatal period. After hydronephrosis is confirmed on postnatal sonogram, a voiding cystourethrogram is performed. The findings of posterior urethral dilatation, as well as bladder neck hypertrophy with bladder wall trabeculation, are consistent with the diagnosis of a posterior urethral valve. Often the valve tissue is visualized at the time of the voiding cystourethrogram.

Once the diagnosis of PUV has been established, the child should undergo prompt relief of the obstruction. Rarely is upper urinary tract diversion necessary for stabilization of the child. There is concern that this

can interrupt normal cyclical bladder filling, and may affect bladder function and development (Lome et al., 1972; Tanagho, 1974). Vesicostomy has proven useful, but this is an invasive surgical procedure which will require a second procedure for closure. Small minirigid cystourethroscopes enable safe, early, primary valve ablation for most boys, including those born prematurely (Smith et al., 1996).

There are three types of urethral valves described, two of which have clinical significance. Type I valves arise near the verumontanum and have a classic 'spinnaker' appearance to the leaflets when filled with urine. A type III valve is located distal to the verumontanum and is diaphragmatic in appearance.

Once the child is stable and intervention has been planned, there are several endoscopic approaches. One technique is to engage the valve tissue without the use of any optical system, using a hook-type device. Optical endoscopic cold knife, electrosurgical incision, and laser treatment are also possible. All modalities appear to be equally effective for the relief of valvular obstruction.

The valve leaflets are ablated laterally at the 5 and 7 o'clock positions. If there is residual obstructing tissue anteriorly, this will need to be incised. For type III diaphragmatic valve obstruction, a stellate incision is most effective. It is important to avoid injury to the external urinary sphincter, and to control the depth of incision to prevent urethral wall injury and subsequent stricture formation.

A catheter is left indwelling and can be removed on the following day. A pull-out voiding cystourethrogram can be performed to document satisfactory valve ablation.

Anterior urethral valves

Anterior urethral valves occur much less frequently than PUV, and are usually associated with a congenital urethral diverticulum (Williams and Retik, 1969; Tank, 1987). The dorsal margin of the diverticulum becomes distended with fluid, resulting in obstruction of the urethral lumen. Treatment involves incising the midline anterior lip of obstructing tissue. Additional urethral reconstructive procedures may be necessary, but initial management through endoscopic incision may be sufficient (van Savage et al., 1997). Postoperatively, patients are treated similarly to those with a posterior urethral valve.

Calculi

Bladder

The term lithotomy was coined in 276 BC by the Greek surgeon Ammonious of Alexandria. Several centuries later, the Roman, Celsus provided a detailed description of the lithotomy procedure in a young child (Wangensteen and Wangensteen, 1978). Virtually every ancient society has described the surgical removal of bladder calculi. Open cystolithotomy remains part of the practice of pediatric urology to this day. There are, however, instances when the endoscopic removal of such calculi is warranted. Bladder calculi in children are a well-known complication of bladder augmentation (Khoury et al., 1977; Kronner et al., 1998). They are related to urinary stasis, mucous production and bacteriuria, each of which have an important role in the formation of bladder calculi. The removal of all stone fragments is essential to prevent any nidus for stone regrowth.

The cystoscopic removal of bladder calculi is somewhat limited by the caliber of the urethra in young children. All forms of intracorporeal lithotripsy have proven effective for the management of bladder calculi (Razui et al., 1996; Teichman et al., 1997). The most potentially damaging devices to the wall of the augmented bladder include electrohydrolic lithotripsy and the holmium laser lithotriptors. It is important not to allow either one of these energy sources to come in near or direct contact with the bladder wall. Electrohydrolic lithotripsy may result in perforation of the augmented bladder, if the procedure is performed in a distended bladder or if a stone is wedged against the augmented portion. Another potential complication includes gross hematuria from bladder wall irritation which may necessitate catheterization postoperatively.

Percutaneous removal of bladder calculi has also been demonstrated to be an effective technique (van Savage et al., 1996; Elder, 1997). This is a more invasive procedure that involves a percutaneous suprapubic puncture for direct visualization of the calculi, as well as vacuum suction removal. If the urethra is not patent, a second suprapubic puncture is necessary for both visualization and removal of the calculi. This technique appears well suited for stones up to 1 cm in size, or multiple stones less than 1 cm.

The bladder is filled until it is palpable. A small gauge needle is used to confirm both position and depth in order to approach the bladder percutaneously. A 14 G needle is introduced which allows placement of a 0.038 inch (0.97 mm) guidewire into the bladder. The tract is dilated over the wire to a size equal to that of the largest stone in millimeters multiplied by 3 (an 8 mm stone requires at least a 24 Fr sheath). If intracorporeal lithotripsy is required, EHL, ultrasonic ballistic, or laser have proven suitable. The stones and any fragments are then removed using suction tubing attached to a vacuum device. Postoperative bladder drainage is necessary for 5–7 days.

Ureter and intrarenal collecting system

Debate continues regarding the most efficacious treatment of ureteral and renal calculi in children. Each case needs to be individualized in order to choose the best form of treatment with regard to extracorporeal shockwave lithotripsy versus retrograde ureteroscopy versus an antegrade percutaneous approach. Shockwave lithotripsy for calculi in the renal calyces and proximal ureter is the least invasive form of therapy offering reasonable stone-free rates of greater than 80% with minimal complications (Newman et al., 1986; Kroovand et al., 1987; Frick et al., 1988; Marberger et al., 1989; Thornhill et al., 1990; Ali Farsi et al., 1994; Myer et al., 1995). It can be done as an outpatient procedure. Problems include higher retreatment rates and the potential need for ancillary procedures to achieve stone-free status. Even though many centers have documented safety for use within the pediatric population, there is always concern over the long-term effect on renal function (Nijman et al., 1989; Frick et al., 1991; Lottman et al., 1998; Lifshitz et al., 1998; Willis et al., 1999). In addition, it is difficult to perform shockwave lithotripsy over the bony pelvis, and distal stones in young females are a relative contraindication owing to the location of the female genital organs.

As technology has improved, retrograde ureteroscopic stone extraction throughout the entire urinary tract has slowly become adapted for use within the pediatric population. Published reports have shown excellent results, with the successful removal of over 100 calculi from the pediatric ureter (Ritchey et al., 1988; Caione et al., 1990; Hill et al., 1990; Thomas et al., 1993b; Scarpa et al., 1995; Shroff and Watson, 1995; Kurzrock et al., 1996; Lim et al., 1996; Smith et al., 1996; Al Busaidy et al., 1997; Minevich Erousseau and Wacksman, 1997; Jayanthi et al.,

1999). Several of these patients were adolescents and could be physically considered adults, although over one-half of the total stones have been removed from prepubertal patients. There are reports documenting the successful removal of stones in children as young as 6 months (Al Busaidy *et al.*, 1997).

Advantages of ureteroscopy include negligible retreatment rates with near 100% stone-free status after one procedure (Kapoor *et al.*, 1992; Grasso *et al.*, 1995a). Both shockwave lithotripsy and ureteroscopy require general anesthesia in the pediatric population. A fear regarding increased complications in the pediatric population has not been documented in the literature. This may be because current reports are being presented from centers experienced with endourology. Since endourology is an important part of today's urologic training, this trend should continue as further numbers are gathered. Most studies have not included routine postoperative evaluation with a voiding cystourethrogram. In one study, in which the ureter was dilated to at least 11.5 Fr for placement of the rigid ureteroscope, there was no documented reflux on postoperative voiding cystourethrogram (VCUG) (Caione *et al.*, 1990). Other series in which ureteral dilation has been performed have documented cases of postoperative reflux, none of which has become clinically significant (Al Busaidy *et al.*, 1997).

For intrarenal stones greater than 1 cm, or multiple small calculi, and in children with urinary tract malformations or previous reconstruction, a percutaneous approach may be more suitable (Fig. 9.24). A percutaneous tract can be used for the management of ureteral stones by utilizing antegrade ureteroscopy. This is a more invasive form of therapy for ureteral stones and may therefore be subplanted by primary retrograde ureteroscopy. Ureteropelvic junction obstruction with associated stones can also be managed in an antegrade fashion.

The most common presenting symptoms for stones within the urinary tract in children include abdominal pain in 40–75%, gross or microscopic hematuria in 25–40%, and symptoms attributable to UTIs in 10–30% (Choi *et al.*, 1987; Polinsky *et al.*, 1987; Milliner and Murphy, 1993; Cohen *et al.*,

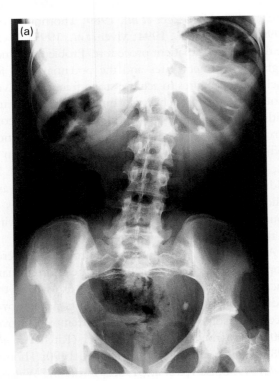
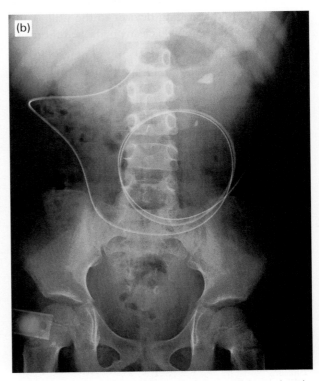

Figure 9.24 (*a*) Multiple left renal calculi and (*b*) large solitary pelvic stones may be treated using a 'mini-perc' technique. The left distal ureteral stone (*a*) was treated with retrograde ureteroscopy, while the proximal ureteral stone (*b*) was removed with antegrade ureteroscopy at the time of the percutaneous procedure.

1996). It has been demonstrated in adult series that stones less than 4 mm will pass spontaneously 80% of the time. Stones between 4 and 6 mm have a 59% passage rate while stones over 6 mm will pass only 21% of the time. This yields an overall spontaneous passage rate of approximately 55% (Ueno *et al.*, 1997). Similar stone passage rates are seen in children. Some studies suggest that the rate of passage depends on the stones' position within the ureter. Stones in the proximal ureter were found to pass approximately 22% of the time, compared with 46% and 71% for those in the middle and distal third of the ureter (Morse and Resnick, 1991). Conservative expectant therapy should be undertaken unless there are clinical signs of uncontrolled pain or vomiting, or signs of urosepsis.

When performing ureteroscopy for stones within the ureter or renal collecting system, access is gained as discussed previously. A safety wire is always left in place to avoid losing access to the ureter in case of iatrogenic injury during stone manipulation. In the young male child, it is important to inspect the urethral meatus periodically throughout the procedure to prevent harm to the glans penis. It is also important to keep in mind that most ureteroscopes have a graduated tapered shaft and that the most proximal end may not be adequately accommodated by the small male urethra. The bladder should be emptied after placement of the initial guidewire so that it will not become overdistended. Saline irrigant should be used and can be attached to a single, spring-loaded syringe pumping system, if needed. Irrigation is used sparingly to clear the operative field to prevent proximal migration of calculi.

A minirigid ureteroscope should be used for distal and mid-ureteral calculi. It may also be successfully passed into the proximal ureter in young females. Flexible ureteroscopy is often needed for proximal ureteral calculi and for those contained within the renal collecting system (Fig. 9.25). If there is significant ureteral wall edema with stone impaction, then either *in situ* laser lithotripsy or disimpaction with dislodgment of the stone into the proximal dilated ureter should be performed. The holmium laser lithotriptor can fragment all stones, and most fragments are small enough to pass spontaneously (Teichman *et al.*, 1998) (Fig. 9.26). The tip of the laser probe needs to be visualized during the procedure in order to prevent local tissue injury or guidewire damage. This author prefers the use of graspers to remove calculi from the ureter owing to the ease with which a stone fragment can be disengaged if it becomes lodged within a narrowed portion of the ureter. If a stone fragment becomes displaced outside the ureteral wall as a result of perforation, further attempts at extraction of the migrated calculus should be abandoned (Lopez-Alcina *et al.*, 1998). If multiple fragments are removed, at least one should be retrieved for crystallographic analysis. During the procedure, the remaining fragments may be deposited in the bladder, which eliminates the need for complete withdrawal of the ureteroscope. A dual-lumen catheter is helpful for replacing a working wire over which the flexible ureteroscope may be guided back into the proximal ureter.

In the early experience of endoscopy, most if not all children had postoperative stents or temporary catheters after endoscopic manipulation. In one recent report, only 26% of patients had a stent placed,

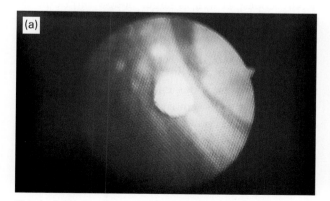

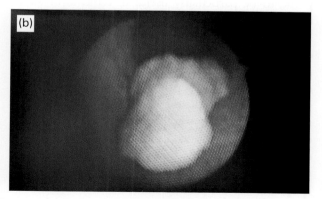

Figure 9.25 Flexible ureteroscopic view of a papillary tip calculus (*a*) with surrounding evidence of nephrocalcinosis in an active metabolic stone-forming adolescent. Large intrarenal stones (*b*) can be successfully treated by retrograde flexible ureteroscopy in a single setting.

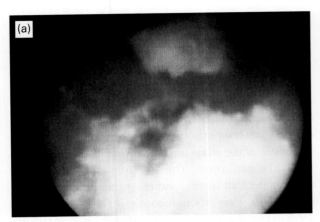
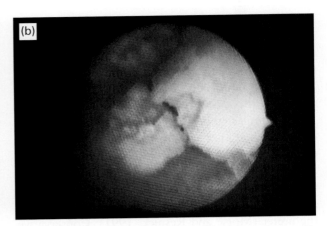

Figure 9.26 A large ureteral calculus (*a*) may be reduced in volume before removal by smoothing the edges with the holmium laser, leaving dust debris (foreground) which will pass spontaneously. Alternatively, a large stone (from Figure 9.25b) may be precisely cleaved by the laser fiber (lower left corner) into small enough fragments which can be removed individually.

and there was no significant sequelae associated with non-stenting (Kurzrock *et al.*, 1996). Certainly, if there is perforation or significant ureteral wall edema, a stent should be placed. It is this author's preference to leave a dangler retrieval string attached to a double pigtail stent to facilitate removal without anesthesia (Fig. 9.27).

The 'mini-perc' technique is most appropriate for stones less than 2 cm or multiple small calculi contained within the renal collecting system pelvis. This procedure becomes more tedious with larger stone burdens because of the inability to remove significant amounts of stone either through the small hollow ultrasound probes or through fragmentation with laser, ballistic, or electrohydrolic lithotripsy. The author has not found the 4.5 Fr hollow ultrasound probe to be particularly useful in removal of stone debris during lithotripsy. Therefore, holmium laser lithotripsy, which permits precise cleavage of the calculus into fragments suitable for removal through a percutaneous sheath is preferred. A 9 Fr mini-rigid endoscope with two separate channels enables active suction removal of dust debris during laser lithotripsy. Stone fragments over 2 mm are removed with a 3 or 4.5 Fr three-pronged grasper. A flexible pediatric cystoscope can be used to visualize completely the entire intrarenal collecting system at the end of the procedure. This should be introduced as far down the ureter as possible to look for any migrated stone particles. If the procedure was uncomplicated and there do not appear to be significant residual frag-

ments, either endoscopically or radiographically, a 5 Fr open-ended catheter is placed into the renal pelvis and secured at the level of the skin at the termination of the procedure. This is left in place temporarily until a postoperative plain X-ray the following morning reveals no fragments. It is not placed to drainage unless the patient experiences significant pain due to obstruction from an unrecognized stone particle or leakage around the tube. The author does not routinely leave indwelling ureteral stents after uncomplicated percutaneous nephrostolithotomy.

For larger stone burdens and any degree of stone branching into the calyces, it is more prudent to perform this procedure with a larger percutaneous tract of approximately 24 Fr. This enables the use of larger nephroscopes, as well as larger hollow ultrasonic or ballistic probes that may decrease the time needed for stone removal. A nephrostomy tube should be placed to drainage at the conclusion of the procedure and can be removed before discharge from the hospital if no further percutaneous endoscopic procedures are planned. Prior to its removal, a trial of tube clamping or an antegrade nephrostogram should be performed to demonstrate adequate resolution of any postoperative edema at the level of the UPJ.

Most children require only a single session for complete calculus removal. For a large staghorn calculus, initial percutaneous debulking followed by shockwave lithotripsy with an additional percutaneous procedure may be the most effective way to

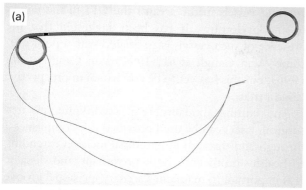

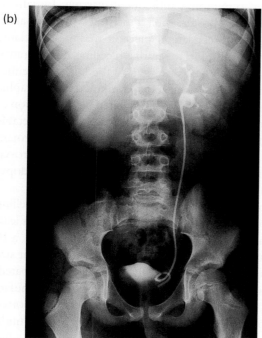

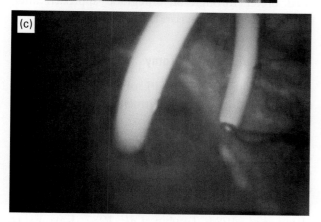

Figure 9.27 (a) Double pigtail ureteral stent with a string attached facilitates removal without anesthesia. To help prevent postoperative stent irritation, (b) there should be no stent redundancy, and endoscopically (c) the stent should curl away from the trigone of the bladder.

accomplish a stone-free condition (Burns and Joseph, 1993; Chandhoke, 1996). Blood loss requiring transfusion and sepsis appear to be the most significant postoperative complications in children, but fortunately these are an uncommon occurrence (Woodside *et al.*, 1985; Boddy *et al.*, 1987; Callaway *et al.*, 1991; Dushinski *et al.*, 1997b). Most children will have a low-grade fever postoperatively, which is of no concern unless there is documented infection at the time of the procedure (Cadeddu *et al.*, 1998). Routine perioperative intravenous antibiotic coverage is recommended. Bleeding during the procedure is minimized by gentle technique and the avoidance of levering the nephroscope during the procedure. Additional prospective studies are needed to demonstrate the advantages of a 'mini-perc' over the standard, large-caliber percutaneous approach.

While the correct surgical management of stones within the intrarenal collecting system is continually debated, it is appropriate to say that shockwave lithotripsy and endourologic procedures have all but replaced open surgical procedures.

Shockwave lithotripsy is considered the first-line treatment for renal stones less than 1 cm. For stones greater than 1.5 cm or for those that exhibit any degree of branching into the calyces, a percutaneous approach should be considered part of the treatment strategy. If a stone is felt to be very dense with increased opacity on plain X-ray or is associated with abnormal renal anatomy, such as a narrowed infundibulum or calyceal diverticulum, than a primary endourologic approach is recommended.

Percutaneous access should be guided towards a renal position that enables successful completion of the procedure. This involves either a superior or middle pole calyx allowing direct access to the UPJ, and the ability to perform antegrade ureteroscopy for migrated stone fragments. Complex urinary calculi may require multiple percutaneous access sites for successful treatment.

Ureteropelvic junction obstruction

The pathophysiology and evaluation of the child with UPJ obstruction are discussed in Chapter 20. Traditionally, UPJ obstruction in the pediatric population has been corrected by open pyeloplasty with greater than 90% success. The endourologic management of this condition in adults is now considered by some to be the first option for treatment. Compared with an open surgical procedure, there is decreased morbidity and a comparable degree of success in adults. These benefits have not been demonstrated in any conclusive form in the pediatric population. It is this author's opinion that in infants and toddlers, open surgical repair should be considered the primary treatment modality for children with primary UPJ obstruction.

Balloon rupture

The quickest and simplest endourologic procedure for correction of UPJ obstruction is active balloon dilation. While technically less challenging, the overall success rate has been disappointing. In a series of published reports in children the overall success is 62% for primary and 66% for secondary obstruction (Doraiswamy, 1994; Tan et al., 1995; Sugita et al., 1996; Wilkinson and Aozmy, 1996). Whether the ureter remained stented postoperatively or not did not appear to have a significant effect on the overall outcome.

Endopyelotomy

Arthur Smith is credited for coining the phrase 'endopyelotomy' when discussing the endourologic incision of the UPJ. The procedure is a modification of the 'ureterotomie externe' which was originally described by Albarran (1903). The technique was later popularized by Davis (1943) in his descriptive analysis of the intubated ureterotomy. These techniques involved a longitudinal incision made outside the ureter extending into the internal ureteral lumen. A stent was placed for several weeks during ureteral regeneration. Early studies demonstrated that a period of approximately 6 weeks is required for complete ureteral smooth muscle formation with return of active peristalsis (Davis et al., 1948; Davis, 1958). The duration of postoperative indwelling stent placement is based on these studies and therefore is suggested for 4–6 weeks.

The success of endopyelotomy in both adults and children appears to be related to several preoperative factors. Many agree that in a kidney demonstrating severe (grade IV) hydronephrosis or split renal function less than 25%, the outcome for endopyelotomy is significantly reduced (Thomas et al., 1993a; Van Gangh et al., 1994; Gupta et al., 1997; Figenshau and Clayman, 1998). More controversial is the role of crossing vessels in the area of the UPJ in the failure of endopyelotomy. It has been suggested that the presence of such vessels is associated with a poor outcome (Van Gangh et al., 1994; Van Cangh et al., 1996), but this has yet to be confirmed in prospective clinical trials.

Any cutting modality (e.g. cold knife, electrosurgical, laser) can be used provided it accomplishes a through-and-through longitudinal incision extending to healthy urothelium both proximally and distally. It is important to maintain a solitary incisional groove in order to minimize subsequent scarring. Initially, it was felt that a posteriolateral incision would be safest, although a direct lateral incision may be associated with less risk of intraoperative bleeding. Preoperative vascular radiologic assessment of the UPJ, with either endoluminal ultrasound or computed tomographic (CT) angiography, is recommended before incision of a secondary UPJ obstruction because of unpredictable postsurgical anatomy (Figenshau and Clayman, 1998). However, no prospective study has proven their utility for either primary or secondary endopyelotomy.

A postoperative ureteral stent remains indwelling for a period of 4–6 weeks. Stent size should be at least 7 Fr, although if the ureter is of sufficient caliber, a 10 Fr stent may be more beneficial. Optimum stent size and duration postoperatively continue to be debated. Several tapered endopyelotomy stents are manufactured, although ureteral necrosis has been reported after placement of a 14 Fr tapered stent into an undilated ureter through an antegrade approach after endopyelotomy (Sutherland et al., 1992).

Technique of endopyelotomy

After the diagnosis of UPJ obstruction has been made, an individualized treatment strategy needs to be discussed. It is important to mention to parents that the gold standard for repair of UPJ obstruction is an open pyeloplasty. From all published data on the endourologic incisional management of UPJ obstruction in children, there is an overall success rate of 81% for primary and 87% for secondary UPJ obstructions (King et al., 1984; Towbin et al., 1987; Kavoussi et al., 1991; Tan et al., 1993; Bolton et al., 1994; Faerber et al., 1995; Bogaert et al., 1996; Netto et al., 1996; Capolicchio et al., 1997; Duschinsky et al., 1997a; Schenkman and Tarry, 1998; Young et al., 1999). Discussion of the risks for any procedure is mandatory when obtaining informed consent. These risks include bleeding, the possibility of open surgical correction, and the potential for loss of renal function. Prior to any endourologic procedure there should be documentation of sterile urine, and perioperative intravenous antibiotics should be administered. The routine preoperative assessment for crossing vessels in the area of the UPJ may not be necessary, although it is recommended before undertaking correction of secondary obstruction.

Retrograde endopyelotomy

After induction of general anesthesia the patient is placed in the dorsal lithotomy position. Routine cystoscopic examination is performed and a retro-grade ureteropyelogram obtained. Use of a 5 Fr open-ended catheter is helpful to gauge the caliber of the ureteral orifice. A guidewire is then advanced into the renal pelvis and confirmed using fluoroscopy. The bladder is emptied before removal of the cystoscope.

There are two distinctly different techniques for performing retrograde endopyelotomy. The first involves a balloon cutting device and is performed under fluoroscopy. The second uses direct endoscopic visualization with either flexible or rigid ureteroscopy and surgical incision.

The Acucise (Applied Urology, Laguna Hills, CA, USA) balloon cutting device has a 10 Fr profile which may require active ureteral dilation for retrograde placement (Fig. 9.28). It is passed over a 0.028 inch (0.71 mm) guidewire, and when fully inflated the balloon is 24 Fr in diameter. The length of the active cutting wire is approximately 3 cm and requires a pure cutting current of 50–75 W. The maximum inflation volume of the balloon is 2.2 ml. Radiopaque markers located on the catheter body assist in proper positioning of the balloon across the UPJ.

As the catheter is advanced towards the UPJ it is imperative that the cutting wire be fluoroscopically visualized and oriented in the desired direction. This may require varying the angle of the C-arm unit if the desired position is not directly lateral. Contrast can be instilled through a side port to delineate the area for incision. Once proper positioning has been confirmed, the balloon is inflated with approximately 1 cm of contrast material demonstrating 'waisting' at the narrowed segment. The electrical current is then applied while simultaneously inflating the balloon to its maximum volume. This should be performed quickly under fluoroscopic imaging, and if successful the waist disappears. The balloon is left inflated for 5–10 min, then deflated and removed. Extravasation of contrast material should be confirmed before placement of an indwelling stent (Fig. 9.29). A bladder catheter is left in place overnight and removed the next morning before discharge.

The direct ureteroscopic treatment of UPJ obstruction has been described for adults, and is this author's preferred approach for endopyelotomy. This technique uses either flexible or rigid instrumentation as well as electrosurgical or holmium laser incision. Advantages of this approach include direct visualization of the area as well as confirmation

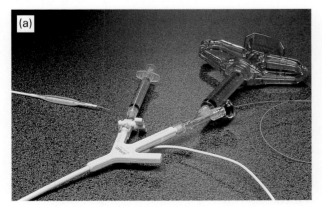
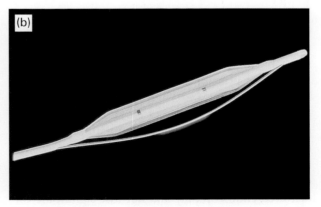

Figure 9.28 The Acucise (Applied Urology, Laguna Hills, CA, USA) balloon cutting device; (*b*) close-up view. The active cutting portion of the wire is the distance between the two radiopaque markers.

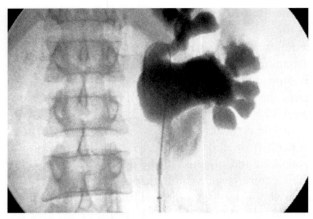

Figure 9.29 Extravasation of contrast from the incised ureteropelvic junction should be visualized to confirm a deep enough incision.

of a transmural incision exposing retroperitoneal adipose tissue. After incision, active balloon dilation using either a 15 or 18 Fr balloon catheter is performed to disrupt any remaining fibrous bands. Contrast extravasation is confirmed and a ureteral stent is placed and left indwelling for 4–6 weeks. A postoperative bladder catheter is removed on the following day.

Incontinence and vesicoureteral reflux

The endoscopic treatment of urinary incontinence as well as VUR is intriguing because of the minimally invasive nature of the technique. Berg (1973) described the use of injectable polytetrafluoroethylene (Teflon) paste for the correction of surgically incurable urinary incontinence. In 1981 this form of therapy was expanded to the correction of primary VUR (Matouschek, 1981). Since these initial reports, ongoing clinical studies have tried to define proper patient selection, as well as the most suitable injectable material.

The basic principle is the same for the correction of both incontinence and VUR. The treatment goal is submucosal bulking of either the subureteric space or proximal urethra resulting in coaptation to prevent retrograde flow of urine up the ureter, or to increase urethral resistance to prevent the passive flow of urine out of the bladder. The ideal agent needs to be delivered endoscopically and not lose significant volume or effectiveness over time. It is important that this material be biocompatible as well as non-anti-

genic, non-migratory, and non-carcinogenic. The search is ongoing for an agent which meets all of these requirements.

Technique

Vesicoureteral reflux

After induction of anesthesia, the patient is placed in the dorsal lithotomy position and administered a broad-spectrum antibiotic. The ureteral orifices are identified and an 20–24 G needle is placed through a working channel at least 5 Fr size. In some instances it may be helpful first to place a 3 Fr catheter into the ureteral orifice in order to tent-up the ureter to facilitate proper needle placement. The bevel of the needle is placed anteriorly and the bladder mucosa is punctured precisely at the 6 o'clock position several millimeters distal to the ureteral orifice. The needle is then advanced proximally until positioned posterior to the ureteral orifice (Fig. 9.30). It is important to avoid multiple puncture sites as this increases the risk for local extravasation of injected material. Once the bulking agent is delivered, the needle should be maintained in position for several minutes to allow the injected material to settle into position. The patient is generally sent home on the same day.

Incontinence

There are three specific methods for the placement of bulking agents in the treatment of urinary incontinence. The patient is placed in the dorsal lithotomy position and antibiotic prophylaxis is administered. Multiple injection sites are needed for adequate coaptation, but typically they should first be directed at the 4 and 8 o'clock positions.

The periurethral approach is best suited to the treatment of women with urinary incontinence. Because of a shortened urethra, it is difficult to deliver the needle cystoscopically. During cystoscopic visualization, the needle is directed through the skin periurethrally towards the lumen of the urethra until reaching the submucosal space just distal to the bladder neck. It is important to maintain the integrity of the urethral mucosa to prevent extravasation of bulking material. Generally, a 20 gauge spinal needle is used.

The transurethral approach involves the use of a cystoscope with at least a 5 Fr working channel. The

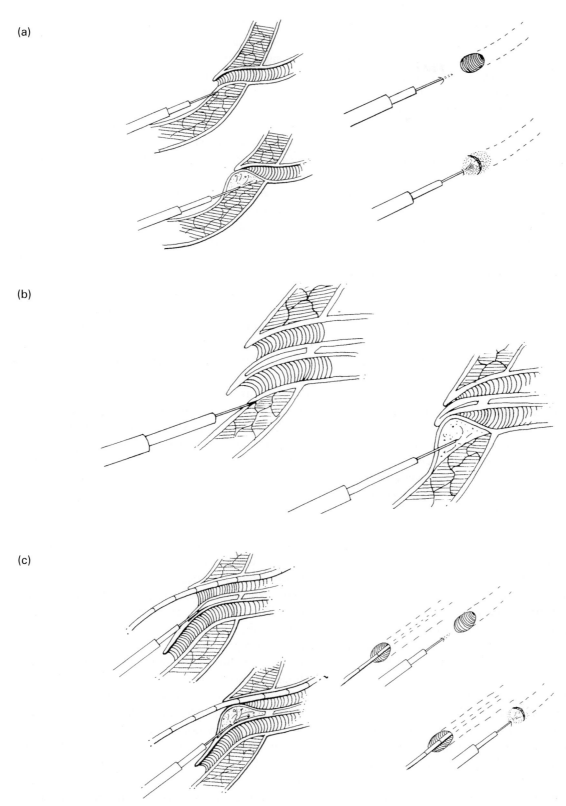

Figure 9.30 (*a*) Endoscopic injection of single refluxing system; (*b*) if the ureteral orifices of a duplex system are close in proximity, coaptation can be done through implantation beneath both ureters; (*c*) if the duplex orifices are spread apart, a catheter may aid the procedure. (After Ortenberg, 1998.)

bevel should be directed towards the lumen and the urethral submucosal space is penetrated at the 4 and 8 o'clock positions with subsequent injection of the bulking material. Other sites are used as necessary to complete adequate coaptation. Once the material is injected, the cystoscope should not be advanced into the bladder because of the potential effect of disrupting the urethral coaptation. At the conclusion of the procedure, a small feeding tube may be used to drain the bladder.

The percutaneous antegrade injection of the bladder neck is a technique described as a better delivery method in those patients with non-compliant urethral tissue due to previous surgical procedures. Antegrade cystoscopy can be performed through a previous suprapubic tract or a percutaneous cystotomy can be performed under retrograde cystoscopic guidance. This approach has been described for postprostatectomy incontinence and has limited indications in children.

Results

It is important to remember that, for the endoscopic treatment of both incontinence and reflux, desired outcome may not be achieved with one treatment. The type of agent used may also have significant effects on long-term outcome. For vesicoureteral reflux, grades I–IV have faired better than most grade V reflux. Reflux associated with neuropathic bladders may have a less successful outcome due to the inherent bladder-wall abnormalities (Engel et al., 1997). Incontinent children with areflexic neuropathic bladders with good compliance and low leak-point pressure have improved outcomes (Chernoff et al., 1997; Silveri et al., 1998). Children with either primary epispadias or exstrophy with epispadias may have better results if they have not had a prior bladder neck procedure (Capozzi et al., 1995; Duffy and Ransley, 1998).

Teflon is the most widely studied agent for both incontinence and reflux. In 1973, Berg described his technique for correction of urinary incontinence in postsurgical patients. This was expanded for use in primary vesicoureteral reflux, which was first reported in 1981 by Matouschek, and later popularized by Puri and O'Donnell. In a recent report with over 12 000 refluxing ureters of grade I–IV, there was a 75% resolution with one injection followed by 12% after two, and 2% after three or four injections. An additional 6% improved to grade I, requiring no further treatment. Only 4.5% could not be corrected or were significantly downgraded, and then went on to reimplantation. Only 0.3% required reimplantation due to vesicoureteral junction obstruction after Teflon injection.

At follow-up of more than 2 years in more than 90% of patients, reflux was noted to occur in only 2.8% (Puri and Granata, 1998). Similarly, Teflon has been noted as a good endoscopic agent for correction or improvement of incontinence. Unfortunately, reports of particle migration, embolization and the formation of granulomas at the site of injection in both animals and humans have curtailed the widespread use of Teflon as an injectable agent within the USA (Malizia et al., 1984; Aaronson et al., 1993). However, it continues to be used in many centers in the remaining portions of the world.

Biodegradable glutaraldehyde crosslinked bovine collagen (GAX-collagen) is a commercially available solution of type I and type III collagen. This agent has been approved in the USA for use as an injectable agent for incontinence. Problems with the collagen are its biodegradable properties, which result in loss of volume over time and the development of serum antibodies and its unknown correlation to autoimmune diseases (Cukier et al., 1993; Leonard et al., 1998). Therefore, results are not as promising as in agents such as Teflon. Several studies have reported results of between 60 and 80% cure rate after 1 year (Frey et al., 1995; Frankenschmidt et al., 1997). Follow-up is limited and several have reported the need for repeat injections. Incontinence treatment is, unfortunately, less encouraging, with fewer than 50% of children showing any long-term durable improvement (Chernoff et al., 1997; Sundaram et al., 1997; Silveri et al., 1998). Not only is the increased cost of numerous repeat injections a concern, but the risk of treatment failure with subsequent possible renal damage is also worrying.

'Deflux' is a one-to-one mixture of dextranomer microspheres suspended in a sodium hyaluronan solution, making it a non-immunogenic biodegradable bulking agent (Stenberg and Lackgren, 1995). It has been used primarily for vesicoureteral reflux and is not approved for clinical use within the USA. Because of their larger particle size of greater than 80 μm, there is limited risk of circulatory migration (Stenberg et al., 1997). Initial animal studies have shown retention of approximately 77% of injected volume in the pig. It is felt that the local recruitment of fibroblast and collagen-producing cells with subsequent ingrowth of blood vessels is responsible for producing a significant bulking effect. The viscous material can be delivered through a 3.5 Fr needle. Initial short-term results are promising, although long-term effects still remain unanswered.

Macroplastique is a 40:60 mixture by volume of polydimethylsiliozane particles suspended in a water-soluble polyvinylpyrrolidone hydrogel solution and has been used for the treatment of both vesicoureteral reflux and urinary incontinence (Buckley *et al.*, 1991; Shulman, 1994). Once again, results have been encouraging, but approximately 5% of the particles are less than 80 μm. The risk of migration has hampered its widespread use (Buckley *et al.*, 1991; Henly *et al.*, 1995).

Polyvinyl alcohol has been studied, but due to potential tumorigenic effects, further work has been discontinued. Injectable bioglass has been shown in laboratory animals to also be feasible, but no clinical work has been presented (Walker *et al.*, 1992).

Several autologous materials have been tested (Kershan and Atala, 1999). The first substance tried was autologous fat, although problems with significant loss of volume have not made this a durable source for endoscopic treatment of incontinence or reflux. The use of autologous collagen, as well as chondrocytes, which are harvested from the hyaline cartilage of the auricular surface, hold some promise for the future. Autologous smooth muscle cells, which have been collected from the bladder have been used as a bulking agent.

One other non-autologous system that may hold promise is the detachable self-sealing membrane balloon system for both reflux and incontinence (Atala *et al.*, 1992; Yoo *et al.*, 1997). Clinical trials are currently underway for urinary incontinence and ongoing laboratory work is being pursued for the treatment of vesicoureteral reflux.

Calyceal diverticula

Calyceal diverticula are non-secreting, urothelial-lined cavities that communicate with the collecting system through a narrow forniceal channel. The abnormality was first described by Rayer in 1841 and he felt that it represented either a cyst or localized hydronephrosis. Their reported incidence is from 2.1 to 4.5 per 1000 intravenous pyelograms. It is felt to be congenital in origin, but some have proposed VUR as a main cause. Two types have been described. Type I are common, are usually adjacent to a minor calyx, and are less likely to produce symptoms. Type II diverticula communicate directly with the renal pelvis or adjacent major calyx. While type I are usually less than 1 cm in size, type II are usually larger and therefore are more likely to have associated symptoms. The incidence is similar for both children and adults, and there appears to be no predilection for either gender. They are bilateral in only approximately 3% (Johnson, 1969; Middleton and Pfister, 1974; Timmons *et al.*, 1975; Siegel and McAlister 1979).

Approximately 50% of calyceal diverticula contain stones and approximately 30% are symptomatic (Timmons *et al.*, 1975). The most common complaint is pain, but they are also associated with infection and hematuria. Intervention is considered for chronic pain, gross hematuria, urolithiasis, recurrent infections, or progressive renal damage. Calyceal diverticula are often visualized on intravenous pyelography, and CT scans with delayed contrast images are also quite helpful (Fig. 9.31). Retrograde ureteropyelography is also effective for demonstrating diverticula, but this is more invasive and generally not necessary as a primary diagnostic tool.

Open surgical techniques have been supplanted by less invasive forms of therapy. Shockwave lithotripsy has been advocated as primary therapy, but the overall symptom-free and stone-free percentage is 60 and 23, respectively (Psihramis and Dretler, 1987; ritchie *et al.*, 1990). Shockwave lithotripsy

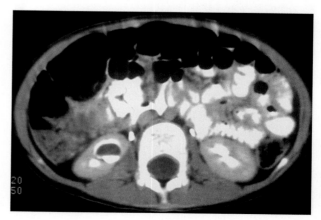

Figure 9.31 Layering of contrast is seen in a right calyceal diverticulum on delayed CT scan.

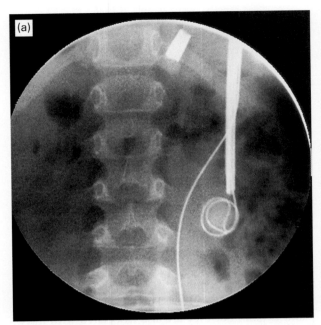
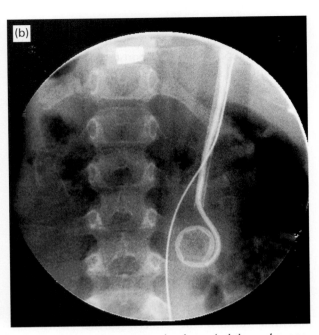

Figure 9.32 (*a*, *b*) A lower pole calyceal diverticulum in a 5-year-old girl was best treated using a 'mini-perc' procedure. A closed stent was left indwelling for 2 weeks through the percutaneous site.

seems most appropriate for diverticula containing stones less than 1 cm and that have a patent neck, which would allow for postlithotripsy drainage (Streem and Yost, 1992).

Endourologic approaches for the treatment of calyceal diverticula include direct or indirect percutaneous puncture, retrograde ureteroscopic access, and laparoscopic unroofing. There are minimal data on the treatment of children, so most outcomes are based on adult patient experience. Percutaneous treatment is the most widely used and the most successful of the three modalities, with a stone-free rate of approxi-

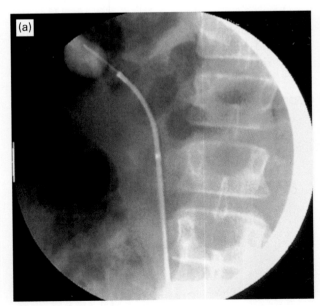
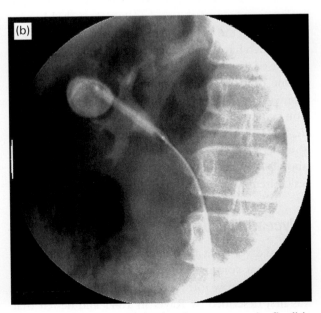

Figure 9.33 (*a*, *b*) Mild and upper pole diverticula can be successfully approached using retrograde flexible ureteropyeloscopy in a 12-year-old girl.

mately 94% and symptom-free rate of 93% (Jones *et al.*, 1991; Shalhave *et al.*, 1998) (Fig. 9.32). In patients treated ureteroscopically, there is an 80% stone-free and 85% symptom-free rate (Grasso *et al.*, 1995b; Batter and Dretler, 1997; Baldwin *et al.*, 1998) (Fig. 9.33). Recently, there have been two case reports of the laparoscopic unroofing of peripherally and located diverticula with thinned parenchyma overlying the cavity (Ruckle and Segura, 1994; Hoznek *et al.*, 1998). The ureteroscopic approach is well suited for diverticula contained within the upper portion of the kidney, which permits easier access, and those which contain stones smaller than 1 cm.

Debate continues over the optimal treatment of the diverticular wall and neck. It is suggested by some that fulguration of the diverticular cavity and incision of the diverticular neck versus dilation may result in better outcome for complete obliteration. Depth of incision should be minimal to avoid the deeper pericalyceal vessels which are typically found in the anteroposterior plane. After balloon dilation, a drainage catheter is placed across the neck of the diverticulum. This is generally left indwelling for several weeks to permit calyceal decompression with subsequent obliteration.

References

Albarran J (1903) Operations plastiques et anastomoses dan la traitment des retentions de viem. Theses, Paris.

Al Busaidy SS, Pren AR, Medhat M (1997) Pediatric ureteroscopy for ureteric calculi: a 4-year experience. *Br J Urol* **80**: 797–801.

Ali Farsi HM, Mosli HA, Alzemonty M *et al.* (1994) *In situ* extracorporeal shock wave lithotripsy (ESWL) for the management of primary ureteric calculi in children. *J Pediatr Surg* **29**: 1315–6.

Allen JS, Summers JL, Wilkerson SE (1972) Meatal calibration in newborn boys. *J Urol* **107**: 499.

Aslan P, Kuo RL, Hazel K *et al.* (1999) Advances in digital imaging during endoscopic surgery. *J Endourol* **13**: 251–5.

Bagley DH (1992) The use of flexible ureteropyeloscopy. *Adv Urol* **5**: 95–9.

Bagley DH (1993) Intrarenal access with the flexible ureteropyeloscope. Effects of active and passive tip defection. *J Endourol* **7**: 221–4.

Baldwin DD, Beaghler MA, Ruckle HC *et al.* (1998) Ureteroscopic treatment of symptomatic caliceal diverticular calculi. *Tech Urol* **4**: 92–8.

Barlow DE (1990) Fiberoptic instrument technology. In: TR (ed.) *Small animal endoscopy*. St. Louis: CV Mosby Co.

Batter SJ, Dretler SP (1997) Ureterorenoscopic approach to the symptomatic caliceal diverticulum. *J Urol* **158**: 709–13.

Berg S (1973) Polytef augmentation urethroplasty. Correction of surgically incurable urinary incontinence by injection technique. *Arch Surg* **107**: 379–81.

Bloom DA, Morgan RJ, Scardino PL (1989) Thomas Hillier and the percutaneous nephrostomy. *Urology* **33**: 346–50.

Blyth B, Passerini-Glazel G, Camuffo C *et al.* (1993) Endoscopic incision of ureteroceles: intravesical vs. ectopic. *J Urol* **149**: 556–60.

Boddy SM, Kellett MJ, Fletcher MS *et al.* (1987) Extracorporeal shock wave lithotripsy and percutaneous nephrolithotomy in children. *J Pediatr Surg* **22**: 223–7.

Bogaert GA, Kogan BA, Mevorach RA *et al.* (1996) Efficacy of retrograde endopyelotomy in children. *J Urol* **156**: 734–7.

Bolton DM, Bogaert GA, Mevorach RA *et al.* (1994) Pediatric ureteropelvic junction obstruction treated with retrograde endopyelotomy. *Urology* **44**: 609–13.

Bozzini P, Lichtleiter J (1806) Der pract. Arzneykunde und Wundarzneykunst. C.W. Hufeland, **24**: 107.

Burns JR, Joseph DB (1993) Combination therapy for a partial staghorn calculus in an infant. *J Endourol* **7**: 469–71.

Bush IM, Goldbert E, Javadpour N *et al.* (1970) Ureteroscopy and renoscopy: a preliminary report. *Chicago Med School Q* **30**: 46–9.

Cadeddu JA, Chen R, Bishoff J *et al.* (1998) Clinical significance of fever after percutaneous nephrolithotomy. *Urology* **52**: 48–50.

Caione P. DeGennard M, Capozza M *et al.* (1990) Endoscopic manipulation of ureteral calculi in children by rigid operative ureteroscopy. *J Urol* **144**: 484–5.

Callaway TW, Lingaroh G, Basata S, Sylven M (1991) Percutaneous nephrolithotomy in children. *J Urol* **148**: 1067–8.

Capolicchio G, Homsy YL, Houle AM *et al.* (1997) Long-term results of percutaneous endopyelotomy in the treatment of children with failed open pyeloplasty. *J Urol* **158**: 1534–7.

Chandhoke PS (1996) Cost-effectiveness of different treatment options for staghorn calculi. *J Urol* **156**: 1567–71.

Chaussy C, Fuchs G, Kahn R *et al.* (1987) Transurethral ultrasonic ureterolithotripsy using a solid wire probe. *Urology* **29**: 531–2.

Choi H, Snyder HM III, Duckett JW (1987) Urolithiasis in childhood: current management. *J Pediatr Surg* **22**: 158–64.

Cohen TD, Ehreth J, King LR, Preminger GM (1996) Pediatric urolithiasis: medical and surgical management. *Urology* **47**: 292–303.

Cussen LJ (1971). The morphology of congenital dilation of the ureter: intrinsic ureteral lesions. *Aust. NZ J Surg* **41**: 185–94.

Davis DM (1943) Intubated ureterotomy, new operation for ureteral and ureteropelvic stricture. *Surg Gynecol Obstet* **76**: 513–23.

Davis DM (1958) The process of ureteral repair: a recapitulation of the splinting question. *J Urol* **79**: 215–23.

Davis DM, Strong GH, Drake WM (1948) Intubated ureterotomy: experimental work and clinical results. *J Urol* **59**: 851–62.

Desai M, Ridhorkar V, Patel S *et al.* (1999) Pediatric percutaneous nephrolithotomy: assessing impact of technical innovations on safety and efficacy. *J Endourol* **13**: 359–64.

De'Sormeaux AJ (1865) Del'endoscope et de ses application au diagnostic et au traitment des affections del'urethre et de la vessie. Paris.

Doraiswamy N (1994) Retrograde ureteroplasty using balloon dilation in children with pelvicureteric obstruction. *J Pediatr Surg* **29**: 937–40.

Dretler SP, Bhatta KM (1991) Clinical experience with high power (140 MJ), large fiber (320 micron) pulsed dye laser lithotripsy. *J Urol* **146**: 1228–31.

Duschinsky J, Plaire J, Lingeman JE (1997a) Antegrade endopyelotomy in the pediatric population. World Congress of Endourology, Edinburgh, UK.

Dushinski JW, Plair JC, Lingeman JE (1997b) Percutaneous nephrolithotomy in the pediatric population. *J Endourol* **11**: S133.

Elder JS (1997) Percutaneous cystolithotomy with endotracheal tube tract dilation after urinary tract reconstruction. *J Urol* **157**: 2298–300.

Erhard MJ, Bagley DM (1995). Urologic applications of the holmium laser: preliminary experience. *J Endourol* **9**: 383–6.

Faerber G, Ritchey M, Bloom DA (1995) Percutaneous endopyelotomy in infants and young children after failed open pyeloplasty. *J Urol* **154**: 1495–7.

Fernstrom I, Johansson B (1976) Percutaneous pyelolithotomy: a new extraction technique, *Scand J Urol Nephrol* **10**: 257–9.

Figenshau RS, Clayman RV (1998) Endourologic options for management of ureteropelvic unction obstruction in the pediatric patient. *Urol Clin North Am* **25**: 199–209.

Frick J, Kohle R, Kunit G (1988) Experience with extracorporal shock wave lithotripsy in children. *Eur Urol* **14**: 181–3.

Frick J, Sarica K, Kohle G *et al.* (1991) Long-term follow-up after extracorporeal shock wave lithotripsy in children. *Eur Urol* **19**: 225–9.

Goodman TM (1977). Ureteroscopy with a pediatric cystoscope in adults. *Urology* **9**: 394.

Goodwin WE, Casey WC, Woolf W (1955) Percutaneous trocar (needle) nephrostomy in hydronephrosis. *JAMA* **157**: 891–4.

Gow JG (1998) Harold Hopkins and optical systems for urology an appreciation. *Urology* **1**: 152–7.

Grasso M (1996a) Experience with the holmium laser as an endoscopic lithotrite. *Urology* **48**: 199–203.

Grasso M (1996b) Flexible fiberoptic ureteropyeloscopy. In: Smith AD, Badlani GH, Bagley DH *et al.* (eds) *Smith's textbook of endourology*. St Louis: Quality Medical Publishing.

Grasso M, Bagley DH (1994a) A 7.5/8.2 F actively deflectable, flexible ureteroscope: a new device for both diagnostic and therapeutic upper urinary tract endoscopy. *Urology* **43**: 435–41.

Grasso M, Bagley DH (1994b) Endoscopic pulsed-dye laser lithotripsy: 159 consecutive cases. *J Endourol* **8**: 25–7.

Grasso M, Beaghler M, Loisides P (1995a) The case for primary endoscopic management of upper urinary tract calculi: II. cost and outcome assessment of 112 primary ureteral calculi. *Urology* **45**: 372–6.

Grasso M, Lang G, Loisides P *et al.* (1995b) Endoscopic management of the symptomatic caliceal diverticular calculus. *J Urol* **153**: 1878–81.

Gregory E, Simmons D, Weinburg JJ (1988) Care and sterilization of endourologic instruments. *Urol Clin North Am* **15**: 541–6.

Gupta M, Yuncay OL, Smith AD (1997) Open surgical exploration after failed endopyelotomy: a 12–year perspective. *J Urol* **157**: 1613–9.

Haupt G, Pannek J, Herde T *et al.* (1995) The lithovac: new suction device for the Swiss lithoclast. *J Endourol* **9**: 375–7.

Helal M, Black T, Lockhart J, Figueroa TE (1997) The Hickman peel-away sheath: alternative for pediatric percutaneous nephrolithotomy. *J Endourol* **11**: 171–2.

Hill DE, Segura JW, Patterson DE, Kramer SA (1990) Ureteroscopy in children. *J Urol* **144**: 481–3.

Honey RJ (1998) Assessment of a new tipless nitinol stone basket and comparison with an existing flat-wire basket. *J Endourol* **12**: 529–31.

Hoznek A, Herard A, Ogiez N *et al.* (1998) Symptomatic caliceal diverticula treated with extraperitoneal laparoscopic marsupialization fulguration and gelatin resorcinol formaldehyde glue obliteration. *J Urol* **160**: 352–5.

Huffman JL, Bagley DH, Lyon ES (1988) *Ureteroscopy*. Philadelphia, PA: WB Saunders.

Hulbert JC, Reddy PK, Gonzalez R *et al.* (1985) Percutaneous nephrostolithotomy: an alternative approach to the management of pediatric calculus disease, *Pediatrics* **76**: 610–12.

Jackman SV, Hedican SP, Peters CA, Docimo SG (1998) Percutaneous nephrolithotomy in infants and preschool age children: experience with a new technique. *Urology* **52**: 697–701.

Jayanthi VR, Arnold PM, Koff SA (1999) Strategies for managing upper tract calculi in young children. *J Urol* **1162**: 1234–7.

Johnson DE (1969) Calyceal diverticulum: report of 31 cases with reference to associated anomalies. *South Med J* **62**: 220–2.

Jones JA, Lingeman JE, Steidle CP (1991) The rules of extracorporeal shock wave lithotripsy and percutaneous nephrostolithotomy in the management of pyelocaliceal diverticula. *J Urol* **146**: 724–7.

Kapoor DA, Leech JE, Yap WT *et al.* (1992) Cost and efficacy of extracorporeal shock wave lithotripsy versus ureteroscopy in the treatment of lower ureteral calculi. *J Urol* **148**: 1095–6.

Kavoussi LR, Meretyk S, Dierks SM *et al.* (1991) Endopyelotomy for secondary ureteropelvic junction obstruction in children. *J Urol* **145**: 345–9.

Khoury AE, Salomon M, Doche R *et al.* (1997) Stone formation after aligmentation cystoplasty: the role of intestinal mucus. *J Urol* **158**: 1133–7.

King LR, Coughlin PW, Ford KK *et al*. (1984) Initial experiences with percutaneous and transurenteric ablation of postoperative ureteral strictures in children. *J Urol* **131**: 1167–70.

Kronner KM, Casale AJ, Cain MP *et al*. (1998) Bladder calculi in the pediatric augmented bladder. *J Urol* **160**: 1096–8.

Kroovand RL, Harrison LH, McCullough DL (1987) Extracorporeal shock wave lithotripsy in children. *J Urol* **138**: 1106–8.

Kuo RL, Delvecchio FC, Preminger GM (1999). Use of a digital camera in the urologic setting. *Urology* **53**: 613–6.

Kurzrock EA, Huffman JL, Hardy BE, Fugelso P (1996) Endoscopic treatment of pediatric urolithiasis. *J Pediatr Surg* **31**: 1413–6.

Lifshitz DA, Lingeman JE, Zafar FS *et al*. (1998) Alterations in predicted growth rates of pediatric kidneys treated with extracorporeal shock wave lithotripsy. *J Endourol* **12**: 469–75.

Lim DJ, Walker RD, Ellsworth PI *et al*. (1996) Treatment of pediatric urolithiasis between 1984 and 1994. *J Urol* **156**: 702–5.

Litvak AA, Morris JD, McRoberts JW (1976) Normal size of the urethral meatus in male children. *J Urol* 736–8.

Loisides P, Grasso M, Bagley DH (1995) Mechanical impactor employing nitinol probes to fragment human calculi: fragmentation efficiency with flexible endoscope deflection. *J Endourol* **9**: 371–4.

Lome LG, Howat JM, Williams DI (1972) The temporarily defunctionalized bladder in children. *J Urol* **107**: 469–72.

Lopez-Alcina E, Broseta E, Oliver F *et al*. (1998) Paraureteral extrusion of calculi after endoscopic pulsed-dye laser lithotripsy. *J Endourol* **12**: 517–21.

Lottman HB, Archambaud F, Hellal B *et al*. (1998) Technetium-dimercaptosuccinic acid renal scan in the evaluation of potential long-term renal parenchymal damage associated with extracorporeal shock wave lithotripsy in children. *J Urol* **159**: 521–4.

Lyons ES, Kyker JS, Schoenbert HW (1978) Transurethral ureteroscopy in women: a ready addition to urologic armamentarium. *J Urol* **119**: 35–6.

Lyons ES, Banno JJ, Schoenberg HW (1979) Transurethral ureteroscopy in men using juvenile pediatric cystoscopy equipment. *J Urol* **122**: 152–3.

Marberger M, Turk C, Steinkogler I (1989) Piezoelectric extracorporeal shock wave lithotripsy in children. *J Urol* **142**: 349–52.

Marshall VF (1964) Fiberoptics in urology. *J Urol* **9**: 110–11.

Matouschek E (1981) Die Behandlung Des Vesikorenalen. Refluxes durch transurethrale einspritzung von teflonpast. *Urologe-Augable A* **20**: 263–4.

Middleton AW Jr, Pfister RC (1974) Stone-containing pyelocalical diverticulum: embryogenic, anatomic, radiologic and clinical characteristics. *J Urol* **111**: 2–6.

Milliner DS, Murphy ME (1993) Urolithiasis in pediatric patients. *Mayo Clin Proc* **68**: 241–8.

Minevich E, Rousseau MB, Wacksman J *et al*. (1997) Pediatric ureteroscopy: technique and preliminary results. *J Pediatr Surg* **32**: 571–4.

Monfort G, Morrison-Lacombe G, Coquet M (1985) Endoscopic treatment of ureteroceles revisited. *J Urol* **133**: 1031–3.

Morse R, Resnick M (1991) Ureteral calculi: natural history and treatment in an era of advanced technology. *J Urol* **145**: 263–5.

Mulvaney W (1953) Attempted disintegration of calculi by ultrasonic vibration. *J Urol* **70**: 704–6.

Mulvaney WP, Beck CW (1968) The laser beam in urology. *J Urol* **99**: 112–5.

Myers DA, Mobley TB, Jenkins KM *et al*. (1995) Paediatric low energy lithotripsy with the lithostar. *Br J Urol* **153**: 453–7.

Netto NR, Ikari O, Esteves SC *et al*. (1996) Antegrade endopyelotomy for pelviureteric junction obstruction in children. *Br J Urol* **78**: 607–12.

Newman DM, Coury T, Lingeman JE *et al*. (1986) Extracorporeal shock wave lithotripsy experience in children. *J Urol* **136**: 238–40.

Nijman RJM, Ackaert K, Scholtmeijer RJ *et al*. (1989) Long-term results of extracorporeal shock wave lithotripsy in children. *J Urol* **142**: 609–11.

Nitze M (1891) *Das Operation Skystoskop*. Vorlaufige Mitteilung, Centr. bl. Chir, **18**: 993.

Ortenberg J (1998) Endoscopic treatment of vesicoureteral refluxin children. *Urol Clin North Am* **25**: 151–6.

Pearle MS, Sech SM, Cobb CG *et al*. (1998) Safety and efficacy of the alexandrite laser for the treatment of renal and ureteral calculi. *Urology* **51**: 34–8.

Pfister C, Ravasse P, Barret E *et al*. (1998) The value of endoscopic treatment for ureteroceles during the neonatal period. *J Urol* **159**: 1006–9.

Piergiovanni M, Desgrandclamps F, Cochand-Priollet B *et al*. (1994) Ureteral and bladder lesion after ballistic, ultrasonic, electrohydraulic or laser lithotripsy. *J Endourol* **8**: 293–9.

Polinsky MS, Kaiser BA, Baluarte HJ (1987) Urolithiasis in children. *Pediatr Clin North Am* **34**: 683–710.

Poon M, Beaghler M, Baldwin D (1997) Flexible endoscopic defectability: changes using a variety of working instruments and laser fibers. *J Urol* **11**: 247–9.

Preminger GM (1996) Video imaging and documentation. In: Smith AD, Badlani GH, Bagley DH *et al*. (eds) *Smith's textbook of endourology* St Louis: Quality Medical Publishing, 29–59.

Psihramis KE, Dretler SP (1987) Extracorporeal shock wave lithotripsy of caliceal diverticula calculi. *J Urol* **138**: 707–11.

Razui HA, Song TY, Denstedt JD (1996) Management of vesical calculi: comparison of lithotripsy devices. *J Endourol* **10**: 559–63.

Rich MA, Keating MA, Snyder HM III, Duckett JW (1990) Low transurethral incision of single system intravesical ureteroceles in children. *J Urol* **144**: 120–1.

Ritchey M, Patterson DE, Delalis PP, Segura JW (1988) A case of pediatric ureteroscopic lasertripsy. *J Urol* **139**: 1271–4.

Ritchie AWS, Parr MJ, Moussa SA, Tolley DA (1990) Lithotripsy for calculi in caliceal diverticula? *Br J Urol* **66**: 6–8.

Rupel E, Brown R (1955) Nephrostomy in hydronephrosis. *JAMA* **157**: 891–4.

Ruckle HC, Segura JW (1994) Laparoscopic treatment of stone filled, caliceal diverticulum: a definitive minimally invasive therapeutic option. *J Urol* **151**: 122–4.

Scarpa RM, DeLisa A, Porru D *et al*. (1995) Ureterolithotripsy in children. *Urology* **46**: 859–62.

Schenkman EM, Tarry WF (1998) Comparison of percutaneous endopyelotomy with open pyeloplasty for pediatric UPJ obstruction. *J Urol* **159**: 1013–5.

Schulze H, Haupt G, Piergiovanni M *et al*. (1993) The Swiss lithoclast: a new device for endoscopic stone disintegration. *J Urol* **149**: 15–8.

Shalhave AL, Soble JJ, Nakada SY *et al*. (1998) Long-term outcome of caliceal diverticula following percutaneous endosurgical management. *J Urol* **160**: 1635–9.

Shepherd P, Thomas R, Harmon EP (1988) Urolithiasis in children: innovations in management. *J Urol* **140**: 790–2.

Shroff S, Watson GM (1995) Experience with ureteroscopy in children. *Br J Urol* **75**: 395–400.

Siegel MJ, McAlister WH (1979) Calyceal diverticula in children: unusual features and complications. *Radiology* **131**: 79.

Smith C, Gosalbez R, Parrott TS *et al*. (1994) Transurethral puncture of ectopic ureteroceles in neonates and infants. *J Urol* **152**: 2110–12.

Smith DP, Jerkins GR, Noe HN (1996) Urethroscopy in small neonates with posterior urethral valves and ureteroscopy in children with ureteral calculi. *Urology* **47**: 908–10.

Spencer-Barthold J (1998) Editorial: Individualized approach to the prenatally diagnosed ureterocele. *J Urol* **159**: 1011–12.

Streem SB, Yost A (1992) Treatment of caliceal diverticular calculi with extracorporeal shock wave lithotripsy: patient selection and extended follow-up. *J Urol* **148**: 1043–6.

Sugita Y, Clarnette T, Huston J (1996) Retrograde balloon dilation for primary pelvi-ureteric junction stenosis in children. *Br J Urol* **77**: 587–9.

Sutherland RS, Pfister RR, Koyle MA (1992) Endopyelotomy associated ureteral necrosis: complete ureteral replacement using the Boari flap. *J Urol* **148**: 1490–2.

Takagi T, Go T, Takayasu H, Aso Y (1971) Fiberoptic pyeloureteroscopy. *Surgery* **70**: 661–3.

Tan HL, Najmaldin A, Webb DR (1993) Endopyelotomy for pelvi-ureteric junction obstruction in children. *Eur Urol* **24**: 84–8.

Tan H, Roberts J, Grattan-Smith D (1995) Retrograde balloon dilation in ureteropelvic obstructions in infants and children: early results. *Urology* **46**: 89–91.

Tanagho EA (1974) Congenitally obstructed bladder: fate after prolonged defunctionalization. *J Urol* **111**: 102–9.

Tank ES (1986) Experience with endoscopic incision and open unroofing of ureteroceles. *J Urol* **136**: 241–2.

Tank ES (1987) Anterior urethral valves resulting from congenital urethral diverticula. *Urology* **30**: 467–9.

Teichman JMH, Rogenes VJ, McIver BJ, Harris JM (1997) Holmium:Yttrium–aluminum–garnet laser cystolithotripsy of large bladder calculi. *Urology* **50**: 44–8.

Teichman JM, Vassar GJ, Bishoff JT, Bellman GC (1998) Holmium:YAG lithotripsy yields smaller fragments than lithoclast, pulsed dye laser or electrohydraulic lithotripsy. *J Urol* **159**: 16–23.

Ten CL, Fhong P, Preminger GM (1998) Laboratory and clinical assessment of pneumatically driven intracorporeal lithotripsy. *J Endourol* **12**: 163–9.

Thomas R, Cherry R, VandenBerg T (1993a) Long term efficacy of retrograde ureteroscopic endopyelotomy. *J Urol* **149**: 276A.

Thomas R, Ortenberg J, Lee BR, Harmon EP (1993b) Safety and efficacy of pediatric ureteroscopy for management of calculus disease. *J Urol* **149**: 1082–4.

Thornhill JA, Moran K, Mooney EE *et al*. (1990) Extracorporeal shock wave lithotripsy monotherapy for paediatric urinary tract calculi. *Br J Urol* **65**: 638–40.

Timmons JW Jr, Malek RS, Hattery RR, Deweerd JH (1975) Caliceal diverticulum. *J Urol* **114**: 6–9.

Towbin RB, Wacksman J, Ball WS (1987) Percutaneous pyeloplasty in children: experience in three patients. *Radiology* **163**: 381–4.

Ueno A, Kawamura T, Ogawa A *et al*. (1977) Relation of spontaneous passage of calculi to size. *Urology* **10**: 544–6.

Van Cangh PJ, Neea S, Galeon M *et al*. (1996) Vessels around the ureteropelvic junction: significance and imaging by conventional radiology. *J Endourol* **10**: 111–9.

Van Gangh PJ, Wilmart JF, Opsomer RJ *et al*. (1994) Long term results and late recurrence after endoureteropyelotomy: a critical analysis of prognostic factors. *J Urol* **151**: 934–7.

Van Savage JG, Khoury AE, McLorie GA, Churchill BM (1996) Percutaneous vacuum vesicolithotomy under direct vision: a new technique. *J Urol* **156**: 706–8.

Van Savage JG, Khoury AE, McLorie GA, Bagley DJ (1997) An algorithm for the management of anterior urethral valves. *J Urol* **158**: 1030–2.

Vassar GJ, Chan KF, Teichman JM *et al*. (1999) Holmium:YAG lithotripsy: photothermal mechanism. *J Endourol* **13**: 181–90.

Wangensteen OH, Wangensteen SD (1978) Lithotomy and lithotomies. In: *The rise of surgery from empiric craft to scientific discipline*. Minneapolis, MN: University of Minnesota Press, 71–80.

Watson G, Murray S, Dretler SP, Parrish JA (1987) The pulsed dye laser for fragmentation of urinary calculi. *J Urol* **138**: 195–8.

Weber HN, Miller K, Ruschoff K *et al*. (1991) Alexandrite laser lithotriptor in experimental and first clinical application. *J Endourol* **5**: 51–5.

Wilkinson A, Aozmy A (1996) Balloon dilation of the pelvi-ureteric junction in children: early experience and pitfalls. *Pediatr Radiol* **26**: 882–6.

Williams DI, Retik AB (1969) Congenital valves and diverticula of the anterior urethra. *Br J Urol* **41**: 228–34.

Willis LR, Evan AP, Connors BA *et al.* (1999) Relationship between kidney size, renal injury and renal impairment induced by shock wave lithotripsy. *J Am Soc Nephrol* **10**: 1753–62.

Woodside JR, Stevens GF, Stark GL*et al.* (1985) Percutaneous stone removal in children. *J Urol* **134**: 1166–7.

Young HH, McKay RW (1929) Congenital valvular obstruction of the prostatic urethra. *Surg Gynecol Obstet* **48**: 509–11.

Young JD, Gigenshau RS, Coplen DE, Clayman RV (1999) *Pediatric endopyelotomy: the Washington University experience*. Dallas, TX: Society of Pediatric Urology.

Yutkin L (1955) *Electrohydraulic lithotripsy*. English translation for US Department of Commerce, Office of Technical Services. Dic 62–15184 MDL 1207/1–2.

Urinary tract infections in children   10

H. Gil Rushton and Hans G. Pohl

Introduction

During the 1990s many new insights have been gained into the etiology and pathophysiology of urinary tract infections (UTIs) in children. The role of bacterial virulence in the etiology of urinary tract infections has assumed greater importance; several genetically encoded bacterial virulence factors have been identified that enhance the potential of uropathogenic bacteria to cause symptomatic disease. These include the ability of certain strains of bacteria to adhere or attach to human uroepithelium. Interacting with these virulence factors is a multitude of host defense factors operating at every level of the urinary tract. These complex host–parasite interactions determine an individual's susceptibility to urinary infection.

Epidemiology

UTIs in children may be symptomatic or asymptomatic. Symptomatic infections may be confined to the bladder (cystitis), or they may involve the upper collecting system (ureteritis, pyelitis), or extend into the renal parenchyma (pyelonephritis). Age, gender, race, circumcision status, the method of detection, and presentation all influence the prevalence of symptomatic versus asymptomatic urinary infection.

Overall, the incidence of neonatal bacteriuria has been reported as 1–1.4% (O'Dougherty, 1968; Littlewood et al., 1969; Abbott, 1972). The male-to-female ratio in infants is the opposite to that seen in older children. From a compilation of screening studies of healthy newborns reviewed by Stamey (1980), 1.5% of boys versus only 0.13% of girls had bacteriuria (Stamey, 1980). However, the actual incidence of UTI during infancy has probably been under-

estimated in the past, partly because of the difficulty in diagnosing UTI in this age group. In a three-year prospective study of 3581 infants (aged 0–1 year) in Goteborg, Sweden, asymptomatic bacteriuria was confirmed by suprapubic aspiration of urine in 2.5% of boys and 0.9% of girls (Jodal, 1987). Symptomatic urinary infection occurred equally often in both sexes (1.2% of boys and 1.1% of girls). Overall, 3.7% of boys and 2% of girls had positive urine cultures during the first year of life. The male predominance noted in the Goteborg study during the first few months of life has also been reported by others (Bergstrom et al., 1972; Drew and Acton, 1976; Ginsburg and McCracken, 1982; Majd et al., 1991). Uncircumcised infant boys are eight to ten times more likely to have symptomatic urinary infection than their circumcised counterparts (Wiswell et al., 1985).

During preschool and school age, the male-to-female ratio observed in neonates is reversed, making screening bacteriuria more prevalent in girls (Bergstrom et al., 1972; Drew and Acton, 1976) (Table 10.1). In several large studies of school-age children the aggregate risk of screening bacteriuria has been reported to be 0.7–1.95% of girls and 0.04–0.2% of boys (Kunin, 1970; Savage, 1973; Saxena et al.,

Table 10.1 Gender ratio of urinary tract infections

Age range	Females	Males
Neonate	0.4	1
1–6 months	1.5	1
6–12 months	4.0	1
1–3 years	10.0	1
3–11 years	9.0	1
11–16 years	2.0	1

(From Belman and Kaplan, 1981, modified from Winberg et al., 1974.)

Table 10.2 The Clinical history and symptoms of 109 children with 'screening' bacteriuria

History/symptoms	Prevalence (%)
All symptoms (excluding nocturnal enuresis)	70
Urgency	54
Frequency	53
Nocturnal enuresis	51
Diurnal enuresis	47
Previous urinary tract infection	20
Dysuria	13
Unexplained fever	7
Flank pain	4
Nocturia	4

(Modified from Savage, et al., 1973.)

1974; Newcastle Asymptomatic Bacteriuria Research Group, 1975; Lindberg et al., 1975a). However, in as many as one-third of these children a prior history of UTI or voiding symptoms could be elicited (Table 10.2). Based on an average annual incidence figure of 0.4%, Kunin (1964) estimated that bacteriuria will develop in approximately 5% of girls prior to graduation from high school. Additional data collected by Kunin (1970) revealed that infection will recur in up to 80% of all white girls and 60% of black girls within 5 years.

In a prospective population-based study of symptomatic UTI's in children living in Goteborg, Sweden, Winberg et al. (1974) estimated that the aggregate risk for symptomatic UTI up to the age of 11 years was at least 3% for girls and 1.1% for boys. In an update of a previous study, the incidence of culture documented UTIs was twice as high as previously estimated, affecting 7.8% of girls and 1.6% of boys during the first 6 years of life (Hellstrom et al., 1991). To confirm these findings, Marild and Jodal (1998) recently performed a retrospective population-based study of 41 000 children of Goteborg, Sweden. The cumulative incidence rate of symptomatic UTIs was 6.6% for girls and 1.8% for boys. These data probably do not reflect an increasing incidence of UTIs since the publication of the earliest report, but instead a greater detection rate. In these epidemiologic studies, the incidence of febrile UTIs was greater in infant boys and girls than in children over 2 years of age. Gender differences in the incidence rates of first-time febrile and non-febrile UTIs were most evident in children greater than 2 years old. Girls greater than 2 years old were much more likely to present with first time UTI, both with and without fever, compared with their age-matched male counterparts (Fig. 10.1a, b).

Once treated, infants with symptomatic urinary infections are at risk for recurrent infection (26%), usually in the first 3 months of follow-up. In older girls the risk for recurrence following symptomatic urinary infection is as high as 40–60% within 18 months. This risk persists into adulthood (Bergstrom et al., 1972). In one study, 60 girls with childhood bacteriuria followed into adulthood (9–18-year follow-up) were compared with 38 non-bacteriuric controls (Gillenwater et al., 1979). During pregnancy, a significantly greater incidence of bacteriuria was diagnosed in the group with the history of positive urine cultures in childhood (63.8%) than in the controls (26.7%). Interestingly, the propensity for urinary infection persisted in the children born to bacilluric women, whereas none of the children born to healthy controls demonstrated urinary infection.

Further evidence supporting a lifelong risk for symptomatic urinary infection in individuals presenting during childhood is reported by the Goteborg Childhood UTI Research Group. These authors followed 111 women with renal scarring or recurrent UTIs. Febrile UTIs were more prevalent than non-febrile UTIs during the first 10 years of life but continued to occur into the third decade. Although the prevalence of febrile UTIs diminished in adulthood, women with renal scarring during childhood were significantly more likely to have subsequent febrile UTIs. Overall, the median incidence of symptomatic UTIs was seven per individual (Martinell et al., 1990; Martinell et al., 1996a).

Bacteriology

The organisms that colonize the urinary tract are specifically adapted towards this purpose. Research has identified specific virulence factors that determine an organism's pathogenic potential, thus differentiating strains commonly associated with asymptomatic bacteriuria, cystitis, or acute pyelonephritis. However, uropathogenic strains do not rigorously conform to predicted behavior. Rather, a few general principles are applicable, such as the presence of surface molecules important for adhesion and toxins that assist tissue invasion.

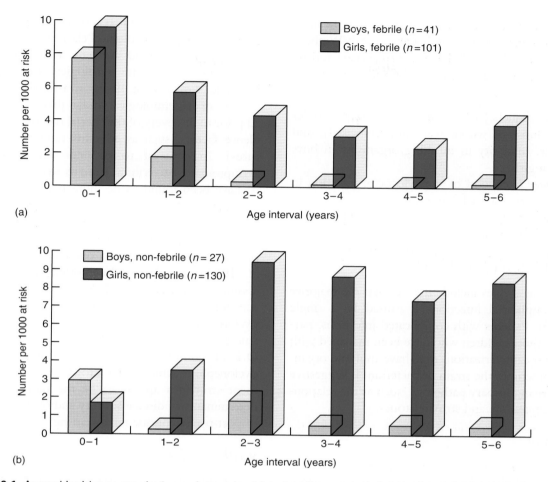

Figure 10.1 Annual incidence rate in 1 year intervals of febrile urinary tract infection in children studied during a 20-month period between 1979 and 1981. (*a*) Incidence of febrile infections in boys compared with girls. (*b*) Incidence of non-febrile infections in boys compared with girls. (Adapted from Marild and Jodal, 1998.)

A large family of Gram-negative, aerobic bacilli known as Enterobacteriaciae causes the majority of uncomplicated UTIs. Included in this family are the species *Escherichia, Klebsiella, Enterobacter, Citrobacter, Proteus, Providencia, Morganella, Serratia,* and *Salmonella*. Of these, *E. coli* is by far the most frequently isolated organism, being responsible for approximately 80% of UTIs. This family of bacteria is generally characterized by a negative reaction to the oxidase test and the capacity to ferment glucose and reduce nitrates to nitrite. *Pseudomonas* is also a Gram-negative, aerobic bacillus but is distinct and unrelated to Enterobacteriaciae. Most *Pseudomonas* recovered from the urine are of relatively low virulence and do not tend to invade tissue unless host defense mechanisms are compromised.

The most common Gram-positive organisms found in UTIs are *Staphylococcus* and *Enterococcus*.

Anaerobic fecal flora rarely produces UTIs despite being 100–1000 times more abundant than *E. coli* in stools (Brook, 1981). Occasionally, unusual or fastidious organisms may produce infections that are difficult to detect because they do not grow well in commonly used culture media. For example, *Haemophilus influenza* has been reported to cause urinary infections (Granoff and Roskes, 1974), as well as epididymo-orchitis in infant males (Rytand and Spreiter, 1981). Other unusual organisms include *Salmonella* sp. and *Shigella*. Although *Lactobacilli, Corynebacteria* and alpha-*Streptococcus* may rarely cause UTIs, they probably should be considered contaminants unless they are found in cultures of specimens obtained by suprapubic aspiration or by catheterization.

The bacteriologic findings in the Goteburg study suggest that 'the [predisposing] environmental conditions in the periurethral region and the host defense mechanisms vary with age and sex' (Winberg *et al.*, 1974). This study identified four characteristic bacteriologic trends in childhood urinary tract infections:

1 a high frequency of *Proteus* sp. infections in older boys (most of whom were uncircumcised), and greater variability in infecting organisms in boys than in girls;
2 a greater likelihood of staphylococcal infection in adolescence, especially in girls;
3 a greater frequency of *E. coli* urinary infection in neonatal boys than in girls of that age;
4 a decreased frequency of *Klebsiella* urinary infection in older children (Table 10.3).

Other general rules include the fact that the majority of uncomplicated infections is caused by a single organism. Patients with complicated infections, particularly those children who have been managed with long-term catheterization, may have multiple organisms. Sometimes the strain of bacterium is suggestive of underlying urinary pathology, such as the relationship of *Proteus* sp. and struvite stones.

Serology

Escherichia coli, the most common species of uropathogens, can be typed serologically by three major groups of antigenic structures capable of producing specific antibodies. There are more than 150 O (cell-wall) antigens, more than 50 H (flagellar) antigens,

and approximately 100 K (capsular) antigens. Not all strains are typable. Serological classification in UTI is restricted mainly to O antigens. Early studies had attempted to correlate serological markers with increased virulence or tissue invasiveness. Most of these were epidemiological studies that were conducted prior to discovery of the special role of specific virulence factors, such as adhesins (attachment structures). In contrast to patients with cystitis or asymptomatic bacteriuria, patients with pyelonephritis have been found to be more frequently infected with certain O typable strains and strains having certain K antigens. Eight O antigen types (O1, O2, O4, O6, O7, O18, O25, and O75) were the cause of 80% of cases of pyelonephritis in one report (Lindberg *et al.*, 1975b). Another study reported that *E. coli* possessing five K antigens (K1, K2, K3, K12, and K13) accounted for 70% of isolates from patients with pyelonephritis (Kaijser, 1977). These earlier serologic studies have been extended to identify more specific O:K:H combination serotypes characteristic of pyelonephritogenic strains. However, specific attachment structures appear to be the more important determinants of disease severity and of the likelihood of post-pyelonephritic renal scarring.

Virulence factors

The term 'virulence' simply refers to the ability of microorganisms to cause disease. The concept of uropathogenic bacteria refers to certain strains that are selected from the fecal flora, not by chance or preva-

Table 10.3 Infecting bacteria (%) isolated from 'first-time' urinary infection in children catergorized by age and gender

Infecting organism	All neonates (n = 73)	Females (%)		Males[a] (%)	
		1 month to 10 years[b] (n = 30)	10–16 years (n = 30)	1 month to 10 years (n = 62)	10–16 years (n = 42)
E. coli	57% (females) 83% (males)	83%	60%	85%	33%
Klebsiella	11	4	0	2	2
Proteus sp.	0	3	0	5	33
Enterococcus	3	2	0	0	2
Staphylococcus	1	4	30	0	12
Other, mixed or unknown	9	11	10	8	17

(Modified from Winburg *et al.*, 1974.)
[a]Males not routinely circumcised in Scandinavia.
[b]No difference between girls 1 month to 1 year old and 1 to 10 years old.

lence, but because of the presence of specific virulence factors that enhance colonization of the uroepithelium. Other virulence factors aid in persistence of bacteria in the urinary tract and provide these organisms with the capacity to induce inflammation of the urethra, bladder, or renal parenchyma. Specific, recognized *E. coli* virulence factors include but are not limited to (1) adherence to uroepithelial cells, (2) high quantity of K antigen in the capsule of the bacteria, (3) hemolysin production, (4) colicin production, (5) the ability of bacteria to acquire iron, and (6) resistance to serum bactericidal activity. Studies of pyelonephritogenic strains of *E. coli* reveal the presence of a limited number of bacterial clones that possess specific virulence factors that are expressed only in certain O groups (Vaisanen-Rhen *et al.*, 1984).

Adherence

Bacterial adherence or attachment is an essential initiating step in all infections. Perineal colonization by uropathogenic bacteria has been found to precede clinical UTI in women and children at risk for UTI (Fussell *et al.*, 1977; Glauser *et al.*, 1978; Gillenwater, 1981; Fussell *et al.*, 1988). Tissue invasion, inflammation, and cell damage are secondary events. Utilizing specialized structures (adhesins), uropathogenic bacteria, especially *E. coli*, can attach to specific receptor sites on the uroepithelium and can also bind in a non-specific manner by electrostatic and hydrophobic factors. By virtue of such attachment, virulent strains of bacteria can ascend into the upper urinary tract even in the absence of structural abnormalities such as vesicoureteral reflux (VUR).

Specific attachment (bacterial tropism) to uroepithelial cells is mediated by adhesins localized either in an outer coat of capsule or on specialized structures. Collectively known as fimbria, these attachment structures are capable of recognizing and attaching to receptors located on uroepithelial cells and to some constituents of the basement membrane. Several different types of fimbria have been identified. Type-1 fimbria mediate agglutination between bacteria and cells in culture. Since this agglutination can be competitively inhibited by a mannose-rich solution, these fimbria are termed mannose sensitive. Other fimbria attach to uroepithelial cells in the presence of soluble mannose and are termed mannose resistant (Fig. 10.2). Uropathogenic bacteria rely on both mannose-

sensitive type 1 fimbria and mannose-resistant type 2 (also termed P-fimbria) to colonize the urinary tract. In addition to type 1 and P-fimbria, uropathogenic bacteria possess several other adhesins, both fimbrial and non-fimbrial. Unfortunately, little epidemiological evidence exists to clarify the role of these additional 'novel' adhesins on *E. coli* (S-fimbria, FIC-fimbria, S/FIC-related fimbria), *Klebsiella* (MR/K HA) and *Proteus* sp. (MR/P HA, PMF, ATF, NAF, UCA) in the pathogenesis of UTI.

In addition to promoting attachment, type-1 fimbria mediate bacterial invasion into the uroepithelial cells, thus protecting bacteria from antibiotics that do not penetrate the cell's membrane, such as aminoglycosides (Malvey *et al.*, 1998). In fact, viable internalized bacteria can be isolated from uroepithelial cells 48 hours after infection, and may account for recurrent infection by the same bacterial strain (Fig. 10.3). Once type-1 fimbriated *E. coli* attach, the uroepithelial cells undergo apoptosis (programmed cell death) that results in bladder mucosal ulceration.

Although the entire urothelial surface, including the upper urinary tract, contains glycoprotein receptors for type 1 fimbria, no evidence exists that implicates type 1 fimbria directly in the pathogenesis of pyelonephritis. However, it has been demonstrated in experimental models and clinical studies that once pyelonephritis occurs, the presence of type 1 fimbria significantly increases a strain's ability to persist in the urinary tract and to stimulate inflammation (Hagberg *et al.*, 1983; Marild *et al.*, 1989a; Connell *et al.*, 1996).

Clinical and experimental studies have shown that pyelonephritic *E. coli* frequently possess fimbriae that can recognize and agglutinate erythrocytes of the P-1 blood group. Hence, this type of pili has been termed P-fimbria. The P-fimbria are mannose-resistant adhesins that attach to the carbohydrate portion [alpha-D-galactopyranosyl-(1-4)-beta-D-galacotpyranoside] of the glycolipid antigen in the P blood group series, which is also expressed by human uroepithelial cells (Kallenius *et al.*, 1980; Leffler and Svanborg-Eden, 1980). The components of P-fimbria are encoded by 11 genes in the pap gene cluster, of which pap E, F, and G encode for the adhesin subunits.

Further research has identified that not all P-fimbria are alike. Proteins located at the tip (G-tip proteins or tip adhesins) determine the fimbria's specific attachment properties. Three classes have been identified, of which only class II and class III

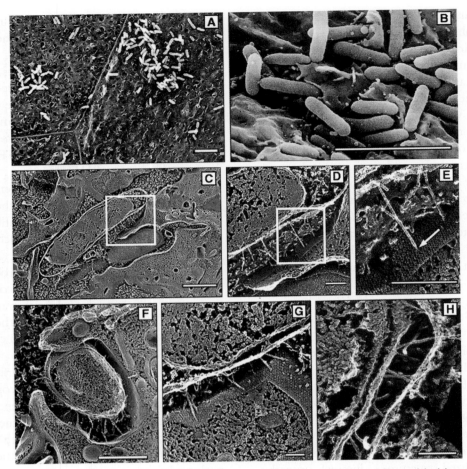

Figure 10.2 Type 1 pilus-mediated bacterial adherence to the bladder epithelium. Mouse bladders were processed for (a, b) scanning electron microscopy (SEM) and high resolution EM at 2 h after infection with E. coli NU14. The boxed areas in (c) and (d) are shown magnified in (d) and (e), respectively. The arrow in (e) indicates the FimH-containing tip. In (h), type 1 pili span from the host cell membrane on the right to the bacterium on the left. Scale bars = 5 μm (a, b), 0.5 μm (c, f), and 0.1 μm (d–h). (From Malvey et al., 1998.)

P-fimbria have uropathogenic potential. *In vitro* studies have found that the class III P-fimbria bind receptors found in higher density on bladder uroepithelium. In contrast, class II tip adhesins may be more important in the evolution of acute pyelonephritis by virtue of an increased density of class II-specific receptors located on the uroepithelium of the upper urinary tract (Lomberg *et al.*, 1989). A recent study described a statistically significant greater likelihood of clinical and histologic indicators of acute pyelonephritis in primates inoculated with class II fimbriated *E. coli* than in primates inoculated with class III fimbriated *E. coli* (James-Ellison *et al.*, 1997).

Epidemiological studies in children have provided considerable evidence that the presence of P-fimbriae on *E.coli* is a significant virulence factor, particularly in upper urinary tract infections. These studies have shown that 76–94% of pyelonephritogenic strains of *E.coli* are P-fimbriated compared with 19–23% of cystitis strains, 14–18% of strains isolated from patients with asymptomatic bacteriuria, and 7–16% of fecal isolate strains (Vaisanen-Rhen, 1984; Kallenius *et al.*, 1984). Other evidence supporting the importance of P-fimbria in causing upper UTIs comes from animal model studies. Inoculation of the bladders of non-refluxing primates with P-fimbriated *E. coli* resulted in pyelonephritis in 66% of animals. In contrast, pyelonephritis was not seen in any of the monkeys inoculated with non-P-fimbriated *E. coli* (Roberts *et al.*, 1985).

In addition to their role in the pathogenesis of pyelonephritis through attachment to renal epithelial cells, P-fimbria function to promote intestinal

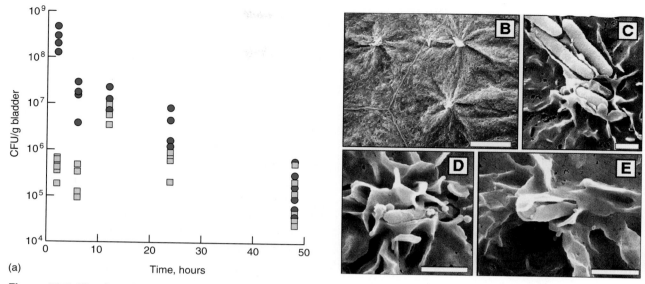

Figure 10.3 Kinetics of bacterial reduction in NU14–infected bladders and the persistence of intracellular bacteria. (a) The total numbers of bacteria per gram of mouse bladder (circles) and the numbers of gentamicin-protected bacteria (boxes) were examined per time point. (B–E) Bacteria in various stages of internalization into superficial cells at 2 h after infection with NU14 were detected by scanning electron microscopy (SEM). Scale bars = 10 μm (b) and 1 μm (c–e). (From Malvey et al., 1998.)

carriage by the host, as well as enhancing perineal colonization (see host factors) and persistence in the urinary tract. Although the data regarding intestinal carriage and perineal colonization (see host factors) by P-fimbriated *E. coli* strongly implicate the P-fimbria in the pathogenesis of infection, the data regarding bacterial persistence are less clear.

Although fimbria appear to be the primary method by which bacteria colonize the urinary tract, there is also attachment to non-exposed 'receptors' located in the interstitium. Secondary binding to fibronectin occurs by means of fimbria encoded by pap, papG, sfa, afa, and prsG DNA sequences, a feature also more common in pyelonephritogenic strains than in strains causing cystitis or asymptomatic bacteriuria (Johanson et al., 1993; Daigle et al., 1994). Other adhesins may play a protective role by preventing UTI through competitive binding. For example, S-fimbria and type 1 fimbria bind to Tamm–Horsfall protein and low molecular weight substances, respectively. Once bound, clearance of bacteria by periodic shedding of these soluble bacteria–protein complexes in the urine offers a theoretical advantage by reducing the number of infecting organisms.

Some data suggest that an organism's phenotype is variable, first facilitating colonization of the uroepithelium, then undergoing specific changes to evade

eradication by the host's immune response (Roberts, 1996a). For example, some type 1 bacteria reach the renal parenchyma (as in the case of VUR). These bacteria, however, must then escape type 1 fimbria-specific neutrophil receptors. *In vitro* studies have demonstrated that neutrophils elicit a more severe inflammatory response in the presence of type 1 fimbriated strains than when in the presence of a mutant strain lacking the type 1 fimbria (Connell et al., 1996). Phase variation to non-type-1 fimbriated strains is known to occur, thereby conferring a potentially protective advantage. Despite this apparently unified view of bacterial virulence, several studies also exist to challenge any attempt to simplify the complex interaction between bacteria and host (Bartkova et al., 1994; Perngini and Vidotto, 1996). In fact, the appearance of P-fimbriated strains in the periurethral region of girls at risk for cystitis does not inevitably result in urinary infection (Schlager et al., 1995). Thus, bacterial virulence properties should not be the sole focus of blame in the development of urinary tract infection. Host risk factors are probably of equal, if not greater, significance.

Despite its significance, bacterial adherence is only one of several factors believed to play a role in infection. Other bacterial virulence factors and host defense factors may play an even greater role in tissue invasion and inflammation. In an experimental study in mice, the presence of P-fimbriae was necessary for colonization of the upper urinary tract but did not produce tissue invasion unless combined with other virulence factors (O'Hanley *et al*., 1985). Similarly, in a clinical study that employed dimercaptosuccinic acid (DMSA) renal scans to document acute inflammatory parenchymal damage in children with febrile UTI, no difference in the prevalence of P-fimbriated *E. coli* was found in children with an abnormal scan compared with those who had a normal scan (Majd *et al*., 1991). Likewise, renal scarring has been reported to be more common following pyelonephritis caused by non-*E. coli* organisms compared with those caused by P-fimbriated *E. coli* (Lomberg *et al*., 1989; Rushton *et al*., 1992).

Other virulence factors

1 *Endotoxin*: a lipolysaccharide present in the bacterium's cell wall, endotoxin, is responsible for initiating the acute inflammatory response common to Gram-negative infections. This same inflammatory response that eradicates the bacteria probably also leads to post-pyelonephritic scarring.

2 *K antigen*: capsular polysaccharides afford K antigen specificity to *E. coli*. K antigen has been shown to shield bacteria from complement lysis and phagocytosis and to enhance the persistence of bacteria in the kidneys of experimental mice (Horowitz and Silverstein, 1980; Svanborg-Eden *et al*., 1987; Blanco *et al*., 1994; Siegfrid *et al*., 1994; Blanco *et al*., 1996). It is more commonly isolated from children with clinical pyelonephritis than in those from children with cystitis or healthy controls (Kaijser, 1973; Blanco *et al*., 1994; Siegfrid *et al*., 1994; Blanco *et al*., 1996).

3 *Hemolysins:* Cytotoxic proteins, such as hemolysins, are another recognized virulence property capable of damaging renal tubular cells *in vitro*. Hemolytic strains of *E. coli* produce more severe experimental pyelonephritis in mice (Waalwijk *et al*., 1983).

4 *Colicin*: another protein elaborated by pyelonephritogenic *E. coli*, colicin, kills other bacteria in the vicinity of the *E. coli* producing it. The colicin V plasmid is also thought to encode for an iron uptake system that further promotes the survival and pathogenicity of colicin-producing organisms (Williams, 1979).

5 *Iron-binding capacity*: most bacteria require iron for optimal growth and metabolism, and have developed mechanisms to acquire iron when there is limited supply. Mediated by such proteins as aerobactin, iron-binding capacity has also been shown to be associated with increased virulence in epidemiological studies (Carbonetti *et al*., 1986; Jacobson *et al*., 1988a).

6 *Serum resistance*: in the presence of fresh human serum, many strains of *E. coli* are killed following activation of complement. Serum resistance to such killing action is another property that has been related to virulence of Gram-negative bacteria both in UTIs and Gram-negative bacteremia (Olling *et al*., 1973; McCabe *et al*., 1978).

Although these virulence factors have been considered separately, their effect appears to be additive. In contrast to those with cystitis or asymptomatic bacteriuria, the majority of bacterial isolates in patients with non-reflux acute pyelonephritis express three or four virulence properties (Lomberg *et al*., 1989). The frequency of P-fimbriae and other virulence factors is significantly lower in patients who have VUR (Figs. 10.4, 10.5). This would appear logical since, in the presence of reflux, virulence properties such as adherence are not necessary for bacteria to reach the upper urinary tract. It has been suggested that efforts aimed at interfering with 'virulent' bacteria , such as by vaccination, may be of less value in patients with recurrent pyelonephritis and reflux, the group in whom renal scars are more likely to develop. Furthermore, others have not demonstrated a significant difference in virulence traits among pyelonephritogenic strains in patients with and without reflux (Arthur *et al*., 1989).

Renal scarring

Regardless of their role in the etiology of UTI, some studies suggest that there may be a paradoxical relationship between bacterial virulence, defined by P-fimbriated binding, and renal scarring. In one study of patients with recurrent pyelonephritis, virulent clones expressing P-fimbria occurred significantly less often in those who developed scarring (22%) than in those who did not develop renal scars (62%) (Lomberg *et al*., 1989). Although the frequency of scarring among girls with VUR was 57% in contrast to 8% of those without reflux, this alone did not explain the selection of bacteria of low virulence in

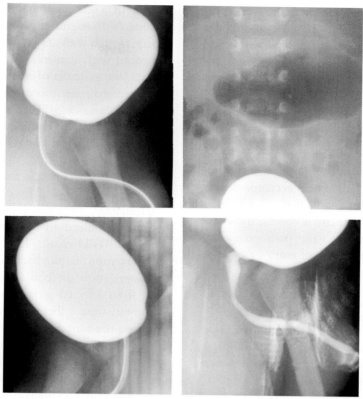

Figure 10.4 Voiding cystourethrogram demonstrating the absence of vesicoureteral reflux and obstructive pathology (posterior urethral valves, ureterocele) in an uncircumcised infant boy with acute pyelonephritis confirmed by [^{99m}Tc]DMSA renal scan.

those patients with scar development. Lomberg *et al.* (1989) concluded that reduced host resistance was essential for the tendency towards renal scarring after acute pyelonephritis.

Other evidence supports the hypothesis that bacteria with greater virulent potential, as measured by the presence of adhesins, may elicit a more rigorous host inflammatory response than less virulent clones and are thus cleared more rapidly. An alternative

explanation would be that children infected with more virulent bacteria present earlier with symptoms such as fever, resulting in more prompt diagnosis and treatment. Observations in patients with bladder dysfunction and asymptomatic bacteriuria have demonstrated a low prevalence of P-fimbriated *E. coli* (less than 20%), suggesting that the presence of specific attachment structures may not be necessary for bacterial persistence in the urinary tract (Hagberg *et al.*,

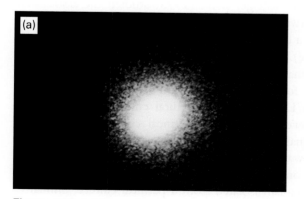
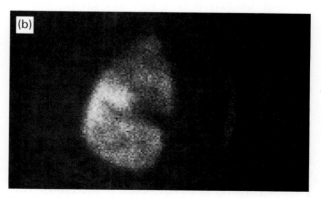

Figure 10.5 (*a*) Isocystogram demonstrating the absence of vesicoureteral reflux in a child with (*b*) [^{99m}Tc]DMSA renal scan documented acute pyelonephritis (upper and lower poles are affected).

1981; Svanborg-Eden *et al.*, 1987). Moreover, coincident with an inflammatory response, P- and type 1 fimbriated *E. coli* were demonstrated to be cleared more rapidly than non-fimbriated strains from individuals with bladder abnormalities (Anderson *et al.*, 1991).

Host defense factors

Interacting with bacterial virulence properties is an equally important and complex number of mechanical, hydrodynamic, anti-adherence, receptor-dependent and immunologic host factors that affect an individual's susceptibility to UTI. By necessity, these factors are closely interrelated to the pathogenesis of UTIs, beginning with the route of entry of bacteria into the urinary tract.

Perineal factors

Hematogenous seeding of the urinary tract is an uncommon source of urinary infection in children. When this is the cause of a renal infection, a cortical abscess rather than classic pyelonephritis is more likely to occur. Considerable clinical and experimental evidence has clearly established an ascending or retrograde urethral route of entry of bacteria in the majority of UTIs. The same bacterial strains causing urinary infections can be found on perineal cultures prior to bladder invasion. This is in contrast to negative perineal cultures in healthy controls (Stamey *et al.*, 1971; Stamey, 1973; Leadbetter and Slavins, 1974; Bollgren and Winburg, 1976a). The usual organisms originate from fecal flora that colonize the perineum (Gruneberg, 1969).

An infant's initial exposure to uropathogenic bacteria occurs at the time of birth, and infants born to bacilluric mothers have a four-fold greater risk of UTIs (Gareau *et al.*, 1959; Patrick, 1967). It has been postulated that other host defense factors mature during the first year of life, resulting in a decrease in both periurethral colonization and frequency of UTI. Overall, the quantities and species of colonizing bacteria in the periurethral area diminish during the first year of life until few remain at the age of 5 years. Meanwhile, normal periurethral flora may even be protective against urinary infection by competitive interference with attachment of uropathogenic bacteria (Chan *et al.*, 1984; Chan *et al.*, 1985). This potential protective effect can be altered by the administration of antimicrobial agents, given for any

reason. In a study of children with first-time acute pyelonephritis, significantly more children had recently been treated with antibiotics, usually for non-UTIs, compared with controls (Marild *et al.*, 1989b). In general, the genitalia of infant boys are more heavily colonized than are those of infant girls and, when colonized, boys carry *E. coli* more frequently than do girls. These data concur with Winburg's epidemiological findings that boys younger than 6 months are at greater risk than their female counterparts and that UTI occurs less frequently with advancing age.

Ultimately, an infant's own intestinal tract may become colonized by bacteria with uropathogenic potential. Wold *et al.* (1992) reported on 13 girls with asymptomatic bacteriuria who underwent characterization of fecal flora. Resident strains isolated from affected girls more commonly expressed P-fimbria, were adherent to colonic epithelium in a mannose-resistant fashion, and were one of several uropathogenic serotypes present when compared with transient strains of *E. coli*. Plos *et al.* (1995) confirmed these findings in a prospective review of fecal isolates from children with UTIs. Affected children demonstrated intestinal colonization with P-fimbriated *E. coli* more frequently than healthy controls both during infection (86% vs 29%) and during infection-free intervals (40% vs 29%) (Plos *et al.*, 1995).

Since Bollgren and Winburg's original work in 1976 in school-aged girls with a history of recurrent UTIs, three additional studies have reported on the natural history of periurethral colonization. Despite the widely accepted concept of an ascending route of infection, the mere presence of uropathogenic bacteria on the perineum did not portend symptomatic UTI. Schlager *et al.* (1995) studied the association between periurethral colonization and recurrent UTI in a cohort of seven toilet-trained girls (3–6 years of age). Each girl underwent weekly periurethral and urinary cultures during a 6-month period immediately following their first UTI. Almost half (43%, 53/122) of the periurethral cultures were positive; however, a positive perineal culture was obtained equally as often in the absence of urinary infection as it was prior to a symptomatic recurrence. Moreover, in only one of the four recurrences was the causative organism isolated from a perineal culture. Similarly, although heavy periurethral colonization has been reported in 75–80% of healthy infants and toddlers of both sexes (Bollgren and Winburg, 1976b), only 1–3% become infected (Winberg *et al.*, 1974). In a study similar to Schlager's, Brumfitt *et al.* (1987) found that perineal colonization by the responsible organism did not precede the symptomatic recurrent UTI in up to 34% of the adult women studied. These data may reflect the transient nature of bacterial species colonizing the perineum. Alternatively, these findings may reflect the short time course between initiation of perineal colonization and symptomatic UTI by uropathogenic bacteria in certain individuals.

Although it is not unreasonable to suspect that an abrupt change in the expression of certain key virulence factors might precipitate ascent from the perineum to the bladder, some data exist to refute this hypothesis. Schlager *et al.* (1995) characterized the expression of six virulence factors among *E. coli* colonizing the bladder in the absence of symptoms and those causing symptomatic UTI in seven girls. Although P-fimbria were commonly identified in infecting species of *E. coli*, none of the six virulence factors, including P-fimbria, accurately predicted which colonizing species would ultimately cause symptomatic infection. Thus, although sufficient evidence exists to support bacterial ascent into the bladder from the perineum as the mode of entry, the facilitating events in that mechanism remain poorly understood.

Prepuce

A hematogenous route of infection, rather than ascent into the urinary tract from the perineum, has been suggested in the newborn. This proposal was based on the more frequent finding of bacteremia associated with UTI in this age group (Ginsburg and McCracken, 1982). However, others have not substantiated a higher incidence of bacteremia in neonates compared with other infants and children with febrile UTIs (Hellstrom *et al.*, 1991; Majd *et al.*, 1991). Furthermore, the increased risk for UTI (including pyelonephritis) in uncircumcised boys compared with both girls and circumcised boys provides additional convincing support for an ascending route of infection even during the first several months of life. In fact, over 90% of boys with febrile UTIs during the first year of life are uncircumcised (Ginsburg and McCracken, 1982; Rushton and Majd, 1992a). Wiswell *et al.* (1985) initially found a 20-fold

higher rate of UTI among infant boys who were not circumcised than among those who were (4.12% vs 0.21%). Subsequently, two larger cohort studies by the same investigator, encompassing 637 097 infants, found that the rate of UTI among uncircumcised boys to be less than that originally described, but still significantly greater (10-fold) than the incidence of UTI among those circumcised (Wiswell *et al.*, 1987; Wiswell and Hachey, 1993) (Table 10.4). Rushton and Majd (1992a) prospectively found that 92% of boys under 6 months of age hospitalized with febrile UTIs were uncircumcised compared with 49% of a control group of infant boys hospitalized with febrile respiratory infections.

Evidence exists to implicate the prepuce as a reservoir for uropathogenic bacteria. Wijesina *et al.* prospectively cultured the periurethral flora before and after circumcision in 25 boys. Before circumcision 52% (13/25) of the boys were colonized by potentially uropathogenic organisms as opposed to none of the boys after circumcision. Other studies have demonstrated that uropathogenic P-fimbriated *E. coli* adhere well to the mucosal surface of the prepuce, whereas non-pathogenic *E. coli* do not (Fussell *et al.*, 1988).

One must wonder what differs in neonatal boys, recognizing that the incidence of pyelonephritis declines throughout childhood despite the persistence of foreskin and periurethral colonization. In a retrospective study, Kim (1996) suggested that the increased risk of UTI in neonates might be related to the inability to retract the foreskin. However, many boys cannot retract their prepuces until adolescence. Despite this conflicting evidence, the periurethral area of the uncircumcised infant is a closed space harboring bacteria with the potential to cause serious urinary infection in some boys (Fussell *et al.*, 1988;

Table 10.4 Incidence of urinary tract infection (UTI) in female and circumcised and uncircumcised male infants (0–1 year old) born in US army hospitals (1974–83)

	Total no.	No. with UTI	Rate per 1000
All males	217 116	661	3.0
Circumcised	175 317	193	1.1
Uncircumcised	41 799	468	11.2
Females	205 212	1164	5.7

(Modified from Wiswell and Roscelli, 1986.)

Roberts, 1996b). Consequently, circumcision may help to prevent UTI in male infants by removal of the mucosal surface necessary for bacterial adherence to occur. However, since even in uncircumcised boys the incidence of UTI is low, the debate regarding routine circumcision as a preventive health measure is likely to continue. Justification for circumcision in boys who have other risk factors for UTI, such as antenatally detected hyrdronephrosis, posterior urethral valves, megaureters, or high-grade VUR, is more easily argued.

Urethra

The short urethra in girls appears to be the most obvious explanation for the increased relative incidence of UTIs in girls compared with boys after the first 6–12 months of life. Narrowed urethral caliber, historically blamed as the pre-eminent factor influencing susceptibility to lower UTIs in girls, does not play a role. It has long been established that the intrinsic urethral luminal size is not significantly narrower in those girls who are bacteriuric than in those who never have been infected (Graham et al., 1967; Immergut and Wahman, 1968). In fact, both of these studies demonstrated that the urethral diameter was slightly larger in infected groups than in those never infected. Consequently, there is no role for urethral dilation or cystoscopic procedures in the routine management of childhood UTIs.

Other commonly held misconceptions related to the etiology of UTIs are that improper wiping techniques and bubble baths predispose to urinary infections. There is no evidence to support these myths. The strongest evidence against improper wiping techniques being a cause of UTIs is that over 95% of non-toilet-trained infants never develop urinary infection despite daily exposure to soiled diapers. Although bubble baths may occasionally cause dysuria from local meatal or vaginal irritation, there is no association with bacterial cystitis. More important for urethral ascent into the bladder is the ability of uropathogenic bacteria to attach to uroepithelial cells. Similar to the findings with periurethral cells (Kallenius and Winberg, 1978), increased adherence of bacteria to uroepithelial cells has been demonstrated in children prone to urinary infections (Svanborg-Eden and Jodal, 1979). This implies a difference in host receptor density or affinity that influences an individual's susceptibility to infection.

Blood factors

Antiadherence

Epidemiological and in vitro data support the hypothesis that some blood group antigens behave as bacterial receptors in addition to their long-recognized role in determining red cell phenotypes. Of the many carbohydrate antigens, the role of ABH, Lewis antigens (Le^a, Le^b, Le^x, and Le^h), P, Kell, Duffy, MNS, and Kidd systems in host susceptibility to urinary infection is becoming better understood. Blood group antigens can be found on the surfaces of many epithelial cells in the body, including vaginal and uroepithelial cells, and as secreted antigens in mucus as well as on erythrocytes (Markus, 1969; Hakomori and Kobata, 1974). Presumably, bacterial colonization of epithelial surfaces is facilitated by cell-surface-bound antigens, while secreted antigens mitigate against colonization by virtue of competitive inhibition.

Individuals belong to one of two distinct phenotypes based on the expression of ABH and Lewis antigens on cell surfaces and in secretions (Table 10.5). The secretor phenotype is characterized by ABH antigens in saliva, Le^b and Le^y antigens on epithelial cell surfaces, and Le(a$^-$b$^+$) erythrocytes. Non-secretors have mucus devoid of ABH antigens, express Le^a and Le^x antigens on epithelial cells, and have Le(a$^+$b$^-$) erythrocytes. Those with Le(a$^-$b$^-$) erythrocytes can be secretors or non-secretors depending on the presence of ABH antigens in secretions (Navas et al., 1993).

Since bacterial attachment to glycoprotein (type 1 fimbria) or glycolipid (P-fimbria) receptors is a critical step in colonization and tissue invasion, respectively, an individual's risk for UTI may be influenced by the composition of surface receptors available for

Table 10.5 Distribution of antigens in secretions and on epithelial cells and erythrocytes in the secretor and non-sectretor phenotypes

	Secretor	Non-secretor
Secretions (saliva, mucus)	ABH antigens	No ABH antigens
Epithelial cell	Le^{b+}, Le^{y+}	Le^{a+}, Le^{x+}
Erythrocytes	Le^{a-}, Le^{b+}	Le^{a+}, Le^{b-}
	Le^{a-}, Le^{b-}	Le^{a-}, Le^{b-}

bacterial attachment. Observations by Schaeffer *et al.* (1994) in healthy women found that the profile of antigen expression on vaginal cells and in vaginal mucus correlated with the ABO phenotype and secretor status. They also noted that individuals within the same blood group phenotype expressed different amounts of ABH and Lewis antigens. Moreover, longitudinal analysis demonstrated that the level of expression of these antigens fluctuated over time. However, using quantitative immunohistochemical techniques, Schaeffer's group did not identify an association between a particular phenotype and a positive history of UTI when controlling for secretor status (Navas *et al.*, 1994). Thus, despite the appealing hypothesis that some individuals may be more susceptible to bacterial colonization by virtue of genetically determined cell-surface antigens, these data do not support this notion in adult women.

In children, similar associations between blood group phenotypes and the risk of UTI have been sought. Sheinfeld *et al.* (1990) studied the expression pattern of blood group antigens in 72 tissue specimens from children who underwent urologic surgery for anatomic abnormalities of the urinary tract. Sixty-six per cent (48/72) had a history of UTI and the remainder served as controls. Although an increased susceptibility to UTI was noted among non-secretors compared with secretors, the high risk of UTI was most likely to be a consequence of the prevalence of structural abnormalities in this study population. Jantausch *et al.* (1994) performed a more extensive analysis of blood group antigens in seven different systems and found that only the Le(a⁻b⁻) phenotype correlated with a positive history of febrile UTIs in children, yielding a three-fold relative risk. Albarus *et al.* (1997) sought to confirm the association between blood group phenotypes and the susceptibility to childhood febrile UTIs. In a well-matched case–control study of children with a febrile UTI during the first year of life, no such association existed. If blood group phenotypes and secretor status do not influence the risk of UTI, as some data might suggest, then perhaps the susceptibility to UTI is mediated by urinary or epithelial factors that are as yet unidentified.

Urinary inhibitory factors

Although urine commonly provides the appropriate environmental conditions for successful bacterial growth, several constituents within urine have been identified that inhibit bacterial growth. Normally, the pH of urine fluctuates between 4.6 and 7.2 in accordance with physiologic needs. Since the optimal pH range for bacterial growth is between 6 and 7, increases in urine acidity can limit bacterial growth. Extremes of urine osmolarity also can inhibit bacterial growth by virtue of the limited nutrients available to support replication in dilute urine (hypoosmolarity) or of the dehydration that ensues in concentrated urine (hyperosmolarity). Tamm–Horsfall protein, a glycoprotein secreted by luminal cells of the ascending loop of Henle, may also be protective. This glycoprotein has been shown to contain abundant mannose residues and is identical to uromucoid. *In vitro* studies have shown adherence of large numbers of *E. coli* with type 1 fimbria to uroepithelial cells coated with uromucoid, in contrast to poor adherence to uroepithelial cells devoid of uromucoid (Chick *et al.*, 1981). It has been postulated that free Tamm–Horsfall protein in the urine may trap *E. coli* possessing type 1 fimbria, thereby inhibiting attachment to uroepithelium. Two studies have demonstrated such binding between type 1 and S-fimbria and Tamm–Horsfall protein (Orskov *et al.*, 1980; Parkinnen *et al.*, 1983). Tamm–Horsfall protein has also been demonstrated to bind to neutrophils and it is believed that this interaction mediates recognition of bacterial invasion by neutrophils (Toma *et al.*, 1994). A study of UTIs in infants revealed a significantly lower mean concentration of Tamm–Horsfall protein in those with documented *E. coli* infections than in healthy controls (Israele *et al.*, 1987).

Dysfunctional elimination

One of the most important host risk factors for recurrent UTIs is voiding dysfunction. Common voiding disorders in children prone to UTI range from the small-capacity, unstable bladder characterized by frequency, urgency, posturing, and wetting to the infrequent voider ('lazy bladder syndrome') characterized by very infrequent voiding, a large-capacity bladder, overflow incontinence (wet despite a large bladder capacity), and constipation. The prevalence of some of these symptoms is listed in Table 10.6. Numerous reports have linked dysfunctional voiding and recurrent UTIs in children (Hinman, 1974; Allen, 1977; van Goll and Tanagho, 1977; Koff *et al.*, 1979; Koff and Murtagh, 1983; Hansson *et al.*, 1990; Snodgrass,

Table 10.6 Prevalence of symptoms characteristic of dysfunctional elimination in 7–8 year-old school-children: results of Danish Epidemiological Questionnaire Survey

	Girls (%)	Boys (%)
Urge symptoms	20	21
Day wetting	13	9
Night wetting	13	22
Nocturia	7	6
Encopresis	5	8
Emptying difficulties	8	7

(From Hanson *et al.*, 1997.)

1991; Hansson, 1992). Attention has also been focused on the association between dysfunctional voiding and the presence of VUR in infants and children with recurrent UTIs (Koff *et al.*, 1979; Mayo and Burns, 1990). The predisposition to recurrent UTIs and VUR in children with dysfunctional voiding is related to the presence of residual volume resulting from inadequate emptying of the bladder, increased intravesical pressure created by uninhibited bladder contractions, and bladder overdistension from infrequent voiding habits (van Gool, 1995). The elimination of bacteria from the bladder by frequent and complete emptying plays a significant role in preventing infection (Cox and Hinman, 1961). In a group of girls followed with asymptomatic bacteriuria (ABU), the incidence of recurrent bacteriuria correlated directly to bladder emptying. The average residual volume in those with ABU was 23.7 ml, whereas the mean residual volume in normal controls was 1.1 ml. On follow-up, recurrent bacteriuria was present in 75% of those with more than 5 ml of residual urine compared with only 17% of those with less than 5 ml of residual urine (Lindberg *et al.*, 1975a). The establishment of normal voiding habits in these children has been shown to reduce the incidence of recurrent UTIs (Loening-Baucke, 1997; De Paepe *et al.*, 1998; Schulman *et al.*, 1999).

Paramount to identifying the dysfunctional voider is a thorough voiding history. Squatting, delayed or infrequent micturition, urgency, constipation and/or encopresis are significant symptoms which frequently can be elicited in 50–94% of children with UTI (Hinman, 1974; Koff *et al.*, 1979; Van Gool *et al.*, 1984; Seruca, 1989; Snodgrass, 1991; Hjalmas, 1992; Van Gool *et al.*, 1992; Williams *et al.*, 1994).

Hellstrom *et al.* (1991) reported an abnormal voiding history in up to 49% of girls presenting between 3 and 5 years of age with their first UTI. Specifically, the presence of daytime urinary symptoms strongly correlated with the risk for subsequent infection. In a related study of the same children, Hansson (1992) found that more girls with 'covert' bacteriuria had urodynamic evidence of dysfunctional bladders compared with controls. Wan *et al.* (1995) evaluated the relationship between toileting habits and anatomic abnormalities that predispose to infection in 101 children with UTI (77 girls and 24 boys). Ninety per cent of the children without structural abnormalities demonstrated dysfunctional elimination as a contributing factor to their urinary infections, compared with 40% of those patients found to have a structural abnormality such as VUR.

Similarly, there is a definite correlation between constipation and urinary incontinence, VUR, and recurrent UTIs in children (Neumann *et al.*, 1973; O'Regan *et al.*, 1985). Constipation classically is characterized by infrequent bowel movements that are large caliber and firm. This may be associated with perineal and/or abdominal pain from colonic distension. Paradoxically, children with constipation may be referred for encopresis (fecal soiling), a manifestation of the elimination of loose stool around feces impacted within the rectal vault. Unfortunately, physical examination of the constipated child is unreliable and often a soft abdomen or an empty rectal vault is encountered even when significant constipation is present radiographically. Likewise, the diagnosis of constipation can be difficult in children under 5 years who are unable to provide an accurate history.

A growing body of evidence suggests that constipation is an important facet of disordered elimination that, if appropriately managed, can help reduce the number of recurrent UTIs and promote resolution of VUR. Although this theoretically may be the result of mechanical factors related to compression of the bladder and bladder neck by a hard mass of stool, it is more likely to be due to the frequent coexistence of constipation with dysfunctional voiding and incomplete bladder emptying. In an epidemiological questionnaire surveying 1557 Danish children aged 7–8 years (863 girls, 728 boys, 6 gender unknown) the overall prevalence of encopresis was 13.9% (5.6% girls, 8.3% boys) (Hanson *et al.*, 1997) (Table 10.7). Among the girl respondents, 75 had a history of UTI and 13% of these suffered from encopresis versus

Table 10.7 Difference in micturition symptoms in girls with and without prior urinary tract infection (UTI)

Symptoms	Prior UTI (n = 75) (%)	No history of UTI (n = 723) (%)	p-Value
Day wetting	29.3	12.9	< 0.0002
Bed wetting	25.3	12.4	< 0.002
Prolonged voiding	33.3	17.8	< 0.002
Incomplete emptying	32.0	17.3	< 0.002
Poor stream	29.3	15.8	< 0.003
Manual compression of abdomen	17.3	7.3	< 0.003
Staccato voiding	30.6	17.4	< 0.006
Straining	17.3	8.6	< 0.02
Does not reach the toilet	40.0	27.9	< 0.03
Encopresis	13.3	6.0	<0.03

(Modified from Hansen *et al.*, 1997.)

only 6% of the girls without UTIs. Moreover, in a prospective study of 234 chronically constipated children, approximately one-third of the children demonstrated associated daytime incontinence (24%) and night-time incontinence (34%), reflecting the degree to which bowel and bladder elimination disorders are interrelated (Loening-Baucke, 1997). The resolution of constipation resulted in disappearance of daytime and night-time incontinence in a majority of children (89% and 63%, respectively). Most significant was the impact on the frequency of UTIs (approximately 10% of total) that completely disappeared in children without structural abnormalities.

Chronic constipation also plays a role in the etiology of recurrent UTIs in children with primary VUR. Recently, Koff *et al.* (1998) demonstrated that up to 50% of the children with VUR who might otherwise be considered normal have significant disorders of elimination (Table 10.8). Of the dysfunctional elimination symptoms, chronic constipation was the most prevalent in the presence of recurrent UTIs. Of those studied who had VUR, dysfunctional elimination sig-

nificantly increased the risk of breakthrough UTIs resulting in more frequent reimplantation surgery in these children. In addition, it took 1.5 years longer for primary VUR to resolve in children with dysfunctional elimination (constipation included) than in those without any elimination symptoms, despite a lower mean grade of reflux in those with dysfunctional elimination.

Upper urinary tract factors

Receptors

Bacterial adherence, particularly by P-fimbria on certain strains of *E. coli*, appears to be particularly significant in the pathogenesis of upper UTIs. As discussed earlier, a special class of glycosphingolipids, possessing Gal 1–4 Gal oligosaccharide, acts as receptors for P-fimbriated *E. coli* (Kallenius *et al.*, 1980; Leffler and Svanborg-Eden, 1980). These receptors are antigens in the P-blood group system. It is felt that host susceptibility to bacterial adherence is conferred by the P1 blood group phenotype, since this group is overrepresented in children with recurrent pyelonephritis in contrast to normal controls (Lomberg *et al.*, 1983; Tomisawa *et al.*, 1989). However, this overrepresentation of the P1 blood group phenotype is seen only in patients with pyelonpheritis who do not have associated VUR (Lomberg *et al.*, 1983). Despite the tenuous association between non-secretor status and an increased susceptibility to UTI, apparently as a result of diminished secretion of anti-adherence factors, a recent study has identified the presence of specific

Table 10.8 Prevalence of elimination symptoms among 143 children with primary vesicoureteral reflux

Symptom	Prevalence (%)
Constipation	23
Bladder instability	19
Infrequent voiding	16

(From Koff *et al.*, 1998.)

attachment structures for *E. coli* in non-secretors. Stapleton *et al.* (1998) identified glycosphingolipids on vaginal and renal epithelial cells that bind each of the three major classes of *E. coli* adhesins. Of the glycosphingolipids studied, sialosyl galactosyl globoside was determined to be the preferred binding receptor for uropathogenic *E. coli*. Thus an individual's risk for UTI may be more strongly influenced by the presence of receptors for bacterial attachment than by the absence of blocking antigens.

Vesicoureteral reflux

Numerous reports have documented that VUR is present in 25–50% (average 35%) of children with culture documented UTIs (Smellie *et al.*, 1975). In contrast, in a survey of the literature Bailey (1973) reported an incidence of VUR in children without UTI of only 0.4–1.8%. Similar findings were reported by Ransley (1978), who compiled voiding cystograms in 535 children without a history of UTI and found VUR in only seven children (1.3%). VUR, when present, continues to be the most significant host risk factor in the etiology of childhood pyelonephritis. The risk for both acute pyelonephritis and subsequent renal scarring is directly related to the severity of VUR. In one prospective study of children with febrile UTIs, approximately 80% of patients with VUR demonstrated changes consistent with acute pyelonephritis on [technetium-99m (^{99m}Tc)]DMSA renal scans, including 100% of patients with moderate to severe reflux (grades III–V/V) (Majd *et al.*, 1991). In contrast, only 60% of patients without demonstrable reflux had evidence of acute pyelonephritis on the DMSA scan. Kidneys associated with moderate or severe reflux were twice as likely to demonstrate abnormalities on DMSA scans (67%) compared with kidneys with mild (32%) or no reflux (34%). In a compilation of 10 published clinical studies of children with febrile UTIs, DMSA renal scan abnormalities have been reported in 50–80% of children (Rushton, 1997). When VUR was present, approximately 80–90% of patients had abnormal studies, including almost all with moderate or severe VUR.

The presence of VUR appears to compensate for decreased virulence of *E. coli* in patients with recurrent pyelonephritis (Lomberg *et al.*, 1989). When there is reflux of infected urine from the bladder into the upper urinary tract, bacteria do not require special virulence properties, such as cellular attaching ability, to ascend from the bladder to the kidney. In one study of girls with recurrent pyelonephritis, infections were caused by P-fimbriated *E. coli* in only 36% of those with VUR compared with 71% of those without VUR (Lomberg *et al.*, 1989). Despite the important role that VUR plays when it is present, studies of children with febrile UTIs have reported that the majority of patients (60–68%) with abnormal DMSA renal scans demonstrating acute pyelonephritic changes do not have demonstrable VUR at the time of investigation (Rushton, 1997).

In children with dysfunctional voiding, the presence of residual urine and elevated voiding pressures during UTI is more likely to result in significant post-pyelonephritic renal scarring than anticipated for the grade of VUR present. Perhaps because of more frequent breakthrough infections while on antibacterial prophylaxis, these children have been found to be at greater risk for progressive renal scarring (up to 44%) (Naseer and Steinhardt, 1997).

Obstruction

Urinary obstruction may occur at the ureteropelvic junction, the ureterovesical junction, or the posterior urethra in boys with valves. Patients with obstruction may present with severe infection. Ectopic ureters, with or without associated ureteroceles, also represent obstructed pathology. However, such anomalies are present in only a minority of children with UTIs. In fact, recent prospective studies of children presenting with first-time febrile UTIs have reported significant obstructive uropathy in fewer than 1% (Hobermann and Wald, 1997). Perhaps this lower incidence is due in part to the increased detection of hydronephrosis on prenatal ultrasonography prior to the development of clinical infection. The increased predisposition to infection pesumably results from impairment of urinary flow with resultant stasis that compromises bladder and renal defense mechanisms. Both obstruction and high-grade reflux result in an increase in the residual volume of urine in the bladder or dilated urinary tract, permitting the multiplication of bacteria in the urine (Cox and Hinman, 1961). Obstruction also inhibits the mechanical washout or flushing effect associated with ureteral peristalsis and effective micturition and may alter other local defense factors as well. All of these factors result in increased susceptibility of the parenchyma to infection and damage.

Heredity

Evidence that heredity plays a role in determining individual susceptibility to UTI is accumulating. The daughters of mothers who had been bacteriuric in childhood show a higher incidence of UTI, and female siblings also tend to show a higher incidence of bacteriuria (Fennell *et al.*, 1977; Gillenwater *et al.*, 1979). Children with first-time pyelonephritis significantly more often have relatives with a history of UTI than do controls (Marild *et al.*, 1989b). Racially dependent differences in the prevalence of UTIs and in the rate of bacteriuria have also been reported. Kunin *et al.* (1964) reported a 1.2% bacteriuria prevalence rate in white girls compared with a rate of 0.5% in black girls in the same age group. In a retrospective review, the number of black girls evaluated following UTI who were found to have VUR was one-third that of white girls at an institution where equal number of black and white girls were hospitalized (Askari and Belman, 1982). This observation was subsequently confirmed by a prospective study of patients admitted to the same institution with febrile UTIs (Majd *et al.*, 1991). Experimental UTI in mice is also significantly influenced by heredity, as evidenced by a slower response to treatment in certain strains of inbred mice compared with others that resolve the UTI more rapidly (Hopkins *et al.*, 1998). These same studies have also demonstrated that the acute inflammation and acquired immune response (antibody production) that follow urinary infection differ among genetically different strains of mice. As stated, '[this] result strongly suggests that the presence or absence of specific host genes will determine how effectively an *E. coli* UTI will be resolved.'

Immunity

The immunologic response to urinary tract infection has been studied at both the kidney and bladder level. Understanding the immune response to infection is particularly important because immunization is currently being explored as a possible means of preventing recurrent UTIs. The antibody response to infection has also been used diagnostically to localize the level of urinary infection to the upper or lower urinary tract (Thomas *et al.*, 1974; Hellerstein *et al.*, 1978).

Antibody response

The focus of most of the clinical and experimental immunologic studies of urinary tract infection has been the immune response to pyelonephritis. During acute pyelonephritis a systemic antibody response occurs with antibody production primarily against the O antigen of the infecting bacteria. A diminshed response is seen toward the K antigen (Kaijser, 1973; Hanson *et al.*, 1977). Counteracting bacterial adherence to host epithelial cells are protective antibodies that may be acquired passively (from mother to fetus) or actively through previous exposure to infection. Conversely, in the absence of protective antibodies some individuals are at greater risk for UTI (Hopkins *et al.*, 1995). Antibodies of the immunoglobulin M (IgM), IgG, IgA, and secretory IgA (sIgA) type have all been demonstrated in the serum and urine of children and experimental animals with acute pyelonephritis (Sohl-Akerlund *et al.*, 1979; Mattsby-Baltzer *et al.*, 1981). High IgG, IgA, and secretory IgA antibody levels have also been found in the urine of girls with pyelonephritis (Sohl-Akerlund *et al.*, 1979). The presence of antibodies within the renal parenchyma enhances bacterial opsonization, the process by which bacteria are coated by proteins, leading to further phagocytosis.

An antibody response to pili has also been found following pyelonephritis (Rene and Silverblatt, 1982). Secretory IgA directed against pili have been recovered from the urine of patients with acute pyelonephritis and have been shown to prevent *in vitro* adherence of *E. coli* to human uroepithelial cells (Svanborg-Eden and Svennerholm, 1978). Mannose-specific interactions between *E. coli* and the carbohydrate moiety of secretory IgA have been reported (Wold *et al.*, 1988). Secretory IgA, when bound to the uroepithelium, may thus offer a receptor site for bacteria. When excreted, it may result in competitive inhibition of binding.

With regard to the immune response of the bladder to urinary infection, a systemic circulating antibody response to cystitis is not seen (Clark *et al.*, 1971; Sohl-Akerlund *et al.*, 1979). However, an elevation of secretory IgA antibody in the urine has been observed in children with UTI, suggesting local antibody production (Uehling and Steihm, 1971; Sohl-Akerlund *et al.*, 1979). A more recent study reported a decreased excretion rate of secretory IgA in uninfected children with a history of symptomatic infections compared with healthy controls. However, when these girls were subsequently studied at the time of symptomatic UTI, secretory IgA excretion rates were significantly higher than in controls (Fleidner *et al.*,

1986). Other evidence supporting a role for secretory IgA as a host defense factor comes from animal studies. Attempts at local immunization of the urinary tract have shown that intravesical immunization is effective against experimentally induced ascending UTI in rats (Kaijser et al., 1983). The presence of secretory IgA in the urine following local bladder or vaginal immunization has been shown to decrease adherence to uroepithelial cells in this experimental model (Uehling et al., 1978; Uehling et al., 1982).

The urine of newborns has nearly undetectable levels of sIgA that increase during the first year of life, particularly in breastfed compared with non-breastfed infants. Case–control studies have identified a diminished incidence of UTI in breastfed infants, presumably related to soluble substances that are absorbed enterically and excreted into the urine. Using high-performance liquid chromatography to purify oligo-saccharides in breast milk, Coppa et al. (1990) identified low molecular weight, neutral oligosaccharides that significantly decreased adhesion between human uroepithelial cells and E. coli isolated from an infant with UTI. In addition, breast milk contains T- and B-lymphocytes, cytokines, growth factors and, most importantly, antibodies that may act synergistically to decrease the breastfed infant's risk of UTI.

No differences have been noted in the levels of urinary sIgA among boys and girls and thus impaired immunity does not explain the higher incidence of UTI in infant boys compared with girls. Instead, the predominance of UTI in infant boys is likely to reflect local periurethral factors (especially among uncircumcised boys) (James-Ellison et al., 1997).

Cell-mediated immunity

The protective role, if any, of cell-mediated immunity in UTI is controversial (Hahn and Kaufmann, 1981). T- and B-lymphocytic response is seen in the kidney during experimental pyelonephritis (Hjelm, 1984). However, others have shown a depressed cell-mediated response during the early phase of renal infection when bacterial replication is maximal (Miller et al., 1978). Although such studies have documented cell-mediated host responsiveness to bacterial infection, they have not defined the role of this process in the pathogenesis of UTI. There is no strong clinical evidence to support abnormality of cell-mediated immunity in patients prone to UTI. Experimental UTI in mice has demonstrated no increased susceptibility to

E. coli in athymic animals (with dysfunctional cellular immune systems) and normal controls (Svanborg-Eden et al., 1984). Similarly, in patients with compromised immune systems, an increased susceptibility to UTIs has not been reported. Studies to define the role of the immune response in UTI are obviously needed.

Further evidence supports a role for the uroepithelial cell in immunity against uropathogenic bacteria. Normally, uroepithelial cells have the capacity to produce cytokines when exposed to bacteria in vivo and in cell culture systems. While some cytokines are secreted to serve as chemoattractants for inflammatory cells, others are not secreted and may play a role in the uroepithelial cells' inherent response to invasion by pathogenic bacteria.

The specific stimulus for uroepithelial cell cytokine production and release appears to be components of P- and type 1 fimbria, since urinary levels of interleukin-6 (IL-6) are significantly greater in the presence of adhering bacteria and adhesin-positive P-fimbria (Hedges et al., 1992; Agace et al., 1993; Svensson et al., 1994). Further in vitro studies have determined that, in response to direct contact between bacterial fimbria and receptors located on the uroepithelial cell membrane, the uroepithelial cell is able to suppress bacterial growth (Mannhardt et al., 1996). Moreover, using human uroepithelial cells in culture, Mannhardt et al. (1996) have demonstrated that, in individuals with a history of recurrent UTIs, a transmembrane defect impedes signal transduction within the urothelial cell, thus rendering the cell incapable of responding to bacterial attachment. These data lend support to the concept that the most important arm of cellular immunity in the urinary tract may not be T- and B-cells, as classically described, but instead the inherent ability of the uroepithelium to respond to bacterial invasion.

Vaccine

Much of the significance of clarifying the immune response to UTI relates to the possibility of developing an effective vaccine to prevent urinary infections. Experimental evidence has accumulated to suggest that this may be possible in the near future. Protection against experimental ascending pyelonephritis in rats has been demonstrated using isolated capsular antigen to stimulate antibody production directed at K antigen (Kaijser et al., 1983). Similarly, immunization with E. coli P-fimbria in both mice and confers protection against ascending pyelonpheritis, presumably by interfering with adherence of the organism to the uroepithelium (Roberts *et al.*, 1984; Pecha *et al.*, 1989). Immunization of rats with purified type 1 fimbria also affords substantial protection against experimental ascending pyelonephritis (Silverblatt *et al.*, 1982). Thankavel *et al.* (1997) have identified the specific subunit region within the FimH determinant of type 1 fimbria that is responsible for attachment to uroepithelial cells. Antibodies directed specifically against this region of only 25 amino acids, and not other regions on FimH or FimA subunits of type 1 fimbria, reduced experimental pyelonephritis in mice. Some evidence suggests a potential role for immunization with hemolysins as well (O'Hanley *et al.*, 1985).

Recent clinical investigations have demonstrated the efficacy of acquired immunity as prophylaxis against recurrent UTIs in women and children. Both vaginal and intramuscular immunization with inactivated uropathogenic bacteria has resulted in significantly increased levels of sIgA (Uehling *et al.*, 1997). In a small trial involving only 10 girls with recurrent UTIs and an equal number of healthy controls, intramuscular immunization also resulted in significantly fewer recurrences in the vaccinated girls (Nayir *et al.*, 1995). Although these results are promising, the full value of such vaccines to prevent pyelonephritis will be critically assessed only by appropriately controlled, large clinical trials.

Diagnosis of urinary tract infection

UTI can be reliably diagnosed only by urine culture. Symptoms of dysuria, urgency, frequency, and enuresis are non-specific and may be the result of vulvitis, urethritis, dysfunctional voiding, or non-specific causes, such as dehydration associated with febrile illness. In 34 children with lower urinary symptoms alone, urine culture demonstrated significant bacteriuria in only 18%; 40% of those with sterile urine had upper respiratory tract infection. Similarly, Heale *et al.* found that of 378 children with specific urinary complaints, only 14.3% had urinary infection. Thirty-three per cent with flank pain, frequency, and/or dysuria and 31.5% with the recent onset of wetting had UTI, whereas only 4.2% with chronic nocturnal enuresis were infected. Of those without specific complaints, 4.4% had UTI (there was little difference from those who were wet only at night).

Urinalysis

Although routine urinalysis can be helpful in calling attention to those who might be infected, the association of inflammatory cells in the urine by itself is at best only about 70% reliable (Pryles and Eliot, 1965; Corman *et al.*, 1982; Ginsburg and McCracken, 1982). The finding of significant pyuria on routine urinalysis varies with the volume of urine centrifuged and examined, the force and duration of centrifugation, the volume in which cells are resuspended, and observer error (Stamm, 1983). Urine microscopy for bacteria significantly improves the reliability of urinalysis for the detection of urinary infection, particularly when one combines this with examination of urinary sediment for pyuria (Robins *et al.*, 1975). Jenkins *et al.* reviewed approximately 40 publications reporting urine microscopy for bacteria and found a wide variation in methodology and diagnostic criteria. They concluded that the least reliable method was examination of unstained, uncentrifuged urine. When stained, centrifuged urine was examined, the sensitivity using the criteria of one or more organisms per oil immersion field was greater than 95% when compared with urine culture growing $\geq 10^5$ colony-forming units (cfu) per ml. The specificity was at least 95% when more than five organisms per oil immersion field were viewed. Hoberman *et al.* (1994) compared quantitative urine cultures with an enhanced urinalysis for the detection of pyuria and bacteriuria in urine specimens obtained by catheterization in children presenting with fever. The data obtained demonstrated that UTI is best defined by more than 10 leukocytes/mm^3 on urinalysis combined with urine cultures yielding more than 50 000 cfu/ml. In contrast, dipstick determination for the presence of leukocyte esterase and nitrite yielded sensitivities of only 52.9% and 31.4%, respectively, in detecting clinically significant bacteriuria (greater than 50 000 cfu/ml). In both this and another study of febrile infants, the findings of urinalysis were compared with the results of [^{99m}Tc]DMSA renal scans. Both studies concluded that acute pyelonephritis in febrile infants is almost always associated with the finding of pyuria on urinalysis (Hoberman *et al.*, 1994; Landau *et al.*, 1994).

Partly as a result of the technique and operator-dependent variability with urine microscopy, a number of enzymatic methods for detection of bacteriuria or pyuria has been developed. The two most popular are the leukocyte esterase and the nitrite reductase tests. These studies are inexpensive, rapid, and easy to perform.

Leukocyte esterase test

The leukocyte esterase dipstick test demonstrates the presence of pyuria by histochemical methods that specifically detect esterases in the neutrophils. When compared with chamber count methods, studies have reported sensitivity as high as 88–95% for the detection of pyuria using a cut-off of 10 or more leukocytes/mm^2 (Gillenwater, 1981; Kusumi et al., 1981). However, in a study that evaluated 110 children with fever and positive urine cultures, the leukocyte esterase test had sensitivities of only 52.9% and 66.7% in detecting $\geq$ 10 and $\geq$ 20 leukocytes/mm^3, respectively (Poyles and Eliot, 1965). Furthermore, one would not anticipate this test to be any more sensitive than the finding of pyuria alone for the identification of children with positive urine cultures.

Nitrite test

Bacteria convert urine nitrate to nitrite. The nitrite method employs reagent paper impregnated with sulfanilic acid and α-naphthylamine, which form a red azo dye when in contact with nitrite. Thus, a positive colorimetric assay implies the presence of bacteria in the bladder. However, a relatively long incubation period (4 hours) is required for conversion of nitrate to nitrite. For this reason, the first-morning urine sample in a toilet-trained child is the best specimen to test. A single test on a randomly collected urine specimen was reported to have a sensitivity of only 29.2–44% on 790 urine specimens using dipsticks from two manufacturers. However, the specificity was 98% when the test was positive (James et al., 1978; Landau et al., 1994). This test is not a reliable office screening method when used alone (Kusumi et al., 1981).

Combining the leukocyte test and the nitrite test on a single dipstick has improved the accuracy to detect or exclude UTI. In a review of rapid methods to detect UTIs, Pezzlo (1988) reported a sensitivity of 78–92% and a specificity of 60–98% when using the combination test (Pezzlo, 1988). However, the accuracy is affected by the probability of the patient being infected based on clinical findings (Pezzlo, 1988; Bolann et al., 1989). Accordingly, urine culture may be omitted when the dipstick test is negative only when there is limited suspicion for UTI based on clinical symptoms. Conversely, urine culture should be obtained in any patient suspected of having a UTI or in whom the dipstick test is positive.

Others have evaluated the role of urinary N-acetyl-β-glucosaminidase (NAG) (a renal tubular enzyme thought to be a marker of tubular damage) and β_2-microglobulin (β_2M) (a low molecular weight circulating protein with increased fractional excretion in children with tubulointerstitial disease) in the diagnosis of pyelonephritis in febrile children. Unfortunately, urinary marker elevation has been found both in children with febrile UTIs and in children with sterile urine who had severe renal scarring associated with high-grade VUR, making these markers unreliable for the diagnosis of acute pyelonephritis (Jantausch et al., 1994; Miyakita and Puri, 1994; Tomlinson et al., 1994).

Urine culture

In the pre-toilet-trained group, the urine specimen is often obtained by applying a collection bag. The results are reliable only when the specimen is negative. Contamination is directly related to the length of time the bag is in place. If a specimen has not been obtained within 30 min of application, reliability begins to decrease. Removing the appliance and plating or refrigerating the urine immediately after the child voids is paramount. Having the parent apply the bag before leaving for the physician's office in an effort to shorten the wait is acceptable only when the cultured specimen is negative. When confirmation of voided urine or immediate treatment is necessary, bladder catheterization or suprapubic aspiration (SPA) should be employed. A feeding tube (8–10 Fr) inserted only a few centimeters into the bladder is ideal for catheterization. In girls and boys who can void on command, midstream specimens are more reliable than bag-collected specimens.

SPA has achieved popularity in some centers. Young children are particularly favorable candidates for SPA because of the abdominal location of their urinary bladders. However, the procedure cannot be expected to be successful when the bladder is empty. This is the major drawback of SPA. If urine is not obtained initially, time should not be wasted in a sick child who requires antibiotic treatment. Urethral catheterization should be done. SPA is performed after first cleaning the suprapubic area with an antiseptic solution. A 21–25 gauge needle is inserted perpendicular to the patient in the midline one finger-breadth above the symphysis. Although a local anesthetic can first be infiltrated, this appears unnecessary and may actually cause more pain than a quick in-and-out aspiration. It is practical to apply a U-bag to the perineum before cleaning the abdomen. In many cases the child voids during preparation for aspiration, obviating the necessity for the procedure if the voided urine is immediately plated or refrigerated.

It has often been stated that 'any number of bacteria' obtained by suprapubic aspiration is significant. Since the bladder is a reservoir and this method of collection depicts the number of bacteria in that reservoir, one should not anticipate colony counts significantly different from those properly collected by other means. Ginsburg and McCracken (1982) found ≥ 100 000 cfu/ml in 96% and 40 000–80 000 in the remaining 4% of 100 febrile infants with bacteriuria demonstrated on SPA. None showed fewer than 40 000 colonies. Nelson and Peters (1965) had previously reported similar results in a study of premature and term infants. Hoberman *et al.* (1994) recently reported the results of positive urine cultures on specimens obtained by catheterization in 110 febrile infants < 2 years old. Of 110 urine cultures with ≥ 10 000 cfu/ml, 92 (84%) had ≥ 100 000 cfu/ml, 10 (9%) had 50 000–99 000 cfu/ml, and only 8 (7%) had 10 000–49 000 cfu/ml. Furthermore, urine specimens with 10 000–49 000 were much more likely to yield Gram-positive or mixed organisms than specimens with >50 000 cfu/ml. These authors concluded that UTI is best defined by ≥ 10 leukocytes/mm^3 and colony counts of ≥50 000 on catheterized specimens. Thus colony counts from the bladder < 50 000 cfu/ml are suspect regardless of the manner in which the urine was collected.

Clinical presentation and localization

As one would anticipate, the classic signs and symptoms for UTI are usually lacking in the very young. Instead, non-specific symptoms, such as irritability, poor feeding, failure to gain weight, vomiting, and diarrhea, may be the only signs suggestive of an underlying problem (Table 10.9). In one study of children with symptomatic urinary infections, only 9% of 78 infants were initially referred with a suspected diagnosis of UTI (Smellie *et al.*, 1964). Often absent in neonates, fever is present in most infants between 1 and 12 months old who present with symptomatic UTIs (Winberg *et al.*, 1974; Jodal, 1987; Marild and Jodal, 1998). In fact, UTIs have recently been described as one of the most common serious bacterial illnesses among febrile infants and young children, with a reported prevalence ranging from 4.1–7.5% (Hoberman *et al.*, 1994). In one study of 945 infants who presented to a pediatric ER with fever, the overall prevalence of UTI was 5.3% (Hoberman *et al.*, 1993). The prevalence was highest in Caucasian girls, 17% of whom had a positive urine culture. In contrast, the prevalence of UTI among African–American girls was only 3.5% and among boys it was 2.5%. Another prospective study reported urinary tract infection in 7.5% of 442 infants (less than 8 weeks of age) presenting to the emergency room with fever ≥ 38.1°C, only half of whom had abnormal urinalyses suggestive of UTI (>5 white blood cells per high-power field or any bacteria present) (Crain and Gershel, 1990). Thus, a urine specimen for culture, preferably collected by catheterization, should be obtained routinely whenever a non-verbal, non-toilet-trained child presents with unexplained fever.

As the child becomes verbal and is toilet-trained, urinary tract symptomatology is more easily detected. Fever continues to be relatively common in toddlers with first-time symptomatic infection. However, fever is not as frequently associated with recurrent and/or long-standing infection. In older children urgency, frequency, enuresis, and dysuria are common presenting symptoms. Failure to become toilet trained at the proper age may occasionally herald

Table 10.9 Prominent symptoms in neonatal non-obstructive urinary tract infection: combined results of four studies (*n* = 255)

Symptom	Prevalence (%)
Failure to thrive or weight loss	51
Fever	41
Jaundice	12
Cyanosis/pallor	30
Vomiting	35
Diarrhea	29
Convulsions/CNS symptoms	20

underlying chronic lower urinary infection. Although urinary tract symptoms such as vaginal pain, urinary frequency, dysuria, and enuresis are common following childhood sexual abuse, actual urinary infection is not (Klevan and De Jong, 1990).

There are few population-based studies of symptomatic UTIs in childhood. The classic epidemiologic study by Winberg *et al.* (1974) was carried out between 1960 and 1966 in Goteborg, Sweden. The special organizational structure of that city's pediatric medical care has afforded unique opportunities to perform ongoing epidemiologic studies of UTIs in children. Jodal (1987) reported a follow-up prospective epidemiologic study conducted in Goteborg from

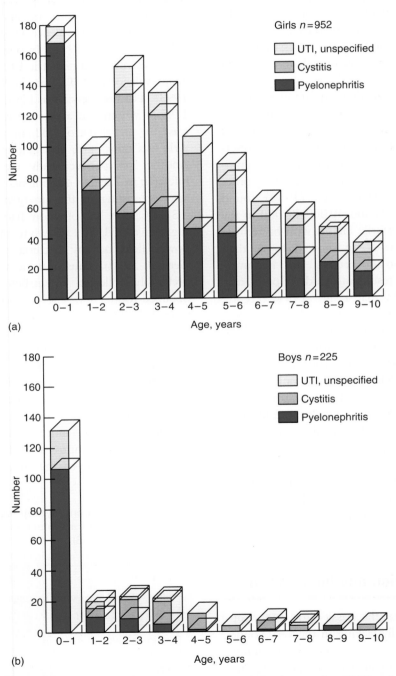

Figure 10.6 Children with first-time diagnosis of urinary tract infection at the Children's Hospital in Goteborg, Sweden, according to age and clinical diagnosis. (Reprinted from Jodal, 1994, with permission.)

1970 to 1979. There were 952 females and 225 males (4.2:1) below age 10 years of age who were treated for a first-time symptomatic urinary infection (Fig. 10.6). Of the 225 boys, 59% presented during the first year of life. The number of boys diagnosed in the higher age groups was low, especially over the age of 5 years. The number of first infections in girls was also highest in the first year of life (19%). A gradual decrease in number of girls with first-time infections was associated with increasing age. In both girls and boys, febrile infections, presumed to be pyelonephritis, predominated during the first year of life. Acute cystitis was most commonly seen between 2 and 5 years of age in both sexes, with a marked peak frequency in girls during the third year of life. As expected, infections during infancy were the most difficult to characterize as pyelonephritis or cystitis.

Cystitis

Acute cystitis in children is rarely associated with significant long-term morbidity. Typical symptoms that accompany acute cystitis in toilet-trained children include dysuria, frequency, urgency, and/or secondary-onset enuresis. Fever and systemic complaints are generally not a feature of the clinical picture. As previously mentioned, however, these same irritative lower tract symptoms are often seen in the absence of bacterial cystitis, mandating that a specimen for urine culture be obtained prior to institution of therapy.

Although the recurrence rate of lower UTIs is high, most cases can be considered little more than a nuisance and recurrences tend to decrease or disappear by adolescence. However, it is worth noting that many children prone to recurrent lower UTIs have voiding dysfunction, particularly infrequent voiding. Typically, these children do not void for 1 or 2 hours after awakening in the morning and then may void only two or three times throughout the day. Consequently, bladder capacity is abnormally large and bladder emptying is often incomplete. Often these children also have chronic constipation, including encopresis in some. Other children with recurrent cystitis have underlying bladder instability associated with urinary frequency, urgency, urge incontinence, and posturing associated with a reduced functional bladder capacity. Girls with a history of UTI are significantly more likely to report a variety of chronic

voiding disturbances compared with girls without a history of UTI (Hellstrom et al., 1991; Hansen et al., 1997) (Table 10.7). In some cases, recurrent UTIs may be a precipitating factor to the child's voiding disturbance. Conversely, primary bladder instability may itself contribute to an increased susceptibility to UTIs. In contrast to daytime voiding disorders, isolated bedwetting is rarely associated with a history of previous UTI (Hellstrom et al., 1991).

Approximately 10% of susceptible girls will have a recurrent infection shortly after completion of a course of antibiotic therapy. These children have chronic symptoms of bladder instability. Squatting or posturing in response to unstable bladder contractions is common in this group. Many have voiding dyssynergia associated with high voiding pressures and incomplete bladder emptying. Some also have chronic inflammatory changes of the bladder. Historically, endoscopic evaluation of these children often revealed multiple raised 'cysts' in the area of the bladder neck and trigone. Histologically, submucosal lymphoid follicles were present. Clinically, this entity has been termed cystitis cystica, although the histologic appearance suggests it would be more accurately referred to as cystitis follicularis. The presence of these follicles suggests an immunologic response to chronic infection (Uehling and King, 1973). It should be noted that treatment of these children is no longer predicated on the basis of these endoscopic findings. Rather, treatment is determined by the recurrence rate of infection and the type of underlying voiding and bowel disorder.

Asymptomatic bacteriuria

The natural history and uroradiographic findings in patients with asymptomatic or covert bacteriuria vary according to the age of the patient and prior episodes of symptomatic infections. Screening bacteriuria does not necessarily represent asymptomatic bacteriuria, as approximately one-third of school-aged girls with screening bacteriuria have a prior history of symptoms related to the urinary tract and some have had previous symptomatic UTIs. It is unclear whether the prognosis is any different for children who have primary asymptomatic bacteriuria than for those in whom asymptomatic bacteriuria develops following treatment of a symptomatic infection.

A study of asymptomatic and symptomatic bacteriuria in infants under 1 year of age reveals interesting differences in the two populations (Jodal, 1987). In two of 50 patients with asymptomatic bacteriuria, clinical acute pyelonephritis developed within 2 weeks of detection. The others remained free of symptoms. In 46 (92%) of the patients with asymptomatic bacteriuria, mild reflux (grades I–II) was found, occurring in only 11% (5/46). Of 45 left untreated, 36 spontaneously cleared the bacteriuria and eight others became abacteriuric following antibiotic treatment for other reasons. Although asymptomatic recurrences developed in six (12%), no pyelonephritic recurrences occurred in this group during follow-up of at least 1 year. Follow-up urography, done in 36, did not reveal any evidence of renal scarring. In contrast, among 40 infants with symptomatic infections, one patient had a significant ureteropelvic junction obstruction and 14 of 39 (36%) had VUR, including three with grade III or greater. Fourteen of 40 (35%) experienced recurrences, including six with acute pyelonephritis and three with cystitis, whereas asymptomatic bacteriuria was noted in five. It was concluded that infants with asymptomatic bacteriuria represent a low-risk group with a tendency spontaneously to become abacteriuric, usually within a few months.

Considerable variation in uroradiographic findings has been reported in school-aged children found to have bacteriuria on screening. These studies have reported VUR in 19–35% and renal scarring in 10–26% (Kunin et al., 1964; Savage et al., 1973; Linberg et al., 1975a; McLachlan et al., 1975; Newcastle Asymptomatic Bacteriuria Research Group, 1975). However, many of these children had a prior history of symptomatic UTIs and others undoubtedly had infections during infancy that were overlooked or misdiagnosed. Although recurrent infections following treatment occur in up to 80%, the risk for development of acute pyelonephritis in a girl older than 4 years of age with untreated asymptomatic bacteriuria is small and seems to be associated with a change in bacterial strain, perhaps as a result of antibiotic treatment (Kunin, 1970; Lindberg et al., 1978c). Follow-up by the Cardiff–Oxford Bacteriuria Study Group revealed that those school-children who presented initially with a radiographically normal urinary tract remained normal in spite of persistent asymptomatic bacteriuria (Cardiff–Oxford Bacteriruia Study Group, 1978). Only in those children who had previous renal scarring did new scars or progression of scarring develop, and all of

these children had VUR. Other studies have shown that asymptomatic bacteriuria is associated with low-virulence bacterial strains lacking the ability to adhere and cause symptoms (Svanborg-Eden et al., 1976; Svanborg-Eden and Svennerholm, 1978; Kallenius et al., 1981). Furthermore, there is considerable evidence that these organisms may be commensal with the host and may even protect against infection by more virulent strains (Linshaw, 1996).

Pyelonephritis

Pathophysiology of acute pyelonephritis

Acute pyelonephritis represents the most serious type of UTI in children. It is not only responsible for greater acute morbidity, but it also has the potential for causing irreversible damage. Acute pyelonephritis in older children typically presents with fever and flank pain or tenderness associated with pyuria and positive urine culture. In the majority of cases, laboratory evaluation reveals an elevated serum white blood cell count (WBC), erythrocyte sedimentation rate (ESR), and/or C-reactive protein (CRP). However, when compared directly with localization studies such as DMSA renal scans, these clinical and laboratory parameters are associated with high false-positive and/or false-negative rates (Rushton, 1997). This is particularly true in neonates and young infants, an age group at greatest risk for renal scarring following pyelonephritis. Neonates in particular present with non-specific symptoms such as irritability, poor feeding, failure to thrive, vomiting and diarrhea (Table 10.9). When one considers that approximately one-half of all children with febrile UTIs present during the first year of life, the importance of early and accurate diagnosis becomes obvious.

Experimental studies by Roberts and others have found that bacterial adherence to uroepithelium elicits an inflammatory cascade proportional to the virulence of the infecting organism. The same acute inflammatory response that is responsible for the eradication of bacteria is also responsible for the damage to renal tissue and subsequent renal scarring (Roberts, 1991). Through a series of experimental studies using the primate model, Roberts has developed a unified theory of the chain of events involved in the process that ultimately leads to renal scarring (Fig. 10.7). The initiating event is bacterial inoculation of the renal parenchyma that elicits both immune and inflammatory responses. Whereas the immune response can be stimulated by live or heat-killed bacteria, the acute inflammatory response occurs only following inoculation by live bacteria (Robert *et al.*, 1982). Since heat-killed bacteria do not cause renal scarring, it appears that it is the acute inflammatory response that is more important as a cause for the subsequent development of permanent renal damage. Potent cytokines induce chemotaxis of granulocytes and cellular and humoral mediated bacterial killing.

Studies have also reported that focal ischemia may be a consequence of acute pyelonephritis. Kaack *et al.* (1986) showed that granulocyte aggregation within capillaries leads to vascular occlusion. Renal ischemia is then evidenced by a transient rise in circulating renin levels. Hill and Clark (1972) found evidence of marked cortical vasoconstriction in areas of acute inflammation in rabbits with acute renal infection, with inflammatory cells obstructing the peritubular capillaries. Androulakakis *et al.* (1987) found microvascular changes in acute pyelonephritis in pigs

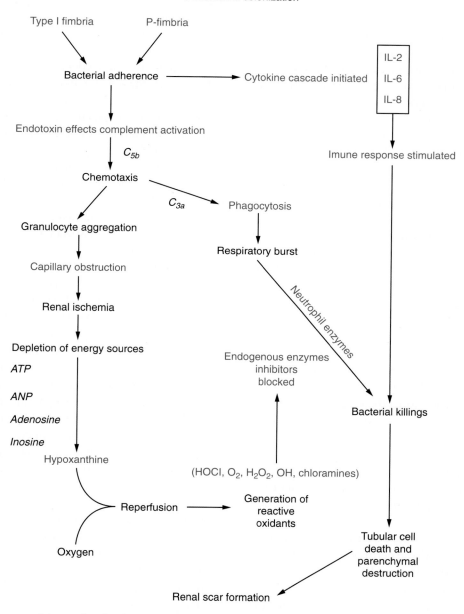

Figure 10.7 Diagram of the pathophysiologic events (from bacterial adherence to renal scar formation) that are characteristic of acute pyelonephritis. (Modified from Roberts, 1995.)

using microradiological and stereomicroscopic techniques. Focal ischemia in areas involved by the acute inflammatory response was evidenced by compression of glomeruli, small peritubular capillaries, and vasa rectae, presumably from interstitial edema. Using the microsphere technique, Majd and Rushton (1992) evaluated renal blood flow changes associated with acute pyelonephritis in the refluxing piglet model. Focal renal blood flow was decreased in sites of acute pyelonephritis identified by diminished uptake of DMSA and subsequently confirmed by histopathology. Uninvolved areas of the affected kidneys demonstrated normal blood flow comparable to that of the contralateral normal kidney.

Since host-derived cytotoxins are central in the genesis of tissue suppuration, investigators have tried to understand and modify the inflammatory response. Granulocytes kill bacteria, releasing toxic enzymes (lysozymes) both within the granulocyte and into the lumen of renal tubules, which causes renal cell damage. The respiratory burst, a phenomenon universal to acute inflammatory responses, generates oxygen radicals (superoxides) that have classically been felt to mediate bacterial killing, as well as that of granulocytes and surrounding tubular cells (Roberts *et al.*, 1983).

The role of reactive oxidants, inducible nitric oxide (iNOS) and tissue-destructive proteinases in the acute inflammatory response has only recently been elucidated (Weiss, 1989). In an extensive review of the literature spanning 70 years, Weiss (1989) proposes that neutrophil-derived superoxide and oxygen radicals are merely highly reactive intermediates in the production of toxic chlorinated oxidants (e.g. hypochlorous acid and chloramines). If these chlorinated oxidants are the true mediators of tissue destruction, then inhibiting their generation should lessen tissue injury. In fact, *in vitro* models have demonstrated that cellular destruction could be prevented in the presence of specific inhibitors of the H_2O_2–halide-myeloperoxidase system, effectively preventing HOCl (hypochlorous acid) generation (Weiss, 1989). Despite this compelling evidence, Weiss' enthusiasm for HOCl as the sole agent in inflammation-mediated tissue destruction is tempered by the fact that living tissue perfused with HOCl solutions remains viable (Dakin, 1915). However, evidence suggests that the primary role for HOCl and chloramines is to neutralize circulating enzyme inhibitors that prevent the untimely digestion of host tissues by neutrophils. These oxidants have mild direct cytotoxic effects. Thus, in the absence of significant inflammation, any enzymes released from neutrophilic lysosomes are immediately inactivated. However, once stimulated, the neutrophil can release the aforementioned oxidants into its immediate surroundings and can create a microenvironment capable of inactivating enzyme inhibitors, activating latent neutrophil-derived enzymes, and rapidly degrading microbes, host cells, and connective substratum (Ginsburg and Kohen, 1995). Tubular cell death releases the toxic inflammatory agents into the interstitium, causing further damage.

Oxygen radicals are also produced by cell reaction during reperfusion of ischemic tissue. Focal parenchymal ischemia, resulting from intravascular granulocyte aggregation and edema, occurs with bacterial infection of the renal parenchyma (Roberts *et al.*, 1983; Kaack *et al.*, 1986; Roberts, 1991). In ischemic tissue, hypoxanthine is produced during anaerobic metabolism of adenosine monophosphate. During reperfusion, hypoxanthine in the presence of xanthine oxidase and oxygen yields superoxides and hydrogen peroxide (Roberts *et al.*, 1982). Treatment with allopurinol, an inhibitor of xanthine oxidase, protects against tissue damage from reperfusion injury and from that associated with bacteria in the renal parenchyma (Robert *et al.*, 1982).

It appears that the interstitial damage associated with the acute inflammatory response of pyelonephritis results from ischemia-related injury and from toxic enzymes. In addition, bacterial virulence factors, such as hemolysins and lipopolysaccharides, work in concert with neutrophil-derived mediators to disrupt cellular membranes and degrade the extracellular matrix. The inflammatory process extends through the renal interstitium, thus contributing to the damage that ultimately results in irreversible renal scarring.

Recently, the impact of adjunctive corticosteroids on postinflammatory renal scarring was evaluated in the treatment of experimental pyelonephritis in the refluxing piglet model. Following induction of acute pyelonephritis as confirmed by DMSA scintigraphy, animals were randomized to receive either standard antibiotic therapy or antibiotics and prednisolone (2 mg/kg, daily). Two months later, DMSA scintigraphy was repeated and kidneys were harvested for gross and microscopic examination. The risk of focal scarring corresponded to the severity of the initial acute pyelonephritic lesion, based on the percentage of renal parenchyma involved. In kidneys with mild and moderate acute pyelonephritic lesions, antibiotics alone were equally effective in preventing scarring when compared to treatment with antibiotics and steroids. However, severe pyelonephritic lesions were three times as likely to heal without scarring in animals treated with antibiotics in conjunction with steroids as compared to antibiotics alone (Pohl *et al.*, 1999).

Detection of acute pyelonephritis

The diagnosis of acute pyelonephritis traditionally has been made on the basis of the classic signs and symptoms of fever and flank pain or tenderness asssociated with pyuria and positive urine culture. However, accurate diagnosis based solely on these parameters is often difficult, particulary in neonates and infants (Busch and Huland, 1984; Majd *et al.*, 1991). Despite the fact that the majority of patients (50–80%) with fever and systemic clinical findings consistent with acute pyelonephritis have abnormal DMSA scan findings, there is still a high false-positive and/or negative rate based on routine clinical and laboratory parameters, including fever, elevated WBC, elevated CRP, elevated ESR, and the presence of VUR (Rushton, 1997).

Direct techniques have been used to localize the level of UTI to the upper or lower urinary tract. These include split-urine cultures collected by ureteral catheterization (Stamey *et al.*, 1965), bladder washout (Fairley *et al.*, 1971), and thin-needle aspiration of renal pelvic urine under ultrasonic guidance. Although these efforts may accurately localize infection to the upper or lower urinary tract, they are invasive and do not assess the extent of renal parenchymal involvement.

Renal cortical scintigraphy with [99mTc]DMSA has emerged as the imaging agent of choice for the detection and evaluation of acute pyelonephritis and renal scarring in children. Early clinical reports showed that renal cortical scintigraphy using [99mTc]DMSA or glucoheptonate was significantly more sensitive than intravenous urography (IVU) and renal sonography in the detection of acute pyelonephritis (Handmaker, 1982; Traisman *et al.*, 1986; Sty *et al.*, 1987). Subsequently, to evaluate the true sensitivity and specificity of renal cortical scintigraphy, experimental studies in an animal model were conducted using strict histopathologic criteria as the standard of reference (Rushton *et al.*, 1988; Parkhouse *et al.*, 1989). In these two contemporary investigations, pyelonephritis was created in young piglets by surgically inducing unilateral

VUR of infected urine. Typical DMSA renal scan findings of acute pyelonephritis included focal areas of diminished uptake of DMSA with preservation of the renal contour (Fig. 10.8). The DMSA scan was determined to be highly sensitive and reliable for the detection and localization of experimental acute pyelonephritis, with a sensitivity of 87–89% and specificity of 100% in both. When individual pyelonephritic lesions were analyzed, DMSA scan findings correlated with histopathologic changes with an overall agreement rate of 89–94%. Those lesions not detected were microscopic foci of inflammation not evident on gross examination and not associated with significant parenchymal damage.

Not only is DMSA scintigraphy highly sensitive and specific for the diagnosis of acute pyelonephritis, but it also provides important information regarding renal function and the extent of renal parenchymal inflammation. Documentation of renal parenchymal damage associated with acute pyelonephritis is fundamental to understanding the roles of infection and VUR in the etiology of pyelonephritis and renal scarring.

Spect

The application of single photon emission computerized tomography (SPECT) to DMSA scintigraphy reportedly further enhances the sensitivity of DMSA in the detection of acute pyelonephritis (Tarkington *et al.*, 1990; Itoh *et al.*, 1991; Itoh *et al.*, 1995). In clinical studies, a greater number of defects have been

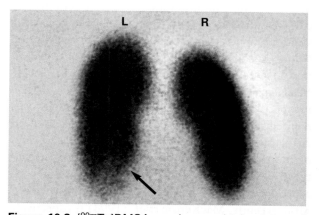

Figure 10.8 [99mTc]DMSA renal scan obtained 1 week after introduction of infection in young pig with experimentally produced left vesicoureteral reflux. Focal decrease in uptake with preservation of renal contour is noted in left lower pole (*arrow*). Pathologic examination confirmed left lower pole pyelonephritis. (Reprinted from Rushton and Majd, 1992, with permission.)

detected by SPECT than by standard pinhole imaging. In these clinical trials, histopathologic confirmation of the abnormal findings demonstrated by renal scintigraphy was not possible. To evaluate further the accuracy of SPECT imaging in the detection of acute pyelonephritis, SPECT was compared with pinhole imaging of DMSA renal scans for the detection and localization of acute pyelonephritis in 16 piglets (32 kidneys) with bilateral reflux of infected urine (Majd *et al.*, 1996). Animals were evaluated with both imaging modalities immediately before being killed at 1, 2, 3, and 10 days following the introduction of infection into their bladders. The overall sensitivity for detection of affected renal zones with histologic evidence of pyelonephritis was 86% for pinhole imaging and 91% for SPECT. The specificity was 95% for pinhole imaging and 82% for SPECT. Overall accuracy for the presence or absence of kidney involvement was 88% for both (Fig. 10.9). Thus, SPECT imaging appears to be slightly more sensitive than standard pinhole imaging, but its application may result in more false-positive findings. Furthermore, it is easier to differentiate acute inflammatory changes from chronic renal scarring with pinhole imaging. Whether pinhole or SPECT imaging is used depends to some extent on the availability and experience of the imaging unit.

Other imaging studies used to detect pyelonephritis

Sonography and intravenous pyelography

Several recent clinical studies have clearly demonstrated that renal sonography is not as reliable as DMSA scintigraphy for the detection of acute pyelonephritis (Bjorgvinsson *et al.*, 1991; Melis *et al.*, 1992; Shanon *et al.*, 1992; Tasker *et al.*, 1993; Benador *et al.*, 1994; MacKenzie *et al.*, 1994; Yen *et al.*, 1994). In one prospective study of 91 children with culture-documented febrile UTIs, DMSA renal scans showed changes consistent with acute pyelonephritis in 63% of the patients (Bjorgvinsson *et al.*, 1991). In contrast, sonography revealed changes consistent with acute pyelonephritis in only 39% of the same patients. More recently, MacKenzie *et al.* (1994) prospectively compared the results of renal sonograms with DMSA renal scans in 112 children with their first documented, symptomatic UTI. Although ultrasound was particuarly effective in detecting dilatation of the collecting system and renal swelling, it failed to detect over one-half of those patients with abnormal DMSA

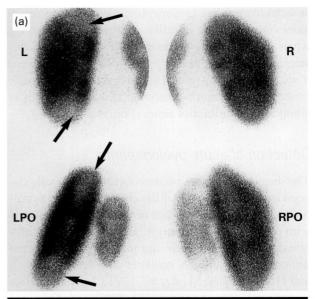

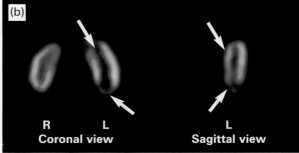

Figure 10.9 (*a*) Posterior and posterior oblique pinhole and (*b*) Coronal and sagital SPECT images of [^{99m}Tc]DMSA renal scan in a young pig with bilateral vesicoureteral reflux and acute left pyelonephritis 48 h after introduction of E. coli broth into the bladder. Photopenic lesions in the left upper and lower poles are demonstrated by both modalities (*arrows*).

scans demonstrating photon-deficient areas consistent with the acute inflammatory changes of pyelonephritis (Fig. 10.10). Intravenous pyelography has been shown to be very insensitive for the detection of acute pyelonephritis (Silver *et al.*, 1976).

Other renal isotopes

The usefulness of an early [^{99m}Tc]mercaptoacetytriglycine (MAG-3) renal scan in predicting renal alterations seen on DMSA renal scans was evaluated by Piepz *et al.* (1992). These investigators concluded that the accuracy of the MAG-3 renal scan was population dependent. When the DMSA scan was normal or very abnormal, the MAG-3 image correctly reflected the findings of the DMSA renal scan. However, when the DMSA abnormalities were less pronounced, the early MAG-3 scan failed to detect about one-half of the cases.

[^{99m}Tc]Glucoheptonate has also been used in the detection of the acute inflammatory changes associated with acute pyelonephritis (Traisman *et al.*, 1986; Sty *et al.*, 1987; Sreenarasimhaiah and Alon, 1995). Although the sensitivity and specificity of ^{99m}Tc-labelled glucoheptonate and DMSA have not been directly compared, certain observations can be made. Approximately 60% of the administered dose of [^{99m}Tc]DMSA is tightly bound to the proximal tubular cells, and only a small amount is excreted slowly in the urine. Consequently, DMSA allows for excellent visualization of the renal parenchyma without interference from retained tracer in the collecting systems. In contrast, only about 20% of the administered dose of [^{99m}Tc]glucoheptonate is firmly bound to the tubular cells. Most of the administered dose is excreted in the urine, which allows for moderately good visualization of the renal collecting systems on the early images. This additional information makes glucoheptonate the preferred agent of some clinicians (Sreenarasimhaiah and Alon, 1995). However, the quality of the delayed renal cortical images is clearly better with DMSA.

Magnetic resonance imaging, computed tomographic scans, and power Doppler sonography

The use of MRI with UTIs has also been reported. In a clinical study on the detection of acute pyelonephritic damage in children, the sensitivity and specificity of gadolinium-enhanced MRI was equal to that of [^{99m}Tc]DMSA scanning (Lonergan *et al.*, 1998). In a more recent animal study, SPECT imaging using DMSA was compared with spiral CT scanning (pre- and postcontrast), gadolinium-enhanced MRI, and power Doppler sonography in 35 infected piglets with 70 refluxing kidneys (Majd *et al.*, 2001). The imaging modalities were interpreted independently and compared in a blinded fashion with histopathologic findings. SPECT DMSA, spiral CT, and MRI were equally sensitive and reliable in the detection and localization of acute pyelonephritis (Figs. 10.11, 10.12). Power Doppler sonography was significantly less accurate. Undoubtedly, with increased experience and enhanced applications, clinical use of spiral CT and MRI is likely to gain popularity in the evaluation of the pediatric urinary tract.

Evaluation of the child with urinary tract infection

Controversy continues to exist regarding when and how a child with documented UTI should be evaluated. A recent systematic overview of the literature to assess the evidence on which current recommendations for routine diagnostic imaging are based found that there were no controlled trials or analytic

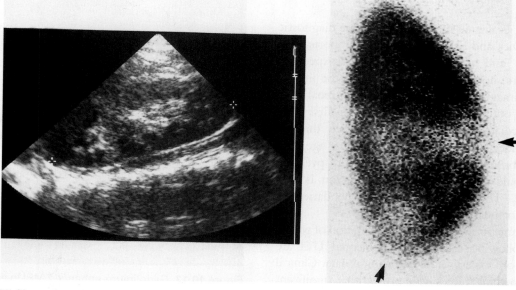

Figure 10.10 Normal sonogram and grossly abnormal [^{99m}Tc]DMSA renal scan of right kidney showing large midzone and moderate lower pole photopenic lesions characteristic of acute pyelonephritis in a 4-year-old girl who presented with her first documented febrile UTI (*arrows*). VCUG was negative for vesicoureteral reflux.

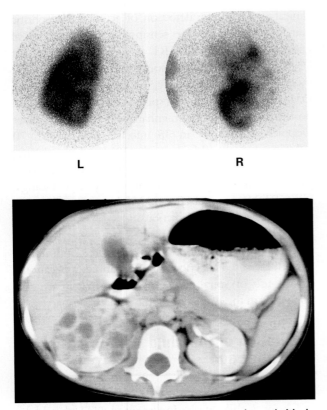

L   R

Figure 10.11 Severe multifocal acute pyelonephritis in the right kidney is well demonstrated on both a [99mTc]DMSA renal scan and CAT scan in a 3-year-old girl with her first febrile UTI. Photopenic areas on DMSA scan correspond to attenuated hypodense lesions on CAT scan. Note diffuse right renal swelling on CAT scan.

with VUR and recurrent UTIs than in those with reflux who have had only a single infection (Winberg *et al.*, 1975; Smellie *et al.*, 1981). Similarly, Jodal (1987) reported a strong association between the number of pyelonephritic episodes and the incidence of renal scarring. Recurrence of UTI within 1 year of a preceding infection occurs in approximately 30% of girls with one, 60% with two, and 75% with three prior infections (Winberg *et al.*, 1974). Furthermore, the non-specificity of signs and symptoms that typically accompany urinary infection in infants and toddlers often makes it impossible to determine whether an infection actually represents the first episode (Winberg *et al.*, 1974). Additional justification for early evaluation is based on the high yield of uropathology obtained from the evaluation of children with culture documented UTIs. Cystography in Caucasian girls with symptomatic UTIs consistently demonstrate the presence of VUR in approximately 30–50% of cases (Smellie *et al.*, 1975; Jodal, 1987), regardless of whether the study is requested by pediatric subspecialists (urology/nephrology) or other clinicians (pediatricians, family practitioners, adult urologists) (Sargent and Stringer, 1995). The exception is found in African–American girls with UTI in whom the relative incidence of VUR is about one-third that of Caucasian girls (Askari and Belman, 1982; Majd *et al.*, 1991).

studies that evaluated the need for routine diagnostic imaging (Dick and Feldman, 1996). All reports were descriptive and the majority was retrospective. Furthermore, none provided evidence of the impact of routine imaging on the development of renal scars and clinical outcomes in children with their first UTI.

Most pediatric urologists would agree that all children under 5 years of age, boys of any age, and all with febrile UTI or documented acute pyelonephritis should be evaluated when infection is first recognized. The key to this recommendation is adequate documentation of UTI.

The arguments in favor of early evaluation of young children following their first documented UTI are based on both experimental and clinical data. Clinical and experimental studies have proved that significant renal scarring can occur after a single UTI (Ransley and Risdon, 1981; Smellie *et al.*, 1985). A higher incidence of renal scarring has been reported in children

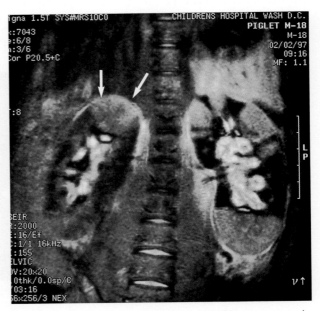

Figure 10.12 Gadolinium-enhanced MRI in a young pig with bilateral vesicoureteral reflux demonstrates multiple acute pyelonephritic lesions in both kidneys as evidenced by bright parenchymal lesions (*arrows*).

Unfortunately, other clinical parameters have proven unreliable in distinguishing those children with UTI who also have VUR (Van Gool *et al.*, 1992). All of the aforementioned factors offer a convincing argument to pursue early evaluation of young children following their first documented UTI. Waiting until a child has had two or more UTIs before proceeding with evaluation clearly increases the risk that permanent scarring, which might have otherwise been prevented, may occur.

History

Evaluation of the child with a UTI should always begin with a careful history. Because bladder emptying plays an important role in the etiology and prevention of UTI, a careful voiding history is an essential component of the work-up of toilet-trained children with UTIs (Koff, 1991). Many of these children also have associated constipation that may only be detected when specific questions are directed towards the patient and parents. Family history should also be obtained since heredity appears to play a role in an individual's predisposition toward infection, as evidenced by familial studies showing an increased incidence of bacteriuria in female siblings (Fennell *et al.*, 1977). Similarly, a significant familial risk for VUR has been demonstrated when a sibling or parent has a history of having reflux (Jerkins and Noe, 1982).

Physical examination

Physical examination of the child presenting with UTI should include palpation for flank masses, bladder distension, and/or abdominal masses caused by fecal impaction. Although genital examination in boys should exclude significant meatal stenosis, this is an extremely rare cause of UTI. Considering the epidemiological evidence demonstrating an increased risk for UTI in uncircumcised boys, the circumcision status is of particular importance in male infants. Abnormal genital findings in girls include vulvovaginitis or the presence of labial adherence that might predispose the child to perineal colonization by bacteria. More often labial adherence increases the risk for contamination of 'clean-catch' urine specimens for culture. In children with a significant history of voiding dysfunction associated with constipation and/or encopresis, a brief neurologic examination should include evaluation of perineal sensation, of peripheral reflexes in the lower extremities, and of the lower back for sacral dimpling or cutaneous abnormalities that suggest an underlying spinal abnormality (occult spinal dysraphism). Rectal examination for fecal impaction may be indicated if the history suggests severe constipation or encopresis.

Imaging

Recommended imaging studies for a child with a history of a culture-documented UTI are based, to some extent, on the experience of the radiologist and the availability of imaging modalities. Age, gender, race, and the type and frequency of UTIs must also be taken into consideration. For many years, the emphasis on the investigation of the child with UTI has centered on diagnosis of VUR. More recently, some authors have suggested that the emphasis should be focused on whether the child has renal scarring or is at risk for renal scarring (Verber *et al.*, 1988; Verboven *et al.*, 1990; Gleeson and Gordon, 1991; Haycock, 1991; Ditchfield *et al.*, 1994; MacKenzie, 1996). They argue that if there is no evidence of renal damage at the time of the infection, then it is not necessary to evaluate for VUR as the risk for future renal scarring is minimal. Consequently, these authors have recommended that the initial evaluation in children older than 1–2 years should be of the kidney, including sonography to exclude surgical conditions that predispose to infection and DMSA scintigraphy to detect acute pyelonephritic inflammation. With this approach, cystography is reserved for infants under 1–2 years and older children with abnormal DMSA scan findings or recurrent UTIs. In contrast, most American urologists, pediatricians, and radiologists still recommend that the evaluation of infants and toddlers should always include a cystogram to detect the presence of VUR, ureteroceles, a posterior urethral valve in boys, or bladder wall thickening and a sonogram to look for obstruction, hydronephrosis, or other congenital malformations (Nash and Siegele, 1996; AAP Committee on Quality Improvement, 1999). Whether or not one accepts the recommendation that DMSA scintigraphy should precede voiding cystourethrography in the evaluation of children with UTIs is determined in part by the goal of management of these patients. For those whose ultimate goal of treatment is the cessation of VUR, when present, then voiding cystourethrography will continue to be the initial study of choice. For others, whose primary goal is the detection and future prevention of pyelonephritis and new renal damage, DMSA scintigraphy may well replace voiding cystourethrography as the initial investigation of children with symptomatic urinary tract infections. It should be recognized that, to date, no studies have analyzed the relative advantages of any specific imaging approach with regard to documentation of their impact on the development of renal scars or other clinical outcomes (Dick and Feldman, 1996).

Timing of evaluation

The timing of evaluation is often a concern of the urologist, radiologist, and pediatrician. Many recommend that children requiring hospitalization should at least be screened for obstruction with a sonogram before discharge. For patients evaluated with cystography, it has been suggested that this be delayed by 4–6 weeks following the acute infection to avoid demonstrating transient mild reflux secondary to inflammatory changes of the ureterovesical junction. However, it is rare for reflux to be detected during infection and then disappear after treatment (Gross and Lebowitz, 1981; Craig et al., 1997). Furthermore, since the significance of reflux is greatest at the time of bacterial infection, demonstration of even transient reflux may be very meaningful. One potential disadvantage of obtaining a cystogram early in the course of a febrile infection is that ureteral dilatation secondary to the effect of endotoxins may result in overestimation of the grade of reflux (Roberts, 1975; Hellstrom et al., 1987). Never-

theless, a prolonged waiting period is not necessary. The cystogram usually can be performed whenever the patient is no longer symptomatic and when the urine is sterile (Lebowitz and Mandell, 1987). Regardless of when studies are performed, antibiotic prophylaxis should be maintained until that time, particularly in infants or in children with a previous febrile UTI, in order to prevent reinfection (Smellie et al., 1985; Lebowitz and Mandell, 1987).

For patients evaluated with DMSA renal scintigraphy, the timing of the study is in part determined by the reason for the study. If one is attempting to document acute pyelonephritic inflammatory changes, the DMSA renal scan is best obtained early within the first several days of the acute episode (Stokland et al., 1996). However, if the primary goal is to document irreversible renal scarring after an episode of infection, then the study should be delayed for 6 months following the acute infection since transient acute changes on DMSA scans can persist for up to 5 months before resolving (Jakobsson and Svensson, 1997).

Cytography

Both direct and indirect cystographic techniques are used. Direct cystography involves filling the bladder by urethral catheterization or percutaneous suprapubic infusion. Both standard contrast medium and radiolabeled nuclides are satisfactory. In boys, contrast cystography is preferred because it provides for visualization of the urethra and for grading reflux (Fig. 10.13).

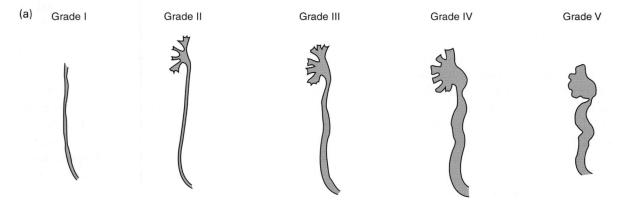

(a)　Grade I　　　Grade II　　　Grade III　　　Grade IV　　　Grade V

Figure 10.13 (a) International classification of vesicoureteral reflux: grade I, ureter only; grade II, ureter, pelvis, calyces, no dilatation, normal calyceal fornices; grade III, mild or moderate dilatation and/or tortuosity of ureter, and mild or moderate dilatation of the pelvis, but no or slight blunting of the fornices; grade IV, moderate dilatation and/or tortuosity, of ureter and mild dilatation of renal pelvis and calyces, complete obliteration of sharp angle of fornices but maintenance of papillary impressions in majority of calyces, grade V, gross dilatation and tortuosity of ureter, gross dilatation of renal pelvis and calyces, papillary impressions are no longer visible in majority of calyces. (Modified from International Reflux Committee, 1981.) (b) Shown opposite.

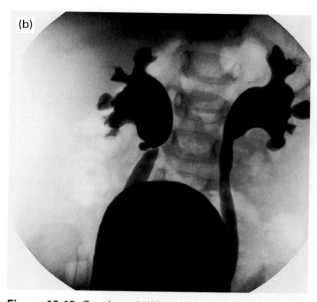

(b)

Figure 10.13 Continued. (*b*) Voiding cystogram shows grade III vesicoureteral reflux on the right with moderate dilatation and tortuosity of ureter, moderate dilatation of the pelvis, but slight blunting of the fornices. Grade IV reflux is seen on the left with similar dilatation of the ureter and pelvis but with obliteration of sharp angle of fornices. Papillary impressions are maintained in the majority of the calyces.

It is also more reliable for detecting duplication, ureteral ectopia with or without ureteroceles, posterior urethral valves, bladder trabeculation, bladder diverticula, and foreign bodies. Many also prefer its use for the initial examination in girls because the grade of reflux can be determined. Several methods for grading are used. The International Reflux Study method is most widely accepted (International Reflux Committee, 1981). A disadvantage of standard contrast cystography is the high gonadal radiation dose that it entails, particularly with multiple studies or fluoroscopic monitoring. The addition of digital fluoroscopy reduces gonadal radiation exposure (Cleveland *et al.*, 1991). Using a low-dose fluoroscopic system with a computer-based video-frame grabber, the ovarian radiation dose has been reported to compare favorably to radionuclide cystography (Diamond *et al.*, 1996).

Direct radionuclide cystography allows continuous monitoring for reflux throughout the study without additional radiation exposure. It is reported to be more sensitive than contrast cystography for the diagnosis of reflux (Conway *et al.*, 1972; Nasrallah *et al.*, 1982; Jaya *et al.*, 1996). Whereas precise grading of VUR is lim-

ited, it usually can be categorized as mild, moderate, or severe (Fig. 10.14). Although radionuclide cystography has been criticized for being unable to detect grade I/V VUR, a recent study found that direct radionuclide cystography demonstrated VUR to the renal pelvis in all 17 kidneys with grade I/V VUR on contrast cystography (Saraga *et al.*, 1996). The radiation dose from radionuclide cystography reportedly is 50–200 times lower than that with standard techniques using contrast cystography, making it ideal for the follow-up of children with VUR and for following the results of antireflux surgery (Willi and Treves, 1985).

Indirect radionuclide cystography uses [^{99m}Tc]diaminotetraethylpentacetic acid (DTPA), which is excreted by glomerular filtration. The presence of reflux can be assumed when radioisotope counts increase in the renal areas after voiding. Indirect cystography is less reliable for the detection of VUR than direct radionuclide cystography, with false-negative rates ranging from 22 to 51% (Majd *et al.*, 1983; De Sadeleer *et al.*, 1994). More recently, indirect radionuclide cystography using [^{99m}Tc]MAG-3 was also reported to be unreliable for the detection of VUR, missing approximately two-thirds of refluxing kidneys (De Sadeleer *et al.*, 1994) (Fig. 10.15).

Upper tract imaging

Recommendations for evaluating the upper urinary tract in children presenting with UTI also vary from institution to institution. The ideal study should be painless, safe, cost-effective, and associated with minimal or no radiation, and yet should be capable of detecting clinically significant structural malformations as well as renal scarring. Unfortunately, such an all-encompassing study does not exist.

One approach is to first screen all patients with a history of UTI with a renal–bladder sonogram (Kangarloo *et al.*, 1985). In children, sonography has been found to be as sensitive as intravenous pyelography (IVP) for the detection of any significant renal abnormality except for uncomplicated duplication anomalies and focal renal scarring (Horgan *et al.*, 1984; Jequier *et al.*, 1985; Kangarloo *et al.*, 1985; Leonidas *et al.*, 1985). Sonography is painless, noninvasive, simple to perform, radiation free, and independent of renal function. It is critical that appropriate images of the ureters, bladder, and true pelvis be routinely obtained in order to detect the presence of ureteroceles or dilated ureters secondary to ureteral

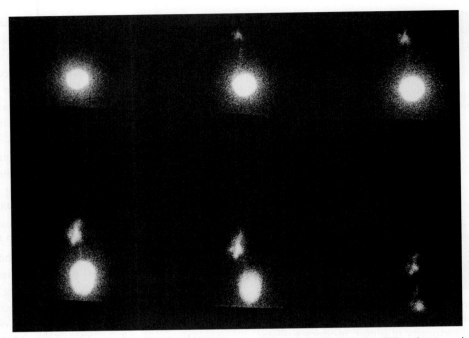

Figure 10.14 Isotope cystogram demonstrates mild left vesicoureteral reflux during filling (*top row*) which becomes moderate reflux when the bladder is full and during voiding (*bottom row*).

ectopia, ureterovesical junction obstruction, or severe VUR. To do so, the bladder should be full during the examination. Postvoiding residual urine can also be demonstrated at the completion of the study. Hydronephrosis revealed by sonography that is not the result of reflux, is best evaluated with diuretic renography using [99mTc]DTPA or [99mTc]MAG-3 (Majd, 1992). When combined with the findings of the renal–bladder sonogram, the site of obstruction can be reliably determined in almost all cases. Occasionally,

due to massive hydronephrosis or poor renal function, further evaluation becoms necessary and can best be accomplished with percutaneous antegrade pyelography and pressure-perfusion studies (Whitaker test) (see Chapter 20).

Considering the very low incidence of surgically significant hydronephrosis presenting as UTI, some authors have questioned the role of sonography in the investigation of UTIs in children, recommending instead a cortical renal scan as the initial upper tract

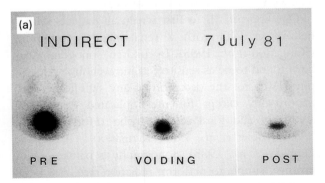

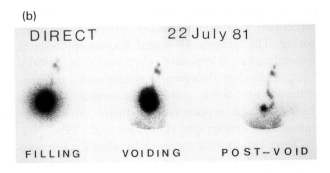

Figure 10.15 (*a*) False-negative indirect radionuclide cystogram in a 6-year-old girl. Images before and after voiding demonstrate no evidence of vesicoureteral reflux. (*b*) Selected images from a direct radionuclide cystogram in the same patient obtained 2 weeks after the indirect study show moderate reflux on the right during filling and voiding, and after voiding. (Reprinted from Majd *et al.*, 1985, with permission.)

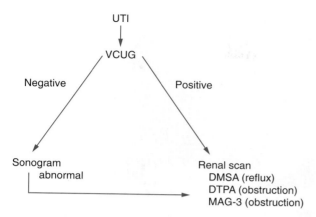

Figure 10.16 Algorithm for evaluation of children with urinary tract infection. (Adapted from Rushton, 1992, with permission.)

study of choice (MacKenzie *et al.*, 1994; Mucci and Macguire, 1994; Sreenarasimhaiah and Alon, 1995; Alon and Ganapathy, 1999). Still other authors have suggested a tailored approach to the evaluation of children with UTI, beginning with a voiding cystogram (Blickman *et al.*, 1985; Ben-Ami *et al.*, 1989). If no reflux is present, a renal ultrasound scan is done to exclude hydronephrosis or other upper tract malformations. Otherwise, if reflux is demonstrated, the next study would be a renal cortical scan to detect renal scarring (Fig. 10.16). This approach seems reasonable for the majority of cases.

In clinical practice, the use of DMSA scintigraphy is best reserved for those occasions when it will influence management. DMSA scintigraphy can be helpful in the initial evaluation and follow-up of patients with VUR. For example, not all patients with VUR and breakthrough UTIs require immediate surgical intervention, particulary those with asymptomatic bacteriuria (Hansson *et al.*, 1989c) (Fig. 10.17). In contrast, when new renal damage associated with a breakthrough UTI is objectively demonstrated by DMSA scintigraphy, antireflux surgery should be seriously considered (Fig. 10.18). Likewise, DMSA scintigraphy is important in the initial evaluation of infants with prenatally detected VUR, as many of these patients will have significant congenital reflux nephropathy.

DMSA scintigraphy is also particulary helpful for establishing the correct diagnosis of pyelonephritis in situations when the diagnosis is unclear based on clinical and laboratory findings, such as in neonates and young infants. Not infrequently, the diagnosis in these young children is obscured by improper urine collection techniques or the institution of antibiotics before a urine culture is obtained. Other difficult diagnostic situations include children with neuropathic bladders managed by clean intermittent catheterization (Cohen *et al.*, 1990; Ottolini *et al.*, 1995). These children are usually chronically bacteriuric, therefore, the diagnostic significance of a positive urine culture at the time of a febrile episode is lost.

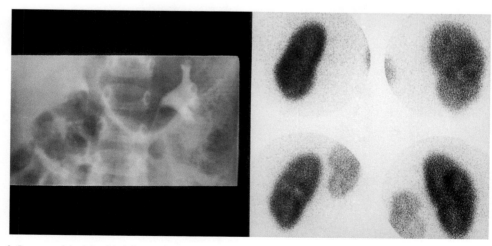

Figure 10.17 A 3-year-old girl with bilateral grade II vesicoureteral reflux (*left*) developed a breakthrough febrile UTI while on antibiotic prophylaxis. A [⁹⁹ᵐTc]DMSA renal scan (*right*) at the time of the infections did not demonstrate any evidence of pyelonephritis or scarring. Her prophylaxis was changed and repeat isotope cystogram 1 year later revealed complete resolution of her reflux.

(a)

(b)

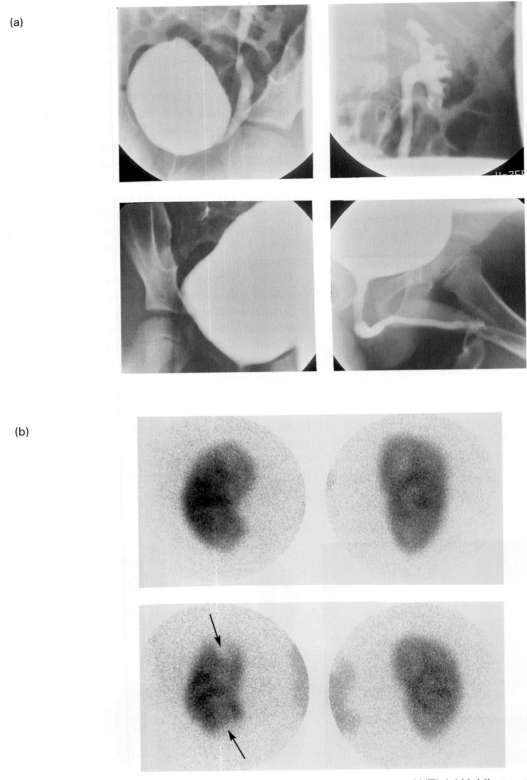

Figure 10.18 A 2-year-old girl presented with her first culture documented UTI. (*a*) Voiding cystogram demonstrates left grade III vesicoureteral reflux. (*b*) (*Top*) Initial [99mTc]DMSA renal scan was normal. (*Bottom*) Repeat [99mTc]DMSA renal scan following a breakthrough febrile UTI reveals acute pyelonephritic changes in the left upper and lower poles (*arrows*). Left ureteral reimplantation was performed.

Renal scarring

Partly because most renal scars that are detected in children with prior UTI(s) have become established by the time of initial evaluation, the pathogenesis of renal scarring remains controverisal (McLachlan *et al.*, 1975; Newcastle Asymptomatic Bacteriuria Research Group, 1975; Smellie *et al.*, 1981). Furthermore, it has become increasingly clear that the term renal scarring has been applied to the end result of more than one type of pathophysiological process, including both abnormalities that are congenital and those that are acquired postnatally. Although the vast majority of renal scarring associated with VUR is detected during the evaluation of children with UTI, recent studies of prenatally detected hydronephrosis secondary to high-grade VUR have also confirmed cases of congenital functional abnormalities documented by DMSA renal scintigraphy, even in the absence of infection (Gordon, 1990; Najmaldin *et al.*, 1990; Anderson and Rickwood, 1991; Sheridan *et al.*, 1991; Burge *et al.*, 1992; Crabbe *et al.*, 1992) (Fig. 10.19). The correlation between the severity of VUR and renal scarring is well established (Bellinger and Duckett, 1984; Bisset *et al.*, 1987; Jodal, 1987; Skoog *et al.*, 1987). Furthermore, a higher prevalence of renal scarring has been reported in children with secondary VUR associated with functional or anatomical bladder outlet obstruction, including posterior urethral valves and neuropathic bladders, than in children with primary VUR (Rushton *et al.*, 1992). Lumping renal sequelae from all of these pathophysiologic entities under the terms

'renal scarring' or 'reflux nephropathy' has hampered attempts at understanding the pathogenic mechanisms involved.

The critical role that infection plays in the pathogenesis of renal scarring associated with reflux was clarified in Ransley and Risdon's classic experimental studies of VUR in piglets in 1978. They demonstrated that, in the face of VUR and normal voiding pressures, renal scarring occurs only when urinary infection is present. Reflux in the absence of infection caused renal changes only when bladder outlet resistance was increased, so that obstruction, not reflux, was the pathophysiologic explanation for renal damage. It was suggested that the portions of the kidney at risk for scarring are those susceptible to pyelotubular backflow (intrarenal reflux), based on papillary morphology and configuration (Figs. 10.20, 10.21).

Clinically, new or progressive scarring is almost always associated with a history of UTI. Experimental studies and clinical experience have shown that a single episode of pyelonephritis can lead to significant renal damage (Fig. 10.22) (Ransley and Risdon, 1981; Smellie *et al.*, 1983). Furthermore, a clear association between the number of pyelonephritic attacks and incidence of renal scarring has been reported (Fig. 10.23) (Smellie *et al.*, 1985; Jodal, 1987; Martinell *et al.*, 1996b). Both experimental and clinical studies have also shown that some renal scarring can be prevented or diminished by early antibiotic treatment of acute pyelonephritis (Figs. 10.24) (Glauser *et al.*, 1978; Ransley and Risdon, 1981; Winberg *et al.*, 1982; Winter *et al.*, 1983). Further-

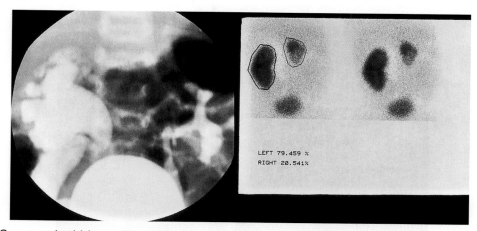

Figure 10.19 One-month-old boy with prenatally detected hydronephrosis. (*Left*) Voiding cystogram shows right grade V (note intrarenal reflux) and left grade III vesicoureteral reflux. (*Right*) [99mTc]DMSA scan reveals a hypoplastic right kidney with markedly reduced differential renal function. He had been on antibiotic prophylaxis since birth and urine cultures were negative.

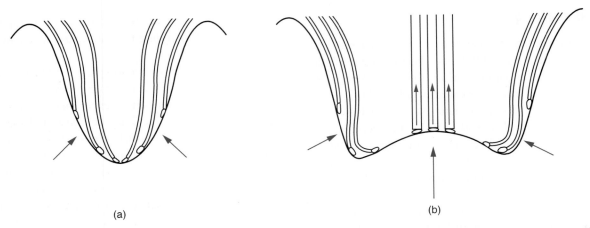

(a)   (b)

Figure 10.20 Papillary configuration in intrarenal reflux. (*a*) Convex papilla (non-refluxing): crescentric or slit-like orifices of collecting ducts opening obliquely onto the papilla. (*b*) Concave or flat papilla (refluxing papilla): round, gaping orifices of collecting ducts opening at right angles onto flat papilla. (Reprinted Ransley, 1977, with permission.)

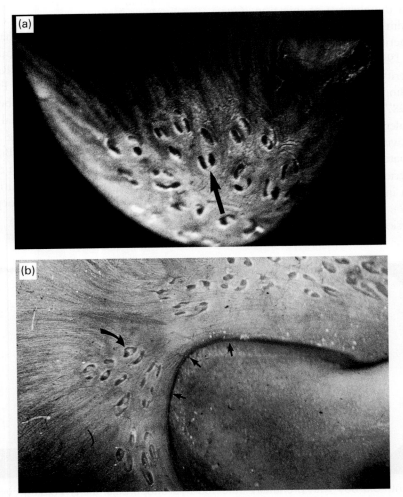

Figure 10.21 (*a*) Non-refluxing simple papilla with convex conical configuration and slit-like orifices of collecting ducts (*arrow*). (*b*) Refluxing compound papilla with concave configuration (arrows) and gaping oval to round orifices of collecting ducts (*curved arrow*). (Reprinted from Rushton *et al.*, 1988, with permission.)

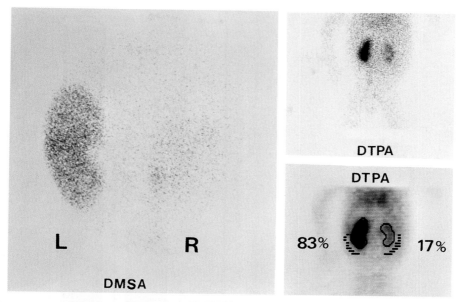

Figure 10.22 A 9-month-old girl hospitalized with her first febrile UTI. VCUG demonstrated right grade IV vesicoureteral reflux. Sonography showed moderate right hydronephrosis. (a) Initial [99mTc]DMSA renal scan at the time of hospitalization demonstrates marked diffuse decreased uptake (function) in the right kidney, consistent with acute pan-pyelonephritis. (b) Follow-up [99mTc]DTPA renal scan 1 month later shows partial recovery of function, but the kidney is contracted and scarred with a differential function of only 17%. (Reprinted from Rushton, 1992, with permission.)

more, when reflux is present, progressive renal scarring can be successfully prevented by keeping the patient free of infection (Edwards *et al.*, 1977; Bellinger and Duckett, 1984; Skoog *et al.*, 1987). Based on all of the above, it is clear that infection, not reflux alone, is a prerequisite for acquired renal scarring.

Congenital renal scarring associated with reflux

Severe reflux may be associated with significant renal dysplasia thought to result from abnormal induction of the nephrogenic cord during embryogenesis (Mackie and Stephens, 1975; Sommer and Stephens, 1981). Several reports have described DMSA scan renal functional abnormalities in patients with primary VUR detected prenatally (Najmaldin *et al.*, 1990; Gordon *et al.*, 1990; Anderson and Rickwood, 1991; Sheridan *et al.*, 1991; Burge *et al.*, 1992; Crabbe *et al.*, 1992). The reported incidence of renographic abnormalities in these studies has varied widely, ranging from 17 to 60% (Anderson and Rickwood, 1991; Sheridan *et al.*, 1991; Crabbe *et al.*, 1992). Many of these infants were evaluated by renal scintigraphy before any known episodes of infection, confirming that the functional abnormalities present at birth represent a congenital fetal nephropathy rather than a secondary acquired

abnormality. In one study, nephrectomy specimens in a few of these severely scarred kidneys with minimal function demonstrated severe dysplasia and growth arrest (Anderson and Rickwood, 1991). This would suggest that both congenital and acquired scarring may occur in the same kidney.

Imaging of renal scarring

In the past, the primary imaging modality for the detection of renal scarring was the IVP. However, limitations of the IVP have actually hindered understanding of the pathogenesis of renal scarring. Although relatively sensitive for the detection of renal scarring, the IVP is very insensitive in the detection of acute pyelonephritis (Silver *et al.*, 1976). Furthermore, pyelographic evidence of new renal scarring may take 2 or more years to develop after a documented UTI (Filly *et al.*, 1974; Smellie *et al.*, 1985). Consequently, this has forced investigators to speculate retrospectively about the etiology of renal scarring.

In contrast, DMSA renal cortical scintigraphy is capable of detecting both the acute inflammatory changes of pyelonephritis and renal scarring. Several studies comparing the DMSA renal scan to the IVP in

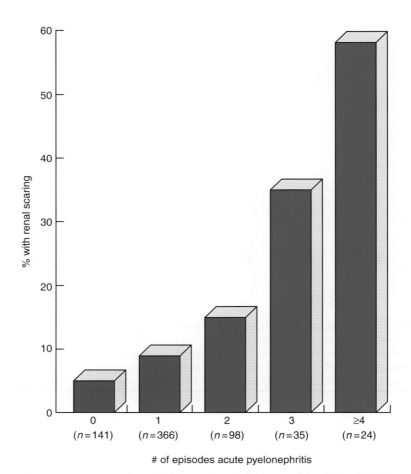

Figure 10.23 Relationship of renal scarring to number of episodes of acute pyelonephritis. (Adapted from Jodal, 1987.)

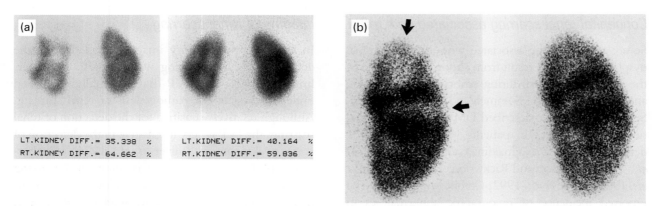

Figure 10.24 (a) [99mTc]DTPA renal scan in a 3.5–year-old girl with left grade IV vesicoureteral reflux and multiple recurrent UTIs. (*Left*) Multifocal acute pyelonephritis is demonstrated in the upper and lower poles and mid-zone of the left kidney. (*Right*) Follow-up [99mTc]DMSA renal scan 1 year later reveals significant improvement in function of the left kidney. (Reprinted with permission from Rushton, 1994.) (b) (*Left*) [99mTc]DMSA renal scan in 4.5-year-old girls with acute pyelonephritis evidenced by typical changes of photopenia with preservation of the renal contour in the upper pole and mid-zone of the right kidney (*arrows*). (*Right*) Repeat DMSA renal scan 15 months later demonstrates complete resolution of acute inflammatory changes without residual scarring or loss of cortex. (Reprinted from Rushton and Majd, 1992, with permission.)

the detection of renal scarring have demonstrated a greater sensitivity with isotope imaging, especially in younger children (Merrick *et al.*, 1980; Stoller and Kogan, 1986; Goldraich *et al.*, 1987; Monsour *et al.*, 1987; Farnsworth *et al.*, 1991; Elison *et al.*, 1992; Shanon *et al.*, 1992). Merrick *et al.* (1980) compared the findings of IVP to DMSA scans in 79 children who had proven UTI and had been followed for a period of 1–4 years (Merrick *et al.*, 1980). The sensitivity of IVP for the detection of renal scars was 80% and the specificity was 92%, whereas cortical scintigraphy had a sensitivity of 92% and a specificity of 98%. When both IVP and DMSA scintigraphy demonstrate scars, an excellent correlation on a site-by-site basis has been reported (Merrick *et al.*, 1980; Goldraich *et al.*, 1987; Monsour *et al.*, 1987; Farnsworth *et al.*, 1991; Stokland *et al.*, 1998). When compared with histology in an animal model, the sensitivity of the DMSA scan for the detection of renal scarring in 60 piglets with reflux and infected urine was 85% and the specificity was 97% (Arnold *et al.*, 1990). Thus, DMSA renal cortical scintigraphy offers a superior opportunity to study the progression of renal damage or functional loss from the time of the initial insult until either complete healing or irreversible scarring develops.

Studies that have compared ultrasonography with DMSA scintigraphy for the detection of renal scarring have consistently reported greater sensitivity with DMSA renal scans (Shanon *et al.*, 1992; Tasker *et al.*, 1993; MacKenzie *et al.*, 1994). In one study, Yen *et al.* (1994) compared sonography, IVP, and both planar and SPECT DMSA renal scintigraphy in the evaluation of 130 children with UTI (42 patients), VUR (37 patients), and unilateral or bilateral small kidneys (51 patients). SPECT imaging of DMSA scans detected the highest number of defects, followed by planar imaging.

Renal scars detected by DMSA scintigraphy appear as focal or generalized areas of diminished uptake of radioisotope associated with loss or contraction of functioning renal cortex. This may appear as thinning or flattening of the cortex in some kidneys, while in others renal scars appear as classic discrete wedge-shaped parenchymal defects (Fig. 10.25). In more severe cases, generalized damage may be associated with multifocal or diffusely scarred kidneys and reduced differential renal function. In contrast, defects associated with acute pyelonephritis are more typically characterized by focal areas of diminished uptake but

with preservation of the normal renal contour (Fig. 10.26). Although it is often possible for an experienced observer to distinguish acute from chronic lesions, it should be recognized that this differentiation may be less apparent in those kidneys with acute pyelonephritis superimposed on pre-existent renal scarring.

New or acquired scarring

Until recently, a common assumption was that VUR was an absolute prerequisite for new or acquired renal scarring. This mindset was further perpetuated by earlier investigations of new or acquired renal scarring, most of which focused retrospectively on patients with known VUR. However, in one earlier study which selected patients on the basis of infection alone, only one-half of the 37 children who formed new renal scars had VUR (Winter *et al.*, 1983).

Several investigators have now evaluated the evolution of the acute inflammatory changes associated with pyelonephritis using serial DMSA renal scans (Rosenberg *et al.*, 1992; Rushton and Majd, 1992b; Wallin and Bajc, 1993; Stokland *et al.*, 1994; Jakobsson and Svensson 1997). The interval from the initial DMSA scan obtained at the time of acute infection until the repeat scan ranged from 3 months to 2 years. Acute DMSA renal scan defects persisted as renal scarring in 36–52% of kidneys. The sites of new renal scarring corresponded exactly to those sites of acute pyelonephritis seen on the initial DMSA renal scans, confirming the primary role of the acute inflammatory response to infection in the etiology of acquired renal scarring (Fig. 10.27). Contralateral

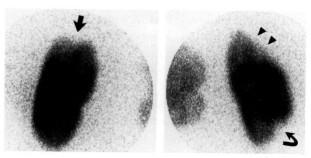

Figure 10.25 [⁹⁹ᵐTc]DMSA renal scan in a 7–year-old girl 7 months after her first documented febrile UTI. A VCUG revealed bilateral grade II vesicoureteral reflux. Renal scarring is present in both kidneys. The left upper pole is flattened (*arrow*). There is a wedge-shaped defect in the right lower pole (*curved arrow*) and thinning of the right upper pole (*arrow heads*). (Reprinted from Rushton, 1994, with permission.)

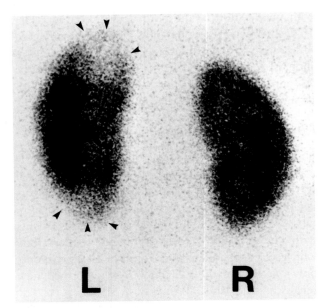

Figure 10.26 [99mTc]DMSA renal scan demonstrates typical changes of acute pyelonephritis in the upper and lower poles of the left kidney. Diminished uptake of isotope is seen with an intact renal cortical outline without volume loss or contraction (*arrows*). (Reprinted from Cohen *et al.*, 1990, with permission.)

normal kidneys and initially uninvolved areas of abnormal kidneys have almost always remained normal on follow-up DMSA renal scans. Surprisingly, reflux has been present in only 25–50% of kidneys that developed new renal scarring. This is attributable in part to the fact that the majority of patients (63–75%) with acute inflammatory changes on the initial DMSA renal scans did not have VUR. Nevertheless, in one prospective study of 38 kidneys with initially abnormal DMSA scans, scarring developed in six of 15 (40%) kidneys with associated VUR and in 10 of 23 (42%) kidneys without demonstrable reflux (Rushton *et al.*, 1992). Similar findings have been observed by others (Jakobsson *et al.*, 1994). These observations provide convincing clinical evidence that renal parenchymal infection, rather than VUR, is the prerequisite for acquired (postnatal) renal scarring. Once bacteria have invaded the renal parenchyma, the inflammatory response appears similar and the propensity for renal scarring is equally as great whether or not reflux is present.

Despite these findings, the importance of VUR (particularly grades III or higher) as a risk factor for renal scarring should not be discounted. Clearly, patients with moderate and severe reflux are much

more likely to develop acute pyelonephritic damage than children with mild or no reflux (Majd *et al.*, 1991; Jakobsson *et al.*, 1992). Furthermore, although 62% of the kidneys with postpyelonephritic renal scarring in one study were drained by non-refluxing ureters, renal scarring was still significantly more common in those kidneys with grade III or higher VUR compared with kidneys with mild or no reflux (Jakobsson *et al.*, 1994). Thus, the increased propensity for scarring in patients with higher grades of VUR is attributable in part to the increased risk of these kidneys for acute inflammatory damage at the time of the initial infection (Majd *et al.*, 1991; Jakobsson *et al.*, 1992; Melis *et al.*, 1992). Coupled with this, reflux (pyelotubular backflow of urine from the pelvis into the collecting ducts) of infected urine or scarring of adjacent papillae may transform marginally competent, non-refluxing papillae into papillae that do reflux, thereby predisposing the kidney to greater pyelonephritic damage (Ransley and Risdon, 1978; Majd *et al.*, 1991). Indeed, in one study that attempted to quantitate the area of acute pyelonephritic parenchymal damage, the presence of grade ≥ III reflux was associated with a significantly greater frequency of kidneys demonstrating large defects (defined as >10% of the kidney demonstrating DMSA uptake <2 SD of

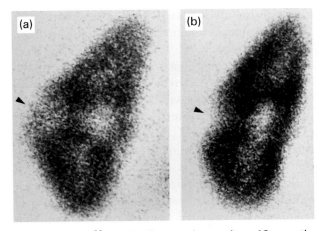

Figure 10.27 [99mTc]DMSA renal scan in a 13–month-old girl with an acute febrile UTI. (*a*) Left posterior oblique view on the initial DMSA scan demonstrates acute pyelonephritis of the midzone of the left kidney evidenced by a photopenic lesion with preservation of the renal contour (*arrow*). (*b*) Follow-up DMSA renal scan reveals progression to renal scar in the exact same site characterized by contraction and loss of functioning renal cortex (*arrow*). (Reprinted from Rushton *et al.*, 1992, with permission.)

the control kidney) compared with kidneys with no VUR ($p < 0.02$) (Jakobsson *et al.*, 1992). Thus, when present, moderate or severe reflux (grade $\geq$ III) remains the most significant host risk factor for acute pyelonephritis and renal scarring.

Other risk factors for the development of renal scarring include associated bladder pathology, regardless of whether reflux is present. In one study, the frequency of new renal scarring was significantly higher in kidneys associated with overt bladder pathology than in those with normal bladders (86% vs 32%; $p = 0.028$) (Rushton and Majd, 1992b). Marked bladder thickening and trabeculation, suggesting either functional or anatomical bladder outlet obstruction, was present in 67% of the patients with bladder pathology who developed new scarring. Urodynamic evaluation of children with neuropathic bladders associated with spina bifida has demonstrated that increased intravesical pressure may lead to upper tract deterioration, with or without VUR (McGuire and Woodside, 1981). Animal studies have also shown an increased propensity for renal scarring when infection and reflux occur in the presence of bladder outlet obstruction (Ransley and Risdon, 1978).

Two studies have also analyzed the association of various clinical and bacteriologic parameters with the development of new renal scarring (Rushton and Majd, 1992b; Jakobsson *et al.*, 1994). In both studies children who developed new renal scars were actually older at the time of acute pyelonephritis, although the difference was statistically significant in only one (Stokland *et al.*, 1994). An elevated WBC at the time of the initial infection was not associated with renal scarring. When comparing those patients with and without new scarring, no significant differences were noted in race, gender, duration of fever, maximum temperature, or acute inflammatory signs (CRP, ESR) at the time of the acute pyelonephritic episode. *Escherichia coli* was cultured from the urine of 88–95% of the patients in both studies. Interestingly, new scarring occurred in 33–41% of patients infected with *E. coli* compared with 100% of patients in both studies who were infected with other bacteria. In one study no significant association was found between bacterial virulence factors (hemolysin, colicin, P-fimbriae) and renal scarring, although colicin production was found almost twice as often in the bacteria isolated from patients with new renal scarring (Rushton *et al.*, 1992). In a more recent report of 157 children evaluated with a DMSA renal scan 1 year after their

first-time symptomatic UTI, children with high levels of CRP, high fever, and dilating vesicoureteral reflux had an increased risk of renal scarring up to 10 times higher than children with normal or slightly elevated CRP levels, no or mild fever, and no reflux (Stokland *et al.*, 1996).

Sequelae of renal scarring

Hypertension

Renal scarring is reported to be a common cause of hypertension in children and young adults (Llyod-Still and Cottom 1967; Gill *et al.*, 1976; Londe, 1978; Wanner *et al.*, 1985). The risk of hypertension in patients with renal scarring varies based on the length of follow-up and severity of scarring. In follow-up studies of children with renal scarring, approximately 6–13% of children with scarring will develop hypertension (Heale *et al.*, 1977; Wallace *et al.*, 1978; Beetz *et al.*, 1989; Goonasekera *et al.*, 1996; Martinell *et al.*, 1996b). In some cases, it may be associated with progressive renal insufficiency (Jacobson *et al.*, 1989). A report of an older cohort of 294 patients (mean age at presentation 17.3 years) with reflux nephropathy noted that the risk of hypertension increased with age and length of follow-up (Zhang and Bailey, 1995). Whereas 8.5% of these patients had hypertension at presentation, 38% became hypertensive later on (mean age 34.2 years). Hypertension was significantly more common in those with severe bilateral parenchymal scarring. Similarly, in another series 13% (ll/83) of children with renal scarring were hypertensive at initial evaluation and another 17% (14/83) developed hypertension over the next 4–20 years (Smellie and Normand, 1979).

The development of hypertension is clearly related to the severity of renal scarring and is more often observed in patients with a history of recurrent episodes of pyelonephritis associated with moderate or severe VUR (Haele *et al.*, 1977; Jacobson *et al.*, 1989). The actual risk for hypertension in children with milder degrees of scarring is unknown, but is undoubtedly less. The etiology of hypertension associated with renal scarring is controversial. Some investigators report no evidence that the renin–angiotensin–aldosterone (RAS) system contributes (Bailey *et al.*, 1978; Bailey *et al.*, 1984), whereas, others report that it does (Holland *et al.*, 1975; Luscher *et al.*, 1985; Savage *et al.*, 1987; Jacobson *et al.*, 1988b). Despite these controversies, most would agree that the risk for hypertension in patients with severe renal scarring is significant, and long-term follow-up is mandatory, since hypertension may take 10–20 years to develop.

Renal insufficiency

The actual risk of renal insufficiency secondary to postpyelonephritic renal scarring is unknown. The annual incidence of new patients presenting with end-stage renal disease (ESRD) associated with reflux nephropathy in Australia and New Zealand between 1985 and 1989 was 3.9 and 4.89 per million of the population, respectively (Disney, 1991). Overall, this represented 7% of all new cases of ESRD starting treatment during this period, including 24% in the teenage group. In a more recent study of 102 patients with ESRD seen at a pediatric hospital over a 10-year period, only three had reflux nephropathy, including one patient with no history of UTI and another with a single, afebrile UTI (Sreenarasimhaiah and Hellerstein, 1998). Only one child with grade II–III bilateral reflux had a history of recurrent UTIs.

Studies have shown that the incidence of renal insufficiency in patients with postpyelonephritic renal scarring increases with age. The incidence of renal insufficiency in a report by Martinell *et al.* (1996b) of 30 adults who were diagnosed with severe renal scarring as children was 10%. Another study of an older cohort of 294 patients (mean age at presentation 17.2 years) with reflux nephropathy found a 2% incidence of renal insufficiency [defined as a glomerular filtration rate (GFR) < 40–69 ml/min] at presentation which increased to 24% at last follow-up (mean age 34.2 years). The more extensive the renal scarring, the higher proportion with renal insufficiency (Jacobson *et al.*, 1989). Most patients (90–100%) with reflux nephropathy and ESRD have focal segmental glomerulosclerosis, almost always associated with proteinuria (Zimmerman *et al.*, 1973, Kincaid-Smith, 1975; Bhathena *et al.*, 1980; Torres *et al.*, 1980).

Treatment

The obvious goals of treatment of UTI are symptomatic relief and the prevention of new or progressive renal damage, especially in infants and young children who appear to be at greatest risk for renal scarring. Initial treatment, ideally, should be based on *in vitro* sensitivity studies. Frequently, such testing is not done or treatment is instituted before the results are available. Fortunately, because the common uropathogens are susceptible to multiple antibiotics and the response to antibiotics correlates best with urine levels which are usually more highly concentrated than serum levels (Stamey *et al.*, 1974), high cure rates have been reported in most therapeutic trials.

Uncomplicated lower urinary tract infection

Agents that have been used successfully for acute, uncomplicated lower urinary infections include sulfonamides, trimethoprim–sulfamethoxazole (TMP–SMX), nitrofurantoin, trimethoprim, and oral cephalosporins (see Appendix). Unfortunately, ampicillin and amoxicillin are used commonly by primary healthcare physicians. High intestinal levels of these two antibiotics often result in the rapid development of resistant enteric organisms, which then become the reinfecting bacteria. The emergence of resistant strains to ampicillin or amoxicillin has limited its efficacy in treating urinary infections compared with other antibiotics (Russo *et al.*, 1989–91). Resistance rates to ampicillin–amoxicillin have been recently reported to be as high as 54% in children with their first documented symptomatic UTI (Craig *et al.*, 1998). This drawback of the synthetic penicillins has been diminished by the relatively recent combination of clavulinic acid with amoxicillin (Augmentin). Clavulinic acid inhibits the bacterial β-lactamase enzymes, which render the β-lactamic antibiotics ineffective. This combination has proved effective in eradication of UTIs in children, even when *in vitro* susceptibility testing demonstrated resistance to amoxicillin alone (Al Roomi *et al.*, 1984; Ruberto *et al.*, 1989). However, ampicillin–clavulinic acid is associated with a high incidence of side-effects, is expensive, and is no more effective than the usual drugs.

The fluoroquinolones have been shown to have a wide spectrum of activity that includes most Gram-positive and Gram-negative organisms, including *Pseudomonas aeruginosa* and *Proteus* (Barry *et al.*, 1997). These are bactericidal agents and are believed to work by inhibiting the essential bacterial enzyme deoxyribonucleic acid (DNA) gyrase, which is essential for DNA replication in bacterial cells (Hooper *et al.*, 1987). Concern regarding arthropathic effects, based on animal studies showing cartilage toxicity, has prevented its approval for use in children (Schluter, 1986). However, the same experimental toxic effects have been reported with all quinolones, including nalidixic acid, which is licensed for use and has been used in children for decades (Bouissou et al., 1978). A retrospective match-controlled study of naildixic acid in 11 children treated for 10–600 days with follow-up examination 3–12 years later did not reveal any differences in arthropathic effects compared with controls (Schaad and Wedgwood-Krucko, 1978). Furthermore, clinical evidence of cartilage toxicity has not been reported in a study of more than 100 children with cystic fibrosis treated with varying courses of high-dose ciprofloxacin (Ball, 1986). Despite the lack of clinical evidence demonstrating cartilage toxicity in children, the use of fluoroquinolones in growing children generally should be avoided until definitive studies have been performed.

Duration of treatment

The optimal duration of treatment of acute, uncomplicated, lower UTIs in children is controversial. Several randomized, controlled studies have been published reporting the efficacy of single-dose or short-course antimicrobial therapy in children. The potential advantages of short-course therapy include decreased costs, improved compliance, decreased antibiotic-related side-effects, and decreased effect on the fecal flora.

In 1988, Moffatt et al. reported a methodologic analysis by four independent reviewers of 14 randomized, controlled trials of short-course antimicrobial therapy for uncomplicated lower UTIs in children. Short-course therapy varied in these 14 studies. Conventional therapy ranged from 7 to 10 days. In two, short-course therapy was less effective. One study compared single-dose versus 10-day amoxicillin therapy (Avner et al., 1983), and one compared 1-day versus 10-day cefadroxil therapy (McCracken et al., 1981). The other 12 studies showed no difference in outcome. The authors concluded that there was insufficient evidence to recommend short-course therapy for UTIs in children.

In a more recent review article published by Khan (1994), the findings in 12 of these reports were re-evaluated by pooling the data on 320 infants and children. He reported that single-dose therapy achieved an overall cure rate of 89% (63–100%), defined as a negative follow-up culture at 1 week and the lack of a

subsequent recurrence of the same organism. However, the response varied with the antimicrobial agents. Intramuscular aminoglycosides, used in 178 (56%), achieved the highest cure rate (96%), followed by TMP–SMX or a sulfa drug (90%). The cure rate of amoxicillin was significantly lower (75%; $p < 0.01$). Another large clinical study investigated single-dose versus multidose antibiotic therapy in 132 children with a culture-documented (first-time) acute UTI. There was no difference in the bacteriologic cure rate for single-dose (93%) versus multidose regimens (96%), but recurrence rates at 10–12 days or 28–37 days after treatment were significantly higher in the single-dose group (20.5%) compared with the 3-day (5.6%) and 7-day (8%) groups (Madrigal et al., 1988).

Two other studies have compared relatively short 3-day versus conventional 10-day courses of antibiotics for treatment of uncomplicated UTIs in children. In one prospective, randomized, open multicenter study of 264 girls aged 1–15 years, similar results were observed when short-course treatment with either 3 days of sulfamethizole or pivmecillinam was compared with 10 days of sulfamethizole (Petersen, 1991). Specifically, there was no difference in the number of girls with no or insignificant growth on urine cultures after treatment, or in the recurrence-free interval after treatment among the three groups. In another study of 10 children, no difference in initial cure or subsequent relapse rates was found in children treated with 3-day therapy versus 10 days using either cotrimoxazole or nitrofurantoin (Ruberto et al., 1984).

Based on the available data, it appears reasonable to treat acute, uncomplicated lower tract infections in children with a relatively short 3-day course of antibiotics. However, young children with their first infection or those with febrile infections should then continue to receive low-dose antimicrobial prophylaxis until radiographic evaluation is completed.

Asymptomatic bacteriuria

Treatment of true asymptomatic bacteriuria does not appear to be necessary if the urinary tract is otherwise normal (Eichenwald, 1986; White, 1987; Hansson et al., 1989a). The risk for pyelonephritis in infants and young girls with untreated asymptomatic bacteriuria is small, and many demonstrate spontaneous remission (Winberg et al., 1974; Jodal, 1987). In a prospective follow-up of 50 infants with initial screening bacteriuria, 37 were followed for a minimum of 6 years (Wettergren *et al.*, 1990). Of the original 50, two infants developed pyelonephritis within 2 weeks after bacteriuria was diagnosed. In 45, bacteriuria was left untreated. Spontaneous clearance was observed in 36, while in eight clearance followed treatment with antibiotics for respiratory infections. Recurrence of bacteriuria was observed in 10 of 50 children, of whom one had pyelonephritis. No child had more than one recurrence. Follow-up urography in 36 of 50 children after a median of 32 months showed no evidence of renal damage in any of them.

In contrast to infants with screening bacteriuria, treatment of school-aged girls with asymptomatic bacteriuria is followed by high recurrence rates of up to 80% (Kunin, 1970). Most are caused by new strains, which may carry the risk of being more virulent (McGeachie, 1966; Bergstrom *et al.*, 1967). In contrast, when left untreated, spontaneous changes of strain are uncommon (Hansson *et al.*, 1989a).

Several studies in the 1970s reported that non-treatment of asymptomatic bacteriuria was associated with normal growth of kidneys without the development of new scars, provided the urinary tract initially appeared normal radiographically (Savage *et al.*, 1975; Cardiff–Oxford Bacteriruia Study Group, 1978; Lindberg *et al.*, 1978c; Newcastle Asymptomatic Bacteriuria Research Group, 1981). In a 4-year follow-up by the Cardiff–Oxford Bacteriuria Study Group (1978) in children aged 5–12 years with untreated covert bacteriuria, new or progressive renal scarring did not occur unless VUR was present. Similarly, the presence of asymptomatic bacteriuria in the absence of VUR is not a risk factor for renal scarring in children with neuropathic bladders who perform clean intermittent catheterization (Ottolini *et al.*, 1995).

Hansson *et al.* (1989b) compared retrospectively treatment versus non-treatment of asymptomatic bacteriuria in older girls (median age 8 years) with pre-existent renal scarring. Many also had mild grade I–II/V VUR. Of 21 girls who were given a short course of antibiotics, 17 acquired a new infection within a year, including seven with pyelonephritic recurrences. Of 23 girls treated with antibiotic prophylaxis for 2–3 years, one-half developed breakthrough infections, and recurrences after completion of long-term prophylaxis were as common as after short-term treatment. Overall, in girls who received short- or long-term antibiotic treatment, 14 patients developed 21 episodes of acute pyelonephritis during a total of 140 patient years of observation. In contrast, asymptomatic bacteriuria was left untreated in 29 girls for a total of 74 patient years of observation. Only one patient developed acute pyelonephritis.

Based on this information it is reasonable that true asymptomatic bacteriuria, particularly in older girls, be left untreated (Svanborg-Eden and Svennerholm, 1978; Linshaw, 1996). However, in the presence of VUR, the risks of non-treatment of asymptomatic bacteriuria has not been clearly established, particularly in infants and younger children. It should also be recognized that bladder dysfunction is commonly found in girls with so-called asymptomatic bacteriuria, including detrusor instability, infrequent voiding and incomplete emptying (Hansson *et al.*, 1990). This explains in part the marked tendency for recurrent infection after treatment of asymptomatic bacteriuria with antibiotics alone. Treatment of the underlying voiding dysfunction is key to the successful long-term management of these patients.

Pyelonephritis

The child with suspected pyelonephritis requires a greater degree of assurance of immediate therapeutic success, since the degree of scarring and renal damage resulting from an infection may be influenced by the rapidity of effective therapy (Glauser *et al.*, 1978; Ransley and Risdon, 1981; Windberg *et al.*, 1982; Winter *et al.*, 1983; Smellie *et al.*, 1994). Oral medication can be initiated in older children who are not septic or vomiting as long as good compliance is ensured. Trimethoprim-sulfamethaxosole can be anticipated to be effective in most cases. Cephalosporins are also a good choice for initial therapy in the febrile child who does not require parenteral therapy. New third-generation cephalosporins such as cefixime offer the advantage of once-daily dosing and have been shown to be as effective as twice-daily TMP–SMX (Dagan *et al.*, 1992; Hoberman *et al.*, 1999). Treatment can be changed to include less expensive agents when the antibiotic sensitivities become available.

Although most would concur with a 10–14 day course of antibiotic therapy for pyelonephritis, there is considerable controversy over the need for hospitalization and treatment with parenteral antibiotics versus outpatient therapy with oral drugs. In a recent survey of 445 general practitioners, 143 pediatricians, and 45 pediatric nephrologists, there were significant differences in the recommendation for initial hospitalization by the general practitioners and pediatricians (17%) compared with the pediatric nephrologists (69%) (Cornu *et al.*, 1994). The pediatric nephrologists were evenly split between single and combined antibiotic therapy, whereas general practitioners and pediatricians preferred monotherapy. Intravenous antibiotics were preferred by 78% of the pediatric nephrologists compared with only 23–27% of pediatricians and general practitioners. This may suggest a greater concern and/or awareness on the part of the nephrologists regarding the potential for renal damage associated with pyelonephritis in children. However, in a recent prospective randomized clinical trial of 306 children 1–24 months old with febrile UTIs, outpatient treatment with oral third-generation cephalosporins was equally effective when compared with initial treatment with intravenous antibiotics. There was no significant difference in treatment success, duration of fever, or subsequent renal scarring on DMSA scans (Hoberman *et al.*, 1999).

Clearly, there is a need for controlled therapeutic trials for UTI in children with old and new drugs in different dosages and for varying lengths of treatment. These trials should categorize patients into different age groups such as: (1) neonates aged 0–28 days; (2) infants aged 1 month to < 2 years; (3) older children ≥ 2 years; and (4) adolescents (Helwig, 1994). Meanwhile, until such clinical trials are conducted, non-toxic children and infants > 3 months of age can be treated as outpatients as long as compliance is not an issue. It is reasonable to initiate therapy with 1–2 days of a long-acting, third-generation cephalosporin, such as ceftriaxone, administered intramuscularly, followed by 10–14 days of oral antibiotics and prophylaxis until evaluated. Ceftriaxone is active against most Gram-negative uropathogens and it achieves very high levels in both the urine and renal parenchyma following single daily doses. This approach virtually assures compliance and adequate antimicrobial coverage until the urine culture and sensitivity results are known. Alternatively, if compliance does not seem to be a problem, initial therapy with appropriate, broad-spectrum oral antibiotics may be as effective in the treatment of acute pyelonephritis and in the prevention of irreversible renal damage (Hoberman *et al.*, 1999).

In contrast, the toxic child and infants < 3 months of age with suspected acute pyelonephritis should be considered candidates for immediate hospitalization and parenteral therapy. In these patients combination therapy, including an aminoglycoside and ampicillin, are appropriate choices until the urine culture results are known. Alternatively, one of the newer third-generation cephalosporins may be used, but these are more expensive and do not provide comprehensive coverage of Gram-positive organisms, including *Enterococcus*. Parenteral antibiotic therapy should be continued for 7–10 days in neonates, although oral outpatient therapy to complete a full 10–14 day course can be substituted in patients > 2 months when afebrile for 24–48 h. Follow-up specimens for urine culture should be obtained at the completion of therapy, and prophylaxis should be instituted until evaluation of the urinary tract is completed.

Renal abscess

In the past, the majority of rebal abscesses, a rare form of renal infection, were not caused by ascending infection. Historically, *Staphylococcus aureus* has been the offending agent as a result of hematogenous seeding from a peripheral cutaneous site of origin (Rote *et al.*, 1978), or seeding of the contused renal parenchyma after blunt abdominal trauma (Vachvanichsanong *et al.*, 1992). Diagnosis is often delayed in these patients because urine cultures are negative in most. With the advent of early recognition and effective therapy, the frequency of staphylococcal bacteremia and renal abscesses has decreased. More cases of Gram-negative infections in the presence of VUR or other anatomic abnormalities of the urinary tract are now being seen (Timmons and Perlmutter, 1976).

Most patients with a renal abscess present with high fever, leukocytosis, and an elevated ESR, often accompanied by flank pain. A variety of imaging techniques has been used to diagnose renal abscesses, including IVP and angiography (Koehler, 1974), gallium-67 scintigraphy (Kumar *et al.*, 1975; Hopkins *et al.*, 1976), sonography, and CT (Gerzof and Gale, 1982; Wippermann *et al.*, 1991) (Fig. 10.28). The classic treatment of renal abscess has been surgical drainage in addition to appropriate antibiotic therapy. However, improved antibiotics and diagnostic techniques, together with the ability to obtain culture by percutaneous aspiration or drainage under ultrasonic

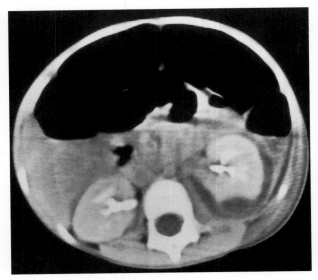

Figure 10.28 CT scan reveals a filling defect in upper pole of left kidney consistent with a renal abscess in a child with flank pain and fever. (Reprinted from Rushton, 1992, with permission.)

control, have often obviated the neccesity for surgical intervention. In seven patients reported by Schiff *et al.* (1977), 10 days of parenteral antibiotic treatment alone followed by an additional 2 weeks of appropriate oral therapy was successful. However, in a review of the literature performed by Steele *et al.* (1990), 62% (16/23) of the children with renal abscesses ultimately required surgical intervention. Unfortunately, no controlled data exist that rigorously compare the resolution rate between children treated with antibiotics alone and those treated with antibiotics and drainage. Currently, most cases of renal abscess initially can be managed without intervention, percutaneous drainage being reserved for persistent infection (Fig. 10.29). Children who are immunocompromised through malnutrition or infection with the human immunodeficiency virus are at particular risk for developing recurrent renal abscesses (Brandeis *et al.*, 1995) and abscesses containing unusual organisms (e.g. *Listeria monocytogenes*) (Gomber *et al.*, 1998). In these circumstances, early and more aggressive surgical or percutaneous intervention is often necessary to eradicate the infection.

Antibacterial prophylaxis

Long-term, continuous antibiotic prophylaxis is recommended in children with VUR (particularly under 8 years of age) and those with frequent symptomatic

recurrences. Antibiotic prophylaxis should also be considered in young children (under the age of 1 year) with non-reflux acute pyelonephritis when acute or chronic renal damage is documented by cortical scintigraphy. These children, in particular, appear to have bacterial virulence–host defense factors that place them at significance risk for pyelonephritic damage.

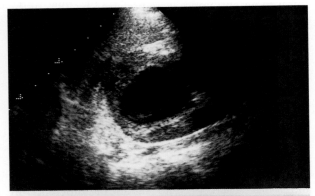

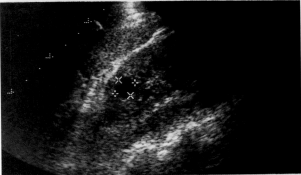

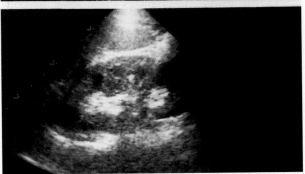

Figure 10.29 Sonogram in a 16–year-old girl who presented with fever and flank pain. (*Top*) Sonolucent mass in the left upper pole consistent with a renal abscess. Needle aspiration under sonographic guidance yielded purulent material that grew E. coli. Following 2 weeks of parenteral and 4 weeks of oral antibiotic therapy, sonograms 7 weeks later (*middle*) and 17 weeks later (*bottom*) show progressive resolution of abscess cavity. (Reprinted from Rushton, 1992, with permission.)

In children with VUR, prophylaxis is usually continued until the reflux spontaneously resolves or is surgically corrected. Some advocate stopping prophylaxis in children older than 7 or 8 years of age who have mild or even moderate (grades I–III) VUR, particularly when there is no evidence of prior renal scarring (Belman, 1995). If infection recurs during that time and reflux persists, correction shoud be considered for those with clinical or DMSA scan-documented pyelonephritis. Regardless of whether reflux is present, girls with a history of recurrent UTIs should be advised of the importance of surveillance urine cultures during pregnancy because they are at increased risk for pyelonephritis. In one review, a group of 41 women who had UTIs in childhood were followed through 65 pregnancies (Martinell *et al.*, 1990). They were compared with age-matched controls. Of those with a history of childhood UTIs, 19 had renal scarring and 22 did not. The incidence of bacteriuria was higher in those with renal scarring (47%) than in those without (27%), but both were significantly greater (p <.001 and <0.01, respectively) than in controls without a history of UTI (2%). This is true regardless of whether or not reflux is present (Gillenwater *et al.*, 1979). Even those who underwent successful surgical correction of reflux during childhood continue to be at increased risk for pyelonephritis during pregnancy (Austenfeld and Snow, 1988; Mansfield *et al.*, 1995; Bukowski *et al.*, 1998).

Children with recurrent pyelonephritis and those with frequent recurrent symptomatic lower UTIs (three in 6 months, four in a year) should also be considered for prophylaxis for a minimum of 6–12 months, even in the absence of VUR. Periodic urine specimens for culture should be obtained every 3–6 months to monitor the success of prophylaxis. Medication should then be reinstituted for an additional 12 months if infection recurs within 3 months of discontinuation. It is not necessary to discontinue treatment to obtain urine specimens for culture. When breakthrough infection occurs, the offending organism will be resistant to the current agent. Therefore, the culture media will not be sterilized by the excreted drugs.

Although prophylaxis effectively prevents infection, it cannot be expected to reduce the recurrence rate of urinary infection after therapy has been discontinued. In one trial using TMP–SMX, all of the children were treated for 2 weeks and then were randomized to receive no treatment or 6 months of prophylaxis (Stansfeld, 1975). Although prophylaxis was highly effective in preventing infection, the rate of recurrent infection after stopping prophylaxis was virtually identical to that observed after 2 weeks of treatment. Similarly, Smellie *et al.* (1976) reported a high recurrence rate (42%) in children with a history of recurrent urinary infections following discontinuation of long-term antimicrobial prophylaxis. In those with cystitis cystica (cystitis follicularis), 80% experience recurrences within 1 year after 6–12 months of continuous prophylaxis (Belman, 1978). Nevertheless, it is helpful to achieve an infection-free period in those children with a history of multiple, symptomatic urinary infections. During this period, aggressive efforts should be made to improve the voiding and bowel habit patterns in those children who have clinical and/or urodynamic evidence of dysfunctional voiding, a common finding in this difficult group of patients.

Antimicrobials with proved efficacy in the prevention of recurrent urinary infections include nitrofurantoin (Smellie *et al.*, 1978), TMP–SMX or TMP–sulfadiazine (Smellie *et al.*, 1976; Hansson *et al.*, 1989b), and TMP alone (Lidin-Janson *et al.*, 1980; Smellie *et al.*, 1982; White, 1987). Brendstrup *et al.* (1990) compared prophylaxis with nitrofurantoin versus trimethoprim alone in a double-blind study in 130 children. Nitrofurantoin demonstrated superior efficacy in those chldren with abnormal urography and/or reflux. However, no differences were seen in children without urinary tract abnormalities. Nitrofurantion did not alter the pattern of resistance of intestinal bacterial flora, while trimethoprim significantly increased the percentage of trimethoprim resistant bacteria during prophylaxis. Side-effects, primarily gastrointesinal, were more frequent in the nitrofurantion group (37%) compared with the trimethoprim group (21%) ($p = 0.05$). The authors recommended nitrofurantoin as the first choice for prophylaxis in children with recurrent UTI and urinary tract abnormalities. Pure SMX is less effective, and synthetic penicillins are particularly poor prophylactic agents because of the frequent emergence of resistant organisms.

Prophylactic doses are generally lower than those used to treat acute infection. Smellie *et al.* (1976, 1978) effectively used SMX, 10 mg, plus TMP, 2 mg/kg per day, or nitrofurantoin, 1–2 mg/kg per day in one or two doses (Smellie *et al.*, 1976; Smellie *et al.*, 1978). The present authors' practice is to administer one-third to one-half of the therapeutic dose once daily. Alternatively, intermittent prophylaxis with low-dose TMP–SMX every other day has also been reported to be effective both in children with VUR and in preadolescent girls with recurrent infection (Harding *et al.*, 1975; Hori *et al.*, 1997). In difficult cases of children who develop breakthrough UTIs on single-drug antimicrobial prophylaxis, double prophylaxis with nitrofurantoin and TMP–SMX has been shown to be effective in reducing recurrences. In one study of 31 girls with recurrent breakthrough infections on single-drug therapy, 68% had VUR, 49% had voiding dysfunction, and 26% had both (Smith and Elder, 1994). When treated with double-drug prophylaxis, the rate of infection was reduced from 17.4 UTIs/100 patient months to 3.6 UTIs/100 patient months ($p < 0.001$). These patients were also treated with anticholinergics and a voiding program.

Treatment in renal failure

The dynamics of antibiotic detoxification and excretion are usually deranged in the child with renal failure. Antibacterial doses need to be adjusted in such patients to avoid adverse reactions. Certain drugs, i.e. those that are dependent on renal function for efficacy, are useless in these patients. The frequency of administration of those drugs that are effective in the face of renal failure, rather than their dosages, should be modified based on the degree of renal insufficiency.

Specific therapy

In addition to appropriate antimicrobial therapy, other factors must be taken into consideration in patient management. Voiding frequency and control of constipation are the two most common variables that are readily modifiable and may be the most important in effecting changes in susceptibility to infection, particularly for children who are infrequent voiders. Establishing a voiding schedule in children may be extremely difficult and may provoke conflict in the parent–child relationship. The physician can interject his or her influence by explaining the treatment goal to the child and requesting that a regular voiding pattern be instituted and maintained. Children should be told that they will be reminded by their parents to void regularly and that they should follow this request even if they do not feel the urge to void at that time. Multialarm wrist watches can be a useful and inexpensive reminder for older school-aged children.

The mainstay of treatment of children with recurrent UTIs and underlying bladder instability involves the long-term use of anticholinergic medicine, primarily oxybutynin (Ditropan). Other anticholinergic and antispasmodic agents include hyoscyamine (Levsinex) and tolterodine (Detrol). Koff and Murtagh (1983) reported that after initial clearing of urinary infection, 31 of 58 (58%) children with recurrent UTIs and uninhibited bladder contractions who were treated with anticholinergics alone maintained sterile urine. The necessity for long-term antibiotic prophylaxis in these patients is then determined by the frequency of subsequent recurrences and/or the presence of VUR. For children older than 6 years, the usual dosage of oxybutynin is 2.5–5 mg, given two or three times daily. A new long-acting formulation, Ditopan XL, is now available which only requires once-daily dosing. The usual dose for hyoscyamine in this age child is one 0.375 mg time cap twice daily. Although not yet approved for children in the US, tolterodine has been used successfully with doses of 1–2 mg twice daily. Reportedly, tolterodine has a more specific action on the bladder and is associated with fewer side-effects. Comparative efficacy among these medications has not been established in children. Timed voidings should always be used in conjunction with anticholinergic therapy.

In more difficult cases of voiding dysfunction with detrusor–sphincter dyssynergia, pelvic floor relaxation biofeedback therapy has been used successfully in the treatment of recurrent UTIs (Sugar and Firlit, 1982). In a recent report, 42 girls with recurrent UTIs and urodynamically confirmed dysfunctional voiding were treated with a multimodal approach involving pelvic floor relaxation biofeedback, a voiding and drinking schedule, anticholinergics in those with bladder instability, and antibiotic prophylaxis (De Paepe *et al.*, 1998). This combined therapeutic approach was effective in preventing recurrent UTIs in 35 (83%).

For constipation, an intensive therapeutic approach is often required. Initially, in severe cases, enemas given for several days may be necessary to disrupt a high fecal impaction and relax an overstretched colon. Increased intake of fiber and fluid and regular toilet habits must then be instituted. In refractory cases, regular use of a fiber-based laxative may be necessary. In most cases, these are long-term requirements, and failure to continue this regimen generally results in recurrence of both constipation and UTI (Yazbeck *et al.*, 1982). A study of 234 constipated and encopretic children found that urinary infection was present in 11%, daytime urinary incontinence in 29%, and nocturnal incontinence in 34% (Loening-Baucke, 1997). During follow-up of at least 12 months after initiation of treament for constipation, recurrent UTIs were effectively prevented in all patients who had no anatomic abnormality of the urinary tract. Daytime urinary incontinence resolved in 89% and nocturnal incontinence resolved in 63% of patients.

Urinary stasis for any other reason needs to be addressed if infection cannot be otherwise controlled with antibiotic prophylaxis. Causes may include severe reflux with secondary poor bladder emptying (megacystis–megaureter syndrome), dilatation in the absence of obstruction, bladder diverticula, or residual ureteral stumps. Since otherwise unexplained urinary infection is so common, it is incumbent upon the physician to document the influence of any of these entities on infection before recommending surgical correction. For example, a specimen for culture may be obtained by needle aspiration of a dilated, non-obstructed upper collecting system to ascertain its involvement prior to surgical revision.

Tuberculosis

The advent of effective antituberculosis agents has made genitourinary tuberculosis an uncommon occurrence in the Western world. In 1984, 21 197 cases were reported in the United States and nearly 2000 people died of the disease (Weinberg and Boyd, 1988). The infection rate in children living in the United States whose parents were born in this country ranges between one and two cases per 10 000 per year. Genitourinary tuberculosis accounts for approximately one-fifth of the cases of extrapulmonary tuberculosis (Weinberg and Boyd, 1988).

Tuberculosis in children occurs most often in lower socioeconomic groups. Case rates are higher in black children and other minorities than in white children. Transmission of tuberculous infection from mother to infant via the placenta or amniotic fluid has been reported in 130 to 200 patients (Smith and Marquis, 1981).

Pathogenesis

Mycobacterium tuberculosis, the tubercle bacillus, is a slow-growing, acid-fast organism that is usually acquired through inhalation of respiratory droplets from an infected person. Renal tuberculosis is always preceded by a focus of infection in some other organ system, usually pulmonary (Cotran *et al.,* 1989). The tubercle bacilli gain access to the kidneys by means of hematogenous dissemination, and therefore renal infection must be considered bilateral in nature.

Pathology

Genitourinary tuberculosis occurs in 4 to 15 per cent of patients with tuberculosis (Cinman, 1982; Cos and Cockett, 1982); it accounts for 73% of the cases of extrapulmonary tuberculosis (García-Rodriguez *et al.,* 1989). Renal tuberculosis is a late and uncommon complication of pulmonary disease, and occurs less than 4–5 years after primary infection. Predisposing conditions, such as malnutrition, diabetes mellitus, and chronic corticosteroid administration, play a significant role in the development of genitourinary tuberculosis. Like all blood-borne renal infections, the tuberculous bacillary emboli are deposited initially in the glomerular and cortical arterioles and cause small tubercles to develop. These tubercles undergo necrosis, with eventual caseation and cavitation of sloughed material into the calyceal walls at the papillary tips. The lesions may extend throughout the renal parenchyma and cause total destruction of the renal pyramids. Rupture of the bacilli into the calyx and collecting system results in extension of disease to other calyces, renal pelvis, ureter, and bladder.

Local progression results in fibrosis causing stenosis at the calyceal neck, infundibulum, ureteropelvic junction, mid-ureter, and ureterovesical junction. Ureteral fibrosis results in straightening and shortening of the ureter and ultimately produces the classic gaping ureteral orifice with vesicoureteral reflux. Alternatively, ureteral stricture may produce hydroureteronephrosis and ultimately a nonfunctioning 'autonephrectomized' kidney (Murphy *et al.,* 1982). Involvement of the bladder by tuberele bacilli causes ulceration and bleeding with destruction of the vesical mucosa.

Tuberculosis of the genital tract is uncommon in both sexes before puberty. In males, involvement of the genital tract usually occurs either hematogenously or through retrograde passage of infected urine through the posterior urethra in the prostatic ducts. Tuberculous epididymitis or epididymo-orchitis can occur in early childhood and may be the initial method of presentation. The fallopian tubes are involved in approximately 90%, the endometrium in 50%, the ovaries in 20–30%, and the cervix in 2–4% of females with genital tuberculosis (Smith and Marquis, 1981).

Symptoms

The majority of young children with genitourinary tuberculosis have no symptoms during the initial infection (Ehrlich and Lattimer, 1971). Due to the lag time between pulmonary infection and the clinical onset of renal tuberculosis, symptoms of frequency, dysuria, hematuria, and pyuria occur late in the course of disease, when the lesions ulcerate through the calyces and renal pelvis, and tubercle bacilli are disseminated to the bladder. Genitourinary tuberculosis must be suspected in children with sterile pyuria, draining sinuses, and those with a history of tuberculosis elsewhere in the body. One child with a tuberculous vesicovaginal fistula and total urinary incontinence has been reported (Singh *et al.*, 1988). With treatment of the tuberculosis, the fistula closed and the incontinence was corrected.

Diagnosis

Microscopic hematuria and pyuria are usually present. Routine urine specimens for culture are often negative; however, 15–20% per cent of patients with tuberculous bacilluria may have coexistent bacterial infection. The diagnosis of genitourinary tuberculosis is suggested by the demonstration of acid-fast bacilli in the stained urinary sediment and is confirmed by culture, usually guinea pig inoculation. Collection of fresh morning urine specimens appears to be just as accurate as 24-hour urinary concentrates in providing the diagnosis (Kenney *et al.*, 1960). The acid-fast tubercle bacilli are discharged intermittently, and therefore at least three separate specimens should be collected for study. Tetracycline and sulfa medications exert mild bacteriostatic effects on tuberculosis cultures, and these drugs should be discontinued before urine collection (Lattimer *et al.*, 1960). Skin tests for tuberculosis (PPD) are usually positive except in cases of overwhelming infection or with human immunodeficiency virus (HIV) infection. The erythrocyte sedimentation rate (ESR) may be increased, and anemia may be seen in advanced disease.

Plain films of the abdomen may reveal punctate calcification overlying the renal parenchyma (Hartman *et al.*, 1977). In approximately 10% of patients with renal tuberculosis, calculi are present. The earliest radiograph-

ic findings on the excretory urogram is minimal calyceal dilatation or erosion of the papillary tip. As the infection proceeds, there is increased destruction of the calyces. With advanced disease, there may be cavitation and cicatricial deformity of the collecting system, progressing to pyonephrosis and nonfunction. Conversely, a normal excretory urogram does not rule out active genitourinary tuberculosis. In patients with hydroureteronephrosis or non-functioning renal units, ureteral catheterization may be helpful for selective urinary collection and retrograde pyelography may be necessary to provide accurate delineation of pyelocalyceal architecture.

Cystoscopic examination reveals only minimal inflammatory changes in the early stages of disease. With coalescence of the tubereles, there may be areas of white or yellow raised nodules with a halo of hyperemia. With advanced localized disease, bladder capacity may become markedly diminished, with fixed and incompetent ureteral orifices, mucosal ulceration, and diffuse cystitis.

Treatment

The advent of short-course chemotherapy has changed the surgical management of genitourinary tuberculosis (Gow, 1986). The current recommendation is for surgery to restore function or to remove irreparable disease. Surgery can be performed 6 weeks after the start of chemotherapy.

Antituberculosis drugs inhibit multiplication of tubercle bacilli and arrest the course of disease progression. Various antituberculosis agents are currently available (American Academy of Pediatrics, 1988; Glassroth *et al.*, 1980; Smith and Marquis, 1981). The efficacy of combination chemotherapy compared with single-drug administration has been well documented and treatment with orally administered agents is as effective as parenteral drug administration.

Isoniazid

The dosage of isoniazid (INH) is 10–20 mg/kg of body weight per day, up to 300 mg daily, given in one dose. The drug is the most effective of the antituberculosis agents available and remains the keystone of all therapeutic regimens. Isoniazid is metabolized in the liver and is excreted primarily through the kidney. It is available in liquid form (50 mg/5 ml) and in tablets, which may be dissolved in fruit juice or water; this makes drug administration easier in infants and young children. Peripheral neuritis is the most common side effect and is probably caused by inhibition of pyridoxine metabolism. Neurotoxic side effects have not been reported in children younger than 11 years of age, and thus pyridoxine supplementation is not recommended unless nutrition is inadequate. Hepatotoxicity, which is seen often in older patients, rarely occurs in children.

Rifampin

The dosage of rifampin is 10–20 mg/kg/day, up to 600 mg daily. Rifampin is extremely effective and virtually nontoxic for administration in children. Rare cases of minor hepatic and renal dysfunction and thrombocytopenia have been reported. This drug is indicated for the initial treatment of genitourinary tuberculosis and for cases requiring re-treatment. Rifampin is excreted in the bile and urine and may cause orange discolouration of urine, tears, and sweat. In older females taking rifampin, contraceptive drugs should be avoided because rifampin changes the kinetics of the estrogen component.

Ethambutol

The dosage of ethambutol is 15–20 mg/ kg/day, up to 2500 mg daily, divided into two to three doses. This is an extremely effective antituberculosis drug, which has replaced *p*-aminosalicylic acid for use in most adults. It is rapidly absorbed and excreted in the urine. Optic neuritis is a major toxic effect of ethambutol, and monthly visual examinations are required. This drug is not recommended for use in small children who are not able to cooperate in examination of visual acuity and color vision.

Streptomycin

The dosage of streptomycin is 20–40 mg/kg/day given intramuscularly, up to 1000 mg daily. Although streptomycin is still a useful drug for the treatment of genitourinary tuberculosis, the risk of eighth nerve damage prohibits use of this medication for longer than 12 weeks.

p-Aminosalicylic acid (PAS)

The dosage of PAS is 200 mg/kg/day, up to 10 g daily. PAS is an effective bactericidal drug for the treatment of renal tuberculosis when used in combination with other antituberculosis medications. However, PAS is not effective when used alone. Major side effects are gastrointestinal problems, including nausea, vomiting, diarrhea, and anorexia. It is best to give PAS after meals and in the form of sodium and potassium PAS to decrease gastrointestinal irritability.

Pyrazinamide

The dosage of pyrazinamide is 30 mg/kg/day, up to 2 g/day. The drug is bactericidal, seldom hepatotoxic, and well tolerated by children.

Ethionamide

The dosage of ethionamide is 15–20 mg/kg/day, up to a maximum of 1 g/day. The drug is well tolerated by children, is bacteriostatic, and occasionally is useful for drug-resistant cases. A physician experienced with this drug should be consulted prior to its use.

Other drugs

Cycloserine, kanamycin, and capreomycin may be useful in treating drug-resistant cases of genitourinary tuberculosis.

Specitic therapy for genitourinary tuberculosis

The accepted treatment for genitourinary tuberculosis is triple-drug chemotherapy administered daily for 2 years (Wechsler and Lattimer, 1975). Short-course chemotherapy (6-month treatment regimen) has been advocated in an attempt to (1) increase patient compliance, (2) decrease the cost of medication, (3) lower drug toxicity, and (4) produce an equally successful regimen comparable with the standard therapy (Fox, 1979; Gow, 1986). Short-course chemotherapy must include rifampin as one of the drugs (Weinberg and Boyd, 1988).

The recommendation of the American Academy of Pediatrics for treatment of genitourinary tuberculosis is 9 months of INH and rifampin. In the first 2 months of therapy, a third drug should be added. This may include pyrazinamide, streptomycin, or ethambutol in children older than 5 years of age. If the infection is associated with HIV infection, treatment should include three drugs and may need to be longer than 9 months (American Academy of Pediatrics, 1988).

The majority of relapses occur within the first 2 years. Females in the childbearing years should avoid pregnancy until therapy is completed (Gow and Barbosa, 1984). Women who are delivered of a baby while they have genitourinary tuberculosis may infect the infant with tuberculosis (Schaaf *et al.*, 1989).

With the rapid bactericidal activity of drugs like rifampin, recent recommendations call for 1-year follow-up unless calcification is seen on abdominal radiographs (Weinberg and Boyd, 1988). If calcification is present, long-term follow-up is required to be sure that the disease does not progress. During the follow-up period, urinalysis is performed every 2 months. The upper urinary tracts should be monitored prior to, during, and after treatment to assess for obstruction because strictures are common.

Surgical therapy in patients with genitourinary tuberculosis is essentially of historical significance (Flechner and Gow, 1980; Wong and Lau, 1980). The results of chemotherapy are so impressive that surgical intervention is limited to exceptional cases, such as ureteral stricture (Murphy *et al.*, 1982), ureterovesical junction reconstruction, or augmentation cytoplasty in children with small contracted bladders (Zinman and Libertino, 1980).

Xanthogranulomatous pyelonephritis

Xanthogranulomatous pyelonephritis is an atypical form of severe chronic renal parenchymal infection characterized by unilateral destruction of parenchyma and accumulation of lipid-laden macrophages (xanthoma cells) either surrounding abscess cavities or as discrete yellow nodules. More than 50 cases of xanthogranulomatous pyelonephritis have been reported in children (Watson *et al.*, 1982; Yazaki *et al.*, 1982; Goodman *et al.*, 1998). The age of presentation has ranged from infancy to 16 years. Most patients present with non-specific symptoms of chronic infection, including weight loss, recurrent fever, failure to thrive, pallor, and lethargy (Watson *et al.*, 1982), although those with the focal form often appear healthy (Yazaki *et al.*, 1982). A palpable abdominal mass is present in approximately one-third of cases. Bacterial specimens for culture can be obtained from the urine or renal abscess in the majority of cases, with *Proteus* being the most common organism isolated.

Both diffuse and focal forms of the disease have been reported, with the focal form being more common in children than in adults (Schulman and Denis, 1977; Watson *et al.*, 1982). The pathologic and radiologic differences between focal and diffuse xanthogranulomatous pyelonephritis have been described (Bagley *et al.*, 1977). Radiologic evaluation in the diffuse form of the disease often reveals non-function of the entire kidney. Calcification or stones may be present, although this is less common in the focal form of the disease. Characteristic sonographic or CT appearances of xanthogranulomatous pyelonephritis also have been reported (Subramanyam *et al.*, 1982). However, these features are non-specific and often mimic neoplasia or other forms of chronic inflammatory renal parenchymal disease. Consequently, the correct diagnosis is seldom made preoperatively (Malek and Elder, 1978). Nephrectomy is curative, although partial nephrectomy may be adequate in focal disease, assuming that the diagnosis can be established. No incidence of recurrence in the contralateral kidney has been reported.

Appendix: antibacterial agents

Sulfonamides

Sulfonamides act by competitively blocking the conversion of para-aminobenzoic acid to dihydrofolic acid (Feingold, 1963). About 75% of the oral dose is absorbed. Free sulfonamide is excreted into urine by filtration and tubular secretion. Although high tissue levels are not achieved, excellent urine levels result. Sulfonamides are most effective against *E. coli* but may also be effective against other Gram-negative and Gram-positive organisms.

Sulfonamides are well tolerated by children, are inexpensive, and produce few side-effects. They affect the gastrointestinal flora when used for long-term prophylaxis but are effective agents for short-term acute therapy of uncomplicated infections. They displace protein-bound bilirubin and hence in the neonate have the potential to interfere with bilirubin excretion and cause jaundice. Once the infant has passed through the period of physiologic jaundice, these agents can be used safely. Some patients are allergic to sulfa, but fortunately most reactions are of a minor cutaneous nature, such as urticaria. There have been some problems with major hypersensitivity reactions, such as the Stevens–Johnson syndrome, but these are rare. The most widely used agent is sulfisoxazole employed in a dose of 120–150 mg/kg of body weight per day, given acutely in four to six divided doses orally (Behrman and Vaughan, 1987).

Trimethoprim–sulfamethoxazole

The trimethoprim–sulfamethoxazole (TMP–SMX) combination is useful both in the management of simple cystitis and for long-term antibacterial prophylaxis. This combination has a diminished effect on bowel flora and offers the advantage of trimethoprim entering vaginal secretions in the adult female (Stamey *et al.*, 1977). This latter characteristic appears to be of particular utility in its effectiveness as a prophylactic agent. Trimethoprim has also been shown *in vitro* to induce phase variation of fimbriated *E. coli* to a non-fimbriated state (Vaisanen *et al.*, 1982). This and the high concentration in vaginal secretions work to prevent vaginal and periurethral colonization with organisms that could potentially cause urinary tract infection. Trimethoprim interferes with dihydrofolic acid reductase, and sulfa blocks the conversion of para-aminobenzoic acid to dihydrofolic acid. The combination is effective against many Gram-negative as well as Gram-positive organisms. It is well absorbed, attains high levels in both serum and urine, and is well tolerated by children. Neutropenia and thrombocytopenia are not uncommon with its use. However, the clinical significance of these changes is unknown (Asmar *et al.*, 1981).

The combination is available as a suspension containing 40 mg of trimethoprim and 200 mg of sulfamethoxazole per 5 ml. The dose employed in children over 2 months of age is TMP 6–12 mg and SMX 30–60 mg/kg per day, in two divided doses (Behrman and Vaughan, 1987).

Nitrofurantoin

Nitrofurantoin is quite useful in the treatment of simple cystitis and is also a very effective agent for long-term, low-dose prophylaxis. It is thought to interfere with early stages of the bacterial Krebs cycle (AMA, 1971). It is well absorbed from the gastrointestinal tract and has minimal effect on bowel flora. Tissue levels are low because it is excreted almost entirely in the urine by glomerular filtration. Urinary levels tend to be quite high. Urinary alkalinization increases urine levels, whereas acidification increases tissue levels. It works well against most *E. coli* and enterococci but is not particularly effective against *Klebsiella*, *Proteus*, or *Pseudomonas*.

Nausea and vomiting are frequent troublesome side-effects in children; however, these can be minimized by administering the agent immediately after a meal or by using nitrofurantoin macrocrystals sup-plied in capsule form. For the small child, the contents of the capsule can be emptied and administered in mashed potatoes, apple sauce, pudding or yogurt.

In neonates nitrofurantoin has the potential to cause a hemolytic anemia because of glutathione instability. Consequently, it should not be used in this age group. In addition, the drug is ineffective in patients with significant renal impairment. Other side-effects are rare but include peripheral neuropathy and pulmonary infiltrates. The usual dose in children older than 3 months of age is 5–7 mg/kg per day given orally with food in three or four divided doses (Behrman and Vaughan, 1987).

Nalidixic acid

Nalidixic acid is an antibacterial agent that produces high urinary levels and is effective against Gram-negative organims. It is especially effective against *Proteus*. Previous negative reports regarding the effectiveness of this agent can probably be accounted for by inadequate dosage (Stamey and Bragonzi, 1976). Nalidixic acid is readily absorbed from the gastrointestinal tract and is well tolerated by children. It is rapidly inactivated by the liver. It is thought to interfere with DNA synthesis. The development of pseudotumor cerebri has been reported as a complication of its use in children (Anderson *et al.*). Nalidixic acid is available in both tablet and suspension form. The recommended dose is 55 mg/kg per day in four divided doses (Behrman and Vaughan, 1987).

Methenamine mandelate and methenamine hippurate

These agents are readily absorbed from the intestinal tract and remain inactive until they are excreted by the kidney and concentrated in the urine. Methenamine in an acid urine is converted to the bactericidal agent formaldehyde; however, this conversion takes a minimum of 2 hours to achieve adequate bactericidal levels. Mandelic and hippuric acids are urinary acidifiers that have some additional inherent but weak antibacterial agent. The efficacy of methenamine may be enhanced further by supplementary urinary acidification, such as with ascorbic acid. Both can cause dysuria when administered in high doses, and methenamine mandelate has on rare occasions produced hemorrhagic cystitis (Ross and Conway, 1970). The recommended dose for these agents initially is 100 mg/kg per day given orally in four divided doses, followed by 50 mg/kg per day in four divided doses (Behrman and Vaughan, 1987).

Penicillin

The penicillins as a class are probably the most widely used antibiotics. All act by blocking mucopeptide synthesis in the cell walls so that the bacterium is unprotected from its high internal osmotic pressure. This effect occurs only in growing cells.

- *Penicillin G*: extremely high urine levels can be achieved with penicillin G in patients with normal renal function, and under those circumstances this drug may be very effective against both *E. coli* and *Proteus*. Its major toxic effect is allergy manifested by rash or anaphylaxis.
- *Ampicillin* is the most widely used penicillin in the treatment of UTI. It is not well absorbed from the gastrointestinal tract; therefore, high fecal levels occur and diarrhea is common. High serum and urine concentrations are achievable. This agent should not be administered to patients with a known history of penicillin allergy. The usual dose is 50–100 mg/kg per day given every 6 hours. It can be administered either orally or intravenously (Behrman and Vaughan, 1987).
- *Amoxicillin* is a derivative of ampicillin that is absorbed more readily and therefore produces less diarrhea. It is administered orally in a dose of 20–40 mg/kg per day every 6–8 hours (Behrman and Vaughan, 1987).
- *Carbenicillin* is an agent that may be useful in the treatment of *Pseudomonas* and indole-positive *Proteus*; however, its usefulness is often diminished by the emergence of resistant strains. It is available as tablets and as a parenteral solution. When it is used parenterally for urinary tract infection in children, the usual dose is 50–200 mg/kg per day given every 4 hours; for severe infections, the dose can be increased to 400–500 mg/kg per day (Kunin, 1987). The oral form is not predictably effective in children.
- *Ticarcillin* is available for parenteral therapy only. Like carbenicillin, it is active against *Pseudomonas* and indole-positive *Proteus*, which may be resistant to other drugs. It is often used with an aminoglycoside for a synergistic effect. This combination may also delay the emergence of resistant strains. Sodium overload is less likely to occur with ticarcillin than with carbenicillin. The usual dose in children for treatment of urinary tract infection is 50–100 mg/kg per day given every 4–6 hours. In life-threatening infections, the dose can be increased to 200–300 mg/kg per day (Kunin, 1987).
- *Piperacillin* has essentially the same antimicrobial spectrum as carbenicillin and ticarcillin, but is more effective on a weight basis. Piperacillin may have some advantage in allowing lower doses and therefore less sodium load compared with carbenicillin and ticarcillin. The dosage in children is 50 mg/kg per day given every 4–6 hours (Kunin, 1987).

Cephalosporins

Cephalosporins are usually effective against most of the Gram-negative and many of the Gram-positive pathogens. Excretion is by both glomerular filtration and tubular secretion. Although there can be some cross-reactivity in patients who are allergic to penicillin, in general these agents can be cautiously administered to patients with penicillin allergy.

Oral drugs

Oral cephalexin, a first-generation cephalosporin, is well absorbed from the gastrointestinal tract and can be given in a dose of 25–50 mg/kg per day every 6 hours (Behrman and Vaughan, 1987). Cefaclor, a second-generation oral cephalosporin, is somewhat more active against gram-negative bacteria but is more expensive than cephalexin. The dosage is 20–40 mg/kg per day given every 8 hours (Behrman and Vaughan, 1987). Other oral cephalosporins include cephradine (first generation) and cefadroxil (second generation). A newer, third-generation cephalosporin for oral administration, cefixime, is also available. In addition to broader coverage of Gram-negative organisms, an advantage of cefixime is a prolonged half-life, allowing for once or twice daily dosage. The recommended dose for children is 8 mg/kg per day in one or two divided doses (Drug Newsletter, 1989).

Parenteral drugs

Numerous cephalosporins are available for parenteral use. The first-generation cephalosporins (cephalothin, cefazolin, cepharadine, cephapirin) are useful agents for urinary infections caused by most strains of *E. coli*, *Klebsiella*, and *Proteus*, but not *Pseudomonas*. As with all cephalosporins, they are inactive against enterococci. The second-generation parenteral cephalosporins (cefamandole, cefoxitin) are more active than the first-generation agents against many enteric Gram-negative bacteria, but not *Pseudomonas*. Cefoxitin is the most active cephalosporin against anaerobes, including *Bacteroides fragilis*. A number of new third-generation cephalosporins (cefoperazone, cefotaxime, ceftazidime, ceftriaxone) have been developed because of their relatively greater activity against Gram-negative bacteria. Although most retain some activity against Gram-positive bacteria, they are much less active than first-generation cephalosporins for staphylococci or other Gram-positive bacteria. Ceftriaxone has a longer half-life, allowing for once or twice daily dosage. It is also more active than cefoperazone against most Gram-negative bacteria.

Other cephalosporins

There are so many new cephalosporins that it is difficult to choose among them. It is recommended that the physician become familiar with the use of one oral and one parenteral drug in each generation. Dosage in children varies with each cephalosporin.

Aminoglycosides

The aminoglycosides are well tolerated by children and are of special utility in the treatment of complicated Gram-negative UTI. They interfere with protein synthesis by binding proteins of the bacterial ribosomes.

- *Gentamicin* is probably the most widely used of the aminoglycosides in children and is especially effective against *Pseudomonas*. The usual pediatric dose is 5–7.5 mg/kg per day parenterally in two divided doses, depending on age (Behrman and Vaughan, 1987). It achieves high tissue concentration and can be ototoxic, particularly to the vestibular cells. Nephrotoxicity also occurs in a small percentage of patients and should be monitored for by checking serum creatinine periodically during the course of therapy. Nephrotoxicity occurs particularly frequently when gentamicin is given in combination with cephalosporins. Both ototoxicity and nephrotoxicity are usually transient.
- *Tobramycin* has the advantage of particular efficacy against *Pseudomonas*. It is said to be less nephrotoxic than gentamicin (Kurnin, 1980). The dosage

is 4–7.5 mg/kg per day given every 8–12 hours, depending on age (Behrman and Vaughan, 1987).
- *Amikacin*: this newer aminoglycoside was developed to improve activity against emerging resistant strains of *Pseudomonas*. As with other aminoglycosides, it is potentially both nephrotoxic and ototoxic. The dosage is 15–22.5 mg/kg per day given every 8–12 hours, depending on age (Behrman and Vaughan, 1987).

Tetracyclines

Tetracyclines should not be used in children under 8 years of age because they stain the permanent teeth. The need for tetracycline is extremely unusual in modern-day pediatrics.

References

AAP Committee on Quality Improvement (1999) Practice parameter: the diagnosis, treatment and evaluation of the initial urinary tract infection in febrile infants and children. *Pediatrics* **103**: 843–52.

Abbott GD (1972) Neonatal bacteriuria: a prospective study in 1,460 infants. *BMJ* **i**: 267–9.

Agace W, Hedges S, Ceska M *et al*. (1993) IL-8 and the neutrophil response to mucosal Gram negative infection. *J Clin Invest* **92**: 780–5.

Al Roomi LG, Sutton AM, Cockburn F, McAllister TA (1984) Amoxycillin and clavulanic acid in the treatment of urinary infection. *Arch Dis Child* **59**: 256–9.

Albarus MH, Salzano FM, Goldraich NP (1997) Genetic markers and acute febrile urinary tract infection in the first year of life. *Pediatr Nephrol* **11**: 691–4.

Allen TD (1977) The non-neurogenic bladder. *J Urol* **117**: 232.

Alon US, Ganapathy S (1999) Should renal ultrasonography be done routinely in chldren with first urinary tract infection? *Clin Pediatr* **38**: 21–5.

American Academy of Pediatrics (1988) *Report of the Committee on Infectious Diseases*, 21st ed. Elk Grove Village, IL, American Academy of Pediatrics.

American Medical Association (1971) *AMA drug evaluations*. Chicago, IL: AMA.

Anderson P, Engberg I, Lidin-Janson G *et al*. (1991) Persistence of *Escherichia coli* bacteriuria is not determined by bacterial adherence. *Infect Immun* **59**: 2915–21.

Anderson PAM, Rickwood AMK (1991) Features of primary vesicoureteric reflux detected by prenatal sonography. *Br J Urol* **67**: 267.

Androulakakis PA, Ransley PG, Risdon RA *et al*. (1987) Microvascular changes in the early stage of reflux pyelonephritis: an experimental stusy in the pig kidney. *Eur Urol* **13**: 219.

Arnold AJ, Brownless SM, Carty HM, Rickwood AM (1990) Detection of renal scarring by DMSA scanning – an experimental study. *J Pediatr Surg* **25**: 391–3.

Arthur M, Johnson CE, Rubin RH *et al.* (1989) Molecular epidemiology of adhesin and hemolysin virulence factors amon uropathogenic *Escherichia coli*. *Infect Immun* **57**: 303.

Askari A, Belman AB (1982) Vesicoureteral reflux in black girls. *J Urol* **127**: 747–8.

Asmar BI, Maqbool S, Dajani AS (1981) Hematologic abnormalities after oral trimethoprim–sulfamethoxazole therapy in children. *Am J Dis Child* **135**: 1100–3.

Austenfeld MS, Snow BW (1988) Complications of pregnancy after reimplantation for vesicoureteral reflux. *J Urol* **140**: 1103.

Avner ED, Ingelfinger JR, Herrin JT *et al.* (1983) Single-dose amoxicillin therapy of uncomplicated pediatric urinary tract infections. *J Pediatr* **102**: 623–7.

Bagley FH, Stewart AM, Jones PF (1977) Diffuse xanthogranulomatous pyelonephritis in children: an unrecognized variant. *J Urol* **118**: 434.

Bailey RR (1973) The relationship of vesico-ureteric reflux to urinary tract infection and chronic pyelonephritis-reflux nephropathy. *Clin Nephrol* **1**: 132.

Bailey RR, Lynn KL, McRae CU (1984) Unilateral reflux nephropathy and hypertension. *Contrib Nephrol* **39**: 116.

Bailey RR, McRae CU, Maling TMJ *et al.* (1978) Renal vein renin concentration in the hypertension of unilateral reflux nephropathy. *J Urol* **120**: 21.

Ball P (1986) Ciprofloxacin: an overview of adverse experiences. *J Antimicrob Chemother* **18** (Suppl D): 187.

Barry HC, Ebell MH, Hickner J (1997) Evaluation of suspected urinary tract infection in ambulatory women: a cost–utility analysis of office-based strategies. *J Family Pract* **44**: 49–60.

Bartkova G, Ciznar I, Lehotska V *et al.* (1994) Characterization of adhesion associated surface properties of uropathogenic *Escherichia coli*. *Folia Microbiol* **39**: 373.

Beetz R, Schulte-Wissermann H, Trojger J *et al.* (1989) Long-term follow-up of children wiht surgically treated vesciorenal reflux: postoperative incidence of urinary tract infections, renal scars and arterial hypertension. *Eur Urol* **16**: 366–71.

Behrman RF, Vaughan VCI (1987) *Nelson Textbook of pediatrics*. 13th edition. Philadelphia, PA: WB Saunders Co.

Bellinger MF, Duckett JW (1984) Vesicoureteral reflux: a comparison of non-surgical and surgical management. In: *Contributions to Nephrology. Reflux Nephropathy Update 1983* Volume 39.

Belman AB (1978) Clinical significance of cystitis cystica in girls: results of a retrospective study. *J Urol* **127**: 7474.

Belman AB (1995) A perspective on vesicoureteral reflux. *Urol Clin N Am* **22**: 139–50.

Belman AB, Kaplan GW (1981) *Genitourinary problems in pediatrics*. Philadelphia, PA: WB Saunders Co.

Ben-Ami T, Rozin M, Hertz M (1989) Imaging of children with urinary tract infection: a tailored approach. *Clin Radiol* **40**: 64.

Benador D, Benador N, Slosman DO *et al.* (1994) Cortical scintigraphy in the evaluation of renal parenchymal changes in children with pyelonephritis. *J Pediatr* **124**: 17–20.

Bergstrom T, Larson H, Lincoln K, Winberg J (1972) Studies of urinary tract infections in infancy and childhood. XII. Eighty consecutive patients with neonatal infection. *J Pediatr* **80**: 858–66.

Bergstrom T, Lincoln K, Orskov F *et al.* (1967) Studies of urinary tract infections in infancy and children. VIII Reinfection vs relapse in recurrent urinary tract infections: evaluation by means of identification of infecting organisms. *J Pediatr* **72**: 13.

Bhathena DB, Weiss JH, Holland NH *et al.* (1980) Focal and segmental glomerulosclerosis in reflux nephropathy (chronic pyelonephritis). *Am J Med* **68**: 886.

Bisset GS III, Strife JL, Dunbar JS (1987) Urography and voiding cystourethrography: findings in girls with urinary tract infection. *AJR Am J Roentgenol* **148**: 479–82.

Bjorgvinsson E, Majd M, Eggli DK (1991) Diagnosis of acute pyelonephritis in children: comparison of sonography and 99m-Tc DMSA scintigraphy. *AJR Am J Roentgenol* **157**: 539.

Blanco M, Blanco JE, Alonso MP, Blanco J (1994) Virulence factors and O groups of *Escherichia coli* strains isolated from cultures of blood specimens from urosepsis and non urosepsis patients. *Microbiologia* **10**: 249.

Blanco M, Blanco JE, Alonso MP, Blanco J (1996) Virulence factors and O groups of *Escherichia coli* isolates from patients with acute pyelonephritis, cystitis, and asymptomatic bacteriuria. *Eur J Epidemiol* **12**: 191.

Blickman JG, Taylor GA, Lebowitz RL (1985) Voiding cystourethrography: the initial radiologic study in children with urinary tract infection. *Radiology* **156**: 659–62.

Bolann BJ, Sandberg S, Digranes A (1989) Implications of probability anaylisis for interpreting results of leukocyte esterase and nitrite test strips. *Clin Chem* **35**: 1663.

Bollgren I, Winburg J (1976a) The periurethral aerobic bacterial flora in girls highly susceptible to urinary infections. *Acta Paediatr Scand* **65**: 81.

Bollgren I, Winburg J (1976b) The periurethral aerobic bacterial flora in healthy boys and girls. *Acta Paediatr Scand* **65**: 74.

Bouissou H, Caujolle DCF *et al.* (1978) Tissus cartilagineux et acide nalidixique. *C R Acad Sci (Paris)* **23**: 1743.

Brandeis JM, Baskin LS, Kogan BA *et al.* (1995) Recurrent *Staphylococcus aureus* renal abscess in a child positive for the human immunodeficiency virus. *Urology* **46**: 246–8.

Brendstrup L, Hjelt K, Perertsen KE *et al.* (1990) Nitrofurantoin versus trimethoprim prophylaxis in recurrent urinary tract infection in childhood. A randomized, double-blind study. *Acta Paediatr Scand* **79**: 1225–34.

Brook I (1981) Anaerobes as a cause of urinary tract infection in children [Letter]. *Lancet* **i**: 835.

Brumfitt W, Gargan RA, Hamilton-Miller JM (1987) Periurethral enterobacterial carriage preceding urinary infection [published erratum appears in *Lancet* 1987; **i**: 994]. *Lancet* **i**: 824–6.

Bukowski TP, Betrus GG, Aquilina JW, Perlmutter AD (1998) Urinary tract infections and pregnancy in women who underwent antireflux surgery in childhood. *J Urol* **159**: 1286–9.

Burge DM, Griffiths MD, Malone PS, Atwell JD (1992) Fetal vesicoureteral reflux: outcome following conservative postnatal management. *J Urol* **148**: 1743–5.

Busch R, Huland H (1984) Correlation of symptoms and results of direct bacterial localization in patients with urinary tract infections. *J Urol* **132**: 282–5.

Carbonetti NH, Boonchai S, Paary SH *et al.* (1986) Aerobactin-mediated iron uptake by *Escherichi coli* isolates from human extraintestinal infections. *Infect Immun* **51**: 966.

Cardiff–Oxford Bacteriruia Study Group (1978) Sequelae of covert bacteriuria in school children. *Lancet* **i**: 889.

Chan RCY, Bruce AW, Reid G (1984) Adherence of cervical, vaginal and distal urethral normal microbial flora to human uroepithelial cells and inhibition of adherence of gram-negative uropathogens by competetive exclusion. *J Urol* **131**: 596.

Chan RCY, Reid G, Irvin RT *et al.* (1985) Competetive exclusion of uropathogens from human uroepithelial cells by *Lactobacillus* whole cells and cell wall fragments. *Infect Immun* **47**: 84.

Chick S, Harver MJ, MacKenzie R *et al.* (1981) Modified method for for studying bacterial adhesion to isolated uroepithelial cells and uromucoid. *Infect Immun* **34**: 256.

Cinman AC (1982) Genitourinary tuberculosis. *Urology* **20**: 353.

Clark H, Ronal AR, Turck M (1971) Serum antibody response in renal versus bladder bacteria. *J Infect Dis* **123**: 539.

Cleveland RH, Constantinou C, Blickman J *et al.* (1991) Voiding cysoturethrography in children: value of digital fluoroscopy in reducing radiation dose. *Am J Radiol* **158**: 137.

Cohen RA, Rushton HG, Belman AB *et al.* (1990) Renal scarring and vesicoureteral reflux in children with myelodysplasia. *J Urol* **144**: 541–54.

Connell I, Agace W, Klenem P *et al.* (1996) Type-1 fimbrial expression enhances *E. coli* virulence for the urinary tract. *Proc Natl Acad Sci USA* **93**: 9827.

Conway JJ, King LR, Belman AB (1972) Detection of vesicoureteral reflux with radionuclide: a comparison study with roentgenographic cystography. *AJR Am J Roentgenol* **115**: 720.

Coppa GV, Gabrielli O, Giorgi P *et al.* (1990) Preliminary study of breastfeeding and bacterial adhesion to uroepithelial cells. *Lancet* **335**: 569–71.

Corman LI, Forsage WS, Kotchmar GS (1982) Simplified urinary microscopy to detect significant bacteriuria. *Pediatrics* **70**: 133.

Cornu C, Cochat P, Collet J-P *et al.* (1994) Survey of the attitudes to management of acute pyelonephritis in children. *Pediatr Nephrol* **8**: 275.

Cos LR and Cockett ATK (1982) Genitourinary tuberculosis revisited. *Urology* **20**: 111.

Cotran RS, Kumar V and Robbins SL (1989) *Robbins Pathologic Basis of Disease*, 4th ed. Philadelphia, WB Saunders Co, 1989, pp 374–80.

Cox CE, Hinman F (1961) Experiments with induced bacteriuria, vesical emptying, and bacterial growth on the mechanisms of bladder defense to infection. *J Urol* **86**: 739.

Crabbe DC, Thomas DF, Gordon AC *et al.* (1992) Use of ^{99m}technetium-dimercaptosuccinic acid to study patterns of renal damage associated with prenatally detected vesicoureteral reflux. *J Urol* **148**: 1229–31.

Craig JC, Irwig LM, Knight JF *et al.* (1998) Symptomatic urinary tract infection in preschool Australian children. *J Paediatr Child Health* **34**: 154–9.

Craig JC, Knight JF, Sureshkumar P *et al.* (1997) Vesicoureteric reflux and timing of micturating cystourethrography after urinary tract infection. *Arch Dis Child* **76**: 275–7.

Crain EF, Gershel JC (1990) Urinary tract infections in febrile infants younger than 8 weeks of age. *Pediatrics* **86**: 363–7.

Dagan R, Einhorn M, Lang R *et al.* (1992) Once daily cefixime compared with twice daily trimethoprim–sulfamethoxazole for urinary tract infection in infants and children. *Pediatr Infect Dis J* **11**: 198–203.

Daigle F, Harel J, Fairbrother JM *et al.* (1994) Expression and detection of pap-, sfa-, and afa-encoded fimbrial adhesin systems among uropathogenic *Escherichia coli*. *Can J Microbiol* **40**: 286.

Dakin HD (1915) On the use of certain antiseptic substances in the treatment of infected wounds. *BMJ* **ii**: 318–20.

De Paepe H, Hoebeke P, Renson C *et al.* (1998) Pelvic-floor therapy in girls with recurrent urinary tract infections and dysfunctional voiding. *Br J Urol* **81** (Suppl 3): 109–13.

De Sadeleer C, DeBoe V, Keuppens F *et al.* (1994) How good is technetium-99m mercaptoacetyltryglycine indirect cystography? *Eur J Nucl Med* **21**: 223–27.

Diamond DA, Kleinman PK, Spevak *et al.* (1996) The tailored low-dose fluoroscopic voiding cystogram for familial reflux screening. *J Urol* **155**: 681–2.

Dick PT, Feldman W (1996) Routine diagnostic imaging for childhood urinary tract infections: a systematic overview. *J Pediatr* **128**: 15–22.

Disney APS (1991) Reflux nephropathy in Australia and New Zealand: prevalence, incidence and management – 1975–1989. *Second CJ Hodson Symposium on Reflux Nephropathy*. Christ Church, New Zealand: Design Printing Services, 53–9.

Ditchfield MR, De Campo JF, Cook DJ *et al.* (1994) Vesicoureteral reflux: an accurate predictor of acute pyelonephritis in childhood urinary tract infection? *Radiology* **190**: 413–15.

Drew JH, Acton CM (1976) Radiological findings in newborn infants with urinary infection. *Arch Dis Child* **51**.

Drug Newsletter (1989) *Facts and Comparisons* Div. 8:56 edition. St Louis, MO: JB Lippincott Co.

Edwards D, Normand IC, Prescod N *et al.* (1977) Disappearance of vesicoureteric reflux during long-term prophylaxis of urinary tract infection in children. *BMJ* **2**: 285–8.

Ehrlich RM, Lattimer JK (1971) Urogenital tuberculosis in children. *J Urol* **105**: 461.

Eichenwald HF (1986) Some aspects of the diagnosis and management of urinary tract infection in children and adolscents. *Pediatr Infect Dis J* **5**: 760.

Elison BS, Taylor D, Van Der Wall H *et al.* (1992) Comparison of DMSA scintigraphy with intravenous urography for the detection of renal scarring and its correlation with vesicoureteral reflux. *J Urol* **69**: 294.

Fairley KF, Carson NE, Gutch RC *et al.* (1971) Site of infection in acute urinary-tract infection in general practice. *Lancet* **ii**: 615–18.

Farnsworth RH, Rossleigh MA, Leighton DM *et al.* (1991) The detection of reflux nephropathy in infants by ^{99m}technetium dimercaptosuccinic acid studies. *J Urol* **145**: 542–6.

Feingold DS (1963) Antimicrobial chemotherapeutic agents: the nature of their action in selected toxicity. *N Engl J Med* **269**: 900.

Fennell RS, Wilson SG, Garin EH *et al.* (1977) Bacteriuria in families of girls with recurrent bacteriuria. *Clin Pediatr* **16**: 1132.

Filly R, Friedland GW, Govan DE, Fair WR (1974) Development and progression of clubbing and scarring in children with recurrent urinary tract infections. *Radiology* **113**: 145–53.

Flechner SM and Gow JG (1980) Role of nephrectomy in the treatment of non-functioning or very poorly functioning unilateral tubercutous kidney. *J Urol* **123**: 822.

Fleidner M, Mehls O, Rauterberg EW *et al.* (1986) Urinary SIgA in children with urinary tract infection. *J Pediatr* **109**: 416.

Fox W (1979) The chemotherapy of pulmonary tuberculosis: a review. *Chest* **76**: 785.

Fussell EN, Kaack MB, Cherry R *et al.* (1977) Bacteriuria in families of girls with recurrent bacteriuria. *Clin Pediatr* **16**: 1132.

Fussell EN, Kaack MB, Cherry R, Roberts JA (1988) Adherence of bacteria to human foreskins. *J Urol* **140**: 997–1001.

García-Rodriguez IA, García Sanchez IE, Gómez-García AC, *et al.* (1989) Extrapulmonary tuberculosis in a university hospital in Spain. *Eur J Epidemiol* **5**: 154.

Gareau FE, Mackel DC, Boring JR *et al.* (1959) The acquisition of fecal flora by infants from their mothers during birth. *J Pediatr* **54**: 313.

Gerzof SG, Gale ME (1982) Computed tomographic and ultrasonography for diagnosis and treatment of renal and retroperitoneal abscesses. *Urol Clin N Am* **9**: 1.

Gill DG, Mendes da Costa B, Cameron JS *et al.* (1976) Analysis of 100 children with severe and persistent hypertension. *Arch Dis Child* **51**: 951.

Gillenwater JY, Harrison RB, Kunin CM (1979) Natural history of bacteriuria in schoolgirls. A long-term case-control study. *N Engl J Med* **301**: 396–9.

Gillenwater JYJ (1981) Detection of urinary leukocytes by chemstrip-1. *J Urol* **125**: 383.

Ginsburg CM, McCracken GH Jr (1982) Urinary tract infections in young infants. *Pediatrics* **69**: 409–12.

Ginsburg I, Kohen R (1995) Cell damage in inflammatory and infectious sites might involve a coordinated 'cross-talk' among oxidants, microbial haemolysins and ampiphiles, cationic proteins, phospholipases, fatty acids, proteinases, and cytokines (an overview). *Free Rad Res* **22**: 489–517.

Glassroth I, Robins AG and Snider DE Jr (1980) Letter to the editor. *N Engl J Med* **303**: 940.

Glauser MP, Lyons JM, Brande AI (1978) Prevention of chronic experimental pyelonephritis by suppression of acute suppuration. *J Clin Invest* **61**: 403.

Gleeson FV, Gordon I (1991) Imaging in urinary tract infection. *Arch Dis Child* **66**: 1282–3.

Goldraich NP, Ramos DL, Goldraich JH *et al.* (1987) Urography versus DMSA scan in children with vesicoureteral reflux. *Pediatr Nephrol* **3**: 1.

Gomber S, Revathi G, Krishna A, Gupta A (1998) Perinephric abscess (presenting as abdominal pain) due to *Listeria monocytogenes*. *Ann Trop Paediatr* **18**: 61–2.

Goodman TR, McHugh K, Lindsell DR (1998) Paediatric xanthogranulomatous pyelonephritis. *Int J Clin Pract* **52**: 43–5.

Goonasekera CD, Shah V, Wade AM *et al.* (1996) 15–year follow-up of renin and blood pressure in reflux nephropathy. *Lancet* **347**: 640–3.

Gordon AC, Thomas DFM, Arthur AJ *et al.* (1990) Prenatally diagnosed reflux: a follow-up study. *Br J Urol* **65**: 407.

Gordon I (1990) Urinary tract infection in paediatrics: the role of diagnostic imaging. *Br J Radiol* **63**: 507–11.

Gow JG (1986) Genitourinary tuberculosis. In *Campbell's Urology*, Vol. 1, 5th ed. (edited by PC Walsh, RF Gittes, AD Perlmutter *et al.*). Philadelphia, WB Saunders Co, pp. 1037–69.

Gow IG and Barbosa S (1984) Genitourinary tuberculosis: a study of 1117 cases over a period of 34 years. *Br J Urol* **56**: 449.

Graham JB, King LR, Kropp KA *et al.* (1967) The significance of distal urethral narrowing in young girls. *J Urol* **97**: 1045.

Granoff DM, Roskes S (1974) Urinary tract infection due to hemophilus influenzae, type b. *J Pediatr* **84**: 414–16.

Gross GW, Lebowitz RL (1981) Infection does not cause reflux. *AJR Am J Roentgenol* **137**: 929–32.

Gruneberg RN (1969) The relationship of infecting organisms to fecal flora in patients with symptomatic urinary infection. *Lancet* **ii**: 766.

Hagberg L, Hull R, Hull S *et al.* (1983) Contribution of adhesion to bacterial persistence in mouse urinary tract. *Infect Immun* **40**: 265–72.

Hagberg L, Jodal U, Korkonen T *et al.* (1981) Adhesion, hemagglutination, and virulence of *Escherichia coli* causing urinary tract infections. *Infect Immun* **31**: 564–70.

Hahn H, Kaufmann SHE (1981) The role of cell-mediated immunity in bacterial infections. *Rev Infect Dis* **3**: 1221.

Hakomori SI, Kobata A (1974) Blood group antigens. In: *The antigens*. Volume 2. New York: Academic Press, 79–140.

Handmaker H (1982) Nuclear renal imaging in acute pyelonephritis. *Semin Nucl Med* **12**: 246.

Hansen A, Hansen B, Dahm TL (1997) Urinary tract infection, day wetting and other voiding symptoms in seven- to eight-year-old Danish children. *Acta Pediatr* **86**: 1345–9.

Hanson LA, Ahlstedt S, Fasth A *et al*. (1977) Antigens of *Escherichia coli*, human immune response, and the pathogenesis of urinary tract infections [Review]. *J Infect Dis* **136** (Suppl): S144–9.

Hansson S (1992) Urinary incontinence in children and associated problems. *Scand J Urol Nephrol* **141**: 47.

Hansson S, Caugant D, Jodal U, Svanborg-Eden C (1989a) Untreated asymptomatic bacteriuria in girls: I. – Stability of urinary isolates. *BMJ* **298**: 853–5.

Hansson S, Hjalmas K, Jodal U *et al*. (1990) Lower urinary tract dysfunction in girls with asymptomatic or covert bacteriuria. *J Urol* **143**: 333.

Hansson S, Jodal U, Noren L (1989b) Treatment vs. non-treatment of asymptomatic bacteriuria in girls with renal scarring. In: *Host–parasite interactions in urinary tract infections*. Chicago, IL: University of Chicago Press, 289–91.

Hansson S, Jodal U, Noren L *et al*. (1989c) Untreated bacteriuria in asymptomatic girls with renal scarring. *Pediatrics* **84**: 964.

Harding GK, Ronald AR, Boutros P, Lank B (1975) A comparison of trimethorprim–sulfamethoxazole with sulfamethoxazole alone in infections localized to the kidneys. *Can Med Assoc J* **112**(13 Spec No.): 9–12.

Hartman GW, Segura JW and Hattery RR (1977) Infectious diseases of the genitourinary tract. In *Emmett's Clinical Urography: An Atlas and Textbook of Roentgenologic Diagnosis*, Vol 2, 4th ed. (edited by DM Witten, GH Myers Jr, DC Utz). Philadelphia, WB Saunders Co, pp. 898–918.

Haycock GB (1991) A practical approach to evaluating urinary tract infection in children. *Pediatr Nephrol* **5**: 401–2.

Heale WF, Weldone DP, Hewstone AS (1977) Reflux nephropathy: presentation or urinary infection in children. *Med J Aust* **1**: 1138.

Hedges S, Svensson M, Svanborg C (1992) Interleukin-6 response of epithelial cell lines to bacterial stimulation *in vitro*. *Infect Immun* **60**: 1295–301.

Hellerstein S, Kennedy E, Nussbaum L, Rice K (1978) Localization of the site of urinary tract infections by means of antibody-coated bacteria in the urinary sediments. *J Pediatr* **92**: 188–93.

Hellstrom A, Hanson E, Hansson S *et al*. (1991) Association between urinary symptoms at 7 years old and previous urinary tract infection. *Arch Dis Child* **66**: 232–4.

Hellstrom M, Jodal U, Marild S, Wettergren B (1987) Ureteral dilatation in children with febrile urinary tract infection or bacteriuria. *AJR Am J Roentgenol* **148**: 483–6.

Helwig H (1994) Therapeutic strategies for urinary tract infections in children. *Infection* **22** (Suppl): 12.

Hill GS, Clarck RL (1972) A comparative angiographic, microangiographic, and histologic study of experimental pyelonephritis. *Invest Radiol* **7**: 33.

Hinman F. Urinary tract damage in children who wet. *Pediatrics* **54**: 143–50.

Hjalmas K (1992) Functional daytime incontinence: definitions and epidemiology. *Scand J Urol Nephrol* **141** (Suppl): 39.

Hjelm EM (1984) Local cellular immune response in ascending urinary tract infection: occurrence of T-cells, immunoglobulin-producing cells, and Ia-expressing cells in rat urinary tract tissue. *Infect Immun* **44**: 627.

Hoberman A, Chao HP, Keller DM *et al*. (1993) Prevalence of urinary tract infection in febrile infants. *J Pediatr* **123**: 17–23.

Hoberman A, Wald ER, Hickey RW *et al*. (1999) Oral versus initial intravenous therapy for urinary tract infections in young febrile children. *Pediatr* **104**: 74–86.

Hoberman A, Wald ER, Reynolds EA *et al*. (1994) Pyuria and bacteriuria in urine specimens obtained by catheter from young children with fever. *J Pediatr* **124**: 513–19.

Hobermann A, Wald ER (1997) Urinary tract infections in young febrile children. *Pediatr Infect Dis* **16**: 11–17.

Holland NH, Kotchen T, Bhathena D (1975) Hypertension in children with chronic pyelonephritis. *Kidney Int* **8**: S243.

Hooper DC, Wolfson TS, Ng EY *et al*. (1987) Mechanism of action and resistance to ciprofloxacin. *Am J Med* **82** (Suppl 4A): 12.

Hopkins GB, Hall RL, Mende CW (1976) Gallium-67 scintigraphy for the diagnosis and localization of perinephric abscesses. *J Urol* **115**: 126.

Hopkins WJ, Gendron-Fitzpatrick A, Balish E, Uehling DT (1998) Time course and host response to *Escherichia coli* urinary tract infection in genetically distinct mouse strains. *Infect Immun* **66**: 2798–802.

Hopkins WJ, Xing Y, Dahmer LA, Balish E, Uehling DT (1995) Western blot analysis of anti-*Escherichia coli* serum immunoglobulins in women susceptible to recurrent urinary tract infections. *J Infect Dis* **172**: 1612–16.

Horgan JG, Rosenfeld NS, Weiss RM *et al*. (1984) Is renal ultrasound a reliable indicator of nonobstructed duplication anomaly? *Pediatr Radiol* **14**: 388.

Hori C, Hiraoka M, Tsukahara H *et al*. (1997) Intermittent trimethoprim–sulfamethoxazole in children with vesicoureteral reflux. *Pediatr Nephrol* **11**: 328–30.

Horowitz MA, Silverstein SC (1980) Influence of *Escherichia coli* capsule on complement fixation and on phagocytosis and killing by human phagocytes. *J Clin Invest* **65**: 82.

Immergut MA, Wahman GE (1968) The urethral caliber of female children with urinary tract infection. *J Urol* **99**: 189.

International Reflux Committee (1981) Medical versus surgical treatment of primary vesicoureteral reflux. *Pediatrics* **67**: 392.

Israele V, Darabi A, McCracken GH Jr (1987) The role of bacterial virulence factors and Tamm-Horsfall protein in the pathogenesis of *Escherichia coli* urinary tract infection in infants. *Am J Dis Child* **141**: 1230–4.

Itoh K, Asano Y, Tsukamoto E *et al*. (1991) Single photon emission compured tomography with Tc-99m-dimercaptosuccinic acid in patients with upper urinary tract infection and/or vesicoureteral reflux. *Ann Nucl Med* **5**: 29–34.

Itoh K, Yamashita T, Tsukamoto E *et al*. (1995) Qualitative and quantitative evaluation of renal parenchymal damage by 99mTc-DMSA planar and SPECT scintigraphy. *Ann Nucl Med* **9**: 23–8.

Jacobson SH, Eklof O, Eriksson CG *et al*. (1989) Development of hypertension and uraemia after pyelonephritis in childhood: twenty-seven year follow-up. *BMJ* **299**: 703.

Jacobson SH, Kjellstrend CM, Lins LE (1988b) Role of hypervolaemia and renin in the blood pressure control of patients with pyelonephritic renal scarring. *Acta Med Scand* **224**: 47.

Jacobson SN, Hammarlind M, Lidelfeldt KJ et al. (1988a) Incidence of aerobactin-positive *Escherichia coli* strains in patients with symptomatic urinary tract infection. *Eur J Clin Microbiol Infect Dis* **7**: 630.

Jakobsson B, Berg U, Svensson L (1994) Renal scarring after acute pyelonphritis. *Arch Dis Child* **70**: 111.

Jakobsson B, Nolstedt L, Svensson L et al. (1992) 99mTc-dimercaptosuccinic acid (DMSA) in the diagnosis of acute pyelonephritis in children: relation to clinical and radiological findings. *Pediatr Nephrol* **6**: 328–34.

Jakobsson B, Svensson L (1997) Transient pyelonephritic changes on 99m-technetium-demrcaptosuccinic acid scan for at least five months after infection. *Acta Paediatr* **86**: 803–7.

James GP, Paul KL, Fuller JB (1978) Urinary nitrate in urinary tract infection. *Am J Clin Pathol* **70**: 671.

James-Ellison MY, Roberts R, Verrier-Jones K et al. (1997) Mucosal immunity in the urinary tract: changes in sIgA, FSC, and total Iga with age and in urinary tract infection. *Clin Nephrol* **48**: 69–78.

Jantausch BA, Criss VR, O'Donnell R et al. (1994) Association of Lewis blood group phenotypes with urinary tract infection in children. *J Pediatr* **124**: 863–8.

Jaya G, Bal CS, Padhy AK et al. (1996) Radionuclide studies in the evaluation of urinary tract infections in children. *Ind Pediatr* **33**: 635–40.

Jequier S, Forbes PA, Negrady MB (1985) The value of ultrasound as a screening procedure in first documented urinary tract infections in children. *J Ultrasound Med* **4**: 393.

Jerkins GR, Noe HN (1982) Familial vesicoureteral reflux: a prospective study. *J Urol* **128**: 7743.

Jodal U (1987) The natural history of bacteriuria in childhood. **1**: 713.

Jodal U (1994) Urinary tract infection in children. In: Holliday M, Barratt TM, Avner ED (eds) *Pediatric Nephrology*. 3rd edition. Baltimore, MD: Williams and Wilkins.

Johanson M, Plos K, Machlund BI et al. (1993) Pap, papG, and prsG DNA sequences in *Escherichia coli* from the fecal flora and the urinary tract. *Microb Pathogen* **15**: 121.

Kaack MB, Dowling KJ, Patterson GM, Roberts JA (1986) Immunology of pyelonephritis: E. coli causes granulocytic aggregation and renal ischemia. *J Urol* **136**: 1117.

Kaijser B (1973) Immunology of *Escherichia coli*: k antigen and its relation to urinary-tract infection. *J Infect Dis* **127**: 670–7.

Kaijser B (1977) Immunology of *Escherichia coli* K antigen and its relation to urinary tract infections in children. *Lancet* **i**: 633.

Kaijser B, Larsson P, Olling S (1983) Protection against ascending *Escherichia coli* pyelonephritis in rats and significance of local immunity. *Infect Immun* **20**: 78.

Kallenius G, Mollby R, Svenson SB et al. (1981) Occurrence of p-fimbriated escherichia coli in urinary tract infections. *Lancet* **ii**: 1369–72.

Kallenius G, Mollby R, Svensson SB et al. (1980) The pK antigen as receptor for the hemagglutination of pyelonephritogenic *Escherichia coli*. *FEMS Microbiol Lett* **7**: 297.

Kallenius G, Winberg J (1978) Bacterial adherence to periurethral epithelial cells in girls prone to urinary-tract infections. *Lancet* **ii**: 540–3.

Kangarloo H, Gold RH, Fine RN et al. (1985) Urinary tract infection in infants and children evaluated by ultrasound. *Radiology* **154**: 367–73.

Kenney M, Loechel AB and Lovelock FJ (1960) Urine cultures in tuberculosis. *Am Rev Respir Dis* **82**: 564.

Khan AJ (1994) Efficacy of single-dose therapy of urinary tract infection in infants and children: a review. *J Natl Med Assoc* **86**: 690–6.

Kim KK (1996) Preputial condition and urinary tract infections. *J Korean Med Sci* **11**: 332.

Kincaid-Smith P (1975) Glomerular lesions and atrophic pyelonephritis in reflux nephropathy. *Kidney Int* **8**: S81.

Klevan JL, De Jong AR (1990) Urinary tract symptoms and urinary tract infection following sexual abuse. *Am J Dis Child* **144**: 242–4.

Koehler PR (1974) The roentgen diagnosis of renal inflammatory masses – special emphasis on angiographic changes. *Radiology* **112**: 257.

Koff SA (1991) A practical approach to evaluating urinary tract infections in children. *Pediatr Nephrol* **5**: 398–400.

Koff SA, Lapides J, Piazza DH (1979) Association of urinary tract infection and reflux with uninhibited bladder contractions and voluntary sphincteric obstruction. *J Urol* **122**: 373–6.

Koff SA, Murtagh DS (1983) The uninhibited bladder in children: effect of treatment on recurrence of urinary infection and on vesicoureteral reflux resolution. *J Urol* **130**: 1138–41.

Koff SA, Wagner TT, Jayanthi VR (1998) The relationship among dysfunction elimination syndromes, primary vesicoureteral refluz and urinary tract infections in children. *J Urol* **160**: 1019–22.

Kumar B, Coleman RE, Anderson PO (1975) Gallium citrate Ga-67 imaging in patients with suspected inflammatory processes. *Arch Surg* **110**: 1237.

Kunin CM (1970) The natural history of recurrent bacteriuria in schoolgirls. *N Engl J Med* **282**: 1443–8.

Kunin CM (1987) *Detection, prevention and management of urinary tract infections*. 4th edition. Philadelphia, PA: Lea and Febiger.

Kurnin GD (1980) Clinical nephrotoxicity of tobramycin and gentamicin: a prospective study. *JAMA* **244**: 1808.

Kusumi Rk, Glover PJ, Kunin CM (1981) Rapid detection of pyuria by leukocyte esterase activity. *JAMA* **254**: 1653.

Landau D, Turner ME, Brennan J, Majd M (1994) The value of urinalysis in differentiating acute pyelonephritis from lower urinary tract infection in febrile infants. *Pediatr Infect Dis* **13**: 777.

Lattimer JK, Vasquez G, Wechsler H (1960) New drugs for treatment of genitourinary tuberculosis: a comparison of efficacy. *J Urol* **83**: 493.

Leadbetter G Jr, Slavins S (1974) Pediatric urinary tract infections: significance of vaginal bacteria. *Urology* **3**: 581.

Lebowitz RL, Mandell J (1987) Urinary tract infection in children: putting radiology in its place. *Radiology* **165**: 1–9.

Leffler H, Svanborg-Eden C (1980) Chemical identification of a glycoshpingolipid receptor for *Escherichia coli* attaching to human urinary tract epithelial cells and agglutinating human erythrocytes. *FEMS Microbiol Lett* **8**: 127.

Leonidas JC, McCauley RG, Klauber GC, Fretzayas AM (1985) Sonography as a substitute for excretory urography in children with urinary tract infection. *AJR Am J Roentgenol* **144**: 815–19.

Lidin-Janson G, Jodal U, Lincoln K (1980) Trimethoprim-och nitrofurantoin for profylax mot UVI hos barn. *Recip Reflex Suppl VI*: 38.

Lindberg U, Bjure J, Hangstvedt S *et al.* (1975a) Asymptomatic bacteriuria in school girls. III. Relation between residual urine volume and recurrence. *Acta Paediatr Scand* **64**: 437.

Lindberg U, Claesson I, Hanson LA *et al.* (1975b) Asymptomatic bacteriuria in school girls: I. Clinical and laboratory findings. *Acta Paediatr Scand* **64**: 425.

Lindberg U, Claesson I, Hanson LA *et al.* (1978c) Asymptomatic bacteriuria in schoolgirls: VIII. Clinical course during a three-year follow-up. *J Pediatrics* **92**: 194.

Lindberg U, Hanson LA, Lidin-Janson G *et al.* (1975c) Asymptomatic bacteriuria in school girls: II. Differences in *E. coli* causing asymptomatic and symptomatic bacteriuria. *Acta Paediatr Scand* **64**: 432.

Linshaw M (1996) Asymptomatic bacteriuria and vesico-ureteral reflux in children. *Kidney Int* **50**: 312.

Littlewood JM, Kite P, Kite BA (1969) Incidence of neonatal urinary tract infection. *Arch Dis Child* **44**: 617.

Lloyd-Still J, Cottom D (1967) Severe hypertension in childhood. *Arch Dis Child* **42**: 34–9.

Loening-Baucke V (1997) Urinary incontinence and urinary tract infection and their resolution with treatment of chronic constipation of childhood. *Pediatrics* **100**: 228–32.

Lomberg H *et al.* (1989) Properties of *Escherichia coli* in patients with renal scarring. *J Infect Dis* **159**: 579–82.

Lomberg H, Hanson LA, Jacobsson B *et al.* (1983) Correlation of p blood group, vesicoureteral reflux, and bacterial attachment in patients with recurrent pyelonephritis. *N Engl J Med* **308**: 1189–92.

Londe S (1978) Cause of hypertension in the young. *Pediatr Clin N Am* **25**: 55–65.

Lonergan GJ, Pennington DJ, Morrisson JC *et al.* (1998) Childhood pyelonephritis: comparison of gadolinium-enhanced MR imaging and renal vortical scintigraphy for diagnosis. *Radiology* **207**: 377–85.

Luscher TF, Wanner C, Hauri D *et al.* (1985) Curable renal parenchymatous hypertension: current diagnosis and management. *Cardiology* **72** (Suppl): 33–45.

MacKenzie JR (1996) A review of renal scarring in children. *Nucl Med Commun* **17**: 176–90.

MacKenzie JR, Fowler K, Hollman AS *et al.* (1994) The value of ultrasound in acute urinary tract infection. *Br J Urol* **74**: 240.

Mackie GG, Stephens FD (1975) Duplex kidneys: a correlation of renal dysplasia with position of the ureteral orifice. *J Urol* **114**: 2743.

Madrigal G, Odio CM, Mohs E *et al.* (1988) Single dose antibiotic therapy is not as effective as conventional regimens for management of acute urinary tract infections in children. *Pediatr Infect Dis J* **7**: 316.

Majd M (1992) Nuclear medicine in pediatric urology. In: *Clinical pediatric urology*. 3rd edition. Philadelphia, PA: WB Saunders.

Majd M, Kass EJ, Belman AB (1983) The accuracy of the indirect (intravenous) radionuclide cystogram in children. *J Nucl Med* **24**: 23.

Majd M, Kass EJ, Belman AB (1985) Radionuclide cystography in children: comparison of direct (retrograde) and indirect (intravenous) techniques. *Ann Radiol* **28**: 322–8.

Majd M, Blask ARN, Markle BM *et al.* (2001) Acute Pyelonephritis: Comparison of diagnosis with 99m Tc-DMSA SPECT, Spiral CT, MR imaging and power doppler US in an experimental pig model. *Radiology* **218**: 101–108.

Majd M, Rushton HG (1992) Renal cortical scintigraphy in the diagnosis of acute pyelonephritis. *Semin Nucl Med* **22**: 98–111.

Majd M, Rushton HG, Chandra R *et al.* (1996) ^{99m}Tc-DMSA renal cortical scintigraphy for the detection of experimental acute pyelonephritis in piglets: comparison of planar (pinhole) and SPECT imaging. *J Nucl Med* **37**: 1731–4.

Majd M, Rushton HG, Jantausch B, Wiedermann BL (1991) Relationship among vesicoureteral reflux, p-fimbriated *Escherichia coli*, and acute pyelonephritis in children with febrile urinary tract infection. *J Pediatr* **119**: 578–85.

Malek RS, Elder JS (1978) Xanthogranulomatous pyelonephritis: a critical analysis of 26 cases of the literature. *J Urol* **119**: 589.

Malvey MA, Lopez-Bondo Y, Wilson C *et al.* (1998) Induction and evasion of host defenses by type-1 piliated uropathogenic *Escherichia coli*. *Science* **282**: 1494–7.

Mannhardt W, Becker A, Putzer M *et al.* (1996) Host defense within the urinary tract. I. Bacterial adhesion initiates an uroepithelilal defense mechanism. *Pediatr Nephrol* **10**: 568–72.

Mansfield JT, Snow BW, Cartwright PC, Wadsworth K (1995) Complications of pregnancy in women after childhood reimplantation for vesicoureteral reflux: an update with 25 years of followup. *J Urol* **154**: 787–90.

Marild S, Jodal U (1998) Incidence rate of first-time symptomatic urinary tract infection in children under 6 years of age. *Acta Paediatr* **87**: 549–52.

Marild S, Jodal U, Mangelus L (1989b) Medical histories of children with acute pyelonephritis compared with controls. *J Pediatr Infect Dis* **8**: 511.

Marild S, Jodal U, Orskov I *et al.* (1989a) Special virulence of *Escherichia coli* O1:K1:H7 clone in ascute pyelonephritis. *J Pediatr* **115**: 40–5.

Markus DM (1969) The ABO and Lewis blood group system. Immunocytochemistry, genetics and relation to human disease. *N Engl J Med* **280**: 994.

Martinell J, Jodal U, Lidin-Janson G (1990) Pregnancies in women with and without renal scarring after urinary infections in childhood. *BMJ* **300**: 840–4.

Martinell J, Lidin-Janson G, Jagenburg R *et al.* (1996a) Girls prone to urinary infections followed into adulthood. Indices of renal disease. *Pediatr Nephrol* **10**: 139–42.

Martinell J, Lidin-Janson G, Jagenburg R *et al.* (1996b) Girls prone to urinary infections followed into adulthood. Indices of disease. *Pediatr Nephrol* **10**: 139–42.

Mattsby-Baltzer I, Claesson I, Hanson LA *et al.* (1981) Antibodies to lipid a during urinary tract infection. *J Infect Dis* **144**: 319–28.

Mayo ME, Burns MW (1990) Urodynamic studies in enuresis and the non-neurogenic bladder. *Br J Urol* **65**: 641.

McCabe WR, Kaijser, B, Olling S *et al.* (1978) *Escherichia coli* in bacteremia: K and O antigens and serum sensitivity of strains from adults and neonates. *J Infect Dis* **138**: 33–41.

McCracken GH Jr, Ginsburg CM, Namasonthi V, Petruska M (1981) Evaluation of short-term antibiotic therapy in children with uncomplicated urinary tract infections. *Pediatrics* **67**: 796–801.

McGeachie J (1966) Recurrent infection of the urinary tract: reinfection or recrudescence? *BMJ* i: 952.

McGuire EJ, Woodside JR (1981) Diagnostic advantages of fluoroscopic monitoring during urodynamic evaluation. *J Urol* **125**: 830–4.

McLachlan M, Mellor S, Verrier-Jones E *et al.* (1975) Urinary tract infection in school girls with covert bacteriuria. *Arch Dis Child* **50**: 253.

Melis K, Vandevivere J, Hoskens C *et al.* (1992) Early 99m Tc-dimercaptosuccinic acid scintigraphy insympptomatic first time urinary tract infection. *Acta Pediatr* **85**: 430.

Merrick MV, Uttley WS, Wild SR (1980) The detection of pyelonephritic scarring in children by radioisotope imaging. *Br J Radiol* **53**: 544–56.

Miller TE, Scott L, Stewart E *et al.* (1978) Modification by suppressor cells and serum factors of the cell-mediated immune response in experimental pyelonephritis. *J Clin Invest* **61**: 864.

Miyakita H, Puri P (1994) Urinary levels of N-acetyl-beta-D-glucosaminidase – a simple marker for predicting tubular damage in higher grades of vesicoureteric reflux. *Eur Urol* **25**: 135.

Moffatt M, Embree J, Grimm P, Law B (1988) Short-course antibiotic therapy for urinary tract infections in children. A methodological review of the literature. *Am J Dis Child* **142**: 57–61.

Monsour M, Azmy AF, MacKenzie JR (1987) Renal scarring secondary to vesicoureteric reflux. Critical assessment and new grading. *Br J Urol* **32**: 375–8.

Mucci B, Macguire B (1994) Does routine ultrasound have a role in the investigation of children with urinary tract infection? *Clin Radiol* **49**: 324–5.

Murphy DM, Fallon B, Lane V *et al.* (1982) Tuberculous stricture of ureter. *Urology* **20**: 382.

Najmaldin A, Burge DM, Atwell TD (1990) Reflux nephropathy secondary to intrauterine vesocioureteric reflux. *J Pediatr Surg* **25**: 387.

Naseer SR, Steinhardt GF (1997) New renal scars in children with urinary tract infections, vesicoureteral reflux and voiding dysfunction: a prospective evaluation. *J Urol* **158**: 566–8.

Nash MA, Siegele RL (1996) Urinary tract infections in infants and children. *Adv Pediatr Infect Dis* **11**: 403–8.

Nasrallah PF, Sreeramulu N, Crawford J (1982) Clinical applications of nuclear cystography. *J Urol* **128**: 550.

Navas EL, Venegas MF, Duncan JL *et al.* (1993) Blood group antigen expression on vaginal and buccal epithelial cells and mucus in secretor and nonsecretor women. *J Urol* **149**: 1492.

Navas EL, Venegas MF, Duncan JL *et al.* (1994) Blood group antigen expression on vaginal cells and mucus in women with and without a history of urinary tract infections. *J Urol* **152**: 345–9.

Nayir A, Evare S, Sinin A *et al.* (1995) The effects of vaccination with inactivated uropathogenic bacteria in recurrent urinary tract infections in children. *Vaccine* **13**: 987–90.

Nelson JD, Peters PC (1965) Suprapubic aspiration of urine in preterm and term infants. *Pediatrics* **36**: 132.

Neumann PZ, DeDomenico IJ, Nogrady MB (1973) Constipation and urinary tract infection. *Pediatrics* **52**: 241–5.

Newcastle Asymptomatic Bacteriuria Research Group (1975) Asymptomatic bacteriuria in school children in Newcastle-upon-Tyne. *Arch Dis Child* **50**: 90.

Newcastle Asymptomatic Bacteriuria Research Group (1981) Asymptomatic bacteriuria in school children in Newcastle-upon-Tyne: a 5–year followup. *Arch Dis Child* **56**: 585–92.

O'Doherty NJ (1968) Urinary tract infection in the neonatal period and later in infancy. In: *Urinary tract infection*. London: Oxford University Press.

O'Hanley P, Lark D, Falkow S, Schoolnik G (1985) Molecular basis of *Escherichia coli* colonization of the upper urinary tract in BALB/C mice. *J Clin Invest* **75**: 347.

O'Regan S, Yazbeck S, Schick E (1985) Constipation, bladder instability, urinary tract infection syndrome. *Clin Nephrol* **23**: 152.

Olling S, Hansson LA, Holmgren JU *et al.* (1973) The bactericida; effect of normal human serum on E. coli strains from normals and from patients with urinary tract infections. *Infect Immun* **1**: 24.

Orskov I, Ferencz A, Orskov F (1980) Tamm-Horsfall protein or uromucoid is the normal urinary slime that traps Type-1 fimbriated *Escherichia coli*. *Lancet* ii: 887.

Ottolini MAC, Schaer CM, Rushton HG *et al.* (1995) Relationship of asymptomatic bacilluria and renal scarring in children with neuropathic bladders who are practicing intermittent catheterization. *J Pediatr* **127**: 368.

Parkhouse HF, Godley ML, Cooper J *et al.* (1989) Renal imaging with 99m-Tc-labelled DMSA in the detection of acute pyelonephritis: an experimental study in the pig. *Nucl Med Commun* **30**: 1219.

Parkinnen J, Virkola R, Korhonen TK (1983) *Escherichia coli* strains binding neuraminyl a2–3 galalctosides. *Biochem Biophys Res Commun* **11**: 456–61.

Patrick MJ (1967) The influence of maternal renal infection on the foetus and infant. *Arch Dis Child* **42**: 208.

Pecha B, Low D, O'Hanley P (1989) Gal-Gal pili vaccines prevent pyelonephritis by piliated *E. coli* in a murine model. *J Clin Invest* **83**: 2102.

Perngini MK, Vidotto MC (1996) Frequency of pap and pil operons in *Escherichia coli* stratins associated with urinary infections. *Braz J Med Biol Res* **29**: 351.

Petersen KE (1991) Short term treatment of acute urinary tract infections in girls. Copenhagen Study Group of Urinary Tract Infections in Children. *Scand J Infect Dis* **23**: 213–20.

Pezzlo M (1988) Detection of urinary tract infection by rapid methods. *Clin Microbiol Rev* **1**: 268.

Piepsz A, Pintelon H, Verboven M *et al.* (1992) Replacing 99mTcm-DMSA for renal imaging? *Nucl Med Commun* **13**: 494–6.

Plos K, Connell H, Jodal U *et al.* (1995) Intestinal carriage of p fimbriated *Escherichia coli* and the susceptibility to urinary tract infection in young children. *J Infect Dis* **171**: 625–31.

Pohl HG, Rushton HG, Park J-S *et al.* (1999) Adjunctive oral corticosteroids reduces renal scarring: The piglet model of reflux and acute experimental pyelonephritis. *J Urol* **162**: 815.

Pryles CV, Eliot CR (1965) Pyuria and bacteriuria in infants and children: the value of pyuria as a diagnostic criterion of urinary tract infections. *Am J Dis Child* **110**: 628.

Ransley PG (1977) Intrarenal reflux: anatomical, dynamic and radiological studies. Part I. *Urol Res* **5**: 61.

Ransley PG (1978) Vesicoureteral reflux: continuing surgical dilemma. *Urology* **12**: 246.

Ransley PG, Risdon RA (1978) Reflux in renal scarring. *Br J Radiol* 51 Suppl **14**: 1.

Ransley PG, Risdon RA (1981) Reflux nephropathy: effects of antimicrobial therapy on the evolution of the acute pyelonephritic scar. *Kidney Int* **20**: 733.

Rene P, Silverblatt FJ (1982) Serological response to *Escherichia coli* in pyelonephritis. *Infect Immun* **37**: 749.

Roberts JA (1975) Experimental pyelonephritis in the monkeys: III. Pathophysiology of ureteral malfunction induced by bacteria. *Invest Urol* **13**: 117.

Roberts JA (1995) Mechanisms of renal damage in chronic pyelonephritis (reflux nephropathy). In: *Current Topics in Pathology*. Heidelberg: Springer.

Roberts JA (1991) Etiology and pathophysiology of pyelonephritis. *Am J Kidney Dis* **17**: 1.

Roberts JA (1996a) Factors predisposing to urinary tract infections in children. *Pediatr Nephrol* **10**: 517.

Roberts JA (1996b) Neonatal circumcision: an end to the controversy? *S Med J* **89**: 167–71.

Roberts JA, Hardaway K, Kaack B *et al.* (1984) Prevention of pyelonephritis by immunization with p-fimbria. *J Urol* **131**: 602.

Roberts JA, Ruth JK, Dominique GL *et al.* (1982) Immunology of pyelonephritis in the primate model: effect of superoxide dismutase. *J Urol* **128**: 1394.

Roberts JA, Suarez GM, Kaack B *et al.* (1985) Experimental pyelonephritis in the monkey VII: ascending pyelonephritis in the absence of vesicoureteral reflux. *J Urol* **133**: 1068.

Roberts KB, Charney E, Sweren RJ *et al.* (1983) Urinary tract infection in infants with unexplained fever: a collaborative study. *J Pediatr* **103**: 864–7.

Robins DG, Rogers KB, White RHR (1975) Urine microscopy as an aid to detection of bacteriuria. *Lancet* i: 476.

Rosenberg AR, Rossleigh MA, Brydon MP *et al.* (1992) Evaluation of acute urinary tract infection in children by dimercaptosuccinic acid scintigraphy: a prospective study. *J Urol* **148**: 1746–9.

Ross R Jr, Conway GF (1970) Hemorrhagic cystitis following an accidental overdosage of methenamine mandelate. *Am J Dis Child* **119**: 86.

Rote AR, Bauer SB, Retik AB (1978) Renal abscess in children. *J Urol* **119**: 254.

Ruberto U, D'Eufemia P, Ferretti L, Giardini O (1984) Effect of 3– vs 10–day treatment of urinary tract infections. *J Pediatr* **104**: 483–4.

Ruberto U, D'Eufemia P, Martino F *et al.* (1989) Amoxycillin and clavulanic acid in the treatment of urinary tract infections in children. *J Int Med Res* **17**: 168.

Rushton HG (1992) Genitourinary infections: nonspecific infections. In: Kelalis PP, King LR, Belman AB (eds) *Clinical Pediatric Urology*. 3rd edition. Philadelphia, PA: WA Saunders Co.

Rushton HG (1994) Reflux versus nonreflux pyelonephritis: is there a difference? In: Gonzales ET, Paulson DF (eds) *Problems in urology. Advances in pediatric urology*. Volume 8. Philadelphia, PA: JB Lippincott Co., 473–94.

Rushton HG (1997) The evaluation of acute pyelonephritis and renal scarring with technetium 99m-dimercaptosuccinic acid renal scintigraphy: evolving concepts and future directions. *Pediatr Nephrol* **11**: 108.

Rushton HG, Majd M (1992a) Pyelonephritis in male infants: how important is the foreskin? *J Urol* **148**: 733.

Rushton HG, Majd M (1992b) Dimercaptosuccinic acid renal scintigraphy for the evaluation of pyelonephritis and scarring: a review of experimental and clinical studies. *J Urol* **148**: 1726–32.

Rushton HG, Majd M, Chandra R, Yim D (1988) Evaluation of 99m-technetium-dimercaptosuccinic acid renal scans and experimental acute pyelonephritis in piglets. *J Urol* **140**: 1169–74.

Rushton HG, Majd M, Jauntausch B *et al.* (1992) Renal scarring following reflux and non-reflux pyelonephritis in children: evaluation with 99m-technetium dimercaptosuccinic acid distribution patterns in acute pyelonephritis. *J Urol* **147**: 1327–32.

Russo RM, Gururaj VJ, Laude TA *et al.* (1989–91) The comparative efficacy of cephalexin and sulfisoxazole in acute urinary tract infection in children. *Clin Pediatr* **16**: 83–4.

Rytand DA, Spreiter S (1981) Prognosis in postural (orthostatic) proteinuria: forty to fifty-year follow-up of six patients after diagnosis by thomas addis. *N Engl J Med* **305**: 618–21.

Saraga M, Stanicic A, Markovic V (1996) The role of direct radionuclide cystography in the evaluation of vesicoureteral reflux. *Scand J Urol Nephrol* **30**: 367–71.

Sargent MA, Stringer DA (1995) Voiding cystourethrography in children with urinary tract infection: the frequency of vesicoureteric reflux is independent of the specialty of the physician requesting the study. *AJR Am J Roentgenol* **164**: 1237–41.

Savage DCL, Howie G, Adler K, Wilson MI (1975) Controlled trial of therapy in covert bacteriuria in childhood. *Lancet* i: 358–61.

Savage DCL, Wilson MI, McHardy M *et al.* (1973) Covert bacteriuria of childhood: a clinical and epidemiological study. *Arch Dis Child* **48**: 8.

Savage JM, Koh CT, Shah V *et al.* (1987) Five year prospective study of plasma renin activity and blood pressure in patients with longstanding reflux nephropathy. *Arch Dis Child* **62**: 678.

Savage JP (1973) The deleterious effect of constipation upon the reimplanted ureter. *J Urol* **109**: 501–3.

Saxena SR, Collis A, Laurence BM (1974) Bacteriuria in preschool children. *Lancet* ii: 517.

Schaad UB, Wedgwood-Krucko J (1978) Nalidixic acid in children: a retrospective matched controlled study for cartilage toxicity. *Infection* **15**: 165.

Schaeffer AJ, Navas EL, Venegas MF *et al.* (1994) Variation of blood group antigen expression on vaginal cells and mucus in secretor and nonsecretor women. *J Urol* **152**: 859–64.

Schaaf HS, Smith I, Donald PR *et al.* (1989) Tuberculosis presenting in the neonatal period. *Clin Pediatr* (Phila) **28**: 474.

Schiff M Jr, Glickman M, Weiss RM *et al.* (1977) Antibiotic treatment of renal carbuncle. *Ann Intern Med* **8**: 305.

Schlager TA, Whittam TS, Hendley JO *et al.* (1995) Comparison of expression of virulence factors by *Escherichia coli* causing cystitis and *E. coli* colonizing the periurethra of healthy girls. *J Infect Dis* **172**: 772–7.

Schluter G (1986) Toxicology of ciprofloxacin. *First International Ciprofloxacin Workshop, Proceedings*, 61.

Schulman CC, Denis R (1977) Xanthogranulomatous pyelonephritis in childhood (Letter). *J Urol* **117**: 398.

Schulman SL, Quinn CK, Plachter N, Kodman-Jones C (1999) Comprehensive management of dysfunctional voiding. *Pediatrics* **103**: 31.

Seruca H (1989) Vesicoureteral reflux and voiding dysfunction: prospective study. *J Urol* **142**: 494.

Shanon A, Feldman W, McDonald P *et al.* (1992) Evaluation of renal scars by technetium-labeled dimercaptosuccinic acid scan, intravenous urography, and ultrasonography: a comparative study. *J Pediatr* **120**: 399–403.

Sheinfeld J, Cordon-Cardo C, Fair WR *et al.* (1990) Association of type 1 blood group antigens with urinary tract infections in children with genitourinary structural abnormalities. *J Urol* **144**: 469–73, Discussion 474.

Sheridan M, Jewkes F, Gough DCS (1991) Reflux nephropathy in the 1st year of life – the role of infection. *Pediatr Surg Int* **6**: 214.

Siegfrid L, Kmetkova M, Pazovd H *et al.* (1994) Virulence associated factors in *Escherichia coli* strains isolated from cultures of blood specimens from urospesis and non-urosepsis patients. *Microbiologia* **10**: 249.

Silver TM, Kass EJ, Thornbury JR *et al.* (1976) The radiological spectrum of acute pyelonephritis in adults and adolescents. *Radiology* **118**: 65.

Silverblatt FJ, Weinstein R, Rene P (1982) Protection against experimental pyelonephritis by antibodies to pili. *Scand J Infect Dis* **33**: 79.

Singh A, Fazal AR, Sinha SK *et al.* (1988) Tuberculous vesicovaginal fistula in a child. *Br J Urol* **62**: 615.

Skoog SJ, Belman AB, Majd M (1987) A nonsurgical approach to the management of primary vesicoureteral reflux. *J Urol* **138**: 941–6.

Smellie J, Edwards D, Hunter N *et al.* (1975) Vesicoureteral reflux and renal scarring. *Kidney Int* **8** (Suppl): 65.

Smellie JM, Bantock HM, Thompson BD (1982) Co-trimoxazole and the thyroid [Letter]. *Lancet* ii: 96.

Smellie JM, Gruneberg RN, Leakey A, Atkin WS (1976) Long-term low-dose co-trimoxazole in prophylaxis of childhood urinary tract infection: clinical aspects. *BMJ* ii: 203–6.

Smellie JM, Hodson CJ, Edwards D *et al.* (1964) Clinical and radiological features of of urinary infection in childhood. *BMJ* ii: 1222.

Smellie JM, Katz G, Gruneberg RN (1978) Controlled trial of prophylactic treatment in childhood urinary-tract infection. *Lancet* ii: 175–8.

Smellie JM, Normand ICS (1979) Reflux nephropathy in childhood. In: *Reflux nephropathy*. New York: Masson, 14–20.

Smellie JM, Normand ICS, Katz G (1981) Children with urinary infection: a comparison of those with and without vesicoureteric reflux. *Kidney Int* **20**: 717.

Smellie JM, Poulton A, Prescod NP (1994) Retrospective study of children with renal scarring associated with reflux and urinary infection. *BMJ* **308**: 1193–6.

Smellie JM, Preece MA, Paton AM (1983) Somatic growth in girls receiving low dose prophylactic co-trimoxazole. *BMJ Clin Res Ed* **287**: 875.

Smellie JM, Ransley PG, Normand IC *et al.* Development of new renal scars: a collaborative study. *BMJ Clin Res Ed* **290**: 1957–60.

Smith EM, Elder JS (1994) Double antimicrobial prophylaxis in girls with breakthrough urinary tract infections. *Urology* **43**: 708–12.

Smith MHD and Marquis IR (1981) Tuberculosis and other myco-bacterial infections. In *Textbook of Pediatric Infectious Diseases*. Vol 1. (edited by RD Feigin and ID Cherry.) Philadelphia, WB Saunders Co, pp. 1016–60.

Snodgrass W (1991) Relationship of voiding dysfunction to urinary tract infection and vesicoureteral reflux in children. *Urology* **38**: 341.

Sohl-Akerlund A, Ahlstedt S, Hanson LA *et al.* (1979) Antibody responses in urine and serum against *Escherichia coli* in childhood urinary tract infections. *Acta Path Microbiol* **87**: 29.

Sommer JT, Stephens FD (1981) Morphogenesis of nephropathy with partial ureteral obstruction and vesicoureteric reflux. *J Urol* **125**: 67.

Sreenarasimhaiah S, Hellerstein S (1998) Urinary tract infections per se do not cause end-stage kidney disease. *Pediatr Nephrol* **12**: 210–13.

Sreenarasimhaiah V, Alon US (1995) Uroradiologic evaluation of children with urinary tract infection: are both ultrasonograpy and renal cortical scintigraphy necessary? *J Pediatr* **127**: 373–7.

Stamey TA (1973) The role of introital bacteria in recurrent urinary infections. *J Urol* **109**: 467.

Stamey TA (1980) Urinary infections in infancy and childhood. In: *Pathogenesis and treatment of urinary tract infections*. Baltimore, MD: Williams and Wilkins.

Stamey TA, Bragonzi J (1976) Resistance to nalidixic acid: a misconception due to underdosage. *JAMA* 236.

Stamey TA, Condy M, Mihara G (1977) Prophylactic efficacy of nitrofurantoin macrocrystals and trimethoprim–sulfamethoxazole in urinary infections: biologic effects on the vaginal and rectal flora. *N Engl J Med* **296**: 780.

Stamey TA, Fair WR, Timothy MM et al. (1974) Serum versus urinary antimicrobial concentrations in cure of urinary-tract infections. *N Engl J Med* **291**: 1159–63.

Stamey TA, Govan DE, Palmer JM (1965) The localization and treatment of urinary tract infections: the role of bactericidal levels as opposed to serum levels. *Medicine* **44**: 1.

Stamey TA, Timothy M, Millar M et al. (1971) Recurrent urinary infections in adult women. The role of introital enterobacteria. *Calif Med* **115**: 1.

Stamm WE (1983) Measurement of pyuria and its relationship to bacteriuria. *Am J Med* **75** (Suppl): 53.

Stansfeld JM (1975) Duration of treatment for urinary tract infections in children. *BMJ* **iii**: 65–6.

Stapleton AE, Stroud MR, Hakomori SI, Stamm WE (1998) The globoseries glycosphingolipid sialosyl galactosyl globoside is found in urinary tract tissues and is a preferred binding receptor *in vitro* for uropathogenic *Escherichia coli* expressing pap-encoded adhesins. *Infect Immun* **66**: 3856–61.

Steele BT, Petrou C, de Maria J (1990) Renal abscesses in children. *Urology* **36**: 325–8.

Stokland E, Hellstrom M, Hansson S et al. (1994) Reliability of ultrasonography in identification of reflux nephropathy in children. *BMJ* **309**: 235–9.

Stokland E, Hellstrom M, Jacobsson B et al. (1996) Renal damage one year after first urinary tract infection: role of dimercaptosuccinic acid scintigraphy. *J Pediatr* **129**: 815–20.

Stokland E, Hellstrom M, Jacobsson B et al. (1998) Evaluation of DMSA scintigraphy and urography in assessing both acute and permanent renal damage in children. *Acta Radiol* **4**: 447–52.

Stoller ML, Kogan BA (1986) Sensitivity of ^{99m}technetium-dimercaptosuccinic acid for the diagnosis of chronic pyelonephritis: clinical and theoretical considerations. *J Urol* **135**: 977–80.

Sty JR, Wells RG, Starshak RJ, Schroeder BA (1987) Imaging in acute renal infection in children. *AJR Am J Roentgenol* **148**: 471–7.

Subramanyam BR, Megibow AJ, Raghavendra BN et al. (1982) Diffuse xanthogranulomatous pyelonephritis: analysis by computed tomography and sonography. *Urol Radiol* **4**: 5.

Sugar EC, Firlit CF (1982) Urodynamic biofeedback: a new therapeutic approach for childhood incontinence/infection (vesical voluntary sphincter dyssynergia). *J Urol* **128**: 1253–8.

Svanborg-Eden C, Briles D, Hagberg L et al. (1984). Genetic factors in host resistance to urinary tract infection. *Infection* **12**: 118–23.

Svanborg-Eden C, Eriksson B, Hanson LA (1977) Adhesion of *Escherichia coli* to human uroepithelial cells *in vitro*. *Infect Immun* **21**: 767–74.

Svanborg-Eden C, Hagberg L, Hull R et al. (1987) Bacterial virulence versus host resistance in the urinary tracts of mice. *Infect Immun* **55**: 124.

Svanborg-Eden C, Hanson CA, Jodal U et al. (1976) Variable adherence to normal human urinary tract epithelial cells of *Escherichia coli* strains associated with various forms of urinary infection. *Lancet* **ii**: 490.

Svanborg-Eden C, Jodal U (1979) Attachment of *Escherichia coli* to sediment epithelial cells from UTI prone and healthy children. *Infect Immun* **26**: 837.

Svanborg-Eden C, Svennerholm AM (1978) Secretory immunoglobulin A and G antibodies prevent adhesion of *Escherichia coli* to human urinary tract epithelial cells. *Infect Immun* **22**: 790.

Svensson M, Lindstedt R, Radin N et al. (1994) Epithelial glycosphingolipid expression as a determinant of bacterial adherence and cytokine production. *Infect Immun* **62**: 4404–10.

Tarkington MA, Fildes RD, Levin K et al. (1990) High resolution single photon emission computerized tomography (SPECT) 99m-technetium-dimercaptosuccinic acid renal imaging: a state of the art technique. *J Urol* **144**: 598–600.

Tasker AD, Lindsell DR, Moncrieff M (1993) Can ultrasound reliably detect renal scarring in children with urinary tract infection? *Clin Radiol* **47**: 177–9.

Thankavel K, Madison B, Ikeda T et al. (1997) Localization of a domain in the FimH adhesin of *Escherichia coli* type 1 fimbriae capable of receptor recogniction and use of a domain-specific antibody to confer protection against experimental urinary tract infection. *J Clin Invest* **100**: 1123–36.

Thomas V, Shelokov A, Forland M (1974) Antibody coated bacteria in the urine and the site of urinary tract infection. *N Engl J Med* **290**: 588.

Timmons JW, Perlmutter AD (1976) Renal abscess: a changing concept. *J Urol* **115**: 299.

Toma G, Bates J, Kumar S (1994) Uromodulin (Tamm-Horsfall protein) is a leukocyte adhesion molecule. *Biochem Biophys Res Commun* **200**: 275–82.

Tomisawa S, Kogure T, Kuroume T et al. (1989) P blood group and proneness to urinary tract infections in Japanese children. *Scand J Infect Dis* **21**: 403.

Tomlinson PA, Smellie JM, Prescod N et al. (1994) Differential excretion of urinary proteins in children with vesicoureteric reflux and reflux nephropathy. *Pediatr Nephrol* **8**: 21.

Torres VE, Velosa JA, Holley KE *et al*. (1980) Progression of vesicoureteral refllux nephropathy. *Ann Intern Med* **92**: 776–84.

Traisman ES, Conway JJ, Traisman HS *et al*. (1986) The localization of urinary tract infection with 99m Tc glucoheptonate scintigraphy. *Pediatr Radiol* **16**: 403.

Uehling DT, Hopkins WJ, Balish E *et al*. (1997) Vaginal mucosal immunization for recurrent urinary tract infection: phase II clinical trial. *J Urol* **157**: 2049–52.

Uehling DT, Jensen J, Balish E (1982) Vaginal immunization against urinary tract infection. *J Urol* **128**: 1382.

Uehling DT, King LR (1973) Secretory immunoglobulin A excretion in cystitis cystica. *Urology* **1**: 305.

Uehling DT, Mizutani K, Balish E (1978) Effect of immunization on bacterial adherence to urothelium. *Invest Urol* **16**: 145.

Uehling DT, Steihm ER (1971) Elevated urinary secretory IgA in children with urinary tract infection. *Pediatrics* **47**: 40–6.

Vachvanichsanong P, Dissaneewate P, Patrapinyokul S *et al*. (1992) Renal abscess in healthy children: report of three cases. *Pediatr Nephrol* **6**: 273–5.

Vaisanen V, Lounatama R, Korhonen TK (1982) Effects of sublethal concentrations of antimicrobial agents on the hemagglutination adhesion, and ultrastructure of pyelonephritogenic *Escherichia coli* strains. *Antimicrob Agents Chemother* **22**: 120.

Vaisanen-Rhen VE *et al*. (1984) P-fimbriated clones among uropathogenic strains of *Escherichia coli*. *Infect Immun* **43**: 149.

Van Gool J, Tanagho E (1977) External sphincter activity and urinary tract infections in girls. *Urology* **10**: 348.

van Gool JD (1995) Dysfunctional voiding: a complex of bladder/sphincter dysfunction, urinary tract infections and vesicoureteral reflux. *Acta Urol Belg* **63**: 27–33.

Van Gool JD, Kuitjin RH, Donekerwolcke RA *et al*. (1984) Bladder-sphincter dysfunction, urinary infection and vesicoureteral reflux with special reference tocognitive bladder training. *Contrib Nephrol* **39**: 190.

Van Gool JD, Vijverberg MA, de Jong TP (1992) Functional daytime incontinence: clinical and urodynamic assessment. *Scand J Urol Nephrol* **141**: 58.

Verber IG, Strudley MR, Meller ST (1988) 99mtc dimercaptosuccinic acid (DMSA) scan as first investigation of urinary tract infection. *Arch Dis Child* **63**: 1320–5.

Verboven M, Ingels M, Delree M, Piepsz A (1990) 99m Tc-DMSA scintigraphy in acute urinary tract infection in children. *Pediatr Radiol* **20**: 540–2.

Waalwijk C, MacLaren DM, deGraaf J (1983) *In vivo* function of hemolysin in the nephropathogenicity of *Escherichia coli*. *Infect Immun* **42**: 245.

Wallace DMA, Rothwell DL, Williams DI (1978) The long-term follow-up of surgically treated vesicoureteral reflux. *Br J Urol* **50**: 479–84.

Wallin L, Bajc M (1993) Typical technetium dimercaptosuccinic acid distribution patterns in acute pyelonephritis. *Acta Paediatr* **82**: 1061–5.

Wan J, Kaplinsky R, Greenfield S (1995) Toilet habits of children evaluated for urinary tract infection. *J Urol* **154**: 797–9.

Wanner C, Lusher T, Groth H *et al*. (1985) Unilateral parenchymatous kidney disease and hypertension: results of nephrectomy and medical treatment. *Nephron* **41**: 250–7.

Watson AR, Marsden HB, Cendron M *et al*. (1982) Renal pseudotumors caused by xanthogranulomatous pyelonephritis. *Arch Dis Child* **57**: 635.

Wechsler H and Lattimer JK (1975) An evaluation of the current therapeutic regimen for renal tuberculosis. *J Urol* **113**: 760.

Weinberg AC and Boyd SD (1988) Short-course chemotherapy and role of surgery in adult and pediatric genitourinary tuberculosis. *Urology* **31**: 95.

Weiss SJ (1989) Tissue destruction by neutrophils. *N Engl J Med* **320**: 365–75.

Wettergren B, Hellstrom M, Stokland E, Jodal U (1990) Six year follow up of infants with bacteriuria on screening. *BMJ* **301**: 845–8.

White RHR (1987) Management of urinary tract infection. *Arch Dis Child* **62**: 421.

Willi UV, Treves ST (1985) *Radionuclide voiding cystography*. New York: Springer, 105–20.

Williams MA, Noe HN, Smith RA (1994) The importance of urinary tract infection in the evaluation of the incontinent child. *J Urol* **151**: 188–90.

Williams PH (1979) Novel iron uptake system specified by Col V plasmids: an important component in the virulence of invasive strains of *Escherichia coli*. *Infect Immun* **26**: 295.

Winberg J, Andersen HJ, Bergstrom T *et al*. (1974) Epidemiology of symptomatic urinary tract infection in childhood. *Acta Paediatr Scand* **252** (Suppl): 1.

Winberg J, Bergstrom T, Jacobsson B (1975) Morbidity, age, and sex distribution, recurrences and renal scarring in symptomatic urinary tract infection in childhood. *Kidney Int* **8**: S101.

Winberg J, Bollgren I, Kallenius G *et al*. (1982) Clinical pyelonephritis and focal renal scarring. A selected review of pathogenesis, prevention, and prognosis. *Pediatr Clin N Am* **29**: 801–14.

Winter AL, Hardy BE, Alton DJ *et al*. (1983) Acquired renal scars in children. *J Urol* **129**: 1190–4.

Wippermann CF, Schofer O, Beetz R *et al*. (1991) Renal abscesses in childhood: diagnostic and therapeutic progress. *Pediatr Infect Dis J* **10**: 446–50.

Wiswell TE, Enzenauer RW, Holton ME *et al*. (1987) Declining frequency of circumcision: implications for changes in the absolute incidence and male to female sex ratio of urinary tract infections in early infancy. *Pediatrics* **79**: 338–42.

Wiswell TE, Hachey WE (1993) Urinary tract infections and the uncircumcised state: an update. *Clin Pediatr* **32**:130–4.

Wiswell TE, Roscelli JD (1986) Corroborative evidence for the decreased incidence of urinary tract infections in circumcised male infants. *Pediatrics* **78**: 96.

Wiswell TE, Smith FR, Bass JW (1985) Decreased incidence of urinary tract infections in circumcised male infants. *Pediatrics* **75**: 901–3.

Wold AE, Caugant DA, Lidin-Janson G *et al*. (1992) Resident *E. coli* strains frequently dispaly uropathogenic characteristics. *J Infect Dis* **165**: 46.

Wold AE, Mestecky J, Svanborg-Eden C (1988) Agglutination of *E. coli* by secretory IgA-a result of interaction between bacterial mannose-specific adhesins and immunoglobulin carbohydrate? *Monogr Allergy* **24**: 307.

Wong SH and Lau WY (1980) The surgical management of non-functioning tuberculous kidneys. *J Urol* **124**: 187.

Yazaki T, Ishikawa S, Ogawa Y *et al.* (1982) Xanthogranulomatous pyelonephritis in childhood: case report and review of English and Japanese literature. *J Urol* **127**: 80–3.

Yen TC, Chen WP, Chang SL *et al.* (1994) A comparative study of evaluating renal scars by 99m-Tc-DMSA planar and SPECT renal scans intravenous urography, and ultrasonography. *Ann Nucl Med* **8**: 147–52.

Zhang Y, Bailey RR (1995) A long term follow up of adults with reflux nephropathy. *N Z Med J* **108**: 142–4.

Zimmerman SW, Uehling DT, Burkholder PM (1973) Vesicoureteral reflux nephropathy: evidence for immunologically mediate glomerular injury. *Urology* **2**: 534–38.

Zinman L and Libertino IA (1980) Antirefluxing ileocecal conduit. *Urol Clin North Am* **7**: 503.

Fungal, parasitic, and other inflammatory diseases of the genitourinary tract

11

William A. Kennedy II and Linda M. Dairiki Shortliffe

Fungal infections of the urinary tract

Candidiasis

Pediatric fungal inflammations of the genitourinary tract are becoming more common with both the increasing number of preterm infants surviving aggressive intensive care unit management and the increasing number of immunocompromised children living with either malignancies, human immuno-deficiency virus (HIV), or solid organ and bone marrow transplantation. Preterm neonates are often intubated for weeks, receiving long-term hyperalimentation and broad-spectrum antibiotics. Baley *et al.* (1981) report that systemic candidiasis will develop in as many as 4% of those weighing 1500 g and 10% of those weighing 1000 g. Prolonged survival of profoundly immunocompromised pediatric patients has likewise led to the emergence of fungal infections as the major cause of mortality and morbidity in advanced disease states. *Candida* is the leading bloodstream isolate from children hospitalized with opportunistic infections (Muller *et al.*, 1999).

Candida albicans is a yeast that belongs to the comensal flora of the mouth, intestinal tract, vagina, and skin. *Candida* is the most common of the opportunistic mycoses. Systemic disease occurs almost exclusively in patients with impaired host resistance. Conditions that predispose to candidemia include contamination of intravenous catheters, long-term antibiotic therapy, steroid administration, immuno-suppressive agents, cytotoxic drug therapy, burns, and open surgical wounds (Stone *et al.*, 1974).

The diagnosis of candiduria is made by urine culture. In the neonate, urine is obtained by catheterization or suprapubic bladder aspiration, or by percutaneous renal aspirate if renal candidiasis is suspected. Colony counts of greater than 10 000 *Candida* per 1 ml of urine signify infection (Krozinn *et al.*, 1978).

Colony counts of 15 000/ml in midstream voided urine in males or straight catheterized specimen in females suggest renal *Candida* infection (Wise *et al.*, 1976). Urine specimens taken from indwelling catheters may have colony counts as high as 100 000/ml with no relationship to upper tract candidal infection.

Pediatric patients with renal candidiasis present with symptoms of urosepsis. Ureteral obstruction due to fungus ball infestation has been reported (Schonebeck *et al.*, 1970). Anuria in infants can result from bilateral pelvic fungus balls (Eckstein *et al.*, 1982). Radiologic evaluation of these patients with ultra-sound may demonstrate unilateral or bilateral hydro-nephrosis with an intrapelvic mass. Renal scintigraphy generally demonstrates that the involved kidney exhibits poor function. In patients with localized candidal cystitis, symptoms often consist of urinary urgency, frequency, and dysuria, or may be asymptomatic.

The treatment of candidiuria is dependent on the extent of the infection. Candiduria that occurs in otherwise healthy children after long-term broad-spectrum antibiotic therapy should clear spontaneously after the antibiotic has been stopped. Symptomatic infections limited to the bladder may be controlled and eradicated by urinary alkalinization and/or intermittent instillation or irrigation with a solution of amphotericin B (5% in sterile water, shielded from light) via a three-way bladder catheter (Wise *et al.*, 1982). Candidiuria confined to the upper collecting system may require treatment with oral 5-flucytosine or nephrostomy irrigation with amphotericin solution; however, 5-flucytosine should not be used in children with azotemia or bone marrow depression. Infants with obstructing renal fungus balls may require surgical removal via pyelotomy or percutaneous aspiration, followed by nephrostomy tube irrigation. Alkalay *et al.* (1991) reported the therapeutic use of forced diuresis with furosemide to clear fungus balls from the renal pelvis.

Fluid intake and furosemide therapy were adjusted to keep the urine output at a level of 4 ml/kg per hour.

The treatment of choice for systemic candidiasis is intravenous amphotericin B with or without the addition of 5-flucytosine. Amphotericin B is nephrotoxic and must be carefully titrated to obtain appropriate serum levels. Peak serum levels should be twice the mean inhibitory concentration for the infectious organism and trough levels should be equal to the mean inhibitory concentration. The duration of therapy is dependent on the extent of the disease; however, administration is often required for several weeks to eradicate systemic infections. Toxic side-effects include fever, nausea and vomiting, generalized malaise, and renal failure. Monitoring of serum creatinine every other day is necessary.

Other antifungal medications exist for the treatment of candidiasis. These include fluconazole, which has less associated nephrotoxicity than amphotericin B and is therefore preferred by some physicians. Its use has steadily increased in such closed populations as the neonatal nursery. Amphotericin continues to be the gold standard of treatment in the management of neonatal candidiasis as the incidence of fluconazole resistance will probably increase given its recent widespread use (Rowen and Tate, 1988).

Aspergillosis

Aspergillosis refers to a group of diseases caused by mycelial fungus of the genus *Aspergillus*. Aspergillosis is the second most common fungal infection in immunocompromised children (Walmsley *et al.*, 1993). *Aspergilli* are distributed worldwide, and spores are readily isolated from soil and decaying plants. Outbreaks of invasive disease usually occur among groups of immunocompromised children as a result of exposure to aerosolized spores at large construction sites near hospitals. Once the infection is acquired from inhalation of airborne spores, it is widely disseminated through hematogenous spread. The organisms may also be introduced through operative wounds, or indwelling foreign bodies such as intravenous or urinary catheters.

Microscopic hematuria and pyuria are often present in patients with aspergillosis. The fungi may be identified as branched septate hyphae on potassium hydroxide preparations of infected urine. Results of urine cultures are often inconclusive and multiple cultures may be required to make a diagnosis. Obstruc-tive uropathy resulting from an aspergilloma in the renal pelvis may be the initial mode of presentation (Eisenberg *et al.*, 1977). Invasive aspergillosis of the renal parenchyma is characterized by focal micro-abscess formation and occasional papillary necrosis.

Treatment of invasive aspergillosis remains high-dose intravenous amphotericin B. In patients with fungus balls in the renal pelvis, upper tract irrigation through a nephrostomy tube is indicated. Percutaneous or open surgical removal of obstructing aspergillomas is sometimes necessary.

Coccidioidomycosis

Coccidioidomycosis is an infection caused by the dimorphic fungus *Coccidioides immitis*, found in the soil of the western hemisphere. Endemic areas in the USA are confined to the south-western states, including Texas, New Mexico, Arizona, and southern California.

Genitourinary involvement occurs with disseminated disease. Autopsy studies (Conner *et al.*, 1975) of patients with disseminated coccidioidomycosis indicate that renal involvement occurs in approximately 60% of cases. Fungal involvement of the kidney is confined to the cortex as small miliary granulomas or microabscesses. Large, obstructive lesions within the renal pelvis do not occur as with other fungal infections. The radiographic findings of advanced renal coccidioidomycosis are similar to those of renal tuberculosis. They include infundibular stenosis, blunted or sloughed calyces, and calcified granulomas.

Antifungal chemotherapy is indicated for those at high risk for severe coccidioidomycosis and those with recognized disseminated disease. Currently available antifungal agents for use in treatment of coccidioidomycosis include amphotericin B, fluconazole, and ketoconazole. In the pediatric patient with rapidly progressing coccidioidomycosis, it is generally agreed that amphotericin B is the drug of choice.

Parasitic infections of the urinary tract

Schistosomiasis

Schistosomiasis is a parasitic disease that infects more than 200 million individuals, primarily children and young adults. Urinary schistosomiasis, or bilharziasis, is a vascular parasitic infection caused by the blood fluke *Schistosoma haematobium*. The disease is endemic in Egypt but can also be found in areas of Africa, Asia, South America, and the Caribbean. Prevalence is increasing in many areas, as population density increases and new irrigation projects provide broader habitats for vector snails. Rare cases are seen in the USA and always originate from an endemic area.

Humans are infected through contact with water contaminated with cercariae, the free-living infective stage of the parasite. These organisms emerge from infected snails and penetrate the intact human skin. The cercariae change into schistosomula in the subcutaneous tissues and then migrate to the portal circulation where they reach sexual maturity. Adult worms then migrate to the perivesical and periureteral venous plexus. Upon fertilization, female worms deposit eggs in the small venules which eventually reach the lumen of the urinary tract. Eggs are passed into freshwater, where they hatch, infect freshwater snails, and begin the cycle anew (Fig. 11.1).

Humans become infected with *Schistosoma* after coming into contact with contaminated water. Children of any age are most at risk through activities such as swimming, bathing, and drinking contaminated water. Acute schistosomiasis occurs between 3 and 9 weeks after infection and coincides with deposition of eggs in the bladder wall. The classic findings are terminal hematuria and dysuria. Bleeding can be so severe as to result in anemia. During the inactive phase of the infection, fibrosis and contracture of the bladder and distal ureter occur. The disease process is insidious and gross hydroureteronephrosis with renal insufficiency may occur before clinical symptoms appear.

Vester *et al.* (1997) defined the prevalence of schistosomiasis infection in an endemic region of Mali by screening 824 villagers. Infection ranged from 77% in adolescents to 51% in adults older than 40 years of age. Intensity of infection was generally low, with

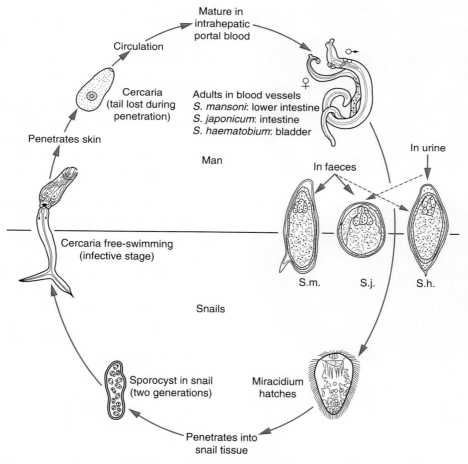

Figure 11.1 The life cycle of the schistosome. (From US Department of Health & Human Services, Public Health Services Publications, US Government Printing Office, Washington, DC, 1964, with permission.)

91% excreting fewer than 100 ova per 10 ml urine. Bladder wall enlargement and irregularities, bladder masses, and dilatation of the upper tracts were found ultrasonographically in approximately one-third of the individuals. Bladder lesions were more frequent in children than adults and correlated well with the intensity of the infection in younger age groups. The prevalence of urinary tract pathology dropped significantly with age, suggesting that either spontaneous resolution of urinary tract pathology occurs or the incidence in that population is increasing.

Schistosoma eggs produce a pronounced eosinophilic infiltrate within the bladder wall. As the disease progresses, collagen infiltration of the bladder occurs. There is deposition of calcareous material with ultimately sclerosis of the bladder due to calcification. Mucosal hyperplasia, squamous metaplasia and epithelial dysplasia of the urothelium may occur at any stage of the disease process. Involvement of the trigone and bladder neck is most pronounced. Eventual bladder neck fibrosis may lead to outlet obstruction. Stasis of urine and urinary infections may lead to vesical calculi while chronic bladder irritation predisposes these patients to squamous cell carcinoma. Vesicoureteral reflux (VUR) is reported in up to 50% of affected individuals as a result of fibrosis of the intramural ureter (Hanash and Bissada, 1982).

The diagnosis of schistosomiasis is established by the presence of terminal-spined eggs in the urine. A 24-hour urine collection with microscopic examination of the sediment is recommended. If infection is suspected and evaluation of the urine is negative, then cystoscopy and bladder biopsy may be necessary. Peripheral blood examination will usually show eosinophilia. Anemia may be associated with longstanding infection due to destruction of erythrocytes by the blood fluke.

Calcification of the bladder wall presenting an eggshell appearance on plain film of the lower abdomen is classic for chronic urinary schistosomiasis (Fig. 11.2). Hydronephrosis secondary to a ureteral stricture may be found on imaging studies of the urinary tract. On cystoscopic evaluation of the bladder, bilharzial tubercles predominate over the trigone and posterior bladder wall (Hanash and Bissada, 1982). Overdistension of the bladder results in bleeding. In patients with chronic disease, fibrosis and calcification of the tubercles in the submucosa form dull, granular 'sandy patches' that resemble grains of sand under water.

Various drugs are available for the treatment of urinary schistosomiasis, most of which carry significant side-effects. Management of children with schistosomiasis should be based on an appreciation of the intensity of the infection and the extent of the disease. The current drug of choice is praziquantel, which is effective against all species of *Schistosoma*. It is administered orally as a single or divided dose of 40–60 mg/kg per day (King and Mahmoud, 1989).

Surgical intervention in schistosomiasis should be reserved until the effects of medical management can be assessed. Fibrosis and contracture of the bladder may require autoaugmentation, intestinal augmentation, or bladder replacement. Bilharzial strictures of the lower ureter can produce obstructive uropathy. Extensive fibrosis of the ureteral wall and the bladder mucosa usually precludes ureteroneocystotomy by traditional submucosal tunneling. Bazeed *et al.*

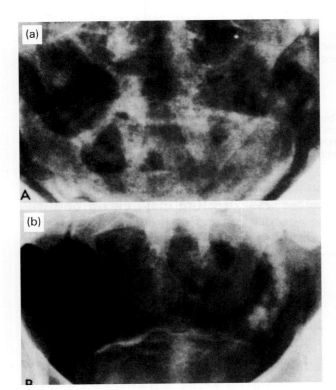

Figure 11.2 (*a*) Plain film shows curvilinear calcification of the bladder and both distal ureters. (*b*) There are numerous calculi in the left ureter. (From Hanash BA, Bissada NK, Lewall DB *et al.*: Genito-urinary schistosomlasis (bilharziasis): Part 2, Clinical, parasitologic, immunologic, and radiologic diagnosis. *King Faisal Specialist Hosp Med J* **1**: 119, 1981. By permission of the King Faisal Specialist Hospital and Research Centre.)

(1982) suggest a method of partial flap ureteroneocystotomy to alleviate distal obstruction. They report improvement or stabilization of the upper tracts in 83% of individuals. VUR may develop in as many as 30% of these individuals after surgery.

Echinococcosis

Echinococcosis is the most prevalent human cestode infection in the world. It is commonly called hydatid cyst disease. There is virtually no part of the human anatomy that is immune from hydatid cyst disease. It is caused by the dog tapeworm *Echinococcus granulosus*. Although uncommon in the USA, it is endemic in the sheep-raising areas of the world such as Argentina, Australia, Spain, and Greece.

Humans are an intermediate host for the larval eggs of the adult tapeworm. The adult tapeworm lives in the intestinal tracts of dogs and sheds larval eggs that are excreted in dog feces. Humans, as well as sheep, cattle, and pigs, may accidentally ingest these larval eggs through orofecal contamination. Dogs initially acquire the disease by swallowing the parasite scolex, which have become encysted in the liver or lungs of sheep, thus completing the life-cycle of this parasitic worm.

In humans, the larval eggs pass through the intestinal wall and are widely disseminated throughout the body. Dissemination may occur by direct, vascular, or lymphatic invasion (Angulo *et al.*, 1998). The primary organ affected in humans is the liver. Genitourinary involvement has been documented in the kidney, ureter, bladder, prostate, and epididymis (Halim and Vaezzadeh, 1980). The most common location for hydatid cyst disease in humans is the kidney. It is estimated that approximately 3% of all echinococcal infection involves the kidney (Silber and Moyad, 1972).

The largest series of pediatric echinococcosis was reported by Auldist and Myers (1974), who document 114 cases of hydatid cyst disease. Children of all ages were infected; however, manifestations of the disease were infrequently evident in children under 5 years of age. This is probably a result of the slow growth pattern of the hydatid cyst. The growth rate of hydatid cysts is estimated at 1 cm/year (Blanton, 1996). The cyst is typically very large at the time of initial presentation. The most common site of genitourinary infestation in the pediatric population is also the kidney. Hydatid cysts of the kidney usually present as a painful flank mass. Microscopic hematuria is present in the majority of the cases. Acute flank pain may be caused by rupture of the hydatid cyst into the collecting system. The passage of scolices (daughter cysts) may be associated with gross hematuria and urinary obstruction (Gilsanz *et al.*, 1980).

Sonography has proved to be the most valuable tool in the diagnosis of hydatid disease. Hydatid cysts are easily uncovered on ultrasonographic evaluation of the abdomen in children. The coexistence of hydatid disease in other organs assists in the diagnosis. Plain films or computed tomography (CT) of the abdomen and pelvis may also reveal calcification within the walls of these cysts. The diagnosis of echinococcosis is usually suspected when there is a history of contact with sheep dogs in an edemic area of the world.

As humans are infected with only an intermediate stage of *Echinococcus*, the actual parasite cannot be routinely recovered from any easily accessible body fluid. If the hydatid cyst has ruptured into the collecting system, the recovery of scolices from the urine is pathognomonic for genitourinary echinococcosis. Serological studies can also be useful in confirming the diagnosis of echinococcosis. Apt and Knierim (1970) report that eosinophilia is present in one-third of children affected with echinococcosis. Indirect hemagglutination and enzyme-linked immunosorbent assay (ELISA) are the most sensitive immunologic methods of diagnosing human hydatidosis; however, a false-positive reaction from other parasitic infections is possible (Angulo *et al.*, 1998). Immunoelectrophoresis to detect specific antibodies against antigens isolated from hydatid cyst fluid is currently the most specific method for diagnosing echinococcosis (Babba *et al.*, 1994).

Albendazole is the preferred drug for medical management of cystic hydatidosis. This drug therapy (15 mg/kg per day divided into three doses for 28 days) may be repeated for as many as four courses with 15 day drug-free intervals. A positive response is seen in 40–60% of pediatric patients treated (Blanton, 1996). Ultrasonographic indications of successful therapy include flattening of the cyst, increase in echogenicity, and detachment of membranes from the cyst capsule. The factors predictive of success with chemotherapy are age of the cyst (<2 years), low internal complexity of the cyst, and small size (Todorov *et al.*, 1992).

Although previously thought to be contraindicated because of the risk of anaphylaxis, percutaneous drainage of cysts under ultrasound guidance during albendazole therapy has become increasingly successful for complete resolution of cystic disease. Spillage of cyst fluid is uncommon during aspiration. Nevertheless, systemic anaphylactic reactions are always possible with spillage of cyst fluid.

Surgical therapy is also an option for solitary lesions or failed medical management. Considerable care must be taken at the time of surgical resection to ensure that there is no rupture of the cyst or spillage of cyst fluid during removal, as viable protoscolices may contaminate the surgical field. Each of these is capable of forming a secondary cyst wherever it lodges. There is also the risk of developing anaphylaxis as a result of spillage of cyst fluid at the time of surgical resection.

Enterobiasis

Pinworm infestation (enterobiasis) is caused by the nematode *Enterobius vermicularis*. Humans are infected by ingesting eggs that are carried on fingernails, clothing, or bedding. The adult worm lives in the large intestines of humans. The gravid adult female worm migrates at night to the rectum and deposits her eggs in the perianal and perineal skin. Perianal irritation during oviposition by female worms induces scratching. Eggs carried underneath the fingernails promote reinfection and dissemination of the disease to others. The peak age of infection is between 5 and 14 years.

Enterobiasis has been implicated as a factor in acute and chronic urinary tract infections (UTIs). In a study of female children, Kropp *et al.* (1978) demonstrated that 22% of girls with documented UTIs had pinworm infestations, compared with only 5% of an age-matched control population. They also reported that the recovery of pinworms from the perianal region is higher in girls with enteric organisms present on a swab of their introitus.

Definitive diagnosis is established by either finding the parasitic eggs or recovering worms. Eggs can be easily detected by pressing adhesive tape against the perianal region early in the morning. The tape is then applied to a glass slide and examined under low-power magnification. These repeated examinations are generally recommended to make a negative diagnosis.

Drug therapy should be given to all infected individuals. A single dose of pyrantel pamoate (11 mg/kg or maximum dose of 1 g) with a repeat dose at 2 weeks is the drug treatment of choice. Mebendazole (100 mg dose) with a repeat dose at 2 weeks is an alternative treatment. Neither is recommended in children under 2 years of age. Kropp *et al.* (1978) reported a greater than 50% success rate in eradicating multiple recurrent UTIs in girls with concomitant pinworm infestation when the infestation is definitively treated.

Other inflammatory diseases of the urinary tract

Chlamydial infection

Chlamydia are obligate intracellular bacteria that are distinguished by a unique developmental cycle. They possess their own DNA and RNA, contain ribosomes, and have a cell wall. *Chlamydia*, however, lack the ability to generate adenosine triphosphate and are therefore considered an energy parasite. *Chlamydia* alternate between an infectious metabolically inactive extracellular form, the elementary body (EB) and a non-infectious, metabolically active form, the reticulate body (RB). It is the EB that binds to specific receptor proteins on the cell membrane and enters the cell by endocytosis. Within 12 hours of cellular ingestion, the EB differentiates into the RB form and undergoes binary fission. This results in the typical intracytoplasmic inclusion bodies characteristic of a chlamydial infection. After approximately 36 hours, the RB differentiates back into an EB and is then released from the cell by a process of exocytosis.

Chlamydia trachomatis is the only one of the four chlamydial species that commonly infects the human genitourinary tract and also causes ocular disease. *Chlamydia trachomatis* is thought to be responsible for the majority of non-gonococcal urethritis and pelvic inflammatory diseases in adolescents. Rettig and Nelson (1981) also documented the coexistence of *Chlamydia* in boys with anogenital gonorrhea.

Chlamydial infections in children can be divided into two categories: perinatally transmitted infections and sexually transmitted infections in older children. Cervical chlamydial infections are found in approximately 25% of pregnant women. Active chlamydial infections at the time of pregnancy may be transmitted to the infant at the time of vaginal delivery. The risk of transmission from mother to child is about 50% (Hammerschlag, 1996). Conjunctivitis and pneumonia are the most common perinatally transmitted chlamydial infections. Genitourinary sites of perinatal transmission include the vagina and urethra. Perinatally transmitted vaginal, urethral, or rectal infections may persist for 3 years with minimal or no symptoms; therefore, the presence of *Chlamydia* in a young child is not an absolute indication of child abuse.

The most common chlamydial infections in older infants and children include vaginitis in girls and urethritis and epididymitis in boys. In boys, the most common symptom of chlamydial urethritis is a clear mucoid urethral discharge. It may or may not be associated with urinary urgency and frequency. In girls, acute inflammatory changes in the vagina or cervix may lead to mucopurulent discharge.

The definitive diagnosis of chlamydial infection includes isolation by culture of the organism from the urethra in boys and endocervical region in girls. Several non-culture methods have also been approved by the US Food and Drug Administration (FDA) that include a direct fluorescent antibody test or an enzyme immunoassay. Newer tests for the diagnosis of chlamydial infections use a DNA probe and a polymerase chain reaction assay. These two assays have not yet been approved for testing in children.

Antibiotics are the mainstay of therapy for chlamydial infections in children. These antimicrobials, usually sulfonamides, erythromycin, and tetracyclines, are typically given for 10–14 days. Tetracyclines should not be administered to children under the age of 8 years because of the resulting dental discoloration that may occur.

Viral cystitis

Viral cystitis causes irritative voiding symptoms and hematuria in infants and children. In the toilet-trained and older child, it is characterized by severe urinary frequency, urgency, incontinence and gross hematuria with a negative urine culture for bacteria. Severe hemorrhagic viral cystitis is seen more frequently in pediatric patients undergoing bone-marrow transplantation (Shields *et al.*, 1985). Viral cystitis also commonly occurs in the child infected with the human immunodeficiency virus (HIV). Viral infections can often be life threatening in these immunocompromised patients.

The usual causative viruses are adenovirus types 11 and 21, influenza A, and cytomegalovirus (Mufson

and Belshe, 1976). Studies of acute hemorrhagic cystitis in Japanese and American children revealed adenovirus type 11 as the most common cause. It was noted that 51% of the Japanese children and 23% of the American children had adenoviriuria during their episode of hemorrhagic cystitis. In both populations male outnumbered female patients by a ratio of nearly 2–3:1 (Mufson and Belshe, 1976). Viral shedding may continue throughout the duration of the illness and may last from 4 days to 2 weeks. Herpes zoster involving the bladder may also cause bladder irritative symptoms.

The diagnosis of adenoviral cystitis can be made by the immunofluorescence of adenoviral antigen in exfoliated bladder epithelial cells in the urine of these patients. However, this test is not commonly done (Belshe and Mufson, 1974). Since viral cystitis is not an ascending infection, routine voiding cystourethrography (VCUG) as part of the evaluation is not necessary if the diagnosis is confirmed. Radiographic changes within the bladder are remarkable and often resemble that of a bladder sarcoma. Ultrasonography may show a diffusely thickened bladder wall (Fig. 11.3) with areas of mucosal changes that suggest tumor. These changes usually resolve within 2–3 weeks. If complete resolution of sonographic bladder

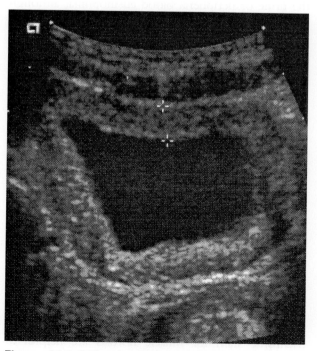

Figure 11.3 Diffusely thickened bladder wall of a 6-year-old boy with adenovirus cystitis.

wall changes occurs, then cystoscopy is unnecessary. These infections are self-limited and supportive care with hydration is often all that is necessary.

The immunocompromised pediatric patient may require additional management. The use of Ribavirin, an intravenous antiviral agent, has been suggested for treatment of acute adenovirus hemorrhagic cystitis (Jurado *et al.*, 1995). If treatment with aggressive fluid hydration and forced diuresis with furosemide has failed to control symptoms of hemorrhagic cystitis, some clinicians have advocated the instillation of prostaglandin E_1 into the bladder for up to 7 days (Trigg *et al.*, 1990) before resorting to chemical fulgaration with alum or formalin for those with intractable bleeding.

Eosinophilic cystitis

Eosinophilic cystitis is a rare inflammatory disorder of the urinary bladder that is characterized by severe, unremitting irritative voiding symptoms. These include dysuria, frequency, lower abdominal pain, and hematuria (Okafo *et al.*, 1985). Children may present with a palpable suprapubic mass on physical examination that occasionally is mistaken for a pelvic sarcoma (Thijissen and Gerridzen, 1990). Often the child will have a history of allergies. Eosinophils in the urine or peripheral blood eosinophilia, although diagnostically helpful, are frequently not found (Thauscher and Shaw, 1981).

Imaging studies of the bladder usually begin with sonography. Focal thickening of the bladder wall may be evident as well as hydronephrosis and hydroureter if the lesion affects the region of the ureteral orifice. These findings are similar to those of bladder sarcoma (Champion and Ackles, 1966). The definitive diagnosis is established by cystoscopy and bladder biopsy. Cystoscopic findings include erythematous, velvety, raised plaques. The mucosa is often edematous with areas of ulceration (Littleton *et al.*, 1982). Eosinophilic cystitis in children affects all parts of the bladder. Urethral involvement has been seen in only one reported case (Sujka *et al.*, 1992).

Biopsy findings demonstrate a classic eosinophilic infiltration of the lamina propria and muscle layers of the bladder. There may be muscle necrosis or significant muscle fibrosis. Giemsa stain for eosinophils and trichrome stain for muscle fibrosis are helpful in making the diagnosis (Hellstrom *et al.*, 1979). Electron microscopy is also a useful diagnostic aid. If eosinophils are degenerating, ultrastructural examination may be the only way to document their presence.

The true etiology of eosinophilic cystitis remains unknown. An immonoglobulin E (IgE)-mediated allergic cause has been suggested given the strong allergic histories of the patients. Food allergens, drugs, and other substances have been implicated (Wenzl *et al.*, 1964). It has been postulated that various inciting agents such as bacteria and foreign protein act as antigenic stimuli in the bladder to produce an eosinophilic infiltration. The antigens form immune complexes resulting in the release of lysosomes that break down bladder tissue and result in inflammation.

The treatment of eosinophilic cystitis involves removing the antigenic stimulus if present and identifiable. Identification of the antigenic stimulus may be difficult in a pediatric population. In a cohort of eight pediatric patients with eosinophilic cystitis, an identifiable cause could be found in only one case (parasitic infection). The role of antihistamines and steroids is unclear. Sutphin and Middleton (1984) reported that, of eight patients with biopsy-proven eosinophilic cystitis, only two received antihistamines and steroids. These individuals showed resolution of their symptoms and radiographic findings within 2 weeks. The other untreated pediatric patients also resolved their symptoms; however, the mean interval to resolution was greater than 7 weeks. The prognosis for children with eosinophilic cystitis is generally very good. Almost all reported cases in the literature resolved within 12 weeks.

Despite the apparent self-limited course of eosinophilic cystitis, it should be kept in mind that recurrence of this disease is possible. Documented recurrences have been reported several years after the initial event (Axelrod *et al.*, 1991). It has been hypothesized that local surgical trauma to the bladder or an anesthetic agent may be the cause for recurrence. A recommendation for pretreatment with steroids and antihistamines prior to bladder surgery has been made for patients with a previous history of eosinophilic cystitis (Axelrod *et al.*, 1991).

Malacoplakia

Malacoplakia is an unusual benign granulomatous condition that was first recognized by Michaelis and Gutmann (1902). It has been postulated that the cause is the defective digestion of phagocytosed bacteria due to an intracellular abnormality of macrophage function (Curran, 1987). Microscopically, malacoplakia consists of large macrophages mixed with lymphocytes and plasma cells. Michaelis–Gutmann bodies are evident on histological evaluation. They are rounded intracytoplasmic inclusions with a concentric 'owl-eye' appearance (Fig. 11.4). The Michaelis-Gutmann bodies contain incompletely digested bacterial components mineralized with iron and calcium phosphate salts.

In an affected adult population, malacoplakia involves the bladder in about 40% (Long and Althausen, 1989). Conversely, in a pediatric population, a wide variety of organs such as the tongue, gastrointestinal tract, lungs, brain, adrenal, and retroperitoneum may be involved. Although Witherington *et al.* (1984) described a case of bladder malacoplakia in a child with recurrent UTIs, VUR, and a selective IgA deficiency, in general renal malacoplakia occurs more frequently in children and may involve one or both kidneys.

Pediatric genitourinary malacoplakia occurs in the setting of recurrent urinary tract infections, usually with *Escherichia coli* (Long and Althausen, 1989). Renal malacoplakia is suspected in the pediatric patient when response to traditional antimicrobial therapy does not occur. These patients often have persistent nephromegaly without abscesses demonstrated by either ultrasonography or CT. Diagnosis is usually confirmed by renal biopsy (either open or percuta-

neous) showing chronic parenchymal inflammation with Michaelis–Gutmann bodies. Recent reports (Kapasi *et al.*, 1998) have confirmed the feasibility of diagnosis by cytologic evaluation of a renal fine-needle aspirate.

Previously, bilateral renal malacoplakia in the pediatric population was considered a fatal disease. Unilateral disease was frequently treated with nephrectomy. Honjo *et al.* (1997) suggest a conservative treatment plan consisting of an immunomodulating regime. Patients should receive antimicrobial therapy with an antimicrobial agent with intracellular activity (e.g. trimethoprim–sulfamethoxasole) as well as immunomodulating pulse therapy with methylprednisolone and intravenous granulocyte colony-stimulating factor (G-CSF). If a patient is on immunosuppressive therapy, they recommend appropriate reductions. With the advent of such treatment nephrectomy may no longer be mandatory in renal malacoplakia and the disease is no longer fatal in the pediatric population.

Other inflammatory diseases of the genitourinary tract

Epididymitis

Epididymitis has traditionally been thought of as a rare occurrence in the pediatric population. It results from an inflammatory reaction of the epididymis. This may be secondary to an infectious agent or a chemical irritant. However, often the etiology is not identified. Infection with bacteria or viral organisms is thought to be the cause of epididymitis in many of these boys, but in the majority, culture-proven UTIs are not documented (Quist, 1956). The retrograde passage of sterile urine into the epididymis may also incite an inflammatory reaction. Epididymal infection may therefore occur as a result of passage of urine from the bladder through the ejaculatory ducts (Megalli *et al.*, 1972), hematogenous spread from a systemic infection, or direct extension from pre-existing orchitis.

Boys with epididymitis usually present with scrotal pain and edema. They are exquisitely tender to palpation in the region of the epididymis and the vas deferens. A reactive hydrocele may also be present. The differential diagnosis of epididymitis in a child must always include testicular torsion, torsion of an appendix testis, and idiopathic scrotal edema. The

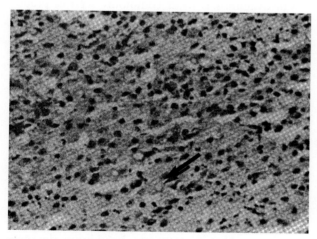

Figure 11.4 Bladder biopsy from a 2.5-year-old boy with *E. coli* urinary tract infection and hematuria. Inflammatory reaction with Michaelis–Gutmann body (*arrow*) seen in the lamina propria. (From Witherington *et al.*, 1984, with permission.)

onset of pain in boys with epididymitis is often more insidious than in boys with torsion of the testis or appendix testis. Careful physical examination, along with imaging studies, such as Doppler sonography or radionuclide testicular scanning, often aid in making the correct diagnosis. If a definitive diagnosis of epididymitis cannot be arrived at, surgical exploration may be required to exclude testicular torsion.

The use of urinalysis in making the diagnosis of epididymitis would seem to be a valuable discriminator; however, it is often inconclusive. Gislason et al. (1980) showed that only 24% of patients with epididymitis had greater than 10 white blood cells per high-powered field at the time of presentation. Urinalysis has also been reported to be abnormal in 10% of boys who present with testicular torsion (Ransler and Allen, 1982). Urine cultures are also unrewarding in making the diagnosis of epididymitis, as only 12.5% were positive in the cohort of boys with epididymitis that wasstudied retrospectively by Gislason et al. (1980).

The evaluation of a boy with epididymitis should not end once the diagnosis has been confirmed. This relatively rare problem in children is often enigmatic in its etiology. In prepubertal boys, bacterial infection in the epididymis may result from an anatomic defect such as a posterior urethral valve or an ectopic ureter draining into the seminal vesicle or vas deferens (Seigel et al., 1987). Urologic investigational procedures after resolution of the inflammation should be performed. Urologists vary widely in their recommendations for radiologic examinations. Most agree that, at a minimum, evaluation with a sonogram of the kidneys and bladder should be performed. Excretory urography would be the imaging study of choice to identify an ectopic ureter draining to a seminal vesical, while a VCUG would demonstrate urethral anomalies and reflux of urine into the ejaculatory ducts. If epididymitis is associated with a documented bacterial UTI, both VCUG and sonography should be performed.

The consideration of dysfunctional voiding has been proposed as an etiology for epididymitis in older boys (Bukowski et al., 1995). External sphincter spasm is thought to facilitate retrograde urine flow through the vas deferens. In their report of 56 boys with epididymitis, nearly 25% had dysfunctional voiding tendencies as the etiology of their epididymitis. Therefore, the addition of a detailed voiding history and the use of non-invasive urodynamic testing with uroflow, patch electromyography, and ultrasonographic residual urine assessment has been advocated for the evaluation of boys over the age of 5 years who present with non-bacterial epididymitis. It appears that congenital urologic anomalies are less frequently a cause of epididimitis in the absence of documented bacterial infection.

The treatment of acute epididymitis includes scrotal support and elevation, and analgesic and anti-inflammatory medications. If a bacterial infection is likely, an antibiotic may be started after obtaining a urine culture. Once the acute infection is treated, then age-appropriate studies to determine the etiology of the epididymitis should be undertaken.

Vulvovaginitis

Vulvovaginal inflammation is the most common gynecological complaint of the prepubertal girl. Most cases are initially treated by the primary care physician, with referral to the pediatric urological specialist only when symptoms persist.

The majority of neonatal girls has a profuse, thick vaginal discharge during the newborn period that is primarily a response to the perinatal stimulation of circulating maternal hormones. This is and should not be mistaken for a pathologic process. At puberty, both the vulvar and vaginal tissues are once again stimulated by circulating estrogens, and therefore swelling and discharge may once again be expected.

Vulvovaginitis is most commonly seen in prepubertal females between the ages of 2 and 7 years. The child is typically brought to the physician with complaints of discharge, discomfort, pruritus, and often urinary symptoms such as burning with voiding. The parents frequently note a discharge present in the child's diaper or undergarments. An abnormal odor and/or redness of the vulva may also be described.

There are several reasons why young girls are particularly susceptible to vulvovaginitis. Anatomically, the vulva of the young girl is relatively unprotected, lacking the labial fat pads and pubic hair of the postpubertal girl. Vulvar skin is also thin, sensitive, and easily irritated by minor trauma. In addition, the vaginal mucosa is thin and unstimulated by estrogen in this age group. The vaginal cavity in these prepubertal girls is also an excellent culture medium for bacteria, with its neutral pH and warm, moist environment.

These obvious structural and biological differences make the vulvovaginal environment of prepubertal girls particularly sensitive to inflammation. In addition, children tend to have poor hygiene habits when compared with adolescents. They do not practise good handwashing and often play in areas that expose them to dirt and sand creating chronic irritation of the vulva. The presence of a foreign body or suspected sexual abuse must also be considered in the list of risk factors for vulvovaginitis in the prepubertal girl (Farrington, 1997).

In evaluating the young child with vulvovaginitis, the preceding risk factors should be kept in mind. A complete history and detailed perineal examination must be performed. The history should include information concerning the onset of the condition and any therapies previously instituted for treatment. A history of potential chemical irritants should be elicited (e.g. bubble baths, soaps, powders). A previous surgical history and family history of diabetes, eczema, or contact sensitivities should also be addressed. The child's social setting should specifically be reviewed for information regarding potential child abuse (e.g. primary caregiver, day care, contact with older children). The physical examination should look for evidence of chronic illness, dermatologic problems, or traumatic injury. Most girls can be comfortably examined in the frog-leg position without the aid of sedation. Some sexual abuse experts recommend a knee–chest position for a complete examination. Cultures may be obtained by a sterile saline-moistened swab or a saline flush of the vaginal introitus. If bleeding or malodorous discharge raises the issue of a foreign body, then formal vaginoscopy may need to be undertaken under anesthesia. If a persistent and continuous watery flow from the vaginal introitus is present, then an ectopic ureter may enter the differential diagnosis. In this situation, excretory urography will assist in confirming the diagnosis.

The treatment of vulvovaginitis depends entirely on the etiology of the inflammation. Non-specific vaginitis accounts for the majority of these prepubertal cases of vulvovaginitis. It is thought to involve alterations in the normal flora of the vagina resulting in vulvar and distal vaginal inflammation. The vagina of a prepubertal girl is typically colonized with the same variety of bacteria as observed in older women. It may be appropriate to request colony counts on all organisms recovered from culture, as overgrowth by one particular organism may warrant antimicrobial therapy directed at that organism. Routine treatment of non-specific vaginitis is usually directed towards improved hygiene, avoidance of irritating stimuli, and techniques to promote drying of the vulva, such as wearing loose-fitting clothes at night.

Specific vaginitis in prepubertal girls may be the result of infections with *Candida albicans* and *Enterobius vermicularis* (pin worms). Treatments of these infections have been previously outlined. Other causes of specific vaginitis include sexually transmitted organisms such as gonorrhea, chlamydia, and herpes. The treatment of these infections is outlined in Table 11.1. These organisms may be acquired during passage of the newborn through the birth canal, or may result from sexual abuse or the simple sharing of infected underclothing. The age at presentation, along with social history and physical examination, will suggest the etiology.

Malodorous discharge with associated vaginal bleeding should alert the clinician to the possibility of the presence of a foreign body within the vagina. Eighty per cent of all foreign bodies present within the vagina are wads of toilet tissue lodged in the vaginal vault (Henderson and Scott, 1966). This may result in both an abacterial and non-specific inflammatory response. Various other foreign bodies have been recovered, including coins, safety pins, pen tops, fruit pits, and small toys (Hepp and Everhart, 1950). The probability of foreign bodies being recovered from the vagina of prepubertal girls presenting with vulvovaginitis is 4% (Paradis and Willis, 1985). The inflammatory response associated with the presence of the foreign body resolves with the removal of the object.

Table 11.1 Treatment of specific vulvovaginitis

Specific infection	Treatment
Gonorrhea	Penicillin G 100 000 IU/kg i.m. preceded by probenecid 25 mg/kg If allergic: Tetracycline* 40 mg/kg for 7 days
Chlamydia	Tetracycline* 40 mg/kg p.o. for 7 days
Gardnerella vaginalis	Metronidazole 15 mg/kg p.o.
Herpes	Acyclovir 1200 mg/day p.o. for 7–10 days

*Not to be used in children under 8 years old.

Idiopathic scrotal and penile edema

It is well known that acute scrotal swelling in children may primarily be due to conditions such as testicular torsion, torsion of the appendix testis, epididymoorchitis, acute hydrocele, or incarcerated inguinal hernia. There is, however, a lesser known clinical entity called idiopathic scrotal edema, that is characterized by painful scrotal swelling. This is a distinct clinical entity and may be responsible for up to 20% of cases of acute scrotal inflammation (Quist, 1956). It typically presents in boys between the ages of 1 and 14 years (Kaplan, 1977).

The largest single series of idiopathic scrotal edema is reported by Evans and Snyder (1977), in which they retrospectively review 30 cases in 26 patients over an 8 year study period. These boys usually exhibit a sudden 1 day onset of unilateral or bilateral scrotal wall erythema and swelling which is minimally tender. The edema may frequently extend onto the anterior abdominal wall or the perineum. The child is frequently afebrile with a normal urinalysis and normal peripheral white blood cell count. Occasionally, eosinophilia is present. When examined early in the process of scrotal swelling, the spermatic cord and testes should feel normal. Characteristically, the clinical findings resolve in 1–2 days. In Kaplan's (1977) report on six patients the edema was confined to the superficial layers of the scrotum, although it may extend to the penis. Lau and Ong (1981) report that a similar benign and self-limiting condition of the penis exists which is suspected to be a variant of idiopathic scrotal edema.

If the diagnosis is uncertain, radionuclide testicular scanning or Doppler ultrasonography may be necessary to exclude testicular pathology. Although, on physical examination this can often be achieved by manipulation of the testis into the superficial inguinal pouch where it can be noted to be palpably normal and non-tender. In the rare instance when diagnostic uncertainty continues to exist, scrotal exploration to rule out testicular pathology will reveal a normal testis and epididymis with the inflammation confined to the scrotal wall.

There has been much speculation on the etiology of acute, idiopathic scrotal edema. Infection with cellulitis was thought to be the etiology until multiple studies revealed negative cultures, no elevation of the peripheral white blood cell count and normal urinalysis and culture (Evans and Snyder, 1977). The process is also self-limiting and resolves without the use of antibiotics. Insect bites were entertained as a cause, but the lack of a lesion characteristic of a bite has made this less likely. Allergy has also be suggested as an etiology, especially given the presence of eosinophilia in selected cases. In no case, however, has a particular allergen been identified, and the majority of these patients is not characterized as having an allergic diasthesis (Kaplan, 1977).

Evans and Snyder (1977) suggest that idiopathic scrotal edema bears a strong resemblance to idiopathic angioedema, which is characterized by a localized painless swelling of the subcutaneous tissue of various body parts. The overlying skin is usually normal in color and temperature, but slightly reddened. The chief sensation is one of distension. The individual lesion may persist from 1 to 3 days. Angio edema results from a dilation of small blood vessels with a transudation of fluid through the capillaries. These vascular changes are believed to be mediated by a local derangement of histamine release. Recommended therapy consists of reassurance and perhaps a short course of antihistamines.

Interstitial cystitis

Interstitial cystitis is a chronic, debilitating bladder disease of unknown etiology that is seldom reported to occur in children. The first report of the disease was made by Skene in 1878. Since that initial report only a handful of manuscripts have documented this disease process in the pediatric population (Chenoweth and Clawater, 1960; Farkas et al., 1976; Close et al., 1996).

Patients with interstitial cystitis typically have severe sensory urgency with urinary frequency, and bladder pain is often temporarily alleviated with voiding. Cystoscopy after hydrodistension in these patients will show mucosal changes varying from petechial hemorrhage to regions with classic Hunner's ulcers. (Hunner, 1918). Middle-aged women comprise the majority of patients with interstitial cystitis.

Chenoweth and Clawater (1960) were the first to report on interstitial cystitis in children. In their series of seven cases they describe the presenting signs and symptoms as day and night frequency of urination, abdominal pain, decreased bladder capacity, and negative urinalysis and culture. In addition, these children were described as being extremely, nervous and tense, resting poorly, crying frequently and having poor appetites. Farkas *et al.* (1976) report that the pediatric cases of interstitial cystitis are more common in adolescent girls.

Close *et al.* (1996) reported the first large retrospective analysis of interstitial cystitis in the pediatric population, distinguishing this group of patients from the hundreds of individuals who present with voiding dysfunction. They characterized a group of 16 individuals who presented over a 12 year period. Unlike previous reports they described less of a female preponderance, with 70% girls and 30% boys in the study population. The most common presenting symptom was urinary frequency and urgency (88%), followed by abdominal pain relieved by voiding (81%). All patients had negative urinalyses and urine cultures.

Diagnostic evaluation of pediatric patients suspected of having interstitial cystitis consists of cystoscopy with hydrodistension. Close *et al.* (1996) reported that all patients had diffuse glomerulations and terminal hematuria after hydrodistension (60–70 cmH$_2$O for 1–2 min). Bladder biopsies obtained in select cases revealed chronic inflammation with lymphocytic infiltrate. No mast cells or eosinophils were noted. Urodynamic evaluation demonstrated early bladder filling sensation with no evidence of involuntary bladder contractions. Bladder capacity was also significantly reduced in these individuals. Poor bladder compliance was only documented in approximately 40% of patients (Close *et al.*, 1996).

Treatment of interstitial cystitis in children is met with the same disappointing results as in adults. Bladder distension may temporarily alleviate symptoms (Chenoweth and Clawater, 1960; Farkas *et al.*, 1976; Close *et al.*, 1996). Repeated hydrodistensions were required in 50% of the patients reported by Close *et al.* (1996). In rare circumstances chlorpactin instillations have been used with temporary and incomplete relief of symptoms (Chenoworth and Clawater, 1960). Although bladder augmentation with intestine has been reported (Farkas *et al.*, 1976) as a treatment option, inflammatory changes consistent with interstitial cystitis have been found in the bowel segment on follow-up, as well as recurrence of symptoms. Surgical management of this disease in children should be considered only when all other treatment options have failed and the diagnosis has been absolutely confirmed.

References

Alkalay AL, Srugo I, Blifeld C *et al.* (1991) Noninvasive medical management of fungus ball uropathy in a premature infant. *Am J Perinatol* **8**: 1330–2.

Angulo JC, Escribano J, Diego A *et al.* (1998) Isolated retrovesical and extrarenal retroperitoneal hydatidosis: clinical study of 10 cases and literature review. *J Urol* **159**: 76–82.

Apt W and Knierim F (1970) An evaluation of the diagnositic tests for hydatid disease. *Am J Trop Med Hyg* **19**: 943–6.

Auldist AW and Myers NA (1974) Hydatid disease in children. *Aust NZJ Surg* **44**: 402–7.

Axelrod SL, Ring KS, Collins MH *et al.* (1991) Eosinophilic cystitis in children. *Urology* **37**: 549–52.

Babba H, Messsdi A, Masmoudi S *et al.* (1994) Diagnosis of human hydatidosis: comparison between imaginery and six serologic techniques. *Amer J Trop Med Hyg* **50**: 64–8.

Baley JE, Annable WL, Kliegman RM (1981) Candida endopthalmitis in the premature infant. *J Pediatr* **98**: 458–61.

Bazeed MA, Ashamalla A, Abd-Alrzek AA *et al.* (1982) Partial flap ureteroneocystostomy for bilharzial strictures of the lower ureter. *Urology* **20**: 237–41.

Belshe RB and Mufson, MA (1974) Identification by immunofluorescence of adinoviral antigen in exfoliated bladder epithelial cells for patients with acute hemorrhagic cystitis. *Proc Soc Exp Biol Med* **146**: 754–8.

Blanton R (1996) Echinococcosis. In *Nelson Textbook of Pediatrics* (edited by RE Behrman, RM Kliegman and AM Arvin). Philadelphia, WB Saunder Co., pp. 995–7.

Bukowski TP, Lewis AG, Reeves D *et al.* (1995) Epididymitis in older boys. dysfunctional voiding as an etiology. *J Urol* **154**: 762–5.

Champion RH and Ackles RC (1966) Eosinophilic cystitis. *J Urol* **96**: 729–32.

Chenoweth CV and Clawater EW (1960) Interstitial cystitis in children. *J Urol* **83**: 150–2.

Close CE, Carr ME, Bums MW *et al.* (1996) Interstitial cystitis in children. *J Urol* **156**: 860–2.

Conner WT, Drach GW and Bucher WC (1975) Genitourinary aspects of disseminated coccidioidomycosis. *J Urol* **113**: 82–8.

Curran FT (1987) Malakoplakia of the bladder. *Br J Urol* **59**: 559–63.

Eckstein C, Koss EJ and Koft SA (1982) Anuria in a newborn secondary to bilateral ureteropelvic fungus balls. *J Urol* **127**: 109–10.

Eisenberg RL, Hedgcock MW and Shanser JD (1977) Aspergillus mycetoma of the renal pelvis associated with UPJ obstruction. *J Urol* **118**: 466–7.

Evans JP and Snyder HM (1977) Idiopathic scrotal edema. *Urology* **9**: 549–51.

Farkas A, Waisman J and Goodwin WE (1976) Interstitial cystitis in adolescent girls. *J Urol* **118**: 837–9.

Farrington PF (1997) Pediatric vulvovaginitis. *Clin Obs Gyn* **40**: 135–40.

Gislason T, Noronha RF and Gregory JG (1980) Acute epididymitis in boys. a 5 year retrospective study. *J Urol* **124**: 533–4.

Gilsanz V, Lozano F and Jimenez J (1980) Renal hydatid cysts: communicating with the collecting system. *AJR* **135**: 357–61.

Halim A and Vaezzadeh K (1980) Hydatid disease of the genitourinary tract. *Br J Urol* **52**: 75–8.

Hammerschlag MR (1996) Chlamydia In *Nelson Textbook of Pediatrics* (edited by RE Behrman, RM Kliegman and AM Arvin). Philadelphia, WB Saunder Co., pp. 827–32.

Hanash KA and Bissada NK (1982) Genitourinary schistosomiasis, Part I. *King Faisal Specialist Hosp Med J* **1**: 59–64.

Hellstrom HR, Davis BK and Shonnard JW (1979) Eosinophilic cystitis: a study of 16 cases. *Am J Clin Pathol* **72**: 777–84.

Henderson P and Scott R (1966) Foreign body vaginitis caused by toilet tissue. *Am J Dis Child* **111**: 529–32.

Hepp J and Everhart W (1950) Foreign body in the immature vagina. *Am J Surg* **79**: 589–91.

Honjo K, Sato T, Matsuo M *et al.* (1997) Renal malakoplakia in a four week old infant. *Clin Nephrol* **47**: 341–4.

Hunner GL (1918) Elusive ulcer of the bladder: further notes on a rare type of bladder ulcer with a report of 25 cases. *Am J Obst* **78**: 374–95.

Jurado M, Navarro JM, Hemandez J *et al.* (1995) Adenovims-associated haemorrhagic cystitis after bone marrow transplantation successfully treated with intravenous ribavirin. *Bone Marrow Transplant* **15**: 651–2.

Kapasi H, Robertson S and Futter N. (1998) Diagnosis of renal malakoplakia by fine needle aspiration cytology. *Acta Cytologica* **42**: 1419–23.

Kaplan GW (1977) Acute ideopathic scrotal edema. *J Ped Surg* **12**: 647–9.

King CH and Mahmoud AAF (1989) Drugs five years later. Praziquantel. *Ann Intern Med* **110**: 290–96.

Kozinn PJ, Taschdjian CL, Goldberg PK *et al.* (1978) Advances in the diagnosis of renal candidiasis. *J Urol* **119**: 184–7.

Kropp KA, Cichocki GA and Bansal NK (1978) Enterobius vermicularis, introital bacteriology and recurrent UTIs in children. *J Urol* **120**: 480–2.

Lau JTK and Ong GB (1981) Acute idiopathic penile edema. a separate clinical entity. *J Urol* **126**: 704–5.

Littleton RH, Farah RN and Cemy JC (1982) Eosinophilic cystitis: an uncommon form of cystitis. *J Urol* **127**: 132–3.

Long JP and Althausen AF (1989) Malakoplakia: a 25 year experience with a review of the literature. *J Urol* **141**: 1328–31.

Megalli M, Gursel E and Lattimer JK (1972) Reflux of urine into ejaculatory ducts as a cause of recurring epididymitis in children. *J Urol* **108**: 978–9.

Michaelis L and Gutmann C (1902) Uber einschlusse in blasentumoren. *Clin Med* **47**: 208–16.

Mufson MA and Belshe RB (1976) A review of adenovirus in the etiology of acute hemorrhagic cystitis. *J Urol* **115**: 191–4.

Muller FMC, Groll AH and Walsh TJ (1999) Current approaches to diagnosis and treatment of fungal infections in children infected with HIV. *Eur J Pediatr* **158**: 187–99.

Okafo BA, Jones HW, Dow D *et al.* (1985) Eosinophilic cystitis: pleomorphic manifestations. *Can J Surg* **28**: 17–18.

Paradise J and Willis E (1985) Probability of vaginal foreign body in girls with genital complaints. *Am J Dis Child* **139**: 472–6.

Quist O (1956) Swelling of the scrotum in infants and children and nonspecific epididymitis. *J Acta Chir Scand* **110**: 417–21.

Ransler CW and Allen TD: Torsion of the spermatic cord. *Urol Clin North Am* **9**: 245–50.

Rettig PJ and Nelson JD (1981) Genital tract infection with Chlamydia trachomatis in prepubertal children. *J Pediatr* **99**: 206–10.

Rowen JL and Tate JM (1998) Management of neonatal candidiasis. *Pediatr Infect Dis J* **17**: 1007–11.

Schonebeck J, Andersson L, Lingardh G *et al.* (1970) Ureteric obstruction caused by yeast-like fungi. *Scand J Urol Nephrol* **4**: 171–5.

Shields AF, Hackman RC, Fife KH *et al.* (1985) Adenovirus infections in patients undergoing bone marrow transplantation. *NEJM* **312**: 529–33.

Siegal A, Snyder HM and Duckett JW (1987) Epididymitis in infants and boys: underlying urogenital anomalies and efficacy of imaging modalities. *J Urol* **138**: 1100–3.

Silber SJ and Moyad RA (1972) Renal echinococcus. *J Urol* **108**: 669–72.

Skene AJC (1878) Cystitis. In *Diseases of the Bladder and Urethra in Women*. New York, William Wood and Co., pp. 167–72.

Stone HH, Kolb LD, Currie CA *et al.* (1974) Candida sepsis: pathogenesis and principles of treatment. *Ann Surg* **179**: 697–711.

Sutphin MS and Middleton AW (1984) Eosinophilic cystitis in children. a self limited process. *J Urol* **132**: 117–19.

Sujka SK, Fisher JE, Greenfield SP (1992) Eosinophilic cystitis in children. *Urology* **40**: 262–4.

Thauscher JW and Shaw DC (1981) Eosinophilic cystitis. *Clin Pediat* **20**: 741–3.

Thijssen A and Gerridzen RG (1990) Eosinophilic cystitis presenting as invasive bladder cancer: comments on pathogenesis and management. *J Urol* **144**: 977–9.

Trigg ME, O'Reilly J, Morgan D, *et al.* (1990) Prostaglandin El bladder instillations to control severe hemorrhagic cystitis. *J Urol* **143**: 92–4.

Todorov T, Mechkov G, Vutova K *et al.* (1992) Factors influencing the response to chemotherapy for human cystic echinococcosis. *Bull WHO* **70**: 347–58.

Vester U, Kardorflf R, Traore M *et al.* (1997) Urinary tract morbidity due to Schistosoma haematobium infection in Mali. *Kidney Int* **52**: 478–81.

Walmsley S, Devi S, King S *et al.* (1993) Invasive Aspergillus infections in a pediatric hospital. a ten-year review. *Pediatr Infect Dis J* **12**: 673–82.

Wenzl JE, Greene LF and Harris LE (1964) Eosinophilic cystitis. *J Pediatr* **64**: 746–9.

Wise GJ, Goldberg P and Kozinn PJ (1976) Genitourinary candidiasis: diagnosis and treatment. *J Urol* **116**: 778–80.

Wise GJ, Kozinn PJ and Goldberg P (1982) Amphotericin B as a urological irrigant in the management of noninvasive candiduria. *J Urol* **128**: 82–4.

Witherington R, Branan WJ, Wray BB *et al.* (1984) Malakoplakia associated with vesicoureteral reflux and selective immunoglobin A deficiency. *J Urol* **132**: 975–7.

Dysfunctional voiding disorders and nocturnal enuresis

Yves L. Homsy and Paul F. Austin

Introduction

Wetting disorders are mostly considered a nuisance associated with the growing years. Most children outgrow their particular disorder with maturation and wetting is usually tolerated until the child is found to lag behind his or her peers in achieving a state of dryness. By the time persistent wetters are brought to medical attention, they are often found to have developed a clinically significant symptom pattern. Attempts to address the problem do not usually follow a systematic and structured plan. The reason may be that there exists a spectrum of voiding disorders in children. Only recently have these disorders – or dysfunctions – acquired their letters of nobility to be recognized as scientifically founded treatable entities. In this chapter, it is our purpose to offer a classification of voiding disorders and management guidelines.

Historical note

Nocturnal enuresis has been described in early medical texts dating back in antiquity to the Ebers papyrus, with multiple dissertations on causes and remedies across the centuries (Glicklich, 1951). Daytime urinary incontinence, strangely enough, did not attract much attention. At the beginning of the twentieth century, Beer (1915) published the first paper on chronic retention with daytime wetting in children. There were very few publications on childhood voiding disorders prior to the 1970s. It was not until Hinman and Baumann's publication in 1972, followed by Allen's paper on the 'non-neurogenic neurogenic bladder' in 1977, that serious interest was generated in dysfunctional voiding. Until the mid-1970s, urodynamic studies in children were so cumbersome and impractical to perform, for lack of appropriate equipment, that they were not reproducible and therefore had little clinical value. By that time, more sophisticated electronic urodynamic equipment was becoming available and further insight could thus be gained into these heretofore unexplored disorders.

Definitions

Voiding dysfunction is a non-neurological disorder in which the voiding pattern of an individual is noted to deviate from what is expected for his or her particular age group and usually results in one form or another of urinary incontinence. There are several types of voiding dysfunction, each with its own characteristic features.

Enuresis is defined as normal voiding that occurs at an inappropriate time or occurs in a socially unacceptable setting and is involuntary. In general, the term enuresis is used to refer to nocturnal enuresis. However, as there are several subtypes of enuresis, it has become important to characterize the enuretic child so that type-specific therapy may be administered.

In previous pediatric urology texts it was customary to consider nocturnal enuresis and voiding dysfunction as distinct entities and to discuss them in separate chapters. There is, however, sufficient significant overlap in the features of enuresis and voiding dysfunction that they should be advantageously discussed together, pointing out the characteristics of each condition. It is not uncommon for an enuretic child to wet the underclothes during the day, nor is it unusual for a day-wetter to also wet the bed. In both situations involuntary urinary incontinence occurs in inappropriate circumstances. As etiological factors are becoming more clearly understood they are providing more focused therapeutic guidance. Various descriptive terms have made their way into the literature since the 1970s. However, confusion still persists over the appropriate nomenclature of some conditions. In 1997, the International Children's Continence Society generated a report on standardization and definitions for lower urinary tract dysfunction in children (Norgaard *et al.*, 1998).

Development of bladder control

To increase our understanding of abnormal bladder emptying, let us review how bladder control is attained in the developing child. Bladder emptying in the neonate is classically thought to occur as a result of a sacral spinal cord reflex (Muellner, 1960). This primitive spinal micturition reflex occurs when the bladder reaches a critical stretch threshold. Afferent signals are sent to the spinal cord to activate the parasympathetic outflow to the bladder and urethra and inhibit the sympathetic and pudendal storage reflex pathways (de Groat *et al.*, 1981). Consequently, this efferent reaction results in relaxation of the external urinary sphincter with detrusor contraction.

Few reports have described the voiding pattern of infants. Goellner *et al.* (1981) reported that urination in normal newborns occurred about 20 times per day during the first year of life. Similarly, Holmdahl *et al.* (1996) found that infants voided an average of once per hour, with only a slight decrease in the frequency of micturition during the first year of life. With postnatal development, the primitive spinal cord micturition reflex becomes inhibited or modulated by the pontine micturition center in the brainstem via a spinobulbospinal reflex pathway (Noto *et al.*, 1989). In addition, the development of segmental interneurons further modifies the primitive micturition reflex during this neural reorganization (Araki and de Groat, 1997).

As the infant and child mature, there is an increase in bladder capacity and voided volumes and a decrease in voiding frequency (Goellner *et al.*, 1981; Yeung, 1995; Holmdahl *et al.*, 1996). At approximately the age of 2 years, conscious sensation of bladder fullness develops, although the need to void is not yet fully mastered, resulting in 'physiological' urge incontinence (Hjälmås, 1988). It is believed that voluntary control of bladder fullness occurs from 2 to 4 years of age and that by the age of 4 years most children have acquired an adult pattern of voiding (Stein and Susser, 1967). Two large surveys exami-

ning age at the time of toilet training support this concept. Brazelton (1962) reviewed the charts from 1170 children and found that 26% of the parents said that their children achieved daytime continence by the age of 24 months and 52.5% by 27 months. By the age of 30 months, daytime continence rose to 85.3%, with 98% of the children reportedly trained by 36 months. Bloom *et al.* surveyed 1186 children and found the age of toilet training ranged from 0.75 to 5.25 years with a mean of 2.4 years (Brazelton, 1962; Bloom *et al.*, 1993).

There will be variations in attainment of bladder control and these milestones must be individualized. In general, the usual sequence of development of bowel and bladder control is as follows: (1) nocturnal bowel control; (2) daytime bowel control; (3) daytime control of voiding; and (4) nocturnal control of voiding (Rushton, 1995).

Classification of voiding dysfunction

Dysfunctional micturition may be divided into nonneuropathic or functional disorders, known as dysfunctions, and neuropathic disorders that are clearly associated with a neurologic condition such as spina bifida, transverse myelitis, or spinal cord trauma. This chapter will cover the non-neuropathic spectrum of wetting disorders ranging from monosymptomatic nocturnal enuresis to the Hinman and the Ochoa syndromes. Neuropathic disorders are addressed elsewhere in this book.

Dysfunctional voiding disorders may be classified according to their impact on the upper urinary tract. Three categories with 12 distinct types (see Table 12.1) have been identified, each with its own set of characteristics.

The moderate and severe disorders may occur in sufficiently serious forms to cause upper tract damage. Functional infravesical obstruction may result in vesioureteric reflux (VUR) or secondary obstruction at the ureterovesical junction. In both the Hinman and Ochoa syndromes, and in transient urodynamic dysfunction of infancy, some form of inappropriate relaxation of the external urethral sphincter complex seems to be present. The first six voiding disorders, while being relatively benign in that the upper tracts are usually spared, are the cause of much parental anxiety because of their chronicity and the negative effect produced on the child's self-image and social develop-

Table 12.1 Classification of voiding disorders

> A *Minor dysfunctional disorders*
>   Extraordinary daytime urinary frequency
>   syndrome
>   Giggle incontinence
>   Stress incontinence
>   Postvoid dribbling
>   Nocturnal enuresis
>
> B *Moderate dysfunctional disorders*
>   Lazy bladder syndrome
>   Overactive bladder
>   Dysfunctional elimination syndromes
>
> C *Major dysfunctional disorders*
>   Hinman syndrome
>   Ochoa syndrome
>   Transient urodynamic dysfunction of infancy
>   Myogenic detrusor failure

ment. Parents are also worried that there may be something serious that is wrong with the child's kidneys.

Diagnosis

The common denominator in voiding dysfunction is urinary incontinence without any underlying structural or obvious neurologic anomaly. The incontinence may either be diurnal, nocturnal, or both, and may or may not be associated with fecal retention or outright constipation. Careful questioning of the child and parents in as relaxed a manner as possible will often bring forth useful information. Although there is some overlap in the features of many voiding disorders, each has a characteristic pattern that makes it stand out sufficiently from the rest so as to be appropriately identified. Every effort should be made to understand the factors that contribute to each disorder so as to ensure that each factor may be appropriately addressed in the management plan. Ongoing parental/patient education and participation is emphasized. Significant patience is required until parents can fully grasp what is wrong with their child and what is required of them in the therapeutic process. Many are already frustrated with the child's persistent symptoms at the time of presentation. Family dynamics may be so altered in some cases that it may be difficult to initiate an effective therapeutic regimen.

Mild dysfunctional disorders

Extraordinary daytime urinary frequency syndrome

The sudden onset of daytime urinary urgency and frequency every 10–20 min without burning, dysuria, or incontinence characterizes this syndrome. It is seen more commonly in 3–8 year-olds. Typically, there is no nocturia or enuresis, although this may sometimes occur. The urine remains uninfected. A careful history is often all that is necessary to reach a diagnosis, because of the striking symptomatology. Imaging of the upper tracts and bladder is unremarkable and urodynamics are normal. Very few, if any, investigations are necessary other than urinalysis and culture. When the syndrome is suspected, one should refrain from delving into elaborate investigations because of their invasiveness, expense, and low yield. There seems to be an increased incidence of the extraordinary frequency syndrome in the spring and fall, although the etiology remains unknown. A behavioral component may sometimes be incriminated. Anticholinergics are of little help. The syndrome is self-limiting and tends to resolve almost as suddenly as it appeared, anywhere from 2 days to 16 months (average 2.5 months). Although recurrence is possible it is rare (about 3%). Reassurance is therefore the mainstay of therapy (Koff and Byard, 1988; Zoubek *et al.*, 1990).

Giggle incontinence (enuresis risoria)

In this type of incontinence a massive unexpected detrusor contraction causes the bladder to empty completely. The syndrome was recently attributed exclusively to peripubertal girls. Embarrassing wetting episodes occur almost exclusively with laughter but may be associated with exertion. The diagnosis is made mainly from the history. The urine is normal and the upper tracts are not affected. Urodynamics may show mild uninhibited contractions. The condition was believed to be self-limiting until it was recently noticed that it persisted into adulthood. Women learn to live with it by withdrawing from activities that will bring on excessive hilarity, thus avoiding exposure. Treatment includes anticholinergics and sometimes sympathomimetics. Reinberg *et al.* (1996) observed the occurrence of giggle incontinence in boys and girls and its persistence in adult women. They reported a favorable response to methylphenidate (Ritalin) administered in varying dose schedules for 1 to 5 years. Alteration of muscle tone may be precipitated by laughter and is suggestive of a functional relationship to cataplexy, a part of the narcoleptic syndrome complex that may respond to stimulant medication. Another therapeutic modality has been reported consisting of conditioning therapy. Inhibition of the voiding reflex was conditioned after self-administration of a harmless, painless, low-voltage electric shock to the back of one hand when incontinence was induced by laughter. Five children received eight sessions of 45 min duration. The frequency of wetting was reduced by a mean of 89% 1 year after treatment was completed (Elzinga-Plomp *et al.*, 1995).

Stress incontinence

Most commonly encountered in adult women, stress incontinence is not seen in childhood but is rather encountered in teenagers. Affected adolescents are usually athletic. In a large study of 156 nulliparous, college varsity female athletes with a mean age of 19.9 years, the prevalence of incontinence while participating in their sport was 28%. Incontinence induced by jumping, high-impact landings, and running was first noted by 40% of the young women when participating in their sport while in high school. In 17% it was reported to have started in junior high school. The proportion of incontinent subjects participating in different sports was: gymnastics 67%, basketball 66%, tennis 50%, field hockey 42%, track 29%, swimming 10%, volleyball 9%, softball 6%, and golf 0% (Nygaard *et al.*, 1994). The relationship between incontinence and force absorption on impact was assessed by foot arch flexibility. Medial longitudinal arch height was measured in the neutral gait stance and in the maximally dorsiflexed ankle position. The change in arch height between the two gait stances and the prevalence of incontinence showed a statistically significant association when there was decreased foot flexibility ($P = 0.03$) (Nygaard *et al.*, 1996). The mechanics involved in the transmission of impact forces to the pelvic floor may provide further understanding of the pathophysiology and management of stress urinary incontinence in the adolescent.

The upper tracts and bladder do not reveal any anomalies by either imaging or urodynamics. Ambulatory urodynamics was performed during exercise. Needle electromyographic assessment of pelvic floor muscles with simultaneous urethral and bladder pressure measurements revealed no uninhibited contractions during leakage episodes but there was a high prevalence of urethral sphincteric incompetence (Bo *et al.*, 1994). The degree of incontinence is quite minimal and can usually be managed by timely bladder emptying prior to exercising. A response to sympathomimetics may sometimes be obtained.

Postvoid dribbling (vaginal voiding)

Although patients presenting with vaginal voiding have a wetting problem, it occurs in girls only after they have finished urinating. When they get up, urine that has found its way into the lower vagina towards the end of voiding trickles into the underwear. The reflux of urine into the vagina, so frequently seen during voiding cystourethrography (VCUG), is a finding that is usually not accompanied by any symptoms. It is due to the recumbent position that is adopted for the examination and therefore has little clinical significance. Patients with postvoid dribbling often present with labiovulvar erythema and/or leukorrhea, which may cause burning, itching, and skin excoriation. The problem is typically encountered either in very small girls or, paradoxically, in obese girls. In the former, their tiny body habitus causes them to adopt a hairpin configuration on the toilet bowl, with their feet being unsupported during micturition. As the force of the urinary stream decreases towards the end of urination, this position favors the accumulation of a small amount of urine in the introitus and lower vagina. The condition is often diagnosed as a fungal vulvovaginitis that does not respond well to medication, as it is really secondary to a postural problem. Correction of the posture adopted during micturition will usually resolve the condition. Parents are asked to ensure that the child sits astride the narrower front section of the toilet bowl, facing the wall to ensure that the back is erect and the thighs are well separated. Alternatively, a toilet seat adapter or foot supports may be provided, but these may be cumbersome.

In obese girls, vaginal trapping of urine occurs for a different reason. These girls often do not spread their legs sufficiently apart when they void, perhaps because they are restricted by tight jeans or underwear. Asking them to void facing the wall will make them remove any restrictive clothing and their stream is likely to become more realigned towards the vertical than the horizontal. Recognizing that this condition is a functional postural anomaly will probably spare the child interminable treatments with inefficient creams and ointments.

Nocturnal enuresis

Although nocturnal enuresis is a minor dysfunction inasmuch as its effects on renal function are concerned, its etiology and management have remained elusive for many centuries. There has been a recent surge of significant research in this field. In order to avoid distracting the reader's train of thought with an extensive update at this point, nocturnal enuresis is discussed later in detail.

Moderate dysfunctional disorders

Lazy bladder syndrome (large-capacity hypotonic bladder, detrusor hyporeflexia, infrequent voider)

First described by DeLuca et al. (1962), this syndrome is characterized by the manifestation of the desire to void only every 8–12 hours, with incontinence in between.

The child will often not urinate upon awakening and only do so in mid-morning or even later. Bladder infections are frequent and constipation is usually also present. Patients may strain to void. The urinary stream is poor and unsustained and voiding is incomplete. Upper tract dilatation is sometimes found and the bladder is large and smooth-walled. Urodynamics typically demonstrates a large-capacity hypotonic bladder with a variable amount of postvoid residual urine. Outflow obstruction has not been demonstrated. Ruarte and Quesada (1987) studied 636 children without overt neurological disease or outflow obstruction urodynamically and established the incidence at 6.9% of incontinent children. Treatment is oriented to re-education of the bowel and bladder. Management of constipation or lesser degrees of fecal retention must first be diligently addressed with a bowel regimen tailored to the patient's degree of constipation. The management of constipation is pertinent to most forms of voiding dysfunction and will be addressed below in more detail. The administration of oral polyethylene glycol (Mizalax®) or sodium phosphate (Fleet®) enemas for a few days to empty the lower bowel of hard stool, followed by a stool softener and a 30 g fiber diet is beneficial before specific therapy is oriented to the bladder. Bladder retraining is achieved by timed double and triple voiding while constantly ensuring that bowel function is being attended to. Intermittent catheterization is the next step and should be maintained for a few months. After initiating a 6-hourly catheterization schedule, patients will usually start to void on their own without wetting. At that point, catheterization should be performed after voiding to measure residual urine, which will be found to diminish progressively. Encouraging results have recently been obtained with α_1-adrenergic blockers in a variety of conditions associated with poor bladder emptying, including the lazy bladder syndrome (Austin et al., 1999). At present, a trial with α-blockers should be undertaken before resorting to clean intermittent catheterization.

Overactive bladder (bladder instability, urge syndrome, hyperactive bladder, persistent infantile bladder, detrusor hypertonia)

As the most common voiding dysfunction encountered in children, the overactive bladder has a peak incidence between 5 and 7 years. Ruarte and Quesada (1987) found an incidence of 57.4% in a group of 383 incontinent children ranging in age from 3 to 14 years. The gender prevalence was 38.9% in boys and 60.1% in girls.

In children, bladder overactivity is believed to be due to a delay in the acquisition of cortical inhibition over uninhibited detrusor contractions in the course of achieving the mature voiding pattern of adulthood. The site of maturational delay is thought to lie in the reticulospinal pathways of the spinal cord or in the inhibitory center within the cerebral cortex. Cortical control over subcortical centers is normally established between 3 and 5 years of age. The subcortical centers subsequently modulate medullary automatism to achieve voluntary micturition control (Lapides and Diokno, 1970; Buzelin et al., 1988).

A delay in the fine-tuning of vesicosphincteric coordination during micturition will cause uninhibited detrusor contractions to be met with voluntary external urethral sphincter contractions, the control of which is acquired at an earlier age. An increase in intravesical pressure can manifest itself in an array of symptoms that include urgency, urge incontinence, and nocturnal enuresis. Disturbed voiding dynamics predisposes to the establishment of recurrent urinary tract infections (UTIs) and an acquired form of VUR. Reflux occurs in 33–50% of children with overactive bladders and can be associated with significant upper tract dilatation (Koff *et al.*, 1979; Snodgrass, 1991). Several studies have shown that addressing the overactive bladder, or the associated dysfunctional elimination problems when they are present, will triple the rate of reflux resolution in relation to controls (Koff and Murtagh, 1983; Homsy *et al.*, 1985; Seruca, 1989; Snodgrass, 1991; Koff *et al.*, 1998; McKenna *et al.*, 1999).

Constipation may contribute significantly to the symptomatology of the overactive bladder and must be delineated in the course of the patient/family interview (see Dysfunctional elimination syndromes, below).

Signs and symptoms

The overactive bladder manifests itself mainly by daytime urgency and incontinence. It may have a nocturnal component, which causes it to be sometimes confused with the symptoms of nocturnal enuresis. Some nocturnal enuretics also may have episodes of wetting during the day and this overlap is the source of difficulties in diagnosis and management. Nocturnal bladder instability has been demonstrated in about one-third of enuretics (Watanabe, 1994).

The uninhibited or overactive detrusor contraction that triggers bladder overactivity occurs early in the filling phase, causing the pelvic floor to respond by a voluntary contraction, which in turn gives rise to holding maneuvers such as leg crossing, squatting, or Vincent's curtsey. The passive external urethral compression that is achieved in this manner may possibly cause a temporary reflex relaxation of the detrusor, affording momentary relief from the effects of an uninhibited detrusor contraction.

A constant finding in the urge syndrome is a small functional bladder capacity for the child's age. This is due to a state of detrusor hypertonicity resulting from persistent neural overactivity that resolves as the condition improves. It is therefore a good clinical indicator of response to treatment. Functional bladder capacity is readily measured by the use of a measuring cup or urine specimen 'hat' that can be conveniently placed into the toilet bowl. Voided volumes are charted in a voiding diary for 2–3 days on a periodic basis.

The association of constipation or various degrees of fecal retention with the urge syndrome has led to speculation that the frequent voluntary pelvic floor contractions generated to combat incontinence episodes result in constipation. The condition often starts as a benign physiological dysfunction related to maturational delay and later becomes a chronic syndrome that requires an intensification of therapeutic measures (see Dysfunctional elimination syndrome).

Treatment

Several therapeutic modalities are available for the management of the overactive bladder of childhood.

Behavioral therapy

Alteration of behavior through bladder-retraining programs is labor intensive and often requires the involvement of a multidisciplinary team. This approach was used in a 2 week inpatient setting by a Belgian group in a cohort of 108 children with voiding dysfunction resistant to other therapies for more than 1 year. At 12 month follow-up there was a significant decrease in recurrence of UTIs with resolution of diurnal problems in 99/108. Nocturnal continence was attained in 92/108 for at least 3 months. Unfortunately, there were relapses in 28/92 patients. It was not clear whether the patients in that study had a problem with constipation and how aggressively that was addressed (Vandaele *et al.*, 1999).

Electrical stimulation

Biofeedback to retrain the bladder has been used in adults for more than 20 years and has met with reasonable success (Cardozo *et al.*, 1978). This therapeutic modality has also been used in children with varying degrees of sustained positive results (51–83%) (Hellstrom *et al.*, 1987; Jerkins *et al.*, 1987; Hoebecke *et al.*, 1996; Combs *et al.*, 1998; Schulman *et al.*, 1999). Difficulties in maintaining the child's attention are inherent to biofeedback therapy so that long-term results can be quite variable. Recently, a program was developed that makes use of computer games to maintain the child's interest. Game action is controlled by patient pelvic muscle activity and the program was carried out in an outpatient setting with very encouraging results (McKenna *et al.*, 1999).

An overactive bladder results from an overactivation or insufficient cortical inhibition of the micturition reflex. Neuromodulation has shown some success in the management of adults with bladder instability refractory to other forms of treatment (Bower *et al.*, 1998). The micturition reflex may be blocked by pudendal somatic afferent stimulation directly at the sacral cord. In children the use of transcutaneous neuromodulation (TENS) shows promise in the management of detrusor hyperactivity. Twenty-seven out of 40 children were placed on trial therapy for 1 month and showed sufficient response to continue therapy for 6 months with stimulation delivered via surface electrodes to the level of the S_3 foramen for 2 hours every day (Hoebecke *et al.*, 1999). Favorable response rates were seen in 70–75% with this mode of therapy, with a cure rate of 56% at 1 year in this pilot study. Alternatively, the surface electrodes may be placed suprapubically, in which case stimulation is increased to 150 Hz.

Pharmacologic therapy

Propantheline (Probanthin) has long been available as a smooth muscle relaxant of the bowel. Anticholinergic effects were found to extend to the bladder and this agent has been used to treat bladder overactivity for many years. Oxybutynin chloride (Ditropan) then became available and was found to have a more specific action on the bladder, while still having some effect on the bowel. A sustained-release preparation is now available (Ditropan XL). Hyoscyamine preparations are also effective in achieving detrusor relaxation and they are available in different forms, from sublingual to sustained release (Levsin, Levsinex). Glycopyrrolate (Robinul) is also sometimes used.

The newest addition to this group of medications is tolterodine (Detrol). It is an antimuscarinic agent that is relatively selective for the bladder. Tolterodine has been found to have comparable efficacy to oxybutynin in adults and produces less mouth dryness (Abrams *et al.*, 1998). Its safety profile, efficacy, and pharmacokinetics have recently been established in children 5–10 years old with a body weight of 17–39 kg (Hjälmås *et al.*, 1999).

The anticholinergic effects of the medications mentioned above rely on partial blockade of the efferent parasympathetic innervation to the detrusor. Systemic side-effects often preclude the use of sufficiently high doses to combat detrusor overactivity. The periodic intravesical instillation of capsaicin or resiniferatoxin holds promise. They are specific neurotoxins that desensitize the C-fiber afferent neurons, responsible for triggering detrusor overactivty. While the side-effect profile of capsaicin may preclude its use in children, resiniferatoxin, an ultrapotent analog of capsaicin with fewer side-effects, may be more useful (Chancellor and de Groat, 1999).

Dysfunctional elimination syndrome

The common association of fecal elimination disturbances with dysfunctional voiding syndromes led Koff and associates to coin the phrase 'dysfunctional elimination syndromes' (DES). These syndromes comprise functional bowel and/or bladder disorders, including bladder instability, constipation, and infrequent voiding (lazy bladder). The effects of dysfunctional elimination on the upper tract are not negligible. In a group of 143 children thought to have primary VUR, 66 patients (43%) manifested bowel and bladder disturbances. Eighty-two per cent of these children had breakthrough infections and required reimplantation surgery, as opposed to 18% without the syndromes. After reflux resolution, the rate of recurrent UTI remained four times higher in children with DES. Unsuccessful surgical outcomes with reimplantation surgery only occurred in children with DES and high intravesical pressure (Koff *et al.*, 1998). Recurrent UTI is the sounding board that should alert the clinician to screen patients for DES even in the absence of reflux. Parents have a tendency to be more aware of voiding problems in their children than of problems with defecation, as the latter are more subtle in their manifestations.

Major dysfunctional disorders

Hinman syndrome

> *The bladder is the mirror of the soul ...*
> Confucius, 551–479 BC

Severe voiding dysfunction was recognized in the first half of the twentieth century and first reported by Beer (1915). He attributed the condition to 'disharmony between the detrusor and sphincter muscles or relative hypertonicity of the sphincter'. He was right. Laidley (1942) recognized a syndrome of incoordination and called it achalasia of the urinary tract. In 1954 and again in 1969, Williams reported similar cases (Williams, 1954; Williams and Taylor, 1969). Paquin *et al.* (1960) reported on 27 children with a large bladder and symptoms of dysfunctional voiding and called it the megacystis syndrome.

Ambrose and Swanson (1960) noted that in 13 children with what they labeled 'hypertonic-type neurogenic bladders', there was no neurologic lesion. Hinman and Baumann (1972) observed voiding disturbances associated with upper tract damage in two boys aged 8 and 10 years who did not manifest any anatomical obstruction or neurologic stigmata. They did, however, have a psychological disturbance. To emphasize the absence of neurological disease, the term 'non-neurogenic neurogenic bladder' was coined. As this term seemed to cause some confusion the condition became known as the Hinman syndrome in 1986. It must be recognized that urodymamic equipment was rather crude and lacked precision until the mid-1970s. Allen (1977) reported on 21 well-documented cases of 'non-neurogenic neurogenic bladders', of which he described four in detail. He confirmed that this was an acquired disorder and could identify psychopathological features in about one-half of his patients. His vibrant message was that reconstructive surgical procedures were associated with a high failure rate in these patients and that bladder retraining should be the mainstay of therapy. The following features originally characterized the Hinman syndrome: (1) a common age of onset between childhood and puberty of voiding dysfunction in mostly boys without neurologic or obstructive disease; (2) a clinical picture of wetting during the daytime as well as at night with fecal retention and soiling (encopresis); (3) UTI; (4) a spectrum of radiological abnormalities from bladder trabeculation to ureterovesical obstruction or reflux, as well as dilatation of the upper urinary tract and renal damage; (5) no demonstrable neurologic disease; (6) no demonstrable bladder outlet obstruction; (7) failure of surgical reparative procedures; (8) a psychological make-up best described as personality failure; and (9) improvement after re-education and suggestion therapy.

The features have remained the same except that girls are now more often included and pharmacotherapy is being used more than suggestion therapy. Neurologic examination must be normal. Psychologic disturbances are not always evident and their detection, although helpful, is not quintessential to establishing a diagnosis.

Etiology

According to Hinman (1986), 'the syndrome is a functional disorder and it is useful clinically to think of it as a bad habit that develops in children of certain personality types in an unfavorable family setting. The condition is reversible for the same reasons.' Despite extensive attempts to find an underlying lesion by means of state-of-the-art diagnostic methods including computed tomographic (CT) scans and magnetic resonance imaging (MRI), the consensus remains that affected children are neurologically normal. They manifest an inability to inhibit the detrusor reflex as well as overcompensatory activity of the external sphincter/pelvic floor. The warning of an imminent detrusor contraction is either not perceived or ignored. In order to avoid wetting, the child must forcibly contract the external sphincter/pelvic floor. Although this may work initially, the resulting imbalance eventually results in incontinence, an intermittent stream, residual urine, infection, and structural damage to the urinary tract due to high bladder pressure. The varied impact of emotions over micturition have been extensively reviewed in the literature (Galdston and Perlmutter, 1973; Schmitt, 1982). They are mainly related to stress, fright, depression, phobias, confused priorities, trauma associated with toilet training (including fear of falling), excessive parental pressure, and sexual abuse (Koff *et al.*, 1979; Hinman, 1986; Ellsworth *et al.*, 1995).

Diagnosis

Most patients will present with incontinence associated with chronic urinary retention. An intermittent voiding pattern with reduced flow rates and prolonged voiding time can be seen on uroflowmetry. Elevated postvoid residuals may or may not be present. Clinical examination will fail to reveal a neurological abnormality. Renal function is often reduced, with elevations in serum creatinine and reduced clearance. Hypertension may be present.

Renal/bladder sonography will show varying degrees of unilateral or bilateral hydronephrosis with or without dilatation of the ureters. Bladder wall thickening should be assessed and the examination should be repeated after emptying the bladder. This will help to determine whether ureteral dilatatation is secondary to bladder dysfunction rather than an intrinsic ureterovesical junction obstruction. The presence of renal scarring should be noted and monitored by dimercaptosuccinic acid (DMSA) renal scans.

VCUG may show varying grades of reflux, either a trabeculated or an enlarged, decompensated bladder with failure to empty completely. Careful attention to the urethra may yield clues as to the effects of sphincteric overactivity such as posterior urethral dilatation in boys or a 'spinning-top' urethra in girls with poor visualization of the anterior urethra.

Urodynamics may show a variety of patterns depending on the severity and duration of this acquired malfunction. Uroflowmetry usually demonstrates intermittency with reduced flow rates and prolonged voiding as mentioned above. Cystometric findings will depend on the stage of the disease, with uninhibited contractions early on and bladder atony in advanced cases, with myogenic detrusor failure. Initially, detrusor hyperreflexia is associated with sphincteric dyssynergia. The electromyographic tracing differs from that of dyssynergia associated with neurologic bladder disease (as in spinal transection) in the timing of onset of sphincteric contraction (Rudy and Woodside, 1991). With time and as the detrusor decompensates, a broad spectrum of dysfunction may be found. Some cases may show detrusor hypotonia or atony while the sphincter may or may not be hyperactive. Griffiths and Scholtmeijer (1983) thoroughly studied 143 children with detrusor-sphincter dyssynergia and found a variety of patterns of activity both in the detrusor and in the urethra. These authors introduced the concept of consistent urethral overactivity that they found to be significantly more common in children with upper tract changes.

MRI should be performed to rule out cord tethering and other neurologic lesions before reaching a final diagnosis.

Psychological problems may not be evident initially. History taking must ensure that all diagnostic elements pointing toward the diagnosis are present, with an emphasis on the psychosocial and economic status of the patient's family. Unemployment, alcoholism, divorce, sexual abuse, and a dominating or overprotective parent are the rule. Cultural problems in migrant families may be a source of social pressure to which the child is exposed. Paradoxically, in some cases, the child may appear quite happy rather than withdrawn, seeming to have found a way to become articulate and to get attention through the disease (Variam and Dippell, 1995). Psychologic intervention should be introduced at the most opportune time in a collaborative manner among the psychologist, urology nurse/urotherapist, and pediatric urologist.

Treatment

Treatment is multimodal and must be personalized. It is aimed at restoring balanced voiding and at preventing upper tract deterioration. In some cases the impact of psychological factors on the etiology and management may be quite profound (Phillips and Uehling, 1993). In other cases it is less significant.

Hinman considers involuntary wetting from psychological causes the hallmark of the syndrome. He therefore recommends suggestion and hypnosis after psychological evaluation. Allen prefers to focus on bladder retraining with or without intermittent catheterization and resorts to psychotherapy in patients with major psychological disturbances and in those in whom the condition persists into puberty. Biofeedback is now used in the home setting after a few training sessions with experienced personnel.

Drug therapy is guided by urodynamic findings and includes anticholinergics and α-blockers either alone or in combination. Dosage will need careful adjustment and will depend on patient response as determined by periodic imaging and urodynamic evaluation.

Recently, therapy has been tried with botulinum-A toxin in an attempt to cause striated muscle paralysis. Presynaptic release of acetylcholine at the neuromuscular junction is inhibited by the toxin, which binds selectively to specific receptors on the cell surface without causing damage to peripheral nerves. The procedure is widely used in ophthalmology in the management of ocular muscle spasms and strabismus. It has been used to treat vesicosphincteric dyssynergia in patients with spinal cord injury (Schurch et al., 1996). Steinhardt et al. (1997) used it in managing a young girl with dysfunctional voiding who was refractory to other forms of treatment. Repeated injections may be necessary every few months. As the degree of paralysis produced is dose dependent and reversible, this method may eventually find its place in the management of the Hinman syndrome.

It has become clear that therapeutic strategies must be tailored to the individual. Sensate patients may not be compliant with their intermittent catheterization regimen, thus allowing renal function to deteriorate further. However, psychological management may cause delays in the initiation of specific therapy targeted to the urinary tract. It is therefore essential to ensure that the patient receives the full benefit of well-orchestrated multimodal therapy. In some centers major psychological problems are excluded by an adapted psychological history taking that follows the criteria of the DSM-III classification for major behavioral problems (American Psychiatric Association, 1987; Hoebecke *et al.*, 1996). The order in which therapeutic intervention occurs will have to depend on the circumstances. Appropriate timing and close follow-up will allow assessment of the progress being achieved. If the upper tracts continue to deteriorate, then temporary urinary diversion as dictated by the child's age and condition should be considered.

Ochoa (urofacial) syndrome

Similar in many ways to the Hinman syndrome, the urofacial syndrome was first described by Bernardo Ochoa of Medellin, Colombia, in 1979 and it was soon to be named after him (Ochoa and Gorlin, 1987). The prevalence is rather low, and fewer than 200 cases have been identified. The syndrome is of particular interest because, in addition to the features usually found in the Hinman syndrome, it is genetically determined and is associated with an unusual inversion of facial expression when smiling is attempted. The face becomes contorted into a grimace that makes it appear as if the subject is sobbing or crying, thus making it possible to recognize afflicted patients early in life (Ochoa, 1992). In addition, the Ochoa syndrome is characterized by hereditary transmission.

Etiology

Patients with the Ochoa syndrome can be identified as early as the age of 2 years. The consistent relationship between the grimacing expression on their faces when they attempt to smile and their dysfunctional voiding, together with the recessive pattern of inheritance, led Ochoa to hypothesize that the syndrome has an organic rather than acquired etiology. The micturition reflex is processed in the reticular formation of the brainstem, in close anatomical proximity to the origin of the facial nerves. Lesions within the reticular formation are expected to produce functional lesions affecting coordination, rather than paralytic or paretic lesions as when the nuclei are involved, making it more difficult to localize the site of the lesion with precision.

Genetics

It was originally suggested by Elejalde (1979) that the mode of inheritance was autosomal dominant with variable expressivity and incomplete penetrance. The subsequent discovery of many additional families with the features of the syndrome with several siblings affected, normal parents, and parental consanguinity made it clear that inheritance was autosomal recessive (Cardozo *et al.*, 1978).

The urofacial syndrome (UFS) gene was mapped recently in the immunology laboratories of the University of Florida, using a genome screen and a combination of homozygosity-mapping and DNA-pooling strategies in families from Colombia. The gene was mapped to a genomic interval of approximately 1 cM on chromosome region 10q23–24 (Wang *et al.*, 1997). Subsequently, genetic homogeneity of the syndrome was demonstrated through homozygosity mapping in American patients of Irish heritage. The precise location of the gene within the UFS critical region and its genomic structure were determined (Wang *et al.*, 1999).

Clinical features

As already mentioned, the urologic features resemble those of the Hinman syndrome. They are, however, detected earlier because, as the syndrome runs in families, patients are screened sooner, particularly if they exhibit the characteristic grimacing.

Management

Bladder re-education is the mainstay of therapy, with a combination of anticholinergics, antibacterials, and attempts at relaxing the external sphincter region. α-blockers may play a role in this endeavor. Intermittent catheterization or temporary vesicostomy may be needed in some patients. As with the Hinman syndrome, constipation constitutes a major problem and must be vigorously addressed.

Transient urodynamic dysfunction of infancy

It was first shown by Sillén *et al.* (1992) that high-grade reflux in infancy can be accompanied by very high voiding pressures. These authors recently reported an increased spontaneous resolution rate of high-grade reflux in infants with smaller bladder capacities who manifested hypercontractility (27% in grades V and 40% in grades III–IV) (Sillén *et al.*, 1999a). Yeung *et al.* (1997) reported on a number of infants with antenatally detected hydronephrosis associated with thick-walled bladders. At birth, the neonates, mainly boys, were found to have high-grade reflux without any detectable infravesical obstruction despite carefully performed cystography and cystoscopy. Post-mortem dissections were performed, focusing on the bladder neck and external urinary sphincter in 23 cadaver specimens of human fetuses, neonates, infants, and young boys and girls. The findings revealed that the human external urinary sphincter can first be identified at 20–21 weeks of gestation as a complete ring of undifferentiated striated muscle. As differentiation progresses, the sphincter changes its ring-like appearance to assume a horseshoe or omega configuration. This is the classic appearance of the external sphincter in adults. The hypothesis was developed that high intravesical pressures encountered in early life may be related to the ring-shaped configuration of the sphincter (Kokoua et al., 1993). The normalization of intravesical pressures associated with improvement or spontaneous reflux resolution seems to coincide with the period at which the external sphincter assumes the split-ring, omega configuration. The 'splitting' of the sphincter appears to progress from caudal to rostral. It was also postulated that the configuration change from ring to omega possibly decreases outflow resistance and intravesical pressures. Clinical support for this theory may be found in several studies (Sillén et al., 1992; Yeung et al., 1997; Sillén et al., 1999a).

In addition, a study by Chandra et al. (1996) demonstrated high voiding pressures in 39 male and 22 female infants undergoing urodynamics in the course of investigation for UTI and/or reflux. Abnormal voiding was more frequently detected in males (97%) than in females (77%), including high voiding pressures ($>40 \, cmH_2O$) in 92% of the male and 66% of the female infants. Follow-up urodynamics of the 15 infants revealed spontaneous resolution of detrusor hyperreflexia and decreased voiding pressure in 14. Chandra et al. coined the term 'transient urodynamic dysfunction of infancy' to describe voiding abnormalities that predispose infants to UTI and reflux but improve spontaneously (Chandra, 1995; Chandra et al., 1996). Yeung et al. (1998) compared urodynamic patterns in infants with primary grade III–V VUR with those in infants with normal lower urinary tracts. They found abnormal urodynamic patterns in 24 of 42 refluxing infants (57%). The spectrum of detected abnormalities included unstable bladders with small voided volumes in seven infants, markedly dyssynergic patterns in 10, obstruc-

tive patterns in two, and inadequate voiding dynamics in five. The most severe manifestations of this clinical entity were described by Jayanthi et al. (1997) in five male and two female patients. It appears possible to identify patients at risk noninvasively by observing their free voiding pattern on a 4 hour observation basis. Low-capacity voiders void frequently and in small amounts, whereas high-capacity voiders void large volumes at infrequent intervals and have increased residuals. These findings were confirmed urodynamically by Sillen et al. (1999b).

Myogenic detrusor failure

Myogenic detrusor failure occurs as end-stage bladder decompensation. It is frequently seen in patients with neuropathic bladders. In the non-neuropathic context of voiding dysfunction it can be encountered in patients with the Hinman and Ochoa syndromes. It can also be seen in patients with posterior urethral valves (PUV) who were treated in infancy. As this altered detrusor state takes time to develop, patients have typically reached early adolescence by the time it is recognized. Some of them will have achieved balanced voiding but may carry a moderate amount of residual urine. They may thus be prone to develop recurrent UTIs. Hydronephrosis is the result of the earlier hyperreflexic state of the detrusor before decompensation and usually remains stable. These patients may require intermittent catheterization or α-blocker therapy.

Defecation and micturition: are they related?

Man should strive to have his intestines relaxed all the days of his life.

Moses Maimonides, AD 1135–1204

Normal defecation

The stimulus for defecation is initiated by rectal distension. The rectum normally distends when peristaltic activity propels feces from the sigmoid colon into the rectum, stimulating sensory receptors in the rectal wall that will allow the sensation of distension to be perceived and recognized. Perception of rectal distension (through sensory ascending fibers) causes a voluntary temporary contraction of the striated external sphincter and puborectalis muscles. Voluntarily maintaining this contraction will cause the rectum to adapt to the increased volume and the sense of fecal urgency disappears until the arrival of another fecal bolus. Distension of the rectal wall will generate a nervous impulse that is transmitted distally through its wall via the myenteric plexus, activating the rectosphincteric relaxation reflex and causing smooth muscle relaxation in the internal anal sphincter. The degree of relaxation is in proportion to the fecal volume and the speed at which the rectum is distended. An increase in intra-abdominal pressure lowers the pelvic floor, thereby increasing intrarectal pressure. Relaxation of the external sphincter allows the fecal bolus to be expelled.

Fecal retention, constipation, and voiding dysfunction

It is difficult to quantify degrees of constipation other than in the most overt forms. There are several forms of constipation that are secondary to diseases such as Hirschsprung's disease or anal stenosis. The most common variety encountered in children is functional constipation. This motility disorder usually sets in after the age of toilet training. Whether it is due to 'overlearning' of control over excretory functions, or to other factors such as insufficient fiber intake, is not quite clear. The memory of painful defecation is one of the factors that has been incriminated. There has been recent interest in the study of childhood functional gastrointestinal disorders (FGIDs) for which criteria have been defined by a multinational taskforce (Rasquin-Weber et al., 1999).

Because the bladder and rectosigmoid are anatomical neighbors, their innervation shares a common circuitry and it is not unusual that disturbances in lower urinary tract function might also affect bowel function and vice versa (Issenman et al., 1999). This association is not new, as Swenson (1952) showed that constipation and megaureter appeared to be etiologically linked. Shopfner (1968) reported 39 constipated children aged 5–13 years in whom fecal retention was radiologically demonstrable who also had a high incidence of enuresis (54%), bladder wall irregularity (31%), hydronephrosis (31%), and reflux (20%). It is widely accepted that organic constipation in diseases such as Hirschsprung's disease, congenital anal stenosis, and ectopic-anterior anus are often seen in

association with urinary tract pathology such as hydroureteronephrosis and UTI. Several studies now confirm that functional constipation is closely related to dysfunctional voiding disorders, recurrent UTIs, and possibly VUR (O'Regan et al., 1985; Yazbeck et al., 1987; Koff et al., 1998). Incomplete pelvic floor relaxation may result in hesitancy, a weak or interrupted stream, holding maneuvers, and bladder decompensation with large postvoid residuals. By the same token, fecal retention will also be present with an enlarged rectal ampulla and leakage of stool manifested by encopresis, soiling, or 'skid-marks' in the underwear, and persistence of a large amount of fecal material in the rectal ampulla, despite a recent bowel movement. The constipated fecal mass that is stored in the rectosigmoid may exert sufficient pressure on the bladder wall to prevent it from fully expanding, thus effectively reducing functional bladder capacity. In addition, the stimulation of stretch receptors within the bladder wall by the extrinsic fecal mass may trigger detrusor contractions of various amplitudes and thus sustain a vicious cycle. This scenario may have some parallels with the bladder disturbances seen during pregnancy as the uterus expands. Drawing from this comparison and from the fact that urinary problems are invariably relieved with the termination of pregnancy, it would seem wise to start therapy in patients with dysfunctioned elimination with the management of constipation. During the course of therapy, as regularity improves and stool becomes softer in consistency, patients will soon report voiding less frequently and in larger amounts. If total dryness is not achieved and bladder capacity is still below the expected norm for age, an anticholinergic may be added. It is preferable to administer anticholinergics only after ensuring that bowel function is optimal. The risks of increasing fecal retention, a well-known side-effect of anticholinergic medication, may be avoided and further bladder hyperactivity thus prevented (Homsy, 1997).

It is usually easy to check for fecal retention non-invasively in the course of physical examination by asking the child to breathe deeply while gently massaging the abdominal musculature over the left iliac fossa to relax it, thus detecting distension of the sigmoid colon when present. Abdominal palpation can be less revealing in obese or older individuals. An abdominal X-ray or pelvic sonogram will confirm suspicions of possible fecal retention. Rectal manometric studies have shown that children would normally tolerate rectal balloon inflation to about 20 ml before feeling an urge to defecate. Constipated children will easily tolerate volumes of 120 ml or more before feeling a vague urge to do so (O'Regan *et al.*, 1985). A gradual loss in muscle tone in the bowel wall promotes further stagnation of hardening stool and bowel dilatation. Firmly addressing the constipation issue should be the first step towards the restoration of adequate smooth muscle tone to the dilated rectosigmoid, thus helping it to recuperate its propulsive function. This process is long and tedious, taking a few months to a few years. It must be viewed as a rehabilitative effort with all the patience and dedication that are invariably required in rehabilitative therapy. In a study reported in 1997 by Loening-Baucka, of 234 constipated children, 29% had daytime incontinence, 34% had night-time incontinence, and 11% had UTIs. After 1 year, constipation was relieved in only 52%. However, all patients stopped having recurrent UTIs, and 89% were cured of their daytime incontinence and 63% of their night-time incontinence.

Management of constipation

There are several effective regimens for the management of constipation. Many are based on the individual health professional's preferences. They must be tailored to the patient's needs, which can be quite variable as to circumstances, degree of fecal retention/constipation and likelihood of compliance to prescribed therapy. It is important to bear in mind that the management of chronic constipation is based on two principles: (1) empty the rectum; and (2) keep it empty.

For many years, the authors have relied on initiating therapy with the administration of sodium phosphate (Fleet®) enemas for disimpaction and complete emptying of the rectum and colon. The process usually takes several days. In some patients it can take several weeks, particularly when stool is visualized up to the cecum on plain X-rays of the abdomen. Although enemas are effective, they are not sufficiently popular to ensure compliance. We have recently had appreciable success with the administration of polyethylene glycol 3350 (Miralax®), now available in oral form. The powder is dissolved in a glass of water. The iso-osmotic solution is transparent and has no detectable taste, so that it has been well accepted by children. It is neither absorbed nor metabolized; its

osmotic activity and electrolyte concentration result in almost no net absorption or excretion of ions or water. Taken once daily, effective disimpaction occurs gently over several days. It is not currently recommended for use beyond 2 weeks. However, studies are starting to indicate that oral polyethylene glycol is safe to use for longer periods in children. We believe that this medication holds much promise in the management of chronic constipation. The effect of both polyethylene glycol and enemas on the bowel is threefold: (1) bowel disimpaction from hard stool; (2) restoration of normal propulsive muscle tone to the distended bowel wall musculature; and (3) avoidance of abdominal cramps that may be associated with oral laxative/stool softener intake in the presence of impaction. Some families have difficulty accepting enema administration over a prolonged period. After disimpaction, it is important to keep the bowel empty by using an oral laxative that is safe to use over a long period of time, such as milk of magnesia. It may take up to 1 year to allow the bowel to regain its normal peristaltic activity and diameter. Children tolerate the concentrated form of milk of magnesia better because they can ingest effective doses in smaller quantities. At the same time the child must become accustomed to the intake of a high-fiber diet. The American Dietetic Association recommends a daily intake of 20–35 g of fiber per day in the general population. In children, the recommended amount is reached by the formula: *age in years + 5 = recommended daily fiber intake in grams*. As these are the recommended amounts for normal individuals, they should probably be increased in constipated subjects. Compliance may become a problem, particularly with picky eaters. It is admittedly difficult to consistently maintain a high-fiber diet in childhood. Therefore diet must be supplemented with hyperosmolar agents (milk of magnesia and Lactulose®, which are safe for long-term administration and do not produce dependency). They may be incorporated into ingenious recipes to make them more palatable and ensure compliance. It must be made clear at the outset that therapy must be continued for between 6 months and 1 year and often longer. Lack of compliance is often seen to cause a recurrence of wetting after an initial period of improvement (Parker, 1999). An excellent up-to-date clinician's guide to laxatives may be found in an issue of *Pediatric Annals* entirely devoted to pediatric constipation and encopresis (Lowe and Parks, 1999).

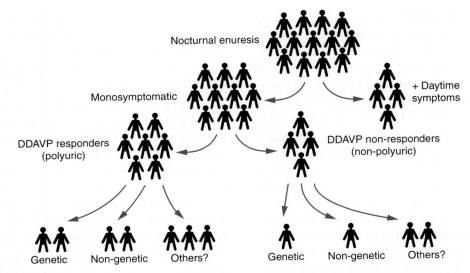

Figure 12.1 Different subtypes of nocturnal enuresis based on pathophysiological findings. (From Djurhuus and Rittig, 1998, with permission.)

Nocturnal enuresis

Terms and definitions

Recently, standardization and definitions have been established for lower urinary tract dysfunction in children (Nørgaard *et al.*, 1998). Nocturnal enuresis may be divided into different subtypes (see Fig. 12.1).

1 *Primary nocturnal enuresis (PNE)*: monosymptomatic bedwetting in individuals who have never been dry at night for an uninterrupted period of time of at least 6 months. It may be polyuric or non-polyuric and should not be associated with daytime voiding symptoms.

2 *Nocturnal enuresis with daytime symptoms*: minimal daytime symptoms may coexist such as frequency, urge syndrome, or occasional dampness. Patients will often wet the bed more than once during the night, which may result from a reduced bladder capacity. This element must be taken into consideration as it is probably the most confusing single issue in diagnosis and management. If it is not sufficiently stressed during questioning, therapy may be misdirected.

3 *Familial nocturnal enuresis*: monosymptomatic bedwetting in individuals with first-degree relatives who have (had) the same condition.

4 *Onset nocturnal enuresis*: monosymptomatic bedwetting in individuals who have been dry at night for an uninterrupted period of 6 months or more. The term 'secondary enuresis' has been used in the past to describe onset nocturnal enuresis and also those patients who have nocturnal enuresis due to some underlying organic etiology, such as polyuria from diabetes insipidus.

Importance

Nocturnal enuresis is among the most common urologic complaints in children. It is estimated to occur in up to 15% of 5-year-old (Forsythe and Redmon, 1974) and 10% of 7-year-old children (Hellstrom *et al.*, 1990). The relatively high incidence must be conveyed to parents and children to reassure them that those affected are not 'abnormal' or 'defective'. Persistent enuresis can cause a high level of stress and anxiety in affected children and their families (Moffatt, 1994). It is an embarrassing problem that may inhibit the development of confidence and a positive self-image. Several studies have reported improved self-esteem in patients who have undergone successful treatment of nocturnal enuresis (Moffatt *et al.*, 1987; Hägglöf *et al.*, 1997).

Another negative impact of enuresis is the economic burden for the families as well as on healthcare systems worldwide (Nørgaard and Andersen, 1994). Pugner and Holmes (1997) recently reported on the total cost of having an enuretic child from case studies in five countries and analysed different treatment methods. Comparisons were made between treatments that included desmopressin, enuresis alarm, and no treatment other than the use of diapers. Besides the costs of each therapeutic modality, the authors also estimated the direct and indirect costs to the family. Interestingly, in those case studies where the child had three or more wet nights per week, the no-treatment group incurred the highest overall cost burden.

When evaluating enuretic children, it is important to empathize with the family. They need to know of the common occurrence of PNE in the general population, and that there is a spontaneous resolution rate of approximately 15% per year with approximately 99% of children becoming dry by 15 years of age (Beer, 1915). Before taking a thorough medical history (including a voiding and elimination history) and performing a physical examination, the treating practitioner should have a clear understanding of the various etiologies of nocturnal enuresis in order to reassure the child and families that there are many reasons for the enuresis and that their child is not being stubborn or demonstrating defiant behavior.

Etiology

Enuresis has been attributed to an overall multifactorial delay or a maturational lag in several spheres, namely: (1) bladder function; (2) the circadian rhythm of antidiuretic hormone (ADH) secretion; and (3) sleep/arousal mechanisms. The most convincing argument for developmental delay is that, if left untreated, almost all enuretics eventually develop complete control. The role that genetic and hereditary factors may play in developmental delay is not clear at the moment. The importance of recognizing the etiological factors mentioned above is that therapeutic measures should first seek to address the factor that appears to predominate in each case. If this does not resolve the problem, combination therapy, addressing the next most important contributory factor, may be necessary for a successful outcome. Genetically determined forms of enuresis are amenable to treatment by conventional methods.

Delay in functional bladder maturation

As mentioned previously, bladder volume increases with age and many studies of enuretics have reported urodynamic findings of small-capacity bladders as well as 'infantile-like' bladders with instability (Firlit et al., 1978; McGuire and Savastano, 1984). These, and other studies, reinforced the predominant thinking that a high prevalence of bladder instability was responsible for enuretic episodes. Unfortunately, many of these studies were flawed as the populations studied were not homogeneous and included patients with overt bladder instability and daytime wetting.

Nørgaard et al. (1989) subsequently performed daytime and night-time urodynamics in 31 children who had nocturnal enuresis only. In this report, only a 16% incidence of bladder instability was found out of a total of 102 cystometrograms during daytime urodynamics. The incidence of bladder instability, however, increased to approximately 50% with night-time urodynamics. The occurrence of bladder instability was equally likely to lead to arousal and controlled nocturnal voiding as to involuntary voiding (nocturnal enuresis). Furthermore, enuresis occurred when the nocturnal bladder volume reached the maximal bladder capacity and was characterized by a normal coordinated mature voiding episode with complete emptying.

Despite the normal bladder capacity and coordinated micturition event demonstrated by Nørgaard et al., other authors have found that functional bladder capacity is important in the pathogenesis of enuresis. Watanabe et al. (1994) reported that detrusor overactivity during sleep has been observed in a significant number of enuretics. Other studies by Eller et al. (1997) and Rushton et al. (1996) have documented that functional bladder capacity is a strong predictor of response to desmopressin with nocturnal enuresis. This importance of bladder capacity was also supported by the Aarhus group, who found that patients with desmopressin-resistant monosymptomatic nocturnal enuresis had a smaller functional and maximal bladder capacity and more frequent daytime micturitions compared with normal children (Kirk et al., 1995). Furthermore, Watanabe and Kawauchi (1995) observed that bladder capacity is not fixed and can change with varying circumstances. It was seen to change with respect to daytime or night-time as well during different states of arousal during sleep. The difference between arousal bladder capacity and the bladder capacity at enuresis was significantly lower in the enuretic patients than in non-enuretics.

Supporting the concept that an adequate bladder capacity is important for nocturnal bladder control,

Yeung *et al.* recently reported that children with refractory monosymptomatic primary nocturnal enuresis commonly had bladder dysfunction, including a small functional capacity and detrusor instability during sleep. In summary, there are subgroups of enuretics who do not have polyuria and seem to have a decreased bladder capacity or an element of latent bladder instability that is contributing to the enuretic event. Furthermore, these bladders change or mature with time.

Those enuretics who present with daytime wetting should not be considered as monosymptomatic nocturnal enuretics but rather as nocturnal enuretics with daytime symptoms. Some of these patients may not actually wet themselves during the day but may only have some frequency, which could remain undetected by the parents. When they are made to keep a voiding diary for 2 or 3 days, preferably at weekends, many of them will manifest a small functional bladder capacity. The formula Age (in years) + 2 = Bladder capacity (in ounces) is used to determine the expected capacity for age (Koff, 1982). Night-time bladder instability was demonstrated in approximately one-third of nocturnal enuretics, some of whom had some frequency or urgency by day (Watanabe, 1994). This type of patient may benefit from therapy oriented towards increasing bladder capacity first, i.e. anticholinergics.

Delay in development of circadian antidiuretic hormone secretion

Urine production normally decreases at night because of the circadian rhythm of secretion by the posterior pituitary of the antidiuretic hormone arginine vasopressin (AVP or ADH) (George *et al.*, 1975). Loss of the normal increase in night-time ADH production will result in relative nocturnal polyuria, which can exceed the functional capacity of the bladder, resulting in an enuretic episode. Rasmussen *et al.* (1996) demonstrated that nocturnal enuresis can be provoked in normal healthy children by increasing nocturnal urinary output. Although nocturnal polyuria (Poulton, 1952) and abnormal levels of ADH (Puri, 1980) had been implicated as a cause for nocturnal enuresis, it was not until the work from the Danish group in Aarhus that a nocturnal ADH deficiency was demonstrated as an etiologic factor. In their 1985 landmark article, nocturnal urine production was shown to be equal to or in excess of daytime

urine production in some enuretic children (Nørgaard *et al.*, 1985). Nocturnal polyuria was attributed to a deficiency in the normal surge of night-time ADH production in these children and thus provided an objective physiologic explanation for nocturnal enuresis. The Aarhus group substantiated this finding by demonstrating significant lower nocturnal levels of serum ADH with large amounts of poorly concentrated urine in enuretic children when compared with normal subjects (Rittig *et al.*, 1989). These studies were critical in adding a new perspective to the etiology and management of nocturnal enuresis. A novel physiologic explanation for nocturnal enuresis was provided that prompted further interest and research regarding other pathophysiologic etiologies.

Some of the newer research findings associated with ADH or vasopressin include the association of aquaporins. Aquaporins are proteins that mediate transmembrane water transport in a variety of tissues including the kidney, and have been implicated in the pathophysiology of nocturnal enuresis. Aquaporin 2 (AQP2) is located at the apical membrane of the renal collecting ducts and is stimulated by ADH to reabsorb water. In animal studies, Frøkiær and Nielson (1997) reported low levels of AQP2 in association with extreme polyuria in vasopressin-deficient rats. Furthermore, treatment with vasopressin resulted in a threefold increase in AQP2 levels. They surmised that nocturnal enuresis may partly be due to a lack of vasopressin-mediated AQP2 expression which resolves after treatment with desmopressin.

ADH is primarily released from the posterior pituitary in response to changes in extracellular fluid osmolality, but may also be released by other stimuli including trauma, pain, anxiety, drugs, and anesthetics (Guyton, 1971). Kawauchi *et al.* (1993) reported, in a small clinical study, that serum ADH levels decreased in patients who had their urine diverted by Foley catheters and were further lowered after cystectomy and ileal conduit diversion. In addition, they reported an increase in ADH levels in patients with full bladders during cystometry and theorized that ADH secretion may be influenced by bladder fullness or stretch. The study by Ohne (1995) supported this theory by demonstrating an increased activity of ADH in the hypothalamus via upregulated expression of c-Fos in vasopressin neurons in the presence of urethral obstruction. Finally, two recent reports have implicated a 'vesicorenal' reflex in that bladder fullness may affect renal production of urine (Schmidt *et al.*, 1995; Hvistendal *et al.*, 1997). Vasopressin receptors have been found in the bladders of Sprague–Dawley rats (Thibonnier *et al.*, 1986). Their presence in the human bladder might contribute in some way to the activation of ADH secretion. To the authors' knowledge, however, they have not been identified in the human bladder. Despite these potential mechanisms relating urine production and ADH control, it is apparent that there are other complex physiologic processes involved in nocturnal enuresis.

Sleep/arousal mechanisms

A strong association between sleep and nocturnal enuresis has been historically cited throughout the literature (Broughton, 1968; Kales and Kales, 1974). Many enuretics have been noted to be deep sleepers and difficult to arouse, which is often believed to be the cause for their nocturnal enuresis. These earlier studies, however, failed to compare the ability to awaken enuretic children compared with normal controls. Controlled sleep studies subsequently demonstrated that there was no difference in the degree of arousal among children with or without nocturnal enuresis (Boyd, 1960; Graham, 1973). Nevertheless, a recent study reported that when enuretic and non-enuretic children are exposed to the same auditory stimulus during sleeping, the enuretic children were more difficult to arouse (Wolfish *et al.*, 1997).

Early sleep studies reported that nocturnal enuresis occurred during the stage of deep sleep (Pierce *et al.*, 1961). However, other studies have demonstrated that enuresis may occur during light sleep or when the child is awake (Ritvo *et al.*, 1969). More sophisticated sleep studies have documented that enuretic events occur randomly throughout the night in proportion to the amount of time spent in each sleep stage (Kales *et al.*, 1977; Mikkelson *et al.*, 1980). Nørgaard *et al.* (1989) examined whether the quality of sleep is altered by bladder filling during night-time cystometric measurements and concluded that sleep in enuretic children is mostly unaltered by bladder filling.

The issue is a controversial one, and Watanabe and associates have provided a significant amount of data regarding sleep and arousal with nocturnal enuresis. In their original report of simultaneous electroencephalographic (EEG) and cystometric (CMG) monitoring of 204 enuretic children, they classified three types of EEG and CMG patterns associated with nocturnal enuresis (Fig. 12.2) (Watanabe and Azuma, 1989). Type I enuresis is reflected by light sleep on EEG monitoring and complete stability of the bladder. Type IIa enuretics differ in that they have a deep sleep EEG pattern rather than a light sleep pattern but still have bladder stability. Type IIb enuretics are similar to type IIa enuretics with a deep sleep EEG pattern, but they differ from both type I and type IIa by having bladder instability on cystometric measurement. Subsequent evaluation of 1033 enuretic patients demonstrated a prevalence of 58% with type I, 10% with type IIa, and 32% with type IIb patterns.

When Watanabe examined sleep patterns in 15 healthy infants, he discovered that type IIa enuresis was normal in infants until approximately 2 years of age (Watanabe, 1995). With maturation, only type I enuresis was seen in the older children. He postulated that persistence of type IIa enuresis may be associated with a delay in the development of the child's arousal response to bladder distension. Furthermore, type IIb enuresis may represent a pathologic condition. Watanabe also noted that there was a transition from deep sleep to light sleep when the bladder was full, which he elucidated in a rat experiment.

Anatomic and physiologic studies have shown that at least four arousal networks are present in the brain, each using a different transmitter: (1) the locus coeruleus which uses noradrenaline as its transmitter; (2) the raphe nuclei which use serotonin; (3) the tuberomammillary nucleus which uses histamine; and (4) the laterodorsal tegmental nucleus which uses acetylcholine as its transmitter. Of these networks, the noradrenaline-activating neurons originating in the locus coeruleus (located at the bottom of the fourth cerebral ventricle) are believed to be the most important activating mechanism for arousal (Kayama and Koyama, 1993; Watanabe, 1998). Thus, deep sleep and difficulty in arousal may be governed by different mechanisms and the relationship of each to nocturnal enuresis remains to be defined.

Recent evidence has suggested that vasopressin exerts a stimulatory effect in the central nervous system (CNS). DiMichele *et al.* (1996) found in a rat model that desmopressin and vasopressin lowered dopamine levels in the CNS, with a subsequent increase in locomotor activity. Desmopressin may thus not only affect urine production but may also stimulate arousal during sleep.

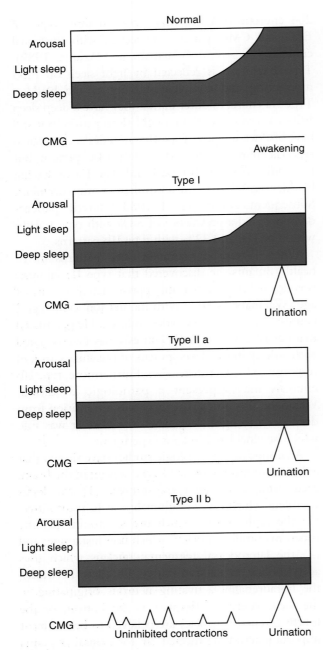

Figure 12.2 Classification of enuresis by overnight simultaneous monitoring of EEG and CMG. (From Imada *et al.*, 1998, with permission.)

Genetic/hereditary factors

The genetic or hereditary causes of nocturnal enuresis have been well documented (Hallgren, 1957). Bakwin (1973) reported in a large survey that when one parent of a child had a history of enuresis there was a 44% incidence in their children. When both parents had a history of enuresis, 77% of the children were enuretic. If neither parent had a history of enuresis then only 15% of the children had enuresis. Fergusson *et al.* (1986) also reported that a family history of enuresis was predictive of the age of attainment of urinary control in a large survey of 1265 children. Several studies in twins have also documented the genetic component of nocturnal enuresis.

Using molecular biology techniques, validation of the genetic influence on nocturnal enuresis has recently been accomplished. Eiberg *et al.* (1995) were the first to report an unidentified enuresis gene (*ENUR1*) in chromosome region 13q using linkage analysis. In this study, the *ENUR1* gene demonstrated a high autosomal dominant penetrance in families where enuresis was prevalent over multiple generations. Arnell *et al.* (1997) then demonstrated genetic linkage (*ENUR2*) of nocturnal enuresis in chromosome 12q. In the 392 analysed families, nocturnal enuresis was dominant in 43%, recessive in 9%, and sporadic in 48%. Finally, further linkage analysis by Eiberg (1998) has recently identified chromosome 22 as another genetic vehicle for nocturnal enuresis (*ENUR3*). Despite these known chromosomes with genetic linkage to nocturnal enuresis, there is still no specific gene identified in these chromosome regions. Many candidate genes exist and these studies are just the beginning in the exploration of the molecular and genetic influence on nocturnal enuresis. Furthermore, there is a wide variation in the phenotypic expression of these genes, which reflects the genetic heterogeneity of nocturnal enuresis (von Gontard *et al.*, 1998).

In addition to the genetic predilection for nocturnal enuresis, there is a strong genetic linkage of the response of enuretics towards therapy. Hogg and Husmann (1993) reported a 91% response rate of patients with nocturnal enuresis to desmopressin therapy if there was a positive family history of PNE. In contrast, they found that when there was no family history of PNE, the response to desmopressin was only 7% in effecting a cure. Despite this finding of a genetic component in the prediction of desmopressin response in enuretics, other studies have not demonstrated that a positive family history is predictive of the response to desmopressin (Monda and Husmann, 1995; Rushton *et al.*, 1995). A recent report suggests that there is also a subgroup of nocturnal enuretics who have a strong family history of non-responsiveness towards desmopressin (Schaumburg *et al.*,

1999). As mentioned before, these studies emphasize the heterogeneous population seen in nocturnal enuretics and the variable genetic influence within these groups.

Evaluation

Children with monosymptomatic PNE do not need an extensive work-up. A careful history and physical examination will generally identify that the enuresis is truly monosymptomatic. In particular, a detailed family history of PNE is beneficial in establishing a genetic pattern. Questions on the history of relevant surgery, previous UTIs, hematuria, neurologic problems or congenital anomalies should be included. The elimination history, including bladder and bowel function, physical examination, and keeping a voiding diary are essential prerequisites that are no different to those outlined previously for the evaluation of other voiding dysfunctions. The physical examination and urinalysis will identify any children with secondary enuresis due to a urologic or neurologic disease. Basically, unless a child has an abnormal examination or a complicated enuresis history, e.g. severe voiding dysfunction, encopresis, or UTIs, imaging and urodynamic studies are not warranted.

Treatment

After verifying that a child has PNE, treatment options should be presented to both the parent and the child, with particular attention to the parent and child's motivation. Therapy is rarely necessary before the age of 6 years, which is usually the time when the child enters elementary school and there is heightened socialization, including sleep-over visits. After counseling about regular voiding and drinking habits, there are basically three major treatment options: (1) pharmacologic therapy; (2) behavioral modification therapy; or (3) observation. Therapy must be individualized with the child and parent and should be directed at the most probable etiological cause. Combination therapy is sometimes necessary, particularly in resistant cases. When therapeutic modalities are combined they should be added sequentially so that the effect of each may be assessed. Alternative therapeutic methods such as hypnotherapy and acupuncture have not been subjected to controlled studies, although they may have a place in management.

Pharmacological therapy

Pharmacological therapy typically entails using imipramine or DDAVP (1-deamino-[8-D-arginine]-vasopressin). Anticholinergics such as oxybutynin reduce or abolish uninhibited bladder contractions and may be particularly beneficial in patients who have daytime frequency or day-wetting associated with an unstable bladder. In the non-polyuric form of enuresis, anticholinergics may be of help when functional bladder capacity is reduced. Otherwise, anticholinergics have little effect in the management of monosymptomatic PNE.

Imipramine

Imipramine hydrochloride (Tofranil) is a widely used tricyclic antidepressant that has been used to treat enuresis since 1960 (MacLean, 1960). The exact pharmacologic mechanism of action of imipramine is not completely known, but it is thought to have an anticholinergic and antispasmodic effect at the bladder body and a sympathomimetic effect at the bladder outlet. Imipramine was also thought to alter sleep and arousal. However, subsequent studies have demonstrated that this mechanism is not responsible for its prevention of enuresis (Kales *et al.*, 1977; Mikkelson *et al.*, 1980).

The initial response to imipramine is usually good and studies have reported as many as 50% of enuretics achieving dryness (Blackwell and Currah, 1973). The cure rate, however, varies widely. Blackwell and Currah (1973) analysed eight double-blinded, controlled studies and reported a combined 25% long-term cure rate once the imipramine was discontinued. The dose of imipramine commonly prescribed is 25 mg for patients 6–8 years old and 50 mg for older children and adolescents, given at bedtime with fluid restriction. The dosage can also be determined by the child's weight, at 0.9–1.5 mg/kg per day. However, one study reported that this regimen achieved therapeutic levels in only 30% of the patients (Jorgensen *et al.*, 1980). Typically, imipramine is given 1–2 hours before bedtime and treatment is short term at 3–6 months. After that period the child should be weaned by reducing the dose and then the frequency (e.g. every 2–3 nights over 3–4 weeks) of medication.

Side-effects limit the usage of imipramine and include daytime sedation, anxiety, insomnia, dry mouth, nausea, and adverse personality changes.

Overdose can result in fatal cardiac arrhythmias, hypotension, respiratory distress, and convulsions. Parents should be warned about these side-effects, particularly if there are small children in the home who could possibly tamper with this medication. The use of this drug has decreased dramatically, and because of its side-effects and dangers, it should be used only in select circumstances with proper warnings and precautions.

Desmopressin/DDAVP

A significant number of enuretics can be controlled by the administration of desmopressin, an analog synthetic substitute of ADH. The reported response rate is 40–70% (Wille, 1986; Klauber, 1989). The cure rate, however, does not exceed 30% after 1 year (Hjälmås et al., 1998). A linear correlation has been shown to exist between bladder capacity and response to desmopressin (Eller et al., 1998; Rushton et al., 1996). The probability of success was higher than 75% when bladder capacity was above 65% of age-adjusted expected capacity (Fig. 12.3). In the presence of normal bladder capacity, dry nights may be achieved in up to 90% (Tanguay et al., 1992). Desmopressin has a rapid onset of action and is useful to control symptoms for the duration of therapy when candidates are carefully selected. Relapses are common upon cessation of the medication. Patients must, therefore, be warned that although the enuresis may be controlled they should not expect to be cured by the medication. A spontaneous resolution rate of 15% per year is known to occur in enuresis. Cure in responders is expected when the child's own circadian

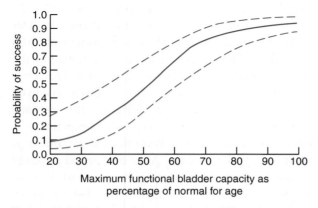

Figure 12.3 Estimated success probability of reponse to DDAVP treatment as a function of bladder capacity (with 95% confidence limits). (From Eller et al., 1998, with permission.)

rhythm becomes established. Desmopressin has only a few minor side-effects related to nasal irritation when the spray is used, but intestinal cramps have been reported. It must be remembered that desmopressin is an antidiuretic and that hyponatremic seizures from water intoxication have been reported. Patients should therefore be kept on the dry side in the evening and warned never to take the medication in the morning. An effective regimen is to start with the lowest dose (10 µg for the spray and 0.2 mg for the tablets) administered at bedtime. The dose should be increased one week later to 20 µg/0.4 mg if there has been no response and then to 30 µg/0.6 mg, with the objective of maintaining the patient on the smallest most effective dose. Only a handful of patients will respond to a higher dose (Eller et al., 1998) if they did not respond initially. Alternatively, therapy may be started with the higher dose and titrated downwards every week until the effective dosage is reached. Although desmopressin is quite effective in controlling bedwetting, there are only a few long-term outcome studies available. The Swedish Enuresis Trial (SWEET) addresses this question. Out of 399 monosymptomatic enuretics, 245 decreased their number of wet nights by more than half over a period of 4 weeks on 20–40 µg of desmopressin. These enuretics were selected for long-term therapy (1 year) with 1-week interruptions every 3 months to avoid overtreatment. Approximately one-third (77/245) of patients became dry off medication at the end of the study, while roughly another third (73/245) who were still on medication had reduced their number of wet nights to fewer than 10%. Another 51 children had halved the number of nights on which they were wet. No serious adverse effects were reported (Hjälmås et al., 1998).

Conditioning therapy

Small, user-friendly enuretic alarm devices have replaced the bell-and-pad system. They consist of a metallic clip that is attached to the underclothes. The clip is connected by a wire to a battery-powered alarm that is worn on the wrist or shoulder. The alarm rings when the underclothes become moist with the first drops of urine. The child must be taken to the bathroom to complete urination in the toilet in an awake state. The use of enuresis alarm systems provides a permanent cure in over 90% of bedwetters in motivated families. The relapse rate is approximately

25–30% after using a device for 6–8 weeks following the last enuretic episode. In case of a relapse, another cycle of device use will result in further cure rates in the same range. Bladder capacity was found to increase by approximately 30% following a 6-week treatment period regardless of whether patients became dry or not (Hansen and Jorgensen, 1995). Overlearning, by forcing fluids at bedtime by increments of 30–60 g every evening, will increase the chances of success, as will cleanliness training and retention control training. Houts *et al.* (1983) developed a program in which children and their parents attended a 1 hour group session during which they were shown how to implement the program at home. The program required minimal professional time and was cost-effective, with an initial success rate of 81% and a 24% relapse rate at 1 year follow-up. There is no substitute for waking the child, and studies document the failure of this approach if the child is not awakened (Houts, 1995). Unquestionably, this method requires motivation on behalf of the child and commitment on behalf of the parents. Overall, conditioning therapy is the single most effective form of therapy (Monda and Husmann, 1995). It is important to select families appropriately before initiating this therapy and to ensure that the enuresis is mono-symptomatic.

Miniaturized ultrasound bladder volume-controlled devices have shown promising results. They are activated when bladder capacity reaches approximately 80% of the typical volume that produces enuresis, so that the child may be spared the actual wetting episode (Pretlow, 1999). These devices must be small enough to be comfortable for smaller children when mounted on an elastic belt that is worn around the abdomen (Petrican and Sawan, 1998).

References

Abrams P, Freeman R, Anderstorm C, Mattiasson A (1998) Tolterodine, a new antimuscarinic agent: as effective but better tolerated than oxybutynin in patients with an overactive bladder. *Br J Urol* **81**: 801–10.

Allen TD (1977) The non-neurogenic neurogenic bladder. *J Urol* **117**: 232–8.

Ambrose SS, Swanson HS (1960) The hypertonic neurogenic bladder in children: its sequelae and management. *J Urol* **83**: 672–5.

American Psychiatric Association (1987) *DSM-III-R: diagnostic and statistical manual of mental disorders*. Washington, DC: APA.

Araki I, de Groat WC (1997) Developmental synaptic depression underlying reorganization of visceral reflex pathways in the spinal cord. *J Neurosci* **17**: 8402–7.

Arnell H, Hjälmås K, Jagervall M *et al.* (1997) The genetics of primary nocturnal enuresis: inheritance and suggestion of a second major gene on chromosome 12q. *J Med Genet* **34**: 360–5.

Austin PF, Homsy YL, Masel JL *et al.* (1999) a-Adrenergic blockade in children with neuropathic and non-neuropathic voiding dysfunction. *J Urol* **162**: 1064–7.

Bakwin H (1973) The genetics of enuresis. In: Kolvin I, MacKeith RC, Meadow SR (eds): *Bladder control and enuresis*. London: Heinemann Medical, 73–7.

Beer E (1915) Chronic retention of urine in children. *JAMA* **65**: 1709–13.

Blackwell B, Currah J (1973) The psychopharmacology of nocturnal enuresis. Chapter 25. In: Kolvin I, MacKieth RC, Meadow SR (eds) *Bladder control and enuresis*. Philadelphia, PA: JB Lippincott, 231–57.

Bloom DA, Seeley WW, Ritchey ML, McGuire EJ (1993) Toilet habits and continence in children: an opportunity sampling in search of normal parameters. *J Urol* **149**: 1087–90.

Bo K, Stien R, Kulseng-Hanssen S, Kristofferson M (1994) Clinical and urodynamic assessment of nulliparous young women with and without stress incontinence symptoms: acase control study. *Obstet Gynecol* **84**: 1028–32.

Bower WF, Moore KH, Adams RD, Shepherd R (1998) A urodynamic study of surface neuromodulation versus sham in detrusor instability and sensory urgency. *J Urol* **160**: 2133–6.

Boyd MM (1960) The depth of sleep in enuretic school children and nonenuretic controls. *J Psychosom Res* **4**: 274–9.

Brazelton TB (1962) A child-oriented approach to toilet training. *Pediatrics* **29**: 121–8.

Broughton RF (1968) Sleep disorders: disorders of arousal? *Science* **159**: 1070–8.

Buzelin JM, Lacerte P, Lenormand L (1988) Ontogénèse de la fonction vésico-sphinctérienne. *J Urol (Paris)* **94**: 211–14.

Cardozo LD, Abrams, PD, Stanton SL, Feneley RCL (1978) Idiopathic bladder instability treated by biofeedback. *Br J Urol* **50**: 521–6.

Chancellor MB, de Groat WC (1999) Intravesical capsaicin and resiniferatoxin therapy: spicing up the ways to treat the overactive bladder. *J Urol* **162**: 3–11.

Chandra M (1995) Reflux nephropathy, urinary tract infection and voiding disorders. *Curr Opin Pediatr* **7**: 164–70.

Chandra M, Maddix H, McVicar M (1996) Transient urodynamic dysfunction of infancy: relationship to urinary tract infections and vesicoureteral reflux. *J Urol* **155**: 673–7.

Combs AJ, Glassberg AD, Gerdes D, Horowitz M (1998) Biofedback therapy for children with dysfunctional voiding. *Urology* **52**: 312–15.

de Groat WC, Nadelhaft I, Milne RJ *et al.* (1981) Organization of the sacral parasympathetic reflex pathways to the urinary bladder and large intestine. *J Auton Nerv Syst* **3**: 135–60.

DeLuca FG, Swenson O, Fisher JH, Loutfi AH (1962) The dysfunctional 'lazy' bladder syndrome in children. *Arch Dis Child* **37**: 117–20.

DiMichele S, Sillén U, Engel JA *et al.* (1996) Desmopressin and vasopressin increase locomotor activity in the rat via a central mechanism: implications for nocturnal enuresis. *J Urol* **156**: 1164–8.

Djurhuus JC, Ritlig S (1998) Current trends, diagnosis, and treatment of enuresis. *Eur Urol* **33** (Suppl 3): 30–3.

Eiberg H (1998) Total genome scan analysis in a single extended family for primary nocturnal enuresis: evidence for a new locus (ENUR3) for primary nocturnal enuresis on chromosome 22q11. *Eur Urol* **33** (Suppl 3): 34–6.

Eiberg H, Berendt I, Mohr J (1995) Assignment of dominant inherited nocturnal enuresis (ENUR1) to chromosome 13q. *Nature Genet* **10**: 354–6.

Elejalde R (1979) Genetic and diagnostic considerations in three families with abnormalities of facial expression and congenital urinary obstruction: 'the Ochoa syndrome'. *Am J Med Genet* **3**: 97–108.

Eller DA, Homsy YL, Austin PF *et al.* (1997) Spot urine osmolality, age and bladder capacity as predictors of response to desmopressin in nocturnal enuresis. *Scand J Urol Nephrol* Suppl **183**: 41–5.

Eller DA, Austin PF, Tanguay S, Homsy YL (1998) Daytime functional bladder capacity as a predictor of response to dermopressin in monosymptomatic nocturnal enuresis. *Eur Urol* **33** (Suppl 3): 25–9.

Ellsworth PI, Merguerian PA, Copening ME (1995) Sexual abuse: another causative factor in dysfunctional voiding. *J Urol* **153**: 773–6.

Elzinga-Plomp A, Boemers TM, Messer AP *et al.* (1995) Treatment of enuresis risoria in children by self-administered electric and imaginary shock. *Br J Urol* **76**: 775–8.

Fergusson DM, Horwood LJ, Shannon FT (1986) Factors related to the age of attainment of nocturnal bladder control: an 8-year longitudinal study. *Pediatrics* **78**: 884–90.

Firlit CF, Smey P, King LR (1978) Micturition urodynamic flow studies in children. *J Urol* **119**: 250–3.

Forsythe WI, Redmon A (1974) Enuresis and spontaneous cure rate: study of 1129 enuretics. *Arc Dis Child* **49**: 259–63.

Frøkiær J, Nielsen S (1997) Do aquaporins have a role in nocturnal enuresis? *Scand J Urol Nephrol* Suppl **183**: 31–2.

Galdston R, Perlmutter AD (1973) The urinary manifestations of anxiety in children. *Pediatrics* **52**: 818–22.

George CP, Messeril FH, Genest J *et al.* (1975) Diurnal variation of plasma vasopressin in man. *J Clin Endocrinol Metab* **41**: 332–8.

Glicklich LB (1951) An historical account of enuresis. *Pediatrics* **8**: 859–62.

Goellner MH, Ziegler EE, Fomon SJ (1981) Urination during the first three years of life. *Nephron* **28**: 174–8.

Graham P (1973) Depth of sleep and enuresis: a critical review. In: Kolvin I, MacKieth RC, Meadow SR (eds) *Bladder control and enuresis*. London: Heinemann Medical, 78–83.

Griffiths DJ, Scholtmeijer RJ (1983) Detrusor/sphincter dyssynergia in neurologically normal children. *Neurourol Urodynam* **2**: 27–9.

Guyton AC (1971) Introduction to endocrinology, the hypophyseal hormones, and the pineal gland. In: Guyton AC (ed.) *Textbook of medical physiology*. Philadelphia, PA: WB Saunders Co., 872–85.

Hägglöf B, Andrén O, Bergström E *et al.* (1997) Self-esteem before and after treatment in children with nocturnal enuresis and urinary incontinence. *Scand J Urol Nephrol* Suppl **183**: 79–82.

Hallgren B (1957) Enuresis. A clinical and genetic study. *Acta Psychiatr Neurol Scand* **114**: 1–159.

Hansen AF, Jorgensen TM (1995) Treatment of nocturnal enuresis with the bell-and-pad system. *Scand J Urol Nephrol* Suppl **173**: 101–2.

Hellstrom AL, Hjälmås, Jodal U (1987) Rehabilitation of the dysfunctional bladder in children: method and 3-year followup. *J Urol* **138**: 847–9.

Hellstrom AL, Hansin E, Hansson S *et al.* (1990) Micturition habits and incontinence in 7-year-old Swedish school entrants. *Eur J Pediatr* **149**: 434–7.

Hinman F Jr (1986) Nonneurogenic neurogenic bladder (the Hinman syndrome) – 15 years later. *J Urol* **136**: 21–9.

Hinman F Jr, Baumann FW (1972) Vesical and ureteral damage from voiding dysfunction in boys without neurologic or obstructive disease. *Trans Am Assoc Genitour Surg* **64**: 116–21.

Hjälmås K (1988) Urodynamics in normal infants and children. *Scand J Urol Nephrol* Suppl **114**: 20–7.

Hjälmås K, Hanson E, Hellstrom AL *et al.* (1998) Long-term treatment with desmopressin in children with primary monosymptomatic nocturnal enuresis: an open multicenter study. Swedish Enuresis Trial (SWEET) Group. *Br J Urol* **82**: 704–9.

Hjälmås K, Hellström AL, Mogren K *et al.* (1999) Safety, efficacy and pharmacokinetics of tolterodine in pediatric patients with overactive bladder. Invited Lecture. In Abstract Book, International Children's Continence Society, 2nd Congress, August 22–24, 1999, Denver, Colorado, USA, 78–9.

Hoebecke P, Vande Walle J, Theunis M *et al.* (1996) Outpatient pelvic-floor therapy in girls with daytime incontinence and dysfunctional voiding. *Urology* **48**: 923–7.

Hoebecke P, De Paepe H, Renson C *et al.* (1999) Transcutaneous neuromodulation in non-neuropathic bladder sphincter dysfunction in children: preliminary results. Presented at the 2nd Congress, International Children's Continence Society, Denver, Colorado, USA, August 22–24, 1999 (Abstract No. 55) 102.

Hogg RJ, Husmann D (1993) The role of family history in predicting response to desmopressin in nocturnal enuresis. *J Urol* **150**: 444–5.

Holmdahl G, Hanson E, Hanson M *et al.* (1996) Four-hour voiding observation in healthy infants. *J Urol* **156**: 1809–12.

Homsy Y (1997) Place de la rétention stercorale. In: Cochat P (ed.) *Enurésie et troubles mictionnels de l'enfant*. Paris: Elsevier, 169–84.

Homsy YL, Nsouli I, Hamburger B *et al.* (1985) Effects of oxybutynin on vesicoureteral reflux in children. *J Urol* **134**: 1168–71.

Houts AC (1995) Behavioral treatments for enuresis. *Scand J Urol Nephrol* Suppl **173**: 83–7.

Houts AC, Liebert RM, Padawer W (1983) A delivery system for the treatment of nocturnal enuresis. *J Abnorm Child Psychol* **11**: 513–19.

Hvistendal J, Kopp U, Scmidt F et al. (1997) Vesico-renal reflex mechanisms modulate urine output and renal blood flow during elevated bladder pressure in the pig. 8th Annual Meeting of the European Society of Paediatric Urology, Rome.

Imada N, Kawauchi A, Tanaka Y, Yamao Y, Watanabe H, Takeuchi Y (1998) Classification based on overnight simultaneous monitoring by electroencephalography and cystometry. Eur Urol 33 (Suppl 3): 45–8.

Issenman RM, Filmer RB, Gorski PA (1999) A review of bowel and bladder control development in children: how gastrointestinal and urological conditions relate to problems in toilet training. Pediatrics 103: 1346–52.

Jayanthi VR, Khoury AE, McLorie GA, Agarwal SK (1997) The nonneurogenic neurogenic bladder of early infancy. J Urol 158: 1281–5.

Jerkins GR, Noe HN, Vaughn WR, Roberts E (1987) Biofeedback training for children with bladder sphincter incoordination. J Urol 138: 1113–15.

Jorgensen OS, Lober M, Christiansen J, Gram LF (1980) Plasma concentration and clinical effect in imipramine treatment of childhood enuresis. Clin Pharmacokinet 5: 386–93.

Kales A, Kales JD (1974) Sleep disorders: recent findings in the diagnosis and treatment of disturbed sleep. N Engl J Med 290: 487.

Kales A, Kales JM, Jacobsen A et al. (1977) Effects of imipramine on enuretic frequency and sleep stages. Pediatrics 60: 431–6.

Kawauchi A, Watanabe H, Kitamore T et al. (1993) The possibility of centripetal stimulation from the urinary bladder for vasopressin excretion. J Kyoto Pref Univ Med 102: 747–52.

Kayama Y, Koyama Y (1993) Brainstem neural mechanisms of sleep and wakefulness. J Physiol Soc Jpn 55: 1–14.

Kirk J, Rasmussen PV, Rittig S, Djurhuus JC (1995) Micturition habits and bladder capacity in normal children and in patients with desmopressin-resistant enuresis. Scand J Urol Nephrol Suppl 173: 49–50.

Klauber GT (1989) Clinical efficacy and safety of desmopressin in the treatment of nocturnal enuresis. J Pediatr 114: 719–22.

Koff SA (1982) Estimating bladder capacity in children. Urology 21: 248.

Koff SA, Byard MA (1988) The daytime urinary frequency syndrome of childhood. J Urol 140: 1280–2.

Koff SA, Murtagh DS (1983) The uninhibited bladder in children: effect of treatment on recurrence of urinary infection and on vesicoureteral reflux resolution. J Urol 130: 1138–41.

Koff SA, Lapides J, Piazza DH (1979) Association of urinary tract infection and reflux with uninhibited bladder contractions and voluntary sphincteric obstruction. J Urol 122: 373–6.

Koff S, Wagner T, Jayanthi V (1998) The relationship among dysfunctional elimination syndromes, primary vesicoureteric reflux and urinary tract infection in children. J Urol 60: 1019–22.

Kokoua A, Homsy Y, Lavigne JF et al. (1993) Maturation of the external urinary sphincter: acomparative histotopographic study in humans. J Urol 150: 617–22.

Laidley JW (1942) Achalasia of the urinary tract in children. Med J Aust 2: 475–9.

Lapides J, Diokno AC (1970) Persistence of the infant bladder as a cause of urinary infection in girls. J Urol 103: 243–8.

Loenig-Baucke V (1997) Urinary incontinence and urinary tract infection and their resolution with treatment of chronic constipation of childhood. Pediatrics 100: 228–32.

Lowe JR, Parks BR (1999) Movers and shakers: a clinician's guide to laxatives. Pediatr Ann 28: 307–10.

McGuire EJ, Savastano JA (1984) Urodynamic studies in enuresis and the non-neurogenic–neurogenic bladder. J Urol 132: 299–302.

McKenna PH, Herndon CDA, Connery S, Ferrer FA (1999) Pelvic floor muscle retraining for pediatric voiding dysfunction using interactive computer games. J Urol 162: 1056–63.

MacLean REG (1960) Imipramine hydrochloride (Tofranil) and enuresis. Am J Psychiatry 117: 551–6.

Mikkelson EJ, Rapoport JL, Nee L et al. (1980) Childhood enuresis. I. Sleep patterns and psychopathology. Arch Gen Psychiatry 37: 1139–44.

Moffatt MEK (1994) Nocturnal enuresis – is there a rationale for treatment? Scand J Urol Nephrol Suppl 163: 55–66.

Moffatt MEK, Kato C, Pless IB (1987) Improvements in self concept after treatment of nocturnal enuresis: a randomized clinical trial. J Pediatr 110: 647–52.

Monda JM, Husmann DA (1995) Primary nocturnal enuresis: a comparison among observation, imipramine, desmopressin acetate and bed-wetting alarm systems. J Urol 154: 745–8.

Muellner SR (1960) Development of urinary control in children: some aspects of the cause and treatment of primary enuresis. JAMA 172: 1256–61.

Nørgaard JP (1989) Urodynamics in enuretics I: reservoir function. Neurourol Urodyn 8: 199–211.

Nørgaard JP, Andersen TM (1994) Nocturnal enuresis – a burden on family economy? Scand J Urol Nephrol Suppl 163: 49–54.

Nørgaard JP, Pedersen EB, Djurhuus JC (1985) Diurnal anti-diuretic-hormone levels in enuretics. J Urol 134: 1029–31.

Nørgaard JP, Hansen JH, Wildschiøtz G et al. (1989) Sleep cystometries in children with nocturnal enuresis. J Urol 141: 1156–9.

Nørgaard JP, van Gool JD, Hjälmås K et al. (1998) Standardization and definitions in lower urinary tract dysfunction in children. Br J Urol 81 (Suppl 3): 1–16.

Noto H, Roppolo JR, Steers WD, de Groat WC (1989) Excitatory and inhibitory influences on bladder activity elicited by electrical stimulation in the pontine micturition center in the rat. Brain Res 492: 99–115.

Nygaard IE, Thompson FL, Svengalis SL, Albright JP (1994) Urinary incontinence in elite nulliparous athletes. Obstet Gynecol 84: 183–7.

Nygaard IE, Glowacki C, Saltzman CL (1996) Relationship between foot flexibility and urinary incontinence in nulliparous varsity athletes. Obstet Gynecol 87: 1049–51.

Ochoa B (1992) The urofacial (Ochoa) syndrome revisited. J Urol 148: 580–3.

Ochoa B, Gorlin RJ (1987) Urofacial (Ochoa) syndrome. Am J Med Genet 27: 661–6.

Ohne T (1995) The increase in c-Fos expression in vasopressin- and oxytocin-immunoreactive neurons in paraventricular and supraoptic nucleus of the hypothalamus following urinary retention. *J Kyoto Pref Univ Med* **104**: 393–403.

O'Regan S, Yazbeck S, Schick E (1985) Constipation, bladder instability, urinary tract infection syndrome. *Clin Nephrol* **23**: 152–4.

Paquin AJ Jr, Marshall VF, McGovern JH (1960) The megacystis syndrome. *J Urol* **83**: 634–9.

Parker PH (1999) To do or not to do? That is the question. *Pediatr Ann* **28**: 283–90.

Petrican P, Sawan MA (1998) Design of a miniaturized ultrasonic bladder volume monitor and subsequent preliminary evaluation on 41 enuretic patients. *IEEE Trans Rehabil Eng* **6**: 66–74.

Phillips E, Uehling DT (1993) Hinman syndrome: a vicious circle. *Urology* **42**: 51–4.

Pierce CM, Whitman RM, Maas JW, Gay ML (1961) Enuresis and dreaming; experimental studies. *Arch Gen Psychiatry* **4**: 166–70.

Poulton EM (1952) Relative nocturnal polyuria as a factor in enuresis. *Lancet* **ii**: 906–8.

Pretlow RA (1999) Treatment of nocturnal enuresis with an ultrasound volume controlled alarm device. *J Urol* **162**: 1224–8.

Pugner K, Holmes J (1997) Nocturnal enuresis: economic impacts and self-esteem preliminary research results. *Scand J Urol Nephrol* Suppl **183**: 65–9.

Puri VN (1980) Urinary levels of antidiuretic hormone in nocturnal enuresis. *Ind Pediatr* **17**: 675–6.

Rasmussen PV, Kirk J, Borup K *et al.* (1996) Enuresis nocturna can be provoked in normal healthy children by increasing the nocturnal urine output. *Scand J Urol Nephrol* **30**: 57–61.

Rasquin-Weber A, Hyman PE, Cucchiara S *et al.* (1999) Childhood functional gastrointestinal disorders. *Gut* **45 (Suppl 2)**: II60–8.

Reinberg Y, Sher PK, Gonzalez R (1996) Treatment of giggle incontinence with methylphenidate. *J Urol* **156**: 656–9.

Rittig S, Knudsen UB, Nørgaard JP *et al.* (1989) Abnormal diurnal rhythm of plasma vasopressin and urinary output in patients with enuresis. *Am J Physiol* **256**: F664–71.

Ritvo ER, Ornitz EM, Gottlieb F *et al.* (1969) Arousal and nonarousal enuretic events. *Am J Psychiatry* **126**: 115–22.

Ruarte AC, Quesada EM (1987) Urodynamic evaluation in children. *Int Perspect Urol* **14**: 114–24.

Rudy DC, Woodside JR (1991) Non-neurogenic neurogenic bladder: the relationship between intravesical pressure and the external sphincter electromyogram. *Neurourol Urodyn* **10**: 169–73.

Rushton HG (1995) Wetting and functional voiding disorders. *Urol Clin North Am* **22**: 75–93.

Rushton HG, Belman AB, Zaontz M *et al.* (1995) Response to desmopressin as a function of urine osmolality in the treatment of monosymptomatic nocturnal enuresis: a double-blind prospective study. *J Urol* **154**: 749–53.

Rushton H, Belman AB, Zaontz M *et al.* (1996) The influence of small bladder capacity and other predictors on the response to desmopressin in the management of monosymptomatic nocturnal enuresis. *J Urol* **156**: 651–5.

Schaumburg HL, Rittig S, Djurhuus JC (1999) Failure of family history to predict response to desmopressin in nocturnal enuresis. Presented at the 2nd Congress, International Children's Continence Society, Denver (Abstract No. 38).

Schmidt F, Jorgensen TM, Djurhuus JC (1995) The relationship between the bladder, the kidneys and the CNS. *Scand J Urol Nephrol* Suppl **173**: 51–2.

Schmitt BD (1982) Daytime wetting (diurnal enuresis). *Pediatr Clin North Am* **29**: 9–20.

Schulman SL, Quinn CK, Plachter N, Kodman-Jones C (1999) Comprehensive management of dysfunctional voiding. *Pediatrics* **103**: E31.

Schurch B, Hauri D, Rodic B *et al.* (1996) Botulinum-A toxin as a treatment of detrusor-sphincter dyssynergia: a prospective study in 24 spinal cord injury patients. *J Urol* **155**: 1023–9.

Seruca H (1989) Vesicoureteral reflux and voiding dysfunction: a prospective study. *J Urol* **142**: 494–8.

Shopfner EC (1968) Urinary tract pathology associated with constipation. *Radiology* **90**: 865–77.

Sillén U, Hjälmås K, Aili M *et al.* (1992) Pronounced detrusor hypercontractility in infants with bilateral gross reflux. *J Urol* **148**: 598.

Sillén U, Bachelard M, Hansson S, Hermansson G (1999a) Bladder dysfunction as a prognostic factor for resolution of high-grade infant vesico-ureteric reflux. Presented at the 10th Annual Meeting of the European Society for Pediatric Urology, Istanbul, Turkey, April 15–17, 1999. *Br J Urol* **83**: 69 (Abstract No. 3).

Sillen U, Hellstrom AL, Hermanson G, Abrahamson K (1999b) Comparison of urodynamic and free voidng pattern in infants with dilating reflux. *J Urol* **61**: 1928–33.

Snodgrass W (1991) Relationship of voiding dysfunction to urinary tract infection and vesicoureteral reflux in children. *Urology* **38**: 341–4.

Stein Z, Susser M (1967) Social factors in the development of sphincter control. *Dev Med Child Neurol* **9**: 692–706.

Steinhardt G, Naseer S, Cruz OA (1997) Botulinum toxin: novel treatment for dramatic urethral dilatation associated with dysfunctional voiding. *J Urol* **158**: 190–1.

Swenson O (1952) A new concept in the pathology of megaloureters. *Surgery* **32**: 367–77.

Tanguay S, Homsy Y, Hamburger B (1992) Desmopressin in nocturnal enuresis – urine osmolality screening and correlation with clinical response. *Dialog Pediatr Urol* **15**: 1–6.

Thibonnier M, Snadjar RM, Rapp JP (1986) Characterization of vasopressin receptors of rat urinary bladder and spleen. *Am J Physiol* **251**: H115–20.

Vandaele J, Vandewalle J, Hoebecke P *et al.* (1999) A multidisciplinary therapeutical approach in a 'voiding school' for therapy-resistant dysfunctional voiding. Presented at the 2nd Congress, International Children's Continence Society, Denver, Colorado, USA, August 22–24, 1999 (Abstract No. 49).

Variam DE, Dippell J (1995) Non-neurogenic neurogenic bladder and chronic renal insufficiency in childhood. *Pediatr Nephrol* **9**: 1–5.

von Gontard A, Eiberg H, Hollmann E *et al.* (1998) Molecular genetics of nocturnal enuresis: clinical and genetic heterogeneity. *Acta Paediatr* **87**: 571–8.

Wang CY, Hawkins-Lee B, Ochoa B *et al.* (1997) Homozygosity and linkage-disequilibrium mapping of the urofacial (Ochoa) syndrome gene to a 1-cM interval on chromosome 10q23–24. *Am J Hum Genet* **60**: 1641–7.

Wang CY, Huang YQ, Shi JD *et al.* (1999) Genetic homogeneity, high resolution mapping and mutation analysis of the urofacial (Ochoa) syndrome and exclusion of the glutamate oxaloacetate transaminase gene (GOT1) in the critical region as the disease gene. *Am J Hum Genlt* **84**: 454–9.

Watanabe H (1995) Sleep patterns in children with nocturnal enuresis. *Scand J Urol Nephrol* Suppl **173**: 37–41.

Watanabe H (1998) Nocturnal enuresis. *Eur Urol* Suppl **3**: 2–11.

Watanabe H, Azuma Y (1989) A proposal for a classification system of enuresis based on overnight simultaneous monitoring of electroencephalography and cystometry. *Sleep* **12**: 257–64.

Watanabe H, Kawauchi A (1995) Is small bladder capacity cause of enuresis? *Scand J Urol Nephrol* Suppl **173**: 37–41.

Watanabe H, Kawauchi A, Kitamori T, Azuma Y (1994) Treatment system for nocturnal enuresis according to an original classification system. *Eur J Urol* **25**: 43–50.

Wille S (1986) Comparison of desmopressin and enuresis alarm for nocturnal enuresis. *Arch Dis Child* **61**: 30–3.

Williams DI (1954) The radiological diagnosis of lower urinary obstruction in the early years. *Brit J Radiol* **27**: 473–80.

Williams DI, Taylor JS (1969) A rare congenital uropathy: vesico-urethral dysfunction with uper tract anomalies. *Br J Urol* **41**: 307–10.

Wolfish NM, Pivik RT, Busby KA (1997) Elevated sleep arousal thresholds in enuretic boys: clinical implications. *Acta Pediatr* **86**: 381–4.

Yazbeck S, Schick E, O'Regan S (1987) Relevance of constipation to enuresis, urinary tract infection and reflux. A review. *Eur Urol* **13**: 318–21.

Yeung CK (1995) The normal infant bladder. *Scand J Urol Nephrol* Suppl **173**: 19–23.

Yeung CK, Godley ML, Dhillon HK *et al.* (1997) The characteristics of primary vesicoureteric reflux in male and female infants with prenatal hydronephrosis. *Br J Urol* **80**: 319–27.

Yeung CK, Godley ML, Dhillon HK *et al.* (1998) Urodynamic patterns in infants with normal lower urinary tracts or primary vesico-ureteric reflux. *Br J Urol* **81**: 461–7.

Zoubek T, Bloom DA, Sedman AB (1990) Extraordinary urinary frequency. *Pediatrics* **85**: 112–4.

Neuropathology of the lower urinary tract

Stuart B. Bauer

13

Introduction

At least 25% of the more severe clinical problems in pediatric urology are caused by neurologic lesions that affect lower urinary tract function. The advent of clean intermittent catheterization (CIC), introduced in the early 1970s by Lapides (Lapides *et al.*, 1972), and the refinements in the techniques of urodynamic studies in children (Gierup and Ericson, 1970; Blaivas *et al.*, 1977; Blaivas, 1979) dramatically changed the way these children were managed (Smith, 1972). As a result, there is now a greater understanding of the pathophysiology of the many diseases that primarily affect children. Functional assessment of the lower urinary tract is currently an essential element in the evaluation process and is as important as X-ray visualization in characterizing and managing these abnormal conditions (McGuire *et al.*, 1981). Urodynamic testing is discussed in Chapter 14.

Assessment

Initially, all children with overt or suspected neuropathic bladder dysfunction should undergo evaluation:

1 History:
   - birth and development
   - bowel and bladder habits
   - pattern of incontinence.
2 Physical examination:
   - spine
   - lower extremities:
       reflexes
       muscle mass and strength
       sensation
       gait
       perineal sensation/tone/reflexes.
3 Laboratory:
   - urine analysis/culture
   - urine specific gravity
   - serum creatinine level.
4 Radiography:
   - renal sonography
   - voiding cystourethrography
   - spine radiograph (ultrasound <3 months of age; magnetic resonance imaging >3 months).
5 Urodynamics:
   - flow rate
   - residual urine
   - cystometrogram
   - external urethral sphincter electromyography
   - static/filling/voiding urethral pressure profile.

Of paramount importance in the work-up of children with neuropathic bladder dysfunction are the history and physical examination. The child's voiding habits prior to any injury and the current pattern of bladder emptying should be delineated. It is imperative to note whether the child voids voluntarily, spontaneously, or only with a Credé maneuver. Does the child have periods of dryness between voiding, or is there constant urinary leakage? Is the incontinence characterized by urgency and an inability to reach the toilet on time? Does the urine flow with a good stream or only dribble out during emptying? Does leakage occur with crying or laughing? Has the child had a urinary infection? How much urine is produced each day? What is the pattern of bowel function?

A careful assessment is made of perianal and perineal sensation, anal sphincter tone, and the presence of bulbocavernosus and anocutaneous reflexes. The bulbocavernosus reflex is elicited by placing one's finger just at or slightly inside the external anal sphincter and briskly squeezing the glans penis or compressing the clitoris. If the reflex is present, the external anal sphincter should contract. The anocutaneous reflex is elicited by scratching the pigmented skin directly adjacent to the anal opening, which results in a contraction of the perianal muscle. In children with suspected neuropathic bladder dysfunction, complete evaluation of the back, including looking for agenesis of the sacrum or a cutaneous manifestation of an underlying occult spinal dysraphism, is an important diagnostic aid (Mandell *et al.*, 1981; Bauer, 1983; Satar *et al.*, 1997). Examination of the lower extremities, comparing muscle mass and strength of each leg, eliciting deep tendon reflexes, pinpointing sensory losses, and observing the gait, may provide clues to the presence of an occult spinal dysraphism affecting not only the sacral but also the lumbar cord.

Classification of neuropathic bladder

The classification of neuropathic bladder dysfunction used in this chapter is that which has been adopted by the Urology Section of the American Academy of Pediatrics in conjunction with the Urodynamic Society's classification, and, most recently, with the International Continence Society.

Under normal conditions, all portions of the lower urinary tract (detrusor, bladder neck, and external sphincter mechanism) function as a coordinated unit for adequate storage and efficient evacuation of urine. When a neurourologic lesion exists, these components usually fail to act in unison. A classification has been adopted based on dysfunction of a specific area of the vesicourethral unit rather than on a specific etiology:

1 Storage:
  (a) detrusor tone
    ■ normal
    ■ increased
        non-elastic
        overactive
        hyperreflexic
        decreased
  (b) urethral closing mechanism
    ■ incompetent
        bladder neck
        external sphincter
        non-reciprocal
        periodic hypoactivity.
2 Evacuation:
  (a) detrusor contraction
    ■ normoactive
    ■ underactive

        areflexic (non-reactive)
        hypoactive (unsustained)
  (b) urethral closing mechanism
    ■ non-synchronous
        bladder neck
        external sphincter.

Improper storage may be related to an alteration in detrusor function or an inadequate urethral closure mechanism. The bladder may have increased tone secondary to loss of elasticity of the muscle, overactivity from excessive or unopposed sympathetic discharges, or hyperreflexia due to a central nervous system (CNS) lesion above the sacral cord, the brainstem, or cerebral cortex, that prevents the normal inhibitory centers from influencing the sacral reflex arc. Incontinence may occur with any one of these conditions despite a normal level of resistance in the bladder neck and urethra. Alternatively, incontinence may occur when the bladder neck and external sphincter areas do not provide adequate resistance during filling of the bladder or do not generate a reciprocal increase in outflow resistance as the bladder fills or abdominal pressure is raised. An injury to the spinal cord or nerve roots affecting the sympathetic, parasympathetic, or sacral somatic nervous system may alter both bladder neck and urethral tone. Periodic relaxation of the external urethral sphincter during filling of the bladder, the result of loss of CNS inhibition, may also lead to urinary incontinence.

Incomplete evacuation of the bladder may be due to a hypoactive or an areflexic detrusor muscle. A CNS lesion affecting the parasympathetic efferents may be responsible. However, non-synchronous relaxation of the bladder neck or external urethral sphincter area mechanisms (dyssynergia) (Fig. 13.1) resulting from a lesion in the CNS above the sacral cord, for example the pontine center or the cerebral cortex, can produce a similar effect. Myogenic failure occurs as the detrusor muscle hypertrophies and then decompensates owing to persistent bladder outflow resistance. Eventually, this mechanism may produce an overflow type of incontinence.

In general, medical treatment of neuropathic bladder dysfunction is based on the functional impairment produced by the specific neurourologic defect (see Table 13.1). Inadequate storage capacity may be enhanced by lowering detrusor tone or abolishing uninhibited contractions with anticholinergic medication, such as oxybutynin, glycopyrrolate,

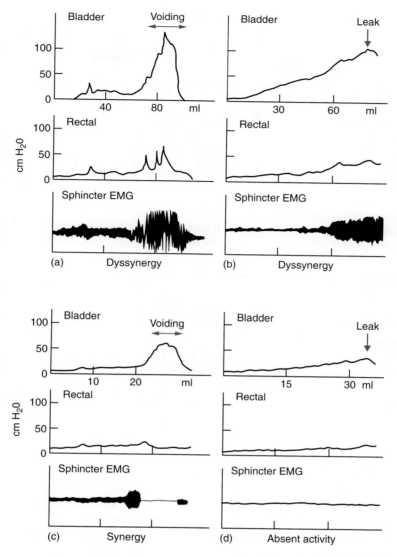

Figure 13.1 Various patterns of urodynamic findings in newborns with myelodysplasia. Note that a hypertonic detrusor with a non-relaxing sphincter (*b*) is also labeled dyssynergy. (From Bauer, 1988.)

hyoscyamine, tolteridine, or propantheline. These drugs block cholinergic receptor sites in the detrusor muscle, diminishing its tone and suppressing involuntary contractions of the bladder. Other drugs, for example flavoxate, act directly on the smooth muscle cells and lower detrusor tone without affecting contractility. Failure of drug therapy to increase bladder capacity and lower detrusor tone results in the need for augmentation cystoplasty to enhance bladder storage capability. This procedure is appropriate as long as bladder outflow resistance is normal or increased.

If inadequate urethral resistance is the primary reason for impaired storage of urine, the bladder neck mechanism or the external sphincter area, or both, may be responsible. α-Sympathomimetic agents, such as ephedrine sulfate, pseudoephedrine, and phenyl-propanolamine, stimulate α₁-receptors concentrated in the bladder neck area to enhance the tone of the muscles in this region. No drugs are commercially available that will increase the tone of denervated skeletal muscle in the external sphincter region.

Incomplete emptying of the bladder may also be due to an areflexic bladder, unsustained detrusor contractions, or uncoordinated activity at the bladder neck or external sphincter area. Emptying may be facilitated by α-sympatholytic agents, or skeletal muscle relax-

Table 13.1 Drug therapy in neuropathic bladder dysfunction

Type	Minimum dosage	Maximum dosage
Cholinergic		
Bethanechol (Urecholine)	0.7 mg/kg t.i.d.	0.8 mg/kg q.i.d.
Anticholinergic		
Propantheline (Pro-Banthine)	0.5 mg/kg b.i.d.	0.5 mg/kg q.i.d.
Oxybutynin (Ditropan)	0.2 mg/kg b.i.d.	0.2 mg/kg q.i.d.
Glycopyrrolate (Robinul)	0.01 mg/kg b.i.d.	0.03 mg/kg t.i.d.
Hyoscyamine (Levsin)	0.03 mg/kg b.i.d.	0.1 mg/kg q.i.d.
Tolteridine (Detrol)	0.01 mg/kg b.i.d.	0.04 mg/kg b.i.d.
Sympathomimetic		
Phenylpropanolamine (alpha) (Ornade)	2.5 mg/kg b.i.d.	2.5 mg/kg t.i.d.
Ephedrine (alpha) (Ephedrine)	0.5 mg/kg b.i.d.	1.0 mg/kg t.i.d.
Pseudoephedrine (alpha) (Sudafed)	0.4 mg/kg b.i.d.	0.9 mg/kg t.i.d.
Sympatholytic		
Prazosin (alpha) (Minipress)	0.05 mg/kg b.i.d.	0.1 mg/kg t.i.d.
Phenoxybenzamine (alpha)	0.3 mg/kg b.i.d.	0.5 mg/kg t.i.d.
Propranolol (beta)	0.25 mg/kg b.i.d.	0.5 mg/kg b.i.d.
Doxazosin (alpha) (Cardura)	0.01 mg/kg q.d.	0.02 mg/kg q.d.
Smooth muscle relaxant		
Flavoxate (Urispas)	3.0 mg/kg b.i.d.	3.0 mg/kg t.i.d.
Dicyclomine (Bentyl)	0.1 mg/kg t.i.d.	0.3 mg/kg t.i.d.
Other		
Imipramine (Tofranil)	0.7 mg/kg b.i.d.	1.2 mg/kg t.i.d.

ants. Although conflicting reports have been published regarding the efficacy of bethanechol, it does seem to improve emptying of the bladder in most instances. It should be administered with α-sympatholytic agents because bethanechol also increases urethral resistance at the bladder neck. α-Sympatholytic agents, such as phenoxybenzamine or prazosin, act primarily in the bladder neck area, whereas diazepam and baclofen diminish skeletal muscle tone at the external sphincter region to lower outlet resistance to voiding.

Most neurologic conditions affecting vesicourethral function in children, including myelomeningocele, lipomeningocele, sacral agenesis, and occult lesions, are congenital neurospinal dysraphisms:

1 Neuropathic:
  (a) spinal cord
    (i) congenital
      ■ neurospinal dysraphism
      ■ other anatomic
    (ii) acquired
      ■ trauma
      ■ tumor
      ■ infection
      ■ vascular
      ■ miscellaneous
  (b) supraspinal cord
    ■ anatomic/congenital
    ■ trauma
    ■ tumor
    ■ infection
    ■ vascular
    ■ degenerative
    ■ miscellaneous
    ■ temporary
  (c) peripheral
    ■ trauma
    ■ tumor
    ■ degenerative
    ■ Guillain–Barré syndrome

2 Non-neuropathic:
  ■ anatomic
  ■ myopathic
  ■ psychological
  ■ endocrinologic
  ■ toxic

Occasionally, bladder dysfunction is seen in conjunction with other neurologic lesions. Cerebral palsy is an acquired non-progressive form of dysfunction occurring in the perinatal period as a consequence of cerebral anoxia from a variety of conditions.

Children without obvious neurologic disease may have a voiding abnormality on a functional or maturational basis. Most children gain urinary control before the age of 5 years. Persistent day and night incontinence without a prolonged period of dryness or the recurrence of nocturnal wetting lasting into puberty are indications for urodynamic evaluation in neurologically normal children. Although an overwhelming number have normal findings, a significant percentage may have a dysfunctional voiding state. The types of abnormality are discussed separately along with individual approaches to therapy.

Neurospinal dysraphisms

Myelodysplasia

The most common etiology of neuropathic bladder dysfunction in children is secondary to abnormal spinal column development. Formation of the spinal cord and vertebrae begins around the 18th day of gestation. The canal closes from a cephalad to caudal direction and is complete by 35 days. Although the exact mechanism causing a dysraphic state is unknown at present, numerous factors have been implicated. The incidence has been reported to be 1 per 1000 births in the USA (Stein *et al.*, 1982), but there has been a definite decrease in this occurrence (Laurence, 1989). Two explantations are possible for this phenomenon: with the advent of prenatal screening many families are electing to terminate their pregnancies when they have affected fetuses (Palomaki *et al.*, 1999), and the addition of folic acid supplements to the diet of women of child-bearing age has reduced the incidence of spina bifida by more than 50% (MRC Vitamin Study Group, 1991; AAP Committee on Genetics, 1999). If spina bifida is already present in one member of a family, there is a 2–5% chance of a second sibling being born with the same condition (Scarff and Fronczak, 1981). The incidence doubles when more than one family member has a neurospinal dysraphism (Table 13.2).

Table 13.2 Familial risk of myelodysplasia in the USA per 1000 live births

Relationship	Incidence
General population	0.7–1.0
Mother with one affected child	30–50
Mother with two affected children	100
Patient with myelodysplasia	40
Mother older than 35 years	30
Sister of mother with affected child	10
Sister of father with affected child	3
Nephew who is affected	2

Adapted from Kroovand (1986).

Pathogenesis

Myelodysplasia is an all-inclusive term used to describe the various abnormal conditions of the vertebral column that affect spinal cord function. More specific labels regarding each abnormality include the following:

- a meningocele occurs when just the meninges extend beyond the confines of the vertebral canal without any neural elements contained inside it;
- a myelomeningocele implies that neural tissue, either nerve roots and/or portions of the spinal cord, have evaginated with the meningocele;
- a lipomyelomeningocele denotes that fatty tissue has developed with the cord structures and both are protruding into the sac.

Myelomeningocele accounts for over 90% of all the open spinal dysraphic states (Stark, 1977). Most spinal defects occur at the level of the lumbar vertebrae, with the sacral, thoracic, and cervical areas being affected in decreasing order of frequency (Table 13.3) (Bauer *et al.*, 1977). An overwhelming number of meningoceles is directed posteriorly, but on rare

Table 13.3 Spinal level of myelomeningocele

Location	Incidence (%)
Cervical–high thoracic	2
Low thoracic	5
Lumbar	26
Lumbosacral	47
Sacral	20

Adapted from Kroovand (1986).

occasions, the meningocele may protrude anteriorly, particularly in the sacral area. Usually the meningocele is made up of a flimsy covering of transparent tissue, but it may be open and leaking cerebrospinal fluid (CSF). For this reason, urgent repair is necessary, with sterile precautions being followed in the interval between birth and closure. In 85% of affected children there is an associated Arnold–Chiari malformation, in which the cerebellar tonsils have herniated down through the foramen magnum, obstructing the fourth ventricle and preventing the CSF from entering the subarachnoid space surrounding the brain and spinal cord.

The neurologic lesion produced by this condition can be quite variable. It depends on what neural elements, if any, have everted with the meningocele sac. The bony vertebral level often gives little or no clue as to the exact neurologic level or lesion that is produced. The height of the bony level and the highest extent of the neurologic lesion may vary from one to three vertebrae in one direction or another (Bauer *et al.*, 1977). There may be differences in function from one side of the body to the other at the same neurologic level, and from one neurologic level to the next, as a result of asymmetry of affected neural elements. In addition, 20% of affected children have a vertebral bony or intraspinal abnormality occurring more cephalad from the vertebral defect and meningocele, which can affect function in those additional portions of the cord as well. Children with thoracic and upper lumbar meningoceles often have complete reconstitution of their spine in the sacral area and these individuals will frequently have intact sacral reflex arc function involving the sacral spinal roots. In fact, it is more likely for children with upper thoracic or cervical lesions to have just a meningocele and no myelocele. Finally, the differential growth rates between the vertebral bodies and the elongating spinal cord add a factor of dynamicism in the developing fetus that further complicates the picture (Pontari *et al.*, 1995). Superimposed on all this is the Arnold–Chiari malformation, which may have profound effects on the brainstem and pontine center areas involved in the control over lower urinary tract function.

Thus, the neurologic lesion produced by this condition influences lower urinary tract function in a variety of ways and cannot be predicted just by looking at the spinal abnormality or the neurologic function of the lower extremities. This wide spectrum of dysfunction is evident when looking at babies with sacral level lesions (Dator *et al.*, 1992). Even careful assessment of the sacral area may not provide sufficient information to make a concrete inference. Therefore, urodynamic evaluation in the neonatal period is now performed at most pediatric centers in the USA because it not only provides a clear picture of the function of the sacral spinal cord and lower urinary tract but also has predictive value regarding babies at risk for future urinary tract deterioration and progressive neurologic change (McGuire *et al.*, 1981; VanGool *et al.*, 1982; Bauer *et al.*, 1984; Sidi *et al.*, 1986; Kaefer *et al.*, 1999).

Newborn assessment

Ideally, it would be best to perform urodynamic testing immediately after the baby is born, but the risk of spinal infection and the urgency for closure has not made this a viable option at this time. In a 1990 study, however, preoperative testing was accomplished, and it showed that fewer than 5% of children experience a change in their neurologic status as a result of the spinal canal closure (Kroovand *et al.*, 1990). Therefore, renal ultrasonography and a measurement of residual urine are performed as early as possible after birth, either before or immediately after the spinal defect is closed, with urodynamic studies delayed until it is safe to transport children to the urodynamic suite and place them on their backs or sides for the test. For infants who cannot empty their bladder following a spontaneous void, intermittent catheterization is begun, even before urodynamic studies are conducted. The normal bladder capacity in the newborn period is between 10 and 15 ml; thus, an acceptable residue of urine is less than 5 ml. Other tests that should be performed in the neonatal period include a urine analysis and culture, and determination of the serum creatinine level (Bauer, 1991).

Once the spinal closure has healed sufficiently, either excretory urography or renal ultrasonography and renal scintigraphy are performed to reassess upper urinary tract architecture and function. Following this, voiding cystourethrography (VCUG) and a urodynamic study are conducted. These studies fulfill several objectives (McGuire *et al.*, 1981; Bauer, 1984b; Bauer *et al.*, 1984; Sidi *et al.*, 1986):

■ They provide baseline information about the radiologic appearance of the upper and lower urinary tract, as well as the condition of the sacral spinal cord and the CNS.

- The studies can then be compared with later assessments, so that early signs of deteriorating urinary tract drainage and function, or of progressive neurologic denervation, can be detected.
- They help to identify babies at risk for urinary tract deterioration as a result of detrusor hypertonicity or outflow obstruction from detrusor sphincter dyssynergy, which then allows prophylactic measures to be initiated before the changes actually take place.
- They help the physician to counsel parents with regard to their child's future bladder and sexual function.

Findings

Ten to 15 per cent of newborns have an abnormal radiographic appearance to their urinary tract when first evaluated (Bauer, 1985); 3% have hydrouretero-nephrosis secondary to spinal shock, probably from the closure procedure (Chiaramonte *et al.*, 1986), whereas 10% have abnormalities that developed *in utero* as a result of abnormal lower urinary tract function in the form of outlet obstruction.

Urodynamic studies in the newborn period have shown that 57% of infants with myelomeningocele have bladder contractions. This is especially true in children with upper lumbar or thoracic lesions who have sparing of the sacral spinal cord, 83% of whom have detrusor contractions (Keating *et al.*, 1987). Forty-three per cent have an areflexic bladder, and compliance during bladder filling is either good (25%) or poor (18%) in this subgroup (Bauer *et al.*, 1984). Electromyographic assessment of the external urethral sphincter demonstrates an intact sacral reflex arc with no evidence of lower motor neuron denervation in 47% of newborns, whereas partial denervation is seen in 24% and complete loss of sacral cord function is noted in 29% (Spindel *et al.*, 1987).

Combining bladder contractility and external sphincter activity results in three categories of lower urinary tract dynamics: synergic; dyssynergic, with and without detrusor hypertonicity; and complete denervation (see Fig. 13.1) (Bauer *et al.*, 1984; Sidi *et al.*, 1986). Synergy is characterized by complete silencing of the sphincter during a detrusor contraction or when capacity is reached at the end of filling. Voiding pressures are usually within the normal range. Dyssynergy occurs when the external sphincter fails to decrease, or actually increases its activity during a

detrusor contraction or a sustained increase in intravesical pressure, as the bladder is filled to capacity (Blaivas *et al.*, 1986). Frequently, a poorly compliant bladder with high intravesical pressure is seen in conjunction with a dyssynergic sphincter, resulting in a bladder that empties only at high intravesical pressures (Sidi *et al.*, 1986; VanGool *et al.*, 1982). Complete denervation is noted when no bioelectric potentials are detectable in the region of the external sphincter at any time during the micturition cycle or in response to a Credé maneuver or sacral stimulation.

Categorizing lower urinary tract function in this way has been extremely useful because it has defined which children are at risk for urinary tract changes, who should be treated prophylactically, who needs close surveillance, and who can be followed at greater intervals without fear of deterioration. On initial assessment or subsequent studies, 71% of newborns with voiding dyssynergy had urinary tract deterioration within the first 3 years of life, whereas only 17% of synergic voiders and 23% with completely denervated bladders developed similar changes (Fig. 13.2). The infants in the synergic group whose upper tracts deteriorated did so only after they converted to a dyssynergic pattern of sphincter function. Among the infants with complete denervation, the only babies with hydronephrosis were those who had elevated levels of urethral resistance, presumably due to fibrosis of the skeletal muscle component of the external sphincter. Thus, it appears that outlet obstruction is a major contributor to the

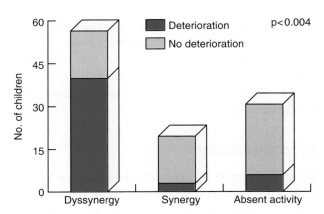

Figure 13.2 Urinary tract deterioration is related to outflow obstruction and most often associated with dyssynergy. Children with synergy converted to dyssynergy and patients with complete bladder denervation developed fibrosis with a fixed high-outlet resistance in the external sphincter, before any changes occurred in the urinary tract. (From Bauer, 1988.)

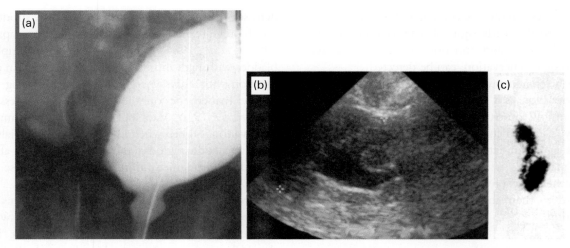

Figure 13.3 (*a*) Voiding cystourethrography in a newborn girl with dyssynergy and elevated voiding pressures demonstrated no reflux and a smooth-walled bladder. Her initial renal echogram was normal. She was started on clean intermittent catheterization and oxybutynin (Ditropan) but did not respond. Within 1 year, she had right hydronephrosis (*b*) and severe reflux on a radionuclide cytogram (*c*).

development of urinary tract deterioration in these children (Fig. 13.3). Bladder tonicity plays an important but somewhat less critical role in this regard (McGuire *et al.*, 1981), although detrusor compliance seems to be worse in children with high levels of outlet resistance (Ghoniem *et al.*, 1989). This combination of parameters (poor compliance and high outlet resistance) is very provocative for the development of hydro-ureteronephrosis (McLorie *et al.*, 1986; Steinhardt *et al.*, 1986), whereas detrusor-sphincter dyssynergia is a significant factor in the onset of vesicoureteral reflux (VUR) (Seki *et al.*, 1999) (Fig. 13.3). Bloom *et al.* (1990) noted an improvement in compliance when outlet resistance was lowered following gentle urethral dilation in these children; however, the reasons for this are unclear and the long-term effect of this maneuver on ultimate continence and upper urinary tract function remains uncertain.

Recommendations

Because expectant treatment has revealed that infants with outlet obstruction in the form of detrusor-sphincter dyssynergy are at considerable risk for urinary tract deterioration, the idea of prophylactically treating the children has emerged as an important alternative. When CIC is begun in the newborn period, it becomes easy for parents to master, even in uncircumcised boys, and for children to accept as they grow older (Joseph *et al.*, 1989). Complications of meatitis, epididymitis, or urethral injury are rarely encountered, and symptomatic urinary infection occurs in fewer than 30% (Kasabian *et al.*, 1992).

CIC alone or in combination with anticholinergic agents, when detrusor filling pressures are greater than 40 cmH$_2$O and voiding pressures reach levels higher than 80–100 cmH$_2$O, has resulted in only an 8–10% incidence of urinary tract deterioration (Fig. 13.4). (Geraniotis *et al.*, 1988; Kasabian *et al.*, 1992; Edelstein *et al.*, 1995). This represents a significant drop in the occurrence of detrimental changes compared with the group of children followed expectantly (McGuire *et al.*, 1981; Bauer *et al.*, 1984; Sidi *et al.*, 1986). Oxybutynin hydrochloride is administered in a dose of 1.0 mg per year of age, every 12 hours, in order to help lower detrusor filling pressure. In neonates or children younger than 1 year of age, the dose is lowered to below 1.0 mg in relation to the child's age at the time and increased proportionately as he or she approaches 1 year. No side-effects were seen when oxybutynin was administered according to this schedule (Joseph *et al.*, 1989; Kasabian *et al.*, 1992). When a hyperreflexic or hypertonic bladder fails to respond to these measures, augmentation cystoplasty may be required. However, the need for this operative modality in children managed proactively has been substantially reduced to 17%, as compared to a 41% incidence in children followed expectantly (Kaefer *et al.*, 1999) (Fig. 13.4). Furthermore, the use of vesicostomy drainage has been almost completely eliminated.

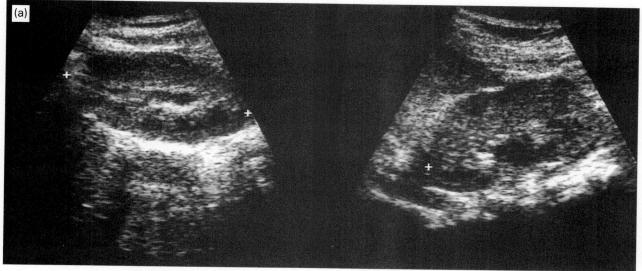

Right kidney   Left kidney

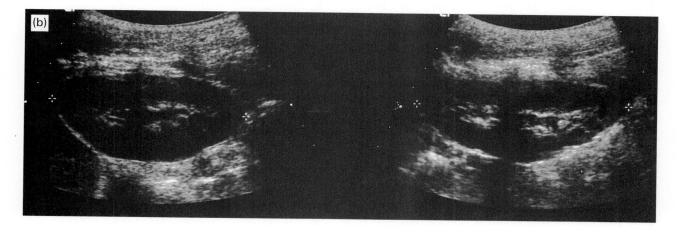

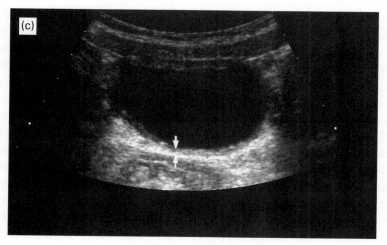

Figure 13.4 Another newborn boy with detrusor sphincter dyssynergia was successfully treated with clean inter-mittent catheterization and oxybutynin. Over a 14 year period his kidneys have remained normal by renal ultrasound (a, b) and his bladder wall has not increased its thickness (c).

Neurologic findings and recommendations

The neurourologic lesion in myelodysplasia is a dynamic disease process with changes taking place throughout childhood (Epstein, 1982; Reigel, 1983; Venes and Stevens, 1983), especially in early infancy (Spindel *et al.*, 1987), and then at puberty (Begger *et al.*, 1986), when the linear growth rate accelerates again. When a change is noted on neurologic, orthopedic, or urodynamic assessment, radiologic investigation of the CNS often reveals: (1) tethering of the spinal cord; (2) a syrinx or hydromyelia of the cord; (3) increased intracranial pressure due to a shunt malfunction; or (4) partial herniation of the brainstem and cerebellum. Children with completely intact or only partially denervated sacral cord function are particularly vulnerable to progressive changes. Magnetic resonance imaging (MRI) is the test of choice because it reveals anatomic details of the spinal column and CNS. However, it is not a functional study, and when used alone, it cannot provide exact information with regard to a changing neurologic lesion.

Sequential urodynamic testing on a yearly basis, beginning in the newborn period and continuing until 5 years of age, provides the means for carefully following these children to detect signs of change, thus offering the hope that early detection and neurosurgical intervention may help to arrest or even reverse a progressive pathologic process. Changes occurring in a group of newborns followed in this manner involved both the sacral reflex arc and the pontine–sacral reflex interaction (Spindel *et al.*, 1987; Lais *et al.*, 1993) (Fig. 13.5). Most children who change tend to do so in the first 3 years of life (Fig. 13.6). Twenty-two of 28 children who exhibited a worsening in their neurologic picture underwent a second neurosurgical procedure. Half had a beneficial effect from the surgery, with 11 of these 22 showing improvement in urethral sphincter function (Lais *et al.*, 1993).

As a result of these developments, all babies with myelodysplasia should be observed according to the guidelines set forth in Table 13.4. It is not enough to look at just the radiographic appearance of the urinary tract; critical scrutiny of the functional status of the lower urinary tract is important as well. In addition to the reasons cited above, it may be necessary to repeat the urodynamic study when the upper urinary tract dilates secondary to impaired drainage from a hypertonic detrusor or urinary incontinence occurs after a prolonged period of dryness on intermittent catheterization and medical therapy.

Management of reflux

VUR occurs in 3–5% of newborns with myelodysplasia, usually in association with detrusor hypertonicity and/or dyssynergia. It is rare to find reflux in any neonate with a spinal cord lesion without dyssynergy or poor compliance (Bauer, 1984a; Geraniotis *et al.*, 1988). If left untreated, the incidence of reflux in these at-risk infants increases with time until 30–40% are afflicted by 5 years of age (Bauer, 1984a), with even higher levels noted in older children (Seki *et al.*, 1999).

In children with mild to moderate grades of reflux (I–III), who void spontaneously or who have complete lesions with little or no outlet resistance and empty their bladder completely, management consists of antibiotic prophylaxis to prevent recurrent infection. When these children have high-grade reflux (grade IV or V), intermittent catheterization is begun to ensure complete emptying. Children who cannot empty their bladders spontaneously, regardless of the grade of reflux, are catheterized intermittently to ensure complete emptying. Children with detrusor hypertonicity, with or without hydroureteronephrosis, are also treated with oxybutynin to lower intravesical pressure and ensure adequate upper urinary tract decompression. When reflux has been managed in this manner, a dramatic response has resulted, with reflux resolving in 30–55% of individuals (Kass *et al.*, 1981; Bauer, 1984a; Joseph *et al.*, 1989; Flood *et al.*, 1994). Although bacteriuria can be seen in as many as 56% of children on intermittent catheterization, generally it is not harmful except in the presence of high-grade reflux because symptomatic urinary infection and renal scarring rarely occur with the lesser grades of reflux (Kass *et al.*, 1981; Cohen *et al.*, 1990).

Credé voiding is to be avoided in children with reflux, especially those with a reactive external sphincter. Under these conditions, the Credé maneuver results in a reflex response of the external sphincter that increases urethral resistance and raises the pressure needed to expel urine from the bladder (Barbalias *et al.*, 1983) (Fig. 13.7). This has the effect of aggravating the degree of reflux and increasing upper tract dilatation. Vesicostomy drainage (Duckett, 1974; Mandell *et al.*, 1981), used much less frequently today than in previous years, is reserved for (1) those infants who have such severe reflux that intermittent catheterization and anticholinergic medication fail to improve upper urinary tract drainage; or (2) those children whose parents cannot adapt to the catheterization program.

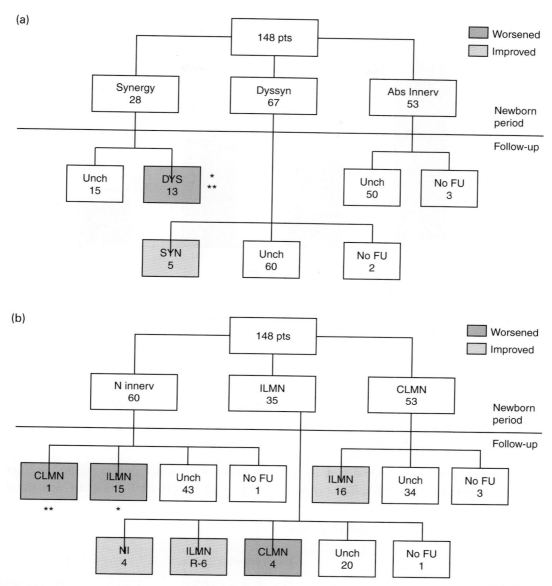

Figure 13.5 (*a*) Pontine–sacral reflux arc changes that occurred in a group of children with myelodysplasia followed with sequential urodynamic studies between the newborn period and 3 or more years of age. Dyssyn = dyssynergy; Abs Innerv = absence of innervation; Unch = unchanged; DYS = dyssynergy; FU = follow-up; Syn = synergy; * = one patient who changed from normal innervation to partial and then complete denervation; ** = four patients who changed from normal innervation to partial denervation. (*b*) Sacral reflex arc pathway changes that occurred in the same group of children. N innerv = normal innervation; ILMN = incomplete lower motor neuron; CLMN = complete lower motor neuron; Unch = unchanged; FU = follow-up; N = normal; * = four of 15 patients who changed from synergy to dyssynergy; ** = one patient who changed from synergy to dyssynergy.

The indications for antireflux surgery today are not very different from those for children with normal bladder function and include recurrent symptomatic urinary infection while on adequate antibiotic therapy and appropriate catheterization techniques, persistent hydroureteronephrosis despite effective emptying of the bladder and lowering of intravesical pressure, severe reflux with an anatomic abnormality at the ureterovesical junction, and reflux persisting into puberty. In addition, children with any grade of reflux who are being considered for implantation of an artificial urinary sphincter or any other procedure designed to increase bladder outlet resistance should have the reflux corrected

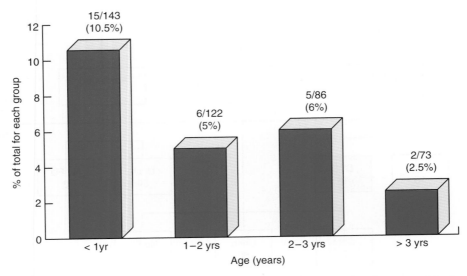

Figure 13.6 Propensity for deterioration in external urethral sphincter innervation is greatest in the first year of life with a decreasing incidence noted subsequently. (From Bauer, 1988.)

at the time of or prior to the anti-incontinence surgery.

Jeffs *et al.* (1976) noted that antireflux surgery could be very successful in children with neuropathic bladder dysfunction as long as it is combined with measures to ensure complete bladder emptying. Since the advent of intermittent catheterization, success rates for antireflux surgery have approached 95% (Kass *et al.*, 1981; Woodard *et al.*, 1981; Bauer *et al.*,

1982; Kaplan and Firlit, 1983) (see Chapter 25). Unilateral reflux does not warrant bilateral reimplantation because the incidence of contralateral reflux postoperatively is insignificant (Bauer *et al.*, 1982).

Continence

Urinary continence is becoming an increasingly important issue to deal with at an early age as parents

Table 13.4 Surveillance in infants with myelodysplasia[a]

Sphincter activity	Recommended tests	Frequency
Intact — synergic	Postvoiding residual	Every 4 months
	IVP or renal echo	Every 12 months
	UDS	Every 12 months
Intact — dyssynergic[b]	IVP or renal echo	Every 12 months
	UDS	Every 12 months
	VCUG or RNC[c]	Every 12 months
Partial denervation	Postvoiding residual	Every 4 months
	IVP or renal echo	Every 12 months
	UDS[d]	Every 12 months
	VCUG or RNC[c]	Every 12 months
Complete denervation	Postvoiding residual	Every 6 months
	Renal echo	Every 12 months

[a]Until the age of 5 years.
[b]Patients on intermittent catheterization and anticholinergic agents.
[c]If detrusor hypertonicity or reflux already present.
[d]Depending on degree of denervation.
IVP = intravenous pyelography; echo = sonography; UDS = urodynamic study; VCUG = voiding cystourethrography; RNC = radionuclide cystography.

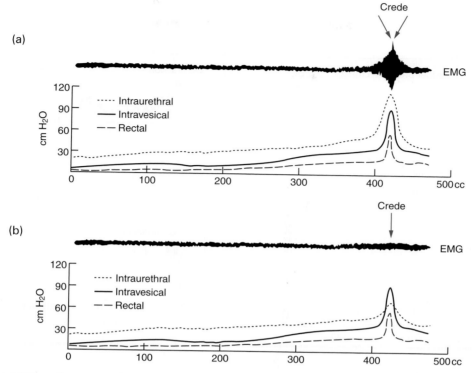

Figure 13.7 (a) When the external sphincter is reactive, a Credé maneuver produces a reflex increase in electro-myographic (EMG) activity of the sphincter and a concomitant rise in urethral resistance, resulting in high voiding pressure. (b) A child whose sphincter is denervated and non-reactive will not have a corresponding rise in EMG activity, urethral resistance, or voiding pressure. A Credé maneuver here will not be detrimental. (From Bauer, 1988.)

try to mainstream their handicapped children. Initial attempts at achieving continence include CIC and drug therapy designed to maintain low intravesical pressure and a reasonable level of urethral resistance (Figs. 13.8, 13.9). Although this approach can be conducted on a trial-and-error basis, it is more efficient to have exact treatment protocols based on specific urodynamic findings. As a result, urodynamic testing is performed if initial attempts with CIC and oxybutynin fail to achieve continence. Without urodynamic studies, it is hard to know whether (1) a single drug is effective, (2) the drug dosage should be increased, (3) a second drug should be added to the regimen, or (4) alternative methods of treatment should be employed.

If urodynamic testing reveals that urethral resistance is inadequate to maintain continence because there is either a failure of the sphincter to react to increases in abdominal pressure or a drop in resistance with bladder filling, then α-sympathomimetic agents are added to the regimen (see Table 13.1).

Sexuality

Sexuality in this population has become an increasingly important issue to deal with as more and more individuals have reached adulthood and want either to marry or to have meaningful long-term relationships (Cromer et al., 1990). Few studies are available, however, that look critically at sexual function in these patients.

In one study, researchers interviewed a group of affected teenagers and reported that at least 28% of them had one or more sexual encounters, and almost all had a desire to marry and ultimately bear children (Cromer et al., 1990). In a more recent study (Decter et al., 1997) 57 men were questioned regarding their sexual history: 41 (72%) had erections and 27 of them (66%) had ejaculations. Twenty men said they had had sexual intercourse but only 11 attempted to father children, of whom eight were successful. Overall, 12 men (21%) were married. Another study revealed that 70% of myelodysplastic women were

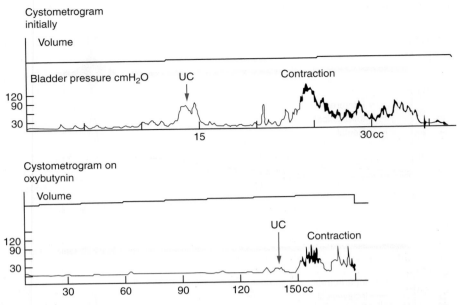

Figure 13.8 Oxybutynin is a potent anticholinergic agent that dramatically delays detrusor contractions and lowers contraction pressure, as demonstrated on these two graphs from a 6-month-old girl with myelodysplasia. UC = uninhibited contraction. (From Bauer, 1988.)

able to become pregnant and have an uneventful pregnancy and delivery, although urinary incontinence in the latter stages of gestation and cesarean section were common (Cass *et al.*, 1986). In the same study, 17% of males claimed that they were able to father children. It is more likely for males to have problems with erectile and ejaculatory function because of the frequent neurologic involvement of the sacral spinal cord, whereas reproductive function in

the female, which is under hormonal control, is not affected. However, the level of the neurologic lesion is not predictive of ultimate sexual function in men (Decter *et al.*, 1997).

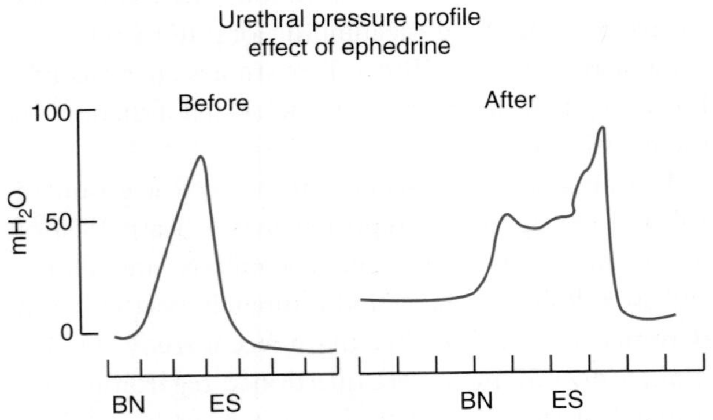

As important as knowing what the precise sexual function is in an individual, sexuality or the ability to interact with the opposite sex in a meaningful and lasting way is just as important. Sexual identity, education, and social mores are issues that have been taken out of the realm of secrecy and are now openly discussed and taught to handicapped people (Woodhouse, 1998; Palmer *et al.*, 1999). Boys reach puberty at an age similar to that for normal males, whereas breast development and menarche tend to start as much as 2 years earlier than usual in myelodysplastic females. The etiology of this early hormonal surge is uncertain, but it may be related to pituitary function changes in girls secondary to their hydrocephalus (Hayden, 1985).

Lipomeningocele and other spinal dysraphisms

Diagnosis

A group of congenital defects affects the formation of the spinal column but does not result in an open vertebral canal (James and Lassman, 1972). These occult spinal dysraphisms include:

Figure 13.9 α-Sympathomimetic agents potentially have their greatest effect in the bladder neck region where the highest concentration of α-receptor sites exist. They can raise outlet resistance and improve continence in many individuals. (From Bauer, 1988.)

- lipomeningocele
- intradural lipoma
- diastematomyelia
- tight filum terminale
- dermoid cyst/sinus
- aberrant nerve roots

- anterior sacral meningocele
- cauda equina tumor.

These lesions may be very subtle with no obvious outward signs. But, in more than 90% of cases, the children manifest a cutaneous abnormality overlying the

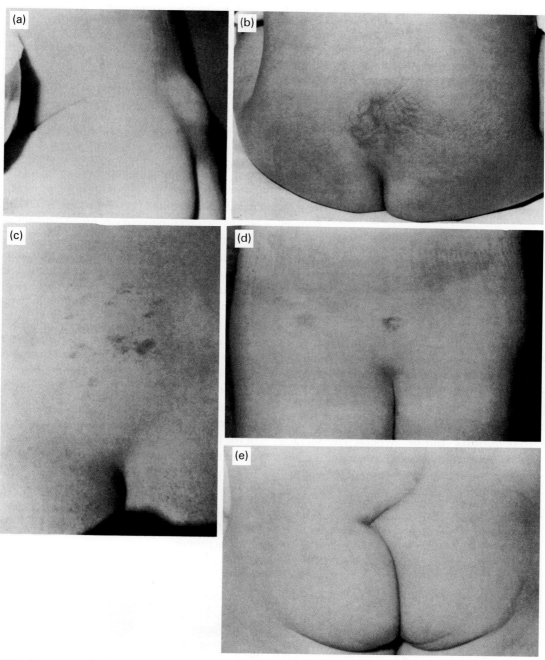

Figure 13.10 Cutaneous lesions occur in 90% of children with various occult dysraphic states. These lesions may vary from a small lipomeningocele (*a*) to a hair patch (*b*), a dermal vascular malformation (*c*), a dimple (*d*), or an abnormal gluteal cleft (*e*).

lower spine (Anderson, 1975). This may vary from a small dimple or skin tag to a tuft of hair, a dermal vascular malformation, or a very noticeable subcutaneous lipoma (Fig. 13.10). In addition, on careful inspection of the legs, one may note a high arched foot or feet, alterations in the configuration of the toes, with hammer or claw digits being seen, a discrepancy in muscle size and strength between the legs with weakness at the ankle, and/or a gait abnormality, especially in older children, as a result of shortness of one leg (Dubrowitz *et al.*, 1965; Weissert *et al.*, 1989). Absent perineal sensation and back pain are not uncommon symptoms in older children or young adults (Yip *et al.*, 1985; Linder *et al.*, 1982; Weissert *et al.*, 1989). Lower urinary tract function is abnormal in 40% of affected individuals (Mandell *et al.*, 1980).

The child may experience difficulty with urinary control (especially during the pubertal growth spurt), urinary retention, recurrent urinary infection, and/or fecal soiling after an initial period of dryness.

Findings

When these children are evaluated in the newborn or early infancy period, the majority have a perfectly normal neurologic examination. Urodynamic testing, however, will reveal abnormal lower urinary tract function in about one-third of the babies younger than the age of 18 months (Keating *et al.*, 1988; Satar *et al.*, 1997) (Fig. 13.11). These studies may provide the only evidence for a neurologic injury involving the lower spinal cord (Keating *et al.*, 1988; Foster *et al.*, 1990). When present, the most likely abnormality is an upper motor neuron lesion characterized by detrusor hyperreflexia and/or hyperactive sacral reflexes, with mild forms of detrusor-sphincter dyssynergy being noted rarely. Lower motor neuron

signs with denervation potentials in the sphincter, or detrusor areflexia, occur in only 10% of young children.

In contrast, practically all individuals in the group older than 3 years of age who have not been operated upon or have been belatedly diagnosed as having an occult dysraphism will have either an upper motor neuron and/or lower motor neuron lesion on urodynamic testing (92%) (Fig. 13.11), or neurologic signs of lower extremity dysfunction (Yip *et al.*, 1985; Kondo *et al.*, 1986; Keating *et al.*, 1988; Satar *et al.*, 1995). There does not seem to be a preponderance for one type of lesion over the other (upper versus lower motor neuron); each occurs with equal frequency, and often the child manifests signs of both (Hellstrom *et al.*, 1986; Kondo *et al.*, 1986).

Pathogenesis

The reason for this difference in neurologic findings may be related to (1) compression on the cauda equina or sacral nerve roots by an expanding lipoma or lipomeningocele (Yamada *et al.*, 1983), or (2) tension on the cord from tethering secondary to differential growth rates between the bony and neural elements (Dubrowitz *et al.*, 1965). Under normal circumstances, the conus medullaris ends just below the L-2 vertebra at birth and should recede upwards to T-12 by adulthood (Barson, 1970). When the cord does not 'rise' secondary to one of these lesions, ischemic injury may ensue (Yamada *et al.*, 1981). Correction of the lesion in infancy has resulted in not only stabilization but also improvement in the neurologic picture in some instances (Fig. 13.12). Sixty percent of the babies with abnormal urodynamic findings preoperatively reverted to normal postoperatively, with improvement noted in 30%, whereas 10% worsened

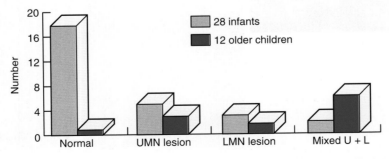

Figure 13.11 Most newborns with a covered spinal dysraphism have normal lower urinary tract function, whereas older children tend to have both upper and lower motor neuron lesions. UMN = upper motor neuron; LMN = lower motor neuron; U + L = upper and lower motor neuron.

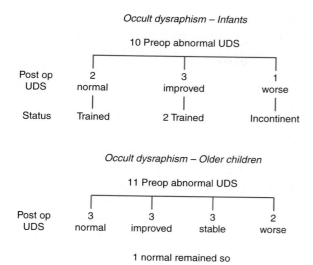

Figure **13.12** Potential for recoverable function is greatest in infants [six of 10 (60%)] and less in older children [three of 11 (27%)]. The risk of damage to neural tissue at the time of exploration to those with normal function is small [two of 19 (11%), not shown].

with time. In the older child, there is a less dramatic change following surgery, with only 27% becoming normal, 27% improving, 27% stabilizing, but 19% worsening with time (Keating *et al.*, 1983) (Fig. 13.12). Older individuals with hyperreflexia tend to improve, while those with areflexic bladders do not (Hellstrom *et al.*, 1986; Kondo *et al.*, 1986; Flanigan *et al.*, 1989). Finally, fewer than 5% of the children operated on in early childhood developed secondary tethering when observed for several years, suggesting that early surgery has both a beneficial and sustaining effect with these conditions.

As a result of these findings, it is apparent that urodynamic testing may be the only way to document that an occult spinal dysraphism is affecting lower spinal cord function (Keating *et al.*, 1988; Khoury *et al.*, 1990). Some investigators have shown that posterior tibial somatosensory evoked potentials are even a more sensitive indicator of tethering and should be an integral part of the urodynamic evaluation (Roy *et al.*, 1986). The implication of this recommendation is that early detection and intervention are associated with both a reversibility to the lesion that is lost in the older child (Yamada *et al.*, 1981, 1983; Tami *et al.*, 1987; Kaplan *et al.*, 1988) and a degree of protection from subsequent tethering, which seems to be a frequent occurrence when the lesion is not dealt with expeditiously in infancy (Seeds and Jones, 1986).

Recommendations

Both MRI (Tracey and Hanigan, 1990) and urodynamic testing should be conducted in everyone who has a questionable skin or bony abnormality of the lower spine (Packer *et al.*, 1986; Campobasso *et al.*, 1988; Hall *et al.*, 1988). If the child is younger than 4–6 months of age, ultrasonography may be useful to image the spinal canal before the vertebral bones have had a chance to ossify (Raghavendra *et al.*, 1983; Scheible *et al.*, 1983). In the past, these conditions were usually treated by removing only the superficial skin lesions without dissecting further into the spinal canal to remove or repair the entire abnormality. Today, most neurosurgeons advocate laminectomy and removal of the intraspinal process as completely as possible without injuring the nerve roots or cord as soon as feasible after the diagnosis is made, in order to release the tethering and to prevent further injury that might ensue with subsequent growth (Linder *et al.*, 1982; Kondo *et al.*, 1986; Kaplan *et al.*, 1988; Foster *et al.*, 1990).

Sacral agenesis

Sacral agenesis has been defined as absence of part or all of two or more lower vertebral bodies. Although the etiology of this condition is still uncertain, teratogenic factors may play a role in that insulin-dependent mothers have a 1% chance of giving birth to a child with this disorder. In addition, 16% of children with sacral agenesis have a diabetic mother (Passarge and Lenz, 1966; Guzman *et al.*, 1983), although it may only have been gestational, insulin-dependent diabetes. Sacral agenesis has been reproduced in chicks when exposed as embryos to insulin (Landauer, 1945; White and Klauber, 1976). Maternal insulin–antibody complexes have been noted to cross the placenta, and their concentration in the fetal circulation is directly correlated with macrosomia (Menon *et al.*, 1990). It is possible that a similar cause-and-effect phenomenon is occurring in sacral agenesis.

Diagnosis

The diagnosis is often delayed until failed attempts at toilet training bring the child to the attention of a physician. Sensation, including perianal dermatomes, is usually intact, and lower extremity function is normal (Koff and DeRidder, 1977; Jakobson *et al.*, 1985). Because these children have normal sensation and little or no orthopedic deformity involving the lower

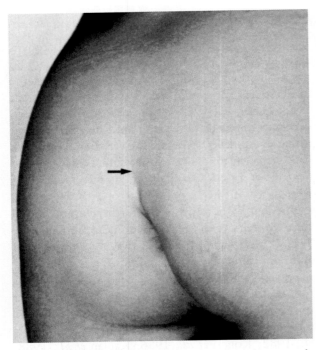

Figure 13.13 Characteristically, the gluteal crease is short and seen only inferiorly (*below arrow*) as a result of the flattened buttocks in sacral agenesis.

extremities (although high arched feet and/or claw or hammer toes may be present), the underlying lesion is often overlooked. In fact, 20% of children escape detection until the age of 3 or 4 years, when parents begin to question their ability to train their child (Guzman *et al.*, 1983). The only clue, requiring a high index of suspicion, is flattened buttocks and a low short gluteal cleft (Bauer, 1990) (Fig. 13.13). Palpation of the coccyx will detect the absent vertebrae (White and Klauber, 1976). The diagnosis is most easily confirmed with a lateral film of the lower spine, because this area is often obscured by the overlying gas pattern on an anteroposterior projection (White and Klauber, 1976; Guzman *et al.*, 1983) (Fig. 13.14). MRI has been used to visualize the spinal cord in these cases, and a sharp cut-off of the conus opposite the T-12 vertebra seems to be a consistent finding (Fig. 13.15).

Urodynamic findings

When urodynamic studies are undertaken, almost an equal number of individuals will manifest an upper or lower motor neuron lesion (35% versus 40%, respectively), whereas 25% have no signs of denervation at all (Guzman *et al.*, 1983). The upper motor neuron lesion is characterized by detrusor hyperreflexia, exaggerated

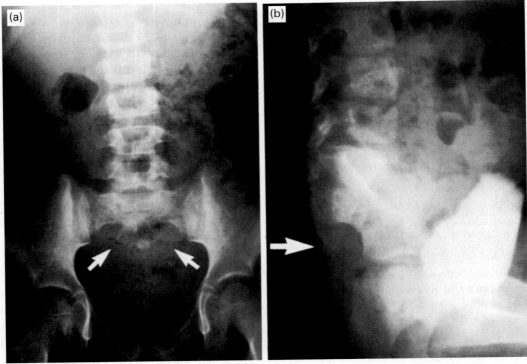

Figure 13.14 The diagnosis is easily confirmed on an anteroposterior (*a*) or lateral (*b*) film of the spine (the latter is performed if bowel gas obscures the sacral area).

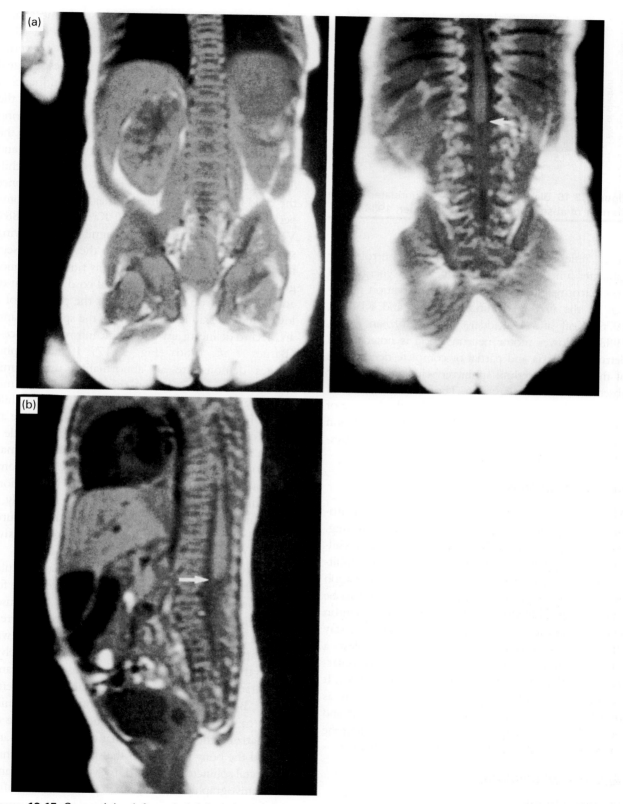

Figure 13.15 Coronal (*a, left and right*) and sagittal (*b*) magnetic resonance images in a 6-month-old girl with sacral agenesis at S-1 reveal a squared lower limit of the cord adjacent to T-12 (*arrow*). Note a solitary right kidney (*a, left*).

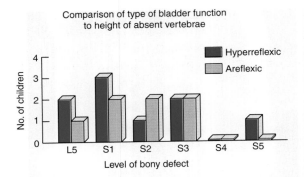

Figure 13.16 Bladder contractility is unrelated to the number of absent vertebrae. (From Bauer, 1988.)

sacral reflexes, absence of voluntary control over sphincter function, detrusor-sphincter dyssynergy, and no electromyographic evidence of denervation potentials in the urethral sphincter (White and Klauber, 1976; Koff and DeRidder, 1977; Guzman et al., 1983). A lower motor neuron lesion is noted when detrusor areflexia and partial or complete denervation of the external urethral sphincter with diminished or absent sacral reflexes are seen. The number of affected vertebrae does not seem to correlate with the type of motor neuron lesion present (Fig. 13.16). The lesion usually appears to be stable without signs of progressive denervation.

Recommendations

Management depends on the specific type of neuro-urologic dysfunction seen on urodynamic testing. Anticholinergic agents should be given to those children with upper motor neuron findings of uninhibited contractions, whereas intermittent catheterization and α-sympathomimetic medication may need to be initiated in individuals with lower motor neuron deficits who can neither empty their bladder nor stay dry between catheterizations. The bowel manifests a similar picture of dysfunction and needs as much characterization and treatment as the lower urinary tract. It is important to identify these individuals as early as possible so that they can be rendered continent and out of diapers at an appropriate age, thus avoiding the social stigmata of fecal and/or urinary incontinence.

Associated conditions

Imperforate anus

Imperforate anus is a condition that can occur alone or as part of a constellation of anomalies that has been called the VATER or VACTERL syndrome (Barry and Auldist, 1974). This mnemonic stands for all of the organs that possibly can be affected (V = vertebral, A = anal, C = cardiac, TE = tracheo-esophageal fistula, R = renal, L = limb). Urinary incontinence is not common unless the spinal cord is involved or the pelvic floor muscles and/or nerves are injured during the imperforate anus repair. A plain film of the abdomen and an ultrasonic image of the spine and kidneys are obtained in the neonatal period in all children regardless of the level of the rectal atresia, once the child has either stabilized or has had a colostomy performed (Tunnell et al., 1987; Karrer et al., 1988). Vertebral bony anomalies often signify an underlying spinal cord abnormality. Because the vertebral segments have not fully calcified at this time, ultrasonography can readily image the spinal cord. Any hint of an abnormality on these studies or the presence of a lower midline skin lesion overlying the spine warrants an MRI to delineate any pathologic intraspinal process (Barnes et al., 1986) (Fig. 13.17). If radiographic images demonstrate an abnormality, urodynamic studies are conducted soon thereafter. Urodynamic studies are also indicated before repair in the child with a high imperforate anus who has undergone an initial colostomy. Abnormal findings may provide a reason to explore and treat any intraspinal abnormality in order to improve the child's chances of becoming continent of both feces and urine; in addition, they furnish a baseline for comparison, especially if incontinence should become a problem in the future, particularly in those children needing extensive surgery for their imperforate anus.

Electromyographic studies of the perianal musculature at this time help to define the optimal location for the future anus. Before the Peña operation, which uses a posterior midline approach, was developed to correct a high imperforate anus, rectal incontinence was thought to be due to an injury involving the pelvic nerves that innervate the levator ani muscles (Williams and Grant, 1969; Parrott and Woodard, 1979; Peña, 1986). Because the dissection is confined to the midline area, this procedure has reduced the chance of traumatizing the nerve fibers that course laterally and around the bony pelvis from the spine to the urethral and rectal sphincter muscles. Urodynamic and perianal electromyographic (EMG) studies are repeated after the imperforate anus repair, if fecal and/or urinary continence has not been achieved by a reasonable age or if urinary incontinence develops secondarily.

Thirty to 45 per cent of these children have a spinal abnormality even though they may not have any other associated anomalies (Uehling *et al.*, 1983; Carson *et al.*, 1984). This abnormality may range from tethering of the spinal cord secondary to an intraspinal dysraphism, which produces an upper motor neuron type of dysfunction involving the bladder and external urethral sphincter, to an atrophic abnormality of the conus medullaris, which leads to a partial or complete lower motor neuron lesion

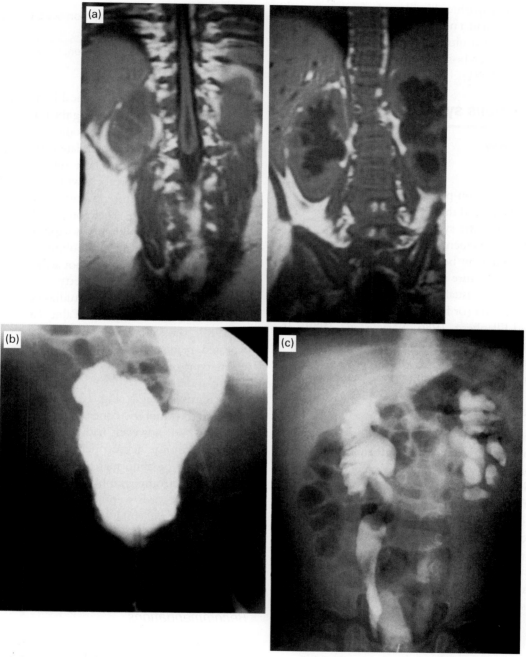

Figure 13.17 (*a, right and left*) This 1-year-old girl with an imperforate anus and bony vertebral abnormalities has bilateral hydronephrosis and a tethered cord on this MRI scan. (*b*) Her voiding cystourogram reveals significant trabeculation and reflux on the left, whereas her excretory urogram (*c*) demonstrates bilateral hydronephrosis secondary to the reflux on the left and a ureterovesical junction obstruction on the right. Her urodynamic study manifested detrusor hypertonicity and dyssynergy.

involving the lower urinary tract (Greenfield and Fera, 1991). In these circumstances, urinary and fecal incontinence might be the child's only complaints. Because lower extremity function may be totally normal, an examination of the legs alone can be misleading (Carson *et al.*, 1984). In one review, 20% of children with neuropathic bladder dysfunction and imperforate anus had a normal bony spine, suggesting that postnatal spinal ultrasonography should be performed in all newborns with imperforate anus (Sheldon *et al.*, 1991).

Central nervous system insults

Cerebral palsy

Etiology

Cerebral palsy is a non-progressive injury to the brain in the perinatal period that produces a neuromuscular disability or a specific symptom complex of cerebral dysfunction. Its incidence is approximately 1.5 per 1000 births but may be increasing as more smaller and younger premature infants are surviving in intensive care units. It is usually due to a perinatal infection or period of anoxia (or hypoxia) that affects the CNS (Nelson and Ellenberg, 1986; Naeye *et al.*, 1989). It most commonly appears in babies who were premature, but it may be seen following a seizure, infection, or intracranial hemorrhage in the neonatal period.

Diagnosis

Affected children have delayed gross motor development, abnormal fine motor performance, altered muscle tone, abnormal stress gait, and exaggerated deep tendon reflexes. These findings can vary substantially from being very obvious to exquisitely subtle with no discernible lesion present unless a careful neurologic examination is performed. Among the more overtly affected individuals, spastic diplegia is the most common of the five types of dysfunction that characterize this disease, accounting for nearly two-thirds of the cases.

Findings

Most children with cerebral palsy develop total urinary control. Incontinence is a feature in some, but the exact incidence has never been truly determined (McNeal *et al.*, 1983; Decter *et al.*, 1987). The presence of incontinence is not related to the extent of the physical

Table 13.5 Lower urinary tract function in cerebral palsy[a]

Type of dysfunction	No. (%)
Upper motor neuron lesion	49 (86)
Mixed upper and lower motor neuron lesion	5 (9.5)
Incomplete lower motor neuron lesion	1 (1.5)
No urodynamic lesion	2 (3)

[a]The study included 57 children.

impairment, although the physical handicap may prevent the individual from reaching the toilet before he or she has an episode of wetting. Some children have such a severe degree of mental retardation that they are not trainable, but the majority have sufficient intelligence to learn basic societal protocol with patient and persistent handling. Oftentimes, continence is achieved at a later than expected age. Therefore, urodynamic evaluation is reserved for children who appear trainable and do not seem to be hampered too much by their physical impairment, but who have not achieved continence by later childhood or early puberty.

One review of urodynamic studies performed in 57 children with cerebral palsy (Table 13.5) (Decter *et al.*, 1987), revealed that 49 (86%) presented with the expected picture of a partial upper motor neuron lesion type of dysfunction, with exaggerated sacral reflexes, detrusor hyperreflexia, and/or detrusor-sphincter dyssynergia (Fig. 13.18), even though they manifested voluntary control over voiding. Six of the 57 (11%), however, had evidence of both upper and lower motor neuron denervation with detrusor areflexia and/or abnormal motor unit potentials on sphincter electromyographic assessment (Table 13.6). When their records were analysed on a retrospective basis, most of the children who exhibited these latter findings had experienced an episode of cyanosis in the perinatal period (Table 13.7). Thus, a lower motor neuron lesion may be seen in addition to the expected upper motor neuron dysfunction.

Recommendations

Treatment usually centers around abolishing the uninhibited contractions with anticholinergic medication, but residual urine volume must be monitored closely to ensure complete evacuation with each void. Intermittent catheterization may be required for those who cannot empty their bladders.

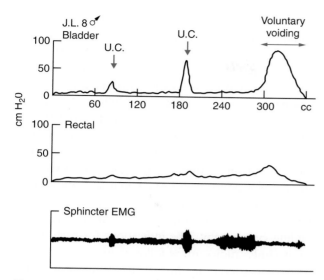

Figure 13.18 An 8-year-old boy with spastic diplegia has a typical partial upper motor neuron lesion-type bladder with uninhibited contractions (UCs) associated with increased sphincter activity but normal voiding dynamics at capacity. Wetting is due to these contractions when unaccompanied by the heightened sphincter activity. (From Bauer, 1988.)

Traumatic injuries to the spine

Despite the exposure and potential for a traumatic spinal cord injury, this condition is rarely encountered in children. When an injury does occur, it is most likely to happen as a result of a motor vehicle accident, a gunshot wound, or a diving incident (Cass *et al.*, 1984). It has also occurred iatrogenically following surgery to correct scoliosis, kyphosis, or other intra-

Table 13.6 Urodynamic findings in cerebral palsy[a]

Finding	Number
Upper motor neuron	
Uninhibited contractions	35
Detrusor-sphincter dyssynergy	7
Hyperactive sacral reflexes	6
No voluntary control	3
Small-capacity bladder	2
Hypertonia	2
Lower motor neuron	
Excessive polyphasia	5
Increased amplitude and increased duration potentials	4

[a]The study included 57 children; some exhibited more than one finding.

Table 13.7 Perinatal risk factors in cerebral palsy

Factor	UMN	LMN
Prematurity	10	1
Respiratory distress/arrest/apnea	9	2
Neonatal seizures	5	
Infection	5	
Traumatic birth	5	
Congenital hydrocephalus	3	
Placenta previa/abruption	2	2
Hypoglycemia with or without seizures	2	
Intracranial hemorrhage	2	
Cyanosis at birth	1	3
No specific factor noted	15	

UMN = upper motor neuron lesion; LMN = lower motor neuron lesion.

spinal problems as well as congenital aortic arch anomalies or patent ductus arteriosus (Cass *et al.*, 1984). Newborns are particularly prone to hyperextension injuries during a high forceps delivery (Adams *et al.*, 1988; Lanska *et al.*, 1990). The lower urinary tract dysfunction that ensues is not likely to be an isolated event but, rather, it is usually associated with loss of sensation and paralysis of the lower limbs. Radiologic investigation of the spine may not reveal any bony abnormality, even though momentary subluxation of osseous structures due to the high elasticity of vertebral ligaments can result in a neurologic injury (Pollack *et al.*, 1988). Myelography and computed tomography (CT) will show swelling of the cord below the level of the lesion (Adams *et al.*, 1988; Lanska *et al.*, 1990). Often, what appears initially as a permanent lesion turns out instead to be a transient phenomenon. Although sensation and motor function in the lower extremities may be restored relatively soon, the dysfunction involving the bladder and rectum may persist for a considerable period.

If urinary retention occurs immediately following the injury, an indwelling Foley catheter is passed into the bladder and left in place for as short a period as possible, until intermittent catheterization can be started safely on a regular basis (Guttmann and Frankel, 1966; Barkin *et al.*, 1983). When the child starts voiding again, the timing of catheterization can be such that it is used as a means of measuring the residual urine volume after a spontaneous void. Residual urine volumes of 25 ml or less are considered safe enough to allow for a reduction in the frequency and even cessation of the catheterization program

(Barkin *et al.*, 1983). If there is no improvement in the urinary tract function after 2–3 weeks, urodynamic studies are conducted to determine whether or not this condition is the result of spinal shock or actual nerve root or spinal cord injury. Detrusor areflexia is not uncommon under these circumstances (Iwatsubo *et al.*, 1985). EMG recording of the sphincter often reveals normal motor units without fibrillation potentials, but absent sacral reflexes and a non-relaxing sphincter with bladder filling, a sign that transient spinal shock has occurred (Iwatsubo *et al.*, 1985). The outcome from this condition is guarded but good, inasmuch as most cases resolve completely as edema of the cord in response to the injury subsides, leaving no permanent damage (Iwatsubo *et al.*, 1985; Fanciullacci *et al.*, 1988).

Most permanent traumatic injuries involving the spinal cord produce an upper motor neuron type lesion with detrusor hyperreflexia and detrusor-sphincter dyssynergia. The potential danger from this outflow obstruction is obvious (Donnelly *et al.*, 1972). Substantial residual urine volumes, high pressure reflux, urinary infections, and their sequelae are the leading cause of long-term morbidity and mortality in spinal cord-injured patients. Urodynamic studies will identify those patients at risk (Barkin *et al.*, 1983). Early identification and proper management may prevent the signs and effects of outlet obstruction before they become apparent on X-ray examination of the urinary tract (Pearman, 1976; Ogawa *et al.*, 1988).

Functional voiding disorders

Enuresis is defined as inappropriate voiding at an age when urinary control is expected. It is difficult, however, to say when this should occur. Studies of large groups of children have provided some guidelines for expectations, but there are no absolute milestones for the individual child (Bellman, 1966; Fergusson *et al.*, 1986). Girls tend to become trained before boys, and daytime continence is achieved before night-time control. It is rare to achieve control before 18 months of age (Yeats, 1973). Thereafter, urinary control is gained by approximately 20% of children for each year of life up to 4.5 years, with a smaller percentage of the population attaining complete continence every year after that. By the age of 10, about 5% of children still have some nocturnal wetting, but this diminishes to 2% after puberty (MacKeith *et al.*, 1973).

The evaluation of the incontinent child begins with a comprehensive history, including details of the mother's pregnancy and delivery, family history of enuresis, developmental milestones, school performance, fine and gross motor coordination, previous continence, social setting and sibling interaction, parental expectations, and characterization of the wetting episodes. If there is a suspicion of an ectopic ureter in a girl (someone who voids normally but is constantly damp both day and night), then excretory urography is performed. Boys who have a question of outflow obstruction (urgency or urge incontinence with enuresis beyond the age of 5) are evaluated by voiding cystography. The indications for performing urodynamic studies are as follows: any suspicion of a neurologic condition, diurnal incontinence with no associated pathology, fecal and urinary incontinence at any age, persistent voiding difficulties long after a urinary infection has been treated, recurrent urinary infection despite continuous antibiotics, and bladder

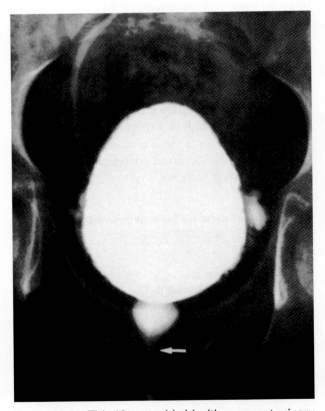

Figure 13.19 This 10-year-old girl with recurrent urinary tract infections has spasm of the sphincter during voiding with narrowing in the distal urethra demonstrated on this voiding cystourethrogram (*arrow*). Note grade II/V right-sided reflux.

trabeculation and/or 'sphincter spasm' on voiding cystography (Fig. 13.19).

When urodynamic studies are performed on a group of children who have these findings without an obvious systemic neurologic disorder, a spectrum of voiding pattern abnormalities emerges (Bauer *et al.*, 1980):

- small-capacity bladder
- detrusor hyperreflexia
- infrequent voider–lazy bladder syndrome
- psychologic non-neuropathic bladder (Hinman syndrome)

Classification and a detailed description of these disorders help one to understand and treat each condition specifically.

Small-capacity hypertonic bladder

Children with recurrent urinary infection without an anatomic abnormality may have symptoms of voiding dysfunction, including frequency, urgency, urge incontinence, staccato voiding, nocturia and/or enuresis, and dysuria, long after the infection has cleared. Sometimes, persistence of these symptoms with their associated abnormal voiding dynamics can lead to repeated infections (Hansson *et al.*, 1990).

An inflammatory reaction in the bladder wall may produce an irritability that affects the sensory threshold and increases the need to void sooner than anticipated. If the detrusor muscle is affected as well, the increased irritability may lead to instability of the muscle and eventually to poor compliance (Mayo and Burns, 1990). When the child attempts to hold back urination because it is either painful or inappropriate to void, he or she may actually tighten or only partially or intermittently relax the external sphincter

muscle during voiding, producing a form of outflow obstruction and disrupting the laminar flow pattern that normally exists (Tanagho *et al.*, 1971; VanGool and Tanagho, 1977; Hansson *et al.*, 1990) (Fig. 13.20). This stop-and-start (staccato) voiding (Fig. 13.21) is a prominent pattern of dysfunction in girls leading to recurrent infection (Borer *et al.*, 1999) because bacteria can be carried back up into the bladder from the meatus as a result of the 'milk-back' phenomenon occurring within the urethra when urination is interrupted in this manner (Webster *et al.*, 1984). Theoretically, if unrecognized or left untreated in young girls, this may become the forerunner of interstitial cystitis seen in many adult females and may even be the precursor of prostatitis in males.

Radiologic investigation often reveals a normal upper urinary tract, but the bladder may be small and have varying degrees of trabeculation on routine excretory urography or a thickened wall on ultrasonography (Bauer *et al.*, 1980; Lebowitz and Mandell, 1987). During the voiding phase of cystourethrography, the posterior urethra may show signs of intermittent dilatation at its upper end, with a uniform narrowing occurring toward the external sphincter region. In girls, this 'spinning-top' deformity has raised the question of an obstructed meatus (Tanagho *et al.*, 1971; VanGool and Tanagho, 1977) (see Fig. 13.19), whereas in boys, it has often been mistaken for posterior urethral valves. This appearance is due to failure of complete relaxation of the external sphincter and persistence of a relative obstruction at the distal end of the posterior urethra in an attempt by the child to suppress voiding (Saxton *et al.*, 1988) and has no correlations with meatal size.

Urodynamic studies demonstrate a bladder of small capacity (when adjusted for age) and elevated detrusor pressure during filling (Bauer *et al.*, 1980;

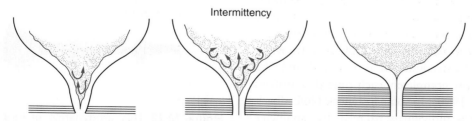

Intermittency

Figure 13.20 Non-laminar flow secondary to periodic tightening and relaxation of the external sphincter leads to eddy current and the 'milk-back' phenomenon, which can carry bacteria colonized at the urethral meatus up into the bladder and cause infection of the residual urine.

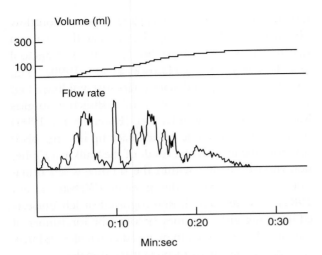

Figure 13.21 Staccato voiding is seen in this 8-year-old girl with recurrent infection.

VanGool and Tanagho, 1977) (Fig. 13.22). At capacity, the child has an uncontrolled urge to void and sometimes cannot suppress urination, despite contracting the external sphincter. The bladder contraction is usually sustained, with pressures reaching higher than normal values. Emptying may not always be complete despite these high pressures. The baseline sphincter EMG activity is normal at rest, but there may be complex repetitive discharges (pseudomyotonia) (Dyro *et al.*, 1983) or periodic relaxation of the muscle during filling, contributing to the sense of urgency or actual incontinent episodes. During voiding, the sphincter may relax intermittently or even completely at first, but then contract in response to discomfort, preventing complete emptying (Hansson *et al.*, 1990; Rudy and Woodside, 1991) (Fig. 13.22).

Treatment is based on trying to eliminate the recurrent infections, minimize any possible environmental influences that predispose the individual to infection, and improve the child's voiding pattern and bathroom habits. Girls should learn to take showers instead of baths, or at least to bathe alone without other siblings, wipe from front to back, try to completely relax when they void so that a steady stream is produced, and take the time to empty completely each time they urinate (Hansson *et al.*, 1990). In some instances, biofeedback training to teach individuals to relax the sphincter when they void has been used with success (Masek, 1985). In addition to antibiotics, antispasmodic/anticholinergic agents are administered.

Detrusor hyperreflexia

Children with long-standing symptoms of daytime frequency, urgency, or sudden incontinence and squatting, in addition to nocturia and/or enuresis, may have detrusor hyperreflexia. Vincent's curtsy, a characteristic posturing by these children in an attempt to prevent voiding, is a commonly described behavior pattern (Vincent, 1966; Kondo *et al.*, 1983). The child's parents or siblings often relate a personal history of delayed control over micturition. These affected family members may compensate for their own abnormality by displaying continued daytime frequency or nocturia, or both. Although the child's physical examination may be normal, hyperactive deep tendon reflexes in the lower and/or upper extremities, ankle clonus, posturing with a stress gait, or difficulty with tandem walking, and mirror movements (similar motion in the contralateral hand when the individual is asked rapidly to pronate and supinate one hand) may be evident. Left-handedness, left-footedness, or left-eyed-

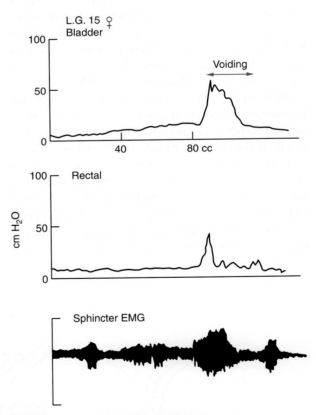

Figure 13.22 This urodynamic picture in a teenage female with recurrent infections reveals a small-capacity bladder and a hypertonic sphincter that relaxes only partially during voiding.

ness in a family in which all other members are right-handed may signify crossed dominance from a previously unrecognized perinatal insult. Attention deficit disorders, poor writing ability and/or incoordination, and learning difficulties are more commonly encountered in these children as well. Carefully questioning the parents about perinatal events or reviewing birth history records may uncover such an insult that has affected the CNS system and caused these findings.

X-ray evaluation usually reveals no abnormality other than a mildly trabeculated or thick-walled bladder. Urodynamic studies demonstrate uninhibited contractions of the bladder during filling, which the child may or may not sense and/or abolish by increasing the activity of the external urethral sphincter (Bauer *et al.*, 1980; Rudy and Woodside, 1991) (see Fig. 13.18). Alternatively, periodic relaxation of the sphincter, the initial phase of an uninhibited contraction, that leads to a sense of urgency or to an episode of leaking, may be the only clue to a hyperreflexic bladder (Fig. 13.23). During filling, capacity may be reached sooner than expected, at which time a normal detrusor contraction occurs with a sustained relaxation of the sphincter, resulting in complete emptying. Some children will not be able to suppress this contraction even though the bladder has not been filled to capacity. Sometimes, uninhibited contractions may only be elicited following a cough or strain, or when the child assumes a change in posture (Kondo *et al.*, 1983). The uninhibited contractions

are thought to be responsible for the symptoms (McGuire and Savastano, 1984).

These findings may be the result of a cerebral insult, however mild, in the neonatal period, but they are linked more commonly to delayed maturation of the reticulospinal pathways and the inhibitory centers in the midbrain and cerebral cortex. Thus, total control over vesicourethral function may be lacking (MacKeith *et al.*, 1973; Mueller, 1960; Yeats, 1973). Several investigators have found a similar urodynamic picture in a significant number of adults with nocturnal enuresis and/or daytime symptoms (Torrens and Collins, 1975). Parents who exhibit the same behavior pattern as their children may have a genetically determined delayed rate of CNS maturation.

On occasion, children with profound constipation develop uninhibited contractions of the bladder and urinary incontinence secondary to them (O'Regan *et al.*, 1985). The etiology of this condition is unclear, but treatment of the bowel distention has resulted in a dramatic improvement in the bladder dysfunction (O'Regan *et al.*, 1986) (see Chapter 12).

Sometimes, repeated urinary infection may produce an identical urodynamic picture. Detrusor hyperreflexia occurs as a result of the inflammatory response in the bladder wall that irritates the receptors located in the submucosa and/or detrusor muscle layers (Koff and Murtagh, 1983). Therefore, all these children should be screened for infection. It has been postulated that a hyperactive detrusor may lead to inappropriate voiding. When the child realizes what is happening, he or she tightens the sphincter to reverse this process, which shuts the distal urethra first and the bladder neck second, causing the 'milk-back' phenomenon and the potential for urinary infection, as presented in the previous discussion, to occur (as previously presented) (Koff and Murtagh, 1983; Webster *et al.*, 1984).

Anticholinergic medication and imipramine alone or in combination have been used successfully to manage this condition (Kondo *et al.*, 1983). Recently, biofeedback training using computer technology has been employed successfully in achieving continence and in reducing the need for medication in children refractory to anticholinergic medication (McKenna *et al.*, 1999; Yamanishi *et al.*, 2000). If infection is present, it should be eradicated and antibacterial prophylaxis should be employed (Buttarazzi, 1977; Firlit *et al.*, 1978; Kass *et al.*, 1979; Bauer *et al.*, 1980; Mayo and Burns, 1990).

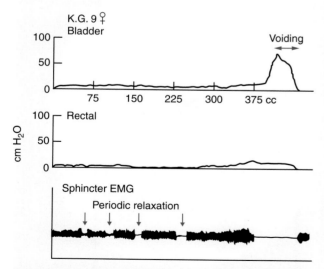

Figure 13.23 Some children only manifest periodic relaxation of the sphincter without a rise in detrusor pressure as an early phase of a hyperreflexic bladder producing urgency and incontinence.

The infrequent voider: lazy bladder syndrome

Most children urinate four or five times per day, and defecate daily or at least every other day. Some children, primarily girls, may void only twice a day, once in the morning (either at home or after they are in school), and again at night (DeLuca *et al.*, 1962). It is not uncommon to find children who do not void at all while in school. These children exhibited normal voiding patterns as infants, but after toilet training, they learned to withhold micturition for extended periods. As a result, a few develop a fear of strange bathrooms or mimic their mother's pattern of infrequent urination and defecation (Bauer *et al.*, 1980). Others have experienced an aversive event or had an infection associated with dysuria around the time of training, which led to the infrequent pattern of micturition. Some children are excessively neat or have a fetish for cleanliness that causes them to avoid bathrooms. Often, they only void enough to relieve the pressure to urinate and do not empty their bladder completely. The decrepit conditions in many school bathrooms predispose children, mainly girls, to limit the number of times that they relieve themselves during the school day; consequently, they become infrequent voiders all of the time.

The infrequent voiding and incomplete emptying produce an ever-increasing bladder capacity and a diminished stimulus to urinate (Webster *et al.*, 1984). The chronically distended bladder is at risk for urinary infection and/or overflow or stress incontinence. Sometimes, these signs are the first manifestations of the abnormal voiding pattern. When the child is carefully questioned, the aberrant micturition is easily detected. More often, the problem is diagnosed following VCUG or radionuclide cystography performed for an assessment of urinary tract infection. A larger than normal capacity (for age) and/or a high residual urine volume on initial catheterization is noted. When the child is questioned about his or her voiding habits this infrequent pattern of elimination is detected (Webster *et al.*, 1984) (Fig. 13.24a, b). The cystogram, however, usually reveals a smooth-walled bladder without reflux.

Urodynamic studies demonstrate a very large-capacity, highly compliant bladder with either normal,

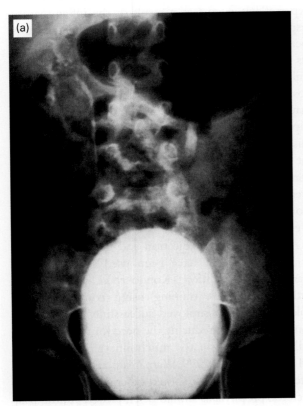
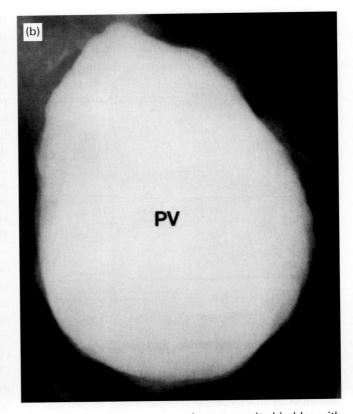

Figure 13.24 (*a*) Excretory urogram in a girl who urinates infrequently, demonstrates a large-capacity bladder with a normal upper urinary tract. (*b*) Her postvoiding (PV) residual is quite large.

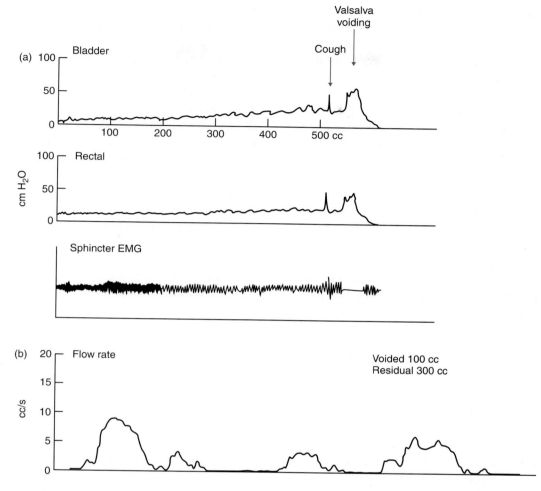

Figure 13.25 (*a*) Urodynamic evaluation reveals a very-large-capacity, low-pressure bladder. She empties entirely by straining after relaxing the sphincter with no apparent detrusor contraction. EMG = electromyography. (*b*) Her intermittent urinary flow rate is characteristic of this effort to empty and leads to a considerable volume of residual urine.

unsustained, or absent detrusor contractions (Bauer *et al.*, 1980) (Fig. 13.25a). Straining to void is a common form of emptying. Sphincter EMG reveals normal motor unit potentials at rest and normal responses to various sacral reflexes, bladder filling, and attempts at emptying. The urinary flow rate may be intermittent, with sudden peaks coinciding with straining, or it may be normal but short lived, secondary to an unsustained detrusor contraction (Webster *et al.*, 1984). Unless strongly encouraged, the child will not completely empty his or her bladder during voiding (Bauer *et al.*, 1980) (Fig. 13.25b). This picture is consistent with myogenic failure from chronic distention (Koefoot *et al.*, 1981).

Changing the child's voiding habits is the first approach to therapy. Keeping to a rigid schedule of toileting and encouraging the child to empty each time he or she voids are mandatory (Masek, 1985). Behavioral therapy techniques to encourage compliance are helpful. Rarely, intermittent catheterization may be necessary to allow the detrusor muscle to regain its contractility and ability to empty. Antibiotics are needed when urinary infection is present and are continued until the voiding pattern improves.

Psychological non-neuropathic bladder (Hinman syndrome)

Hinman (1974) described an apparent 'syndrome' of voiding dysfunction that mimics neuropathic bladder disease but may be a learned disorder. At first, this syndrome was believed to be caused by an isolated neurologic lesion (Johnston and Farkas, 1975; Williams *et al.*, 1975; Mix, 1977), but now it is felt to be an acquired abnormality (Hinman, 1974; Allen, believe; Allen and Bright, 1978; Bauer *et al.*, 1980). It is produced by an active contraction of the sphincter during voiding, creating a degree of outflow obstruction. Some investigators think that this phenomenon may be the result of persistence of the transitional phase of gaining control in which the child learns to prevent voiding by voluntarily contracting the external urethral sphincter (Allen, 1977; Rudy and Woodside, 1991). Others believe that this pattern results from the child's normal response to uninhibited contractions (McGuire and Savastano, 1984). This behavior becomes habitual because the child has difficulty in distinguishing between involuntary and voluntary voiding; as a consequence, the inappropriate sphincter activity occurs all the time (Bauer *et al.*, 1980). Jayanthi *et al.* (1997) report similar findings in a group of younger children, newborn to 30 months of age. All were managed by vesicostomy, with spontaneous improvement after vesicostomy closure in some.

These children have urgency, urge and/or stress incontinence, infrequent voluntary voiding, intermittent urination associated with straining, recurrent urinary infection, and irregular bowel movements, with fecal soiling in between (Bauer *et al.*, 1980). Most striking is the similarity in the pattern of family dynamics that is disclosed on carefully observing and questioning (Allen and Bright, 1978). Hinman syndrome can be diagnosed as follows:

1 Clinical features:
- day and night wetting
- encopresis/constipation/impaction
- recurrent urinary tract infections
- parental characteristics
    domineering/exacting
    divorce
    alcoholism
    punishments (mental and physical) inflicted
       for wetting
- previous surgery
    ureteral reimplantation
    bladder neck plasty
    diversion.
2 Radiologic features:
- hydronephrosis, with or without pyelonephritis
- reflux: III/V in degree

- large-capacity, trabeculated bladder
- large residual urine volume
- posterior urethra sometimes dilated with narrowing at external sphincter
- heavily loaded colon
3 Urodynamic features:
- elevated detrusor filling and voiding pressures
- ineffective detrusor contractions
- high resting sphincter electromyography
- unsustained sphincter relaxation during voiding
- large residual volume
4 Treatment (individualized):
- bladder retraining
    behavioral modification
    double voiding
    biofeedback techniques for sphincter relaxation
- drugs
    oxybutynin
    flavoxate
    bethanechol
    prazosin
    diazepam
- bowel reregulation program
    stool softeners
    bulking agents
    laxatives, enemas

The parents, especially the father, tend to be domineering, exacting, unyielding, and intolerant of weakness or failure. Divorce and alcoholism are common threads that only exacerbate the situation. Wetting is perceived as immature, defiant, and/or purposeful behavior that the parents feel must be counteracted with stern reprimands. The children are often punished, both mentally and physically, for their ineptness. Confusion, depression, and withdrawal for fear of wetting with its added punitive response become the children's prevalent attitudes because they do not know how to, nor can they prevent this provocative behavior. They try to withhold urination and defecation further by keeping the sphincter muscle tight, aggravating the situation. Thus, wetting becomes more commonplace, and abdominal pain from chronic constipation is likely.

X-ray evaluation reveals profound changes within the urinary tract. Hydroureteronephrosis with or without pyelonephritic scarring from recurrent infection occurs in two-thirds of the children (Bauer *et al.*, 1980) (Fig. 13.26). Fifty per cent have severe VUR. Nearly every child has a grossly trabeculated, large-capacity bladder with a considerable postvoiding residual urine volume (Fig. 13.26b). Voiding films show either persistent or intermittent narrowing in the region of the external sphincter in almost half of the children (Fig. 13.26c). Finally, the scout film from the excretory urogram displays considerable

fecal material in the colon, consistent with chronic constipation.

Urodynamic studies demonstrate a large-capacity bladder with poor compliance, uninhibited contractions, and either high-pressure or ineffective detrusor contractions during voiding (Kass *et al.*, 1979; Bauer

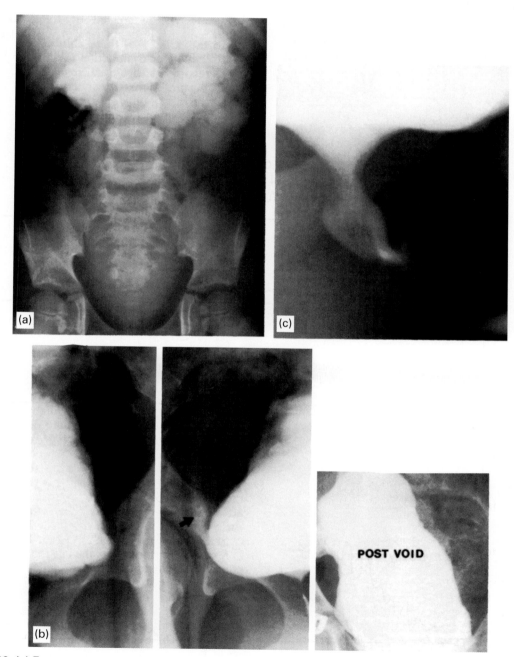

Figure 13.26 (*a*) Excretory urogram in a 14-year-old male with daytime and night-time incontinence and encopresis. Note the impression of a faintly opacified distended bladder. (*b*) His voiding cystourethrogram reveals trabeculation, mild right vesicoureteral reflux (*arrow*), and a large postvoiding residual urine volume. (*c*) A film during voiding demonstrates intermittent relaxation of the external sphincter area.

et al., 1980) (Fig. 13.27a). Sometimes, Valsalva voiding is needed to empty the bladder. The urinary flow rate is often intermittent as a result of the failure of the external sphincter to relax completely throughout voiding (Fig. 13.27b). The bethanechol supersensitivity test may be positive; in the past, this response led to the belief that these children had neuropathic bladder dysfunction (Williams *et al.*, 1975). EMG recordings, however, reveal normal external urethral sphincter innervation and exclude the possibility of a sacral spinal cord lesion. The sphincter fails to relax completely and may actually tighten episodically once voiding commences (Rudy and Woodside, 1991); this finding, along with the uninhibited contractions, suggests an upper motor neuron lesion, but usually, no other signs are present to confirm this urodynamic hypothesis. MRI has failed to reveal any intraspinal process as a cause for the voiding dysfunction in these children (Hinman, 1986).

The dyssynergy created by the incoordination between the bladder and sphincter muscles leads to high voiding pressures initially and, later, to ineffec-

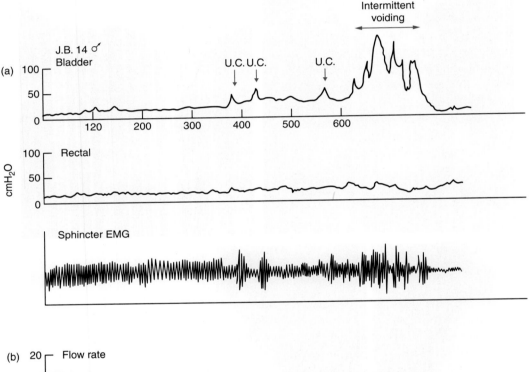

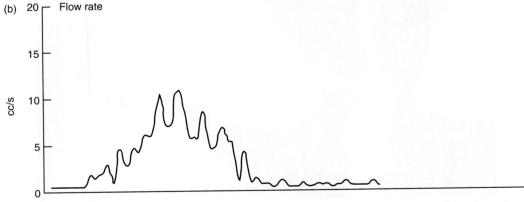

Figure 13.27 (*a*) Uninhibited detrusor contractions (UC) and increases in external urethral sphincter electromyography (EMG) activity are noted as the bladder is filled. During voluntary voiding, very high bladder pressures (above 100 cmH$_2$O) are generated owing to increased activity and then intermittent relaxation of the external sphincter. (*b*) The urinary flow rate reflects the voiding pattern seen on urodynamic evaluation.

tive detrusor contractions (Rudy and Woodside, 1991). Depending on which point of the spectrum one is at, a low or intermittent flow rate and either a minimal or significant postvoiding residual urine volume are noted.

Before this 'syndrome' was recognized and the pathophysiology elucidated, many children underwent multiple operations to improve bladder emptying and correct VUR. Failure of these procedures to succeed led to urinary diversion in a number of instances. Some of these individuals were eventually able to be undiverted at an older age after they outgrew the conditions that caused their dysfunction in the first place. Today, an entirely different approach is taken. Treatment is focused on improving the child's ability to empty the bladder and bowel and alleviating the psychosocial pressures that contribute to the aggravation of the voiding dysfunction (Masek, 1985, Hinman, 1986). A frequent emptying schedule accompanied by biofeedback techniques to relax the sphincter during voiding, anticholinergic drugs to abolish uninhibited contractions, and improved bowel emptying regimes are instituted (Bauer *et al.*, 1980). Despite these measures, intermittent catheterization may be needed in children who fail to respond and in those individuals who require immediate decompression of their upper urinary tract (Snyder *et al.*, 1982). In some cases, the outflow obstruction may have produced severe renal damage and even chronic kidney failure, which must be managed accordingly.

Psychotherapy is an integral part of the rehabilitative process to re-educate both the child and the parents in appropriate voiding habits. Punishments are stopped and a reward system is initiated in order to improve the child's self-image and confidence (Masek, 1985).

References

AAP Committee on Genetics (1999) Folic acid for the prevention of neural tube defects. *Pediatrics* **104**: 325.

Adams C, Babyn PS, Logan WJ (1988) Spinal cord birth injury: value of computed tomographic myelography. *Pediatr Neurol* **4**: 109.

Allen TD (1977) The non-neurogenic bladder. *J Urol* **117**: 232.

Allen TD, Bright TC (1978) Urodynamic patterns in children with dysfunctional voiding problems. *J Urol* **119**: 247.

Anderson FM (1975) Occult spinal dysraphism: a series of 73 cases. *Pediatrics* **55**: 826.

Barbalias GA, Klauber GT, Blaivas JG (1983) Critical evaluation of the Credé maneuver: a urodynamic study of 207 patients. *J Urol* **130**: 720.

Barkin M, Dolfin D, Herschorn S *et al.* (1983) The urologic care of the spinal cord injury patient. *J Urol* **129**: 335.

Barnes PD, Lester PD, Yamanashi WS, Prince JR (1986) MRI in infants and children with spinal dysraphism. *Am J Radiol* **147**: 339.

Barry JE, Auldist AW (1974) The Vater syndrome. *Am J Dis Child* **128**: 769.

Barson AJ (1970) The vertebral level of termination of the spinal cord during normal and abnormal development. *J Anat* **106**: 489.

Bauer SB (1983) Urodynamics in children: indication and methods. In: Barrett DM, Wein AJ (eds) *Controversies in neuro-urology*. New York: Churchill Livingstone, 193–202.

Bauer SB (1984a) Vesico-ureteral reflux in children with neurogenic bladder dysfunction. In: Johnston EH (ed.) *International perspectives in urology*, Vol. 10. Baltimore, MD: Williams & Wilkins, 159–77.

Bauer SB (1984b) Myelodysplasia: newborn evaluation and management. In: McLaurin RL (ed.) *Spina bifida: a multi-disciplinary approach*. New York: Praeger, 262–7.

Bauer SB (1985) The management of spina bifida from birth onwards. In: Whitaker RH, Woodard JR (eds) *Paediatric urology*. London: Butterworths, 87–112.

Bauer SB (1988) Early evaluation and management of children with spina bifida. In: King LR (ed.) *Urologic surgery in neonates and young infants*. Philadelphia, PA: WB Saunders, 252–64.

Bauer SB (1990) Urodynamics in children. In: Ashcraft KW (ed.) *Pediatric urology*. Orlando, FL: Grune & Stratton, 49–76.

Bauer SB (1991) Evaluation and management of the newborn with myelomeningocele. In: Gonzales ET, Roth DVR (eds) *Common problems in urology*. St. Louis, MO: Mosby Year Book, 169–80.

Bauer SB, Labib KB, Dieppa RA *et al.* (1977) Urodynamic evaluation in a boy with myelodysplasia and incontinence. *Urology* **10**: 354.

Bauer SB, Retik AB, Colodny AH *et al.* (1980) The unstable bladder of childhood. *Urol Clin North Am* **7**: 321.

Bauer SB, Colodny AH, Retik AB (1984) The management of vesico-ureteral reflux in children with myelodysplasia. *J Urol* **128**: 102.

Bauer SB, Hallet M, Khoshbin S *et al.* (1984) The predictive value of urodynamic evaluation in the newborn with myelodysplasia. *JAMA* **152**: 650.

Begger JH, Meihuizen de Regt MJ, Hogen Esch I *et al.* (1986) Progressive neurologic deficit in children with spina bifida aperta. *Z Kinderchir* **41** (Suppl 1): 13.

Bellman N (1966) Encopresis. *Acta Paediatr Scand* **70** (Suppl 1): 1.

Blaivas JG (1979) A critical appraisal of specific diagnostic techniques. In: Krane RJ, Siroky MB (eds) *Clinical neuro-urology*. Boston, MA: Little, Brown & Co., 69–110.

Blaivas JG, Labib KB, Bauer SB, Retik AB (1977) Changing concepts in the urodynamic evaluation of children. *J Urol* **117**: 777.

Blaivas JG, Sinka HP, Zayed AH *et al.* (1986) Detrusor-sphincter dyssynergia: a detailed electromyographic study. *J Urol* **125**: 545.

Bloom DA, Knechtel JM, McGuire EJ (1990) Urethral dilation improves bladder compliance in children with myelomeningocele and high leak point pressures. *J Urol* **144**: 430.

Borer JG, Butler A, Zurakowski D *et al.* (1999) predominant urodynamic patterns in girls with recurrent urinary tract infection. Presented at the American Urological Meeting, Dallas TX, May 3, 1999. Abstract No. 622.

Buttarazzi PJ (1977) Oxybutynin chloride (Ditropan) in enuresis. *J Urol* **118**: 46.

Campobasso P, Galiani E, Verzerio A *et al.* (1988) A rare cause of occult neuropathic bladder in children: the tethered cord syndrome. *Pediatr Med Chir* **10**: 641.

Carson JA, Barnes PD, Tunell WP *et al.* (1984) Imperforate anus: the neurologic implication of sacral abnormalities. *J Pediatr Surg* **19**: 838.

Cass AS, Luxenberg M, Johnson CF, Gleich P (1984) Management of the neurogenic bladder in 413 children. *J Urol* **132**: 521.

Cass AS, Bloom BA, Luxenberg M (1986) Sexual function in adults with myelomeningocele. *J Urol* **136**: 425.

Chiaramonte RM, Horowitz EM, Kaplan GA *et al.* (1986) Implications of hydronephrosis in newborns with myelodysplasia. *J Urol* **136**: 427.

Cohen RA, Rushton HG, Belman AB *et al.* (1990) Renal scarring and vesicoureteral reflux in children with myelodysplasia. *J Urol* **144**: 541.

Cromer BA, Enrile B, McCoy K *et al.* (1990) Knowledge, attitudes and behavior related to sexuality in adolescents with chronic disability. *Dev Med Child Neurol* **32**: 602.

Dator DP, Hatchett L, Dyro FM *et al.* (1992) Urodynamic dysfunction in walking myelodysplastic children. *J Urol* **148**: 362.

Decter RM, Bauer SB, Khoshbin S *et al.* (1987) Urodynamic assessment of children with cerebral palsy. *J Urol* **138**: 1110.

Decter RM, Furness PD, Nguyen TA *et al.* (1997) Reproductive understanding, sexual functioning and testosterone levels in men with spina bifida. *J Urol* **157**: 1466.

DeLuca FG, Swenson O, Fisher JH, Loutfi AH (1962) The dysfunctional 'lazy' bladder syndrome in children. *Arch Dis Child* **37**: 117.

Donnelly J, Hackler RH, Bunts RC (1972) Present urologic status of the World War II paraplegic: 25-year follow-up comparison with status of the 20-year Korean War paraplegic and 5-year Vietnam paraplegic. *J Urol* **108**: 558.

Dubrowitz V, Lorber J, Zachary RB (1965) Lipoma of the cauda equina. *Arch Dis Child* **40**: 207.

Duckett JW (1974) Cutaneous vesicostomy in childhood. *Urol Clin North Am* **1**: 485.

Dyro FM, Bauer SB, Hallett M, Khoshbin S (1983) Complex repetitive discharged in the external urethral sphincter in a pediatric population. *Neurourol Urodynam* **2**: 39.

Edelstein RA, Bauer SB, Kelly MD *et al.* (1995) Long-term urologic response of neonates with myelodysplasia treated proactively with intermittent catheterization and anticholinergic therapy. *J Urol* **150**: 1500.

Epstein F (1982) Meningocele: pitfalls in early and late management. *Clin Neurosurg* **30**: 366.

Fanciullacci F, Zanollo A, Sandri S, Catanzaro F (1988) The neuropathic bladder in children with spinal cord injury. *Paraplegia* **26**: 83.

Fergusson DM, Hons BA, Horwood LJ, Shannon FT (1986) Factors related to the age of attainment of nocturnal bladder control: an eight year longitudinal study. *Pediatrics* **78**: 884.

Firlit CF, Smey P, King LR (1978) Micturition: urodynamic flow studies in children. *J Urol* **119**: 250.

Flanigan RF, Russell DP, Walsh JW (1989) Urologic aspects of tethered cord. *Urology* **33**: 80.

Flood HD, Ritchey ML, Bloom DA *et al.* (1994) Outcome of reflux in children with myelodysplasia managed by bladder pressure monitoring. *J Urol* **152**: 1574.

Foster LS, Kogan BA, Cogan PH, Edwards MSB (1990) Bladder function in patients with lipomyelomeningocele. *J Urol* **143**: 984.

Geraniotis E, Koff SA, Enrile B (1988) Prophylactic use of clean intermittent catheterization in treatment of infants and young children with myelomeningocele and neurogenic bladder dysfunction. *J Urol* **139**: 85.

Ghoniem GM, Bloom DA, McGuire EJ, Stewart KL (1989) Bladder compliance in meningocele children. *J Urol* **141**: 1404.

Gierup J, Ericsson NO (1970) Micturition studies in infants and children: intravesical pressure, urinary flow and urethral resistance in boys with intravesical obstruction. *Scand J Urol Nephrol* **4**: 217.

Greenfield SP, Fera M (1991) Urodynamic evaluation of the imperforate anus patient: a prospective study. *J Urol* **146**: 539.

Guttmann L, Frankel H (1966) The value of intermittent catheterization in the early management of traumatic paraplegia and tetraplegia. *Paraplegia* **4**: 63.

Guzman L, Bauer SB, Hallett M *et al.* (1983) The evaluation and management of children with sacral agenesis. *Urology* **23**: 506.

Hall WA, Albright AL, Brunberg JA (1988) Diagnosis of tethered cord by magnetic resonance imaging. *Surg Neurol* **30** (Suppl 1): 60.

Hansson S, Hjalmas K, Jodal U, Sixt R (1990) Lower urinary tract dysfunction in girls with untreated asymptomatic or covert bacteriuria. *J Urol* **143**: 333.

Hayden P (1985) Adolescents with meningomyelocele. *Pediatr Rev* **6**: 245.

Hellstrom WJ, Edwards MS, Kogan BA (1986) Urologic aspects of the tethered cord syndrome. *J Urol* **135**: 317.

Hinman F (1974) Urinary tract damage in children who wet. *Pediatrics* **54**: 142.

Hinman F (1986) Non-neurogenic bladder (the Hinman syndrome) fifteen years later. *J Urol* **136**: 769.

Iwatsubo E, Iwakawa A, Koga H *et al.* (1985) Functional recovery of the bladder in patients with spinal cord injury –

prognosticating programs of an aseptic intermittent catheterization. *Acta Urol Jpn* **31**: 775.

Jakobson H, Holm-Bentzen M, Hald T (1985) Neurogenic bladder dysfunction in sacral agenesis and dysgenesis. *Neurourol Urodynam* **4**: 99.

James CM, Lassman LP (1972) *Spinal dysraphism: spina bifida occulta*. New York: Appleton-Century-Crofts.

Jayanthi VR, Khoury AE, McLorie CA et al. (1997) The non-neurogenic neurogenic bladder of early infancy. *J Urol* **158**: 1281–5.

Jeffs RD, Jones P, Schillinger JF (1976) Surgical correction of vesico-ureteral reflux in children with neurogenic bladder. *J Urol* **115**: 449.

Johnston JH, Farkas A (1975) Congenital neuropathic bladder: practicalities and possibilities of conservational management. *Urology* **5**: 719.

Joseph DB, Bauer SB, Colodny AH et al. (1989) Clean intermittent catheterization in infants with neurogenic bladder. *Pediatrics* **84**: 78.

Kaefer M, Pabby A, Kelly M et al. (1999) Improved bladder function after prophylactic treatment of high risk neurogenic bladder in newborns with myelodysplasia. *J Urol* **162**: 1068.

Kaplan WE, Firlit CF (1983) Management of reflux in myelodysplastic children. *J Urol* **129**: 1195.

Kaplan WE, McLone DG, Richards I (1988) The urologic manifestations of the tethered spinal cord. *J Urol* **140**: 1285.

Karrer FM, Flannery AM, Nelson MD Jr et al. (1988) Anal rectal malformations: evaluation of associated spinal dysraphic syndromes. *J Pediatr Surg* **23**: 45.

Kasabian NG, Bauer SB, Dyro FM et al. (1992) The prophylactic value of clean intermittent catheterization and anticholinergic medication in newborns and infants with myelodysplasia at risk of developing urinary tract deterioration. *Am J Dis Child* **146**: 840.

Kass EJ, Diokno AC, Montealegre A (1979) Enuresis: principles of management and results of treatment. *J Urol* **121**: 794.

Kass EJ, Koff SA, Lapides J (1981) Fate of vesico-ureteral reflux in children with neuropathic bladders managed by intermittent catheterization. *J Urol* **125**: 63.

Keating MA, Bauer SB, Krarup C et al. (1987) Sacral sparing in children with myelodysplasia. Presented at the Annual Meeting of the American Urological Association, Anaheim, May 18, 1987.

Keating MA, Rink RC, Bauer SB et al. (1988) Neuro-urologic implications of changing approach in management of occult spinal lesions. *J Urol* **140**: 1299.

Khoury AE, Hendrick EB, McLorie GA et al. (1990) Occult spinal dysraphism: clinical and urodynamic outcome after division of the filum terminale. *J Urol* **144**: 426.

Koefoot RB, Webster GD, Anderson EE, Glenn JF (1981) The primary megacystis syndrome. *J Urol* **125**: 232.

Koff SA, DeRidder PA (1977) Patterns of neurogenic bladder dysfunction in sacral agenesis. *J Urol* **118**: 87.

Koff SA, Murtagh DS (1983) The uninhibited bladder in children. Effect of treatment on recurrence of urinary infection and vesico-ureteral reflux. *J Urol* **130**: 1158.

Kondo A, Kobayashi M, Otani T et al. (1983) Children with unstable bladder: clinical and urodynamic observation. *J Urol* **129**: 88.

Kondo A, Kato K, Kanai S, Sakakibara T (1986) Bladder dysfunction secondary to tethered cord syndrome in adults: is it curable? *J Urol* **135**: 313.

Kroovand RL, Walsh PC, Gittes RF (1986) Myelomeningocele. In: Walsh PC et al. (eds) *Campbell's urology*. 5th edition. Philadelphia, PA: WB Saunders, pp. 2193–216.

Kroovand RL, Bell W, Hart LJ, Benfeld KY (1990) The effect of back closure on detrusor function in neonates with myelodysplasia. *J Urol* **144**: 423.

Lais A, Kasabian NG, Dyro FM et al. (1993) Neurosurgical implications of continuous neuro-urological surveillance of children with myelodysplasia. *J Urol* **150**: 1879.

Landauer W (1945) Rumplessness of chicken embryos produced by the injection of insulin and other chemicals. *J Exp Zool* **98**: 65.

Lanska MJ, Roessmann U, Wiznitzer M (1990) Magnetic resonance imaging in cervical cord birth injury. *Pediatrics* **85**: 760.

Lapides J, Diokno AC, Silber SJ, Lowe BS (1972) Clean intermittent self-catheterization in the treatment of urinary tract disease. *J Urol* **107**: 458.

Laurence KM (1989) A declining incidence of neural tube defects in U.K. *Z Kinderchir* **44** (Suppl 1): 51.

Lebowitz RL, Mandell J (1987) Urinary tract infection in children: putting radiology in its place. *Radiology* **165**: 1.

Linder M, Rosenstein J, Sklar FH (1982) Functional improvement after spinal surgery for the dysraphic malformations. *Neurosurgery* **11**: 622.

McGuire EJ, Savastano JA (1984) Urodynamic studies in enuresis and non-neurogenic bladder. *J Urol* **132**: 299.

McGuire EJ, Woodside JR, Borden TA, Weiss RM (1981) The prognostic value of urodynamic testing in myelodysplastic patients. *J Urol* **126**: 205.

McKenna PH, Herndon CDA, Connery S et al. (1999) Pelvic floor muscle retraining for pediatric voiding dysfunction using interactive computer games. *J Urol* **162**: 1056.

MacKeith RL, Meadow SR, Turner RK (1973) How children become dry. In: Kolvin I, MacKeith RL, Meadow SR (eds) *Bladder control and enuresis*. Philadelphia, PA: JB Lippincott, 3–15.

McLorie GA, Perez-Morero R, Csima AL, Churchill BM (1986) Determinants of hydronephrosis and renal injury in patients with myelomeningocele. *J Urol* **140**: 1289.

McNeal DM, Hawtrey CE, Wolraich ML, Mapel JR (1983) Symptomatic neurogenic bladder in a cerebral-palsied population. *Dev Med Child Neurol* **25**: 612.

Mandell J, Bauer SB, Hallett M et al. (1980) Occult spinal dysraphism: a rare but detectable cause of voiding dysfunction. *Urol Clin North Am* **7**: 349.

Mandell J, Bauer SB, Colodny AH, Retik AB (1981) Cutaneous vesicostomy in infancy. *J Urol* **126**: 92.

Masek BJ (1985) Behavioral management of voiding dysfunction in neurologically normal children. *Dialog Pediatr Urol* **8**: 7.

Mayo ME, Burns MW (1990) Urodynamic studies in children who wet. *Br J Urol* **65**: 641.

Menon RK, Cohen RM, Sperling MA *et al.* (1990) Transplacental passage of insulin in pregnant women with insulin-dependent diabetes mellitus. *N Engl J Med* **323**: 309.

Mix LW (1977) Occult neuropathic bladder. *Urology* **10**: 1.

MRC Vitamin Study Group (1991) Prevention of neural tube defects: results of the Medical Research Council Vitamin Study. *Lancet* **338**: 131.

Mueller SR (1960) Development of urinary control in children. *JAMA* **172**: 1256.

Naeye RL, Peters EC, Bartholomew M, Landis R (1989) Origins of cerebral palsy. *Am J Dis Child* **143**: 1154.

Nelson KB, Ellenberg JH (1986) Antecedents of cerebral palsy. *N Engl J Med* **315**: 81.

Ogawa T, Yoshida T, Fujinaga T (1988) Bladder deformity in traumatic spinal cord injury patients. *Acta Urol Jpn* **34**: 1173.

O'Regan S, Yazbeck S, Schick E (1985) Constipation, unstable bladder, urinary tract infection syndrome. *Clin Nephrol* **5**: 154.

O'Regan S, Yazbeck S, Hamburger B, Schick E (1986) Constipation: a commonly unrecognized cause of enuresis. *Am J Dis Child* **140**: 260.

Packer RJ, Zimmerman RA, Sutton LN *et al.* (1986) Magnetic resonance imaging of spinal cord diseases of childhood. *Pediatrics* **78**: 251.

Palmer JS, Kaplan WE, Firlit CF (1999) Sexuality of the spina bifida male and female: anonymous questionnaire. Presented at Section on Urology of AAP, Washington DC, October 9, 1999 (Abstract No. 13).

Palomaki GE, Williams JR, Haddow JE (1999) Prenatal screening for open neural-tube defects in Maine (Letter). *New Engl J Med* **340**: 1049.

Parrott T, Woodard J (1979) Importance of cystourethrography in neonates with imperforate anus. *Urology* **13**: 607.

Passarge E, Lenz K (1966) Syndrome of caudal regression in infants of diabetic mothers: observations of further cases. *Pediatrics* **37**: 672.

Pearman JW (1976) Urologic follow-up of 99 spinal cord injury patients initially managed by intermittent catheterization. *Br J Urol* **48**: 297.

Peña A (1986) Posterior sagittal approach for the correction of anal rectal malformations. *Adv Surg* **19**: 69.

Pollack IF, Pang D, Sclabassi R (1988) Recurrent spinal cord injury without radiographic abnormalities in children. *J Neurosurg* **69**: 177.

Pontari MA, Keating M, Kelly M *et al.* (1995) Retained sacral function in children with high level myelodysplasia. *J Urol* **154**: 775.

Raghavendra BN, Epstein FJ, Pinto RS *et al.* (1983) The tethered spinal cord: diagnosis by high-resolution real-time ultrasound. *Radiology* **149**: 123.

Reigel DH (1983) Tethered spinal cord. *Concepts Pediatr Neurosurg* **4**: 142.

Roy MW, Gilmore R, Walsh JW (1986) Evaluation of children and young adults with tethered spinal cord syndrome: utility of spinal and scalp recorded somatosensory evoked potentials. *Surg Neurol* **26**: 241.

Rudy DC, Woodside JR (1991) Non-neurogenic neurogenic bladder: the relationship between intravesical pressure and the external sphincter EMG. *Neurourol Urodynam* **10**: 169.

Satar N, Bauer SB, Shefner J *et al.* (1995) Effects of delayed diagnosis and treatment in patients with occult spinal dysraphism. *J Urol* **154**: 754.

Satar N, Bauer SB, Scott RM *et al.* (1997) Late effects of early surgery on lipoma and lipomeningocele in children less than one year old. *J Urol* **157**: 1434–7.

Saxton HM, Borzyskowski M, Mundy AR, Vivian GC (1988) Spinning top deformity: not a normal variant. *Radiology* **168**: 147.

Scarff TB, Fronczak S (1981) Myelomeningocele: a review and update. *Rehab Literature* **42**: 143.

Scheible W, James HE, Leopold GR, Hilton SW (1983) Occult spinal dysraphism in infants: screening with high-resolution real-time ultrasound. *Radiology* **146**: 743.

Seeds JW, Jones FD (1986) Lipomyelomeningocele: prenatal diagnosis and management. *Obstet Gynecol* **67** (Suppl): 34.

Seki N, Akazawa K, Senoh K *et al.* (1999) An analysis of risk factors for upper urinary tract deterioration in patients with myelodysplasia. *Br J Urol* **84**: 679.

Sheldon C, Cormier M, Crone K, Wacksman J (1991) Occult neurovesical dysfunction in children with imperforate anus and its variants. *J Pediatr Surg* **26**: 49.

Sidi AA, Dykstra DD, Gonzalez R (1986) The value of urodynamic testing in the management of neonates with myelodysplasia: a prospective study. *J Urol* **135**: 90.

Smith ED (1972) Urinary prognosis in spina bifida. *J Urol* **108**: 115.

Snyder H McC, Caldamone AA, Wein AJ, Duckett JW Jr (1982) The Hinman syndrome – alternatives for treatment. Presented at the Annual Meeting of the American Urological Association, Kansas City, May 16, 1982.

Spindel MR, Bauer SB, Dyro FM *et al.* (1987) The changing neuro-urologic lesion in myelodysplasia. *JAMA* **258**: 1630.

Stark GD (1977) *Spina bifida: problems and management.* Oxford, Blackwell Scientific Publications.

Stein SC, Feldman JG, Freidlander M *et al.* (1982) Is myelomeningocele a disappearing disease? *Pediatrics* **69**: 511.

Steinhardt GF, Goodgold HM, Samuels LD (1986) The effect of intravesical pressure on glomerular filtration rates in patients with myelomeningocele. *J Urol* **140**: 1293.

Tami S, Yamada S, Knighton RS (1987) Extensibility of the lumbar and sacral cord. Pathophysiology of the tethered cord in cats. *J Neurosurg* **66**: 116.

Tanagho EA, Miller EA, Lyon RP (1971) Spastic striated external sphincter and urinary tract infection in girls. *Br J Urol* **43**: 69.

Torrens MJ, Collins CD (1975) The urodynamic assessment of adult enuresis. *Br J Urol* **47**: 433.

Tracey PT, Hanigan WC (1990) Spinal dysraphism: use of magnetic resonance imaging in evaluation. *Clin Pediatr* **29**: 228.

Tunnell WP, Austin JC, Barnes TP, Reynolds A (1987) Neuroradiologic evaluation of sacral abnormalities in imperforate anus complex. *J Pediatr Surg* **22**: 58.

Uehling DT, Gilbert E, Chesney R (1983) Urologic implications of the VATER syndrome. *J Urol* **129**: 352.

VanGool JD, Kuijten RH, Donckerwolcke RA, Kramer PP (1982) Detrusor-sphincter dyssynergia in children with myelomeningocele: a prospective study. *Z Kinderchir* **37**: 148.

VanGool JD, Tanagho EA (1977) External sphincter activity and recurrent urinary tract infection in girls. *Urology* **10**: 348.

Venes JL, Stevens SA (1983) Surgical pathology in tethered cord secondary to meningomyelocele repair. *Concepts Pediatr Neurosurg* **4**: 165.

Vincent SA (1966) Postural control of urinary incontinence. The curtsy sign. *Lancet* ii: 631.

Webster GD, Koefoot RB, Sihelnik S (1984) Urodynamic abnormalities in neurologically normal children with micturition dysfunction. *J Urol* **132**: 74.

Weissert M, Gysler R, Sorensen N (1989) The clinical problem of the tethered cord syndrome – a report of 3 personal cases. *Z Kinderchir* **44**: 275.

White RI, Klauber GT (1976) Sacral agenesis: analysis of twenty-two cases. *Urology* **8**: 521.

Williams DI, Grant J (1969) Urologic complications of imperforate anus. *Br J Urol* **41**: 660.

Williams DI, Hirst G, Doyle D (1975) The occult neuropathic bladder. *J Pediatr Surg* **9**: 35.

Woodard JR, Anderson AM, Parrott TS (1981) Ureteral reimplantation in myelodysplastic children. *J Urol* **126**: 387.

Woodhouse CJR (1998) Sexual function in boys born with exstrophy, myelomeningocele and micropenis. *Urology* **52**: 3.

Yamada S, Zincke DE, Sanders D (1981) Pathophysiology of 'tethered cord syndrome.' *J Neurosurg* **54**: 494.

Yamada S, Knierim D, Yonekura M *et al.* (1983) Tethered cord syndrome. *J Am Paraplegia Soc* 6 (Suppl 3): 58.

Yamanishi T, Yasuda, K. Murayama N *et al.* (2000) Biofeedback training for detrusor overactivity in children. *J Urol* **164**: 1686–90.

Yeats WK (1973) Bladder function in normal micturition. In: Kolvin I, MacKeith RL, Meadow SR (eds) *Bladder control and enuresis*. Philadelphia, PA: JB Lippincott, 28–41.

Yip CM, Leach GE, Rosenfeld DS *et al.* (1985) Delayed diagnosis of voiding dysfunction: occult spinal dysraphism. *J Urol* **124**: 694.

Urodynamics of the lower and upper urinary tract

14

William E. Kaplan

Introduction

Many of the patients evaluated by a pediatric urologist have urinary tract dysfunction requiring urodynamic studies. Although the majority of urodynamics performed involves the assessment of lower tract function, there are select patients who need upper tract dynamic studies.

Most children referred for urodynamic studies already have a specific pathologic diagnosis (spinal dysraphism, spinal cord injury, cerebral pathology, etc.) but require a more definitive neurologic classification for appropriate therapy. Many patients with voiding dysfunction require urodynamics to determine whether their urinary problems are neurologic or functional in origin. In addition, patients are referred for urodynamics when other diagnostic studies, e.g. radiographic or isotopic, are equivocal.

The expansion of pediatric urodynamics in the late 1970s and early 1980s came about because of the need to understand the volume–pressure relationships of the urinary tract. The introduction of clean intermittent catheterization in the 1970s (Lapides *et al.*, 1972) opened the creative gates for the management of children with dysfunctional storing and emptying of their urinary tracts. However, correct characterization of the pathology by urodynamics was critical at this juncture.

Adult diagnostic techniques needed modification for children, and what began with work on flow rates by Gierup *et al.* (1969), progressed to sophisticated flow and electromyographic (EMG) studies by Blaivis *et al.* (1977), and to the introduction of surface monitoring of the pelvic floor by Maizels and Firlit (1979). An additional valuable contribution of correct filling rates by Joseph in 1992, and sedation techniques, emphasized the importance of a more focused approach to children.

There is still controversy regarding the diagnostic methodology best suited for upper tract pathology. The child with idiopathic hydronephrosis with preservation of renal function and no symptoms creates the greatest diagnostic dilemma. Standard imaging techniques are usually adequate for patients with normal renal function. However, when renal function becomes impaired, renal perfusion studies may offer a more significant diagnostic role. It is clear that the physiology of the upper tract does not exist in isolation, and although pure upper tract obstruction [e.g. well-defined ureteropelvic junction (UPJ) obstruction] is associated with pressure elevation with less dependence on lower tract function, the relationship of lower to upper tract pressure equilibrium must constantly be in the forefront of any diagnostic study. The fact that bladder pressure must be 'in the loop' in any diagnostic study emphasizes how important bladder dynamics has become in modern pediatric urology. The ability to assess and manage bladder function and pressure has contributed to the burgeoning of numerous surgical, pharmacologic, and neuromodulating techniques that are best used to manage the child with neurourologic dysfunction.

This chapter will focus on pediatric urodynamic studies that best categorize neuropathology and help to define the best treatment modalities.

Historical features

The basics of pediatric urodynamics are no different from any form of good medicine. A thorough

Table 14.1 Evaluation of children who wet

History	Prenatal, congenital history
	Voiding characteristics
	Bladder and bowel function
Physical examination	Abdomen and perineum
	Spine
	Lower extremities:
	Reflexes
	Gait
	Physical structure
Laboratory	Urinalysis/culture
	Chemistry: urine/serum
Radiography	Ultrasonography: renal/bladder
	Voiding cystography
	Flat plate abdomen/spine (AP and lateral)
Urodynamics	Flow/bladder capacity
	Cystometry
	Pelvic muscle evaluation: pads/needle
	Compliance: LPP/VLPP and PSBV

AP = anteroposterior; LPP = leak point pressure; VLPP = valsalva leak point pressure; PSBV = pressure specific bladder volume.

history and physical examination must precede any diagnostic study (Table 14.1). In patients in whom the general diagnosis is clear, e.g. spinal cord trauma or myelomeningocele, the historic diagnostic dilemma will not be a challenge. However, in those patients with urinary tract dysfunction and no obvious neurological abnormality, all clinical acumen must come into play.

An accurate voiding history is most important. The patient's age and expectations of urinary control may dictate the concerns over voiding habits. However, even in infants, the pattern of wet and dry diapers can be significantly diagnostic. Newborns presenting with constant dribbling or signs of overflow incontinence may have been subjected to a traumatic delivery, e.g. hyperextension injury to the cervical spinal cord. Infants of diabetic mothers have an increased risk of neural tube defects. Infants of mothers with substance abuse are at increased risk for hydronephrosis. These are only a few examples demonstrating that a thorough prenatal and obstetric history is essential in determining whether urodynamics studies are indicated and tailoring such studies to the uropathology (Mahalik et al., 1980; Chasnoff et al., 1988; Phelan et

al., 1997). Historic information, such as prematurity or global delay in physical or mental capabilities, is significant. Although this information may not aid in therapy, it may help to explain to parents how similar delays in gaining urinary control occur. Infants with irregular bowel habits (diarrhea or constipation) in association with urinary symptomatology should be cause for careful evaluation.

As the child matures, urinary tract infections (UTIs) or incontinence may become the primary symptoms. van Gool et al. (1992) proposed the use of a standardized questionnaire that would address common themes in the child with dysfunctional voiding. Frequency of wetting, voiding characteristics, and the presence of urgency are the main focus of the questionnaire. The concept of a standardized approach is valid, although in a large practice, the similarity of the patients in any given day may ensure a routine history.

The use of a voiding diary or 12-hour home pad test may also be helpful (Hellstrom et al., 1986; Mattsson, 1994). In practice, results can be misinterpreted easily if less than fastidious notes are kept, or if the pads are not attended to in a prompt manner. Parents often experience great anxiety when the 'volume in' does not equate with the exact 'volume out' by these measuring techniques. The quality of the flow rate and whether a child is always wet despite effective voiding are important historic features. The male child with a poor flow rate would be suspect for posterior urethral valves, whereas the female with paradoxical incontinence (continuously damp while voiding normally) would be expected to have an ectopic ureter. In the older child, the history must include details on bowel habits, as it is clear that constipation has a direct relationship to urinary control, as well as urinary infections (Loening-Baucke, 1997; Koff et al., 1998).

Physical examination

Prior to urodynamic studies, a thorough physical examination is essential. Patients may exhibit evidence of delayed gross motor development or abnormal fine motor skills consistent with global abnormalities from *in utero* or birthing issues. In these children, a complete neurologic examination by a pediatric neurologist, including muscle tests and nerve conduction velocity, may be indicated.

A routine systematic approach including having the child completely undressed from head to toe (although covered with a warm blanket and with a nurse and parent in attendance) will help to reveal general congenital defects that might contribute to syndromes that involve the urinary tract. Following the general assessment, most of the pertinent pathology will be found below the umbilicus. The abdomen should be palpated for stool, although significant fecal retention can exist with a soft abdomen and an empty rectal vault.

The back, perineum, and lower extremities should be examined critically. During examination of the back, all midline abnormalities should be cause for concern. However, there is less importance if a simple dimple can be grasped with the tip of the coccyx. Obvious or subtle mid-line skin tags, tufts of hair, or vascular malformations may indicate underlying spinal malformations, e.g. lipomas, and spinal magnetic resonance imaging (MRI) is then indicated. A short or abnormal gluteal cleft may indicate an underlying sacral dysgenesis or agenesis. A flattened buttock suggests deficient gluteal muscle tone, consistent with an anorectal malformation or caudal regression syndrome (Fig. 14.1).

Rectal tone, perianal sensation, and the presence or absence of a bulbocavernosus reflex should be noted. A digital rectal examination confirms the presence of stool and rules out rare prostatic lesions. The vaginal introitus should be inspected to rule out significant labial adherence or urethrovaginal abnormalities. In the male, the meatus should be observed, and if uncircumcised, the foreskin either retracted gently or pulled forward, so that the meatus can be inspected down the tunnel of foreskin.

The lower musculoskeletal system should be examined and any discrepancy in muscle tone or muscle mass should be noted. It is essential to remove the shoes and socks to discover a high arched foot or hammer claw digits, consistent with a true neurologic abnormality (Fig. 14.2). A gait disturbance is noted easily in barefoot children as they walk up and down the corridor. The author recently saw an incontinent child who was a star rollerblader, but on barefoot gait analysis was noted to have severe ankle weakness and intoeing. This could have been masked by the above-the-ankle rollerblades. Subsequent MRI revealed a tethered spinal cord. Finally, the deep tendon reflexes should be evaluated. Exaggerated reflexes are consistent with cerebral palsy.

At the first office visit, a urinalysis (glucose and specific gravity) flow rate and postvoid residual measured by ultrasound should be accomplished. In children with a normal renal/bladder sonogram, and no history of significant UTIs, the majority of patients will be started on a timed voiding program, with attention to bowel habits, and a brief course of anticholinergic medication. In the remaining patients, a more thorough work-up including radiographic evaluation and urodynamic studies is indicated.

Radiographic evaluation

Radiographic examination is used selectively. All patients undergo a renal and bladder sonogram with postvoid imaging to evaluate bladder emptying and the effects of bladder fullness on upper tract dilatation. If UTIs are an issue, a voiding cystourethrogram is warranted. A conventional X-ray voiding cystourethrogram (VCUG) is performed to evaluate the bladder, outlet, and urethra. This study can document whether there is significant stool in the colon. Children with both fecal and urinary incontinence should have lumbosacral images. In patients with clearly abnormal studies, spinal MRI is performed (Fig. 14.3).

Lower urinary tract urodynamics

A complete voiding history should precede urodynamic evaluation. A parental questionnaire includes the details of the foregoing discussion. This can be accomplished at the time of the examination, but the study can be best tailored if the staff is made aware of significant problems by telephone or mail consultation prior to the office appointment. All outside studies should accompany the family to the laboratory.

In the majority of cases, the child with a non-neurogenic voiding abnormality will be old enough to cooperate, tolerating a precystometrogram flow study followed by a cystometrogram with patch electrodes and a postvoid study. Typically, the child with neurogenic disease comes to the laboratory on a clean intermittent catheterization program and is being evaluated because of increasing dysfunction (tethered cord, shunt malfunction). Voiding studies become less important and needle electrode myography may be

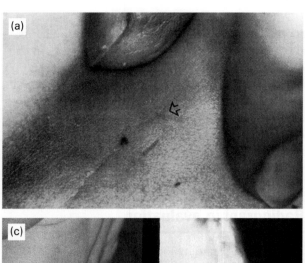

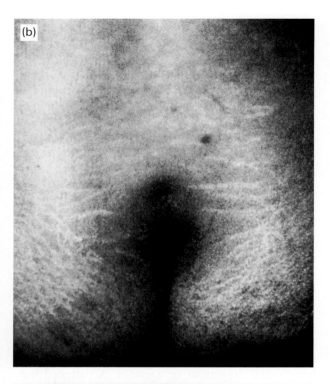

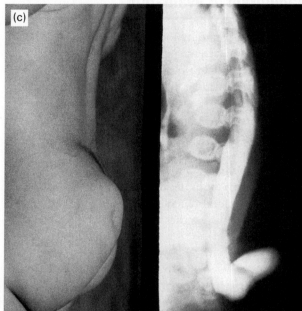

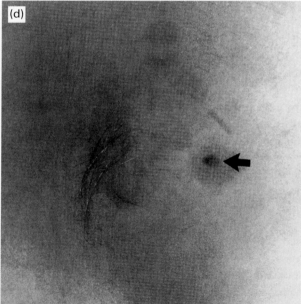

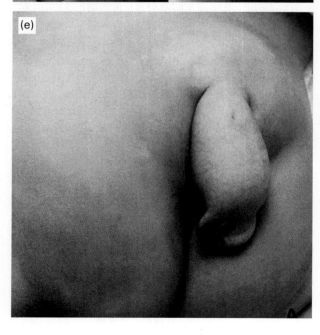

Figure 14.1 Cutaneous lesions discovered on midline spinal examination: (*a*) dermal sinus tract (*open arrow*) in infant who developed meningitis shortly after birth; (*b*) a subtle fullness of one buttock and mild scoliosis in a child with incontinence and subsequently discovered to have a lipoma; (*c*) an obvious sinus tract and lipoma in infant with lipomeningocele; (*d*) a sinus (*arrow*) and associated hairy patch characteristically associated with a flat capillary hemangioma; (*e*) an unusual appendage and dermal sinus tract.

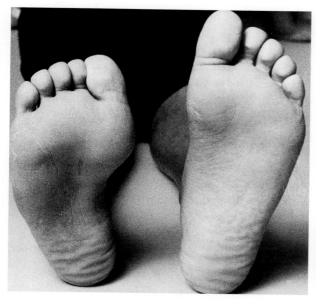

Figure 14.2 Leg length and foot asymmetry in a 10-year-old child with spina bifida.

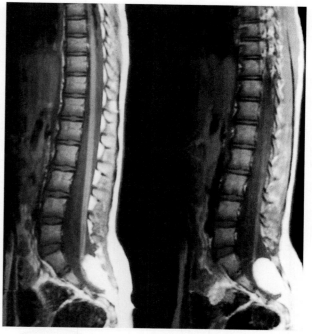

Figure 14.3 Lumbosacral MRI, T_1 weighted, indicates a long tethered spinal cord. The elongated (bowstring) cord ends in the lipoma rather than at L_3.

more important. In all instances, a relatively clean rectum will result in a more accurate study.

It is most important that the child is comfortable, and that the laboratory is child friendly (posters, movies, books, stickers, etc.) and temperature controlled. All voidings should be as private as possible. For the older child, a separate room with a flowmeter and a one-way mirror to observe voidings can be helpful. Given enough time and patience, most studies can be completed successfully with reproducible results. Meperidine, 1 mg/kg, can be given to an extremely anxious child, although this is not common practice (Table 14.2) (Ericsson *et al.*, 1971).

Table 14.2 Urodynamic studies

Urodynamic study	Purpose: to evaluate:
Uroflow/residual urine	Voiding function sensation, storage, emptying of the bladder
Cystometry	Coordination/function of muscular outlet
Pelvic floor/external sphincter EMG	Bladder/outlet function
Leak point pressure: Bladder Stress (VLPP)	Storage pressure Competence of bladder neck/proximal urethra
Videourodynamics	Anatomy and function of bladder and outlet (simultaneously)

EMG = electromyogram; VLPP = valsalva leak point pressure.

Urinary flow rate and bladder capacity

The urinary flow rate measurement is a simple non-invasive study that is defined as the voided volume per unit time (ml/s) (Figs. 14.4, 14.5). This study can evaluate incontinence secondary to problems in storage or emptying. Reliability comes from repeated studies (at least two) and is related to voided volume. Bladder capacity (BC) should be based on age rather than body surface. Although the linear formula of Berger *et al.* (1983) and Koff (1983) [BC (oz) = Age + 2] has been the most frequently used to estimate bladder capacity, it is clear that bladder growth from a newborn (especially in the first years) to 13 years is not linear. Kaefer *et al.* (1997) responded to this chal-lenge with their non-linear formulae of [BC (oz) = 2 × age (years) + 2] for children less than 2 years of age and [BC (oz) = Age (years) ÷ 2 + 6] for those older than 2 years. In all of these studies normal children were used to gain data. It has been shown previously that children less than 14 years of age with spina bifida and neuropathic bladders do not exhibit similar growth rates to normal children. In fact, on comparing bladder growth in a small group of patients with spina bifida to the linear formula of Berger, bladders of patients with spina bifida grew half as well as those without neurologic abnormalities (Kaplan *et al.*, 1989). Thus, in order to calculate normal flow patterns and rates, one must first know the expected bladder capacity in order to determine whether the

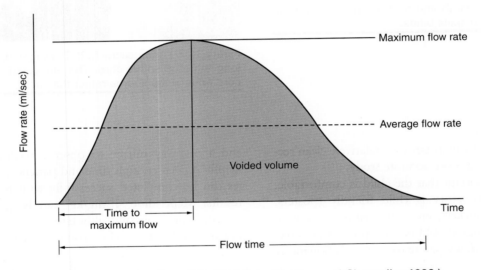

Figure 14.4 Idealized diagram of urine flow. (Modified from Blaivass and Chancellor 1996.)

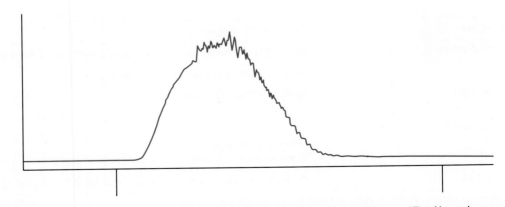

Figure 14.5 Normal uroflow in a 12-year-old male: maximum = 38 ml/s, average = 17 ml/s, volume = 222 ml.

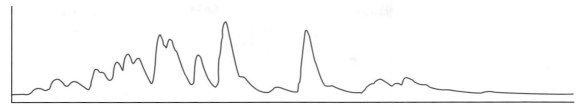

Figure 14.6 Abnormal uroflow in an 8-year-old male with abdominal straining and no detrusor activity.

voiding volume is within the expected range. Accurate determination of the flow rate/voided volume is a common problem, particularly in the anxious child or in the child who voids frequently in small volumes. In general, voided volumes of less than 50% expected capacity should be suspect (Mattsson and Spångberg, 1994; Szabo and Fegyvernski, 1995). The bladder is best filled by forcing oral fluids on the way into the laboratory or by intravenous hydration. Multiple voids can be spontaneous, but Lasix administration can be helpful to ensure repeated measurements.

Critical features of the flow rate include the shape of the curve, maximum flow rate, and average flow rate. In a study of 180 schoolchildren aged 7–16 years, 98% had a bell-shaped flow pattern (Mattsson and Spångberg, 1994) (Fig. 14.4). The shape of the curve had no relationship to voided volume, but the other parameters were volume dependent. Although the maximum flow, average flow, and time to maximum flow can be of diagnostic interest, the shape of the flow appears to be the best screening parameter. Repeated deviations from the bell-shaped curve should prompt further studies (Fig. 14.6). Estimation of residual urine can be an important clue to overall bladder function. Except in infants, the child's bladder should empty to completion with each void. There are multiple pitfalls when evaluating for retained urine. An anxious child in a foreign setting will not void efficiently. Furthermore, children with significant reflux may often harbor residual urine just after voiding. Thus, while complete evacuation can be helpful to know, an elevated postvoid residual may not signify important pathology. A bladder scan with ultrasound or placement of a catheter just prior to the cystometrogram will determine the residual urine.

Cystometry

Cystometry is the pressure–volume study of the bladder that examines both the storage and the voiding phase of micturition (Figs 14.7, 14.8). Both of these aspects of bladder function have been examined as the key to bladder health in relationship to upper tract drainage. An accurate assessment of bladder storage begins in a calm laboratory setting with the necessary techniques to decrease patient anxiety. Gentle passage of an age-appropriate catheter is then performed. Male newborns usually require a 5 Fr feeding tube connected to a three-way stopcock which allows for both measuring pressure and fluid instillation. Care should be taken to avoid an overly large catheter in newborns, which can obstruct the urethra and produce an abnormally high leak point pressure, as

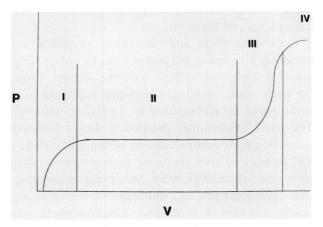

Figure 14.7 Cystometrogram indicating four phases and filling and detrusor activity: I, initial vesical pressure with early filling; II, stable tonus limb; III, increase in tonus at full vesicoelastic expansion; IV, voiding. (Modified from Dmochowski, 1996.)

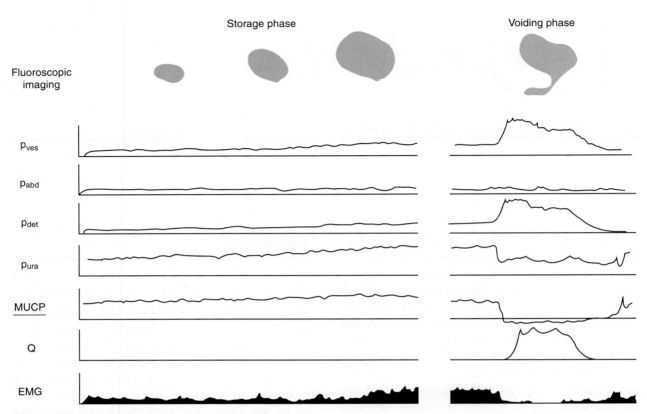

Figure 14.8 Idealized urodynamic tracing with accompanying fluoroscopic images. p_{ves} = intravesical pressure; p_{abd} = abdominal pressure; p_{det} = detrusor pressure; i.e. the $p_{ves} - p_{abd}$; p_{ura} = urethral pressure; MUCP = maximal urethral closure pressure; Q = urinary flow; EMG = surface electromyography. (Modified from Abrams *et al.*, 1998.)

the fluid tries to leak around the catheter (Decter and Harpster, 1992). In older children, a 7–10 Fr catheter can be used. **Latex-free materials** are essential for the spina bifida population, as they are prone to severe latex allergy and reactions.

Both intravesical and abdominal pressures are recorded. The abdominal pressure can be obtained by inserting a pressure catheter into the rectum. These are easily made by tying a latex-free finger cot to a small plastic tube connected to a pressure monitor. The rectal (abdominal) pressure is then subtracted from the intravesical pressure to obtain a true detrusor pressure. These are basic measurements taken with a two-channel recorder. Membrane or microtip transducer catheters and multichannel recorders are readily available if so desired. The equipment can vary; however, direct, hands on, expert observation is probably more important than the size and complexity of the equipment. Straining, crying, and gross movements need to be noted and subtracted to obtain accurate detrusor pressures. The pressure

transducer should be level with the symphysis pubis.

Saline that is warmed from a range of body to room temperature should be used. Carbon dioxide is not recommended. Joseph (1992) noted that a change in detrusor pressure, as well as maximum detrusor pressure, were adversely affected by increasing the rate of filling from slow (approximately 2% of estimated bladder capacity, 0–10 ml/min) to medium fill (approximately 20% of estimated bladder capacity, 10–100 ml/min). In general, it is recommended to fill at less than 10 ml/min in children.

An EMG should be performed at the same time as detrusor pressure evaluation. The electrodes can be surface pads, wires, or concentric needles. In children with neurogenic disease and lack of perineal sensation, recording from the external sphincter/perineal floor is often performed. In the male, a concentric needle can be placed directly into the bulbocavernosus muscle by aiming towards the bulb of the urethra. For the external sphincter, the needle is placed through the perineal skin just below the bulb of the urethra. A finger in the rectum will help to guide the needle. In females the external sphincter is identified by a needle placed just lateral to the urethral meatus and advanced < 1 cm. To capture correctly individual motor action potentials, both an audio channel and oscilloscope are needed. This study is best performed by a trained neurophysiologist. It is the most accurate method to diagnose the degree of denervation of the urethral sphincter and establish the diagnosis of detrusor-sphincter dyssynergia (Fig. 14.9). It should be noted, however, that in the majority of children, surface pad electrodes will give excellent information about a composite view of muscle activity.

In select circumstances, a urethral pressure profile can be performed. Saline can be infused at a rate of 2 ml/min while the catheter is slowly withdrawn at 2 mm/s. The urethral pressure profile measures the passive resistance of a particular point in the urethra. To obtain dynamic information of the outlet during voiding, micturition urethral pressure profilometry should be performed. This study is done in mid-voiding cycle to help eliminate the transient responses of the bladder neck and external sphincter during micturition. In some sophisticated laboratories, micro-tipped transducer catheters can be used rather than saline infusion.

Videourodynamics is a technique that simultaneously combines the evaluation of the anatomy of the lower tract with recorded urodynamic studies (Fig. 14.10). It is especially useful to delineate the bladder outlet during storage and voiding and to identify the causes of incontinence. In the incontinent patient without uninhibited contractions noted on the cystometrogram, the position and function of the bladder neck and proximal urethra can be evaluated under fluoroscopy to determine whether the urethra's incompetence or mobility is the etiology of the wetting. Videofluoroscopy can also be used to evaluate bladder compliance in relation to vesicoureteral reflux. That is, reflux may act as a 'pop-off valve' for elevation in detrusor pressure, and knowledge of the timing of reflux relative to bladder pressure can be important for proper management with clean intermittent catheterization and anticholinergics. The technique is the same as standard cystometry except that the infusant is radiographic contrast. A triple-lumen urethral catheter is slowly withdrawn and a urethral pressure profile can be performed. The radio-opaque marker that identifies the urethral port is positioned at the point of highest urethral pressure. Under fluoroscopic control, the bladder, bladder neck, and urethra are visualized while the pressure is recorded. The first leak through the bladder neck can

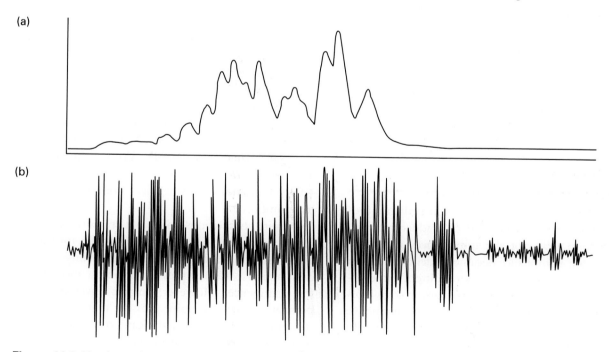

(a)

(b)

Figure 14.9 Urodynamics tracing in incontinent child with vesicosphincter dyssynergia. (*a*) Uroflow; (*b*) electromyogram

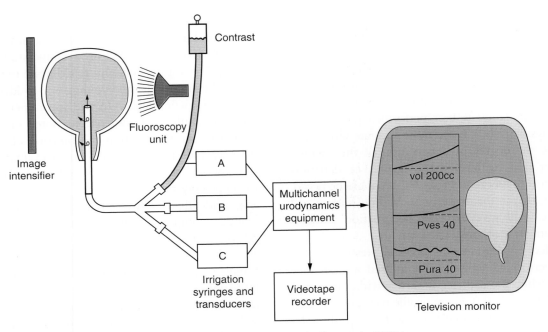

Figure 14.10 Videourodynamic equipment. (Modified from McGuire *et al.*, 1996.)

be seen and recorded. McGuire used videourodynamics and the abdominal leak point pressure [(ALPP), also called the stress leak point pressure] to diagnose correctly the incontinent older patient with detrusor instability/ineffective outlet, as well as the pediatric patient with complex causes of incontinence. Videourodynamics can easily evaluate the neurologically normal child with pseudosphincter dyssynergia and help in the diagnostic dilemma of the child with neurogenic disease and decreased compliance, detrusor-sphincter dyssynergia and areflexic emptying (McGuire *et al.*, 1996) (Fig. 14.11).

Compliance

Since the late 1970s great advances in pediatric urology have occurred in the field of bladder management. A firm grasp of the importance of bladder health or 'safe' compliance became evident coincident with the introduction of clean intermittent catheterization by Lapides. The interest in neurourology blossomed with non-surgical as well as reconstructive techniques introduced to reconfigure bladder compliance. McGuire (1989), Houle *et al.* (1993) and McGuire *et al.* (1996) described two complementary studies to evaluate lower tract function and health.

McGuire popularized the concept of the leak point pressure. The leak point pressure is the detrusor pressure at which leakage occurs through the outlet. It is dependent on the resistance to flow. Without fluoroscopy the point of resistance will not be evident. It is measured by performing a slow fill cystometrogram, noting the pressure at which the leak occurs around the catheter per urethra. It has been shown in several centers that in the myelodysplastic population, children with leak point pressures of greater than 40 cmH$_2$O are at greater risk for upper tract damage (hydronephrosis and reflux) than patients who have leak point pressures less than 40 cmH$_2$O (McGuire *et al.*, 1981; Bauer *et al.*, 1984). Although many treatment programs are based on this 'magic number' of 40, the limitations of a single leak point pressure need recognition.

Despite its relationship to outlet resistance, measurement of leak point pressure can be misleading when used to evaluate continence capability. Specifically, a high leak point pressure implies a good chance for continence. However, in the myelodysplastic population, the leak point pressure may be high but still not correlate with significant continence in the presence of a fixed but open bladder outlet.

The stress leak point pressure measurement was an innovation to help in the assessment of continence

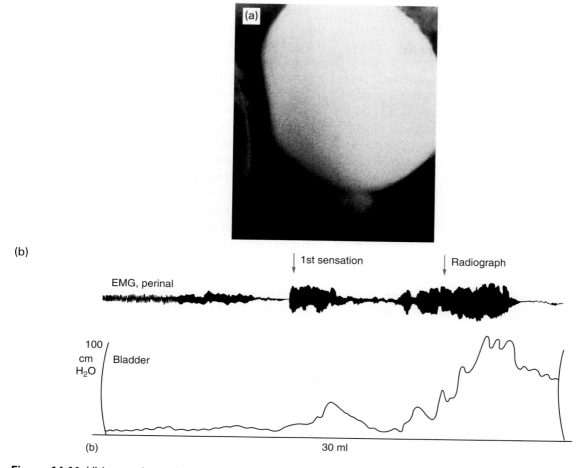

Figure 14.11 Videourodynamic study to indicate detrusor external sphincter dyssynergia. Note: detrusor contraction and simultaneous perineal EMG activity. The video indicates the dysfunctional void.

capability. The stress leak point pressure is slightly different from the simple bladder leak point pressure and can be determined without fluoroscopy. This value is obtained by slowly filling the bladder and having the child strain as if to have a bowel movement. The lowest pressure is then noted during which leakage first occurs. The child can also be asked to cough vigorously while the pressure is measured. It is a reproducible urodynamic test that can evaluate the capability of the outlet in both the open and poorly functioning state (e.g. the myelodysplastic child) as well as in the marginally to fully resistive mode. The stress leak point pressure can help to determine whether outlet reconstructive procedures are needed to achieve urinary continence (Wan *et al.*, 1993).

The leak point pressure is an accurate measure of bladder storage. However, Houle proposed that bladder storage characteristics might be better assessed by observing the volume at which a child can safely store urine, i.e. pressure-specific bladder volume. Houle indicated that in normal children, 99% of bladder capacity can be stored at less than 30 cmH$_2$O. Thus, a safe pressure of 20–30 cmH$_2$O was chosen and the volume noted which kept the pressure in that range (Houle *et al.*, 1993; Landau *et al.*, 1994). This is a most useful judge of compliance. Therapeutic interventions can be implemented based on this safe storage pressure. Voiding and catheterization diaries for patients may be obtained and evacuation schedules or additions of medications (anticholinergics) adjusted accordingly. If conservative measures do not consistently allow the bladder to store in a safe zone, augmentation or neuromodulation procedures are used (Fig. 14.12). It seems prudent and it is easy to obtain the leak point pressures, both simple and stress, as well as the pressure-specific bladder volume. However, it is unclear whether these data alone should be used as a basis to intervene prophylactically or must be interpreted in conjunction with imaging (e.g. renal and bladder sonography). Both programs have their staunch advocates. Suffice it to say that accurate studies performed in a consistent and timely manner can only benefit the current population of children and give guidance for future cost-effective management.

Upper tract urodynamics

The issue of flow and pressure extends to the upper urinary tract. There is a variety of modalities to evaluate the functional patency of the upper tract. As in most aspects of medicine, the more tests that are available to evaluate a single subject, the more likely it

is that no one test is the gold standard. At both ends of the spectrum, one would hope that clear-cut obstruction versus non-obstruction would be evident by studies including serial ultrasonography, diuretic excretory urography, retrograde pyelography, or diuretic renography. Urodynamics of the upper tract is given credence when any or all of these studies become equivocable. Although the invasive Whitaker study (as originally described) would have promise as being the gold standard, it also is fraught with interpretive error. However, as in the case of the static leak point pressure, stress leak point pressure, and pressure-specific bladder volume, a variety of methods exist to evaluate the response of the upper urinary tract to flow and pressure.

The classic antegrade perfusion test as applied by Whitaker (1979a) based on the work of Kiil (1957) and Backlund and Reuterskold (1969), is well known. Simply, the test requires the infusion of saline into the renal pelvis at a constant flow rate, and the

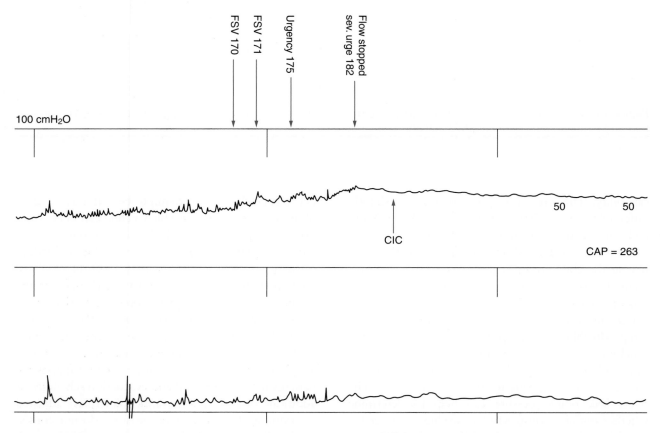

Figure 14.12 Urodynamic study to show poorly compliant neuropathic bladder pressure at capacity is 62 cmH$_2$O and patient-recorded typical catheterization volumes (CIC) that were at elevated pressures (70 cmH$_2$O). Failure at conservative management resulted in augmentation.

pressure from the pelvis is then recorded. The access to the pelvis is typically percutaneously (in the preoperative evaluation); however, open access is certainly possible (Fig. 14.13).

Why would one feel compelled to go to the bother and expense of this invasive test? There is a select group of patients and circumstances where diuretic renography will not be diagnostic, i.e. in the child in whom renal function is so compromised that the renal parenchyma cannot adequately handle the introduced isotope, technetium-99m-diaminotetraethylpentacetic acid ([^{99m}Tc]DTPA) (O'Reilly *et al.*, 1979). The technique of the renogram, as well as the timing of the diuretic administration, and upper tract compliance can also influence the results. The diuretic renogram, even under ideal conditions, cannot evaluate renal pelvic pressure. Thus, in the proper setting, the effort involved in a urodynamic evaluation of the upper tract is indicated.

The patient is sedated and often anesthetized, and a catheter is inserted into the bladder and attached to a three-way stopcock. The patient is placed prone, but prior to renal pelvic access, the 22-gauge access catheter is infused at 10 ml/min to determine the resistance of the catheter itself. Both the infusion and bladder catheters are connected to pressure transducers and leveled to the renal pelvis and superior border of the symphysis pubis, respectively. For the classic Whitaker pressure–flow study, a motor-driven syringe pump is used to infuse fluid at a constant rate of 10 ml/min. The study can be repeated at 5 and 2 ml/min. If there is a sudden and rapid rise in renal pressure, the catheter may be abutting against the wall of the pelvis, and needs adjustment. If the bladder pressure rises significantly, the stopcock should be opened and the bladder drained. The issue of bladder fullness is critical, because as the bladder fills and its pressure elevates, it can result in greater emptying pressure of the ureter and pelvis. The bladder pressure, as well as the infusion pressure through the infusant catheter and tubing, need to be subtracted from the pelvic pressure (Smyth *et al.*, 1991). The pelvic or absolute pressure, minus the bladder and tubing pressure, equals the relative pressure. In simple terms, two groups of patients emerge: those with relative pressures below 15 cmH$_2$O and those with relative pressures greater than 22 cmH$_2$O. In the ideal, the

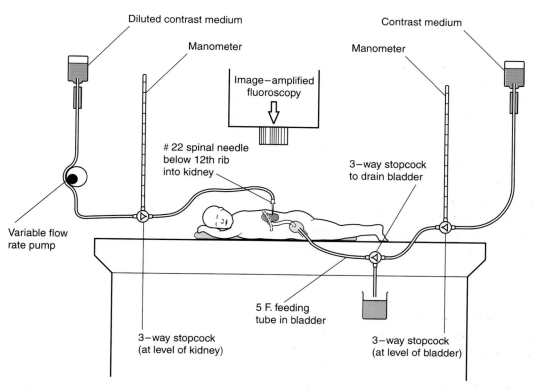

Figure 14.13 Whitaker test. Percutaneous puncture of renal pelvis and measurement of renal and bladder pressure. (Modified from King and Levitt, 1986.)

Table 14.3 Summary of the Whitaker test

Kidney pressure	Normal	Raised	Raised	Raised
Relative pressure (cmH$_2$O) (Pelvic–tubing–bladder)	<15	>22	<15	>22
Bladder pressure	Normal	Normal	Raised	Raised
Result	Unobstructed	Obstructed	Non-compliant bladder	Non-compliant bladder and obstruction

test can indicate obstruction (>22 cmH$_2$O), no obstruction (<15 cmH$_2$O) and the general site of obstruction. That is, if the renal pelvic pressure and bladder pressure drop by emptying the bladder, the bladder is the culprit and bladder management is needed, i.e. to improve bladder compliance by surgical or non-surgical means. If the relative pressure is subtracted from the absolute pressure and the result is over 12–15 cmH$_2$O, there is some degree of ureteral obstruction (Whitaker, 1979b) (Table 14.3). There are several concerns regarding the absoluteness of Whitaker's relative pressure. In the original description, Whitaker noted that the fullness of pelvis and ureter could be noted if radio-opaque contrast was used for the infusant. This equilibrium/fullness factor, however, may be somewhat arbitrary. To assess the pressure correctly, the system needs to be full. The infusion rate has also come under question. Fung *et al.* (1995) tweaked the nomogram collector, by suggesting that the original Whitaker test may be made more accurate by infusing a volume more individualized for patient size and glomerular function rather than the standard rate of 10 ml/min (Chapter 20). Mortensen *et al.* (1983) found, in the pig, large enough overlaps in the relative pressure, so as to call into question the concern over a 12–15 cmH$_2$O pressure. Forthcoming were debates over constant flow versus constant pressure studies. The constant pressure technique is likened to the pressure-specific bladder volume work. That is, it may be critical to know the pressure required to produce flow across the system, as the pressure should be the final determinate of upper tract health. In the human one-kidney model, keeping pressure constant by elevating the infusant solution to known levels and measuring flow could be accomplished. However, in the child with two kidneys, measuring output from the studied kidney only is still a challenge (Ripley and Somerville, 1982; Woodbury *et al.*, 1989). Finally, a variety of influences on the urinary tract can significantly alter the renal pelvis emptying pressure, e.g. pharmacotherapy (principally anticholinergics), infections, and reflux (Fichtner *et al.*, 1998; Cowan and Shortliffe, 1998; Angell *et al.*, 1998).

The expanded subject of the pressure-flow study, renogram, prediction of pathology, and prediction of renal salvage is beyond the scope of this technical chapter. However, for the moment, although the most complex diagnostic dilemmas may not be totally solved by urodynamics of the upper tract (however one chooses to execute the study), in the very select patient with poor renal function and a dilated system, a carefully planned diagnostic attack should also include the capability to perform a reproducible evaluation of the pressure–flow characteristics of the system (Chapter 20).

References

Abrams P, Khoury S, Wein A (1998) WHO Publication. Geneva: World Health Organization, 353–401.

Angell SK, Pruthi RS, Shortliffe LMD (1998) The urodynamic relationship of renal pelvic and bladder pressures, and urinary flow rate in rats with congenital vesicoureteral reflux. *J Urol* 160: 150–6.

Backlund L, Reuterskold AG (1969) The abnormal ureter in children. I. Perfusion studies of the wide non-refluxing ureter. *Scand J Urol Nephrol* 3: 219–28.

Bauer SB, Hallett N, Khoshbin *et al.* (1984) Predictive value of urodynamic evaluation in newborns with myelodysplasia. *JAMA* 252: 650–2.

Berger RM, Maizels M, Moran GC *et al.* (1983) Bladder capacity (ounces) equals age (years) plus 2 predicts normal bladder capacity and aids in diagnosis of abnormal voiding patterns. *J Urol* 129: 347–9.

Blaivass J, Chancellor M (eds) (1996) *Atlas of urodynamics.* Baltimore, MD: Williams and Wilkins.

Blaivas JG, Labib KB, Bauer SB, Retik AB (1977) changing concepts in the urodynamic evaluation of children. *J Urol* 117: 778–81.

Chasnoff IJ, Chisum GM, Kaplan WE (1988) Maternal cocaine use and genitourinary tract malfunctions. *Teratology* **37**: 201–4.

Cowan BF, Shortliffe LMD (1998) Oxybutynin decreases renal pelvic pressures in normal and infected rat urinary tract. *J Urol* **160**: 882–6.

Decter R, Harpster L (1992) Pitfalls in determination of leak point pressure. *J Urol* **148**: 588–91.

Dmochowski R (1996) Cystometry. *Urol Clin North Am* **23**: 243–51.

Ericsson NO, Hellstrom B, Negardth A, Rudhe U (1971) Micturition urocystography in children with myelomeningocele. *Acta Radiol Diagn* **11**: 321–36.

Fichtner J, Boinlau FG, Lewy JE, Shortliffe LMD (1998) Oxybutynin lowers elevated renal pelvic pressures in a rat with congenital unilateral hydronephrosis. *J Urol* **160**: 887–91.

Fung LCT, Khoury AE, McLorie GA *et al.* (1995) Evaluation of pediatric hydronephrosis using individualized pressure flow criteria. *J Urol* **154**: 671–6.

Gierup J, Ericksson NO, Okmain L (1969) Micturition studies in infants and children: technique. *Scand J Urol Nephrol* **3**: 1–8.

Hellstrom A-L, Andersson K, Hjälmås K, Jodal U (1986) Pad tests in children with incontinence scared. *J Urol Nephrol* **20**: 47–50.

Houle A, Gilmour RF, Churchill BM *et al.* (1993) What volume can a child normally store in the bladder at a safe pressure. *J Urol* **149**: 561–4.

Joseph DB (1992) The effect of medium-fill and slow-fill saline cystometry on detrusor pressure in infants and children with myelodysplasia. *J Uro* **147**: 444–6.

Kaefer M, Zurakowski D, Bauer SB *et al.* (1997) Estimating normal bladder capacity in children. *J Urol* **158**: 2261–4.

Kaplan WE, Richards TW, Richards I (1989) Intravesical transurethral bladder stimulation to increase bladder capacity. *J Urol* **142**: 600–2.

Kiil F (1957) *The function of the ureter and renal pelvis.* Oslo: Oslo University Press.

King LR, Levitt SB (1986) Vesicoureteral reflux, megaureter and ureteral reimplantation. In: *Campbell's urology.* 5th edition. Philadelphia, PA: WB Saunders, 2031–88.

Koff SA (1983) Estimating bladder capacity in children. *Urology* **21**: 248.

Koff SA, Wagner TT, Jayanthi VR (1998) The relationship among dysfunctional elimination syndromes, primary vesicoureteral reflux and urinary tract infections in children. *J Urol* **160**: 1019–22.

Landau EH, Churchill BM, Jayanthi VR *et al.* (1994) The sensitivity of pressure specific bladder volume versus total bladder capacity as a measure of bladder storage dysfunction. *J Urol* **152**: 1578–81.

Lapides J, Diokno AC, Silber SJ, Lowe BS (1972) Clean intermittent self catheterization in the treatment of urinary tract disease. *J Urol* **107**: 458–61.

Loening-Baucke V (1997) Urinary incontinence and urinary tract infection and their resolution with treatment of chronic constipation of childhood. *Pediatrics* **100**: 228–32.

McGuire EJ, Woodside JR, Barden TA, Weiss RM (1981) Prognostic value of urodynamic testing in myelodysplastic patients. *J Urol* **126**: 205–9.

McGuire EJ, Cespedes RD, O'Connell HE (1996) Leak point pressures. *Urol Clin N Am* **23**: 253–62.

Mahalik MP, Gautieri RF, Mann DE Jr (1980) Teratogenic potential of cocaine hydrochloride in CF-1 mice. *J Pharm Sci* **69**: 703–6.

Maizels M, Firlit CF (1979) Pediatric urodynamics: clinical comparison of surface versus needle pelvic floor/external sphincter electromyography. *J Urol* **122**: 518–22.

Mattsson SH (1994) Voiding frequency, volumes and intervals in healthy school children. *Scand J Urol Nephrol* **28**: 1–11.

Mattsson S, Spångberg A (1994) Urinary flow in healthy school children. *Neurourol Urodyn* **13**: 281–96.

Mortensen J, Kjurhuus JD, Laursen H, Bisballe S (1983) The relationship between pressure and flow in the normal pig renal pelvis. *Scand J Urol Nephrol* **17**: 369–72.

O'Reilly PH, Lawson RS, Shields RA (1979) Ideopathic hydronephrosis. *J Urol* **121**: 153–5.

Phelan SA, Mariko I, Loeken MR (1997) Neural tube defects in embryos of diabetic mice. Role of the Pax-3 genes and apoptosis. *Diabetes* **46**: 1189–97.

Ripley SH, Somerville JJF (1982) Whitaker revisited. *Br J Urol* **54**: 594–8.

Smyth TB, Shortliffe LMD, Constantinou CE (1991) The effect of urinary flow and bladder fullness on renal pelvic pressure in a rat model *J Urol* **146**: 592–6.

Szabo L, Fegyvernski S (1995) Maximum and average urine flow rates in normal children – the Miskolc nomograms. *Br J Urol* **76**: 16–20.

van Gool JD, Hjälmås K, Tamminen-Möbius T, Olbing H (1992) On behalf of the international reflux study in children: historical clues to the complex of dysfunctional voiding, urinary tract infection and vesicoureteral reflux. *J Urol* **148**: 1699–702.

Wan J, McGuire EJ, Bloom DA, Ritchie ML (1993) Stress leak point pressure: a diagnostic tool for incontinent children. *J Urol* **150**: 700–2.

Whitaker RH (1979a) The Whitaker test. *Urol Clin North Am* **6**: 529–39.

Whitaker RH (1979b) An evaluation of 170 diagnostic pressure flow studies on the upper urinary tract. *J Urol* **121**: 602–4.

Woodbury PW, Mitchell ME, Scheidler DM *et al.* (1989) Constant pressure perfusion: a method to determine obstruction in the upper urinary tract. *J Urol* **142**: 632–5.

Operations on the bladder outlet

15

Anthony J. Casale

Introduction

Surgery to correct urinary incontinence began in 1852 with a procedure to divert the ureters into the sigmoid colon of a boy with exstrophy (Simon, 1852). Our understanding of the physiology and cause of urinary incontinence has grown slowly over the twentieth century and more has been learned since the mid-1970s than in prior medical history. Early surgeons did not have the necessary technology to define the physiology of the bladder neck but they were keen observers of anatomy. As early as 1906 the German surgeon Trendelenburg had suggested division of the symphysis pubis to gain access for surgical narrowing of the bladder outlet in epispadias patients with the goal of improving urinary control. Hugh Hampton Young was the first American urologist to identify abnormal anatomy of the bladder neck as the cause of urinary incontinence and devise surgery to correct it in 1908. In 1919, Young presented his original procedure to provide continence in patients with bladder outlet incompetence.

By examining these patients with early cystoscopes and at the time of open surgery, Young noted that the bladder neck and proximal urethra were enlarged and funnel shaped. The remainder of the bladder appeared healthy. He surmised that if he could restore the bladder neck and proximal urethra to a more normal appearance, then function would improve. He excised a wedge of mucosa from the posterior urethra and bladder below the trigone and narrowed the muscle with a single layer of sutures.

Since Young's bold procedure, surgery for the weak bladder outlet, has progressed from the goal of re-creating normal anatomy to that of constructing continence mechanisms that bear no resemblance to the normal bladder outlet. Other developments in urinary tract reconstruction, such as intermittent catheterization, bladder augmentation, and continent catheterizable stomas, have made new procedures to repair the weak bladder outlet possible and offer additional solutions to problems that early surgeons saw as incurable.

Indications and evaluation

Urinary incontinence may be the result of bladder outlet inadequacy in conditions such as epispadias, exstrophy, cloacal exstrophy, traumatic injuries of the urethra and bladder neck, urogenital sinus, bilateral ectopic ureters, and neuropathology. Indications for bladder outlet surgery in these diseases include evidence that weakness of the outlet is the cause of incontinence and the failure of maximal medical therapy to correct the problem.

The bladder outlet includes the bladder neck and proximal urethra. Together, they may be considered as a unit and normally function as a sphincter in both boys and girls. There is no identifiable anatomic sphincter but a mixture of smooth and striated muscle, intracellular matrix, and mucosal factors that combine to make up a functional sphincter (Blaivas et al., 1998). Compression of the urethral lumen and the resultant outlet resistance depends on several factors. Among the components that make up the normal sphincter mechanism are smooth and striated muscle tone and contractions, elastic properties of the urethra, mechanical forces transmitted from the abdomen, and structural support of the posterior urethral wall and bladder neck against which the urethra is compressed with increased abdominal pressure. The conditions that cause incontinence in children often present inadequacies in several if not all of these.

In health, the bladder neck provides a variable resistance to the flow of urine through the urethra.

The resistance increases as the pressure rises with bladder filling. It also increases reflexively with increased abdominal pressure due to coughing or valsalva, and decreases dramatically when the patient begins to void. For the bladder neck to maintain continence it must be able to generate pressure within the lumen that is greater than the pressure within the bladder at all times except during voiding.

There are several methods to evaluate the competency of the bladder outlet. Just as Young noted, the cystoscopic appearance of the bladder neck reflects its function. When viewed from the proximal urethra, the posterior lip of the bladder neck should be elevated above the level of the urethra and the base of the bladder. The bladder neck should close easily when fluid flow through the cystoscope is stopped. While these observations are helpful they are by no means completely reliable in predicting continence.

The bladder outlet may also be evaluated by imaging with a radiographic cystogram. A competent

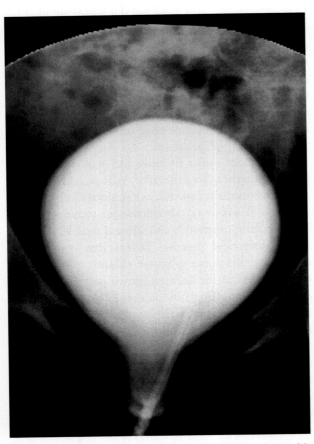

Figure 15.1 Voiding cystourethrogram of a patient with an open bladder neck throughout filling with contrast. The bladder neck is funneled during the entire study.

bladder outlet appears closed as the bladder is filled and contrast should not leak into the urethra. The incompetent bladder outlet may remain open and funnel shaped during the filling process or may open with valsalva or suprapubic pressure (Gonzalez and Sidi, 1985) (Fig. 15.1). Lateral views of the cystogram may reveal the lack of adequate elevation and suspension of the posterior bladder outlet.

Urodynamic studies of the bladder are invaluable in determining causes of incontinence. Bladder leak point pressure and sphincter electromyography (EMG) are commonly used to measure bladder neck function. Leak point pressure is simply the pressure within the bladder at which fluid begins to leak through the bladder outlet into the urethra. Sphincter EMG is the measurement of electrical activity of the striated muscle of the sphincter. The sphincter EMG is most helpful in evaluating coordination of the detrusor and sphincter and may be of some benefit in documenting neural innervation of the sphincter in incontinent children. It is seldom helpful in children who are candidates for bladder outlet surgery.

Bladder leak point pressure is the most reliable objective study in children incontinent due to bladder outlet dysfunction. Low leak point pressures indicate incompetence of the bladder outlet and may cause incontinence independent of detrusor function. McGuire et al. (1981) defined the importance of leak point pressure in children with myelodysplasia and neuropathic bladders when he found that high leak point pressures greater than 40 cmH_2O resulted in upper tract deterioration due to reflux and hydronephrosis. Children with pressures less than 40 cmH_2O were protected from such changes but were prone to leak urine easily owing to weak bladder outlet. He also found that the radiographic appearance of an open bladder neck did not correlate well with measured leak point pressures.

McGuire found that most children with myelomeningocele have fixed bladder outlet resistance that is located distal to the bladder neck and does not vary with either filling or leaking. When these children were treated with intermittent catheterization and anticholinergic medications, patients with closed bladder necks on cystography were uniformly continent, while only 60% of those with an open bladder neck became continent. This finding was independent of leak point pressure, indicating its limits in predicting continence in all patients.

Leak point pressure should be measured with a small urethral catheter (5 or 7 Fr) and the water should be infused with a pump rather than gravity. The technique should be standardized for each measurement, since Decter and Harpster (1992) demonstrated that measured values of leak point pressures in children vary with catheter size and with rate and method of infusion. Patients should be encouraged to cough and sit or stand if possible to measure leak point pressures in a dynamic, more normal, setting. The volume at which leaking begins is important because it reflects the functional capacity of the bladder and prognosis for continence.

Other urodynamic measurements are critical in diagnosing the cause of incontinence. Bladder pressures and volumes indicate storage capacity of the bladder and must be adequate for continence. Compliance may be considered the inverse of stiffness and is a helpful indicator of bladder adaptability. Poorly compliant bladders tend to produce higher pressures with lower volumes of urine, making patients more prone to upper tract deterioration and incontinence (Ghoniem et al., 1989). Detrusor measurements in children with completely incompetent bladder necks may be performed by inflating the balloon of a Foley catheter at the bladder neck and pulling it down to occlude the bladder outlet (Woodside and McGuire, 1982). It is fruitless to consider treatment of bladder outlet incompetence unless the bladder has adequate volume and pressure characteristics for the storage of urine.

Another important part of the examination of the causes of incontinence in children who are candidates for bladder outlet procedures is the voiding/catheterizing diary. Unlike radiographic and urodynamic examinations, these diaries represent the level of incontinence during normal activity. Some parameters, such as functional storage capacity of the bladder, may be quite different than tests may imply. Patients can measure voided/catheterized amounts of urine obtained, the times that the bladder is emptied, when incontinence occurs, the degree of incontinence, and activities associated with leaking. This information, along with urodynamic data, examination by cystogram, and cystoscopy, may be needed to define the cause or causes of incontinence.

If incontinence is found to be due to incompetence of the bladder outlet the physician has two basic treatments available, medical and surgical. Medical treatment should always be exhausted completely before considering surgical therapy. This is important, not only because some patients will become dry with medical management alone, but also to demonstrate that the family is committed and willing to comply with the rigorous medical management that accompanies most surgical procedures to create continence.

Medical therapy

Patients found to have inadequate bladder outlet resistance may be treated with various non-surgical modalities. Some therapy helpful in incontinent adults has no role in children. Pelvic floor exercises, biofeedback, and electric stimulation of the bladder outlet have not been helpful in children with incontinence secondary to anatomic and neuropathic conditions.

Some medications are used to stimulate muscles of the weak bladder outlet. These medications are α-sympathomimetic agents and include ephedrine and ephedrine-like compounds (Sudafed®). Their mechanism of action is to stimulate the large number of α-adrenergic receptor sites found in the proximal urethra and bladder neck, and to cause smooth muscle contraction (Andersson, 1993). These compounds produce troublesome side-effects in some patients, including hypertension, anxiety, and palpitations. Results have not been predictably reliable in children who have severe anatomic and neurologic defects at the bladder outlet. The author has had little success with medical stimulation of the bladder outlet to improve continence.

Other medical therapies include clean intermittent catheterization (CIC) to empty the bladder completely on a prearranged schedule. This procedure remains the single most important contribution to the treatment of incontinence in children. In children with neuropathic bladders, intermittent catheterization alone will provide continence in 19–24% (Hilwa and Permutter, 1978; Purcell and Gregory, 1984). The addition of anticholinergic medications, which lower bladder pressures and inhibit detrusor contractions, to CIC programs raised the continence rates to 68–89% (Mulcahy et al., 1977; Wang et al., 1988). It is important to recognize that continence has been defined differently by various authors in the past and while most patients gain some social or daytime continence with medical therapy, complete dryness is possible in less than one-third. Even if bladder outlet function is marginal, continence may be improved by maximizing other aspects, such as bladder storage capacity, with medication and emptying the bladder regularly with catheterization.

Procedures to increase bladder outlet resistance

Once the bladder outlet has been identified as a cause of incontinence and medical therapy has been exhausted without acceptable improvement, the next option is a surgical procedures to enhance bladder outlet resistance. This may be accomplished by three basic methods: procedures to change the suspension, support, or angle of the bladder outlet, procedures to compress the lumen of the bladder outlet, either with an external compression device or by injection of material under the mucosa, and procedures to reconfigure the bladder outlet into a more efficient continence valve.

Procedures to suspend the bladder outlet

Since the beginning of the twentieth century inadequate support or elevation of the bladder neck and proximal urethra have been identified as causes of urinary incontinence (Blaivas, 1994). Inadequate suspension contributes to incontinence by making the bladder outlet too mobile, allowing it to descend into the pelvis. Normal suspension of the posterior bladder outlet is necessary to provide resistance from below to counter increased abdominal pressures from above and thus to compress the lumen. Suspension of the bladder outlet may be accomplished in several ways, including procedures that fasten the existing periurethral fascia to the anterior pelvic wall and procedures that reinforce the posterior bladder outlet with a sling made of fascia or some other external material.

In 1949, Marshall, Marchetti, and Krantz (MMK) introduced a procedure to improve stress incontinence by surgically elevating and suspending the bladder neck and proximal urethra (Marshall *et al.*, 1949). The procedure is based on sewing the anterior vaginal fascia just lateral to the urethra and bladder neck to the cartilaginous portion of the symphysis pubis (Fig. 15.2). These sutures suspend and support the bladder

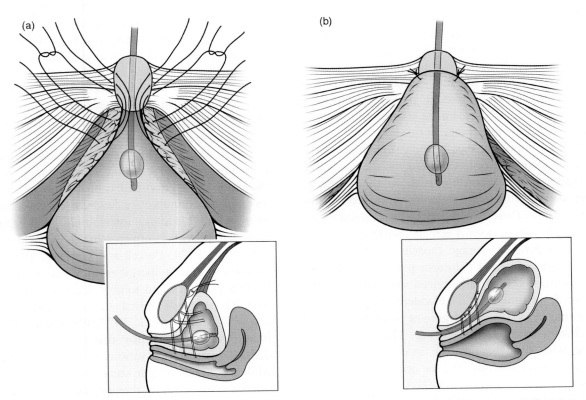

Figure 15.2 The Marshal–Marchetti–Krantz procedure elevates and suspends the bladder outlet including the proximal urethra by sewing the anterior vaginal fascia to the underside of the symphysis pubis. These are permanent sutures and re-create the posterior angle of the bladder neck. The concept of bladder neck suspension is still a cornerstone in incontinence surgery. (*a*) Placement of sutures between the anterior vaginal fascia and underside of the pubis. (*b*) Suspension and elevation of the bladder outlet.

outlet and re-create its posterior angle. The MMK procedure was, for many years, the gold standard of incontinence surgery and the concept is still critical in correcting these problems. Burch's procedure to suspend the bladder outlet from Cooper's ligament was another form of suspension that gained wide acceptance (Burch, 1961). Both suspension surgeries produce cure rates of greater than 90% in patients with pure stress incontinence (Webster and Khoury, 1998). Today, suture suspension of the bladder outlet in children is used usually as an adjunct procedure with other incontinence surgery and helps to produce continence in up to 88% of patients (Raz *et al.*, 1988a; Freedman *et al.*, 1984).

Pereya in 1959 (Pereya and Ledherz, 1967), Stamey (1973), and Raz (1981) developed proce-

dures that were also designed to elevate and suspend the weak bladder outlet. They supported and elevated the bladder neck using sutures from the perivesical and periurethral fascia to the rectus abdominal fascia. These procedures were clear advances because they could be done through small incisions using long needles to place the suspension sutures (Fig. 15.3). The surgeons could confirm correct suture placement at the time of the procedure with the cystoscope and the patients suffered minimal discomfort.

McGuire improved on a concept introduced by Goebell (1911) of suspending the bladder outlet with a sling of fascia or muscle. McGuire developed a method of passing an isolated strip of rectus fascia beneath the bladder neck and reattaching it to the anterior abdominal wall at the insertion of the rectus fascia and the

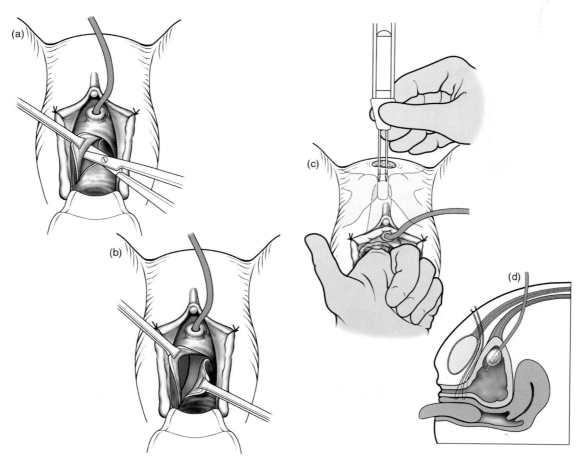

Figure 15.3 The Raz sling suspension uses long needles to pass permanent sutures from the anterior rectus fascia to suspend the bladder outlet from the anterior abdominal wall. The sutures support and elevate the bladder outlet and re-create the normal position and anatomy of the posterior bladder neck. They are dependent on the strength of the fascia surrounding the bladder neck and posterior urethra. (*a, b*) Exposure of the anterior vaginal fascia on either side of the bladder outlet. (*c*) Passing a needle from the anterior abdominal fascia to the vaginal incision in order to place sutures. (*d*) Suture suspension of the bladder outlet.

pubis (McGuire and Lytton, 1978) (Fig. 15.4). Slings may improve continence by compressing the urethra, elevating the bladder outlet into the abdomen, or by providing a stable point against which the urethra is compressed during increases in abdominal pressure. This fascial sling and its variations have proven valuable for children with bladder outlet incompetence (McGuire *et al.*, 1986). The use of fascia under the bladder neck is more reliable in these children than sutures alone, which must rely on the strength of the native fascia adjacent to the bladder neck and proximal urethra to hold the suspension sutures.

The most popular form of bladder outlet sling suspension in children involves a long strip of rectus fas-

cia that is passed around the bladder outlet and sewn to the anterior abdominal wall fascia on each side. This suspension depends completely on the fascia to support the bladder outlet and is done entirely through a lower abdominal incision (Fig. 15.5).

Bladder neck suspension, usually in the form of a rectus fascia sling, has been most helpful in girls with myelomeningocele on intermittent catheterization (Woodside and Borden, 1982). The female urethra is more easily manipulated in this way and results have been good in this population, with continence rates of 78–90% (Bauer *et al.*, 1989; Elder, 1990; Gormley *et al.*, 1994). The success rate in males in the present author's hands has been considerably lower than in

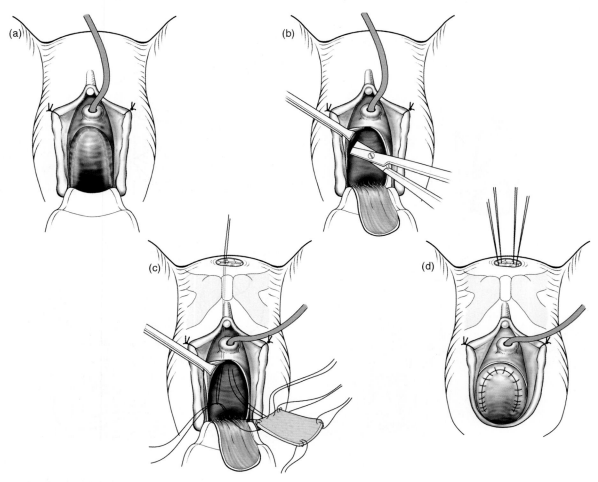

Figure 15.4 McGuire developed a suspension procedure that uses long sutures from the anterior abdominal wall to support a short strip of fascia. This fascia is passed posterior to the bladder outlet and supports and elevates the bladder outlet. This procedure provides more uniform support the posterior bladder neck and does not rely on the native fascia around the bladder neck and urethra. (*a*) Vaginal incision to expose anterior vaginal fascia. (*b*) Dissection on either side of the bladder outlet. (*c*) Placement of the sling. (*d*) Sutures that elevate and suspend the bladder outlet.

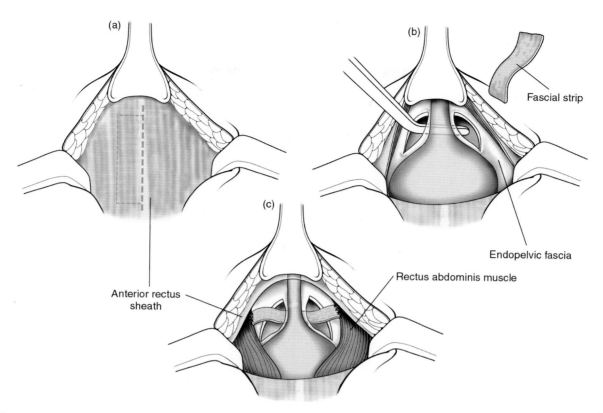

(a)

(b)

Fascial strip

(c)

Endopelvic fascia

Rectus abdominis muscle

Anterior rectus sheath

Figure 15.5 Fascial slings may be harvested from the anterior rectus fascia at the time of open surgery and used to suspend the bladder outlet from the anterior abdominal wall. (*a*) A single strip of fascia can be taken from the lateral aspect of a midline incision and (*b*) passed behind the bladder outlet. (*c*) Each end of the sling can then be sewn to the anterior rectus fascia on each side to elevate and support the bladder neck and urethra.

females when suspension is used alone, although some authors report good experiences (Raz *et al.*, 1988b; Kakizaki *et al.*, 1995; Ludlow *et al.*, 1995). The combination of slings with other bladder neck, surgery such as narrowing the outlet, has been successful for some surgeons (Herschorn and Randomski, 1992).

Fascial sling suspension of the bladder outlet is not without complications. Decter (1993) reported erosion of the sling into the bladder and late degeneration of detrusor compliance after sling placement. Often patients have difficulty in catheterizing through the urethra after sling placement owing to the altered angle of the urethra. The sling has been known to break during physical activity, acutely returning the child to a state of incontinence. As with many other procedures to improve bladder outlet resistance, augmentation cystoplasty has often been required to provide a large, low-pressure reservoir for optimal continence.

Procedures to compress the weak bladder outlet

Surgery to compress the bladder neck externally can take one of two forms; variable or fixed. Since the normal bladder neck offers variable outlet resistance this form is the most desirable so that the resistance can be relaxed to allow voiding or easy catheterization. The artificial urinary sphincter developed by Scott in 1972 has been valuable in the management of incontinence for many years (Scott *et al.*, 1974).

Artificial urinary sphincter

The artificial urinary sphincter is a hydraulic device that is comprised of three parts: an inflatable cuff that surrounds and compresses the bladder neck and posterior urethra or bulbous urethra, a pressure-generating balloon, and a pump control module (Fig. 15.6). The artificial sphincter enables the patient to deflate the cuff and reduce the compression of the bladder

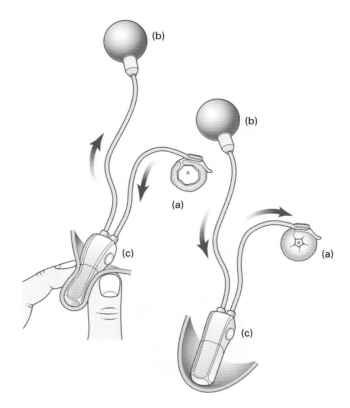

Figure 15.6 The artificial urinary sphincter is a mechanical device comprised of three components: (*a*) an inflatable cuff, (*b*) a pressure-regulating reservoir balloon, and (*c*) a control pump. It functions by using hydraulic pressure to inflate the cuff that compresses the urethra and provides continence. By squeezing the pump (implanted in the scrotum or labium) the patient can manually deflate the cuff and allow voiding or catheterization through the urethra. The pressure in the balloon then restores pressure throughout the system and reinflates the cuff in 3 min.

neck at will. The pump is placed in the scrotum or labium and the entire device is contained within the body. Continence rates are close to 90% after placement of the device (Gonzalez *et al.*, 1995; Levisque *et al.*, 1996).

The bladder neck and most proximal urethra is the preferred site of placement in children (Fig. 15.7). The usual minimal age for placement of artificial sphincters is 6 years for boys and 8 or 9 years for girls (Barrett and Licht, 1998). The pressure exerted on the urethra is regulated by the balloon/reservoir. Most children need 61–70 cmH$_2$O pressure to control the bladder outlet safely. The device is not activated after surgery as cuff pressure may cause erosion of the cuff into the bladder. The sphincter may be activated after 6–8 weeks with less risk of erosion (Barrett and Furlow, 1981).

Initially, there were concerns that performing intermittent catheterization through the implanted sphincter could cause damage to the tissue compress-

ed by the cuff and lead to erosion. Sphincters were only placed in patients who could void, but as many as 50% of children cannot void efficiently after sphincter placement, making catheterization nevertheless necessary (Gonzalez *et al.*, 1989). Barrett and Furlow (1982, 1984) reported a series of children with neuropathic bladders who could not void after artificial sphincter surgery and found that intermittent catheterization could be performed safely if the cuff was deflated to pass the catheter. Continence was satisfactory and no patients suffered erosion due to catheterization. It appears that the ability to void may deteriorate with time, particularly in boys with neuropathic bladders. Gonzalez *et al.* (1995) reported that 74% of patients followed for a mean of 8 years after sphincter placement ultimately required intermittent catheterization. Upsizing the sphincter cuff size in adolescent boys who suffer delayed voiding failure after sphincter placement has not been successful in restoring the ability to void (Kaefer *et al.*, 1997).

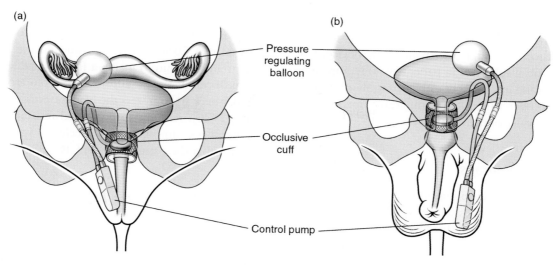

(a)   (b)

Pressure
regulating
balloon

Occlusive
cuff

Control pump

Figure 15.7 Placement of the artificial urinary sphincter in children is at the bladder neck and proximal urethra. Unlike in adults, the bulbous urethra is not an advisable site in children because of cuff size and the risk of erosion.

Historically, there has been a higher rate of reoperation with artificial sphincters than with bladder outlet reconfiguration (Sidi *et al.*, 1987). This risk appears to be lessening with better technique and newer devices. Kryger *et al.* (1999) reported an average of 0.03 revisions per year with the newest model and 70% of children who had sphincters placed since 1987 have not required revision. The long-term survival of the artificial sphincter in children in two large series is approximately 60%, with device infection and erosion being the most common reasons for loss. Eventually, all devices will wear out and fail, requiring replacement, but if complications can be avoided the mean survival of the new devices in children is over 12 years (Levisque *et al.*, 1996). The newest model (AS 800), with a narrow backing cuff, was developed in 1988. It had a mechanical failure rate of 7.6%, a non-mechanical failure rate of 9%, and a sphincter survival rate of 92% in 184 adult patients with a mean follow-up of 40.8 months (Elliott and Barrett, 1998).

Roth and others reported an important complication of artificial sphincter placement in 1986 when they discovered that some patients suffered late deterioration of the upper urinary tracts (Bauer *et al.*, 1986; Roth *et al.*, 1986; Kronner *et al.*, 1998). This deterioration was due to two factors: a failure to void efficiently in some patients and the new development of detrusor hypertonicity in others. Deterioration of detrusor function after sphincter placement remains a serious problem and there is currently no reliable

method to predict which patients will undergo these changes or the timetable for risk (Light and Pietro, 1986). Because of this threat it is necessary to follow patients with artificial sphincters with periodic upper tract imaging and urodynamics indefinitely after placement of the sphincter.

Augmentation cystoplasty, as either a simultaneous procedure with artificial sphincter placement or carried out at a later date, is necessary in approximately 30% of children (Barrett *et al.*, 1993; Levisque *et al.*, 1996). Augmentation increases storage volume and decreases storage pressures of the bladder due to poor compliance or hypercontractatility of the detrusor. Augmentation performed at the same time as sphincter placement has been associated with an increased risk of device infection if colon and small bowel are used (Light *et al.*, 1995). Apparently, augmentation with stomach does not present an increased risk of infection of the device (Miller *et al.*, 1998).

Patient selection for artificial urinary sphincter is important. While there has been an increased risk of erosion with girls who had prior bladder neck surgery, Bosco *et al.* (1991) demonstrated that the risk to girls and boys is similar if they have not had prior bladder surgery. The condition of the bladder outlet that will be compressed with the cuff is critical, and prior bladder neck surgery or excessive scarring increases the risk of erosion. The artificial urinary sphincter is the only method of producing variable bladder outlet resistance and thereby allowing volitional voiding. Candidates are children who have the ability to void prior to surgery and the potential to do so after placement of the device. Use of the artificial sphincter in patients who require augmentation and intermittent catheterization offers little advantage over other less complicated methods to increase bladder outlet resistance.

Bladder outlet wraps

There have been a few attempts to compress the bladder neck with a fixed resistance and these have usually been in conjunction with bladder neck reconstruction surgery. Silicone rubber sheaths have been placed around the narrowed bladder neck, but in early series over 60% eroded into the lumen and required removal (Kropp *et al.*, 1993). Quimby *et al.* (1996) presented a large series of 94 patients treated with silicone sheaths used in conjunction with a Young–Dees–Leadbetter bladder neck reconstruction. The authors continued to modify their technique until the erosion rated dropped to 7% in 35 patients. This improvement was attributed to using omentum to wrap the sheath and using a single-layer short silicone wrap. Satisfactory continence in this group was achieved in 72% with this method. Walker *et al.* (1995) described a procedure to wrap and compress the bladder neck circumferentially with rectus fascia, with good results (Fig. 15.8). Some of his patients also needed bladder neck narrowing at the

same time. Unlike with silicone rubber, there were no erosions by the fascia, and postsurgery urodynamics showed that 70% of patients could not be made to leak at any pressure. Finally, a flap of bladder detrusor has been harvested and used to wrap around the bladder neck to compress the bladder neck (Kurzrock *et al.*, 1996). Any increase in fixed resistance at the bladder neck almost always precludes voiding and requires that the patient rely on CIC.

Injection therapy of the bladder outlet

Several substances have been injected under the mucosa of the bladder neck in order to increase intraluminal pressure generated by the weak bladder outlet and provide continence. The first substance used in significant numbers of patients was polytetrafluoroethelyene paste or polytef (Berg, 1973). Politano popularized its use in adults and eventually applied the concept to children (Politano *et al.*, 1974; Vorstman *et al.*, 1985). They reported 86% success rates in patients who were incontinent from bladder neck surgery and 50% in patients with neuropathic bladders. Injection therapy was relatively easy to perform and required no incision, so it could be done on an outpatient basis. Unfortunately, particles of polytef were found to migrate to other organs in animal studies and particles were found in pulmonary granulomas in a human after periurethral injection (Mittleman and Marraccini, 1983; Malizia *et al.*,

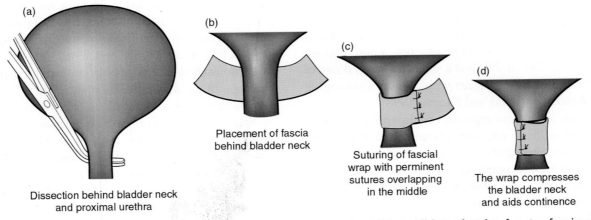

(a) Dissection behind bladder neck and proximal urethra

(b) Placement of fascia behind bladder neck

(c) Suturing of fascial wrap with perminent sutures overlapping in the middle

(d) The wrap compresses the bladder neck and aids continence

Figure 15.8 Walker described a fascial wrap of the bladder outlet in incontinent children. A strip of rectus fascia was harvested and wrapped around the bladder outlet and sewn together with permanent sutures. This provides consistent compression of the open bladder outlet and constant outlet resistance. Some patients with wide bladder outlets required bladder neck narrowing.

1984). Safety concerns have caused its abandonment in the USA. Other agents have been used, including autologus fat and collagen. Gonzalez de Garibay *et al.* (1989) reported periurethral injection of fat obtained from liposuction of the abdominal wall. Initial success in treating incontinence was never as good as with polytef and the effects diminished with time because the fat did not survive owing to poor neovascularity (Bartynski *et al.*, 1990). Eventually, 80–90% of the injected fat was absorbed by the local tissue.

The most common agent used today is gluteraldehyde cross-linked collagen. It is used in the same manner as polytef paste and is injected beneath the mucosa through a needle passed through a cystoscope (Fig. 15.9). The success in treating children with incontinence has been inconsistent with around 50–88% considered to have a good result and 20–63% becoming dry (Wan *et al.*, 1992; Perez *et al.*, 1996). Bombalaski *et al.* (1996) reported a large series of collagen injections in children. They reported a 22% cure rate of incontinence in 40 children with improvement in another 54%. Of those patients with a mean follow-up of 4.5 years, the cure or improvement rate remained stable over time. They had greater success in exstrophy/epispadias patients than in with those with neuropathic bladders.

These findings have limited injection therapy for incontinent children in most pediatric urologists' hands to patients who have had failed bladder neck reconstruction surgery. Up to 50% of these patients may become dry with injection therapy, but some require multiple injections (Ben-Chaim *et al.*, 1995). This is a simple outpatient procedure but the collagen may degrade with time and its effects diminish. The limited success and potential degradation should be explained to the patient and family. In addition, 2.5% of patients are allergic to the collagen from dietary exposure and a further 0.9% may develop late hypersensitivity (Strothers and Goldenberg, 1998). Preoperative skin testing is necessary to establish that the patient does not have antibodies to the collagen and is less likely to react to the injection.

Surgical reconfiguration of the bladder outlet

Young–Dees–Leadbetter procedure

In 1922 Young presented a refined procedure to reconfigure the wide bladder neck and posterior urethra in epispadias patients who were incontinent owing to an incompetent bladder outlet. Young had

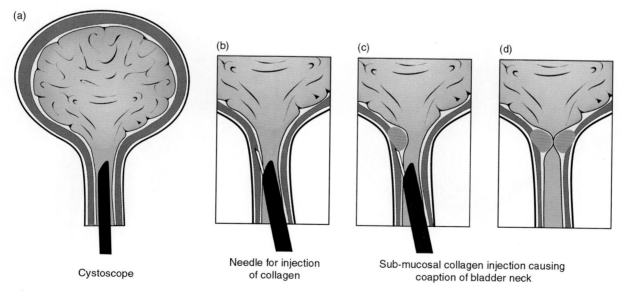

(a) Cystoscope

(b) Needle for injection of collagen

(c)(d) Sub-mucosal collagen injection causing coaption of bladder neck

Figure 15.9 Injection of the bladder neck with various materials such as polytef paste and collagen solutions has been used with more success in adults than in children. The needle is passed through a cystoscope and the material is injected submucosally either from the urethra or from a suprapubic approach. The material provides passive pressure to help to occlude the bladder outlet.

altered his approach from narrowing the posterior bladder outlet to narrowing the anterior urethra and bladder neck. He excised a full-thickness strip of tissue from the funnel-like neck of the bladder and

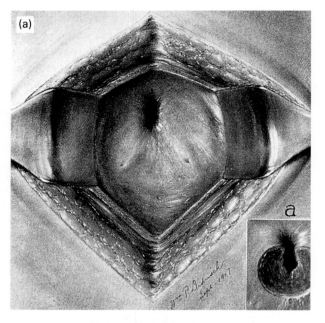

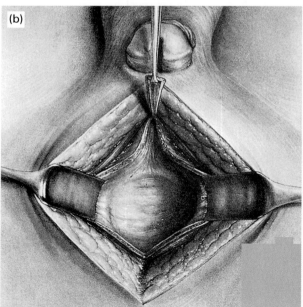

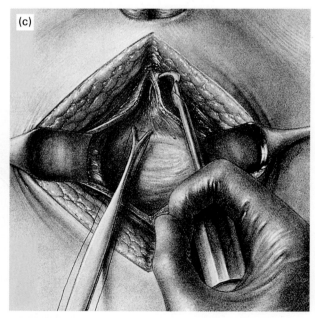

reapproximated the sides with a single row of chromic catgut sutures to create a more normal appearance (Fig. 15.10). Ureterosigmoidostomy diversion was the accepted surgical treatment of incontinence due to epispadias and exstrophy prior to Young's procedure (Culp, 1973). Young was pleased with the results of his procedure and reported, 'No fistula, no stricture, perfect urinary control, sexual powers normal'. For over 25 years after Young first presented his method to reconfigure the bladder neck for in epispadias, his procedure remained the best surgical treatment for urinary incontinence due to a weak bladder outlet.

Dees (1949) improved on Young's procedure by extending the posterior urethral flap into the bladder and removing the mucosa from the muscle on the lateral aspect of this flap (Fig. 15.11). This posterior strip of urethra and bladder was then closed in two layers, mucosa and muscle, to form a neourethra. While Young had been content to narrow the proximal urethra and bladder neck, Dees changed the position of the bladder neck itself. He created a long neourethra from tissue that normally

Figure 15.10 Young's original bladder neck repair was essentially an excision and narrowing of the outlet. He excised a full-thickness strip of mucosa and muscle from the bladder neck and proximal urethra and closed it with a single row of sutures to create a more normal appearing bladder neck when viewed from within the bladder. This, in essence, lengthened the urethra and placed the bladder neck higher in the pelvis. (*a*) The open bladder outlet viewed from above. (*b*) Excision of the strip of mucosa and muscle. (*c*) Narrowing of the bladder outlet using Young's instrument to pass suture.

would have been the posterior bladder wall. The result was to move the bladder outlet higher into the pelvis and provide a longer, more muscular, urethra.

Leadbetter (1964) advanced this concept further by extending the posterior bladder flap even higher into the bladder. This was made possible by moving the ureters from their normal location to a more cranial position further from the urethra and original bladder neck. The position of the ureters had been the limiting factor when Dees created his neourethra and moved the bladder neck above its natural location. Leadbetter moved the ureters out of the way by mobilizing them and reimplanting them transversely across the posterior bladder wall well above the trigone.

By extending the neourethra higher in the bladder, Leadbetter was also presented with a wider strip of bladder to use for his neourethra. A narrow strip of mucosa was left in the central portion of the neo-

urethra. This was tubularized, all of the mucosa lateral to the this strip was excised, and the two flaps of muscle lateral to the neourethra were then wrapped over the mucosa in an overlapping fashion, providing addition muscular support to the neourethra and bladder neck (Fig. 15.12). With few changes today, the Young–Dees–Leadbetter (YDL) bladder neck repair remains the gold standard of bladder neck reconstruction. Continence has been obtained in 78% of patients with neuropathic bladders and in 80% in exstrophy patients (Gearhart and Jeffs, 1998; McMahon *et al.*, 1996; Donnahoo *et al.*, 1999). It must be noted that augmentation cystoplasty was necessary to obtain this degree of continence in 90% of the neuropathic bladder children in the author's series and in 50% of the exstrophy–epispadias patients in the Mayo Clinic series.

Disadvantages of the YDL bladder neck reconstruction include loss of significant bladder capacity due to the use of bladder wall tissue to create the

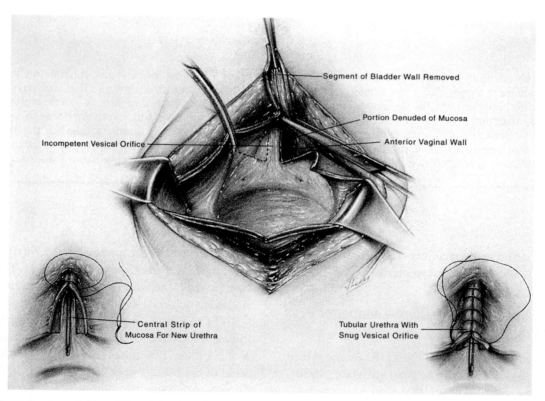

Figure 15.11 Dee's revision of Young's procedure extended the posterior urethral flap into the bladder and allowed a longer neourethra. He removed the mucosa from the muscle on the lateral aspect of this flap and, after closing the central flap of mucosa into a tube, he closed the muscle over the mucosa in a second layer. This provided additional muscle around the neourethra.

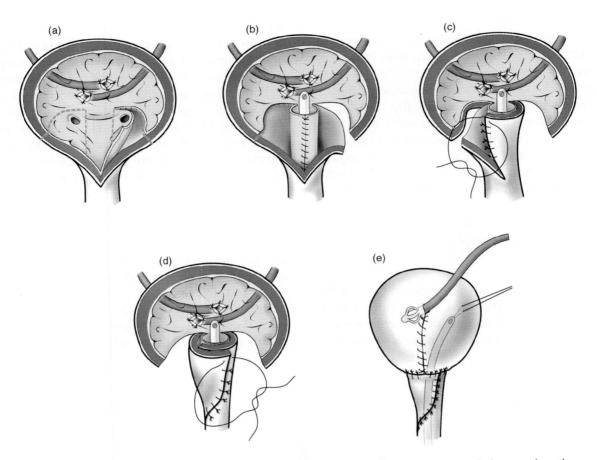

Figure 15.12 Leadbetter further improved upon the Young–Dee's bladder neck repair by moving the ureters to a new location higher along the posterior bladder wall and away from the urethra. This maneuver allowed the posterior bladder strip to be even longer and produce a long neourethra and a much higher bladder neck. (*a, b*) Leadbetter removed the mucosa from the triangular flaps of bladder muscle on each side of the mucosal strip that was to be used for the neourethra. (*c*) After rolling the strip into a tube for the neourethra he closed the lateral muscle flaps over the neourethra in layers to provide even more muscle at the bladder outlet. (*d*) Muscle is rotated over the neo-urethra in an overlapping fashion. (*e*) Dependable bladder drainage is necessary.

urethral continence mechanism. The neourethra may be tortuous and difficult to catheterize.

Variations of the Young–Dees–Leadbetter procedure

There are many variations to the YDL, among which Mollard's is closest to the original (Mollard, 1980). He creates a 7 cm long urethral strip which is wide enough to close over a 10 Fr catheter and removes the mucosa from the triangular muscle flaps lateral to the strip. He then incises one of the periurethral muscular flaps vertically parallel to the strip and rotates it

horizontally across the midline in order to develop an anterior bladder neck angle (Fig. 15.13). His procedure has been applied mostly to exstrophy patients and he has achieved a 70% continence rate.

Koff's variation on the YDL also varies from the original in its use of the periurethral muscle flaps (Koff, 1990). His initial incision is on the lateral aspect of the bladder neck rather than the midline and this produces a single long muscle flap on one side of the bladder. After he moves the ureters cephalad, Koff strips the mucosa from the long muscle flap, leaving a midline strip of urethra and bladder to tubularize for the neourethra. The long muscle flap is then wrapped

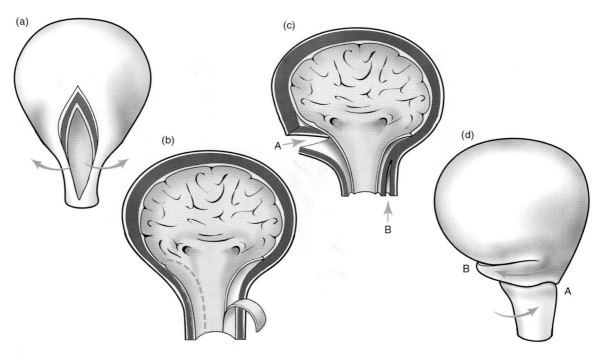

Figure 15.13 Mollard's variation of the Young–Dees–Leadbetter procedure is similar in the construction of the neourethra from a long posterior strip of urethra and bladder. It differs in that one of the two triangular flaps is incised vertically and parallel to the neourethra. This flap is then rotated horizontally across the midline to create an angle of the anterior bladder neck. (*a*) The bladder is opened in the mid-line. (*b*) The mucosa lateral to the central urethal strip is excised. (*c*) The two lateral muscle flaps are incised, one vertically and one horizontally. (*d*) One flap (*B*) is rotated horizontally across the repair to create an anterior bladder neck.

around the neourethra, producing what he has termed 'the cinch' (Fig. 15.14). Koff reports 80% continence rates, mostly in exstrophy patients. All of the patients have had significant difficulties in voiding. Forty per cent of the children required bladder augmentation and intermittent catheterization. Bladder capacity is lost to a similar degree as in the YDL procedure.

Mitchell returned to Young's original concept of a narrowed neourethra without added muscular support (Jones *et al.*, 1993). He noted that overlapping bladder muscle flaps used to create more outlet resistance made the bladder smaller by reducing the bladder itself. Mitchell's procedure is the only bladder neck repair that does not decrease bladder capacity as the anterior bladder and urethral flap is incorporated into the bladder (Fig. 15.15). He mobilized a triangular full-thickness flap of anterior urethra and bladder neck and then narrowed the bladder outlet. The flap was then rotated cephalad and integrated into the bladder. All patients voided spontaneously

and continence was achieved in 64% of a mixed group of children with neuropathic bladders and exstrophy.

Some other variations on the YDL have been developed, including Koyle's Thiersch–Duplay type tubularization of the posterior bladder wall (Koyle, 1998). This procedure isolates and rolls a strip of mucosa into a tube in situ and then closes muscle and mucosa over the tube by rolling in the lateral tissue (Fig. 15.16). He calls this the reverse Kropp or Ppork repair and has achieved 82% continence in neuropathic bladder patients. There may be problems with catheterization per urethra, so all of these patients had alternative access for bladder catheterization via a catheterizable stoma.

Arap *et al.* (1980) presented the most radical variation on the YDL posterior-tube bladder neck repair for use in the most severe cases of exstrophy with tiny bladder plates. His procedure is performed in two stages. The first stage is creation of a colon conduit with an antirefluxing ureterocolonic anastamosis. The

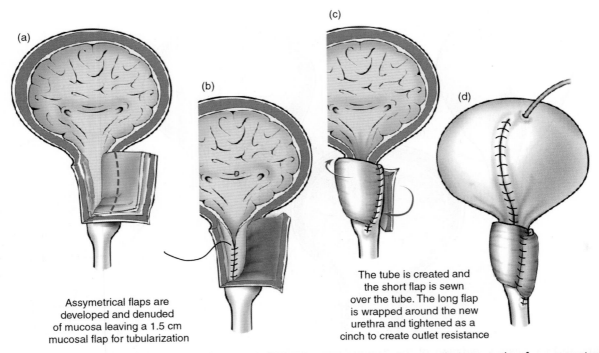

Assymetrical flaps are
developed and denuded
of mucosa leaving a 1.5 cm
mucosal flap for tubularization

The tube is created and
the short flap is sewn
over the tube. The long flap
is wrapped around the new
urethra and tightened as a
cinch to create outlet resistance

Figure 15.14 Koff's variation of the Young–Dees–Leadbetter procedure also creates the neourethra from a posterior flap of urethra and bladder and covers it with a flap of demucosalized muscle. The construction of this flap is different to other repairs that rely on two flaps. Koff makes a lateral incision of the bladder neck instead of opening the midline. This creates a single long flap on one side of the neourethra. The flap is then wrapped around the neourethra and sewn to itself with permanent sutures. It acts as a constant compression of the bladder outlet. (*a*) The bladder outlet is opened on one side. (*b*) A midline mucosal strip is tubularized and the mucosa is dissected from the reamining muscle flap. (*c, d*) The muscle flap is then rotated around the bladder outlet.

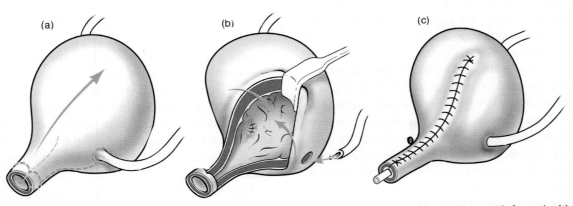

Figure 15.15 Mitchell returned to Young's original concept of a narrowed bladder neck that is not reinforced with additional muscle layers. His repair mobilizes a triangular flap of anterior bladder and urethra based on the bladder-side blood supply and then rotates the flap into the bladder. It is the only repair that does not decrease bladder volume. (*a*) An incision is made across the anterior urethra, extending up along the posterior lateral wall of the bladder outlet on each side. (*b*) The flap of bladder and urethra is rotated back into the bladder. (*c*) The incision is closed in the midline.

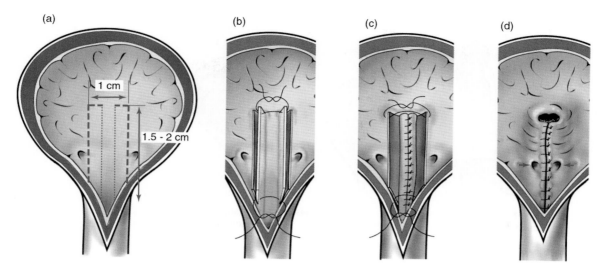

Figure 15.16 Koyle presented a bladder neck reconfiguration that isolates a strip of posterior mucosa in the posterior midline of the bladder. This strip is then rolled into a tube creating a neourethra. Finally, the neourethra is covered with flaps of muscle and mucosa that have been mobilized lateral to the neourethra. (*a*) A mucosal flap is outlined. (*b*) The flap is then tubularized. (*c*) A second layer of muscle is closed. (*d*) Lateral mucosa is closed over the tube.

second procedure creates a tube in the same manner as the YDL but uses the entire bladder except for the dome, which is left open as a wide funnel (Fig. 15.17). The previously created colon conduit is then reconfigured as a reservoir and attached to the funneled bladder plate. Arap reported a 75% continence rate with patients voiding frequently. Intermittent catheterization has provided continence and allowed a long dry interval in the author's limited experience with the Arap procedure.

Tanagho bladder neck repair

In 1968, Tanagho was studying the function and anatomy of bladder muscle when he noticed 'a condensation of circle fibers above the internal meatus' (Tanagho and Smith, 1968). He then designed the first anterior bladder tube repair for incontinence and perfected it in dogs (Tanagho *et al.*, 1969). Three years later he presented his experience in patients including postprostatectomy adults (Tanagho and Smith, 1972).

Tanagho intended to capture the muscle fibers of the anterior bladder and incorporate them into the bladder neck. He created a bladder-based flap from the anterior bladder just proximal to the urethra and rolled it into a tube for the neourethra (Fig. 15.18).

He then divided the urethra from the original bladder neck and anastomosed the neourethra to the native urethra end to end. The effect of this maneuver was to lengthen the urethra and to create a new, more cephalad bladder neck.

He achieved a 72% continence rate and patients voided well. He compared his long-term results in 50 patients to the YDL procedure performed in 25 patients and found a 70% success with the Tanagho anterior bladder tube compared with 52% with the YDL posterior tube (Tanagho, 1981). One advantage of Tanagho's bladder-based anterior flap included its applicability to short urethras, as demonstrated by Diamond and Ransley (1987) in urogenital sinus patients. The Tanagho repair is most commonly used in this situation today. Disadvantages include the necessity to divide the bladder from the urethra, possibly resulting in difficult catheterization, and loss of bladder volume.

Kropp bladder neck repair

In 1972, Lapides made a contribution that changed forever our attitude and approach to incontinence surgery (Lapides *et al.*, 1972). His introduction of CIC controlled infection, decreased bladder pressure, and made many patients continent without further

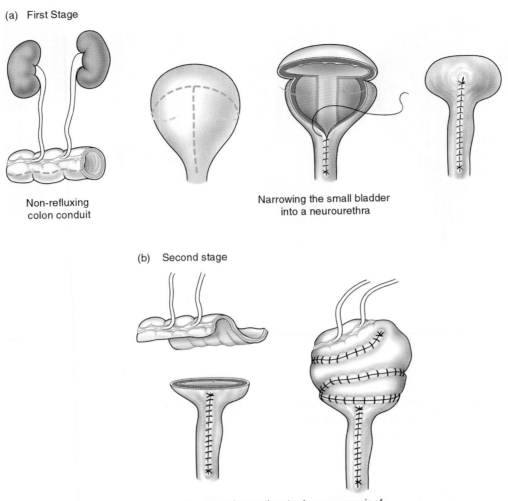

(a) First Stage

Non-refluxing
colon conduit

Narrowing the small bladder
into a neourethra

(b) Second stage

Creation of a continent urinary reservoir of
bowel and using the tubularised bladder as urethra

Figure 15.17 Arap's staged bladder reconstruction is the most radical reconfiguration of the bladder outlet. In the first stage the ureters are transplanted from the bladder plate to a non-refluxing anastamosis into a colon conduit. The second procedure creates a neourethra from the entire bladder except for the dome that is left open as a wide funnel. The colon conduit is then reconfigured as a reservoir and sewn to the funneled bladder.

surgery (Cass *et al.*, 1984). CIC made voiding an option rather than a requirement, and changed the goals and results of incontinence surgery.

Kropp was the first surgeon to develop a new bladder neck reconstruction designed to take full advantage of CIC (Kropp and Angwafo, 1986). The goals of the surgery had changed. Dryness was foremost and voiding was no longer a consideration. CIC had been used in patients with other forms of bladder neck reconstruction before this, but they were all procedures that allowed the patient to void, at least in theory. The Kropp operation was the first to preclude voiding.

The Kropp procedure uses a full-thickness flap of anterior bladder muscle. This flap is based on the urethra, unlike Tanagho's flap which is based on the bladder. The full-thickness bladder flap is isolated from the bladder and rolled into a tube of the same diameter as the urethra. The tube is then implanted in a submucosal tunnel in the midline of the posterior bladder wall between the ureters (Fig. 15.19).

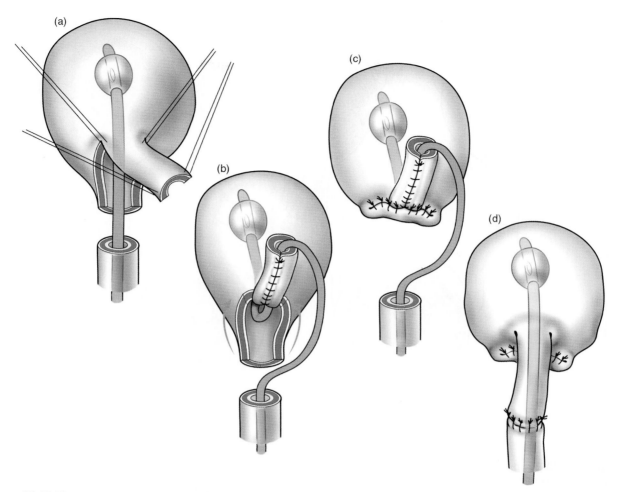

Figure 15.18 Tanagho's procedure created a neourethra from a strip of the anterior bladder neck and bladder. This allowed the creation of an angle at the posterior bladder neck. It required complete separation of the bladder from the urethra and a reanastmosis of the neourethra to the native urethra. (*a*) The bladder outlet is divided from the urethra and an anterior bladder-based tube is formed. (*b*) The flap is tubularized. (*c*) The posterior bladder is closed. (*d*) The tube is sewn to the urethra.

Advantages of Kropp's reconstruction included a very high continence rate of 80–94% (Belman and Kaplan, 1989; Nill *et al.*, 1990). Kropp's strict definition of continence was complete dryness or rare leakage. The reoperation rate was high in the original series but most secondary procedures involved the storage function of the bladder and only 20% required additional surgery to the bladder outlet. To facilitate storage and to compensate for the bladder volume lost in construction of the tube, Kropp now suggests that all patients undergo a simultaneous bladder augmentation. Since high urethral resistance is created, there is a high risk of bladder rupture if catheterization is not performed

on a timely basis. There have also been problems catheterizing through the repair, but the improvement of leaving lateral attachments at the bladder neck intact and not completely separating the neourethra from the bladder has minimized this difficulty.

In 1997, Snodgrass reported a series of 22 children treated with the modified Kropp procedure described by Belman and Kaplan (1989). Snodgrass created a urethral-based flap of anterior bladder wall and rolled it into a tube. He did not divide the bladder neck from the remainder of the bladder. The posterior bladder mucosa is then incised in the midline to create a trough and the tube is laid in this trough with

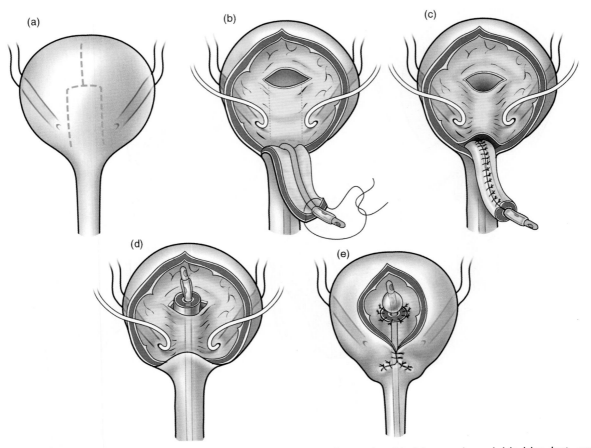

Figure 15.19 Kropp also creates a neourethra from a flap of anterior bladder neck and bladder but, unlike Tanagho, Kropp's flap is based on the urethra. The flap is tubularized and then placed in a submucosal tunnel created along the midline of the posterior bladder wall. (*a*) An anterior urethral-based flap is mobilized. (*b, c*) The flap is tubularized. A submucosal tunnel is made in the posterior bladder wall. (*d, e*) The tube is placed in the tunnel.

the mucosa closed over the tube (Fig. 15.20). No attempt is made to tunnel the tube. He reported a 91% continence rate, defined as dry intervals of 3 hours. Snodgrass notes that these patients are socially continent and will have slight leakage when catheterization is delayed. Bladder augmentation was performed in 91% of his patients at the same time of bladder outlet surgery. Just as in the original Kropp procedure, voiding is impossible.

Pippi Salle bladder neck repair

Pippi Salle developed a bladder outlet repair for incontinence by creating a neourethra composed of both anterior and posterior bladder flaps (Pippi Salle *et al.*, 1994). This tubularized continence mechanism is made of two separate flaps. Both anterior and posterior strips of bladder are isolated and the anterior flap is completely mobilized as a flap based on the urethra. The posterior flap is outlined with two parallel mucosal incisions and the posterior bladder muscle is left intact. The anterior bladder flap is then flipped down to oppose the posterior flap at the level of the posterior bladder wall. The two flaps are sewn together creating a neourethra, which extends above the level of the ureters (Fig. 15.21). Mucosa on either side of the strip of posterior bladder wall is mobilized and the muscle from the anterior strip is sewn to the muscle of the posterior bladder. The complete-thickness bladder tube is then covered with the previously mobilized bladder mucosa just lateral to the tube.

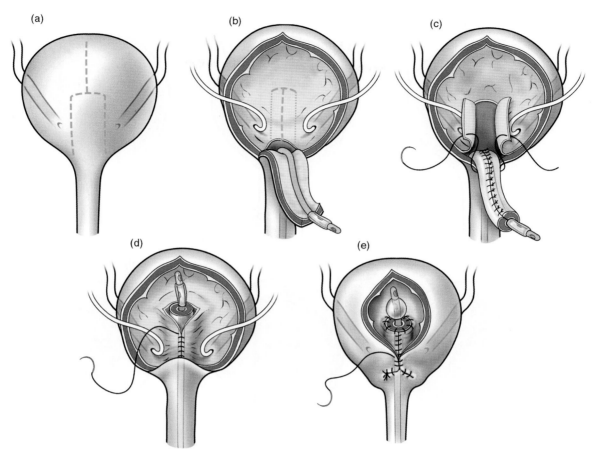

Figure 15.20 The Snodgrass variation of the Kropp procedure lays the Kropp tube in a trough instead of a tunnel. Construction of the tube is identical to Kropp.

The Pippi Salle repair produces continence rates of 80% and this repair is easy to catheterize primarily because the posterior wall remains intact (Rink *et al.*, 1994). Bladder volume is decreased by the use of bladder wall to create the continence mechanism. This repair also requires the patient to catheterize, as voiding is impossible. McLorie and Khoury (1998) warned of the potential danger of damaging its blood supply when isolating the long, thin anterior bladder flap.

Bladder neck closure

The ultimate bladder neck reconfiguration is complete closure of the bladder outlet. Today, after years of experience, most but not all bladder necks can be made continent. Those that cannot be repaired can be closed. The concept of bladder neck closure was made a viable option in 1980 when Mitrofanoff constructed the continent appendicovesicostomy and combined it with bladder neck closure in patients with neuropathic bladders (Fig. 15.22). Duckett and Snyder (1986) presented variations on bladder neck closure and continent stomas and Van Savage *et al.* (1996) presented a series of 46 children with closure of the bladder neck. After division of the urethra, both stumps are closed with two layers of absorbable sutures.

In general, bladder neck closure is a procedure of last resort and is used after other more flexible options in bladder neck reconstruction have been exhausted (Gearhart *et al.*, 1995; Hensle *et al.*, 1995). The indications for bladder neck closure are intractable urinary incontinence resistant to maximal medical management and other surgical procedures. Patients usually have failed previous incontinence surgery or suffer

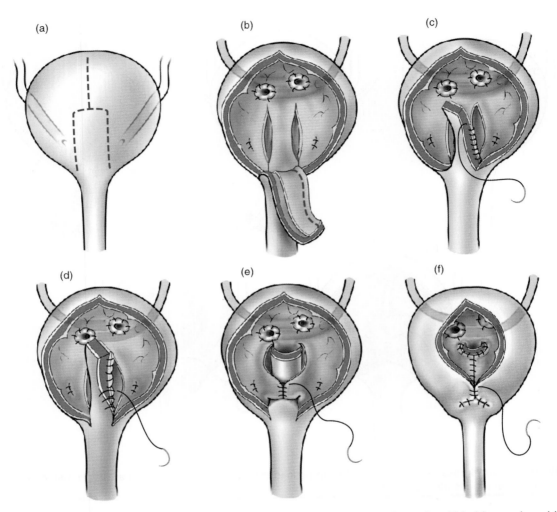

Figure 15.21 Pippi Sallee creates a neourethra from an anterior and a posterior strip of bladder neck and bladder. The two are sewn together but only the anterior flap is mobilized completely. The posterior flap is isolated but not mobilized from the posterior bladder wall. The neourethra is then covered with mucosa and some muscle which is mobilized on each side. (*a*) An anterior bladder flap is mobilized. (*b*) A posterior bladder mucosal flap is mobilized. (*c*) The mucosa of the anterior and posterior flaps are sewn together. (*d*) the muscle of the flaps is sewn together. (*e, f*) The bladder mucosa in closed over the neo-urethra.

from a primary condition that projects failure. The obvious advantage is complete urethral continence in as many as 96%. Eighty-nine per cent have stable upper urinary tracts and no bladder capacity is lost in the creation of the continence mechanism (Jayanthi *et al.*, 1995). Disadvantages include a complete life-long reliance on an extra-anatomical method of bladder emptying and no pressure pop-off valve. Sixty per cent of patients with closed bladder necks require additional surgery for complications including fistulas, stones, augmentation, ruptures, and other revisions.

The Mitrofanoff principle

Mitrofanoff's contribution, now termed the Mitrofanoff principle, has had a profound effect on incontinence surgery in children. His development of alternative continent bladder access through a continent stoma has relieved the necessity for the patient either to void efficiently or to catheterize through the reconstructed bladder neck. There have been other alternatives to Mitrofanoff's original use of appendix for extra-anatomical access to the bladder. Other options for continent bladder access include ureter,

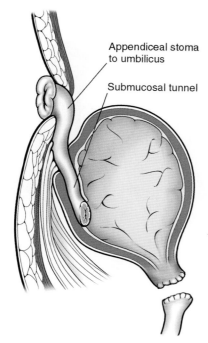

Figure 15.22 Mitrofanoff used a continent catheterizable stoma to empty the bladder. By implanting the appendix into the bladder in a continent manner he allowed efficient bladder emptying without relying on the urethra. This allowed him to close the bladder neck surgically, leaving the appendix as the only access with which to empty the bladder.

fallopian tube, bladder tubes, and tubularized bowel (Casale, 1991; Yang, 1993; Monti *et al.*, 1997). With the recent interest in the Malone antegrade colonic enema (MACE) for patients with neuropathic bowel and bladder (see Chapter 18), the appendix has been used more often as access to the colon (Malone *et al.*, 1990). Tubularized ileum and Yang/Monti tubes have been the most dependable and flexible method of bladder access for patients in whom the appendix is not available (Cain *et al.*, 1998)(Fig. 15.23). Casale (1999) developed a longer ileal tube for patients with a greater distance between the bladder and skin (Fig. 15.24). Today, an easily accessible, continent, catheterizable access for emptying the bladder is available for almost all patients.

Catheterizable abdominal stomas may promote continence by avoiding manipulation of the reconstructed bladder neck. In some cases, they encourage patient compliance with intermittent catheterization because catheterizing through an abdominal stoma is easier, more appealing, and less time consuming than urethral catheterization for many patients. Regular catheterization keeps bladder pressures low and minimizes stress on reconstruction done at the bladder neck. Stomas allow the surgeon to be more aggressive in creating resistance at the bladder outlet because the

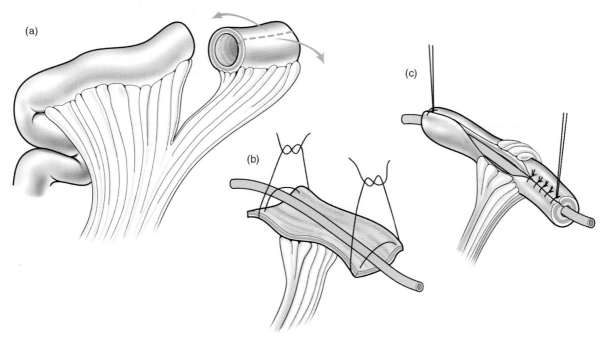

Figure 15.23 Monti popularized a concept originally described by Yang, who created a catheterizable tube from small bowel. (*a*) A 3–4 cm section of bowel is isolated on its mesentery and split on the antimesenteric border. (*b*) It is then closed along the transverse axis, 90° from the original. (*c*) This doubles the length of tube produced from a piece of bowel. The tube may then be implanted into the bladder for continent catheterizable access.

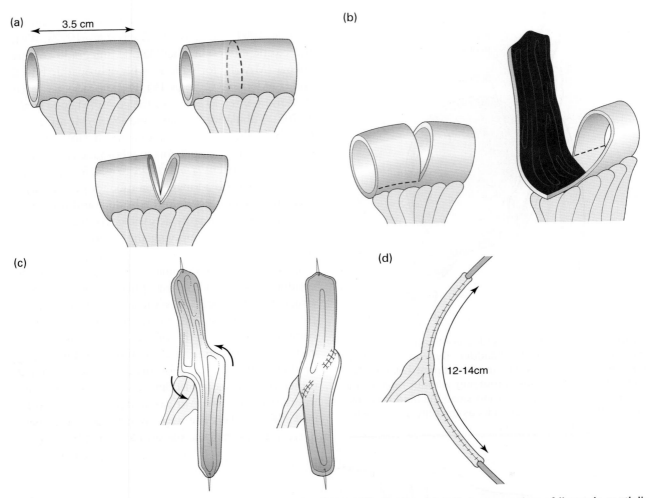

Figure 15.24 Casale presented a variation of the reconfigured ileal tube. (*a*) A 3–4 cm section of ileum is partially split into two rings, leaving the bowel over the mesentary intact. (*b*) The two rings are then split on opposite sides, allowing the bowel to be unfolded into a much longer flap. (*c*) Corners of bowel along the mesentary are sewn along the long axis of the flap and it is tubularized. (*d*) The longer tube allows more flexibility in placement of the anastomosis, mesentary, and stoma.

urethra will not be needed as the primary access for catheterization. The combination of continent stomas and bladder augmentation has allowed patients who have suffered multiple failed continence surgeries to become continent (Gearhart *et al.*, 1991).

Indicators for success

The definition of continence has changed over the years and is open to interpretation by each surgeon. 'Social continence' was felt to be adequate in the past, and if a child used several continence pads per day but was free of diapers most pediatric urologists consid-

ered their treatment successful. Society's tolerance of wetness has changed over the years, perhaps in response to the change in public policy in the 1970s to mainstream the education of children with disabilities. In more modern reviews, surgeons have been more specific in defining successful continence. Dryness, without the odor of urine, has become the expected goal. This evolution of the definition of success makes comparing results from different eras and series difficult.

The effectiveness of procedures to treat the weak bladder outlet cannot be judged easily. Ultimate success is based on continence, but other criteria, such as the ability to void and the need for additional surgery to attain continence, such as bladder augmentation, must be taken into the equation. It is unfair to compare procedures that allow voiding with those that prevent the ability to void by design.

Of the procedures that allow voiding, the YDL and its variations, and the Tanagho have been the most successful, allowing 70–100% to urinate spontaneously. However, voiding after this type of surgery is seldom normal as these procedures usually produce a fixed resistance at the weak bladder neck. Voiding is often accomplished with abnormally high bladder pressures that are generated by valsalva. These pressures are necessary to overcome the static increased bladder outlet resistance. Even if the patient is able to void for a period of several years the detrusor may eventually fail and intermittent catheterization may then be required. Many procedures produce 75% continence rates but are often dependent on intermittent catheterization and chronic detrusor relaxation achieved with medication or augmentation.

The artificial urinary sphincter would seem the best alternative for the patient who can void prior to surgery as it provides a variable resistance at the bladder neck and should allow voiding at more physiologic pressures. Long-term studies of sphincters in children reveal that most patients eventually require intermittent catheterization because of inadequate emptying due to detrusor failure. The other complications of inevitable reoperation and potential secondary detrusor hyperreflexia are additional negatives with this device. If the patient does have the potential to void over a long period the artificial sphincter is the best option. Around 80% of patients will be continent over a long period with the sphincter, although most require intermittent catheterization. Augmentation rates of 30–35% in long-term selective studies are lower than with other bladder procedures.

Of the procedures that prevent voiding by design and rely on intermittent catheterization, the slings are the most simple and dependable in females and produce 80% continence rates with good durability. The Pippi Salle bladder neck reconstruction produces 80% continence, while the Kropp procedure produces the highest continence rate, approaching 100%. Bladder neck closure is also very dependable but leaves the patient reliant on only one bladder access, an extra-anatomical continent stoma with no pop-off valve.

When choosing a bladder neck procedure, one must have specific goals in mind relating to the patient's potential to void. Patients with neuropathic bladders from sacral agenesis, myelomeningocele, and spinal cord trauma have poor potential to void regardless of bladder outlet resistance. Patients with epispadias and some with exstrophy have better detrusor function as a group and have the best potential to void.

If the goals of surgery are to have the patient dry and voiding the artificial sphincter would seem the best choice, followed by the YDL procedure or variations. If the surgical goals are to have the patient dry and to catheterize through the bladder neck and urethra, then the Kropp or Pippi Salle procedure or the artificial sphincter allows continence with easy catheterization in most cases. If the goals are to have the patient dry and the bladder neck and urethra are not important for voiding or catheterization because a continent stoma is available, then bladder neck closure is a good option.

Another measure of success that has been used to judge bladder neck surgery is the need for bladder augmentation to achieve continence. On the surface, it would seem that the YDL and its variations and the Tanagho procedures are superior because series of these procedures report augmentation rates of 0–40%. This compares with Kropp's reported augmentation rate of 78%, bladder neck closure of 61–80%, and rates of 80% with the Pippi Salle. Closer inspections of the series reveal that the patient groups are not comparable. Studies with the lowest augmentation rates (15–20%) are consistently made up of mostly epispadias, exstrophy, and urogenital sinus patients, while the series with high augmentation rates (70–90%) usually include a significant number with neuropathic bladders. The need for augmentation is much more a function of the underlying condition and the pathophysiology of the detrusor, rather than being a result of bladder outlet incompetence or corrective surgery.

Conclusions and recommendations

Patients found to have incontinence due to bladder outlet incompetence as demonstrated by leak point pressures, cystograms, and/or cystoscopic examinations should always be treated with all available medical options needed to improve continence. CIC, anticholinergic medication, α-adrenergic medications, control of constipation, and control of infection should be utilized. If these methods fail and the patient and family have the sufficient motivation and understanding of what continence procedures require, then the urologist may explore the surgical options.

The patient and family should play a vital role in the decision-making process and they must understand the consequences of having surgery to increase leak point pressure. The surgeon makes a profound change in the physiology of the urinary tract and in doing so depends on the patient and family to perform the management required by this change. Whether it is performing intermittent catheterization, emptying the bladder on schedule with an artificial sphincter, or taking medication, the success of the surgery and the health of the child depend on their willingness and ability to comply.

Once the child, family, and surgeon agree to perform a procedure to increase resistance at the bladder neck there are many good options. The choice of procedure depends on the goals of surgery and the particular surgeon's preferences. It is important to approach each patient individually, and children with incontinence who require surgical management are often complex with other health and social concerns. In general, however, one can look at the underlying pathology and goals of surgery and recommend procedures that are good management options.

If the child can void to completion prior to surgery and has a condition that may allow long-term voiding, then the artificial sphincter or the YDL procedure is a good option. The conditions that leave children with relatively isolated bladder outlet incompetence and adequate detrusor function include epispadias, bilateral ectopic ureters, some surgical injuries to the bladder neck, and urogenital sinus anomalies. As a rule, artificial sphincters should not be used if there has been prior bladder neck reconstruction, such as in exstrophy closure, because of the risk of erosion. The rare child with pure stress incontinence may be treated with suspension of the bladder outlet using any of the procedures used for adult stress incontinence such as described by McGuire or Raz. Slings may be used in children who void, but should be applied loosely.

Patients with exstrophy are still treated with the YDL or one of the variations. New urodynamic data suggest that procedures such as the YDL that surgically alter the trigone may lead to worsening of detrusor function. Kaefer et al. (1999) studied epis-padias patients and Diamond et al. (1999) reviewed exstrophy patients before and after bladder neck surgery, and both studies showed that most patients suffer a deterioration of filling and voiding dynamics. Most developed high pressures, increased contractility, and diminished capacity, while some bladders increased in size and developed poor contractility. Only 25% of 30 exstrophy patients maintained normal detrusor function after their bladder outlet resistance was surgically increased. Whether the detrusor functional changes observed are the result of surgical trauma to the bladder or increased demands on the bladder to retain urine and cycle, or are predetermined by different levels of dysfunction inherent in each exstrophy bladder has yet to be determined.

The newest development in exstrophy surgery is to perform the entire repair, including closure, bladder neck reconfiguration, and urethroplasty, as a single procedure in the newborn period (Grady et al., 1999) (see Chapter 27). The author continues to perform staged repairs, with the bladder outlet repair done at age 3 years. For the past 2 years he has been adding a continent umbilical urinary stoma at the time of bladder outlet repair. This allows the child to void per urethra but also offers easy access to check residual urine or to perform intermittent catheterization without violating the repaired bladder outlet if the child cannot void adequately. The surgeon should elevate and suspend the bladder neck and urethra at the same time as a bladder outlet reconfiguration such as the YDL is performed.

In patients who cannot void adequately prior to surgery and who have poor potential for good detrusor function there are more options. These children, for the most part, have neuropathic bladders from myelodysplasia or other neurologic conditions. They will be dependent on CIC to empty the bladder. In girls, the fascial sling has become the treatment of choice because of its simplicity and reliability. In boys, there are many options but the author currently uses either the YDL or Kropp procedure. If the plan calls for intermittent catheterization through the repaired bladder neck in a boy the Pippi Salle is preferred because it is easy to catheterize. At this time, almost all patients have simultaneous creation of a continent catheterizable abdominal stoma. This allows easy access to the bladder and there is no need to worry about routine urethral catheterization or trauma to the repaired bladder outlet.

The majority of children with neuropathic incontinence at the bladder outlet will also have bladders with limited detrusor function and storage capacity. Most children today undergo a simultaneous augmentation cystoplasty to create a large, low-pressure, storage reservoir. There is no question that augmentation alone will improve continence in this patient population even if the bladder outlet is weak (Cher and Allen, 1993). However, in the author's experience, augmentation alone has not provided reliable continence even in patients with reasonable bladder outlet resistance. For this reason, in most cases of reconstruction for incontinence, the surgeon should maximize both bladder outlet resistance and the storage capacity of the bladder.

Procedures to improve resistance at the incompetent bladder outlet have been advanced greatly since the 1970s by the development of associated procedures such as bladder augmentation. Two singular contributions in this field came from Lapides, with his concept of CIC, and Mitrofanoff, whose novel idea to create a continent catheterizable stoma allowed a non-urethral method of bladder emptying. Finally, the predictors of success in bladder outlet reconstruction remain unchanged despite these advances. They are sufficient resistance at the bladder outlet, a low-pressure reservoir of adequate size, and a reliable means to empty the bladder efficiently.

References

Andersson K (1993) Pharmacology of lower urinary tract smooth muscles and penile erectile tissues. *Pharmacol Rev* **45**: 253–308.

Arap S, Giron A, Menezes de Goles G (1980) Initial results of the complete reconstruction of bladder exstrophy. *Urol Clin North Am* **7**: 477–88.

Barrett D, Furlow W (1981) Implantation of a new semi-automatic artificial genitourinary sphincter. Experience with patients utilizing a new concept of primary and secondary activation. *Prog Clin Biol Res* **78**: 375–86.

Barrett D, Furlow W (1982) The management of severe urinary incontinence in patients with myelodysplasia by implantation of the AS 791/792 urinary sphincter device. *J Urol* **128**: 484–6.

Barrett D, Furlow W (1984) Incontinence, intermittent self-catheterization and the artificial genitourinary sphincter. *J Urol* **132**: 268–9.

Barrett D, Licht M (1998) Implantation of the artificial genitourinary sphincter in men and women. In: Walsh P, Retik A, Vaughn E, Wein A (eds) *Campbell's urology*. Volume 7. Philadelphia, PA: WB Saunders, 1121–34.

Barrett D, Parulkar B, Kramer S (1993) Experience with AS 800 artificical sphincter in pediatric and young adult patients. *Urology* **42**: 431–6.

Bartynski J, Marion M, Wang T (1990) Histopathologic evaluation of adipose autografts in a rabbit ear model. *Otolaryngology* **102**: 314–21.

Bauer S, Reda E, Colodny A, Retik A (1986) Detrusor instability: a delayed complication in association with the artificial sphincter. *J Urol* **135**: 1212–15.

Bauer S, Peters C, Colodny A *et al.* (1989) The use of rectus fascia to manage urinary incontinence. *J Urol* **142**: 516–19.

Belman A, Kaplan G (1989) Experience with the Kropp anti-incontinence procedure. *J Urol* **141**: 1160–2.

Ben-Chaim J, Jeffs R, Peppas D, Gearhart JL (1995) Submucosal bladder neck injections of glutaraldehyde cross-linked bovine collagen for the treatment of urinary incontinence in patients with the exstrophy/epispadias complex. *J Urol* **154**: 862–4.

Berg S (1973) Polytef augmentation urethroplasty. *Arch Surg* **107**: 379–81.

Blaivas J (1994) Pubovaginal slings. In: Kursh ED, McGuire EJ (eds) *Female urology*. Philadelphia, PA: JB Lippincott Co., 235.

Blaivas J, Romanzi L, Heritz D (1998) Urinary incontinence: pathophysiology, evaluation, treatment overview, and non-surgical management. In: Walsh P, Retik A, Vaughn E, Wein A (eds) *Campbell's urology*. Volume 7. Philadelphia, PA: WB Saunders, 1007–36.

Bombalaski M, Bloom D, McGuire E, Panzl A (1996) Glutaralyde cross-linked collagen in the treatment of urinary incontinence in children. *J Urol* **155**: 699–702.

Bosco P, Bauer S, Colodny A *et al.* (1991) The long-term results of artificial sphincters in children. *J Urol* **146**: 396–9.

Burch J (1961) Urethrovaginal fixation to Cooper's ligament for correction of stress incontinence, cystocele, and prolapse. *Am J Obstet Gynecol* **81**: 281–90.

Cain M, Casale A, Rink R (1998) Initial experience utilizing a catheterizable ileovesicostomy (Monti procedure) in children. *Urology* **52**: 870–3.

Casale A (1991) Continent vesicostomy: a new method utilizing only bladder tissue (Abstract 72). Presented at the 60th Annual Meeting of the American Academy of Pediatrics, New Orleans, 1991.

Casale A (1999) A long continent ileovesicostomy made of a single piece of bowel. *J Urol* **162**: 1743–5.

Cass A., Luxenberg M, Gleich P *et al.* (1984) Clean intermittent catheterization in the management of neurogenic bladder in children. *J Urol* **132**: 526–8.

Cher M, Allen T (1993) Continence in the myelodysplastic patient following enterocystoplasty. *J Urol* **149**: 1103–6.

Culp O (1973) Treatment of epispadias with and without urinary incontinence: experience with 46 patients. *J Urol* **100**: 120–5.

Decter R (1993) Use of the fascial sling for neurogenic incontinence: lessons learned. *J Urol* **150**: 683–6.

Decter R, Harpster L (1992) Pitfalls in determination of leak point pressure. *J Urol* **148**: 588–91.

Dees J (1949) Congenital epispadias with incontinence. *J Urol* **62**: 513–22.

Diamond D, Ransley P (1987) Use of the anterior detrusor tube in managing urogenital sinus anomalies. *J Urol* **138**: 1057–9.

Diamond D, Bauer S, Dinlecn C *et al.* (1999) Normal urodynamics in patients with bladder exstrophy: are they achievable? *J Urol* **162**: 841–5.

Donnahoo K, Rink R, Cain M, Casale A (1999) The use of the Young–Dees–Leadbetter bladder neck repair in patients with neurogenic incontinence. *J Urol* **161**: 1946–9.

Duckett J, Snyder H (1986) Continent urinary diversion: variations on the Mitrofanoff principle. *J Urol* **136**: 58–62.

Elder J (1990) Periurethral and puboprostatic sling repair for incontinence in patients with myelodysplasia. *J Urol* **144**: 434–7.

Elliott D, Barrett D (1998) Mayo Clinic long-term analysis of the functional durability of the AMS 800 artificial urinary sphincter: a review of 323 cases. *J Urol* **159**: 1206–8.

Freedman E, Singh G, Donnell S *et al.* (1994) Combined bladder neck suspension and augmentation cystoplasty for neuropathic incontinence in female patients. *Br J Urol* **73**: 621–4.

Gearhart J, Canning D, Jeffs R (1991) Failed bladder neck reconstruction: options for management. *J Urol* **146**: 1082–4.

Gearhart J, Jeffs R (1998) Management of the exstrophy–epispadias complex and urachal anomalies. In: Walsh P, Retik A, Vaughn E, Wein A (eds) *Campbell's urology.* Volume 7. Philadelphia, PA: WB Saunders, 1939–40.

Gearhart J, Peppas D, Jeffs R (1995) The application of continent urinary stomas to bladder augmentation or replacement in the failed exstrophy reconstruction. *Br J Urol* **75**: 87–90.

Ghoniem G, Bloom D, McGuire E, Stewart K (1989) Bladder compliance in myelomeningocele children. *J Urol* **141**: 1404–6.

Goebell R (1911) Zur operativen beseritigung der angerborenen incontinentia vesical. *Ztsch Gynak* **2**: 187.

Gonzalez R, Sidi A (1985) Preoperative prediction of continence after enterocystoplasty or undiversion in children with neurogenic bladder. *J Urol* **134**: 705–7.

Gonzalez R, Koleilat N, Austin C, Sidi A (1989) The artificial sphincter AS800 in congenital urinary incontinence. *J Urol* **142**: 512–15.

Gonzalez R, Merino F, Vaughn M (1995) Long term results of the artificial urinary sphincter in male patients with neurogenic bladder. *J Urol* **154**: 769–70.

Gonzalez de Garibay A, Jimeno C, York M *et al.* (1989) Endoscopic autotransplantation of fat tissue in the treatment of urinary incontinence in the female. *J Urol* **95**: 363–6.

Gormley E, Bloom D, McGuire E, Ritchey M (1994) Pubovaginal slings for the management of urinary incontinence in female adolescents. *J Urol* **152**: 822–5.

Grady R, Carr M, Mitchell M (1999) Complete primary closure of bladder exstrophy. Epispadias and bladder exstrophy repair. *Urol Clin North Am* **26**: 95–109.

Hensle T, Kirsch A, Kennedy W, Reiley E (1995) Bladder neck closure in association with continent urinary diversion. *J Urol* **154**: 883–5.

Herschorn S, Randomski S (1992) Fascial slings and bladder neck tapering in the treatment of male urologic incontinence. *J Urol* **147**: 1073–5.

Hilwa N, Perlmutter A (1978) The role of adjunctive drug therapy for intermittent catheterization and self-catheterization in children with vesical dysfunction. *J Urol* **119**: 551–4.

Jayanthi V, Churchill B, McLorie G, Khoury A (1995) Concomitant bladder neck closure and Mitrofanoff diversion for the management of intractagble urinary incontinence. *J Urol* **154**: 886–8.

Jones J, Mitchell M, Rink R (1993) Improved results using a modification of the Young–Dees–Leadbetter neck repair. *Br J Urol* **555**: 555–61.

Kaefer M, McLaughlin K, Rink R *et al.* (1997) Upsizing of the artificial urinary sphincter cuff to facilitate spontaneous voiding. *Urology* **50**: 106–9.

Kaefer M, Andler R, Bauer S *et al.* (1999) Urodynamic findings in children with isolated epispadias. *J Urol* **162**: 1172–5.

Kakizaki H, Shibata T, Shinno Y *et al.* (1995) Fascial sling for the management of urinary incontinence due to sphincter incompetence. *J Urol* **153**: 644–7.

Koff S (1990) A technique for bladder neck reconstruction in exstrophy: the cinch. *J Urol* **144**: 546–9.

Koyle M (1998) Flap valve techniques in bladder neck reconstruction. *Dialog Pediatr Urol* **21**: 6: 6.

Kronner K, Rink R, Simmons G *et al.* (1998) Artificial urinary sphincter in the treatment of urinary incontinence: preoperative urodynamics do not predict the need for future bladder augmentation. *J Urol* **160**: 1093–5.

Kropp K, Angwafo F (1986) Urethral lengthening and reimplantation for neurogenic incontinence in children. *J Urol* **135**: 533–6.

Kropp B, Rink R, Adams M *et al.* (1993) Bladder outlet reconstruction: fate of the silacone sheath. *J Urol* **150**: 703–4.

Kryger J, Spencer Barthold J, Fleming P, Gonzalez R (1999) The outcome of artificial sphincter placement after a mean 15-year follow-up in a paedric population. *Br J Urol Int* **83**: 1026–31.

Kurzrock E, Lowe P, Hardy B (1996) Bladder wall pedicle wraparound sling for neurogenic urinary incontinence in children. *J Urol* **155**: 305–8.

Lapides J, Diokno A, Silber S *et al.* (1972) Clean intermittent catheterization in the treatment of urinary tract disease. *J Urol* **107**: 458–61.

Leadbetter G Jr (1964) Surgical correction of total urinary incontinence. *J Urol* **91**: 261–4.

Levisque P, Bauer S, Atala A *et al.* (1996) Ten year experience with the artificial urinary sphincter in children. *J Urol* **156**: 625–8.

Light K, Pietro T (1986) Alteration in detrusor behavior and the effect on renal function following insertion of the artificial urinary sphincter. *J Urol* **136**: 632–5.

Light J, Lapin S, Vohra S (1995) Combined use of bowel and the artificial urinary sphincter in reconstruction of the lower urinary tract: infectious complications. *J Urol* **153**: 331–3.

Ludlow J, Keating M, Wahle G *et al.* (1995) Fascial slings in children – the gender gap. *J Urol* **153**: 279A, (Abstract 201).

McGuire E, Lytton B (1978) Pubovaginal sling for stress incontinence. *J Urol* **119**: 82–4.

McGuire E, Wang C, Usitalo H, Savastano J (1986) Modified pubovaginal sling in girls with myelodysplasia. *J Urol* **135**: 94–6.

McGuire E, Woodside J, Borden T, Weis R (1981) Prognostic value of urodynamic testing in myelodysplastic patients. *J Urol* **126**: 205–9.

McLorie G, Khoury A (1998) Anterior bladder wall flap (Sallee procedure). *Dialog Pediatr Urol* **21**: 6: 5.

McMahon D, Cain M, Husmann D, Kramer S (1996) Vesical neck reconstruction in patients with the exstrophy–epispadias comlex. *J Urol* **155**: 1411–13.

Malizia A Jr, Reiman H, Meyers R *et al.* (1984) Migration and granulomatatous reaction after periurethral injection of polytef (Teflon). *JAMA* **251**: 3277–81.

Malone P, Ransley P, Kiely E (1990) Preliminary report: the antegrade continence enema. *Lancet* **336**: 1217–18.

Marshall V, Marchetti A, and Krantz K (1949) The correction of stress incontinence by simple vesico-urethral suspension. *Surg Gynecol Obstet* **88**: 509–18.

Miller E, Mayo M, Kwan D, Mitchel M (1998) Simultaneous augmentation cystoplasty and artificial urinary sphincter placement: infection rates and voiding mechanisms. *J Urol* **160**: 750–3.

Mitrofanoff P (1980) Cystostomie continente trans-appendiculaire dans le traitement des vesses neruologiques. *Chir Pediatr* **21**: 297–305.

Mittleman R, Marraccini J (1983) Pulmonary Teflon granulomas following periurethral teflon injection for urinary incontinence. *Arch Pathol Lab Med* **107**: 611–12.

Mollard P (1980) Bladder reconstruction in exstrophy. *J Urol* **124**: 525–.

Monti P, Lara R, Dutra M, De Carvalho J (1997) New techniques for construction of efferent conduits based on the Mitrofanoff principle. *Urology* **49**: 112–15.

Mulcahy J, James H, McRoberts J (1977) Oxybutynin chloride combined with intermittent clean catheterization in the treatment of myelomeningocele patients. *J Urol* **118**: 95–6.

Nill T, Peller P, Kropp K (1990) Management of urinary incontinence by bladder tube urethral lengthening and submucosal reimplantation. *J Urol* **144**: 559–63.

Pereya A, Ledherz T (1967) Combined urethrovesical suspension and vaginal urethroplasty for correction of urinary stress incontinence. *Obstet Gynecol* **30**: 537–46.

Perez L, Smith E, Parrott T *et al.* (1996) Submucosal bladder neck injection of bovine dermal collagen for stress urinary incontinence in the pediatric population. *J Urol* **156**: 633–6.

Pippi Salle J, De Fraga J, Amarante A *et al.* (1994) Uretheral lengthening with anterior bladder wall flap for urinary incontinence: a new approach. *J Urol* **152**: 803–4.

Politano V, Small M, Harper J, Lynn C (1974) Periurethral teflon injection for urinary incontinence. *J Urol* **111**: 180–3.

Purcell M, Gregory J (1984) Intermittent catheterization: evaluation of complete dryness and independence in children with myelomeningocele. *J Urol* **132**: 518–20.

Quimby G, Diamond D, Mor Y *et al.* (1996) Bladder neck reconstruction: long-term followup of reconstruction with omentum and silicone sheath. *J Urol* **156**: 629–32.

Raz S (1981) Modified bladder neck suspension for female stress incontinence. *Urology* **17**: 82–5.

Raz S, Ehrlich E, Zeidman E *et al.* (1988a) Surgical treatment of the incontinent female patient with myelomeningocele. *J Urol* **139**: 524–7.

Raz S, McGuire E, Ehrilch R *et al.* (1988b) Fascial sling to correct male neurogenic sphincter incompetence: the McGuire/Raz approach. *J Urol* **139**: 528–31.

Rink R, Adams M, Keating M (1994) The flip-flap technique to lengthen the urethra (Sallee procedure) for treatment of neurogenic urinary incontinence. *J Urol* **152**: 799–802.

Roth D, Vyas P, Kroovand R, Perlmutter A (1986) Urinary tract deterioration associated with the artificial urinary sphincter. *J Urol* **135**: 528–30.

Scott F, Bradley W, Timm G (1974) Treatment of urinary incontinence by an implantable prosthetic urinary sphincter. *J Urol* **112**: 75–80.

Sidi A, Reinberg Y, Gonzalez R (1987) Comparison of artificial sphincter implantation and bladder neck reconstruction in patients with neurogenic urinary incontinence. *J Urol* **138**: 1120–2.

Simon J (1852) Ectropia vesicae (absence of the anterior walls of the bladder and pubic abdominal parietes); operation for directing the orifices of the ureters into the rectum; temporary success; subsequent death; autopsy. *Lancet* ii: 568.

Snodgrass W (1997) A simplified Kropp procedure for incontintnce. *J Urol* **158**: 1049–52.

Stamey T (1973) Endoscopic suspension of the vesical neck for urinary incontinence. *Surg Gynecol Obstet* **136**: 547–54.

Strothers L, Goldenberg S (1998) Delayed hypersensitivity and systemic arthralgia following transurethral collagen injection for stress urinary incontinence. *J Urol* **159**: 1507–9.

Tanagho E (1981) Bladder neck reconstruction for total urinary incontinence: 10 years of experience. *J Urol* **125**: 321–4.

Tanagho E, Smith D (1968) Mechanism of urinary continence. I. Embryologic, anatomic and pathologic considerations. *J Urol* **100**: 640–6.

Tanagho E, Smith D (1972) Clinical evaluation of a surgical technique for the correction of complete urinary incontinence. *J Urol* **107**: 402–11.

Tanagho E, Smith D, Meyers F, Fisher R (1969) Mechanism of urinary continence. II. Technique for surgical correction of incontinence. *J Urol* **101**: 305–13.

Trendelenburg F (1906) The treatment of ectopia vesicae. *Ann Surg* **44**: 281–9.

Van Savage J, Khoury A, McLorie G, Churchill B (1996) Outcome analysis of Mitrofanoff principle applications using appendix and ureter to umbilical and lower quadrant stomal sites. *J Urol* **156**: 1794–7.

Vorstman B, Lockhard J, Kaufman M, Politano V (1985) Polytetrafluoroethylene injection for urinary incontinence in children. *J Urol* **133**: 248–50.

Walker R, Flack C, Hawkins-Lee B *et al.* (1995) Rectus fascial wrap: early results of modification of the rectus fascial sling. *J Urol* **154**: 771–4.

Wan J, McGuire E, Bloom D, Ritchey M (1992) The treatment of urinary incontinence in children using glutaraldehyde cross-linked collagen. *J Urol* **148**: 127–30.

Wang S, McGuire E, Bloom D (1988) A bladder pressure management system for myelodysplasia – clinical outcome. *J Urol* **140**: 1499–1502.

Webster G, Khoury J (1998) Retropubic suspension surgery for female sphincteric incontinence. In: Walsh P, Retik A, Vaughn E, Wein A (eds) *Campbell's urology*. Volume 7. Philadelphia, PA: WB Saunders, 1095–102.

Woodside J, McGuire E (1982) Technique for detection of detrusor hypertonia in the presence of urethral sphincteric incompetence. *J Urol* **127**: 740–3.

Woodside J, Borden T (1982) Pubovaginal sling procedure for the management of urinary incontinence in a myelodysplastic girl. *J Urol* **127**: 744–6.

Yang W (1993) Yang needle tunneling technique in creating antireflux and continent mechanisms. *J Urol* **150**: 830–4.

Young H (1919) An operation for the cure of incontinence of urine. *Surg Gynecol Obstet* **28**: 84–90.

Young H (1922) An operation for the cure of incontinence associated with epispadias. *J Urol* **7**: 1–32.

16

Bladder augmentation: current and future techniques

Bradley P. Kropp and Earl Y. Cheng

Introduction

The surgical management of the child with a neuropathic bladder can be a formidable task, but major advances in surgical technique have been made in recent decades. The ability to augment the capacity of the bladder with a piece of reconfigured bowel in conjunction with clean intermittent catheterization (CIC) has dramatically altered our ability to form a compliant urinary reservoir that protects the integrity of the upper urinary tract and promotes urinary continence. Conventional enterocystoplasty uses detubularized segments of small or large bowel. Despite the functional success of intestinocystoplasty, clinical experience has demonstrated that numerous complications can result from the incorporation of small and large bowel and their associated heterotopic epithelium into the urinary tract. To avoid some of these deleterious side-effects of the use of bowel for bladder augmentation, several procedures have now been developed to augment the bladder without the use of bowel, including gastrocystoplasty, autoaugmentation, seromuscular enterocystoplasty, and ureterocystoplasty. In addition, recent advances in tissue engineering techniques have increased the possibility of regenerating new bladder tissue that is clinically useful for augmentation purposes. This chapter will review the relevant surgical anatomy and physiology, advantages and disadvantages, surgical technique, and clinical results of conventional enterocystoplasty and each of the alternative procedures that avoid the use of bowel. These are summarized in Table 16.1. Since the care of the child with a neuropathic bladder can be complex and requires individualization that is dependent on the desires of the patient and family, familiarity with each of these procedures is extremely important for the pediatric urologist when considering augmentation cystoplasty.

Indications and preoperative assessment

Enterocystoplasty is performed when there is a need to enlarge and/or decrease the storage pressure in the native bladder, when the native bladder becomes an inadequate reservoir owing to abnormal bladder wall dynamics. This can result from a host of conditions including spina bifida, spinal cord trauma, posterior urethral valves, dysfunctional voiding, radiation, and infectious or other chronic inflammatory processes. Enterocystoplasty is intended to relieve high-pressure and low-capacity characteristics. There are two major indications for enterocystoplasty. The first is the presence or risk of upper tract deterioration secondary to a poorly compliant bladder. The second indication is when the bladder is a causative factor in urinary incontinence. All patients who are being considered for enterocystoplasty should be thoroughly studied with preoperative urodynamics and initially treated by medical alternatives such as anticholinergic medications and/or intermittent catheterization. It is extremely important that patients understand that, in most instances, enterocystoplasty will not result in normal voiding and a lifelong commitment to intermittent catheterization will be required (Gleason *et al.*, 1972).

Lapides' landmark studies in the early 1970s, demonstrating that intermittent catheterization can be performed safely and effectively in children (Lapides *et al.*, 1972, 1976), have had the single greatest impact on the ability to perform enterocystoplasties in children. If a patient is not dedicated to performing lifelong intermittent catheterization, then a non-continent form of urinary diversion should be chosen instead of enterocystoplasty.

The goals of enterocystoplasty are to change the native bladder environment by reducing storage pressure and increasing volume. A thorough preoperative evaluation will help to determine which type of

Table 16.1 Advantages and disadvantages of procedures for bladder augmentation

Procedure	Advantages	Disadvantages
Intestinocystopasty	Extremely complaint tissue Availability of tissue Proven long-term clinical efficacy	Heterotopic epithelium Mucus Infections Stones Hyperchloremic metabolic acidosis Malignant transformation Spontaneous rupture

Gastrocystoplasty	Compliant tissue with easily definable
	   submucosal plane for reimplantation
	Minimal mucus and stone formation
	Acid buffering in renal insufficiency patients
		Hematuria dysuria
		Hypochloremic hypokalemic metabolic
		   alkalosis

Autoaugmentation	Preservation of native urothelium Avoids bowel Technically less demanding procedure Extraperitoneal procedure Does not preclude future conventional enterocystoplasty	Inability to predict success preoperatively
Seromuscular enterocystoplasty	Preservation of native urothelium Muscle-backed mucosa	Technically demanding procedure Inability to predict success preoperatively
Ureterocystoplasty	Preservation of native urothelium Muscle-backed mucosa Compliant tissue Avoids bowel	Limited patient population Large surgical incision(s)

augmentation is most appropriate and beneficial for each child. Major factors that must be addressed before proceeding with enterocystoplasty include: (1) assessment of renal function; (2) absence or presence of reflux and/or ureteral dilatation; (3) determination of outlet resistance; (4) history of bowel dysfunction; (5) need for a continent catheterizable stoma; (6) physical and mental capacity to perform intermittent catheterization; and (7) previous urinary diversion. Since there is currently no perfect bladder augmentation applicable to all children, all of the above factors must be considered in order to make the most suitable and best choice for the patient and his or her family.

Renal function

Renal function can be assessed by measurement of serum creatinine, using one of several methods to calculate estimated creatinine clearance, 24-hour urine collection or estimation of glomerular filtration rate via a radioisotope renal scan. The authors prefer to obtain a serum creatinine and nuclear renal scan before any type of bladder augmentation. In patients with abnormal renal function, a 24-hour urine collection for volume and creatinine clearance is also performed. The information obtained from this assessment may make one segment of bowel or an alternative procedure more attractive or appropriate than others. For example, in a patient with chronic renal insufficiency, a gastrocystoplasty is often a better choice than intestinocystoplasty because fewer urinary wastes are absorbed and electrolyte disturbances such as metabolic acidosis are reduced.

Reflux and ureteral dilatation

The presence of reflux and/or massive ureteral dilatation is an important preoperative determinant. When massive ureteral reflux is present, the exact bladder capacity and compliance may be difficult to assess. Occlusion of the ureteral orifices with balloon catheters can be helpful in assessing these parameters. An anesthetic is usually required to place these catheters.

Although reflux has been reported to resolve spontaneously after enterocystoplasty (Nasrallah and Aliabadi, 1991), antireflux surgery should be considered at the time of reconstruction, especially if reflux occurs at low intravesical pressures. In patients who have low to moderate grade reflux in association with high intravesical pressures and poor bladder compliance, enterocystoplasty alone without ureteral reimplantation can be considered, as the reflux tends to resolve with reduction of intravesical pressure.

In cases where there is ureteral dilatation in the absence of reflux, a very low-pressure reservoir must be constructed so that adynamic ureters can propel the urine into the bladder. Although not well documented in the literature, clinical experience strongly suggests that dilated ureters with walls that do not coapt are not capable of generating a peristaltic wave of greater than 40 cmH$_2$O. Thus, dilated ureters are likely to require very low intravesical pressures, well below 40 cmH$_2$O, for proper efflux of urine into the bladder.

Preoperative assessment of native bladder wall dynamics can be extremely difficult in patients who have a neuropathic bladder with an open bladder neck and low outlet resistance. In these patients who leak from an empty bladder, cyclical filling and distension of the bladder do not occur. The bladder has not been stretched under physiologic conditions. When performing preoperative urodynamics in these patients, a balloon catheter can be snugged down into the bladder neck to prevent leakage and bladder capacity, and compliance can be evaluated. This technique has been reported to be a good predictor of the need for future augmentation (de Badiola et al., 1992). However, Kronner et al. (1988a) demonstrated that preoperative urodynamics in such patients do not necessarily correlate well with eventual bladder outcome. They concluded that preoperative assessment of bladder capacity and compliance could not reliably predict which patients would eventually require enterocystoplasty after outlet resistance had been increased. Since preoperative urodynamics do not appear to be accurate in patients with an open bladder neck, the decision to perform an enterocystoplasty in conjunction with a bladder neck procedure should be based on preoperative discussions regarding the risks and benefits of immediate versus delayed enterocystoplasty.

Previous urinary diversion

As with patients with low outlet resistance, those with a defunctionalized bladder secondary to previous urinary diversion who are being considered for undiversion or transplantation are also difficult to assess preoperatively with regard to the need for bladder augmentation. In patients with a vesicostomy, urodynamics can be performed by occluding the vesicostomy with the balloon from the urodynamic catheter. For the same reasons previously described for patients with a poor outlet, interpretation of these urodynamic findings and assessment of their significance may be difficult. In posterior urethral valve (PUV) patients who have previously had

urinary diversion and subsequently undergo renal transplantation, there are good data showing that the native bladders re-expand and regain function irrespective of preoperative urodynamic findings (Firlit, 1976; MacGregor et al., 1986; Serrano et al., 1996). Currently, there are few data on outcomes in patients with neuropathic bladders associated with spina bifida after primary closure or undiversion without enterocystoplasty.

In the defunctionalized bladder not associated with spina bifida, some authors feel that bladder cycling may help to determine whether a bladder is adequate for closure without augmentation (MacGregor et al., 1986; Serrano et al., 1996). A gastrotomy button placed in the vesicostomy to facilitate bladder cycling can be used in these patients (de Badiola et al., 1996). The authors' experience has been that preoperative bladder cycling can be helpful in some patients, at least in increasing bladder capacity. However, urodynamic results remain difficult to interpret in many. In general, we favor undiversion without augmentation when there is doubt as to whether augmentation will be required. Secondary enterocystoplasty can always be performed in patients in whom the bladder does not eventually attain adequate bladder compliance and capacity following undiversion or transplantation. It should be emphasized that this approach is only recommended for patients with a defunctionalized bladder not associated with spina bifida, since such patients usually do poorly following vesicostomy closure. Reliable follow-up also needs to be assured in all patients following undiversion.

Bowel function

A thorough evaluation of bowel function, including a history of constipation or diarrhea, must be carried out prior to enterocystoplasty. Postoperative bowel dysfunction can occur in up to 50% of patients who have undergone enterocystoplasty (N'Dow et al., 1998). In addition, King (1987) found that removal of the ileocecal segment in children with spina bifida causes severe diarrhea in approximately 10% of patients. Therefore, before undertaking urinary reconstruction, discussion with the patient and family should include potential gastrointestinal complications. The type of augmentation should be chosen with these potential complications in mind.

Ability to catheterize

Since most patients who undergo enterocystoplasty will not be able to void completely and will require lifelong intermittent catheterization, one should consider the formation of a catheterizable stoma at the time of the augmentation. This is especially important in patients who are sensate or are in wheelchairs. Clinical experience has shown that when both the native urethra and a catheterizable stoma are present, the majority of patients will choose to use the catheterizable stoma. In addition, assessment of the physical and mental capacities of the patient and family must be undertaken to make sure that they will be able to perform intermittent catheterization on a regular schedule.

Families want to believe that their child will become continent after enterocystoplasty and that the kidneys will be protected. However, the amount of time and effort that will be required is often not appreciated preoperatively. Therefore, all must understand the risks and benefits of enterocystoplasty prior to surgery and the lifelong commitment to a relatively rigorous schedule of intermittent catheterization. Since there are many potential problems associated with failure to catheterize, including spontaneous bladder rupture and death, urinary reconstruction should be deferred until the patient has the physical and mental maturity needed to care for him or herself.

Intestinocystoplasty

Small bowel

Currently, ileum is the most commonly used bowel segment for enterocystoplasty. The abundant supply of small bowel, easy workability, mobility, reliable blood supply, and compliance of the reconfigured ileum have led most reconstructive surgeons to choose ileum over other bowel segments. Although the jejunum can be used for urinary reconstruction, the high incidence of metabolic complications (hyponatremic, hypochloremic, and hyperkalemic acidosis) associated with use of this segment make it less desirable and thus it is rarely used. The major contraindications to the use of ileum are a history of short gut syndrome, inflammatory bowel disease, pelvic and/or abdominal radiation and significant renal insufficiency. Under these conditions alternative segments such as stomach are more appropriate.

Anatomy and physiology

The proximal two-fifths of the small bowel proper is jejunum and the distal three-fifths is ileum. The coils of mid-ileum usually lie in the pelvis, while the terminal 30 cm of ileum, the most commonly used portion for enterocystoplasty, usually rise out of the pelvis to lie in close relationship to the cecum and the ascending colon.

The mesentery of the small bowel attaches to the posterior abdominal wall. The 'root' of the small bowel mesentery runs obliquely across the abdomen. As the root of the mesentery runs obliquely from left to right, it crosses, in order, the abdominal aorta, the vertebral column, and the third portion of the duodenum. The mid-portion of the small bowel has the longest mesentery, whereas the segments of the small bowel closest to the cecum and the duodenojejunal flexure have the shortest. Therefore, in patients in whom the mesentery is short, a segment of ileum 30 cm or more above the ileocecal valve will be the most mobile and will reach the furthest into the pelvis.

The arterial supply to the entire small bowel is derived from the superior mesenteric artery (Fig. 16.1). There are usually 12–16 branches of the superior mesenteric artery running to the jejunum and ileum and entering the small bowel at its mesenteric border. The ileocolic artery is the most distal segment of this vessel. It is found in the right lower abdominal quadrant, where it gives off branches that supply the terminal ileum, the cecum and appendix, and the proximal ascending colon. Venous drainage of the

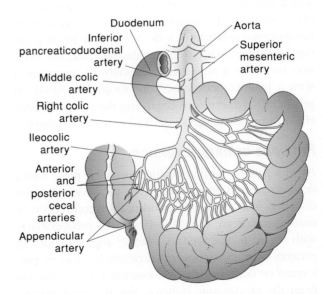

Figure 16.1 Arterial blood supply to the small intestine. The portion of the ileum with the longest mesentary that is commonly used for intestinocystoplasty is around 20–30 cm proximal to the ileocecal valve. (Adapted from Lindner, 1989, with permission.)

small bowel occurs through multiple mesenteric channels that coalesce to form the superior mesenteric vein. It is this abundant and redundant blood supply that makes the use of different segments of ileum available for urinary reconstruction.

The small intestine is innervated from the autonomic plexuses grouped around the 'take-off' of the superior mesenteric artery from the aorta. These plexuses include preganglionic parasympathetic nerves from the vagus as well as postganglionic sympathetic fibers from the celiac plexus. The submucosa of the small intestine contains the nerve plexus of Meissner. Between the longitudinal and circular muscle of the small bowel is the intramuscular myenteric (Auerbach's) plexus, consisting of non-myelinated nerve fiber plus numerous ganglion cells.

The bowel wall is made up of an outer serosal coat, two layers of muscle (outer longitudinal smooth muscle and inner circular smooth muscle), a submucosal layer, and a mucous membrane composed of a single layer of columnar epithelial cells. Since the muscle and epithelial layers are relatively thin, the plane between these layers is difficult to establish surgically, therefore tunneling procedures for ureters and catheterizable stomas may be quite difficult in small bowel.

The physiology of the small and large intestine involves an intricate balance of water and electrolyte shifts. The major mechanisms of intestinal transport of water and electrolytes are illustrated in Figure 16.2. Water and electrolyte movement varies throughout the length of the bowel. These changes can be accounted for by both structural and functional differences between the small and large bowel. The major structural difference between the small and large bowel involves the 'tight' junctions that join the epithelial cells (Fig. 16.2). These tight junctions have characteristic permeabilities and ionic conductance that form the basis for paracellular ion and water movement (Powell, 1987). Because such junctions are tightest in the colon and more permeable or leaky in the proximal small bowel, paracellular movement may account for a significant portion of water and electrolyte transport in the small bowel, and not play as an important role in the colon.

Although paracellular movement accounts for some of the bidirectional water and electrolyte transport, most of these shifts are thought to occur via transcellular mechanisms that occur through the intestinal absorptive cell. A characteristic example of the intestinal absorptive mechanism is the Na^+/K^+-

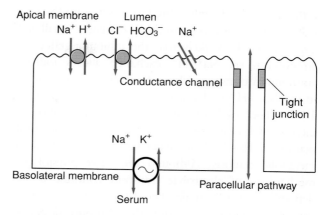

Figure 16.2 Intestinal transport mechanisms. Sodium absorption in both the small and large bowel is transcellular and occurs via a Na^+–H^+ exchanger on the apical membrane and a Na^+–K^+ pump on the basolateral membrane. The colon has an additional pathway of entry for Na^+ via conductance channels which allows for non-coupled sodium absorption. Chloride and bicarbonate transport is coupled which is pertinent in the development of metabolic acidosis following intestinocystoplasty. Water and electrolyte movement also occurs via paracellular pathways associated with tight junctions between the cells. Paracellular movement occurs more in the ileum than in the colon owing to leakier tight junctions. (Adapted from Lindner, 1989, with permission.)

ATPase enzyme, which is located on the basolateral membrane. This pump maintains low intracellular sodium concentrations and thus creates an electrochemical gradient for sodium absorption as well as passive transport of other electrolytes and water.

Sodium entry in the small bowel is accomplished by way of an Na^+–H^+ countertransport system in the apical membrane. In addition, a significant portion of the sodium entry into the colon also occurs via electrogenic Na^+ conductance channels that allow for non-coupled sodium absorption. The presence of this channel in the colon probably accounts for its ability to transport Na^+ and water against large gradients.

Chloride is absorbed throughout the entire small and large bowel. Bicarbonate is absorbed in large quantities in the jejunum but secreted in the ileum and colon. Chloride absorption in exchange for HCO_3^- secretion plays a large role in the transport of these electrolytes in the ileum and colon. Na^+–H^+ exchange and Cl^-–HCO_3^- exchange occur together. The net result is the electroneutral absorption of Na^+ and Cl^-.

Metabolic acidosis may develop whenever urine is in contact with ileal or colonic mucosa. The mechanism by which this hyperchloremic metabolic acidosis occurs is thought to be directly related to ammonium (NH_4^+) reabsorption that can occur along the entire small and large bowel. It is likely that the inhibitory effect of ammonium on Na^+–H^+ exchange allows ionized ammonium transport where it substitutes for sodium in the Na^+–H^+ exchanger (Stampfer and McDougal, 1997). The result of this ammonium absorption is increased Cl^- absorption in order to maintain electrical neutrality. This leads to hyperchloremia and eventual metabolic acidosis. Although the exact physiologic mechanisms of electrolyte transport continue to be defined, it must be remembered that the major function of the intestine, regarding this transport, does not change when intestine is used for urinary reconstruction. Continued fluid and electrolyte fluxes account for the majority of the physiologic problems associated with the use of intestine in the urinary tract.

Advantages and disadvantages

Ileum is the most commonly used bowel segment for bladder augmentation. The advantages that are obtained with use of ileum are: (1) large quantity available; (2) ease in handling and reconfiguration; (3) predictable and abundant blood supply; (4) most compliant segment of bowel; (5) moderate mucus production compared to colon; (6) less severe metabolic complications than colon or stomach; and (7) fewer gastrointestinal complications than cecum.

The disadvantages in using ileum include: (1) occasional short mesentery that cannot reach the pelvis; (2) possible development of diarrhea and vitamin B_{12} deficiency when the most distal ileum is used; (3) difficulty with creation of submucosal tunnels; and (4) metabolic acidosis; as well as (5) bowel obstruction; (6) stone formation; (7) mucus production; (8) urinary tract infections (UTIs); and (9) tumor formation, all of which are risks with large bowel segments as well.

Large bowel

Through the early 1980s, the cecum and sigmoid colon were more commonly used than ileum for enterocystoplasty. However, because of the shorter mesenteries, increased mucus production, and difficulty with configuration associated with large bowel, ileum has come to be the preferred segment of bowel for enterocystoplasty for most surgeons. Nevertheless, detubularized large bowel is still used for simple bladder augmentation in select patients.

Anatomy and physiology

Anatomically, the large bowel can be divided into five sections: (1) the cecum and vermiform appendix; (2) the ascending colon and the hepatic flexure; (3) the transverse colon and mesocolon; (4) the splenic flexure and descending colon; and (5) the sigmoid colon.

The colon is 1.4–1.7 m in length. Its diameter is greatest on the right side and gradually decreases as it approaches the sigmoid colon. The diameter of the sigmoid colon is often no wider than a loop of terminal ileum. The large bowel is made up of five distinct layers: serosa, muscularis externa, submucosa, muscularis mucosa, and mucosa. The outer serosal coat is a component of the peritoneum and normally completely covers the cecum, the appendix, and the transverse and sigmoid colon segments. The muscularis externa of the large bowel is composed of a complete inner circular and incomplete outer longitudinal layer of smooth muscle. The submucosa is composed of areolar tissue and lies between the muscularis externa and the muscularis mucosa. This layer contains the blood and lymphatic vessels supplying the bowel and is also the most important layer when developing an anastomosic site. The thin muscularis mucosa is made up of circular and longitudinal smooth muscle. The mucosa is composed of a layer of simple columnar epithelium containing goblet cells and is smooth and devoid of villi.

The muscle layers of the colon are notably different from those of the stomach, small intestine, and rectum. Longitudinal smooth muscle covers the large bowel incompletely. The longitudinal fibers are arranged in three narrow but distinct bands called teniae coli. The teniae of the cecum and ascending colon have a constant position relative to the bowel circumference. One band lies on the ventral surface of the colon while the other two lie medial and lateral to the ventral band. The teniae of the transverse colon are less constant in position. Near the rectosigmoid junction the teniae become quite indistinct. The unique anatomy of the teniae facilitates reimplantation of ureters, appendix, and catheterizable stomas to create a reliable flap-valve continence mechanism. The deep circular muscular coat of the colon wall is visible between the longitudinal muscle fibers of the teniae. Contractions of the colon produce a pouching or saculations of the bowel between the teniae. These pouchings, or haustra, are randomly distributed and are easily noted on gross examination and visible on X-ray studies.

Cecum and vermiform appendix

The cecum measures approximately 6 cm in length and lies caudal to the entrance of the ileum into the colon. It is the thinnest portion of the colon. The cecum is normally mobile. In over 90% of individuals it is completely covered with peritoneum and possesses no mesentery. In some patients, such as children with spina bifida and ventroperitoneal shunts, the cecum can become fused with the posterior abdominal wall. This in turn causes foreshortening of the peritoneal attachments, resulting in the cecum becoming more superiorly located in the right colic gutter (Hedican *et al.*, 1999).

The terminal 14 cm of ileum, the cecum, appendix, and the ascending colon are supplied by the ileocolic artery, which is the terminal segment of the superior mesenteric artery. The ileocolic artery ends just proximal to the ileocecal junction and then divides into four major branches. The most superior branch, the colic artery, passes to the ascending colon, anastomosing with the descending branches of the right colic artery initiating the right colic portion of the marginal artery of Drummond or mesenteric arcade (Fig. 16.3.).

The three bands of teniae coli originate at the base of the appendix. The appendix varies in length from 2 to 20 cm with an average of 9 cm. In the majority of patients, the appendix is held in position by the posterior inferior ileocecal fold. In about 5% of patients, the mesentery of the appendix runs directly from the posterior peritoneum in the region of the ileocecal junction onto the midportion of the appendix, at which point it is usually joined by the appendicular artery, a branch of the ileocolic artery. The appendicular artery arises either as a branch of the posterior cecal artery or directly from the main ileocolic trunk. It may also arise from the ileal branch of the ileocolic artery. Regardless of its site of origin the appendicular artery will usually pass dorsal to the most distal segment of the terminal ileum before it enters the mesoappendix.

Ascending colon and transverse colon

The ascending colon occupies most of the right side of the abdominal cavity and extends from the cecum to the hepatic flexure. The blood supply to the ascending colon comes from the colic branches of the

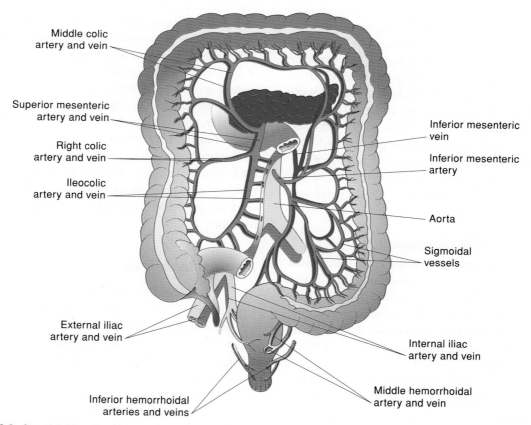

Figure 16.3 Arterial blood supply to the large bowel. Preservation of the marginal artery is extremely important when isolating portions of colon for intestinocystoplasty. (Adapted from Lindner, 1989, with permission.)

ileocolic artery, the right colic artery, and the right branches of the middle colic artery. The right colic artery is the most variable vessel in the colon and is absent in 5–7% of people. The transverse colon receives blood from the left colic artery; however, the major supplier is the middle colic artery which is a more direct branch of the superior mesenteric artery.

Sigmoid colon

The sigmoid colon frequently has an S-shape, and is divided into a fixed superior and a mobile inferior portion. The fixed portion of the sigmoid colon begins at the level of the iliac crest. The mobile portion of the sigmoid colon begins at the medial border of the left psoas major muscle and ends where it joins the rectum. The length, location of loops, degree of redundancy, relationship to other structures, and mobility of the sigmoid colon are markedly variable. It is very common in the spina bifida population to encontour sigmoid colon so enlarged and redundant that the mobile portion crosses the midline and lies anterior to the cecum.

The inferior mesenteric artery is the major vessel to the left transverse colon, the splenic flexure, the left colon, the sigmoid colon, and the rectum. The left colic artery is the first branch of the inferior mesenteric artery and runs in the direction of the superior half of the descending colon. The ascending branch of the left colic artery runs superiorly and parallel with the left colon contributing to the marginal artery of Drummond. The descending branch of the left colic artery supplies the fixed segment of the sigmoid. The sigmoid arteries, which are second branches of the inferior mesenteric, supply the lower portion of the descending colon, the sigmoid colon, and a small segment of the upper rectum.

Advantages and disadvantages

The ileocecal segment and cecum have been used extensively in reconstructive urology. One major advantage of these segments is utilization of the portion of bowel that has the largest diameter resulting in a capacious and compliant reservoir that often fits the bladder base neatly. It has a well-defined blood supply that is reliable. The modified ileocecal valve can also be used as an antireflux or continence mechanism.

The major disadvantage in using the ileocecal segment is related to the loss of the ileocecal valve in the intestine. Patients with neurologic disorders or short gut may have an increased incidence of diarrhea and difficulty with fecal continence following removal of this segment from the intestinal tract. In addition, it is not available in the cloacal exstrophy population who have little or no hindgut. The ileocecal segment also reabsorbs urinary wastes, which may result in hyperchloremic acidosis. Finally, cecum usually produces more mucus than the ileum, which can lead to increased infections and stone formation.

The major advantage in using sigmoid colon is the redundancy that is present, especially in the spina bifida population. The mobile portion of the sigmoid is so redundant in such children that it often lies in the right lower quadrant. It can be easily opened and reconfigured into a U-shape to increase compliance. The thicker muscle can be used to create an antireflux ureteral anastomosis as well as for placement of a tunneled continent catheterizable stoma such as the appendix.

The major disadvantage in using the sigmoid colon is the reduced ability to create a large-capacity, compliant reservoir. The diameter of the sigmoid may be only as large as the ileum. In this circumstance, a segment of colon at least 20–28 cm is required to create an adequately sized reservoir. This amount of sigmoid colon can occasionally be difficult to obtain in the non-spina bifida population. Mucus production from the sigmoid is increased compared with small bowel. This may increase the potential for the development of UTI and bladder stones. In the Indiana series the highest spontaneous perforation rate occurred among those with sigmoid cystoplasties (Rink et al., 1995). However, this has not been observed in other large series. Finally, hyperchloremic acidosis is more common when the sigmoid colon is used, compared with other bowel segments. Frequently, patients will need lifelong alkalizing agents, but this is also true after cecocystoplasty or ileocystoplasty (Di Benedetto and Monfort, 1997).

Surgical technique

The goals of bladder augmentation are to provide a large-capacity, low-pressure urinary reservoir. Hinman (1988) and Koff (1988), in particular, have documented the importance of detubularization and reconfiguration of the small and large bowel to facilitate maximum gains in capacity and compliance. Detubularization of bowel segments prevents synchronous contractions of the circular muscle of the gut. Since the radius of the reservoir is directly related to the volume, a greater radius in the augmented blad-

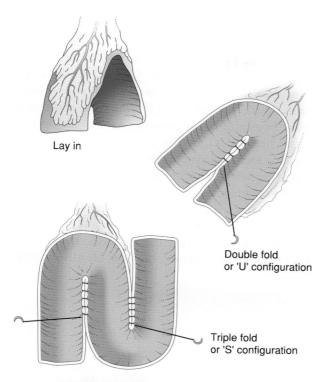

Figure 16.4 The detubularized ileum can be reconfigured in numerous ways. Each additional fold increases the potential radius of the augmented bladder. (Adapted from Rink and Adams, 1988, with permission of W.B. Saunders.)

der translates into a larger low-pressure reservoir. The diameter of the reconfigured bowel segment increases with the number of folds that are incorporated during the reconfiguration (Fig. 16.4). Regardless of the bowel segment used for augmentation, detubularization and reconfiguration should always be employed.

Ileocystoplasty

Enterocystoplasty is very reliable in lowering storage pressures and expanding the capacity of the non-compliant bladder. Ureteral implantations and procedures to increase outlet resistance can safely be undertaken at the same time. However, not every augmentation is completely successful. This may be related to the bladder having a great tendency to re-form itself, turning the augmentation into a diverticulum with a relatively small opening. To prevent this, the bladder should be bivalved ('clamshelled') from the bladder neck ventrally to the trigone posteriorly. Alternatively, when the bladder is small and thick walled, the 'star' modification can be performed (Keating *et al.*, 1996) (Fig. 16.5). The star procedure involves open-

ing the bladder in the sagittal plane. A second incision is then made in the coronal plane. If ureteral reimplantation or bladder neck reconstruction is being performed, the second incision is not made until after these procedures are completed. The authors will also occasionally employ an upside-down U-shaped or a Boari flap modification for the initial bladder opening when a catheterizable stoma is being positioned at the umbilicus. In severely diseased bladders from tuberculosis, schistosomiasis, interstitial cystitis, and rarely bladder exstrophy, supratrigonal bladder excision is sometimes necessary, as in neuropathic bladders when the walls are very thick. Whatever type of bladder opening is used, the goal is the same: to provide a wide bladder plate to which the bowel segment can be sewn, thus preventing a narrow anastomosis or hourglass deformity that might result in the augmentation becoming a diverticulum.

When using ileum for enterocystoplasty, the segment chosen should be at least 15 cm proximal to the ileocecal valve to prevent vitamin B_{12} malabsorption, diarrhea due to malabsorption of bile salts, and potential injury to the blood supply to the cecum. Guidelines on the length of ileum required to obtain the appropriate size and shape of the augmentation vary (Koff, 1988; Rink and Mitchell, 1990). Most commonly, an ileal segment between 20 and 35 cm in length is used. However, a slightly longer segment may be required in an older child or an individual with a severely diseased and contracted bladder.

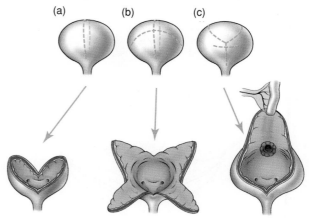

Figure 16.5 The native bladder can be opened in several ways: (*a*) bivalved in a 'clam'-like fashion with full extension of the incision into the bladder neck to prevent an hourglass deformation of the augmented bladder; (*b*) the 'star' modification; (*c*) a 'U' incision to create a flap of bladder that can be used for tunneling when creating a continent catheterizable stoma to the umbilicus.

Prior to harvesting the ileal segment, it is important to ensure the mesentery reaches well down into the pelvis. Extensive mobilization of the mesentery is sometimes required if it is foreshortened. This is most common in the spina bifida population, often secondary to spinal abnormalities and the intraperitoneal adhesions that occur from the ventriculoperitoneal shunt. Once the appropriate bowel segment has been selected, the bowel is divided between straight clamps. The authors prefer to perform a single-layer hand-sewn ileoileostomy. A two-layer hand-sewn or a stapled anastomosis can also be used. Closure of the mesenteric window with interrupted permanent sutures then completes the anastomosis. The isolated ileal segment is detubularized along its antimesenteric border after thorough intraluminal irrigation with normal saline. The ileal segment is then reconfigured into a U, S, or W (Fig. 16.6).

After opening the native bladder as described above, the reconfigured bowel segment is anastomosed to the bladder with a full-thickness absorbable suture beginning at the posterior apex of the opened native bladder. Once the posterior aspect of the running, locking anastomosis has been completed, a second running, locking suture beginning at the bladder neck apex is begun and carried along the lateral aspect to meet the previous suture. Before final closure of the anastomosis, a suprapubic tube is brought out through the native bladder wall. After completion of the augmentation, the bladder is inflat-

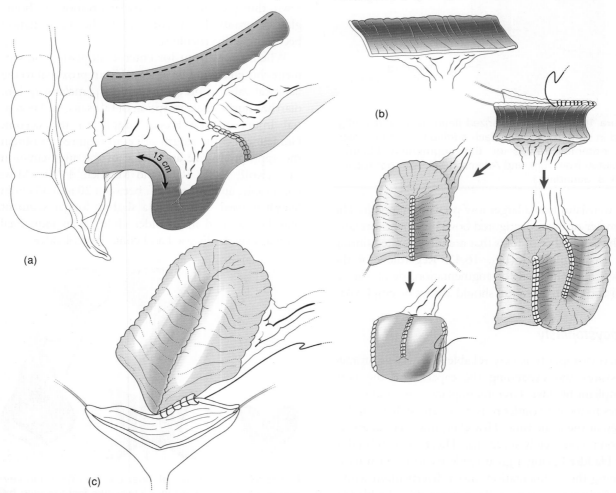

Figure 16.6 Ileocystoplasty. (*a*) A dependent portion of the ileum that is 20–30 cm long and a minimum of 15 cm proximal to the ileocecal valve is isolated and detubularized. Bowel continuity is reestablished with an end-to-end ileoileostomy. (*b*) Depending on the size of the ileal segment, it can be reconfigured and folded in several ways including the U, S, and W (not illustrated) configurations. In addition, the edges of the reconfigured bowel can be sewn together to create a cup patch. (*c*) The anastomosis of the reconfigured bowel to the native bladder begins in the posterior apex of the opened bladder. (Adapted from Rink and Adams, 1988, with permission of W.B. Saunders.)

ed and a water-tight anastomosis confirmed by irrigation. A penrose or closed suction drain is usually left in place along the posterior and anterior aspects of the bladder. The bowel is then examined to confirm its integrity and the abdomen is closed in an anatomic fashion using heavy, running, absorbable sutures.

Ileocecocystoplasty and cecocystoplasty

The ileocecal segment and cecum have frequently been used for augmentation cystoplasty. The cecum alone is rarely used. Simple detubularization and reconfiguration can be performed. The terminal ileum can be detubularized and incorporated into the cecal segment to increase total volume (Fig. 16.7). Continuity of the bowel is reestablished with an end-to-side ileocolostomy. The reconfigured ileocecal segment is then anastomosed to the bivalved bladder with a single or double layer of running, locking, absorbable suture. Alternatively, the terminal ileum can be used for ureteral replacement when the ureters are short or the ileum can be tapered and used as a continent catheterizable stoma.

Sigmoid cystoplasty

The sigmoid colon easily reaches the bladder and can be used for augmentation cystoplasty. It is especially valuable when reimplantation of ureters or a catheterizable stoma is not possible in the native bladder because the sigmoid musculature can easily be separated from the muscosa facilitating tunneling. Twenty cm of sigmoid is usually sufficient to achieve an adequate capacity after the segment is reconfigured. It is important to detubularize the sigmoid in order to prevent high-pressure

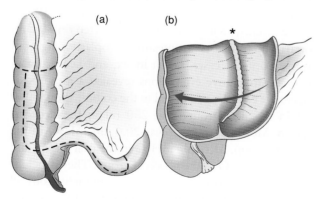

Figure 16.7 Ileocecocystoplasty: the ileum and cecum are isolated as a single unit (*a*) and reconfigured to form a 'cup' for augmentation (*b*). * = suture line between ileum and cecum. (Adapted from Rink and Adams, 1988, with permission of W.B. Saunders.)

coordinated contractions. Several techniques of sigmoid reconfiguration have been described (Fig. 16.8). The authors prefer the U or S configuration because of simplicity and the possibility of significant contractile activity that may result from the method described by Mitchell (Rink, 1999) (Fig. 16.8c). When the sigmoid segment has been isolated, colon continuity is re-established with a single-layer, hand-sewn, end-to-end colocolostomy. The reconfigured sigmoid segment is then anastomosed to the native bladder in a similar fashion as described for ileum.

Postoperative care

Following enterocystoplasty, parenteral antibiotics are continued for 48 hours unless the intraoperative urine culture is positive. Then, a full 7 days of culture-sensitive coverage is used. A nasogastric tube is left in place until bowel function returns. Urinary drainage is maintained through the suprapubic tube and a secondary catheter through either the native urethra or the appendicovesicostomy (when performed). Diligent observation is needed during the immediate postoperative period to ensure that obstruction of the catheters does not occur secondary to blood clots or mucus. Daily bladder irrigations are important to decrease mucus build-up in the bladder, which can lead to infection, stone formation, and inefficient emptying. Bladder irrigations can begin immediately after surgery with 30 ml three times a day. This is increased to 60 ml twice a day after discharge. Both the suprapubic tube and secondary catheter are left to gravity drainage for 2–3 weeks. The suprapubic tube is then plugged and the patient begins intermittent catheterization. Before this, a cystogram can be performed to ensure adequate healing and the absence of extravasation; however, it is not absolutely necessary. Adequate emptying of the bladder with catheterization can be confirmed by checking residual urine via the indwelling suprapubic tube. Once the patient demonstrates proficiency at performing intermittent catheterization, the suprapubic tube is removed. Daily irrigations to clear the bladder of mucus are then recommended. Patients are told to catheterize every 2–3 hours during the daytime and once at night for the next few weeks. The time interval between catheterizations is gradually lengthened depending on the compliance of the augmented bladder and the gradually increasing storage volumes. In general, adequate stretching of the augmented bladder occurs within 6 months so that most patients

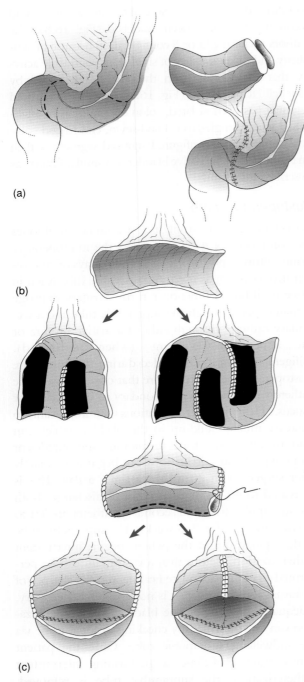

Figure 16.8 Sigmoid cystoplasty. (*a*) A portion of sigmoid colon is isolated. (*b*) The sigmoid can then be reconfigured in a similar fashion as is performed for ileocystoplasty with detubularization and folding back on itself. (*c*) Alternatively, the colonic segment can be closed at both ends, opened along the antimesenteric border and then anastomosed to the bladder. This latter method is less optimal owing to the persistence of high intraluminal pressures following augmentation. (Adapted from Rink and Adams, 1988, with permission of W.B. Saunders.)

need only catheterize approximately four to six times during the day to stay dry and maintain safe filling pressures. If a patient is going to attempt spontaneous voiding, one should wait until at least 3 months after surgery and then follow postvoid residuals to ensure adequate emptying. Radiographic imaging of the augmented bladder and the upper urinary tract is performed approximately 3 months postoperatively.

Results of ileocystoplasty and colocystoplasty

Bladder capacity and compliance

The most common preoperative urodynamic finding in the pediatric patient with a neuropathic bladder in need of bladder augmentation is a small-capacity, poorly compliant bladder with or without evidence of hyperreflexia and bladder instability. Both small and large bowel segments, when detubularized and reconfigured, have been found to provide adequately compliant tissue for enterocystoplasty that ameliorates or eliminates these adverse characteristics (Goldwasser *et al.*, 1987). Flood *et al.* (1995) reported on 22 augmentation cystoplasties performed over a period of 8 years. Mean age at surgery was 37 years, with a range of 2–82 years. The major indication for augmentation cystoplasty was reduced bladder compliance. A detubularized ileal augmentation was performed in 67% of the patients, 30% had a detubularized ileocecocystoplasty, and the remainder had detubularized sigmoid augmentation. Mean follow-up was 37 months. Bladder capacities increased from a preoperative mean of 108 ml to 438 ml postoperatively. Excellent or improved results by all parameters were achieved in 95% of these patients (Flood *et al.*, 1995). More recently, Kilic *et al.* (1999) reported on 30 children who underwent intestinocystoplasty. Sigmoid was used in 11 cases, ileum in six, and ileocecum in two. Postoperative evaluations revealed a mean postoperative capacity of 237 ml in the colonic group, 240 ml in the ileal group, and 250 ml in the ileocecal group. Mean compliance was 20.6 ml/cmH$_2$O in the colonic group, 21.6 ml/cmH$_2$O in the ileal group, and 25.5 ml/cmH$_2$O in the ileocecal group. They concluded that ileal, ileocecal, and colonic augmentations all provided high-volume reservoirs of similar compliance.

It is apparent that all segments of intestine, when appropriately reconfigured, can adequately increase the capacity of the native bladder. However, enterocystoplasty does not guarantee that the bladder will be free of hyperreflexia. Robertson *et al.* (1991) reported the persistence of hyperreflexia in 23% of patients after enterocystoplasty and documented regular phasic contractions in 77% of the augmented bladders despite bowel detubularization. It should be mentioned that in a majority of the patients in this series an ileocecal segment was used. Recently, Pope *et al.* (1998) reported on 19 of 323 patients who had undergone primary enterocystoplasty but required a secondary augmentation owing to the persistence of high pressures. Twelve of the 19 patients had had colocystoplasties (14% of the total colocystoplasties), four had gastrocystoplasties (10% of the total gastrocystoplasties), and two had undergone ileocystoplasty. Cecum was used in one (1%). It is apparent in this large series that colocystoplasties are more likely to allow high storage pressures to persist. However, it must be noted that not all of the colocystoplasties were completely detubularized but instead reconfigured after the ends were closed with the colon opened along the antimesenteric border. Given this, it is difficult in this series to compare colon to ileum that was reconfigured into an S or W shape. Nevertheless, these studies emphasize the importance of careful functional and urodynamic follow-up in patients after enterocystoplasty, since some will require anticholinergics or secondary augmentation due to failure of the original procedure to improve bladder capacity and compliance adequately.

In summary, it appears that both small and large bowel, when detubularized, can be used for cystoplasty to provide a compliant and large-capacity reservoir. However, the large bowel may retain increased contractile activity despite detubularization (Goldwasser *et al.*, 1987; Rink *et al.*, 1995). It appears that detubularized ileum has less energetic phasic contractions than colon and therefore has potentially less risk for persistent high storage pressures (Pope *et al.*, 1998). Given these advantages of ileum over colon, it is the authors' preference to use ileum whenever possible when performing simple enterocystoplasty.

Metabolic issues

Electrolytes

The major function of intact small and large bowel is to absorb food, fluid, and electrolytes. When urine is stored in the bowel for prolonged periods there is increased absorption of urinary solutes, which increases the risk of metabolic derangement. Koch and McDougal (1985) hypothesized that ammonium reabsorption plays a key role in the development of hyperchloremic metabolic acidosis in patients following intestinocystoplasty. In support of this hypothesis, Stampfer and McDougal (1997) demonstrated in a rat model that ammonium inhibits the sodium/hydrogen exchanger, resulting in ionized ammonium transport where it substitutes for sodium in the exchanger. This then leads to the increased absorption of chloride to maintain electrolyte neutrality, resulting in the development of hyperchloremic metabolic acidosis. In patients with normal renal function, serum electrolytes are usually unaffected by enterocystoplasty (Mitchell and Piser, 1987; Salomon *et al.*, 1997; Kockum *et al.*, 1999). However, in patients with impaired renal function metabolic acidosis can be profound. Careful preoperative evaluation and judicious use of bowel is recommended in patients with chronic renal insufficiency (Stampfer *et al.*, 1997). A gastric segment or cutaneous diversion may be safer. Owing to the electrolyte problems that can often develop in patients with significant renal insufficiency, the authors recommend gastrocystoplasty rather than conventional enterocystoplasty in this patient population.

Bone growth

Impaired bone growth and demineralization are major concerns related to prolonged acidosis. Demineralization occurs secondary to the increased excretion of titratable acid (bony buffers). Hochstetler *et al.* (1997) demonstrated in a rat model that animals with ileocystoplasty, when given an acid challenge, developed bone demineralization and decreased bone growth that can be corrected with bicarbonate therapy. Mundy and Nurse (1992) reported an average of 20% reduction in growth potential in three of six children who had colocystoplasties. However, no decrease in growth potential was noted in 10 children who had ileocystoplasties. They concluded that bone growth impairment after colocystoplasty was more likely than after ileocystoplasty. Recently, however, two reports demonstrated no impairment of bone growth or demineralization in children and adults after urinary reconstruction with various bowel segments (Stein *et al.*, 1998; Kockum *et al.*, 1999). Further longitudinal studies will be required to clarify this issue. Therefore, until such studies are available, close observation for the development of acidosis and the treatment of any electrolyte abnormalities following intestinocystoplasty with bicarbonate therapy is recommended.

Bowel dysfunction

Bowel dysfunction is known to occur occasionally after enterocystoplasty. Diarrhea can develop after resection of large segments of ileum, removal of the ileocecal valve, and extensive colonic resections. The incidence of bowel dysfunction following enterocystoplasty in all patients, including adults, has been reported to be between 10 and 54% (Singh and Thomas, 1997; N'Dow et al., 1998; Herschorn and Hewitt, 1998). In the spina bifida population, the incidence is approximately 20%. Since the overall incidence of bowel problems in children with spina bifida is further increased when the ileocecal valve is removed, one should try to avoid the use of ileocecal segments for augmentation in this patient population. Osmotic diarrhea has been theorized to occur after removal of the ileocecal valve, which results in a decreased transit time within the intestine (King et al., 1987). Careful preoperative screening of patients with spina bifida with regard to their bowel habits is extremely important.

The diarrhea that develops postoperatively can be osmotic or secretory in nature. Secretory diarrhea is thought to occur because of decreased resorption of bile salts and subsequent fat malabsorption resulting in steatorrhea. Barrington et al. (1995) reported on 14 patients who developed bowel difficulties after enterocystoplasty. They showed a direct correlation in many of these patients between their diarrhea and interruption of the enterohepatic circulation of bile acids. They also found that these patients can be identified by using bowel frequency charts and can be treated with anion-exchange resins.

Vitamin B$_{12}$ deficiency

Concerns regarding the development of vitamin B$_{12}$ deficiency following small bowel resection or the use of small bowel for urinary reconstruction are well documented. The distal ileum is the major site of vitamin B$_{12}$ absorption. It has previously been reported that up to 35% of patients will develop vitamin B$_{12}$ deficiency following the construction of a Kock pouch, which uses about 80 cm of small bowel (Akerlund et al., 1989). Despite theoretical and legitimate concerns about the development of vitamin B$_{12}$ deficiency in children following ileocystoplasty, it has yet to be reported in the literature. Stein et al. (1998) reported on 51 children who had undergone such reconstructions, but no significant drop in vitamin B$_{12}$ levels was noted following surgery. From the available published data, it appears that the use of shorter segments of ileum, about 35 cm, as used for the Camey type 1 enterocystoplasty and conventional ileocystoplasty in children, does not place the patient at significant risk for vitamin B$_{12}$ deficiency, even in the long term (Salomon et al., 1997).

Despite the lack of evidence of any vitamin B$_{12}$ deficiencies developing in children undergoing enterocystoplasty, the authors recommend harvesting small bowel segments that are at least 15 cm away from the ileocecal valve. The B$_{12}$ receptor sites are clustered in the most terminal portion of the ileum. If large amounts of small bowel are required for reconstruction of the bladder, periodic vitamin B$_{12}$ levels should be obtained postoperatively. Alternatively, a vitamin B$_{12}$ injection can be given prophylactically 3 years after enterocystoplasty. There is no evidence that the use of sigmoid colon for augmentation places patients at risk for vitamin B$_{12}$ deficiency.

Mucus production and stone formation

Mucus production and bladder stone formation are both complications related to the use of the gastrointestinal tract for urinary reconstruction. All segments of bowel produce mucus. However, mucus production from the ileum is less than from the colon (Rink and Adams, 1998). This has been confirmed clinically by several authors (Hendren and Hendren, 1990; Rink et al., 1995). Mucus in the urinary tract is associated with an increased risk of infection (Bruce et al., 1984). Mucus production also increases during an acute infection resulting in poor bladder emptying, especially when small catheters are used to drain the bladder (Rink and Mitchell, 1990). Clinically, mucus production appears to decrease over time following ileocystoplasty. This is probably because of villus atrophy that occurs in the ileum. Colonic epithelium does not appear to undergo this type of change. Significant mucus production in colonic augmentations continues throughout the life of the patient.

The risk of stone formation after enterocystoplasty ranges between 7 and 52% (Blyth et al., 1992; Palmer et al., 1993; Brough et al., 1998; Kaefer et al., 1998) (Kronner et al., 1998b). The usual stone composition reported is magnesium ammonium phosphate (struvite), although several other stone compositions have been reported. Since the majority of stones is struvite in origin, it appears that chronic bacteriuria with urease-producing organisms may have a contributory role. However, it is also clear that the presence of mucus has an important role in the development of bladder stones following intestinocystoplasty. Mucus may serve as a biofilm that can harbor bacteria and promote further growth in a protected environment. Khoury *et al.* (1997) have also demonstrated that the mucus from stone formers has increased levels of calcium, phosphate, and magnesium, and an increase in the calcium to phosphate ratio, compared with non-stone formers. This increased calcium to phosphate ratio may be clinically important in predicting which patients are at risk for stone formation. Given these findings, it appears that mucus has strong lithogenic properties and is a nidus for stone formation. Daily irrigation of the augmented bladder to prevent excess mucus build-up is important in reducing the risk of stone formation in the augmented bladder. However, Brough *et al.* (1998) did not observe a decreased incidence of stone formation when they instituted a regular bladder washout program in children following intestinocystoplasty.

Palmer *et al.* (1993) identified an additional risk factor for the development of bladder stones in the augmented bladder. They noted the presence of hypocitraturia in some of their stone-forming patients. Treatment with oral potassium citrate returned urinary citrate levels to within normal values and no recurrent calculi were then seen.

Bladder calculi in the augmented bladder are amenable to both open surgery and endoscopic management (Blyth *et al.*, 1992; Palmer *et al.*, 1993; Palmer *et al.*, 1994; Docimo *et al.*, 1998; Kronner *et al.*, 1998b). Neither procedure appears to have a clear advantage at this time. An open procedure is usually simpler when the stones are large, although new energy sources for the endoscopic treatment of stones, such as the holmium laser, may enhance the ability to manage bladder stones non-invasively. Treatment of bladder calculi needs to be individualized. Factors that should influence the surgical approach include: number and size of calculi, previous bladder outlet procedure, availability of endoscopic equipment, availability of energy sources, and the surgeons experience with endoscopic techniques.

Infections

Bacteriuria following enterocystoplasty is the rule since these patients are being intermittently catheterized. If the bladder is not emptied completely, symptomatic UTI may result. It is not known whether one type of bowel segment is at greater risk for the development of UTIs than another. Hirst (1991) reported the presence of bacteriuria in 50% of sigmoid augmentations, whereas only 25% of ileocystoplasties had bacteriuria at any one time. In a series of 231 augmentation patients, Rink *et al.* (1995) reported a symptomatic UTI rate of 22.7% following ileocystoplasty, 17.3% following sigmoid cystoplasty, 12% following cecocystoplasty, and 8% following gastrocystoplasty. They reported an overall 14% incidence of febrile UTIs with no statistical difference in the incidence between the various bowel segments. It appears that all augmented bladders are at risk for infection.

Tumors

Many fear that there may be an increased risk of malignancy in bladders after enterocystoplasty, as is the case after conventional ureterosigmoidostomy. Adenocarcinoma is the predominant tumor that develops after ureterosigmoidostomy, found most frequently at the site of the ureteral orifice. The latency period for tumor formation in the ureterosigmoidostomy patients range between 3 and 53 years, with a mean of 26 years. It is estimated that there is a 7000-fold increase risk of developing adenocarcinoma following ureterosigmoidostomy. It is with great trepidation that we enter the new millennium with hundreds of children having received enterocystoplasties without knowing whether there is an increased risk for the development of cancer. Filmer and Spencer (1990) reported on 14 patients with tumor formation in the augmented bladder. Nine of these patients had ileocystoplasty and, colon was used in five. The exact etiology and pathogenesis of these tumors are unknown but they seem analogous to cancers occurring after uterosigmoidostomy. Nurse and Mundy (1989) studied 34 patients who had undergone augmentation cystoplasty or colonic substitution cystoplasty. A high incidence of histologic abnormalities in the intestinal segment was reported to occur along the anastomotic suture line and in the remaining bladder. Such abnormalities were directly correlated with heavy mixed bacterial growth in the urine and high levels of urinary n-nitrosamines. The association of chronic bacteriuria and elevated n-nitrosamines with these histologic changes remains to be elucidated. Shokeir *et al.* (1995) showed that all bowel segments exposed to urine, regardless of their position (bladder or ureteral substitution), are at risk for malignant changes, and that urine cytologies may be a useful diagnostic tool in this setting. More recently, Barrington et al. (1997a) reported on four patients who developed tumors in augmented bladders. All of the tumors were adenocarcinomas and were located on the bladder side of the anastomosis. It was concluded that these tumors were derived from the native urothelium. It was also demonstrated that transitional epithelium could undergo intestinal mucosal-like changes throughout the exposed native urothelium, including the renal pelvis, which was observed in one patient who had vesicoureteral reflux (VUR).

Barrington et al. (1996a) showed that there are elevated levels of transforming growth factor-beta (TGF-β) in the enterocystoplasty population. It is believed that TGF beta increases cellular proliferation and/or phagocytic activity, producing nitrosamines and oxygen free radicals. It has been demonstrated that urinary TGF-β levels can be decreased with the administration of pentosan polysulfate sodium (Barrington et al., 1996b). Therefore, if further research demonstrates elevated TGF-β as a risk factor, potential treatment options would be available. Barrington et al. (1997b) have also demonstrated a decreased serum level of selenium, a free oxygen radical scavenger, in the neuropathic bladder population. These may be possible reasons for augmented bladders being at increased risk for tumor formation.

The issue of potential malignancy in augmented bladders cannot be overlooked or ignored. This is a potentially disastrous complication for children in whom one hopes to provide a surgically reconstructed bladder that will last for life. Future research is needed to determine the true risk of tumor formation, which children are at greatest risk, and whether premalignant changes can be detected endoscopically or with urine markers or cytology. Although the incidence of tumor formation following enterocystoplasty is unknown, lifelong follow-up and yearly cystoscopic evaluation and urine cytologies from the augmented bladder should be considered beginning 10 years after the augmentation. All malignant tumors reported have occurred after this time lapse (Filmer and Spencer, 1990).

Perforation

Many complications can occur following enterocystoplasty. However, no complication is more potentially devastating or life threatening than unsuspected spontaneous bladder perforation. Although the exact incidence of perforation is not known, nearly every large series of enterocystoplasties includes at least one patient (Rink and Adams, 1998; Elder et al., 1988; Glass and Rushton, 1992; Rosen and Light, 1991; Sheiner and Kaplan, 1988; Rushton et al., 1988; Anderson and Rickwood, 1991; Bauer et al., 1992). Amongst these reports, seven deaths have been directly attributed to such perforation (Couillard et al., 1993). Most of these deaths were due, at least in part, to delay in diagnosis. Therefore, a high index of suspicion is needed in any patient with a history of enterocystoplasty who presents with abdominal pain.

It is not known whether one type of bowel is particularly prone to perforation after cystoplasty. Rink (1999) reported a higher incidence of spontaneous perforations in sigmoid cystoplasties. They initially felt that the sigmoid colon was inherently at greater risk for perforation, but they now feel that this higher incidence may be more directly related to their initial technique of sigmoid detubularization. Others have reported that the highest incidence of perforation occurred when ileum was used (Bauer et al., 1992). It appears that no segment of bowel, tubularized or detubularized, is immune from this complication.

The etiology of bladder perforation is unknown. Initially, perforations were thought either to be linked to traumatic catheterization or as a consequence of failure to catheterize on a timely basis (Elder et al., 1988; Rushton et al., 1988). However, perforation has been reported in patients who do not perform intermittent catheterization (Rosen and Light, 1991). Another contributing factor in bladder perforation may be vascular compromise in the bowel wall. Crane et al. (1991) reported that specimens from perforated bladders demonstrated histologic evidence of bowel wall ischemia. Also supporting the theory of bowel wall ischemia is an arterial perfusion study in a canine augmentation model, where a decrease in blood flow to the bowel wall was seen when the reservoir was overdistended and intravesical pressures were increased (Essig et al., 1991). The perfusion change was most striking at the antimesenteric border in the detubularized bowel. In addition to overdistension, high pressures due to bladder hyperreflexia may lead to an increased risk of perforation. Bauer et al. (1992) noted the presence of postoperative hyperreflexia in 40% of their patients who suffered a spontaneous perforation.

Some authors have suggested that a low urethral resistance is protective against both the high pressures associated with bladder hyperreflexia and failure to empty the reservoir on a timely basis (Anderson and Rickwood, 1991). However, Jayanthi *et al.* (1995) reported on 28 patients who underwent complete bladder neck ligation in conjunction with enterocystoplasty with a catheterizable stoma. In this series the one bladder perforation that occurred was associated with blunt trauma and was not spontaneous in origin. Therefore, achieving total urinary continence surgically without a pop-off valve mechanism does not in itself increase the risk for spontaneous rupture.

There does not appear to be one single etiology or risk factor that makes some more prone to bladder perforation than others. Multiple factors are probably involved. Repetitive overdistension secondary to poor compliance, bladder hyperreflexia, and chronic infection all appear to place the augmented bladder at increased risk for spontaneous perforation.

The diagnosis of bladder perforation can be difficult at times and a high index of suspicion is required to make the diagnosis quickly. Most pediatric patients who undergo enterocystoplasty are neurologically impaired. Lower abdominal sensation is diminished, therefore, the clinical presentation may be non-specific. Nausea, vomiting, fever, oliguria, and possibly referred pain to the shoulder secondary to diaphragmatic irritation may be presenting complaints.

On physical examination the abdomen is distended, with pain and irritation above the level of anesthesia. It may be difficult to distinguish pyelonephritis from a spontaneous bladder perforation. Thus, a standard or computed tomographic (CT) cystogram is recommended in any patient with an augmented bladder who presents with the above symptoms. Although the diagnostic role of a cystogram has been questioned in the past (Sheiner and Kaplan, 1988; Rushton *et al.*, 1988), it is the most specific diagnostic radiographic test (Rosen and Light, 1991; Bauer *et al.*, 1992). Braverman and Lebowitz (1991) have recommended fluoroscopy during the filling phase to make sure that the bladder is completely distended in order to diagnosis the perforation accurately. Residual contrast in the abdomen after the bladder has been drained establishes the diagnosis. Alternatively, an abdominal CT scan can be diagnostic and is helpful in demonstrating the extent of the extravasation.

When spontaneous perforation of the augmented bladder is suspected clinically and/or confirmed radiographically, immediate treatment is required. Catheter drainage, fluid resuscitation and broad-spectrum antibiotics should be started immediately. In a stable patient, non-operative management with catheter drainage, antibiotics, and serial physical evaluations may be all that is needed (Slaton and Kropp, 1994). This non-operative approach should be used only in selected patients in whom a small rupture is suspected. In the majority of patients, immediate exploration and closure of the bladder leak is safer. Intra-abdominal lavage, and irrigation and placement of intra-abdominal drains should then be done. Finally, all patients with an augmented bladder must be educated on the potentially lethal complications associated with delay in diagnosis of a spontaneous perforation. They should be instructed to inform a treating physician that they have an augmented bladder, and are at some risk for bladder perforation.

Surgical alternatives to intestinocystoplasty

As discussed above, bladder augmentation with small and large bowel segments may result in electrolyte abnormalities, UTIs, mucus production, stones, and tumor formation. Most long-term complications are attributable to the presence of intestinal mucosa in a urinary tract reservoir for urine storage. In an effort to avoid the unwanted effects of enterocystoplasty, several alternative surgical procedures have been developed. These include gastrocystoplasty, ureterocystoplasty, autoaugmentation, and seromuscular enterocystoplasty.

Gastrocystoplasty

Gastric tissue was first reported to be applied to the urinary tract in 1956 when Sinaiko described the use of a stomach segment for urinary diversion. Leong and Ong (1972, 1975) subsequently reported the successful use of stomach for augmentation of the bladder in both dogs and humans. More recently, Mitchell and colleagues have modified Leong's original techniques for gastrocystoplasty and popularized its use in pediatric patients (Piser *et al.*, 1987; Adams *et al.*, 1988).

Anatomy and physiology

Anatomically, the stomach can be divided into five

parts: the lesser curvature, greater curvature, fundus, body and antrum. The layers of the gastric wall include the outer serosal coat, a muscular coat, the submucosal layer, and the epithelium. The muscular coat consists of smooth muscle fibers oriented in a longitudinal, circular, and an oblique fashion. The epithelium of the gastric mucosa consists of a single layer of tall columnar epithelial cells and smaller acid-secreting cells. Loose areolar tissue in the submucosa lies between the mucosal and muscular layers. This loosely arranged layer allows technically simple separation of the mucosa from underlying muscle, permitting implantation of ureters in an antireflux fashion and tunneling of continent catheterizable stomas.

The entire arterial supply of the stomach is based on branches of the celiac artery, including the gastric, splenic, and hepatic arteries (Fig. 16.9). The right and left gastroepiploic arteries supply the greater curvature and are pertinent for use in gastrocystoplasty. The gastroepiploic arteries arise from the right gastric and splenic arteries, respectively. They usually do not anastomose directly but are connected through small arterial branches.

The main physiologic function of the stomach is to digest food mechanically and chemically. Given this, the muscle of the stomach functionally contracts in a manner that is different from the rest of the intestinal tract in that it acts to churn its contents as opposed to moving the bolus of food along a peristaltic wave. This unique pattern of contractility may be the cause of the phasic contractions that are seen in the augmented bladder following gastrocystoplasty.

The stomach chemically digests food through the secretion of acid. The exact mechanisms responsible for the control of acid secretion from the stomach are still not completely understood. Current evidence suggests that parietal cells, which are mainly located in the body of the stomach, secrete acid in response to gastrin that is released from G cells located in the antral mucosa. G cells, in turn, are stimulated to release gastrin by direct contact of the mucosa with food, antral distension, and vagal stimulation. Acid secretion can also be stimulated by acetycholine and histamine. The latter is important in that acid secretion from gastric segments following gastrocystoplasty can be inhibited with H_2 receptor blockers.

In addition to the stomach's ability to secrete chloride, other metabolic properties of importance include its barrier function to ammonium and chloride reabsorption. The combination of hydrogen ion

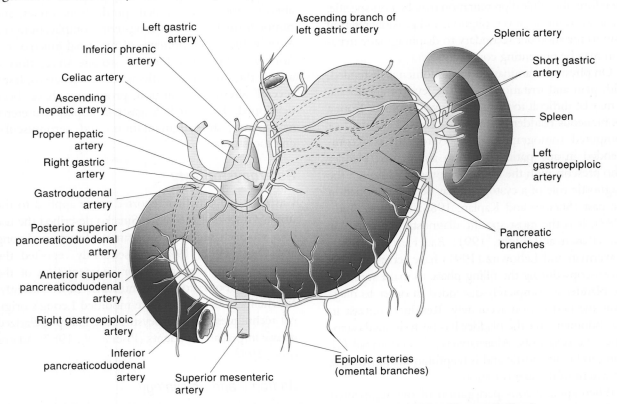

Figure 16.9 Arterial blood supply to the stomach. (Adapted from Lindner, 1989, with permission.)

and chloride secretion predisposes patients to the development of hypochloremic, hypokalemic, and metabolic alkalosis following gastrocystoplasty. However, this secretion of acid is beneficial in patients who have chronic acidosis associated with renal insufficiency.

Advantages and disadvantages

Surgically, the stomach is relatively thick and easy to work with. Use of stomach for bladder augmentation has clear advantages in patients with renal insufficiency owing to its ability to secrete acid. This allows for buffering of systemic acidosis and reduces the need for bicarbonate supplementation. The resultant acid urine also appears to decrease the incidence of bacteriuria. In comparison to other intestinal segments, there is decreased mucus production and stone formation. The inherent musculature of the gastric segment may offer an additional advantage over small and large bowel by increasing the possibility for spontaneous voiding. This may result in more efficient emptying, less residual urine, and decreased need for intermittent catheterization (Sheldon *et al.*, 1995; Kajbafzadeh *et al.*, 1995). Lastly, gastrocystoplasty can potentially be accomplished laparoscopically, which offers significant advantages in more rapid patient recovery following surgery (Docimo *et al.*, 1995).

The main disadvantage of gastrocystoplasty that currently limits its widespread use in children with neuropathic bladders is the high incidence of hematuria–dysuria syndrome (HDS). This is most troublesome in patients who have a sensate urethra and perineum. Given this, caution should be exercised in selecting patients who are sensate and are at risk for incontinence (i.e. bladder exstrophy) when other enteric segments are available. This also applies when considering gastrocystoplasty in a patient with end-stage renal disease in need of transplantation, since ulcer formation and perforation of defunctionalized bladders have been reported (Reinberg *et al.*, 1992).

Postoperative studies suggest that gastrocystoplasty results in a less compliant and capacious reservoir than that usually achieved with conventional enterocystoplasty. Gastrocystoplasty may therefore be less useful in patients with a very small, non-compliant bladder plate (El-Ghoneimi *et al.*, 1998; Kilic *et al.*, 1999).

Surgical technique

The original gastrocystoplasty, as described by Leong and Ong (1972, 1975), used the antrum of the stom-

ach. Since incorporation of antral tissue may increase cyclical secretion of acid because of antral distension during bladder filling, more recent forms of gastrocystoplasty (Adams *et al.*, 1988; Dewan *et al.*, 1995a) favor utilization of a wedge taken from the greater curvature of the stomach that incorporates more body and less antrum (Fig. 16.10). Depending on the individual vascular supply, this wedge of tissue may be based on either the right or left gastroepiploic artery. There is usually a vascular window between these arteries that defines which artery is dominant. Since the right gastroepiploic artery is longer and dominant in the majority of cases, this is more commonly used. A 10–15 cm length of stomach along the greater curvature is chosen, with special care being taken to minimize inclusion of antral tissue. Branches of the gastroepiploic artery that are not directly supplying the

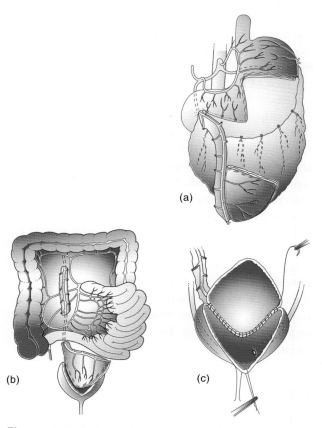

(a)

(b)

(c)

Figure 16.10 Gastrocystoplasty. (*a*) A wedge of stomach is isolated along the greater curvature of the stomach with its blood supply based on either the right or left gastroepiploic artery. (*b*) The flap is brought through the mesentaries of the small and large bowel or retroperitonealized following complete mobilization of the small and large bowel. (*c*) The flap is then anastomosed to the bivalved bladder.

wedge to be harvested are ligated. The wedge of stomach is isolated with the use of bowel clamps or an automatic stapler. The authors prefer the latter. The apex of the gastric wedge should be at least 1 cm below the lesser curvature to prevent injury to the vagus nerve and the right gastric vessels. Before isolation of the gastric wedge, it is advisable to ligate branches of the right gastric artery near the apex of the wedge, since failure to do this can result in significant blood loss (Rink, 1994). A flap of greater omentum must also be mobilized along with the gastric wedge. The stomach is then closed in two layers. Alternatively, Raz *et al.* (1993) have described a technique using an automatic stapler to harvest a gastric segment along the greater curvature of the stomach without opening the stomach.

Once the gastric segment is isolated, it is retroperitonealized by bringing it through the mesenteries of the transverse colon and small bowel. Special care should be taken to close these defects in the mesentery to prevent internal intestinal herniation. Alternatively, the right colon and duodenum can be mobilized up to the root of the small bowel mesentery, which allows placement of the gastric segment and its trailing vascular supply entirely in the retroperitoneal space. After the segment has been relocated inferiorly into the pelvis, it is rotated 90° to straighten the mesentery and vessels. The staples are then removed and the posterior tip of the stomach is sutured to the posterior aspect of the bivalved bladder using a running, interlocking 3-0 polyglactin suture.

Postoperatively, the augmented bladder should be adequately drained with a suprapubic tube and urethral catheter. A nasogastric suction tube is maintained for 3–5 days postoperatively. Following removal of the nasogastric tube and resumption of oral intake, the patient should be encouraged to eat small, frequent meals for the first few weeks to months.

Results

The urodynamic results of gastrocystoplasty are somewhat variable. Most authors report that it is useful in increasing capacity and compliance, similar to large and small bowel (Kurzrock *et al.*, 1998a). In studies that have analysed both preoperative and postoperative urodynamics, gastrocystoplasty has been shown to increase bladder capacity by approximately 150–200% (Kurzrock *et al.*, 1998b; Atala *et al.*,

1993)(Gosalbez *et al.*, 1993a). However, it should be noted that there is a wide range of results reported with regard to increased bladder capacity following gastrocystoplasty (Kilic *et al.*, 1999; Dewan *et al.*, 1995a; Kurzrock *et al.*, 1998a; Atala *et al.*, 1993; Gosalbez *et al.*, 1993a; Bogaert *et al.*, 1994). In a recent series comparing the urodynamic findings and clinical outcomes following augmentation with stomach versus intestine, it was shown that both stomach and intestine are efficacious in improving compliance, but that the use of ileum and colon results in a higher volume reservoir. Intestinal segments appear to expand more readily following augmentation than does stomach (Kilic *et al.*, 1999). Some of the differences in the literature regarding improvements in capacity and compliance following gastrocystoplasty may be in part explained by the variable amounts of stomach that have been harvested in individual patients. However, less volume expansion seems inherent to gastric segments when compared with ileum and colon.

A unique postoperative urodynamic finding after gastrocystoplasty is the presence of low-amplitude, rhythmic contractions during bladder filling. These contractions are usually less than 30 cmH$_2$O (Adams *et al.*, 1988; Bogaert *et al.*, 1994). However, contractions greater than 30 cmH$_2$O have been noted to be present in 10% of patients (Atala *et al.*, 1993) (Gosalbez *et al.*, 1993a; Bogaert *et al.*, 1994).

Taken together, experience with gastrocystoplasty demonstrates that it is clearly an effective procedure in providing improvements in bladder compliance and capacity. However, in comparison to ileum and colon, stomach often results in a reservoir that is less capacious and perhaps less compliant.

Hematuria–dysuria syndrome (HDS) is unique to gastrocystoplasty. HDS is defined as the presence of pain in the bladder, suprapubic, or genital area, coffee-brown or bright-red hematuria in the absence of infection, skin irritation or excoriation, and painful urination or pain with catheterization. HDS occurs in up to one-third of patients and is the major factor that has limited the more widespread use of gastrocystoplasty in children requiring enterocystoplasty. In the largest series to date, Nguyen *et al.* (1993) reported that 36% of patients following gastrocystoplasty had some element of this syndrome. Other retrospective series have reported the incidence of HDS to be as low as 2% and as high as 50% (Di Benedetto and Monfort, 1997; Kurzrock *et al.*, 1998a). The disparity in these numbers probably relates to the make-up of the patient populations. HDS is much more prevalent in patients who have a sensate urethra and perineum, whereas it is less common in patients who are insensate, as in patients with neuropathic bladders secondary to spina bifida or spinal cord injury. Despite the relatively high incidence of HDS following gastrocystoplasty, most patients respond well to either H_2 receptor blockers or hydrogen ion pump blockers such as omeprazole (Kinahan *et al.*, 1992). In some patients, alkaline irrigation of the bladder can also be used effectively (Mitchell, 1994).

The etiology of HDS is not entirely clear. Bogaert *et al.* (1995) demonstrated that the gastric mucosa in the augmented bladder is stimulated in the same way as the native stomach. With this in mind, some authors have proposed that hypergastrinemia may be a causative or major contributing factor in patients with HDS. The association of hypergastrinemia and HDS has been demonstrated in several patients (Gosalbez *et al.*, 1993a; Kinahan *et al.*, 1992; Gosalbez *et al.*, 1993b; Ortiz and Goldenberg, 1995; Plawker *et al.*, 1995). Despite this association, there has never been a direct correlation between this syndrome and aciduria and/or hypergastrinemia (Kurzrock *et al.*, 1998a; Nguyen *et al.*, 1993).

Another potential complication associated with the use of stomach is peptic ulcer disease of the gastric patch with subsequent perforation (Reinberg *et al.*, 1992). It has been postulated that *Helicobacter pylori* infection may be an important etiologic factor in patients who develop ulcerative changes in the gastric portion of the augmented bladder (Celayir *et al.*, 1997). Although patients are at significant risk for the development of HDS following gastrocystoplasty and other related complications associated with acid secretion by the stomach segment, it is rarely necessary to remove the gastric patch. Medical management of these problems is usually successful.

The beneficial effects of gastrocystoplasty in patients with reduced renal function and systemic acidosis are well documented (Adams *et al.*, 1988; Sheldon *et al.*, 1995). However, the metabolic losses of acids and chloride may be overabundant, resulting in significant hypochloremic, hypokalemic, and metabolic alkalosis in some. This metabolic imbalance has been severe enough to warrant hospitalization in up to 7% of patients with gastrocystoplasty (Kurzrock *et al.*, 1998a, 1998b). The precise mechanisms responsible for the development of a severe form of hypo-

chloremic, hypokalemic alkalosis have not been precisely or sequentially elucidated. Significant risk factors appear to be recent viral illness associated with vomiting and other gastrointestinal losses, urinary concentrating defect (Adams *et al.*, 1988), renal insufficiency (McDougal, 1992), and the absence of acidosis prior to gastrocystoplasty.

As is the case with HDS, the development of hypergastrinemia following gastrocystoplasty has been postulated, although not definitively proven, to play a significant etiologic role in the development of metabolic alkalosis (Kinahan *et al.*, 1992; Gosalbez *et al.*, 1993b; Plawker *et al.*, 1995). Clinical management of patients with hypochloremic, hypokalemic alkalosis includes aggressive intravenous rehydration with normal saline, replenishment of sodium and chloride, and use of H_2 receptor blockers. Once again, it is unusual to have an electrolyte abnormality that is so severe and unresponsive to medical therapy that removal of the gastric segment becomes necessary.

In comparison to conventional enterocystoplasty with small and large bowel, the incidence of bacteriuria, mucus production, and the development of bladder stones are significantly less following gastrocystoplasty (Kaefer *et al.*, 1998; Adams *et al.*, 1988; Bogaert *et al.*, 1994; Lewis *et al.*, 1995; Palmer *et al.*, 1998). The combination of decreased mucus, acidic urine, and the potential for spontaneous voiding (thus eliminating the need for intermittent catheterization) may be responsible for this decreased incidence.

Autoaugmentation

Autoaugmentation, also known as vesicomyotomy and vesicomyectomy, was introduced by Cartwright and Snow (1989a,b). This is a novel approach to bladder augmentation that aims to enlarge bladder capacity and improve bladder compliance without using a patch graft or opening the bladder. In essence, this procedure creates a large bladder diverticulum by removal of the bladder muscle from the dome. The most important advantage for this procedure is the avoidance of intestinal epithelium with its associated complications. The native urothelium is preserved. The major drawback of autoaugmentation is that experience has failed to identify the most appropriate patients for this procedure. Mixed results have been obtained clinically with regard to symptomatic and postoperative urodynamic improvement in the autoaugmented bladder. Evaluation of the available data indicates that there is no direct correlation between preoperative urodynamic findings and success. It works well in some patients while it fails in others. Nevertheless, it appears that this procedure is best suited for patients with reduced compliance in combination with a near normal preoperative bladder capacity (Cartwright and Snow, 1999; Duel *et al*., 1998; Snow and Cartwright, 1996). However, it should be noted that autoaugmentation has been successful in some patients with a small-capacity, poorly compliant bladder (Cartwright and Snow, 1989b, 1999).

Despite the problems in predicting surgical success preoperatively, it seems reasonable to consider autoaugmentation as an option in most patients in whom conventional enterocystoplasty is needed. One exception may be children with failed bladder exstrophy repair, those who have had multiple previous bladder operations, and patients with small capacities. Autoaugmentation in these children is more difficult technically and results in general have been poor (Snow and Cartwright, 1996; Cartwright and Snow, 1999).

Anatomy and physiology

Autoaugmentation preserves the native bladder urothelium. The metabolic and physiologic properties of this urothelium following autoaugmentation are not well studied, although available data suggest that no significant changes occur. Following autoaugmentation, the mucosal herniation has been shown in both experimental animals and humans to have evidence of collagen deposition, neovascularity, variable inflammatory changes, and occasional muscle fibers (Snow and Cartwright, 1996; Dewan *et al*., 1994a, 1995b). No significant metaplastic or dysplastic changes in the native urothelium have been reported.

Advantages and disadvantages

The primary advantage of autoaugmentation over conventional enterocystoplasty is preservation of the patient's native urothelium in the augmented segment. This avoids the complications associated with enterocystoplasty related to the presence of heterotopic epithelium in contact with the urine noted previously. Technically, autoaugmentation is an extraperitoneal procedure that can be performed through a Pfannenstiel incision and avoids the complications of transperitoneal bowel surgery. Although autoaugmentation is

performed without a formal cystotomy, other bladder procedures such as ureteral reimplantation and appendicovesicostomy can be carried out (intravesically or extravesically) at the same time. Lastly, it is important to note that autoaugmentation does not preclude further augmentation procedures if unsuccessful.

The main disadvantage of autoaugmentation is the inability to predict which patients will do well with this technique. An additional concern is the theoretical risk of bladder rupture that has been demonstrated in animal studies (Rivas *et al*., 1996; Chancellor *et al*., 1996). Although perforation of the autoaugmented bladder has been reported in only one patient (Ahmed *et al*., 1998a), the overall increased risk of bladder rupture compared with other types of bladder augmentation has yet to be defined.

Surgical technique

Patients should receive a full bowel preparation preoperatively and be counseled on the possible need to perform an alternative type of augmentation if intraoperative findings dictate that autoaugmentation is not technically feasible. Specifics regarding the technique of autoaugmentation have been well described by Snow and Cartwright (1996). The procedure is usually performed through a Pfannenstiel incision and is done extraperitoneally. Once the bladder is mobilized, the peritoneal covering is entirely detached. Snow and Cartwright advocate the performance of intraoperative urodynamics, both before and after the autoaugmentation. Although not definitive, intraoperative urodynamics can be useful in making an assessment of potential success. It also assists in establishing the maximum volume following autoaugmentation to which the bladder can be safely distended during the immediate postoperative period.

Once initial intraoperative urodynamics is completed, the bladder is filled and a needle-tipped electrocautery is used to divide the detrusor musculature from the underlying epithelium (Fig. 16.11). This is usually started ventrally in a vertical fashion. The plane between the underlying epithelium and the overlying muscle is then identified and further developed using both blunt and sharp dissection. Special care is taken to avoid tears in the urothelium, since this can be difficult to repair in some cases and urinary extravasation postoperatively is associated with inflammation. Inability to distend the bladder postoperatively may result in contraction. When perforation does occur, it should be repaired with fine, absorbable suture. Removal of overlying muscle fibers continues until the detrusor musculature is removed from at least one-half of the bladder. Optimally, as much musculature is removed as possible. At this juncture, intraoperative urodynamics is repeated once again. If there is minimal to no improvement in bladder capacity and/or compliance, autoaugmentation should be abandoned and conventional enterocystoplasty undertaken following excision of the redundant bladder epithelium.

After autoaugmentation is completed, either one can excise the detached detrusor musculature or the remaining lateral bladder muscle can be attached to the psoas muscles. However, neither of these steps has been found to be essential for success (Johnson *et al.*, 1994; Snow and Cartwright, 1996). Postoperatively, a urethral catheter and penrose drain are left in place. Suprapubic tubes are avoided as the bladder should be watertight. Experience has shown that bladder distension during initial healing is important for surgical success. This can be accomplished either by intermittent distension of the bladder to the capacity that was determined appropriate intraoperatively or by maintaining catheter drainage with constant bladder distension at an intravesical pressure of 20–40 cmH$_2$O. The catheter can generally be removed in 1–2 weeks. It is recommended that a cystogram be performed before catheter removal to exclude urinary extravasation.

Recently, several authors have demonstrated that successful bladder autoaugmentation can be accomplished laparoscopically (Ehrlich and Gershman, 1993; Braren and Bishop, 1998; Britanisky *et al.*, 1995; McDougall *et al.*, 1995). Although a laparoscopic approach is feasible, further experience is necessary to determine whether this approach is successful and cost-effective.

Results

The efficacy of autoaugmentation in improving bladder capacity and compliance has been varied. Cartwright and Snow (1999) have reported follow-up of greater than 1 year in 30 patients, 19 of whom had a neuropathic bladder secondary to spina bifida. All patients had preoperative urodynamic evidence of reduced bladder compliance and detrusor hyperreflexia. While clinical success has been dramatic in some, the overall results have been less impressive. One-

third of the patients had a significant increase in bladder capacity, an additional third were unchanged, while one-third had loss of capacity. Evaluation of bladder compliance revealed that 60% had an improvement in compliance by greater than 50% compared with preoperative measurements, 20% had a 20–50% improvement, and the remainder did not change significantly. Following autoaugmentation, the majority of patients remained on intermittent catheterization, although 20% demonstrated the ability to void spontaneously. Seven of these 30 patients have required secondary enterocystoplasty.

Snow and Cartwright have re-evaluated preoperative parameters in these patients in an effort to identify specific factors that would help to prognosticate eventual outcome following autoaugmentation. Unfortunately, they were unable to identify any such factors. However, certain generalizations can be made from this analysis. Autoaugmentation appears to be poorly suited to patients with a history of bladder exstrophy or multiple prior bladder operations, since in these patients it is difficult to develop a plane between the bladder muscle and mucosa. Results have also been relatively poor in these groups. The ideal candidate is the patient with a near normal bladder capacity but reduced compliance.

Since the original publications, several other centers have reported their experiences with autoaugmentation in children. Stothers *et al.* (1994) performed autoaugmentations in 12 pediatric patients. They observed a mean increase in bladder capacity of 40% and a mean decrease in leak point pressure of 33%. Skobejko-Wlodarska *et al.* (1998) have reported on the use of autoaugmentation in 21 children with spina bifida and found a modest increase in bladder capacity in two-thirds of patients and significant improvements in bladder compliance in another two-thirds.

The experience with autoaugmentation in the adult population appears to be more predictable and consistently favorable than the results described thus far in children. Stohrer *et al.* (1995, 1997) reported on 50 adult patients from their spinal cord injury center. In patients with neuropathic hyperreflexive bladders that were refractory to medical therapy, bladder autoaugmentation was found to increase mean bladder capacity from 121 to 406 ml with concomitant improvements in bladder compliance. McGuire and colleagues (Leng *et al.*, 1999) recently compared the efficacy of enterocystoplasty to autoaugmentation in

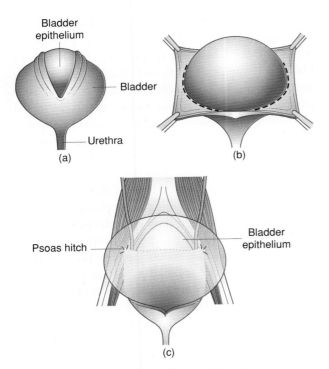

Figure 16.11 Autoaugmentation. (*a*) The detrusor muscle is incised in the midline and a plane is established between the muscle and the underlying mucosa. (*b*) This plane is further developed and a large mouth diverticulum is created. (*c*) The remaining detrusor muscle is fixed posteriorly to prevent its coaptation. (Adapted from Cartwright and Snow, 1989, with permission.)

adults. They reported on over 60 patients undergoing either autoaugmentation or conventional enterocystoplasty. There were no significant differences in postoperative urodynamic parameters between enterocystoplasty and autoaugmentation in patients with refractory detrusor instability, interstitial cystitis, radiation cystitis, and other forms of neuropathic bladder. An important finding was that enterocystoplasty was uniformly superior to autoaugmentation in patients with a history of myelodysplasia. The overall improvement in the results of autoaugmentation in adults may be related to differences in the bladder disease processes and patient population. Autoaugmentation is mostly performed in children with a neuropathic bladder from congenital causes, while in adults the neuropathic bladder is usually an acquired condition. It may be that autoaugmentation is more successful in adults because surgery is undertaken earlier in the disease process prior to irreversible histologic and functional changes in the bladder wall.

Seromuscular enterocystoplasty

Seromuscular enterocystoplasty combines autoaugmentation with a demucosalized flap of colon or stomach. The removal of the gastrointestinal mucosa results in a denuded seromuscular flap that can be placed over the exposed bladder mucosa of an autoaugmented bladder. The use of a demucosalized segment of bowel for bladder augmentation was first described by Shoemaker in 1955 (Shoemaker, 1955; Shoemaker and Marucci, 1955). He was able to show that seromuscular bowel flaps, when placed into the bladder wall with the denuded side either inward or reversed, such that the serosa faced the lumen of the bladder, were re-epithelialized by urothelium. Unfortunately, subsequent long-term studies in small and large animals have consistently demonstrated that seromuscular bowel segments alone scar and contract (Cheng *et al.*, 1994; Oesch, 1988; Salle *et al.*, 1990; de Badiola *et al.*, 1991). Histologic evaluation suggests that the scarring is due to either the trauma associated with the demucosalization process, a prolonged inflammatory response in the denuded bowel before the hoped-for urothelial re-epithelialization, or both.

The intention of seromuscular enterocystoplasty is to combine the advantages of conventional enterocystoplasty with those of autoaugmentation while avoiding the potential specific adverse effects of each procedure. Ideally, a muscle-backed augmentation flap that is lined with urothelium should result. Contraction of the seromuscular flap is hopefully avoided by rapid adherence of the native urothelium to the demucosalized gastrointestinal segment. Clinical experience thus far suggests that the success of this procedure is limited by the same factors that give rise to inconsistent results with autoaugmentation. Failures may relate to patient selection, preoperative bladder characteristics, postoperative inflammatory changes in the augmented segment, non-union of the bladder mucosa and seromuscular flap, or a combination of these factors. Given the present data, it appears that seromuscular enterocystoplasty is best suited to the patient who is considered an optimal candidate for autoaugmentation alone, that is, one with a relatively large bladder capacity. Further experience is needed to confirm this notion.

Anatomy and physiology

Seromuscular enterocystoplasty has been accomplished with both stomach and colon. Since the plane between the mucosa and the underlying seromuscular segment is difficult to establish in small bowel, ileum has not been used in this procedure. The metabolic consequences of seromuscular enterocystoplasty are presumed to be minimal, since the native urothelium is kept intact. This assumption is supported in part by animal studies (Denes *et al.*, 1997). Histology from these studies reveals that the urothelium covering the seromuscular flap appears normal (Dewan *et al.*, 1994b)(Buson *et al.*, 1994). Whether or not late metaplastic changes will occur in the bladder urothelium when it is placed in direct contact with a seromuscular segment of bowel is not known. It has been well documented that stromal–epithelial interactions in other individual organs are important for normal cell growth and function (DiSandro *et al.*, 1998; Baskin *et al.*, 1996). The stroma of the bowel segment may adversely affect the overlying growth and function of the bladder urothelium in the long term.

Advantages and disadvantages

The advantages of this procedure are similar to those of autoaugmentation, with the most important being preservation of the native urothelium. This avoids the aforementioned complications associated with the interposition of heterotopic intestinal epithelium in the urinary tract. Since it has been shown that partial re-epithelialization of the seromuscular segment with enteric epithelium can occur, it is not clear that these problems will totally be avoided. This is especially important when considering the long-term risk of tumor formation, since the presence of any intestinal mucosa is clearly worrisome. An advantage of seromuscular enterocystoplasty over autoaugmentation alone is the provision of adequate muscle backing of the augmented segment. This may potentially reduce the risk of scarring and fibrosis and may lessen the risk of spontaneous perforation.

There are currently two major disadvantages to this procedure. It is a technically demanding procedure and much more labor intensive than conventional augmentation cystoplasty or autoaugmentation alone. In addition, clinical experience is limited and the available published results are mixed with regard to postoperative urodynamic improvements. Postoperative distension of the augmented bladder is important for the success of this procedure. Thus, some authors have advocated routinely increasing bladder outlet resistance with seromuscular enterocystoplasty and

the avoidance of concomitant intravesical procedures when possible (Duel *et al.*, 1998).

Surgical technique

Seromuscular enterocystoplasty is initially begun by performing an autoaugmentation as described above. A section of stomach or colon is then isolated for use as the seromuscular flap (Fig. 16.12). The most difficult and technically demanding portion of this procedure is demucosalization of the flap. It has been suggested that the muscularis mucosa which is contained in the submucosa needs to be removed in addition to the enteric mucosa to prevent regrowth of intestinal mucosa and flap contracture. Dewan *et al.* (1997) reported that this plane can readily be identified intraoperatively. Removal of the mucosa and submucosa is accomplished with sharp dissection and the use of electrocautery. Usually, the mucosa can be progressively peeled away from the underlying muscle once the proper plane has been established. Some authors have recommended occlusion of the arterial blood supply during this dissection to decrease blood loss and facilitate visualization (Carr *et al.*, 1999). Once the seromuscular flap has been demucosalized, the flap is placed on top of the bladder mucosa that has been exposed by the autoaugmentation.

Adherence of the bladder mucosa to the raw surface of the seromuscular flap is critical to the long-term success of this operation. Several techniques have been suggested to facilitate this process. A small, flat Jackson–Pratt drain has been used to prevent the formation of a hematoma or seroma between the urothelium and the seromuscular flap that could prevent adherence between the two surfaces. Multiple mattress sutures can also be used. As with autoaugmentation, postoperative distension of the bladder with intermittent irrigation or constant distension of the bladder to 20–30 cmH$_2$O has been used. Carr *et al.* (1999) used a Helmstein balloon in the bladder postoperatively to produce partial distension and compaction of the urothelium against the denuded muscle. A suprapubic tube is then placed for postoperative urinary drainage.

Results

The clinical results of seromuscular enterocystoplasty have been mixed and unpredictable. Initial reports by Dewan and Gonzalez in both animal models and

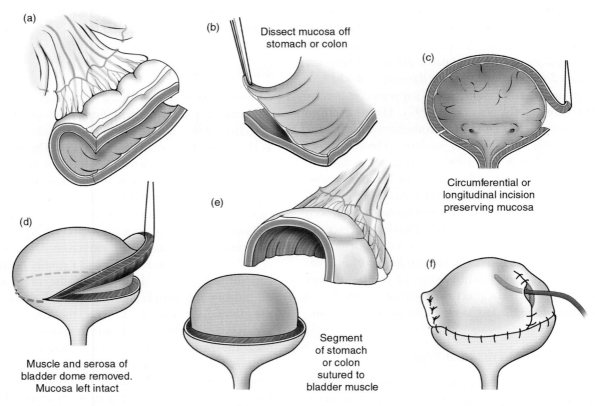

Figure 16.12 Seromuscular enterocystoplasty. (*a*) A portion of stomach or colon is isolated. (*b*) The mucosa is removed with sharp dissection. (*c, d*) An autoaugmentation is then performed resulting in an exposed diverticulum of bladder mucosa. (*e*) The demucosalized flap of stomach or colon is laid on top of the exposed mucosa and anastomosed to the edges of bladder muscle. (*f*) A drain can be placed in between the flap and the mucosa to facilitate adherence of the two surfaces. (Adapted from Buson *et al.*, 1994, with permission.)

humans have been encouraging (Dewan *et al.*, 1994b; Buson *et al.*, 1994; Dewan and Stefanek, 1994; Gonzalez *et al.*, 1995). In a series of 16 patients undergoing seromuscular colocystoplasty using sigmoid colon, bladder capacity was increased to almost 2.5 times the preoperative volume and end filling pressures decreased by approximately 50% (Gonzalez *et al.*, 1995). Dewan and Stefanek (1994) have reported on five patients undergoing seromuscular gastrocystoplasty. Four of the five patients had urodynamic evidence of improved bladder capacity and compliance during the first postoperative year. Despite these initial encouraging results, it is important to note that the follow-up in these series has been relatively short, and approximately 25% of patients have eventually required a secondary operation due to either complications related to the seromuscular flap (contracture) and/or failure to improve adequately bladder capacity and/or compliance.

A more recent report of 13 patients after seromuscular gastrocystoplasty (Carr *et al.*, 1999) describes variable results, at best. The mean follow-up was 50 months. Five patients had a good outcome with regard to objective urodynamic and subjective clinical improvement. Four patients were found to have a 'fair' outcome in that they had some objective improvement, while the remaining four patients had a poor result and required reaugmentation. Evaluation of preoperative urodynamic and radiographic data in these patients again demonstrated that it was not possible to predict preoperatively which patients would do well after seromuscular gastrocystoplasty.

Recurrent or persistent colonic mucosa has been found in several patients after seromuscular colocystoplasty. In a series of seromuscular colocystoplasty patients, three out of ten patients who had subsequent biopsies during follow-up had evidence of residual colonic mucosa. Whether this partial intestinal regrowth is progressive or clinically relevant remains to be determined. As mentioned above, it has been suggested and supported by animal studies that removal of the submucosa may prevent re-epithelialization of the seromuscular flap with islands of native enteric mucosa. This can be accomplished without compromising flap integrity (Dewan *et al.*, 1997).

Ureterocystoplasty

The use of ureteral tissue for bladder augmentation was first described in 1992 (Mitchell *et al.*, 1992; Wolf and Turzan, 1993). Since then, its use in children has become more popular (Churchill *et al.*, 1993; Bellinger, 1993, 1998). For many reasons native ureter is the best tissue available for augmentation cystoplasty. It is autologous, lined with urothelium, backed by muscle, distensible, and compliant. However, few patients in need of bladder augmentation have widely dilated ureters available for such use. Patients who are candidates for ureterocystoplasty should have either a non-functional renal unit that can be removed making the ureter and renal pelvis available, or a functional renal unit that is associated with a massively dilated, tortuous, and elongated ureter (Churchill *et al.*, 1993; Gosalbez and Kim, 1996). The lower ureter can then be used for augmentation while kidney drainage is re-established either by reimplantation of the straightened upper ureter into the bladder or by transureteroureterostomy. An example of an ideal candidate is one with vesicoureteral reflux and dysplasia (VURD) syndrome from PUV. Ureterocystoplasty is also appropriate in patients with end-stage renal failure on dialysis who are awaiting transplantation and are in need of augmentation owing to bladder dysfunction.

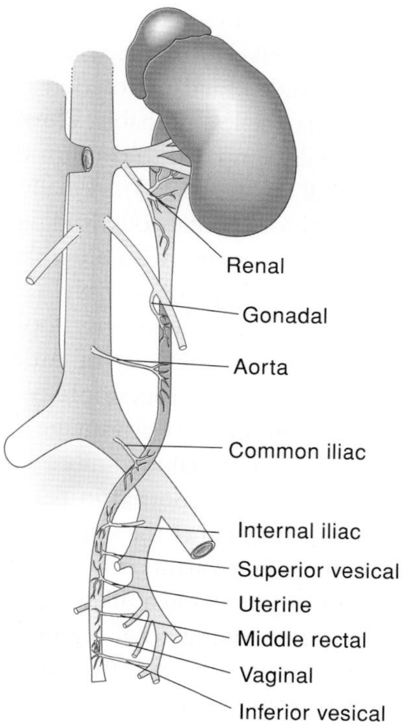
Renal
Gonadal
Aorta
Common iliac
Internal iliac
Superior vesical
Uterine
Middle rectal
Vaginal
Inferior vesical

Figure 16.13 Arterial blood supply to the ureter. (Adapted from Lindner, 1989, with permission.)

Anatomy and physiology

Preservation of the ureteral blood supply is paramount when performing ureterocystoplasty. The normal ureter receives its blood supply from branches of numerous vessels including the aorta and renal, gonadal and common iliac arteries (Fig. 16.13). The upper ureter receives its blood supply medially while the lower ureter receives it posterolaterally. There are extensive anastamosing plexuses in the adventitia of the ureter that are important to preserve if viability of the ureter is to be maintained. Careful attention to these vessels allows for long segments of ureter to be mobilized without vascular compromise. Ureteral urothelium is contiguous with the urothelium from the bladder and has similar physiologic characteristics. Peristalsis of the ureter depends on autonomic innervation and input from intrinsic pacemaker sites in the minor calyces of the renal collecting system (Kabalin, 1998). Although the ureter is detubularized and its inherent innervation is disrupted with ureterocystoplasty, it appears that the ureteral tissue still maintains some ability to contract. Clinical experience and postoperative urodynamics demonstrate that the ureter remains very compliant.

Advantages and disadvantages

There are several advantages in using the ureter for augmentation. As is the case with autoaugmentation, the major advantage of ureterocystoplasty is that the native urothelium is preserved, thereby avoiding the specific potential problems associated with the use of bowel. Unlike some cases following autoaugmention, the full-thickness opened ureter does not tend to shrink with time, unless the vascular supply is compromised. In patients with end-stage renal disease, the procedure can be performed extraperitoneally, thus preserving the peritoneum for future peritoneal dialysis. When needed, concomitant procedures in the bladder may also be performed. It seems likely that the risk of tumor formation will be avoided, and perforation of the augmented bladder may be less probable. However, long-term follow-up will be needed to confirm these possibilities (Churchill *et al.*, 1993). Finally, there is increased potential for spontaneous voiding postoperatively, especially in patients who are able to empty their bladders adequately preoperatively.

The main disadvantage of ureterocystoplasty is that it is only applicable in a minority of patients. More recently, the use of ureterocystoplasty has been expanded in an attempt to take advantage of this valuable tissue and make it available to more surgical candidates. Its use has been reported in patients with a duplex system in which either the upper or lower pole is non-functioning (Ben-Chaim *et al.*, 1996). In patients with a duplex system and a dilated ureter in conjunction with a functioning renal segment, drainage of that segment can be accomplished with an ipsilateral pyeloureterostomy or a ureteropyelostomy with preservation of the distal portion of the ureter for augmentation. Ahmed *et al.* (1998b) also described the tandem use of bilateral megaureters for ureterocystoplasty.

Efforts are being made to produce dilated ureters in an attempt to make ureterocystoplasty available to more patients. Lailas *et al.* (1996) have demonstrated in a rabbit model that a temporary cutaneous ureterostomy can be used to perform hydrostatic distension of the ureter with subsequent successful ureterocystoplasty. Others have reported that placement of a tissue expander in pig ureters adequately dilates the ureter (Ikeguchi *et al.*,1998; Stifelman *et al.*, 1998).

Surgical technique

Patients undergoing ureterocystoplasty should have a full bowel preparation and sterilization preoperatively in case the ureter is not suitable for augmentation. The procedure can be performed either through a midline incision with transperitoneal approach to the urinary tract or via two incisions such as is used for nephroureterectomy (Reinberg *et al.*, 1995). The latter approach is extraperitoneal. This may be advantageous in patients with severe renal insufficiency who may subsequently require peritoneal dialysis. A nephrectomy is performed initially, preserving the renal pelvis. The upper portion of the ureter and renal pelvis are then mobilized (Fig. 16.14). Efforts

should be made to preserve as much renal pelvis as possible since this increases the surface area of the augmentation. One should include any available periureteral tissue to protect the network of vessels within the ureteral adventitia. Although the blood supply from the lower ureter (which is derived posterolaterally) can maintain the viability of the upper ureter via this adventitial network, efforts should also be made to preserve collaterals from the gonadal vessels and the main renal vessels. These vessels supply the renal pelvis and upper ureter directly and their preservation helps to ensure adequate vascular supply to the upper portion of the ureter. As Churchill *et al.* (1995) have noted, preservation of the upper ureteral blood supply is most important when previous reconstructive surgery has compromised the collaterals involving the distal ureter.

Following mobilization of the renal pelvis and ureter, the ureter is detubularized and reconfigured to form a patch. The bladder is then opened. The bladder incision extends from the ipsilateral ureteral orifice to the contralateral ventral quadrant of the bladder. The incision is carried through the ipsilateral ureteral orifice so that it unroofs the intravesical ureter and meets the detubularization incision in the ureter. This allows

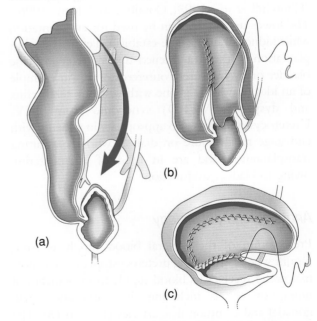

Figure 16.14 Ureterocystoplasty. A standard nephrectomy is performed with preservation of the renal pelvis. (*a*) The proximal ureter is mobilized with preservation of the medial blood supply. (*b*) The ureter is then detubularized with the incision for detubularization connecting with the off-center cystostomy. (*c*) The ureter is folded on itself and anastamosed to the opened bladder.

the bladder to be opened sufficiently for ureterocystoplasty without much risk of an hourglass deformity. Alternatively, to preserve vascularity, the incision can stop short of the orifice, maintaining the normal configuration of the distal ureter for a few centimeters (Wolf and Turzan, 1993). Once the bladder is adequately opened, the reconfigured ureteral segment is sutured to the defect in the bladder creating a wide anastomosis. Prior to closure, a suprapubic tube is placed through the native bladder, and left indwelling for 2–3 weeks. Postoperative care is essentially the same as for routine enterocystoplasty except that daily irrigation for mucus is not required.

Results

Over 30 children undergoing ureterocystoplasty have been reported since 1992. Despite the relatively small numbers, the encouraging results have led to enthusiasm for this technique. Most prefer to use ureter instead of intestinal segments whenever adequate ureteral tissue is available. The largest published series is that of Churchill et al. (1993), in which ureterocystoplasty was performed in 16 patients. Thirteen patients had adequate urodynamic data available postoperatively for evaluation, 12 of whom had excellent results. As a group, there was a 218% increase in bladder capacity, a 284% increase in pressure-specific bladder capacity, and a 227% increase in bladder compliance. In a follow-up to this study, Landau et al. (1994) compared the urodynamic results between patients treated with ileocystoplasty and those with ureterocystoplasty. They report no significant differences in the postoperative mean increase in bladder capacity and pressure-specific bladder volume. Both procedures resulted in excellent functional results. Hitchcock et al. (1994) described similar excellent short-term results in eight patients. The main drawback is the limited number of patients with severe enough ureteral dilitation to be candidates for this procedure. Novel techniques to make ureterocystoplasty more readily available are currently being developed. However, it may be possible to use the ureter even when it is not significantly dilated. This approach has been reported in one patient with long-term follow-up pending (McKenna and Bauer, 1995).

Tissue-engineered bladder

The complications associated with using various portions of the gastrointestinal tract for genitourinary reconstruction in both adults and children which have been described in detail earlier in this chapter have stimulated the development of tissue-engineering techniques for bladder reconstruction through bladder regeneration. Current research efforts are focussed on the development of biodegradable materials which are well characterized with predictable behavior that can be used as alternatives to gastrointestinal segments for bladder reconstruction. Although attempts at bladder reconstruction via bladder regeneration are not new (Tizzoni and Poggi, 1888), the major obstacle has been the unavailability of a biomaterial, either permanent or biodegradable, that will function as a suitable scaffold to allow the process of regeneration to occur either naturally or with the addition of cultured cells. The ideal graft material is one that would be replaced by the host tissue, provide a low-pressure reservoir, and serve as a scaffold for regeneration of the bladder wall with normal functional characteristics. If a suitable graft material were developed, the need for autogenous tissue and the associated complications of intestinal segments could be eliminated. Currently, two types of tissue-engineering technology have been shown to induce bladder regeneration in preliminary studies. These are unseeded and seeded technologies.

Unseeded technology

The first technique currently being investigated for bladder regeneration is unseeded technology. This involves the use of tissue matrix grafts that are biodegradable, acellular, collagen based, autologous, or xenogenic (Kropp et al., 1995b; Sutherland et al., 1996; Piechota et al., 1998a). This technology involves placement of the graft into the wall of the host bladder. The body then provides the needed environment for subsequent cell growth and tissue generation. This represents an unseeded bladder regenerating process.

Thus far, the major obstacle to unseeded tissue-engineering technology has been the inability to develop an optimal biomaterial that will act as a suitable scaffold for the 'natural' process of regeneration. Synthetic non-biodegradable materials such as silicone, rubber, polytetrafluoroethylene, and polypropylene have been tried with unsuccessful results because of host–foreign body reactions (Bohne et al., 1955, 1957; Kudish 1957; Swinney et al., 1961; Ashkar and Heller, 1967). As a consequence of these failures with non-biodegradable materials, synthetic biodegradable materials were developed. It is anticipated that these grafts will allow the host bladder adequate time for regeneration but dissolve before the onset of foreign body reactions. These materials have been used experimentally and have shown less graft encrustation and fewer infectious complications than non-biodegradable materials. However, graft shrinkage still limits the potential clinical utility of these materials (Agishi et al., 1975). Non-synthetic biodegradable materials such as placenta, amnion, and pericardium have been investigated and have shown a clear ability to host bladder regeneration (Scott et al., 1988; Kambic et al., 1992; Gorham et al., 1984; Fishman et al., 1987). However, despite initial encouraging laboratory results, none of these materials has been found to be suitable for clinical use. The reasons for this are not entirely clear. It can only be speculated from the available literature that long-term experimental results with these biodegradable materials did not replicate the initial results and, therefore, clinical trials were not undertaken.

Recently, new types of biodegradable material have been developed that have shown tremendous potential for the induction of bladder regeneration with unseeded tissue-engineering technology. These materials are acellular extracellular matrix (ECM) grafts that are derived from various different organs. The graft is made acellular by a mechanical process that lyses the cells and/or by detergent and enzymatic extraction. These types of ECM grafts have been derived from full-thickness bladder and stomach and the submucosal layer of small intestine (Kropp et al., 1995b; Probst et al., 1997; Reddy et al., 1999).

The most thoroughly studied collagen-based ECM graft for bladder augmentation and urinary reconstruction using unseeded technology is small intestinal submucosa (SIS) (Kropp, 1998). SIS is a xenogenic membrane derived from pig small intestine in which the mucosa is mechanically removed from the inner surface and the serosa and muscularis are mechanically removed from the outer surface. This results in a thin, translucent membrane (0.1 mm wall thickness) composed mainly of the submucosal layer of the intestinal wall. Production of SIS is reminiscent of the manufacture of sausage casing. This unique material has been shown to function well as an arterial or venous graft, with rapid replacement by native tissues and evidence of tissue-specific regeneration (Badylak et al., 1989; Lantz et al., 1990, 1992).

SIS grafts have been shown to promote full-thickness bladder regeneration in both rat and canine animal models (Kropp, 1995a). The regenerated bladder tissue is composed of all three layers of the normal bladder wall (urothelium, smooth muscle, and serosa). In addition, the regenerated segment is contractile, compliant, and functionally innervated. Urodynamic studies in a long-term canine augmentation model have demonstrated that the SIS augmented bladder maintains normal bladder capacity and compliance for at least 15 months postoperatively (Kropp et al., 1996a). In vitro muscle strip studies on the regenerated portions of the bladders also demonstrate contractility and compliance that is similar to normal bladder (Kropp et al., 1996b).

SIS has been shown to be non-immunogenic, with over 1000 cross-species transplants and direct challenge testing elucidating no response (Badylak, 1994; Metzger et al., 1996). In addition, SIS is unique from other biomaterials that have been studied thus far in that it contains a combination of active intrinsic growth factors, cytokines, structural proteins, glycoproteins, and proteoglycans that may assist in cell migration, cell-to-cell interaction, and cell growth and differentiation during the regenerative process (Badylak, 1996; Voytik-Harbin et al., 1997; Hodde et al., 1996). These inherent elements within SIS may prove to be vital to the regenerative process. Further research is needed to identify the functional importance of each of these elements and factors.

Similar types of acellular ECM grafts to SIS have also been shown to induce bladder regeneration. Preliminary work by Sutherland et al. (1996) and Piechota et al. (1998b) demonstrated that successful morphologic and functional regeneration of the rat urinary bladder can be accomplished with homologous bladder acellular matrix grafts (BAMG). Reddy et al. (1999) also reported on partial bladder substitution with porcine bladder acellular matrix allografts (BAMA) in a porcine model. They demonstrated that the regenerated urothelium with BAMA was multilayered and that there was also histologic evidence of organized smooth muscle regeneration and neoangiogenesis at 30 days.

The above experience with SIS and other similar ECM-derived biomaterials clearly demonstrates that bladder regeneration using unseeded tissue-engineering technology is feasible without the complications of graft shrinkage, incrustation, and infection. These observations have significant clinical ramifications. The ability to augment the bladder without the use of bowel or other native host tissue would eliminate many of the complications of conventional enterocystoplasty and would simplify the technical aspects of this operation. Further research into the individual composition of the various biomaterials, the cell-to-cell interactions, and the growth factors (Sutherland *et al.*, 1996; Pope *et al.*, 1997) that are involved in the bladder regenerative process will be required before clinical use of these grafts.

Seeded technology

The second type of tissue-engineering technology, the seeded technique, involves the use of biodegradable materials that act as cell-delivery vehicles for cultured cells from the patient. This technique has been applied to the urinary bladder. Initially, this process is begun by harvesting native bladder tissue for the establishment and expansion of primary cultures of both bladder smooth muscle and epithelial cells. Cilento *et al.* (1994) demonstrated that it is possible to expand a bladder epithelial cell culture from a single biopsy specimen such that the cultured cells could cover a surface area of over 400 m^2 within 8 weeks. Once the cells are grown, they are seeded on a biodegradable membrane *in vitro* and then transplanted back into the host for continuation of the regenerative process. Atala *et al.* (1992) demonstrated the successful use of non-woven polyglycolic acid polymer sheets that allow the seeded growth of rabbit and human bladder epithelium and smooth muscle cells. Further work demonstrated that these cell–polymer constructs could then be implanted into athymic mice, with the subsequent formation of organized layers of bladder epithelial and smooth muscle cells. Yoo *et al.* (1998) and Oberpenning *et al.* (1999) reported on the feasibility of dog bladder augmentation using allogenic bladder submucosa or polyglycolic acid polymers seeded with urothelial and smooth muscle cells. Organized bladder histology was noted in the regenerated bladder tissue. More importantly, the regenerated bladder tissue was found to increase bladder capacity and was urodynamically compliant.

It is clear that bladder regeneration is possible using both unseeded and seeded tissue-engineering technologies. Further advances in current techniques will eventually revolutionize urologic reconstructive surgery as we know it today. Additional work is need-ed before clinical application of these techniques. All of the animal studies performed thus far have been in animals with a normal bladder. It is not known whether normal or abnormal bladder regeneration can be achieved with either unseeded or seeded technology in an animal or a patient with a neuropathic bladder. Active research is currently being done to investigate this vital question. Studies are also needed to understand the differences between the unseeded and seeded approaches and the resultant regenerated bladder, such that the best aspects of each technology may be used to achieve a superior result. It is likely that future chapters on bladder augmentation will discuss the use of intestinal segments as a historical footnote, while the major focus will be on the indications and methods for various types of tissue-engineering technologies.

References

Adams MC, Mitchell ME, Rink RC (1988) Gastrocystoplasty: an alternative solution to the problem of urological reconstruction in the severely compromised patient. *J Urol* **140**: 1152–6.

Agishi T, Nakazono M, Kiraly RJ *et al.* (1975) Biodegradable material for bladder reconstruction. *J Biomed Mater Res* **9**: 119–31.

Ahmed S, Sripathi V, Sen S (1998a) Perforation of an autoaugmented bladder. *Aust NZ J Surg* **68**: 617–19.

Ahmed S, Neel KF, Sen S (1998b) Tandem ureterocystoplasty. *Aust NZ J Surg* **68**: 203–5.

Akerlund S, Delin K, Kock NG *et al.* (1989) Renal function and upper urinary tract configuration following urinary diversion to a continent ileal reservoir (Kock pouch): a prospective 5 to 11-year followup after reservoir construction. *J Urol* **142**: 964–8.

Anderson PA, Rickwood AM (1991) Detrusor hyper-reflexia as a factor in spontaneous perforation of augmentation cystoplasty for neuropathic bladder. *Br J Urol* **67**: 210–12.

Ashkar L, Heller E (1967) The silastic bladder patch. *J Urol* **98**: 679–83.

Atala A, Vacanti JP, Peters CA *et al.* (1992) Formation of urothelial structures *in vivo* from dissociated cells attached to biodegradable polymer scaffolds *in vitro*. *J Urol* **148**: 658–62.

Atala A, Bauer SB, Hendren WH, Retik AB (1993) The effect of gastric augmentation on bladder function. *J Urol* **149**: 1099–102.

Badylak SF (1994) The immunogenic response of SIS (personal communication).

Badylak SF (1996) Speculation (with a little evidence) for the foles of cell proliferation, differentiation, neovascularization, and environmental stressors in SIS-induced remodeling. In: *First SIS Symposium*, Orlando, FL, 1996.

Badylak SF, Lantz GC, Coffey A, Geddes LA (1989) Small intestinal submucosa as a large diameter vascular graft in the dog. *J Surg Res* **47**: 74–80.

Barrington JW, Fern-Davies H, Adams RJ *et al.* (1995) Bile acid dysfunction after clam enterocystoplasty. *Br J Urol* **76**: 169–71.

Barrington JW, Fraylin L, Fish R *et al.* (1996a) Elevated levels of basic fibroblast growth factor in the urine of clam enterocystoplasty patients. *J Urol* **155**: 468–70.

Barrington JW, Fulford S, Fraylin L (1996b). Reduction of urinary basic fibroblast growth factor using pentosan polysulphate sodium. *Br J Urol* **78**: 54–6.

Barrington JW, Fulford S, Griffiths D, Stephenson TP (1997a) Tumors in bladder remnant after augmentation enterocystoplasty. *J Urol* **157**: 482–5; Discussion 485–6.

Barrington JW, Jones A, James D (1997b) Antioxidant deficiency following clam enterocystoplasty. *Br J Urol* **80**: 238–42.

Baskin LS, Hayward SW, Sutherland RA *et al.* (1996) Mesenchymal–epithelial interactions in the bladder. *World J Urol* **14**: 301–9.

Bauer SB, Hendren WH, Kozakewich H *et al.* (1992) Perforation of the augmented bladder. *J Urol* **148**: 699–703.

Bellinger MF (1993) Ureterocystoplasty: a unique method for vesical augmentation in children. *J Urol* **149**: 811–13.

Bellinger MF (1998) Ureterocystoplasty update. *World J Urol* **16**: 251–4.

Ben-Chaim J, Partin AW, Jeffs RD (1996) Ureteral bladder augmentation using the lower pole ureter of a duplicated system. *Urology* **47**: 135–7.

Blyth B, Ewalt DH, Duckett JW, Snyder HMd (1992) Lithogenic properties of enterocystoplasty. *J Urol* **148**: 575–7; Discussion 578–9.

Bogaert GA, Mevorach RA, Kogan BA (1994) Urodynamic and clinical follow-up of 28 children after gastrocystoplasty. *Br J Urol* **74**: 469–75.

Bogaert GA, Mevorach RA, Kim J, Kogan BA (1995) The physiology of gastrocystoplasty: once a stomach, always a stomach. *J Urol* **153**: 1977–80.

Bohne AW, Osborn RW, Hettle PJ (1955) Regeneration of the urinary bladder in the dog, following total cystectomy. *Surg Gynecol Obstet* **100**: 259–64.

Bohne AW, Urwiller KL (1957) Experience with urinary bladder regeneration. *J Urol* **77**: 725–32.

Braren V, Bishop MR (1998) Laparoscopic bladder autoaugmentation in children. *Urol Clin North Am* **25**: 533–40.

Braverman RM, Lebowitz RL (1991) Perforation of the augmented urinary bladder in nine children and adolescents: importance of cystography. *AJR Am J Roentgenol* **157**: 1059–63.

Britanisky RG, Poppas DP, Shichman SN *et al.* (1995) Laparoscopic laser-assisted bladder autoaugmentation. *Urology* **46**: 31–5.

Brough RJ, O'Flynn KJ, Fishwick J, Gough DC (1998)

Bladder washout and stone formation in paediatric enterocystoplasty. *Eur Urol* **33**: 500–2.

Bruce AW, Reid G, Chan RC, Costerton JW (1984) Bacterial adherence in the human ileal conduit: a morphological and bacteriological study. *J Urol* **132**: 184–8.

Buson H, Manivel JC, Dayanc M *et al.* (1994) Seromuscular colocystoplasty lined with urothelium: experimental study. *Urology* **44**: 743–8.

Carr MC, Docimo SG, Mitchell ME (1999) Bladder augmentation with urothelial preservation. *J Urol* **162**: 1133–6; Discussion 1137.

Cartwright PC, Snow BW (1989a) Bladder autoaugmentation: partial detrusor excision to augment the bladder without use of bowel. *J Urol* **142**: 1050–3.

Cartwright PC, Snow BW (1989b) Bladder autoaugmentation: early clinical experience. *J Urol* **142**: 505–8; Discussion 520–1.

Cartwright PC, Snow BW (1999) Autoaugmentation cystoplasty. In: Dewan PA, Mitchell ME (eds) *Bladder augmentation*. London: Edward Arnold, 83–92.

Celayir S, Goksel S, Unal T, Buyukunal SN (1997) *Helicobacter pylori* infection in a child with gastric augmentation. *J Pediatr Surg* **32**: 1757–8.

Chancellor MB, Rivas DA, Bourgeois IM (1996) Laplace's law and the risks and prevention of bladder rupture after enterocystoplasty and bladder autoaugmentation. *Neurourol Urodyn* **15**: 223–33.

Cheng E, Rento R, Grayhack JT *et al.* (1994) Reversed seromuscular flaps in the urinary tract in dogs. *J Urol* **152**: 2252–7.

Churchill BM, Aliabadi H, Landau EH *et al.* (1993) Ureteral bladder augmentation. *J Urol* **150**: 716–20.

Churchill BM, Jayanthi VR, Landau EH *et al.* (1995) Ureterocystoplasty: importance of the proximal blood supply. *J Urol* **154**: 197–8.

Cilento BG, Freeman MR, Schneck FX *et al.* (1994) Phenotypic and cytogenetic characterization of human bladder urothelia expanded *in vitro*. *J Urol* **152**: 665–70.

Couillard DR, Vapnek JM, Rentzepis MJ, Stone AR (1993) Fatal perforation of augmentation cystoplasty in an adult. *Urology* **42**: 585–8.

Crane JM, Scherz HS, Billman GF, Kaplan GW (1991) Ischemic necrosis: a hypothesis to explain the pathogenesis of spontaneously ruptured enterocystoplasty. *J Urol* **146**: 141–4.

de Badiola F, Manivel JC, Gonzalez R (1991) Seromuscular enterocystoplasty in rats. *J Urol* **146**: 559–62.

de Badiola FI, Castro-Diaz D, Hart-Austin C, Gonzalez R (1992) Influence of preoperative bladder capacity and compliance on the outcome of artificial sphincter implantation in patients with neurogenic sphincter incompetence. *J Urol* **148**: 1493–5.

de Badiola FI, Denes ED, Ruiz E *et al.* (1996) New application of the gastrostomy button for clinical and urodynamic evaluation before vesicostomy closure. *J Urol* **156**: 618–20.

Denes ED, Vates TS, Freedman AL, Gonzalez R (1997) Seromuscular colocystoplasty lined with urothelium protects dogs from acidosis during ammonium chloride loading. *J Urol* **158**: 1075–80.

Dewan PA, Stefanek W (1994) Autoaugmentation gastrocystoplasty: early clinical results. *Br J Urol* **74**: 460–4.

Dewan PA, Stefanek W, Lorenz C, Byard RW (1994a) Autoaugmentation omentocystoplasty in a sheep model. *Urology* **43**: 888–91.

Dewan PA, Lorenz C, Stefanek W, Byard RW (1994b) Urothelial lined colocystoplasty in a sheep model. *Eur Urol* **26**: 240–6.

Dewan PA, Chacko J, Ashwood P (1995a) Gastrocystoplasty: technical and metabolic characteristics of the most versatile childhood bladder augmentation modality (Letter; Comment). *J Pediatr Surg* **30**: 1531–2.

Dewan PA, Owen AJ, Stefanek W *et al.* (1995b) Late follow up of autoaugmentation omentocystoplasty in a sheep model. *Aust N Z J Surg* **65**: 596–9.

Dewan PA, Close CE, Byard RW *et al.* (1997) Enteric mucosal regrowth after bladder augmentation using demucosalized gut segments. *J Urol* **158**: 1141–6.

Di Benedetto V, Monfort G (1997) Stomach versus sigmoid colon in children undergoing major reconstruction of the lower urinary tract. *Pediatr Surg Int* **12**: 393–6.

DiSandro MJ, Li Y, Baskin LS *et al.* (1998) Mesenchymal–epithelial interactions in bladder smooth muscle development: epithelial specificity. *J Urol* **160**: 1040–6; Discussion 1079.

Docimo SG, Moore RG, Adams J, Kavoussi LR (1995) Laparoscopic bladder augmentation using stomach. *Urology* **46**: 565–9.

Docimo SG, Orth CR, Schulam PG (1998) Percutaneous cystolithotomy after augmentation cystoplasty: comparison with open procedures. *Tech Urol* **4**: 43–5.

Duel BP, Gonzalez R, Barthold JS (1998) Alternative techniques for augmentation cystoplasty. *J Urol* **59**: 998–1005.

Ehrlich RM, Gershman A (1993) Laparoscopic seromyotomy (auto-augmentation) for non-neurogenic neurogenic bladder in a child: initial case report. *Urology* **42**: 175–8.

Elder JS, Snyder HM, Hulbert WC, Duckett JW (1988) Perforation of the augmented bladder in patients undergoing clean intermittent catheterization. *J Urol* **140**: 1159–62.

El-Ghoneimi A, Muller C, Guys JM *et al.* (1998) Functional outcome and specific complications of gastrocystoplasty for failed bladder exstrophy closure. *J Urol* **160**: 1186–9.

Essig KA, Sheldon CA, Brandt MT *et al.* (1991) Elevated intravesical pressure causes arterial hypoperfusion in canine colocystoplasty: a fluorometric assessment. *J Urol* **146**: 551–3.

Filmer RB, Spencer JR (1990) Malignancies in bladder augmentations and intestinal conduits. *J Urol* **143**: 671–8.

Firlit CF (1976) Use of defunctionalized bladders in pediatric renal transplantation. *J Urol* **116**: 634–7.

Fishman IJ, Flores FN, Scott B *et al.* (1987) Use of fresh placental membranes for bladder reconstruction. *J Urol* **138**: 1291.

Flood HD, Malhotra SJ, O'Connell HE *et al.* (1995) Long-term results and complications using augmentation cystoplasty in reconstructive urology. *Neurourol Urodyn* **14**: 297–309.

Glass RB, Rushton HG (1992) Delayed spontaneous rupture of augmented bladder in children: diagnosis with sonography and CT. *AJR Am J Roentgenol* **158**: 833–5.

Gleason DM, Gittes RF, Bottaccini MR, Byrne JC (1972) Energy balance of voiding after cecal cystoplasty. *J Urol* **108**: 259–64.

Goldwasser B, Barrett DM, Webster GD, Kramer SA (1987) Cystometric properties of ileum and right colon after bladder augmentation, substitution or replacement. *J Urol* **138**: 1007–8.

Gonzalez R, Buson H, Reid C, Reinberg Y (1995) Seromuscular colocystoplasty lined with urothelium: experience with 16 patients. *Urology* **45**: 124–9.

Gorham S, McCafferty I, Baraza R, Scott R (1984) Preliminary development of a collagen membrane for use in urological surgery. *Urol Res* **12**: 295–9.

Gosalbez R Jr, Woodard JR, Broecker BH *et al.* (1993a) The use of stomach in pediatric urinary reconstruction. *J Urol* **150**: 438–40.

Gosalbez R Jr, Woodard JR, Broecker BH, Warshaw B (1993b) Metabolic complications of the use of stomach for urinary reconstruction. *J Urol* **150**: 710–12.

Gosalbez R Jr, Kim CO Jr (1996) Ureterocystoplasty with preservation of ipsilateral renal function. *J Pediatr Surg* **31**: 970–5.

Hedican SP, Schulam PG, Docimo SG (1999) Laparoscopic assisted reconstructive surgery. *J Urol* **161**: 267–70.

Hendren WH, Hendren RB (1990) Bladder augmentation: experience with 129 children and young adults. *J Urol* **144**: 445–53; Discussion 460.

Herschorn S, Hewitt RJ (1998) Patient perspective of long-term outcome of augmentation cystoplasty for neurogenic bladder. *Urology* **52**: 672–8.

Hinman F Jr (1988) Selection of intestinal segments for bladder substitution: physical and physiological characteristics. *J Urol* **139**: 519–23.

Hirst G (1991) Ileal and colonic cystoplasties. In: Rowland RB (ed.) *Problems in urology*. Hagerstown: JB Lippincott, **223**.

Hitchcock RJ, Duffy PG, Malone PS (1994) Ureterocystoplasty: the 'bladder' augmentation of choice. *Br J Urol* **73**: 575–9.

Hochstetler JA, Flanigan MJ, Kreder KJ (1997) Impaired bone growth after ileal augmentation cystoplasty. *J Urol* **157**: 1873–9.

Hodde JP, Badylak SF, Brightman AO, Voytik-Harbin SL (1996) Glycosaminoglycan content of small intestinal submucosa: a bioscaffold for tissue replacement. *Tissue Eng* **2**: 209–17.

Ikeguchi EF, Stifelman MD, Hensle TW (1998) Ureteral tissue expansion for bladder augmentation. *J Urol* **159**: 1665–8.

Jayanthi VR, Churchill BM, McLorie GA, Khoury AE (1995) Concomitant bladder neck closure and Mitrofanoff diversion for the management of intractable urinary incontinence. *J Urol* **154**: 886–8.

Johnson HW, Nigro MK, Stothers L (1994) Laboratory variables of bladder autoaugmentation in an animal model. *Urology* **44**: 260–3.

Kabalin JN (1998) Surgical anatomy of the retroperitoneum, kidneys, and ureters. In: Walsh PC, Retik AB, Vaughn ED,

Wein AG (eds) *Campbell's urology*. 7th edition. Philadelphia, PA: WB Saunders, 49–89.

Kaefer M, Hendren WH, Bauer SB *et al*. (1998) Reservoir calculi: a comparison of reservoirs constructed from stomach and other enteric segments. *J Urol* 1998; **160**: 2187–90.

Kajbafzadeh AM, Quinn FM, Duffy PG, Ransley PG (1995) Augmentation cystoplasty in boys with posterior urethral valves. *J Urol* **154**: 874–7.

Kambic H, Kay R, Chen JF *et al*. (1992) Biodegradable pericardial implants for bladder augmentation: a 2.5-year study in dogs. *J Urol* **148**: 539–43.

Keating MA, Ludlow JK, Rich MA (1996) Enterocystoplasty: the star modification. *J Urol* **155**: 1723–5.

Khoury AE, Salomon M, Doche R *et al*. (1997) Stone formation after augmentation cystoplasty: the role of intestinal mucus. *J Urol* **158**: 1133–7.

Kilic N, Celayir S, Elicevik M *et al*. (1999) Bladder augmentation: urodynamic findings and clinical outcome in different augmentation techniques. *Eur J Pediatr Surg* **9**: 29–32.

Kinahan TJ, Khoury AE, McLorie GA, Churchill BM (1992) Omeprazole in post-gastrocystoplasty metabolic alkalosis and aciduria. *J Urol* **47**: 435–7.

King L (1987) Protection of the upper tracts in children. In: King LR, Stone AR, Webster GD (eds) *Bladder reconstruction and continent urinary diversion*. Chicago, IL: Year Book Medical Publishers, **127**.

King LR, Webster GD, Bertram RA (1987) Experiences with bladder reconstruction in children. *J Urol* **138**: 1002–6.

Koch MO, McDougal WS (1985) The pathophysiology of hyperchloremic metabolic acidosis after urinary diversion through intestinal segments. *Surgery* **98**: 561–70.

Kockum CC, Helin I, Malmberg L, Malmfors G (1999) Pediatric urinary tract reconstruction using intestine. *Scand J Urol Nephrol* **33**: 53–6.

Koff SA (1988) Guidelines to determine the size and shape of intestinal segments used for reconstruction. *J Urol* **140**: 1150–1.

Kronner KM, Rink RC, Simmons G *et al*. (1998a). Artificial urinary sphincter in the treatment of urinary incontinence: preoperative urodynamics do not predict the need for future bladder augmentation. *J Urol* **160**: 1093–5; Discussion 1103.

Kronner KM, Casale AJ, Cain MP *et al*. (1998b) Bladder calculi in the pediatric augmented bladder. *J Urol* **160**: 1096–8; Discussion 1103.

Kropp BP (1998) Small-intestinal submucosa for bladder augmentation: a review of preclinical studies. *World J Urol* **16**: 262–7.

Kropp BP, Badylak S, Thor KB (1995a) Regenerative bladder augmentation: a review of the initial preclinical studies with porcine small intestinal submucosa. *Adv Exp Med Biol* **385**: 229–35.

Kropp BP, Eppley BL, Prevel CD *et al*. (1995b) Experimental assessment of small intestinal submucosa as a bladder wall substitute. *Urology* **46**: 396–400.

Kropp BP, Rippy MK, Badylak SF *et al*. (1996a) Regenerative urinary bladder augmentation using small intestinal submucosa: urodynamic and histopathologic assessment in long-term canine bladder augmentations. *J Urol* **155**: 2098–104.

Kropp BP, Sawyer BD, Shannon HE *et al*. (1996b) Characterization of small intestinal submucosa regenerated canine detrusor: assessment of reinnervation, *in vitro* compliance and contractility. *J Urol* **156**: 599–607.

Kudish HG (1957) The use of polyvinyl sponge for experimental cystoplasty. *J Urol* **78**: 232.

Kurzrock EA, Baskin LS, Kogan BA (1998a) Gastrocystoplasty: is there a consensus? *World J Urol* **16**: 242–50.

Kurzrock EA, Baskin LS, Kogan BA (1998b) Gastrocystoplasty: long-term followup. *J Urol* **160**: 2182–6.

Lailas NG, Cilento B, Atala A (1996) Progressive ureteral dilation for subsequent ureterocystoplasty. *J Urol* **156**: 1151–3.

Landau EH, Jayanthi VR, Khoury AE *et al*. (1994) Bladder augmentation: ureterocystoplasty versus ileocystoplasty. *J Urol* **152**: 716–19.

Lantz GC, Badylak SF, Coffey AC *et al*. (1990) Small intestinal submucosa as a small-diameter arterial graft in the dog. *J Invest Surg* **3**: 217–27.

Lantz GC, Badylak SF, Coffey AC *et al*. (1992) Small intestinal submucosa as a superior vena cava graft in the dog. *J Surg Res* **53**: 175–81.

Lapides J, Diokno AC, Silber SJ, Lowe BS (1972) Clean, intermittent self-catheterization in the treatment of urinary tract disease. *J Urol* **107**: 458–61.

Lapides J, Diokno AC, Gould FR, Lowe BS (1976) Further observations on self-catheterization. *J Urol* **116**: 169–71.

Leng WW, Blalock HJ, Fredriksson WH *et al*. (1999) Enterocystoplasty or detrusor myectomy? Comparison of indications and outcomes for bladder augmentation. *J Urol* **161**: 758–63.

Leong CH, Ong GB (1972) Gastrocystoplasty in dogs. *Aust N Z J Surg* **41**: 272–9.

Leong CH, Ong GB (1975) Proceedings: gastrocystoplasty. *Br J Urol* **47**: 236.

Lewis AG, Gardner B, Gilbert A *et al*. (1995) Relative microbial resistance of gastric, ileal and cecal bladder augmentation in the rat. *J Urol* **154**: 1895–9.

Lindner H (1989) *Clinical anatomy*. Norwalk, CT: Appleton and Lange.

MacGregor P, Novick AC, Cunningham R *et al*. (1986) Renal transplantation in end stage renal disease patients with existing urinary diversion. *J Urol* **135**: 686–8.

McDougal WS (1992) Metabolic complications of urinary intestinal diversion. *J Urol* **147**: 1199–208.

McDougall EM, Clayman RV, Figenshau RS, Pearle MS (1995) Laparoscopic retropubic auto-augmentation of the bladder. *J Urol* **153**: 123–6.

McKenna PC, Bauer MB (1995) Bladder augmentation with ureter. *Dialog Pediatr Urol* **18**: 4–5.

Metzger DW, Moyad TF, McPherson T, Badylak SF (1996) Cytokine and antibody responses to xenogeneic SIS transplants. In: *First SIS Symposium*, Orlando, FL, 1996.

Mitchell ME (1994) Gastrocystoplasty. In: Hinman FJ (ed.)

Atlas of pediatric urologic surgery. Philadelphia, PA: WB Saunders, **473**.

Mitchell ME, Piser JA (1987) Intestinocystoplasty and total bladder replacement in children and young adults: follow-up in 129 cases. *J Urol* **138**: 579–84.

Mitchell ME, Rink RC, Adams MC (1992) Augmentation cystoplasty implantation of artificial urinary sphincter in men and women and reconstruction of the dysfunctional urinary tract. In: Walsh PC, Retik AB, Stamey TA, Vaughn ED (eds) *Campbell's urology*. 6th edition. Philadelphia, PA: WB Saunders, 2654–716.

Mundy AR, Nurse DE (1992) Calcium balance, growth and skeletal mineralisation in patients with cystoplasties. *Br J Urol* **69**: 257–9.

Nasrallah PF, Aliabadi HA (1991) Bladder augmentation in patients with neurogenic bladder and vesicoureteral reflux. *J Urol* **146**: 563–6.

N'Dow J, Leung HY, Marshall C, Neal DE (1998) Bowel dysfunction after bladder reconstruction. *J Urol* **159**: 1470–4; Discussion 1474–5.

Nguyen DH, Bain MA, Salmonson KL (1993) The syndrome of dysuria and hematuria in pediatric urinary reconstruction with stomach. *J Urol* **150**: 707–9.

Nurse DE, Mundy AR (1989) Assessment of the malignant potential of cystoplasty. *Br J Urol* **64**: 489–92.

Oberpenning F, Meng J, Yoo JJ, Atala A (1999) *De novo* reconstitution of a functional mammalian urinary bladder by tissue engineering. *Nat Biotechnol* **17**: 149–55.

Oesch I (1988) Neourothelium in bladder augmentation. An experimental study in rats. *Eur Urol* **14**: 328–9.

Oldwasser B, Barrett DM, Webster GD, Kramer SA (1987) Cystometric properties of ileum and right colon after bladder augmentation, substitution or replacement. *J Urol* **138**: 1007–8.

Ortiz V, Goldenberg S (1995) Hypergastrinemia following gastrocystoplasty in rats. *Urol Res* **23**: 361–3.

Palmer LS, Franco I, Kogan SJ *et al.* (1993) Urolithiasis in children following augmentation cystoplasty. *J Urol* **150**: 726–9.

Palmer LS, Franco I, Reda EF *et al.* (1994) Endoscopic management of bladder calculi following augmentation cystoplasty. *Urology* **44**: 902–4.

Palmer LS, Palmer JS, Firlit BM, Firlit CF (1998) Recurrent urolithiasis after augmentation gastrocystoplasty. *J Urol* **159**: 1331–2.

Piechota HJ, Dahms SE, Nunes LS (1998a) *in vitro* functional properties of the rat bladder regenerated by the bladder acellular matrix graft. *J Urol* **159**: 1717–24.

Piechota HJ, Dahms SE, Probst M *et al.* (1998b) Functional rat bladder regeneration through xenotransplantation of the bladder acellular matrix graft. *Br J Urol* **81**: 548–59.

Piser JA, Mitchell ME, Kulb TB *et al.* (1987) Gastrocystoplasty and colocystoplasty in canines: the metabolic consequences of acute saline and acid loading. *J Urol* **138**: 1009–13.

Plawker MW, Rabinowitz SS, Etwaru DJ, Glassberg KI (1995) Hypergastrinemia, dysuria–hematuria and metabolic alkalosis: complications associated with gastrocystoplasty. *J Urol* **154**: 546–9.

Pope JC, Davis MM, Smith ER Jr *et al.* (1997) The ontogeny of canine small intestinal submucosa regenerated bladder. *J Urol* **158**: 1105–10.

Pope JC, Keating MA, Casale AJ, Rink RC (1998) Augmenting the augmented bladder: treatment of the contractile bowel segment. *J Urol* **160**: 854–7.

Powell DW (1987) Intestinal water and electrolyte transport. In: Johnson LR (ed.) *Physiology of the gastrointestinal tract*. 2nd edition. New York: Raven Press, **1267**.

Probst M, Dahiya R, Carrier S, Tanagho EA (1997) Reproduction of functional smooth muscle tissue and partial bladder replacement. *Br J Urol* **79**: 505–15.

Raz S, Ehrlich RM, Babiarz JW, Payne CK (1993) Gastrocystoplasty without opening the stomach. *J Urol* **150**: 713–15.

Reddy PP, Barrieras DJ, Wilson G (2000) Regeneration of functional bladder substitutes using large segmented acellular matrix allografts in a porcine model. *J Urol* **164**: 936–41.

Reinberg Y, Manivel JC, Froemming C, Gonzalez R (1992) Perforation of the gastric segment of an augmented bladder secondary to peptic ulcer disease. *J Urol* **148**: 369–71.

Reinberg Y, Allen RC Jr, Vaughn M, McKenna PH (1995) Nephrectomy combined with lower abdominal extra-peritoneal ureteral bladder augmentation in the treatment of children with the vesicoureteral reflux dysplasia syndrome. *J Urol* **153**: 177–9.

Rink R, Mitchell M (1990) Role of enterocystoplasty in reconstructing the neurogenic bladder. In: Gonzales E, Roth D (eds) *Common problems in pediatric urology*. St. Louis, MO: Mosby Year Book, 192–204.

Rink RC (1994) Gastrocystoplasty. In: Hinman FJ (ed.) *Atlas of pediatric urologic surgery*. Philadelphia, PA: WB Saunders, 472–3.

Rink RC (1999) Bladder augmentation. Options, outcomes, future. *Urol Clin North Am* **26**: 111–23, viii–ix.

Rink RC, Adams MC (1998) Augmentation cystoplasty. In: Walsh PC, Retik AB, Vaughan ED, Wein AJ (eds) *Campbell's urology*. 7th edition. Philadelphia, PA: WB Saunders, 3167–89.

Rink RC, Hollensbe D, Adams MC (1995) Complications of bladder augmentation in children and comparison of gastrointestinal segments. *AUA Update Series* **14**: 122–7.

Rivas DA, Chancellor MB, Huang B *et al.* (1996) Comparison of bladder rupture pressure after intestinal bladder augmentation (ileocystoplasty) and myomyotomy (autoaugmentation). *Urology* **48**: 40–6.

Robertson AS, Davies JB, Webb RJ, Neal DE (1991) Bladder augmentation and replacement. Urodynamic and clinical review of 25 patients. *Br J Urol* **68**: 590–7.

Rosen MA, Light JK (1991) Spontaneous bladder rupture following augmentation enterocystoplasty. *J Urol* **146**: 1232–4.

Rushton HG, Woodard JR, Parrott TS *et al.* (1988) Delayed bladder rupture after augmentation enterocystoplasty. *J Urol* **140**: 344–6.

Salle JL, Fraga JC, Lucib A *et al.* (1990) Seromuscular enterocystoplasty in dogs. *J Urol* **144**: 454–6; Discussion 460.

Salomon L, Lugagne PM, Herve JM *et al.* (1997) No evidence

of metabolic disorders 10 to 22 years after Camey type I ileal enterocystoplasty. *J Urol* **157**: 2104–6.

Scott R, Mohammed R, Gorham SD *et al.* (1988) The evolution of a biodegradable membrane for use in urological surgery. A summary of 109 *in vivo* experiments. *Br J Urol* **62**: 26–31.

Serrano DP, Flechner SM, Modlin CS *et al.* (1996) Transplantation into the long-term defunctionalized bladder. *J Urol* **156**: 885–8.

Sheiner JR, Kaplan GW (1988) Spontaneous bladder rupture following enterocystoplasty. *J Urol* **140**: 1157–8.

Sheldon CA, Gilbert A, Wacksman J, Lewis AG (1995) Gastrocystoplasty: technical and metabolic characteristics of the most versatile childhood bladder augmentation modality. *J Pediatr Surg* **30**: 283–7; Discussion 287–8.

Shoemaker WC (1955) Reversed seromuscular grafts in ureinart tract reconstruction. *J Urol* **74**: 453.

Shoemaker WC, Marucci HD (1955) The experimental use of of seromuscular grafts in bladder reconstruction: preliminary report. *J Urol* **73**: 314.

Shokeir AA, Shamaa M, el-Mekresh MM, el-Baz M, Ghoneim MA (1995) Late malignancy in bowel segments exposed to urine without fecal stream. *Urology* **46**: 657–61.

Sinaiko ES (1956) Artificial bladder from segment of stomach and study effect of urine on gastric secretion. *Surg Gynecol Obstet* **102**: 433–8.

Singh G, Thomas DG (1997) Bowel problems after enterocystoplasty. *Br J Urol* **79**: 328–32.

Skobejko-Wlodarska L, Strulak K, Nachulewicz P, Szymkiewicz C (1998) Bladder autoaugmentation in myelodysplastic children. *Br J Urol* **81 (Suppl 3)**: 114–16.

Slaton JW, Kropp KA (1994) Conservative management of suspected bladder rupture after augmentation enterocystoplasty. *J Urol* **152**: 713–15.

Snow BW, Cartwright PC (1996) Bladder autoaugmentation. *Urol Clin North Am* **23**: 323–31.

Stampfer DS, McDougal WS (1997) Inhibition of the sodium/hydrogen antiport by ammonium ion. *J Urol* **157**: 362–5.

Stampfer DS, McDougal WS, McGovern FJ (1997) The use of in bowel urology. Metabolic and nutritional complications. *Urol Clin North Am* **24**: 715–22.

Stein R, Lotz J, Andreas J *et al.* (1998) Long-term metabolic effects in patients with urinary diversion. *World J Urol* **16**: 292–7.

Stifelman MD, Ikeguchi EF, Hensle TW (1998) Ureteral tissue expansion for bladder augmentation: a long-term prospective controlled trial in a porcine model. *J Urol* **160**: 1826–9.

Stohrer M, Kramer A, Goepel M *et al.* (1995) Bladder autoaugmentation – an alternative for enterocystoplasty: preliminary results. *Neurourol Urodyn* **14**: 11–23.

Stohrer M, Kramer G, Goepel M *et al.* (1997) Bladder autoaugmentation in adult patients with neurogenic voiding dysfunction. *Spinal Cord* **35**: 456–62.

Stothers L, Johnson H, Arnold W *et al.* (1994) Bladder autoaugmentation by vesicomyotomy in the pediatric neurogenic bladder. *Urology* **44**: 110–13.

Sutherland RS, Baskin LS, Hayward SW, Cunha GR (1996) Regeneration of bladder urothelium, smooth muscle, blood vessels and nerves into an acellular tissue matrix. *J Urol* **156**: 571–7.

Swinney J, Tomlinson BE, Walder DN (1961) Urinary tract substitution. *Br J Urol* **33**: 414–27.

Tizzoni G, Poggi A (1888) Die Wiederherstellung der Harnblase: experimentelle Untersuchungen. *Centralbl Chir* **15**: 921.

Voytik-Harbin SL, Brightman AO, Kraine MR *et al.* (1997) Identification of extractable growth factors from small intestinal submucosa. *J Cell Biochem* **67**: 478–91.

Wolf JS Jr, Turzan CW (1993) Augmentation ureterocystoplasty. *J Urol* **149**: 1095–8.

Yoo JJ, Meng J, Oberpenning F, Atala A (1998) Bladder augmentation using allogenic bladder submucosa seeded with cells. *Urology* **51**: 221–5.

Urinary diversion

17

R.C. Rink and Mark P. Cain

Introduction

The past two decades have seen tremendous advances in lower urinary reconstruction in children. The majority of congenital urologic abnormalities can now be addressed by primary reconstruction without the need to divert the urine. These reconstructions can often be performed even in the smallest of neonates. Thus, the need for permanent conduit diversion with the storage receptacle outside the body as a bag has dwindled, and is now used primarily in children who will never be independent. When permanent urinary diversion is required it is nearly always of the continent variety with an internal storage receptacle constructed that is then emptied by intermittent catheterization. This chapter will primarily focus on these continent urinary reservoirs (CURs).

Some urologic problems remain, primarily severe urinary obstruction in the neonate, for which definitive reconstruction may not initially be appropriate. In this group temporary diversion may become necessary. Intubated diversions are generally reserved for patients requiring a short duration (weeks to a few months) of urinary drainage. These may be especially useful in the setting of an unstable or a small premature child who requires relief of obstruction, or when renal function cannot be adequately assessed without first alleviating the obstruction. These non-continent urinary diversions will be briefly discussed.

Temporary urinary diversion

Temporary intubated diversions

Urethral catheter

The simplest and most frequently used form of intubated urinary diversion is the urethral catheter. The most common urologic condition managed initially with a urethral catheter in the neonate is a posterior urethral valve (PUV). A 5 or 8 Fr feeding tube may be used to drain the bladder temporarily prior to valve fulguration. In any male with a dilated posterior urethra, the catheter will occasionally coil in the prostatic urethra and inadequately drain the bladder. In this situation a small lacrimal duct probe can be used as a catheter guide. It can also be helpful to elevate the posterior urethra by pushing anteriorly with the index finger in the rectum. Whenever the catheter is difficult to pass, it is helpful to obtain an abdominal radiograph, after injecting a small amount of contrast through the catheter, to ensure its proper position in the bladder. In the older child who requires bladder drainage, a 6 or 8 Fr balloon (Foley) catheter is a reasonable alternative, there being less chance of inadvertent removal of this catheter compared with a feeding tube. Intermittent catheterization is another option for children with urinary retention and has proven to be safe in even the small neonate.

Complications of urethral catheters in children are primarily related to improper placement or prolonged use, and include urethral injury, urethritis or meatitis, urinary tract infection (UTI), urethral stricture, and bladder stones.

Suprapubic cystotomy (percutaneous)

In the rare circumstance when a urethral catheter is contraindicated or cannot be placed, a suprapubic cystotomy tube will provide short- or long-term bladder drainage. Percutaneous cystotomy is very useful in the infant or child with urethral trauma or following a reconstructive procedure for epispadias or complex hypospadias. Many preassembled kits are available that rely on either the Seldinger technique or a trocar, with the catheter placed either simultaneously with the trocar (Stamey percutaneous suprapubic catheter set, Cook Urologic; Fig. 17.1) or through it (Cystocath suprapubic drainage system, dow corning; Fig. 17.2). A full bladder is a prerequisite to percutaneous

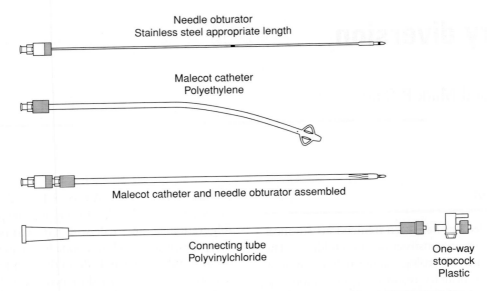

Needle obturator
Stainless steel appropriate length

Malecot catheter
Polyethylene

Malecot catheter and needle obturator assembled

Connecting tube
Polyvinylchloride

One-way
stopcock
Plastic

Figure 17.1 Diagram of Stamey Malecot percutaneous suprapubic tube set (Cook Urological, Spencer, IN, USA).

catheter placement and can be confirmed sonographically. If necessary, the bladder can be filled with a small urethral catheter or by percutaneously placing a small angiocatheter or spinal needle into the bladder for localization, and filling the bladder until it is palpable. When attempting to place a suprapubic tube in the awake child, conscious sedation and infiltration of the skin and fascia with 1% lidocaine can be used to prevent anxiety and pain. It is helpful to establish the distance from the skin to the bladder lumen with a small needle to prevent injury to any structure posterior to the bladder. The trocar is passed with gentle pressure until urine is obtained and the catheter is passed 1–2 cm beyond the trocar. Alternatively, the percutaneous

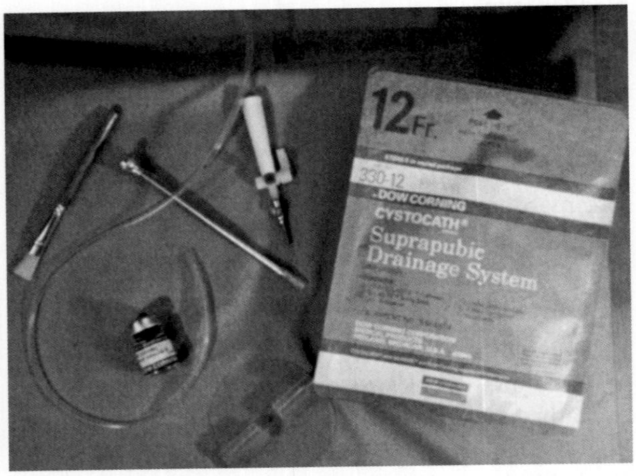

cystotomy tube and obturator are passed together into the bladder until urine is obtained, then the catheter is advanced over the obturator. A recently described technique using the light from a flexible cystoscope to help to localize the position of the bladder dome may allow percutaneous tube cystotomy in the more difficult cases (Alagiri and Seidmon, 1998). It is often safest to use the site of a prior suprapubic tract that is fixed to the posterior abdominal fascia to place suprapubic tubes in patients who have undergone previous urologic reconstructive procedures. The catheter is fixed to the skin with permanent suture. These tubes are designed for temporary bladder drainage, and long-term use has been associated with bladder wall thickening and contracture, UTI, bladder stones, and upper urinary tract dilatation (Belman, 1985; Duckett and Ziylan, 1995).

Surgically placed cystotomy

Because of the relative ease and safety of percutaneous cystotomy tube placement, open suprapubic tube placement is almost always used as a part of a more extensive reconstructive procedure, or for placement of a large-bore drainage tube following urethral or bladder trauma. Open placement is also necessary at times when a patient has had prior extensive pelvic procedures that may have resulted in bowel adhesions to the anterior dome of the bladder.

With the patient in the supine position, the perivesical space is exposed using either a low transverse

Figure 17.2 Trocar type of percutaneous suprapubic catheter set (Dow Corning Cystocath, Midland, MI, USA).

abdominal incision or a low vertical midline incision (for those that may later undergo a transabdominal reconstructive procedure). After selecting an appropriate mobile portion near the bladder dome, stay sutures are placed and a small cystotomy is made. If a Foley catheter is to be used for the suprapubic tube, it is first brought through a small skin incision and then through the rectus fascia and muscle. After the tube has been placed in the bladder it is pulled to the dome of the bladder. Bladder muscle adjacent to the tube is secured to the posterior fascial wall with absorbable suture. The suprapubic tube is sutured to the skin with permanent suture and taped to the abdominal wall.

Ureteral stents

Ureteral stents are frequently used for temporary upper tract drainage following reconstruction, trauma, or stone surgery in children. There are two general options available, either an entirely internal stent or a ureteral stent with the end brought out through the skin or via the urethra (external). External stents have traditionally been used more frequently in children following open surgery as they do not require an anesthetic for removal, and do not carry the same risk of proximal migration found with internal stents. A magnetically tipped stent has been developed that allows retrieval without anesthesia (Mykulak *et al.*, 1994), but this has not been widely used. Other problems have frequently been associated with JJ stents in children (Slaton and Kropp, 1996) including:

- encrustation/stone formation
- infection
- proximal migration
- stent fragmentation
- discomfort/bladder spasms
- requirement of anesthesia for removal of stent.

Internal stents can be placed either at the time of open surgery, endoscopically, or by means of an antegrade approach through a percutaneous nephrostomy tract. Endoscopic placement of internal stents is often difficult because of the small size of the working port of pediatric cystoscopes.

Percutaneous nephrostomy

The improvements in the availability and expertise of pediatric interventional radiologists have led to percutaneous nephrostomy tube drainage almost complete-

ly replacing the need for isolated open nephrostomy tube placement in children. Common indications for nephrostomy tube drainage in children include obstruction, renal/ureteral calculi, pyonephrosis, fungal bezoar, or for a diagnostic Whitaker study. Although general anesthesia will often be required in the young or uncooperative child, the procedure can frequently be performed with sedation only (Stanely and Diament, 1986), and has been reported in unstable neonates with only local anesthesia while in their incubators in the intensive care unit (Morelli *et al.*, 1997). The technique most commonly used is the Seldinger technique. A small needle is advanced into the renal pelvis using computerized tomography (CT), ultrasound, or fluoroscopic guidance. A small guidewire is then passed into the renal pelvis and the tract is dilated until a nephrostomy tube can be easily advanced. Multiple types of nephrostomy tubes are commercially available, most of which rely on a pigtail curl to maintain their position within the renal pelvis. It is critical that broad-spectrum intravenous antibiotics be initiated before tube placement, especially in the child with obstruction and infection, as any manipulation may precipitate an episode of urosepsis. Complications directly related to the procedure are rare (Farrell and Hicks, 1997; Papanicolaou, 1998) and include:

- hemorrhage
- urosepsis
- arteriovenous fistula/pseudoaneurysms
- urinary extravasation
- pneumothorax
- bowel injury
- air embolism.

Percutaneous nephrostomy tube placement and irrigation with antifungal agents have become the optimal treatment for neonates with obstructing fungal bezoars (Bell *et al.*, 1993; Bartone *et al.*, 1998). In addition to draining the obstruction and providing access for intermittent irrigation of the obstructed collecting system, the fungal ball can be fragmented with the guidewire at the time of tube placement, which will lead to more rapid clearance of the fungal debris.

Open nephrostomy tube

Open placement of a nephrostomy tube is indicated in instances when percutaneous nephrostomy is technically not possible, or carries too great a risk. These include low platelet count, solitary kidney, abnormal renal position following a complicated reconstruction of the renal pelvis and exploration for renal trauma when significant injury to the ureter or pelvis has occurred. The kidney is exposed through a small flank incision and mobilized until the renal pelvis is identified. After the pelvis has been secured with stay sutures a small pyelotomy is made and a clamp is passed into an inferior, dilated calyx. A small nephrotomy is made, and the Malecot catheter is advanced into the renal pelvis as shown in Figure 17.3. The catheter is secured to the renal capsule with a purse-string chromic suture. The nephrostomy tube is brought out through a stab incision in the skin and secured with sutures. A small Penrose drain is left in the renal fossa. Some newer catheters come pre-assembled as either simple nephrostomy catheters or nephrostents, often with an attached trocar that can be advanced in a retrograde fashion out of the selected calyx.

Temporary non-intubated diversion

Cutaneous vesicostomy

Cutaneous vesicostomy continues to be the most widely used and simplest method of temporary decompression of the obstructed urethra or bladder outlet. Most commonly it is used for patients with a neuropathic bladder or PUV. In multiple series temporary diversion with vesicostomy has resulted in significant improvement in urinary tract dilatation, stabilization of renal function, and decrease in the frequency and severity of febrile UTIs (Noe and Jerkins, 1985; Krahn and Johnson, 1993; Duckett and

Ziylan, 1995; Hutton and Thomas, 1998). The introduction of clean intermittent catheterization (CIC) in early infancy has limited the role of vesicostomy in some centers, and has provided equivalent long-term results (Edelstein et al., 1995). One concern regarding temporary cutaneous vesicostomy is potential impairment in bladder function due to inadequate cycling of the detrusor during the period of diversion. Jayanthi et al. (1995) reported on a large group of patients who underwent cutaneous vesicostomy and eventual bladder closure. They found no significant alteration in bladder capacity or function. These findings were also supported in a series of patients with PUV managed with either valve ablation or urinary tract diversion, with no evidence of bladder dysfunction based on urodynamic findings in those who had diversion with vesicostomy (Kim et al., 1996).

Two basic techniques are described for cutaneous vesicostomy in children. The procedure described by Lapides involves creation of extensive skin flaps to allow a tension-free anastomosis of the bladder to the skin, and a very wide stoma that is less prone to stenosis (Lapides et al., 1960). This procedure was initially intended as a semi-permanent form of vesicostomy in the adult patient, where the bladder position is deeper in the pelvis. Because of the complexity of both creating and taking down the Lapides vesicostomy there is limited application for the majority of pediatric patients. The more popular technique for vesicostomy in children was described by Blocksom (1957) and modified by Duckett et al. (1995), as outlined in Figure 17.4. The key technical points are: adequate mobilization of the bladder dome for a ten-

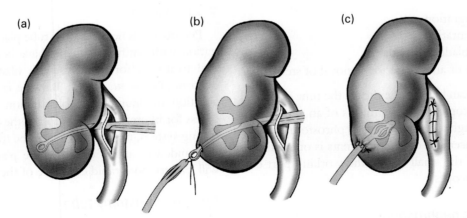

(a)   (b)   (c)

Figure 17.3 Technique for open nephrostomy. A small Randall forcep or right angle clamp is passed through an inferior calyx via a small pyelotomy incision. The renal capsule is incised with electrocautery and the catheter is advanced into the calyx. The catheter is secured to the renal capsule with absorbable suture. The pyelotomy is closed with either running or interrupted, absorbable suture.

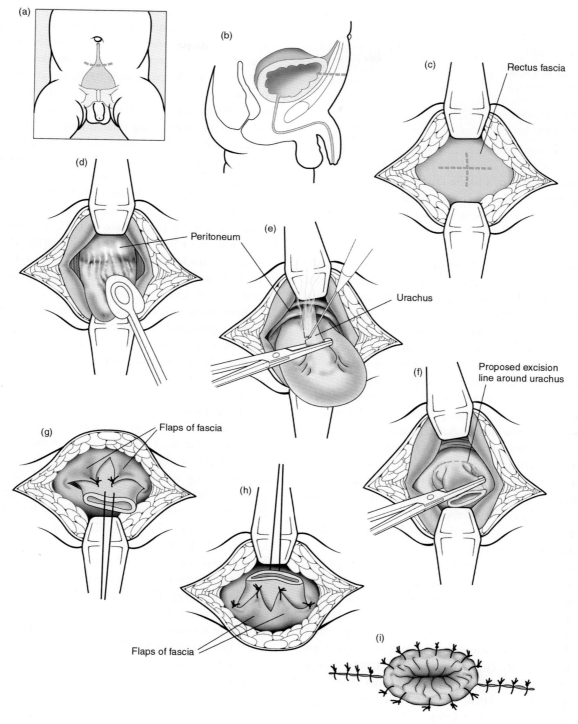

Figure 17.4 Technical points for Blocksom vesicostomy. (*a, b*) A small transverse skin incision is made midway between the pubis and umbilicus. (*c*) The rectus fascia is opened vertically and horizontally and the muscle is retracted laterally. (*d*) Stay sutures are placed in the bladder and the peritoneum is bluntly mobilized superiorly, exposing the bladder dome. (*e*) The urachus is identified and divided. The urachal segment is mobilized until it reaches the skin without tension. (*f*) The urachus is excised, ensuring an adequate caliber opening into the bladder (22–24 Fr). (*g*) The detrusor is circumferentially secured to the rectus fascia. (*h*) The lateral edges of the fascia are closed, allowing easy passage of a 22–24 Fr sound. (*i*) The bladder mucosa and detrusor are secured to the skin, and the lateral skin edges are closed in layers.

Table 17.1 Complications of cutaneous vesicostomy

Complication	Frequency (%)
Stomal prolapse	9–17
Stomal stenosis	3–12
Peristomal dermatitis	3–14
Stone formation	3–7
Parastomal hernia	3–4

From Skoog (1995).

sion-free anastomosis to the fascia and skin, use of the dome of the bladder to create the stoma, and creating an adequate caliber stoma (at least 22 Fr) that is flush with the skin (Duckett and Ziylan, 1995; Skoog, 1998).

Common problems following vesicostomy are listed in Table 17.1. The majority of complications that lead to stomal revision are secondary to technical errors of stomal placement, inadequate stomal diameter, or primary bladder pathology that results in an extremely thick-walled bladder that is difficult to mobilize to create an adequate caliber stoma.

Bladder prolapse through the vesicostomy stoma is usually due to placement of the stoma too inferior, allowing the more mobile posterior bladder wall to evert through the stoma. Acute prolapse can be managed with manual decompression and bladder drainage with a catheter through the vesicostomy until the edema subsides. Rarely, the prolapsed bladder will incarcerate, requiring emergency reduction under anesthesia. Revision of the vesicostomy by moving the stoma to a more superior position in the dome of the bladder will prevent recurrence.

The patient with stomal stenosis will often present with either UTI or worsening hydronephrosis. Stenosis is thought to occur secondary to excess tension on the skin anastomosis or too small a fascial opening, and is more frequent in patients with very thick-walled bladder or patients with prune belly syndrome (Duckett and Ziylan, 1995; Skoog, 1998). Simple revision with creation of a wider caliber stoma and occasional use of a small V-shaped skin flap to disrupt the circumferential stomal ring will usually correct the problem and prevent recurrence.

Cutaneous ureterostomy

The indications and need for temporary and permanent urinary diversion with cutaneous ureterostomy or pyelostomy have been significantly reduced over the past several decades. Advances in percutaneous and endoscopic techniques, new options for managing the obstructed urinary tract, and the ability to perform these procedures even in the smallest neonates or infants have all contributed to the trend away from cutaneous upper tract diversion. In addition, we now have a better understanding of the pathophysiology and natural history of the dilated ureter in childhood. Observation with radiographic surveillance has replaced surgical intervention in many instances. There are still clear indications for ureterostomy to decompress massively dilated upper tracts, for example in the neonate or infant who is not a candidate for reconstruction because of size or UTI, or when there is a question of functional adequacy in the involved kidney. In this latter instance, an interval of diversion may help one to decide between reconstruction and nephrectomy (Cendron, 1995).

Controversy still exists with respect to the benefit of more proximal diversion in patients with PUV who have persistent severe hydronephrosis and azotemia despite ablation of the valve or diversion by vesicostomy. Earlier studies suggested that proximal diversion would result in relief of relative obstruction at the ureterovesical junction and improve eventual glomerular filtration rate and somatic growth potential (Krueger et al., 1980; Joyner and Khoury, 1999). More recent studies have challenged this concept, demonstrating no difference in eventual renal outcome in children who are managed with primary valve ablation compared with patients who underwent upper tract diversion (Reinberg et al., 1992b; Smith et al., 1996). Those who oppose routine proximal diversion think that the improved renal function following diversion is attributable to normal transitional nephrology that occurs with or without proximal diversion (Smith et al., 1996; Tietjen et al., 1997). In a study of 26 patients managed with bilateral high diversion for PUV, Tietjen et al. (1997) reported renal dysplasia on biopsy in 85% and true ureterovesical junction obstruction based on Whitaker studies in only 4%.

The benefits in favor of upper tract diversion include the ability to perform renal biopsy for determining prognosis, the ability to monitor accurately the function of each kidney individually, and allowing time to decide on eventual reconstruction. Potential problems of ureterostomy relate to the need for a more complex reconstructive procedure at a later date, the potential for impaired ureteral vascularity, and difficulty in covering the stoma with an appliance as the child grows.

The techniques for proximal diversion have not changed over the past several decades. There is still some debate over the preferred technique (Cendron, 1995), i.e. whether a pyelostomy, loop, or Y-ureterostomy should be performed. The Y-ureterostomy, as described by Sober (1973), maximizes flow to the bladder, allowing greater preservation of bladder cycling. This avoids the potential later problem of carrying out a complex lower tract reconstructive procedure into a small, defunctionalized bladder. Regardless of the technique used, adhering to three basic operative principles is critical for a successful outcome (Rink and Keating, 1993): (1) during mobilization the ureter should only be manipulated with fine stay sutures and not grasped with forceps; (2) ureteral mobilization should be minimized to preserve maximal blood supply, yet be adequate to allow a tension-free skin anastomosis; and (3) kinking of the ureter or compression by the abdominal wall at the stomal site must be avoided.

Techniques for high ureterostomy are illustrated in Figure 17.5. All of these procedures can be accomplished through a subcostal incision, which allows mobilization of the ureter proximally to the renal pelvis and creation of a tension-free anastomosis to the skin. The loop ureterostomy is preferred by some surgeons because of the greater simplicity of the procedure. This makes it more applicable to the sick infant (Gonzales, 1998). Closure of the ureterostomy and lower urinary reconstruction are often staged but can be safely carried out at the time of reconstruction of the lower urinary tract if there is careful attention to the periureteral vasculature.

Distal, end ureterostomy is useful in patients with obstructed megaureters or ectopic ureters who are not candidates for immediate reconstruction. In addition to the potential benefit of recovery of renal function, decompressing the ureter may allow the ureteral diameter to decrease sufficiently that tapering of the ureter is not required at eventual reimplantation. The surgical approach is usually through a low transverse muscle-splitting incision that allows access to the retroperitoneum. The ureter is carefully mobilized to the level of the bladder hiatus and transected, taking care to preserve the periadventitial and retroperitoneal blood supply. The ureter can be brought out either in the lateral margin of the incision or in the midline. In cases of bilateral obstruction the ureters can be joined with a transureteroureterostomy and brought out as a single stoma (Gonzales, 1992). A V-shaped skin flap can be used to prevent stomal stenosis, but this occurs infrequently with a dilated ureter (Pfeffer and Caldamone, 1992).

Cutaneous pyelostomy

Cutaneous pyelostomy is an excellent option for upper tract diversion but is only useful in patients with a dilated extrarenal pelvis. The advantages of this procedure are the minimal disturbance of ureteral blood supply during both formation and closure and direct urine drainage from the kidney. The surgical approach is through a flank incision or a dorsal lumbotomy (Joyner and Khoury, 1999). The renal pelvis is mobilized and exteriorized superior to the ureteropelvic junction through the skin incision, taking care to avoid angulation (Fig. 17.6).

Conduit urinary diversion

With the advances made in reconstruction for urinary continence, the indications for permanent, non-continent urinary diversion in children have continued to decline. Initial enthusiasm for conduit diversion several decades ago has been tempered by long-term follow-up that has demonstrated significant problems with renal deterioration (Schwarz and Jeffs, 1975; Shapiro et al., 1975; Pitts and Muecke, 1979; Elder et al., 1983; Husmann et al., 1989; Koch et al., 1992). Despite the associated risks to the kidney, conduit diversion still remain the best option for a small subset of children. Patients with limited ability to care for themselves, and children with malignancies who have undergone extensive pelvic/abdominal radiation or who have limited life expectancy may be candidates for non-continent urinary diversion. As opposed to recommendations in the adult population (Grune and Taylor, 1996; McDougal, 1998), renal failure in children is not an absolute indication for conduit diversion, as most children will be candidates for renal transplantation and will have a better eventual outcome with primary bladder reconstruction.

Virtually any section of small or large intestine can be used to create a urinary conduit; however, ileum and colon are most frequently selected. Some surgeons prefer using colon conduits in children because of the lower incidence of late deterioration associated with

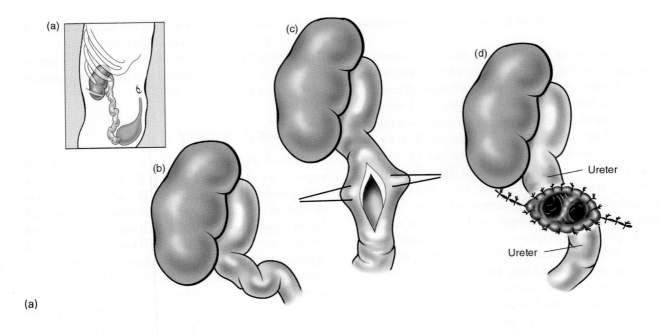

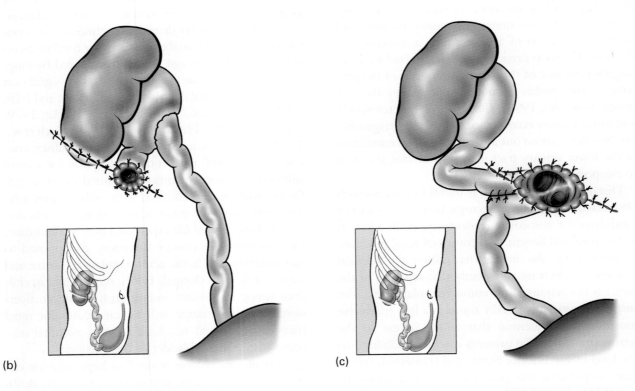

Figure 17.5 Various options for high cutaneous ureterostomy; (*a*) loop ureterostomy; (*b*) Sober ureterostomy; (*c*) ring ureterostomy. Care is taken with each technique to preserve the medial blood supply and create a tension-free skin anastomosis.

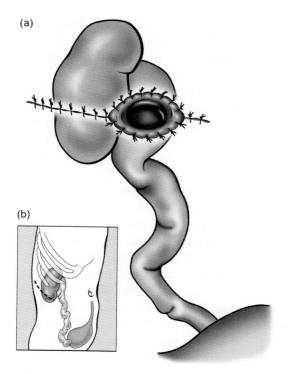

(a)

(b)

Figure 17.6 Cutaneous pyelostomy. (*a*) The renal pelvis is approached through a subcostal, posterior flank or dorsal lumbotomy incision. The kidney and dilated renal pelvis are mobilized until the renal pelvis can reach the skin without tension. (*b*) The renal pelvis is opened widely and secured to the skin with interrupted, absorbable sutures.

the non-refluxing ureterocolonic anastomosis (Elder *et al.*, 1983; Husmann *et al.*, 1989). In addition, the ability to incorporate the colon segment into a continent reservoir at a later date without the need to revise the ureteral anastomosis is advantageous (McLaughlin and Rink, 1998). Jejunal conduits carry an unacceptably high risk of severe metabolic problems and are mentioned only for historic reference. The primary electrolyte problem with incorporating jejunum into the urinary tract is hypochloremic, hyponatremic, and hyperkalemic metabolic acidosis, as well as relative hypovolemia (McLaughlin and Rink, 1998).

The important technical aspects of creating a conduit are similar whether using ileum or colon. This begins with an appropriate mechanical and antibiotic bowel preparation, which may need to be altered based on specific patient needs in the pediatric population. For example, the child with myelomeningocele frequently has significant chronic constipation, and will require initiation of the mechanical preparation 3–4 days earlier than patients with normal bowel motility. The standard pediatric bowel

preparation involves admission to the hospital on the day before surgery for intravenous antibiotics to sterilize the urinary tract and whole gut lavage with a polyethylene glycol solution (GoLYTELY) via nasogastric tube until the rectal effluent is clear. Another key aspect of the preoperative preparation is identifying an appropriate location for the stoma, which is most effectively done with the input of an enterostomal therapist with the child awake before surgery. Several locations should be identified that allow optimal fitting of the appliance with the patient in the sitting, standing, or supine position. This is critical for the wheelchair-bound patient who may have significant abdominal girth.

Although the incidence of postoperative complications may differ slightly for colon or ileal conduits, the types of associated problems are very similar and can be divided into early or late complications (Table 17.2). Both ureteroenteric and stomal complications are generally related to surgical technique, representing the most common problems leading to reoperation. The general principles of minimal handling of the ureter, maintaining maximal adventitial blood supply, minimizing mobilization, preventing angulation of the ureter, and securing a mucosa-to-mucosa watertight anastomosis with fine sutures will decrease the potential for postoperative problems. The use of ureteral stents has been shown to decrease significantly anastomotic leaks (Regan and Barrett, 1985), a complication that increases the risk of late stricture. Suspected ureteral leaks should be promptly investigated and if present treated by insertion of a percutaneous nephrostomy tube and antegrade stent place-

Table 17.2 Complications of ileal and colon conduits

	Frequency (%)	
Early complications	Ileal conduit	Colon conduit
Bowel obstruction	10	4
Urinary leak	3	5
Pyelonephritis	12	13
Late complications		
Stomal stenosis/parastomal hernia	24	20
Renal deterioration	18	15
Metabolic acidosis	16	5
Ureteroenteric stricture	8	9
Renal calculi	7	5

From McDougal (1998)

ment. Continuous drainage of the conduit with a Foley catheter after surgery may also help to minimize extravasation.

Ureteral strictures may take several years before they become evident (Levy and Arsdalan, 1994), reinforcing the need for long-term, periodic radiographic surveillance. Treatment of strictures at the ureteroenteric anastomosis can initially be attempted with endourologic techniques. However, regardless of the technique used (balloon dilation alone versus incision and dilation), approximately 50% will eventually require open revision (Levy and Van Arsdalan, 1994; Razvi *et al.*, 1996).

Stomal problems may vary from a minor nuisance (bleeding, dermatitis) to more life-threatening complications such as stomal obstruction with UTI:

- bleeding
- bowel necrosis
- dermatitis
- parastomal hernia
- stomal prolapse
- stomal stenosis
- stomal retraction
- loop obstruction (early/late).

Problems with local skin irritation can be minimized by creating an everted nipple or loop stoma, so that the appliance can be fitted snuggly to the adjacent skin. Stomal stenosis and parastomal hernia are the most common problems that require surgical revision. The risk of these complications can be minimized by bringing the bowel through an adequately sized defect without angulation, securing the conduit to the fascia in four quadrants, and creating a nipple stoma (Fitzgerald *et al.*, 1997). It was initially thought that colon conduits had a lower incidence of stomal stenosis than ileal conduits, but this has not been supported in more contemporary series (Webster, 1995).

Tumor within the bowel segment has been reported in both ileal and colon conduits (Filmer and Spencer, 1990). Although the risk for malignancy is unknown, it should be significantly lower than for ureterosigmoidostomy, where urine and stool are mixed.

Technique for ileal conduit

The abdomen is opened through a midline incision and the ureters are identified through incisions in the posterior peritoneum at the level of the iliac bifurca-

tion. The left ureter is mobilized and brought across the midline in a retroperitoneal tunnel, taking care to avoid angulation. A 10–15 cm segment of ileum is selected that has an adequate vascular arcade, and the mesentery to this segment is isolated. The mesentery of the distal end of the segment is mobilized to allow this end to be brought up to the skin as the stoma. The last 15 cm of distal ileum should be avoided, as this segment of ileum is important for iron and vitamin B_{12} absorption. The bowel segment is harvested and bowel continuity is restored using a side-to-side stapled or end-to-end hand-sewn anastomosis. The mesenteric defect is closed with permanent suture. The proximal end of the conduit is closed in two layers (after removing the staples if a stapling device was used to harvest the segment), and secured to the sacral promontory. Ureteroileal anastomoses are carried out using either the Bricker (1950) or Wallace (1970) technique (Fig. 17.7a, b), and the proximal end of the loop is retroperitonealized. The distal segment of the loop is brought out at the predetermined site for the stoma, and an everting nipple or loop stoma is created (Fig. 17.8).

Technique for colon conduit

The colon conduit is constructed in a similar fashion to the ileal conduit with the exception of the ureteral anastomosis, which is usually created in a non-refluxing manner using the tenia (Leadbetter technique) (Fig. 17.9). Alternatively, a submucosal tunnel may be created (Goodwin technique) (McDougal, 1998). Both techniques are facilitated by injecting saline or dilute epinephrine under the mucosa to minimize bleeding and aid in the dissection. Because of the added risk of ureteral obstruction within the submucosal tunnel, stenting the ureteral anastomosis is recommended.

Most commonly a sigmoid segment will be used to create the conduit (Fig. 17.10), but in children with a history of pelvic radiation or inadequate ureteral length the transverse colon should be used.

Ileocecal conduit

By using the non-refluxing properties of the ileocecal valve, the ileocecal conduit provides an alternative to the tunneled ureteral reimplantation (and the associated risks) used to achieve a non-refluxing ureteral anastomosis with other colon conduits. The ileocecal

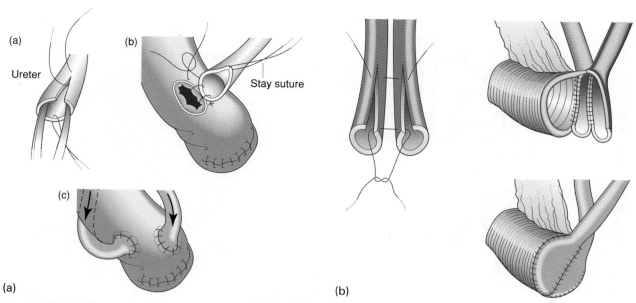

Figure 17.7 (*a*) The Bricker technique for ureterointestinal anastomosis. The ureter is spatulated, and following excision of a small ellipse of intestine, the anastomosis is secured with fine interrupted absorbable sutures. The external stent is placed across the anastomosis and brought out through the stoma. Both ureters are secured using an end-to-side anastomosis. (*b*) The Wallace procedure for ureteroileal anastomosis. The ureters are spatulated and joined at their medial borders using running or interrupted absorbable sutures. The lateral edges of both ureters are then secured to the conduit in an end-to-end anastomosis.

conduit can later be incorporated into a ureterosigmoidostomy with reduced risk of cancer, as the ileocecal valve will prevent the direct contact of feces and urine at the site of the ureteral anatomosis. The greatest concern in using this segment for urinary diversion is the theoretical risk of diarrhea and fecal incontinence in the myelomeningocele patient who may

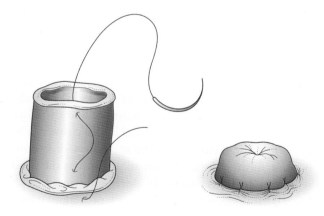

Figure 17.8 An everted stomal nipple is optimal for creating a snuggly fitting appliance. This is created by placing sutures between the skin/subcutaneous tissue, lateral bowel serosa, and distal edge of the stoma.

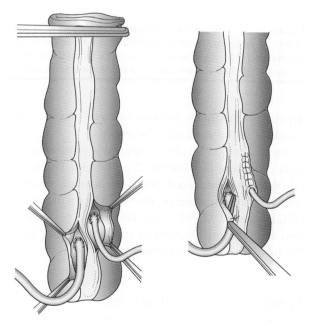

Figure 17.9 The non-refluxing ureterocolonic anastomosis described by Leadbetter. A submucosal tunnel is created by incising the tenia to create a submucosal trough, the ureter is anastomosed to the colonic mucosa, and the muscularis loosely closed over the ureter with absorbable suture.

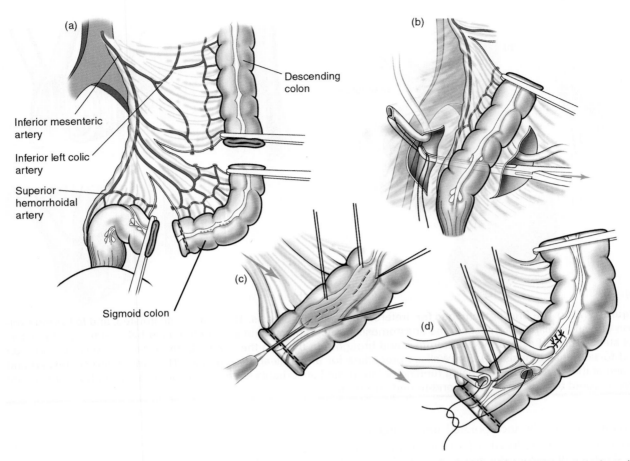

Figure 17.10 Surgical technique for creation of a sigmoid colon conduit. (*a*) A segment of colon is isolated, maintaining a wide mesenteric pedicle. (*b*) The ureters are mobilized through posterior incisions in the peritoneum and transected. The right ureter is brought across the midline in a retroperitoneal tunnel. (*c*) The tenia is incised to create a tunnel. (*d*) The ureters are anastomosed as illustrated in Figure 17.7.

depend on the intact ileocecal valve to prevent rapid transit of liquid stool into the colon.

The technique involves isolating a portion of the right colon and distal ileum (Fig. 17.11). The ileocecal valve is reinforced with permanent plication sutures that intussuscept the valve into the cecum (Williams *et al.*, 1997). The ureters are reimplanted into the proximal portion of the ileum using either the Bricker or Wallace technique.

Continent urinary diversion

Continent urinary diversion has generally meant that a storage receptacle for urine has been created from the gastrointestinal tract which is then emptied by intermittent catheterization through a channel created that does not use the native urethra. A neobladder has been

defined as replacement of the urinary bladder by a gastric or an intestinal segment, which is anastomosed to the native urethra allowing the patient to empty by spontaneous voiding. While neobladders have become extremely popular in adults who have undergone cystectomy for cancer, the use of these is virtually unheard of in the pediatric population, and therefore neobladders will not be considered in this chapter. The exact lines of separation of these various diversions become further blurred by situations such as the child who has had his native bladder augmented with bowel, has undergone a bladder neck procedure which does not allow voiding, and empties by a catheterizable channel to the abdominal wall. This, in effect, would be a CUR, but is certainly not what most readers view as a standard CUR. For the purposes of this chapter we will not consider the use of the native bladder or urethra in the discussion of CURs.

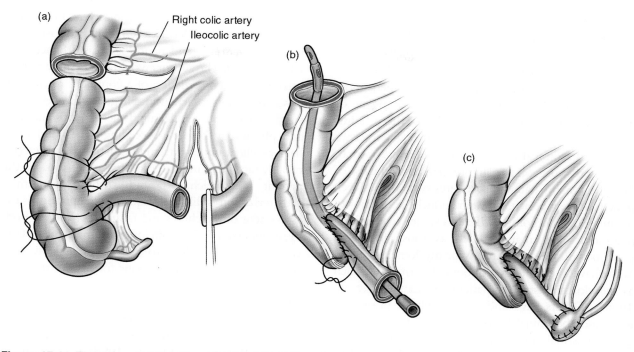

Figure 17.11 The non-refluxing ileocecal conduit as described by Zinman and Libertino. (*a*) The ileocecal segment is harvested based on the ileocolic artery. (*b*) The ileocecal valve is intussuscepted into the cecum with permanent sutures. (*c*) The terminal ileum is plicated into the cecum also with permanent sutures. The ureters are anastomosed to the proximal ileal segment using either the Bricker or the Wallace technique.

Continent urinary diversion is not new, in fact, urinary diversion with a continence mechanism was first introduced in 1851 by Simon, who performed ureterosigmoidostomy on a 13-year-old boy with bladder exstrophy (Simon, 1852). While several other efforts at continent diversion were attempted, no significant advances were made until nearly 100 years later when Gilcrest and Merricks created the first modern-day reservoir by making a cecal bladder with continence based on the ileocecal valve, with the ileal 'urethra' brought to the abdominal wall (Gilcrest *et al.*, 1950). Gilcrest *et al.*, reported good success with this, but others had difficulty in duplicating their results, and intermittent catheterization was not well accepted at the time (Harper *et al.*, 1954; Wells, 1956). Gilcrest continued to use this method and was able to achieve continence in 37 of 40 patients (Sullivan *et al.*, 1973; Merricks, 1987). Bricker (1950) tried a similar reservoir at the time but could not achieve continence and therefore abandoned these efforts and popularized his well-known ileal conduit, which became widely accepted as the diversion of choice. Thus, continent diversion lay largely dormant for the next 30 years, but ultimately formed the basis for some of the procedures used currently.

Urologic historians will record the 1980s and 1990s as the era of continent urinary diversion, as there was an explosion of growth and refinement of these reconstructive techniques during this period. This has been an area of significant cross-pollination between adult and pediatric urologists to provide the current state of the art. Several factors have allowed this to occur. Most significant was Lapides' introduction of CIC (Lapides *et al.*, 1972). Reliable urodynamic evaluation in children by Blavis *et al.* (1977) and improved pediatric anesthesia allowed long reconstructive cases. Hendren's work with dilated ureters and reconstruction, and his demonstration that the previously diverted urinary tract could be refunctionalized allowed further progress in this area in children (Hendren, 1969, 1970, 1973). Without question, CIC was the key component as reconstruction no longer required volitional voiding. A storage vesical alone could be created with emptying reliably achieved by CIC.

Bricker's ileal conduit was the mainstay of urinary diversion for over 20 years but with the acceptance of CIC there was great interest in Kock's early work with a continent urinary ileal reservoir, which he adapted from his continent ileostomy (Kock *et al.*,

1982). The Kock pouch, which was refined and popularized by Skinner's team, rekindled interest in continent diversion (Skinner *et al.*, 1984, 1987, 1989). Over 40 types of CUR have now been described. Gastrointestinal CURs have gained most acceptance in the adult population as a means of diversion following cystectomy. In these adult patients, the urinary tract and gastrointestinal tract are usually anatomically and neurologically normal, allowing the surgeon to plan preoperatively the use of one of the many named procedures such as the Kock pouch, Indiana pouch, or Mainz pouch. The majority of children undergoing CURs has severe anatomic or neurologic abnormalities such as those found in patients with classic exstrophy or myelomeningocele. Some have a combination of both abnormalities, such as the cloacal exstrophy patient (McLaughlin *et al.*, 1995a). Others have undergone multiple prior urologic and abdominal procedures and have associated gastrointestinal anomalies such as short-gut syndrome. In these situations, creation of a standard named CUR may not be possible. For example, the cloacal exstrophy patient may not have an ileocecal valve or the colonic segment may have been discarded, excluding the possibility of constructing an Indiana or a Mainz pouch. The short-gut syndrome patient does not have an adequate length of ileum necessary to create a Kock pouch. In those who have had a prior appendectomy, the appendix is not available as a catheterizable channel, negating a Penn pouch. These anatomic and neurologic abnormalities do not prevent continent urinary diversion in children, but they require the surgeon to have a fertile imagination and depth of knowledge of all options available, as well as a good understanding of the concepts necessary to provide a reliable reservoir.

Patient selection and preoperative evaluation

Before proceeding with continent urinary diversion a number of factors must be considered. First and foremost, the urinary tract should be maintained intact in children whenever possible. In general, continent urinary diversion in children is performed in order to achieve continence or protect the upper urinary tract. One should exhaust medical management, including CIC and pharmacologic manipulation, before turning to surgical therapy. If medical management fails, the vast majority can be treated by reconstructing their native bladder by intestinocystoplasty and/or reconstruction of the bladder neck. Only in the most severe forms of anatomic and neurologic disturbances is a CUR selected. The authors would not hesitate to proceed with the construction of a continent reservoir if it was necessary to achieve their goals. However, the surgical team must understand the patient's anatomy and physiology before proceeding. The child must have excellent upper extremity function to catheterize reliably and the mental capacity to do so. If the patient is wheelchair bound, orthotopic urethral catheterization is difficult. Equally as important is the assessment of the child's and family motivation. Both must understand that a lifelong commitment to CIC is required and failure to catheterize reliably may result in urinary infection, stone formation, reservoir perforation, or renal deterioration, even in the face of a technically perfect operation.

Preoperatively, the overall renal function should be determined by measuring serum creatinine and electrolytes. Benson and Olsson (1998) noted that no patient should have a reservoir created if their creatinine clearance is < 60 ml/min. It is now well known that urinary solutes are reabsorbed from the urine in contact with the bowel mucosa. With the incorporation of ileum or colon into the urinary tract, chloride and ammonium are absorbed and sodium and bicarbonate are excreted (Fig. 17.12). This was first noticed by Ferris and Odel (1950) in patients with ureterosigmoidostomy. Children with normal renal function generally tolerate this well, but in those with renal insufficiency, a severe metabolic acidosis may occur (Ferris and Odel, 1950; Demos, 1962; Koch and McDougal, 1985). Mitchell and Piser (1987) noted that the chloride level increased and the bicarbonate level decreased in every patient following intestinocystoplasty at their institution. Rink *et al.* (1995) later reviewed 231 patients and found 16% to have a serum chloride level above the normal range. Those patients with severe elevations all had colonic segments in their urinary tract. Others have reported similar findings following CURs (Allen *et al.*, 1985; McDougal, 1986; Asken, 1987; Thoroff *et al.*, 1987; Boyd *et al.*, 1989). These changes would be expected to be most severe in CURs where the entire storage surface area is enteric. Nurse and Mundy (1989) demonstrated that following intestinocystoplasty, the blood gas values may be abnormal even with normal serum chloride levels. This chronic systemic acidosis may also have a profound effect on overall linear

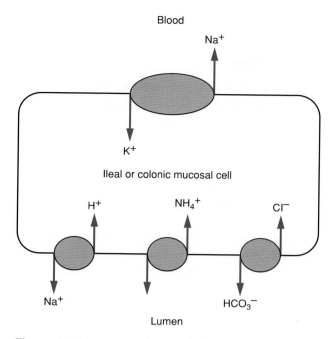

Blood

Na⁺

K⁺

Ileal or colonic mucosal cell

H⁺   NH₄⁺   Cl⁻

Na⁺   HCO₃⁻

Lumen

Figure 17.12 Ileal and colonic mucosa absorb ammonium, hydrogen, and chloride, while secreting sodium and bicarbonate.

growth of the child by interfering with bony buffers (Hall *et al.*, 1991). Although measuring growth in some of the population undergoing CURs, such as children with myelomeningocele, is difficult, several authors have noted that linear growth is impaired following cystoplasties (Mundy and Nurse, 1992; Wagstaff *et al.*, 1992). Children with acidosis following a CUR should be started on bicarbonate therapy. It may be reasonable to do this even in those who have been able to maintain normal acid–base balance, but this is controversial.

Many children undergoing creation of a CUR have renal tubular dysfunction from primary urinary obstruction resulting in a severe urine concentrating defect. The end result may be the excretion of very large volumes of urine. Therefore, a 24-hour urine for volume should always be checked preoperatively. The reservoir must be made large enough to handle the patient's urine output adequately at low pressures to allow emptying no more frequently than every 4 hours. Graphs and guidelines have been developed to predict the length of a bowel segment needed to achieve a certain volume (Rink and Mitchell, 1990). However, these graphs may prove cumbersome and are not routinely used (Rink, 1999). Even if renal and

bowel function are normal it is better to err on making the reservoir too large rather than too small.

Liver function testing should also be carried out as suggested by McDougal (1992). Hyperammonemia can occur in patients with large or small intestine incorporated into the urinary tract when hepatic dysfunction is present, as these segments absorb ammonium.

Radiographic evaluation of the urinary tract is always needed preoperatively. Intravenous pyelography is now used infrequently in children but can be very helpful in preoperative evaluation for a CUR as it will provide some functional information, but more importantly allows visualization of the ureteral anatomy as well as peristaltic activity. Hensle and Ring (1991) noted that tapering and reimplanting scarred, aperistaltic ureters often results in obstruction. More accurate renal function measurements may be obtained by radionuclide renal scanning. Since the native bladder and urethra are not used, voiding cystography is less helpful in these patients, although the presence of reflux is important as the refluxing scarred ureter is also fraught with complications in reconstruction (Rink and Adams, 1998). If the patient has had previous urinary diversion then a retrograde contrast study of the conduit (loop-o-gram) should be done to define anatomy.

Stomal location should also be determined before the operative procedure. While this is less important for continent diversion than conduit diversion, where a stomal appliance is required, it is still important to be certain the child will be able to pass the catheter easily. Skin folds and areas of abdominal wall scarring should be avoided. It is best if the patient can visualize the stoma. The stoma may be placed in an orthotopic location to allow catheterization of a normal urethral meatus, but in most patients this is not warranted. In a study by Horowitz *et al.* (1995), patients who had the opportunity to catheterize either their native urethra or an abdominal wall stoma overwhelming preferred the latter.

Finally, and not least important, latex allergy precautions must be observed in all patients with spinal dysrhaphism.

Principles of continent urinary diversion

The ideal reservoir (1) preserves the function of the upper urinary tract, (2) avoids reservoir–ureteral reflux and ureteral obstruction, (3) avoids urinary infection, and (4) has a reliable continence mechanism that would allow spontaneous voiding. As noted previously, spontaneous voiding by a voluntarily controlled native sphincter mechanism is essentially never achieved except following ureterosigmoidostomy or cystectomy in the neurologically intact patient. All other types of reservoirs require CIC. However, the remaining goals can be achieved by following the three principles of CURs: (1) creation of a high-capacity, low-pressure reservoir; (2) creation of a reliable antireflux mechanism; and (3) creation of a reliable continence mechanism that allows easy catheterization.

Creation of a compliant reservoir

When considering the creation of the reservoir portion of the CUR a number of questions must be answered. What is the underlying diagnosis? What tissues are available to use as a storage vesical? What are the pros and cons of each gastrointestinal segment and are there contraindications in the child to the use of a particular segment? Once the segment is chosen, how long should that segment be and how should it be configured? Is the reservoir amenable to creating a reliable continence and antireflux mechanism? Each child is unique and the answers to these questions may differ in various cases. Often, in children undergoing a CUR, the surgeon encounters what is similar to a puzzle. The urinary tract must be taken apart and then reconstituted in such a way that all principles are achieved.

When the bowel is maintained in its native tubular shape and used as a reservoir, very high reservoir pressures may be generated by the intestinal contractile activity. Fowler (1988) noted that intact cecum used as a reservoir may generate pressures of 60–90 cmH_2O at high volumes. Peristaltic waves generating pressures as high as 75–100 cmH_2O have been found in the tubular ileal Camey procedure (Camey et al., 1991). Kock (1969), in his early work, found that both large and small bowel could generate pressures as high as 100 cmH_2O when used in a closed loop. Light and Engelman (1985) demonstrated a mean maximum pressure of 90 cmH_2O in ileocecal and intact cecal segments used for augmentation. They felt that the entire large bowel was capable of creating significant intraluminal pressures. These high pressures can result in urinary leakage and upper urinary tract deterioration, and may even contribute to perforation (Pope et al., 1999). In what is now a landmark

paper, McGuire et al. (1981) reported a striking difference between myelodysplastic patients who leaked per urethra at <40 cmH_2O and those with pressures >40 cmH_2O. No patient in the former group had reflux or ureteral dilatation, whereas 68% had reflux and 81% dilatation in the latter. It is now well accepted that intravesical (intrareservoir) pressures must be maintained <40 cmH_2O.

Both Hinman (1988) and Koff (1988) demonstrated the advantages of detubularizing the intestinal segment and reconfiguring it into as near a sphere as possible. Detubularization will result in ineffective, asynchronous contractile activity. Reconfiguration will also increase the reservoir capacity (Fig. 17.13). The volume of a cylinder is proportional to the square of the radius ($v = \pi r^2 \times L$), whereas the volume of a sphere ($v = 4/3\pi r^3$) is proportional to the cube of the radius. The result is that the more closely the reservoir resembles a sphere, the greater the eventual radius for any given bowel segment, maximizing its capacity. Furthermore, from LaPlace's law ($T = Pr$), the larger the radius (r), the greater the wall tension (t), and the more it will enlarge over time. Compliance also increases by reconfiguring and detubularizing the bowel segment. The surgeon must understand that while detubularization and reconfiguration should always be done, contractile activity is not totally abolished by these maneuvers. In fact, Lytton and Green (1994) found contractions up to 60–110 cmH_2O in patients with detubularized right colon bladder substitutions. Although the pressures diminished with time, Sidi et al. (1986) noted average peak pressures of 41 cmH_2O following cup-patch sigmoid cystoplasties. In a comparison of the

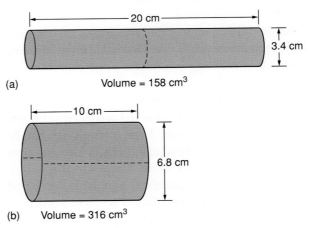

(a) Volume = 158 cm³

20 cm

3.4 cm

(b) Volume = 316 cm³

10 cm

6.8 cm

Figure 17.13 The effect of reconfiguring a cylinder to a sphere. The volume doubles (Hinman, 1988).

cystometric properties of ileum and right colon, mean maximal contractile pressures were 63 cmH$_2$O for tubular right colon and 42 cmH$_2$O for detubularized colon (Goldwasser *et al.*, 1986). Even more impressive was the effect noted by detubularizing ileum, where the mean maximal pressures were 81 cmH$_2$O in the tubularized versus 28 cmH$_2$O in the detubularized state. Clinically significant contractions (> 40 cmH$_2$O at volumes < 200 ml) were observed in only 10% of the right colon and none of the ileal segments. Ileal segments were thought to be urodynamically superior, but only at large volumes. Cecal reservoirs were thought to have higher pressures than ileal reservoirs at corresponding volumes and ten times greater motor activity (Berglund *et al.*, 1987). This has very important clinical significance. The reservoir must be made large enough to allow catheterization at 4 hour intervals at low intrareservoir pressures regardless of the volume of urine made by any given patient. If upper tract deterioration or urinary leakage occurs, urodynamics must be repeated to determine whether significant contractile activity persists. In the authors' augmentation cystoplasty population another segment of bowel had to be added in 19 of 323 patients owing to persistent contractile activity of the initial bowel segment (Pope *et al.*, 1998). Twelve of 87 undergoing colocystoplasty (13.8%), and four of 30 undergoing gastrocystoplasty (10.3%) required a secondary augmentation bowel segment, while only two of 145 ileocystoplasties (1.4%) did. The authors agree with Goldwasser and Webster (1986) that ileum is the least contractile intestinal segment, with cecum intermediate and sigmoid and stomach being the most contractile (Pope and Rink, 1999).

Choice of bowel segment

While some of the metabolic and contractile properties of the gastrointestinal tract have been discussed above, there remains a number of advantages and disadvantages of each segment (Table 17.3). Several studies have reported on experience with the various gastrointestinal segments used in reconstructing the lower urinary tract (Rink and McLaughlin, 1994; Rink *et al.*, 1995; Pope and Rink, 1999; Rink, 1999). The majority of data in children comes from augmentation cystoplasty rather than complete reservoir construction.

Ileum, as noted previously, when reconfigured will provide the most compliant, least contractile segment. Mucus production, while greater than stomach, is less than with sigmoid or cecum and tends to decrease with time (Kulb *et al.*, 1986). Hyperchloremic acidosis occurs with small and large bowel but seems to be

Table 17.3 Advantages and disadvantages of each segment

Segment	Advantages	Disadvantages
Ileum	Most compliant Less mucus	Diarrhea Vitamin B$_{12}$ deficiency Short mesentery Hyperchloremic acidosis Poor muscle backing
Sigmoid	Readily mobilized Easily implanted Good muscle backing	Unit contractions Lower compliance Mucus Hyperchloremic acidosis Perforation risk
Ileocecal	Valve as antireflux/continence mechanism Good capacity reservoir Constant blood supply	Diarrhea Not always available Contractile
Stomach	Short gut/radiation Chloride pump Minimal mucus Few infections Ease of implantation Good muscle backing	Hypochloremic alkalosis Rhythmic contractions Hematuria/dysuria

less significant with ileum. Except in instances of short gut syndrome, as in cloacal exstrophy, there is generally an abundance of ileum available for reservoir construction and for the creation of catheterizable channels. If short ureters are present a 'tail' of ileum extending from the pouch can be used to bridge the gap. However, at times the mesentery is short, making an anastomosis to an orthotopic catheterization site difficult.

The ileum is responsible for vitamin B_{12} absorption, which occurs in the terminal portion. If possible, the distal 15 cm of ileum should be preserved. Resection of long segments of ileum have resulted in B_{12} deficiency but may take several years to become clinically manifest as a megablastic anemia and neuropathy, as B_{12} stores may last for years (Rowland, 1991; Rink and McLaughlin, 1994; Sheldon and Snyder, 1996). Akerlund et al. (1989) noted this problem in patients following Kock pouch construction. Canning et al. (1989) found no patient with B_{12} deficiency in 26 patients evaluated following bladder augmentation using ileum. However, this group was followed for only 3 years. Resection of large segments of ileum has also been found to result in diarrhea and to increase the risk of cholelithiasis (Steiner and Morton, 1991; Sheldon and Snyder, 1996). Roth et al. (1995) reported the occurrence of chronic diarrhea in 11% of patients who had a CUR constructed from ileum. Baker and Gearhart (1998) noted that if > 100 cm of ileum is resected, steatorrhea and cholethiasis can develop.

The cecum and ileocecal segments have been the most widely used tissues for CUR construction. The ileocecal segment has a constant, reliable blood supply that allows easy mobilization and placement of the pouch in the pelvic inlet, when necessary. The large cecal size makes for an excellent reservoir and the ileocecal valve can be used as either a continence or an antireflux mechanism. The appendix is also available for use as a continence mechanism. This segment is used in several of the most popular reservoirs, i.e. the Indiana pouch, Florida pouch, Mainz pouch, and Penn pouch.

The ileocecal segment has been less frequently used in children as the majority undergoing CURs have a neuropathic component. In this group of patients, the ileocecal valve seems to be important in maintaining fecal continence. Removal of the ileocecal valve has reportedly led to diarrhea in 10% of children (King, 1987). Gonzalez and Cabral (1987) reported that a patient required replacement of the ileocecal valve to reverse or correct intractable diarrhea. Roth et al. (1995) noted that 23% of patients having an ileocecal reservoir had chronic diarrhea. Furthermore, in cloacal exstrophy patients the colonic segment may have been absent or discarded at the time of previous surgery and thus not available for use. Cecal incorporation into the urinary tract may lead to hyperchloremic metabolic acidosis as well as significant mucus production.

The sigmoid colon has been extensively used in lower urinary reconstruction in children. It is often quite enlarged and redundant in the spinal dysraphism population, allowing it to reach easily any portion of the abdomen or pelvis. Its mucosa can be easily dissected to provide submucosal tunnels for antireflux or continence mechanisms. While it seemingly has a number of advantages, it has the disadvantages of significant contractile activity in spite of detubularization and reconfiguration (Pope et al., 1998). It also has the greatest mucus production (Kulb et al., 1986) and highest rates of bacteriuria (Hirst, 1991), and is most likely to result in significant hyperchloremic metabolic acidosis. In the authors' hands, when used to augment the bladder it has resulted in the highest spontaneous bladder perforation rate (Pope et al., 1999). However, this latter problem was not found in the Boston series (Bauer et al., 1992). This difference may be in the means of reconfiguration. The authors no longer simply close the two ends of the segment (Mitchell, 1986) and open the antimesenteric border, but rather recommend complete reconfiguration of the sigmoid.

The use of the stomach in lower urinary reconstruction in children was popularized with the initial report by Adams et al. (1988). It was rapidly incorporated into the surgeon's armamentarium because of a number of demonstrable advantages. Stomach has excellent muscle backing and submucosal tunnels can be created in a manner similar to native bladder to allow ureteral reimplantation or tunneled continence mechanisms (Adams et al., 1995). The stomach was also thought to be an ideal tissue for those who had undergone pelvic radiation as it is generally outside the irradiated field. Bladder calculi, which have been a significant problem with the use of intestinal segments, have nearly been non-existent with the use of the stomach (Kaefer et al., 1995; Kronner et al., 1998). Kaefer et al. (1995) found that only two of 70 patients developed stones with the use of stomach, compared with 30 of 137 with stones following the use of other enteric segments. Perhaps most importantly, the stomach differs metabolically from the other intestinal segments (Piser *et al.*, 1987). Gastric mucosa secretes chloride, which may be beneficial in those with azotemia (Piser *et al.*, 1987; Kennedy *et al.*, 1988). Serum chloride has been noted to decrease and bicarbonate increase following the use of stomach in the urinary tract (Adams *et al.*, 1988; Ganesan *et al.*, 1991). This net chloride excretion has led to a decrease in bacteriuria (Rink *et al.*, 1995) and, along with less mucus production, probably plays a significant role in the lower incidence of stone formation.

Unfortunately, the popularity of the stomach has waned somewhat as two unique problems have been noted: profound hypochloremic metabolic alkalosis (in five of 37 patients) and the hematuria–dysuria syndrome (HDS) found in approximately one-third of patients following gastrocystoplasty (Castro-Diaz *et al.*, 1992; Reinberg *et al.*, 1992a; Atala *et al.*, 1993; Gosalbez *et al.*, 1993; Nguyen *et al.*, 1993; Ngan *et al.*, 1993; Rink *et al.*, 1995). The dysuria may be quite debilitating in those with sensation and is worse in those with oliguria (Sheldon *et al.*, 1995). If a reservoir is to be constructed from stomach, the continence mechanisms must be 100% reliable, as severe skin excoriation may occur with urinary leakage (Nguyen *et al.*, 1993; Ngan *et al.*, 1993; Rink and Adams, 1998). Stomach should be avoided if a period of anuria is anticipated, as the urine is necessary to buffer the gastric acid production, thus preventing ulceration and perforation (Castro-Diaz *et al.*, 1992). Pharmacologic therapy with H_2 blockers and hydrogen ion pump blockers may be helpful in reducing acid production (Kinahan *et al.*, 1992).

Another disadvantage of stomach is its contractile activity. Rhythmic contractions are reported in all large series, occurring in up to 62% of patients (Atala *et al.*, 1993; Gosalbez *et al.*, 1993; Adams *et al.*, 1995). This is partly due to the small wedge segment of stomach initially used. Larger, more rhomboid segments, have improved the urodynamics but contractility can remain a problem necessitating a secondary augmentation (Rink and Adams, 1996; Pope *et al.*, 1998).

No gastrointestinal segment will make the perfect bladder. Each segment has its own advantages and disadvantages, which must be weighed prior to CUR construction in relation to each patient. As noted previously, the anatomy and innervation are frequently abnormal and often the tissues are scarred from prior

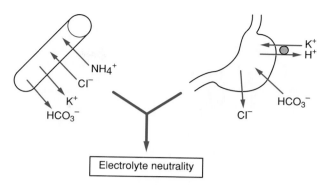

Figure 17.14 The effect of combining intestine with stomach. Electrolyte neutrality is achieved.

surgery. Any segment can work well if used correctly. Recently, stomach in combination with intestinal segments has been used to create a metabolically neutral reservoir (Lockhart *et al.*, 1993; McLaughlin *et al.*, 1995a; Austin *et al.*, 1997; Austin *et al.*, 1999a). The hypochloremic alkalosis associated with stomach is offset by the hyperchloremic acidosis associated with small and large bowel usage creating a more 'balanced' reservoir (Fig. 17.14). Only a relatively small (8 × 4 cm) gastric segment is necessary to achieve neutrality. Lockhart *et al.* (1994) have demonstrated that larger segments may result in HDS. In 12 patients with long-term follow-up, 11 have normalized their mean serum HCO_3 levels. Serum pH levels have also been corrected, and only one patient has had persistent metabolic acidosis (Austin *et al.*, 1999a). Gastroileal composite reservoirs seem to provide many advantages but take longer to construct as a second anastomosis is necessary and there is potentially significant blood loss.

Creation of an antireflux mechanism

The second of the three principles of CUR construction is the creation of a reliable antireflux mechanism. While the necessity for this can be debated in the adult patient when a low-pressure, large reservoir has been constructed, it is widely agreed that this is very important in the pediatric population. The historic aspects and the various mechanisms were reviewed by Walker (1994). Antireflux mechanisms today are generally based on intraluminal or extraluminal tunnel techniques or by the creation of nipples by intussusception. These techniques are similar to those that are used to provide continence mechanisms, so will only be briefly discussed here.

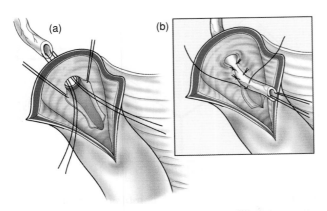

Figure 17.15 LeDuc reimplant. (*a*) A mucosal sulcus is created in the ileum. (*b*) The ureter is brought into the bowel segment and placed in the sulcus between the mucosal edges which are tacked to the ureter. (Adapted from LeDuc *et al.*, 1987, with permission.)

Tunneling techniques into bowel have been modified over the years by a number of surgeons, but all have their basis in the original technique introduced by Coffey (1911) (see the technique described for antireflux under colon conduit description). Developing submucosal tunnels in small intestine can be quite difficult. Two techniques to create ileal tunnels are worthy of mention. LeDuc *et al.* (1987) described an intralumenal tunneling technique, whereby a 3 cm mucosal sulcus is created. The ureter is brought through the bowel wall, placed in this sulcus, and secured. The intestinal mucosal edges are sutured to the ureteral adventitia and, with time, the mucosa will cover the ureter to create a tunnel with muscle backing (Fig. 17.15). Abol-Enein and Ghoneim (1994) described an ingenious technique using a serosal tunnel, which is easily constructed and appears to reliably prevent reflux (Fig. 17.16).

Nipple valves are generally constructed by intussuscepting ileum or using the ileocecal valve. These techniques will be covered under continence mechanisms as the technique is the same. The ureters are

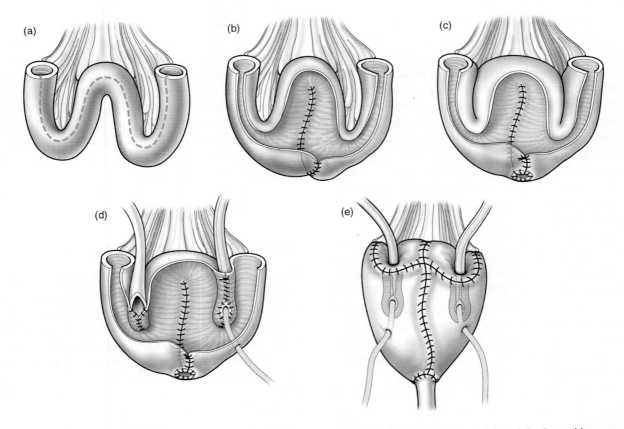

Figure 17.16 Abol-Enein, Ghoneim reimplant. (*a, b*) A W-shaped ileal segment is fashioned and the bowel is opened on the antimesenteric border. (*c, d*) Two serous lined troughs are created and the ureters are placed in the troughs with the ureteral meatus anastomosed to the intestinal mucosa. (*e*) The free bowel edges are closed over the ureter, creating a serosal lined tunnel. (Adapted from Abol-Enein and Ghoneim, 1994, with permission.)

implanted by direct anastomosis to the bowel proximal to the nipple valve. As a general rule, antireflux intestinal nipple valves have had more complications than tunneling techniques and are more difficult to construct. In the authors' experience there has been nearly a 50% incidence of reflux noted on long-term follow-up in those in whom a reinforced intussuscepted ileocecal valve was used as the antireflux mechanism. Therefore, other techniques are currently being used. A split cuff nipple valve using ureter has been reported by several authors, and is very easily constructed and surprisingly reliable (Turner-Warwick and Ashken, 1967; Goldwasser and Webster, 1986; Stone and MacDermott, 1989) (Fig. 17.17). Stone and MacDermott (1989) noted mild reflux in only one of 35 ureters, all of whom had at least a 2 year follow-up. This is particularly useful in the dilated ureter where tunneling techniques are more likely to lead to ureteral obstruction.

Regardless of the antireflux mechanism, the results have been good. Walker (1994) noted success rates only slightly worse than reimplantation into native bladder. Most interesting is the report by Lockhart *et al.* (1991), where 165 of 201 ureters were anastomosed end to side with no effort made to prevent reflux. Neither reflux nor obstruction occurred in 87%. Tunneled reimplantations have successfully prevented reflux in greater than 95% of patients.

Creation of a continence mechanism

The final and most important principle of CUR construction is the creation of a reliable continence mechanism that is easily catheterizable. The creation of the perfect reservoir with no reflux is of no value to the child who continually leaks urine onto the abdominal wall. Equally disastrous is having difficulty in catheterizing the completely continent reservoir, which puts the child at risk for reservoir perforation. As Benson and Olsson (1999) have observed, the integrity or failure of the continence mechanism determines the success or failure of the diversion. Numerous techniques have been described to provide continence but they all fall basically into one of the following categories: nipple valves, plicated valves, flap valves, and hydraulic valves. Some techniques use a combination of these valve mechanisms. Examples of each type will be demonstrated. The interested reader should be aware of two excellent reviews of continence mechanisms by Sagalowski (1992) and Austin and Lockhart (1998).

Nipple valves are generally created by intussuscepting an intestinal segment to create a sphincteric compression mechanism. These nipples are used in many of the most popular CURs. An ileal nipple is used in the Kock pouch (Fig. 17.18) and the Mainz pouch (Fig. 17.19). An ileocecal nipple is used in the pouch

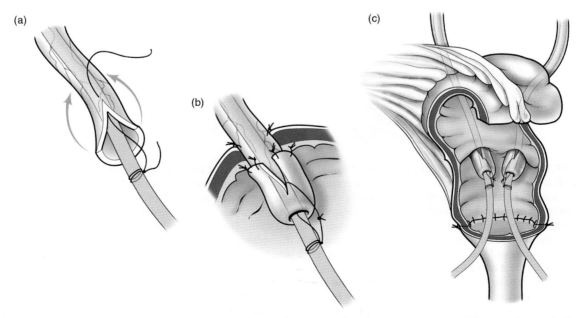

(a)

(b)

(c)

Figure 17.17 Split cuff nipple, created by spatulating and everting the ureter over a stent. They are brought through the bowel wall and secured. (Adapted from Goldwasser and Webster, 1986, with permission.)

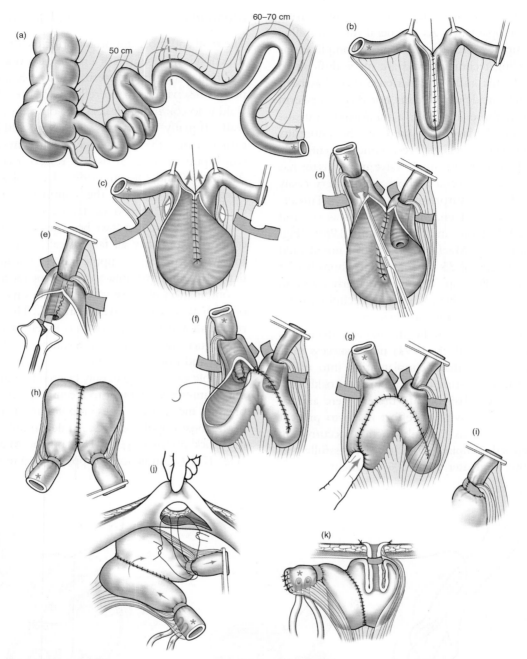

Figure 17.18 Kock pouch (continent ileal reservoir). (*a*) Bowel segment measuring 60–70 cm is isolated approximately 50 cm from the ileocecal valve and positioned as the letter U with the terminal end directed towards the head of the patient and the bottom of the U towards the left side of the patient. (*b*) The legs of the U are united at the antimesenteric border with continuous 3–0 polygylcolic acid sutures. (*c*) The intestine is divided adjacent to the suture line and the incision is continued for 3 cm on afferent limb. The mucous membrane is sutured with continuous 3–0 polyglycolic acid sutures. Openings are made in mesentery supplying the future base of the nipple valves. (*d*) Intussusception of the afferent and efferent segments into the future reservoir. (*e*) The nipple valves are secured with staples. (*f*) The reservoir is closed with two continuous inverting 3–0 polyglycolic acid sutures. (*g*–*h*) The reservoir is brought into its final position by pushing the corners of the reservoir downwards between mesenteric leaves. (*i*) A fascia of Marlex mesh encircles the base of the nipple valve, and the ends are approximated with three or four non-absorbable sutures. The reservoir wall is sutured to the cylinder with 3–0 polyglycolic acid sutures. (*j*) The cylinder at the efferent segment is attached to the opening and anterior rectus sheath with non-absorbable sutures. (*k*) The completed continent ileal reservoir.

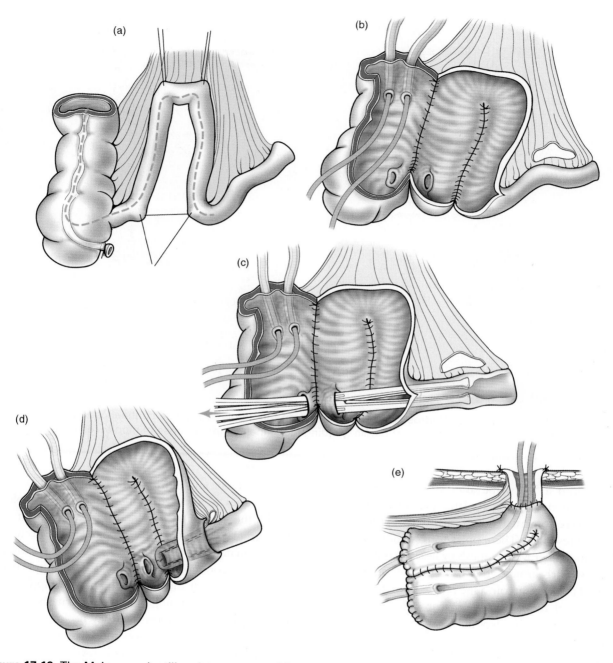

Figure 17.19 The Mainz pouch utilizes intussuscepted ileum pulled through the ileocecal valve (*c*) as the continence mechanism.

described by Mansson. When the nipple valve is within the lumen of the reservoir the principle of equilibration pressures adds further to continence. Unfortunately, the intrareservoir pressure that compresses the nipple to provide continence also applies forces to evert, flatten, or destabilize the nipple (Fig. 17.20). Because of the nipple's tendency to fail over time, many ingenious methods to stabilize the nipple

have been reported. Hendren (1980) described dissecting the mesentery off the ileum to be intussuscepted and scarifying it to provide internal fixation. The Kock pouch has been modified many times from its original application as a continent ileostomy (Kock, 1973). The procedure reported in the first 12 patients involved the use of 60–70 cm ileum for the reservoir (Kock *et al.*, 1982). The middle 40 cm was

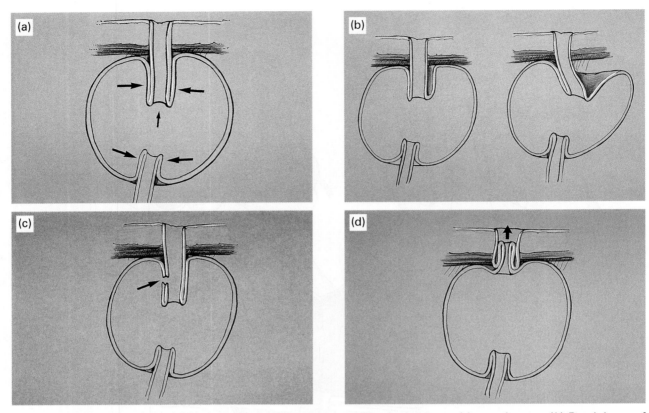

Figure 17.20 Nipple valves. (*a*) Hydrostatic forces exerted on the nipple to provide continence. (*b*) Breakdown of nipple, yielding incontinence. (*c*) Fistula of nipple, yielding incontinence. (*d*) Prolapse of nipple, resulting in inability to catheterize.

folded into a 'U' shape after being opened on its antimesenteric border. In later patients, the nipple valves were constructed by intussuscepting the ileum into the reservoir. The nipples were stabilized by stapling and either Marlex mesh or fascia was positioned as a cylinder around the base of the nipples and secured to the reservoir. One nipple was used for continence and the other to prevent reflux. The Kock pouch has since been popularized by Skinner, who made further modifications. There appears to be a steep learning curve, but in Skinner's hands the results have been reported to be excellent (Skinner *et al.*, 1989): 16% suffered early complications and late complications have been noted in 22% of 531 patients, with the vast majority involving the efferent nipple (Skinner *et al.*, 1989). The large amount of ileum required (78 cm), the complexity of the procedure, and the requirement for two nipples with stapling and collar fixation have deterred its widespread use in children. But it does provide the least contractile and most compliant reservoir, with pouch capacities ultimately over 700 ml (Benson and Olsson,

1998). Hanna and Bloiso (1987) achieved success in a small series in children. But modified the nipple to avoid the use of staples and Marlex. Benson and Olsson (1998) noted that nipple failure occurs in approximately 15% in the best of hands, with the three most common complications of the nipple being pinhole fistulae at the base of the nipple, nipple valve prolapse, and shortening of the nipple length. Because of this high complication rate they no longer recommend its routine use (Benson and Olsson, 1999).

The ileocecal valve is commonly used as a continence mechanism with the cecum acting as the reservoir. However, in its native form it is functionally adequate in only 25% of the population (Cohen *et al.*, 1968). Rendelmen *et al.* (1958) found that at 25 cmH$_2$O, the valve is incompetent in 25%. This incompetence increases such that only 7% are continent at 50 cmH$_2$O pressure (Rendelmen). Reinforcement to achieve continence was achieved by Zinman and Libertino (1975) by wrapping the cecum around the ileum. Intussusception of the ileocecal valve as a nipple to enhance its continence is the basis for the pouch described by Mansson *et al.*

(1990). The Mainz pouch (mixed augmentation with ileum and cecum) uses tunneled ureteral implants to prevent ureteral reflux and an unusual nipple valve for continence with the reservoir created by combining detubularized cecum and ileum (Fig. 17.19). The ileum is intussuscepted to create a nipple, which is then pulled through the ileocecal valve and secured by stapling. Continence rates have been greater than 95% and reservoir capacities greater than 600 ml in 179 patients, 41 of whom were children (Thuroff *et al.*, 1986; Thuroff *et al.*, 1988; Hohenfellner *et al.*, 1990). Again, owing to nipple complications and the difficulty in constructing them, the Mainz group no longer uses the nipple but instead an *in situ* appendix, which is buried in the cecum, as the continence mechanism (Fig. 17.21). Stein *et al.* (1995) reported 374 patients undergoing a Mainz pouch in which 116 had the appendix as the continence mechanism, with 6.7% having early complications and 25% late complications. All of the incontinence occurred with use of the nipple valves. None of the appendiceal efferent stomas was incontinent. Gerharz *et al.* (1997) compared the two continence mechanisms in the Mainz pouch (96 appendiceal stomas, 106 ileal nipples) and noted that 17% of the appendiceal stomas required 23 reinterventions with all but two being for stenosis. Nipple valves required a second operation in 12.3%, but the revisions were much simpler in the appendiceal group and this has become their preferred method. If the appendix is not available a Lampel tube of cecum (Fig. 17.22(A)) or submuscular tube (Fig. 17.22(B)) is now used

(Lampel *et al.*, 1995). The Mainz group also looked at vitamin. A, B, B_2, B_6, D, and E and folic acid levels, as well as bone density, after these diversions and all were within normal limits (Stein *et al.*, 1998). Vitamin B_{12} levels and bone density were normal in the 51 children but dropped significantly in adults. They recommend checking B_{12} levels after 4 years.

The appendix has also been used by others to create an intussuscepted nipple as a continence mechanism for a right colon pouch (Tillen *et al.*, 1987; Issa *et al.*, 1989; Bissada, 1993). There is only minimal intussusception in the Bissada technique (Bissada, 1993), but Issa *et al.* (1989) reinforced this with a mesh wrap similar to the ileal nipple in the Kock pouch. Tillen *et al.* (1987) reinforce the appendix only if leakage is demonstrated after filling the cecum to 60 cmH$_2$O.

An interesting nipple valve was developed by Benchekroun (1982; Benchekroun *et al.*, 1989) and modified by Guzman *et al.* (1989). The ileum is inverted into itself to create an 'inkwell' system whereby urine enters between the walls and compresses the inner layer for continence (Fig. 17.23). Benchekroun *et al.* (1989) reported 136 patients with 75% continence after the initial operation. Another 17.6% achieved continence after revision. The results with this technique by the Hopkins group were not nearly as good and after initially recommending this procedure they have now abandoned it, as stomal stenosis in children and destabilization are problems (Sanda *et al.*, 1988; Leonard *et al.*, 1990). This hydraulic nipple valve, while ingenious, has not gained wide acceptance.

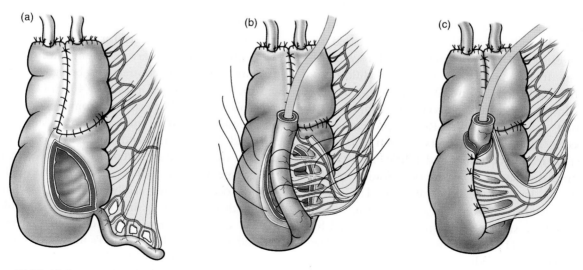

Figure 17.21 Mainz pouch with appendix. (*a*) The cecum has been patched with ileum. A seromuscular incision is made in the tenia. (*b*) Mesenteric windows are made in the mesoappendix. (*c*) The appendix is placed in the submucosal tunnel and the cecum is closed over it, avoiding the appendiceal vasculature.

(A)

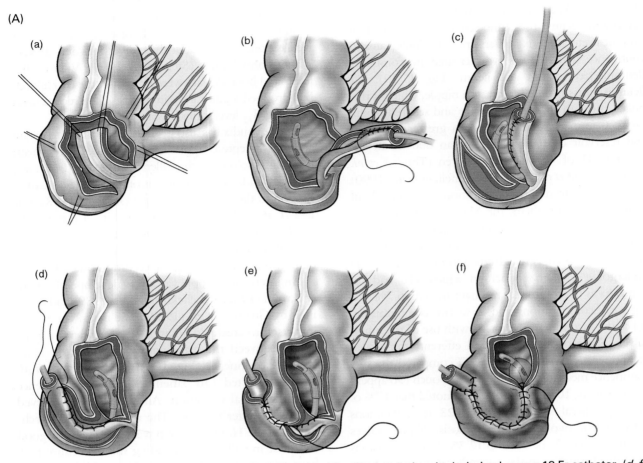

Figure 17.22 (*A*) Lampel tube. (*a–c*) A full-thickness bowel flap is elevated and tubularized over a 18 Fr catheter. (*d–f*) It is then placed in a submucosal subtineal tunnel and the bowel wall is closed. (*B*) *Continued opposite.*

Plication techniques have been widely accepted as reliable continence mechanisms and have been popularized by the Indiana group in what has become known as the Indiana pouch. This pouch is based on a modification of Gilcrest and Merrick's cecoileal reservoir. It has undergone several modifications since the initial report in 1985 (Rowland *et al.*, 1985). In this procedure the cecum is detubularized and used as the reservoir. Reflux prevention is obtained by tunneling the ureters into the tenia or by the LeDuc technique (Rink and Bihrle, 1990). The continence mechanism is based on plication of the ileum to the level of the ileocecal valve. The native ileocecal valve is reinforced by Lembert sutures (Fig. 17.24). A very similar technique has been used by Lockhart *et al.* (1990) in the Florida pouch. The advantage of this procedure is its ease of construction, using techniques familiar to all urologists. Carroll and Presti (1992) compared plicated versus stapled ileal segments and noted that mean contraction pressures

were higher in the stapled group (63 ± 27 cmH$_2$O vs 41 ± 21 cmH$_2$O). They have previously shown that contractions in the ileal segment always precede or are concomitant with cecal reservoir contractions (Carroll *et al.*, 1989). Mean reservoir volumes were 675 ml, with mean reservoir contractions being 24 cmH$_2$O and mean plicated ileal pressures 40 cmH$_2$O in the reservoir. As would be expected from these data, continence rates have been quite good. Rowland (1995) reviewed several series and noted that one of 176 patients (0.6%) required repair of the efferent limb for leakage. Canning (1998), however, reported that leakage occurs more readily with this mechanism than with nipples. Ring and Hensle (1992) achieved a 95% continence rate in 29 children undergoing the Indiana pouch. In Rowland's most recent report, five of the last 81 patients had incontinence secondary to high reservoir pressures (Rowland, 1996). Patching the cecal reservoir with ileum may correct this.

Koff *et al.* (1989) reported a technique to provide

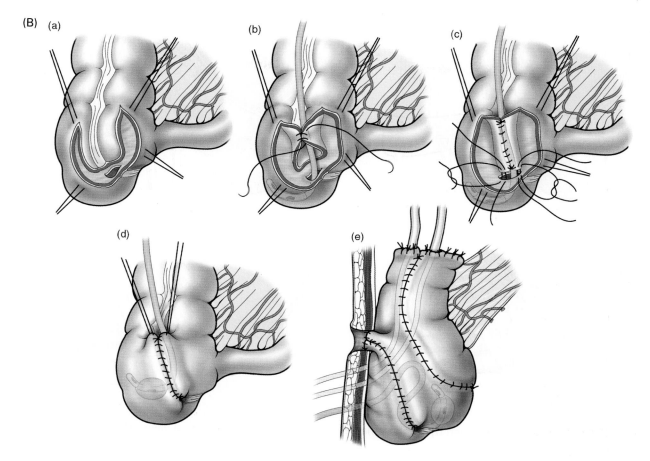

Figure 17.22 (*B*) *Continued.* Lampel seromuscular tube. (*a, b*) The elevated seromuscular layer is tubularized over an 18 Fr catheter and (*c*) anastomosed at its base to the mucosal opening. (*d*) The bowel wall is closed over the tube and (*e*) brought to the umbilicus as a catheterizeable stoma. (Reprinted from Lampel *et al.*, 1995.)

hydraulic compression to the efferent ileal limb of the Indiana pouch (Koff *et al.*, 1989). A segment of ileum is used to wrap around the efferent limb and is anastomosed to the cecal pouch. While this would increase resistance further, it adds complexity to an

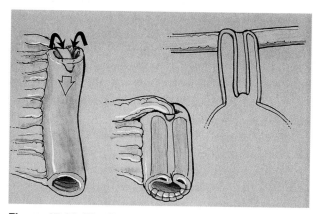

Figure 17.23 The Benchekroun ileo-nipple.

otherwise easily performed procedure that already has a high continence rate. Koff's approach has not gained widespread use.

Without question, the most commonly used continence mechanism in children is based on the flap-valve principle as introduced by Mitrofanoff. Mitrofanoff (1980) reported the use of the appendix to tunnel into the neuropathic bladder (similar to a ureteral reimplantation to prevent reflux) to provide a continent catheterizable stoma into the native bladder. The procedure was popularized by Duckett and Snyder (1986), who extended the use of this technique to create a continent ileocecal pouch, the Penn pouch (Duckett and Snyder, 1987) (Fig. 17.25). Since these early reports many authors from around the world have reported their experience using not only appendix but also ureter, tapered ileal, colonic or gastric tubes, fallopian tubes, and vas deferens (Monfort *et al.*, 1984; Bihrle *et al.*, 1991; Cendron

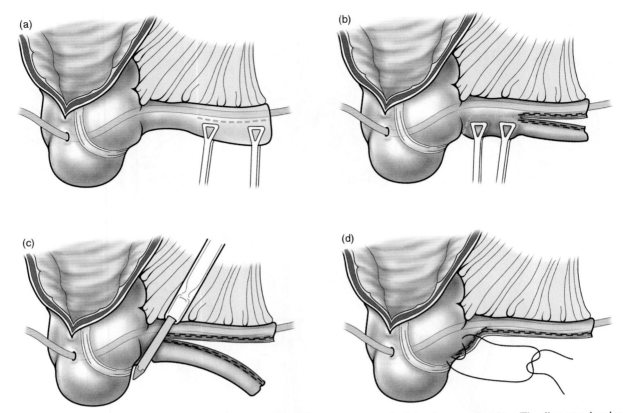

Figure 17.24 Continence is achieved by plcating the ileum to the level of the ileocecal valve. The ileocecal valve is reinforced (*d*)

and Gearhart, 1991; Dykes *et al.*, 1991; Keating *et al.*, 1993; Sumfest *et al.*, 1993; Hasan *et al.*, 1994; Woodhouse and MacNeily, 1994; Kaefer and Retik, 1997; Suzer *et al.*, 1997). The continence mechanism is based on placing a supple tube in a submucosal tunnel with a 5:1 ratio of length to tube diameter. Firm muscle backing of the tube prevents reflux (Fig. 17.26). It was initially thought that the tube itself must also be muscular, but bladder urothelium, colonic mucosa, and preputial skin alone have all been used successfully (Perovic, 1996; Sen and Ahmed, 1998; Casale and Rink, 1999).

This is a relative simple procedure using techniques familiar to pediatric urologists. It is also particularly useful in children who, as noted previously, often are not candidates for use of the ileocecal valve or long segments of ileum. Kaefer and Retik (1997) reviewed several series and found that continence rates ranged from 86 to 96%. The most common complication reported is stomal stenosis. Khoury *et al.* (1996) noted stomal stenosis in 5–57% of patients and described a technique of placing the stoma at the umbilicus. The

Mainz group concluded that stomal stenosis is slightly higher when placed at the umbilicus. A higher risk for stenosis has also been seen when using the appendix compared with tapered ileum (Fichtner *et al.*, 1997; Kaefer *et al.*, 1999). The Great Ormond Street group has reported a decrease in the incidence of stomal stenosis using a VQZ skin-flap technique (Kajbafzadeh *et al.*, 1995) (Fig. 18.3). At a minimum, a skin flap should be placed into the spatulated tube. In the authors' last 100 patients in whom the Mitrofanoff principle has been applied there is a 99% continence rate. Stomal stenosis has occurred in 12% (5/57 appendix, 1/22 ileum, and 6/21 bladder) (Cain *et al.*, 1999). In the Boston experience five of 50 patients leaked at the stomal level (Kaefer and Retik, 1997). Five had stomal stenosis, and one an appendiceal stricture.

Since the introduction of the MACE procedure (Malone antegrade colonic enema), which used the appendix brought to the skin for irrigation of the cecum, it has become necessary to find other tissue to form a catheterizable urinary stoma. The recent description of the Yang–Monti technique (Yang,

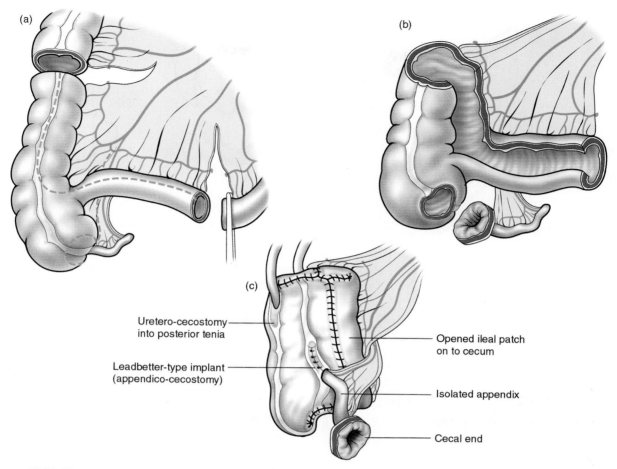

Uretero-cecostomy into posterior tenia

Leadbetter-type implant (appendico-cecostomy)

Opened ileal patch on to cecum

Isolated appendix

Cecal end

Figure 17.25 The Penn pouch. (*a*) The ileocecal segment is isolated and incised on its antimesenteric border; the ureters are implanted into the colonic segment. (*b*) The appendix is isolated in its mesentery. (*c*) The ileocecal segments are joined and the appendix is implanted into the cecum; the cecal end is brought to the skin as a catheterizable stoma.

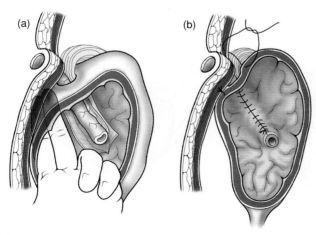

Figure 17.26 Appendivesicostomy is performed by tunneling the appendix submucosally into the bladder. (Reprinted from Keating *et al.*, 1993.)

1993; Monti *et al.*, 1997), which uses only 2 cm of reconfigured ileum to form a tube has been a great advance and has been used successfully (Cain *et al.*, 1998) (Fig. 17.27). Tunneling of these tubes into colon or stomach is easily accomplished but is difficult in ileum. A seromuscular trough for implantation has been described (Keating *et al.*, 1993) and Plaire *et al.* (1999) have described a serosal reimplant similar to the Abol–Enein, Ghoneim ureteral reimplant (Fig. 17.16). It is now clear that the Mitrofanoff principle is a major advance and that virtually any supple tube placed in a tunnel that has adequate muscular backing will successfully provide continence.

Complete gastric reservoirs have been popularized by Mitchell's group (Austin *et al.*, 1999a). They recently described three techniques to provide continence

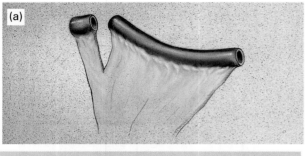

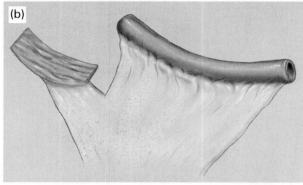

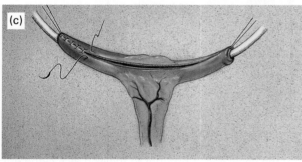

Figure 17.27 Yang-Monti. (*a*) A 2 cm segment of small bowel is isolated on its mesentery. (*b*) It is opened on its antimesenteric border. (*c*) The segment is retubularized by closing it in a longitudinal fashion (see also Figs. 15.23 and 15.24).

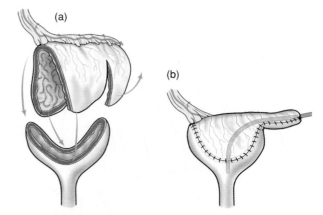

Figure 17.28 Gastric continence mechanisms. (*a*) A gastric wedge is harvested from greater curvature of stomach with anterior strip mobilized for tubularization. (*b*) The anterior strip is tubularized with two sutured layers over a 12 Fr catheter. The proximal end is formed into nipple for the continence mechanism. (From Close and Mitchell, 1997.)

(Close and Mitchell, 1997) (Figs. 17.28 and 17.29). Two of these are based on the Mitrofanoff principle and one on a nipple valve. Stomach is very receptive to tunneled reimplants for either antireflux or continence mechanisms. To reduce acidity, stomach may be used in combination with ileum as the reservoir, rather than stomach alone, applying a Yang–Monti ileal tube tunneled into the stomach as the continence mechanism (Austin *et al.*, 1997, 1999a, b). This prevents the peristomal irritation sometimes seen with gastric tubes (Bihrle *et al.*, 1991; Close and Mitchell, 1997).

The only reservoir that provides a volitional continence mechanism, which also happens to be the first

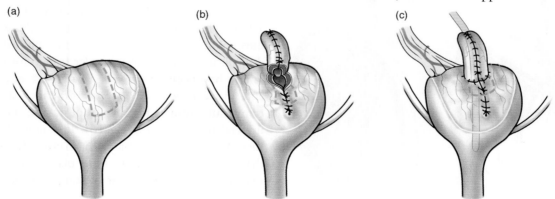

Figure 17.29 Gastroileal pouch with a Monti tube. (*a*) The flap to be tubularized is indicated on existing gastrocystoplasty. (*b*) The flap is raised and tubularized, and the bladder defect is closed. (*c*) Creation of a continent nipple valve by intussusception of gastric tissue as a cuff around the base of the gastric tube. (From Close and Mitchell, 1997.)

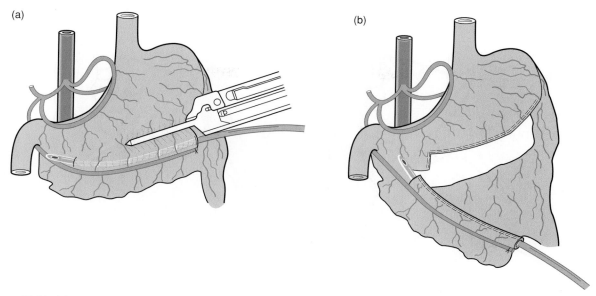

Figure 17.30 (*a*) An isolated gastric tube is harvested with GIA-90 stapler over 12F catheter. (*b*) Mobilized isolated gastric tube is ready for placement into augmented bladder or reservoir.

continent reservoir, is the ureterosigmoidostomy (Simon, 1952). Since its introduction over 60 modifications have been proposed. Because of problems with upper tract deterioration, occasional incontinence, acidosis, and the risk for adenocarcinoma it has been largely abandoned. However, the opportunity for controlled continence without CIC continues to make it very attractive. It cannot be used in spinal dysraphism as a neurologically intact anal sphincter is required. In children it has been used almost exclusively in the exstrophy population when continence cannot be achieved with bladder neck surgery. It has been suggested that oatmeal enemas be given preoperatively to check anal continence (Spirnak and Caldamoni, 1986). Classically, ureterosigmoidostomy has been done by simply tunneling the ureters into the rectum. However, the risk of cancer at the anastomotic site and night-time incontinence led surgeons to pursue other efforts to provide more of a reservoir effect and avoid direct contact of the ureters with the stool. Development of neoplasms seems to require urine to be in contact with stool and bowel mucosa (Crissey *et al.*, 1980; Daher *et al.*, 1988). Of 94 children with ureterosigmoidostomy followed at the Children's Hospital of Boston, seven developed adenocarcinoma of the colon, four of whom died (Rink and Retik, 1991). Rink and Retik (1991) proposed that an ileocecal conduit be initially constructed and the conduit later anastomosed to the intact sig-

moid by end-to-side colocolostomy. Kock *et al.* (1988) described a 'valved-rectum' with the colon intussuscepted at the rectosigmoid junction to prevent reflux of rectal contents and an ileal patch anastomosed to the anterior rectal wall. This allowed the rectal capacity to increase from 200 to 700 ml with maximal pressures of only 24 cmH$_2$O and minimal metabolic disturbances.

A hemi-Kock pouch anastomosed to the rectum has also been described, but the complexity of creating the colonic nipple in these two procedures make them less attractive. The sigma rectum (Mainz pouch II) has been proposed from the group from Mainz as a means of lowering the very high pressures in the intact rectosigmoid colon without the need for nipples or augmentation (Fisch *et al.*, 1993) (Figs. 17.30 and 17.31). Continence was achieved in 40 of 47 patients, with voiding five times per day, and extracolonic pressures remained low. The results in 34 patients of the Mainz II were reported by Gerharz *et al.* (1988). All were continent during the day. One had night-time soiling and had creation of an ileal conduit due to recurrent septicemia. One ureteral obstruction led to a nephrectomy and two had mild hyperchloremic acidosis. While lower pressures with the new procedures should reduce the risk for upper tract changes, the risk for adenocarcinoma still weighs heavily when contemplating any type of ureterocolonic diversion.

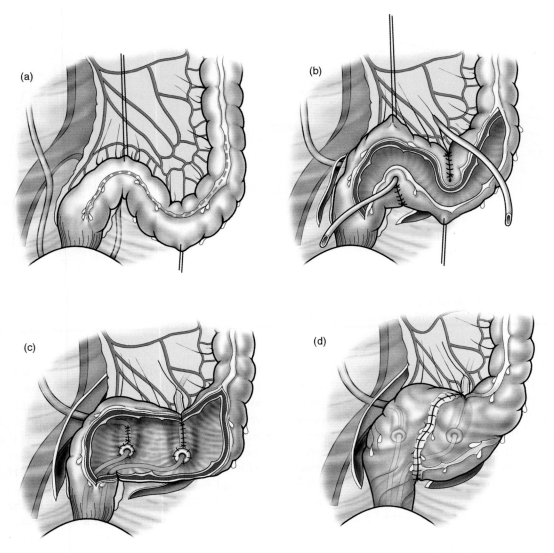

Figure 17.31 The Mainz pouch II (sigma rectum) has been presented as a means of reconstructing a low-pressure ureterosigmoidostomy. The ureters are implanted in the detubularized portion of the sigmoid.

Postoperative care

In the early postoperative interval ureteral drainage is provided by stents which are left indwelling for at least 1 week. Antibiotics are given until all tubes are removed. H_2 blockers are given temporarily if stomach is used. The reservoir is drained by a large-bore silastic tube for 3 weeks. The reservoirs are irrigated three times a day for the first 3 weeks and then slowly decreased to daily, for the rest of the patient's life. A pouch-o-gram is obtained before removal of the stents. The indwelling reservoir drainage tube is maintained until the patient and family demonstrate that they can easily and reliably catheterize the stoma and empty the reservoir. Demonstration of complete emptying is mandatory to prevent long-term problems of infection, stone formation, incontinence, and perforation, and to maintain stable renal function.

Renal and pouch sonography, abdominal radiographs, and serum creatinine and electrolytes are all obtained 3 months postoperatively, repeated at 6 month intervals, twice, and yearly thereafter. Vitamin B_{12} levels should be checked in the long term and somatic growth monitored. Endoscopic evaluation of the pouch should be carried out annually starting at 5–10 years postoperatively.

Summary

Tremendous advances have been made in lower urinary tract reconstruction in children. The entire urinary tract can now be completely replaced. Bladders can be constructed that are continent, ureters can be replaced with antireflux mechanisms easily achieved, and kidneys can be transplanted. Direct cutaneous diversion is generally only used as a temporary means to provide drainage. Non-continent diversion is only used in children who are incapable of independent care. It is ideal to maintain the native urinary tract intact and reconstructive efforts should be directed to achieve this. If this cannot be achieved a CUR should be provided. The limits of reconstruction are based only on the surgeon's imagination and skills. As long as the principles of CUR construction outlined in this chapter are met, a successful surgical result can almost always be achieved. True success, however, will always require the cooperation of a well-motivated child and equally motivated parents. Furthermore, this type of major reconstruction necessitates that the surgeon be surrounded by dedicated personnel who function as a team for the betterment of the health of these children.

References

Abol-Enein H, Ghoneim MA (1994) A novel uretero-ileal reimplantation technique: the serous lined extramural tunnel. A preliminary report. *J Urol* **151**: 1193–7.

Adams MC, Mitchell ME, Rink PC (1988) Gastrocystoplasty: an alternative solution to the problem of urological reconstruction in the severely compromised patient. *J Urol* **140**: 1152–6.

Adams MC, Bihrle R, Rink RC (1995) The use of stomach in urologic reconstruction. *AUA Update Series* **27**: 218–33.

Akerlund S, Delin K, Kock NG *et al.* (1989) Renal function and upper urinary tract configuration following urinary diversion to a continent ileal reservoir (Kock pouch): a prospective 5- to-11 year follow up after reservoir construction. *J Urol* **142**: 964–8.

Alagiri M, Seidmon EJ (1998) Percutaneous endoscopic cystostomy for bladder localization and exact placement of a suprapubic tube. *J Urol* **159**: 963–4.

Allen T, Peters PC, Sagalowsky A (1985) The Camey procedure: preliminary results in patients. *World J Urol* **3**: 167.

Asken MH (1987) Urinary cecal reservoir. In: King LR, Stone AR, Webster GD (eds) *Bladder reconstruction and continent urinary diversion.* Chicago, IL: Yearbook Medical Publishers, 288–351.

Atala A, Bauer SB, Hendren WH *et al.* (1993) The effect of gastric augmentation on bladder function. *J Urol* **149**: 1099–102.

Austin PF, DeLeary G, Homsey YL *et al.* (1997) Long term metabolic advantages of a gastrointestinal composite urinary reservoir. *J Urol* **158**: 1704–8.

Austin PF, Lockhart JL (1998) Continence mechanisms in urinary reconstruction. *AUA Update Series* **29**: 226–31.

Austin PF, Rink RC, Lockhart JL (1999a) The gastrointestinal composite urinary reservoir in patients with myelomeningocele and exstrophy: long-term metabolic follow up. *J Urol* **162**: 1126–8.

Austin PF, Lockhart JL, Rink RC (1999b) The gastrointestinal composite reservoir. *Dialog Pediatr Urol* **22**: 7, 8.

Baker LA, Gearhart JP (1998) Continent urinary diversion. *Prog Paediatr Urol* **1**: 67–79.

Bartone JJ, Hurwitz RS, Rojas EL, Steinberg E (1998) The role of percutaneous nephrostomy in the management of obstructing candidiasis of the urinary tract in infants. *J Urol* **140**: 338–41.

Bauer SB, Hendren WH, Kozakewich H *et al* (1992) Perforation of the augmented bladder. *J Urol* **148**: 699–703.

Bell DA, Rose SC, Starr NK *et al.* (1993) Percutaneous nephrostomy for nonoperative management of fungal urinary tract infections. *J Vasc Intervent Radiol* **4**: 311–15.

Belman AB (1985) Temporary diversion. In: Kelalis PP, King LR, Belman AB (eds) *Clinical pediatric urology.* Philadelphia, PA: WB Saunders, 582.

Benchekroun A (1982) Continent cecal bladder. *Br J Urol* **54**: 505–6.

Benchekroun A, Essakalli N, Faik M *et al.* (1989) Continent urostomy with hydraulic valve in 136 patients. 13 years of experience. *J Urol* **142**: 46–51.

Benson MC, Olsson CA (1998) Continent urinary diversion. In: Walsh PC, Retik AB, Vaughn ED, Wein AJ, (eds) *Campbell's urology.* 7th edition. Philadelphia, PA: WB Saunders 3190–245.

Benson MC, Olsson CA (1999) Continent urinary diversion. *Urol Clin North Am* **26**: 125–47.

Berglund B., Kock NG, Nrlen L, Philipson MB (1987) Volume capacity and pressure characteristics of the continent ileal reservoir used for urinary diversion. *J Urol* **137**: 29–34.

Bihrle R, Klee LW, Adams MC *et al.* (1991) Transverse colon–gastric tube composite reservoir. *Urol* **37**: 36–40.

Bissada NK (1993) A new continent ileocolonic urinary reservoir: the Charleston pouch with minimally altered *in-situ* appendix stoma. *Urol* **41**: 524–6.

Blavis JG, Labib KB, Bauer SB *et al* (1977) Changing concepts in the urodynamic evaluation of children. *J Urol* **117**: 778–81.

Blocksom BH (1957) Bladder pouch for prolonged tubeless cystostomy. *J Urol* **78**: 398–401.

Boyd SD, Schiff WM, Skinner DG *et al.* (1989) Prospective study of metabolic abnormalities in patients with continent Koch pouch urinary diversion. *Urology* **33**: 85–8.

Bricker EM (1950) Bladder substitution after pelvic evisceration. *Surg Clin North Am* **30**: 1511–21.

Cain MP, Casale AJ, King SJ, Rink RC (1999) Appendico-vesicostomy and newer alternatives for the Mitrofanoff procedure: results in the last 100 patients at Riley Children's Hospital. *J Urol* **162**: 1749–52.

Cain MP, Casale AJ, Rink RC (1998) Initial experience utilizing a catheterizable ileovesicostomy (Monti procedure) in children. *Urology* **52**: 870–3.

Camey M, Richard F, Botto H (1991) Ileal replacement of bladder. In: King LS, Stone AR, Webster GD (eds) *Bladder reconstruction and continent urinary diversion*. St. Louis, MO: Mosby Yearbook, 389–410.

Canning DA, Perman JA, Jeffs RD, Gearhart JP (1989) Nutritional consequences of bowel segments in the lowery urinary tract. *J Urol* **142**: 509–11.

Canning DC (1998) Continent urinary diversion. In: King LR (ed.) *Urologic surgery infants and children*. Philadelphia, PA: WB Saunders, 139–61.

Carroll PR, Presti JC Jr (1992) Comparison of plicated and stapled continent ileocecal stoma. *Urology* **40**: 107–9.

Carroll PR, Presti JC Jr, McAninch JW *et al.* (1989) Functional characteristics of the continent ileocecal urinary reservoir: mechanisms of continence. *J Urol* **142**: 1032–6.

Casale AJ, Rink RC (1999) Continent vesicostomy. *Dialog Pediatr Urol* **22**: 5–6.

Castro-Diaz D, Froemming C, Manivel JC *et al.* (1992) The influence of urinary diversion on experimental gastrocystoplasty. *J Urol* **148**: 571–4.

Cendron M (1995) Discussion; temporary cutaneous urinary diversion in children. *Dialog Pediatr Urol* **18**: 1–8.

Cendron M, Gearhart JP (1991) The Mitrofanoff principle: technique and application in continent urinary diversion. *Urol Clin North Am* **18**: 615–21.

Close CE, Mitchell ME (1997) Continent gastric tube; new techniques and long term follow up. *J Urol* **157**: 51–5.

Coffey RC (1911) Physiologic implantation of the severed ureter or common bile duct Into the intestine. *JAMA* **56**: 397–403.

Cohen S, Harris LD, Levitan, R (1968) Manometric characteristics of the human ileocecal junctional zone. *Gastroenterology* **54**: 72–75.

Crissey MM, Steele GD, Gittes RF (1980) Rat model for carcinogenesis in ureterosigmoidostomy. *Science* **207**: 1079.

Daher N, Gantier R, Abourachid H (1988) Rat colonic carcinogenesis after ureterosigmoidostomy: pathogenesis and immunohistological study. *J Urol* **139**: 1331–6.

Demos MP (1962) Radioactive electrolyte absorption studies of small bowel, comparison of different segments for use in urinary diversion. *J Urol* **88**: 638–93.

Duckett JW, Snyder HM III (1986) Continent urinary diversion: variations on the Mitrofanoff principle. *J Urol* **135**: 58.

Duckett JW, Snyder HM III (1987) The Mitrofanoff principle in continent urinary reservoirs. *Semin Urol* **5**: 55–62.

Duckett JW, Ziylan O (1995) Uses and abuses of vesicostomy. *AUA Update Series* **14**: 130–5.

Dykes EH, Duffy PG, Ransley PG (1991) The use of the Mitrofanoff principle in achieving clean intermittent catheterization and urinary continence in children. *J Pediatr Surg* **26**: 535–8.

Edelstein RA, Bauer SB, Kelly MD *et al.* (1995) The long term urologic response of neonate with myelodysplasia treated proactively with intermittent catheterization and anticholinergic therapy. *J Urol* **154**: 1500–4.

Elder DD, Moisey CU, Rees RWM (1983) A long term follow up of the colonic conduit operation in children. *Br J Urol* **55**: 629–31.

Farrell TA, Hicks ME (1997) A review of radiologically guided percutaneous nephrostomies in 303 patients. *J Vasc Intervent Radiol* **8**: 769–74.

Ferris DO, Odel HM (1950) Electrolyte pattern of the blood after bilateral ureterosigmoidostomy. *JAMA* **142**: 634–40.

Fichtner J, Fischer R, Hohenfellner R (1997) Appendiceal continence mechanisms in continent urinary diversion. *World J Urol* **157**: 635–7.

Filmer RB, Spencer JR (1990) Malignancies in bladder augmentation and intestinal conduits. *J Urol* **143**: 671–8.

Fisch M, Wammack R, Muller SC, Hohenfellner R (1993) The Mainz pouch II (sigma rectum pouch). *J Urol* **149**: 258–63.

Fitzgerald J, Malone MJ, Gaertner RA, Zinman LN (1997) Stomal construction, complication, and reconstruction. *Urol Clin North Am* **24**: 729–33.

Fowler JE Jr (1988) Continent urinary reservoirs. *Surg Ann* **20**: 201–25.

Ganesan GS, Mitchell ME, Adams MC *et al.* (1991) Use of stomach for reconstruction of the lower urinary tract in patients with compromised renal function. New Orleans: Presented at the American Academy of Pediatrics Meeting, 1991.

Gerharz EW, Kohl U, Weingartner K *et al.* (1997) Complications related to different continence mechanism in ileocecal reservoirs. *J Urol* **158**: 1709–13.

Gerharz EW, Kohl UN, Weingartner K *et al.* (1988) Experience with the Mainz modification of ureterosigmoidostomy. *Br J Urol* **85**: 1512–6.

Gilcrest RK, Merricks JW, Hamlin HH, Rieger IT (1950) Construction of a substitute bladder and urethra. *Surg Gynecol Obstet* **90**: 752–60.

Goldwasser B, Barrett DM, Webster GD, Kramer SA (1986) Cystometric properties of ileum and right colon after bladder augmentation, substitution or replacement. *J Urol* **138**: 1007–8.

Goldwasser B, Webster GD (1986) Augmentation and substitution enterocystoplasty. *J Urol* **135**: 215–24.

Gonzalez ET (1992) Posterior urethral valves and other urethral anomalies. In: Walsh PC, Retik AB, Vaughan ED, Wein AJ (eds) *Campbell's urology*. Philadelphia, PA: WB Saunders, 865–903.

Gonzalez ET (1998) Posterior urethral valves and other urethral anomalies. In: Walsh PC, Retik AB, Vaughan ED, Wein AJ (eds) *Campbell's urology*. Philadelphia, PA: WB Saunders, 2069–91.

Gonzalez R, Cabral BHP (1987) Rectal continence after enterocystoplasty. *Dialog Pediatr Urol* **10**: 3–4.

Gosalbez R, Woodard JR, Broecker BH *et al.* (1993) The use of stomach in pediatric urinary reconstruction. *J Urol* **150**: 438–40.

Grune MT, Taylor RJ (1996) Aspects of urinary diversion: the current role of conduits. *AUA Update Series* 15: 166–71.

Guzman JM, Montes de Oca L, Gonzalez R *et al.* (1989) Modified Benchekroun technique for continent ileal stoma. *J Urol* 142: 1431–3.

Hall MC, McDougall NS, Kock MD (1991) Metabolic consequences of urinary diversion through intestinal segments. *Urol Clin North Am* 18: 725–35.

Hanna MK, Bloiso G (1987) Continent diversion in children: modification of Kock pouch. *J Urol* 137: 1206–8.

Harper JGM, Berman MH, Hertzberg HD *et al* (1954) Observations on the use of the cecum as a substitute urinary bladder. *J Urol* 71: 600–2.

Hasan ST, Marshall C, Neal DE (1994) Continent urinary diversion using the Mitrofanoff principle. *Br J Urol* 74: 454–9.

Hendren WH (1969) Operative repair of megaureter in children. *J Urol* 101: 491–507.

Hendren WH (1970) A new approach to infants with severe obstructive uropathy: early complete reconstruction. *J Pediatr Surg* 5: 184–99.

Hendren WH (1973) Reconstruction of previously diverted urinary tract in children. *J Pediatr Surg* 8: 135–50.

Hendren WH (1980) Reoperative ureteral reimplantation: management of the difficult case. *J Pediatr Surg* 15: 770–86.

Hensle TW, Ring KS (1991) Urinary tract reconstruction in children. *Urol Clin North Am* 18: 701–15.

Hinman F Jr (1988) Selection of intestinal segments for bladder substitution: physical and physiologic characteristics. *J Urol* 139: 519–23.

Hirst G (1991) Ileal and colonic cystoplasties. *Prob Urol* 5: 223.

Hohenfellner R, Riedmiller H, Thuroff JW (1990) Commentary: the MAINZ pouch. In: Whitehead ED (ed.) *Current operative urology*. Philadelphia, PA: JB Lippincott, 168.

Horowitz M, Kuhr CS, Mitchell ME (1995) The Mitrofanoff catheterizable channel: patient acceptance. *J Urol* 153: 771–2.

Husmann DA, McLorie GA, Churchill BM (1989) Nonrefluxing colonic conduits: a long term life table analysis. *J Urol* 142: 1201–3.

Hutton KA, Thomas DF (1998) Selective use of cutaneous vesicostomy in prenatally detected and clinically presenting uropathies. *Eur Urol* 33: 405–11.

Issa MM, Oesterling JE, Canning DA, Jeffs RD (1989) A new technique of using *in-situ* appendix as a catheterizable stoma in continent urinary reservoirs. *J Urol* 141: 1385–7.

Jayanthi VR, McLorie GA, Khoury AE, Churchill BM (1995) The effect of temporary cutaneous diversion on ultimate bladder function. *J Urol* 154: 889–92.

Joyner BD, Khoury AE (1999) The role of urinary diversion in childhood: temporary, continent, or otherwise. In: Gonzalez ET, Bauer S (eds) *Pediatric urology practice*. Baltimore, MD: Lippincott, Williams and Wilkins, 687–704.

Kaefer M, Hendren WH, Bauer SB *et al* (1995) Reservoir calculi. A comparison of reservoirs constructed from stomach and other enteric segments. *J Urol* 160: 2187–90.

Kaefer M, Retik AB (1997) The Mitrofanoff principle in continent urinary reconstruction. *Urol Clin North Am* 24: 795–811.

Kaefer M, Rink RC, Cain MP, Casale AJ (1999) Stomal stenosis: is ileum the ideal substrate for efferent limb construction? Presented at the American Academy of Pediatrics, Washington, DC, October, 1999.

Kajbafzadeh AM, Duffy PG, Carr *et al* (1995) A review of 100 Mitrofanoff stomas and reports of the VQZ technique for prevention of complications at the stomal level. ESPU, Toledo, Spain, 1995.

Keating MA, Kropp BP, Adams MC *et al.* (1993) Seromuscular trough modification in construction of continent urinary stomas. *J Urol* 150: 734–6.

Keating MA, Rink RC, Adams MC (1993) Appendicovesicostomy: a useful adjunct to continent reconstruction of the bladder. *J Urol* 149: 1091–4.

Kennedy HA, Adams MC, Mitchell ME *et al.* (1988) Chronic renal failure in bladder augmentation stomach versus sigmoid in the canine model. *J Urol* 140: 1138–40.

Khoury AE, VanSavage JG, McLorie GA, Churchill BM (1996) Minimizing stomal stenosis in appendicovesicostomy using the modified umbilical stoma. *J Urol* 155: 2050–1.

Kim YH, Horowitz M, Cojmbs A *et al.* (1996) Comparative urodynamic findings after primary valve ablation, vesicostomy or proximal diversion. *J Urol* 156: 673–6.

Kinahan TJ, Khoury AE, McLorie G *et al.* (1992) Imepregal in post-gastrocystoplasty metabolic alkalosis and aciduria. *J Urol* 147: 435–7.

King LR (1987) Protection of the upper urinary tracts in children. In: *Bladder Reconstruction and Continent Urinary Diversion*. King LR, Stone AR, Webster GD (eds) Chicago, IL: Yearbook Medical Publishers, 127.

Koch MO, McDougal WS, Hall MC *et al.* (1992) A comparison of myelomeningocele patients managed by clean intermittent catheterization and urinary diversion. *J Urol* 147: 1343–74.

Koch, MO, McDougal WS (1985) The pathophysiology of hyperchloremic metabolic acidosis after urinary diversion through intestinal segments. *J Urol* 134: 162–4.

Kock NG (1969) Internal 'reservoir' in patients with permanent ileostomy. Preliminary observations on a procedure resulting in fecal 'continence' in five ileostomy patients. *Arch Surg* 99: 223–31.

Kock NG (1973) Continent ileostomy. *Prog Surg* 12: 180.

Kock NG, Ghoneim NNNA, Lycke KG (1988) Urinary diversion to the augmented and valved rectum: preliminary results with a novel surgical procedure. *J Urol* 140: 1375–9.

Kock NG, Nelson AE, Nelsson LO *et al* (1982) Urinary diversion via a continent ileal reservoir: clinical results in 12 patients. *J Urol* 128: 469–475.

Koff SA (1988) Guidelines to determine size and shape of intestinal segments used for reconstruction. *J Urol* 140: 1150–1.

Koff SA, Cirulli C, Wise HA (1989) Clinical and urodynamic features of a new intestinal urinary sphincter for continent urinary diversion. *J Urol* 142: 293–6.

Krahn CG, Johnson HW (1993) Cutaneous vesicostomy in the young child: indications and results. *Urology* **41**: 558–63.

Kronner KM, Casale AJ, Cain MP *et al.* (1998) Bladder calculi in the pediatric augmented bladder. *J Urol* **160**: 1096–8.

Krueger RP, Hardy BE, Churchill BM (1980) Growth in boys with posterior urethral valves: primary valve resection vs upper tract diversion. *Urol Clin North Am* **7**: 265–72.

Kulb TB, Rink RC, Mitchell ME (1986) Gastrocystoplasty in azotemic canines. Presented at the American Urological Association, North Central Section Meeting, Palm Springs, FL, 1986.

Lampel A, Hohenfellner M, Schultz-Lampel D, Thuroff JW (1995) *In situ* tunneled bowel flap tubes: 2 new techniques of a continent outlet of MAINZ pouch cutaneous diversion. *J Urol* **153**: 305–18.

Lapides J, Ajemian EP, Lichtwardt JR (1960) Cutaneous vesicostomy. *J Urol* **84**: 609.

Lapides J, Diokno AC, Gould FR *et al* (1972) Clean intermittent self-catheterization in the treatment of urinary tract disease. *J Urol* **107**: 458–61.

LeDuc A, Camey M, Teillac P (1987) An original antireflux ureteroileal implantation technique. Long term follow up. *J Urol* **137**: 1156–8.

Leonard MP, Gearhart JP, Jeffs RD (1990) Continent urinary reservoirs in pediatric urological practice. *J Urol* **144**: 330–3.

Levy JB, Van Arsdalan KN (1994) Ureteral and ureteroenteral strictures. *AUA Update Series* **13**: 230–5.

Light JK, Engleman UH (1985) Reconstruction of the lower urinary tract. Observations on bowel dynamics and the artificial urinary sphincter. *J Urol* **133**: 594–7.

Lockhart JL, Davies R, Cox C *et al.* (1993) The gastroileal pouch: an alternative continent urinary reservoir for patient with short bowel, acidosis and/or extensive pelvic radiation. *J Urol* **150**: 46–50.

Lockhart JL, Figurevoa TE, Persky L (1994) Metabolic advantages and disadvantages of different stomach preparation for urinary reservoir construction. *J Urol* **151**: 240A (Abstract 52).

Lockhart JL, Pow-Sang JM, Persky L *et al.* (1991) Results, complications, and surgical indications of the Florida pouch. *Surg Gynecol Obstet* **173**: 289–96.

Lockhart JL, Pow-Sang JM; Persky L, Kahn P *et al.* (1990) A continent colonic reservoir: the Florida Pouch. *J Urol* **144**: 864–7.

Lytton B, Green DF (1994) Urodynamic studies in patients undergoing bladder replacement surgery. *J Urol* **141**: 1394–7.

Mansson W, Davidsson T, Colleen S (1990) The detubularized right colonic segment as urinary reservoir: evolution of technique for continent diversion. *J Urol* **144**: 1359–61.

McDougal WS (1986) Bladder reconstruction following cystectomy by uretero-ileo-colourethrostomy. *J Urol* **135**: 698–701.

McDougal WS (1998) Use of intestinal segments and urinary diversion. In: Walsh PC, Retik AB, Vaughan ED, Wein AJ (eds). *Campbell's urology*. Philadelphia, PA: WB Saunders, 3121–61.

McDougal WS (1999) Metabolic complications of urinary intestinal diversion. *J Urol* **147**: 1199–208.

McGuire EJ, Woodside JR, Border TA, Weiss RM (1981) Prognostic value of urodynamic testing in myelodysplastic patients. *J Urol* **26**: 205–9.

McLaughlin K, Rink RC (1998) Bladder and prostate rhabdomyosarcoma. In King LR (ed.) *Urologic surgery in infants and children*. Philadelphia, PA: WB Saunders, 168–79.

McLaughlin KP, Rink RC, Adams MC *et al.* (1995a) Stomach in combination with other intestinal segments in pediatric lower urinary tract reconstruction. *J Urol* **154**: 1162–8.

McLaughlin KP, Rink RC, Kalsbeck JE *et al.* (1995a) Cloacal exstrophy: the neurological implications. *J Urol* **154**: 782–4.

Merricks JW (1987) A continent substitute bladder and urethra. In: King LR, Stone AR, Webster GD (eds) *Bladder reconstruction and continent urinary diversion*. Chicago, IL: Yearbook Medical Publishers, 179–203.

Mitchell ME (1986) Use of bowel in undiversion. *Urol Clin North Am* **13**: 349.

Mitchell ME, Piser JA (1987) Intestinocystoplasty and total bladder replacement in children and young adults: follow up in 129 cases. *J Urol* **138**: 579–84.

Mitrofanoff P (1980) Cystostomie continent trans-appendiculaire dans le traitement des vessies neurologiques. *Chir Pediatr* **21**: 297.

Monfort G, Guys JM, Lacombe M (1984) Appedicovesicostomy: an alternative urinary diversion in the child. *Eur Urol* **10**: 361–3.

Monti PR, Lara RC, Dutra MA *et al* (1997) New techniques for construction of efferent conduits based on the Mitrofanoff principle. *Urology* **49**: 112–15.

Morelli G, Gelipetto R, Biver P *et al.* (1997) Use of new nephrostomy catheter for treatment of renal neonatal candidiasis. *Eur Urol* **32**: 485–6.

Mundy AR, Nurse DE (1992) Calcium balance, growth and skeletal mineralization in patient with cystoplasties *J Urol* **69**: 257–9.

Mykulak DJ, Herskowitz M, Gladberg KI (1994) Use of magnetic internal ureteral stents in pediatric urology; retrieval without routine requirement for cystoscopy and general anesthesia. *J Urol* **152**: 976–7.

Ngan JHK, Lau JLT, Lim STK *et al.* (1993) Long term results of antral gastrocystoplasty. *J Urol* **149**: 731–4.

Nguyen DH, Bain MA, Salmonson KL *et al.* (1993) The syndrome of dysuria and hematuria in pediatric urinary reconstruction with stomach. *J Urol* **150**: 707–9.

Noe HN, Jerkins GR (1985) Cutaneous vesicostomy experience in infants and children. *J Urol* **134**: 301–3.

Nurse DE, Mundy AR (1989) Metabolic complications of cystoplasty. *Br J Urol* **63**: 165–70.

Papanicolaou N (1998) Urinary tract imaging and intervention: basic principles. In: Walsh PC, Retik AB, Vaughn ED, Wein AG (eds) *Campbell's urology*. Philadelphia, PA: WB Saunders, 170–260.

Perovic S (1996) Continent urinary diversion using preputial penile or clitoral skin flap. *J Urol* **155**: 1402–6.

Pfeffer DM, Caldamone AA (1992) Management of the dilated ureter in children. In: Fowler JE (ed.) *Urologic surgery*. Boston, MA: Little, Brown and Co., 221–7.

Piser JA, Mitchell ME, Kulb TB *et al.* (1987) Gastrocystoplasty and colocystoplasty in canines: the metabolic consequences of acute saline and acid loading. *J Urol* **138**: 1000.

Pitts WR, Muecke EC (1979) A 20 year experience with ileal conduits: the fate of the kidneys. *J Urol* **122**: 154–7.

Plaire JC, Grady RW, Mitchell EM (1999) The serosal lined tunnel principle in the creation of a continent catheterizable channel. Presented at the AUA Meeting, Dallas, TX, 1999 (Abstract 757).

Pope JC IV, Rink RC (1999) Surgical options in the management of the neurogenic bladder. In *Pediatric Urology Practice*. (Eds ET Conzalez and SB Bauer.) Lippincott, Williams and Wilkins, Philadephia, 401–19.

Pope JC, Albers P, Rink RC *et al.* (1999) Spontaneous rupture of the augmented bladder from silence to chaos. Presented at the European Society of Pediatric Urology, Istanbul, Turkey, 1999.

Pope JC, Keating MA, Casale AJ, Rink RC (1998) Augmenting the augmented bladder. Treatment of the contractile bowel segment. *J Urol* **160**: 854–7.

Razvi HA, Martin TV, Sosa RE, Vaughan ED (1996) Endourologic management of complications of urinary intestinal diversion. *AUA Update Series* **15**: 174–9.

Regan JB, Barrett DM (1985) Stented versus non-stented ureteroileal anatomoses: is there a difference with regard to leak and stricture? *J Urol* **14**: 1101–3.

Reinberg Y, deCastano I, Gonzalez R (1992b) Influence of initial therapy on progression of renal failure and body growth in children with posterior urethral valves. *J Urol* **148**: 532–3.

Reinberg Y, Manivel JC, Froemming C *et al.* (1992a) Perforation of the gastric segment of an augmented bladder secondary to peptic ulcer disease. *J Urol* **148**: 369–71.

Rendelman DF, Anthony JE, Davis C Jr *et al.* (1958) Reflux pressure studies on the ileocecal valve of dogs and humans. *Surgery* **44**: 640–3.

Ring KS, Hensle TW (1992) Urinary diversion. In: Kelalis P, King LE, Belman AB (eds) *Clinical pediatric urology* 865–903.

Rink RC (1999) Bladder augmentation: options, outcomes, future. *Urol Clin North Am* **26**: 111–23.

Rink RC, Adams MC (1996) Augmentation cystoplasty. In: Marshall FF (ed.) *Textbook of Operative Urology*. Philadelphia, PA: WB Saunders, 914–26.

Rink RC, Adams MA (1998) Augmentation cystoplasty. In: Walsh P, Retik AB, Vaughn ED, Wein A (eds) *Campbell's urology*. Philadelphia, PA: WB Saunders, **19**: 3162–89.

Rink RC, Bihrle R (1990) Continent urinary diversion in children and the Indiana pouch. *Prob Urol* **4**: 663–75.

Rink RC, Keating MA (1993) Cutaneous ureterostomy. In: Fowler J (ed.) *Urologic surgery*. Boston, MA: Little Brown and Co., 315–20.

Rink RC, McLaughlin KP (1994) Indications for enterocystoplasty and choice of bowel segment. *Prob Urol* **8**: 389–403.

Rink RC, Mitchell ME (1990) Role of enterocystoplasty in reconstructing the neurogenic bladder. In: Gonzalez ET, Roth D (eds) *Common problems in pediatric urology*. St. Louis, MO: Mosby Yearbook, 192–204.

Rink RC, Retik AB (1991) Ureteroileocecal sigmoidostomy and avoidance of carcinoma of the colon. In: King LR, Stone AR, Webster GD (eds) *Bladder reconstruction and continent urinary diversion*. St. Louis, MO: Mosby Yearbook, 221–7.

Rink RC, Hollensbe DW, Adams MC *et al.* (1995) Complications of bladder augmentation and gastrointestinal segments. *AUA Update Series* **14**: 122.

Roth S, Semjonow A, Waldner M, Hertle L (1995) Risk of bowel dysfunction with diarrhea after continent urinary diversion with ileal and ileocecal segments. *J Urol* **154**: 1696–9.

Rowland RG (1991) Intestine for bladder augmentation and substitution. In: King LR, Stone AR, Webster ED (eds) *Bladder reconstruction and continent urinary diversion*. St. Louis, MO: Mosby Yearbook, 12–28.

Rowland RG (1995) Complications of continent cutaneous reservoirs and neobladder–series using contemporary techniques. *AUA Update Series* **14**: 202–7.

Rowland RG (1996) Present experience with the Indiana pouch. *World J Urol* **14**: 92–8.

Rowland RG, Mitchell ME, Bihrle R (1985) The cecoileal continent urinary reservoir. *World J Urol* **3**: 185.

Sagalowsky AI (1992) Mechanisms of continence in continent urinary diversions. *AUA Update Series* **11**: 34–9.

Sanda MC, Jeffs RD, Gearhart JP (1988) Evaluation of outcomes with the ileal hydraulic continent diversion: reevaluation of the Bechekroun catheterizable stoma. *World J Urol* **14**: 108–111.

Schwarz GR, Jeffs RD (1975) Ileal conduit urinary diversion in children, computer analysis of follow up from 2–16 years. *J Urol* **114**: 285–8.

Sen S, Ahmed S (1998) Construction of continent catheterizable urinary conduit from an isolated segment of colon. *Aust NZ J Surg* **68**: 367–8.

Shapiro SR, Lebowitz R, Colodny AH (1975) Fate of 90 children with ileal conduit urinary diversion a decade later: analysis of complications, pyelography, renal function and bacteriology. *J Urol* **114**: 289–95.

Sheldon CA, Gilbert A, Wacksman J *et al.* (1995) Gastrocystoplasty; technical and metabolic characteristics of the most versatile childhood bladder augmentation modality. *J Pediatr Surg* **30**: 283–8.

Sheldon CA, Snyder HM III (1996) Principles of urinary tract reconstruction. In: Gillenwater JY, Grayhack JT, Howards SS, Duckett JW (eds) *Adult and pediatric urology*. St. Louis, MO: Mosby, 2317–410.

Sidi AA, Reinberg Y, Gonzalez R (1986) Influence of intestinal segment and configuration on the outcome of augmentation enterocystoplasty. *J Urol* **136**: 1201–4.

Simon J (1952) Ectropia vesicae (absence of the anterior walls of the bladder and pubic abdominal parietes); operation for directing the orifices of the ureters into the rectum; temporary success; subsequent death, autopsy. *Lancet* ii: 568.

Skinner DG, Boyd SD, Lieskovsky G (1984) Clinical experience with the Kock continent ileal reservoir for urinary diversion. *J Urol* **132**: 1101–7.

Skinner DG, Lieskovsky G, Boyd S (1987) Continuing experience with the continent ileal reservoir (Kock pouch) as an alternative to cutaneous urinary diversion: an update after 250 cases. *J Urol* **137**: 1140–5.

Skinner DG, Lieskovsky G, Boyd S (1989) Continent urinary diversion. *J Urol* **141**: 1323–4.

Skoog SJ (1998) Pediatric vesical diversion. In: Graham SD (ed.) *Glenn's urologic surgery*. Philadelphia, PA: Lippincott-Raven, 872–8.

Slaton JW, Kropp KA (1996) Proximal ureteral stent migration; an avoidable complication? *J Urol* **155**: 58–61.

Smith GHH, Canning DA, Schulman SL et al. (1996) The long term outcome of posterior urethral valves treated with primary valve ablation and observation. *J Urol* **155**: 1730–4.

Sober I (1973) Pevioureterostomy-en-Y. *J Urol* **107**: 473–5.

Spirnak, JP, Caldamone AA (1986) Ureterosigmoidostomy. *Urol Clinics North Am* **13**: 285–94.

Stanely P, Diament MJ (1986) Pediatric percutaneous nephrostomy: experience with 50 patients. *J Urol* **135**: 1223–6.

Stein R, Lotz J, Andreas J, Fisch M et al. (1998) Long-term metabolic effects in patients with urinary diversion. *World J Urol* **16**: 292–7.

Stein R, Matani Y, Doi Y (1995) Continent urinary diversion using the MAINZ pouch I technique – ten years later. *J Urol* **153**: 251.

Steiner MS, Morton RA (1991) Nutritional and gastrointestinal complications of the use of bowel segments in the lower urinary tract. *Urol Clin North Am* **18**: 743–54.

Stone AR, MacDermott JPA (1989) The split cuff ureteral nipple reimplantation technique. Reliable reflux prevention from bowel segments. *J Urol* **142**: 707–9.

Sullivan H, Gilchrist RK, Merricks JW (1973) Ileocecal substitute bladder long-term follow up. *J Urol* **190**: 43–5.

Sumfest JM, Burns MW, Mitchell ME (1993) The Mitrofanoff principle in urinary reconstruction. *J Urol* **150**: 1875.

Suzer O, Vates AL, Freedman CA et al. (1997) Results of the Mitrofanoff procedure in urinary tract reconstruction in children. *Br J Urol* **79**: 279–82.

Thoroff JW, Alken P, Hohenfellner R (1987) The MAINZ pouch (mixed augmentation with ileum 'n' zecum) for bladder augmentation and continent diversion. In: King LR, Stone AR, Webster GD (eds) *Bladder reconstruction and continent diversion*. Chicago, IL: Yearbook Medical Publishers, 252.

Thuroff JW, Alken P, Reidmiller H et al. (1988) 100 cases of MAINZ pouch: continuing experience and evolution. *J Urol* **140**: 283–8.

Thuroff JW, Alken P, Riedmiller H et al. (1986) The MAINZ pouch (mixed augmentation ileum and cecum) for bladder augmentation and continent diversion. *J Urol* **136**: 17–26.

Tietjen DN, Gloor JM, Husmann DA (1997) Proximal urinary diversion in the management of posterior urethral valves; it is necessary? *J Urol* **158**: 1008–10.

Tillem SM, Kessler OJ, Hanna MK (1987) Long-term results of lower urinary tract reconstruction with the ceco-appendiceal unit. *J Urol* **157**: 1429–33.

Turner-Warwick RT, Ashken MN (1967) The functional results of partial, subtotal and total cystoplasty, with special reference of ureterocaecocystoplasty selective sphincterotous and cystocystoplasty. *Br J Urol* **39**: 3.

Wagstaff KE, Woodhouse CJ, Puffy GP et al. (1992) Delayed linear growth in children with enterocystoplastics. *Br J Urol* **69**: 314–17.

Walker RD (1994) Antireflux mechanisms in continent urinary diversion. *AUA Update Series* **13**: 294–9.

Wallace DM (1970) Ureteroileostomy. *Br J Urol* **42**: 529–34.

Webster GD (1995) Conduit urinary diversion. In: Webster GD, Goldwasser B (eds) *Urinary diversion*. Oxford: Isis Medical Media, 318–29.

Wells CA (1956) The use of the intestine in urology: omitting ureterocolonic anastomosis. *Br J Urol* **28**: 335–50.

Williams O, Vereb MJ, Libertino JA (1997) Incontinent urinary diversion. *Urol Clin North Am* **24**: 735–44.

Woodhouse CRJ, MacNeily AE (1994) The Mitrofanoff principle: expanding upon a versatile technique. *Br J Urol* **74**: 447–53.

Yang W (1993) Yang needle tunneling technique in creating antireflux and continent mechanisms. *J Urol* **150**: 830–4.

Zinman L, Libertino JA (1975) Ileocecal conduit for temporary and permanent urinary diversion. *J Urol* **113**: 317–23.

The Malone antegrade continence enema (MACE)

18

Martin A. Koyle and Padraig S.J. Malone

Introduction

At first glance it may seem strange to devote a chapter in a textbook of pediatric urology to bowel care. However, congenital anomalies of the bowel and urinary tract frequently coexist and constipation by itself may produce significant bladder dysfunction leading to incontinence and urinary tract infection (Malone, 1995a). The pediatric urologist must be conversant with these bowel problems and play an active role in their management. Both systems should always be assessed simultaneously, and with present surgical techniques, it is the urologist who is often best placed to treat both urinary and fecal incontinence synchronously.

The first antegrade continence enema (ACE) or Malone (MACE) procedure was performed in 1989, in an attempt to treat the intractable fecal incontinence associated with conditions such as spina bifida and anorectal malformation. Koyle subsequently introduced the technique in North America in 1991 (Koyle et al., 1995). Malone et al. (1994) reported that 53% of young adults with spina bifida suffered from fecal incontinence, and similar results were reported by Holschneider (1988) in patients with anorectal anomalies, many of whom also had neuropathic bladder dysfunction (Sheldon et al., 1991).

The MACE combined three well-recognized surgical principles: complete colonic emptying could produce fecal continence (Shandling and Gilmour, 1987); colonic emptying could be achieved by intraoperative antegrade colonic irrigation (Radcliffe and Dudley, 1983); and the Mitrofanoff principle for clean intermittent catheterization, applied to the cecum, allowed access for such colonic irrigation (Mitrofanoff, 1980). The combination of these principles, applied to the colon, provided continent intermittent catheter access to the cecum or proximal colon for the administration of antegrade enemas while the patient sat on the toilet. This produced colonic emptying and fecal continence. The preliminary series was reported by Malone et al. (1990) and, subsequently, numerous reports have been published so the procedure is now practiced widely around the world (Squire et al., 1993; Griffiths and Malone, 1995; Koyle et al., 1995; Malone, 1995a; Toogood et al., 1995; Dick et al., 1996; Gerharz et al. 1997). Many modifications have been introduced following the original description (Malone, 1995b), both to simplify the procedure and to reduce the high complication rates initially reported (Squire et al., 1993). This chapter will review the techniques in current use, patient selection and preparation, the enema regimens, and the most recent results.

Patient selection and preparation

All conservative measures must be tried before resorting to the MACE. The underlying diagnosis is important, as it influences the success rate. In the Southampton experience, patients with a neuropathic bowel and an anorectal malformation had a success rate of 73%, compared with 38% for patients with chronic idiopathic constipation (Curry et al., 1998). The Colorado experience similarly showed that those whose primary bowel problem is constipation fare worse than those with other elimination problems. These results have been mirrored by the wider experience in the UK, where a success rate of 91% was also reported for patients with Hirschsprung's disease (Curry and Malone, 1999). The age at operation was also important. In Southampton there was a 70% failure rate for patients under 5 years of age, compared with 24% for those aged over 5 years, a highly significant difference (Curry et al., 1988). This was independent of the underlying diagnosis, and probably reflected the inability of a child under 5 years of age to sit on a toilet for up to 1 hour before emptying is complete. Patient and caregiver motivation was vital in determining the success. A lack of compliance with the washout regimen was a major contributory factor to failure in two patients in the Southampton series and seven patients in the Colorado experience. Detailed preoperative counseling and continued postoperative support, ideally provided by a nurse specialist, are essential to ensure adequate and continued motivation, without which the MACE is doomed to failure. It is an advantage to introduce the potential patient to a child and family with a functioning MACE prior to the surgical procedure.

In summary, the ideal patient for a MACE should be over 5 years of age, have a diagnosis of neuropathic bowel, an anorectal malformation or Hirschsprung's disease, be well motivated with a dedicated family, and have tried and failed all conservative measures first.

Operative technique

An aggressive preoperative bowel preparation is essential to facilitate the initial postoperative enema. A cleanout from below is often necessary, especially in the patient in whom constipation is the primary problem. Broad-spectrum prophylactic antibiotics which cover bowel bacteria are always administered perioperatively. In most instances, since coincidental urinary tract reconstruction is performed, a lower midline or Pfannenstiel is selected, depending on the patient's body habitus, prior surgical scars, and preference. In the patient in whom a MACE only is indicated, without a urinary operation, a laparoscopic approach or an appendectomy incision can be employed.

It has been reported that it is not necessary to construct an antireflux mechanism, and some surgeons simply pull the appendix out to an abdominal stomal site. This may be done using a laparoscopic approach. Both authors have attempted not using an antireflux mechanism on a number of occasions and, in the majority of such cases, the stoma was incontinent of flatus and/or stool. Therefore, it is recommended that an antireflux mechanism be routinely constructed. It is no longer necessary to disconnect the appendix from the cecum and reimplant it as one would for a continent appendicovesicostomy, as initially had been proposed by Malone. Rather, the *in situ* appendix can be folded over with the cecal wall wrapped around it to produce the antireflux mechanism. This is an adapta-

tion of the technique originally described for the Mainz pouch urinary reservoir (Gerharz *et al.*, 1997). The procedure is performed in slightly different ways by the two authors. Koyle simply wraps the cecal wall around the folded appendix using permanent sutures, similar to the technique for a Nissen fundoplication. Malone continues to produce a submucosal tunnel along one of the taenia and inlays the appendix into this, finally closing the seromuscular layer over it with absorbable sutures (Fig. 18.1). Both authors recommend catching the serosa of the appendix wall with covering sutures in order to prevent it from pulling out of the tunnel. The mesentery of the appendix is fenestrated to prevent the wrap from compromising the blood supply to the appendix. Longer term follow-up is required before it can be stated which technique is better, but at the present time both are performing satisfactorily without significant long-term leakage. Once the antireflux mechanism has been constructed, the cecum or colon is sutured to the posterior aspect of the anterior abdominal wall to ensure that the conduit is not lying free in the peritoneal cavity, as this can lead to kinking and difficulties with catheterization.

The technique needs to be modified if simultaneous MACE and appendicovesicstomy procedures are being performed. If the appendix is long enough and the vascular anatomy is suitable, it is possible to split the appendix, and both authors have done this successfully. If the appendix is not suitable to split, or if it is absent, another technique must be instituted. The tubularized cecal or colonic flap (Kiely *et al.*, 1994) is no longer recommended because of the unacceptably high complication rates associated with this technique (Koyle *et al.*, 1995). There are two alternatives to the appendix worthy of serious consideration. The first is the Monti procedure (Monti *et al.*, 1997). This is an ingenious technique in which a segment of ileum is harvested on its pedicle and detubularized transversely on its antimesenteric border (see Chapter 15). The rectangular patch is tubularized along its longitudinal axis to create a catherizable conduit of approximately 7 cm in length. The internal valvulae coniventes run in the longitudinal direction of the conduit, thus facilitating easy catheterization. Both ends of the conduit are free of mesentery and this makes the creation of the antireflux mechanism easy. When a Monti conduit is used, the Mitrofanoff flap valve principle is followed and a submucosal tunnel is created along one of the taenia which is wrapped around it. This is similar to the original description of the MACE (Malone, 1995b). If the patient is obese, it is possible to use two segments of ileum or colon and produce a 14 cm conduit ('The Full Monti') which is long enough for virtually all patients. Experience with this technique is very encouraging and it is the procedure of choice when the appendix is not available (Sugarman *et al.*, 1998).

The other technique worthy of consideration is the use of a cecostomy tube and cecal button. Shandling *et al.* (1996) described a technique for the percutaneous placement of a cecal tube that could be changed at a later date to a low-profile cecal button (similar to a gastrostomy button), which is then used to administer the enema. Eleven patients in the Colorado series manage their MACEs using a button with results similar to those using an appendiceal MACE (Fig. 18.2). Three of the patients had sloughing of cecal tubes formed when the appendix was absent and were subsequently salvaged with a button. Two children/caretakers refused to catheterize their stomas and thus the buttons are being used semipermanently in these cases. The final six patients have had stomal stenosis develop on at least one occasion and the families have preferred the non-operative but-

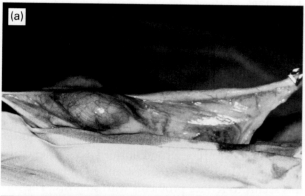
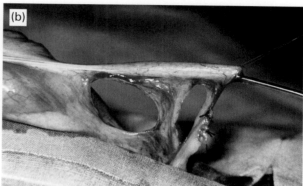
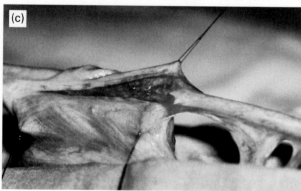
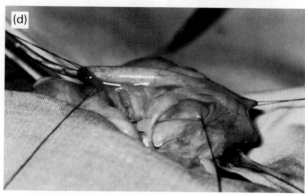
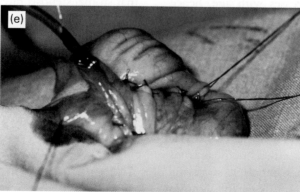

Figure 18.1 *In situ* formation of the MACE: (*a*) *in-situ* appendix attached to the cecum; (*b*) fenestrated appendix mesentery; (*c*) submucosal tunnel along one of the taenia; (*d*) appendix folded into the tunnel; (*e*) completed tunnel (note the short length of appendix).

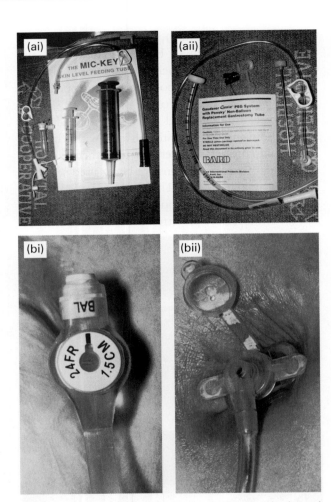

Figure 18.2 (*a*) Mic-Key (Ballard Corporation) and Genie (Bard) button kits. (*b*) i, Mic-Key button in right lower quadrant MACE stoma; ii, Genie in umbilical stoma.

ton option to that of repair under anesthesia. The greatest worry has been erosion or skin problems, as the abdominal wall girth increases with age, hence close follow-up is mandatory. The tubes are unsightly and occasionally leakage around the tube will occur that leads to embarrassment. In a survey of 300 MACE procedures performed in the UK, 19 cecal buttons were used and they worked well in most cases (Curry and Malone, 1999). Chait *et al.* (1997) placed buttons percutaneously under local anesthesia with good results. Fonkulsrud *et al.* (1998) placed Broviac silastic intravenous catheters rather than buttons using an open technique. They reported successful results in a series of 24 patients. Longer follow-up is required before the button can be routinely advocated in place of an intestinal conduit.

By adopting these newer techniques, complications

such as incontinence of the conduit or difficulties with catherterization are rare. Currently, it is easy to perform simultaneous MACE and Mitrofanoff urinary diversion, offering patients the chance of complete continence for the first time (Roberts *et al.*, 1995).

The remaining aspect of operative technique is the construction and placement of the stoma. The most common complication of the MACE is stomal stenosis, reaching 55% in the Southampton series (Curry *et al.*, 1998). In the majority of these patients, stenosis could be managed with simple dilation, but 6/31 (19%) patients have required surgical revision. To date, 22% of the Colorado group required surgical revision for stenosis. When comparing the location of the stoma in the right lower quadrant versus the umbilicus, there was no difference. However, in patients with dual stomas, a Mitrofanoff urinary conduit and a MACE, the stenosis rate was twice as frequent in the MACE group. The Mitrofanoff urinary stoma is catheterized approximately four to six times a day, but the MACE may be intubated as infrequently as once every second or third day. Patients are now advised to intubate the stoma twice a day, and this seems to reduce problems with stenosis. The initial description of the MACE advocated a cutaneous V-flap, but both centers are now using modifications of the Ransley VQZ-flap (Fig. 18.3) when the MACE is positioned in a location other than the umbilicus. This flap has been shown to reduce significantly stomal problems in the Mitrofanoff procedure and better success is also anticipated with the MACE group (Malone *et al.*, 1999). This method uses two separate skin flaps and can be constructed on the abdominal wall (Fig. 18.3) or in the umbilicus (Fig. 18.4). Follow-up is too short, but the impression is that stomal stenosis rates are considerably lower. The conduit is left intubated for a period of 2 weeks (Southampton) to 4 weeks (Denver) postoperatively before intermittent catheterization is begun. The ideal MACE should use the *in situ* appendix or the Monti conduit with an antireflux mechanism. A two-flap cutaneous stoma should be placed either on the abdominal wall or in the umbilicus.

The enema regimen

The first enema is given via the indwelling catheter when bowel activity returns, usually around the 3rd to 5th postoperative day. In those patients whose pri-

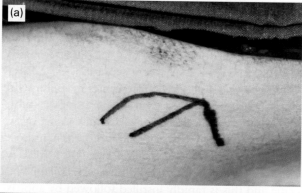

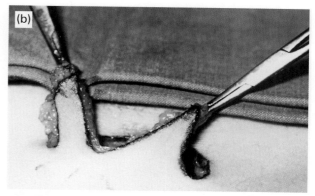

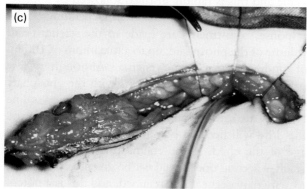

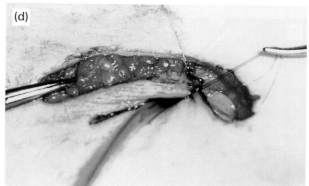

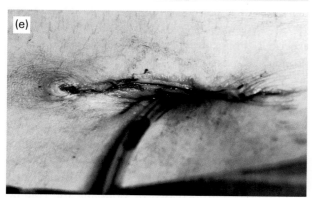

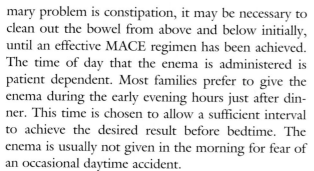

Figure 18.3 VQZ right lower quadrant stoma: (*a*) multiflap abdominal stoma; (*b*) the two mobilized skin flaps; (*c*) V-flap sutured into the posterior aspect of the fish-mouthed conduit; (*d*) the second flap sutured to the anterior wall of the conduit; (*e*) the complete stoma.

mary problem is constipation, it may be necessary to clean out the bowel from above and below initially, until an effective MACE regimen has been achieved. The time of day that the enema is administered is patient dependent. Most families prefer to give the enema during the early evening hours just after dinner. This time is chosen to allow a sufficient interval to achieve the desired result before bedtime. The enema is usually not given in the morning for fear of an occasional daytime accident.

Many enema regimens are used in different centers performing the MACE, and patients frequently modify them to suit their own particular needs. One of the most important points is to advise patients not to expect immediate success. Each individual regimen

usually takes up to 1 month and is established by trial and error. In the Southampton series (Curry *et al.*, 1998), many children did not achieve a steady state or a successful MACE for periods of up to 6 months. It is necessary to counsel patients about this preoperatively, as early disappointment can lead to complete failure. Many patients experience a degree of rectal leakage within the first few hours of the washout, but this is rarely a major problem. While the washout regimen is being established, it is vital to maintain regular contact with the nurse specialist. Initially, daily washouts are recommended, but once the patients are comfortable with the procedure, they may attempt to decrease the frequency to alternate days. Once a steady state has been achieved, there is no benefit

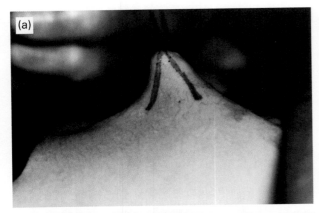

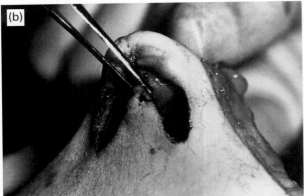

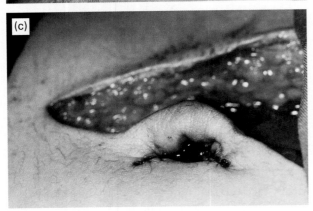

Figure 18.4 V flap umbilical stoma: (*a*) everted umbilicus; (*b*) mobilized V-flap; note that this produces a second anterior flap; (*c*) V-flap sutured into the posterior wall of the conduit, completing the stoma.

from interfering with the regimen. In the Southampton and Colorado series, the mean time taken to perform the washout was 39 min (range 20–60 min) and 34 (11–68 min), respectively. It is essential that patients and caregivers are aware of the time commitment that is required and be prepared to devote this time to bowel care, because if they do not, the MACE will fail. Because patients have to sit on

the toilet for a long time, one of the complications encountered is pressure sores on the buttocks. It is possible to obtain padded toilet seat covers and their use is recommended, particularly for the neuropathic patient with reduced or absent sensation.

The enema given differs from center to center, with most centers in the UK favoring the use of a stimulant, while those in the USA use mainly saline or tap water. In Southampton, the common regimen uses a phosphate enema (Fletchers, Pharmax, UK). Initially, 50 ml of enema solution is diluted to 100 ml with saline and this is rapidly instilled followed by approximately 500 ml of additional saline. Depending on the response, adjustments are made to the strength and volume of the phosphate, up to a maximum of 100 ml of undiluted phosphate enema. Although a few patients achieve successful results with the phosphate alone, the majority requires the additional saline lavage. Care must be taken when using phosphate and the dose will need to be adjusted depending on the age of the child. If the enema does not produce a result, a second one should *not* be given, as phosphate toxicity may occur if it is retained, and this is a potentially life-threatening complication (Hunter *et al.*, 1993). Three patients in the Southampton series have experienced phosphate toxicity. If the enema does not produce an immediate result, patients should be advised to wait 1 hour and then perform a further saline lavage. If that is unsuccessful, they should be admitted to a hospital for a retrograde enema and observation. However, care must be taken irrespective of the agent used, as there are anecdotal reports of deaths occurring when too much salt was added to tap water. In Colorado, tap or salt water is instituted at 50 ml/day and increased by doubling the volume every 3 days until reliable evacuation occurs. If there is no success after reaching 500–600 ml, alternatives are sought, includng mineral oil, Go-lytely® or Fleet's enema through the Mitrofanoff, or altering the frequency of the enema.

Several difficulties have been experienced during establishment of the MACE. The most common problem has been pain during the enema, which occurred in 58% of patients in the Southampton series (Curry *et al.*, 1998). In the majority of patients, the pain subsided during the first 3 months, but it persisted and was a major contributory cause for the failure of the MACE in three patients. Strategies for the reduction of pain include lowering the concentration of the phosphate, reducing the rate of the infusion, using an antispasmodic prior to the enema (Colovac®, Solvary, UK), or changing the enema agent to a liquorice root solution, which produces less peristalsis than the phosphate. Three inches (7.5 cm) of liquorice root or 5 ml of commercially available liquorice granules is microwaved with 100 ml of saline until the mixture boils. It is allowed to cool to room temperature and then diluted with a further 200 ml of saline prior to administration. It is also possible to vary the concentration of the liquorice, depending on the response and whether the patient experiences pain. Many patients in the UK are now successfully using this regimen and it seems to produce much less pain. It is also possible to use many of the other laxatives, such as bisacodyl or docusate sodium, by instilling them directly into the colon via the MACE. In North America, where balanced fluids are used primarily, pain has been less of a problem. Usually, reducing the volume of infusate or the route of administration alleviates the problem.

Despite regular washouts, some patients become constipated and this produces pain and washout failure. Under these circumstances, a Fletchers' arachis oil retention enema (Pharmax, UK) can be instilled 12 hours before the washout, providing there is no history of peanut allergy. In Southampton, saline enemas by themselves have been tried, but this seems to lengthen the time taken to achieve a successful washout, and the authors continue to recommend a stimulant such as phosphate or liquorice.

One of the problems encountered with the MACE is the time taken for the enema to pass and achieve a result, over 1 hour in some cases. In the Southampton series (Curry et al., 1998) the most common cause of failure was the inability to pass the enema, which occurred in 9/12 (75%) cases that failed. Malone has recently been placing the conduit more distally in the colon (transverse/descending) in some patients, and proposes that this speeds up emptying and may also reduce the washout failure rate. In Colorado, if the passage time is greater than 45 min, compliance and hence success have been reduced. The constipated, as opposed to the incontinent group, clearly comprise the majority of these patients.

In summary, many different enema regimens exist, but they are all established in the individual patient by a process of trial and error and may take up to 6 months to stabilize. The frequency of the enema should not be less than alternate days and patients should be prepared to spend up to 1 hour on each enema.

Results

The results of the MACE have been classified as follows (Curry et al., 1998):

- full success: totally clean or minor rectal leakage on the night of the washout;
- partial success: clean but significant rectal leakage, occasional major leak, still wearing protection, but perceived by the parent or child to be improved;
- failure: regular soiling or constipation persisted, no perceived improvement, and the procedure was abandoned, usually to a colostomy.

Curry et al. (1998) reported on 31 patients with a mean follow-up of over 3 years. The MACE failed in 12/31 (39%) patients, including five of the eight patients treated for chronic idiopathic constipation and the one patient with Hirschsprung's disease. When patients with neuropathic bowel and anorectal malformation were analysed separately, partial and full success rates were 75% and 70%, respectively. Curry and Malone (1999) reported on a survey of MACEs performed by members of the British Association of Paediatric Surgeons (BAPS), in which 300 cases were identified and the success rates were dependent on the original diagnosis (Table 18.1).

The overall success rate, including full and partial success, for this large national series was 79%. It is also interesting to note that complication rates were lower than in the earlier historical series. In particular, the stomal stenosis rate was down to 30%. With the widespread adoption of newer techniques for stoma construction, it is likely that future series will continue to demonstrate a decrease in stomal problems.

Shankar et al., (1998) assessed the results of 40 patients who had an ACE more objectively by using a quality of life improvement (QOLI) score. A score of 5 denoted a perfect result, and the mean score for all

Table 18.1 The MACE: success and failure based on original diagnosis

Diagnosis	Full success (%)	Partial success (%)	Failure (%)
Spina bifida	63	21	16
Anorectal	72	17	11
Hirschsprung's disease	82	9	9
Constipation	52	10	38
Other	44	25	31

patients was 3.5. They found the score to be significantly lower in wheelchair-dependent patients with spinal dysraphism (2.5) than in all other mobile patients (4). By using this objective measurement, the MACE has been shown to be successful.

Conclusion

Despite the relatively high complication rates, the MACE offers almost 80% of patients with neuropathic bowel and anorectal malformation a chance to be clean. When successful, the MACE transforms patient's lives, and does not interfere with the final option of a colostomy should that become necessary. No patient should undergo lower urinary tract reconstruction without a complete bowel assessment and, if necessary, a simultaneous MACE should be carried out. A simultaneous procedure does not jeopardize the success of either individual component. The reconstructive urologist is the best person to manage the bowel, as the operative techniques involved are those routinely employed in lower urinary reconstruction. Furthermore, the infrastructure should be in place for meticulous follow-up. This combined approach should enhance the quality of life for these unfortunate patients.

References

Chait PG, Shandling B, Richards HF (1997) The cecostomy button. *J Pediatr Surg* **32**: 849–51.

Curry JL, Malone PS (1999) The MACE procedure: UK experience. *J Pediatr Surg*

Curry JL, Osborne A, Malone PS (1998) How to achieve a successful Malone antegrade continence enema. *J Pediatr Surg* **33**: 138–41.

Dick AC, McCallion WA, Brown S, Boston VE (1996) Antegrade colonic enemas. *Br J Surg* **83**: 642–3.

Fonkalsrud EW, Dunn JCY, Kawaguchi AE (1998) Simplified technique for antegrade continence enemas for fecal retention and incontinence. *J Am Coll Surg* **187**: 456–60.

Gerharz EW, Vik V, Webb G, Woodhouse CRJ (1997) The *in situ* appendix in the MACE (Malone antegrade continence enema) procedure for faecal incontinence. *Br J Urol* **79**: 985–6.

Griffiths DM, Malone PS (1995) The Malone antegrade continence enema. *J Pediatr Surg* **30**: 68–71.

Holschneider AM (1988) Function of the sphincters in anorectal malformations and postoperative evaluation. In: Stephens FD, Smith ED (eds) *Anorectal malformations in children: an update*. Volume 24. New York: Birth Defects Foundation, 425–45.

Hunter MF, Ashton MR, Roberts JP *et al.* (1993) Hyperphosphataemia following enemas in childhood: prevention and treatment. *Arch Dis Child* **68**: 233–4.

Kiely EM, Adde-Ajai N, Wheeler RA (1994) Caecal flap conduit for antegrade continence enemas. *Br J Surg* **81**: 1215.

Koyle MA, Waxman SW, Duque M *et al.* (1995) Applications and modification of the Malone antegrade continence enema for neurogenic and structural fecal incontinence and constipation. *J Urol* **154**: 759–61.

Malone PS (1995a) The management of bowel problems in children with urological disease. *Br J Urol* **76**: 220–5.

Malone PS (1995b) The Malone procedure for antegrade continence enema. In: Spitz L, Coran A (eds) *Rob and Smith's operative surgery, pediatric surgery*. London: Chapman and Hall, 459–67.

Malone PS, Ransley PG, Kiely EM (1990) The antegrade continence enema: preliminary report. *Lancet* **336**: 1217–18.

Malone PS, Wheeler RA, Williams JE (1994) Continence in patients with spina bifida: long term results. *Arch Dis Child* **70**: 107–10.

Malone PSJ, Curry JI, Osborne A (1999) The antegrade continence enema procedure why, when and how? *World J Urol* **16**: 274–8.

Mitrofanoff P (1980) Cystostomie continente transappendiculare dans le traitement des vessies neurologiques. *Chir Pediatr* **21**: 297–305.

Monti PR, Lara RC, Dutra MA, DeCarvalho JR (1997) New techniques for construction of efferent conduits based on the Mitrofanoff principle. *Urology* **49**: 112–15.

Radcliffe AG, Dudley HAF (1983) Intraoperative antegrade irrigation of the large intestine. *Surg Gynecol Obstet* **156**: 721–3.

Roberts JP, Moon S, Malone PS (1995) Treatment of neuropathic urinary and faecal incontinence with synchronous bladder reconstruction and the antegrade continence enema procedure. *Br J Urol* **75**: 386–9.

Shandling B, Gilmour RF (1987) The enema continence catheter in spina bifida: successful bowel management. *J Pediatr Surg* **22**: 271–3.

Shandling B, Chait PG, Richards HF (1996) Percutaneous caecostomy: a new technique in the management of fecal incontinence. *J Pediatr Surg* **31**: 534–7.

Shankar KR, Losty PD, Kenny SE *et al.* (1998) Functional results following the antegrade continence enema procedure. *Br J Surg* **85**: 980–2.

Sheldon C, Cormier M, Crone K, Wacksman J (1991) Occult neurovesical dysfunction in children with imperforate anus and its variants. *J Pediatr Surg* **26**: 49–54.

Squire R, Kiely EM, Carr B *et al.* (1993) The clinical application of the Malone antegrade colonic enema. *J Pediatr Surg* **28**: 1012–15.

Sugarman ID, Malone PS, Terry TR, Koyle MA (1998) Transversely tubularized ileal segments for the Mitrofanoff or Malone antegrade continence enema procedures: the Monti principle. *Br J Urol* **81**: 253–6.

Toogood GJ, Bryant PA, Dudley NE (1995) Control of faecal incontinence using the Malone antegrade continence enema procedure: a critical appraisal. *Pediatr Surg Int* **10**: 37–9.

Anomalies of the kidney

19

Michael Ritchey

Embryology

Anomalies of the urogenital tract are among the most common of all organ systems. It has been estimated that almost 10% of the population has some type of urogenital anomaly (Dees, 1941), but this prevalence was derived from symptomatic patients evaluated with excretory urograms. Using real-time ultrasonography as a screening test in healthy infants, Steinhardt *et al.* (1988) found that 3.2% of infants had an abnormality of the genitourinary tract and half of these required surgical intervention.

A complete understanding of the embryologic development of the urinary tract is a prerequisite for the evaluation and management of a child with a congenital genitourinary malformation. The development of the urinary tract can be divided into two segments, the nephric system and the vesicourethral system (Gray and Skandalakis, 1972; Parrott *et al.*, 1994).

There are three stages in the formation of the nephric system. The two intermediate stages are the pronephros, which completely disappears, and the mesonephros. Although the mesonephros undergoes degeneration, its duct persists and extends caudally to communicate with the anterior cloaca. Vestigial remnants of the mesonephric tubules occur in both sexes and are associated with the reproductive tract. Early in the 4th to 5th weeks, the ureteral bud begins to develop from the distal end of the mesonephric duct near its junction with the cloaca. The cranial end of the ureter then ascends to meet the nephrogenic cord of the intermediate mesoderm. This begins to develop into the metanephros and continues its cephalad migration. The cranial end of the ureteral bud begins a series of branchings to form the renal pelvis, the calyces, and a portion of the collecting ducts (Osathanondh and Potter, 1963). This branching is associated with the simultaneous differentiation of the metanephrogenic cap, which becomes arranged around the branching collecting ducts, and ascends. The ascent of the kidneys occurs in part due to true migration and also secondary to differential somatic growth of the lumbar portion of the body. They reach their final level by the end of the 8th week of fetal life (Fig. 19.1). The kidney also undergoes axial rotation medially of 90° during the 7th and 8th weeks before

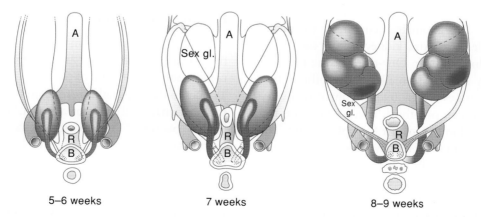

5–6 weeks 7 weeks 8–9 weeks

Figure 19.1 Ascent and rotation of kidneys during fetal life. The normal rotation of the kidney from facing forward to facing medially is shown. A, aorta; R, rectum; B, bladder; Sex gl, sex gland. (From Campbell, 1951.)

it assumes its final position. During ascent, each kidney receives its blood supply from the neighboring vessels. Initially, this is from the middle sacral artery, then the common iliac and inferior mesenteric arteries, and finally the aorta. Failure of inferior arteries to be reabsorbed on a timely basis may be one cause of ureteropelvic junction (UPJ) obstruction. Different renal anamalies encountered may be the result of an arrest in development or a malformation.

Anomalies in number

Supernumerary kidney

A supernumerary kidney is an uncommon anomaly with no more than 60 cases reported in the literature (Wulfekuhler and Dube, 1971; Antony, 1977; N'Guessan and Stephens, 1983). The embryologic basis shares some similarities with that found in ureteral duplication. There are either two ureteral buds arising from the mesonephric duct, leading to double ureters, or a branching of the ureteral bud, which results in a bifid collecting system. It is believed that the two ureteral buds then join two separate metanephros or that a splitting of the nephrogenic blastema occurs. This later develops into twin metanephros after induction by the two ureteral buds. It is not believed to be necessary for the two ureteral buds to be widely divergent (N'Guessan and Stephens, 1983).

The supernumerary kidney is caudal to the ipsilateral kidney in 60% of cases (Fig. 19.2). When the supernumerary kidney is associated with complete ureteral duplication, the supernumerary kidney is more likely to be cranial. There is generally one extra kidney, but as many as five separate renal masses have been reported. This anomaly occurs more frequently on the left side. The extra kidney has its own renal capsule and blood supply. One-third of the time the supernumerary kidney is smaller and exhibits other pathologic changes (e.g. hydronephrosis, pyelonephritis) in another one-third. Renal function is frequently decreased in the smaller hypoplastic unit. The ureter of the anomalous kidney joins the ipsilateral ureter about as commonly as it enters the bladder separately, but only rarely is the ureter ectopic.

Most cases are diagnosed after the third decade of life. Presenting complaints are usually related to urinary obstruction or infection. Patients may experience pain or fever or may be found to have an abdominal

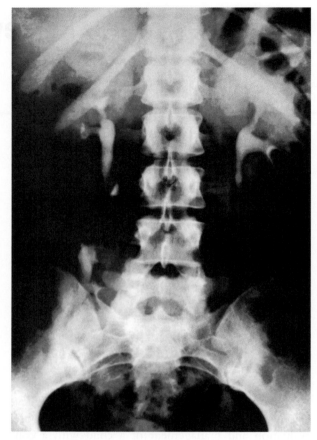

Figure 19.2 Excretory urogram of right supernumerary kidney, which lies opposite the fourth and fifth lumbar vertebrae.

mass on examination. However, many patients remain asymptomatic throughout life and 20% of reported cases were discovered at autopsy (Carlson, 1950).

Unilateral renal agenesis

Renal agenesis results from a failure of induction of the metanephric blastema by the ureteral bud. This could result from failure of the ureteral bud or wolffian duct to develop, failure of the ureteral bud to reach the blastema, or absence or abnormality of the metanephric blastema. The reported incidence of this condition varies between series of patients collected from either clinical or autopsy data. Doroshow and Abeshouse (1961) estimated that unilateral renal agenesis (URA) is found in one of every 1100 autopsies. The clinical incidence found on excretory urogram is one in 1500, suggesting that most cases are diagnosed during life (Longo and Thompson, 1952). There is a slight male predominance, and the condition occurs more frequently on the left side. This male predominance may reflect the earlier differentiation of the wolffian duct that takes place close to the time of ureteral bud formation. The ureteral bud is more likely to be influenced by abnormalities of the wolffian duct than that of the müllerian duct, which occurs later.

Associated anomalies

The ipsilateral ureter is absent in 50–87% of cases (Collins, 1932; Ashley and Mostofi, 1960) and only partially developed in others (Fig. 19.3). On cystoscopy, a hemitrigone will be present in patients with complete ureteral agenesis. Fifteen per cent of cases show anomalies of the contralateral kidney, with malrotation and ectopia most commonly discovered (Longo and Thompson, 1952). Limakeng and Retik (1972) found an increased incidence of contralateral abnormality if there was a hypoplastic ureter associated with the absent kidney. The ipsilateral adrenal was found to be absent on autopsy in 8% of patients with

URA (Ashley and Mostofi, 1960). One report noted ipsilateral agenesis of the adrenal in two of seven patients with URA examined with abdominal ultrasonography (Nakada *et al.*, 1988).

The most commonly associated abnormalities are those of the genitalia. Fortune (1927) noted genital anomalies in 69% of females and 21% of males. Other authors report a 20–40% incidence of genital anomalies for both sexes (Doroshow and Abeshouse, 1961; Thompson and Lynn, 1966). This lower incidence is seen in clinical series. These patients were studied with cystoscopy, excretory urography, and physical examination, with many abnormalities of the internal genitalia going undetected. In the female, such anomalies often assume greater clinical importance, leading to earlier evaluation and diagnosis of the absent kidney. The most common problems involve the uterus and vagina. There is often a unicornuate or bicornuate uterus (Fig. 19.4), and the ipsilateral horn and fallopian tube may be rudimentary or absent (Schumacker, 1938). A duplex uterus can result from incomplete midline fusion of the müllerian ducts and may be associated with a duplicated or septate vagina (Fortune 1927). Complete absence or hypoplasia of the vagina, the Mayer–Rokitansky–Kuster–Hauser syndrome, is frequently associated with agenesis of the kidney (Downs *et al.*, 1973; Griffin *et al.*, 1976). Unilateral renal agenesis is associated with several other syndromes, including Turner, Poland (Mace *et al.*, 1972), and Klippel–Feil syndromes (Moore *et al.*, 1975).

Most of the genital anomalies in female patients with URA are asymptomatic. Obstruction of the lower genital tract can occur, leading to hydrocolpos or hematocolpos. Patients present with a pelvic mass

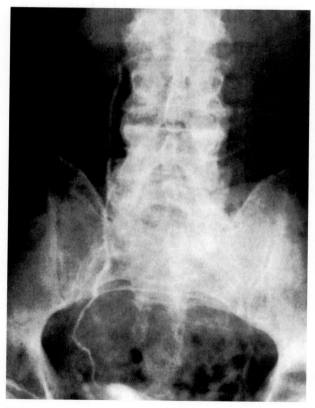

Figure 19.3 Retrograde ureterogram in a patient with known unilateral renal agenesis demonstrating hypoplastic ureter to the level of the renal fossa.

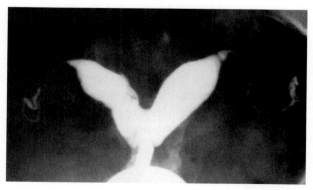

Figure 19.4 Bicornuate uterus seen on hysterosalpingogram with filling of both fallopian tubes. The vagina was normal in this patient with an absent right kidney.

or pain (Yoder and Pfister, 1976) and fail to menstruate at puberty. Patients with complete müllerian arrest will require vaginal construction to achieve adequate sexual function but will be infertile.

In the male, ipsilateral absence of the vas deferens, seminal vesicle, and ejaculatory duct approaches an incidence of 50% (Charney and Gillenwater, 1965) in those with true agenesis. Conversely, in those patients presenting with an absent vas, renal agenesis is infrequently discovered. Goldstein and Schlossberg (1988) used computed tomography (CT) to evaluate 26 men with absence of the vas deferens. Unilateral renal agenesis was noted in only four men, in all of whom the seminal vesicle was absent. An earlier report had suggested a higher incidence of associated renal agenesis in men with absence of the vas deferens (Ochsner et al., 1972). Cysts of the seminal vesicle associated with URA or dysgenesis and an ectopic ureter have also been reported (Roehrborn et al., 1986). The ipsilateral testis is usually present. Collins (1932) found the testis absent in fewer than 1% of patients in his series, although Radasch (1908) reported a 7% incidence of absence of the ipsilateral testis associated with URA.

Approximately 25–40% of patients with URA have other associated congenital anomalies. In such patients, the organ systems most frequently involved include cardiovascular (30%), gastrointestinal (25%), and musculoskeletal (14%) (Emanuel et al., 1974). Malformations of the lower rectum and anus and abnormalities of the lower spine may be found in both sexes. This may represent a regional disturbance causing maldevelopment of structures arising from the posterior portion of the cloaca and the adjacent mesonephric duct. Duhamel (1961) describes this as the 'caudal regression syndrome.' The fact that the genital defects in the male are most severe near the bladder and diminish toward the testes supports the theory of a disturbance in the caudal portion of the embryo involving the wolffian duct. There is a greater frequency of such genital malformations in the female, with the caudal portion of the müllerian ducts (uterus and vagina) more likely to be malformed. The müllerian duct develops later than the wolffian duct. Hence, its chance of being involved in malformations is greater (Fortune, 1927).

Diagnosis

Absence of the kidney may be suspected on a plain film of the abdomen if the gas pattern of the splenic

or hepatic flexure of the colon is displaced into the renal fossa (Mascatello and Lebowitz, 1976; Curtis et al., 1977). This finding is non-specific and is also noted in patients in whom the kidney has been surgically removed. The diagnosis can be confirmed on excretory urography, which reveals an absent kidney and compensatory hypertrophy of the contralateral kidney. Sonography can also establish the diagnosis, but the hypertrophied adrenal gland can be mistaken for a small kidney (McGahan and Myracle, 1986). In these cases, the adrenal gland loses its 'Y' and 'V' configuration and becomes flatter and more elliptical in shape. Renal sonography has been recommended for screening of parents and siblings of children born with renal agenesis. In this group, Roodhooft et al. (1984) reported a 9% incidence of asymptomatic renal malformations, with URA being the most common abnormality found. Sonography, and more recently magnetic resonance imaging (MRI), are useful for examining the internal genital structures in females with a diagnosis of renal agenesis. In general, the uterus and cervix can be visualized in both infants and older girls.

Radionuclide scanning is helpful in confirming the diagnosis of renal agenesis. It is the most sensitive study for identifying small, poorly functioning kidneys and is particularly sensitive for identifying those that are ectopically located (Pattaras et al., 1999). Renal arteriography is rarely indicated in the evaluation of the patient with URA.

The majority of congenital solitary kidneys are diagnosed in children younger than 5 years. This is primarily due to prenatal sonography. Recent follow-up of children with multicystic dysplastic kidneys with serial renal ultrasonography shows that complete disappearance of the dysplastic kidney can occur (Pedicelli et al., 1986; Avni et al., 1987). Some cases of URA diagnosed in past years were in fact spontaneous regression of a multicystic dysplastic kidney (see Chapter 21). Due to an increased incidence of contralateral ureteral abnormalities, vesicoureteral reflux should be ruled out in this group (Song et al., 1995).

Prognosis

For years, physicians have assumed that patients with a normal solitary kidney were not at increased risk for future urologic problems (Dees, 1960). However, experimental evidence suggests that hyperfiltration of remnant nephrons in animals may have an adverse effect on renal function, depending on the number of nephron units remaining. (Shimamura and Morrison, 1975; Hostetter *et al.*, 1981). There are also several reports of focal glomerulosclerosis occuring in humans with URA (Kiprov *et al.*, 1981; Gutierrez-Millet *et al.*, 1986). Whether restriction of dietary protein or other measures to lower glomerular pressures should be recommended in the child with a solitary kidney in an attempt to prevent future glomerular injury is unclear, and will probably remain so for some time.

Bilateral renal agenesis

The incidence of bilateral renal agenesis (Potter's syndrome) is approximately 1 in 4000 births (Potter, 1965). There is a slight male predominance (the male: female ratio is 2.5:1). A familial tendency has been reported (Rizza and Downing, 1971), and the risk of recurrence in subsequent pregnancies is 2–5%. These infants have a characteristic facies (Fig. 19.5) that is found in conditions in which there is an absence of intrauterine renal function. The most constant finding is a prominent epicanthal fold that extends onto the cheek. The skin of these infants is very loose, particu-

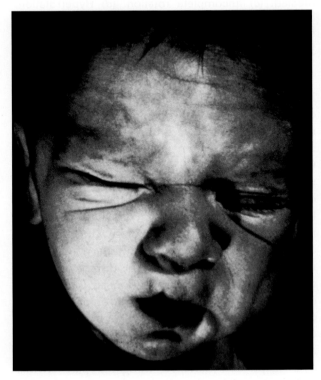

Figure 19.5 Potter facies. (Courtesy of Dr Catherine Poole, University of Miami, Florida.)

larly over the hands. Oligohydramnios during pregnancy is profound, except in rare instances. This causes intrauterine compression of the fetus, which results in other characteristic external features, including bowed legs and clubbed feet. The most significant sequelae of oligohydramnios is pulmonary hypoplasia. This is the result of compression of the thoracic cage, preventing lung expansion, lack of pulmonary fluid stenting the airways, or absence of renal factors, such as proline production (Adzick *et al.*, 1984).

Approximately 40% of such infants are stillborn, and the remainder rapidly succumb to respiratory failure associated with the pulmonary hypoplasia unless aggressively treated. This poor prognosis has led to the recommendation of termination of the pregnancy if the diagnosis is made early in gestation.

The antenatal ultrasonogram of a fetus with bilateral renal agenesis reveals either oligohydramnios or anhydramnios, absence of the kidneys, and non-visualization of the bladder. Because fetal imaging is very difficult in severe oligohydramnios, non-visualization of the urinary bladder is a more reliable indication of fetal renal non-function than the inability to identify the fetal kidneys. The bladder area is examined intermittently over a 2 hour interval, and if the urinary bladder is not seen during this time, 10 mg of furosemide is administered to the mother (Wladimiroff, 1975). Persistent failure to image the bladder confirms fetal anuria. Caution must be used in accepting the antenatal diagnosis of bilateral renal agenesis because false-positive diagnoses have been made (Romero *et al.*, 1985).

The ureter is also absent in 90% of cases and only partially developed in the remaining individuals (Ashley and Mostofi, 1960). The bladder is either absent or severely hypoplastic as a result of the absence of urine flow. The adrenal glands are usually present in their normal position, but are flat (Davidson and Ross, 1954). External genital development is generally normal except when bilateral renal agenesis occurs in the sirenomelic monster. Testicular absence has been reported in up to 10% (Ashley and Mostofi, 1960), but the vasa are present in most cases. This suggests that in some, the cause relates to abnormal development of the urogenital ridge in early fetal life. The presence of the vasa suggests that this anomaly is not due to failure of the wolffian duct to develop. The organs most often abnormal in the female are derived from the müllerian structures. In both sexes, there is an increased incidence of gastrointestinal malformations, with imperforate anus the most common problem, and an increased incidence of spina bifida. This suggests that a regional disturbance affecting the posterior portion of the cloaca and the adjacent mesonephros and müllerian ducts is resposible for bilateral renal agenesis in some (Potter, 1965).

Anomalies of rotation

Incomplete rotation, or malrotation, is most commonly associated with an ectopic or fused kidney, but may also occur in kidneys that ascend completely. The normal orientation of the adult kidney is a medial position of the renal pelvis, with the calyces pointing laterally. The fetal kidneys undergo a 90° rotation during the 6th to 8th weeks of embryonic development, which results in this position (see Fig. 19.1). The rotation of the fetal kidney has been proposed to be the result of differential growth, with more tubules being formed on the ventrolateral side than on the dorsomedial side (Priman, 1929). This theory does not explain all of the abnormalities of rotation. Weyrauch suggested that the ureteral bud makes more lateral contact with the renal blastema. This may explain an anomalous initial position of the kidney, but does not explain normal renal rotation. Campbell (1970) reported only 17 cases of renal malrotation among 32 834 autopsies on adults. Smith and Orkin (1985) found an incidence of 1 in 390 and stated that malrotation accounts for 10% of upper urinary tract anomalies. The true incidence of this type of anomaly is probably understated because in many patients there are no clinical manifestations.

The different types of malrotation are depicted in Figure 19.6. The most common is an incomplete rotation, or non-rotation. The renal pelvis is anterior or between the fetal anterior and normal medial position in the adult. Other major types of anomalous rotation are reverse rotation and hyperrotation (excessive rotation) in which the kidney faces laterally (Weyrauch, 1939). These are exceedingly rare (Fig. 19.7). In reverse rotation, the renal pelvis rotates laterally and the renal vessels cross the kidney anteriorly to reach the hilum (Fig. 19.8). In excessive rotation, the kidney rotates more than 180° but less than 360°. The pelvis faces laterally, but the renal vessels are carried posteriorly to the kidney. Less severe hyperrotation may leave the renal pelvis in a dorsal position (Parrott *et al.*, 1994).

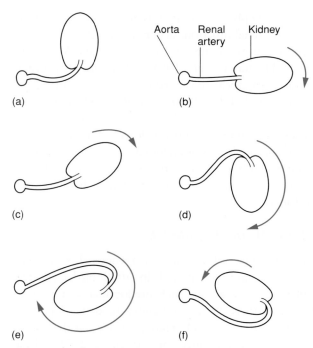

Figure 19.6 Rotation of the kidney during its ascent from the pelvis. The left kidney (with its renal artery) and the aorta are viewed in transverse section to show normal and abnormal rotation during its ascent to the adult site. (*a*) Primitive embryonic position, hilus faces ventrad (anterior). (*b*) Normal adult position, hilus faces mediad. (*c*) Imcomplete rotation. (*d*) Hyperrotation, hilus faces dorsad (posterior). (*e*) Hyperrotation, hilus faces laterad. (*f*) Reverse rotation, hilus faces laterad. (From Parrott *et al.*, 1994.)

Malrotation is usually discovered incidentally during imaging. The condition may be unilateral or bilateral. When symptoms occur, they are most often related to intermittent hydronephrosis and consist of abdominal pain often associated with vomiting. Obstruction may be secondary to compression of the ureter from an anomalous accessory vessel or other obstructive lesions that also occur in normally rotated kidneys. It is important to establish the correct diagnosis and to exclude other pathologic conditions that can produce similar distortion of the kidney. The upper third of the ureter may be displaced laterally and the renal pelvis may appear elongated, suggesting obstruction or effacement by an extrinsic mass. The calyces are often distorted even without any associated obstruction. Gross inspection of the kidney may also reveal an unusual appearance with a discoid or oval shape and flattened elongated parenchyma. Persistent fetal lobulations are often present. Additional diagnostic imaging, such as retrograde pyelo-

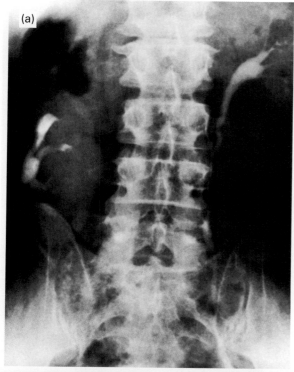

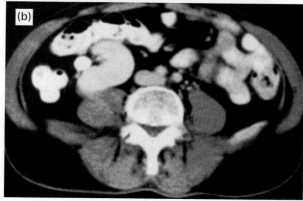

Figure 19.7 An example of excessive rotation of the right kidney. (*a*) Excretory urogram; (*b*) Computed tomographic scan.

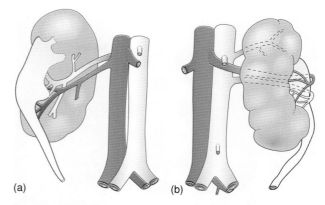

Figure 19.8 Abnormal renal rotation. (*a*) Reverse rotation; (*b*) hyperrotation. (Adapted from Weyrauch, 1939.)

graphy, sonography, or CT, may be necessary to confirm the diagnosis. Treatment of malrotation is reserved for alleviation of associated obstruction, calculi, or infection secondary to poor drainage.

Anomalies of ascent

Renal ectopy

Renal ectopy is the term used to describe a kidney that lies outside the renal fossa. As stated previously,

the kidney migrates cephalad early in gestation to arrive at its normal position. Failure of the kidney to complete its ascent can be due to a number of factors: abnormality of the ureteral bud or metanephric blastema, genetic abnormalities, teratogenic causes, or anomalous vasculature acting as a barrier to ascent (Malek *et al.*, 1971). During ascent, the kidney receives its blood supply from the middle sacral artery, iliac artery, and finally the aorta. The anomalous blood supply that is invariably present is dependent on the final position of the kidney and is probably not the cause of the malposition. However, the blood vessels are frequently short, rendering surgical mobilization or a change of renal position very difficult.

The incidence of renal ectopy in post-mortem studies varies from 1 in 500 (Campbell, 1930) to 1 in 1290 (Thompson and Pace, 1937). The incidence of ectopic kidney is higher in autopsy series than in clinical studies, suggesting that many cases remain unrecognized (Thompson and Pace, 1937; Malek *et al.*, 1971). There is a slight predilection for the left side, and 10% of cases are bilateral. Simple renal ectopy refers to a kidney that remains in the ipsilateral retroperitoneal space. The most common position is in the pelvis (sacral or pelvic kidney) opposite the sacrum or below the aortic bifurcation (Thompson and Pace, 1937). The lumbar or iliac ectopic kidney is one that is fixed above the crest of the ileum but below the level of L-2 and L-3 Malrotation often accompanies renal ectopy (Fig. 19.9). Crossed renal ectopy refers to a kidney that crosses the midline (see discussion on anomalies of fusion later in the text).

The differentiation between a ptotic kidney and renal ectopia can be difficult, but there are several dis-

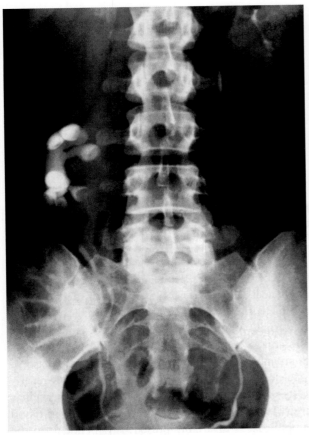

Figure 19.9 Malrotated ectopic kidney opposite lower lumbar vertebrae.

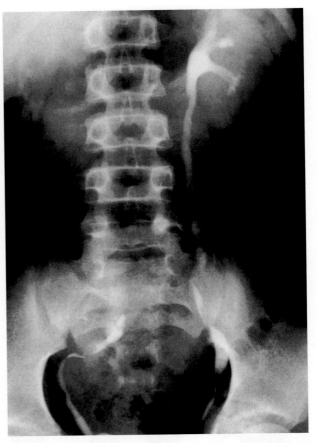

Figure 19.10 Ectopic right pelvic kidney with relatively short ureter.

cerning features. The length of the ureter may be helpful. In renal ectopy ureteral length corresponds to the location of the kidney (Fig. 19.10); in a ptotic kidney, the ureter appears redundant. The ptotic kidney is mobile and usually can be manipulated into its normal position.

Diagnosis

Most cases of renal ectopy recognized in childhood are associated with symptoms attributed to either the genitourinary or gastrointestinal system. Patients have vague abdominal pain or renal colic secondary to ureteropelvic junction obstruction or stone formation. Often these abnormalities are incidentally found when the child is evaluated following a urinary tract infection (UTI). The ectopic kidney may also be noted incidentally in the evaluation of the other associated anomalies. Modern imaging techniques have increased the frequency of diagnosis of these lesions. For example, in a child undergoing cardiac catheteri-

zation, the renal abnormality may be detected on fluoroscopy of the abdomen. Less often, the ectopic kidney can be detected as an abdominal mass on physical examination.

Pelvic kidneys may be difficult to recognize on excretory urography because they overlie bony structures. Oblique films may be quite helpful in visualizing the pelvic kidney (Fig. 19.11). However, most can be identified by radionuclide scan (Pattaras *et al.*, 1999). Whenever a kidney is absent on excretory urography, the pelvic area should be carefully examined for evidence of a ureter from an extopic kidney. Voiding cystourethrography (VCUG) is recommended in all children with a diagnosis of pelvic kidney to exclude vesicoureteral reflux (VUR), which is frequently associated with an ectopic kidney (Fig. 19.12) (Kramer and Kelalis, 1984). Poor visualization of the pelvic kidney on excretory urogram may also be due to diminished function secondary to obstruction or other pathologic conditions. Obstruction in the ectopic kidney is often related to a high insertion of the ureter on the renal pelvis (Fig. 19.13). Retrograde pyelography can be used to opacify the collecting system in cases with inadequate excretion of contrast (Fig. 19.14).

Confirmation of the diagnosis of an ectopic kidney may be made with sonography in most cases. The abnormal calyces and pelvis are readily visible on the ultrasound scan. Diuretic renography may be needed to distinguish these abnormal pyelocalyceal patterns from ureteropelvic junction obstruction. The ectopic kidney can be clearly shown on the renal scan, but the gamma camera should be place anteriorly to obtain better images (Fig. 19.15). However, if the kidney is totally non-functional, CT scan may be the best method of localization. Renal arteriography is now seldom performed in the patient with an ectopic kidney (Fig. 19.16). Most often the kidney is supplied by multiple vessels that arise from the distal aorta, aortic bifurcation, or the iliac artery. These can be identified at the time of surgery.

Associated anomalies

The contralateral kidney is abnormal in up to 50% of patients (Malek *et al.*, 1971). There is a 10% incidence of contralateral renal agenesis. Kramer and Kelalis (1984) found associated VUR in 70% of children with a pelvic kidney. The adrenal gland is in its normal position in most cases of renal ectopy. Genital anomalies are also seen quite frequently, with an incidence ranging from 15% in males to 75% in females (Thompson and Pace, 1937; Downs *et al.*, 1973). In males, the most common abnormalities are hypospadias and undescended testes (Malek *et al.*, 1971). Anomalies of the reproductive organs are seen most frequently in the female: duplication of the vagina, bicornuate uterus, and hypoplasia or agenesis of the uterus or vagina are included (Griffin *et al.*, 1976). These abnormalities have significance in that there are often problems with pregnancy, which may necessitate cesarean section (Downs *et al.*, 1973).

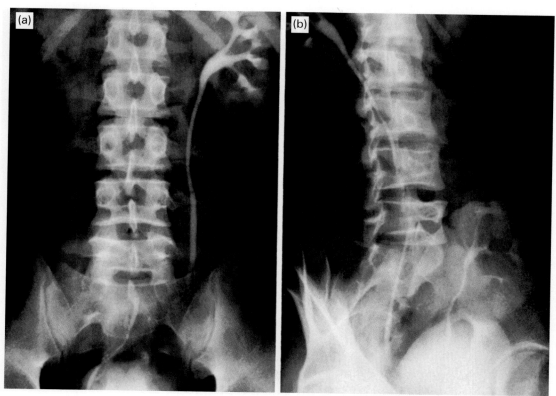

Figure 19.11 Excretory urogram in patient with a right pelvic kidney. (*a*) Only the right ureter is seen overlying the bony structures. (*b*) Oblique film allows much better visualization of the collecting system and renal outline.

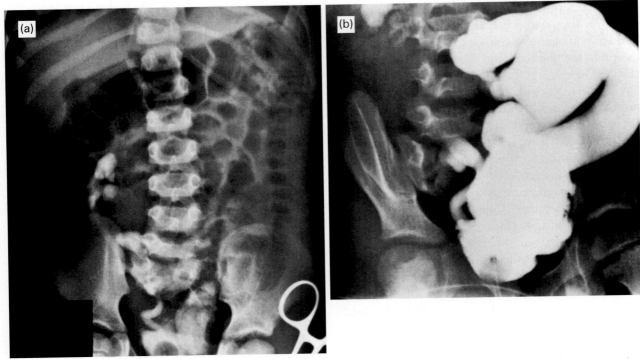

Figure 19.12 Vesicoureteral reflux (VUR) in ectopic kidney. (*a*) Excretory urogram showing dilated left ureter, probably from reflux of contrast medium from the bladder. (*b*) Cystogram showing bilateral VUR, massive into the left system. (From Kelalis *et al.*, 1973. © 1973, The Williams & Wilkins Company, Baltimore.)

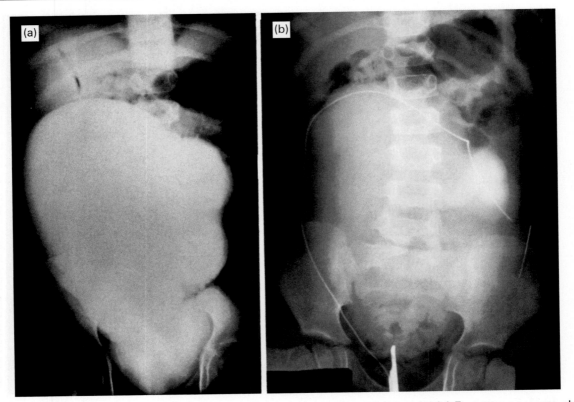

Figure 19.13 Ectopic solitary pelvic kidney in a 6-year-old boy with gross hematuria. (*a*) Excretory urogram showing giant hydronephrosis. (*b*) Retrograde pyelogram showing a catheter in the ureter with high insertion into pelvis.

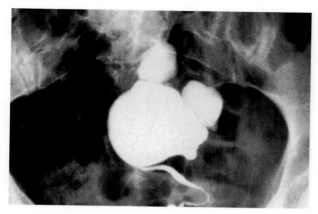

Figure 19.14 Retrograde pyelogram in a patient with a symptomatic ureteropelvic junction obstruction in a left pelvic kidney.

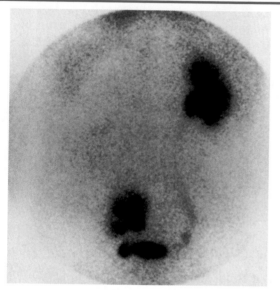

Figure 19.15 Renal scintigram of a right pelvic kidney. The camera was placed anteriorly in this patient with bilateral pyelocaliectasis.

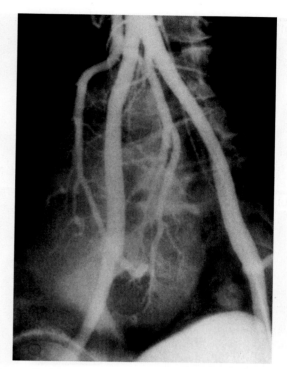

Figure 19.16 Renal arteriogram of a solitary pelvic kidney demonstrating multiple anomalous renal vessels arising from distal aorta and common iliac artery.

Anomalies of other organ systems also occur with increased frequency. Skeletal anomalies occur in up to 50% of children. The most common include asymmetry of the skull, rib abnormalities, dysplastic vertebrae, and absent bones. Cardiovascular lesions were noted in nine of the 21 children studied by Malek *et al.* (1971), and gastrointestinal abnormalities are found in one-third of patients. However, Downs *et al.* (1973) reported a lower incidence of associated extra-genitourinary anomalies.

Management

Many patients with renal ectopy remain undiagnosed

throughout life. Overall, renal disease develops in 40% of patients with a solitary pelvic kidney (Downs *et al.*, 1973). The most common problem is UPJ obstruction. This may be due to the malrotation and high ureteral insertion, or it may be secondary to an anomalous vessel that partially obstructs the collecting system. Treatment should be individualized, but in most cases a transabdominal approach for pyeloplasty is required. The goal of surgery is to achieve dependent drainage, and in some cases ureterocalycostomy may be best. Renal stones may develop in these kidneys (Fig. 19.17). In the past, these were managed with open removal but now are amenable to extracorporeal shockwave lithotripsy (ESWL) or endourologic techniques, particularly if the ureter is dependent. An important consideration in management is that the contralateral kidney is frequently abnormal, so that every effort should be made to salvage renal tissue.

Thoracic kidney

Excessive cranial migration of the kidney results in a thoracic kidney. N'Guessan *et al.* (1984) prefer to call this a 'superior ectopic kidney' because most high kid-

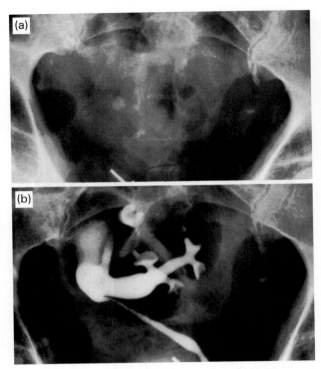

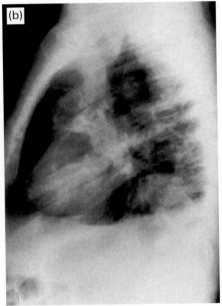

Figure 19.17 Left pelvic kidney. (a) Kidney–ureter–bladder (KUB) study revealed opaque calculus in the true pelvis. (b) Retrograde pyelogram confirmed the stone to be within the renal pelvis of the pelvic kidney.

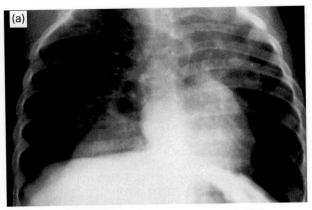

Figure 19.18 Routine roentgenograms of chest in a patient with an intrathoracic kidney.

neys actually lie below the diaphragm. A kidney is intrathoracic when either a portion or all extends above the diaphragm. This accounts for fewer than 5% of renal ectopy with an incidence of 1 in 13 000 autopsies (Campbell, 1930). The left side is more commonly involved and there is a male predominance. In rare instances, the condition can be bilateral (N'Guessan *et al.*, 1984).

Renal ascent is normally complete by the 8th week of gestation. A true intrathoracic kidney may be the result of accelerated ascent prior to diaphragmatic closure or delayed closure of the diaphragmatic anlage, allowing continued ascent (Burke *et al.*, 1967; N'Guessan *et al.*, 1984). The renal vascular supply often arises from the normal site of origin on the aorta (Lundius, 1975), but may arise more superiorly. The kidney appears normal otherwise and generally has completed rotation.

In most cases, the kidney is actually subdiaphragmatic in location. A thin membranous portion of the diaphragm overlying the kidney has been described in patients examined at thoracotomy or necropsy. In the supradiaphragmatic kidney, the ureter and hilar vessels enter through the foramen of Bodchalek. The

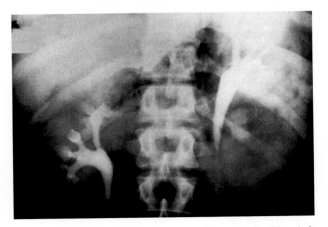

Figure 19.19 Excretory urogram of a patient with a left intrathoracic kidney.

adrenal gland frequently remains caudal to the kidney in its normal location (N'Guessan *et al.*, 1984). A superior ectopic kidney in association with a Bodchalek hernia is uncommon. In this circumstance, there is herniation of other viscera through the diaphragm. The kidney is mobile and can be easily withdrawn from the thorax.

In general, thoracic kidneys function normally and most patients are asymptomatic. The condition is often detected on routine chest radiographs as a suspected mediastinal mass (Fig. 19.18). Excretory urography or CT scans confirm the diagnosis (Fig. 19.19).

Anomalies of fusion

The congenital renal anomaly that produces some of the most bizarre-looking urograms is the result of fusion of two or more kidney masses. Several mechanisms that could lead to this are proposed. As the kidneys ascend out of the pelvis, they cross the umbilical arteries. Malposition of the umbilical arteries may cause the developing nephrogenic blastemas to come together. Fusion of the nephrogenic masses in the midline would result in a horseshoe kidney. If, during ascent, one kidney advances slightly ahead of the other, the inferior pole may come in contact with the superior pole of the trailing kidney. This results in crossed ectopia with fusion. A single nephrogenic mass induced by ureteral buds from both sides may also result in crossed fused renal ectopia (Cook and Stephens, 1977). This latter theory, with the ureters crossing the midline, explains a solitary or bilaterally crossed ectopic kidney. Fusion of the two masses occurs early in embryogenesis, and malrotation is present in all cases.

Horseshoe kidney

The horseshoe kidney represents the most common type of renal fusion. In this anomaly, two renal masses lie on either side of the midline. The lower poles are joined in more than 90% of cases (Fig. 19.20). The isthmus crossing the midline joining the two kidneys may consist of renal parenchyma or fibrous tissue. The horseshoe kidney is usually positioned low in the abdomen, with the isthmus lying just below the junction of the inferior mesenteric artery and aorta. It is postulated that the inferior mesenteric artery obstructs the isthmus and prevents further ascent.

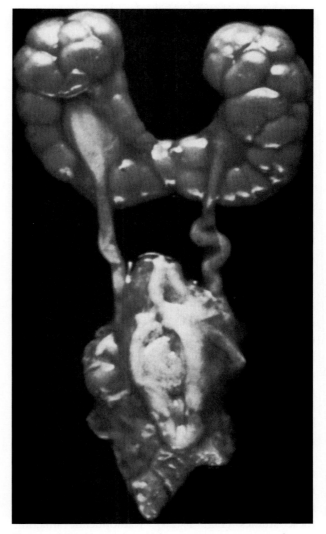

Figure 19.20 Horseshoe kidney, postmortem specimen.

Although the isthmus is usually anterior to the great vessels, it may pass posterior to the aorta and/or inferior vena cava (Dajani, 1966).

The reported incidence of horseshoe kidney varies from 1 in 400 (Glenn, 1959) to 1 in 1800 (Campbell, 1970). The abnormality is more common in males. In autopsy series, this anomaly is found more commonly in children (Campbell, 1970) and is attributed to the high incidence of associated congenital anomalies causing the demise of such children. This is in contrast to the 3.5% incidence of associated congenital malformation in adults discovered to have horseshoe kidneys. Horseshoe kidneys have been reported in identical twins (Bridge, 1960) and in several siblings within the same family (David, 1974).

Diagnosis

The diagnosis of the horseshoe kidney may be suspected from a plain radiograph of the abdomen if one can visualize the renal outlines in their abnormal position. However, it is excretory urography that allows an accurate diagnosis (Fig. 19.21).

Malrotation of the kidney is invariably present. This is attributed to very early fusion of the kidneys before rotation is complete. The renal pelves remain anterior, with the ureters crossing the isthmus. The orientation of the calyces is generally antero-posterior, but the lowermost calyces invariably point towards the midline, medial to the ureter. These lower calyces often overlie the vertebral column. The renal axis appears to be vertical or shifted outward, with the lower poles lying closer together than the upper poles. The course of the ureters is variable, but they often lie anterior to the pelvis. The upper ureter appears to be laterally displaced by a midline mass. Other pertinent urographic findings are low-lying kidneys, and the lower outer border of the kidney appears to continue across the midline. The radiographic appearance of a horseshoe kidney is frequently altered by associated abnormalities such as hydronephrosis and/or diminished renal function (Fig. 19.22).

The diagnosis of a horseshoe kidney can be confirmed by a variety of imaging techniques, including renal sonography, CT, or MRI. The fusion of the kidneys generally can be clearly visualized with any of these studies (Fig. 19.23). Radionuclide imaging (Fig. 19.24) can also be helpful in making the diagnosis when other imaging modalities are inconclusive (Grandone *et al.*, 1985). In the past, renal arteriography was frequently performed, not only to establish the diagnosis of the horseshoe kidney but also to delineate the vascular blood supply. In the majority of cases, there are multiple renal vessels. The blood supply to the isthmus is particularly variable, often supplied by a separate vessel. This may arise from the aorta, common iliac, or inferior mesenteric arteries.

Associated anomalies

There is a frequent association of other anomalies in children with horseshoe kidney. The incidence of these anomalies is much higher if the horseshoe kidney is discovered in the newborn period. Zondek

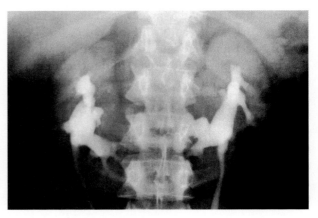

Figure 19.21 Typical appearance of horseshoe kidney on an excretory urogram.

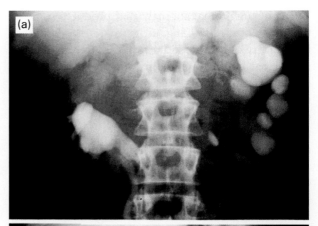

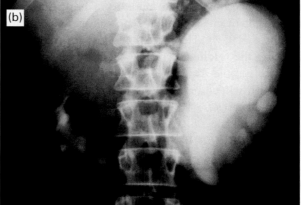

Figure 19.22 Horseshoe kidney. Excretory urograms show severe hydronephrosis with delayed excretion of left renal segment secondary to ureteropelvic obstruction.

and Zondek (1964) examined the post-mortem records of 99 individuals with horseshoe kidneys. Of those infants who were stillborn or who died within

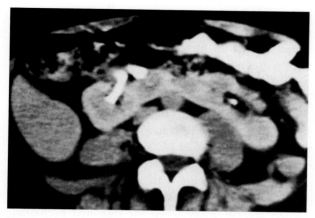

Figure 19.23 Fusion of the lower poles over the great vessels seen on computed tomographic scan.

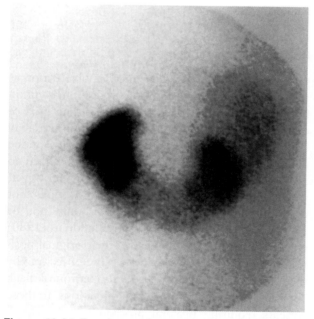

Figure 19.24 Renal scan in a patient with horseshoe kidney showing minimal function of the isthmus.

the first year of life, 78% had malformations of other organ systems. These most commonly involved the central nervous system, gastrointestinal tract, and the skeletal and cardiovascular systems. Boatman *et al.* (1972) reported that one-third of patients with horseshoe kidney had at least one other abnormality.

Horseshoe kidneys have been found with increased frequency with several well-known syndromes, including trisomy 18, which is associated with a 21% incidence of fused kidneys (Boatman *et al.*, 1972;

Warkany *et al.*, 1966). More than 60% of patients with Turner syndrome have renal abnormalities, including horseshoe kidneys, ureteral duplication, or other minor abnormalities (Smith, 1982). One study noted a 7% incidence of horseshoe kidneys in patients with Turner syndrome who were evaluated with renal ultrasound scannng (Lippe *et al.*, 1988). There is also an increased incidence of horseshoe kidneys in patients with neural tube defects (Whitaker and Hunt, 1987).

Other genitourinary abnormalities are also encountered with increased frequency in these patients. Ten per cent of patients have ureteral duplication, and VUR has been found in 10% (Pitts and Muecke, 1975) to 80% of children who undergo evaluation (Fig. 19.25) (Segura *et al.*, 1972). Multicystic dysplasia (Novak *et al.*, 1977) and autosomal dominant polycystic kidney disease have also been reported (Pitts and Muecke, 1975). Hypospadias and undescended testes occur in 4% of the males, bicornuate uterus or septate vagina in 7% of females (Boatman *et al.*, 1972). Retrocaval ureter has been found in association with a horseshoe kidney in six patients (Fernandes *et al.*, 1988).

Prognosis

The presence of a horseshoe kidney does not adversely affect survival. Nearly one-third of patients with a horseshoe kidney remain undiagnosed throughout life (Glenn, 1959; Pitts and Muecke, 1975). Most women are able to go through pregnancy and delivery without adverse effects (Bell, 1946). In those patients with problems, symptoms are most often secondary to hydronephrosis, UTI or urolithiasis. These patients generally present with vague abdominal pain. The finding of abdominal pain and nausea with hyperextension of the spine (Rovsing syndrome) presumably resulting from stretching of the isthmus is uncommon. Operations to divide the isthmus were once performed to relieve pain, but this procedure has no merit (Glenn, 1959; Pitts and Muecke, 1975).

UPJ obstruction is the most common cause of hydronephrosis, occurring in 30% of patients diagnosed during life. The obstruction may be caused by a high ureteral insertion or an anomalous renal vessel. It must be recognized that the calyces may have an abnormal appearance as a result of the malrotation alone and that not all of these kidneys are

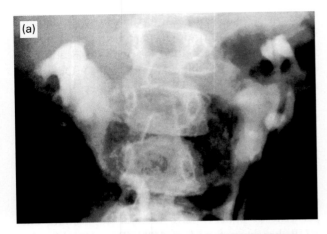

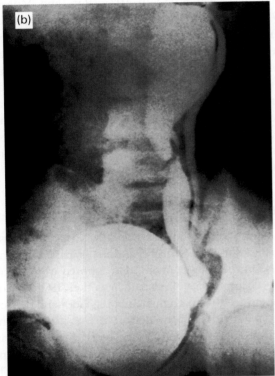

Figure 19.25 Horseshoe kidney. (*a*) Excretory urogram revealing mild hydronephrosis. (*b*) Voiding cystourethrogram demonstrating high-grade vesicoureteral reflux into both segments of a complete ureteral duplication.

obstructed. In addition, the upper urinary tract dilatation may be secondary to VUR (see Fig. 19.25) and should be excluded in all children with a horseshoe kidney.

More than 100 cases of renal malignancy have been reported in patients with horseshoe kidney (Buntley, 1976), with a number of hypernephromas arising from the isthmus (Blackard and Mellinger, 1968). There appears to be an increased incidence of renal pelvic tumors and nephroblastoma compared with that in the general population (Blackard and Mellinger, 1968; Dische and Johnston, 1979). Wilms' tumor is the second most common tumor found in horseshoe kidneys. In a review of National Wilms' Tumor Study patients, Mesrobian *et al.* (1985) found that there was a seven-fold increased risk of a Wilms' tumor developing in patients with a horseshoe kidney. In many cases, the diagnosis of horseshoe kidney was missed preoperatively when the distorted pyelogram was presumed to be secondary to the renal mass. No recommendation was made regarding periodic screening with renal sonography to detect occult malignancies.

Management

Correction of ureteropelvic junction obstruction is the most frequent indication for surgical intervention in a patient with a horseshoe kidney. The goal of dependent drainage following pyeloplasty may be difficult to achieve in these patients. Routine division of the isthmus was once recommended to avoid having the ureter cross the isthmus. However, it has become clear that the isthmus does not contribute to the obstruction and should not be routinely divided. Donahoe and Hendren (1980) report that the kidneys remain in their original position following symphysiotomy because of fixation by the abnormal vasculature. An extraperitoneal flank approach is utilized for unilateral operations. In those patients requiring bilateral procedures, a transperitoneal approach may be preferable in order to allow operation on both sides at once. Extraperitoneal drainage must be assured postoperatively.

Ureterocalycostomy is an excellent alternative to achieve dependent drainage of the dilated urinary tract (Mollard and Braun, 1980). The ureter can be anastomosed to a lower pole calyx, particularly in patients with severe hydronephrosis with thinning of the renal parenchyma.

Urolithiasis develops in 20% of patients with a horseshoe kidney. Stasis secondary to hydronephrosis increases the chance of stone formation, but metabolic factors should not be overlooked (Evans and Resnick, 1981). Most patients with renal stone disease can be managed with ESWL (Smith *et al.*, 1989).

Crossed renal ectopia

Crossed renal ectopia is the second most common fusion anomaly. The ectopic kidney crosses the midline to lie on the opposite side from its ureteral insertion into the bladder (Fig. 19.26). The four varieties of crossed renal ectopia are illustrated in Figure 19.27.

The incidence of crossed ectopia has been placed at 1 in 7000 autopsies (Abeshouse and Bhisitkul, 1959). Crossed renal ectopia with fusion is the most common type and accounts for 85% of the cases. Crossed ectopia without fusion represents fewer than 10% of all cases, and solitary crossed ectopia and bilateral crossed ectopia are exceedingly rare (McDonald and McClellan, 1957; Kakei *et al.* 1976). With all of these abnormalities, there is a slight male predominance and crossing from left to right occurs more frequently than right to left.

There are many variations in the extent of the fusion that can produce bizarre radiographic pictures. Determining the exact type of crossed ectopia may be a difficult task. McDonald and McClellan (1957) described six different varieties of crossed ectopia with fusion (Fig. 19.28). The most common form is unilateral fused type with inferior ectopia, in which the upper pole of the crossed kidney is fused to the lower pole of the normally positioned kidney. The renal pelves remain in their anterior position, representing failure to complete rotation. The second most common type is the sigmoid, or S-shaped, kidney. The crossed kidney is inferior, but both kidneys have completed their rotation so that the two renal pelves face in opposite directions. The fusion of the two kidneys probably occurs later, after axial rotation is completed.

The other four types of fusion are much less common. The lump, or 'cake', kidney and the disk kidney both involve extensive fusion of the two renal masses. In an L-shaped kidney, the crossed kidney assumes a transverse position. The least common type is the superior ectopic kidney, in which the crossed ectopic kidney lies superior to the normal kidney. The two kidneys may also fuse side to side and ascend together to the renal fossa (Fig. 19.29).

Diagnosis

The classification described above was devised to stratify the patients in some logical fashion. There is a

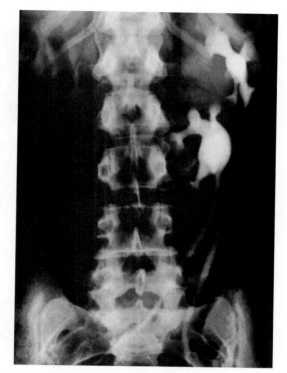

Figure 19.26 Crossed ectopia, with the right kidney crossing midline and fused to the lower pole of the left kidney.

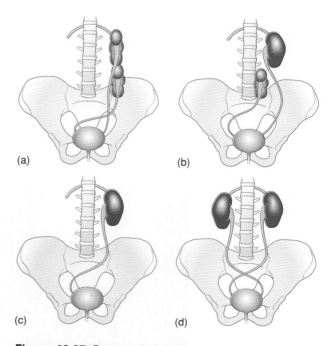

(a)   (b)

(c)   (d)

Figure 19.27 Four varieties of crossed renal ectopia. (*a*) With fusion; (*b*) without fusion; (*c*) solitary; (*d*) bilateral. (Redrawn from McDonald and McClellan, as reproduced by Abeshouse and Bhisitkul, 1959.)

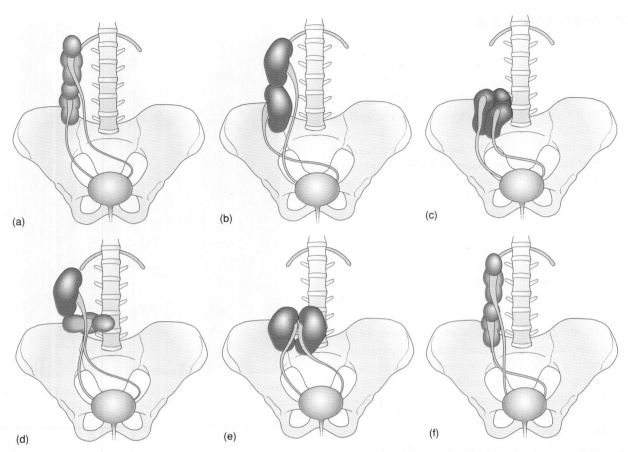

Figure 19.28 Six varieties of crossed renal ectopia with fusion. (*a*) Unilateral fused kidney, superior ectopia; (*b*) sigmoid or S-shaped kidney; (*c*) 'lump' kidney; (*d*) L-shaped kidney; (*e*) 'disk' kidney; (*f*) unilateral fused kidney, inferior ectopia. (Redrawn from McDonald and McClellan, as reproduced by Abeshouse and Bhisitkul, 1959.)

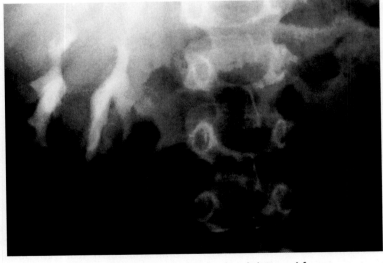

Figure 19.29 Crossed renal ectopy with side-to-side fusion in the right renal fossa.

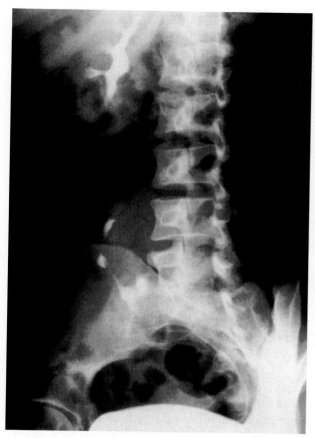

Figure 19.30 Crossed renal ectopy without fusion.

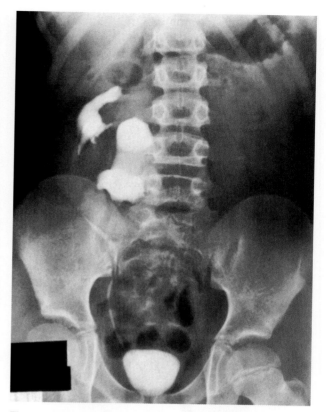

Figure 19.31 Crossed ectopic left kidney is fused to the right kidney, with associated ureteropelvic obstruction.

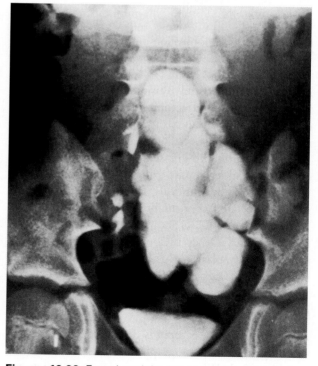

Figure 19.32 Fused pelvic kidney with left hydronephrosis secondary to ureteropelvic obstructiion

spectrum of abnormalities, and it is often difficult to categorize patients based on urographic findings. It can be difficult to distinguish between crossed ectopia with fusion from crossed renal ectopy without fusion. This distinction may be possible on excretory urography if the two renal masses are widely separated (Fig. 19.30). In the past, many cases were confirmed by findings at surgical exploration or necropsy. CT and MRI should enable one to establish the correct diagnosis.

The vascular supply to these kidneys is quite variable. Renal arteriography often demonstrates multiple anomalous branches to both kidneys arising from the aorta, or common iliac artery. Rarely will the renal artery cross the midline to supply the crossed kidney (Rubinstein *et al.*, 1976).

Associated anomalies

There is an increased incidence of malformations of other organ systems, including orthopedic or skeletal anomalies, imperforate anus, and cardiovascular ano-

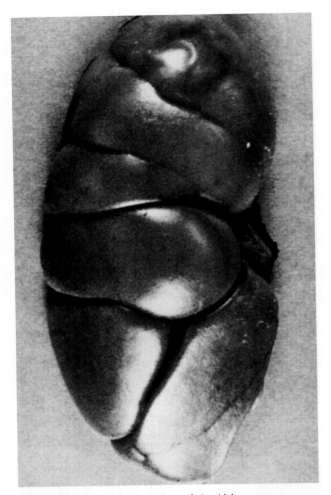

Figure 19.33 Fetal lobulation of the kidney.

and Bhisitkul (1959) reported that one-third of patients had pyelonephritis and one-quarter had hydronephrosis (Fig. 19.31). The calyceal dilatation and distortion may be secondary to the malrotation or the presence of VUR. Urolithiasis has been found in up to one-third of patients (Boatman *et al.*, 1972). Mininberg *et al.* (1971) reported one infant who presented with hypertension secondary to a vascular lesion. Other patients may be found to have an abdominal mass on physical examination or during surgical exploration. It is particularly pertinent in the patient with a fused pelvic kidney (Fig. 19.32) to recognize that this is the total functioning renal parenchyma.

Fetal lobulation

Fetal lobulation is a condition commonly found in children and represents a persistence of normal fetal development (Fig. 19.33). Another term used to describe this is 'renal' lobation because it designates the larger renal lobe (pyramid plus surrounding cortex) rather than the lobule (medullary ray and surrounding glomeruli). Campbell (1970) found fetal lobulation at autopsy in 17.6% of children and in 3.9% of adults. This condition is of no clinical importance, and should be recognized as a variant of normal renal form. Radiographically, it appears as small notches in the renal margin that are placed midway between the calyces.

malies (Abeshouse and Bhisitkul, 1959). In patients with solitary crossed ectopia, there is a higher incidence of genital abnormalities, but this is probably related to the renal agenesis (Kakei *et al.* 1976).

The ureter in the crossed ectopic kidney usually enters the bladder and its orifice is only rarely ectopic (Abeshouse and Bhisitkul, 1959). The most commonly associated abnormality is VUR (Kramer and Kelalis, 1984). VCUG should be performed in all of these patients. Other uncommon problems include multicystic dysplasia (Nussbaum *et al.*, 1987) and renal tumors (Gerber *et al.*, 1980).

Prognosis

Most crossed renal ectopia is discovered incidentally, often by antenatal sonography when two kidneys are not identified. When symptoms do occur, they are often related to infection and obstruction. Abeshouse

References

Abeshouse BS, Bhisitkul I (1959) Crossed renal ectopia with and without fusion. *Urol Int* **9**: 63–91.

Adzick N, Harrison MR, Flake AW *et al.* (1984) Experimental pulmonary hypoplasia and oligohydramnios: relative contributions of lung fluid and fetal breathing movements. *J Pediatr Surg* **19**: 658–65.

Antony J (1977) Complete duplication of female urethra with vaginal atresia and supernumerary kidney. *J Urol* **118**: 877–8.

Ashley DJB, Mostofi FK (1960) Renal agenesis and dysgenesis. *J Urol* **83**: 211–30.

Avni EF, Thova Y, Lalmand B *et al.* (1987) Multicystic dysplastic kidney: natural history from *in utero* diagnosis and postnatal follow-up. *J Urol* **138**: 1420–4.

Bell R (1946) Horseshoe kidney in pregnancy. *J Urol* **56**: 159–61.

Blackard CE, Mellinger GT (1968) Cancer in a horseshoe kidney: a report of two cases. *Arch Surg* **97**: 616–27.

Boatman DL, Kolln CP, Flocks RH (1972) Congenital anomalies associated with horseshoe kidney. *J Urol* **107**: 205–7.

Bridge RAC (1960) Horseshoe kidneys in identical twins. *Br J Urol* **32**: 32–3.

Buntley D (1976) Malignancy associated with horseshoe kidney. *Urology* **8**: 146–8.

Burke EC, Wenzl JE, Utz DC (1967) The intrathoracic kidney: report of a case. *Am J Dis Child* **113**: 487–90.

Campbell MF (1930) Renal ectopy. *J Urol* **24**: 187–98.

Campbell MF (1951) *Clinical pediatric urology*. Philadelphia, PA: WB Saunders, 167–205.

Campbell MF (1970) Anomalies of the kidney. In: Campbell MF, Harrison JH (eds) *Urology*. Volume 2. 3rd edition. Philadelphia, PA: WB Saunders, 1416–86.

Carlson HE (1950) Supernumerary kidney: a summary of fifty-one reported cases. *J Urol* **64**: 224–9.

Charney CW, Gillenwater JY (1965) Congenital absence of the vas deferens. *J Urol* **93**: 399–401.

Collins DC (1932) Congenital unilateral renal agenesia. *Ann Surg* **95**: 715–26.

Cook WA, Stephens FD (1977) Fused kidneys: morphologic study and theory of embryogenesis. *Birth Defects* **13**: 327–40.

Curtis JA, Sadhu V, Steiner RM (1977) Malposition of the colon in right renal agenesis, ectopia, and anterior nephrectomy. *AJR Am J Roentgenol* **129**: 845–50.

Dajani AM (1966) Horseshoe kidney: a review of twenty-nine cases. *Br J Urol* **38**: 388–402.

David RA (1974) Horseshoe kidney: a report of one family. *BMJ* **4**: 571–2.

Davidson WM, Ross GM (1954) Bilateral absence of the kidneys and related congenital anomalies. *J Pathol Bacteriol* **68**: 459–74.

Dees JE (1941) Clinical importance of congenital anomalies of the upper urinary tract. *J Urol* **46**: 659–66.

Dees JE (1960) Prognosis of the solitary kidney. *J Urol* **83**: 550–2.

Dische MR, Johnston R (1979) Teratoma in horseshoe kidneys. *Urology* **13**: 435–8.

Donahoe PK, Hendren WH (1980) Pelvic kidney in infants and children: experience with 16 cases. *J Pediatr Surg* **15**: 486–95.

Doroshow LW, Abeshouse BS (1961) Congenital unilateral solitary kidney: report of 37 cases and a review of the literature. *Urol Surv* **11**: 219–29.

Downs RA, Lane JW, Burns E (1973) Solitary pelvic kidney: its clinical implications. *Urology* **1**: 51–6.

Duhamel B (1961) From the mermaid to anal imperforation: the syndrome of caudal regression. *Arch Dis Child* **36**: 152–5.

Emanuel B, Nachman R, Aronson N et al. (1974) Congenital solitary kidney: a review of 74 cases. *Am J Dis Child* **127**: 17–19.

Evans WP, Resnick MI (1981) Horseshoe kidney and urolithiasis. *J Urol* **125**: 620–1.

Fernandes M, Scheuch J, Seebode JJ (1988) Horseshoe kidney with retrocaval ureter: a case report. *J Urol* **140**: 362–4.

Fortune CH (1927) The pathological and clinical significance of congenital one-sided kidney defect with the presentation of three new cases of agenesia and one of aplasia. *Ann Intern Med* **1**: 377–99.

Gerber WL, Culp DA, Brown RC et al. (1980) Renal mass in crossed-fused ectopia. *J Urol* **123**: 239–44.

Glenn JF (1959) Analysis of 51 patients with horseshoe kidney. *N Engl J Med* **261**: 684–7.

Goldstein M, Schlossberg S (1988) Men with congenital absence of the vas deferens often have seminal vesicles. *J Urol* **140**: 85–6.

Grandone CH, Haller JD, Berdon WE et al. (1985) Asymmetric horseshoe kidney in the infant: value of renal nuclear scanning. *Radiology* **154**: 366.

Gray SW, Skandalakis JE (1972) The kidney and ureter. In: *Embryology for surgeons*. Philadelphia, PA: WB saunders, 443–518.

Griffin JE, Edwards C, Madden JD et al. (1976) Congenital absence of the vagina: the Mayer–Rokitansky–Kuster–Hauser syndrome. *Ann Intern Med* **85**: 224–36.

Gutierrez-Millet R, Nieto J, Praga M et al. (1986) Focal glomerulosclerosis and proteinuria in patients with solitary kidneys. *Arch Intern Med* **146**: 705–9.

Hostetter TH, Olson JL, Rennke HG (1981) Hyperfiltration in remnant nephrons: a potentially adverse response to renal ablation. *Am J Physiol* **241**: F85–93.

Kakei H, Kondo H, Ogisu BI et al. (1976) Crossed ectopia of solitary kidney: a report of two cases and a review of the literature. *Urol Int* **31**: 470–5.

Kiprov DD, Colvin RB, McClusky RT (1981) Focal and segmental glomerulosclerosis and proteinuria associated with unilateral renal agenesis. *Lab Invest* **46**: 275–81.

Kramer SA, Kelalis PP (1984) Ureteropelvic junction obstruction in children with renal ectopy. *Journal d'urologie* **5**: 331–6.

Limakeng ND, Retik AB (1972) Unilateral renal agenesis with hypoplastic ureter: observations on the contralateral urinary tract and report of 4 cases. *J Urol* **108**: 149–52.

Lippe BL, Geffner ME, Dietrich RB et al. (1988) Renal malformation in patients with Turner's syndrome: imaging in 141 patients. *Pediatrics* **83**: 852–6.

Longo VJ, Thompson GJ (1952) Congenital solitary kidney. *J Urol* **68**: 63–8.

Lundius B (1975) Intrathoracic kidney. *AJR Am J Roentgenol* **125**: 678–81.

McDonald JH, McClellan DS (1957) Crossed renal ectopia. *Am J Surg* **93**: 995–1002.

Mace JM, Kaplan JM, Schanberger JE et al. (1972) Poland's syndrome: report of seven cases and review of the literature. *Clin Pediatr* **11**: 98–102.

McGahan JP, Myracle MR (1986) Adrenal hypertrophy: possible pitfall in the sonographic diagnosis of renal agenesis. *J Ultrasound Med* **5**: 265–8.

Malek RS, Kelalis PP, Burke EC (1971) Ectopic kidney in children and frequency of association with other malformations. *Mayo Clin Proc* **46**: 461–7.

Mascatello V, Lebowitz RL (1976) Malposition of the colon in left renal agenesis and ectopia. *Radiology* **120**: 371–6.

Mesrobian HJ, Kelalis PP, Hrabovsky E et al. (1985) Wilms' tumor in horseshoe kidneys: a report from the National Wilms' Tumor Study. *J Urol* **133**: 1002–3.

Mininberg DT, Roze S, Yoon HJ et al. (1971) Hypertension associated with crossed renal ectopia in an infant. *Pediatrics* **48**: 454–7.

Mollard P, Braun P (1980) Primary ureterocalycostomy for severe hydronephrosis in children. *J Pediatr Surg* **15**: 87–91.

Moore WB, Matthews TJ, Rabinowitz R (1975) Genitourinary anomalies associated with Klippel–Feil syndrome. *J Bone Joint Surg* (Am) **57**: 355–7.

Nakada T, Furuta H, Kazama T et al. (1988) Unilateral renal agenesis with or without ipsilateral adrenal agenesis. *J Urol* **140**: 933–7.

N'Guessan G, Stephens FD (1983) Supernumerary kidney. *J Urol* **130**: 649–53.

N'Guessan G, Stephens FD, Pick J (1984) Congenital superior ectopic (thoracic) kidney. *Urology* **24**: 219–28.

Novak ME, Baum NH, Gonzales ET Jr (1977) Horseshoe kidney with multicystic dysplasia associated with ureterocele. *Urology* **10**: 456–8.

Nussbaum AR, Hartman DS, Whitley N et al. (1987) Multicystic dysplasia and crossed renal ectopia. *AJR Am J Roentgenol* **149**: 407–10.

Ochsner MG, Brannan W, Goodier EH (1972) Absent vas deferens associated with renal agenesis. *JAMA* **222**: 1055–6.

Osathanondh V, Potter EL (1963) Development of human kidney as shown in microdissection–3 parts. *Arch Pathol* **76**: 271–302.

Parrott TS, Shandalakis JE, Gray SW (1994) The kidney and ureter. In: JE Shandalakis and SW Gray (eds) *Embryology for surgeons. The embryological basis for the treatment of congenital anomalies*. 2nd edition. Baltimore, MA: Williams and Wilkins, 594–670.

Pattaras JG, Rushton HG, Majd M (1999) The role of ^{99m}technetium dimercapto-succinic acid renal scan in the evaluation of acute ectopic ureters in girls with paradoxical incontinence. *J Urol* **162**: 821–5.

Pedicelli G, Jequier S, Bowen A et al. (1986) Multicystic dysplastic kidneys: spontaneous regression demonstrated with ultrasound. *Radiology* **161**: 23–6.

Pitts WR Jr, Muecke EC (1975) Horseshoe kidneys: a 40 year experience. *J Urol* **113**: 743–6.

Potter El (1965) Bilateral absence of ureters and kidneys: a report of 50 cases. *Obstet Gynecol* **25**: 3–12.

Priman J (1929) A consideration of normal and abnormal positions of the hilum of the kidney. *Anat Rec* **42**: 355–63.

Radasch HE (1908) Congenital unilateral absence of the urogenital system and its relation to the development of the wolffian and müllerian ducts. *Am J Med Sci* **136**: 111–18.

Rizza JM, Downing SE (1971) Bilateral renal agenesis in two female siblings. *Am J Dis Child* **121**: 60–3.

Roehrborn CG, Schneider HJ, Rugendorff EW et al. (1986) Embryological and diagnostic aspects of seminal vesicle cycts associated with upper urinary tract malformation. *J Urol* **135**: 1029–32.

Romero R, Cullen M, Grannum P et al. (1985) Antenatal diagnosis of renal anomalies with ultrasound: III Bilateral renal agenesis. *Am J Obstet Gynecol* **151**: 38–43.

Roodhooft AM, Birnhalz JC, Holmes LB (1984) Familial nature of congenital absence and severe dysgenesis of both kidneys. *N Engl J Med* **310**: 1341–5.

Rubinstein ZJ, Heitz M, Shahin N et al. (1976) Crossed renal ectopia: anaigographic findings in six cases. *AJR Am J Roentgenol* **126**: 1035–8.

Schumacker HB Jr (1938) Congenital anomalies of the genitalia associated with unilateral renal agenesis with particular reference to true unicornuate uterus: report of cases and review of the literature. *Arch Surg* **37**: 586–602.

Segura JW, Kelalis PP, Burke EC (1972) Horseshoe kidney in children. *J Urol* **108**: 333–6.

Shimamura T, Morrison AB (1975) A progressive glomerulosclerosis occurring in partial five-sixths nephrectomized rats. *Am J Pathol* **79**: 95–106.

Smith DW (1982) Turner syndrome. In: DW Smith (ed.) *Recognizable patterns of human malformation. Genetic, embryologic and clinical aspects*. 3rd edition. Philadelphia, PA: WB Saunders, 72

Smith EC, Orkin LA (1945) A clinical and statistical study of 471 congenital anomalies of the kidney and ureter. *J Urol* **53**: 11.

Smith JE, Arsdalen KN, Hanno PM et al. (1989) Extracorporeal shock wave lithotripsy treatment of calculi in horseshoe kidneys. *J Urol* **142**: 683–6.

Song JT, Ritchey ML, Zerin JM, Bloom DA (1995) Incidence of vesicoureteral reflux in children with unilateral renal agenesis. *J Urol* **153**: 1249–51.

Steinhardt JM, Kuhn JP, Eisenberg B et al. (1988) Ultrasound screening of healthy infants for urinary tract abnormalities. *Pediatrics* **82**: 609–14.

Thompson DP, Lynn HB (1966) Genital anomalies associated with solitary kidney. *Mayo Clin Proc* **41**: 538–48.

Thompson GJ, Pace JM (1937) Ectopic kidney: a review of 97 cases. *Surg Gynecol Obstet* **64**: 935–43.

Warkany J, Passarge E, Smith LB (1966) Congenital malformations in autosomal trisomy syndromes. *Am J Dis Child* **112**: 502–17.

Weyrauch HM Jr (1939) Anomalies of renal rotation. *Surg Gynecol Obstet* **69**: 183–99.

Whitaker RH, Hunt GM (1987) Incidence and distribution of renal anomalies in patients with neural tube defects. *Eur Urol* **13**: 322–3.

Wladimiroff JW (1975) Effect of furosemide on fetal urine production. *Br J Obstet Gynecol* **82**: 221–4.

Wulfekuhler WV, Dube VE (1971) Free supernumerary kidney: report of a case. *J Urol* **106**: 802–4.

Yoder IC, Pfister RC (1976) Unilateral hematocolpos and ipsilateral renal agenesis: report of two cases and review of the literature *AJR Am J Roentgenol* **127**: 303–8.

Zondek LH, Zondek T (1964) Horseshoe kidney in associated congenital malformations. *Urol Int* **18**: 347–56.

Anomalies of the renal collecting system: ureteropelvic junction obstruction (pyelocalyectasis) and infundibular stenosis

20

Leo C.T. Fung and Yegappan Lakshmanan

Introduction

In the management of ureteropelvic junction (UPJ) obstruction or infundibular stenosis, the clinician is invariably faced with a range of differential diagnoses, and a wide spectrum in the severity of the condition. In order to present a comprehensive review of UPJ obstruction and infundibular stenosis, this section of the chapter will therefore discuss the broader concept of hydronephrosis, as well as the more specific entities of UPJ obstruction (Figs. 20.1, 20.2) and infundibular stenosis (Fig. 20.3).

Hydronephrosis is defined as dilatation of the urinary collecting system (hydro from Greek *hydor* meaning water, *nephros* meaning kidney, and *osis* meaning condition). It can result from either an impediment in antegrade urinary flow or the retrograde reflux of urine. As vesicoureteral reflux (VUR) is discussed in detail elsewhere in this textbook, this section will be confined to the topics of non-obstructive dilatation and physiologically significant obstruction, and how to distinguish between these conditions.

Of the kidneys that develop hydronephrosis as a result of some form of antegrade obstruction, there is a tremendous variability in natural history. While some undergo progressive and often irreversible renal injury, others remain stable for long periods of time or even improve with growth. For those hydronephrotic kidneys that are found to be in need of treatment, effective surgical treatment is available, resulting in stabilized or improved renal function after successful surgical correction. Given that some hydronephrotic kidneys develop renal injury and others do not, the present controversy in the clinical management of hydronephrosis lies not in how to treat the condition, but rather in differentiating those

kidneys that require surgical treatment from those that do not.

There is currently no consensus on how best to identify those hydronephrotic kidneys that are in need of surgical repair. In order to represent fairly our evolving understanding of the dilated upper urinary

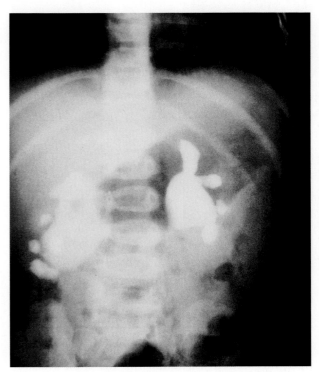

Figure 20.1 Intravenous pyelogram of a 6-month-old boy demonstrating bilateral hydronephrosis compatible with bilateral ureteropelvic junction obstruction. Even though this film was taken only 5 min after the administration of intravenous contrast, there are already well-opacified collecting systems bilaterally, demonstrating prompt excretion of contrast in spite of the presence of bilateral congenital hydronephrosis.

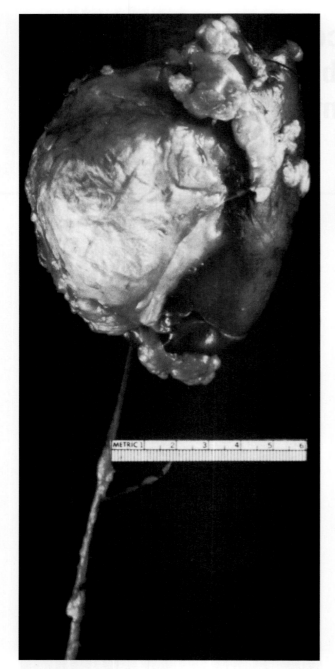

Figure 20.2 Gross specimen: ureteropelvic obstruction.

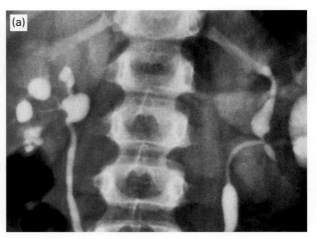

Figure 20.3 Intravenous pyelogram of a 3-year-old boy showing right infundibular stenosis and left infundibulopelvic stenosis.

tract, this section will summarize the latest available information on pathophysiology and natural history, and discuss the strengths and limitations of the various diagnostic modalities available. Recognizing that there may be more than one acceptable way to manage hydronephrosis, the authors' view will be presented as an approach that is in keeping with the known pathophysiology of this condition.

Other obstructive processes distal to the UPJ may share some common features with the material presented here, such as midureteral adynamic segments, obstructive ureteroceles, or ureterovesical junction (UVJ) obstruction. The focus of this section will be confined to the discussion of the dilated collecting system resulting from antegrade obstruction at or proximal to the UPJ, or in other words, pyelocaliectasis.

Ureteropelvic junction obstruction (pyelocaliectasis)

Embryology

During embryogenesis, the mesonephric duct gives rise to the ureteric bud at the time when the mesonephric duct joins the urogenital sinus. Development of the ureteric bud begins at the 5th week of gestation and continues until the 10th week. The ureteric bud migrates in the cephalad direction and progressively branches to give rise to the ureter, UPJ, renal pelvis, major and minor calyces, as well as the collecting ducts. As the ureteric bud migrates cephalad to join the metanephrogenic blastema, the branched collecting ducts induce the blastema to differentiate into individual nephrons, and into the renal parenchyma. The ureteric bud emanates from the wolffian duct and penetrates the blastema at 4–5 weeks of gestation. As the ureteric bud grows cephalad, the metanephric cap becomes progressively larger and rapidly differentiates. The ureteric bud expands within the growing mass of metanephrogenic tissue. While the metanephric blastema is induced to form the renal parenchyma, including the nephrons down to the collecting tubules, the ureteric bud gives rise to the collecting system.

Numerous outgrowths from the renal pelvis push radially into the growing mass and form hollow ducts that branch and rebranch as they push towards the periphery. This branching process allows the ureteric bud to give rise to the ureter, renal pelvis, major and minor calyces and corresponding infundibula, and the primary collecting ducts (Tanagho, 1995). The first three to five generations of branches eventually coalesce and form the renal pelvis and major calyces. The connections that link the first and second series of dichotomous branchings remain unexpanded as the infundibula between the major and minor calyces (Elder, 1992). From the metanephrogenic blastema, the first renal tubules begin to develop at the 7th week of gestation. Functional nephrons are present as early as the 9th week (Kim *et al.*, 1991) and urine production commences by 10–12 weeks. The fetal kidneys become reliably detectable by ultrasonography at 14–15 weeks of gestation (Lawson *et al.*, 1981), and can often be imaged at even earlier gestations.

The UPJ, the renal pelvis and ureter develop into a tubular structure that does not function merely as a conduit. Inner longitudinal and outer circular layers of smooth muscle aligned in a specific configuration enhances its function as an elastic and distensible conduit, in addition to its function as an active peristaltic pump.

Etiology

Obstructive causes of pyelocaliectasis in children include anomalies intrinsic to the UPJ, compression of the collecting system from extrinsic conditions, and obstruction secondary to foreign bodies or mass lesions within the lumen of the collecting system. Aside from foreign bodies, most etiologies result in a relatively constant degree of obstruction, although the degree of dilatation of the collecting system may change dynamically in response to the rate of urine output.

Pyelocaliectasis resulting from an anomaly intrinsic to the UPJ is most commonly associated with a short, narrow, and abnormal segment of the ureter located just at the UPJ that may extend into the proximal ureter. These segments are characterized by underactive or absent peristaltic activity, and decreased capacity for urine transport. For clarity in terminology, these anomalous segments will hereafter be referred to as hypoperistaltic or stenotic segments.

Hypoperistaltic UPJ segments are often evident visually (Fig. 20.4) or may only be identified histologically. When examined at the time of surgical repair, these segments are often narrower in caliber than the adjacent normal distal ureter, and may be somewhat tortuous. Although the lumen is physically patent (Fig. 20.5), it is non-elastic and poorly distensible. Ruano-Gil *et al.* (1975) demonstrated that the ureter is initially a solid cord-like structure that subsequently undergoes canalization during early development. Abnormalities noted at the gross anatomic level are in keeping with their hypothesis that these hypoperistaltic UPJ segments are a result of deformed or incomplete canalization. They might also be the site of compression by temporary renal vessels that are resorbed as the kidney ascends.

On histologic evaluation, muscle bundles responsible for peristaltic activity have been noted to be diminished (Foote *et al.*, 1970) and abnormal in configuration (Murnaghan, 1958) in the hypoperistaltic UPJ segments. These histologic muscle bundle abnormalities may be present with or without disruption of the intercellular relationship between muscle cells on electron microscopy (Gosling and Dixon, 1978; Hanna, 1978). The normal electrical impulse for the propagation of peristalsis along the ureter may be disrupted at the intercellular level. However, even when the electrical impulse is present, the muscle bundles may be insufficient in amount or abnormal in the configuration of circular and longitudinal fibers, and ultimately unable to effect efficient peristaltic contractions. Thus, the diminished capacity for urine transport observed in hypoperistaltic segments

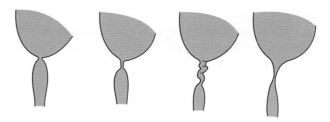

Figure 20.4 Ureteropelvic junction obstruction, secondary to stenosis: simple, segmented, serpiginous, and shelving. (Courtesy of Dr F. Douglas Stephens.)

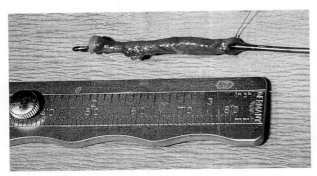

Figure 20.5 Gross specimen: hypoperistaltic/stenotic ureteropelvic junction (marked with suture) and proximal ureter excised from a 3-month-old male infant with severe left hydronephrosis. This long obstructive segment (3.5 cm) was associated with a left differential renal function of 30% and a non-declining curve on lasix nuclear renogram. As is typically encountered, however, the obstructive ureteral segment is patent to probing by a lacrimal probe.

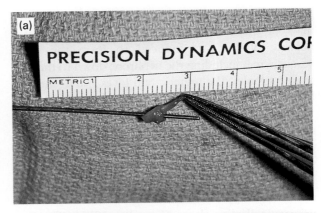

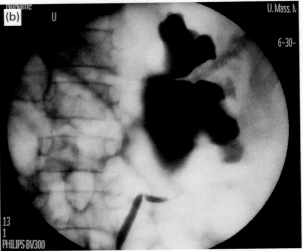

Figure 20.6 A 6-year-old boy presenting with severe intermittent left flank pain, nausea, and vomiting, compatible with recurrent Dietl's crises. (*a*) At the time of pyeloplasty, the excised ureteropelvic junction was seen to contain a 7-mm-long ureteral polyp (held up by foceps) responsible for the intermittent obstruction experienced by the patient. (*b*) A subtle persistent filling defect between the renal pelvis and proximal ureter can be seen on left retrograde pyelography, corresponding to the location of the ureteral polyp.

is likely to be due to the combined effects of diminished luminal size and tortuosity, as well as defects in muscle bundle activity.

Other less frequently seen causes of pyelocaliectasis intrinsic to the UPJ include valves and polyps (Fig. 20.6a, b) located at the proximal ureter or UPJ.

Crossing segmental renal vessels are a relatively common cause of extrinsic compression of the UPJ leading to pyelocaliectasis (Figs. 20.7–20.9a, b), but are less common in neonates who come to require surgery for the correction of UPJ obstruction. At the time of surgical repair, these vessels can be seen to cause a kink in the course of the UPJ and proximal ureter. However, histologic examination often shows features of intrinsic hypoperistaltic segments, including narrow caliber and muscle bundle derangements. It remains unclear whether the compressive force of the vessel induces these intrinsic abnormalities (Allen, 1970), or whether the intrinsic abnormalities and resultant pyelocaliectasis accentuate the appearance of the UPJ kinking around the crossing vessel. From a practical point of view, the surgical correction of UPJ obstruction secondary to a crossing vessel should include both the correction of the ureteral narrowing and the transposition of the UPJ to the side opposite the crossing vessels.

Renal calculi constitute the most common intraluminal foreign bodies causing obstruction at the UPJ. When associated with pre-existing hydronephrosis, such calculi may be secondary to urinary stasis.

Blood clots and debris from infection such as fungal balls can also result in acute obstruction of the UPJ. The etiologies are readily distinguishable from congenital UPJ obstructions by their clinical manifestations and their appearance on imaging studies (Fig. 20.10a, b).

Clinical presentation

UPJ obstruction is always associated with pyelocaliectasis, and such dilatation may persist after the

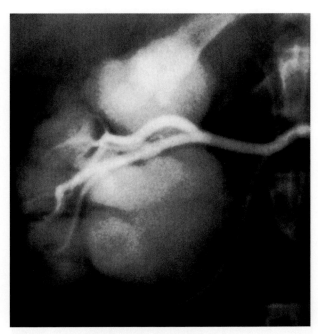

Figure 20.7 Arteriogram revealing aberrant crossing vessel causing ureteropelvic junction obstruction. (Courtesy of Dr E. Everett Anderson.)

obstruction resolves. Dilatation is present in approximately 1 in 1500 newborns. There is a slight male preponderance of approximately 65%. Of the unilateral cases, there is a slightly higher incidence on the left than the right side, with a ratio of 3:2. Kidneys are affected bilaterally in 5–15% of cases. When UPJ obstruction is found in kidneys with duplex collecting systems, the lower moiety is almost always the segment affected, although occasional upper pole obstructions have been reported.

The clinical presentation of UPJ obstruction has changed dramatically since prenatal sonographic screening became widespread. Before the 1980s, UPJ obstructions were detected primarily as a result of clinical signs and symptoms. Presentations included abdominal pain, often associated with vomiting, hematuria with or without relatively minor trauma, urinary tract infection (UTI), abdominal mass (see Fig. 20.13a), and the presence of urinary calculi (see Fig. 20.10a, b). About one-half of the abdominal masses detected in infancy were renal in origin with 40% of these secondary to UPJ obstruction (as quoted by Hashma and King, 1992). In infants under 1 year of age, UTI was the single most common presenting symptom (Johnston *et al.*, 1977), in this large series collected prior to the ultrasonography era.

Other symptoms include failure to thrive, anemia in bilateral cases, sudden-onset of hypertension (Munoz *et al.*, 1977; Grossman *et al.*, 1981), and urinary extravasation (Levitt and Lukzker, 1976). Incidental identification of asymptomatic hydronephrosis on imaging studies performed for other unrelated conditions was uncommon.

Since the 1980s, the widespread use of prenatal sonography has led to the detection of a large number of asymptomatic hydronephrotic kidneys, occurring in approximately 1 in 800 pregnancies. Of these kidneys, approximately one-half are secondary to some degree of UPJ obstruction persisting after birth. In contrast to the pre-1980s era, the majority of hydronephrotic kidneys diagnosed are now asymptomatic. This dramatic switch from predominantly symptomatic to

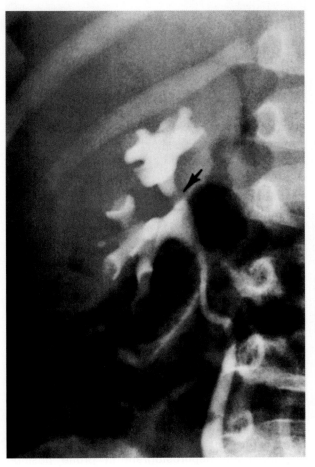

Figure 20.8 Hydrocalycosis resulting from vascular compression in an asymptomatic 2-year-old boy whose bladder was ruptured in a car accident. Excretory urogram shows dilatation of the right upper pole calyx and infundibular compression by renal vessels (*arrow*).

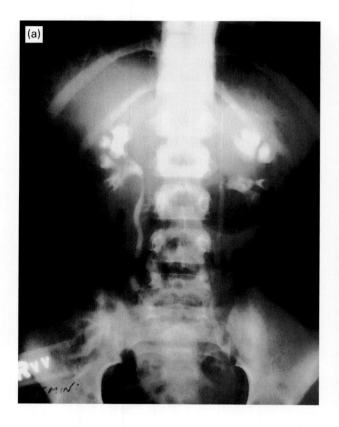

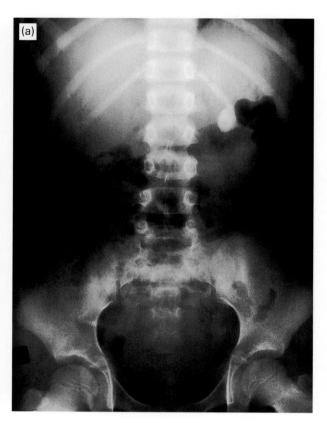

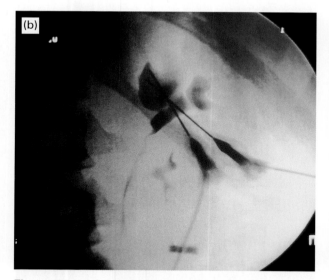

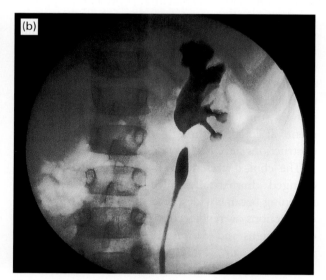

Figure 20.9 (*a*) Intravenous pyelogram showing left upper pole caliectasis in a 3-year-old girl, compatible with obstruction caused by a crossing renal vessel. (*b*) Antegrade nephrostogram in prone position (obtained during a percutaneous pressure–flow study which was positive for significant obstruction) demonstrating a normal left non-dilated collecting system distal to the point of compression by the crossing renal vessel. These observations were subsequently confirmed by intraoperative findings.

Figure 20.10 A 6-year-old girl presenting with microscopic hematuria was found to have a large left renal calculus. (*a*) Kidney, bladder, ureter (KUB) scout film demonstrating radio-opaque left renal calculus. (*b*) Left retrograde pyelogram showing distinct ureteropelvic junction stenotic/hypoperistaltic segment and postobstructive dilatation in the ureter just beyond the obstructive segment. This patient underwent uncomplicated simultaneous open left pyelolithotomy and pyeloplasty.

predominantly asymptomatic presentations has led to heated debates as to which, if any, of these hydronephrotic kidneys require surgical treatment. While clinicians can readily agree upon the need for surgical treatment in the symptomatic patients, the controversy over how to identify asymptomatic kidneys that require surgical treatment remains unresolved and is the focus of this chapter.

While most hydronephrotic kidneys in the young are discovered by sonographic screening, UPJ obstruction in older children and adolescents continues to present symptomatically. Hematuria from minor trauma remains the most common presenting sign in older children. Evaluation of the child with UTI occasionally results in the discovery of an obstructed kidney. Not infrequently, children present with episodic abdominal pain associated with vomiting occurring later in the day or evening. This is the result of intermittent obstruction brought on by a high fluid load. Vomiting is not only a manifestation of the acute renal distension, but also serves to correct the acute obstruction by creating a degree of dehydration that in turn leads to resorption of the intrarenal fluid and decompression of the dilated system. This phenomenon of severe attacks of flank pain, nausea, and vomiting, and even general collapse was described by Dietl and is referred to as Dietl's crisis. It was initially said to be due to partial turning of the kidney upon its pedicle. However, it has now been demonstrated to be secondary to an acute increase in urine output distending the renal pelvis. This in turn kinks the UPJ and worsen the severity of obstruction (Belman, 1991) (see Fig. 20.36a–c), producing a vicious cycle of increasingly severe obstruction.

UPJ obstruction is also often associated with other congenital anomalies, including imperforate anus, contralateral multicystic kidney, congenital heart disease, VATER (vertebral defects, imperforate anus, tracheo-esophageal fistula, and radial and renal dysplasia) syndrome, and esophageal atresia. In patients with these anomalies, screening sonography should be obtained to assess for possible associated urologic anomalies.

Pathophysiology

A clear understanding of the compensatory changes in response to congenital renal obstruction is critical for the correct interpretation of diagnostic information and establishing a sound management plan. While the majority of experimental work on obstruction of the urinary tract has focused on acute obstruction in mature adult animal models, it is now increasingly apparent that congenital hydronephrosis behaves very differently from obstruction in the adult kidneys. First of all, the physiologic profile of congenital hydronephrosis lacks the dramatic swings in renal blood flow, glomerular filtration rate (GFR), and renal pelvic pressure seen in acute obstruction. These parameters can be practically indistinguishable from those of a normal kidney. Secondly, congenital hydronephrosis may have a profound influence on the development of the fetal and infant kidney. Thirdly, unilateral congenital hydronephrosis may exert developmental influence on the contralateral normal kidney.

Renal blood flow, glomerular filtration rate, and renal pelvic pressure

Acute ureteral obstruction has been demonstrated to have a classical triphasic response in renal blood flow and renal pelvic pressure (Moody *et al.*, 1975) (Fig. 20.11). The first phase immediately following acute ureteral obstruction is characterized by an increase in both renal blood flow and renal pelvic pressure lasting for 1–1.5 hours. The second phase then consists of a decrease in renal blood flow, but a continuing rise in renal pelvic pressure up to about 5 hours. During the third phase renal blood flow continues to decrease and renal pelvic pressure then also progressively declines. Thereafter, in subacute and chronic ureteral obstruction, renal blood flow remains decreased and renal pelvic pressure progressively declines back to normal levels. GFR alterations essentially mirror the changes in renal blood flow.

In the extensive experimental literature studying acute renal obstruction, elevation in renal pelvic pressure has uniformly been found to occur first. Changes in renal blood flow and GFR follow. Thus, it appears that elevation in renal pelvic pressure constitutes the initial physical stimulus that triggers the subsequent responses to renal obstruction.

Following an increase in renal pelvic pressure, many of the subsequent alterations observed in acute renal obstruction are attributable to changes in afferent and efferent arteriolar tone. These were initially ascribed to local physical interactions, but have subsequently been shown to be secondary to a whole host of biochemical mediators. A comprehensive review was given by Gulmi *et al.* (1998) of the many molecular mediators

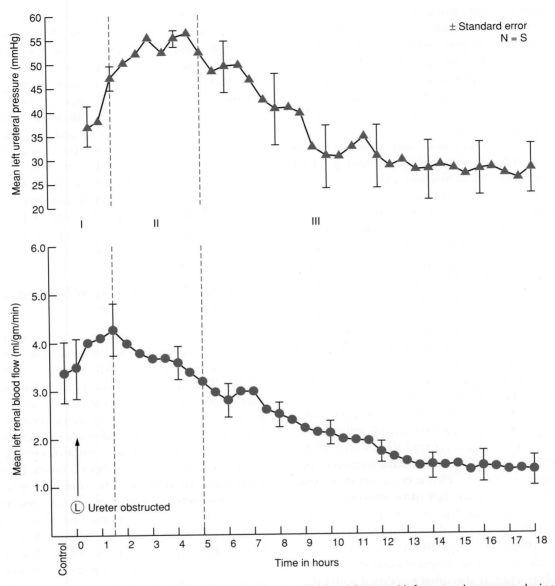

Figure 20.11 The triphasic relationship between ipsilateral renal blood flow and left ureteral pressure during 18 h of left-sided occlusion. The three phases are designated by Roman numerals and divided by vertical dashed lines. In phase I, renal blood flow and ureteral pressure rise together. In phase II, the left renal blood flow begins to decline, whereas ureteral pressure remains elevated and, in fact, continues to rise. Phase III shows the left-sided renal blood flow and ureteral pressure declining together. (Adapted from Moody *et al.*, 1975, with permission.)

implicated, including the arachidonic acid metabolites (eicosanoids), cyclooxygenase pathway metabolites (prostaglandins or prostanoids), the renin–angiotensin system, atrial natriuretic peptide, nitric oxide, endothelin, platelet-activating factor, clusterin, and transforming growth factor-β (TGF-β). The kidney first undergoes preglomerular vasodilation, then postglomerular vasoconstriction, and finally preglomerular vasoconstriction (Gulmi *et al.*, 1998).

As the kidney passes from acute obstruction to the chronic phase, preglomerular vasoconstriction persists along with the attendant decrease in renal blood flow. This decrease in blood flow results in a sustained decrease in GFR. The combination of these events in turn leads to a reduction in the initially elevated renal pelvic pressure, which returns to the normal range. An exception is seen in acute, bilateral complete ureteral obstruction, where the preglomerular vascular tone is in a persistently dilated state, contrary to the preglomerular vasoconstriction seen in unilateral obstruction (Gulmi *et al.*, 1998). As a result, renal pelvic pressure remains elevated in bilateral, acute obstruction during time frames when a reduction would already have been seen in unilateral obstruction (Gulmi *et al.*, 1995). This phenomenon is not fully understood, but is of little relevance to the present discussion, since acute complete bilateral renal obstruction is rarely encountered as part of the usual clinical spectrum of pediatric hydronephrosis.

In analysing the relationship among the various physiologic changes in acute renal obstruction, elevation in renal pelvic pressure appears to be the initial physical stimulus that triggers the compensatory cascade. Changes in renal blood flow then act as the key effector mechanism for subsequent compensatory changes, leading to secondary changes in GFR. These compensatory changes then come full circle, where alterations in renal blood flow and GFR have a direct effect on renal pelvic pressure. By the time renal blood flow and GFR have declined sufficiently for renal pelvic pressure to return to the normal range, the initial alterations triggered by the elevation in renal pelvic pressure abate, and the compensatory changes establish a new equilibrium. While the evidence supporting this sequence of events is derived primarily from experimental models of acute renal obstruction, it appears that these events are expressed, at least in part, in congenital hydronephrosis.

Unlike acute renal obstruction, in congenital hydronephrosis renal pelvic pressures are normal at baseline hydration levels (Fung *et al.*, 1995b) (see Fig. 20.31). Because of the complex interaction between stimuli for renal growth and effects on renal injury, kidneys with congenital hydronephrosis can be seen to have normal, decreased, or even increased renal blood flow (Steckler *et al.*, 1994; Fung *et al.*, 1995d). Thus, a congenitally hydronephrotic kidney with a significant impediment to urine flow can maintain physiologic parameters difficult to distinguish from the normal kidney at baseline conditions. In order to develop strategies effective in accurately detecting those hydronephrotic kidneys that have physiologically significant obstruction, it is important to identify pathophysiologic features to distinguish between significant obstruction and normal function.

The mode of renal injury in obstructed kidneys may provide an important clue for formulating effective diagnostic strategies. While there is evidence that persistently elevated renal pelvic pressure is linked to irreversible renal injury (Fung and Atala, 1996; Fung *et al.*, 1996; Fung and Atala, 1998), there is no conclusive evidence that it is the pressure effect itself that is harmful to the renal cellular elements. However, decreased renal blood flow as part of the compensatory response has been shown to be associated with an upregulation in vascular endothelial growth factor (VEGF), a molecular marker for physiologically significant ischemia at the cellular level (Fung *et al.*, 1996). Thus, the mode of injury for the obstructed kidney appears not to be from the direct pressure effects, but is instead ischemic in nature, resulting from the compensatory response in renal blood flow reduction. From a teleologic point of view, it is unclear what protective advantage is provided to someone with an obstructed kidney by these events. It nevertheless appears that these compensatory responses remain activated until renal pelvic pressure is brought back to normal, even if this is brought about at the expense of decreased renal blood flow, decreased GFR, and even renal cellular ischemia.

Although there is little information as to exactly how the congenitally hydronephrotic kidney consistently maintains normal renal pelvic pressure at baseline hydration, it seems reasonable to presume that the response of a congenitally hydronephrotic kidney to obstruction shares features in common with the acute obstruction models. It would logically follow from this presumption that renal pelvic pressure remains normal in congenitally hydronephrotic kidneys, not so much because the two are unrelated, but because the normal renal pelvic pressure is maintained at the expense of compensatory changes in renal blood flow and GFR, similar to changes noted in the late acute obstruction models. This postulate is supported by the changes in renal pelvic pressure observed in congenitally hydronephrotic kidneys in response to diuresis, compared with normal kidneys.

In a pig model, we have found it to be practically impossible to induce an elevation in renal pelvic pressure in normal collecting systems by instituting a forced diuresis; however, in children with congenital hydronephrosis renal pelvic pressure has been recorded to rise from the normal of less than 10 cmH$_2$O to as high as 63 cmH$_2$O following a furosemide-induced diuresis (Fung *et al.*, 1995c) (see Fig. 20.31). This pattern was similarly observed when rats with congenital hydronephrosis were compared with normal controls (Fichtner *et al.*, 1994). Thus, it appears that renal pelvic pressure is normal in a non-hydronephrotic kidney because the normal collecting system has a huge reserve capacity for handling additional urine flow. In contrast, congenitally hydronephrotic kidneys with significant obstruction are able to maintain normal renal pelvic pressure because they have undergone compensatory changes in renal blood flow and GFR to achieve a new equilibrium. However, there is little or no reserve for handling a diuresis.

This line of reasoning forms the pathophysiologic basis for the diuresis pressure–flow study (described under the Diagnosis section), whereby significantly obstructed kidneys are distinguished from non-obstructed kidneys by their pelvic pressure response to diuresis. Non-obstructed kidneys maintain normal renal pelvic pressures following the induction of diuresis. In contrast, diuresis jolts the obstructed kidney from its compensated state of equilibrium and its initially compensated normal renal pelvic pressure becomes elevated following diuresis.

Developmental influence on the fetal kidney

The degree to which a fetal kidney develops under the influence of obstruction appears to depend on the timing of the onset of obstruction and its degree. While later onset and incomplete obstruction *in utero* lead to hydronephrosis with a varying degree of functional renal impairment, early and complete obstruction results in irreversible renal dysplasia with no functional potential (Glick *et al.*, 1983; 1985). In the spectrum between normal and obvious hydronephrosis, there are also instances when the dilatation can be considered transient or physiological. This may occur as the bladder fills during the increased diuresis of the third trimester. No lasting effects on these kidneys are observed postnatally (Grignon *et al.*, 1986).

It has long been recognized that congenital hydronephrosis represents a spectrum of conditions and severity with the functional potential of the hydronephrotic kidney ranging from complete non-function, as in the case of dysplasia, to entirely normal renal function. More recently, however, the possibility has been raised that congenital hydronephrosis may result in a kidney which functions at a level in excess of normal (Steckler *et al.*, 1994). This phenomenon is termed supranormal differential renal function.

Several clinical series subsequently evaluated the phenomenon of supranormal differential renal function. Fung *et al.* (1995d) studied 16 patients who had a differential renal function of 53% or higher in the unilateral hydronephrotic kidney. While the supranormal differential renal function phenomenon appeared convincing based on the findings of diethylenetriaminepentaacetic acid (DTPA) nuclear renography (mean 58.3%, range 53–66%), the differential renal function observed was less dramatic when these same patients were evaluated using dimercaptosuccinic acid (DMSA) nuclear renography (mean 51.1%, range 42–57%). The results from the DMSA renal scans were not significantly different from the intuitively expected normal differential function of 50%. It was thus concluded that the phenomenon of supranormal differential function appeared to be an artifact specific to DTPA nuclear renal scans, presumably secondary to the presence of background activity preventing an accurate assessment or determination of renal function after isotope had reached the collecting system. These confounding variables would not apply to DMSA renal scans, as delayed images are used for calculating differential renal function, by which time the activity in the dilated collecting system would already have cleared.

Contrary to these findings, Capolicchio *et al.* (1999a) subsequently reported a similar study on 15 patients, defining supranormal differential renal function as greater than 55% of the total. The mean differential renal function on these 15 patients was 55 ± 4% based on DTPA renal scan (range 46–61%) and 55 ± 3% based on DMSA renal scan (range 51–62%). It was concluded in this series that there was no significant difference between the differential renal function assessments performed by DTPA and DMSA renal scans, and that supranormal differential renal function was a real phenomenon.

Kim *et al.* (1999) similarly concluded that supranormal renal function was real. Fourteen patients had differential renal function assessments by DTPA renal scans, and were further assessed by split urinary collection and split creatinine clearance measurements. Supranormal differential renal function was confirmed by split creatinine clearance in two patients, and was shown to be a spurious finding in one. DTPA renal scans had a tendency to overestimate differential renal function in the dilated kidney compared with split creatinine clearance, especially in those kidneys with a significantly reduced renal function.

From these clinical series, it appears that supranormal differential renal function is probably a real but rare phenomenon in unilateral hydronephrosis. It also seems that DTPA renal scans have a tendency to over-estimate differential renal function compared with DMSA renal scans or split urinary creatinine clearances.

Experimental work in fetal sheep by Peters *et al.* (1992b) and Fung and Peters (1995) provides further evidence to support the validity of supranormal differential renal function in unilateral hydronephrosis. Partial unilateral ureteral obstruction of normal fetal kidneys was seen to produce hydronephrotic kidneys of greater weight than the contralateral normal mate or age-matched controls. DNA, RNA, and protein contents were analysed, in order to distinguish hyperplasia from hypertrophy. An increase in DNA content signifies a hyperplastic response, where the net number of cells present was increased. An increase in the ratio of RNA:DNA or protein:DNA signifies that the cells hypertrophied. In these unilaterally partially obstructed fetal sheep kidneys, the increase in weight was secondary to hyperplasia, and there was no evidence of hypertrophy. These findings are in keeping with the concept of supranormal differential renal function being the result of a true increase in size and functional capacity of congenital hydronephrotic kidneys. In the fetus, increased blood flow to the kidneys results as a response to partial obstruction, a difference that supports hyperplasia *in utero*. However, supranormal renal development was seen only in relatively mild, partial, unilateral ureteral obstruction (Fung and Peters, 1995). In more severe obstruction, the hydronephrotic kidneys were observed to have a significantly decreased renal weight and function (Peters *et al.*, 1992a, b).

In the assessment of postnatal differential renal function, it is important for the clinician to be aware that the baseline differential renal function for the hydronephrotic kidney in question may not be the intuitively expected 50%. However, this finding can be the result of poorly done diuretic renography. Guidelines for surgical correction should not be based on an arbitrary threshold, such as when differential renal function is below 40%. Instead, a baseline differential function assessment should be acquired early in the postnatal period, and management should be based on the results of serial repeated evaluations when the diagnosis is equivocal.

Developmental influence on the contralateral normal kidney

Experimental work performed in fetal sheep provides insight into the response of the fetal kidney to obstruction. Unilateral obstruction not only affects the obstructed fetal kidney in unexpected ways, but also has a significant influence on the developmental pattern of the contralateral normal mate (Peters *et al.*, 1992a, b; Fung and Peters, 1995). When the function of the obstructed kidney is significantly impaired, the contralateral kidney becomes larger *in utero* by a combination of hyperplasia and hypertrophy. In contrast, when the partially obstructed kidney has become enlarged by hyperplasia and is supranormal in function, there is evidence that the contralateral normal kidney undergoes an increased rate of cellular deletion by apoptosis, resulting in a net hypoplastic response (Fung and Peters, 1995). Such a hypoplastic response may in turn result in a kidney that has less function than it would otherwise have.

Thus, the identification of a unilateral congenitally hydronephrotic kidney in an infant has prognostic implications different from those in adults. If the hydronephrotic kidney functioned poorly *in utero*, the contralateral normal kidney may have a higher functional potential due to a response which is at least in part hyperplastic in nature. However, if the hydronephrotic kidney is hyperplastic with a degree of supranormal function, the contralateral normal kidney may have a function below the expected 50% level. The burden is thus placed on the clinician to accurately identify and give due consideration to these developmental patterns, so that clinical tests and differential renal function results can be evaluated appropriately and management plans formulated accordingly. It may be difficult to regard a hyperfunctioning kidney as being significantly obstructed, but such a kidney may carry the potential for functional deterioration nonetheless.

Natural history

Based on the preceding discussion, significant obstruction can be defined as an impediment in urine transport resulting in compensatory changes in physiologic renal parameters, including renal pelvic pressure, renal blood flow, and GFR. While such a degree of obstruction is significant in the sense that it is sufficiently severe to produce demonstrable physiological alterations, the question is, what adverse sequelae may follow if the condition remains uncorrected? If surgical correction is necessary, what is the optimal time for performing surgical repair? These questions will be explored in this section by evaluating available information on the natural history of congenital hydronephrosis.

Outcome of unilateral hydronephrosis treated by an observational approach

Before the 1980s, hydronephrosis resulting from UPJ obstruction was evaluated by excretory urography (IVP), unstandardized diuretic renography and the infusion pressure–flow studies (Snyder *et al.*, 1980). Indications for surgical correction were often clearcut and were performed for the amelioration of symptoms. As a result of screening prenatal ultrasonography, the diagnosis of hydronephrosis has increased exponentially. An estimated 1 in 100 pregnancies exhibits at least transient urinary tract dilatation, with approximately 50% above the UPJ (Thomas, 1990) (Fig. 20.12). About one-half of prenatally diagnosed hydronephrosis persists postnatally (Grignon *et al.*, 1986; Mandell *et al.*, 1991). Faced with a large number of infants with asymptomatic hydronephrosis, debate has ensued as to which of these kidneys require surgical correction.

This ability to diagnose hydronephrosis prenatally was initially considered to be an opportunity to detect and correct a congenital abnormality before irreversible renal injury occurred and has led to a marked increase in the number of surgical procedures performed. However, it has became apparent that not all of these congenitally hydronephrotic kidneys develop progressive renal injury if left untreated. A significant number remains functionally stable and drainage has been noted to improve over time in some. This observation prompted several centers to adopt an observational approach to congenital hydronephrosis secondary to UPJ obstruction, where patients were closely monitored, and surgical repair was considered only if unequivocal obstruction or deterioration in renal function occurred (Bernstein *et al.*, 1988; Dejter *et al.*, 1988; Ransley *et al.*, 1990; Koff and Campbell, 1992). The initial concept of observational management was promoted by the notion that the risk of developing significant functional deterioration was relatively low in unilateral hydronephrosis (Koff and Campbell, 1994; Dhillon, 1998).

Koff *et al.* studied a group of 104 patients with a mean follow-up of 21 months. Of the 88 unilateral hydronephrotic kidneys which had initial differential renal function of <40%, six required pyeloplasty after a >10% reduction in renal function, as measured by an estimated GFR derived from DTPA diuretic renography (Shore *et al.*, 1984). The other 16 kidneys with severe unilateral hydronephrosis [grade 4 by Society of Fetal Urology (SFU) classification] all had an obstructive washout pattern on renography and an initial differential renal function of > 40%. Notably, only one kidney required pyeloplasty for worsening function, and all of the other 15 kidneys improved without intervention. Several of Koff's patients were operated upon by others but it is not known whether these kidneys had deteriorated. No compensatory renal hypertrophy was observed in contralateral normal kidneys in the 15 reported patients, providing additional evidence that these unilateral hydronephrotic kidneys were indeed satisfactory in function. In other words, in adhering to the criterion that surgical repair is performed only when differential renal function declined by >10%, six of 88 (6.8%) kidneys with good function initially (≥ 40% differential function) required surgical correction, but only one out of 16 (6.3%) kidneys with poor function (<40% differential function) came to surgery. Thus, in this series only approximately 7% of hydronephrotic kidneys required surgical correction when monitored by an observational approach, regardless of the initial differential renal function status.

The first series to evaluate a non-surgical approach to congenital UPJ obstruction was reported by Ransley *et al.* (1990). This study evaluated 148 hydronephrotic kidneys, with patients accrued between 1980 and 1988. These patients were followed for 5–16 years with serial ultrasonography and DTPA nuclear renal scans. Patients were stratified by poor, moderate, or good differential renal function. In the group of patients with poor ipsilateral renal function (<20%), all ten of the patients received

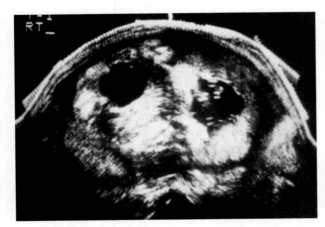

Figure 20.12 Maternal ultrasonogram. Bilateral hydronephrosis secondary to bilateral ureteropelvic junction obstruction.

immediate treatment (seven nephrectomies and three pyeloplasties). In the group with moderately well-preserved ipsilateral renal function (20–39%), there were 28 kidneys in total, of which five remained stable or improved over 5 years without intervention. The remaining 23 kidneys received surgical repair, with 12 improving to good function postoperatively and the other 11 remaining stable without any noticeable improvement when compared with their preoperative functional status. In the last group of 110 unilateral hydronephrotic kidneys considered to have good differential renal function (>40%), six received early pyeloplasty, while 27 others eventually had surgical correction for various indications including worsening function (14), UTI (4), pain (4), social reasons (4), and concentrating defect (1). Surgery was performed within the first 3 years of follow-up in 22 of these 27 kidneys but as late as the age of 9 years in the remainder. In this series, kidneys with poor function received immediate treatment, whereas kidneys with moderate to good renal function were monitored for functional deterioration or symptoms. Of the kidneys treated with an observational approach, 23 out of 28 kidneys (82%) required surgical correction in the group with moderate differential renal function (20–39%), whereas 27 out of 104 kidneys (26%) with good differential function (40%) required surgical correction. These results differ from the series by Koff in that a much higher proportion (25–82%) of hydronephrotic kidneys required surgical correction on the grounds of functional deterioration or symptoms, and the kidneys that functioned relatively poorly to begin with had a higher probability of further functional deterioration, ultimately requiring surgical intervention.

In a third series, unilateral hydronephrotic kidneys were randomized to observation versus surgical repair. This multicenter clinical trial was conducted prospectively by the SFU, studying a total of 32 infants from ten centers (Palmer et al., 1998). Patients studied were all 6 months of age or younger, with unilateral hydronephrosis of grade 3 by SFU classification, and the hydronephrotic kidneys had ≥ 40% differential renal function on standardized nuclear renography (well-tempered renography) (SFU, 1992; Conway, 1992). Once patients were randomized, those in the surgical repair group proceeded to pyeloplasty, whereas the observation group was closely monitored for deterioration. Criteria for the patients in the observation group to require sur-

gery included worsening of isotope washout on well-tempered renogram, increasing grade of hydronephrosis, or >10% loss in differential renal function. Only 19 out of 32 patients were evaluable at 3 years. Of the patients who were initially randomized to the observation arm, four of 16 (25%) came to pyeloplasty. Afterwards, two of these had further loss of renal function. In the surgical repair group, pyeloplasty was found to be effective in improving the anatomic appearance of the hydronephrotic kidneys and in stabilizing differential renal function. During the observation period, however, deterioration in renal function was noted in 25%. It was concluded in this study that for children 6 months old or less, with unilateral hydronephrosis and good function at the time of diagnosis, pyeloplasty provided a superior outcome to observation with regard to preservation of renal function. However, as a group the observational approach spared 12 out of 16 children the need for surgical repair, at least for the duration of the study.

Peters et al. (1987) offered randomization to the parents of 67 babies with severe unilateral hydronephrosis, or allowed the parents to decide what the initial therapy should be. Only five chose randomization; 34 opted for early surgery before 4 months of age, and 28 for observation. Fifty-two were available for a mean follow-up of 2 years (Peters et al., 1987). Resolution of hydronephrosis was seen in only two of 24 in the observation group, and three of this group came to pyeloplasty because of deterioration in renal function. In addition, seven of these elected later surgery to resolve the problem and make follow-up easier. In the surgical group, drainage on the renogram curve was always improved, but three of 28 also had >10% decrease in kidney function.

Summarizing the results from these clinical series in the outcome of unilateral hydronephrotic kidneys monitored by an observational approach, roughly 23% (64/276) of the kidneys monitored were ultimately corrected surgically. Criteria included functional deterioration, evidence for worsening degree of obstruction, or development of symptomatic difficulties. The remainder (approximately 212/276; 77%) continued to have preservation of renal function for the duration of the studies.

While these data represent some of the most comprehensive information available on the natural history of congenital hydronephrosis, they should be interpreted with caution. The numbers are relatively small and the length of follow-up is limited. It is unclear whether more of the patients with ongoing observation will ultimately deteriorate and require surgical intervention, or develop unanticipated adverse long-term sequelae. Furthermore, to conclude that a hydronephrotic kidney does not require surgery because its function has remained stable is somewhat of an oversimplification. Such an approach has not taken into account that those kidneys with reduced function may have potential for improvement after timely surgical intervention.

Optimal timing for surgical intervention

Although there may be a slightly higher risk associated with neonatal surgery compared with surgery performed beyond 6 months of age, numerous reports have attested to the safety of corrective surgery and pediatric anesthesia in the neonate (Perlmutter et al., 1980; Roth and Gonzales, 1983; King et al., 1984b) (Table 20.1). Thus, if neonatal pyeloplasty is deemed necessary, it can be safely carried out by an appropriately equipped pediatric urologic and anesthesia team with a high rate of success.

It is a generally accepted biologic principle that young and developing organs have a higher potential for recovery and regeneration than those of mature adults. In keeping with this principle, one may assume that kidneys that undergo surgical correction may experience a greater degree of improvement in function postoperatively as compared with those corrected after longstanding obstruction. McCrory et al. (1971) were among the first authors to study systematically obstructive uropathies in infants and children from a physiologic point of view. Included were those with bilateral UPJ obstruction and UVJ obstruction, neuropathic bladders secondary to myelomeningocele, posterior urethral valves (PUV), and 'bladder outlet obstruction without anatomically evident lesions at the bladder outlet' associated with low-pressure reflux. Patients were monitored with serial determinations of GFR, as well as renal concentrating ability and acidification capacity. It was concluded that reduced renal function had the capability to return to more normal levels only in infants younger than 6 months of age at the time obstruction was corrected. This study provided the initial evidence that the younger the infant or child at the time of surgical correction of significant renal obstruction, the higher the potential for subsequent improvement in renal function and capacity for renal growth.

Mayor et al. (1975) provided further insight into the relationship between age at the time of treatment and ultimate renal function by studying serial renal function in 24 patients. Pimary diagnoses in these patients were mixed, with either bladder outlet obstruction affecting both kidneys, or high-grade obstruction and/or VUR affecting a solitary kidney. A dramatic pattern emerged. When a patient underwent relief of obstruction before 1 year of age, subsequent GFR increased into the normal range or at least improved as the child grew. When the relief of obstruction took place between 1 and 2 years of age, stable renal function was observed without significant worsening in azotemia, and the kidneys grew in parallel with the child's general growth. If the relief of obstruction took place after the age of 2 years, however, the potential for renal function improvement or renal growth was limited. Successful surgical correction of obstruction stabilized renal function temporarily, but as the child grew, the kidneys were unable to grow and compensate in parallel. These children experienced increasing azotemia, and generally progressed into renal failure as their general growth outstripped the limited capacity of their kidneys to compensate in function. However, since this group did not constitute only patients with pure obstruction, and the clinical history regarding the

Table 20.1 Results of pyeloplasty in early infancy (younger than 3 months of age)

Series	No. of pyeloplasties	Results
King (1988)	24	No re-operation
Flake et al. (1986)	22	All successful
Thorup et al. (1985)	9	Two re-operations, one worse
Hanna and Gluck (1988)	34	No re-operation
Koyle and Ehrlilich (1988)	20	All improved or stable

effects of UTI must also be considered, the significance of this report can be questioned.

The findings by King *et al.* (1984b) in a group of 25 patients were consistent with this emerging trend. Unlike the studies by McCrory *et al.* and Mayor *et al.*, this was a pure group with congenital UPJ obstruction followed after surgical repair. Of the 25 patients, pyeloplasty was carried out between the ages of 1 week and 12.5 months in the 11 younger patients, and in the remaining 14 older patients pyeloplasty was carried out between 5 and 21 years of age. Preoperative and postoperative differential renal function as measured by DTPA renal scans were compared, with follow-up periods of 3 months to 4 years. In the younger group of 11 infants, postoperative improvement in differential renal function ranged from 33 to 625%, with a mean of 154% overall improvement. Notably, a 3-month-old with 5% and a 6-month-old with 4% differential renal function improved to 34 and 29% differential function 3 months postoperatively, respectively, probably enough function to sustain life in the event that the contralateral kidney were lost (Fig. 20.13a–b). However, accurate determination of differential function in largely distended kidneys like this is difficult to determine and initial function was likely grossly underestimated. In contrast, in the group of older patients between 5 and 21 years of age, postoperative differential renal function ranged from a deterioration of 12.5% to an improvement of 45%, with a relatively modest mean overall improvement of 17.7%. The two patients who experienced further deterioration in differential renal function (10 and 12.5% deterioration) in spite of successful surgical correction of obstruction were aged 19 and 21 years, respectively, the two oldest patients in the series.

In keeping with basic biological principles, these series demonstrated that the younger the kidney at the time of relief of obstruction, the more significant the subsequent potential for recovery and growth (Fig. 20.14a–g). The potential for recovery in renal function may be a continuum, most dramatic before 12 months, becoming less noticeable by early childhood, and negligible by adulthood. The developmental physiology of the hydronephrotic kidney and the compensatory response of the contralateral normal kidney appear to provide the underlying explanations for these observations.

In considering the potential for an obstructed kidney to recover, it is important to note that the formation of nephrons is already complete at birth,

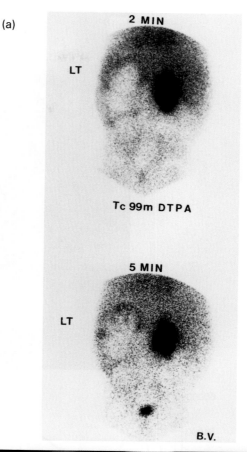

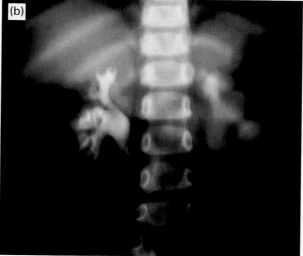

Figure 20.13 A 12.5-month-old boy presenting with a large left-sided abdominal mass. (*a*) Renal scan showing about 4% of total renal function in the obstructed left kidney. The parents, both college graduates, wanted the kidney preserved if feasible. At pyeloplasty, the pelvis held more than 900 ml (measured). The cortex over the dilated calyces was very thin. (*b*) Intravenous pyelogram 6 months after surgery, and *Continued overleaf.*

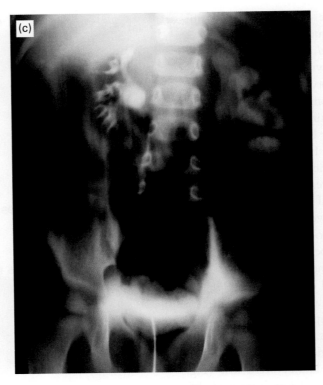

(c)

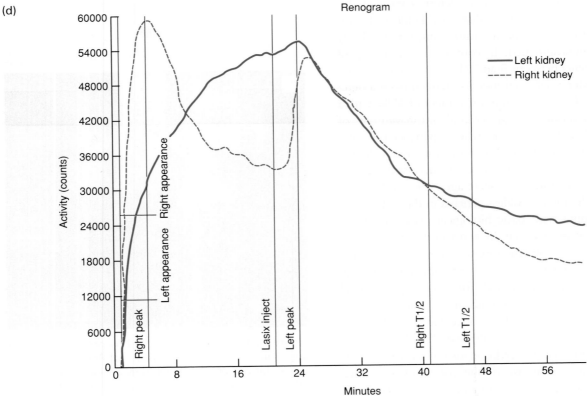

(d)

Figure 20.13 *Continued.* (*c*) 5 years later. (*d*) The renal scan then showed 37% of total renal function in the left kidney. The drainage curve was unequivocally unobstructed. Note that the Lasix was given before all the isotope had accumulated in the collecting system, causing a second peak over the right kidney and worsening the slope of the drainage curve.

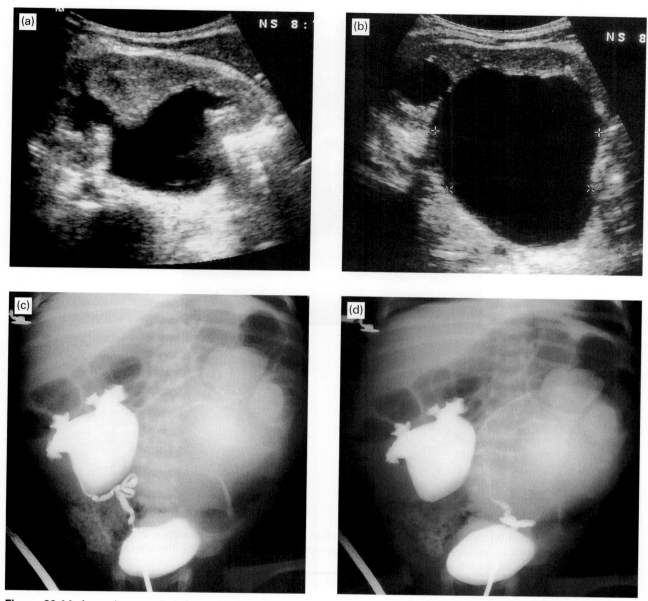

Figure 20.14 A newborn male infant with Noonan's syndrome who was found to have bilateral palpable abdominal masses and bilateral non-palpable testes. Abdominal masses were secondary to bilateral severe hydronephrosis resulting from ureteropelvic junction obstruction. Ultrasonography demonstrated moderate right (*a*) and marked left (*b*) pelvicaliectasis. Bilateral retrograde pyelograms revealed a markedly dilated right renal pelvis (*c*) and an even more massively dilated left renal pelvis (*d*), occupying the entire left flank, crossing the midline, and abutting on the right renal pelvis. At 2 months of age bilateral dismembered pyeloplasties were performed, along with bilateral orchidopexies for his intra-abdominal testes. Intravenous pyelography at 3 months postoperatively. *Continued overleaf.*

but further maturation takes place postnatally. The maturation of nephrons is the most rapid in the first few months of life, and levels off at 2 years of age (Fig. 20.30) (McCrory, 1980). Thus, those kidneys still actively in the process of maturation have the most potential for significant improvement in func-

tion following relief of obstruction, and this potential becomes more limited after the age of 2 years.

In studies on renal growth in infants and children it was found that, when a functioning kidney was removed, usually for Wilm's tumor, the eventual size of the remaining kidney was inversely proportional to

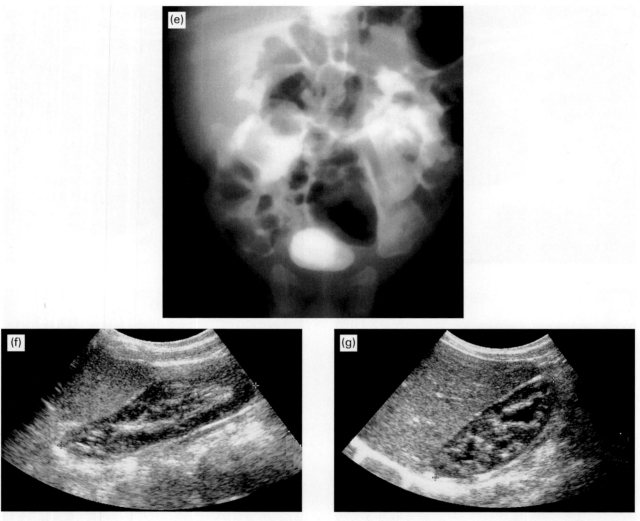

Figure 20.14 *Continued.* (*e*) demonstrated bilateral reduction in dilatation of the collecting systems, especially on the left side. At 2 years' follow-up, ultrasonography reveals complete resolution of right pelvicaliectasis (*f*), and only minimal residual caliectasis on the left (*g*).

the age at nephrectomy up to the age of 4 years (Apenia *et al.*, 1977; Laufer and Griscom, 1971). In other words, the earlier a kidney was removed, the more contralateral hypertrophy could be anticipated. A host of animal experiments in four species has demonstrated that this is so (Larsson *et al.*, 1980). Most dramatically, puppies subjected to 1½ nephrectomy at birth develop normal renal function as the remnant kidney quadruples in mass (Kaufmann *et al.*, 1975). If the 1½ nephrectomy is delayed until 8 weeks of age, the remnant kidney at most doubles in size (Aschinberg *et al.*, 1978).

Compensatory response in the contralateral normal kidney has also been shown to affect the potential for

a unilaterally obstructed kidney to improve after the relief of obstruction. It was believed that if the unilaterally hydronephrotic kidney were left untreated, the contralateral normal kidney would undergo compensatory hypertrophy, thus removing a stimulus for the obstructed kidney to grow even after the obstruction was relieved. This phenomenon was termed 'renal counterbalance' (Hinman, 1923). As there is no functional demand on the fetal kidneys *in utero*, compensatory responses should be in effect only after birth (Laufer *et al.*, 1971). However, it is incompletely understood to what degree compensatory changes may be affected by hyperplasia or hypertrophy *in utero*. It is well established that nephrogenesis takes place between 6 and 36 weeks of gestation and the human kidney can only compensate by maturation and/or hypertrophy beyond this period.

Renal hypertrophy in the contralateral normal kidney occurs rapidly after birth, and is detectable sonographically by an increase in renal size as early as 9 days after birth in babies with unilateral cystic dysplastic kidneys (Chevalier *et al.*, 1984). The process is about half-way to being complete by 4 months, and is complete by about 1 year of age (Laufer *et al.*, 1971). While the relatively limited capacity for renal functional recovery observed in older patients is likely to be multifactorial in nature, it appears that it is due in part to the limitations imposed by the hypertrophy of the contralateral normal kidney. This provides additional support for the concept that recovery of renal function can be maximized by relieving obstruction before compensatory hypertrophy is complete in the contralateral kidney (Dicker and Shirley, 1973; Shirley, 1976).

However, other reports do not support this concept. In a series by MacNeily *et al.* (1993), the authors concluded that no significant recovery in differential renal function was observed postoperatively in the patients studied as a group. Salem *et al.* (1995) compared renal function as determined by nuclear scintigraphy before and after surgical correction of obstruction, and observed only a modest degree of recovery in differential renal function. McAleer and Kaplan (1999) came to a similar conclusion from their patients. There was no statistically significant improvement in differential renal function following pyeloplasty for UPJ obstruction. While the differences were not statistically significant, examination of their raw data presented in a graph format indicated that approximately 26 of 58 patients (45%) in the series had an increased differential renal function postoperatively. Improvements observed ranged from only a few per cent to almost 30% in absolute differential renal function, including one kidney improving from a differential renal function in the low 20s to normal at 49% postoperatively. Thus, this patient group examined as a whole may not show uniformly improved differential renal function postoperatively, but these data indicate that a varying degree of improvement in renal function is certainly possible in a sizeable subgroup of patients.

In a series of 89 patients, Capolicchio *et al.* (1999b) observed a limited degree of improvement in overall differential renal function following surgical correction of UPJ obstruction, but the difference was more marked in the subgroup who had differential renal function of <40% preoperatively, as one would intuitively expect. In this series, children diagnosed as having hydronephrosis prenatally who underwent early pyeloplasty had a higher preoperative differential renal function (8.5% in absolute difference) than children diagnosed postnatally. Children diagnosed postnatally had a mean age of 6.1 years at the time of pyeloplasty. While it is difficult to ascertain whether the prenatally and postnatally diagnosed groups were truly comparable, this observation lends further support to early diagnosis and early intervention providing an opportunity for optimizing long-term renal function.

A series by Chertin *et al.* (1999) stratified 113 patients into two groups: one presenting with prenatally diagnosed hydronephrosis, and a second also with neonatal hydronephrosis who were lost to follow-up and subsequently re-presented with symptomatic UPJ obstruction. Similar to the findings by Capolicchio *et al.* (1999b), it was observed that poor differential function at diagnosis (defined as <30% differential function) was significantly more common in the symptomatic group (56 of 63 patients, 89%) than in the prenatally diagnosed group (six of 50 patients, 12%, $p < 0.05$). A similarly striking difference was seen between the two groups with regard to improvement in postoperative differential renal function. While postoperative differential renal function was improved in 66% of the prenatally diagnosed group with early pyeloplasty, delay in treatment in the symptomatic group was associated with a significantly lower number of patients demonstrating postoperative improvement (16%, $p < 0.05$). It was concluded in this series that meticulous follow-up of prenatally diagnosed hydronephrosis was of critical importance to ensure that no patient suffered the adverse consequences of delayed treatment.

From the relatively divergent spectrum of outcome documented in these series, it is likely that a complex multifactorial process determines the ultimate renal function following surgical relief of UPJ obstruction. While the debate continues regarding whether pyeloplasty can lead to improvement in differential renal function postoperatively, a comprehensive review of currently available data suggests that surgical correction of obstruction does not uniformly result in improved renal function postoperatively, regardless of the age at which surgery is performed. However, improvement in differential renal function can be seen postoperatively in some, including occasional anecdotal reports of presumably non-functional kidneys recovering into essentially normally functioning kidneys postoperatively. There is as yet no reliable method for identifying those kidneys that are capable of postoperative improvement in function. It is reasonable to conclude that early detection and correction of significant UPJ obstruction serve at least to stabilize renal function and reduce the risk of deterioration. In some it may also result in significant recovery or improvement in renal function postoperatively.

Overall, these clinical and experimental data support the proposition that the younger the infant or child at the time of surgical correction of significant obstruction, the higher the potential for subsequent improvement in renal function and capacity for renal growth. The window of opportunity for maximizing ultimate renal functional potential is at its greatest if obstruction is relieved by 3–6 months of age (King *et al.*, 1984b). Thus, diagnostic modalities should ideally provide the clinician with the necessary tools to identify accurately which hydronephrotic kidney will ultimately require surgical intervention, such that surgical correction can take place at the earliest opportunity, preferably by 3–6 months of age.

Hyperfiltration glomerulopathy

Potential for adverse outcome in subclinical renal injury

While it has long been known that one can survive with a solitary kidney or even just part of one kidney, occasional subtle, long-term, adverse consequences have become evident only recently. In caring for the pediatric patient, this potential for long-term deterioration must be kept in mind, so that the treatment given is best, not only for the immediate future, but also for the child's entire lifespan.

Chronic renal insufficiency in humans has been observed almost inevitably to progress to end-stage renal failure (ESRF), regardless of the etiology of the initial renal injury (Brenner *et al.*, 1996). This is believed to be secondary to progressive hyperfiltration injury to the remaining functioning nephrons (Hostetter *et al.*, 1981; Brenner *et al.*, 1982). As the total number of functioning nephrons decreases below a sustainable threshold, the metabolic demands of the body place a progressively larger burden on

each, causing a progressive increase in the glomerular filtration of each individual nephron (single-nephron GFR, or SNGFR). With SNGFR rising above a physiologically safe threshold, pathologic changes begin to occur as a consequence of excessively high glomerular capillary plasma flow rates (Q_A) and mean glomerular capillary hydraulic pressure (P_{GC}) which are, in turn, a result of adaptive reductions in preglomerular and postglomerular arteriolar resistances (Brenner *et al.*, 1996). Progressive glomerular sclerosis and proteinuria then ensue, which further reduces the remaining number of functional nephrons and, in turn, further exacerbate glomerular hypertension and the already elevated SNGFR, thus continuing a vicious cycle until progressive nephron loss and glomerular injury terminate in end-stage renal failure.

The key determinant in developing hyperfiltration injury appears to be a reduction in total functioning nephrons to below a physiologically sustainable threshold. Just as a lower than normal number of nephrons resulting from renal injury of any cause can lead to the development of hyperfiltration injury, people who are born with a lower number of nephrons but have otherwise normal kidneys also appear to be at risk for the development of hyperfiltration injury. The nephron number in the normal population ranges from 800 000 to 1 100 000 or more. Brenner *et al.* (1996) presented several lines of evidence that the nephron endowment at birth is inversely related to the risk of developing hypertension later in life (MacKenzie *et al.*, 1995). If the myriad of potential complications of hypertension can affect individuals who merely have a relatively small congenital endowment of nephrons but otherwise normal kidneys, these same problems can logically also affect the urologic patient who has suffered a loss in nephron number as a result of congenital uropathy. While there are insufficient data to establish a definite association between various congenital uropathies and subsequent long-term adverse outcomes such as hypertension, there are similarly insufficient data to rule out such a possibility. The work of Brenner *et al.* (1996) is very important in pointing out that even entirely subclinical renal anomalies undetectable by current technology may carry the potential to cause significant morbidity in the long term, including glomerular sclerosis, proteinuria, hypertension, and renal failure. Thus, when management decisions are being made in the treatment of congenital hydronephrosis, the clinician needs to weigh the potential risks of surgical correction against, not only clinically measurable renal deterioration, but also the risk of a possible long-term adverse outcome as a result of a reduction in glomerular number.

Among the practical conclusions derived from the work related to hyperfiltration renal injury, clinicians caring for patients with congenital uropathies should be familiar with the finding that appropriate treatment of capillary hyperfiltration and hypertension can limit further renal injury. Dietary protein restriction has been shown to preserve renal function in rats and limit structural injury even when instituted after the onset of established renal injury (Meyer *et al.*, 1987). The appropriate use of antihypertensive medications which are effective in correcting glomerular hypertension has also been shown to slow the progression of experimental renal disease (Brenner *et al.*, 1996). Thus, in caring for patients with urologic disorders, it would be prudent to advise all patients judged to be at risk for having a smaller than normal complement of nephrons to exercise moderation in protein intake, and to have their blood pressure monitored at least annually, so that the onset of hypertension can be detected in a timely fashion and appropriate treatment instituted promptly. Since the hydronephrotic kidney, even when functioning poorly, excretes water well, its presence reduces the risk of hyperfiltration glomerulopathy in the normal mate. Consideration should be given to preserving such kidneys whenever possible, especially in infants and young children.

Summary

At present, approximately 23% of congenitally hydronephrotic kidneys monitored by an observational approach ultimately require surgical intervention because of functional deterioration, worsening degree of obstruction, or development of pain or urinary infection. The remainder often maintain good preservation of renal function for a number of years. Longer term follow-up and follow-up into adulthood are lacking in patients treated by an observational approach, and it is as yet undetermined whether they ultimately reach their full renal functional potential, and whether late obstruction commonly occurs.

In patients who receive surgical intervention, the younger the infant or child at the time of relief of renal obstruction, the higher the potential for subsequent improvement in renal function and capacity for renal growth. The window of opportunity for maximizing ultimate renal functional potential is at its greatest if obstruction is relieved by 3–6 months of age, and certainly within the first year. Even subclinical renal anomalies undetectable by current technology may carry some potential to cause hyperfiltration renal injury over time. Morbidity in the long term includes glomerular sclerosis, proteinuria, and hypertension and its related sequelae.

Thus, when management decisions are being made in the treatment of congenital hydronephrosis, it is overly simplistic only to weigh the risks of surgical correction against clinically measurable renal deterioration. In order to optimize long-term renal function, one should also consider the possibility that successful surgical treatment may result in improvement in renal function beyond its current level, and be mindful of the potential risk of a long-term adverse outcome.

Diagnosis

While most clinicians use similar diagnostic studies for the evaluation of hydronephrosis, there is little overall consensus as to the exact significance of the results of some of the diagnostic studies. In an attempt to make sense of this controversial and somewhat confusing area, this section will discuss the various diagnostic tools in conjunction with relevant pathophysiologic considerations. In order to delineate clearly the strengths and limitations of each of the diagnostic modalities, it is necessary to have a working definition of what constitutes significant obstruction.

Implicit in the preceding discussion on the pathophysiology of congenital hydronephrosis, physiologically significant obstruction will be defined as an impediment in urine transport that leads to compensatory changes in physiologic renal parameters, including but not limited to renal pelvic pressure, renal blood flow, and GFR. However, a kidney identified to have physiologically significant obstruction may not necessarily suffer from functionally significant sequelae. Functionally significant obstruction will be separately defined as an impediment in urine transport which, if untreated, ultimately results in the kidney having less than its full functional potential. It is not always clear whether physiologically significant obstruction leads to functionally significant obstruction. With these working definitions in mind, each diagnostic modality will be discussed according to its ability to delineate the anatomic site of obstruction, to detect physiologically significant obstruction, and to diagnose functionally significant obstruction.

Diagnostic tests that provide images of anatomic detail include ultrasonography, non-contrast computed tomographic (CT) scan, magnetic resonance imaging (MRI) scan, percutaneous antegrade nephrostogram, and retrograde pyelography. Studies performed with intravenous radiographic contrast, such as intravenous pyelography (IVP) or CT scan with intravenous contrast, are primarily useful for obtaining anatomical details, but also provide a limited degree of non-quantitative physiologic information. Diagnostic tools that focus on the measurement of physiologic parameters include nuclear renography with or without the administration of a diuretic agent such as furosemide, percutaneous pressure–flow studies, Doppler studies measuring intrarenal resistive index (RI), and the analysis of urinary markers.

Ultrasonography

Ultrasonography is widely available, and is non-invasive in nature. As a result, it has become the primary initial tool for the identification and evaluation of hydronephrosis both prenatally and postnatally, and is also heavily used in the follow-up assessments of hydronephrosis. Sonography provides excellent images of the renal parenchyma as well as any fluid-filled cavities, such as a urine-filled bladder or a dilated collecting system. While an empty renal pelvis can often be visualized by demonstrating the apposition of renal sinus fat at the renal hilum, a normal ureter cannot be definitively demonstrated by sonography. Thus, the distinction by ultrasonography between pyelocaliectasis alone versus hydroureteronephrosis (where a dilated ureter is also present) may be operator dependent. Sonography is also often limited by its inability to pinpoint the exact level of ureteral obstruction beyond the UPJ (Figs. 20.15a–e, 20.16a–d).

Although sonography is primarily useful in demonstrating anatomic details, functionally significant alterations can at times be inferred from changes in anatomic parameters, such as measurements of contralateral renal lengths and echogenicity of the renal cortex. Parameters related to blood-flow velocity such as the intrarenal resistive index can also be obtained simultaneously while performing ultrasonography. This will be discussed separately.

Prenatal ultrasonography

Routine prenatal obstetric assessment with ultrasonography at 16–20 weeks of gestation has led to large numbers of hydronephrotic kidneys being detected *in utero*. Of the various fetal abnormalities detected by prenatal ultrasonography, hydronephrosis is the most common, accounting for almost 50% of all prenatally identified anomalies (Reddy and Mandell, 1998). Furthermore, about one-half of the hydronephrotic kidneys detected are secondary to

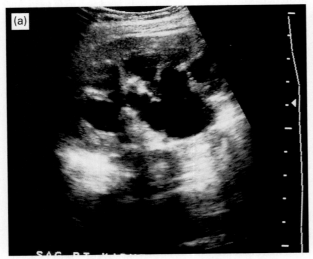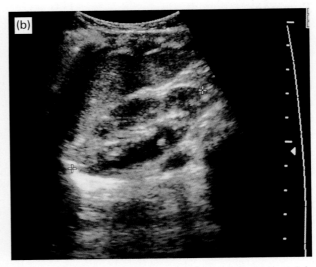

Figure 20.15 Ultrasonography in a 2-month old male infant demonstrating pelvicaliectasis of the right kidney (*a*), and a normal non-dilated left kidney (*b*). (*c*) *Continued opposite*.

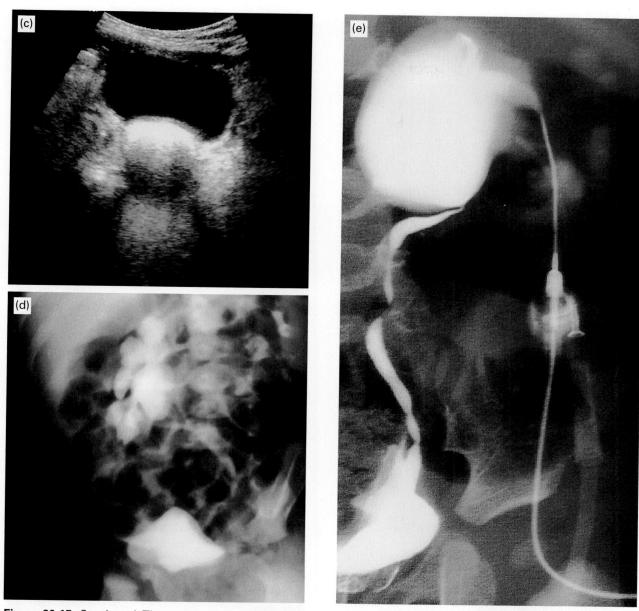

Figure 20.15 *Continued.* The ureters are not visualized in any of ultrasonographic images, including the transverse bladder view (*c*). With the inference that there is no ureteral dilatation, these ultrasonographic findings are compatible with right ureteropelvic junction (UPJ) obstruction. Right (UPJ) obstruction and normal distal ureter were confirmed by intravenous pyelography (*d*) and a right antegrade nephrostogram in prone position obtained during a percutaneous pressure–flow study (*e*).

UPJ obstruction, which may resolve before birth. Of the diagnostic modalities discussed in this section, aside from the limited use of fetal urine analyses, sonography constitutes the sole imaging modality routinely used in the assessment of fetal hydronephrosis. Several sonographic criteria have been developed to stratify the severity of the condition and to predict the outcome of these hydronephrotic kidneys.

A systematic evaluation of fetal hydronephrosis includes the assessment of fetal size and maturity relative to the estimated gestational age, amniotic fluid volume, and gender. The urinary tract is evaluated by measuring bladder volume, size and number of kidneys, the anteroposterior (AP) diameter of the renal pelves, thickness and echogenicity of the renal parenchyma, and the presence of cortical cysts. A

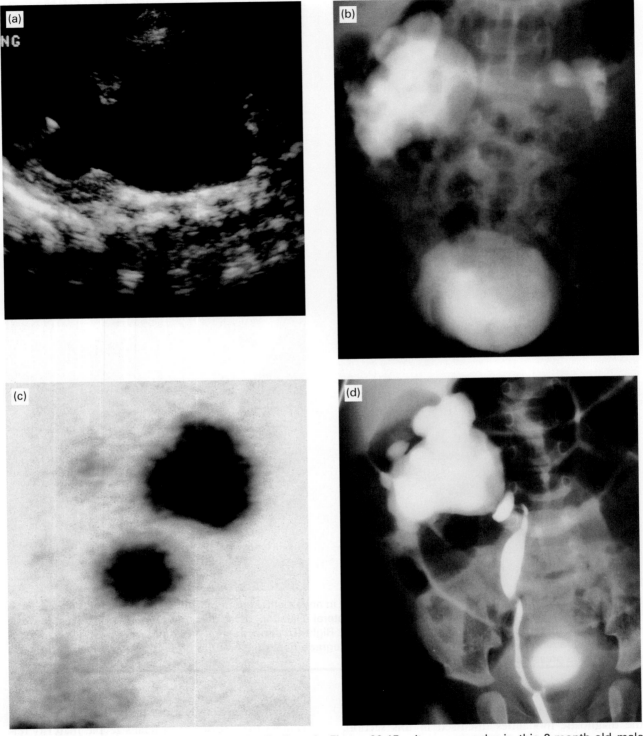

Figure 20.16 Similar to the ultrasonography findings in Figure 20.15, ultrasonography in this 3-month-old male infant revealed right pelvicaliectasis, and the ureters were not visualized (*a*). Intravenous pyelography (*b*) and nuclear renal scan (*c*) were also unable to identify anomalies distal to the ureteropelvic junction (UPJ). Unlike the correct ultrasonographic diagnosis of UPJ obstruction in Figure 20.15, this patient has a right retrocaval ureter. Compression of the proximal ureter just beyond the UPJ can be seen on right retrograde pyelogram (*d*). This case illustrates the principle that the lack of ureteral visualization by ultrasonography cannot always be used as a reliable means to exclude ureteral anomalies distal to the UPJ.

search for the presence of other significant non-urologic congenital anomalies should also be included as part of the evaluation.

The fetal kidneys (Lawson *et al.*, 1981) and bladder (Hobbins *et al.*, 1984) can be reliably visualized by 15 weeks of gestation, and fetal sex can be determined with a high degree of certainty during the second trimester (Birnholz, 1983; Stephens and Sherman, 1983). Since the fetal bladder fills and empties on an approximately hourly cycle, the urinary tract can also be assessed in real time by following the cycling of the bladder. The degree of upper tract dilatation can be examined with the bladder full and empty; the observation of increased upper tract dilatation during active voiding or intermittent hydronephrosis suggests the presence of VUR, and incomplete bladder emptying can suggest the presence of bladder outlet obstruction. If the fetus is confirmed to be male, the differential diagnosis of hydronephrosis includes PUV, as well as other types of urethral and bladder outlet obstruction.

Based on these sonographic parameters, the likelihood of significant obstructive uropathy can be stratified. Decreased amniotic fluid volume prior to the rupture of the amniotic membrane or oligohydramnios, is the best indicator of severe obstructive uropathy. While sonographic estimates for amniotic fluid volume remain inaccurate, severe oligohydramnios is a relatively obvious finding characterized by detecting no area of amniotic fluid greater than 2 cm in diameter (Manning *et al.*, 1981). Since the fetal urine output contributes over 90% of the amniotic fluid volume by the third trimester (Thomas and Smith, 1974), severe oligohydramnios in the absence of an amniotic fluid leak implies a markedly reduced urine output, and suggests the presence of severe obstructive uropathy. However, this is an uncommon finding in fetuses with hydronephrosis.

Diffusely abnormal renal parenchyma associated with bilateral hydronephrosis or a solitary hydronephrotic kidney also raises the concern of severe renal functional impairment. Significant renal parenchymal abnormalities include the presence of severely thinned renal cortex, or increased echogenicity with or without cystic changes secondary to dysplastic parenchymal changes. Hydronephrosis with otherwise well-preserved renal parenchyma is generally anticipated to result in adequate long-term renal function, provided that appropriate treatment is instituted postnatally. Unilateral hydronephrosis with a normal contralateral kidney, a relatively low-risk scenario, is similarly expected to result in good to total long-term renal function.

As ultrasonography provides primarily anatomic detail and not functional or physiologic parameters, attempts have been made over the years to establish morphologic criteria that would lend some degree of insight into the likely ultimate outcome in hydronephrosis. For example, an observation was made that pyelocaliectasis (dilatation of renal pelvis and calices) may indicate significant obstruction as reflected by progressive dilatation and thinning of parenchyma. A prominent extrarenal pelvis is usually a benign normal physiologic variant that does not have the same pathophysiologic significance as when associated with caliectasis (Maizels *et al.*, 1992).

Based on observations relating morphologic configurations to long-term outcome, several methods for grading fetal hydronephrosis have been developed. The AP diameter of the renal pelvis is one such parameter that has been found to be particularly useful as a guide for subsequent evaluation and management (Mandell *et al.*, 1991; Dhillon, 1998). The system suggested by Grignon *et al.* (1986) for fetal evaluation was based on the premise that mild degrees of dilatation resolve spontaneously, and can be considered as a normal physiologic event. The SFU criteria for grading included an empty fetal bladder at the time of sonographic evaluation and a gestational age of at least 20 weeks. In their grading scale, grades 1–5 were defined as:

- grade 1: an increase in the AP diameter of the renal pelvis on the transverse view, up to 10 mm, with no caliectasis;
- grade 2: an AP diameter exceeding 10 mm but with no associated caliectasis;
- grade 3: slight caliectasis, independent of pelvic size;
- grade 4: moderate caliectasis independent of pelvic size, with the cortex greater than 2 mm.;
- grade 5: severe caliectasis with cortical atrophy (less than 2 mm).

In their group of 92 kidneys, on postnatal follow-up studies 3–7 days after birth, the grades of hydronephrosis were unchanged in 72 (78%). Of the remaining 20 hydronephrotic kidneys, 16 progressed (17%) to higher grades. The analysis of outcomes showed good correlation with patients who went on to surgical correction of UPJ obstruction. In patients with grade 1 hydronephrosis, 97% resolved spontaneously.

In grade 2 hydronephrosis, about one-half normalized spontaneously, and 40% were surgically corrected. Sixty-two per cent of grade 3 hydronephrosis, and 100% of kidneys with grades 4 and 5 hydronephrosis had surgical intervention.

The SFU consensus guidelines (SFU, 1988; Maizels *et al.*, 1992) proposed a grading system based on caliectasis and separation of the central renal complex. The renal sinus is normally brightly echogenic from the renal sinus fat, admixed with sonolucent renal pelvis urine and hilar blood. Dilatation of the pelvis with urine causes the central complex to separate to varying degrees. According to this schema hydronephrosis was graded as:

- grade 0: intact central renal complex, normal parenchyma;
- grade 1: slight splitting of central renal complex, normal parenchyma;
- grade 2: central renal complex splitting confined within renal border, normal parenchyma;
- grade 3: wide splitting, pelvis dilated outside renal border and calices uniformly dilated, normal parenchyma;
- grade 4: large dilated calices (may appear convex) with thinning of parenchyma.

The parenchymal thickness was considered thin (grade 4) if it was less than half that of the opposite normal kidney. In cases of bilateral hydronephrosis, <4 mm was used as the cut-off for parenchymal thinning. With the above classification, in their series of 76 children, Maizels *et al.* used grade 3 hydronephrosis to predict obstruction on diuretic renography and demonstrated a sensitivity of 88% and specificity of 95%.

In their retrospective analysis of 177 patients referred for further evaluation of fetal urinary anomalies, Mandell *et al.* (1991) found that UPJ obstruction was the most common postnatal anatomic abnormality (29%), with a large number resolving prenatally (33%) or postnatally (24%). They noted a gradual rise in the renal AP pelvic diameter during gestation in those who came to surgery postnatally. The pelvic diameter representing the group at high risk for surgery was 5 mm at 15–20 weeks, 8 mm at 20–30 weeks, and 10 mm after 30 weeks. Isolated pyelectasis without caliectasis was once again noted to be generally benign, but there was a 10% incidence of progression, underscoring the importance of postnatal follow-up studies regardless of the degree of hydronephrosis.

At the Great Ormond Street Hospital, London (Dhillon, 1998), a group of 110 hydronephrotic kidneys with good renal function is being followed with observation only. In this series, it was found that no child with a postnatal AP pelvic diameter less than 12 mm has required surgery (34 of 104). Of the 76 with AP diameter greater than 12 mm, 27 (36%) had pyeloplasties. Twenty-two of these 27 kidneys had surgery within the first 3 years of postnatal follow-up.

Prenatal ultrasonography alone is generally insufficient for establishing a definitive diagnosis of the cause of the hydronephrosis, requiring more definitive evaluation postnatally. However, prenatal ultrasonography can be invaluable in guiding the most appropriate obstetric and postnatal management. From the above series, it can be seen that the grading scales based on morphologic sonographic criteria are helpful in providing an estimate of the likelihood that significant obstruction is present. Combined with other prenatal sonographic parameters, such as amniotic fluid volume, number of kidneys involved, and the condition of the renal parenchyma, the risk for significant long-term impairment in renal function can be estimated. However, as these morphologic criteria do not directly measure physiologic or functional parameters, it is not surprising that they are not entirely sensitive or specific in predicting physiologically or functionally significant obstruction. Thus, prenatal sonographic assessment of hydronephrosis should only be used as a guide for postnatal evaluation and intervention, and not be regarded as a definitive diagnostic tool. Both serial *in utero* monitoring and postnatal evaluation of prenatally diagnosed hydronephrosis are essential.

Postnatal ultrasonography

Owing to a transient state of dehydration and reduced GFR commonly seen in the immediate postnatal period, the first postnatal ultrasonographic evaluation cannot be considered as an accurate assessment of the degree of collecting system dilatation unless it was performed 48–72 hours after birth. Sonographic parameters used in the postnatal assessment of hydronephrosis are the same as those in the prenatal assessment process.

In unilateral hydronephrosis, the serial measurement of contralateral renal length has been proposed as an indicator of the functional status of the hydronephrotic kidney (Koff *et al.*, 1994; Koff and Peller, 1995). It is reasoned that normal renal function in the hydronephrotic kidney would not induce compensatory hypertrophy in the contralateral kidney, and thus the contralateral renal length would remain within normally expected ranges. However, reduced function in the hydronephrotic kidney can be expected to induce contralateral compensatory hypertrophy and, presumably, longer than normal contralateral renal lengths would be observed. In conjunction with serial differential functions from nuclear medicine renal scans, contralateral renal length measurements have been used as part of a renal growth and function chart to monitor the development of these hydronephrotic kidneys. While this concept may be sound in theory, it is as yet not fully validated, and has some intrinsic limitations (Brandell *et al.*, 1996). First, in the assessment for compensatory hypertrophy, renal length is a one-dimensional estimate of a three-dimensional parameter, i.e., renal parenchymal volume. Secondly, an experimental animal study demonstrated a high degree of variability in renal length measurements as determined sonographically (Ferrer *et al.*, 1997), raising the concern that management decisions based on a relatively small number of serial renal length measurements may be subjected to significant inaccuracies. Advances in three-dimensional ultrasonography may overcome these limitations. Lastly, similar to using differential renal function to determine whether surgical relief of obstruction is necessary, significant alterations in contralateral renal length become apparent only when the obstructed kidney has already lost a significant amount of renal function. Such observations confirm functional deterioration, but cannot be used to detect significant obstruction or to predict the risk of renal function loss prior to deterioration.

Voiding cystourethrography

Voiding cystourethrography (VCUG) is used to assess the presence of vesicoureteral reflux (VUR) and lower urinary tract anomalies. A VCUG should be performed in all children who have hydronephrosis before making the diagnosis of possible UPJ obstruction. Dilatation of the collecting system may be the result of reflux rather than obstruction (Fig. 20.17a–f). In addition, up to 10% of patients with UPJ obstruction also have associated VUR, occasionally severe in degree. Finally, high-grade reflux may lead to secondary UPJ obstruction, wherein the UPJ

becomes kinked as a result of severe tortuosity of the refluxing megaureter (Fig. 20.18a–d).

When UPJ obstruction coexists with mild VUR, a number of findings on VCUG may alert the clinician to the presence of the UPJ obstruction. The degree of pyelocaliectasis is disproportionately greater than the ureteral dilatation seen on VCUG (Fig. 20.19a–c). In addition, the contrast material that gets into the renal pelvis becomes diluted by the fluid in the collecting system and is less dense than that in the ureter.

When upper ureteral obstruction is suspected in association with VUR, it is especially important that when diagnostic studies such as renal scans or excretory urograms are performed the bladder is kept emptied by an indwelling bladder catheter, thereby eliminating the influence of VUR on the interpretation of upper urinary tract drainage or ipsilateral renal function.

Intravenous pyelography (excretory urography)

The IVP is the oldest study used for the evaluation of hydronephrosis (Fig. 20.20). It has the capacity to reveal anatomic details, and also provides some indication of the functional status of the kidneys. Because of its dependence on renal function for visualization of the kidneys and collecting systems, its usefulness is limited in infants. Neonates younger than 2–4 weeks of age have physiologically immature kidneys and tend to have significant intestinal gas, both of which often result in poor renal visualization on IVP. Similarly, kidneys with poor renal function are not well visualized by IVP. In cases where visualization is poor, delayed films may be helpful.

The diagnosis of UPJ obstruction is suggested when the IVP shows dilatation of the renal pelvis and calyces along with non-visualization of the ipsilateral ureter distal to the UPJ. Unlike acute ureteral obstruction, congenital hydronephrosis secondary to UPJ obstruction is generally not associated with a significant delay in excretion of the contrast by the renal parenchyma (see Fig. 20.1). The exception may occur during an episode of Dietl's crisis when acute exacerbation of the obstruction from acute ureteral kinking at the UPJ occurs. Opacification of the renal pelvis may then take much longer than normal owing to the volume of the grossly dilated renal pelvis, and perhaps also to some degree of functional impairment. In order to maximize visualization, delayed imaging is essential. To help to

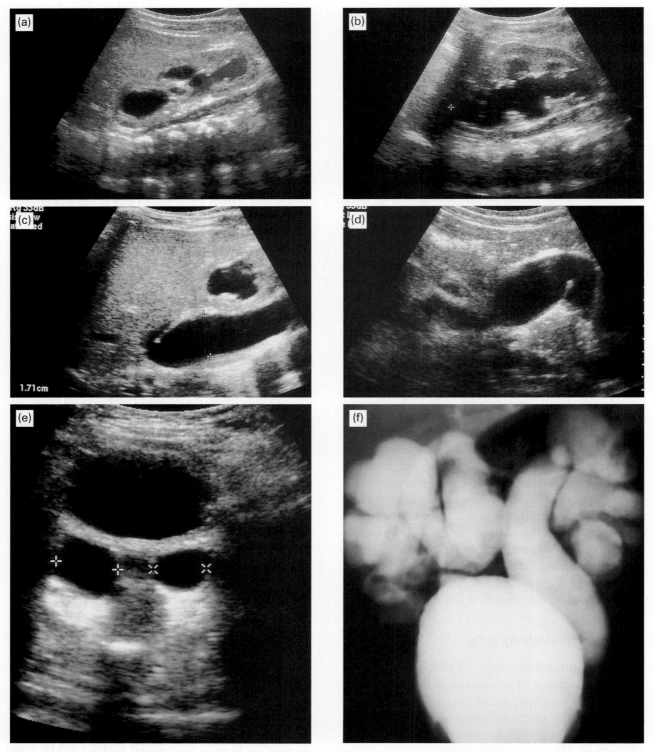

Figure 20.17 A 6-month-old female infant presenting with a febrile urinary tract infection. Ultrasonography revealed bilateral pelvicaliectasis (*a*, right kidney; *b*, left kidney) and bilateral ureteral dilatation (*c*, right ureter; *d*, left ureter; *e*, transverse bladder view showing bilateral dilated ureters). (*f*) Voiding cystourethrogram showed bilateral grade V vesicoureteral reflux (VUR) as the cause of the bilateral hydroureteronephrosis. The detection of ureteral dilatation is an important clue in the evaluation of a dilated collecting system. The presence of ureteral dilatation either indicates antegrade obstruction at a level distal to the UPJ, or it may be the result of VUR.

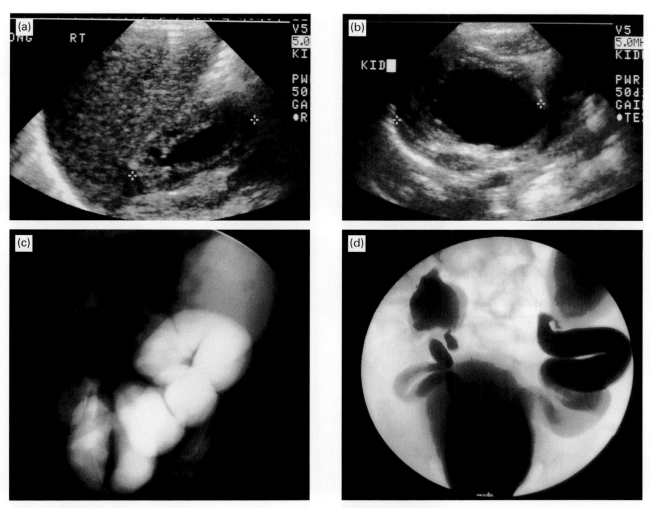

Figure 20.18 This patient had an antenatal ultrasonography diagnosis of bilateral hydronephrosis. At birth he was found to have bilateral anophthalmia, and postnatal ultrasonography confirmed moderate right (*a*) and severe left (*b*) hydronephrosis. (*c*) Voiding cystourethrogram revealed massive bilateral grade V vesicoureteral reflux. (*d*) Bilateral retrograde pyelograms showing tortuous ureters bilaterally, and kinked/obstructive ureteropelvic junction (UPJ) segments compatible with bilateral secondary UPJ obstructions resulting from the ureteral tortuosity.

discern whether the contrast empties from the renal pelvis, the administration of intravenous furosemide (0.5–1.0 mg/kg up to 10 mg) can also be used, referred to as a *diuretic urogram* (Figs 20.21, 20.22). However, renal sonography and nuclear scintigraphy have generally replaced excretory urography in the evaluation of pediatric UPJ obstruction due to the non-invasive and sensitive nature of the former and the objective functional information offered by the latter.

Computed tomographic scan and magnetic resonance imaging

Both computed tomographic (CT) scan and magnetic resonance imaging (MRI) provide highly detailed image slices in the coronal plane, while MRI also offers imaging in the frontal and sagittal planes. These high-resolution two-dimensional image slices can also be reconstructed into three-dimensional images. While these technologies have evolved into the mainstays for the evaluation of many urologic problems, including tumor masses, trauma, and sometimes renal calculi, they do not provide significant advantage in the evaluation of hydronephrosis over other diagnostic modalities discussed in this section (Fig. 20.23a–g).

If hydronephrosis is incidentally noted on a contrast-enhanced CT scan, an abdominal flat plate at the end of the study may be helpful in delineating

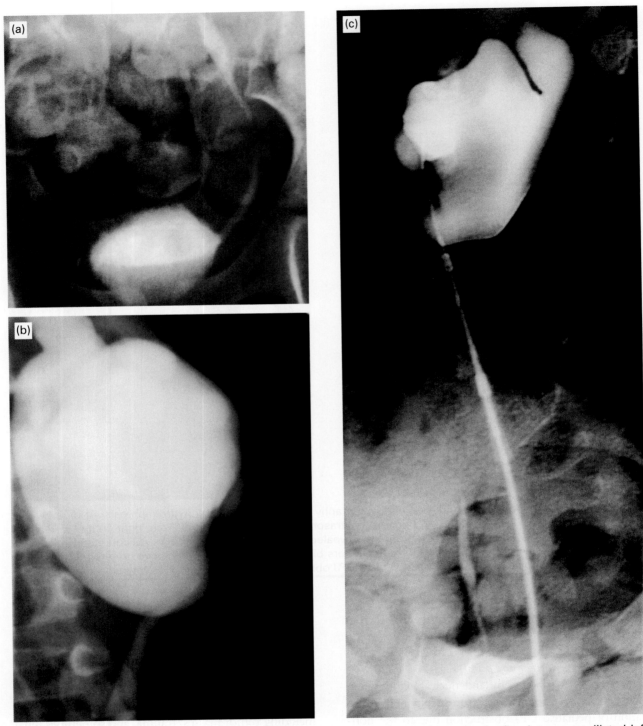

Figure 20.19 Voiding cystourethrogram of a 3.5-year-old girl showing vesicoureteral reflux into a non-dilated left ureter compatible with grade II reflux. (*a*) However, the renal pelvis and calices are disproportionately severely dilated (*b*). This discrepancy in pelvicaliectasis which exceeds the degree of dilatation usually associated with low-grade reflux suggests the concomitant presence of ureteropelvic junction (UPJ) obstruction. A percutaneous diuresis pressure–flow study (*c*, left antegrade nephrostogram in prone position) confirmed high-grade left UPJ obstruction. After the administration of intravenously furosemide, left renal pelvic pressure rose to 63 cmH$_2$O, the highest value recorded at our institution to date. There was no efflux of contrast across the left UPJ, compatible with a Dietl's crisis type of intermittent high-grade UPJ obstruction induced by diuresis.

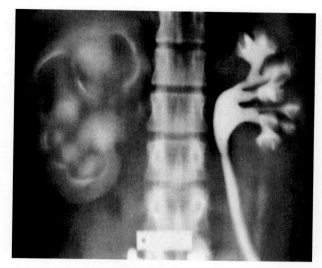

Figure 20.20 Crescent sign of hydronephrosis (IVP).

anatomic detail, providing a planar image of the collecting system similar to that of an IVP.

Retrograde pyelography

Retrograde pyelography remains the best imaging study for demonstrating the anatomic details of the collecting system in a two-dimensional planar view, because of the high-contrast density achievable via the direct retrograde injection of contrast. As the contrast is introduced retrograde, however, non-physiologic distension of the collecting system may occur because

of forcefulness of the injection (Fig. 20.24). The images need to be interpreted with this factor in mind. Once sufficient contrast has been introduced beyond the suspected site of obstruction, the ureteral catheter is removed and the spontaneous reflux of contrast is observed to assess drainage at and distal to the UPJ.

Retrograde pyelography serves an especially important role in instances where antegrade studies, such as IVP and antegrade nephrostogram, fail to demonstrate clearly ureteral anatomy distal to the site of obstruction (see Fig. 20.16a–d).

While the usefulness of retrograde pyelography is well established, the necessity of performing retrograde pyelography prior to pyeloplasty has been a source of controversy. Reviewing 100 pyeloplasties between October 1978 and April 1989, Cockrell and Hendren (1990) concluded that retrograde pyelography should routinely be performed before pyeloplasty unless the ureter distal to the point of obstruction was well visualized by some other means. Presenting the contrary view, Rushton *et al.* (1994) reviewed 108 patients from 1986 to 1992. It was found that sonography and nuclear renal scans were effective in ruling out pathology distal to the UPJ. They encountered no intraoperative problems attributable to not having visualized the ureter beyond the UPJ, and concluded that routine retrograde pyelography was not necessary in the evaluation of the child with UPJ obstruction.

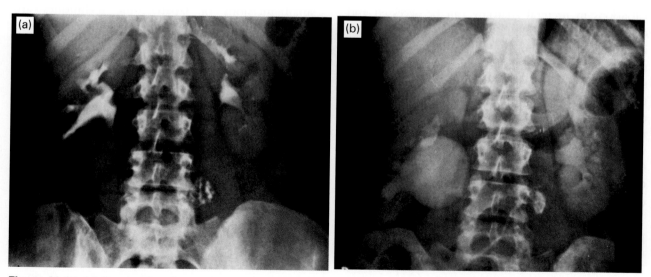

Figure 20.21 (*a*) Conventional excretory urogram; (*b*) same with furosemide. Classic ureteropelvic obstruction on right, clearly demonstrated by the furosemide enhanced diuretic urogram but not by the conventional excretory urogram

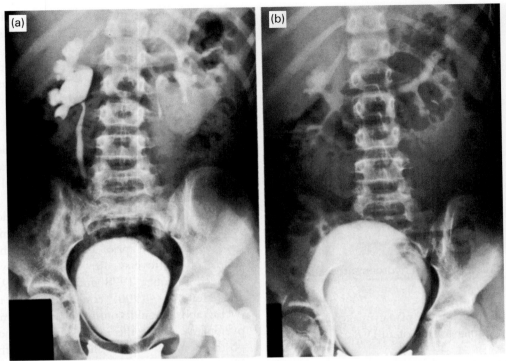

Figure 20.22 (*a*) Excretory urogram showing postoperative right pyeloplasty. There is questionable persisting obstruction. (*b*) Synchronous furosemide study shows prompt drainage. No obstruction is apparent.

While Rushton *et al.* (1994) had a very successful series of pyeloplasties without the routine use of retrograde pyelography, it should be noted that either a subcostal flank or an anterior extraperitoneal incision was used. Although none was reported in this series, variations in ureteral anatomy can be accessed and dealt with successfully by this surgical approach including the previously unrecognized retrocaval ureter. With the recent trend towards minimally invasive surgery, including laparoscopic pyeloplasty, and the revitalized interest in the dorsal lumbotomy approach with its relatively limiting exposure, this may not apply. To address this concern, 146 patients were reviewed from the Toronto Hospital for Sick Children and the University of Massachusetts Medical Center. In six (4.1%) the obstructions were considered unsuitable for the doral lumbotomy approach. These problems were identified only by retrograde pyelography and were missed by other imaging modalities. One ureter was retrocaval (see Fig. 20.16a–d), two had mid ureteral hypoperistaltic segments well below the level of the UPJ, two had very long hypoperistaltic segments spanning two-thirds of the ureteral length, and one had no fewer

than four separate, narrow hypoperistaltic segments (Fig. 20.25).

Retrograde pyelography is not routinely necessary before pyeloplasty, provided that pathology beyond the UPJ has been reliably excluded. However, when small incisions or laparoscopic techniques are employed, it is prudent to delineate ureteral anatomy clearly by an appropriate study before starting the procedure.

Nuclear medicine renography

None of the studies available at this time can predict which kidney will undergo functional deterioration if it remains untreated. However, by its ability to provide a quantitative assessment of differential renal function, nuclear renography comes closest to the goal of detecting functionally significant obstruction.

The characteristics of a nuclear medicine renal scan are dependent on the biological activity of the radionuclide. Agents commonly used for renal evaluation and visualization include technicium-99m-diethylene triamine pentaacetic acid ([99mTc]DTPA), technetium-99m-mercaptoacetyltriglycine ([99mTc]

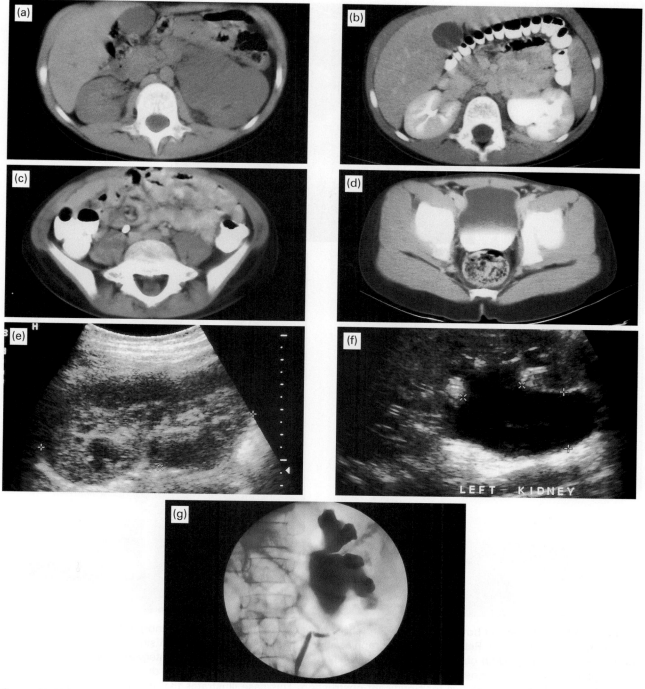

Figure 20.23 A 6-year-old boy presenting with severe intermittent left flank pain, nausea, and vomiting, compatible with recurrent Dietl's crises. A computed tomographic (CT) scan without contrast was initially performed at an outside institution during an acute episode, demonstrating massive left pelvicaliectasis (a). A CT scan with contrast was performed on the following day, after the acute obstructive crisis had subsided. Note that the left pelvicaliectasis is significantly reduced (b). However, there was still no contrast visualized in the left ureter beyond the left ureteropelvic junction (UPJ) (c, d). Ultrasonography images are shown for comparison (e, normal right kidney; f, hydronephrotic left kidney). At the time of pyeloplasty, the excised UPJ was seen to contain a 7-mm-long ureteral polyp responsible for the intermittent obstruction experienced by the patient (see Fig. 20.6). (g) On left retrograde pyelography, a subtle persistent filling defect between the renal pelvis and proximal ureter can be seen, corresponding to the location of the ureteral polyp. Such two-dimensional images can often be more useful in the assessment of hydronephrosis than the axial slices provided by a CT scan.

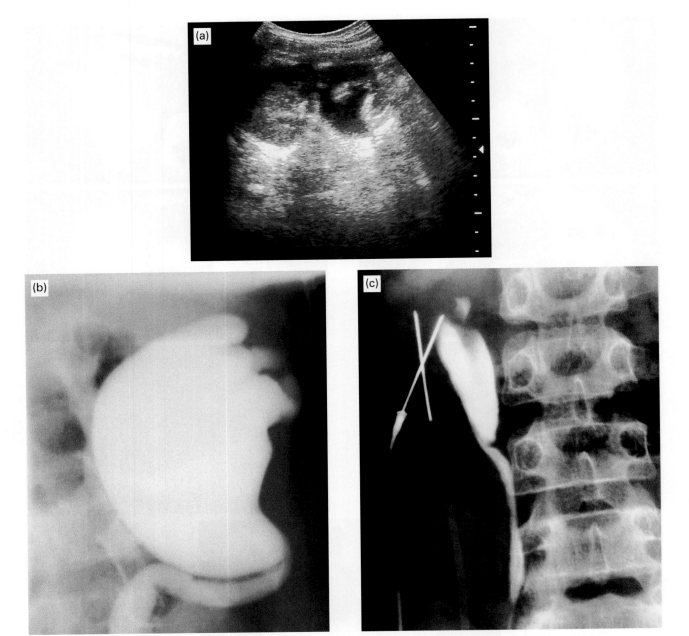

Figure 20.24 An 8-year-old boy presenting with febrile urinary tract infection. Ultrasonography revealed left lower moiety hydronephrosis (*a*). Retrograde pyelography showed findings compatible with significant left lower moiety ureteropelvic junction (UPJ) obstruction, with a laterally placed, kinked UPJ (*b*). On antegrade nephrostography (*c*, left collecting system in prone position), however, the UPJ remains dependent and drains well. A percutaneous pressure–flow study was negative for significant obstruction. This case illustrates that the retrograde distension of the collecting system can produce non-physiologic artifacts.

MAG-3), and technetium-99m-dimercaptosuccinic acid ([^{99m}Tc]DMSA). DTPA and MAG-3 are rapidly concentrated by the kidney and excreted allowing function and drainage estimates, whereas DMSA is a cortical imaging agent used to assess differential function, cortical appearance, and renal scars (see Chapter 6).

Blood-flow agents such as DTPA and MAG-3 are freely filtered through the glomerulus. DTPA is neither secreted nor resorbed by the renal tubules (Kass

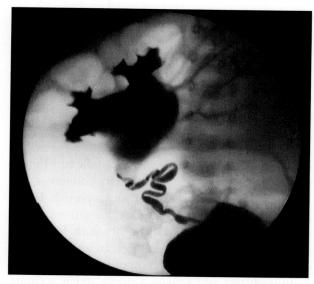

Figure 20.25 A 2-month-old male infant was found to have at least four grossly identifiable stenotic segments along the right ureteropelvic junction and proximal ureter, as shown in this right retrograde pyelogram.

and Fink-Bennett, 1990), whereas MAG-3 is secreted by the tubules. Both are slightly protein bound, resulting an approximately 5% systemic underestimation in the analysis of renal handling. MAG-3 is much more expensive than DTPA, but has the advantage that it gives superior anatomic details on the scan images, and is particularly useful in infants. It can give some information even in the presence of marked renal insufficiency.

Parameters that can be measured on a renal scan performed with these agents include the relative differential renal function of each kidney and the rapidity of clearance of the radioisotope from the collecting system. A good renal scan provides a rough morphologic outline sufficient to distinguish hydronephrosis from hydroureteronephrosis. By calculating the decay curve, an approximate estimate of GFR can also be derived from the renal scan. Clearance of radioisotope from the collecting system can be monitored and the rate of urine excretion can be augmented by the administration of furosemide. When used with furosemide, the study is referred to as a diuretic renogram, or Lasix renal scan. The rapidity of the washout can then be quantitated by determining the rate of decline in radioactivity in the collecting system just proximal to the suspected site of obstruction, expressed as the half-life ($t_{1/2}$) (Fig. 20.26).

In an attempt to optimize Lasix renography results, standardization of various technical aspects of the study has been proposed and generally adapted. In one standardized protocol, referred to as the well-tempered renogram (SFU, 1992; Conway 1992), 10–15 ml/kg of intravenous hydration using a crystalloid solution is infused at the beginning of the study. The appropriate radioisotope (DTPA or MAG-3) is given and 1 mg/kg of intravenous furosemide is administered when the accumulation of radioisotope has plateaued in the collecting system. A urinary catheter is inserted to keep the bladder empty throughout the study. A $t_{1/2}$ of less than 10 min is

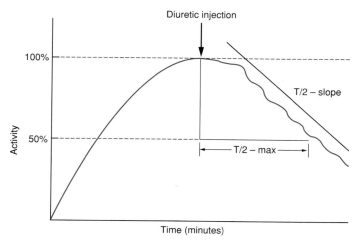

Figure 20.26 The two methods of calculating the drainage half-time. The $T/2_{max}$ measures the time required for half of the tracer to leave the collecting system, with time 0 (zero) being the moment the diuretic is administered. This method of calculation may lead to falsely long half-times. The preferred method is the best linear fit of the washout curve (T/2 linear slope). (Adapted from Kass *et al.*, 1990, with permission.)

considered to be indicative of non-obstructive drainage, between 10 and 20 min is considered inde-terminant, and greater than 20 min is considered to indicate significant obstruction. Visual analysis of the slope of the drainage curve can also provide clues as to the pattern of clearance of radionuclide, an indica-tor of drainage, at the point proximal to the suspect-ed site of obstruction (Fig. 20.27).

Since blood-flow agents such as DTPA and MAG-3 are freely filtered by the glomeruli and quickly reach the collecting system (Kass and Fink-Bennett, 1990), the measurement of differential renal function must be done promptly between 0.5 and 3 min after the injection of the radionuclide. Beyond that, excreted isotope begins to accumulate in the collecting system and no longer reflects true renal accumulation or function.

The Lasix-stimulated scan is the nuclear study of choice to evaluate the dilated system. However, occa-sionally it is desirable to obtain a more accurate mea-sure of cortical function of the involved kidney. DMSA, which is tightly bound to the proximal renal tubule cells, can be used for this purpose. Owing to the lack of significant passage into the urine, DMSA does not accumulate in the collecting system. Fifty per cent of DMSA is localized to the kidneys 1 hour after injection, increasing to 70% by 24 hours (Heyman, 1989; Majd and Rushton, 1992). While this property is desirable for obtaining renal cortical imaging without background activity in the collecting system, it also precludes the possibility of using DMSA to generate drainage curves or washout $t_{1/2}$.

Differential renal function as currently measured in nuclear medicine renography has been the benchmark parameter by which individual renal function has been judged in the presence of hydronephrosis. How-ever, as mentioned above it has its limitations. Alter-native methods for measuring absolute functional renal volume are being developed in an attempt to generate a method that is applicable to bilateral hydronephrosis and solitary kidneys and is accurate even if the contralateral non-hydronephrotic kidney is not normal in size. King *et al.* (1998) developed a method for measuring absolute functional renal vol-ume. This method is a count-based algorithm gen-erated by DMSA three-dimensional single-photon emission computed tomographic (SPECT) scans, which generate a measurement of the functional par-

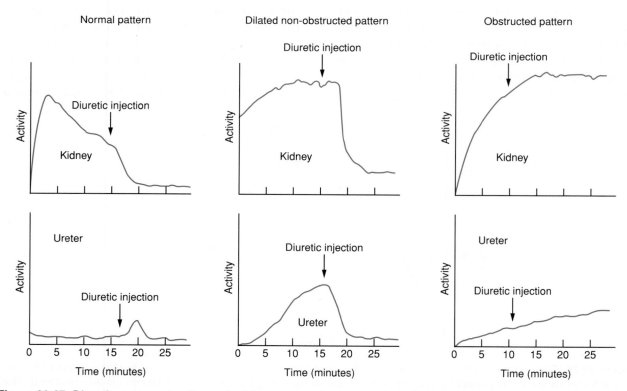

Figure 20.27 Diuretic renography. Reproducible patterns of tracer washout for the kidney and ureter. (Adapted from Koff, 1981, with permission.)

enchymal volume. The volume generated, referred to as the effective functional renal volume (EFRV), has been validated in an *in vitro* model as well as in a porcine *in vivo* model to be within about 5% of the true renal parenchymal volume. While EFRV is currently investigational and not yet validated for clinical use, a method of deriving an absolute measure of renal function by this method or other techniques should greatly enhance our ability to assess the renal function of individual kidneys in hydronephrosis.

Washout half-life

The time required for the radionuclide activity to reduce by one-half, or the washout $t_{1/2}$ calculated from the furosemide-induced diuretic renal scan, has been widely used as a semiquantitative parameter to evaluate drainage from the collecting system. Diuretic renography washout $t_{1/2}$ should be a reasonably accurate indicator of the rate of urinary flow across the suspected site of obstruction. However, there are other physiologic considerations that impact on whether the washout $t_{1/2}$ is a reliable indicator of the severity of the obstruction.

The washout $t_{1/2}$ is to some degree dependent on the compliance and capacity of the collecting system. A small-capacity, low-compliance collecting system would tend to produce relatively short washout $t_{1/2}$, as even a relatively small amount of urine produced would quickly lead to an elevation in collecting system pressure, driving urine across the site of obstruction early in the study. In contrast, a large and highly compliant collecting system would tend to result in a relatively long washout $t_{1/2}$. An example of such a system is the massively distended collecting system where the urine produced results in little change in the collecting system pressure, and seemingly sluggish washout of radionuclide tends to occur even in the absense of significant obstruction. In addition, in this situation the isotope becomes so dispersed that excretion time is prolonged.

In terms of physical properties that govern fluid drainage, obstruction is most appropriately measured by the resistance of the fluid flowing through the conduit. Based on Newtonian physics, resistance is directly proportional to pressure over flow (resistance ∝ pressure/flow). Given that washout $t_{1/2}$ is an indicator of the rate of flow of urine across the suspected site of obstruction, it only measures one of the two variables that determine resistance. Thus, washout $t_{1/2}$

is predictive of the overall conduit resistance only when the pressure within the collecting system remains constant, or if the pressure always varies proportionately to flow. It follows that one needs to account for both pressure and flow simultaneously in order best to determine resistance. Washout $t_{1/2}$, which is an estimate of flow, may therefore be limited in determining the severity of the obstruction (see Fig. 20.33).

Percutaneous pressure–flow study

While hydronephrosis is undoubtedly a highly complex physiologic process, the source of the problem is fundamentally physical in nature. Pressure–flow studies are intrinsically different from imaging studies and nuclear renal scans in that they are designed to provide a measure of the resistance of the collecting system. The pressure–flow study is unique in taking into account both the pressure within the collecting system and the rate of fluid flow.

In any biologic fluid conduit system the resistance of the conduit is directly proportional to pressure over flow (resistance ∝ pressure/flow), modified from the Poiseuille–Hagen law (Holwill and Silvester, 1973), that was originally applied to the flow of Newtonian fluids through rigid tubes. Based on this principle, both pressure and flow must be taken into account simultaneously in order to derive a measurement of the resistance within the conduit.

Pressure–flow studies are relatively invasive procedures, owing to the need to obtain direct access to the lumen of the proximal collecting system to measure the fluid pressure within the system. Insertion of two 22 gauge 2 inch (5 cm) angiocatheters under sonographic guidance and fluoroscopic monitoring has been found to be effective and safe (Figs. 20.28, 20.29a–c). For larger children, the relatively short 2″ angiocathers can be substituted for the longer 22 gauge spinal needles. In children the study is usually carried out under heavy sedation or general anesthesia. The present authors elect to perform all pressure–flow studies in children under general anesthesia. The current percutaneous pressure–flow study protocol at the authors' institution is summarized in Table 20.2. Key concepts of this protocol will be individually discussed in the following sections.

Regardless of what form of percutaneous pressure–flow study is performed, the meaningful interpretation of results depends on an accurate definition

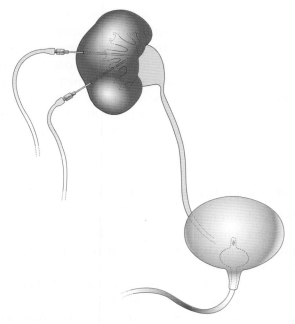

Figure 20.28 Whitaker pressure perfusion test. (Adapted from Wacksman, 1991, with permission.)

of what constitutes the upper limit of normal collecting system pressure. Several studies, both experimental and clinical, have addressed this question. In the rat model, it was found that the proximal renal tubular pressure, intratubular pressure and peritubular capillary pressure all remain constant until the collecting system pressure exceeds the normal renal tubular pressure. In this context, the normal proximal renal tubular pressure was established to be 14.1 ± 0.5 cmH$_2$O in the rat (Brenner *et al.*, 1972). In the human, intrarenal arterial resistance increases acutely once the renal pelvic pressure rises above 14 cmH$_2$O (Fung *et al.*, 1994). Furthermore, Fichtner *et al.* (1994) showed that in the congenitally hydronephrotic rat model, mean renal pelvic pressure was 14.1 ± 1.6 cmH$_2$O under very high urine output with an empty bladder. The mean renal pelvic pressure increased further when

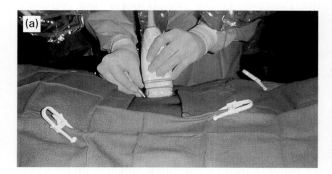

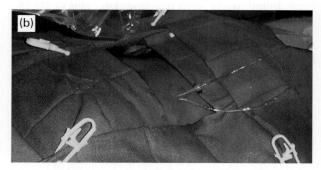

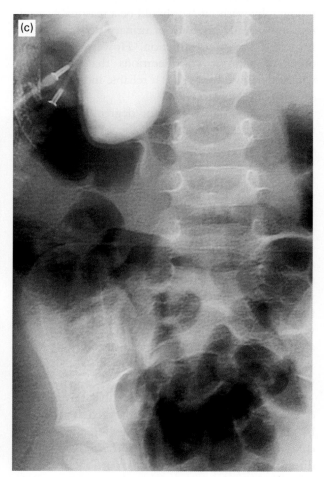

Figure 20.29 For the percutaneous pressure–flow studies performed in children at the authors' institution, all studies are performed under general anesthesia in the prone position. (*a, b*) Two 22 gauge angiocatheters are inserted into the collecting system percutaneously under ultrasonographic guidance. Infusion of contrast verifies satisfactory nephrostomy access (*c*, antegrade nephrostogram in prone position).

Table 20.2 Current percutaneous pressure–flow study protocol at U Mass Memorial Medical Center, Worcester, MA

- Patient is placed under general anesthesia with endotraceal intubation.
- With intravenous access established, antibiotic prophylaxis is given using 40 mg/kg of i.v. cephazolin up to a maximum of 1 g, provided that there is no history of allergic reaction, and hydration is begun with a minimum of 15 ml/kg of a crystalloid solution.
- In supine position, bladder catheter is inserted with the largest caliber catheter that the patient can accept.
- To facilitate placement of percutaneous nephrostomy needles, the bladder catheter may be plugged off at this stage to keep the bladder full and to maximize renal pelvic dilatation.
- The patient is turned to the prone position, and ultrasonographic examination is carried out to plan for nephrostomy access.
- The patient is sterilely prepared and draped. Under untrasonographic guidance, two 22-gauge 2-inch angiocatheters (or other suitable catheters or needles) are inserted percutaneously into the renal pelvis to be examined. The bladder is emptied and the bladder catheter is connected to gravity drainage.
- To verify placement of the nephrostomy access and to establish a means to follow the progress of urine flow, radiographic contrast is injected into the renal pelvis via nephrostomy access. To preserve the baseline renal pelvic pressure dynamics, an equal volume of urine is first aspirated out before the injection of contrast.
- One of the nephrostomy accesses is capped off, and the other is connected to a pressure transducer with no flow going through the nephrostomy.
- The pressure transducer line is zeroed externally to the same level as the tip of the nephrostomy access within the renal pelvis. When connected to the nephrostomy access, the initial pressure reading represents the baseline renal pelvic pressure.
- Furosemide (1 mg/kg i.v., up to a maximum of 10 mg) is given to begin the *diuresis pressure–flow study* component.
- Renal pelvic pressure is continuously monitored for 30 min. Urine output is measured every 5 min to verify satisfactory overall response to i.v. hydration and furosemide. The peak renal pelvic pressure observed in this period determines whether the diuresis pressure–flow study is positive (peak renal pelvic pressure > 14 cmH$_2$O) for significant obstruction.
- During this 30-min interval, fluoroscopy is used intermittently. The renal pelvic pressure at which radiographic contrast is first seen distal to the suspected level of obstruction constitutes the *ureteral opening pressure*.
- If the diuresis pressure–flow study component is strongly positive for significant obstruction (peak renal pelvic pressure markedly above 14 cmH$_2$O), an antegrade nephrostogram is performed to obtain the anatomical details necessary for guiding surgical repair, and the percutaneous pressure–flow study is concluded at this point.
- If the diuresis pressure–flow study component peak renal pelvic pressure is close to or below 14 cmH$_2$O, the *individualized infusion pressure–flow study* is performed next. The other capped off nephrostomy access is connected to an infusion pump, infusing a radiographic contrast solution. The rate of infusion is individually calculated based on patient's age, weight, and height (see Table 20.3) or calculated based on the GFR of the kidney being tested, if known.
- If the resulting renal pelvic pressure is positive for significant obstruction (> 14 cmH$_2$O), an antegrade nephrostogram is performed to obtain the anatomical details necessary for guiding surgical repair, and the percutaneous pressure–flow study is concluded at this point.
- If the resulting renal pelvic pressure is negative for significant obstruction (≤ 14 cmH$_2$O), a supraphysiological rate of infusion is then used (150–200% of the individualized infusion rate) as a measure of the reserve capability of the collecting system to handle additional urine flow.
  Note: Regardless of whether the renal pelvic pressure rises above 14 cmH$_2$O at this point, the pressure–flow study is still considered negative for significant obstruction.
- If a lower tract abnormality, which causes excessively high intravesical pressure, co-exists with the upper tract obstructive site, an initially negative study for significant obstruction (diuresis pressure–flow study) can be further challenged with the bladder filled to the peak naturally occurring intravesical pressure. This is carried out by connecting an intravenous solution drip to the bladder catheter, and the drip chamber is raised to a level that is the same height (in cm) as the peak intravesical pressure (in cmH$_2$O). The desired intravesical pressure being simulated is reached when the drip slows to intermittent drops or stops altogether. The peak renal pelvic pressure recorded in this setting represents a combined effect of both the upper tract obstructive site and the lower tract anomaly on their corresponding upper tract urodynamics.
- Once all necessary urodynamic measurements have been completed, an antegrade nephrostogram is performed to obtain anatomical details necessary for guiding surgical repair. The renal pelvis is aspirated empty and the nephrostomy accesses are removed. The patient is turned back to supine position and awakened from anesthesia. The bladder catheter is removed once significant gross hematuria has been ruled out, and the patient is sufficiently awake to void.
- All patients who have percutaneous pressure–flow studies positive for significant obstruction are covered with oral antibiotic prophylaxis until successful surgical repairs have been achieved.

the bladder was filled. In normal controls mean renal pelvic pressure was below 14 cmH$_2$O under high urine output. With the bladder filled to capacity the highest mean renal pelvic pressure recorded was only 13.2 ± 1.6 cmH$_2$O. These studies suggest that the upper limit of normal renal pelvic pressure is 14 cmH$_2$O, above which undesirable physiologic changes begin to occur.

While these results indicate that renal pelvic pressure above 14 cmH$_2$O produces undesirable physiologic changes, additional evidence indicates that continuous elevation in renal pelvic pressure leads to acute and irreversible renal injury within 24 hours. In a porcine model in which renal pelvic pressure was kept constantly elevated at levels between 20 and 40 cmH$_2$O, urinary levels of N-acetyl-β-D-glucosaminidase (NAG) were found to become elevated, indicative of acute tubular cell membrane disruption (Fung and Atala, 1998). Similar experiments also demonstrated that elevation in renal pelvic pressure led to acute onset of apoptotic cell death, suggestive of a component of irreversible injury (Fung and Atala, 1996). Such tubular disruption and cell death was further found to be associated with decreased renal blood flow and upregulation in vascular endothelial growth factor (VEGF) mRNA levels, an indicator of tissue hypoxia. These changes thus provide evidence that decreased perfusion and tissue hypoxia play an important role when renal pelvic pressure is elevated (Fung et al., 1996). Renal injury was significantly greater in the experimental group with renal pelvic pressure ranging from 20 to 40 cmH$_2$O, when compared with the control animals with renal pelvic pressure of 10 cmH$_2$O or less. Based on these results, the threshold for physiogically safe renal pelvic pressure seems to lie somewhere between 10 and 20 cmH$_2$O. While these experiments did not pinpoint the exact threshold for normal renal pelvic pressure above which renal injury occurs, the data are in keeping with 14 cmH$_2$O as the upper limit of normal renal pelvic pressure, as established in both rat and human studies.

From these lines of evidence, we advocate using 14 cmH$_2$O as the upper limit of physiologically safe renal pelvic pressure, above which undesirable physiological changes and renal injury are expected to occur.

Optimal flow challenge to the collecting system

As urine output can vary tremendously under normal physiological conditions, the collecting system is expected to be able to handle a large range of urine flow rates within physiological limits. Based on the modified Poiseuille–Hagen law, the resistance of a conduit is directly proportional to pressure over flow (resistance ∝ pressure/flow), and an 'obstructed' collecting system with abnormally high resistance would be especially prone to develop elevated pressures when the flow rate is high. In other words, a severely obstructed system with grossly increased resistance to flow would develop elevated pressures with even relatively modest flow challenges. A partially obstructed system with marginally increased resistance to flow may be able to handle lower flow rates, but would develop high pressures when the flow rate increases. A normal collecting system would maintain normal pressures throughout the entire range of physiological flow rates. If the flow challenge is excessively high and exceeds physiological limits, however, even normal collecting systems may become overwhelmed by the unphysiologically high flow challenge, and result in an elevation in pressure within the collecting system.

In selecting a flow rate that would optimally challenge the collecting system in question, the flow rate should reflect the maximum urine output that the kidney in question is capable of generating under normal physiological conditions. By using the maximum urine output possible for the kidney studied, it would ensure that the collecting system is maximally challenged to uncover even more subtle forms of obstruction; yet the flow challenge would remain within physiological confines such that artificially elevated renal pelvic pressures can be avoided from unphysiologically high flow challenges. The maximum physiological urine output that a kidney can generate can be obtained using a calculated estimate (*individualized infusion pressure–flow study*), or can be simulated pharmacologically (*diuresis pressure–flow study*).

Individualized infusion pressure–flow study

The pioneering work in infusion pressure–flow studies was carried out by Whitaker (1978), and the initial form of pressure–flow study was referred to as the 'Whitaker test'. The collecting system was challenged with an externally generated infusion at a known flow rate. Whitaker advocated using a standard infusion rate of 10 ml/min, with the modifier that infusion rates of 2–5 ml/min could be substituted in smaller children, and that an even higher infusion rate of 15 ml/min could be used if a more aggressive flow challenge was deemed useful. Renal pelvic pressures below $10\,cmH_2O$ were interpreted as normal. Pressures $>20\,cmH_2O$ were significant for obstruction and those between 10 and $20\,cmH_2O$ pressure were considered indeterminant. While these concepts were sound in principle, there were few specific guidelines to determine what infusion rate should be used for children of a given age and body size. Further work was therefore undertaken by Fung *et al.* (1995b) in an attempt to provide more specific guidelines such that the infusion rate used would provide physiologically meaningful results.

Adhering to the principle that the infused flow rate should reflect the maximum urine output that the kidney in question is capable of generating under normal physiologic conditions, a method for calculating maximum physiological urine output was devised (Fung *et al.*, 1995b). Three patient parameters form the basis for the calculated estimate of the patient's maximum physiologic urine output: (1) body surface area; (2) age-adjusted 90th percentile GFR; and (3) the maximum percentage of the GFR that one can physiologically diurese. Both surface area (Dubois, 1935) and 90th percentile GFR (ml/min per 1.73 m²) for the patient's age (McCrory, 1972) (Fig. 20.30) can be obtained from population nomograms. Since the renal tubules proximal to the segment sensitive to

antidiuretic hormone reclaim about 80% of the water in the glomerular ultrafiltrate, under non-pathologic conditions the maximum physiologic diuresis cannot exceed approximately 20% of the GFR, even in the complete absence of antidiuretic hormone (Guyton, 1991). The calculation can be summarized as:

Maximum physiological urine output per kidney (ml/min) =

$$\frac{\underset{(m^2)}{\text{Surface area}} \times \underset{(ml/min/1.73\ m^2)}{\text{Age adjusted GFR}} \times \underset{\text{total GFR}}{20\%\ of}}{1.73m^2 \times \text{Number of kidneys}}$$

Since the pressure–flow study is applied to one kidney at a time, the flow rate employed is based on the maximum physiologic urine output per kidney, hence the correction factor 'Number of kidneys'. For a patient with a solitary kidney, compensatory hypertrophy and hyperplasia need to be taken into account. This formula is directly applicable only if the GFR of the solitary kidney has compensated to a level similar to the population-normal total GFR.

For a patient whose total GFR and differential renal function are known, maximum physiologic urine output can be derived directly with this formula. Maximum physiologic urine output for the kidney of interest would then be 20% of the measured total

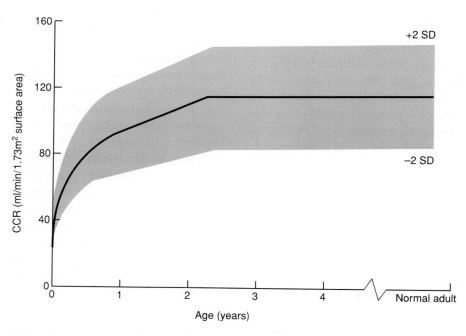

Figure 20.30 Age-adjusted glomerular filtration rate (GFR, in ml/min per 1.73 m²) nomogram (Adapted from McCrory, 1972.)

GFR (ml/min) multiplied by the differential renal function for that kidney (%):

Maximum physiological urine output per kidney (ml/min) =

$$\underset{\substack{\text{Measured GFR} \\ (\text{ml/min})}}{} \times \underset{\substack{20\% \text{ of} \\ \text{total GFR}}}{} \times \underset{\substack{\text{Differential renal} \\ \text{function (\%)}}}{}$$

When these calculations were performed for patients of different ages and body sizes, the appropriate infusion rate corresponding to the respective maximum physiologic urine output per kidney ranged from 0.85 ml/min (appropriate for a 4-week-old infant) to 16.31 ml/min (appropriate for a patient aged 18 years or older). This tremendously wide range underscores the importance of individualizing the infusion rate used for each pediatric patient (Table 20.3). As previously noted, a non-obstructed system should maintain a peak renal pelvic pressure of ≤ 14 cmH$_2$O, whereas a collecting system with significant obstruction develops a peak renal pelvic pressure of > 14 cmH$_2$O. If the renal pelvic pressure remains well below 14 cmH$_2$O at the individualized infusion rate, one can arbitrarily increase the infusion rate by 50% or 100% to challenge the collecting system drainage with a supraphysiologic flow rate to test the reserve capability of that collecting system. However, an elevated renal pelvic pressure (> 14 cmH$_2$O) in this setting is not indicative of physiocologically significant obstruction, as the supraphysiologic infusion rate represents a flow rate that exceeds the urine output that the kidney could normally provide under physiologic conditions.

These modifications from Whitaker's original descriptions form the basis for the individualized infusion pressure–flow study. It is important to note that a urethral catheter is routinely used to keep the bladder empty during all pressure–flow studies to minimize the potential of renal pelvic pressure readings being artificially affected by a full bladder.

Diuresis pressure–flow study

One study explored whether it would be possible to eliminate the need for an external infusion during the pressure–flow study, where the collecting system was instead challenged with a diuresis induced by pharmacologic means, such as the administration of intravenous furosemide. Nephrostomy access was still necessary to measure pressure, as was urethral catheterization. However, in place of an external infusion, the patient received an intravenous bolus of 15 ml/kg of a crystalloid solution followed by 1 mg/kg of furosemide to a maximum of 10 mg. Renal pelvic pressure was monitored continuously for 30 min after the furosemide administration (Fig. 20.31), and urine output was monitored every 5–10 min to ensure that an adequate diuresis had been induced. Similar to the results obtained with percutaneous infusion, a peak renal pelvic pressure of ≤ 14 cmH$_2$O was considered normal, while a peak renal pelvic pressure of > 14 cmH$_2$O was considered to indicate physiologically significant obstruction.

In order to determine if the furosemide-induced diuresis provides a sufficiently rigorous challenge to the collecting system being tested, a series of over 55 patients who received both the individualized infusion and the diuresis pressure–flow studies was analyzed. Peak renal pelvic pressures were found to be similar, agreeing in all but three cases. In these three patients, test results were either borderline positive or borderline negative, with the peak renal pelvic pressures differing by only 2–3 cmH$_2$O. From these data, furosemide-induced diuresis presents a sufficiently rigorous flow challenge to the collecting system, yielding renal pelvic pressure changes comparable to alterations induced by an individualized external infusion (Fung et al., 1995c).

In spite of tailoring infusion rates to individual needs, the individualized infusion still has the drawback that the external infusion is unphysiological. It does not account for changes in renal function, such as decreased GFR, that may limit the kidney's ability to diurese, or renal tubular dysfunction which may result in decreased concentrating ability and increased free water excretion. Furosemide-induced diuresis is more likely to reflect changes in renal functional status, as the flow challenge to the collecting system is generated from endogenous urine output as opposed to an external pump.

The diuresis pressure–flow study is also likely able to reveal the presence of physiologically significant obstruction based on our current understanding of the pathophysiology of renal obstruction. As discussed earlier in this chapter under the pathophysiology section, the congenitally hydronephrotic kidney maintains normal renal pelvic pressure under baseline conditions, and is indistinguishable from the non-obstructed kidney based on renal pelvic pressure measurements. However, the congenitally hydronephrotic kidney with ongoing significant obstruction maintains normal renal pelvic pressure not because of satisfactory drainage, but because of compensatory changes in

Table 20.3 Height, weight, and glomerular filtration rate (GFR) values are obtained from population nomograms[a]

Age (years)	Height (cm)		Weight (kg)		Surface area (m²)		GFR 90th percentile (ml/min/1.73m²)	Maximum physiological urine output per kidney (ml/min)	
	10th percentile	90th percentile	10th percentile	90th percentile	10th percentile	90th percentile		10th percentile	90th percentile
4 weeks	50.5	56.5	3.3	4.8	0.210	0.260	70	0.85	1.05
8 weeks	53.0	60.0	3.9	5.6	0.225	0.290	80	1.04	1.34
12 weeks	55.5	63.0	4.6	6.6	0.250	0.320	90	1.30	1.66
16 weeks	58.0	66.0	5.3	7.5	0.275	0.350	98	1.56	1.98
20 weeks	60.0	68.0	5.9	8.3	0.295	0.375	105	1.79	2.28
0.5	62.5	71.0	6.6	9.4	0.320	0.405	108	2.00	2.53
0.6	64.5	73.0	7.1	10.0	0.340	0.430	111	2.18	2.76
0.7	66.5	75.0	7.5	10.5	0.355	0.445	114	2.34	2.93
0.8	68.0	76.5	7.8	10.9	0.360	0.460	116	2.41	3.08
0.9	69.5	78.5	8.1	11.3	0.380	0.480	118	2.59	3.27
1	74.0	80.0	8.4	11.7	0.400	0.490	120	2.77	3.40
2	80.0	90.0	10.5	14.5	0.470	0.630	138	3.75	5.03
3	88.0	99.0	12.5	17.0	0.540	0.660	144	4.49	5.49
4	94.5	107.0	13.0	19.0	0.560	0.730	144	4.66	6.08
5	101.0	114.5	14.5	21.5	0.630	0.810	144	5.24	6.74
6	107.0	121.0	17.0	24.5	0.700	0.890	144	5.83	7.41
7	112.0	128.0	19.0	28.0	0.760	0.980	144	6.33	8.16
8	117.5	133.5	21.0	31.0	0.820	1.050	144	6.83	8.74
9	123.0	139.0	23.0	35.0	0.870	1.150	144	7.24	9.57
10	128.0	144.5	25.0	40.0	0.930	1.260	144	7.74	10.49
11	133.5	150.0	27.5	44.5	1.000	1.360	144	8.32	11.32
12	138.5	157.0	30.0	51.0	1.070	1.480	144	8.91	12.32
13	143.5	164.0	32.5	59.5	1.140	1.640	144	9.49	13.65
14	152.0	169.0	39.5	64.5	1.300	1.740	144	10.82	14.48
15	154.0	177.0	47.0	68.0	1.420	1.830	144	11.82	15.23
16	154.5	181.0	48.5	71.5	1.450	1.900	144	12.07	15.82
17	154.5	182.5	48.5	73.5	1.450	1.940	144	12.07	16.15
18	154.5	183.0	49.0	74.5	1.460	1.960	144	12.15	16.31
19	154.5	183.0	49.0	75.0	1.460	1.970	144	12.15	16.40

[a]The calculated physiologically maximum urine outputs are provided as rough guidelines for the individualized pressure–flow study infusion rates. N.B.: The maximum urine output estimates tabulated here are expressed as the infusion rate per kidney, representing half of the total calculated urine output estimate. For patients with a solitary kidney, the infusion rate may need to be increased in proportion to its compensatory increase in GFR.

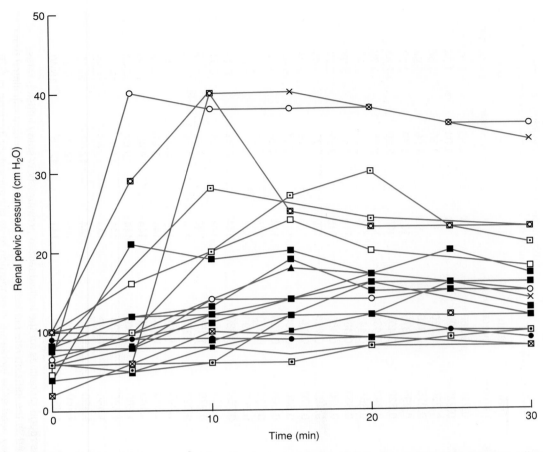

Figure 20.31 Composite graph of a representative group of patients with hydronephrosis undergoing diuresis pressure–flow studies, where renal pelvic pressure is plotted against time. Renal pelvic pressure at time 0 represents baseline pressure. Intravenous furosemide, 1 mg/kg, up to a maximum of 10 mg was given at time 0, and renal pelvic pressure was monitored for 30 min. The furosemide-induced diuresis consitutes the sole form of fluid challenge, and no infusion of fluid takes place during these studies. In the authors' experience studying over 55 hydronephrotic kidneys to date (data not all plotted in this graph in order to maintain clarity), it has been consistently observed that the prediuresis baseline renal pelvic pressures remain relatively low, and do not exceed 10 cmH$_2$O. The highest renal pelvic pressure recorded to date is 63 cmH$_2$O, observed in a patient with ureteropelvic junction (UPJ) obstruction and no evidence of contrast draining across the UPJ throughout the entire pressure–flow study.

renal blood flow and GFR. In this compensatory equilibrium the obstructed kidney has little or no reserve for handling any increase in urine flow and an elevation in renal pelvic pressure ensues upon being challenged by an induced diuresis. Furosemide-induced diuresis is therefore more than just a flow challenge to the collecting system; it is a means of 'agitating' the significantly obstructed kidney into revealing the presence of a compensatory equilibrium. Thus, a positive diuresis pressure–flow study (peak renal pelvic pressure >14 cmH$_2$O) is not merely evidence of a collecting system with an abnormally high resistance to flow, but is also an indication that the kidney being tested is in a compensatory equilibrium state in response to

physiologically significant obstruction, precariously maintaining a normal renal pelvic pressure at baseline conditions at the expense of decreased blood flow and/or GFR.

In a current series of over 55 patients, positive studies correlate with those of patients who are symptomatic or show evidence of renal functional deterioration. These correlations suggest that a positive diuresis pressure–flow study is predictive of functionally significant obstruction. Conversely, those with negative diuresis pressure–flow studies have shown no evidence of deterioration or required surgical intervention for symptomatic complaints at follow-up of 2 years (Fig. 20.32a–d).

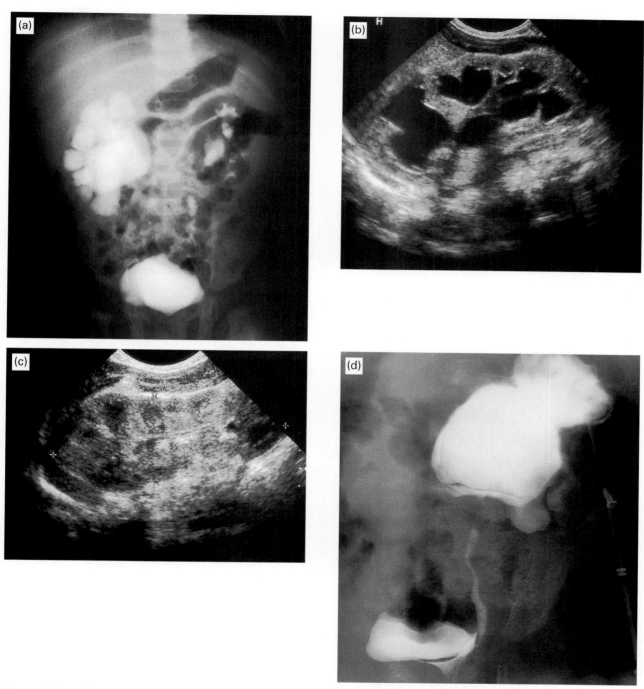

Figure 20.32 Male patient identified as having right hydronephrosis compatible with ureteropelvic junction (UPJ) obstruction, as shown by an intravenous pyelogram (*a*). Ultrasonography demonstrated marked right hydronephrosis with significant thinning of the renal cortex (*b*), and normal left kidney (*c*). A percutaneous pressure–flow study was performed when the patient was 7 weeks of age. (*d*) Right antegrade nephrostogram in the prone position. The pressure–flow study was negative for significant obstruction, where the peak renal pelvic pressure was only 5 cmH$_2$O, well below the upper limit of normal of 14 cmH$_2$O, under both furosemide-induced diuresis and a supra-physiological infusion rate of 200%. Despite significant cortical thinning and pelvicaliectasis, patient was managed with an observational approach in view of the negative pressure–flow study. From his initial right differential renal function of 30%, it spontaneously improved to 52% 1 year later, and further increased to 58% at his 2-year follow-up. It is unclear why his differential renal function increased to beyond 50%, but nevertheless the initial negative pressure–flow study appeared to be reliable in excluding significant UPJ obstruction.

Owing to its invasive nature, it is important to clarify whether the diuresis pressure–flow study reveals uniquely important diagnostic information compared with the more commonly used diuretic renogram. The protocols for the diuresis pressure–flow study and diuretic nuclear renography share the use of a urethral catheter to keep the bladder empty, the infusion of an intravenous crystalloid solution to ensure adequate patient hydration, and the administration of 1 mg/kg of intravenous furosemide to challenge the collecting system with a diuresis.

When 46 hydronephrotic kidneys were studied with both the diuresis pressure–flow study and diuretic nuclear renography, it was found that renal pelvic pressure alterations had little correlation with washout $t_{1/2}$, and that these two variables were essentially independent of each other (Fig. 20.33) (Fung *et al.*, 1995c). Some of the kidneys examined in this study showed evidence of significant obstruction with markedly increased collecting system resistance based on the diuresis pressure–flow study, yet the washout

$t_{1/2}$ was normal. Conversely, some of the kidneys examined showed no evidence of significant obstruction with normal renal pelvic pressure throughout, yet the washout $t_{1/2}$ was grossly elevated.

When basic physical principles are taken into account, however, these results should come as no surprise. Since resistance is directly proportional to pressure over flow, resistance can be assessed only if both pressure and flow parameters are simultaneously taken into account. The diuresis pressure–flow study reflects the status of pressure and flow, whereas diuretic nuclear renography does not measure pressure but provides an indicator of urine flow by the washout $t_{1/2}$. When renal pelvic pressure alterations were found to hold no correlation with washout $t_{1/2}$, it was therefore not because one test was correct and the other faulty. The differences and lack of correlation between the two were simply because the two tests measure intrinsicly different physical parameters, namely resistance to flow as reflected by the peak renal pelvic pressure of diuresis pressure–flow study, and a semi-quantitative

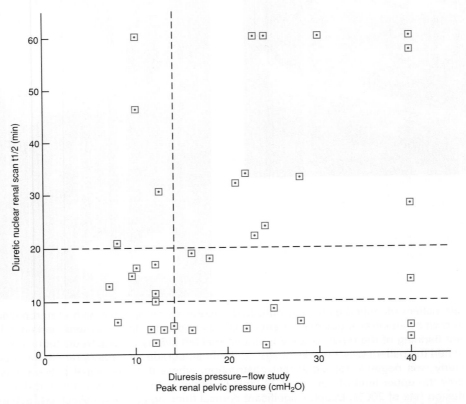

Figure 20.33 Correlation graph depicting diuretic nuclear renal scan $t_{1/2}$ against peak renal pelvic pressure recorded during diuresis pressure–flow studies. While the basic protocols of the two forms of test appear similar, including similar intravenous hydration, furosemide administration, and the use of a bladder catheter, the results of the two tests have little correlation with each other, and these two variables are essentially independent of each other.

measure of the rate of flow by the diuretic nuclear renography washout $t_{1/2}$. When the clinician utitlize these test results to determine the most appropriate course of management, it is therefore important to keep these differences in mind. Significant obstruction in hydronephrosis is fundamentally a result of abnormally high resistance to flow in the collecting system, and the diuresis pressure–flow study is more likely to delineate accurately alterations in resistance based on basic physical principles. The washout $t_{1/2}$ is a semiquantitative measure of rate of flow across the suspected site of obstruction, and should not be used as a substitute for measurements of resistance to flow in the collecting system.

A similar disparity between washout curve results and infusion pressure–flow study results was reported by Dacher *et al.* (1999). However, those that did not correlate were mostly a specific group of postoperative patients with severely dilated collecting systems. Further studies and long-term clinical follow-up will be required to clarify these differences.

At the beginning of a pressure–flow study, contrast is instilled into the renal pelvis to verify proper positioning of the nephrostomy access. Before the instillation of contrast, an equivalent volume of urine should first be aspirated, so that the baseline pressure dynamics of the renal pelvis remain unchanged. With contrast present in the renal pelvis, subsequent renal pelvic pressure changes can then be correlated with dynamic anatomic alterations seen by periodic fluoroscopic monitoring. For example, the pressure at which antegrade contrast is first seen distal to the suspected site of obstruction can be measured. This parameter is defined as the ureteral opening pressure

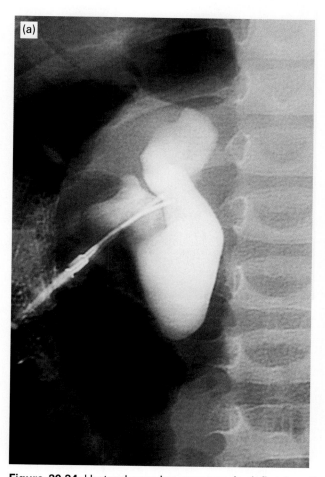
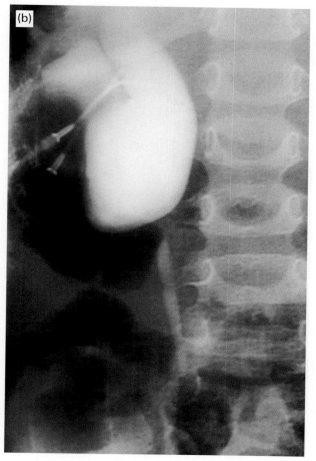

Figure 20.34 Ureteral opening pressure is defined as the pressure at which antegrade contrast is first seen distal to the suspected site of obstruction. In this 4-year-old boy with left hydronephrosis, no contrast was seen to enter the ureter (a; left antegrade nephrostogram in the prone position) until his left renal pelvic pressure reached 17 cmH$_2$O (b). His ureteral opening pressure of 17 cmH$_2$O is compatible with significant ureteropelvic junction obstruction.

(Fung *et al.*, 1998) (Fig. 20.34a, b). In a study of 52 renal units in 43 patients, positive (obstructed) ureteral opening pressures (>14 cmH$_2$O) had a 100% association with a positive individualized infusion pressure–flow study. When the ureteral opening pressure was normal (≤14 cmH$_2$O), however, it was predictive of a negative individualized infusion pressure–flow study in only 57% (Fung *et al.*, 1998).

The antegrade infusion of contrast media is also an effective tool for delineating the anatomic site of obstruction, and for assessing the portion of the ureter distal to the site of obstruction (Fig. 20.35a–d). This can serve as a useful surgical guide. Finally, fluoroscopic monitoring may be helpful in assessing patients with intermittent obstruction secondary to the kinking of the UPJ. On initial infusion, drainage may be relatively efficient. As the flow rate increases, however, the renal pelvis becomes increasingly dilated and the UPJ can be seen to be progressively displaced. This displacement of the UPJ eventually results in the kinking at the UPJ, leading to an acute, high-grade

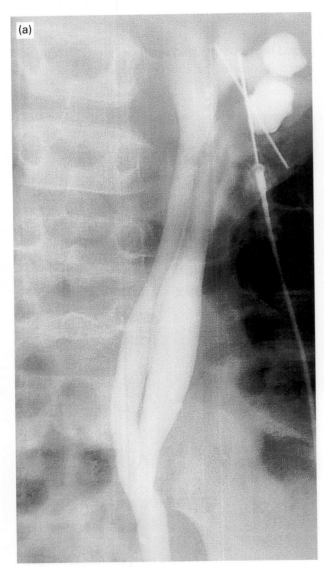

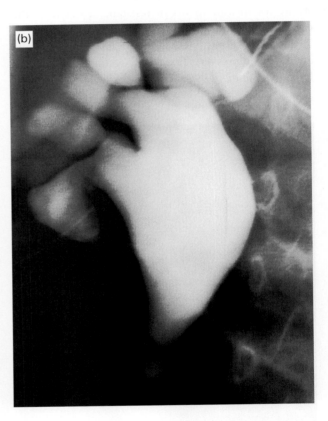

Figure 20.35 Antegrade infusion of contrast media can be an effective tool for delineating the anatomic site of obstruction. (*a*) In this 10-year-old girl, a partial ureteral duplication is well visualized with percutaneous nephrostomy access established to the lower moiety only. (*b*) Possible anomalies at the ureteropelvic junction (UPJ). *Continued opposite.*

obstruction with an elevated intrapelvic pressure. Little or no flow moves through the UPJ. With cessation of infusion or diuresis, the process eventually reverses itself. This may require drainage from the infusion catheter to speed up the decompression process. When intrapelvic volume reaches the threshold at which the UPJ kinking initially occurred, the UPJ can be seen suddenly to open up and renal pelvic pressure returns to normal (Fig. 20.36a–c). See Table 20.2 for a summary of the percutaneous pressure–flow study at the authors' institution.

Diuretic Doppler sonography and intrarenal resistive index

Diuretic Doppler sonography is a non-invasive test wherein the renal unit is stressed by a pharmacologically induced diuresis much like the diuretic pressure–flow study. Instead of monitoring renal pelvic pressure before and after the administration of furosemide, the intrarenal resistive index (RI) is measured at regular intervals during a diuretic Doppler sonography study (Fung et al., 1994). The RI is calculated based on an arterial Doppler waveform (Fig. 20.37), defined as:

$$\text{Resistive index} = \frac{\text{peak systolic velocity} - \text{end diastolic velocity}}{\text{peak systolic velocity}}$$

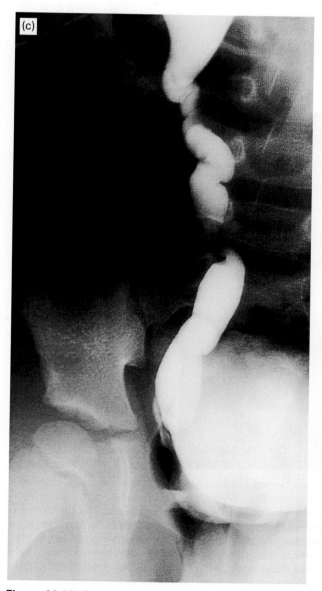

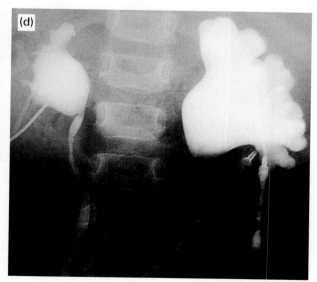

Figure 20.35 *Continued.* (*c*) Possible anomalies at the ureteropelvic junction, midureter and ureterovesical can be seen in this 5.5-year-old boy with a history of posterior urethral valves. (*d*) Bilateral percutaneous pressure–flow studies can also be performed simultaneously

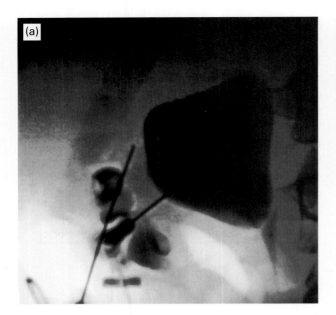

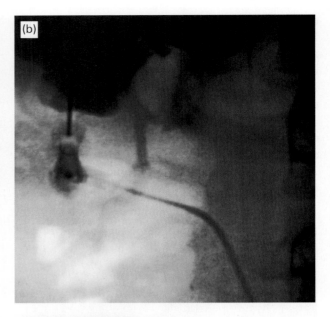

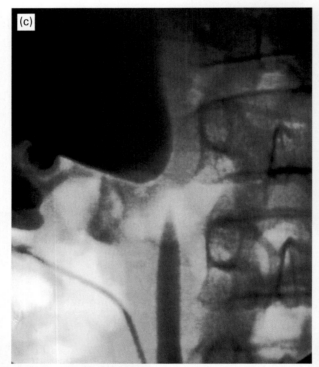

Figure 20.36 This 6-year-old girl was initially misdiagnosed as having chronic gastrointestinal disorder when she presented with recurrent abdominal pain, nausea, and vomiting. When she underwent a percutaneous pressure–flow study to evaluate her left hydronephrosis, contrast was seen to drain promptly across the uretero-pelvic junction (UPJ) into the proximal ureter early in the study (a). As the renal pelvis became progressively more distended, the drainage of contrast across the UPJ ceased entirely (b). Renal pelvic pressure continued to rise sharply, and the pressure–flow study was terminated at 40 cmH$_2$O. No drainage of contrast was seen across the UPJ until fluid was aspirated out of the renal pelvis to decompress the grossly distended collecting system. When the renal pelvis dimensions returned towards its initial baseline, drainage across the UPJ resumed with a gush of contrast into the proximal ureter (c). This pattern of intermittent high-grade obstruction was presumed to be secondary to a kink at the UPJ that was accentuated by the renal pelvis becoming overdistended. Her recurrent abdominal pain, nausea, and vomiting episodes (Dietl's crisis) were successfully corrected by a dismembered pyeloplasty.

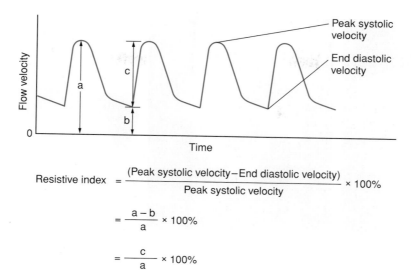

Resistive index $= \dfrac{(\text{Peak systolic velocity} - \text{End diastolic velocity})}{\text{Peak systolic velocity}} \times 100\%$

$= \dfrac{a - b}{a} \times 100\%$

$= \dfrac{c}{a} \times 100\%$

Figure 20.37 Schematic depiction of a typical intrarenal arterial waveform. Parameters and formula used for calculating intrarenal resistive index (RI) are shown. (After Fung *et al.* 1994.)

RI is a measure of arterial resistance (Arima *et al.*, 1979), usually expressed as a percentage. Intrarenal RIs are generally recorded at the arcuate or interlobar arteries (Platt, 1992).

Initial enthusiasm for using intrarenal RI to assess hydronephrosis stemmed from the observation that obstructed kidneys tend to be associated with elevated intrarenal RI (Rodgers *et al.*, 1992). As obstructed kidneys are well documented eventually to develop a compensatory decrease in renal blood flow, it seemed promising that intrarenal RI might reflect this important physiologic compensation. Kidneys that developed acutely rising renal pelvic pressure were observed to also develop a progressive increase in intrarenal RI (Fung *et al.*, 1994). This positive correlation suggested the possibility that instead of monitoring renal pelvic pressure during a relatively invasive diuresis pressure–flow study, intrarenal RI could be monitored non-invasively (Fig. 20.38).

However, when using pressure–flow study results in 30 patients as the standard, no discernible pattern emerged from the diuretic Doppler sonography studies. The reproducibility of any given RI reading was found to be poor, with widely variable measurements from one reading to the next (Fung *et al.*, 1995a).

Urinary markers

The use of urinary markers for the diagnosis of significant renal obstruction is an attractive idea. The test would be non-invasive, requiring only a urine sample to perform. By choosing a specific biochemical marker with proven physiologic associations, the presence of the marker can be used as an indicator of a physiologically significant obstructive process. Various urinary biochemical markers have been evaluated for the diagnosis of significant obstruction, including NAG (Carr *et al.*, 1994), insulin-like growth factor (Cain *et al.*, 1997), and TGF-β_1) (Furness *et al.*, 1999). Urinary electrolytes are also used as an indicator of fetal renal functional status. While some of these markers seem promising, none has been fully validated to be sufficiently sensitive and specific in the diagnosis of physiologically significant obstruction (Furness *et al.*, 1999).

Surgery on the ureteropelvic junction

Introduction to pyeloplasty

The various reconstructive procedures for relieving UPJ obstruction, termed pyeloplasty, follow one of two general principles, either using a flap or by dismembering the UPJ. Flap pyeloplasties enlarge the UPJ by the insertion of tissue from the renal pelvis, while continuity between the ureter and renal pelvis is maintained. Dismembered pyeloplasties involve excision of the obstructing segment. The normal upper ureter is anastomosed to a dependent portion of the renal pelvis. The choice between these two types of procedures depends on the anatomy of the renal

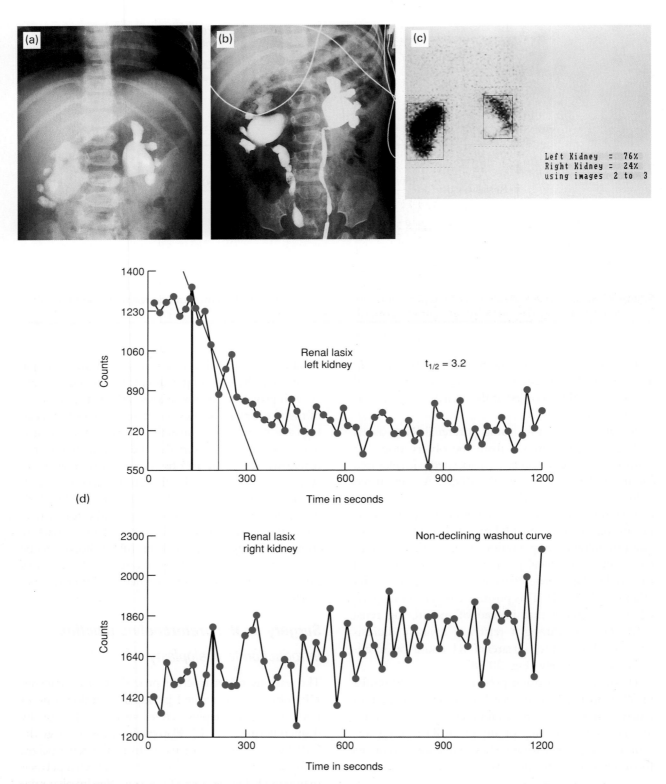

Figure 20.38 This male infant was diagnosed antenatally to have bilateral hydronephrosis. Configuation of the collecting systems are as shown by IVP at 5 min (*a*), and by bilateral retrograde pyelography (*b*). The right kidney had a differential renal function of 24% (*c*), and demonstrated a non-declining washout curve on furosemide nuclear renal scan (*d*) compatible with high grade obstruction. The left kidney had a differential renal function of 76% (*c*) and $t_{1/2}$ of 3.2 min (*d*) compatible with normal non-obstructive drainage. *Continued opposite.*

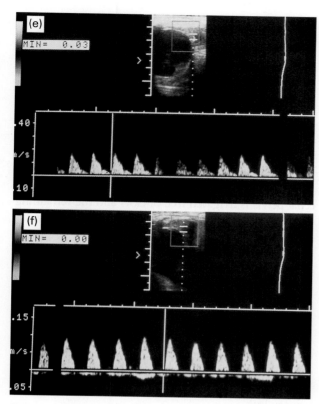

Figure 20.38 *Continued.* Resistive index (RI) of the right kidney was 0.82 (82%) (*e*) at baseline, but rose to 1.00 (100%) with a complete cessation of diastolic flow after the administration of furosemide (*f*).

This dramatic increase in RI is presumably due to the furosemide-induced diuresis causing an increase in renal arterial blood flow as reflected by the elevation in RI. While this case illustrates how changes in RI can non-invasively reflect important alterations in a hydronephrotic kidney with significant obstruction, we subsequently found that there are tremendous variabilities in RI measurements. This poor reproducibility of RI measurements renders it unsuitable for reliably distinguishing non-obstructed from significantly obstructed hydronephrotic kidneys.

pelvis and intraoperative findings. Success rates for procedures suitably chosen and performed range between 95% and virtually 100% (Hendren *et al.*, 1980; Sheldon *et al.*, 1992; Rushton *et al.*, 1994; Austin *et al.*, 2000), with failures primarily due to fibrosis and restenosis of the anastomosis. Re-stenosis of the UPJ is thought to be secondary to urinary extravasation, poor tissue handling and trauma, and/or tissue ischemia.

In order to achieve consistently excellent results, certain principles must be adhered to, regardless of the type of repair chosen. Tissue handling must be atraumatic and the anastomosis must be tension free and dependent. Periureteral vasculature in the adventitia and periadventitial spaces should be preserved to maintain a generous blood supply to the tissue. A watertight closure and good drainage of urine reduce the risk of subsequent fibrosis. This may require an indwelling double pigtail stent or a nephroureteral stent (e.g. KISS stent, Cook Urological Incorporated, Spencer, IN), where the drainage lumen is designed as a trough, rather than with side holes, to minimize the potential for blockage (Ward *et al.*, 1998). A bladder catheter can also be used in the immediate postoperative period to help further reduce the risk of urine leak, particulary in the presence of ipsilateral reflux. In addition, drainage of the perirenal space allows egress of urine from the area around the anastomosis.

An extraperitoneal flank incision allows excellent access to the upper ureter and renal pelvis. A dorsal lumbotomy approach may be used if the anatomy is not complicated. If bilateral UPJ obstructions need repair, these can be performed sequentially or simultaneously. Two separate incisions, dorsal or flank, or a single transperitoneal incision may be used. An oblique subcostal incision extending from the tip of the 12th rib to the lateral rectus border provides good exposure. Electrocautery to divide the muscle layers in the line of the incision minimizes blood loss. The 12th intercostal nerve is carefully preserved and retracted inferiorly. The transversus muscle fibers are separated by blunt dissection after incising the lumbodorsal fascia. The peritoneum extends further posteriorly in infants and children than in adults. Therefore, the Gerota's fascia is opened in the most posterior aspect of the wound after sweeping the peritoneum medially, to avoid an inadvertent peritoneotomy.

The lower pole of the kidney then comes into view. Using a combination of blunt and sharp dissection, the UPJ, distal renal pelvis, and upper ureter are mobilized and cleared of surrounding fat. The upper pole need not be freed completely. The pelvis usually appears as a tense cystic mass. The ureter is on the inferior or medial aspect of the pelvis. Holding sutures are placed on the ureter, 2–3 cm below the UPJ, as well as the renal pelvis, inferiorly and superiorly, approximately 1 cm from the parenchyma. By manipulating these sutures, the anatomy can be fully evaluated to help to decide on a suitable type of tension-free repair.

Dismembered pyeloplasty (Anderson–Hynes)

This type of pyeloplasty can be used for the repair of most UPJ obstructions (Figs. 20.39, 20.40). Once the decision to perform a dismembered procedure has been made, the ureter is transected obliquely proximal to the ureteral stay suture. The medial portion of the redundant renal pelvis is excised with the UPJ, by dividing the pelvis between the stay sutures. Beginning inferiorly, a sweeping cut with a scissors produces a uniform border. The lip on the inferior aspect provides the apex for a dependent ureteral anastomosis. The ureter is spatulated slightly along its lateral border to increase the area of the anastomosis which is accomplished with 5-0 or 6-0 interrupted absorbable sutures with the knots on the outside. The first suture approximates the dependent tongue of renal pelvis to the apex of the spatulated ureter. If there is any tension at the anastomosis, the ureter needs to be further mobilized distally until there is sufficient length to relieve tension. If needed, the kidney can also be further mobilized for eventual inferior nephropexy. However, these maneuvers are seldom necessary.

If a stent is placed, this is done after completion of the back wall of the anastomosis. A double-pigtail stent remains entirely indwelling, while the proximal portion of a nephroureteral stent can be brought out through the parenchyma of the lower pole. To ensure that the distal end of a double-pigtail stent is appropriately positioned in the bladder, as opposed to curling up in the ureter, methylene blue can be instilled into the bladder. In the absence of VUR, reflux of the blue-tinged solution to the renal pelvic via the double-pigtail stent confirms that the distal end of the stent has reached the bladder lumen. However, if the child has pre-existing ipsilateral VUR, this test is unreliable. An abdominal X-ray can be obtained in this case to verify that the distal end of the double-pigtail stent is appropriately curled up in the bladder lumen. Failure to position the distal end of a double-pigtail stent into the bladder can significantly complicate subsequent attempts at cystoscopic stent removal.

After completing the ureteral approximation the renal pelvis is irrigated free of clots and the remaining opening at the superior aspect of the renal pelvis is closed with a running absorbable suture. A drain should be placed over the anastomosis and the incision closed in layers. Postoperative drainage after a watertight anastomosis usually stops in 2–3 days. If it continues beyond 10–14 days the drain should be removed as it may serve as a wick promoting drainage. If drainage then persists placement of a double-pigtail ureteral stent should be instituted. Occasionally, a percutaneous nephrostomy tube may be required to facilitate healing at the site of the urinary leak.

Flap procedures

Y–V (Foley) plasty

This technique is best suited for a high insertion of the ureter into the pelvis or for a small extrarenal pelvis, when resection of excess tissue is not required. A dependent portion of the pelvis is rotated inferiorly as

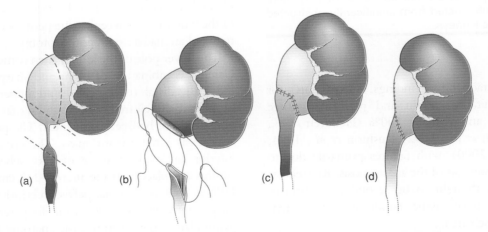

(a)   (b)   (c)   (d)

Figure 20.39 Dismembered pyeloplasty. (*a*) Two alternatives: pelvis may be reduced in size or not. (*b, c*) anastomosis without reduction pyeloplasty or (*d*) with reduction pyeloplasty.

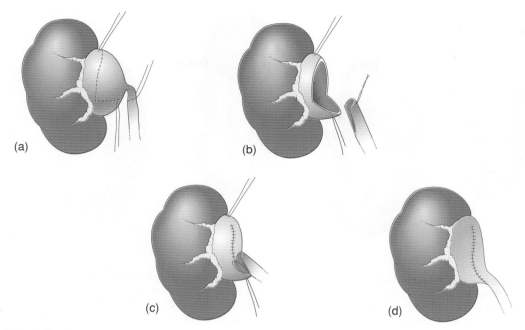

(a)

(b)

(c)

(d)

Figure 20.40 The Hynes–Anderson renal plastic operation. The ureteric catheter is inserted while the lower angle is negotiated in order to prevent both walls from being picked up by the needle.

a simple flap (Figs. 20.41, 20.42). The limbs of the Y are widely separated, one on the anterior and one on the posterior aspect of the renal pelvis. The laterally based portion of the pelvis then drops inferiorly. The lateral border of the ureter is opened longitudinally through the UPJ for at least 1 cm beyond the obstruction into normal ureter (the stem of the Y). The midpoint or apex of the pelvic flap is sutured to the inferior apex of the ureterotomy, converting the incision to a V. The two limbs are then approximated with interrupted sutures as previously described.

Spiral (Culp) flap and vertical (Scardino–Prince) flaps

The spiral and vertical flap pyeloplasties are useful when long, narrow ureteral segments are encountered below the UPJ. This type of obstruction is unusual in children, in whom a second ureteral stricture below the UPJ is uncommon. The length of the spiral flap (Fig. 20.43) is limited only by the size of the dilated pelvis. The flap should be as broad as possible at the base, as much as 2 cm, tapering slightly towards the tip. A flap based medially in a dependent position

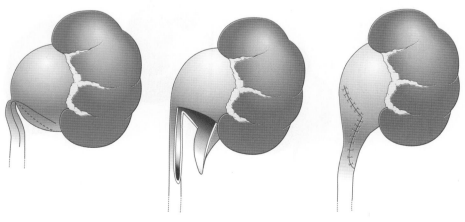

Figure 20.41 Foley Y-V plasty.

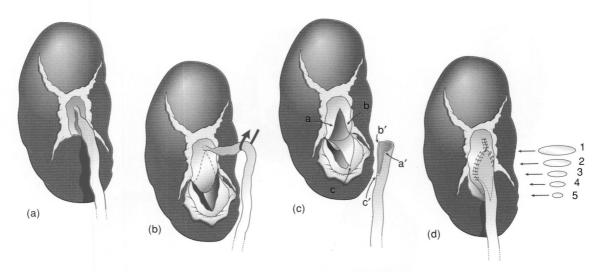

Figure 20.42 Variation of dismembered Foley Y-V-plasty technique for high insertion of a small stenotic ureter in a large but intrarenal pelvis. (*a*) A small renal hilum but large intrarenal pelvis with ureteral stenosis that requires resection. (In cases of extreme ureteral stenosis, it is often not practical to maintain ureteropelvic continuity.) (*b*) Resection of renal parenchyma to expose sufficient pelvis for the flap. The ureter is severed distal to the stenosis. (*c*) Formation of the pelvic flap. Resection of the stenotic ureteral segment with spatulation of the ureter. Approximate a–a', b–b', and c–c' to produce a satisfactory dependent, funneled ureteropelvic segment. (*d*) Anastomosis is completed. Nos. 1–5 illustrate the progressive caliber of the lumen from the pelvis to the ureter through the newly formed ureteropelvic segment. (Adapted from Schaeffer and Grayhack, 1986, with permission.)

near the UPJ can be conveniently extended distally through the stenotic ureter. The spiral flap is especially advantageous when the angle between the ureter and the dependent renal pelvis is greater than 90°. The vertical flap (Fig. 20.44) is used to bridge shorter distances when the angle is 90° or smaller and in cases of high insertion of the ureter.

In flap repairs, the first incision is made in the inferior medial aspect of the posterior renal pelvis and extended through the UPJ to a point 1 cm below the obstruction. A flap is then outlined that will reach the distal ureterotomy without tension. The spiral flap is derived circumferentially from the dilated pelvis, while the vertical flap comes from the anterior or posterior aspect only. To assure vascularity, the length of the flap should be no greater than three times the width of the base. The orientation of the blood vessels on the pelvis should be taken into consideration

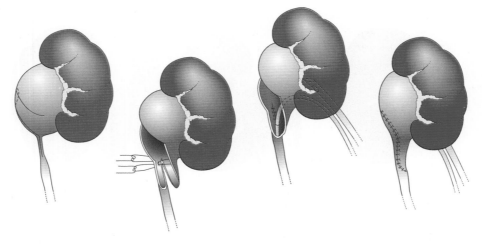

Figure 20.43 Spiral flap.

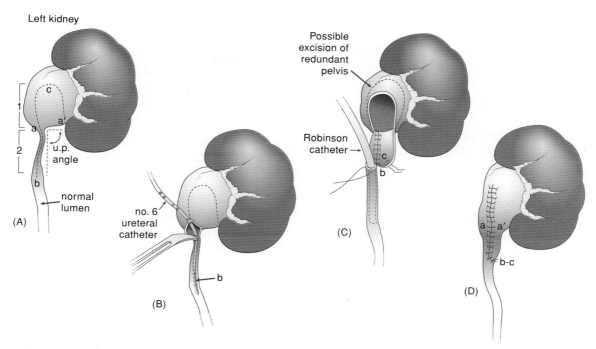

Figure 20.44 Technique of Scardino–Prince vertical flap pyelureteroplasty. (A) This technique is used when the ureteropelvic angle is approximately 90 degrees. (1) The length of the proposed pelvic flap should adequately traverse (2) the segment of ureteral obstruction. The medial and lateral margins at the base of the pelvic flap are (a–a'); (b) is the lower angle of the ureterotomy; (c) is the rounded tip of the pelvic flap. (B) A pyelotomy incision is made in the lower pelvis along the medial border of the proposed pelvic flap incision. A no. 6 ureteral catheter is passed down the ureter. The tip of a hooked blade knife is buried in its wall and, using the catheter as a sliding guide, a clean, precise ureterotomy incision is made. If the stenotic ureteral segment is longer than the available pelvic flap, a Davis intubated ureterotomy operation may be combined with this procedure. If stenting and diversion are required, their selection and placement should be made at this time. (C) A 0000 fixation and retention suture is placed well within the ureteral wall at the lower angle of the ureterotomy. A wide-based pelvic flap is fashioned with sharp plastic scissors, taking care not to 'saw tooth' its margins. The tip of the flap (C) should be rounded to ensure a good blood supply. If necessary, take a somewhat larger flap than needed (wider base). It can always be tailored for excellent approximation. At the time of the incision, a 0000 orientation and traction suture is placed deeply in the tissue at the tip of flap. This ensures accurate subsequent orientation. At times the tip can become distorted by irregular tissue contraction. Equal-margin, interrupted suturing is started at the base of the medial margin of the flap and the lateral ureteral margin and continued down to approximate points (b) and (c). When suturing the pelvic flap to the spatulated ureteral ribbon, an assistant should gently wipe the surface so the mucosal margins can be clearly seen for accurate approximation. (It is difficult to determine the margins of blood-stained mucosa.) Absorbable 5–0 or 6–0 suture should be used.

The ureter is distended to its normal caliber with a Robinson catheter. The tip of the flap is now carefully folded and fitted into the lower angle of the ureterotomy. This is the most vital part of the funnel. At this point, the surgeon should be certain that the ureteral mucosa is engaged with the needle. When working around a catheter this vital layer of the ureteral wall can be easily missed and the tip of the flap may be inadvertently sutured to the outer layers of the ureter. (D) Any redundant pelvis may be excised. The anterior margins are closed, approximating b–c and a–a'. The pelvis and new ureteropeolvic funnel are reconstituted. (Adapted from Schaeffer and Grayhack, 1986, with permission.)

when planning the flap, preserving as many blood vessels as possible. Once the ureter is opened longitudinally, the flap is rotated alongside the open ureter and anastomosed edge to edge, with interrupted sutures at the apex, and running or interrupted sutures along the edges. The proximal or superior edges are positioned first, so that the excess portion of the distal flap can be discarded. After completion of the anastomosis, a drain is positioned near the suture line, within Gerota's fascia, before wound closure.

Ureterocalycostomy

In a ureterocalycostomy, the proximal ureter is anastomosed to a dependent lower pole calyx instead of the renal pelvis (Fig. 20.45). This procedure is generally reserved for situations where dependent renal drainage cannot be established using conventional anastomosis to the renal pelvis, including the horseshoe kidney (Fig. 20.46), repair of a failed pyeloplasty, and other conditions where the renal pelvis is extensively scarred or small in size (Figs. 20.47, 20.48). To gain access to the dependent lower pole calyx, amputation of a portion of the lower pole of the renal parenchyma is necessary. This procedure is therefore best suited for kidneys with a large, dilated lower pole calyx with overlying parenchymal thinning.

Amputation of the lower pole cortex is essential for the success of a ureterocalycostomy. Sufficient cortex must be removed to protect the proximal ureter from entrapment by fibrosis of the remaining renal cortical edge (Hawthorne *et al.*, 1976). The calyx also must be partially mobilized to create a tension-free, mucosa-to-mucosa anastomosis (Flashner and King, 1992). As in any other ureteral procedures, the ureter must be handled with care to minimize tissue trauma, with its adventitia and longitudinal blood supply preserved. At the end of the repair, the anastomosis must be tension free, and there should be no renal cortex remaining at or below the level of the repair.

Available adjacent tissue such as redundant renal capsule, omentum or perinephric fat can be used to cover the repair to minimize postoperative scarring of the repair to the adjacent structures. Stenting of the anastomosis with a double-pigtail stent or nephroureteral stent is advisable and a drain should be used.

Minimally invasive techniques

The benefits of endourologic and laparoscopic techniques for UPJ reconstruction are not as well established in the pediatric population as in adults. Open pyeloplasty is successful, with low morbidity. Furthermore, instrumentation for endourologic procedures is limited for small children. Hence, reported experience has not been extensive. King *et al.* (1984a) reported the initial experience of endoscopic ureteral stricture treatment in children. Other small series have shown success rates of 67–100% with antegrade and retrograde approaches to the UPJ (Cilento and Kaplan, 1998). This is an area that will undoubtedly be further developed in the future.

When considering endourologic intervention, important factors include age, presence of primary or secondary obstruction, degree of hydronephrosis, presence of crossing vessels and the overall and differential renal function (Figenshau and Clayman, 1998). Neonates and infants are not suitable candidates for endourologic intervention owing to difficulty in

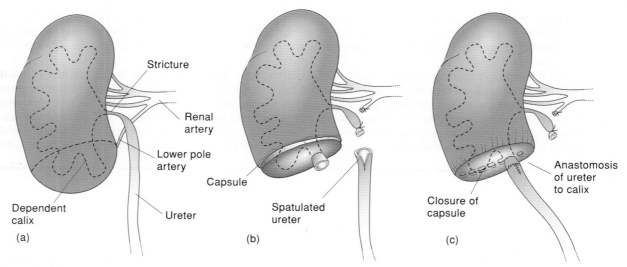

Figure 20.45 Ureterocalycostomy of a kidney with normal parenchyma. Lower pole arterial supply is ligated (*a*), the lower pole is resected (*b*), and anastomosis to the most dependent calyx is accomplished (*c*).

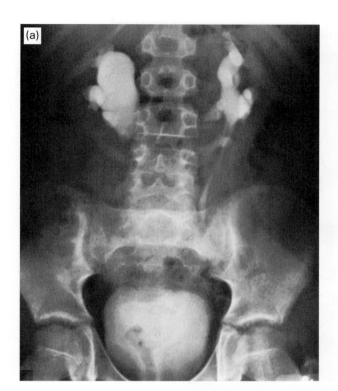

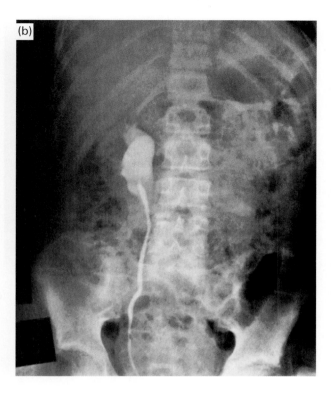

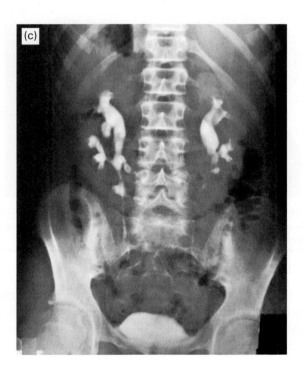

Figure 20.46 Horseshoe kidney with right ureteropelvic obstruction. (*a*) Preoperative excretory urogram. (*b*) Retrograde urogram. High insertion of the ureter into the pelvis. (*c*) Postoperative excretory urogram. Ureterocalycostomy.

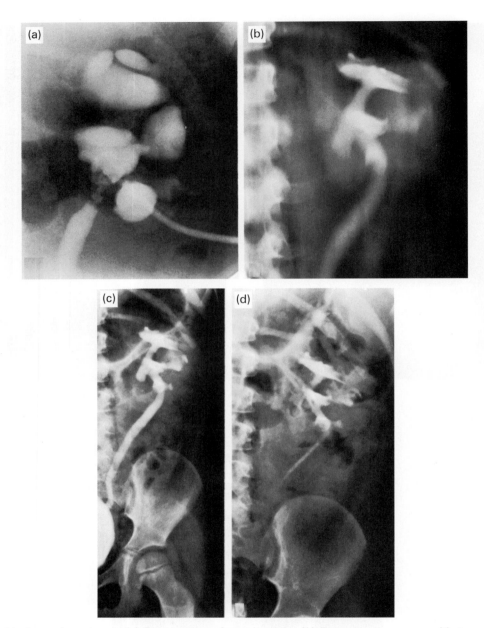

Figure 20.47 Ureterocalycostomy. (*a*) Destruction of renal pelvis. (*b*) Excretory urogram with tomograms clearly shows lower pole partial nephrectomy and ureterocalyceal anastomosis. (*c*) Same patient, 3 months postoperatively. (*d*) Same patient, 9 months postoperatively.

gaining endoscopic control of the UPJ, the need for fluoroscopy with radiation exposure to the spine and abdominal organs, and the possible need for multiple anesthetics. With increasing age, especially in adolescence, the anatomy and caliber more closely resemble the adult and are more suited to endoscopic approaches. In the adolescent patient with mild to moderate hydronephrosis, no evidence of a crossing vessel and split renal function > 25%, endopyeloto-

my has been recommended by Figenshau and Clayman (1998). Children with secondary UPJ obstruction appear to have a better outcome with endopyelotomy compared with those performed for the repair of primary obstruction. The postulated anatomic reason is that after a previous open pyeloplasty, only a short band of tissue at the UPJ remains stenotic and this is likely to be amenable to endoscopic incision.

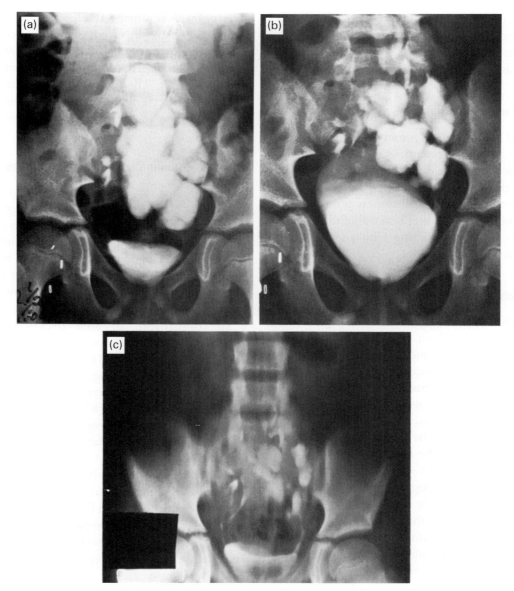

Figure 20.48 Pelvic fused kidney with left ureteropelvic obstruction. (*a*) Preoperative excretory urogram; (*b)* uretero-calycostomy, early postoperative urogram; (*c*) final result at 1 year, postoperative excretory urogram.

Antegrade endopyelotomy

Antegrade endopyelotomy is performed by first obtaining control of the UPJ. The patient is placed prone with legs split on spreader bars while a retrograde pyelogram facilitates percutaneous access through the flank. An appropriately directed incision of the UPJ is achieved under fluoroscopic control. This can be done using the Acucise balloon cutting device (Applied Urology, Laguna Hills, CA, USA) as advocated by Figenshau *et al*. (1996). The incision is performed under fluoroscopy with the Acucise device, provided the caliber of the ureter is adequate (10 Fr). The balloon is positioned across the narrowed segment with the cutting wire directed laterally. The incision in secondary UPJ obstruction can be directed by CT findings to avoid cutting into renal vessels. An indwelling double-pigtail stent (4.8–7 Fr) is placed across the UPJ under direct vision from the renal collecting system into the bladder. A nephrostomy tube is left in place for 2 days.

If the Acucise device cannot be positioned, an antegrade incision may be made with a 2 Fr fine-tipped, right-angle Greenwald electrosurgical probe (Figenshau and Clayman, 1998).

Retrograde endopyelotomy

This method is better suited for an older child or adolescent. The incision is essentially similar to the one described above with the Acucise device, but the procedure is performed entirely in a retrograde manner, with the patient in the dorsal lithotomy position. The patient can be discharged after removal of the bladder catheter the following morning with an indwelling internal ureteral stent.

Balloon dilation and rupture

The retrograde approach can also be used to dilate the UPJ narrowing, without an incision. The balloon is placed across the UPJ and dilated to rupture the UPJ, followed by stent placement. This can be performed on an outpatient basis or with an overnight stay. Of the procedures available, including open pyeloplasty, endopyelotomy, and laparoscopic pyeloplasty, balloon rupture of the UPJ is perhaps the least physiologic procedure. The tissue disruption is uncontrolled and the success of the procedure relies entirely on secondary healing of the UPJ. The results of primary balloon rupture have not been encouraging. Other more successful options are available. Balloon dilation in the treatment of UPJ obstruction is at best limited to opening an obstructed (edematous) anastomosis within several months of an initial repair.

All the above procedures require stent placement and, in children, a brief anesthetic for cystoscopic stent removal 3–6 weeks postoperatively.

Laparoscopic pyeloplasty

The laparoscopic method of pyeloplasty, both dismembered and Y-V-plasty, has been described in adults. Adaptations such as the 'Fenger-plasty' as advocated by Janetschek *et al.* involve transverse closure of a longitudinal incision in a Heineke–Mikulicz fashion with minimal suturing (Chen *et al.*, 1998). These are technically demanding procedures despite advances in suturing techniques, such as the Endo-stitch device (US Surgical Corp, Norwalk, CT, USA).

The primary advantage is early recovery. Reported experiences have involved small numbers of adult patients and even fewer children (Peters *et al.*, 1995; Tan and Roberts, 1996), but no long-term results are available as yet. The present authors' institution has successfully performed laparoscopic dismembered pyeloplasty by a retroperitoneal approach (Fig. 20.49).

Results of minimally invasive techniques

In their extended review of published results of endoscopic approaches to the UPJ, Figenshau and Clayman (1998) found that balloon dilation had only moderate success. In four recent series with a total of 49 patients, the age range was 1 month to 12 years. Forty were for primary obstruction and the overall success rate was 63% at a mean follow-up of 23 months.

In comparison, an 86% overall success was reported for endopyelotomy in eight series with a total of 86 patients (84 done by an antegrade approach). The ages ranged from 2 months to 19 years with a mean follow-up of 32 months. Of these patients, 42 of 51 (81%) had a successful outcome with endopyelotomy as their primary treatment. When used secondarily, 32 of 35 (91%) were successful.

The only series of laparoscopic pyeloplasties to date examined 18 patients (Tan and Roberts, 1996). The age of the patients ranged from 3 months to 15 years (median 17 months). Two procedures failed and one patient is still pending postoperative evaluation. A success rate of 87% was reported.

Infundibular stenosis

Embryology and etiology

Infundibular stenosis is a condition where one or more renal infundibulum is stenotic, resulting in the dilatation of the calyces proximal to the corresponding stenotic infundibula. It can affect renal infundibula in isolation, or it may occur with the concomitant stenosis of the renal pelvis and UPJ (Fig. 20.50). The combined abnormality of infundibular and pelvic stenosis represents the more severe form of the disorder, referred to as infundibulopelvic stenosis. These conditions are a spectrum of anomalies. The stenotic segment can be isolated to a single calyx, affect multi-

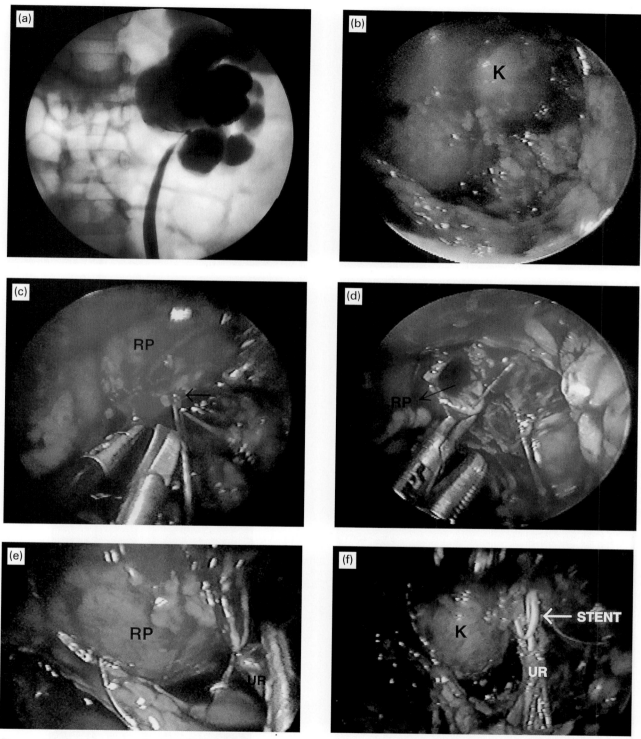

Figure 20.49 Laparoscopic pyeloplasty using retroperitoneal approach is performed in this 3-year-old male. Retrograde pyelography (*a*) demonstrates left hydronephrosis with a lateral insertion of the UPJ. (*b*) Laparoscopy of the retroperitoneal space within Gerota's fascia showed the kidney (labeled 'K'). (*c*) A cut was made into the renal pelvis (RP) and a gush of urine can be seen (*arrow*). (*d*) The UPJ was dismembered, resulting in the visible lumen of the renal pelvis. (*e*) The spatulated apex of the ureter (UR) was sewn with resorable suture to the dependent portion of the renal pelvis, with the use of a vertical renal pelvis flap for increasing its dependency. (*f*) The back-wall of the anastomosis was completed, and a double-pigtail ureteric stent was inserted. (*g*)–(*l*) *Shown overleaf.*

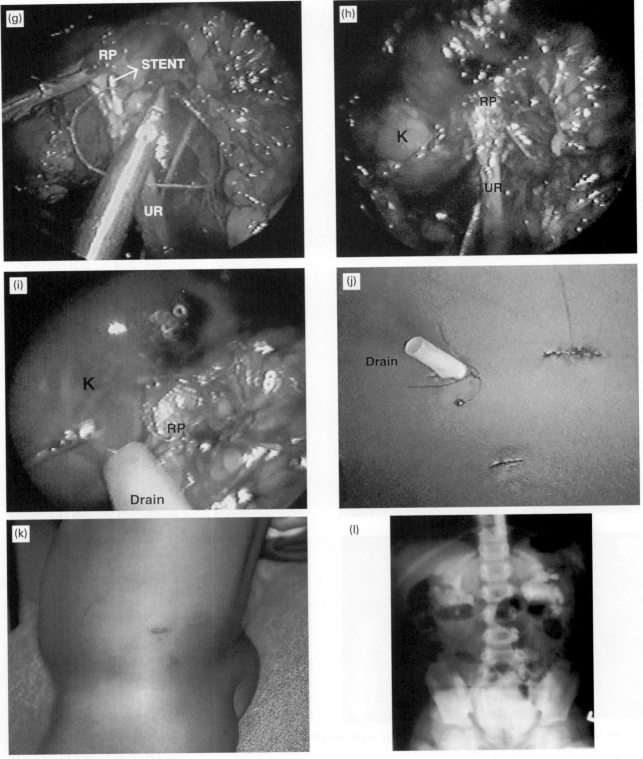

Figure 20.49 *Continued.* (*g*) The front wall of the anastomosis is closed using a running suture. (*h*) The completed anastomosis. (*i*) A penrose drain was placed, exiting one of the three laparoscopic ports (*j*). (*k*) Incisions are well healed by his 6-week follow-up visit. (*l*) Postoperative IVP at 3 months demonstrated a successful pyeloplasty, with a decrease in left collecting system dilation, and contrast was visualized in the distal ureter by the 10 min film.

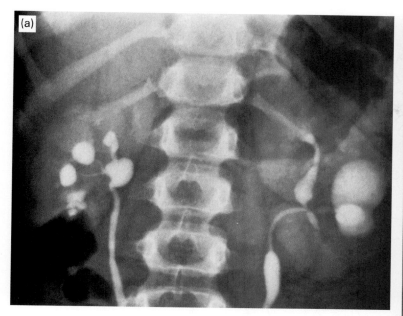

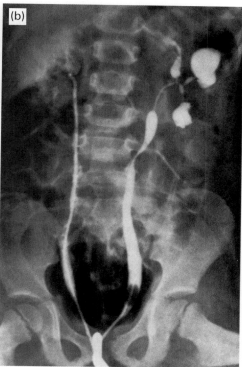

Figure 20.50 Hydrocalycosis and infundibulopelvic stenosis in a 3-year-old boy with bilateral ectopic ureteral orifices (at bladder neck) and other congenital anomalies who presented with urinary infection. The patient remained uninfected on chronic prophylaxis. There were no urographic changes for 5 years. (*a*) Excretory urogram. Right infundibular and left infundibulopelvic stenosis. (*b*) Retrograde ureteropyelogram (bilateral). Mildly dilated left ureter. Note the diffuse tubular backflow on the right.

ple calices, involve the renal pelvis, or even occur bilaterally. When bilateral, the kidneys are generally affected asymmetrically, with infundibular stenosis on one side and infundibulopelvic stenosis on the other (Elder, 1992).

Infundibular stenosis is thought to result from a defect in the timing of the dichotomous branching of the ureteral bud, which in turn leads to interrrupted, premature, or delayed union with the metanephric blastema (Fig. 20.51). The defect occurs early or late. A defect early in the ureteral bud branching process would logically affect the renal pelvis, whereas a later defect may affect only the infundibula. When the junction of the ureteric bud and the metanephric blastema occurs at an anomalous time, the metanephric blastema may lose its potential for normal development. This may then result in abnormal segmental division, hypoplastic development of infundibula and/or pelvis, and cystic dilatation proximal to the hypoplastic stenotic segments (Kelalis and Malek, 1981).

Pathophysiology and clinical considerations

Infundibular or infundibulopelvic stenoses are uncommon disoders. Lucaya *et al.* (1984) reported three affected children out of 11 500 excretory urograms performed over 17 years. Most commonly, the condition is noted following evaluation of the patient with UTI. It may also be identified in association with gross hematuria, polyuria, urethral valves, and UPJ obstruction. There is also a high incidence of associated multiple congenital anomalies involving other organ systems.

More broadly, infundibular stenosis and infundibulopelvic stenosis are part of a spectrum of obstructive renal disease referred to as infundibulopelvic dysgenesis (Boyce and Whitehurst, 1976; Kelalis and Malek, 1981; Uhlenhuth *et al.*, 1990). This concept is supported by the findings of a high incidence of bilateral disease, and its frequent association with contralateral obstruction or multicystic dysplastic kidneys. In this

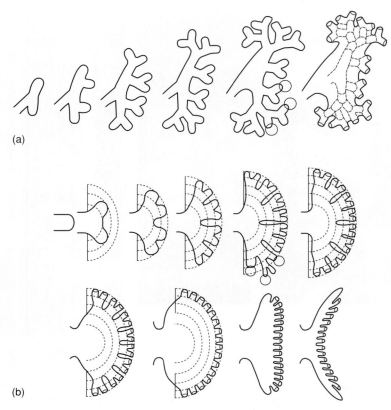

Figure 20.51 (a) Dichotomous branchings of the ureteral bud and dilatation to form the pelvis. Circles indicate possible sites of infundibula between the third, fourth, or fifth generation in the next series of branchings and expansions that give rise to the minor calyces. (b) Development of minor calyx and papillae (*upper row*). Repeated dichotomous branchings for several further generations with resorption of septa form the minor calyx. Circles indicate the generation at which the branch may remain unexpanded, forming a papillary duct. *Lower row*: multiplication and growth of nephrons in the parenchyma cause inversion of the calyx and the papillae. (Adapted from Potter, 1972, with permission.)

spectrum, caliceal diverticula and UPJ obstruction can perhaps be considered as focal forms of this disorder (Fig. 20.52).

Because of its infrequent occurrence, little is known about the exact pathophysiology specific to infundibular stenosis. It can be considered to be within the same spectrum of disorders as UPJ obstruction, sharing the same upstream effects of collecting system dilatation proximal to the level of obstruction. One would anticipate that infundibular stenosis follows a pathophysiologic process similar to that of UPJ obstruction. The same concerns for renal functional deterioration with associated sequelae therefore apply, with the exception that infundibular stenosis can be segmental and the amount of renal parenchyma at risk is proportionally less. While diagnostic modalities used to assess hydronephrosis can also be used in the evaluation of infundibular stenosis, customized localization and special attention to the interpretation of results are required.

Management

There are limited data on the natural history of the disorder, but the combined series of Kelalis and Malek (1981), Malek *et al*. (1975), and Lucaya *et al*. (1984) suggest that the disorder tends to be stable and nonprogressive. Surgical correction therefore appears unnecessary in the majority. Patients with recurrent UTIs should be placed on long-term antibacterial prophylaxis. Periodic long-term follow-up should be initiated to monitor renal function. In the event of functional compromise or subsequent functional deterioration, infundibular reconstruction can be considered.

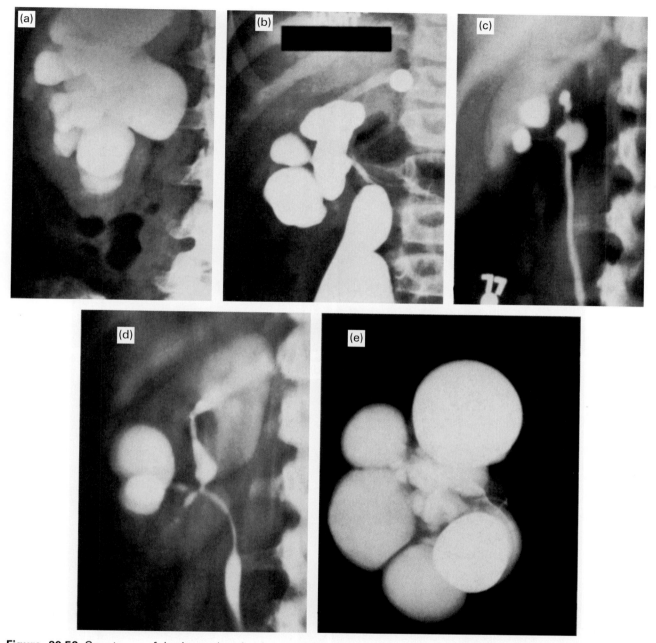

Figure 20.52 Spectrum of hydronephrosis due to (*a*) ureteropelvic junction obstruction; (*b*) pelvic stenosis; (*c*) infundibular stenosis; (*d*) infundibulopelvic stenosis; and (*e*) multicystic dysplastic kidney. (*a*, *b*, and *e* from Kelalis and Malek, 1981, with permission.)

Owing to the rarity and diverse anatomic variations of the disorder, such reconstruction needs to be customized to each patient (Figs. 20.53, 20.54). Principles followed in designing the most appropriate surgical reconstruction are similar to the repair of UPJ obstruction, ureterocalicostomy (Kelalis and Malek, 1981), and the caliceal and infundibuloplasties (cal-iceal anastomosis or calyorrhaphy) (Rocca-Rossetti, 1984), not unlike those performed in the setting of anatrophic nephrolithotomies. In cases where only a small renal segment is affected with otherwise normal renal status, partial nephrectomy is an appropriate option for symptomatic disease. However, renal preserving surgery is generally preferred.

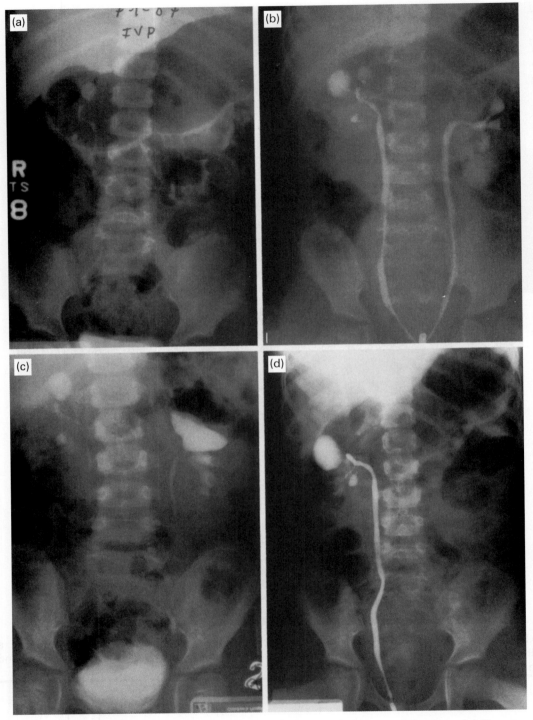

Figure 20.53 The patient is a 2-year-old girl with recurrent febrile urinary tract infections. (*a*) Excretory urogram demonstrates infundibular stenosis involving the upper and lower poles of the right kidney. The left kidney is poorly visualized. (*b*) Bilateral retrograde pyelograms demonstrate the third obstructed calyx in the right kidney and nonvisualization of the obstructed calyx in the left upper pole. The patient underwent left calycopyelostomy. (*c*) One year later, the urogram demonstrates progression of caliectasis in the upper pole of the right kidney and functioning upper pole of the left kidney. Further febrile urinary tract infections subsequently developed. (*d*) With the patient at 5 years of age, the right retrograde pyelogram demonstrates progressive caliectasis of the middle calyx and nonvisualization of the upper pole calyx due to progressive infundibular stenosis. (Courtesy of Ellen Shapiro, MD.)

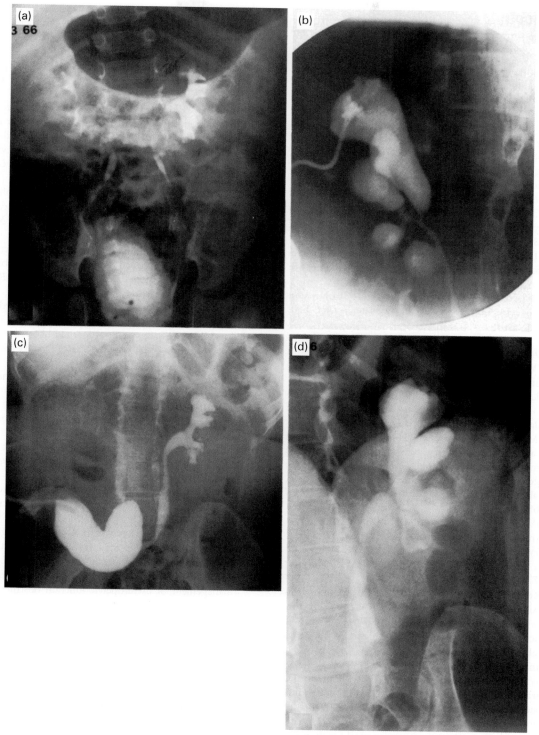

Figure 20.54 The patient is a girl born with myelodysplasia. (*a*) With the patient at 1 year of age, the excretory urogram demonstrates a normal upper urinary tract. The child subsequently underwent ileal conduit because of incontinence. Seventeen years later, a right antegrade nephrostogram (*b*) through the pigtail catheter demonstrates infundibulopelvic stenosis. (*c*) A loopogram demonstrates a normal left kidney. Reconstructive surgery on the right kidney was unsuccessful, and the patient subsequently underwent right nephrectomy. Three years later, a recurrent left pyelonephritis and renal calculi developed. (*d*) The urogram demonstrates severe left infundibulopelvic stenosis and a lower pole calculus.

References

Allen T (1970) Congenital ureteral strictures. *J Urol* **104**: 196.

Aperia A, Borkerger O, Wikstad I *et al.* (1977) Renal growth and function in patients nephrectomized in childhood. *Acta Paediatr Scand* **66**: 185–92.

Arima M, Ishibashi M, Usami M *et al.* (1979) Analysis of the arterial blood flow patterns of normal and allografted kidneys by the directional ultrasonic Doppler technique. *J Urol* **122**: 587.

Aschinberg LC, Koskimies O, Bernstein J *et al.* (1978) The influence of age on the response to renal parenchymal loss. *Yale J Biol Med* **51**: 341–5.

Austin P, Cain M, Rink R (2000) Nephrostomy tube drainage with pyeloplasty: is it necessarily a bad choice? *J Urol* **163**: 1528–30.

Belman AB (1991) Ureteropelvic junction obstruction as a cause for intermittant abdominal pain in children. *Pedr* **88**: 1066–69.

Bernstein GT, Mandell J, Lebowitz RL *et al.* (1988) Ureteropelvic junction obstruction in the neonate. *J Urol* **140**: 1216–21.

Birnholz J (1983) Determination of fetal sex. *N Engl J Med* **309**: 942.

Boyce W, Whitehurst E (1976) Hypoplasia of the major renal conduits. *J Urol* **116**: 352.

Brandell RA, Brock JW III, Hamilton BD *et al.* (1996) Unilateral hydronephrosis in infants: are measurements of contralateral renal length useful? *J Urol* **156**: 188–9.

Brenner BM, Meyer TW, Hostetter TH (1982) Dietary protein intake and the progressive nature of kidney disease: the role of hemodynamically mediated glomerular injury in the pathogenesis of progressive glomerular sclerosis in aging, renal ablation, and intrinsic renal disease. *N Engl J Med* **307**: 652–9.

Brenner BM, Troy JL, Daugharty TM (1972) Pressures in cortical structures of the rat kidney. *Am J Physiol* **222**: 246.

Brenner BM, Lawler EV, MacKenzie HS (1996) The hyperfiltration theory: a paradigm shift in nephrology. *Kidney Int* **49**: 1774–7.

Cain M, Regan T, Mordkin R *et al.* (1997) Alteration in urinary insulin-like growth factor following ureteral obstruction: a potential tool for quantifying acute and chronic obstructive renal injury. American Academy of Pediatrics Annual Meeting (Abstract) 47. New Orleans, LA, November 1, 1997, pp. 109–110.

Capolicchio G, Jednak R, Ding L *et al.* (1999a) Supranormal renographic differential renal function in congenital hydronephrosis: fact, not artifact. *J Urol* **161**: 1290–4.

Capolicchio G, Leonard MP, Wong C *et al.* (1999b) Prenatal diagnosis of hydronephrosis: impact on renal function and its recovery after pyeloplasty. *J Urol* **162**: 1029–32.

Carr M, Peters C, Retik A *et al.* (1994) Urinary levels of renal tubular enzyme N-acetyl-beta-D-glucosaminidase in unilateral obstructive uropathy. *J Urol* **151**: 442.

Chen RN, Moore RG, Kavoussi LR (1998) Laparocopic pyeloplasty: indications, technique and long-term outcome. *Urol Clin North Am* **25**: 323–30.

Chertin B, Fridmans A, Knizhnik M *et al.* (1999) Does early detection of ureteropelvic junction obstruction improve surgical outcome in terms of renal function? *J Urol* **162**: 1037–40.

Chevalier R, Campbell F, Brenbridge A (1984) Nephrosonography and renal scintigraphy in evaluation of new-born with renomegaly. *Urology* **24**: 96.

Cilento BG, Kaplan GW (1998) Ureteropelvic junction obstruction. In: King LR (ed.) *Urologic surgery in infants and children*. Philadelphia, PA: WB Saunders, 18–30.

Cockrell S, Hendren W (1990) The importance of visualizing the ureter before performing a pyeloplasty. *J Urol* **144**: 588–92.

Conway JJ (1992) 'Well tempered' diuresis renography: its historical development, physiological and technical pitfalls and standardized technique protocol. *Semin Nucl Med* **22**: 74.

Dacher J, Pfister C, Thoumas D *et al.* (1999) Shortcomings of diuresis scintigraphy in evaluating urinary obstruction: comparison with pressure flow studies. *Pediatr Radiol* **29**: 742–7.

Dejter SW, Eggli DF, Gibbons DM (1988) Delayed management of neonatal hydronephrosis. *J Urol* **140**: 1305–9.

Dhillon HK (1998) Prenatally diagnosed hydronephrosis: the Great Ormond Street experience. *Br J Urol* **81** (Suppl): **81**: 39.

Dicker SE, Shirley DG (1973) Compensatory renal growth after unilateral nephrectomy in the new-born rat. *J Physiol* **228**: 193–202.

Dubois EF (1935) *Basal metabolism in health and disease*. Philadelphia, PA: Lea & Febiger.

Elder JS (1992) Obstruction: the calyx. In: Kelalis PP, King LR, Belman AB (eds) *Clinical pediatric urology*. Philadelphia, PA: WB Saunders, 683–93.

Ferrer F, McKenna P, Bauer M *et al.* (1997) Accuracy of renal ultrasound measurements for predicting actual kidney size. *J Urol* **157**: 2278–81.

Fichtner J, Boineau FG, Lewy JE *et al.* (1994) Congenital unilateral hydronephrosis in a rat model: continuous renal pelvic and bladder pressures. *J Urol* **152**: 652–7.

Figenshau RS, Clayman RV (1998) Endourologic options for management of ureteropelvic junction obstruction in the pediatric patient. *Urol Clin North Am* **25**: 199–209.

Figenshau SR, Clayman RV, Colberg JW *et al.* (1996) Pediatric endopyelotomy: the Washington University experience. *J Urol* **156**: 2025–30.

Flashner SC, King LR (1992) Ureteropelvic junction. In: Kelalis PP, King LR, Belman AB (eds) *Clinical pediatric urology*. Philadelphia, PA: WB Saunders, pp. 693–725.

Foote J, Blennerhassett J, Wiglesworth F *et al.* (1970) Observations on the ureteropelvic junction. *J Urol* **104**: 252.

Fung LCT, Atala A (1996) Elevation in renal pelvic pressure induces renal apoptotic cell death in a non-obstructive procine model. *J Urol* **155** (Suppl): 314A.

Fung LCT, Atala A (1998) Constant elevation in renal pelvic pressure induces an increase in urinary N-acetyl-beta-D-glucosaminidase in a non-obstructive porcine model. *J Urol* **159**: 212–16.

Fung LCT, Peters CA (1995) Partial unilateral ureteral obstruction in the fetal sheep is associated with a high rate of contralateral apoptotic cell death. American Academy of Pediatrics 1995 Annual Meeting, Abstract. San Francisco, CA, October 15, 1995, **64**: 118–19.

Fung LCT, Steckler RE, Khoury AE et al. (1994) Intrarenal resistive index correlates with renal pelvis pressure. *J Urol* **152**: 607.

Fung LCT, Connolly BL, Chait PG et al. (1995a) Diuretic Doppler sonography: intrarenal resistive index correlates with renal pelvic pressure but with limited reproducibility. American Academy of Pediatrics Annual Meeting, Urology Section Abstract. San Francisco, CA, October 15, 1995, **73**: 129–30.

Fung LCT, Khoury AE, McLorie GA et al. (1995b) Evaluation of pediatric hydronephrosis using individualized pressure–flow criteria. *J Urol* **154**: 671–6.

Fung LCT, Khoury AE, McLorie GA et al. (1995c) Evaluation of renal pelvic pressure changes during diuresis in pediatric hydronephrosis. *J Urol* **153** (Suppl): 377A.

Fung LCT, McLorie GA, Khoury AE et al. (1995d) Contradictory supranormal nuclear renographic differential renal function: Fact or artifact? *J Urol* **154**: 667–70.

Fung LCT, Freeman MR, Atala A (1996) Renal apoptotic cell death induced by acute renal pelvic pressure elevation is associated with up-regulation of medullary VEGF and down-regulation of cortical VEGF. *Am Acad Pediatr* **89** (Suppl): 630.

Fung LCT, Churchill BM, McLorie GA et al. (1998) Ureteral opening pressure: a novel parameter for the evaluation of pediatric hydronephrosis. *J Urol* **159**: 1326–30.

Furness PD, Maizels M, Han SW et al. (1999) Elevated bladder urine concentration of transforming growth factor-β1 correlates with upper urinary tract obstruction in children. *J Urol* **162**: 1033–6.

Glick P, Harrison M, Adzick N et al. (1983) Correction of congenital hydronephrosis *in utero*. III: Early mid-trimester ureteral obstruction produces renal dysplasia. *J Pediatr Surg* **18**: 681.

Glick P, Harrison M, Golbus M et al. (1985) Management of the fetus with congenital hydronephrosis. II: Prognostic criteria and selection for treatment. *J Pediatr Surg* **20**: 376.

Gosling J, Dixon J (1978) Functional obstruction of the ureter and renal pelvis: a histological and electron microscopic study. *Br J Urol* **50**: 145.

Grignon A, Filion R, Filiatrault D et al. (1980) Urinary tract dilatation *in utero*: classification and clinical applications. *Radiology* **160**: 645–7.

Grossman I, Cromie W, Wein A et al. (1981) Renal hypertension secondary to ureteropelvic junction obstruction: unusual presentation and new therapeutic Modality. *Urology* **17**: 69.

Gulmi F, Matthews G, Marion D et al. (1995) Volume expansion enhances the recovery of renal function and prolongs the diuresis and natriuresis after release of bilateral ureteral obstruction: a possible role for atrial natriuretic Peptide. *J Urol* **153**: 1276–83.

Gulmi FA, Felsen D, Vaughan ED Jr (1998) Pathophysiology of urinary tract obstruction. In: Walsh PC, Retik AB, Vaughan ED Jr, Wein AJ (eds) *Campbell's urology*. Philadelphia, PA: WB Saunders, 342–85.

Guyton AC (1991) *Textbook of medical physiology*. Toronto: WB Saunders, 286–97.

Hanna M (1978) Some observations on congenital uretero-pelvic junction obstruction. *Urology* **12**: 151.

Hawthorne N, Zincke H, Kelalis P (1976) Ureterocalicostomy: an alternative to nephrectomy. *J Urol* **115**: 583.

Hendren W, Radhakrishnan J, Middleton A Jr (1980) Pediatric pyeloplasty. *J Pediatr Surg* **15**: 133–44.

Heyman S (1989) An update of radionuclide renal studies in pediatrics. In: *Nuclear medicine annual 1989*. (eds) Freeman LM and Weissmann HS, New York: Raven Press, pp. 179–224.

Hinman F (1923) Renal counterbalance: an experimental and clinical study with reference to the significance of disuse atrophy. *J Urol* **9**: 239–314.

Hobbins J, Romero R, Brannum P et al. (1984) Antenatal diagnosis of renal anomalies with ultrasound I. *Am J Obstet Gynecol* **148**: 868.

Holwill MEJ, Silvester NR (1973) *Introduction to biological physics*. New York: John Wiley & Sons, 59–87.

Hostetter TH, Olson JL, Rennke HG et al. (1981) Hyperfiltration in remnant nephrons: a potentially adverse response to renal ablation. *Am J Physiol* **241**: F85–F93.

Johnston J, Evans J, Glassberg K et al. (1977) Pelvic hydronephrosis in children: a review of 219 personal cases. *J Urol* **117**: 97.

Kass EJ, Fink-Bennett D (1990) Contemporary techniques for the radioisotopic evaluation of the dilated urinary tract. *Urol Clin North Am* **17**: 273–89.

Kaufman JM, Siegel NJ, Hayslett JP (1975) Functional and hemodynamic adaptation to progressive renal ablation. *Circ Res* **36**: 286–93.

Kelalis P, Malek R (1981) Infundibulopelvic stenosis. *J Urol* **125**: 568.

Kim KM, Kogan BA, Massas CA (1991) Collagen and elastin in the obstructed fetal bladder. *J Urol* **146**: 528.

Kim JS, Chung HY, Hee KR et al. (1999) Does the split renal function on DTPA renal scan represent endogenous creatinine clearance ratio in the obstruction of upper urinary tract? *J Urol* **161** (Suppl): 197.

King LR, Coughlin P, Ford K et al. (1984a) Initial experiences with percutaneous and transurethral ablation of postoperative ureteral strictures in children. *J Urol* **131**: 1167–70.

King LR, Coughlin PW, Bloch EC et al. (1984b) The case for immediate pyeloplasty in the neonate with ureteropelvic junction obstruction. *J Urol* **132**: 725–8.

King MA, Narayanan M, Bohyer C et al. (1998) Count-based quantitation of functional renal volume by SPECT imaging. *IEEE Trans Nucl Sci* **45**: 2189–94.

Koff S (1981) Diagnosis of obstruction in experimental hydroureteronephrosis. *Urology* **17**: 570.

Koff SA, Campbell K (1992) Nonoperative management of unilateral neonatal hydronephrosis. *J Urol* **148**: 525–531.

Koff SA, Campbell KD (1994) The nonoperative management of unilateral neonatal hydronephrosis: natural history of poorly functioning kidneys. *J Urol* **152**: 593–5.

Koff SA, Peller PA (1995) Diagnostic criteria for assessing obstruction in the newborn with unilateral hydronephrosis using the renal growth – renal function chart. *J Urol* **154**: 662–6.

Koff SA, Peller PA, Young DC et al. (1994) The assessment of obstruction in the newborn with unilateral hydronephrosis by measuring the size of the opposite kidney. *J Urol* **152**: 596–9.

Larsson L, Aperia A, Wilton P (1980) Effect of normal development on compensatory renal growth. *Kidney Int* **18**: 29–35.

Laufer I, Griscom N (1971) Compensatory renal hypertrophy: absence *in utero* and development in early life. *Am J Roentgenol* **113**: 464–7.

Lawson TL, Foley WD, Li B et al. (1981) Ultrasonic evaluation of fetal kidneys: analysis of normal size and frequency of visualization as related to stage of pregnancy. *Radiology* **138**: 153.

Levitt S, Lutzker L (1976) Urine extravasation secondary to upper urinary tract obstruction. *J Pediatr Surg* **11**: 575.

Lucaya J, Enriquez G, Delgado R et al. (1984) Infundibulo-pelvic stenosis in children. *Am J Roentgenol* **142**: 471.

McAleer IM, Kaplan GW (1999) Renal function before and after pyeloplasty: does it improve? *J Urol* **162**: 1041–4.

McCrory WW (1972) *Developmental nephrology*. Cambridge, MA: Harvard University Press, 79–100.

McCrory WW (1980) Regulation of renal functional development. *Urol Clin North Am* **7**: 243–64.

McCrory W, Shibuya M, Leumann E et al. (1971) Studies of renal function in children with chronic hydronephrosis. *Pediatr Clin North Am* **18**: 445–65.

MacKenzie HS, Brenner BM (1995) Fewer nephrons at birth: a missing link in the etiology of essential hypertension? *Am J Kidney Dis* **26**: 91–8.

MacNeily AE, Maizels M, Kaplan WE et al. (1993) Does early pyeloplasty really avert loss of renal function? A retrospective review. *J Urol* **150**: 769.

Maizels M, Reisman ME, Flom LS et al. (1992) Grading nephroureteral dilatation detected in the first year of life: correlation with obstruction. *J Urol* **148**: 609–14.

Majd M, Rushton HG (1992) Renal cortical scintigraphy in the diagnosis of acute pyelonephritis. *Semin Nucl Med* **22**: 98–111.

Malek R, Aguilo J, Hattery R (1975) Radiolucent filling defects of the renal pelvis: classification and report of unusual cases. *J Urol* **114**: 508.

Mandell J, Blyth BR, Peters CA et al. (1991) Structural genitourinary defects detected *in utero*. *Radiology* **178**: 193–6.

Manning F, Hill L, Platt L (1981) Qualitative amniotic fluid volume determination by ultrasound: antepartum detection of intrauterine growth retardation. *Am J Obstet Gynecol* **139**: 254.

Mayor G, Genton N, Torrado A et al. (1975) Renal function in obstructive nephropathy: long-term effect of reconstructive surgery. *Pediatrics* **56**: 740–7.

Meyer TW, Anderson S, Rennke HB et al. (1987) Reversing glomerular hypertension stabilizes established glomerular injury. *Kidney Int* **31**: 752–9.

Moody T, Vaughan EJ, Gillenwater J (1975) Relationship between renal blood flow and ureteral pressure during 18 hours of total unilateral ureteral occlusion. *Invest Urol* **13**: 246–51.

Munoz A, Pascual Y, Baralt J et al. (1977) Arterial hypertension in infants with hydronephrosis: report of six cases. *Am J Dis Child* **131**: 38.

Murnaghan G (1958) The dynamics of the renal pelvis and ureter with reference to congenital hydronephrosis. *J Urol* **30**: 321.

Palmer LS, Maizels M, Cartwright PC et al. (1998) Surgery versus observation for managing obstructive grade 3 to 4 unilateral hydronephrosis: a report from the Society for Fetal Urology. *J Urol* **159**: 222–8.

Perlmutter AD, Kroovand LR, Lai Y-W (1980) Management of ureteropelvic obstruction in the first year of life. *J Urol* **123**: 535–7.

Peters CA, Lebowitz R, Bauer SB et al. (1987) Renal functional outcomes in prenatally diagnosed severe unilateral ureteropelvic junction obstruction: a prospective study abstract. Section on Urology, American Academy of Pediatricians, 1997 Annual Meeting, San Francisco, CA, 17 October 1987, 67–68.

Peters CA, Carr MC, Lais A et al. (1992a) The fetal kidney: an ovine model of partial ureteral obstruction. *J Urol* **147**: 224A.

Peters CA, Carr MC, Lais A et al. (1992b) The response of the fetal kidney to obstruction. *J Urol* **148**: 503.

Peters CA, Schlussel RN, Retik AB (1995) Pediatric laparoscopic dismembered pyeloplasty. *J Urol* **153**: 1962–5.

Platt J (1992) Duplex Doppler evaluation of native kidney dysfunction: obstructive and nonobstructive disease. *Am J Roentgenol* **158**: 1035.

Potter EL (1972) *Normal and abnormal development of the kidney*. Chicago, IL: Year Book Medical Publishers, 15.

Ransley P, Dhillon H, Gordon I et al. (1990) The postnatal management of hydronephrosis diagnosed by prenatal ultrasound. *J Urol* **144**: 584–7.

Reddy PP, Mandell J (1998) Prenatal diagnosis: therapeutic implications. *Urol Clin North Am* **25**: 171–80.

Rocca-Rossetti S (1984) Reconstructive operations on the intra-renal collecting system. In: Wickham J (ed.) *Intra-renal surgery*. London: Churchill Livingstone, 260.

Rodgers P, Bates J, Irving H (1992) Intrarenal Doppler ultrasound studies in normal and acutely obstructed kidneys. *Br J Rad* **65**: 207.

Roth DR, Gonzales ET (1983) Management of ureteropelvic junction obstruction in infants. *J Urol* **129**: 108–10.

Ruano-Gil D, Coca-Payeras A, Tejedo-Maten A (1975) Obstruction and normal recanalization of the ureter in the human embryo: its relation to congenital ureteric obstruction. *Eur Urol* **1**: 287.

Rushton H, Salem Y, Belman A et al. (1994) Pediatric pyeloplasty: is routine retrograde pyelography necessary? *J Urol* **152**: 604–6.

Salem YH, Majd M, Rushton HG et al. (1995) Outcome analysis of pediatric pyeloplasty as a function of patient age, presentation and differential renal function. *J Urol* **154**: 1889.

Schaeffer AJ, Grayhack JT (1986) Surgical management of ureteropelvic junction obstruction. In: Walsh PC *et al.* (eds) *Campbell's urology*: 5th ed. London, WB Saunders.

Sheldon C, Duckett J, Snyder H (1992) Evolution in the management of infant pyeloplasty. *J Pediatr Surg* **27**: 501–5.

Shirley DG (1976) Developmental and compensatory renal growth in the guinea pig. *Biol Neonate* **30**: 169.

Shore RM, Koff SA, Mentser M *et al.* (1984) Glomerular filtration rate in children: determination from the Tc-99m-DTPA renogram. *Radiology* **151**: 627–33.

Snyder HM, Lebowitz RL, Colodny AH *et al.* (1980) Ureteropelvic junction obstruction in children. *Urol Clin North Am* **7**: 273–90.

Society for Fetal Urology (1992) The 'well tempered' diuretic renogram: a standard method to examine the asymptomatic neonate with hydronephrosis or hydroureteronephrosis. A report from combined meetings of the Society for Fetal Urology and members of the Pediatric Nuclear Medicine Council – The Society of Nuclear Medicine. *J Nucl Med* **33**: 2047–51.

Society for Fetal Urology (1998) A grading schema for infant hydronephrosis. Workshop of Society for Fetal Urology, Boston, MA 1988 (Unpublished proceedings).

Steckler RE, McLorie GA, Jayanthi VR *et al.* (1994) Contradictory supranormal differential renal function during nuclear renographic investigation of hydroureteronephrosis. *J Urol* **152**: 600–3.

Stephens J, Sherman S (1983) Determination of fetal sex by ultrasound. *N Engl J Med* **309**: 984.

Tan H, Roberts J (1996) Laparoscopic dismembered pyeloplasty in children: preliminary results. *Br J Urol* **77**: 909–13.

Tanagho EA (1995) Embryology of the genitourinary system. In: Tanagno EA, McAninch JW (eds) *Smith's general urology*. Norwalk, CT: Appleton & Lange, 17–30.

Thomas D (1990) Fetal uropathy. *Br J Urol* **66**: 225–31.

Thomas I, Smith D (1974) Oligohydramnios, cause of non-renal features of Potter's syndrome, including pulmonary hypoplasia. *J Pediatr* **84**: 811.

Uhlenhuth E, Amin M, Harty J *et al.* (1990) Infundibulopelvic dysgenesis: a spectrum of obstructive renal disease. *Urology* **35**: 334.

Wacksman J (1991) Pyeloplasty. In Glenn JF (ed.) *Urologic surgery*, 4th ed. Philadelphia, PA: JB Lippincott.

Ward MA, Kay R, Ross JH (1998) Ureteropelvic junction obstruction in children: unique considerations for open operative intervention. *Urol Clin North Am* **25**: 211–17.

Whitaker RH (1978) Clinical assessment of pelvis and ureteral function. *Urology* **12**: 146–50.

Multicystic dysplastic kidney

21

John S. Wiener

Introduction

Multicystic dysplastic kidney (MCDK) was recognized by Harley (1864), but most credit Schwartz (1936) with the first true description of the disorder. His initial observations of MCDK remain accurate: 'The outline of the kidney is extremely irregular due to the presence of many cysts varying in size from that of a pea to that of a hen's egg, which are held together like a bunch of grapes by some loose connective tissue.' He described the *classic type* of MCDK; however, there exists a second, rarer form of MCDK known as the *hydronephrotic type*. This latter type can present a diagnostic dilemma since it resembles severe hydronephrosis secondary to ureteropelvic junction (UPJ) obstruction.

Spence (1955) convincingly showed that MCDK was typically a benign unilateral disorder and was distinct from other renal cystic diseases. Despite the similarity in names, multicystic dysplastic kidney disease must never be confused with polycystic kidney disease, a disorder of both kidneys that leads to progressive renal failure. Pathologic examination of polycystic kidneys reveals normal cortex riddled with tiny cysts, whereas, in the multicystic kidney, the cortex is completely replaced with small to large cysts. Likewise, multilocular cysts and simple cortical cysts are completely different entities involving reniform kidneys with normal parenchyma.

Incidence

MCDK is the most common type of renal cystic disease and renal dysplasia in infants. Prior to the era of routine prenatal sonography, MCDK was usually noted only when palpable since patients were rarely symptomatic. Routine fetal sonography has made it possible to detect these kidneys even when they are non-palpable and more closely estimate the true incidence of the disease. Abnormalities of the urinary tract are the most commonly detected fetal anomalies, and MCDK may represent up to 10% of fetal uropathies.(Avni *et al.*, 1986). A review of prenatally-detected urologic anomalies by Gordon *et al.* (1988) has been most often quoted for placing the incidence of unilateral MCDK at 1 in 4300 livebirths. However, MCDK probably becomes more apparent as gestation progresses, so sonography early in pregnancy can miss cases and underestimate the true incidence. A more recent review based on routine fetal sonography revised the estimated incidence of MCDK to 1 in 2400 livebirths (Liebeschuetz and Thomas, 1997). As an aside, only a single case of true unilateral renal agenesis was noted in over 33 000 fetuses, an incidence far less than that quoted for unilateral renal agenesis in adult autopsy series (1 in 1070). The authors hypothesized that many adults with a solitary kidney represent involution of a MCDK rather than true unilateral renal agenesis.

The laterality of MCDK varies among studies. In determining the incidence of bilateral MCDK based on prenatal sonography, Rickwood *et al.* (1992) noted one of 22 cases of MCDK (4.5%) to be bilateral, whereas Gordon *et al.* (1988) found two bilateral cases out of 12 (16.7%) fetuses with MCDK. Of unilateral cases, the left kidney is more commonly affected in most, but not all, large series (Rottenberg *et al.*, 1997; Wacksman, 1998).

Males appear to be more commonly affected with MCDK. In the National Multicystic Kidney Registry in the USA, 56% of affected children are males (Wacksman, 1998). A large review from Great Britain noted that males comprise 73% of MCDK patients (Rickwood *et al.*, 1992).

Pathology

Accurately named, MCDK is characterized by the replacement of normal renal tissue by multiple cysts of varying sizes separated by scant amounts of dysplastic parenchyma. The gross anatomy of the classic type of MCDK was well described by Schwartz's initial report (Schwartz, 1936). In addition, he found the proximal ureter to be atretic. Analysis of the cyst fluid showed 'large amounts of urea,' suggesting that urine production had been present in the kidney at some point. Felson and Cussen (1975) reported four cases of MCDK with small peripheral 'cysts' communicating with a large central 'cyst' which was indistinguishable from a massively dilated renal pelvis and calyces. This uncommon variant of MCDK was termed the hydronephrotic type since it appeared that an atretic ureter had resulted in a severe form of obstructive uropathy. These two variants of MCDK at first seem dichotomous but are likely to represent a spectrum of altered renal development. The classic type of MCDK (Fig. 21.1) results from severe alteration of renal development and bears little resemblance to a normal kidney; whereas, the hydro-nephrotic type (Fig. 21.2) more closely resembles normal renal development and contains some recognizable features of a kidney. This concept of a continuum of maldevelopment is further supported by the demonstration of communication of cysts via constrast injection in all cases of both classic and hydronephrotic MCDK (Glassberg and Kassner, 1998). It had previously been thought that the cysts were completely separate in the classic form of MCDK, but these more recent findings show that the classic form is more similar to hydronephrosis than previously believed.

MCDK vary in total size and in the size of individual cysts. Those with larger cysts tend to have less parenchyma, which has presumably been compressed between the cysts. Smaller MCDK are more solid with smaller cysts and more stroma. The ureter may be atretic or essentially not identifiable, and a renal pelvis is found in cases of the hydronephrotic type.

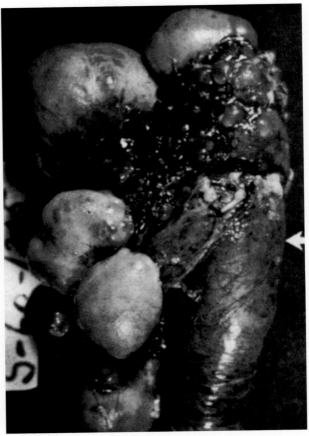

Figure 21.2 Gross appearance of hydronephrotic type of MCDK: cysts of various size surround the dilated renal pelvis. Arrow demonstrates dilated pelvis and proximal ureter.

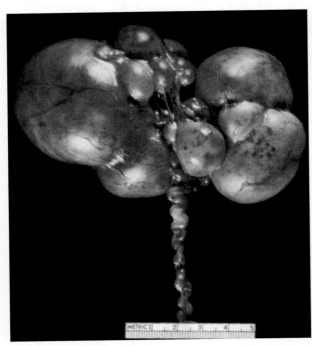

Figure 21.1 Gross appearance of classic type of MCDK: cysts of various size are held together by fibrous tissue. Normal renal tissue and reniform shape are absent. The ureter is tortuous and atretic.

Likewise, the blood supply may be a typical renal pedicle with small vessels or may be totally absent (Parkkulainen *et al.*, 1959).

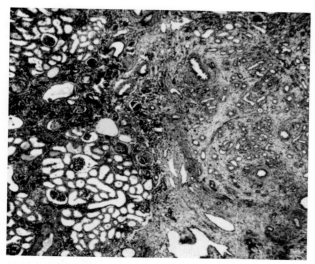

Figure 21.4 High-power microscopic appearance of MCDK: solid tissue demonstrates both mature glomeruli and tubules (*left*) and dysplastic tissue with primitive tubules (*right*).

Despite the varying gross appearance, MCDK share a common microanatomy. The most striking feature is architectural disorganization dominated by cysts. The cysts of varying size are lined by either squamous or cuboidal epithelium (Matsell *et al.*, 1996). Between the cysts are septa of mostly dysplastic renal tissue containing immature glomeruli, primitive tubules, and metaplastic cartilage (Fig. 21.3) In some cases, small islands of mature glomeruli and tubules may be found amongst the dysplastic tissue and may confound the diagnosis of MCDK by demonstrating renal function on radionuclide studies (Fig. 21.4). However, this minimal function is usually found in the medial, rather than peripheral portions, as seen in poorly functioning hydronephrotic kidneys.

Pathogenesis

The etiology of MCDK is most commonly believed to result from early obstruction, as demonstrated by the experimental model of Beck (1971). Beck performed ligation of the ureter in fetal lambs during the first half of gestation and noted uniform renal dysplasia; conversely, ligation during the second half of gestation led only to hydronephrosis in morphologically normal kidneys. Similar experiments were conducted

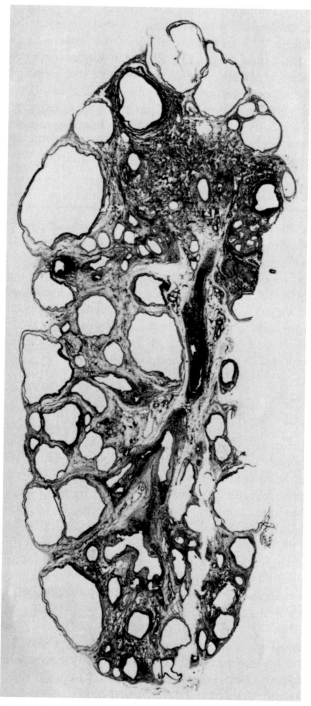

Figure 21.3 Low power microscopic appearance of MCDK: cysts are separated by septa composed of fibrous and dysplastic tissue.

by Glick *et al.* (1983, 1985) in which variable periods and degrees of ureteral obstruction were produced in fetal lambs, and similar conclusions were reached, i.e. early and complete obstruction produced renal dysplasia. Thus, the timing of obstruction may explain the existence of a spectrum of congenital obstructive uropathy. Classic MCDK is at one end of the spectrum presumably caused by early ureteral obstruction, and hydronephrosis secondary to UPJ obstruction lies at the other end of the spectrum, as a result of late obstruction. Hydronephrotic MCDK occupies an intermediate position on the spectrum between the two extremes. Indirect support for this theory of urinary obstruction as a cause of MCDK is the fact that the left kidney is more frequently involved not only with MCDK but also with UPJ obstruction (Glassberg and Filmer, 1992). Studies of ureteral ligation early in gestation in chicks, however, were unable to duplicate the induction of renal dysplasia (Berman and Maizels, 1982).

An alternative hypothesis for the etiology of MCDK is interruption of induction of the metanephric blastema by the migrating ureteric bud in early fetal life. Renal dysplasia has been associated with ureteral ectopia, and Mackie and Stephens (1975) have proposed that ectopic ureters arise from eccentric portions of the Wollfian duct that strike the metanephros cranially or caudally to the optimal central region. This eccentric location of impact leads to failure of induction of the metanephros, and a dysplastic kidney then develops. Critics of this hypothesis note that the ureteral orifice is in a normal position in most cases of MCDK, so ureteral ectopia cannot explain this specific form of renal dysplasia. However, recent studies in mice have shown that altered mesenchymal induction on a molecular rather than an anatomic level can produce renal dysplasia and cyst formation (Dressler *et al.*, 1993; Schuchardt *et al.*, 1994). Disruption of genes known to play a role in ureteric bud branching and early epithelial–mesenchymal induction led to anomalies similar to MCDK.

Detailed histologic and immunohistochemical studies of two human fetal MCDK at 14 and 19 weeks of gestation have produced further insights into the etiology of the disorder and favors the hypothesis of altered mesenchymal induction (Matsell *et al.*, 1996). The most striking finding was the presence of randomly displaced metanephric blastema adjacent to zones of normal nephrogenesis. No cystic dilatation of the ureteral duct or hydronephrosis was noted. At least three different types of cysts were present and appeared to arise from Bowman's space, the proximal tubule, and the collecting duct. This suggests that obstruction was not present but that aberrant induction of the blastema created islands of dysplastic tissue amid normal developing renal tubules. Since the altered induction was not ubiquitous throughout the affected kidney, genetic alteration of nephrogenesis (that would affect all cells) cannot explain development of MCDK. The authors propose that a perturbation of induction of the metanephric blastema by the branching ureteric bud occurs in a non-uniform manner to produce MCDK. Cyst expansion in later fetal life then compresses the normal, functioning renal tissue until little or none remains at birth.

Presentation

In the past, most MCDK cases were diagnosed during the first year of life. Approximately one-third of these were palpable, one-third of the children had anorexia or vomiting secondary to compressive effects of the MCDK, and the remainder presented as a random finding during work-up for urinary tract infection and congenital anomalies (Pathak and Williams, 1964; Rickwood *et al.*, 1992). MCDK have been typically reported to be the second most common cause of palpable abdominal masses in infants (following hydronephrosis) (Raffensperger and Abousteiman, 1968; Wilson, 1982). Compromise of respiratory function by large MCDK has been reported rarely (Triest and Bukowski, 1999). Diagnosis in adolescence or adulthood is also rare and usually a serendipitous finding on imaging studies, but MCDK have been reported to present in older patients with abdominal pain or mass, hematuria, urinary tract infection, or hypertension (Ambrose, 1976; Nakano *et al.*, 1996).

Routine prenatal sonography has dramatically changed the presentation of MCDK so that today prenatal diagnosis is the rule and symptomatic presentations are rare. As recently as 1992, the US National Multicystic Kidney Registry reported that 47% of patients with MCDK presented with a prenatal diagnosis compared with 30% with a palpable mass (Wacksman and Sheldon, 1992). By 1998, cases submitted to the registry with a prenatal diagnosis comprised 71% of the total, and palpable presentations fell to 14% (Wacksman, 1998). Similar figures have been reported in recent series from other countries (Rottenberg *et al.*, 1997; Kessler *et al.*, 1998).

Evaluation

Prenatal imaging

Abnormalities of the urinary tract are detected on pre-natal sonography at a prevalence of 1–3 cases per 1000 livebirths (Greig *et al.*, 1989; Scott and Renwick, 1993). Hydronephrosis is the most common fetal urologic abnormality, followed by MCDK (Avni *et al.*, 1986; Greig *et al.*, 1989). Importantly, MCDK is the most common anomaly found when there is a prenatal misdiagnosis of hydronephrosis (Scott and Renwick, 1993).

The sonographic features of MCDK have been well characterized in postnatal studies and are also useful for prenatal diagnosis (Fig. 21.5). Stuck *et al.* (1982) found the following features in all cases of MCDK: presence of interfaces between cysts, non-medial location of the larger cysts, and absence of an identifiable renal sinus. Nearly all demonstrated a lack of communication between cysts on sonography. The great diagnostic dilemma remains in differentiating hydronephrosis from MCDK, and Sanders and Hartman (1984) have provided useful criteria for differentiation. A reniform shape of the kidney was noted in 91% of hydronephrotic kidneys but only 20% of MCDK. Hydronephrotic kidneys demonstrate visible renal parenchyma surrounding a central cystic component, and longitudinal views show a glove-like pattern with calyces extending from a large central renal

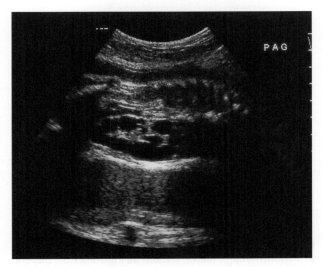

Figure 21.5 Prenatal sonogram of left MCDK: MCDK is present in mid-abdomen beneath (anterior to) spine on longitudal view of fetus. Cysts of various sizes distort normal renal architecture.

pelvis. MCDK, in contrast, have cysts of variable sizes and shapes in a random configuration without visible connections or surrounding parenchyma. A large medial cyst can mimic a dilated renal pelvis and be a source of misdiagnosis on sonography. Other confusing entities include a tortuous megaureter and a prominent gallbladder adjacent to a hydronephrotic or cystic kidney. Simple renal cysts are exceedingly rare in fetuses and, thus, are not a common cause of misdiagnosis. Bilateral MCDK can be seen prenatally and present with oligohydramnios due to absent urine production (Scott and Renwick, 1993). Polycystic kidneys have a greatly different appearance with bilateral enlargement; oligohydramnios may or may not be present. The cysts of infantile polycystic kidney disease (autosomal recessive) are so small that they cannot be detected individually, but a hyperechoic pattern is seen throughout the kidney.

The cysts of MCDK typically enlarge during fetal life as the few functioning tubules produce urine that inflates the cysts. Consequently, it may be impossible to diagnose MCDK prenatally until there is adequate urine production to distend the cysts beyond the threshold of detection. Sixteen weeks after the last menstrual period (LMP) is probably the earliest possible time for detection (Martin *et al.*, 1996; Webb *et al.*, 1997). Cysts have also been noted to shrink and involute during fetal life (Hashimoto *et al.*, 1986; Keski-Nisula *et al.*, 1999). Additional renal anomalies involving or distinct from the MCDK may also be noted on prenatal sonograms (Maayan *et al.*, 1998).

Postnatal imaging

In newborns with a prenatal diagnosis of MCDK, a renal sonogram should be performed prior to discharge from the nursery. The same diagnostic criteria are employed as for prenatal sonography (Fig. 21.6). There is no advantage in delaying sonography in cases suspicious for MCDK because the theoretical issues of relative dehydration and reduced renal function of the newborn have no bearing on the non-functioning MCDK. If there is uncertainty in the diagnosis of MCDK versus hydronephrosis, the radiologic literature suggests obtaining a sonogram at 7–10 days when there is greater urine production to distend an obstructed collecting system (Laing *et al.*, 1984); however, some urologic literature does not support this practice (Docimo and Silver, 1996). One must remain cognizant of the existence of the

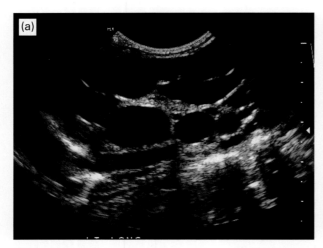
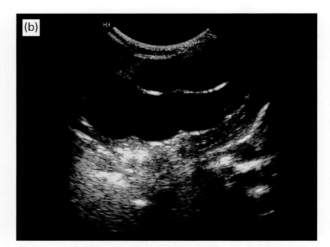

Figure 21.6 Postnatal renal sonogram of left MCDK on the second day of life (same patient as Figure 21.5): longitudinal views of classic type of MCDK with multiple cysts of varying sizes and shapes and fibrous septa.

hydronephrotic form of MCDK, which can mimic UPJ obstruction (Han *et al.*, 1995).

In cases of symptomatic presentation after the newborn period, sonography remains the initial study of choice because it offers quick, accurate imaging of the kidneys and other abdominal structures without the need for radiation or sedation. MCDK can also be detected on other forms of abdominal imaging. Intravenous pyelography shows non-function on the ipsilateral side, and plain films may demonstrate ring-like calcifications of the cyst walls (Ambrose, 1976). Computerized tomography and magnetic resonance imaging show the typical multicystic appearance with little or no renal parenchyma.

Careful evaluation of the contralateral kidney is imperative to exclude abnormalities of the remaining renal tissue. It has been suggested that contralateral compensatory renal hypertrophy may begin *in utero* and can be seen on initial postnatal scans (Rottenberg *et al.*, 1996). The degree of hypertrophy usually rapidly accelerates with age.

Currently MCDK is usually detected by sonography, but it is important to study the function of the involved renal unit as well. This is particularly crucial when anatomic studies are equivocal, as one cannot easily differentiate between the hydronephrotic type of MCDK and true hydronephrosis. Radionuclide imaging provides superior determination of renal function in comparison to intravenous pyelography and should be used exclusively in children (Fig. 21.7). Many advocate the use of technetium-99-m-dimercaptosuccinic acid ([^{99m}Tc]DMSA) scans, but MCDK may

show uptake of DMSA binding to immature renal tubules. [^{99}Tc]MAG-3 (mercaptocetyltriglycine) is more physiological since the tracer is only seen if there is glomerular and/or tubular function. MAG-3 has the added advantage of providing washout data in cases that prove to be UPJ obstruction.

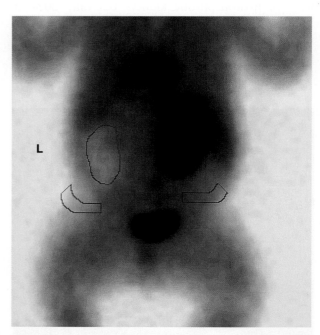

Figure 21.7 Nuclear renogram (MAG-3) of left MCDK at 1 month of age (same patient as Figure 21.5): patient is in the prone position. Tracer is seen in the right kidney and bladder. The photopenic region in the left flank is MCDK displacing tissue with background activity.

Associated findings

It was recognized early that MCDK were found commonly in children with other major anomalies, such as of the cardiac, respiratory, and gastrointestinal systems (Patak and Williams 1964). MCDK have also been associated with rare syndromes linked to single gene alterations (Jankauskiene *et al.*, 1997). Of particular interest to the urologist is that other abnormalities of the urinary tract have been documented in over 50% of cases of MCDK (Atuyeh *et al.*, 1992; Kaneko *et al.*, 1995; Karamzyn and Zerin, 1997).

Contralateral UPJ obstruction had previously been thought to be the most commonly associated urologic anomaly in patients with MCDK, but the increasingly routine use of cystography in the neonatal work-up of MCDK has shown vesicoureteral reflux to be more common. Reflux has been noted in 15–28% of cases; most is contralateral, but a minority is ipsilateral (Atuyeh *et al.*, 1992; Flack and Bellinger, 1993; Selzman and Elder, 1995; Karamzyn and Zerin, 1997). In most the reflux is low grade, but grades IV and V have been reported. Contralateral UPJ obstruction is the next most common concomitant urologic anomaly. Other contralateral obstructive uropathies include ureterovesical junction obstruction, ureteral ectopia, and ureteroceles. MCDK may be present in only a segment of ipsilateral duplication or horseshoe kidney and can be seen in crossed ectopia (Borer *et al.*, 1994; Corrales *et al.*, 1996; Maayan *et al.*, 1998). The demonstration of an absent ipsilateral vas deferens with MCDK suggests that aberrant mesonephric (Wolffian) duct development could be involved in both processes (Drake and Quinn, 1996).

Natural history and complications

Renal function

Bilateral MCDK is not compatible with life due to absent fetal renal function and resulting pulmonary hypoplasia. Most bilateral cases are stillborn and the remainder die in the early postnatal period. Unilateral MCDK, conversely, has an excellent prognosis provided no other serious anomalies are present. With contralateral renal hypertrophy, total creatinine clearance reaches normal levels in most cases, but mean serum creatinine is elevated compared with normal controls (John *et al.*, 1998). Anomalies affecting the contralateral kidney are common and must be aggressively sought and treated to preserve maximal renal function. Obstructive lesions require correction. Vesicoureteral reflux can be managed in the same manner as in patients with two functioning kidneys. Low-grade reflux is followed non-surgically with the patient on a prophylactic antibiotic and usually resolves with growth of the intravesical ureter; high-grade reflux can be followed similarly but may require surgical correction (Selzman and Elder, 1995; Palmer *et al.*, 1997). It has been suggested that reflux has a negative impact on renal hypertrophy, at least during the first year of life, but this finding has not been substantiated (Zerin and Leiser, 1998).

Involution of multicystic dysplastic kidney

Non-operative management of MCDK has helped to define the natural history of the affected kidney. In the latest figures from the National Multicystic Kidney Registry, 18% of MCDK became sonographically non-detectable in the first year of life, 13% in the following 2 years, and 27% in the next 2–5 years (Wacksman, 1998) Conversely, almost one-half are still detectable after 5 years of age and may take up to 20 years to involute. Rottenberg *et al.* (1997) noted a decrease in size in 73% of cases over a mean of 32 months with complete resolution in 40% of the total. There was no change in 9% and an increase in size in 18% (mean of 20.3 mm); the size at presentation did not correlate with the eventual outcome. With an equivalent length of follow-up, similar findings were noted by Strife *et al.* (1993) with a decrease in size in 67%, no change in 19%, and an increase in 10%.

Infection and pain

It has been difficult to document whether persistent MCDK can become a source of infection or pain. With most patients now presenting in infancy, both can be difficult to assess. No patient in the National Multicystic Kidney Registry has required surgery for abscess formation or urinary infection (Wacksman, 1998). An autopsy series of MCDK failed to find any evidence of pyelonephritis in the affected kidneys (Risdon, 1971). Ambrose (1976) reviewed 20 MCDK cases presenting at greater than 11 years of age and had follow-up in only 11. Ten patients presented with pain, and pain was reportedly relieved by nephrectomy in all who had follow-up evaluation. Three had a palpable mass, and one had a urinary tract infection involving the MCDK. The presenting compliants in the remaining patients could not be attributed to their MCDK. Therefore, it remains unclear whether MCDK produces symptoms later in life.

Hypertension

Hypertension has been associated with MCDK, but the incidence of this complication is difficult to ascertain. The first reported case of hypertension in a patient with MCDK cured by nephrectomy was in 1970; pathologic examination revealed hyperplasia of the juxtaglomerular apparatus, suggesting that the hypertension was renin-mediated (Javadpour et al., 1970). Hartman et al. (1986) reviewed nine cases of MCDK with hypertension and found that nephrectomy cured the hypertension in only three (aged 3 weeks, 6 years, and 21 years). Two cases of hypertension in infants with MCDK were shown to be cured by nephrectomy by Susskind et al. (1989). Webb et al. (1997) reported two additional patients with MCDK under 2 years of age who developed hypertension, elevated plasma renin activity, and left ventricular hypertrophy; both the hypertension and ventricular hypertrophy resolved following nephrectomy. In a review of 16 reported cases in the literature, the authors noted that nephrectomy was curative for hypertension in all seven children under 12 years but only in three of nine older individuals (Webb et al., 1997). The authors hypothesized that nephrectomy failed to cure hypertension in older patients because the long-standing hypertension led to irreversible arteriolar changes in the contralateral kidney, producing persistent renin-mediated hypertension even after removal of the MCDK. Emmert and King (1994) reported additional cases of hypertension associated with MCDK and suggested that the incidence of hypertension due to MCDK is underestimated since many cases are not reported and reliable blood pressure measurements can be difficult to obtain in children.

In contrast, others question the validity of these reports and argue that hypertension is rarely associated with MCDK (Gordon et al., 1988; Thomas and Fitzpatrick, 1997). In the initial publication of the National Multicystic Kidney Registry (260 cases), there were four with 'minimal hypertension believed to be unrelated to the multicystic kidney' (Wacksman and Phipps, 1993). The recent report from the registry (660 cases) states 'very few cases reported to the MCK registry have listed hypertension as an associated condition'. (Wacksman, 1998). Further evidence against the role of MCDK in hypertension is the absence of MCDK as a cause in 64 cases of surgically corrected hypertension in series from pediatric centers in Boston (Hendren et al., 1982) and Glasgow (Taylor et al., 1987).

Malignant degeneration

Reports of malignant degeneration are of great concern. At least 12 such malignancies have been reported. The initial report of cancer arising in MCDK was of an atypical embryonal tumor in an adult (Gutter and Hermanek, 1957). Renal cell carcinoma has been documented in five patients aged 15–68 years (Barrett and Wineland, 1980; Burgler and Hauri, 1983; Birken et al., 1985; Shirai et al., 1986; Rackley et al., 1994). Wilms' tumor is the most common renal tumor of childhood and has been associated with MCDK in six children (five in the first year of life and one at 3 years of age) (Uson et al., 1960; Raffensperger and Abousleiman, 1968; Hartman et al., 1986; Muguerza et al., 1996; Homsy et al., 1997). However, the validity of some of these has been questioned due to the possibility of misinterpretation of the diagnosis of malignancy or MCDK (Beckwith, 1997).

Malignancies arising in MCDK are very rare, and determination of the actual risk of malignant degeneration has been difficult. Only one patient in the National Multicystic Kidney Registry has developed Wilms' tumor (at age 10 months) (Wacksman, 1998), and only five with MCDK have been identified in over 7500 children enrolled in the National Wilms' Tumor Study Group (Beckwith, 1997). MCDK have been found to harbor *nephrogenic rests* (abnormal remnants of immature cells) which can serve as precursors of Wilms tumor with greater frequency than normal kidneys (Beckwith, 1996). Nephrogenic rests are present in approximately 0.8–1% of normal newborn kidneys, in 4% of MCDK, and in 20–40% of kidneys resected for Wilms' tumor. This implies that MCDK may have a greater propensity to develop Wilms tumor than normal kidneys, but the nephrogenic rests of MCDK are believed to have a particularly low malignant potential. Beckwith (1996) argues that, if nephrogenic rests are five times more common in MCDK than in normal kidneys, and normal kidneys are estimated to have a 1:10 000 risk of developing Wilms' tumor, then MCDK have at most 1 in 2000 risk of forming Wilms tumor. He concludes that this risk is too low to justify routine nephrectomy to prevent cancer development and raises doubts about the utility of screening patients with MCDK.

Management

The management of symptomatic MCDK is straightforward; fortunately, MCDK are almost never symptomatic. A MCDK that is compromising respiratory function should undoubtedly be removed, but percutaneous cyst aspiration may be a useful adjunct in newborns too fragile to tolerate an operative procedure. It may be difficult to prove MCDK as a cause of pain or gastrointestinal compression, but removal in such cases would appear beneficial. The association between infection and MCDK is tenuous; however, some patients may benefit from nephrectomy, particularly in combination with ureterectomy in cases with ipsilateral vesicoureteral reflux.

The management of asymptomatic MCDK, however, is the one of the most controversial areas in pediatric urology today. The routine use of prenatal sonography has allowed most MCDK to be diagnosed prior to birth, whereas, without this technology, many of these may have never come to clinical recognition. Even palpable MCDK without symptoms rarely require intervention if a secure diagnosis can be made radiographically.

Given the great odds that MCDK will shrink or disappear and the extremely low odds that pain, infection, hypertension, or malignancy will develop, few still recommend routine nephrectomy (Hanna, 1995; Webb *et al.*, 1997). However, the gravity of the latter two complications should not make the clinician complacent in the non-operative management of MCDK. These concerns led the Urology Section of the American Academy of Pediatrics to establish the National Multicystic Kidney Registry in 1986. Although much has been learned, it will take many years until today's childhood cases mature enough to form more definitive guidelines for non-operative management.

Initial work-up

Initially, it is imperative that a clear diagnosis of MCDK be made radiographically. Without a certain diagnosis, exploration is necessary. Reports of Wilms' tumor and mesoblastic nephroma in equivocal cases highlight the need for vigilance on initial and follow-up studies (Minevich *et al.*, 1997). When prenatal sonography is suspicious for MCDK, postnatal renal sonography should be performed early to attempt to differentiate MCDK from hydronephrosis (Fig 21.8). Likewise, sonography is the best initial study upon discovery of a palpable mass in an older child. Voiding cystourethrography should be performed to rule out associated urologic anomalies; if there is delay in performing this study, the newborn should be placed on prophylactic antibiotics (i.e. amoxicillin 15 mg/kg orally once daily) until reflux is excluded. Radionuclide imaging to evaluate function with [^{99}Tc]MAG-3 is preferred because it aids in differentiation between MCDK and obstruction.

Non-operative management

Follow-up renal sonograms are recommended every 3 months during the first year of life and then every 6–12 months until the age 5 years (Wacksman, 1998). The incidence of Wilms' tumor after this age approaches zero, so the likelihood of malignant degeneration diminishes once school age is reached. Parents should be instructed to perform abdominal exams on the child at least monthly to this age because Wilms' tumor can grow very rapidly and become palpable in less than 6 months after a negative sonogram. Reports of other renal malignancies developing from MCDK in adults argue for lifelong radiologic surveillance at some undetermined interval. Suspicious enlargement or development of solid masses in MCDK warrants excision. Blood pressure must also be monitored on a regular basis, and primary care providers must be made aware of the potential for development of hypertension.

Surgical management

If nephrectomy is deemed necessary due to suspicous enlargement, hypertension, mass effect, pain, or infection, there are several options available. Newborns should be allowed to adjust to postnatal life for several months prior to nephrectomy unless Wilms tumor is suspected. These cases are usually technically simple because the kidney can be collapsed by intra-operative decompression of the cysts and the blood vessels are often atretic. Elder *et al.* (1995) reported outpatient nephrectomies for MCDK in children under 5 years

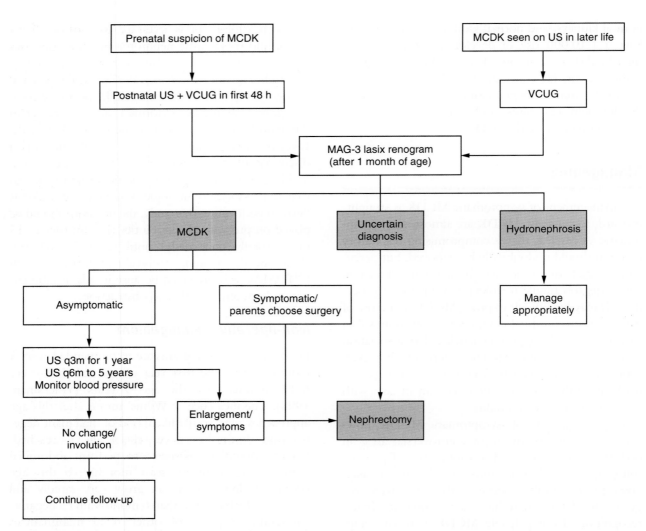

Figure 21.8 Work-up and management of MCDK. MCDK = multicystic dysplastic kidney; US = ultrasound; VCUG = voiding cystourethrogram.

using a 2.5–3.0 cm incision and intercostal nerve block. Transperitoneal laparoscopic nephrectomy has been used for MCDK (Emmert *et al.*, 1994), but potential complications and costs are greater than standard approaches (Colodny, 1995). Laparoscopy through a retroperitoneal approach may avoid intraperitoneal complications, but the cost–benefit ratios remain less favorable in children than adults (Kobashi *et al.*, 1998).

An additional indication for surgery is parental preference. Parents of a child with MCDK must be objectively informed of the potential risks of observation, as well as of the risks of surgery. After weighing the risks and benefits of each, some may elect for surgery, particularly if complicating medical or social factors exist.

Financial concerns

Non-operative management of MCDK with serial sonographic screening has financial costs, as does excision. Perez *et al.* (1998) computed the costs of outpatient nephrectomy alone or as a concomitant procedure and found that it was equivalent to 17–28 ultrasound studies. If one follows the guidelines of follow-up sonograms at 3, 6, 9, and 12 months of age and then every 6 months until 5 years of age, that implies a minimum of 14 scans, but more may be necessary for an indeterminate length of time. Therefore, the costs of operative and non-operative management may not be vastly different.

A less obvious cost to the patient involves the ability to obtain life-insurance later in life. A survey of life insurance companies found that the majority would not issue a policy for a child with MCDK unless the kidney had been removed (Lasalle *et al.*, 1997). Although this may reflect misinformation on the natural history of MCDK among lay persons, it can represent a financial hardship to the patient.

Conclusions

Non-operative management of MCDK seems to be the practice of the majority of those involved in the care of these children and appears to be well justified. Inevitably, a small number of children with MCDK will develop complications, some of which may be life-threatening. However, removal of every MCDK would subject a large number of children to possible surgical and anesthetic complications, some of which may also be life-threatening. Parents must be counseled with the current knowledge of the natural history and complications of MCDK and be allowed to share in the decision-making process. If non-operative management is selected, the clinician must be comfortable with the diagnosis after appropriate imaging and must insure proper follow-up. Currently, it is difficult to estimate the likelihood of potential complications, and only through large multicenter longitudinal studies such as the National Multicystic Kidney Registry can better understanding of this disease be gained.

References

Ambrose SS (1976) Unilateral multicystic renal disease in adults. *Birth Defects* **13**: 349–352.

Atuyeh B, Husmann D, Baum M (1992) Contralateral renal abnormalities in multicystic dysplastic kidney disease. *J Pediatr* **121**: 65–7.

Avni EF, Thoua Y, Lalmand B *et al.* (1986) Multicystic dysplastic kidneys: evolving concepts. *In utero* diagnosis and post-natal follow-up by ultrasound. *Ann Radiol* **29**: 663–8.

Barrett DM, Wineland RE (1980) Renal cell carcinoma in multicystic dysplastic kidney, *Urology* **15**: 152–4.

Beck AD (1971) The effect of intra-uterine urinary obstruction upon development of the fetal kidney. *J Urol* **105**: 784–9.

Beckwith JB (1996) Wilms' tumor in multicystic dysplastic kidneys: what is the risk? *Dialogues Pediatr Urol* **19**(3): 3–5.

Beckwith JB (1997) Comment: Wilms' tumor and multicystic dysplastic kidney disease. *J Urol* **158**: 2259–60.

Berman DJ, Maizels M (1982) Role of urinary obstruction in the genesis of renal dysplasia: a model in the chick embryo. *J Urol* **128**: 1091–6.

Birken G, King D, Vane D *et al*. 1985 Adenocarcinoma arising in a multicystic dysplastic kidney. *J Pediatr Surg* **20**: 619–21.

Borer JG, Glassberg KI, Kassner EG *et al.* (1994) Unilateral multicystic dysplasia in 1 component of a horseshoe kidney: case reports and review of the literature. *J Urol* **152**: 1568–71.

Burgler W, Hauri D (1983) Vitale komplikationen bei multizystischer nierendegeneration (muligzystischer dysplasie). *Urol Int* **38**: 251–6.

Colodny AH (1995) Letter to the editor: The management of multicystic dysplastic kidney in infancy. *Urology* **45**: 1084.

Corrales JG, Elder JS (1996) Segmental multicystic kidney and ipsilateral duplication anomalies. *J Urol* **155**: 1398–401.

Docimo SG, Silver RI (1996) Renal sonography in newborns with prenatally detected hydronephrosis: why wait? *J Urol* **157**: 1387–90.

Drake MJ, Quinn FM (1996) Absent vas deferens and ipsilateral multicystic dysplastic kidney in a child. *Br J Urol* **77**: 756–7.

Dressler GR, Wilkinson JE, Rothenpieler UW *et al.* (1993) Deregulation of Pax-2 expression in transgenic mice generates severe kidney abnormalities. *Nature* **362**: 65–7.

Elder JS, Hladsky D, Selzman AA (1995) Outpatient nephrectomy for non-functioning kidneys. *J Urol* **154**: 712–4.

Emmert GK, King LR (1994) The risk of hypertension is underestimated in the multicystic dysplastic kidney: a personal perspective. *Urology* **44**: 404–5.

Emmert GK, Eubanks S, King LR (1994) Improved technique of laparoscopic nephrectomy for multicystic dysplastic kidney. *Urology* **44**: 422–4.

Felson B, Cussen LJ (1975) The hydronephrotic type of unilateral congenital multicystic disease of the kidney. *Semin Radiol* **10**: 113–23.

Flack CE, Bellinger MF (1993) The multicystic dysplastic kidney and contralateral vesicoureteral reflux; protection of the solitary kidney. *J Urol* **150**: 1873–4.

Glassberg KI, Filmer RB (1992) Renal dysplasia, renal hypoplasia, and cystic disease of the kidney. Chapter 26. In: PP Kelalis, LR King, AB Belman (eds) *Clinical pediatric urology*. 3rd edition. Philadelphia, PA: WB Saunders Co., 1121–84.

Glassberg KI, Kassner EG (1998) *Ex vivo* intracystic contrast studies of multicystic dysplastic kidneys. *J Urol* **160**: 1204–6.

Glick PL, Harrison MR, Noall RA *et al.* (1983) Correction of congenital hydronephrosis in utero. III. Early mid-trimester ureteral obstruction produces mild renal dysplasia. *J Pediatr Surg* **18**: 681–7.

Glick PL, Harrison MR, Globus MS *et al.* (1985) Management of the fetus with congenital hydronephrosis: II. Prognostic criteria and selection for treatment. *J Pediatr Surg* **20**: 376–87.

Gordon AC, Thomas DF, Arthur RJ *et al.* (1988) Multicystic dysplastic kidney: is nephrectomy still appropriate? *J Urol* **140**: 1231.

Greig JD, Raine PAM, Young DG *et al.* (1989) Value of antenatal diagnosis of abnormalities of the urinary tract. *BMJ* **298**: 1417–19.

Gutter W, Hermanek P (1957) Maligner tumor der nierengegend unter dem bilde der knollenniere (nierenblastemcysten). *Urol Int* **4**: 164–82.

Han SJ, Yu CY, Liu GC *et al.* (1995) Ultrasonographic evaluation of multicystic dysplastic kidney. *Kao Hsiung I Hsueh Ko Hsueh Tsa Chih* **11**: 383–9.

Hanna MK (1995) Letter to the editor: The multicystic dysplastic kidney. *Urology* **45**: 171.

Harley G (1864) Congenital cystic disease of the kidney. *Trans Path Soc Lond* **15**: 146–7.

Hartman GE, Smolik LM, Shochat SJ (1986) The dilemma of the multicystic dysplastic kidney. *Am J Dis Child* **140**: 925–8.

Hashimoto BE, Filly RA, Callen PW (1986) Multicystic dysplastic kidney *in utero*: changing appearance on US. *Radiology* **159**: 107–9.

Hendren WH, Kim SH, Herrin JT *et al.* (1982) Surgically correctable hypertension of renal origin in childhood. *Am J Surg* **143**: 432–42.

Homsy YL, Anderson JH, Oudjhane K, Russo P (1997) Wilms' tumor and multicystic dysplastic kidney disease. *J Urol* **158**: 2256–9.

Jankauskiene A, Dodat H, Deiber M *et al.* (1997) Multicystic dysplastic kidney associated with Waardenburg syndrome type 1. *Pediatr Nephrol* **11**: 744–5.

Javadpour N, Chelouhy E, Moncada L *et al.* (1970) Hypertension in a child caused by a multicystic kidney. *J Urol* **104**: 918–21.

John U, Rudnik-Schoneborn S, Zerres K, Misselwitz J (1998) Kidney growth and renal function in unilateral multicystic dysplastic kidney disease. *Pediatr Nephrol* **12**: 567–71.

Kaneko K, SuzukiY, Fukudu Y *et al.* (1995) Abnormal contralateral kidneys in unilateral multicystic kidney disease. *Pediatr Radiol* **25**: 275–7.

Karamzyn B, Zerin M (1997) Lower urinary tract abnormalities in children with multicystic dysplastic kidneys. *Radiology* **203**: 223–6.

Keski-Nisula L, Kiekara O, Kirkinen P (1999) Prenatal collapse of cysts in a dysplastic kidney. *J Clin Ultrasound* **27**: 356–60.

Kessler OJ, Zia N, Livne P, Merlob P (1998) Involution rate of multicystic renal dysplasia. *Pediatrics* **102**: E73.

Kobashi KC, Chamberlin DA, Rajpoot D, Shanberg AM (1998) Retroperitoneal laparoscopic nephrectomy in children. *J Urol* **160**: 1142–4.

Laing FC, Burke VD, Wing VW *et al.* (1984) Postpartum evaluation of fetal hydronephrosis: optimal timing for follow-up sonography. *Radiology* **152**: 423–4.

LaSalle MD, Stock JA, Hanna MK (1997) Insurability of children with congenital urological anomalies. *J Urol* **158**: 1312–15.

Liebeschuetz S, Thomas R (1997) Letter to the Editor: Unilateral multicystic dysplastic kidney. *Arch Dis Child* **77**: 369.

Maayan A, Mashiach R, Kessler OJ *et al.* (1998) Prenatal diagnosis of crossed ectopic multicystic kidney. *Am J Perinatol* **15**: 499–502.

Mackie GG, Stephens FD (1975) Duplex kidneys: a correlation of renal dysplasia with position of the ureteral orifice. *J Urol* **114**: 274–80.

Martin SR, Garel L, Alvarez F (1996) Alagille's syndrome associated with cystic renal disease. *Arch Dis Child* **74**: 232–5.

Matsell DG, Bennett T, Goodyer P, *et al.* (1996) The pathogenesis of multicystic dysplastic kidney disease: insights from the study of fetal kidneys. *Lab Invest* **74**: 883–93.

Minevich E, Wacksman J, Phipps L *et al.* (1997) The importance of accurate diagnosis and early close followup in patients with suspected multicystic dysplastic kidney. *J Urol* **158**: 1301–4.

Muguerza R, Martinez-Urrutia MJ, Lopez Pereira P *et al.* (1996) Multicystic renal dysplasia and Wilms tumor. *Cir Pediatr* **9**: 173–5.

Nakano M, Tada K, Takahashi Y *et al.* (1996) Unilateral multicystic dysplastic kidney in an adult: report of a case. *Hinyokika Kiyo* **42**: 373–6.

Palmer LS, Andros GJ, Maizels M *et al.* (1997) Management considerations for treating vesicoureteral reflux in children with solitary kidneys. *Urology* **49**: 604–8.

Parkkulainen KV, Hjelt L, Sirola K (1959) Congenital multicystic dysplasia of kidney: report of nineteen cases with discussion on the etiology: nomenclature and classification of cystic dysplasia of the kidney. *Acta Chir Scand* **244** (Suppl): 5.

Pathak IG, Williams DI (1964) Multicystic and cystic dysplastic kidneys. *Br J Urol* **36**: 318–31.

Perez LM, Naidu SI, Joseph DB (1998) Outcome and cost analysis of operative versus nonoperative management of neonatal multicystic dysplastic kidneys. *J Urol* **160**: 1207–11.

Rackley RR, Angermeier KW, Levin H *et al.* (1994) Renal cell carcinoma arising in a regressed multicystic dysplastic kidney. *J Urol* **152**: 1543–5.

Raffensperger J, Abousleiman A (1968) Abdominal masses in children under 1 year of age. *Surgery* **63**: 514–20.

Rickwood AMK, Anderson PAM, Williams MPL (1992) Multicystic renal dysplasia detected by prenatal ultrasonography. Natural history and results of conservative management. *Br J Urol* **69**: 538–40.

Risdon RA (1971) Renal dysplasia. I. A clinico-pathological study of 76 cases. *J Clin Pathol* **24**: 57.

Rottenberg GT, DeBruyn R, Gordon I (1996) Sonographic standards for a single functioning kidney in children. *Am J Roentgenol* **167**: 1255–9.

Rottenberg GT, Gordon I, Debruyn R (1997) The natural history of the multicystic dysplastic kidney in children. *Br J Radiol* **70**: 347–50.

Sanders RC, Hartman DS (1984) The sonographic distinction between neonatal multicystic dysplastic kidney and hydronephrosis. *Radiology* **151**: 621–5.

Schuchardt A, D'Agati V, Larsson-Blomberg L *et al.* (1994) Defects in the kidney and enteric nervous system of mice lacking the tyrosine kinase receptor. *Nature* **367**: 380–3.

Schwartz J (1936) An unusual unilateral multicystic dysplastic kidney in an infant. *J Urol* **35**: 259–63.

Scott JES, Renwick M (1993) Urologic anomalies in the Northern Region Fetal Abnormality Survey. *Arch Dis Child* **68**: 22–6.

Selzman AA, Elder JS (1995) Contralateral vesicoureteral reflux in children with a multicystic kidney. *J Urol* **153**: 1252–4.

Shirai M, Kitagawa T, Nakata H, Urano Y (1986) Renal cell carcinoma originating from dysplastic kidney. *Acta Path Jpn* **36**: 1263–9.

Spence HM (1955) Congenital unilateral multicystic kidney. *J Urol* **74**: 693–704.

Stife JL, Souza AS, Kirks DR *et al.* (1993) Multicystic dysplastic kidney in children: US follow-up. *Radiology* **186**: 785–8.

Stuck KJ, Koff SA, Silver TM (1982) Ultrasonic features of multicystic dysplastic kidney: expanded diagnostic criteria. *Radiology* **143**: 217–21.

Susskind MR, Kim KS, King LR (1989) Hypertension and multicystic kidney. *Urology* **34**: 362–6.

Taylor RC, Azmy AF, Young DG (1987) Long term follow up of surgical renal hypertension. *J Pediatr Surg* **22**: 228–30.

Thomas DFM, Fitzpatrick MM (1997) Letter to the editor: Unilateral multicystic dysplastic kidney. *Arch Dis Child* **77**: 368.

Triest JA, Bukowski TP (1999) Multicystic dysplastic kidney as cause of gastric outlet obstruction and respiratory compromise. *J Urol* **161**: 1918–9.

Uson AC, Del Rosario C, Melico MM (1960) Wilms tumor in association with cystic renal disease: report of two cases. *J Urol* **83**: 262–6.

Wacksman J (1998) Multicystic dysplastic kidney. In: TP Ball (ed.) *AUA Update Series*. American Urological Association Office of Education, Houston, TX, Volume 17, 66–71.

Wacksman J, Phipps L (1993) Report of the multicystic kidney registry: preliminary findings. *J Urol* **150**: 1870–2.

Wacksman J, Sheldon CA (1992) Multicystic kidney disease. Chapter 16. In: PP Kelalis, LR King, AB Belman (eds) *Clinical pediatric urology*. 3rd edition. Philadelphia, PA: WB Saunders Co., 772–81.

Webb NJA, Lewis MA, Bruce J *et al.* (1997) Unilateral multicystic dysplastic kidney: the case for nephrectomy. *Arch Dis Child* **76**: 31–4.

Wilson DA (1982) Ultrasound screening for abdominal masses in the neonatal period. *Am J Dis Child* **136**: 147–51.

Zerin JM, Leiser J (1998) The impact of vesicoureteral reflux on contralateral renal length in infants with multicystic dysplastic kidney. *Pediatr Radiol* **28**: 683–6.

Cystic kidney disease

22

Laurence A. Greenbaum

Introduction

Cyst formation is seen in a variety of kidney diseases. Many of these diseases are genetically inherited and many are associated with extrarenal manifestations. They are generally relatively rare diseases, though a few are common enough to cause considerable pediatric morbidity and mortality. Autosomal dominant polycystic kidney disease (ADPKD) is one of the most common human genetic diseases, but its manifestations are usually fairly subtle in pediatric patients. It causes considerable morbidity for adults and it is likely that future therapy of this disease will focus on the pediatric patient.

The last decade has witnessed considerable advances in our understanding of cystic kidney diseases. The defective gene has been cloned in a number of these diseases and this has led to increased understanding of pathogenesis and clarified some important clinical issues. Such genetic studies have also provided increased opportunities for both prenatal and postnatal diagnosis. Increased awareness and understanding of ADPKD has been associated with increased evaluation of asymptomatic children with ADPKD. In the long term this has the potential of identifying a group that may benefit from early medical intervention. In the short term this has created patient anxiety and diagnostic questions that are related more to medical insurance than patient care.

The following cystic kidney diseases are covered in this chapter:

- polycystic kidney disease
    - autosomal recessive polycystic kidney disease
    - autosomal dominant polycystic kidney disease
- cysts of the medulla
    - juvenile nephronophthisis
    - medullary cystic disease
    - medullary sponge kidney
- glomerulocystic kidney disease
    - sporadic glomerulocystic kidney disease
    - familial hypoplastic glomerulocystic kidney disease
    - autosomal dominant glomerulocystic kidney disease
- simple renal cysts
- multilocular cysts
- acquired cystic kidney disease
- syndromes with cystic kidneys
    - tuberous sclerosis
    - meckel syndrome
    - von-Hippel–Lindau disease.

The only exception is the multicystic dysplastic kidney, which is discussed in Chapter 21.

Autosomal recessive polycystic kidney disease

The incidence of autosomal recessive polycystic kidney disease (ARPKD) has been estimated to be from 1 in 6000 to 1 in 55 000 (Cole, 1990; Zerres, 1992). Since ADPKD can present in infancy and ARPKD can present in young adults, the designation ARPKD is more precise than the term 'infantile polycystic kidney disease'. Both the liver and kidneys are affected in ARPKD, with significant variability in severity between patients. Researchers are currently close to identifying the defective gene in this disease. Clinically the prognosis for patients with ARPKD continues to improve.

Genetics

ARPKD is a classic recessively inherited disorder, with unaffected heterozygote parents and a 25% risk of an affected child in subsequent pregnancies. Most, if not all, cases of ARPKD appear to be due to a defect in a gene localized to chromosome 6p (Zerres *et al.*, 1994; Besbas *et al.*, 1998). Mapping of the gene has been done using linkage analysis; current studies are refining the genetic location and searching for the specific gene (Lens *et al.*, 1997; Park *et al.*, 1999). Blyth and Ockenden (1971) suggested that different genetic loci might be responsible for different forms of ARPKD. These authors proposed four phenotypes of ARPKD, with distinct clinical features based on age of presentation and relative severity of hepatic and renal involvement. They argue that the different clinical phenotypes of ARPKD are probably due to different genetic defects. However, affected children within the same family can have very different clinical manifestations (Gang and Herrin, 1986; Kaplan *et al.*, 1988, 1989a; Gagnadoux *et al.*, 1989; Barth *et al.*, 1992). This argues against a need for multiple genetic loci to explain the variable phenotypes. This is confirmed by genetic studies showing that every analyzed case is linked to the same region of chromosome 6p (Zerres *et al.*, 1994; Besbas *et al.*, 1998).

This does not exclude other loci but argues that most cases are due to a single genetic disorder. The variability within families refutes the idea of an absolute correlation between the precise genetic lesion in a family and the patient phenotype. Rather, it seems likely that other background genes (Woo *et al.*, 1997) and/or environmental factors are also important in determining severity.

Pathology

The kidneys are enlarged bilaterally. This enlargement is usually fairly symmetrical and the kidneys retain their reniform shape. Careful examination of the kidney capsule will often reveal opalescent dots, which are due to the termini of dilated collecting ducts below the kidney capsule (Fig. 22.1). Grossly the kidneys have a spongy appearance because of the cystic dilatation of the collecting ducts (Osathanondh and Potter, 1964). Large cysts are unusual in infancy, though there is a gradual increase in cyst size over time (Lieberman *et al.*, 1971). The microscopic

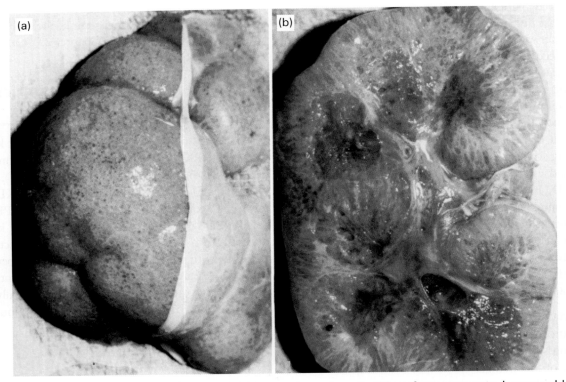

Figure 22.1 (*a*) Subcapsular surface of an autosomal recessive polycystic kidney from a neonate. Innumerable small cysts can be seen beneath the capsule. (*b*) Cross-section of the same kidney. The radial arrangement of the dilated ducts can be seen.

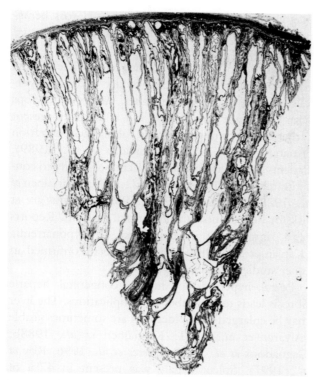

Figure 22.2 Low-power view of the cortex from an autosomal recessive polycystic kidney. Notice the arrangement of dilated ducts, which are perpendicularly oriented to the capsule. (Hematoxylin and eosin, original magnification × 8.)

- abnormal prenatal ultrasound
- enlarged kidneys
- respiratory distress
- failure to thrive
- proteinuria
- pyuria
- hypertension
- renal failure
- hepatomegaly
- esophageal varices
- disease in a sibling.

The majority of patients is diagnosed during the first year of life, with a significant percentage presenting during the first month of life (Lieberman *et al.*, 1971; Isdale *et al.*, 1973; Kääriäinen *et al.*, 1988b; Kaplan *et al.*, 1989a). The most severely affected neonates can have some degree of Potter syndrome due to oligohydramnios. Along with abnormal facies and joint deformities, these children may have respiratory compromise due to pulmonary hypoplasia. Volume overload from renal failure and poor diaphragm function secondary to the enlarged kidneys can also impair respiratory function. Respiratory failure is thus fairly common in neonates (Lieberman *et al.*, 1971; Kääriäinen *et al.*, 1988b; Kaplan *et al.*, 1989a). The importance of the mass effect of the enlarged kidneys has been confirmed by the improvement in respiratory function following unilateral nephrectomy (Bean *et al.*, 1995). Pneumothoraces are probably related to the hypoplasia and the high ventilatory settings that these infants require. Death due to respiratory failure can occur in the first few days of life (Kaplan *et al.*, 1989a).

The kidneys in ARPKD are typically quite large at birth and often increase in size. This causes abdominal distension on physical examination but also has additional important secondary consequences. By limiting diaphragm mobility respiratory function is compromised, adding to the problems described above. In addition, the enlarged kidneys may impair gastric feeding (Bean *et al.*, 1995) and patient mobility. It is important to note, however, that the kidney size can become less impressive over time in some patients, especially those that are receiving chronic dialysis (Lieberman *et al.*, 1971; Gagnadoux *et al.*, 1989).

Chronic renal failure and, ultimately, end-stage renal disease (ESRD) is the usual outcome in ARPKD. Kidney failure may be present at birth

appearance is dominated by the dilated collecting ducts, which are perpendicular to the kidney surface (Fig. 22.2). The cysts are lined with a normal appearing single layer of cuboidal or columnar epithelium (Osathanondh and Potter, 1964). The glomeruli often appear normal in newborns. Over time there is increased interstitial fibrosis and glomerular sclerosis.

These patients also have the typical features of congenital hepatic fibrosis (Landing *et al.*, 1980). There is proliferation and dilatation of bile ducts and fibrosis of portal tracts. The distal portal veins are small, providing a microscopic explanation for the presence of portal hypertension. The absence of hepatocyte destruction correlates with the preservation of liver function (Bernstein, 1987).

Clinical features

There is significant variability in the clinical features and mode of presentation of ARPKD. They include:

(Lieberman *et al.*, 1971; Kääriäinen *et al.*, 1988b), although it more typically develops gradually, with most children not progressing to ESRD until later in childhood or even as young adults (Gagnadoux *et al.*, 1989; Hoyer, 1996). Many patients will actually have some improvement in renal function during the first year of life, followed by a period of stabilization and subsequent decline (Cole *et al.*, 1987; Mattoo *et al.*, 1994). This is probably due to the normal maturation of kidney function. More aggressive therapy in the newborn period might theoretically select for patients with more severe renal involvement, although neonatal presentation is not necessarily a marker for earlier progression to ESRD (Gagnadoux *et al.*, 1989). Patients are at risk for the usual complications of chronic renal failure.

Chronic renal failure, especially untreated, is a potential cause of growth retardation. In addition, poor food intake, due to both renal failure and abdominal distension, may cause malnutrition. Not surprisingly, growth retardation is quite common in ARPKD (Lieberman *et al.*, 1971; Zerres *et al.*, 1996) and some children have severe growth retardation without a clear etiology (Gagnadoux *et al.*, 1989).

Hypertension is very common, probably due to fluid overload. The role of kidney renin production is not clear, with two studies failing to demonstrate increased renin or aldosterone levels (Kaplan *et al.*, 1989a; Gagnadoux *et al.*, 1989). Anywhere from 65 to 78% of patients require antihypertensive therapy (Kääriäinen *et al.*, 1988b; Kaplan *et al.*, 1989a; Gagnadoux *et al.*, 1989; Zerres *et al.*, 1992; Mattoo *et al.*, 1994). The hypertension can be quite severe, causing severe morbidity (Rahill and Rubin, 1972) and even death (Kaplan *et al.*, 1989a; Gagnedoux *et al.*, 1989). Hypertension gradually diminishes in some children and this may permit weaning of antihypertensive medications (Gagnadoux *et al.*, 1989; Jamil *et al.*, 1999).

There is an increased incidence of urinary tract infections (Kääriäinen *et al.*, 1988b; Zerres *et al.*, 1992), which may be related to vesicoureteral reflux and catheterization (Roy *et al.*, 1997), and is more common in girls (Zerres *et al.*, 1996). However, pyuria is often present in the absence of infection (Lieberman *et al.*, 1971) and it appears to be less common in older children (Gagnadoux *et al.*, 1989). Proteinuria may be detected, often intermittently (Kääriäinen *et al.*, 1988b), but it is not of sufficient

magnitude to cause clinical problems. Gross hematuria is quite uncommon but has been reported (Gagnadoux *et al.*, 1989).

Patients can have the typical electrolyte disturbances associated with renal failure such as hyperkalemia and hyperphosphatemia. Acidosis develops with significant renal failure but is at times present earlier owing to impairment in tubular acid excretion (Anand *et al.*, 1975; Gagnadoux *et al.*, 1989). Patients almost always have a decreased ability to concentrate their urine (Anand *et al.*, 1975; Kääriäinen *et al.*, 1988b; Gagnadoux *et al.*, 1989) and thus are at risk for dehydration and nocturnal enuresis. Reports of a significantly increased risk of hyponatremia (Kaplan *et al.*, 1989a) have not been confirmed in other studies (Zerres *et al.*, 1996).

Portal hypertension due to congenital hepatic fibrosis leads to a number of complications. The liver may be enlarged and spider nevi are sometimes visible (Alvarez *et al.*, 1981; Kääriäinen *et al.*, 1988b; Gagnadoux *et al.*, 1989; Zerres *et al.*, 1996; Roy *et al.*, 1997). Splenomegaly was present in 47% of patients over 3 months of age in one series (Kaplan *et al.*, 1989a) and this increased to 60% in children over 1 year of age (Roy *et al.*, 1997). This can be associated with anemia and thrombocytopenia (Alvarez *et al.*, 1981; Roy *et al.*, 1997). Esophageal varices can lead to problems with hematemesis (Alvarez *et al.*, 1981; Jamil *et al.*, 1999) and variceal rupture can be fatal (Kääriäinen *et al.*, 1988b; Kaplan *et al.*, 1989a; Roy *et al.*, 1997). Dilated biliary ducts predispose children with ARPKD to develop cholangitis (Alvarez *et al.*, 1981). This can occur in the neonatal period and it has been fatal in some children (Kääriäinen *et al.*, 1988b). Hepatocyte damage does not occur and synthetic function remains normal (Alvarez *et al.*, 1981; Jamil *et al.*, 1999), though mild abnormalities in liver enzymes are occasionally detected (Kääriäinen *et al.*, 1988b; Zerres *et al.*, 1996).

Some patients initially have predominant liver involvement (Alvarez *et al.*, 1981; Zerres, 1992), with kidney abnormalities discovered as an incidental radiographic finding. Other children have both severe liver and kidney disease at an early age (Gagnadoux *et al.*, 1989). The hypothesis that severe liver disease predicts minimal renal involvement (Blyth and Ockenden, 1971) is no longer accepted (Landing *et al.*, 1980).

It is possible that additional clinical features of ARPKD may be discovered as patients survive further into adulthood. For example, intracranial aneurysms were recently described in a 31-year-old patient with ARPKD (Neumann *et al.*, 1999). While only a case report, this is especially intriguing given the presence of intracranial aneurysms in ADPKD (Chapman *et al.*, 1992).

Radiological features

Intravenous pyelography (IVP) shows enlarged kidneys with a delayed nephrogram (Fig. 22.3) (Chilton and Cremin, 1981; Kääriäinen *et al.*, 1988a). Radial streaks due to contrast in the dilated collecting ducts are usually present in infancy but may not be visible in older children (Isdale *et al.*, 1973). Because of concerns regarding intravenous contrast, a renal sonogram is now the usual front-line diagnostic test. Ultrasound shows enlarged kidneys with increased echogenicity and poor corticomedullary differentiation (Fig. 22.4) (Metreweli and Garel, 1980). A hypoechoic rim is often visible. Older children have increased medullary echogenicity, which may resemble nephrocalcinosis (Gagnadoux *et al.*, 1989). Multiple small cysts may be visible by ultrasound

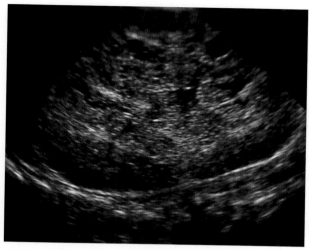

Figure 22.4 Renal ultrasound of a newborn with ARPKD. The kidney is enlarged, with increased echogenicity. A hypoechoic rim is visible. (Courtesy of Dr J. Sty, Children's Hospital of Wisconsin.)

(Gagnadoux *et al.*, 1989) but this is quite variable (Fig. 22.5). Macrocysts are sometimes visible in older children (Metreweli and Garel, 1980; Boal and Teele, 1980; Neumann *et al.*, 1988).

High-quality sonography detects liver abnormalities in approximately 50% of patients (Gagnadoux *et al.*, 1989). It is often possible to detect dilatations of the peripheral intrahepatic biliary ducts and the principle biliary duct. There may also be evidence of portal hypertension (Gagnadoux *et al.*, 1989).

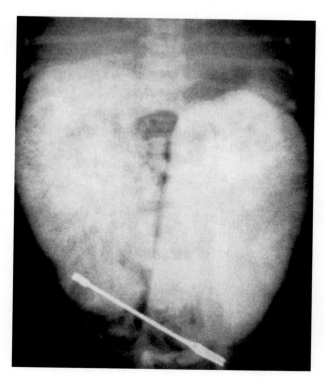

Figure 22.3 IVP from a 2-day-old girl with ARPKD. Notice the sunray appearance of the contrast material and the enormous renal size.

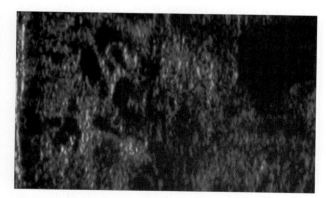

Figure 22.5 High-resolution renal sonogram of the same patient shown in Figure 21.4. With high resolution cysts are seen and the hypoechoic rim is still visible. (Courtesy of Dr J. Sty, Children's Hospital of Wisconsin.)

Diagnosis

The presence of bilaterally enlarged kidneys during the first few years of life is suggestive of ARPKD. The radiologic features as detailed above can be helpful but are not always conclusive. This is especially true in older patients with ARPKD since cysts may have enlarged and thus resemble those seen in ADPKD (Neumann *et al.*, 1988). It is important to investigate the family history; the presence of a sibling with ARPKD is obviously highly suggestive. Consideration must be given to an early presentation of ADPKD and thus it is now common to augment the family history with renal sonograms of the parents, and possibly the grandparents, to rule out this possibility. In one study 6.7% of the patients with neonatally lethal polycystic kidney disease had ADPKD (Kääriäinen *et al.*, 1988b). For inconclusive cases, histological examination of the kidneys or liver is useful. Congenital hepatic fibrosis is always present in ARPKD and is extremely rare in ADPKD (Cobben *et al.*, 1990; Lipschitz *et al.*, 1993). Hepatic sonograms may also demonstrate disease (Gagnadoux *et al.*, 1989). In the histologic evaluation of the kidney, the absence of glomerular cysts supports a diagnosis of ARPKD.

Nephroblastomatosis and bilateral Wilms' tumor are part of the differential diagnosis of bilaterally enlarged kidneys. Transient nephromegaly of the newborn can be confused with ARPKD (Stapleton *et al.*, 1981) but this resolves relatively quickly. A variety of other diseases with renal involvement can also have hepatic manifestations. These include Meckel syndrome (Blankenberg *et al.*, 1987), juvenile nephronophthisis (Boichis *et al.*, 1973), Ivemark's syndrome (Larson *et al.*, 1995), Jeune's syndrome (Brueton *et al.*, 1990), COACH syndrome (Kumar *et al.*, 1996) and Bardet–Biedl syndrome (Pagon *et al.*, 1982).

Prenatal diagnosis

Prenatal sonography often detects abnormalities in a fetus with ARPKD (Habif *et al.*, 1982; Romero *et al.*, 1984; Zerres *et al.*, 1988; Reuss *et al.*, 1990; Zerres, 1992; Bronshtein *et al.*, 1992; Lilford *et al.*, 1992). The kidneys may be hyperechoic (Lilford *et al.*, 1992) and increased in size (Romero *et al.*, 1984; Reuss *et al.*, 1990; Bronshtein *et al.*, 1992). Serial sonograms showing inappropriate increases in kidney length improves diagnostic reliability (Zerres *et al.*,

1988). In addition, some fetuses will have oligohydramnios. However, a precise diagnosis is often impossible prenatally given the limits of current imaging and alternative diagnostic possibilities. Naturally, in a family with a previous child who has ARPKD, the clinical likelihood of this diagnosis is increased. Unfortunately, there have been cases of both false-positive and false-negative diagnoses (Luthy *et al.*, 1985; Lilford *et al.*, 1992). False positives are especially likely in a fetus without a family history of ARPKD or if oligohydramnios is not present (Lilford *et al.*, 1992). Conversely, in a family at risk, a normal prenatal sonogram, especially before the third trimester, should not be used to predict an unaffected child (Luthy *et al.*, 1985; Argubright and Wides, 1987; Reuss *et al.*, 1990; Barth *et al.*, 1992; Zerres *et al.*, 1998). Fetal magnetic resonance imaging (MRI) has also been used to diagnose ARPKD (Nasu *et al.*, 1998).

Linkage analysis can determine whether a fetus has ARPKD in families with a previous affected child (Zerres, 1992). This analysis requires preservation of DNA from the previous child. Such analysis is currently not commercially available but can be performed at research laboratories in both Europe and the USA (Zerres *et al.*, 1998). The clinical course of a previously affected child does not predict the severity of the ARPKD in a subsequent child (Kaplan *et al.*, 1989a; Barth *et al.*, 1992). Parents clearly need genetic counseling regarding this possibility. Supplementing linkage analysis with prenatal imaging studies could theoretically aid in this discussion but it is especially difficult to make outcome predictions based on the fetal sonogram (Barth *et al.*, 1992).

Treatment

The initial management of respiratory distress is quite challenging. In the past many of these children were presumed to have pulmonary hypoplasia and thus therapy was limited. It is now clear that other factors contribute to the respiratory insufficiency. Both unilateral and bilateral nephrectomies, by decreasing the effect of abdominal distension, have been successfully used to improve respiratory function and allow children to wean from respiratory support (Sumfest *et al.*, 1993; Bean *et al.*, 1995). Though providing a less dramatic decrease in abdominal distension, unilateral nephrectomy can be performed without forcing the patient to be placed on dialysis (Bean *et al.*, 1995). It is important to evaluate relative renal function before proceeding with a unilateral nephrectomy, lest the remaining kidney have limited function. Bilateral nephrectomies require that a peritoneal dialysis catheter be placed simultaneously; it is therefore recommended that the kidneys be removed extraperitoneally, paying meticulous attention to the peritoneal membrane (Sumfest et al., 1993).

Reversible causes of respiratory insufficiency such as volume overload, persistent fetal circulation, hyaline membrane disease, infection, and pneumothoraces should be treated before concluding that a patient has irreversible pulmonary failure. The use of more aggressive perinatal support strategies such as surfactant, high-frequency oscillatory ventilation (Bean et al., 1995), extracorporeal membrane oxygenation (ECMO), dialysis, and hemofiltration may also decrease the mortality from respiratory failure.

The massively enlarged kidneys create a variety of problems beyond respiratory distress. Both unilateral and bilateral nephrectomies can have other benefits such as improved tolerance of feedings (Bean et al., 1995) and increased activity in older children. Left nephrectomy, assuming equivalent renal size, may have more benefits for gastric function than right nephrectomy (Bean et al., 1995).

Hypertension should be treated aggressively given that uncontrolled hypertension has been associated with severe complications and even death (Kaplan et al., 1989a). Hypertension is often difficult to control (Zerres, 1992), leading to bilateral nephrectomy and the initiation of peritoneal dialysis in some children (Roy et al., 1997). Hypertension may lessen as the patient ages, allowing successful weaning of antihypertensive medications (Mattoo et al., 1994; Roy et al., 1997).

Chronic renal failure and ESRD are managed using the usual strategies. Patients are treated for electrolyte problems, anemia, and renal osteodystrophy. Tube feedings and growth hormone are often necessary to treat failure to thrive. Dialysis and, ultimately, transplantation are needed when the patient reaches ESRD. Peritoneal dialysis is the preferred modality but hemodialysis can be used if necessary. Both peritoneal dialysis and transplantation may require prior nephrectomies to create sufficient abdominal space.

Complications of portal hypertension need to be addressed (D'Amico et al., 1995). Esophageal varices may require sclerotherapy or placement of a portacaval shunt (Alvarez et al., 1981; McGonigle et al.,

1981), with one patient receiving a shunt as early as 2 years of age (Kaplan et al., 1989a). Cholangitis needs to be treated aggressively with antibiotics. Splenectomy has been performed in children with intractable hypersplenism that causes anemia and thrombocytopenia.

Prognosis

ARPKD is associated with considerable morbidity and mortality. Improved therapy in the newborn intensive care unit and better treatment for chronic renal failure are changing the long-term prognosis. Nevertheless, patients continue to die, with much of the mortality occurring in the first year of life. One study found a 46% survival rate at 15 years; this increased to 79% if patients who died during the first year of life were excluded from the analysis (Kaplan et al., 1989a). Renal failure was the most common cause of death in this series, perhaps suggesting that improved technology will change the long-term outcome. Similar results have been reported by others (Gagnadoux et al., 1989). In another study all 14 patients who survived the first year of life were still alive, though this group had fairly mild disease (Kääriäinen et al., 1988b). Current statistics are limited by the lack of long-term follow-up data for studies in children diagnosed more recently.

There is clearly significant long-term morbidity in these patients as a result of chronic renal failure, systemic hypertension, and portal hypertension. However, patients are continuing to benefit from improvements in both surgical and medical management.

Autosomal dominant polycystic kidney disease

ADPKD, with an incidence of 1:500 to 1:1000, is the most common inherited kidney disease. Although kidney involvement is the major feature for most patients, there are protean extrarenal manifestations, including the potentially life-threatening possibility of a ruptured intracranial aneurysm. Severity varies greatly between patients and symptoms tend to develop over time. Fortunately, most children are asymptomatic and even middle-aged adults may be unaware of their diagnosis. However, some children have severe and occasionally fatal disease. This underscores the importance of avoiding the term 'adult' polycystic kidney disease.

An increasing percentage of children with ADPKD is diagnosed due to a positive family history or because of an incidental finding during an imaging study. This has caused a marked shift in the pediatric patient population, with many patients having no symptoms and requiring very limited intervention.

Genetics

ADPKD is a genetically heterogenous condition; disease occurs owing to mutations in one of at least three separate genetic loci (Table 22.1). Patients with a mutation of the *PKD1* gene (Consortium TEPKD, 1994), which is located on chromosome 16, account for approximately 85% of cases. Most remaining cases are due to a mutation in the *PKD2* gene on chromosome 4 (Mochizuki *et al.*, 1996). The presence of a third locus (*PKD3*) is inferred based on studies showing an absence of genetic linkage to either *PKD1* or *PKD2* in some families with ADPKD (de Almeida *et al.*, 1995; Daoust *et al.*, 1995; Turco *et al.*, 1996), though the evidence for this third locus has been questioned (Paterson and Pei, 1998).

PKD1 encodes for a protein called polycystin, which is a transmembrane protein with multiple extracellular domains (Harris *et al.*, 1995). The *PKD2* gene product, polycystin-2, is also a transmembrane protein and has moderate homology to polycystin (Mochizuki *et al.*, 1996). Polycystin and polycystin-2 appear to interact with each other (Qian *et al.*, 1997; Tsiokas *et al.*, 1997), though their function is not yet known.

The variable development of cyst formation in ADPKD appears to be related to the need for a second inactivating mutation. The kidney cells of patients with the *PKD1* mutation initially have one normal gene for polycystin and one defective gene. Cyst formation occurs when there is a second somatic mutation that inactivates the good gene. This produces a cell that does not produce any normal polycystin. Additional cysts are due to a second mutation in other cells (Qian *et al.*, 1996; Brasier *et al.*, 1997).

Table 22.1 Multiple gene defects causing ADPKD

Gene	Chromosome location	Protein
PKD1	16p	Polycystin
PKD2	4q	Polycystin-2
PKD3	Unknown	Unknown

A similar mechanism takes place in patients with *PKD2* (Koptides *et al.*, 1999; Pei *et al.*, 1999). This helps to explain why cysts appear fairly randomly and increase in number over time.

There is a great deal of variability in the severity of ADPKD, some of which is based on the specific gene affected. Patients with PKD2 have less severe symptoms, including later mean age for the development of ESRD and a decreased incidence of hypertension, urinary tract infections and hematuria (Hateboer *et al.*, 1999). In one study the median age of death or onset of ESRD was 53 and 69 years in patients with PKD1 and PKD2, respectively (Hateboer *et al.*, 1999). Additional sources of variability may involve environmental factors and genetic differences at other loci (Woo *et al.*, 1997). For example, polymorphisms in the angiotensin-converting enzyme (ACE) gene modify renal disease severity in patients with PKD1 (Pérez-Oller *et al.*, 1999).

In some cases of neonatal ADPKD the affected parents have not had early-onset disease (Zerres *et al.*, 1985; Fryns *et al.*, 1986; Kääriäinen *et al.*, 1988b). However, there appears to be an increased likelihood of early disease in affected siblings (Ross and Travers, 1975; Fryns *et al.*, 1986; Kääriäinen, 1987; Kääriäinen *et al.*, 1988b) and other members of the same kindred (Zerres *et al.*, 1985). This may be related to modifying genes (Zerres *et al.*, 1985; Woo *et al.*, 1997). Early-onset disease may be more likely in families with mutations in *PKD1* (Gal *et al.*, 1989).

Pathology

The kidneys are typically enlarged and have random cysts, which can originate from any portion of the nephron (Fig. 22.6). Except for cysts, the renal architecture is initially normal, though as the disease progresses fibrosis and glomerulosclerosis gradually increase.

Clinical features

There are three distinct groups of pediatric patients with ADPKD: asymptomatic children, symptomatic children, and severe neonatal disease. Most children with ADPKD are asymptomatic and increasing numbers of these patients are diagnosed based on a positive family history leading to a screening computed tomograpic (CT) scan or sonogram. Others are diagnosed after kidney cysts are incidentally noted on an imaging study.

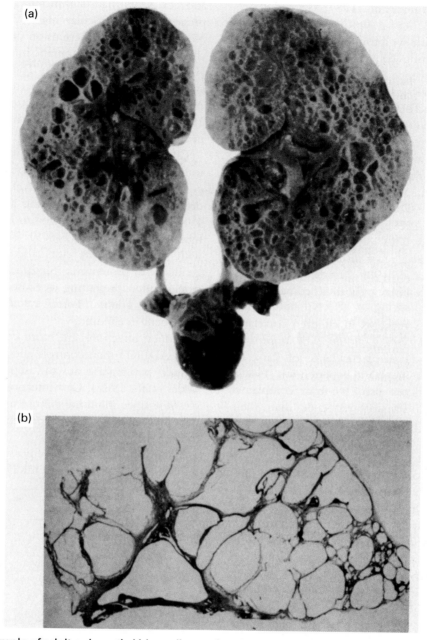

Figure 22.6 (*a*) Example of adult polycystic kidney disease in a 3-month-old infant. Notice the rounded cysts of varying size. (*b*) Low-power view of the same kidney. Foci of normal renal tissue are seen between the grossly dilated tubules. (Reproduced with permission from Blyth and Ockenden, 1971.)

Although children are often asymptomatic, there are numerous reports of severe disease, including neonatally lethal disease (Fryns *et al.*, 1986; Kääriäinen *et al.*, 1988b; Gal *et al.*, 1989). Neonatal mortality is usually due to respiratory failure and is associated with massively enlarged kidneys (Ross *et al.*, 1975; Kääriäinen *et al.*, 1988b; Gal *et al.*, 1989). Some neonates have renal masses but normal renal and respiratory function (Taitz *et al.*, 1987). Other children die of kidney failure during the first year of life. Survivors are at risk for chronic renal failure and some will reach ESRD before adulthood (Gal *et al.*, 1989). However, others, despite their neonatal presentation, will have normal kidney function during childhood (Taitz *et al.*, 1987; Gagnadoux *et al.*, 1989).

Most children with symptomatic ADPKD have a more subtle presenting complaint, typically in late childhood or adolescence (Kääriäinen *et al.*, 1988b; Gagnadoux *et al.*, 1989). Hematuria is quite common in adults with ADPKD (Gabow *et al.*, 1992a) and can manifest in childhood (Kaplan *et al.*, 1977; Sedman *et al.*, 1987; Kääriäinen *et al.*, 1988b; Gagnadoux *et al.*, 1989). Other presenting symptoms include hypertension, abdominal or flank pain, abdominal mass, urinary tract infection, and proteinuria (Table 22.2) (Sedman *et al.*, 1987; Kääriäinen *et al.*, 1988b; Gagnadoux *et al.*, 1989; Fick *et al.*, 1994). The majority of patients who are symptomatic during childhood do not have renal insufficiency as young adults (Gagnadoux *et al.*, 1989) but they may be at a higher risk for early kidney failure (Sedman *et al.*, 1987).

The presence of symptoms in children correlates with the number of cysts. Children with more than ten cysts have an increased incidence of flank or back pain, palpable kidneys, and hypertension (Fick *et al.*, 1994). Such children also have more complaints of palpitations and urinary frequency than their unaffected siblings (Fick *et al.*, 1994).

Recent evidence suggests that hypertension and resultant end-organ damage develop insidiously in older children and young adults with ADPKD. When a group of mostly asymptomatic children were screened, 13% had hypertension (vs 0% of controls) and the hypertensive patients had left ventricular hypertrophy (Ivy *et al.*, 1995). A smaller study using ambulatory blood pressure monitoring found no evidence of hypertension in patients below 15 years, but there was an increase in left ventricular mass (Zeier *et al.*, 1993). In addition, patients between 15 and 25 years had significant increases in blood pressure and ventricular mass (Zeier *et al.*, 1993). Not surprisingly, hypertension is more common in children who are symptomatic in the neonatal period (Kääriäinen *et al.*, 1988b). The renin–angiotensin system is implicated in hypertensive adults with ADPKD and normal renal function (Chapman *et al.*, 1990a), though this mechanism has not been studied in children.

Children with kidney failure are at risk for the typical electrolyte problems of chronic renal insufficiency. Some children with mild ADPKD have a subtle defect in urinary concentrating ability (Gagnadoux, 1989) and this is more common in children with more than ten cysts (Fick *et al.*, 1994). Children with more than ten cysts also have an increased incidence of proteinuria (Sharp *et al.*, 1998). Kidney stones, often presenting as acute flank pain, are increased in adults (Torres *et al.*, 1993), but are infrequent in children.

Kidney infections are more common in patients with ADPKD than controls and complications may include perinephric abscess, septicemia, and death (Sklar *et al.*, 1987). Cyst infection is especially troublesome since the urine culture may be negative and not all antibiotics achieve therapeutic levels in the cyst fluid (Sklar *et al.*, 1987).

There is a large number of possible extrarenal manifestations in adults with ADPKD:

- mitral valve prolapse
- hypertension
- extrarenal cysts
  hepatic cysts
  pancreatic cysts
  ovarian cysts
  testicular cysts

Table 22.2 Presenting complaints in symptomatic children with ADPKD[a]

Symptom	Gagnadoux *et al.* (1989)	Fick *et al.* (1994)	Kääriäinen *et al.* (1987)
Hematuria	3	2	2
Abdominal pain	3	1	1
Hypertension	3	1	0
Renal mass	1	1	0
Frequency	0	2	0
UTI	0	1	1
Proteinuria	0	0	1

[a]Excludes patients with severe neonatal disease.

arachnoid cysts
splenic cysts
pineal cysts
seminal-vesicle cysts
- aortic aneurysms
- intracranial aneurysms
- hernias
- colonic diverticula
- cholangiocarcinoma
- congenital hepatic fibrosis.

Extrarenal problems are less common in childhood. Mitral valve prolapse (MVP) is found in 26% of adults with ADPKD (Hossack et al., 1988). Among a group of children, 12% had MVP (vs 3% of controls) and the incidence increased with age (Ivy et al., 1995). Inguinal hernias are substantially increased in both children (Sedman et al., 1987; Fick et al., 1994) and adults (Modi et al., 1989; Morris-Stiff et al., 1997).

Liver cysts are the most common extrarenal manifestation in adults with ADPKD, with the prevalence increasing with age (Milutinovic et al., 1980; Gabow et al., 1990). Women tend to have more and larger cysts (Everson et al., 1988) and pregnancy is an additional risk factor for women (Gabow et al., 1990). Some adults experience abdominal fullness and pain but cysts almost never impair liver function or cause portal hypertension (Milutinovic et al., 1980; Everson et al., 1988) except in extreme cases (Torres et al., 1994b). Infected liver cysts present with pain, fever, and leukocytosis (Telenti et al., 1990). Liver cysts are rare in children (Milutinovic et al., 1989; Fick et al., 1994). Liver enlargement (Kääriäinen et al., 1988b) has occasionally been described in children. A few patients with ADPKD have congenital hepatic fibrosis (Main et al., 1983; Cobben et al., 1990; Lipschitz et al., 1993) but this liver involvement is usually restricted to one member of the family and thus does not appear to be related to a unique ADPKD gene defect.

Pancreatic cysts are present in only 9% of patients over 30 years of age (Torra et al., 1997) and almost never cause complications (Malka et al., 1998). They are extremely unusual in children (Milutinovic et al., 1989). The claim that ovarian cysts are increased in ADPKD has been questioned in a recent prospective study that did not find an increase among premenopausal women (Stamm et al., 1999). The remaining cystic complications are quite rare (Gabow, 1993).

Ruptured intracranial aneurysms are a significant cause of mortality in adults with ADPKD (Fick et al., 1995). In one study the mean age of bleeding was 39.5 years but 10% of patients were less than 20 years (Chauveau et al., 1994). There are reports of young children with a subarachnoid hemorrhage (Kääriäinen et al., 1988b) and a bleeding arteriovenous malformation (AVM) (Proesmans et al., 1982), and a 12-year-old child who died due to a ruptured intracranial aneurysm (Anton and Abramowsky, 1982). Aneurysms cluster in families (Huston et al., 1993; Ruggieri et al., 1994) and thus a positive family history for intracranial hemorrhage or aneurysm is an important risk factor.

Gender differences in ADPKD include the predisposition to liver cysts in women. The rate of progression to kidney failure is increased in adult males with either PKD1 (Gabow et al., 1992b) or PKD2 (Hateboer et al., 1999). No gender differences among children have been reported (Fick et al., 1994).

Radiological features

Both sonography (Fig. 22.7) and CT scan (Fig. 22.8) are useful for detecting the macroscopic cysts of ADPKD. The number and size of cysts in children increase with age (Fick et al., 1994). Children with more cysts have increased kidney size (Fick et al., 1994). Liver cysts are quite unusual in children (Fick et al., 1994).

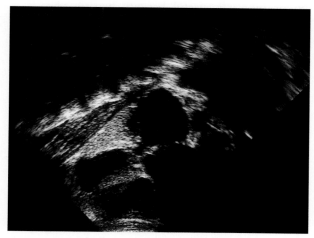

Figure 22.7 Sonogram of an infant with severe ADPKD. The kidneys are enlarged owing to multiple cysts. (Courtesy of Dr J. Sty, Children's Hospital of Wisconsin.)

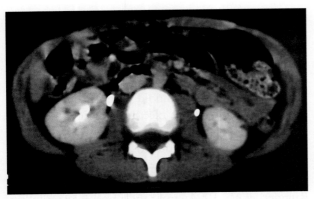

Figure 22.8 Computed tomographic scan of a child with ADPKD. Macroscopic cysts are readily visible. (Courtesy of Dr J. Sty, Children's Hospital of Wisconsin.)

Table 22.3 Sensitivity and specificity of sonography for detecting ADPKD in children

Age	Specificity (%)	Sensitivity (%)
3 months–5 years	89	62
5–10 years	100	82
10–15 years	100	86
15–17.5 years	100	67

Results of ultrasound screening in a group of children with PKD1 by linkage analysis. The presence of a single cyst was interpreted as a positive ultrasound. (Adapted from Gabow et al., 1997).

Diagnosis

Rare, early-onset ADPKD can sometimes be diagnosed by prenatal sonogram (Zerres et al., 1982, 1985; Main et al., 1983; Fryns et al., 1986). Most cases are identified in the last 10 weeks of gestation. The kidneys are large, with increased echogenicity, and cannot easily be distinguished from the kidneys of children with ARPKD. Occasionally, macrocysts are identified (Main et al., 1983). Early diagnosis in a fetus with an affected parent is possible using DNA analysis (Reeders et al., 1986; Novelli et al., 1989).

Even after birth it is often difficult to distinguish early-onset ADPKD from ARPKD. Radiologic studies of the kidneys are often inconclusive. Liver imaging or biopsy is useful because hepatic fibrosis is always present in ARPKD and extremely rare in ADPKD. Kidney pathology is also helpful, given the absence of glomerular cysts in ARPKD. The presence of a parent with ADPKD is the most useful diagnostic clue. However, many parents are unaware of their own disease (Taitz et al., 1987; Gagnadoux et al., 1989) and thus screening imaging studies of 'normal' parents are mandatory. Because of the possibility of a false-negative radiologic study, screening of the grandparents is sometimes useful, especially if the parents are less than 30 years old.

Diagnosis in asymptomatic or mildly symptomatic children is usually accomplished by renal sonography. The sensitivity and specificity of this approach increase with the child's age (Table 22.3). CT scan, though perhaps more sensitive than ultrasound (Levine and Grantham, 1981), is usually not a front-

line approach because of the greater ease of sonography. Unilateral cysts may be the only initial finding in children with ADPKD (Anton and Abramowsky, 1982; Farrell et al., 1984; Porch et al., 1986; Gagnadoux et al., 1989; Fick et al., 1994) and, in the context of a positive family history, even a single cyst is highly suggestive of disease (Gabow et al., 1997). Bilateral cysts are frequently found on later investigation (Fick et al., 1994). For adults, given the increased detection of benign solitary cysts, more stringent criteria are necessary to avoid false positives (Ravine et al., 1994).

The ability to screen patients for mutations in PKD1 or PKD2 is currently not readily available except in a research setting. Because the PKD1 gene is very large and complex, screening for mutations is very difficult. In contrast, linkage analysis is less technically demanding, though it does require testing of multiple family members. Such analysis is especially useful for the evaluation of potential living-related transplant donors who are at risk for disease.

The increasing ability to diagnose ADPKD raises some important issues. Unlike many other genetic diseases, the morbidity and mortality in ADPKD typically occur in older adults and problems are fairly modest in many patients. Nevertheless, among a group of adults at risk for the disease, 97% would like to receive genetic testing (Sujansky et al., 1990). There is also enthusiasm for genetic testing of offspring, with 89% selecting this option (Sujansky et al., 1990). However, knowledge of the presence of this disease has little impact on reproductive decisions. Only 11% of patients do not have children because of the risk of passing the disease to offspring and even fewer (4%) would terminate a pregnancy for ADPKD (Sujansky *et al.*, 1990).

Screening and monitoring

Many children have a parent with ADPKD and therefore have a 50% risk of carrying the defective gene. Undiagnosed, asymptomatic patients may have significant abnormalities such as hypertension, proteinuria, bacteriuria, and an increased creatinine (Zerres *et al.*, 1992). Certainly, at-risk children need periodic screening, with special attention being paid to the blood pressure. A possible algorithm is presented in Figure 22.9. Screening sonograms are not recommended because of concerns regarding obtaining health insurance (Golin *et al.*, 1996). A more aggressive approach will be necessary if an effective early treatment for ADPKD becomes available. Figure 22.9 also presents a basic approach to monitoring the child with a diagnosis of ADPKD, with the caveat that monitoring needs to be customized for the individual patient.

Treatment

Children with severe disease receive standard therapy for chronic renal insufficiency. This should include careful monitoring of nutrition and growth. In adults with moderate renal insufficiency there is no benefit to protein restriction, though there is a marginal slowing in the rate of decline in the glomerular filtration rate (GFR) in patients with severe renal insufficiency (Klahr *et al.*, 1995). Such an approach is not recommended in children because the benefits are minimal and there is potential for adverse effects on growth and development.

Hypertension is fairly common in older children with ADPKD and should be treated. There is no consensus on the ideal class of antihypertensive agent to select for these patients. Despite the pathogenic role of the renin–angiotensin system (Chapman *et al.*, 1990a) and the evidence that ACE inhibitors slow the progression of renal insufficiency in a variety of kidney diseases (Leuis *et al.*, 1993; Maschio *et al.*, 1996), ACE inhibitors, when rigorously tested, do not slow the progression of chronic renal insufficiency in

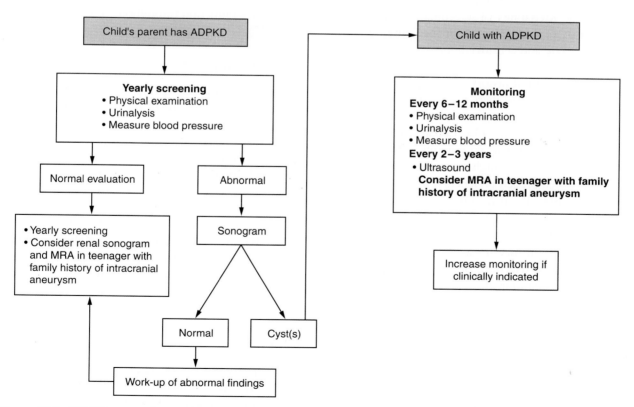

Figure 22.9 ADPKD: screening and monitoring of children. MRA = magnetic resonance angiography.

ADPKD (Maschio *et al.*, 1996). ACE inhibitors reverse left ventricular hypertrophy in hypertensive adults with ADPKD (Ecder *et al.*, 1999) but there is a small risk of precipitating acute renal failure in these patients and thus they must be used cautiously (Chapman *et al.*, 1991). Other agents, such as calcium channel blockers, have also been advocated (Kanno *et al.*, 1996).

The goal of therapy is normalization of blood pressure using standard guidelines (National High Blood Pressure Education Program, 1996). In adults with ADPKD low targets for blood pressure have a deleterious effect on renal function (Klahr *et al.*, 1995).

Urinary tract infections should be treated promptly, with awareness of the increased risk of abscesses and septicemia. Cyst infection requires selection of an antibiotic or antibacterial agent that penetrates the cyst, such as trimethoprim–sulfamethoxazole (Elzinga *et al.*, 1987) or ciprofloxacin (Elzinga *et al.*, 1988); occasionally, cyst aspiration may be necessary (Chapman *et al.*, 1990b). Patients with intractable pain from renal cysts can benefit from either cyst aspiration or surgical unroofing (Bennett *et al.*, 1987).

The possibility of a ruptured intracranial aneurysm is a frightening, albeit rare complication in pediatric patients. The advisability of screening patients is currently debated. Magnetic resonance angiography (MRA) is a safe and sensitive approach for detecting an asymptomatic aneurysm (Huston *et al.*, 1993). However, the natural history of asymptomatic aneurysms is unknown, and there is a need to balance the safety and efficacy of surgical intervention with the risk of aneurysm rupture. One decision analysis supported screening 20-year-old patients with ADPKD (Butler *et al.*, 1996), though others have suggested a less aggressive approach (Wiebers *et al.*, 1992; Chapman *et al.*, 1993). Because of the familial predilection to aneurysm formation (Huston *et al.*, 1993; Ruggieri *et al.*, 1994), screening of older teenagers with a positive family history is a reasonable approach. However, patient selection, timing and frequency of screening continue to evolve.

Prognosis

Most children with ADPKD will have minimal symptoms throughout childhood. The adult course of the disease is extremely variable.

There are currently limited data on the ultimate prognosis for patients diagnosed during childhood.

This is especially true for patients with asymptomatic cysts, and the impact of increased numbers of cysts on the risk of chronic renal failure is unknown. Children who are diagnosed after the neonatal period do not have a decrease in GFR, even in the subgroup with more cysts and symptoms (Fick *et al.*, 1994). In adults, the presence of the *PKD1* gene, younger age at diagnosis, male gender, hypertension, increased left ventricular mass, hepatic cysts in women, three or more pregnancies, gross hematuria, urinary tract infection in men, proteinuria and renal volume are all independently associated with poor renal function (Gabow *et al.*, 1992b; Chapman *et al.*, 1994). Extrapolating these data to children should be done cautiously and, in any case, prediction for the individual patient is impossible. Nevertheless, there seems to be a higher risk of early chronic renal failure when patients have more severe disease as children (Sedman *et al.*, 1987).

Many children diagnosed antenatally have normal renal function (Gagnadoux *et al.*, 1989), though follow-up is relatively limited. The cases diagnosed neonatally frequently have severe, often fatal, disease. These children are at risk for early chronic renal insufficiency and ESRD. However, others maintain normal renal function throughout childhood (Taitz *et al.*, 1987).

Nephronophthisis

Nephronophthisis (NPH), also called juvenile nephronophthisis, is one of the most common genetic causes of chronic renal insufficiency in children (Fivush *et al.*, 1998). The defective gene that is responsible for the majority of cases of NPH has been identified but the genetic basis is not known in all patients, especially those with significant extrarenal disease. NPH, which is recessively inherited, is often grouped with dominantly inherited medullary cystic disease because of an overlapping radiologic and histologic appearance. However, medullary cystic disease is genetically distinct, lacks extrarenal involvement, and usually presents in adulthood. Therefore, it will be considered separately later in this chapter.

Genetics

The majority of cases of NPH is due to mutations in the *NPHP1* gene, which is located on chromosome 2 (Hildebrandt *et al.*, 1997a; Saunier *et al.*, 1997). Patients with an affected *NPHP1* gene are classified as having NPH type 1. The genetic locus has not been identified in other cases; the *NPHP1* gene is not usually the cause of NPH in patients with major extrarenal manifestations such as those patients with Senior–Løken syndrome (see below) (Medhioub *et al.*, 1994). Most patients with NPH type 1 have large chromosomal deletions that affect the *NPHP1* gene (Konrad *et al.*, 1996; Hildebrandt *et al.*, 1997b).

Pathology

Grossly, the kidneys are often small and have a pale finely granular surface (van Collenburg *et al.*, 1978; Waldherr *et al.*, 1982). On light microscopy there is diffuse interstitial fibrosis with a mononuclear cell infiltration (Sherman *et al.*, 1971; Waldherr *et al.*, 1982; Matsubara *et al.*, 1991). Along with tubular atrophy, there is extreme thickening and lamination of the tubular basement membranes (Sherman *et al.*, 1971; Waldherr *et al.*, 1982). Electron microscopy confirms this thickening and also shows splitting of the basement membrane (Waldherr *et al.*, 1982). In a child with a biopsy early in the course of the disease, tubular basement membrane thickening was the only histologic abnormality (Matsubara *et al.*, 1991). Cysts appear to originate from the distal convoluted tubules and collecting ducts (Sherman *et al.*, 1971). The glomeruli may be normal or have periglomerular fibrosis with thickening of Bowman's capsule and glomerular obsolescence eventually develops (Waldherr *et al.*, 1982).

Clinical features

The signs and symptoms of NPH include polyuria and polydipsia, anemia, and growth retardation. Polyuria and polydipsia are due to poor urinary concentrating ability and this can lead to problems such as dehydration, nocturia, and primary or secondary nocturnal enuresis (Waldherr *et al.*, 1982; Clarke *et al.*, 1992; Elzouki *et al.*, 1996). Renal sodium wasting (Waldherr *et al.*, 1982) leads to salt craving in some children (Elzouki *et al.*, 1996). The urinalysis is notable for the absence of abnormalities (van Collenburg *et al.*, 1978; Waldherr *et al.*, 1982; Elzouki *et al.*, 1996), though low levels of proteinuria, usually tubular in origin (Clarke *et al.*, 1992), are sometimes present. Glucosuria is also occasionally present (Tsukahara *et al.*, 1990; Clarke *et al.*, 1992). Probably as a result of the polyuria and salt wasting, hypertension is unusual (van Collenburg *et al.*, 1978), even

in children with ESRD. Symptoms of chronic renal failure, such as fatigue, anorexia and growth retardation, are frequently present (Chamberlin *et al.*, 1977; van Collenburg *et al.*, 1978; Clarke *et al.*, 1992; Elzouki *et al.*, 1996). Symptoms of renal osteodystrophy may be the initial complaint (Chamberlin *et al.*, 1977). Children with NPH have an anemia that is out of proportion to their degree of renal failure and thus often have very low hematocrits and notable pallor (Chamberlin *et al.*, 1977; van Collenburg *et al.*, 1978; Clarke *et al.*, 1992; Warady *et al.*, 1994; Elzouki *et al.*, 1996). The anemia appears to be due to decreased erythropoietin production (Ala-Mello *et al.*, 1996).

The majority of patients with NPH type 1 develop ESRD during childhood at a mean age of about 10–13 years (Waldherr *et al.*, 1982; Hildebrandt *et al.*, 1997b). The defect in urine concentrating ability can lead to severe dehydration and acute renal failure, which may accelerate the development of chronic renal failure (Hildebrandt *et al.*, 1997b). The patients with the *NPHP1* gene defect are clinically indistinguishable from those who are not genetically linked to this locus (Medhioub *et al.*, 1994; Hildebrandt *et al.*, 1997b).

Senior–Løken syndrome is the combination of NPH with congenital amaurosis of Leber, which is also called infantile tapetoretinal degeneration (Senior *et al.*, 1961; Løken *et al.*, 1961). Ocular disease is generally diagnosed in infancy (Valadez *et al.*, 1987). Nystagmus is usually present and there is an absent pupillary response to light. The retina is markedly abnormal on funduscopic examination; findings include arteriolar narrowing, pale optic discs, and granular pigmentation of the fundus (Steele *et al.*, 1980). Most patients are blind or severely visually impaired and have a flat electroretinogram (Clarke *et al.*, 1992). Parents of children with Senior–Løken syndrome are asymptomatic and have a normal ophthalmologic exam but electro-oculographic and electroretinographic studies can sometimes detect abnormalities (Polak *et al.*, 1983). The renal disease in Senior–Løken syndrome is usually similar to NPH type 1, with renal failure typically occurring around the age of 10 years (Valadez *et al.*, 1987).

Some children with NPH have other extrarenal manifestations, including mental retardation (Stanescu *et al.*, 1976; Waldherr *et al.*, 1982; Warady *et al.*, 1994), hepatic fibrosis (Boichis *et al.*, 1973; Stanescu *et al.*, 1976; Delaney *et al.*, 1978; Gidion,

1979; Waldherr *et al.*, 1982; Fernández-Rodriguez *et al.*, 1990), Dandy–Walker syndrome (Warady *et al.*, 1994), cerebellar ataxia (Mainzer *et al.*, 1970; Giedion, 1979), coloboma (Waldherr *et al.*, 1982), and skeletal anomalies (Mainzer *et al.*, 1970; Giedion, 1979; Waldherr *et al.*, 1982; Ellis *et al.*, 1984; Di Rocco *et al.*, 1997). However, there is some question about the rigor of the renal diagnosis in some of these cases (Mendley *et al.*, 1995).

The more common possible extrarenal manifestations of NPH are:

- tapetoretinal degeneration
- liver fibrosis
- skeletal abnormalities
- mental retardation
- cerebellar ataxia.

Most patients with extrarenal manifestations also have tapetoretinal degeneration and thus are part of the Senior–Løken syndrome.

Children with a defect in the *NPHP1* gene usually do not have clinically significant extrarenal involvement, but patients with a defect in the *NPHP1* gene may have ocular findings, including areas of retinal atrophy with flat or low-voltage electroretinograms. However, these patients are usually asymptomatic (Caridi *et al.*, 1998).

Radiological features

By ultrasonography the kidneys are hyperechoic with loss of corticomedullary differentiation, and they are of normal or slightly decreased size (Garel *et al.*, 1984; Blowey *et al.*, 1996; Ala-Mello *et al.*, 1998). Medullary cysts are a hallmark of the disease but they are not always detected sonographically (Garel *et al.*, 1984; Blowey *et al.*, 1996; Elzouki *et al.*, 1996). CT is a more sensitive method for identifying medullary cysts (McGregor *et al.*, 1989) and thin-section CT is recommended (Elzouki *et al.*, 1996).

Diagnosis

The diagnosis of NPH can be challenging, especially in patients without extrarenal manifestations. A history of polyuria and polydipsia, salt craving, disproportionate anemia, a benign urinalysis, and the age of presentation are important clues. The detection of medullary cysts in the setting of chronic renal failure in a child with smallish, echogenic kidneys is virtually diagnostic. The presence of consanguinity or an affected sibling suggests an autosomal recessive disease and thus strongly supports the diagnosis. Renal histology is potentially helpful in uncertain cases. Genetic diagnosis is now possible because screening for a large chromosomal deletion is relatively easy (Konrad *et al.*, 1998) and this will identify approximately 70% of patients with NPH type 1 (Hildebrandt *et al.*, 1997b). Since 30% of patients do not have such a deletion its absence does not rule out the diagnosis. Screening for more subtle point mutations is possible but quite labor intensive at present. Genetic analysis is not yet possible in patients with Senior–Løken syndrome but the classic ocular findings provide support for the diagnosis. All patients should have ocular examinations and liver sonograms to screen for hepatic fibrosis.

Treatment

There is no specific therapy for NPH. Families should be counseled regarding the risk of dehydration due to polyuria. The anemia responds to erythropoietin therapy. Children receive standard therapy for chronic renal insufficiency and ultimately require dialysis and transplantation. The disease does not recur in kidney transplants and thus transplantation is usually quite successful (Steele *et al.*, 1980; Valadez and Firlit, 1987). Appropriate specialist care is necessary in children with extrarenal manifestations.

Medullary cystic disease

Medullary cystic disease (MCD) is frequently grouped with NPH as the juvenile nephronophthisis/medullary cystic disease complex (Strauss and Sommers, 1967). However, MCD is clearly a distinct entity, based on its autosomal dominant inheritance and later onset. (Gardner, 1971). Patients with MCD develop renal failure as young adults (Goldman *et al.*, 1966), although clinical manifestations are sometimes detected in older children (Gardner, 1971; Scolari *et al.*, 1997). In some families the disease is not apparent until a mean age of over 60 years (Christodoulou *et al.*, 1998). Sonograms may show medullary cysts and the histology is similar to NPH. Other similarities between MCD and NPH include the presence of anemia, polyuria, salt wasting, and a fairly benign urinalysis (Goldman *et al.*, 1966; Scolari *et al.*, 1997). Some patients with MCD have hyperuricemia and gouty arthritis (Stavrou *et al.*, 1998; Scolari *et al.*,

1999) but other extrarenal manifestations are rare (Scolari *et al.*, 1997). Genetic loci for MCD have been identified on chromosome 1 (Christodoulou *et al.*, 1998) and chromosome 16 (Scolari *et al.*, 1997), and linkage to the *NPHP1* gene is excluded (Scolari *et al.*, 1998).

Medullary sponge kidney

Medullary sponge kidney (MSK) is predominantly a disease of adults but occasionally presents in childhood (Snelling *et al.*, 1970; Patriquin *et al.*, 1985; Sluysmans *et al.*, 1987). The intrapapillary collecting ducts are dilated and multiple small cysts may be present. Not all renal pyramids are equally affected, providing an explanation for the often asymmetric and focal appearance. This does not appear to be an inherited disease, though a few family clusters have been described (Zawada *et al.*, 1984; Khoury *et al.*, 1988).

The diagnosis of MSK is based on the characteristic changes on intravenous pyelography (IVP), which show stagnation of contrast in one or more renal papillae due to dilatation of the collecting ducts (Fig. 22.10). The resultant image has been described as a 'pyramidal blush' (Palubinskas, 1963). These changes are sometimes misdiagnosed as papillary necrosis (Zawada *et al.*, 1988). CT scan is not as sensitive for making the diagnosis of MSK but it has a superior

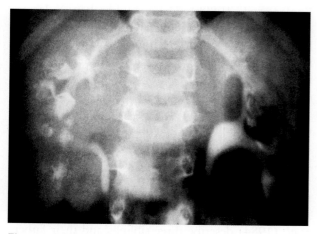

Figure 22.10 Intravenous pyelogram demonstrating bilateral medullary sponge kidneys in a 9-year-old girl who presented with hematuria. Note the characteristic radial stretching and puddling which represent the contrast-filled dilated collecting tubules in this disease. (From Glassberg *et al.*, 1981.)

ability to detect the papillary calcifications that frequently complicate MSK (Patriquin *et al.*, 1985; Ginalski *et al.*, 1991). Sonography also frequently detects this nephrocalcinosis, which may not be visible on a plain film (Patriquin *et al.*, 1985).

Clinically, patients are at increased risk for hematuria, urinary tract infection and nephrolithiasis. There may be an impairment of urinary concentrating ability (Patriquin *et al.*, 1985) or urinary acidification (renal tubular acidosis), but the GFR is normal (Green *et al.*, 1984; Higashihara *et al.*, 1984a). The urinary concentrating defect can lead to complaints of polyuria in a child (Patriquin *et al.*, 1985). The increased risk of nephrolithiasis and nephrocalcinosis (Sage *et al.*, 1982; Parks *et al.*, 1982; Ginalski *et al.*, 1990) is probably secondary to stagnation in the dilated collecting tubules and an increased incidence of hypercalcuria (Higashihara *et al.*, 1988b) and hypocitraturia (Osther *et al.*, 1994). Patients with renal tubular acidosis (RTA) are more likely to have hypercalcuria or hypocitraturia and the acidification defect may be the primary problem (Higashihara *et al.*, 1988b; Osther *et al.*, 1988, 1994). Nevertheless, even patients without a defect in urinary ion excretion have an increased risk of nephrolithiasis (Ginalski *et al.*, 1990), arguing for a contributing role of the dilated tubules (Higashihara *et al.*, 1984b).

The RTA in MSK, when present in a child, can lead to growth retardation (Sluysmans *et al.*, 1987). RTA is sometimes associated with severe potassium wasting and this can lead to symptomatic hypokalemia (Jayasinghe *et al.*, 1984).

Hematuria is usually mild but massive bleeding is occasionally seen (Betts *et al.*, 1992). More commonly, MSK is the explanation for asymptomatic microscopic or gross hematuria, and these are frequent complaints in pediatric cases (Snelling *et al.*, 1970; Patriquin *et al.*, 1985).

The increased risk of urinary tract infection may be related to stasis in the dilated tubules and the presence of stones, which may cause obstruction or act as a nidus of infection. Urinary tract infection in MSK is occasionally complicated by abscess formation (Levine, 1989).

Associated anomalies reported with MSK include hemihypertrophy (Harris *et al.*, 1981; Saypol and Laudone, 1983; Sluysmans *et al.*, 1987; Afonso *et al.*, 1988; Tomooka *et al.*, 1988; Indridason *et al.*, 1996), Caroli's disease (Braga *et al.*, 1994; Mrowka *et al.*, 1996), hyperparathyroidism (Rao *et al.*, 1977;

Maschio *et al.*, 1982), and a variety of miscellaneous disorders (Schoeneman *et al.*, 1984; Khoury *et al.*, 1988; Umeki *et al.*, 1989).

Most patients require limited treatment. Nephrolithiasis is successfully treated by the usual approaches, including extracorporeal shock-wave lithotripsy (ESWL) (Nakada *et al.*, 1993). Patients with MSK and RTA have a good response to alkali therapy, with decreased hypercalcuria and stone formation (Higashihara *et al.*, 1988a, b). Urinary tract infections are treated conventionally, with the caveat that an abscess should be suspected if the patient does not respond (Levine, 1989).

Glomerulocystic kidney disease

Glomerular cysts are present in a variety of diseases:

- syndromes with glomerular cysts
    brachymesomelia–renal syndrome
    oral–facial–digital syndrome
    glutaric acidemia type II
    trisomy 18
    renal retinal dysplasia
    short-rib polydactyly syndrome type II
    tuberous sclerosis
    Zellweger syndrome
- autosomal dominant polycystic kidney disease
- sporadic glomerulocystic kidney disease
- familial hypoplastic glomerulocystic kidney disease
- autosomal dominant glomerulocystic kidney disease.

The diagnosis is made by kidney biopsy. The term glomerulocystic kidney disease (GCKD) is reserved for patients who do not have an underlying disease such as ADPKD. As detailed below, GCKD is not a uniform, well-defined entity; rather, it describes a heterogenous group of patients who have been grouped into categories based on apparent inheritance and kidney size.

Glomerular cysts may be seen in children with a variety of severe, usually inherited, malformation syndromes (Smith *et al.*, 1965; Stapleton *et al.*, 1982; Langer *et al.*, 1983; Kobayashi *et al.*, 1985; Colevas *et al.*, 1988; Saguem *et al.*, 1992; Craver *et al.*, 1993; Montemarano *et al.*, 1995). Many of these patients have accompanying renal dysplasia. Again, these patients have glomerular cysts but do not have GCKD.

Glomerular cysts are seen in ADPKD but most patients also have cysts involving other segments of

the nephron (Fellows *et al.*, 1976; Proesmans *et al.*, 1982; Edwards *et al.*, 1989). However, there are cases of GCKD in children with a strong family history of ADPKD (Ross and Travers, 1975; Dedeoglu *et al.*, 1996). This suggests that, in these patients, GCKD is a variant of ADPKD, with predominance of glomerular cysts. One child had GCKD on initial biopsy but subsequently had pathologic findings consistent with ADPKD (Dedeoglu *et al.*, 1996). It has also been hypothesized that some patients with sporadic GCKD may, in fact, have ADPKD, either due to a new mutation or because of incomplete family studies.

Children with sporadic GCKD have a variable presentation. The kidneys are frequently enlarged at birth, with a loss of corticomedullary differentiation (Fitch *et al.*, 1986; Fredericks *et al.*, 1989). Kidney size may normalize (Fitch *et al.*, 1986) and, occasionally, the medulla is of normal echogenicity despite an echogenic cortex (Fredericks *et al.*, 1989). Renal function may be normal (Fitch *et al.*, 1986; Fredericks *et al.*, 1989) or decreased (McAlister *et al.*, 1979; Cachero *et al.*, 1990). Other cases of sporadic GCKD present in adults; these patients may have mild (Dosa *et al.*, 1984; Romero *et al.*, 1993) or severe (Oh *et al.*, 1986; Egashira *et al.*, 1991; Gonzalez *et al.*, 1994) renal failure, typically with enlarged kidneys.

There is an autosomal dominant form of GCKD that is associated with small (hypoplastic) kidneys and malformed or absent calyces (Rizzonc *et al.*, 1982; Kaplan *et al.*, 1989b). These children have a decreased GFR at birth but then renal function remains fairly stable. Some of these patients have been growth retarded (Kaplan *et al.*, 1989b) and a few have a noticeable prognathism (Rizzoni *et al.*, 1982; Kaplan *et al.*, 1989b).

The remaining families with GCKD have normal or increased kidney size. In one family with apparent autosomal dominant inheritance, kidney size and kidney function are normal but those affected have an abnormal sonogram (Carson *et al.*, 1987). In another family, a 10-year-old girl with an affected father had a mildly depressed GFR (Reznik *et al.*, 1982). Melnick *et al.* (1984) describe three siblings and their father, all of whom have normal kidney size but a decreased GFR. Finally, a large family with GCKD was extensively studied by Sharp *et al.* (1997). These patients were found to have hypertension and renal function ranging from normal to ESRD.

The kidneys are large and echogenic, and pelvocaliectasis and an hypoechoic cortical rim are additional sonographic features. Inheritance is autosomal dominant and linkage analysis indicates that neither the *PKD1* gene nor the *PKD2* gene is responsible for this family's disease (Sharp *et al.*, 1997).

Simple renal cysts

The increased use of radiologic testing has led to the identification of more children with simple cysts, which may be solitary or multiple. The incidence of simple cysts increases with age (Yamagishi *et al.*, 1988; Caglioti *et al.*, 1993; Tsugaya *et al.*, 1995). Fewer than 0.3% of children have simple renal cysts and they are usually not associated with subsequent problems (McHugh *et al.*, 1991). Cysts in children usually do not increase in size and single cysts are commonly located in the right upper pole (McHugh *et al.*, 1991). However, the presence of even a single cyst in the context of an appropriate family history suggests a diagnosis of ADPKD (Gabow *et al.*, 1997). The incidence of simple renal cysts is increased in children with acquired immunodeficiency syndrome (AIDS) (Zinn *et al.*, 1997). Simple renal cysts are rarely detected by fetal ultrasonography and the majority resolve before delivery (Blazer *et al.*, 1999).

Simple renal cysts do not impair renal function (McHugh *et al.*, 1991; Holmberg *et al.*, 1994). They rarely may play a role in causing infection (Limjoco and Strauch, 1966) or hypertension (Churchill *et al.*, 1975; Caglioti *et al.*, 1993; Pedersen *et al.*, 1997). Cysts in children occasionally cause pain (Reiner *et al.*, 1992). Symptomatic cysts can be treated by percutaneous drainage, although they usually recur unless a sclerosing agent is injected. Injection of the cyst with either alcohol (Hanna and Dahniya, 1996; Fontana *et al.*, 1999) or tetracycline (Reiner *et al.*, 1992) prevents recurrence. Surgical marsupialization is rarely necessary. Because cysts frequently occur in the upper pole, it is sometimes difficult to differentiate a cyst from upper pole hydronephrosis due to an obstructed ureterocele or an ectopic ureter. Such a diagnostic dilemma can be resolved by cyst aspiration (Steinhardt *et al.*, 1985; Reiner *et al.*, 1992). Cyst fluid has the same blood urea nitrogen and creatinine concentration as serum (Steinhardt *et al.*, 1985). Most children with simple renal cysts only need routine ultrasound follow-up, unless the cysts are atypical and therefore suggestive of a malignancy.

Multilocular cysts

A multilocular cyst is a unilateral, benign tumor of the kidney. Approximately one-half of the cases occur in children, with the remainder in middle-aged adults (Castillo *et al.*, 1991). Children are more likely to be male, while adults are more likely to be female. Children are usually less than 2 years of age and the most common presenting complaint is an abdominal mass (Austin and Castellino, 1973; Epstein *et al.*, 1978; Castillo *et al.*, 1991). Pathologically, the multilocular cyst is well encapsulated and non-infiltrating. The multiple cysts, which do not communicate, are typically separated by fibrous tissue, though embryonic tissue is sometimes present, especially in pediatric cases. The cysts are well visualized by CT scan or ultrasound. The differential diagnosis includes Wilms' tumor, ADPKD or a multicystic dysplastic kidney. Occasionally, a second multilocular cyst appears months later in the contralateral kidney (Chatten and Bishop, 1977).

Because of the possibility of a cystic Wilms' tumor, surgical resection is recommended (Castillo *et al.*, 1991). Nephrectomy is sometimes the only option but increasing numbers of cases are managed with renal preserving surgery (Chatten and Bishop, 1977; Castillo *et al.*, 1991).

Acquired cystic kidney disease

Kidney failure is sometimes associated with cyst formation in a previously non-cystic kidney. Acquired cystic kidney disease (ACKD) occurs in patients with renal failure, including those on dialysis and postrenal transplantation patients. ACKD occurs in children and the number of cysts increases over time (Leichter *et al.*, 1988; Querfeld *et al.*, 1992; Hogg, 1992; Mattoo *et al.*, 1997; Kyushu Pediatric Nephrology Study Group, 1999). Children with ACKD are at a low risk for gross hematuria and retroperitoneal hemorrhage (Kyushu Pediatric Nephrology Study Group, 1999). More ominously, a small percentage of children develop renal cell carcinoma (Querfeld *et al.*, 1992; Mattoo *et al.*, 1997). Because of this possibility, periodic ultrasound screening of dialysis patients is necessary and children with suspicious lesions should have a nephrectomy.

Syndromes with cystic kidneys

A large number of syndromes is associated with cystic kidneys. These are mostly rare diseases and many are neonatally fatal. The major features of a few prominent entities are reviewed here, with emphasis on those with a defined genetic etiology. A number of additional entities are listed in the section on glomerulocystic disease.

Tuberous sclerosis

Though classified as one of the neurocutaneous syndromes, renal involvement is an important cause of morbidity and mortality in tuberous sclerosis (TS) (Shepherd *et al.*, 1991; Torres *et al.*, 1994a). Patients with TS develop hamartomas in a variety of organs, including angiomyolipomas of the kidneys. The major extrarenal manifestations of TS are:

- neurologic
    - cortical tubers
    - seizures
    - mental retardation
    - intracranial aneurysms
    - retinal hemartoma
- cutaneous
    - hypopigmented macules
    - facial angiofibromas
    - shagreen patch
    - café-au-lait macules
    - molluscum fibrosum pendulum
    - forehead fibrous plaque
    - periungual fibromas
    - confetti-like macules
- cardiac
    - rhabdomyomas
    - Wolf–Parkinson–White syndrome
- bone
    - sclerosis
    - cystic changes
- pulmonary lymphangiomyomatosis.

Most of the features of TS become more prominent over time, except for cardiac rhabdomyomas, which tend to regress during childhood (DiMario *et al.*, 1996). The hypopigmented macules (ash-leaf spots) are especially helpful diagnostically since they are often visible at birth and are eventually present in over 97% of children (Józwiak *et al.*, 1998); use of a Wood's lamp, especially in light-skinned individuals, may aid in their identification. Facial angiofibromas, which may be confused with acne, and Shagreen patches are also extremely common. Neurologic lesions include multiple calcified tubers, disorders of neuron migration, and giant cell astrocytomas. The neurologic manifestations, with both seizures and developmental delay, are often the dominant clinical feature. Tumors of the kidney are the most common cause of malignancy in TS, but a variety of extrarenal cancers is also seen in adults and children (Al-Saleem *et al.*, 1998; Verhoef *et al.*, 1999).

TS is an autosomal dominant condition but two-thirds of the cases are due to new mutations, so most patients will not have a positive family history. There is variable penetrance and thus affected parents usually have mild disease and may be undiagnosed. TS is caused by mutations in either the *TSC1* gene on chromosome 9 (van Slegtenhorst *et al.*, 1997) or the *TSC2* gene on chromosome 16 (European Chromosome 16 Tuberous Sclerosis Consortium, 1993). Both of these genes encode tumor suppressors and the hamartomas arise because of mutations in the normal wild-type gene (Sepp *et al.*, 1996; Carbonara *et al.*, 1996). Intellectual disability is more common in patients with mutations in the *TSC2* gene (Jones *et al.*, 1997; 1999). The *TSC2* gene is located adjacent to the *PKD1* gene on chromosome 16 (Harris *et al.*, 1995). Some children have large chromosomal deletions that affect both the *TSC2* gene and the *PKD1* gene and these children tend to have severe polycystic kidney disease (Harris *et al.*, 1995; Torra *et al.*, 1998). This contiguous gene syndrome is present in the majority of children with early, severe polycystic kidney disease and TS (Sampson *et al.*, 1997).

Angiomyolipomas are the most common renal lesion in TS and are readily seen by CT or ultrasound (Fig. 22.11). Angiomyolipomas are usually not detected in the first few years of life but they are ultimately found in most children with TS and tend to increase in size during childhood (O'Hagan *et al.*, 1996; Ewalt *et al.*, 1998). Larger angiomyolipomas are sometimes associated with pain (Torres *et al.*, 1994a). Hematuria is uncommon (Stillwell *et al.*, 1987); however, retroperitoneal bleeding from angiomyolipomas can be life threatening (Shepherd *et al.*, 1991) and presents with sudden flank pain, a palpable abdominal mass, and symptoms of anemia. Clinical manifestations of angiomyolipomas are relatively uncommon in children (Moolten, 1942; Hendren and Monfort, 1987).

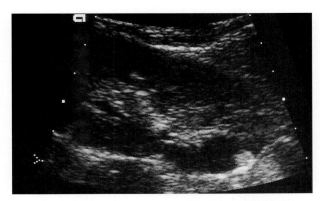

Figure 22.11 Sonogram of a child with angiomyolipomas due to tuberous sclerosis. This case shows the hyperechoic fat (without shadowing) of an angiomyolipoma. (Courtesy of Dr J. Sty, Children's Hospital of Wisconsin.)

Renal cysts (Fig. 22.12) are less common than angiomyolipomas and sometimes disappear on subsequent evaluation (Ewalt *et al.*, 1998). Renal malignancies, including renal cell carcinoma and malignant angiomyolipomas, are a serious concern in TS and both are seen in children, sometimes in early childhood (Al-Saleem *et al.*, 1998; Ewalt *et al.*, 1998).

Both renal cysts and angiomyolipomas cause destruction of normal renal tissue and this can lead to renal failure in both adults (Clarke *et al.*, 1999) and children (Sampson *et al.*, 1997). The risk of renal failure and hypertension (Stapleton *et al.*, 1980) is greater in patients with cystic disease (Anderson and Tannen, 1969; Cree and Nash, 1969). Children with disruption of the contiguous *PKD1* and *TSC2* genes usually have severe cystic disease and are at high risk for hypertension and early kidney failure (Sampson *et al.*, 1997).

The diagnosis of TS is based on the classic clinical features, though genetic analysis is sometimes possible. The possibility of TS should be suspected in a young child with large renal cysts suggestive of early-onset ADPKD. These children may have the contiguous gene syndrome with a deletion affecting both the *PKD1* and *TSC2* genes. A family history of TS is often not present due to variable penetrance and a high rate of new mutations. A search for skin manifestations is usually helpful, though cutaneous manifestations are less prominent or sometimes absent in infants (Józwiak *et al.*, 1998). Young children have fewer cortical tubers than older patients but MRI is quite sensitive for detecting other subtle findings in infancy (Baron and Barkovich, 1999). While MRI is more sensitive, most children have the mineralized subendymal nodules that are visible by CT (Fig. 22.13).

Children with TS require the input of multiple specialists. All children with TS should have a renal sonogram at diagnosis and follow-up studies every 1–3 years, with frequency dictated by the specific clinical situation (Roach *et al.*, 1999). Patients with extensive or rapidly changing lesions require more frequent follow-up. Those with more severe kidney disease may require CT or MRI to screen for malignant changes. Differentiating angiomyolipomas from

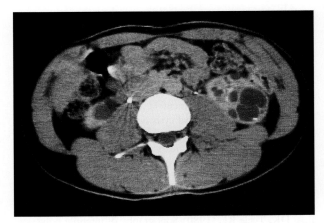

Figure 22.12 Renal computed tomography of a child with cysts due to tuberous sclerosis. Multiple cysts are visible. (Courtesy of Dr J. Sty, Children's Hospital of Wisconsin.)

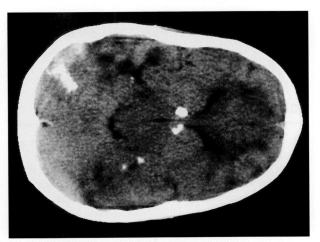

Figure 22.13 Head computed tomography of the same child shown in Figure 21.13. Subendymal calcific densities are present in the region of the foramen magnum. (Courtesy of Dr J. Sty, Children's Hospital of Wisconsin.)

malignancy requires careful comparison of sequential images. Patients with kidney failure are treated with dialysis (Clarke *et al.*, 1999) and transplantation (Balligand *et al.*, 1990). Because of the risk for renal hemorrhage and malignancy there is an argument for bilateral nephrectomies in children who progress to ESRD, especially those with large angiomyolipomas.

Meckel syndrome

Meckel syndrome, sometimes called Meckel–Gruber syndrome, is a lethal autosomal recessive disorder. The most common extrarenal manifestations are posterior encephalocele, polydactyly, and hepatic fibrosis and cysts, but a variety of other findings may also be present (Fraser and Lytwyn, 1981; Salonen, 1984). Cystic dysplasia of the kidneys is present in all cases (Fraser and Lytwyn, 1981; Salonen, 1984). A gene for Meckel syndrome is located on chromosome 17q (Paavola *et al.*, 1995), though there is evidence of genetic heterogeneity (Paavola *et al.*, 1997).

Von-Hippel–Lindau disease

Von-Hippel–Lindau (VHL) disease is a rare autosomal dominant disorder. The most prevalent manifestations are cerebellar hemangioblastoma, retinal angioma, renal cell carcinoma, spinal hemangioblastoma, and pheochromocytoma (Maher *et al.*, 1990; Maddock *et al.*, 1996). Renal cysts are also common but, as in renal cell carcinoma, they are rarely seen in childhood (Maher *et al.*, 1990; Maddock *et al.*, 1996). A mutation in a tumor-suppressor gene, located on chromosome 3, causes VHL disease (Latif *et al.*, 1993).

References

Afonso DN, Oliveira AG (1988) Medullary sponge kidney and congenital hemi-hypertrophy. *Br J Urol* 62: 187–8.

Ala-Mello S, Kivivuori SM, Rönnholm KA *et al* (1996) Mechanism underlying early anaemia in children with familial juvenile nephronophthisis. *Pediatr Nephrol* 10: 578–81.

Ala-Mello S, Jaaskelainen J, Koskimies O (1998) Familial juvenile nephronophthisis. An ultrasonographic follow-up of seven patients. *Acta Radiol* 39: 84–9.

Al-Saleem T, Wessner LL, Scheithauer BW *et al.* (1998) Malignant tumors of the kidney, brain, and soft tissues in children and young adults with the tuberous sclerosis complex. *Cancer* 83: 2208–16.

Alvarez F, Bernard O, Brunelle F *et al.* (1981) Congenital hepatic fibrosis in children. *J Pediatr* 99: 370–5.

Anand SK, Chan JC, Lieberman E (1975) Polycystic disease and hepatic fibrosis in children. Renal function studies. *Am J Dis Child* 129: 810–13.

Anderson D, Tannen RL (1969) Tuberous sclerosis and chronic renal failure. Potential confusion with polycystic kidney disease. *Am J Med* 47: 163–8.

Anton PA, Abramowsky CR (1982) Adult polycystic renal disease presenting in infancy: a report emphasizing the bilateral involvement. *J Urol* 128: 1290–1.

Argubright KF, Wicks JD (1987) Third trimester ultrasonic presentation of infantile polycystic kidney disease. *Am J Perinatol* 4: 1–4.

Austin SR, Castellino RA (1973) Multilocular cysts of kidney. *Urology* 1: 546–9.

Balligand JL, Pirson Y, Squifflet JP *et al.* (1990) Outcome of patients with tuberous sclerosis after renal transplantation. *Transplantation* 49: 515–18.

Baron Y, Barkovich AJ (1999) MR imaging of tuberous sclerosis in neonates and young infants. *AJNR Am J Neuroradiol* 20: 907–16.

Barth RA, Guillot AP, Capeless EL, Clemmons JJ (1992) Prenatal diagnosis of autosomal recessive polycystic kidney disease: variable outcome within one family. *Am J Obstet Gynecol* 166: 560–1.

Bean SA, Bednarek FJ, Primack WA (1995) Aggressive respiratory support and unilateral nephrectomy for infants with severe perinatal autosomal recessive polycystic kidney disease. *J Pediatr* 127: 311–13.

Bennett WM, Elzinga L, Golper TA, Barry JM (1987) Reduction of cyst volume for symptomatic management of autosomal dominant polycystic kidney disease. *J Urol* 137: 620–2.

Bernstein J (1997) Hepatic involvement in hereditary renal syndromes. *Birth Defects Original Article Series* 23: 115–30.

Besbas N, Ozen S, Saatçi U *et al.* (1998) Autosomal recessive polycystic kidney disease: mapping to chromosomal region of 6p21–cen in a Turkish child. *Turk J Pediatr* 40: 245–7.

Betts CD, O'Reilly PH (1992) Profound haemorrhage causing acute obstruction in medullary sponge kidney. *Br J Urol* 70: 449–50.

Blankenberg TA, Ruebner BH, Ellis WG *et al.* (1987) Pathology of renal and hepatic anomalies in Meckel syndrome. *Am J Med Genet* 3 (Suppl): 395–410.

Blazer S, Zimmer EZ, Blumenfeld Z *et al.* (1999) Natural history of fetal simple renal cysts detected in early pregnancy. *J Urol* 162: 812–14.

Blowey DL, Querfeld U, Geary D *et al.* (1996) Ultrasound findings in juvenile nephronophthisis. *Pediatr Nephrol* 10: 22–4.

Blyth H, Ockenden BG (1971) Polycystic disease of kidney and liver presenting in childhood. *J Med Genet* 8: 257–84.

Boal DK, Teele RL (1980) Sonography of infantile polycystic kidney disease. *AJR Am J Roentgenol* 135: 575–80.

Boichis H, Passwell J, David R, Miller H (1973) Congenital hepatic fibrosis and nephronophthisis. A family study. *Q J Med* 42: 221–33.

Braga AC, Calheno A, Rocha H, Lourenço-Gomes J (1994) Caroli's disease with congenital hepatic fibrosis and medullary sponge kidney. *J Pediatr Gastroenterol Nutr* **19**: 464–7.

Brasier JL, Henske EP (1997) Loss of the polycystic kidney disease (PKD1) region of chromosome 16p13 in renal cyst cells supports a loss-of-function model for cyst pathogenesis. *J Clin Invest* **99**: 194–9.

Bronshtein M, Bar-Hava I, Blumenfeld Z (1992) Clues and pitfalls in the early prenatal diagnosis of 'late onset' infantile polycystic kidney. *Prenatal Diagnosis* **12**: 293–8.

Brueton LA, Dillon MJ, Winter RM (1990) Ellis-van Creveld syndrome, Jeune syndrome, and renal–hepatic–pancreatic dysplasia: separate entities or disease spectrum? *J Med Genet* **27**: 252–5.

Butler WE, Barker FGD, Crowell RM (1996) Patients with polycystic kidney disease would benefit from routine magnetic resonance angiographic screening for intracerebral aneurysms: a decision analysis. *Neurosurgery* **38**: 506–15; Discussion 15–6.

Cachero S, Montgomery P, Seidel FG *et al.* (1990) Glomerulocystic kidney disease: case report. *Pediatr Radiol* **20**: 491–3; Discussion 4.

Caglioti A, Esposito C, Fuiano G *et al.* (1993) Prevalence of symptoms in patients with simple renal cysts. *BMJ (Clin Res)* **306**: 430–1.

Carbonara C, Longa L, Grosso E *et al.* (1996) Apparent preferential loss of heterozygosity at TSC2 over TSC1 chromosomal region in tuberous sclerosis hamartomas. *Genes Chromosomes Cancer* **15**: 18–25.

Caridi G, Murer L, Bellantuono R *et al.* (1998) Renal-retinal syndromes: association of retinal anomalies and recessive nephronophthisis in patients with homozygous deletion of the NPH1 locus. *Am J Kidney Dis* **32**: 1059–62.

Carson RW, Bedi D, Cavallo T, DuBose TDJ (1987) Familial adult glomerulocystic kidney disease. *Am J Kidney Dis* **9**: 154–65.

Castillo OA, Boyle ETJ, Kramer SA (1991) Multilocular cysts of kidney. A study of 29 patients and review of literature. *Urology* **37**: 156–62.

Chamberlin BC, Hagge WW, Stickler GB (1977) Juvenile nephronophthisis and medullary cystic disease. *Mayo Clin Proc* **52**: 485–91.

Chapman AB, Johnson A, Gabow PA, Schrier RW (1990a) The renin–angiotensin–aldosterone system and autosomal dominant polycystic kidney disease. *N Engl J Med* **323**: 1091–6.

Chapman AB, Thickman D, Gabow PA (1990b) Percutaneous cyst puncture in the treatment of cyst infection in autosomal dominant polycystic kidney disease. *Am J Kidney Dis* **16**: 252–5.

Chapman AB, Gabow PA, Schrier RW (1991) Reversible renal failure associated with angiotensin-converting enzyme inhibitors in polycystic kidney disease. *Ann Intern Med* **115**: 769–73.

Chapman AB, Rubinstein D, Hughes R *et al.* (1992) Intracranial aneurysms in autosomal dominant polycystic kidney disease. *N Engl J Med* **327**: 916–20.

Chapman AB, Johnson AM, Gabow PA (1993) Intracranial aneurysms in patients with autosomal dominant polycystic kidney disease: how to diagnose and who to screen. *Am J Kidney Dis* **22**: 526–31.

Chapman AB, Johnson AM, Gabow PA, Schrier RW (1994) Overt proteinuria and microalbuminuria in autosomal dominant polycystic kidney disease. *J Am Soc Nephrol* **5**: 1349–54.

Chatten J, Bishop HC (1977) Bilateral multilocular cysts of the kidneys. *J Pediatr Surg* **12**: 749–50.

Chauveau D, Pirson Y, Verellen-Dumoulin C *et al.* (1994) Intracranial aneurysms in autosomal dominant polycystic kidney disease. *Kidney Int* **45**: 1140–6.

Chilton SJ, Cremin BJ (1981) The spectrum of polycystic disease in children. *Pediatr Radiol* **11**: 9–15.

Christodoulou K, Tsingis M, Stavrou C *et al.* (1998) Chromosome 1 localization of a gene for autosomal dominant medullary cystic kidney disease. *Hum Molec Genet* **7**: 905–11.

Churchill D, Kimoff R, Pinsky M, Gault MH (1975) Solitary intrarenal cyst: correctable cause of hypertension. *Urology* **6**: 485–8.

Clarke A, Hancock E, Kingswood C, Osborne JP (1999) End-stage renal failure in adults with the tuberous sclerosis complex. *Nephrol Dialysis Transplant* **14**: 988–91.

Clarke MP, Sullivan TJ, Francis C *et al.* (1992) Senior-Loken syndrome. Case reports of two siblings and association with sensorineural deafness. *Br J Ophthalmol* **76**: 171–2.

Cobben JM, Breuning MH, Schoots C *et al.* (1990) Congenital hepatic fibrosis in autosomal-dominant polycystic kidney disease. *Kidney Int* **38**: 880–5.

Cole BR (1990) Autosomal recessive polycystic kidney disease. In: KD Gardner Jr, J Bernstein (eds) *The cystic kidney*. Boston: Kluwer Academic, 327–50.

Cole BR, Conley SB, Stapleton FB (1987) Polycystic kidney disease in the first year of life. *J Pediatr* **111**: 693–9.

Colevas AD, Edwards JL, Hruban RH *et al.* (1988) Glutaric acidemia type II. Comparison of pathologic features in two infants. *Arch Pathol Lab Med* **112**: 1133–9.

Consortium TEPKD (1994) The polycystic kidney disease 1 gene encodes a 14 kb transcript and lies within a duplicated region on chromosome 16. *Cell* **77**: 881–94.

Craver RD, Ortenberg J, Baliga R (1993) Glomerulocystic disease: unilateral involvement of a horseshoe kidney and in trisomy 18. *Pediatr Nephrol* **7**: 375–8.

Cree JE, Nash FW (1969) Tuberous sclerosis with polycystic kidneys. *Proc R Soc Med* **62**: 327.

D'Amico G, Pagliaro L, Bosch J (1995) The treatment of portal hypertension: a meta-analytic review. *Hepatology* **22**: 332–54.

Daoust MC, Reynolds DM, Bichet DG, Somlo S (1995) Evidence for a third genetic locus for autosomal dominant polycystic kidney disease. *Genomics* **25**: 733–6.

de Almeida S, de Almeida E, Peters D *et al.* (1995) Autosomal dominant polycystic kidney disease: evidence for the existence of a third locus in a Portuguese family. *Hum Genet* **96**: 83–8.

Dedeoglu IO, Fisher JE, Springate JE et al. (1996) Spectrum of glomerulocystic kidneys: a case report and review of the literature. *Pediatr Pathol Lab Med* **16**: 941–9.

Delaney V, Mullaney J, Bourke E (1978) Juvenile nephronophthisis, congenital hepatic fibrosis and retinal hypoplasia in twins. *Q J Med* **47**: 281–90.

DiMario FJJ, Diana D, Leopold H, Chameides L (1996) Evolution of cardiac rhabdomyoma in tuberous sclerosis complex. *Clin Pediatr* **35**: 615–19.

Di Rocco M, Picco P, Arslanian A et al. (1997) Retinitis pigmentosa, hypopituitarism, nephronophthisis, and mild skeletal dysplasia (RHYNS): a new syndrome? *Am J Med Genet* **73**: 1–4.

Dosa S, Thompson AM, Abraham A (1984) Glomerulocystic kidney disease. Report of an adult case. *Am J Clin Pathol* **82**: 619–21.

Ecder T, Edelstein CL, Chapman AB et al. (1999) Reversal of left ventricular hypertrophy with angiotensin converting enzyme inhibition in hypertensive patients with autosomal dominant polycystic kidney disease. *Nephrol Dialysis Transplant* **14**: 1113–16.

Edwards OP, Baldinger S (1989) Prenatal onset of autosomal dominant polycystic kidney disease. *Urology* **34**: 265–70.

Egashira K, Nakata H, Hashimoto O, Kaizu K (1991) MR imaging of adult glomerulocystic kidney disease. A case report. *Acta Radiol* **32**: 251–3.

Ellis DS, Heckenlively JR, Martin CL et al. (1984) Leber's congenital amaurosis associated with familial juvenile nephronophthisis and cone-shaped epiphyses of the hands (the Saldino–Mainzer syndrome). *Am J Ophthalmol* **97**: 233–9.

Elzinga LW, Golper TA, Rashad AL et al. (1987) Trimethoprim-sulfamethoxazole in cyst fluid from autosomal dominant polycystic kidneys. *Kidney Int* **32**: 884–8.

Elzinga LW, Golper TA, Rashad AL et al. (1988) Ciprofloxacin activity in cyst fluid from polycystic kidneys. *Antimicrob Agents Chemother* **32**: 844–7.

Elzouki AY, al-Suhaibani H, Mirza K, al-Sowailem AM (1996) Thin-section computed tomography scans detect medullary cysts in patients believed to have juvenile nephronophthisis. *Am J Kidney Dis* **27**: 216–9.

Epstein L, Wacksman J, Daughtry J, Straffon RA (1978) Multilocular cysts of kidney: a diagnostic dilemma. *Urology* **11**: 573–6.

European Chromosome 16 Tuberous Sclerosis Consortium (1993) Identification and characterization of the tuberous sclerosis gene on chromosome 16. *Cell* **75**: 1305–15.

Everson GT, Scherzinger A, Berger-Leff N et al. (1988) Polycystic liver disease: quantitation of parenchymal and cyst volumes from computed tomography images and clinical correlates of hepatic cysts. *Hepatology* **8**: 1627–34.

Ewalt DH, Sheffield E, Sparagana SP et al. (1998) Renal lesion growth in children with tuberous sclerosis complex. *J Urol* **160**: 141–5.

Farrell TP, Boal DK, Wood BP et al. (1984) Unilateral abdominal mass: an unusual presentation of autosomal dominant polycystic kidney disease in children. *Pediatr Radiol* **14**: 349–52.

Fellows RA, Leonidas JC, Beatty ECJ (1976) Radiologic features of adult type polycystic kidney disease in the neonate. *Pediatr Radiol* **4**: 87–92.

Fernández-Rodriguez R, Morales JM, Martínez R et al. (1990) Senior-Loken syndrome (nephronophthisis and pigmentary retinopathy) associated to liver fibrosis: a family study. *Nephron* **55**: 74–7.

Fick GM, Duley IT, Johnson AM et al. (1994)The spectrum of autosomal dominant polycystic kidney disease in children. *J Am Soc Nephrol* **4**: 1654–60.

Fick GM, Johnson AM, Hammond WS, Gabow PA (1995) Causes of death in autosomal dominant polycystic kidney disease. *J Am Soc Nephrol* **5**: 2048–56.

Fitch SJ, Stapleton FB (1986) Ultrasonographic features of glomerulocystic disease in infancy: similarity to infantile polycystic kidney disease. *Pediatr Radiol* **16**: 400–2.

Fivush BA, Jabs K, Neu AM et al. (1998) Chronic renal insufficiency in children and adolescents: the 1996 annual report of NAPRTCS. North American Pediatric Renal Transplant Cooperative Study. *Pediatr Nephrol* **12**: 328–37.

Fontana D, Porpiglia F, Morra I, Destefanis P (1999) Treatment of simple renal cysts by percutaneous drainage with three repeated alcohol injection. *Urology* **53**: 904–7.

Fraser FC, Lytwyn A (1981) Spectrum of anomalies in the Meckel syndrome, or: Maybe there is a malformation syndrome with at least one constant anomaly. *Am J Med Genet* **9**: 67–73.

Fredericks BJ, de Campo M, Chow CW, Powell HR (1989) Glomerulocystic renal disease: ultrasound appearances. *Pediatr Radiol* **19**: 184–6.

Fryns JP, Vandenberghe K, Moerman F (1986) Mid-trimester ultrasonographic diagnosis of early manifesting adult form of polycystic kidney disease. *Hum Genet* **74**: 461.

Gabow PA (1993) Autosomal dominant polycystic kidney disease. *N Engl J Med* **329**: 332–42.

Gabow PA, Duley I, Johnson AM (1992a) Clinical profiles of gross hematuria in autosomal dominant polycystic kidney disease. *Am J Kidney Dis* **20**: 140–3.

Gabow PA, Johnson AM, Kaehny WD et al. (1990) Risk factors for the development of hepatic cysts in autosomal dominant polycystic kidney disease. *Hepatology* **11**: 1033–7.

Gabow PA, Johnson AM, Kaehny WD et al. (1992b) Factors affecting the progression of renal disease in autosomal-dominant polycystic kidney disease. *Kidney Int* **41**: 1311–19.

Gabow PA, Kimberling WJ, Strain JD et al. (1997) Utility of ultrasonography in the diagnosis of autosomal dominant polycystic kidney disease in children. *J Am Soc Nephrol* **8**: 105–10.

Gagnadoux MF, Habib R, Levy M et al. (1989) Cystic renal diseases in children. *Adv Nephrol Necker Hospital* **18**: 33–57.

Gal A, Wirth B, Kääriäinen H et al. (1989) Childhood manifestation of autosomal dominant polycystic kidney disease: no evidence for genetic heterogeneity. *Clin Genet* **35**: 13–19.

Gang DL, Herrin JT (1986) Infantile polycystic disease of the liver and kidneys. *Clin Nephrol* **25**: 28–36.

Gardner KDJ (1971) Evolution of clinical signs in adult-onset cystic disease of the renal medulla. *Ann Intern Med* **74**: 47–54.

Garel LA, Habib R, Pariente D *et al.* (1984) Juvenile nephronophthisis: sonographic appearance in children with severe uremia. *Radiology* **151**: 93–5.

Giedion A (1979) Phalangeal cone shaped epiphysis of the hands (PhCSEH) and chronic renal disease – the conorenal syndromes. *Pediatr Radiol* **8**: 32–8.

Ginalski JM, Portmann L, Jaeger P (1990) Does medullary sponge kidney cause nephrolithiasis? *AJR Am J Roentgenol* **155**: 299–302.

Ginalski JM, Schnyder P, Portmann L, Jaeger P (1991) Medullary sponge kidney on axial computed tomography: comparison with excretory urography. *Eur J Radiol* **12**: 104–7.

Glassberg KI, Hackett RE, Waterhouse K *et al.* (1981) Congenital anomalies of kidney, ureter and bladder. In: AR Kendall, L Karafin (eds) *Harry S. Goldsmith's Practice of surgery: urology.* Hagerstown, MD: Harper and Row, 1–82.

Goldman SH, Walker SR, Merigan TCJ *et al.* (1966) Hereditary occurrence of cystic disease of the renal medulla. *N Engl J Med* **274**: 984–92.

Golin CO, Johnson AM, Fick G, Gabow PA (1996) Insurance for autosomal dominant polycystic kidney disease patients prior to end-stage renal disease. *Am J Kidney Dis* **27**: 220–3.

Gonzalez JM, Lombardo ME, Truong LD *et al.* (1994) Unusual presentation of glomerulocystic kidney disease in an adult patient. *Clin Nephrol* **42**: 266–8.

Green J, Szylman P, Sznajder II *et al.* (1984) Renal tubular handling of potassium in patients with medullary sponge kidney. A model of renal papillectomy in humans. *Arch Intern Med* **144**: 2201–4.

Habif DVJ, Berdon WE, Yeh MN (1982) Infantile polycystic kidney disease: *in utero* sonographic diagnosis. *Radiology* **142**: 475–7.

Hanna RM, Dahniya MH (1996) Aspiration and sclerotherapy of symptomatic simple renal cysts: value of two injections of a sclerosing agent. *AJR Am J Roentgenol* **167**: 781–3.

Harris RE, Fuchs EF, Kaempf MJ (1981) Medullary sponge kidney and congenital hemihypertrophy: case report and literature review. *J Urol* **126**: 676–8.

Harris PC, Ward CJ, Peral B, Hughes J (1995) Polycystic kidney disease. 1: Identification and analysis of the primary defect. *J Am Soc Nephrol* **6**: 1125–33.

Hateboer N, van Dijk MA, Bogdanova N *et al.* (1999) Comparison of phenotypes of polycystic kidney disease types 1 and 2. European PKD1–PKD2 Study Group. *Lancet* **353**: 103–7.

Hendren WG, Monfort GJ (1987) Symptomatic bilateral renal angiomyolipomas in a child. *J Urol* **137**: 256–7.

Higashihara E, Nutahara K, Tago K *et al.* (1984a). Medullary sponge kidney and renal acidification defect. *Kidney Int* **25**: 453–9.

Higashihara E, Nutahara K, Tago K *et al.* (1984b) Unilateral and segmental medullary sponge kidney: renal function and calcium excretion. *J Urol* **132**: 743–5.

Higashihara E, Munakata A, Hara M *et al.* (1988a) Medullary sponge kidney and hyperparathyroidism. *Urology* **31**: 155–8.

Higashihara E, Nutahara K, Niijima T (1988b) Renal hypercalciuria and metabolic acidosis associated with medullary sponge kidney: effect of alkali therapy. *Urol Res* **16**: 95–100.

Hildebrandt F, Otto E, Rensing C *et al.* (1997a) A novel gene encoding an SH3 domain protein is mutated in nephronophthisis type 1. *Nature Genet* **17**: 149–53.

Hildebrandt F, Strahm B, Nothwang HG *et al.* (1997b) Molecular genetic identification of families with juvenile nephronophthisis type 1: rate of progression to renal failure. APN Study Group. Arbeitsgemeinschaft für Pädiatrische Nephrologie. *Kidney Int* **51**: 261–9.

Hogg RJ (1992) Acquired renal cystic disease in children prior to the start of dialysis. *Pediatr Nephrol* **6**: 176–8.

Holmberg G, Hietala SO, Karp K, Ohberg L (1994) Significance of simple renal cysts and percutaneous cyst puncture on renal function. *Scand J Urol Nephrol* **28**: 35–8.

Hossack KF, Leddy CL, Johnson AM *et al.* (1988) Echocardiographic findings in autosomal dominant polycystic kidney disease. *N Engl J Med* **319**: 907–12.

Hoyer PF (1996) A young adult with so-called infantile cystic kidney disease. *Nephrol Dialysis Transplant* **11**: 377–8.

Huston JD, Torres VE, Sulivan PP *et al.* (1993) Value of magnetic resonance angiography for the detection of intracranial aneurysms in autosomal dominant polycystic kidney disease. *J Am Soc Nephrol* **3**: 1871–7.

Indridason OS, Thomas L, Berkoben M (1996) Medullary sponge kidney associated with congenital hemihypertrophy. *J Am Soc Nephrol* **7**: 1123–30.

Isdale JM, Thomson PD, Katz S (1973) Infantile polycystic disease of the kidneys. *S Afr Med J* **47**: 1892–6.

Ivy DD, Shaffer EM, Johnson AM *et al.* (1995) Cardiovascular abnormalities in children with autosomal dominant polycystic kidney disease. *J Am Soc Nephrol* **5**: 2032–6.

Jamil B, McMahon LP, Savige JA *et al.* (1999) A study of long-term morbidity associated with autosomal recessive polycystic kidney disease. *Nephrol Dialysis Transplant* **14**: 205–9.

Jayasinghe KS, Mendis BL, Mohideen R *et al.* (1984) Medullary sponge kidney presenting with hypokalaemic paralysis. *Postgrad Med J* **60**: 303–4.

Jones AC, Daniells CE, Snell RG *et al.* (1997) Molecular genetic and phenotypic analysis reveals differences between TSC1 and TSC2 associated familial and sporadic tuberous sclerosis. *Hum Molec Genet* **6**: 2155–61.

Jones AC, Shyamsundar MM, Thomas MW *et al.* (1999) Comprehensive mutation analysis of TSC1 and TSC2–and phenotypic correlations in 150 families with tuberous sclerosis. *Am J Hum Genet* **64**: 1305–15.

Józwiak S, Schwartz RA, Janniger CK *et al.* (1998) Skin lesions in children with tuberous sclerosis complex: their prevalence, natural course, and diagnostic significance. *Int J Dermatol* **37**: 911–17.

Kääriäinen H (1987) Polycystic kidney disease in children: a genetic and epidemiological study of 82 Finnish patients. *J Med Genet* **24**: 474–81.

Kääriäinen H, Jääskeläinen J, Kivisaari L et al. (1988a) Dominant and recessive polycystic kidney disease in children: classification by intravenous pyelography, ultrasound, and computed tomography. Pediatr Radiol 18: 45–50.

Kääriäinen H, Koskimies O, Norio R (1988b) Dominant and recessive polycystic kidney disease in children: evaluation of clinical features and laboratory data. Pediatr Nephrol 2: 296–302.

Kanno Y, Suzuki H, Okada H et al. (1996) Calcium channel blockers versus ACE inhibitors as antihypertensives in polycystic kidney disease. Q J Med 89: 65–70.

Kaplan BS, Rabin I, Nogrady MB, Drummond KN (1977) Autosomal dominant polycystic renal disease in children. J Pediatr 90: 782–3.

Kaplan BS, Kaplan P, de Chadarevian JP et al. (1988) Variable expression of autosomal recessive polycystic kidney disease and congenital hepatic fibrosis within a family. Am J Med Genet 29: 639–47.

Kaplan BS, Fay J, Shah V et al. (1989a) Autosomal recessive polycystic kidney disease. Pediatr Nephrol 3: 43–9.

Kaplan BS, Gordon I, Pincott J, Barratt TM (1989b) Familial hypoplastic glomerulocystic kidney disease: a definite entity with dominant inheritance. Am J Med Genet 34: 569–73.

Khoury Z, Brezis M, Mogle P (1988) Familial medullary sponge kidney in association with congenital absence of teeth (anodontia). Nephron 48: 231–3.

Klahr S, Breyer JA, Beck GJ et al. (1995) Dietary protein restriction, blood pressure control, and the progression of polycystic kidney disease. Modification of Diet in Renal Disease Study Group. J Am Soc Nephrol 5: 2037–47.

Kobayashi Y, Hiki Y, Shigematsu H et al. (1985) Renal retinal dysplasia with diffuse glomerular cysts. Nephron 39: 201–5.

Konrad M, Saunier S, Heidet L et al. (1996) Large homozygous deletions of the 2q13 region are a major cause of juvenile nephronophthisis. Hum Molec Genet 5: 367–71.

Konrad M, Saunier S, Calado J et al. (1998) Familial juvenile nephronophthisis. J Molec Med 76: 310–6.

Koptides M, Hadjimichael C, Koupepidou P et al (1999) Germinal and somatic mutations in the PKD2 gene of renal cysts in autosomal dominant polycystic kidney disease. Hum Molec Genet 8: 509–13.

Kumar S, Rankin R (1996) Renal insufficiency is a component of COACH syndrome. Am J Med Genet 61: 122–6.

Kyushu Pediatric Nephrology Study Group (1999) Acquired cystic kidney disease in children undergoing continuous ambulatory peritoneal dialysis. Am J Kidney Dis 34: 242–6.

Landing BH, Wells TR, Claireaux AE (1980) Morphometric analysis of liver lesions in cystic diseases of childhood. Hum Pathol 11: 549–60.

Langer LOJ, Nishino R, Yamaguchi A et al. (1983) Brachymesomelia-renal syndrome. Am J Med Genet 15: 57–65.

Larson RS, Rudloff MA, Liapis H et al. (1995) The Ivemark syndrome: prenatal diagnosis of an uncommon cystic renal lesion with heterogeneous associations. Pediatr Nephrol 9: 594–8.

Latif F, Tory K, Gnarra J et al. (1993) Identification of the von Hippel-Lindau disease tumor suppressor gene. Science 260: 1317–20.

Leichter HE, Dietrich R, Salusky IB et al. (1988) Acquired cystic kidney disease in children undergoing long-term dialysis. Pediatr Nephrol 2: 8–11.

Lens XM, Onuchic LF, Wu G et al. (1997) An integrated genetic and physical map of the autosomal recessive polycystic kidney disease region. Genomics 41: 463–6.

Levine E (1989) Computed tomography of renal abscesses complicating medullary sponge kidney. J Comput Assisted Tomography 13: 440–2.

Levine E, Grantham JJ (1981) The role of computed tomography in the evaluation of adult polycystic kidney disease. Am J Kidney Dis 1: 99–105.

Lewis EJ, Hunsicker LG, Bain RP, Rohde RD (1993) The effect of angiotensin-converting-enzyme inhibition on diabetic nephropathy. The Collaborative Study Group. N Engl J Med 329: 1456–62.

Lieberman E, Salinas-Madrigal L, Gwinn JL et al. (1971) Infantile polycystic disease of the kidneys and liver: clinical, pathological and radiological correlations and comparison with congenital hepatic fibrosis. Med 50: 277–318.

Lilford RJ, Irving HC, Allibone EB (1992) A tale of two prior probabilities – avoiding the false positive antenatal diagnosis of autosomal recessive polycystic kidney disease. Br J Obstet Gynaecol 99: 216–9.

Limjoco UR, Strauch AE (1966) Infected solitary cyst of the kidney: report of a case and review of the literature. J Urol 96: 625–30.

Lipschitz B, Berdon WE, Defelice AR, Levy J (1993) Association of congenital hepatic fibrosis with autosomal dominant polycystic kidney disease. Report of a family with review of literature. Pediatr Radiol 23: 131–3.

Løken AC, Hanssen O, Halvorsen S, Jolster NJ (1961) Hereditary renal dysplasia and blindness. Acta Pediatr 50: 177–83.

Luthy DA, Hirsch JH (1985) Infantile polycystic kidney disease: observations from attempts at prenatal diagnosis. Am J Med Genet 20: 505–17.

McAlister WH, Siegel MJ, Shackelford G et al. (1979) Glomerulocystic kidney. AJR Am J Roentgenol 133: 536–8.

McGonigle RJ, Mowat AP, Bewick M et al. (1981) Congenital hepatic fibrosis and polycystic kidney disease; role of portacaval shunting and transplantation in three patients. Q J Med 50: 269–78.

McGregor AR, Bailey RR (1989) Nephronophthisis-cystic renal medulla complex: diagnosis by computerized tomography. Nephron 53: 70–2.

McHugh K, Stringer DA, Hebert D, Babiak CA (1991) Simple renal cysts in children: diagnosis and follow-up with US. Radiology 178: 383–5.

Maddock IR, Moran A, Maher ER et al. (1996) A genetic register for von Hippel–Lindau disease. J Med Genet 33: 120–7.

Maher ER, Yates JR, Harries R et al. (1990) Clinical features and natural history of von Hippel–Lindau disease. Q J Med 77: 1151–63.

Main D, Mennuti MT, Cornfeld D, Coleman B (1983) Prenatal diagnosis of adult polycystic kidney disease. *Lancet* ii: 337–8.

Mainzer F, Saldino RM, Ozonoff MB, Minagi H (1970) Familial nephropathy associatdd with retinitis pigmentosa, cerebellar ataxia and skeletal abnormalities. *Am J Med* **49**: 556–62.

Malka D, Hammel P, Vilgrain V *et al.* (1998) Chronic obstructive pancreatitis due to a pancreatic cyst in a patient with autosomal dominant polycystic kidney disease. *Gut* **42**: 131–4.

Maschio G, Tessitore N, D'Angelo A *et al.* (1982) Medullary sponge kidney and hyperparathyroidism – a puzzling association. *Am J Nephrol* **2**: 77–84.

Maschio G, Alberti D, Janin G *et al.* (1996) Effect of the angiotensin-converting-enzyme inhibitor benazepril on the progression of chronic renal insufficiency. The Angiotensin-Converting-Enzyme Inhibition in Progressive Renal Insufficiency Study Group. *N Engl J Med* **334**: 939–45.

Matsubara K, Suzuki K, Lin YW *et al.* (1991) Familial juvenile nephronophthisis in two siblings - histological findings at an early stage. *Acta Paediatr Jpn* **33**: 482–7.

Mattoo TK, Khatani Y, Ashraf B (1994) Autosomal recessive polycystic kidney disease in 15 Arab children. *Pediatr Nephrol* **8**: 85–7.

Mattoo TK, Greifer I, Geva P, Spitzer A (1997) Acquired renal cystic disease in children and young adults on maintenance dialysis. *Pediatr Nephrol* **11**: 447–50.

Medhioub M, Cherif D, Benessy F *et al.* (1994) Refined mapping of a gene (NPH1) causing familial juvenile nephronophthisis and evidence for genetic heterogeneity. *Genomics* **22**: 296–301.

Melnick SC, Brewer DB, Oldham JS (1984) Cortical microcystic disease of the kidney with dominant inheritance: a previously undescribed syndrome. *J Clin Pathol* **37**: 494–9.

Mendley SR, Poznanski AK, Spargo BH, Langman CB (1995) Hereditary sclerosing glomerulopathy in the conorenal syndrome. *Am J Kidney Dis* **25**: 792–7.

Metreweli C, Garel L (1980) The echographic diagnosis of infantile renal polycystic disease. *Annal Radiol* **23**: 103–7.

Milutinovic J, Fialkow PJ, Rudd TG *et al.* (1980) Liver cysts in patients with autosomal dominant polycystic kidney disease. *Am J Med* **68**: 741–4.

Milutinovic J, Schabel SI, Ainsworth SK (1989) Autosomal dominant polycystic kidney disease with liver and pancreatic involvement in early childhood. *Am J Kidney Dis* **13**: 340–4.

Mochizuki T, Wu G, Hayashi T *et al.* (1996) PKD2, a gene for polycystic kidney disease that encodes an integral membrane protein. *Science* **272**: 1339–42.

Modi KB, Grant AC, Garret A, Rodger RS (1989) Indirect inguinal hernia in CAPD patients with polycystic kidney disease. *Adv Peritoneal Dialysis* **5**: 84–6.

Montemarano H, Bulas DI, Chandra R, Tifft C (1995) Prenatal diagnosis of glomerulocystic kidney disease in short-rib polydactyly syndrome type II, Majewski type. *Pediatr Radiol* **25**: 469–71.

Moolten SE (1942) Hamartial nature of the tuberous sclerosis complex and its bearing on the tumor problem; report of a case with tumor anomaly of the kidney and adenoma sebaceum. *Arch Intern Med* **69**: 589–623.

Morris-Stiff G, Coles G, Moore R *et al.* (1997) Abdominal wall hernia in autosomal dominant polycystic kidney disease. *Br J Surg* **84**: 615–17.

Mrowka C, Adam G, Sieberth HG, Matern S (1996) Caroli's syndrome associated with medullary sponge kidney and nephrocalcinosis. *Nephrol Dialysis Transplant* **11**: 1142–5.

Nakada SY, Erturk E, Monaghan J, Cockett AT (1993) Role of extracorporeal shock-wave lithotripsy in treatment of urolithiasis in patients with medullary sponge kidney. *Urology* **41**: 331–3.

Nasu K, Yoshimatsu J, Anai T *et al.* (1998) Magnetic resonance imaging of fetal autosomal recessive polycystic kidney disease. *J Obstet Gynecol Res* **24**: 33–6.

National High Blood Pressure Education Program Working Group on Hypertension Control in Children and Adolescents (1996) Update on the 1987 Task Force Report on High Blood Pressure in Children and Adolescents: a working group report from the National High Blood Pressure Education Program. National High Blood Pressure Education Program Working Group on Hypertension Control in Children and Adolescents. *Pediatrics* **98**: 649–58.

Neumann HP, Zerres K, Fischer CL *et al.* (1988) Late manifestation of autosomal-recessive polycystic kidney disease in two sisters. *Am J Nephrol* **8**: 194–7.

Neumann HP, Krumme B, van Velthoven V *et al.* (1999) Multiple intracranial aneurysms in a patient with autosomal recessive polycystic kidney disease. *Nephrol Dialysis Transplant* **14**: 936–9.

Novelli G, Frontali M, Baldini D *et al.* (1989) Prenatal diagnosis of adult polycystic kidney disease with DNA markers on chromosome 16 and the genetic heterogeneity problem. *Prenatal Diagnosis* **9**: 759–67.

Oh Y, Onoyama K, Kobayashi K *et al.* (1986) Glomerulocystic kidneys. Report of an adult case. *Nephron* **43**: 299–302.

O'Hagan AR, Ellsworth R, Secic M *et al.* (1996) Renal manifestations of tuberous sclerosis complex. *Clin Pediatr* **35**: 483–9.

Osathanondh V, Potter EL (1964) Pathogenesis of polycsytic kidneys. *Arch Pathol* **77**: 466–73.

Osther PJ, Hansen AB, Røhl HF (1988) Renal acidification defects in medullary sponge kidney. *Br J Urol* **61**: 392–4.

Osther PJ, Mathiasen H, Hansen AB, Nissen HM (1994) Urinary acidification and urinary excretion of calcium and citrate in women with bilateral medullary sponge kidney. *Urol Int* **52**: 126–30.

Paavola P, Salonen R, Weissenbach J, Peltonen L (1995) The locus for Meckel syndrome with multiple congenital anomalies maps to chromosome 17q21–q24. *Nature Genet* **11**: 213–15.

Paavola P, Salonen R, Baumer A *et al.* (1997) Clinical and genetic heterogeneity in Meckel syndrome. *Hum Genet* **101**: 88–92.

Pagon RA, Haas JE, Bunt AH, Rodaway KA (1982) Hepatic involvement in the Bardet-Biedl syndrome. *Am J Med Genet* **13**: 373–81.

Palubinskas AJ (1963) Renal pyramidal sturcture opacification in excretory urography and its relation to medullary sponge kidney. *Radiology* **81**: 963–70.

Park JH, Dixit MP, Onuchic LF *et al*. (1999) A 1–Mb BAC/PAC-based physical map of the autosomal recessive polycystic kidney disease gene (PKHD1) region on chromosome 6. *Genomics* **57**: 249–55.

Parks JH, Coe FL, Strauss AL (1982) Calcium nephrolithiasis and medullary sponge kidney in women. *N Engl J Med* **306**: 1088–91.

Paterson AD, Pei Y (1998) Is there a third gene for autosomal dominant polycystic kidney disease? *Kidney Int* **54**: 1759–61.

Patriquin HB, O'Regan S (1985) Medullary sponge kidney in childhood. *AJR Am J Roentgenol* **145**: 315–19.

Pedersen JF, Emamian SA, Nielsen MB (1997) Significant association between simple renal cysts and arterial blood pressure. *Br J Urol* **79**: 688–91.

Pei Y, Watnick T, He N *et al*. (1999) Somatic PKD2 mutations in individual kidney and liver cysts support a two-hit model of cystogenesis in type 2 autosomal dominant polycystic kidney disease. *J Am Soc Nephrol* **10**: 1524–9.

Pérez-Oller L, Torra R, Badenas C *et al*. (1999) Influence of the ACE gene polymorphism in the progression of renal failure in autosomal dominant polycystic kidney disease. *Am J Kidney Dis* **34**: 273–8.

Polak BC, van Lith FH, Delleman JW, van Balen AT (1983) Carrier detection in tapetoretinal degeneration in association with medullary cystic disease. *Am J Ophthalmol* **95**: 487–94.

Porch P, Noe HN, Stapleton FB (1986) Unilateral presentation of adult-type polycystic kidney disease in children. *J Urol* **135**: 744–6.

Proesmans W, Van Damme B, Casaer P, Marchal G (1982) Autosomal dominant polycystic kidney disease in the neonatal period: association with a cerebral arteriovenous malformation. *Pediatrics* **70**: 971–5.

Qian F, Watnick TJ, Onuchic LF, Germino GG (1996) The molecular basis of focal cyst formation in human autosomal dominant polycystic kidney disease type I. *Cell* **87**: 979–87.

Qian F, Germino FJ, Cai Y *et al*. (1997) PKD1 interacts with PKD2 through a probable coiled-coil domain. *Nature Genet* **16**: 179–83.

Querfeld U, Schneble F, Wradzidlo W *et al*. (1992) Acquired cystic kidney disease before and after renal transplantation. *J Pediatr* **121**: 61–4.

Rahill WJ, Rubin MI (1972) Hypertension in infantile polycystic renal disease. The importance of early recognition and treatment of severe hypertension in polycystic renal disease. *Clin Pediatr* **11**: 232–5.

Rao DS, Frame B, Block MA, Parfitt AM (1977) Primary hyperparathyroidism. A cause of hypercalciuria and renal stones in patients with medullary sponge kidney. *JAMA* **237**: 1353–5.

Ravine D, Gibson RN, Walker RG *et al*. (1994) Evaluation of ultrasonographic diagnostic criteria for autosomal dominant polycystic kidney disease 1. *Lancet* **343**: 824–7.

Reeders ST, Zerres K, Gal A *et al*. (1986) Prenatal diagnosis of autosomal dominant polycystic kidney disease with a DNA probe. *Lancet* **ii**: 6–8.

Reiner I, Donnell S, Jones M *et al*. (1992) Percutaneous sclerotherapy for simple renal cysts in children. *Br J Radiol* **65**: 281–2.

Reuss A, Wladimiroff JW, Stewart PA, Niermeijer MF (1990) Prenatal diagnosis by ultrasound in pregnancies at risk for autosomal recessive polycystic kidney disease. *Ultrasound Med Biol* **16**: 355–9.

Reznik VM, Griswold WT, Mendoza SA (1982) Glomerulocystic disease – a case report with 10 year follow-up. *Int J Pediatr Nephrol* **3**: 321–3.

Rizzoni G, Loirat C, Levy M *et al*. (1982) Familial hypoplastic glomerulocystic kidney. A new entity? *Clin Nephrol* **18**: 263–8.

Roach ES, DiMario FJ, Kandt RS, Northrup H (1999) Tuberous Sclerosis Consensus Conference: recommendations for diagnostic evaluation. National Tuberous Sclerosis Association. *J Child Neurol* **14**: 401–7.

Romero R, Cullen M, Jeanty P *et al*. (1984) The diagnosis of congenital renal anomalies with ultrasound. II. Infantile polycystic kidney disease. *Am J Obstet Gynecol* **150**: 259–62.

Romero R, Bonal J, Campo E *et al*. (1993) Glomerulocystic kidney disease: a single entity? *Nephron* **63**: 100–3.

Ross DG, Travers H (1975) Infantile presentation of adult-type polycystic kidney disease in a large kindred. *J Pediatr* **87**: 760–3.

Roy S, Dillon MJ, Trompeter RS, Barratt TM (1997) Autosomal recessive polycystic kidney disease: long-term outcome of neonatal survivors. *Pediatr Nephrol* **11**: 302–6.

Ruggieri PM, Poulos N, Masaryk TJ *et al*. (1994) Occult intracranial aneurysms in polycystic kidney disease: screening with MR angiography. *Radiology* **191**: 33–9.

Sage MR, Lawson AD, Marshall VR, Ryall RL (1982) Medullary sponge kidney and urolithiasis. *Clin Radiol* **33**: 435–8.

Saguem MH, Laarif M, Remadi S *et al*. (1992) Diffuse bilateral glomerulocystic disease of the kidneys and multiple cardiac rhabdomyomas in a newborn. Relationship with tuberous sclerosis and review of the literature. *Pathol Res Pract* **188**: 367–73; Discussion 73–4.

Salonen R (1984) The Meckel syndrome: clinicopathological findings in 67 patients. *Am J Med Genet* **18**: 671–89.

Sampson JR, Maheshwar MM, Aspinwall R *et al*. (1997) Renal cystic disease in tuberous sclerosis: role of the polycystic kidney disease 1 gene. *Am J Hum Genet* **61**: 843–51.

Saunier S, Calado J, Heilig R *et al*. (1997) A novel gene that encodes a protein with a putative src homology 3 domain is a candidate gene for familial juvenile nephronophthisis. *Hum Molec Genet* **6**: 2317–23.

Saypol DC, Laudone VP (1983) Congenital hemihypertrophy with adrenal carcinoma and medullary sponge kidney. *Urology* **21**: 510–11.

Schoeneman MJ, Plewinska M, Mucha M, Mieza M (1984) Marfan syndrome and medullary sponge kidney: case report and speculation on pathogenesis. *Int J Pediatr Nephrol* **5**: 103–4.

Scolari F, Valzorio B, Vizzardi V *et al.* (1997) Nephronophthisis-medullary cystic kidney disease complex: a report on 24 patients from 5 families with Italian ancestry. *Contrib Nephrol* **122**: 61–3.

Scolari F, Ghiggeri GM, Casari G *et al.* (1998) Autosomal dominant medullary cystic disease: a disorder with variable clinical pictures and exclusion of linkage with the NPH1 locus. *Nephrol Dialysis Transplant* **13**: 2536–46.

Scolari F, Puzzer D, Amoroso A *et al.* (1999) Identification of a new locus for medullary cystic disease, on chromosome 16p12. *Am J Hum Genet* **64**: 1655–60.

Sedman A, Bell P, Manco-Johnson M *et al.* (1987) Autosomal dominant polycystic kidney disease in childhood: a longitudinal study. *Kidney Int* **31**: 1000–5.

Senior B, Friedmann AI, Braudo JL (1961) Juvenile familial nephropathy with tapetoretinal degeneration: a new oculorenal dystrophy. *Am J Ophthalmol* **52**: 625–33.

Sepp T, Yates JR, Green AJ (1996) Loss of heterozygosity in tuberous sclerosis hamartomas. *J Med Genet* **33**: 962–4.

Sharp CK, Bergman SM, Stockwin JM *et al.* (1997) Dominantly transmitted glomerulocystic kidney disease: a distinct genetic entity. *J Am Soc Nephrol* **8**: 77–84.

Sharp C, Johnson A, Gabow P (1998) Factors relating to urinary protein excretion in children with autosomal dominant polycystic kidney disease. *J Am Soc Nephrol* **9**: 1908–14.

Shepherd CW, Gomez MR, Lie JT, Crowson CS (1991) Causes of death in patients with tuberous sclerosis. *Mayo Clin Proc* **66**: 792–6.

Sherman FE, Studnicki FM, Fetterman G (1971) Renal lesions of familial juvenile nephronophthisis examined by microdissection. *Am J Clin Pathol* **55**: 391–400.

Sklar AH, Caruana RJ, Lammers JE, Strauser GD (1987) Renal infections in autosomal dominant polycystic kidney disease. *Am J Kidney Dis* **10**: 81–8.

Sluysmans T, Vanoverschelde JP, Malvaux P (1987) Growth failure associated with medullary sponge kidney, due to incomplete renal tubular acidosis type 1. *Eur J Pediatrics* **146**: 78–80.

Smith DW, Opitz JM, Inhorn SL (1965) A syndrome of multiple developmental defects including polycystic kidneys and intrahepatic biliary dysgenesis in 2 siblings. *J Pediatr* **67**: 617–24.

Snelling CE, Brown NM, Smythe CA (1970) Medullary sponge kidney in a child. *Can Med Assoc J* **102**: 518–19.

Stamm ER, Townsend RR, Johnson AM *et al.* (1999) Frequency of ovarian cysts in patients with autosomal dominant polycystic kidney disease. *Am J Kidney Dis* **34**: 120–4.

Stanescu B, Michiels J, Proesmans W, Van Damme B (1976) Retinal involvement in a case of nephronophthisis associated with liver fibrosis Senior-Boichis syndrome. *Birth Defects Original Article Series* **12**: 463–74.

Stapleton FB, Johnson D, Kaplan GW, Griswold W (1980) The cystic renal lesion in tuberous sclerosis. *J Pediatr* **97**: 574–9.

Stapleton FB, Bernstein J, Koh G *et al.* (1982) Cystic kidneys in a patient with oral-facial-digital syndrome type I. *Am J Kidney Dis* **1**: 288–93.

Stapleton FB, Hilton S, Wilcox J, Leopold GR (1981) Transient nephromegaly simulating infantile polycystic disease of the kidneys. *Pediatrics* **67**: 554–9.

Stavrou C, Pierides A, Zouvani I *et al.* (1998) Medullary cystic kidney disease with hyperuricemia and gout in a large Cypriot family: no allelism with nephronophthisis type 1. *Am J Med Genet* **77**: 149–54.

Steele BT, Lirenman DS, Beattie CW (1980) Nephronophthisis. *Am J Med* **68**: 531–8.

Steinhardt GF, Slovis TL, Perlmutter AD (1985) Simple renal cysts in infants. *Radiology* **155**: 349–50.

Stillwell TJ, Gomez MR, Kelalis PP (1987) Renal lesions in tuberous sclerosis. *J Urol* **138**: 477–81.

Strauss MB, Sommers SC (1967) Medullary cystic disease and familial juvenile nephronophthisis. *N Engl J Med* **277**: 863–4.

Sujansky E, Kreutzer SB, Johnson AM *et al.* (1990) Attitudes of at-risk and affected individuals regarding presymptomatic testing for autosomal dominant polycystic kidney disease. *Am J Med Genet* **35**: 510–5.

Sumfest JM, Burns MW, Mitchell ME (1993) Aggressive surgical and medical management of autosomal recessive polycystic kidney disease. *Urology* **42**: 309–12.

Taitz LS, Brown CB, Blank CE, Steiner GM (1987) Screening for polycystic kidney disease: importance of clinical presentation in the newborn. *Arch Dis Child* **62**: 45–9.

Telenti A, Torres VE, Gross JBJ *et al.* (1990) Hepatic cyst infection in autosomal dominant polycystic kidney disease. *Mayo Clin Proc* **65**: 933–42.

Tomooka Y, Onitsuka H, Goya T *et al.* (1988) Congenital hemihypertrophy with adrenal adenoma and medullary sponge kidney. *Br J Radiol* **61**: 851–3.

Torra R, Nicolau C, Badenas C *et al.* (1997) Ultrasonographic study of pancreatic cysts in autosomal dominant polycystic kidney disease. *Clin Nephrol* **47**: 19–22.

Torra R, Badenas C, Darnell A *et al.* (1998) Facilitated diagnosis of the contiguous gene syndrome: tuberous sclerosis and polycystic kidneys by means of haplotype studies. *Am J Kidney Dis* **31**: 1038–43.

Torres VE, Wilson DM, Hattery RR, Segura JW (1993) Renal stone disease in autosomal dominant polycystic kidney disease. *Am J Kidney Dis* **22**: 513–19.

Torres VE, King BF, Holley KE *et al.* (1994a) The kidney in the tuberous sclerosis complex. *Adv Nephrol Necker Hospital* **23**: 43–70.

Torres VE, Rastogi S, King BF *et al.* (1994b) Hepatic venous outflow obstruction in autosomal dominant polycystic kidney disease. *J Am Soc Nephrol* **5**: 1186–92.

Tsiokas L, Kim E, Arnould T *et al* (1997) Homo- and heterodimeric interactions between the gene products of PKD1 and PKD2. *Proc Nat Acad Sci* **94**: 6965–70.

Tsugaya M, Kajita A, Hayashi Y *et al.* (1995). Detection and monitoring of simple renal cysts with computed tomography. *Urol Int* **54**: 128–31.

Tsukahara H, Kikuchi K, Mikawa H *et al.* (1990) Juvenile nephronophthisis diagnosed from glucosuria detected by urine screening at school. *Acta Paediatr Jpn* **32**: 548–51.

Turco AE, Clementi M, Rossetti S *et al.* (1996) An Italian family with autosomal dominant polycystic kidney disease unlinked to either the PKD1 or PKD2 gene. *Am J Kidney Dis* **28**: 759–61.

Umeki S, Soejima R, Kawane H (1989) Young's syndrome accompanied by medullary sponge kidney. *Respiration* **55**: 60–4.

Valadez RA, Firlit CF (1987) Renal transplantation in children with oculorenal syndrome. *Urology* **30**: 130–2.

van Collenburg JJ, Thompson MW, Huber J (1978) Clinical, pathological and genetic aspects of a form of cystic disease of the renal medulla: familial juvenile nephronophthisis (FJN). *Clin Nephrol* **9**: 55–62.

van Slegtenhorst M, de Hoogt R, Hermans C *et al.* (1997) Identification of the tuberous sclerosis gene TSC1 on chromosome 9q34. *Science* **277**: 805–8.

Verhoef S, van Diemen-Steenvoorde R, Akkersdijk WL *et al.* (1999) Malignant pancreatic tumour within the spectrum of tuberous sclerosis complex in childhood. *Eur J Pediatrics* **158**: 284–7.

Waldherr R, Lennert T, Weber HP *et al.* (1982) The nephronophthisis complex. A clinicopathologic study in children. *Virchows Arch (Pathol Anat)* **394**: 235–54.

Warady BA, Cibis G, Alon V *et al.* (1994) Senior-Loken syndrome: revisited. *Pediatrics* **94**: 111–12.

Wiebers DO, Torres VE (1992) Screening for unruptured intracranial aneurysms in autosomal dominant polycystic kidney disease. *N Engl J Med* **327**: 953–5.

Woo DD, Nguyen DK, Khatibi N, Olsen P (1997) Genetic identification of two major modifier loci of polycystic kidney disease progression in pcy mice. *J Clin Invest* **100**: 1934–40.

Yamagishi F, Kitahara N, Mogi W, Itoh S (1988) Age-related occurrence of simple renal cysts studied by ultrasonography. *Klin Wochenschr* **66**: 385–7.

Zawada ETJ, Sica DA (1984) Differential diagnosis of medullary sponge kidney. *S Med J* **77**: 686–9.

Zeier M, Geberth S, Schmidt KG *et al.* (1993) Elevated blood pressure profile and left ventricular mass in children and young adults with autosomal dominant polycystic kidney disease. *J Am Soc Nephrol* **3**: 1451–7.

Zerres K (1992) Autosomal recessive polycystic kidney disease. *Clin Invest* **70**: 794–801.

Zerres K, Weiss H, Bulla M, Roth B (1982) Prenatal diagnosis of an early manifestation of autosomal dominant adult-type polycystic kidney disease. *Lancet* **ii**: 988.

Zerres K, Hansmann M, Knöpfle G, Stephan M (1985) Prenatal diagnosis of genetically determined early manifestation of autosomal dominant polycystic kidney disease? *Hum Genet* **71**: 368–9.

Zerres K, Hansmann M, Mallmann R, Gembruch U (1988) Autosomal recessive polycystic kidney disease. Problems of prenatal diagnosis. *Prenatal Diagnosis* **8**: 215–29.

Zerres K, Rudnik-Schoneborn S, Deget F *et al.* (1996) Autosomal recessive polycystic kidney disease in 115 children: clinical presentation, course and influence of gender. Arbeitsgemeinschaft fur Padiatrische, Nephrologie. *Acta Paediatr* **85**: 437–45.

Zerres K, Mücher G, Bachner L *et al.* (1994) Mapping of the gene for autosomal recessive polycystic kidney disease (ARPKD) to chromosome 6p21–cen. *Nature Genet* **7**: 429–32.

Zerres K, Rudnik-Schöneborn S, Deget F (1992) Routine examination of children at risk of autosomal dominant polycystic kidney disease. *Lancet* **339**: 1356–7.

Zerres K, Mucher G, Becker J *et al.* (1998) Prenatal diagnosis of autosomal recessive polycystic kidney disease (ARPKD): molecular genetics, clinical experience, and fetal morphology. *Am J Med Genet* **76**: 137–44.

Zinn HL, Rosberger ST, Haller JO, Schlesinger AE (1997) Simple renal cysts in children with AIDS. *Pediatr Radiol* **27**: 827–8.

Ureteral duplication anomalies: ectopic ureters and ureteroceles

23

Michael A. Keating

Introduction

Ureteral duplications are one of the most common anomalies affecting the genitourinary tract. Variations of incomplete ureteral duplication or complete duplications with normally positioned orifices and normally developed renal moieties comprise the vast majority. As such, they represent no more than radiologic curiosities. Anomalies with clinical implications are much less common, and include ectopic ureters and ureteroceles. Historically, the majority of these probably went unnoticed (Malek *et al.*, 1972). A smaller portion became evident clinically as a consequence of hydronephrosis, vesicoureteral reflux (VUR), or incontinence, either in combination or alone. More recently, antenatal diagnosis has uncovered a plethora of urologic anomalies, including different variants of ureteral duplications, which are asymptomatic. Antenatal detection enables the potential salvage of renal function and the avoidance of illness for some children. For others, perinatal identification has created controversy about the recommendations for their management by introducing a large group of abnor-malities that may have gone undetected in the past.

Despite these decision-making dilemmas, it seems prudent to institute pre-emptive therapy in children diagnosed with urinary tract anomalies. As a consequence, pediatric urologic surgeons must remain familiar with the natural history of duplication anomalies, well versed in the evolving recommendations for their management, and familiar with the variety of surgical techniques available for their solution.

Embryologic considerations

Normal development

A review of normal development provides the basis for understanding the pathophysiology of anomalies of the ureter and, in some cases, aids in their diagnosis and clinical management.

Ureteral development coincides with that of the kidney between 4 and 8 weeks of gestation. The ureteral bud (metanephric duct) projects from the wolffian (mesonephric) duct just proximal to its junction with the cloaca (Fig. 23.1). As the ureteral bud

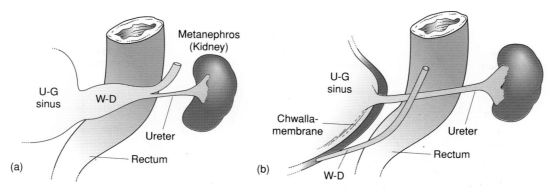

Figure 23.1 Relationships of ureteral bud, wolffian (mesonephric) duct (W-D) and urogential sinus ((U-G). The segment of wolffian duct between urogenital sinus and ureteral bud represents the common excretory duct.

elongates in a cephalad direction, it penetrates the adjacent metanephric tissue and divides into the calyces and collecting ducts. Proper fusion of the bud and nephrogenic blastema is critical to tubular maturation within the renal anlage and ultimate function of the kidney.

The segment of wolffian duct between the cloaca and the take-off of the ureteral bud (the future ureteral orifice) is called the common excretory duct. The migration of tissue that occurs during the excretory duct's incorporation into the urogenital sinus helps to explain the variable relationships that sometimes occur between the ureter(s) and the trigone of the bladder, urethra and genital ducts. Conceptually, these events represent some of the most difficult in uroembryology to understand.

In brief, as the common excretory duct is absorbed into the bladder, the ureteral orifice migrates in a cranial and lateral direction. While this occurs, the excretory duct migrates to the midline and fuses with its contralateral partner to form the primitive trigone, thus explaining the mesodermal origin of the trigone. The orifice of the wolffian duct ends in a caudal and medial position at the utricle. The wolffian (mesonephric) duct ultimately differentiates into the prostate, seminal vesicles, vas deferens, and epididymis in males. In females, the wolffian ducts guide the müllerian ducts into position in the midline, where the latter fuse to form the uterus, proximal vagina, and fallopian tubes. After their involution, wolffian remnants persist in as many as 25% of women as Gartner's duct lying along the anterolateral vaginal wall and uterus, and the epoophoron and oophoron within the broad ligament supporting the fallopian tubes.

Explanations for the variety of anomalies that affect the ureter have their basis in this developmental pro-

gression, although the causes of the initial insult remain unclear (Tanagho, 1976). An alteration in timing seems key.

Abnormal development

Lateral orifice ectopia occurs when the ureteral bud originates from a more caudal position than usual on the mesonephric duct. As a result, the ureteral orifice has more time to be absorbed within the bladder and begin its cranial and lateral migration. As the degree of laterality becomes more exaggerated, the length of submucosal ureter is shortened. In addition, because the common excretory duct is shortened by the premature take-off of the ureteral bud, its mesenchymal contribution to the trigone is blunted. Muscular deficiency of the trigonal–ureteral complex results. Primary reflux becomes a common consequence of lateral ectopia and is thoroughly discussed elsewhere (see Chapter 25).

Caudal ectopia results from an abnormally high take-off of the ureteral bud. This allows less time for the orifice to be absorbed into the bladder. Now more closely positioned to ductal tissue typically destined to become wolffian, the ureter arrives in a medial trigonal or urethral position or is extravesically positioned along the path of wolffian structures or remnants. The location of wolffian remnants helps to explain an important difference in presentation of ectopic ureters between males and females (Fig. 23.2). Ectopic ureters in males are connected to structures that continue to drain into the bladder proximal to the urinary sphincter. Urinary control should be normal. In contrast, ectopic ureters in females that drain outside the bladder or urethra potentially vent into remnants adjacent to the fallopian tube (epoophoron), body of the uterus (paroophoron), and vagina (Gartner's

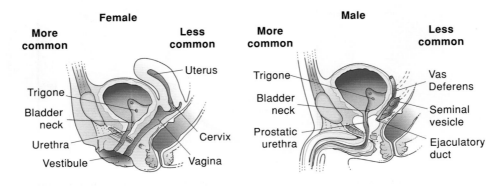

Figure 23.2 Anatomic locations of ectopic ureters.

duct), where they presumably rupture or are absorbed. Since the urinary sphincter is bypassed, incontinence results.

Ureteral duplication occurs when a single ureteral bud branches prematurely during its ascent or when two distinct ureteral buds arise from the wolffian (mesonephric) duct (Fig. 23.3). The clinical significance of these anomalies depends on the location of the buds and their interplay with the developing kidney.

Branching of a single bud after its take-off from the mesonephric duct results in incomplete ureteral duplication. The configurations that can occur range from anomalies as mild as a bifid renal pelvis (late branching) to nearly complete duplications having a common intravesical stem (early branching). The location of the ureteral orifice with incomplete duplications depends on the take-off of the ureteral bud in the sequence cited above. Bifurcations can occur at any level from the bladder to the renal pelvis but are most common in the lower third of the ureter (Lenaghan, 1962). Most buds are normally positioned along the mesonephric duct and, as a consequence, incomplete

duplications are usually radiologic curiosities with little clinical significance.

Complete ureteral duplication occurs when two ureteral buds project from the mesonephric duct, each having a separate interaction with the metanephric blastema. During their early take-off, the buds interact with the primordial kidney in a logical fashion. The most superior/cephalad bud induces the upper portion of the blastema (upper pole), while the lower bud joins the lower pole moiety. However, the ultimate positions of the ureteral orifices are governed by the same enigmatic rules of tissue migration and incorporation into the bladder described for singlets above.

When both buds are close together and project from a normal region along the mesonephric duct, both ureters will generally have normally positioned orifices. When the buds are more widely separated, one or both will be ectopic. If the superior/upper pole bud projects from an abnormally high position along the mesonephric duct, caudal ectopia is the outcome. If the bud to the lower pole originates from a more

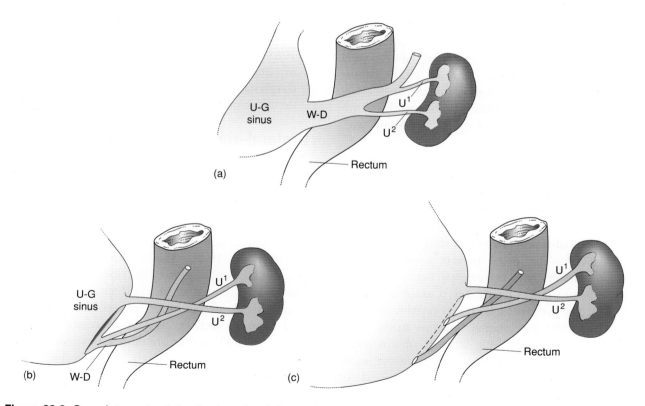

Figure 23.3 Complete ureteral duplication. *Caudal ectopia* (U1) results from abnormally high take-off of ureteral bud, which remains positioned near wolffian duct tissue. *Lateral ectopia* (U2) results from the more caudal position, allowing more time for intravesical migration.

caudal position along the duct, lateral ectopia results. To achieve their ultimate positions, the ureters and their orifices complete a 180° clockwise rotation along their longitudinal axes. These relationships, defined by the Weigert–Meyer law, are unusually consistent (Weigert, 1877; Meyer, 1946). Exceptions have been described but are rare (Lund, 1949; Ahmed and Pope, 1986).

Recent studies using angiotension-2-receptor (AGTR2) gene mutant animals have demonstrated features similar to those of humans with duplication anomalies (Pope *et al.*, 2001). Similarities in renal development, relationships defined by the Weigert–Meyer principle and the theories proposed by Mackie and Stephens, have been correlated with this genetic abnormality. The likelihood that human AGTR2 plays a part in this polygenic mode of inheritence is high.

Ureteroceles

Several theories have been proposed for the development of ureteroceles, though their etiology remains unclear. Some of the more popular are described below.

1 Persistence of Chwalla's membrane, which is a two-layered membrane that transiently separates the caudal end of the wolffian duct from the urogenital sinus (37 days' gestation) (Chwalla, 1927), is possible. Incomplete dissolution of the membrane could account for the cystic dilatation of the terminal ureter and stenosis of the orifice found with ureteroceles.

2 Abnormal muscular development of the terminal ureter has been implicated by a number of studies (Stephens, 1983). Ballooning of the distal ureter could be explained by a deficiency or an absence of its investing muscular layers, a finding shown in over 90% of specimens in one study (Tokunaka *et al.*, 1981). The distal ureters associated with ectopic ureters have consistently better developed musculature than ureteroceles (Caldamone *et al.*, 1984). The ureterocele itself is covered with vesical mucosa while the internal lining is made up of ureteral mucosa. Varying degrees of attenuated smooth muscle and connective tissue are sandwiched between. An element of meatal or perisphincteric obstruction (Stephens, 1971) may also contribute to the dilatation. However, some ureteroceles present without a functioning kidney, suggesting that urinary output is an unnecessary

impetus to distal ureteral ectasia (Passerini *et al.*, 1986). It is also plausible that the kidneys associated with these 'blind ureteroceles' produced urine during an early critical stage in development and that the renal dysmorphism or atrophy was the consequence of distal ureteral obstruction.

3 Abnormal widening of the mesonephric duct may occur in the segment between its insertion at the urogenital sinus and the ureteral bud. This area normally dilates in concert with an undefined stimulus for vesical and urethral expansion. Ureteral migration is presumably completed before this expansion occurs. Proximal extension of the widening process into the distal ureter could result in ureterocele development (Tanagho, 1976). This explanation seems plausible for intravesical ureteroceles, the ureter and orifice of which have migrated appropriately. Late incorporation of the ureteral bud from an abnormally proximal position within this dilated segment is another possibility. This explanation is more compatible with extravesical ureteroceles accompanied by ectopic orifices. Notably, ectopic ureters associated with even more proximal buds are rarely ectatic at their distal ends. They are presumably unaffected by the stimulus that alters the urogenital sinus (Stephens, 1983). As discussed below, the concept of abnormal bud position may also account for the renal dysplasia that accompanies many extravesical ureteroceles.

Ureteral–renal interactions

The ultimate maturation of the renal blastema is dictated by its interaction with the ureteral bud. When this interplay is experimentally altered, the expected transformation of blastema to normal nephron does not occur (Spencer and Maizel, 1987; Sariola *et al.*, 1988). Mackie and Stephens (1975) proposed the mid-region of the elongate metanephric blastema as being most conducive to becoming normal renal parenchyma. Ureteral buds that originate from abnormally cephalic or caudal positions along the wolffian duct are destined to induce polar blastema, which results in cystic dysplasia (Fig. 23.4). This theory offers a ready explanation for the dysplasia and scars found in the absence of reflux. It could also explain why ectopic ureters with urinary insertions (GU-ectopy) are more likely to be associated with functioning renal parenchyma than ectopic

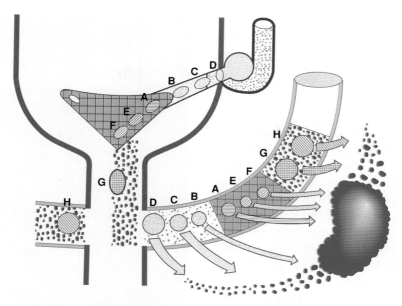

Figure 23.4 In theory, the position of the ureteral bud on the wolffian (mesonephric) duct corresponds to the final position of the ureteral orifice and differentiation of the metanephric blastema. Lateral and caudal ectopia can both result in renal dysplasia.

ureters having wolffian or gynecologic (GYN-ectopy) insertions, where dysplasia is often present (Weiss *et al.*, 1984). Ureteral bud take-off could also explain the difference between the good renal function usually seen with intravesical ureteroceles, and the poor function which occurs with extravesical ureteroceles.

Clinical correlates offers only guarded support of this theory, despite its attractiveness. Most studies generally cite poor renal function in the presence of severe reflux or marked ureteral ectopia (Jee *et al.*, 1993), although the difference between GU- and GYN-ectopy has come into question (Wakhlu *et al.*, 1998). In addition, antenatal detection has added some new wrinkles. In one review of specimens from 50 consecutive patients undergoing heminephrectomies, dysplasia was seen in 70% from ureteroceles and 30% from ectopic ureters (Abel *et al.*, 1997). Each had been diagnosed antenatally and none was felt to have histologic changes that may have benefited from renal preservation surgery. In contrast, in a similar series of 40 consecutive antenatally diagnosed duplication anomalies, only six required heminephrectomy because of poor function. None of these showed evidence of dyplasia (Patil and Mathews, 1995).

Most historic reports cite salvagable renal function in only 20–30% of patients with ureteroceles. This

pales next to the yield of contemporary series, where numbers are inflated by the addition of antenatally diagnosed anomalies and the sensitivity of better diagnostics. The clinical implications are obvious (see Recommendations). Are these renal moieties destined to lose renal function as a consequence of progressive obstruction or infection? Do they benefit from being surgically diverted or endoscopically decompressed? Or is renal parenchyma being preserved that has an intrinsic developmental insult? Nodular renal blastema has been reported in upper pole nephrectomy specimens removed with ectopic ureteroceles (Craver *et al.*, 1986). It is unclear as to whether this is cause for concern. To date, no chronic complications of renal salvage, unrelated to the surgery itself (e.g. hypertension or tumor formation) have been reported.

Nomenclature and classification

Ectopic ureters

The term ectopic ureter refers to a ureter that has migrated with the wolffian duct structures and is more caudally positioned than a normal ureter. Such ureters drain into the urethra, wolffian, or müllerian structures. With duplications to the lower renal pole the ureter, which is often laterally displaced and ectopic in the purest sense, is regarded as orthotopic. Single-system ureters, that are laterally misplaced and reflux as a consequence, are discussed elsewhere (see Chapter 25).

Ureteroceles

Historically, ureteroceles associated with single systems were regarded as orthotopic or simple and considered adult type, despite the fact that some such variants are clearly ectopic and are found in children (Figs. 23.5–23.9). Ureteroceles subtending the upper pole ureter of a duplex system have been described as ectopic and pediatric, although exceptions to both descriptions commonly occur (Glassberg *et al.*, 1984). Gonzales (1992) felt it simplest to describe the anomaly based on the location of its orifice. Other than their association with a single or duplex system, two types of ureteroceles exist; intravesical and extravesical. This definition avoids the confusion associated with the terms ectopic and orthotopic. In addition, such nomenclature reflects the embryologic importance of the ureteral bud/orifice to renal development

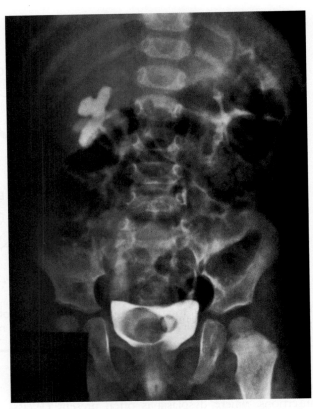

Figure 23.6 Excretory urogram shows bilateral single-system intravesical ureteroceles, right larger than left. Renal function is typically preserved.

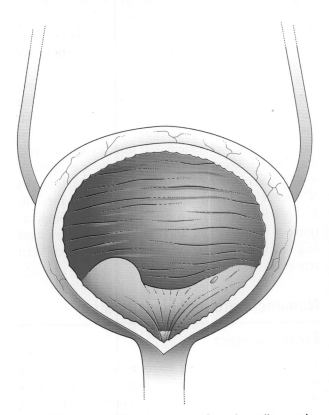

Figure 23.5 Intravesical ureterocele subtending a single ureter. This can also be classified as orthotopic or simple.

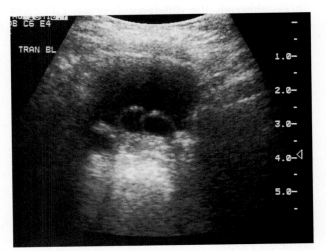

Figure 23.7 Ultrasonic appearance of a similar patient with bilateral intravesical ureteroceles.

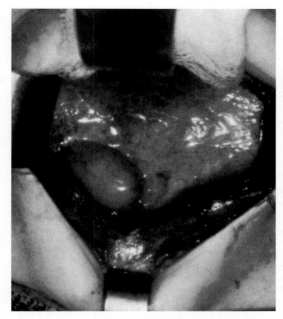

Figure 23.8 Intraoperative photograph of bilateral intravesical single-system ureteroceles.

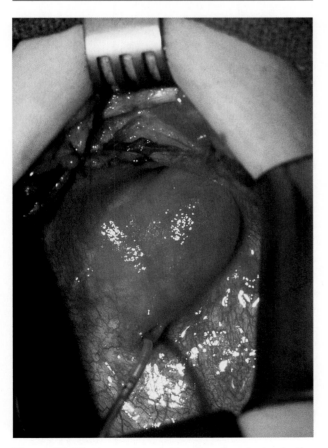

Figure 23.9 Large ureterocele extending towards the bladder neck (top). There is a catheter in the lower pole ureter, which is displaced and freely refluxes.

and distortion of the bladder neck. However, this form of categorization potentially mislabels ureteroceles with an intravesical orifice but an extension into the bladder neck or urethra. Anatomically, these should be considered extravesical.

A variety of other classification schemes has been proposed for ureteroceles, although no system has been adopted universally. Stephens' (1971) categorization can be used to provide additional information about the location and configuration of the orifice of the ureterocele. These factors presumably account for the degree of distortion of the bladder neck and urethra, as well as the extent of renal dysplasia accompanying the anomaly (Table 23.1; Figs. 23.10–23.11).

Characteristics

Ureteral duplications

Duplication is the most common congenital anomaly in the urinary tract; a 0.7% incidence was found in one series of more than 50 000 autopsies (Campbell, 1976). Intravenous urograms demonstrate duplications in 4% of studies, and hydronephrosis and scarring are seen in 27% of these (Caldamone, 1985). Females are affected two to four times more commonly than males. The right and left collecting systems are affected equally, bilateral duplication occurring in 17–33% of cases.

The anomaly is an inheritable defect transmitted in an autosomal fashion having variable penetrance (Atwell *et al.*, 1974). The parents or siblings of a child with a duplex ureter have as much as a one in eight chance of having a similarly affected child (Whitaker and Danks, 1966).

Ectopic ureters

The incidence of ureteral ectopia was approximately 1 in 2000 in one series of autopsies in children. Many remain asymptomatic and a true incidence is difficult to determine (Prewitt and Lebowitz, 1976). Ectopic ureters occur in females two to three times more commonly than in males (Ellerker, 1958; Malek *et al.*, 1972), although as high as 12-fold increases have been cited (Burford *et al.*, 1949). More than 80% of females with ectopic ureters have duplex systems. The majority (75%) in males are singlets (Schulman, 1976; Ahmed and Barker, 1992). Between 70 and 80% of ectopic ureters are associated with complete

Table 23.1 Classification of duplex ureteroceles

Ureterocele	Frequency (%)	Features
Intravesical		
Stenotic	40	Involve a congenitally small ureteral orifice adding an element of obstruction for the upper pole
Non-obstructed	5	The ureteral orifice is large and balloons open without any ureteral obstruction
Extravesical		
Sphincteric	40	The orifice opens outside the bladder and the ureterocele extends into the bladder neck and urethra. The orifice is normal or large and usually opens proximal to the external sphincter. In females, the meatus may open distal to the sphincter. At rest, the bladder neck and sphincter contract on the ureter and orifice, causing obstruction
Sphincterostenotic	5	Similar to sphincteric, but the ureteral orifice is stenotic
Cecoureteroceles	5	A large orifice opens in the bladder but a blind pouch or cecum extends into the submucosa of the urethra. When the cecum distends with urine, urethral obstruction can result
Blind ectopic	5	Similar to sphincteric, with no ureteral orifice

From Stephens (1983).

duplications. Nearly 20% of patients with ureteral ectopy have bilateral involvement (Ellerker, 1958). In one report of nearly 500 ectopic ureters, the posterior urethra and prostatic urethra (57%) were the most common sites of drainage in males. The seminal vesicle (33%) was also commonly involved. More remote terminations at the ejaculatory duct and vas were rare (10%). The urethra and vestibule were the most common drainage sites for 69% of females. Vaginal ectopy occurred in another 25% (Ellerker, 1958).

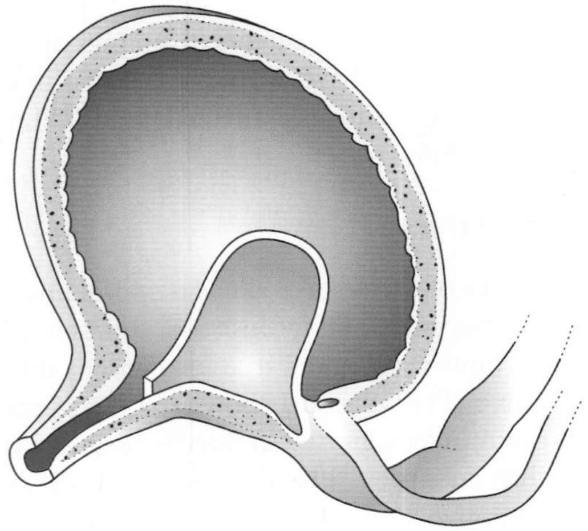

Ureteroceles

The incidence of ureteroceles was as high as 1 in 500 in one autopsy study. They occur in females four times more commonly than in males (Brock and Kaplan, 1978; Mandell *et al.*, 1980). In girls ureteroceles are associated with duplex systems 95% of the time. In contrast, up to 66% of boys have single-system anomalies (Decter *et al.*, 1989). Nearly all appear in Caucasians.

Eighty per cent are associated with the upper pole of a duplex system. The remainder are single-system ureteroceles. Bilateral involvement occurs in 15% of cases (Unson *et al.*, 1961).

Figure 23.10 Sphincteric variant of extravesical ureterocele subtending upper pole ureter of the duplex system. The orifice opens proximal to the external sphincter. Normal contraction of the bladder neck may contribute to ureteral obstruction.

Presentation

Antenatal ultrasonography has dramatically increased the detection of urinary anomalies and, in some cases, has altered our understanding of their natural history.

(a)

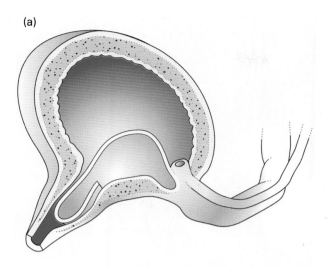

(b)

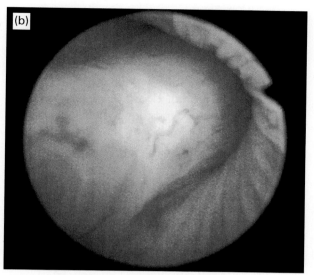

Figure 23.11 (*a*) Cecoureterocele variant of an extravesical ureterocele. Blind-ending extension beneath the submucosa of the urethra can prolapse and/or cause bladder outlet obstruction. (*b*) Cystoscopic appearance of the urethral extension of the cecoureterocele.

Table 23.2 Prenatal diagnosis of hydronephosis and the breakdown of prenatally diagnosed duplex systems

Prenatal diagnosis of hydronephosis (177 cases)[a]	
Hydronephrosis	154
Bilateral hydronephrosis	73
Unilateral hydronephrosis	61
Bladder outlet obstruction	9
Duplex/hydronephrosis	9
Prune-belly syndrome	2
Multicystic dysplastic kidney	10
Autosomal recessive kidney	5
Other	8
Breakdown of prenatally diagnosed duplex systems (39 cases)[b]	
Ureterocele	15
Ectopic ureter	15
Lower pole reflux	6
Lower pole UPJ obstruction	2
Yo-yo reflux	1

[a]Adapted from Mandell J, Blythe B, Peters CA *et al.* (1991) The natural history of structural genitourinary defects detected *in utero. Radiology* **178**: 194.
[b]Adapted from Jee LD, Rickwood AM, Williams MP *et al.* (1993) Experience with duplex system anomalies detected by prenatal ultrasonography. *J Urol* **149**: 808–10.

The yield from routine screening is not insignificant. Abnormalities of the urinary system are detected in approximately 1 in 500 studies, second only to those of the nervous system. The breakdown of diagnoses in typical series is shown in Table 23.2. Notably, ectopic ureters, duplications and ureteroceles can all be detected antenatally. Further evaluation after birth is warranted, even in instances where the anomaly was present earlier in gestation and has presumably resolved (Garmel *et al.*, 1996). In many cases, the exact etiology of hydronephrosis, the most common antenatal finding, cannot be determined until after delivery. Because of the tendency for urinary infections with hydronephrosis, it seems reasonable to keep newborns on a prophylactic antibiotic (amoxicillin) until their anatomy is better defined (see Evaluation, below).

After delivery, an extravesical ureterocele represents the most common cause of bladder outlet obstruction in newborn girls and the second most common cause in boys, after posterior urethral valves (PUV). Prenatal cases of bladder outlet obstruction have also been described (Austin *et al.*, 1998). A true pediatric urologic emergency can result, depending on the degree of obstruction. The diagnosis of an obstructing ureterocele should be considered in any infant, especially a girl, with bladder distension, anuria, or ascites (Gonzalez and Sheldon, 1982). When full-blown prolapse occurs, clinicians will encounter a congested, ecchymotic interlabial mass (Figs. 23.12–15). The mass may have varying hues, depending on the degree of vascular compromise. Since prolapse usually occurs down the posterior wall of the urethra, the meatus will be evident anteriorly and can be catheterized. Cecoureteroceles, the distal projection of which extends down the urethra, have a less protuberant appearance if they reach the perineum. They are rarely ecchymotic since vascular compromise is not an issue (Fig. 23.16). The smooth wall of the round mass helps to differentiate it from the more ominous grapelike sarcoma botryoides. The white mucus-filled peraurethral (Skene's) duct cyst is considered in the differential, as is Gartner's duct cyst. The latter can protrude from the vagina and become infected, and is often associated with an ectopic ureter that is blind ending at its proximal extent or connected to a rudimentary kidney (Currarino, 1982; Rosenfeld and Lis, 1993). When not evident on physical examination, the diagnosis of an obstructing ureterocele (or other urethral obstruction) is suggested by the history of a weak or an intermittent stream.

More commonly, ureteroceles cause unilateral hydronephrosis from ureteral obstruction. In severe cases, an abdominal mass becomes palpable. Patients

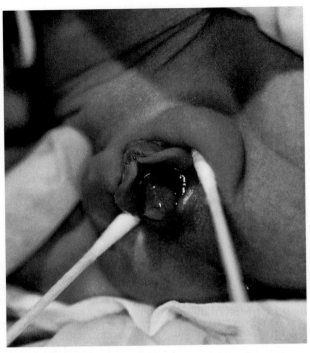

Figure 23.13 After incision at the bedside, the ureterocele is decompressed and retracts into the bladder after a few days. Given the severity of this type of defect, lower urinary tract reconstruction is ultimately warranted in affected infants.

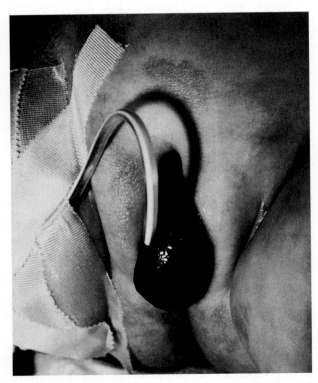

Figure 23.12 Congested and ecchymotic prolapsed ureterocele presenting as an interlabial mass.

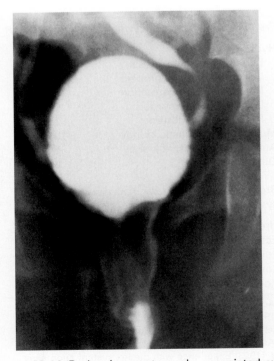

Figure 23.14 Prolapsing ureterocele associated with non-functioning upper pole moiety appears as a filling defect occluding the urethra on excretory urography.

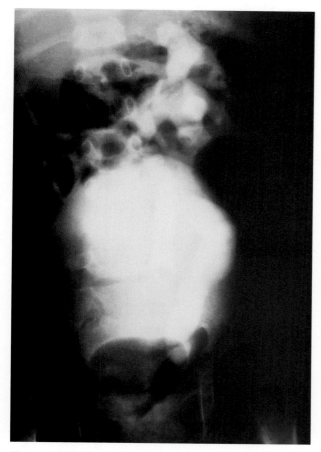

Figure 23.15 Large ureterocele associated with non-functioning right kidney occluding bladder and contralateral kidney. Given the size and position, the prolapse through the urethra of such a variant, especially with urethral extension, is easy to envision.

not recognized antenatally typically present with urinary tract infections (UTIs) (Figs. 23.17 and 23.18). In one series of 58 cases, 90% were identified before the age of 3 years, half of whom presented with UTIs (Caldamone *et al.*, 1984). Non-specific symptoms of failure to thrive and colic also occur.

Flank pain, fever, and abdominal mass are common presentations of ectopic ureters left undetected until a later age (Finan *et al.*, 1987). Ureteroceles can cause irritative voiding symptoms by obstruction or infection but voiding abnormalities accompany ectopic ureters occur far more commonly. In addition, the distal segment of ectopic ureters inserting at the verumontanum can elevate the bladder neck, causing outlet obstruction in boys of any age (Mathews *et al.*, 1999). It is important to remember that ectopic ureters always insert proximal to the urinary sphincter in males. As a result, incontinence does not usually occur in boys with the anomaly. Bilateral single ectopic ureters, associated with bladder neck maldevelopment and lack of sphincter control, are one exception (see below). Another is the frequency and urgency that sometimes results from the trickle of urine into the posterior urethra (Ellerker, 1958). However, the more usual proximal insertions into structures of wolffian origin (seminal vesical, vas, epididymis) present their own problems and ureteral ectopia should be suspected in any infant or child who presents with a culture-proven epididymo-orchitis.

Clinicians should be wary of any girl who reportedly has never been fully toilet trained. These patients

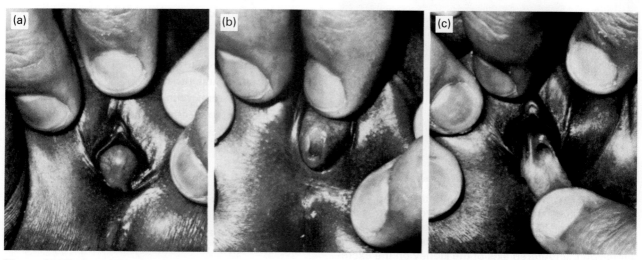

Figure 23.16 A typical cecoureterocele as it presents in (*a*). In (*b*), it is pushed upward, revealing the hymenal ring below. In (*c*) the urethra can be seen above the ureterocele. This ureterocele has a natural pink mucosal coloration, distinguishing it from a periurethral Skene's duct cyst that is yellow-white and mucus-filled.

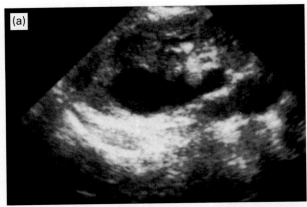

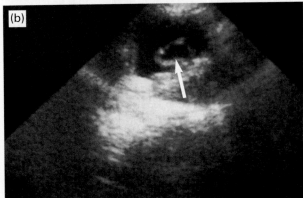

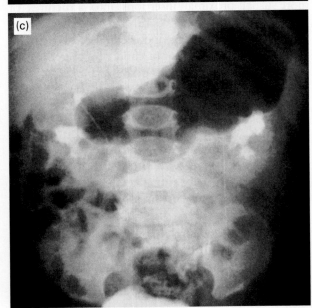

Figure 23.17 A ureterocele in a 3-month-old girl admitted with urinary tract infection. (*a*) Hydronephrosis of the left upper segment. (*b*) Bladder view clearly demonstrates the ureterocele projecting into the bladder (*arrow*). (*c*) Altered axis of the kidney on the excretory urogram suggests the left duplex ureter but does not demonstrate anomaly as effectively as ultrasound, which is often the case in newborns and infants.

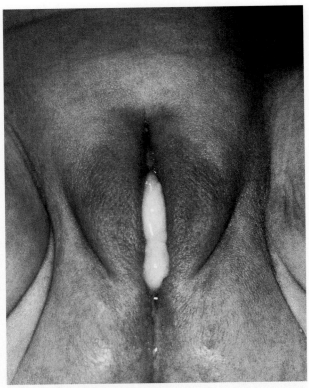

Figure 23.18 Gross pus from the vagina of an infant with an infected ectopic ureter.

must be approached with an open mind, and the possibility of an ectopic ureter always entertained, especially when damp underwear is found on examination. Many have been treated unsuccessfully by a cadre of physicians for bladder dysfunction or presumed psychosocial problems. When the ureter exits along the urethra, the voiding pattern sometimes includes bladder control and spontaneous emptying (from the ureters with normal bladder insertion) followed by an uncontrollable loss of urine as the obstructed system vents secondarily (Fig. 23.19). With vaginal ectopy, continuous wetting in a girl having an otherwise normal micturition pattern and control (in contrast to bladder dysfunction) is a classic presentation for an ectopic ureter (Williams, 1977) (Fig. 23.20 and 23.21). The degree of incontinence depends on the urinary output from the affected kidney. In some cases, small amounts of urine cause sporadic incontinence that occurs only while standing. The latter is commonly mistaken for vaginal voiding or stress incontinence. Table 23.3 summarizes the clinical manifestations of these two ureteral anomalies.

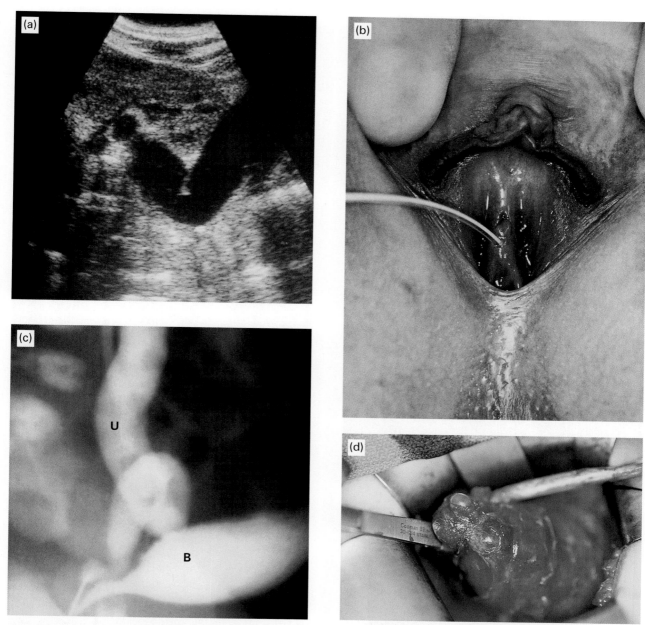

Figure 23.19 Ectopic ureter in a 7-year-old girl with incontinence. (*a*) Sonogram provides a useful screening of such patients and often makes the diagnosis. Shown here is the dilated upper ureter with duplex kidney. Lower pole differentiation is preserved. (*b*) Close physical exam revealed a pinpoint opening (cannulated with a feeding tube). (*c*) Retrograde study of the ectopic ureter. (*d*) At exploration, the megaureter is shown entering the cap of the cystic dysplastic upper pole moiety. (U = ureter; B = bladder.)

Both anomalies can also remain undetected until adulthood (Amitai *et al.*, 1992; Albers *et al.*, 1995). Ectopic ureters in girls that pass through the urinary sphincter but are positioned proximal to the meatus can maintain continence during development. Multiparity can unmask the anomaly, which is often mistaken for stress incontinence. With cases of ectopic ureters that terminate in the male genital tract, prostatitis, seminal vesiculitis, and epididymitis can all occur. Most do not become apparent until the onset of sexual activity. Historically, single-system ureteroceles usually presented during adulthood. An intravesical location, coupled with preserved renal function, allow most to go unnoticed until a later age

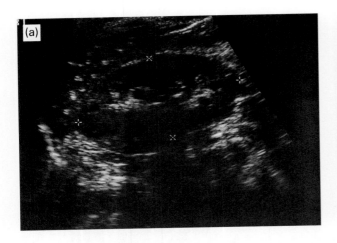

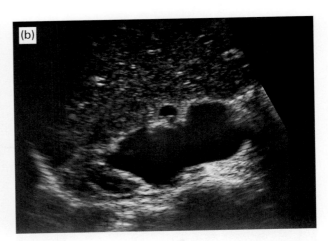

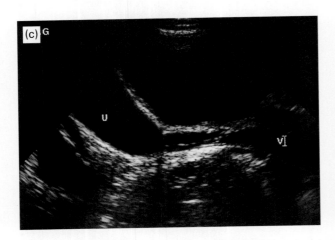

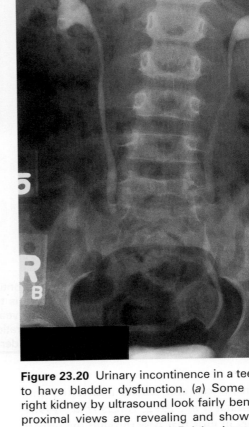

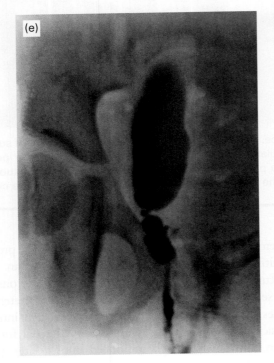

Figure 23.20 Urinary incontinence in a teenage girl felt to have bladder dysfunction. (*a*) Some views of the right kidney by ultrasound look fairly benign. (*b*) More proximal views are revealing and show a superiorly positioned cystic mass. (*c*) Pelvic views demonstrate the ureter entering the vagina. (*d*) Excretory urography shows the duplicated right kidney, with evidence of function to the upper pole. (*e*) Retrograde study of the ectopic ureter.

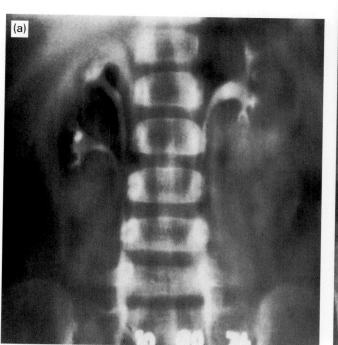

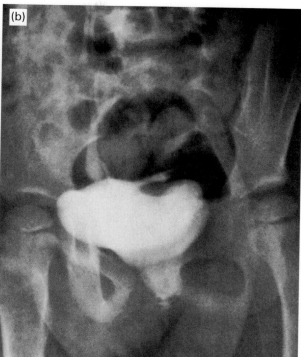

Figure 23.21 Ectopic ureter in a 4-year-old girl with incontinence, demonstrated by excretory urograms. (*a*) Duplication on the right. (*b*) Pooling of the medium into the vagina from the ectopic ureter.

Table 23.3 Clinical presentations

Gender	Features
Ectopic ureters	
Both	Acute or recurrent urinary infection
	Abdominal mass/pain
	Failure to thrive
Females	Continuous dampness with otherwise normal voiding pattern after toilet training
	Vaginal discharge
	Orifice evident along the urethrovaginal septum
Males	Epididymo-orchitis
	Urgency and frequency
	Constipation, pelvic pain, painful ejaculation, epididymitis
Ureteroceles	
Both	Acute or recurrent urinary tract infections
	Hematuria
	Failure to thrive, abdominal or pelvic pain
	Abdominal mass
Females	Prolapsed interlabial mass
	Bladder outlet obstruction
Males	Bladder outlet obstruction

(Fig. 23.22). This accounted for their prior designation as 'adult type', a label since dropped with the advent of antenatal diagnosis. Common presentations still include stones, milk of calcium, and recurrent urinary infection (Golomb *et al.*, 1987).

Evaluation and diagnosis

Ectopic ureters and ureteroceles can present diagnostic dilemmas when it is difficult to determine from which renal moiety they arise. A sonogram and void-

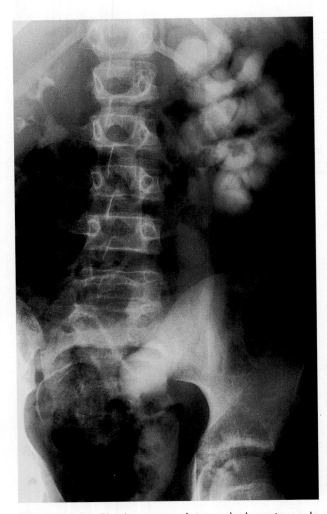

Figure 23.22 Single-system intravesical ureterocele presenting as a urinary tract infection in a 16-year-old. If the impressive dilatation above the small ureterocele represents a progressive change, questions are raised about the natural history of the anomaly and the validity of the expectant treatment of antenatally diagnosed ureteroceles.

ing cystourethrogram (VCUG) are indicated in the initial evaluation of any child suspected of having a ureteral anomaly. Once detected, a functional test (radionuclide renal scan) becomes necessary to the decision-making process when considering the different options in management. Additional studies, for example excretory urography [intravenous pyelography (IVP)] and computed tomography (CT), are also sometimes necessary. Cystoscopy, occasionally in concert with retrograde ureteropyelography (RUP), occasionally completes the evaluation.

Ultrasonography

During initial screening, the differentiation of single from duplex systems is usually possible by ultrasound evaluation. The renal manifestations of ureteroceles and ectopic ureters can be identical. Variable degrees of hydronephrosis of the affected kidney or upper pole moiety depend on the severity of ureteral obstruction (Fig. 23.23). Hyperechoic parenchyma is strongly suggestive of dysplasia. With duplications, the adjacent lower pole can also be hydronephrotic. Reflux (because of lateral ectopia) or obstruction caused by the dilated upper pole ureter must be considered. Hydronephrosis of the lower pole and contralateral kidney may be a direct result of compression by the ureterocele or bladder outlet obstruction.

Ultrasonography should always include a survey of the bladder, where the two anomalies can often be differentiated. Ultrasound is probably the best modality for diagnosing ureteroceles, which usually appear as a cystic protrusion into the posterolateral side of the bladder (Fig. 23.24). The ureter can then be followed deep within the bony pelvis and, in some cases, up to the kidney (Nussbaum *et al.*, 1986; Cremin, 1986). The degree of bladder fullness, however, can reduce the sensitivity of the study. Overdistension causes some ureteroceles to collapse, while an empty bladder will allow a large ureterocele to fill the bladder completely. This gives the impression of a partially full but normal bladder. Ectopic ureters will sometimes also displace the bladder and mimic a ureterocele, the so-called pseudoureterocele (Sumfest *et al.*, 1995) (Figs. 23.25 and 23.26). The muscle wall of the bladder gives a thicker demarcation between its lumen and that of an ectopic ureter than the thin wall of a ureterocele. More typically, the dilated ectopic

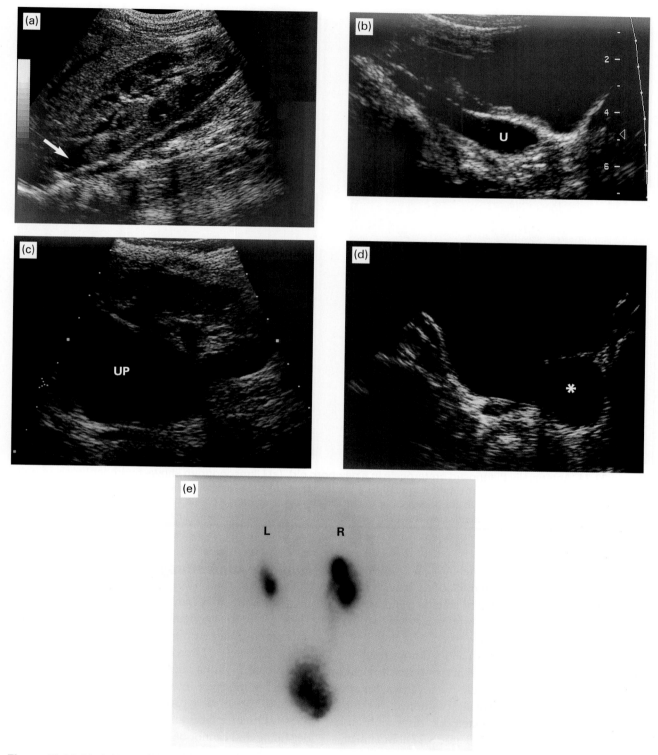

Figure 23.23 Variable appearance of hydronephrosis with duplications. (*a*) Subtle suggestion of obstructed duplication (*arrow*) of the upper pole in a 10-year-old girl with persistent urinary incontinence. (*b*) Dilated ureter shown behind the bladder (U). Urethral ectopy was found to be the cause of wetness. (*c*) Second adolescent girl with similar presentation and vaginal ureteral ectopy. Ultrasound shows markedly dilated upper pole moiety of the left kidney (UP). (*d*) Transverse view of the bladder shows impingement by dilated ureter and pseudoureterocele appearance (*). (*e*) Renal scintigraphy shows deviated axis of the left lower pole and no function of the upper pole.

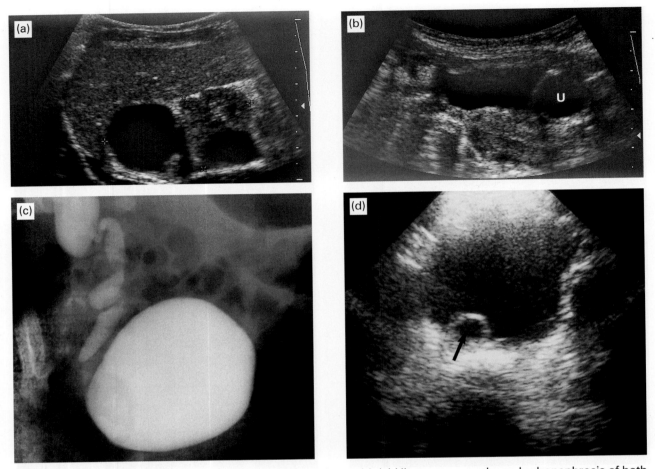

Figure 23.24 Antenatally diagnosed ureterocele in a newborn girl. (*a*) Ultrasonogram shows hydronephrosis of both segments of the right kidney, strongly suggesting a ureterocele. (*b*) Intravesical ureterocele (U) shows on sagittal view of the pelvis. (*c*) Reflux into the lower pole ureter on the right as cause of the hydronephrosis. (*d*) Ultrasonic appearance of a small, intravesical, single-system ureterocele in a different patient (*arrow*).

ureter will taper and terminate into an abnormally inferior position beneath the bladder base. Occasionally, the ureter associated with either anomaly is so tortuous and dilated that it mimics a cystic abdominal mass with multiple septa.

Rarely, these ureteral abnormalities do not result in dilatation of the renal moieties that they affect. Instead, the kidneys associated with single-system anomalies are sometimes small and abnormally positioned, making them difficult to localize (ureterocele disproportion) (Share and Lebowitz, 1989) (Fig. 23.27). In similar fashion, the upper pole variants accompanying duplex variants can be tiny dysplastic remnants crowning otherwise normal kidneys. In both instances, a dilated ureter or ureterocele is still often visualized at the level of the bladder. Additional diagnostics become necessary to define the anatomy more fully.

Voiding cystourethrography

Infant feeding tubes are used to perform this test. These allow for spontaneous voiding and avoid any confusion or distortion offered by the balloons of Foley catheters. Ureteroceles appear as smooth, broad-based filling defects positioned near the trigone. Some evert into the ureter with the bladder full and appear as a diverticulum (Koyanagi *et al.*, 1980). Others efface during the latter stages of bladder filling and cannot be appreciated. Obtaining early images during the filling avoids these problems. An eccentric position may help to define the involved side, although many are centrally located. When laterality cannot be determined and cystoscopy is inconclusive, a cyst puncture with injection of contrast may become necessary.

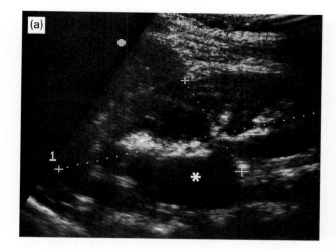

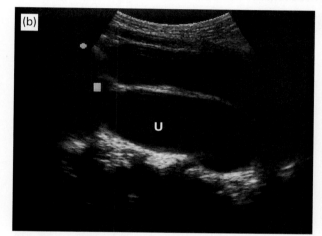

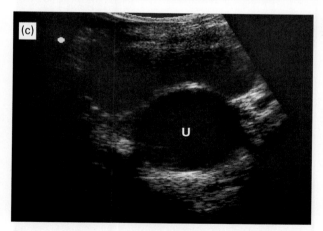

Figure 23.25 Pseudoureterocele appearance of ureter ectopic to the vagina. Ultrasonography in the newborn female with antenatally diagnosed hydronephrosis. (*a*) Upper pole hydronephrosis (∗) with preservation of the lower pole parenchyma. (*b*) Sagittal view of the ureter in the pelvis behind the bladder. (*c*) Psuedoureterocele mimicking the ureterocele on transverse view. Differentiation can usally be made at cystoscopy. Incision is to be avoided with indeterminant cases. (U = ureter.)

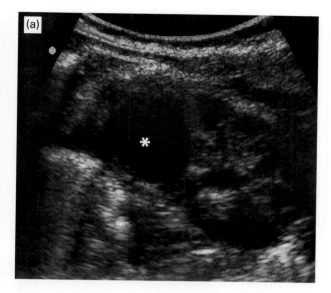

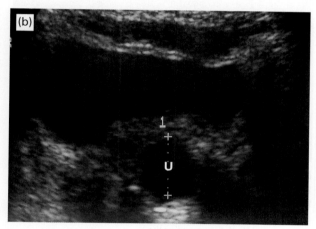

Figure 23.26 Ultrasonic evaluation of antenatally diagnosed hydronephrosis in a newborn girl. (*a*) Markedly hydronephrotic upper pole moiety surrounded by virtually no parenchyma (∗). (*b*) More typical appearance of ectopic ureter (U) en route to the vagina, where the detrusor separating the bladder lumen from the ureter is well developed.

The presence of ipsilateral VUR plays an important role in the management of ureteroceles. Reflux can occur into the ipsilateral lower pole, since the backing required of an effective flap valve is presumably lost with the posteriorly positioned ureterocele (Fig. 23.28). Lateral ectopia, trigonal distortion, and eversion of the ureterocele can also contribute. At times, the ipsilateral reflux can be severe enough that the ureterocele and its duplex kidney are not detected until the time of surgery (Daniels and Allen, 1994). Reflux is also seen in the contralateral system if the

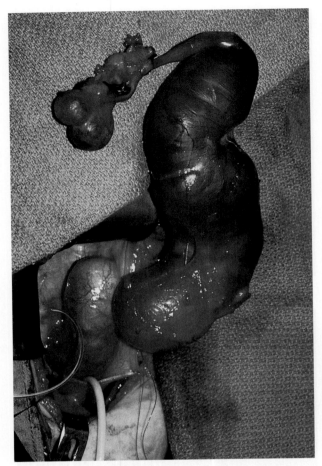

Figure 23.27 Gross example of ureterocele disproportion. Remnant dysplastic cap of tissue as shown are typically associated with massively dilated ureteroceles and ectopic ureters whose renal moiety cannot be appreciated diagnostically.

anomaly is large enough to distort the trigone and opposing submucosal ureteral tunnels. In one series of 148 ureteroceles, ipsilateral reflux was seen in 80 (54%), while contralateral reflux was appreciated in 28% (Senn *et al.*, 1992). Other smaller series have documented similar incidences (Monfort *et al.*, 1992; Rickwood *et al.*, 1992). Reflux into the ureterocele itself is uncommon but can occur (Fig. 23.29).

VUR is a common finding with ectopic ureters (Fig. 23.30). The ipsilateral lower pole ureter refluxes in at least one-half of the cases. Upper pole reflux can also be appreciated depending on the position of the ectopic orifice. Ectopic ureters whose distal extent is positioned within the bladder neck can both reflux and obstruct. Obstruction is intermittent and empty-

ing occurs during voiding, in concert with relaxation of the surrounding musculature. Reflux occurs once the ureter is somewhat emptied and may only be appreciated by performing cyclic (repeated) voiding studies (Wyly and Lebowitz, 1984). Orifices proximal to the bladder neck reflux freely with or without voiding.

Excretory urography

Despite its declining role in the routine evaluation of children with urinary tract problems, excretory urography remains a useful tool in the work-up of certain ureteral anomalies (Figs. 23.31 and 23.32). This is occasionally the case with ureteroceles, when the anatomy is undefinable with ultrasound and renal scintigraphy alone, and is especially true of ectopic

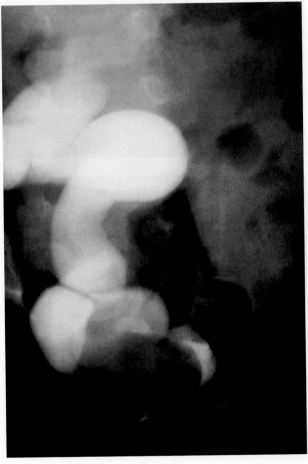

Figure 23.28 Massive reflux into the lower pole ureter. An element of obstruction from the significantly enlarged ureterocele can also contribute to the dilatation.

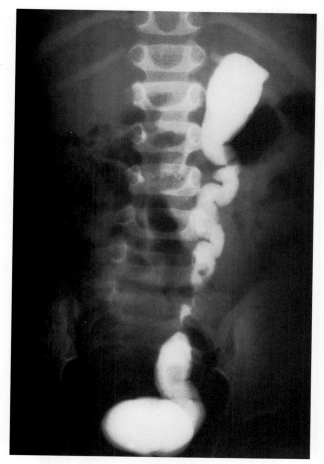

Figure 23.29 Reflux into the ureterocele and upper pole system of the left kidney.

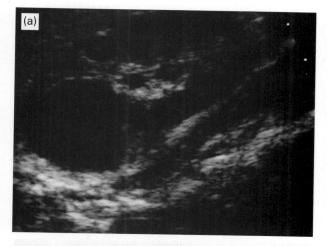

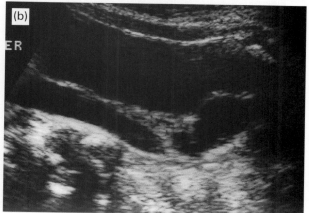

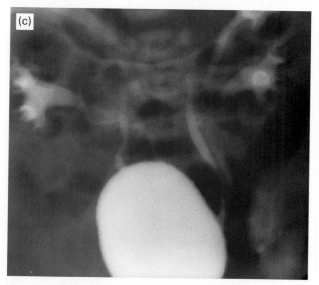

Figure 23.30 Vesicoureteral reflux associated with ectopic ureter to the urethra. (*a*) Duplex right kidney with hydronephrotic upper pole. (*b*) Ectopic ureter behind the bladder could be confused with an ureterocele. (*c*) Voiding cystourethrogram shows reflux into duplicated ureters on the left and the lower pole on the right.

ureters. Many clinicians remain steadfast in their belief that excretory urography remains the definitive diagnostic study for the latter. For girls with infrasphincteric ectopia, who arrive with the classic history of constant urinary dribbling despite being successfully toilet-trained, excretory urography is often the only imaging study necessary to make the diagnosis (Carrico and Lebowitz, 1998) (Figs. 23.33 and 23.34). Radiographic signs of the non-functioning, occult duplications found with ectopic ureters are shown in Table 23.4.

Ureteroceles with minimally functioning upper pole moieties can cause identical upper tract findings. The ureterocele appears as a filling defect within the bladder that gradually fills with contrast from the functioning kidney. When ureteroceles are associated with a functioning kidney they fill with contrast and appear as a 'cobra head' at the ureterovesical junction.

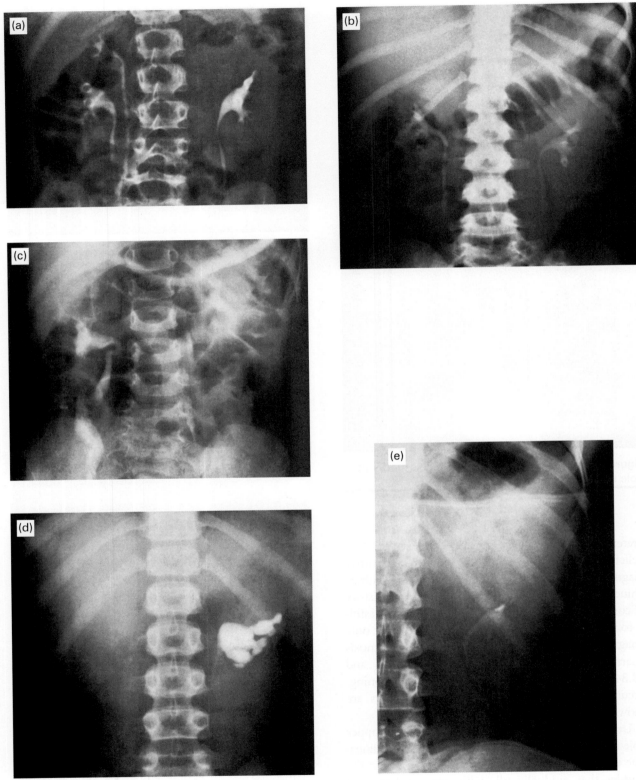

Figure 23.31 Examples of characteristic lateral and downward displacement of lower segment when the functionless upper pole pelvis is dilated. (*a*) Functionless upper left segment. (*b*) Poorly functioning upper right segment and functionless upper left segment. (*c*) Functionless upper right segment and displacement of the lower segment. (*d*) Reflux into displaced lower pole segment. (*e*) Functionless upper left segment simulating mass effect of upper pole.

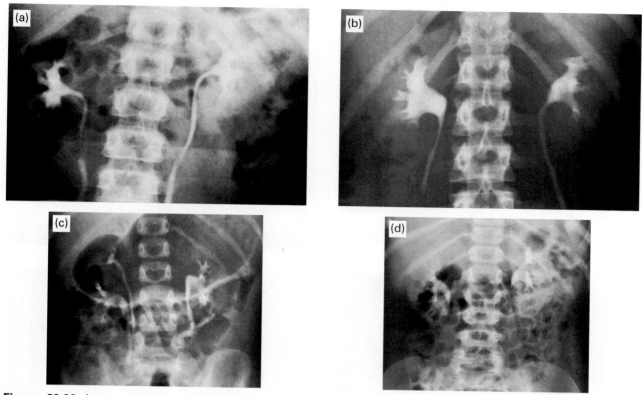

Figure 23.32 Appearance of the lower pole pelvis when the upper pole is functionless and non-dilated. (*a*) Functionless upper right segment. The calyceal system of the lower segment is smaller but relatively normal. (*b*) Functionless upper pole on the left, with decreased number of calyces of the lower segment. (*c*) Functionless upper left segment, with apparent increase in renal substance of the upper pole. The presence of a duplication of the contralateral kidney is often a key to diagnosis. (*d*) Functionless upper right segment, with apparent increase in renal substance thickness on the medial side of the upper pole.

Renal scintigraphy

Radionuclide scans help to quantify the amount of functioning renal parenchyma. This is crucial information when renal salvage is being considered. The degree of obstruction is also assessed, although most ectopic ureters and ureteroceles exhibit delayed drainage because of ureteral dilatation. Technetium-99m-diethylenetriaminepentacetic acid (DTPA) and mercaptoacetyltriglycline (MAG-3) scans fulfill both requirements fairly well. Since (^{99m}Tc)dimercaptosuccinic acid (DMSA) scans are unaffected by obstruction and provide renal tubular labeling, they provide a sensitive assessment of function and are sometimes helpful in detecting occult duplex anomalies and small kidneys associated with ureteral anomalies that are not identified by other techniques (Bozorgi *et al.*, 1998; Pattaras *et al.*, 1999). Because

transitional physiology affects the perinatal kidney's handling of radionuclides, it has been said that renal scans performed early after delivery may not provide an accurate assessment of function. This could contribute to the lower yield of functioning kidneys in historic series when IVPs were obtained in newborns. It could also result in overestimates of the utility of procedures done to alleviate obstructed newborn kidneys, compared to studies that are repeated when the physiology is more conducive to scanning. However, Chung *et al.* (1993), in a landmark paper, reported that the results of diuretic renography in a group of neonates (< 28 days) was as reliable as the results of the repeat studies in the same group of children followed for a mean of 325 days. Comparisons were made in regard to differential renal function, pre- and post-diuretic urine output and drainage half-times.

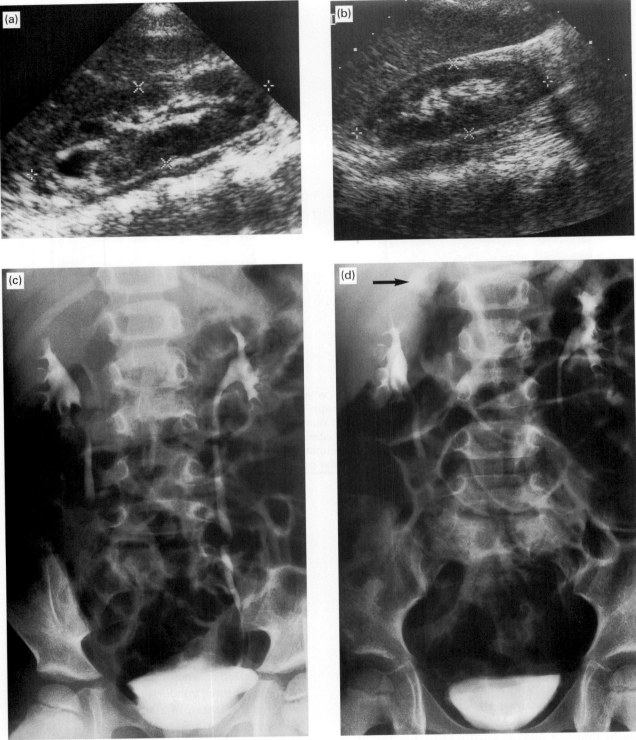

Figure 23.33 Utility of excretory urography. Studies in a 13-year-old girl with continuous wetting were strongly suggestive of an ectopic ureter. Sonograms for the past 7 years read as normal. (*a*) Initial sonogram as a 6-year-old suggests mild upper pole dilatation. (*b*) Current sonogram is essentially unremarkable. Retrieval and review of early excretory urogram confirms the clinical impression. (*c*) Note the deviated axis of the right kidney and ureteral displacement on early sequence of excretory urogram. (*d*) Later film shows delayed uptake of contrast in the upper pole.

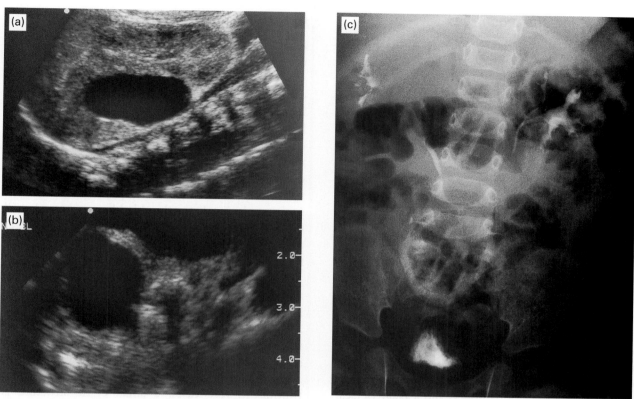

Figure 23.34 An infant boy with urinary tract infection. The role of excretory urography. (*a*) Ultrasonogram initally felt to represent single-system hydronephrotic right kidney. (*b*) Right kidney pelvic view demonstrates a markedly dilated ureter behind the bladder. (*c*) Excretory urography shows displaced lower pole of the right kidney.

Table 23.4 Excretory urography: findings suggesting occult duplex kidney with ectopic ureter

Finding	Features
'Drooping lily sign'	Inferior and lateral displacement of lower pole by minimally or non-functioning upper pole. Delayed films may show function, but most are 'silent'. Axes of the kidneys should normally cross the body of the 10th thoracic vertebra
Lateral displacement of lower pole ureter	Compared with contralateral ureter, differences in the distance from an adjacent vertebral pedicle
'Missing calyx'	Incomplete compliment of calyces with absence of system draining upper pole. A shortened or cut-off infundibulum to the upper pole calyx, which is normally the longest
More upper pole parenchyma than expected with increased renal length	
Duplex kidney on the contralateral side	
Dilated, ectopic ureter appreciated on postvoid film	

Other diagnostic modalities

CT scans may help to define the anatomy of kidneys with collecting systems of bizarre appearance. Duplications in which both ureters and pelves are dilated are one example. CT can also be considered for patients suspected of having ureteral ectopia or ureterocele disproportion but whose poorly functioning renal moiety cannot be defined by other modalities (Hulnick and Bosniak, 1986; Braverman and Lebowitz, 1991) (Fig. 23.35). Magnetic resonance imaging (MRI) can be considered for these types of cases as well, although its role with duplication anomalies has not been well defined (Matsuki *et al.*, 1998). Percutaneous drainage can also be used to vent obstructed kidneys or renal segments that appear salvageable by ultrasound but function poorly. However, the recoverability of function is rare when renal scintigraphy demonstrates little activity.

A variety of dye tests has been used clinically to diagnose ectopic ureters. For example, indigo carmine or methylene blue can be instilled in the bladder with a catheter, which is then removed. Continued evidence of dampness and leakage of clear urine implicates ureteral ectopia. Another test involves placing a dental roll in the vagina. After indigo carmine is given intravenously, the roll will appear blue, provided there is some function to the affected kidney and the child has not stained the roll by spontaneously voiding. The relative invasiveness of such tests, coupled with the increased sensitivities of today's diagnostics, have reduced their utility in most cases.

Cystoscopy

Examples of the cystoscopic appearance of ureteroceles are shown in Figure 23.47. With smaller intravesical ureteroceles, the cystic dilatation expands with each peristalsis, then shrinks as urine drains through its orifice. Not all variants are as easy to appreciate, however. Extravesical variants have ill-defined borders that can undermine the bladder neck and urethra. If the bladder is overfilled, they efface and can even appear as a diverticulum. The orifice of the ureterocele may be difficult to appreciate but is often positioned distal to the bladder neck and will balloon open with the efflux of irrigant. With larger ureteroceles, the adjacent ureteral orifices are also difficult to appreciate because of displacement.

Cystoscopy is less helpful for ectopic ureters, and the ectopic orifice cannot be appreciated more than half the time. Bladder neck and urethral ectopy offer a high yield. Prostatic ectopy sometimes presents as a widened ejaculatory duct that allows easy retrograde study (Schulman, 1976). Examining the vaginal vault along its anterior/lateral aspect for GYN-ectopy is less fruitful. In rare cases, a small cystic structure is identified that can be unroofed and cannulated for retrograde study (Gonzales, 1992). Intravenous indigo carmine is sometimes excreted by even minimally functioning kidneys and can aid in identification. Within the bladder, the hemitrigone on the affected side is often underdeveloped and may be elevated from behind by the dilated ureter. In some cases, the dilated ureter can be palpated on rectal examination. Failure to identify the ectopic insertion

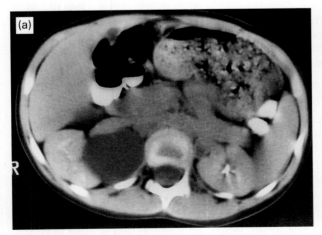 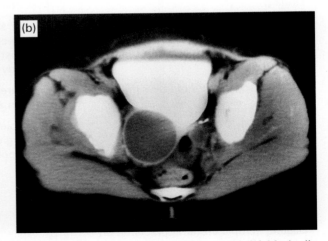

Figure 23.35 Computerized tomography in a female toddler with abdominal pain and palpable mass. (*a*) Markedly dilated ureter displacing the right kidney associated with duplication. (*b*) The ureter is shown behind the bladder.

rarely changes management. In cases where a lower tract approach is planned, the ectopic ureter can be identified outside the bladder or transvesically after incising the trigone on the affected side (see Management, below).

Management considerations

Once the work-up is complete and the diagnosis made, the management of ectopic ureters and ureteroceles is defined by the answers to the following questions.

1 Is the affected ureter(s) a singlet or portion of a duplex system?
2 Is the affected ureter(s) obstructed, refluxing, or both?
3 Are the contralateral and/or ipsilateral ureter(s) and/or the bladder affected by the primary anomaly?
4 What is the status of the kidney or portion of kidney associated with the ureter(s) in question?
5 What is the age and clinical status of the patient?

A description of the experience with various techniques and their technical nuances follow. Simply put, the algorithms in management of these two anomalies historically branched with two main decisions: whether to save or discard the involved kidney and the need or lack thereof to reconstruct the bladder. These remain the mainstays of management for ectopic ureters.

The recommendations for ureteroceles have become controversial, however, with the recent inclusion in the treatment armamentarium of selective puncture. Minimally invasive and a seemingly simple solution, the benefits of cystoscopically decompressing a ureterocele must be weighed against the risks of causing reflux into the involved ureter.

Until recently, the two main areas of contention with ureteroceles dealt with the salvage of functioning upper pole moieties and the need, if any, for removal of ureteroceles subtending upper pole segments after heminephrectomy or proximal ureteral diversion (ureteroureterostomy or ureteropyelostomy) caused their collapse (Fig. 23.36). The introduction of selective puncture offers the obvious third controversy of which ureteroceles to decompress. The answers to these questions are being continually modified by contemporary clinical studies.

A 'cookbook approach' should be avoided when composing algorithms for the management of any urinary abnormality. Each patient requires individualized treatment, since there is often no uniform solution to every urologic anomaly. Nevertheless, trends become apparent in reviewing the literature that allow certain recommendations to be applied to most cases which give the highest likelihood of a favorable outcome.

Recommendations for management
Ectopic ureters
Single system, minimal or non-functioning kidney

Most kidneys (90%) that accompany single-system ectopic ureters do not function appreciably. Nephrectomy is the treatment of choice. In some cases, the question of renal salvage is raised by the appearance of marginal function on nuclear scintigraphy. How much function is enough to warrant ureteral reconstruction rather than ablation of its associated kidney? Nephrectomy is indicated when the creatinine clearance provided by the affected kidney, if it were isolated, would not eliminate the need for dialysis. Using per cent function as a cut-off, like the commonly cited standards of 10 or 15%, may have little meaning, especially if the contralateral kidney exhibits impaired function. In addition, kidneys that function marginally in infancy sometimes assume a progressively smaller portion of overall renal function with interval growth of the child. An intrinsic developmental insult and/or the rules governing renal hypertrophy, where healthy kidneys do not relinquish the additional renal function that they are asked to assume, can be implicated when this occurs.

One area of controversy for some ectopic ureters involves the management of the lower ureteral segment. In cases of wolffian or GYN-ectopy, where an element of obstruction is the rule, the lower ureter need not be removed. Once decompressed, ascending infections of these dry, isolated segments are uncommon and the need for secondary ureterectomies after subtotal ureterectomy is rare. The obstructed ureters found with GU-ectopy typically enter the bladder neck or urethra. These can also remain, although a small number will predispose to recurrent urinary infections that ultimately necessitate their removal. It may be that such systems begin to reflux after the outflow of urine ceases from above (see Cyclic voiding cystourethrography, above).

Refluxing lower ureters have typically been removed in concert with nephrectomy. An extravesical approach through a second lower transverse muscle-splitting (Gibson) incision adds little additional mor-

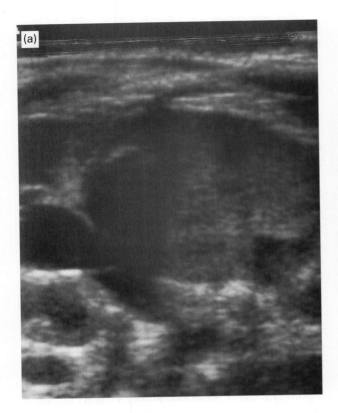

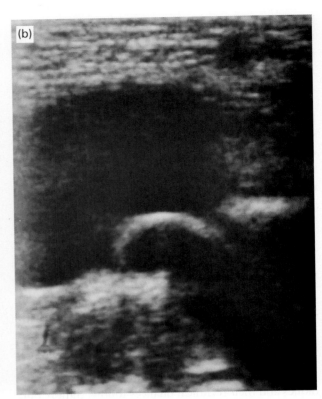

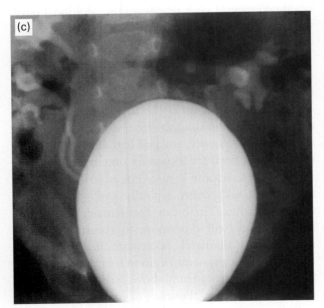

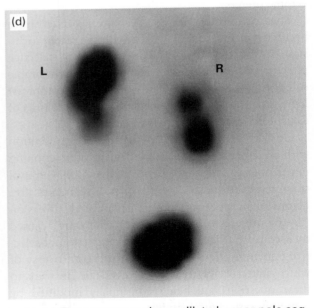

Figure 23.36 Antenatally diagnosed ureterocele in a newborn girl. (*a*) The sonogram shows dilated upper pole segment of the duplex left kidney. (*b*) Pelvic view of the ureterocele projecting within the bladder. (*c*) Cystogram demonstrates reflux into the contralateral duplex ureters and lower pole ureter on the left. (*d*) Renal scan shows preservation of function and hydronephrosis of the left upper pole moiety.

bidity. However, the necessity for a simultaneous approach for these variants has been questioned. In a study by Plaire et al. (1997), secondary surgery for removal of the distal ureter was required in only four of 38 such patients. In cases where a ureteral stump is left, be it refluxing or obstructed, it should be ligated with absorbable sutures following aspiration of urine from the distal end. Urinary fistulae have occurred when presumably obstructed ureteral stumps have been left open and unappreciated reflux commences. However, this will cease with bladder catheter drainage.

Duplex system, minimal or non-functioning upper pole

Heminephrectomy is recommended for the affected upper pole (Smith et al., 1989). The case made for salvage is similar to that in singlets and depends on relative function. Developmentally, the upper 'half' of a normal duplex kidney typically contributes only one-third of that kidney's glomeruli or 16% of overall renal function. The lack of an optimal inductive influence during fetal development combined with an element of obstruction will significantly reduce the contribution of most upper pole moieties drained by ectopic ureters. As in single systems, a subtotal ureterectomy is usually sufficient, taking the ectopic ureter as far distal as possible through a flank incision. When there is reflux into the upper pole and concerns about the ureteral stump, it can be removed through a second incision.

Single system, salvageable function

Reimplantation of the affected ureter is the treatment of choice. It helps to initially identify the ureter outside the bladder, especially when the insertion of the ectopic meatus cannot be localized cystoscopically. Once the ureter is mobilized, a transvesical or an extravesical approach to ureteroneocystostomy can be successfully applied. The distal-most segment that enters the bladder neck/urethra should be avoided with these and other ectopic ureters. The tedious dissection required for their removal risks damaging the urinary sphincter mechanism. Ureteral tailoring is often necessary and can be done using any one of a variety of techniques (see Megaureters).

Duplex system, salvageable function

In cases where the upper pole is obstructed, yet provides significant function, its ureter can be anasto-

mosed to the adjacent lower pole renal pelvis (ureteropyelostomy) or ureter (ureteroureterostomy). The lower ureteral segment can be mobilized to the pelvic brim and excised, and the remainder left alone. Concerns about discrepancy in size between the ectopic and recipient ureter are usually unfounded (Huisman et al., 1987). These operations are no more challenging than the dismembered pyeloplasties required of infants with ureteropelvic junction (UPJ) obstructions. Rates of success should be similar. When technical concerns persist or if the upper pole moiety exhibits signs of cystic dysplasia, a heminephrectomy is recommended. Visualization of the upper pole moiety in assessment of dysplasia is one advantage of this approach. Renal sparing surgeries could probably be used more frequently in this setting. In one study, normal histology was found in 57% of upper pole heminephrectomy specimens removed from ectopic ureters (Smith et al., 1989).

Another option for obstructed systems is to approach the duplication from below. When reflux is present into one or both ureters, a common sheath ureteral reimplantation is the preferred method of treatment (El Ghoneimi et al., 1996). The repair can be technically challenging, especially in smaller infants. In both instances, tailoring of the upper pole ureter usually becomes necessary to achieve the desired length/diameter ratio required of successful ureteroneocystostomy. Revisions are made along the length of ureter opposite the common wall where vascularity is shared by the duplication. When folding techniques cause excessive bulk with larger ureters, excisional tapering is preferred. A psoas hitch is sometimes necessary to gain additional length for the reimplantation. Another option for duplications with an obstructed upper and refluxing lower pole ureter is to perform a proximal diversion of the upper ureter (ureteropyelostomy), discard its remainder, and reimplant the lower pole ureter alone. Although two incisions are required of this approach, it avoids the problems that accompany complex ureteroneocystotomy.

Ureteroceles

Single system, minimal or non-functioning kidney

Nephrectomy is the treatment of choice. Ordinarily, the ureterocele remains collapsed after aspiration and any element of obstruction to the bladder neck or contralateral ureter resolves (Fig. 23.37). The latter may unmask reflux into the contralateral, now

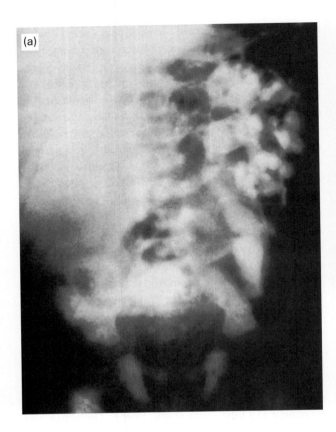

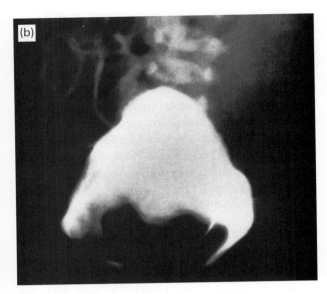

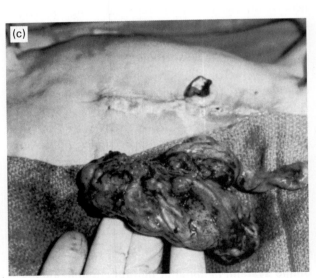

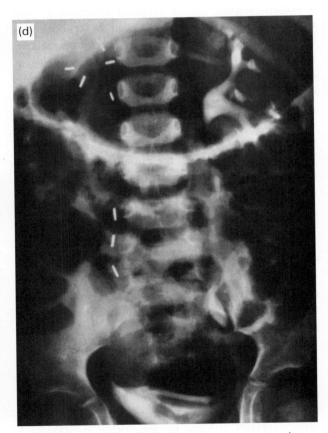

Figure 23.37 Newborn male with a large, single-system ureterocele on the right side. (*a*) Excretory urogram shows poor visualization of the right collecting system and hydronephrosis of the left. (*b*) Cystogram of the same patient shows a large ureterocele filling the bladder and extending through the bladder neck. (*c*) At surgery, the grossly dysplastic hydronephrotic kidney was removed and extravesical dissection of the ureter was completed. (*d*) The postoperative excretory urogram shows significant improvement of the left-sided hydronephrosis and collapse of the ureterocele.

solitary, kidney. With larger ureteroceles a significant reservoir for lower UTIs remains, despite their decompression. Although not well defined in the literature, some of these will require secondary surgery for their removal. Cystoscopic evidence of the open meatus typically accompanying sphincteric or cecoureteroceles may identify those variants particularly at risk for future problems. Simultaneous excision of the ureterocele with bladder reconstruction is not unreasonable, if the age of the patient permits. Conversely, the patient can be followed medically after nephrectomy and repair of the bladder deferred to a later age, if indicated.

Selective cystoscopic puncture is not an option for obstructed ureteroceles associated with a non-functioning kidney. This risks converting the anomaly from one that can be potentially addressed solely from above to one requiring another incision to correct a refluxing ureterocele. Non-selective 'unroofing', as advocated by Tank (1986), remains an option for decompressing obstructed ureteroceles in children who are extremely ill and unable to tolerate open surgery. Interestingly, 50% of renal moieties that showed no function on preoperative excretory urography subsequently demonstrated excretion of contrast after their decompression. These data suggest that some segments may recover function after being vented, but more likely point to the historic shortcomings of excretory urography compared with radionuclide studies in infants with obstructed kidneys. VUR is an expected sequelae of this predecessor of selective puncture (Wines and O'Flynn, 1972). Decompression can also be achieved with percutaneous renal drainage, which is the now preferred method of temporization until the ureterocele can be definitively addressed (O'Brien et al., 1990).

Single system, functioning kidney

The experience with selective incisions and puncture of these ureterocele variants has been encouraging enough that it should be considered the procedure of choice (Monfort et al., 1992; Blythe et al., 1993) (Fig. 23.38). In one recent series, for example, endoscopic decompression was successful in 22 of 25 patients (88%) with single-system intravesical ureteroceles (Husmann et al., 1999). Reflux tends to appear into larger ureteroceles whose detrusor defects provide very little backing to the anomaly. Ureterocele excision, ureteral reimplantation, and correction of any detrusor defects usually become necessary when reflux appears.

Duplex system, minimal or non-functioning upper pole

An upper pole heminephrectomy is indicated but may not finalize the problem (Figs. 23.39 and 23.40). This upper tract approach effectively decompresses the ureterocele, potentially restores trigonal anatomy, and may be the only treatment needed for some patients (Belman et al., 1974; King et al., 1983). In the series reported by Caldamone et al. (1984), seven of 36 patients (19%) needed secondary procedures for persistent reflux (three patients) or bladder outlet obstruction (four patients). VUR appeared in ten cases after decompression, where none was present beforehand. The reflux resolved in three. Long-term follow-up into adulthood is unavailable. Others reported similar rates (about 20%) of persistent reflux into ipsilateral lower pole or contralateral ureters after heminephrectomy alone (Mandell et al., 1980; Mor et al., 1994). In another series of 19 patients reported by Scherz et al. (1989), nine (47%) required intravesical surgery for urinary infection or reflux (Fig. 23.41).

These types of data have led some clinicians to advocate a combined approach where heminephrectomy, ureterocele excision, and ureteral reimplantation are completed with one surgery (Hendren and Mitchell, 1979; Decter et al., 1989). The need for secondary surgeries is far less common with the combined approach. For example, only 14% of patients in the Scherz series (1989) required reoperations for persistent reflux after the combined approach. To its detriment, ureterocele excision and duplex ureteral reimplantation can present a technical tour-de-force in smaller infants and intravesical repairs are unnecessary in perhaps half of these patients. The characteristics of ureteroceles that ultimately require excision and bladder reconstruction remain to be fully defined. Such selection criteria would help identify patients whose problem would be best finalized by the upper tract approach and limit the combined approach to those that truly need it.

The review by Husmann et al. (1995) has been revealing in this regard. Of 87 patients with a ureterocele and non-functioning upper pole treated by heminephrectomy, subtotal ureterectomy, and observation (upper tract approach), 54 (62%) required additional surgery to correct reflux. The need for additional surgery was directly related to the number of renal moieties that originally had VUR present.

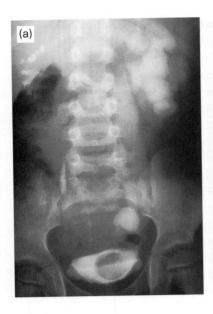
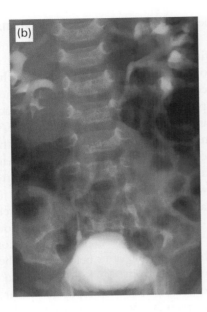
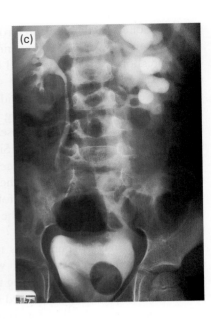
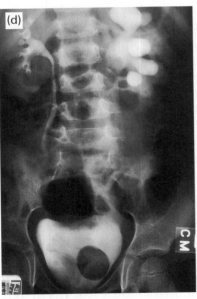
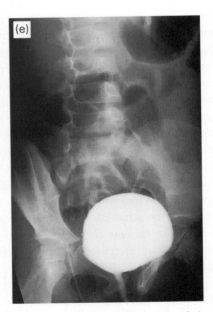

Figure 23.38 (*a*) Single-system intravesical ureterocele causing significant hydroureteronephrosis of the left collecting system. (*b*) After incision, marked improvement in the degree of dilatation is seen. No reflux was present before or after surgery. (*c*) A similar variant with hydronephrosis of the left kidney treated with a selective incision. (*d*) Significant improvement is shown after surgery. (*e*) Voiding cystourethrogram is unremarkable.

When a ureterocele alone was present, 21 of 21 patients required no further surgery. If low-grade reflux (less than III/V) was present into only one ureter, eight of 15 patients (55%) did well with the upper tract approach alone. Finally, and most significantly, when high-grade reflux was seen in one ureter or reflux was associated with more than one moiety, regardless of their grade, surgery became inevitable for 48 of 50 (96%) patients. Ureterocele prolapse is another finding that inevitably portends bladder reconstruction (Gotoh *et al.*, 1988). In addition, the occasional ureterocele that itself refluxes at presentation will, by default, require a combined 'up-and-down' approach for management.

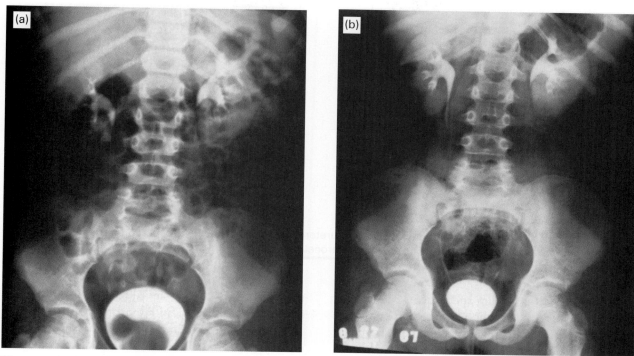

Figure 23.39 (*a*) Preoperative view shows minimally functioning upper pole moiety of the right kidney. (*b*) Postoperative view shows decompression of the ureterocele and an essentially normal right kidney.

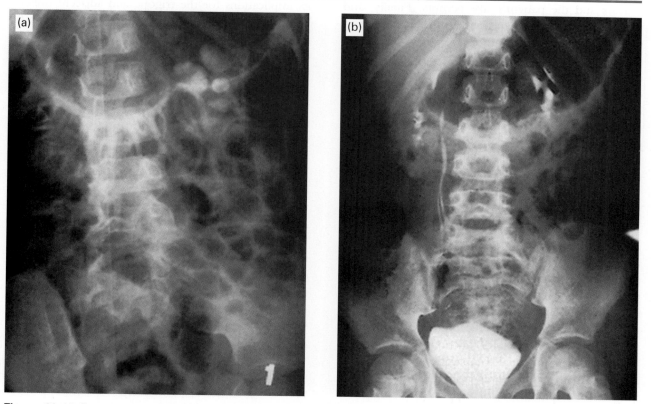

Figure 23.40 Extravesical ureterocele treated by heminephrectomy and subtotal ureterectomy. (*a*) Preoperative excretory urogram shows left-sided anomaly and hydronephrotic lower pole. (*b*) Postoperative view. Preservation of function and appearance of the remaining kidney is often surprisingly good. The ureterocele is fully decompressed.

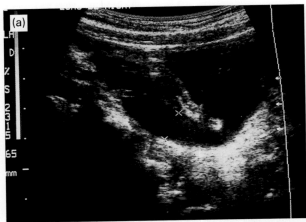
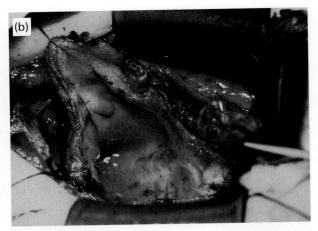

Figure 23.41 (*a*) The stump of the residual ureter and ureterocele remain after heminephrectomy. The patient presented with recurrent urinary infections. (*b*) Large ureterocele opened at surgery.

Given these data, families and patients can be better informed as to the likelihood of needing lower urinary tract surgery if an upper tract approach is initially used. In addition, strong consideration can be given to a complete urinary tract reconstruction if the preoperative work-up returns such ominous prognosticators and the patient's size permits. Finally, and while it might seem an anathema to some, unroofing the ureterocele becomes an option in newborns and small infants who are destined to require 'up-and-down' surgery regardless, because of the significance of their anomaly. Eliminating obstruction significantly reduces the threat of urinary infections and decompression of the ureterocele simplifies the bladder repair (Fig. 23.42). Most children can be effectively managed with antibiotic prophylaxis until they are old enough to have a reconstructive procedure.

Duplex system, functioning upper pole

Like their non-functioning partners, these too can be addressed with an 'upper tract alone' approach. It should be remembered that upper pole duplications optimally contribute approximately 16% of overall renal function. Because of this somewhat marginal contribution, some clinicians recommend heminephrectomies for the majority of functioning duplications. This avoids the potential complications of the reconstruction, risks to the lower pole, and the unknown long-term implications of upper pole retention (Gonzales, 1992). The other option is salvage of the upper pole by creating a ureteropyelostomy or ureteroureterostomy in combination with a subtotal

ureterectomy. No study similar to that cited above for non-functioning duplications treated with an upper tract approach has been reported. Nevertheless, there is every reason to believe that same risk factors for persistent reflux and recurrent urinary infections exist and result from the size and position of the ureterocele and its implications for the trigone and adjacent ureters. With this in mind, the upper tract approach can be reserved for obstructing ureteroceles presenting without reflux into the ipsilateral lower segment, especially in newborns and infants.

It seems reasonable to address the majority of these variants solely at the bladder level, removing the ureterocele and correcting associated reflux, thus eliminating the need for secondary surgery. Such an approach is ideal for the older child whose bladder is large enough to allow a complex reconstruction with a high likelihood of success. The reality is, however, that the majority of ureteroceles are diagnosed antenatally. After birth, such babies remain at significant risk as UTIs associated with obstructions are much more threatening to the child and kidney than those that occur with reflux alone. In addition, the affected kidney potentially incurs progressive damage because of distal ureteral obstruction. As a result, medical management with prophylactic antibiotics should be a short-term approach, allowing for interval growth until a time when the bladder can be safely reconstructed.

Endoscopic treatment provides an effective option for the small child, particularly those who present with a significant UTI. Surgeons should hold realistic expectations for this approach, which rarely provides the final solution for these types of ureteroceles,

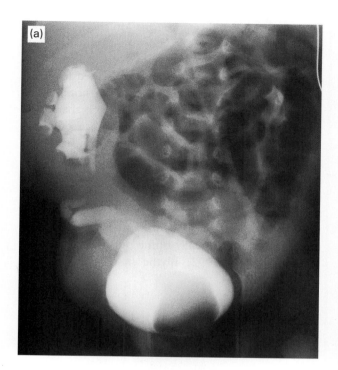

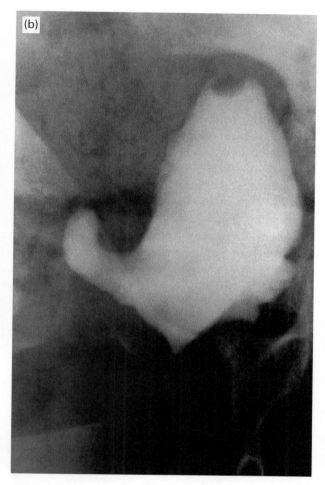

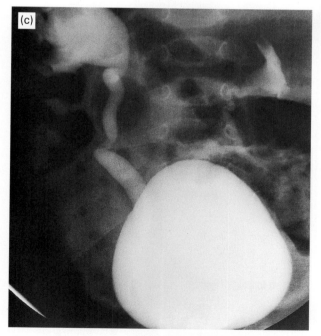

Figure 23.42 A newborn female with urinary tract infection needing a combined approach in the management of a ureterocele. (*a*) Excretory urogram shows a large ureterocele filling the base of the bladder, and non-functioning upper pole of the right kidney. (*b*) Pre-operative cystogram demonstrates eversion of the ureterocele forming a diverticulum, an indication of a significant detrusor defect. No reflux was seen. (*c*) Post-incision cystogram shows bilateral vesicoureteral reflux but decompressed ureterocele. Heminephrectomy and ureterocelectomy were deferred until 1 year of age, since the child remained infection free.

even with selective incision. Instead, the maneuver should be considered a temporizing measure used to vent the obstructed system. This increases the likelihood of success with medical management, thus allowing for additional growth of the child until a definitive bladder reconstruction can be completed. VUR persists or results in the majority of cases. For example, in one series 18 of 21 (86%) patients with extravesical ureteroceles treated endoscopically required additional surgery. In contrast, the results with intravesical variants were strikingly different with 14 of 16 children successfully treated with incision alone (Fig. 23.43) (Pfister *et al.*, 1998). However, in a larger series reported by Husmann *et al.* (1999), the performance of selective incision was discouraging. Ectopic ureteroceles preoperatively

associated with reflux into one or more moieties required further surgery for persistent reflux in 37 of 44 (84%) cases. An identical reoperation rate occurred when heminephrectomy was used for similar variants. Notably, when reflux was not present prior to treatment, incision was more likely than heminephrectomy to result in the appearance of reflux (64% vs 15%). Based on this observation, it would appear that ureteropyelostomy or ureteroureterostomy is the treatment of choice when a salvageable obstructed upper system is not accompanied by lower segment reflux. While success rates with endoscopic incision vary, its weaker performance with extravesical ureteroceles is continually borne out in the literature (Monfort *et al.*, 1992; Blythe *et al.*, 1993) (Figs. 23.44 and 23.45).

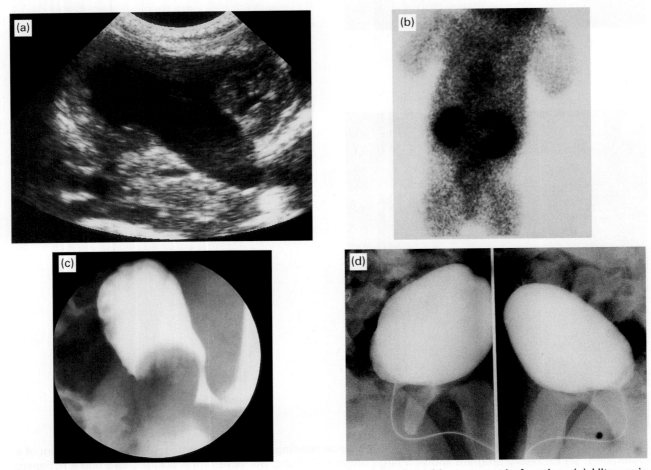

Figure 23.43 Selective incision of duplex system ureterocele with salvagable upper pole function. (*a*) Ultrasonic appearance in a newborn diagnosed antenatally. (*b*) Radionuclide scan shows function to upper pole and filling defect within the bladder. (*c*) Bladder defect during cystogram appears largely intravesical, which may have been a factor in success. (*d*) Postincision cystogram shows no evidence of reflux. Hydronephrosis had virtually resolved.

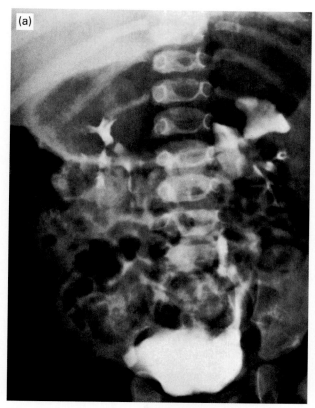
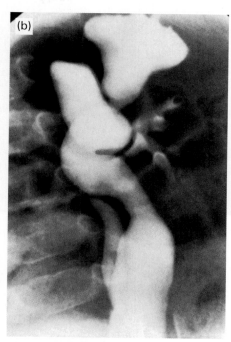

Figure 23.44 Risk of ureterocele incision. (*a*) Duplication of the left kidney associated with the extravesical u. terocele seen on the excretory urography. (*b*) After incision, the previously 'obstructed' system is converted to one that significantly refluxes into both ureters.

Surgical techniques

Although many of these techniques are described elsewhere, observations of their application to the treatment of ectopic ureters and ureteroceles in children deserve comment.

Ureterocele prolapse

The prolapsed ureterocele is not the surgical emergency once supposed. Manual reduction is sometimes possible but, because of the nature of the defect, it is likely to recur. Heminephrectomy to decompress the ureterocele is another option. However, affected bladders will often require secondary reconstructions as well. A simpler solution is to incise the ureterocele at the bedside with a disposable ophthalmic cautery unit. This technique is usually effective and serves the same purpose as cystoscopic incision. In occasional cases, the latter still becomes necessary to treat the intravesical portions of a prolapsing ureterocele that will fail to decompress because of bladder neck obstruction.

Selective cystoscopic incision

The cystoscope is initially passed under vision to avoid traumatizing the ureterocele. For intravesical variants, a distally positioned puncture at the ureterocele's medial base is usually able to decompress the structure, yet preserve enough submucosal length to maintain the characteristics required of an effective flap valve to obviate reflux (Rich *et al.*, 1990) (Figs. 23.46 and 23.47). Cecoureteroceles and sphincteric ureteroceles can be unobstructed by vertically incising the meatus and extending it above the bladder neck (Fig. 23.48). Cutting current is applied across a no. 3 Fr Bugbee electrode or the metal stylet of a ureteral catheter. Both provide a clean, full-thickness

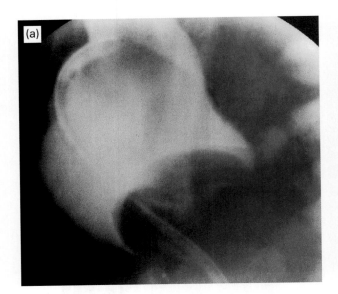

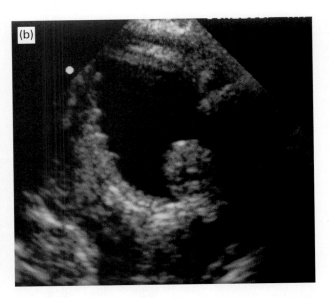

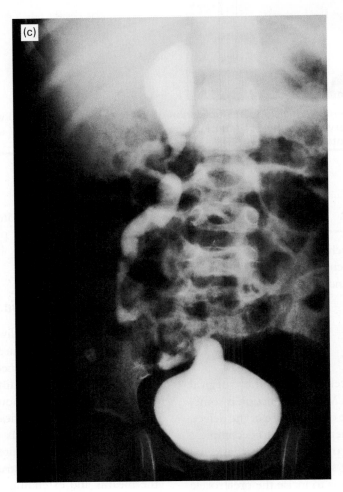

Figure 23.45 (*a*) Large extravesical ureterocele shown during cystography. Both poles functioned and no reflux was seen. (*b*) Successful decompression was seen by ultrasound but (*c*) reflux into the upper pole moiety is documented on postoperative cystogram.

puncture of the ureterocele wall. Aggressive hydration and minimal instillation of irrigation help to keep the ureterocele distended to aid in placement of the puncture. Surgery can be done as an outpatient. A sonogram obtained 10–14 days later should document resolution of hydronephrosis and ureterocele decompression. The decompressed ureterocele typically appears as a pseudomass or mucosal thickening (Keesling *et al.*, 1998). A VCUG done 3 months later demonstrates whether reflux has been created.

Heminephrectomy

The key to success with heminephrectomy at any age, but especially in the infant, is complete and careful mobilization of the kidney. However, the vessels of babies are prone to spasm and intimal tears (Mor *et al.*, 1994) (Fig. 23.49). Therefore, undue traction must be avoided as the organ is gently cleared from the surrounding pararenal fat. It helps to intermittently discontinue the manipulation of smaller kidneys. In cases where vascular spasm persists, topical vasodilatory agents, such as papaverine, can be applied.

In some cases, the vascular pedicle to the upper pole is isolated from that of the lower, making it easily discernable. In others, branching of the two occurs near the renal hilum, making identification of the upper pole vessels more difficult. After the vessels are

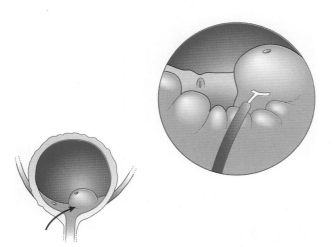

Figure 23.46 Endoscopic incision of the ureterocele with fine bugbee or wire at the medial base of the ureterocele. (Adapted from Rich *et al.*, 1990.)

identified, vessel loops are placed around them. The ureter is transected at its midsection and mobilized superiorly, under the anteriorly positioned renal vessels and used as a handle for traction on the upper pole during its separation from the lower (Fig. 23.50). Upper pole blanching will occur after occlusion of its vessels. Clamps on the lower vessels are avoided. Instead, the kidney is gently grasped between the thumb and index finger to help control bleeding. The rim of renal capsule can be peeled off the upper pole to be used in later closure. The poles are then separated with cautery (high settings) along the line of vascular demarcation (Fig. 23.51).

When a fish-mouthed defect remains in the lower pole, it can be closed with chromic mattress sutures that incorporate parenchyma and capsule. Otherwise, a flap of adjacent fat can be mobilized and tacked into position to cover the defect. Suturing the capsule of the remaining lower pole to the adjacent muscle is also recommended to avoid postoperative torsion. A drain is left in the renal fossa.

Ureteropyelostomy and ureteroureterostomy

The principles of successful ureteropyelostomy and ureteroureterostomy are identical to those of dismembered pyeloplasty: minimal handling of the ureters and maintenance of their orientation. Luminal disparity between the recipient collecting system and upper pole ureter is rarely the cause for concern (Huisman *et al.*, 1987) (Fig. 23.52). In most cases the anastomosis is anterolaterally positioned. Traction sutures define the extent of the ureterotomy or pyelotomy on the recipient ureter or pelvis. A medially oriented oblique incision of the donor ureter is marked to match. Running 6-0 polydiaxanone sutures are used to complete the repair. Urinary drainage tubes are unnecessary, although a drain is left in the region of the repair (Figs. 23.53 and 23.54).

Subtotal ureterectomy

As much of the abnormal ureter as possible should be removed in concert with heminephrectomy or renal salvage procedure. After dividing the ureter, a 12 Fr red rubber catheter is sutured within to provide traction during its dissection. The ureter to the lower pole is identified and minimally handled. Dever

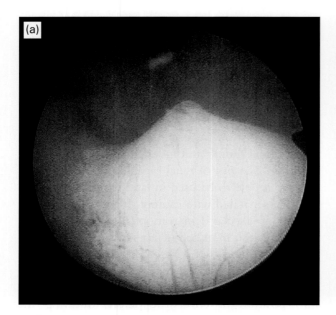

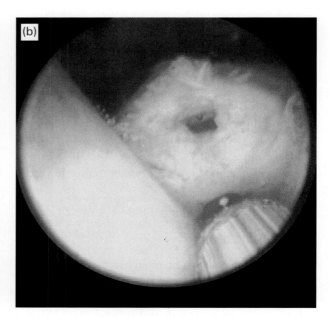

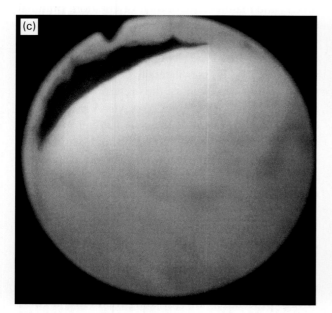

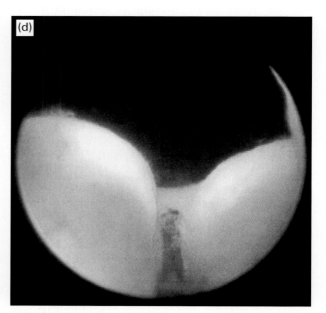

Figure 23.47 (*a*) Cystoscopic appearance of the intravesical ureterocele. (*b*) Ureterocele is decompressed after incision by fine bugbee. (*c*) Extravesical ureterocele is seen occluding the bladder neck. (*d*) Wire is applied at the medial base with the intent of preserving the flap-valve effect.

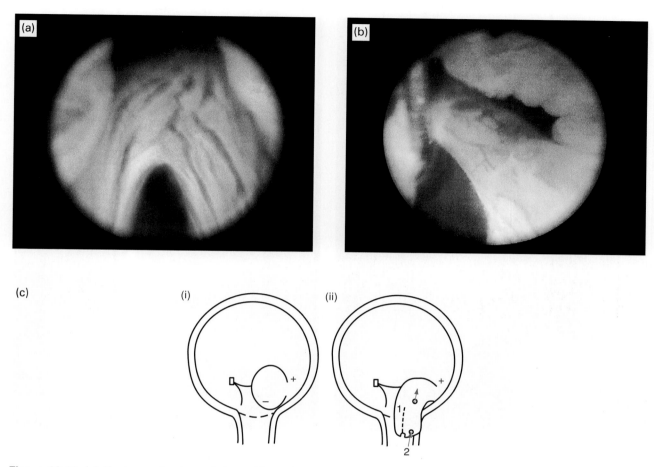

Figure 23.48 (*a*) Cystoscopic view of the sphincteric ureterocele having a widely open orifice (6 o'clock position) distal to the bladder neck. (*b*) Vertical extension by wire eliminates the element of obstruction that accompanies the variant until definitive bladder reconstruction can be done at a later age. (*c*) The diagram depicts the differences in incision between intravesical ureteroceles (*i*) and two methods of dealing with sphincteric varieties (*ii*). (Adapted from Blyth B, Passerini-Glazel G, Camuffo C *et al*. (1993) Endoscopic incision of ureterocele: intravesical versus ectopic. *J Urol* **149**: 556–60.)

retractors are used to lift away the peritoneum as the adventitia and periureteral attachments to the upper ureter are taken down with selective cautery. The dissection is ended near the level of the pelvic brim, where the ureters become more intertwined. Ligation is done with 00 or 000 polyglycolic acid suture after aspiration of the obstructed ureter.

Lower ureterectomy

When it is determined that lower ureterectomy is necessary, a transverse Gibson-type incision is made along a lower abdominal crease. The obliterated hypogastric artery is identified and ligated. This is followed posteriorly until the ureter is encountered

medially. The proximal portion of the ureter is pulled into the wound and acts as a handle during the remainder of the dissection. The ureter should be mobilized from within its adventitial sheath, avoiding the adjacent peritoneum and vas deferens. Once the mobilization is complete, the ureter is ligated and transected just outside the bladder. When ureteral ectopy is being addressed, a catheter is placed to aid in the dissection. The ureter is mobilized to its confluence with the urethra or to just above the pelvic floor, in those that end extravesically, where it is ligated and transected. The distal insertion can be left alone and undue dissection of the sphincter avoided. In the case of duplication, the shared wall of the upper pole ureter is left attached to that of the lower pole,

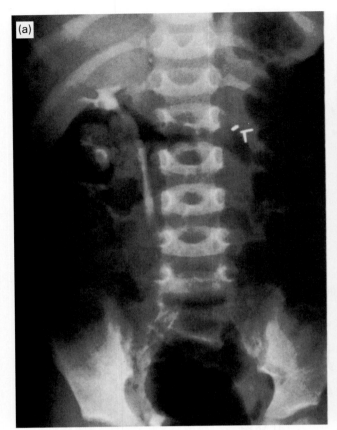

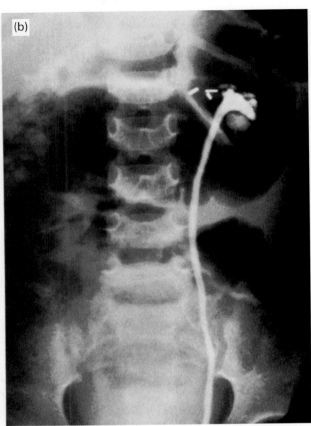

Figure 23.49 Vascular injury with left upper pole heminephrectomy and partial ureterectomy. (*a*) After surgery, failure of contrast excretion by remaining lower pole of the kidney, though the segment had been well vascularized prior to surgery. (*b*) Retrograde pyelogram demonstrates a shrunken, unobstructed lower pole moiety.

avoiding damage to the blood supply. After resecting the ureter at the level of the bladder, several sutures are placed to obliterate its lumen at the hiatus (Fig. 23.55).

Ureterocelectomy

The goals of ureterocele surgery (removal of the ureterocele itself, correction of associated reflux, and repair of any bladder defect) can be achieved by a number of different approaches. A transvesical approach gives the best opportunity to assess the problems associated with the anomaly.

The bladder is opened and the submucosal extent of the ureterocele is appreciated after incising its dome. Laterally and medially, the planes between the ureterocele lining and overlying bladder mucosa are defined. Some bladder mucosa should be preserved for coverage of the resultant defect. As the enucleation/excision is carried posteriorly, the ureterocele

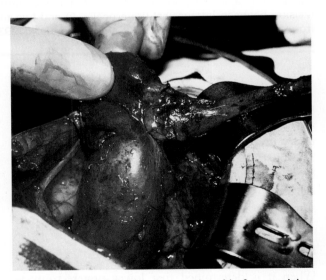

Figure 23.50 Moblization is completed before excising the upper pole segment. The ureter has been transected and carried behind the vessels to the lower pole of the kidney, providing a useful handle and guide to demarcation for heminephrectomy.

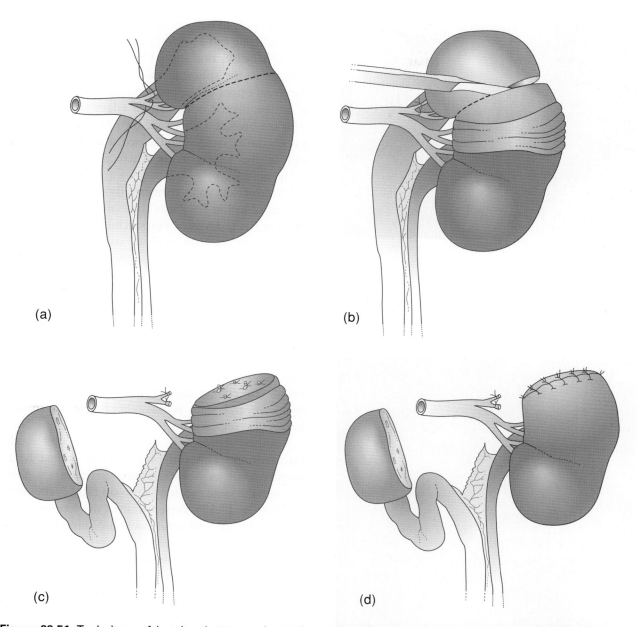

(a)

(b)

(c)

(d)

Figure 23.51 Technique of heminephrectomy (posterior view). (*a*) Vessels to the upper pole are identified and ligated. At this point, the ureter can be fully mobilized from the area of the lower pole hilum and swung posteriorly and superiorly. (*b*) The capsule is peeled away from the upper pole and preserved for closure. A cautery offers less bleeding than the knife. (*c*) Significant vessels are ligated. (*d*) Closure incorporates the capsule and parenchyma.

lining is excised by defining its plane with the underlying detrusor. Proximally, one or both ureters are circumferentially mobilized at their entrance to the bladder. Mobilization is identical to that of ureteroneocystostomy. Lumenal tailoring is usually necessary for the ureter associated with the ureterocele. The bladder defect that remains after the dissection is closed

with interrupted sutures, and ureteral reimplantation is completed with ipsilateral advancement-type (Glenn-Anderson) or cross-trigonal (Cohen) techniques (Fig. 23.56).

Distally, ceco- and sphincteric ureteroceles present a special challenge because of their urethral projections. Flap-valve obstruction of the bladder can result

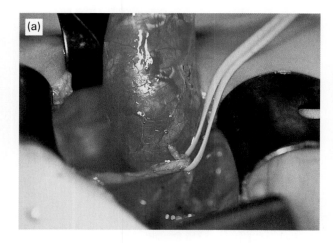

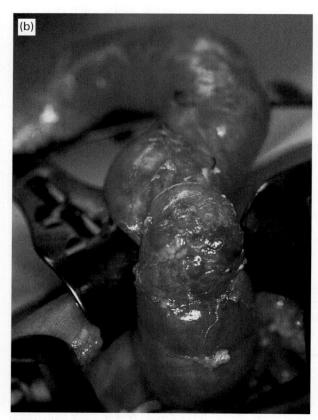

Figure 23.52 (*a*) Disparity in size between the obstructed ureter of the upper pole moiety and the lower ureter (vessel loop) sometimes poses problems for ureteroureterostomy. (*b*) Since the upper pole shown grossly provided only moderate function, a heminephrectomy was performed.

if tissue is left to balloon into the urethra during voiding (Ashcraft and Hendren, 1979). However, extensive distal dissection should be discouraged to avoid damage to the sphincter mechanism. Instead, when the distal extent of the projection can be appreciated, it can be filleted open and its edges trimmed flush with the urethra. Otherwise, the opening to the projection can be defined and closed at the bladder neck, leaving the lumen intact where it rarely poses a problem.

Ureteroceles can be corrected by other approaches. Marsupialization has been successful in some cases, excising the intravesical outpouching of the anomaly and leaving its back wall in continuity with the adjacent bladder as coverage (Scherz *et al.*, 1989) (Fig. 23.57). Reimplantation can be done beneath the marsupialized ureterocele, although it is often necessary to create a trough by incising its mucosa, which is more intimately attached to the posterior musculature than normal bladder. Marsupialization is probably less likely to cause sphincter damage than enucleation. To its detriment, the modification is unable to correct defects in the detrusor and/or sphincter and thus is most applicable to smaller intravesical ureteroceles.

Another approach is to address the ureterocele extravesically. This can be combined with a heminephrectomy or a distal ureteroureterostomy done through the same incision (Kroovand and Perlmutter, 1979) (Fig. 23.58). Preservation of the common wall shared with the ipsilateral lower pole ureter is necessary. A portion of the ureterocele wall can be excised extravesically without opening the bladder mucosa and the detrusor defect closed. In some ways less invasive, this technique cannot address the suburethral extensions found with some ureteroceles without potentially damaging the vagina or urinary sphincter, and may not provide a solution to contralateral or ipsilateral reflux caused by the anomaly.

Laparoscopy

Heminephrectomies, nephrectomies, and ureterectomies can be done laparoscopically. Early reports suggest decreased morbidity compared with open procedures. Magnification also reportedly aids in the dissections (Jordan and Winslow, 1993; Rassweiler *et al.*, 1993; Susuki *et al.*, 1993; Janetschek *et al.*, 1997). To its detriment, prolonged lengths of surgery

(a)

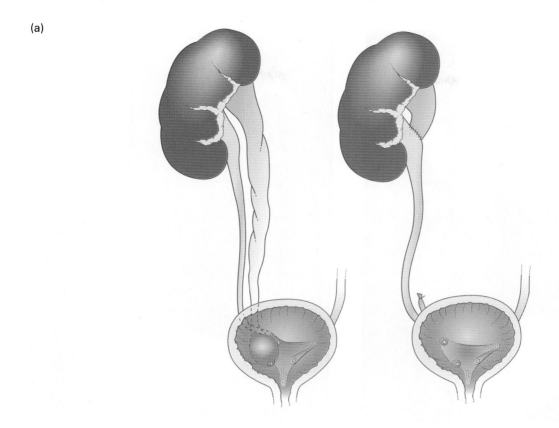

(b)

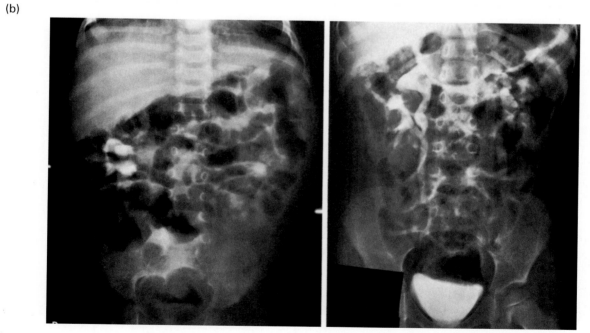

Figure 23.53 (*a*) Pyeloureterostomy and subtotal ureterectomy can be used to treat ureteroceles or ectopic ureters. (*b*) Excretory urography shows bilateral duplication and ectopic ureteroceles. Poorly functioning hydronephrosis of right upper moiety on IUP showed salvageable function by radionuclide scan. (*c*) Excretory urogram after the right pyeloureterostomy and left heminephrectomy shows return of function in the right upper segment and decompression of both ureteroceles below.

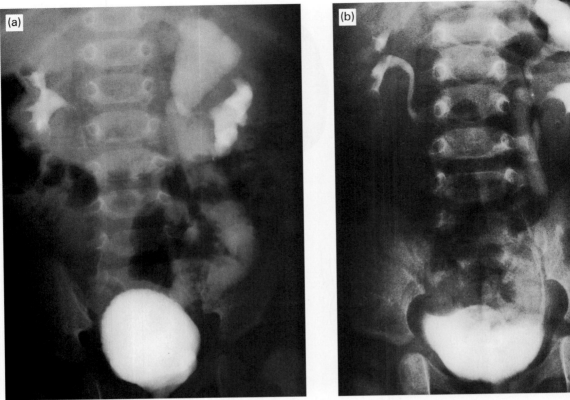

Figure 23.54 A 9-month-old female with intravesical ureterocele. (*a*) Pre-operative excretory urogram shows good function to upper pole. (*b*) Decompression of the upper pole after successful ureteroureterostomy.

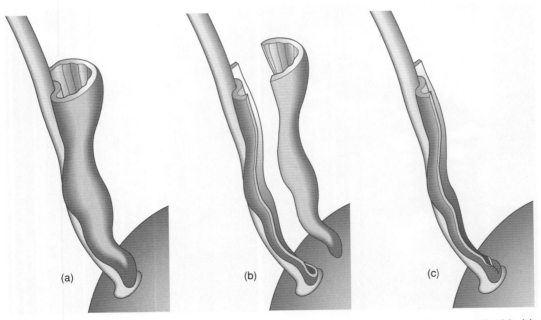

Figure 23.55 Lower ureterectomy. (*a*) It is often difficult to separate the two ureters as they near the bladder. (*b*) The outer wall of the dilated ureter associated with ectopia or ureterocele can be excised to the bladder, preserving a strip of common wall with the lower pole ureter. (*c*) Transfixing sutures obliterate its lumen, with care being taken not to injure the orthotopic ureter. (Adapted from Schlussel R and Retik A (1998) Anomalies of the ureter. In *Campbell's urology*.W.B. Saunders, Philadelphia, Fig. 60.24.)

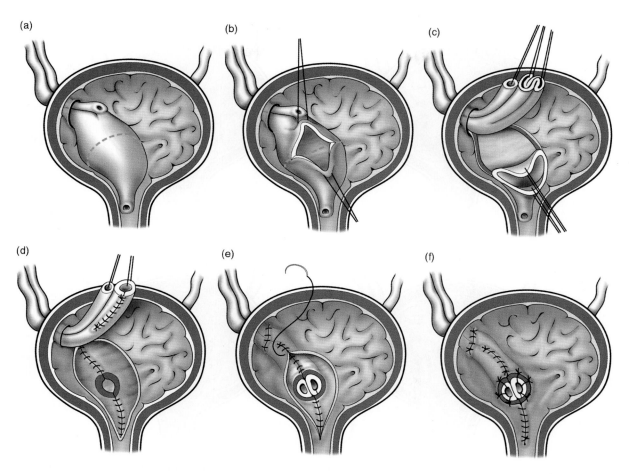

Figure 23.56 Technique for excision of ectopic ureterocele with common sheath reimplantation of both ureters. (*a*) Right-sided ureterocele. Contralateral orifice in close proximity. (*b*) Ureterocele can be opened transversely (as shown). A vertical incision can sometimes offer better visualization of the urethra. In many cases, the mucosa overlying the ureterocele is thinned out and must be discarded. (*c*) The posterior wall is incised and dissected away from the underlying detrusor. The dissection is carried around to the bladder mucosal edges to enable complete removal of the ureterocele. Ureteral orifices are circumscribed and mobilized. (*d*) Ureteral mobilization is completed. The dilated ureter is tapered opposite the common wall. The muscular defect in the bladder is repaired. (*e*) Both ureters are brought through the new hiatus in the bladder wall, though the crosstrigonal method can also be used. The ureters are reimplanted into new tunnels. (*f*) Final appearance. (Adapted from Schlussel R and Retik A (1998) *Anomalies of the ureter.* In *Campbell's urology.* W.B. Saunders, Philadelphia, Fig. 60.36.)

are a concession to the learning curves required of the techniques. Nevertheless, clinicians should expect to see an expanding role for laparoscopy in the management of duplication anomalies as well other urologic anomalies.

Postoperative concerns

An ultrasound examination or functional study is obtained 6–12 weeks after surgery, depending on the procedure used to address the anomaly. These assess the status of salvaged upper pole kidneys or remaining lower pole moieties and effects of surgery on the bladder. Voiding studies are performed 3–6 months after bladder construction to document the adequacy of the repair. Prophylactic antibiotics are taken in the interim. Children with such complex urologic histories require periodic follow-up. The need for more prolonged serial radiographs depends on the remaining urinary configuration. In cases where the anomaly is presumably corrected, a

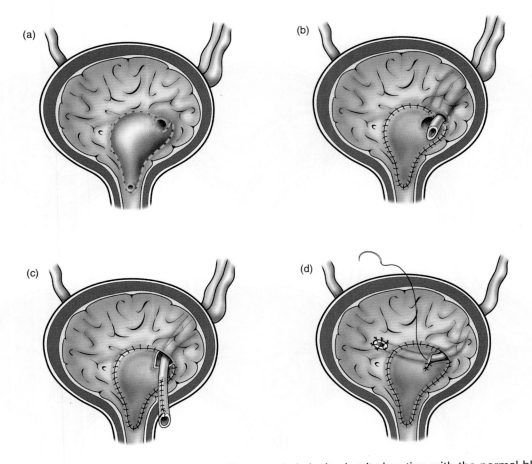

Figure 23.57 Marsupialization of ureterocele. (*a*) Ureterocele is incised at its junction with the normal bladder and sutured to mark the edges and secure hemostasis. (*b*) Completed marsupialization. Mobilization of the duplex ureters is begun as a common sheath. (*c*) Ureteral mobilization is complete and the bladder defect from dissection is repaired. The dilated upper pole ureter has been excised (as shown) or can be tapered opposite to the common wall. (*d*) Crosstrigonal reimplantation is completed beneath the mucosa covering the original base of the ureterocele. (Adapted from Scherz HC, Kaplan GW, Packer MG *et al*. (1989) *J Urol* **142**: 539–40.)

sonogram 2 and 5 years later is probably adequate. Primary physicians may complete periodic checks of the urine, blood pressure, and interval somatic growth. Patients who remain at risk, because of persistent reflux for example, require more frequent evaluation and, if necessary, secondary surgery.

Ureteroceles are particularly challenging in this regard. The length of an adequate trial of medical management for VUR that persists after an upper tract approach or selective incision has not been well defined. Although spontaneous resolution occasionally occurs, it does so at rates significantly lower than those seen with primary reflux. Most bladders are large enough to reconstruct as the child approaches

the first birthday. Although it would seem preferable to address ureteroceles before the onset of toilet training, there may be no optimal age for surgery. Bladder dysfunction appeared in 22 of 33 (67%) of patients whose ectopic ureteroceles were excised and bladders repaired at a mean of 10 months of age. Infrequent voiding, large capacities, and significant postvoid residuals were commonplace. The appearance of voiding dysfunction had no correlation with ureterocele size or location (Abrahamsson *et al*., 1998). Whether these findings are the consequence of surgery or an inherent component of the anomaly is unclear. Regardless, the observation is an important one and may account for the lower rates of success with ureteral reimplantation in these children, when com-

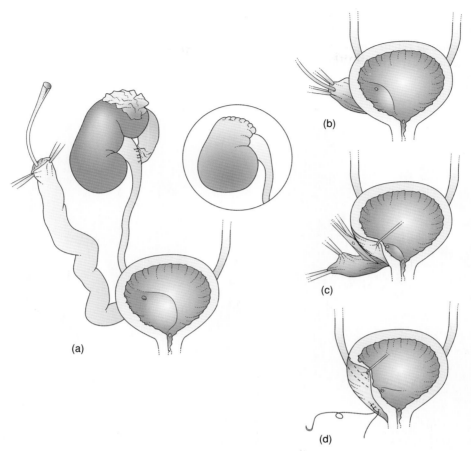

Figure 23.58 (*a*) Technique of extravesical ureterocele excision can be used after either upper pole heminephrectomy or ureteroureterostomy. The remainder of the upper pole ureter is cannulated and approached through the lower incision. (*b, c*) Extravesical dissection can be completed and the detrusor defect repaired. (*d*) In modification, both ureters can be detached to allow for easy separation of their common wall and the lower pole ureter reimplanted using a Lich-type repair after repairing the detrusor defect.

pared with ureteroneocystostomy for primary reflux. Bladder dysfunction should be considered as a contributing factor in any child who continues to have reflux after ureterocele surgery. Urodynamic testing and an assessment of bladder emptying should be obtained before considering any additional surgery.

Related conditions

Bilateral single ectopic ureters

Bilateral single-system ectopic ureters are far more common in girls, who present with significant urologic problems as a consequence. The trigone and bladder neck are wide and poorly defined because of the aberrant insertions of the ureters. These usually drain into the distal urethra, although genital ectopy has also been described. Incompetence of the outlet results, causing a presentation very similar to that of the patient with epispadias. In addition, the bladder is typically small and the detrusor thin-walled, in theory because it has never been required to store urine during development (Fig. 23.59). Renal dysplasia or varying degrees of hydronephrosis are usually present. Reimplantation alone does not correct these glaring bladder abnormalities (Ahmed and Barker, 1992). Augmentation cystoplasty is often required and bladder neck reconstruction becomes necessary to increase outlet resistance. Boys are also occasionally affected by bilateral single-system ectopia, which insert into the prostatic urethra. Bladder dynamics are more favorable, presumably because the better developed external sphincter helps to retain the urine necessary to stimulate bladder capacity (Williams and Lightwood, 1972).

Ureteral triplication

Triplication of the ureter is one of the rarest anomalies in the urinary tract (Parvinen, 1976). The individual take-off of three ureteral buds from the

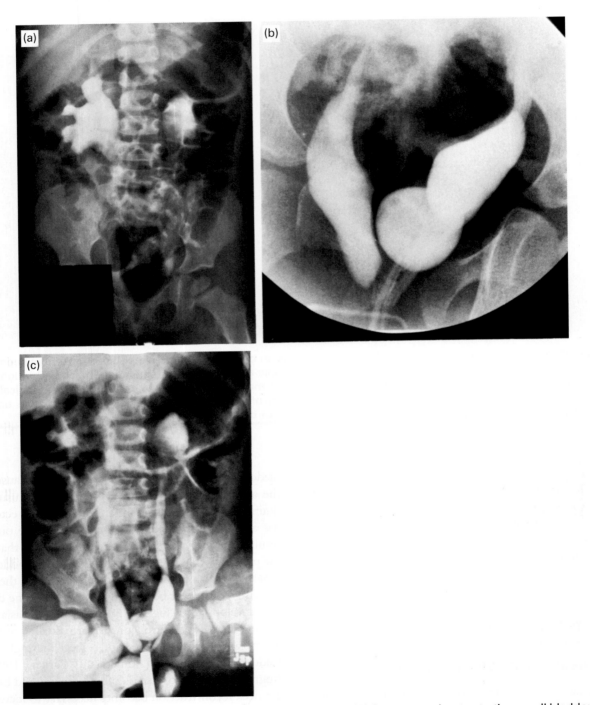

Figure 23.59 Bilateral single ectopic ureters. (*a*) Excretory urogram. (*b*) Cystogram demonstrating small bladder and reflux into ectopic ureters. (*c*) Anatomy is also well demonstrated by injection into the urethral meatus.

wolffian duct or the presence of two buds with early fission of one of the two accounts for the variants of complete or partial triplications that have been described and classified by Smith (1946). The most common is a trifid configuration with all three ureters uniting and draining through a single orifice (Fig. 23.60). Triplicate ureters are more common in females and occur more often on the left side. Common presentations include UTI and/or signs of ureteral obstruction. Ureteral triplications can be associated with ureteroceles, ectopia, and renal fusion anomalies (Pode *et al.*, 1983; Finkel *et al.*, 1983; Gosalbez *et al.*, 1991). The principles in management are similar to those of duplication anomalies.

Lower pole ureteropelvic junction obstruction

Upper ureteral obstructions occasionally involve duplicated ureters at the ureteropelvic junction (Amis *et al.*, 1986). These almost always affect the lower renal pole. Because of their similarity, most problems that affect the ureters of single-system kidneys can affect the lower pole ureters of duplications. The configuration and size of upper pole ureters more closely mimic that of a calyx, making them much less prone to obstruction (Fig. 23.61). Ultrasonography demonstrates lower pole hydronephrosis in the absence of ureteral dilatation. Renal scintigraphy is used to assess function and document obstruction (Fig. 23.62). When the lower pole is salvageable, its pelvis can be

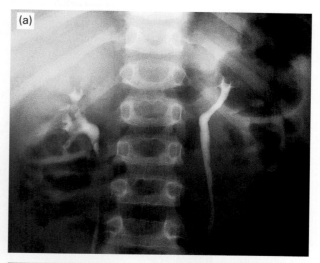

(a)

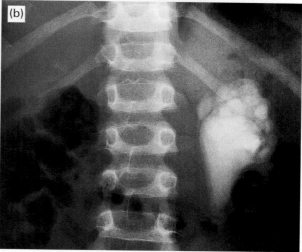

(b)

Figure 23.61 Difference in upper and lower pole configuration shown in different phases of excretory urogram in a teenage boy with left lower pole ureteropelvic junction obstruction. (*a*) Early phase shows upper pole with the appearance of a calyx. (*b*) Later phase shows a typical pelvic appearance of the lower pole. Note the kink from crossing the vessel.

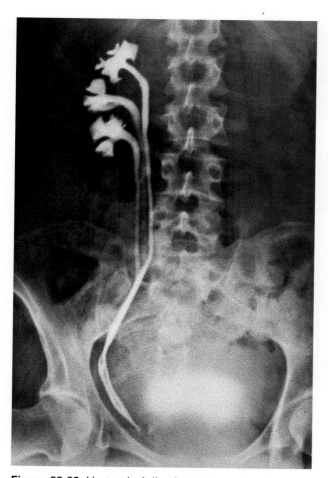

Figure 23.60 Ureteral triplication

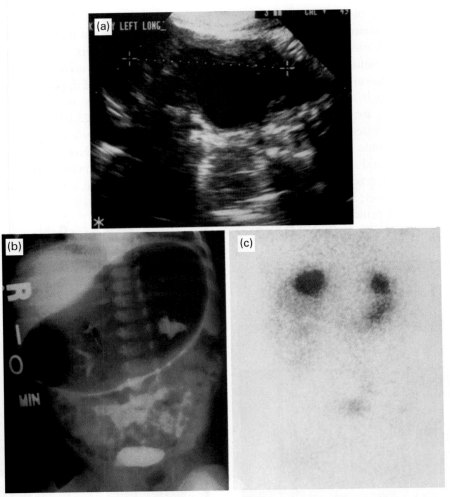

Figure 23.62 Lower pole ureteropelvic junction obstruction diagnosed prenatally. (*a*) Renal sonogram demonstrates lower pole hydronephrosis with better developed renal parenchyma in the upper pole. (*b*) Excretory urography shows opacification of the upper pole structures on the left displaced superiorly and laterally. (*c*) Radioisotope scan demonstrates reduced but salvageable function in the left lower pole.

anastomosed to the adjacent upper pole ureter (pyeloureterostomy) (Fig. 23.63). The remainder of the ureter is ligated above the bifurcation and discarded. A dismembered lower pole pyeloplasty is an alternative approach.

Yo-yo reflux

The phenomenon of yo-yo reflux remains poorly defined and its clinical implications are unclear. Ureteral dilatation of bifurcated ureters was noted in 41% in one series (Kaplan and Elkin, 1968). This raised the question of disordered peristalsis causing partial ureteral obstruction. In theory, antegrade peristalsis

that begins in one ureteral limb initiates a reverse peristalsis in the other once it reaches the junction (Campbell, 1967). High-grade obstruction is rare and an increased tendency to infections seems unlikely (Fig. 23.64). In addition, despite altered to-and-fro peristalsis at its junction, the overall direction of urinary flow is still antegrade. In the rare patient in whom clinically significant yo-yo is suspected, a high ureteroureterostomy is recommended, discarding as much abnormal ureter as possible (Sole *et al.*, 1987) (Fig. 23.65). The preferred option for low-confluence bifurcations is to excise the shared segment and complete a common sheath ureteral reimplantation.

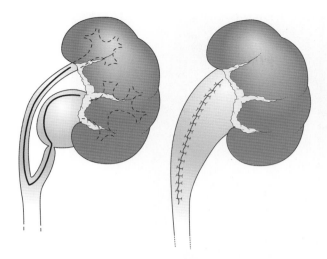

Figure 23.63 Surgical treatment of the lower pole ureteropelvic junction obstruction in incomplete duplication. Joining two systems as shown brings less risk than attempting an isolated dismembered pyeloplasty of the lower system.

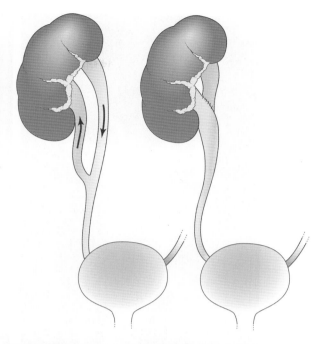

Figure 23.65 A high uretereopyelostomy with elimination of one limb of the yo-yo is occasionally required to treat ureteroureteral reflux.

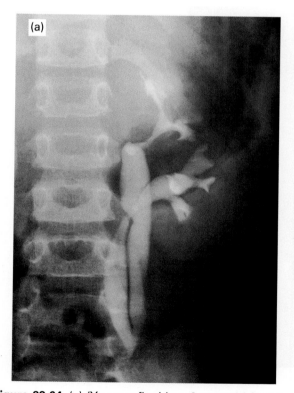

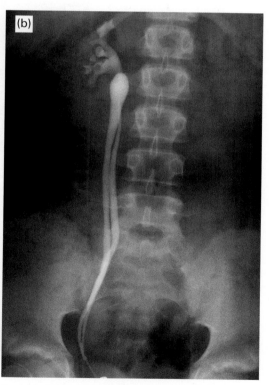

Figure 23.64 (*a*) 'Yo-yo reflux' in a 2-year-old female may contribute to the mild dilatation of the two branches of the incomplete duplication shown. (*b*) Unusual duplication variant in a 4-year-old boy with lower pole ureter ending as a saccular dilatation beneath the normal kidney. While both children are theoretically at risk from to-and-fro peristalsis, both are being followed expectantly and have done well.

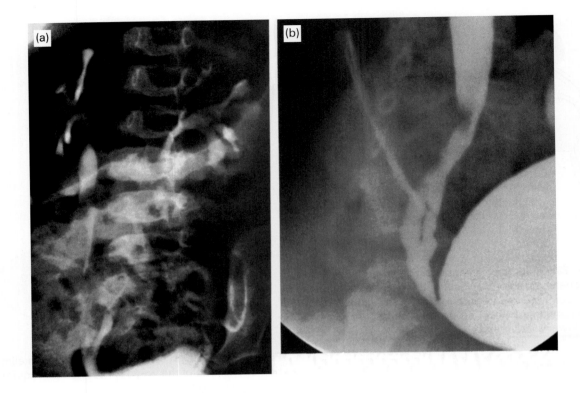

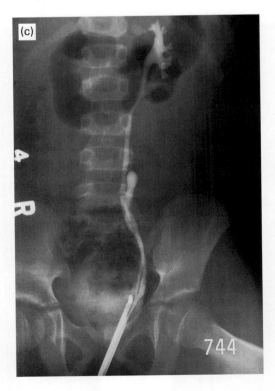

Figure 23.66 Blind-ending bifid ureter. (*a*) Excretory urogram outlines blind-ending bifid ureter on the right side. (*b*) Voiding cystourethrogram shows reflux and bifurcation. (*c*) Retrograde study of similar aborted duplication whose orifice was seen at pre-operative cystoscopy. When encountered unexpectedly, these can be safely reimplanted using a common sheath technique.

Remnant ureters

A blind-ending branch of a bifid ureter is occasionally found in a child, although they are more often discovered in adults. These occur more commonly in females and on the right side. Most are associated with low confluence bifurcations that are prone to reflux, although the anomaly can also occur with complete duplications (Marshall and McLoughlin, 1978; Keane and Fitzgerald, 1987) (Fig. 23.66). Proximally, the ureter ends blindly or may be associated with a small segment of poorly functioning kidney. For larger segments, excision is occasionally warranted. Surgery is usually not indicated unless recurrent infections become problematic in which case common sheath reimplantation is indicated. In occasional cases, an unsuspected duplication is discovered at cystoscopy or even during ureteral reimplantation. The ureter can be cannulated and a retrograde ureteropyelogram obtained. In nearly every case, the surgeon should still proceed with reimplantation unless the segment is short and easily excised. Complications from the retained renal parenchyma associated with remnant ureters have yet to be described.

References

Abel C, Lendon M, Gough DC (1997) Histology of the upper pole in complete duplication – does it affect surgical management? *Br J Urol* **80**: 663–5.

Abrahamsson K, Hansson E, Sillen U *et al.* (1998) Bladder dysfunction: an integral part of the ectopic ureterocele complex. *J Urol* **160**: 1468–70.

Ahmed S, Barker A (1992) Single-system ectopic ureters: a review of 12 cases. *J Pediatr Surg* **27**: 491.

Ahmed S, Pope R (1986) Uncrossed complete ureteral duplication with upper system reflux. *J Urol* **135**: 128.

Albers P, Foster RS, Bihrle R *et al.* (1995) Ectopic ureters and ureteroceles in adults. *Urology* **45**: 870–4.

Amis ES, Cronan JJ, Pfister RD (1985) Lower moiety hydronephrosis in duplicated kidneys. *Urology* **26**: 82.

Amitai M, Hertz M, Jonas P *et al.* (1992) Ectopic ureterocele in adults with a comparison of the anomaly in children. *Urol Radiol* **13**: 181–6.

Ashcraft KW, Hendren WH (1979) Bladder outlet obstruction after operation for ureterocele. *J Pediatr Surg* **14**: 819.

Atwell JD, Cook PL, Howell CJ (1974) Familial incidence of bifid and double ureters. *Arch Dis Child* **49**: 390.

Austin PF, Cain MP, Casale AJ *et al.* (1998) Prenatal bladder outlet obstruction secondary to ureterocele. *Urology* **52**: 1132–5.

Belman AB, Filmer RB, King LR (1974) Surgical management of duplication of the collecting system. *J Urol* **112**: 316.

Blythe B, Passerini-Glaze G, Camuffo G *et al.* (1993) Endoscopic incision of ureteroceles: intravesical versus ectopic. *J Urol* **149**: 556.

Bozorgi F, Connelly LP, Bauer SB *et al.* (1998) Hypoplastic dysplastic kidney with a vaginal ectopic ureter identified by technetium-99m-DMSA scintigraphy. *J Nucl Med* **39**: 113–15.

Braverman RM, Lebowitz RL (1991) Occult ectopic ureter in girls with urinary incontinence: diagnosis by using CT. *AJR Am J Roentgenol* **156**: 365.

Brock WA, Kaplan GW (1978) Ectopic ureteroceles in children. *J Urol* **119**: 800.

Burford CE, Glenn JE, Burford EH (1949) Ureteral ectopia: a review of the literature and 2 case reports. *J Urol* **62**: 211.

Caldamone AA (1985) Duplication anomalies of the upper urinary tract in infants and children. *Urol Clin North Am* **12**.

Caldamone AA, Snyder HM, Duckett JW (1984) Ureteroceles in children: follow-up of management with upper tract approach. *J Urol* **131**: 1130.

Campbell JE (1967) Ureteral peristalsis in duplex renal collecting systems. *Am J Roentgenol Radium Ther Nucl Med* **99**: 577.

Campbell MF (1976) Embryology and anomalies of the urogenital tract. In: Kelalis PP, King LR, Belman AB (eds) *Clinical pediatric urology*. Philadelphia, PA: WB Saunders, 159.

Carrico C, Lebowitz RL (1998) Incontinence due to infrasphincteric ectopic ureter: why the delay in diagnosis and what the radiologist can do about it. *Pediatr Radiol* **28**: 942–9.

Chung S, Majd M, Rushton HG *et al.* (1993) Diuretic renography with evaluation of neonatal hydronephrosis: is it reliable? *J Urol* **150**: 765–8.

Chwalla R (1927) The process of formation of cystic dilation of the vesical end of the ureter and of diverticula at the ureteral ostium. *Urol Cutan Ren* **31**: 499.

Craver R, Dimmick J, Johnson H *et al.* (1986) Congenital obstructive uropathy and nodular renal blastema. *J Urol* **136**: 305–307.

Cremin BJ (1986) A review of the ultrasonic appearances of posterior urethral valves and ureteroceles. *Pediatr Radiol* **16**: 357.

Culp OS (1967) Management of ureteropelvic obstruction. *Bull NY Acad Med* **43**: 355–77.

Currarino G (1982) Single vaginal ectopic ureter and Gartner's duct cyst with ipsilateral renal hypoplasia and dysplasia (or agenesis). *J Urol* **128**: 988.

Daniels MA, Allen TD (1994) Unsuspected ureterocele and ureteral duplication. *J Urol* **152**: 179–81.

Decter RM, Roth DM, Gonzales ET (1989) Individualized treatment of ureteroceles. *J Urol* **142**: 535.

El Ghoneimi A, Miranda J, Truong T *et al.* (1996) Ectopic ureter with complete ureteric duplication: conservative surgical management. *J Pediatr Surg* **31**: 467–72.

Ellerker AG (1958) The extravesical ectopic ureter. *Br J Surg* **45**: 344.

Finan BF, Mollitt DL, Golladay ES *et al.* (1987) Giant ectopic ureter presenting as abdominal mass in infant. *Urology* **30**: 246–7.

Finkel LI, Watts FB Jr, Corbett DP (1983) Ureteral triplication with a ureterocele. *Pediatr Radiol* **13**: 346.

Garmel SH, Crombleholme TM, Cendron M *et al.* (1996) The vanishing fetal ureterocele: a cause for concern? *Prenat Diagn* **16**: 354–6.

Glassberg KI, Braren V, Duckett JW *et al.* (1984) Suggested terminology for duplex systems, ectopic ureters, and ureteroceles.

Golomb J, Korazak D, Lindner A (1987) Giant obstructing calculus in the distal ureter secondary to obstruction by a ureterocele. *Urol Radiol* **9**: 168–70.

Gonzales E (1992) Anomalies of the renal pelvis and ureter. In: Kelalis P, King L, Belman A (eds) *Clinical pediatric urology*. Philadelphia, PA: WB Saunders, 53–579.

Gonzales R, Sheldon CA (1982) Septic obstruction and uremia in newborns. *Urol Clin North Am* **9**: 297.

Gosalbez R Jr, Gosalbez R, Piro C *et al.* (1991) Ureteral triplication and ureterocele: report of 3 cases and review of the literature. *J Urol* **145**: 105–8.

Gotoh T, Koyanagi T, Matsuno T (1988) Surgical management of ureteroceles in children: strategy based on the classification of the ureteral hiatus and the eversion of ureteroceles. *J Pediatr Surg* **23**: 159.

Hartman GW, Hodson CJ (1969) The duplex kidney and related anormalies. *Clin Radiol* **20**: 387–400.

Hendren WH, Mitchell ME (1979) Surgical correction of ureterocele. *J Urol* **121**: 590.

Huisman TK, Kaplan GW, Brock WA *et al.* (1987) Ipsilateral ureteroureterostomy and pyeloureterostomy: a review of 15 years of experience with 25 patients. *J Urol* **138**: 1207–10.

Hulnick DH, Bosniak MA (1986) 'Faceless kidney: CT signs of renal duplicity. *J Comput Assist Tomogr* **10**: 771.

Husmann DA, Ewalt DH, Glenski WJ *et al.* (1995) Ureterocele associated with ureteral duplication and a non-functioning upper pole segment: management by partial nephroureterectomy alone. *J Urol* **154**: 723–6.

Husmann D, Strand B, Ewalt D *et al.* (1999) Management of ectopic ureterocele associated with renal duplication: a comparison of partial nephrectomy and endoscopic decompression. *J Urol* **162**: 1406–9.

Janetschek G, Seibold J, Radmayr C *et al.* (1997) Laparoscopic heminephrectomy in pediatric patients. *J Urol* **158**: 1928–30.

Jee LD, Rickwood AM, Williams MP *et al.* (1993) Experience with duplex system anomalies detected by prenatal ultrasonography. *J Urol* **149**: 808–10.

Jordan GH, Winslow BH (1993) Laparoendoscopic upper pole partial nephrectomy with ureterectomy. *J Urol* **150**: 940.

Keesling CA, O'Hara SM, Chavez DR *et al.* (1998) Sonographic appearance of the bladder after endoscopic incision of ureteroceles. *AJR Am J Roentgenol* **170**: 759–63.

King LR (1989) Urologic surgery in neonates and young infants. Philadelphia, PA: WB Saunders.

King LR, Koglowski JM, Schacht MJ (1983) Ureteroceles in children: a simplified and successful approach to management. *JAMA* **249**: 1461.

Koyanagi T, Hisajima S, Goto T *et al.* (1980) Everting ureterocele: radiographic and endoscopic observation and surgical management. *J Urol* **123**: 538.

Kaplan N, Elkin M (1968) Bifid renal pelves and ureters: radiographic and cineflouroscopic observations. *Br J Urol* **40**: 235.

Keane TE, Fitzgerald RJ (1987) Blind-ending duplex ureter. *Br J Urol* **60**: 275.

Kroovand RL, Perlmutter AD (1979) A one-stage surgical approach to ectopic ureterocele. *J Urol* **122**: 367.

Lenaghan D (1962) Bifid ureters in children: an anatomical, physiological and clinical study. *J Urol* **87**: 808.

Lund AJ (1949) Uncrossed double ureter with rare intravesical orifice relationship: case report with review of the literature. *J Urol* **62**: 22.

Mackie GG, Stephens FD (1975) Duplex kidneys: a correlation of renal dysplasia with position of ureteral orifice. *J Urol* **114**: 274.

Malek RS, Kelalis PP, Burke EC (1972a) Simple and ectopic ureterocele in infancy and childhood. *Surg Gynecol Obstet* **134**: 611.

Malek RS, Kelalis PP, Stickler GB *et al.* (1972b) Observations on ureteral ectopy in children. *J Urol* **107**: 308.

Mandell J, Colodny A, Lebowitz RL *et al.* (1980) Ureteroceles in infants and children. *J Urol* **123**: 921.

Marshall FF, McLoughlin MG (1978) Long blind-ending ureteral duplications. *J Urol* **120**: 626.

Mathews R, Jeffs RD, Maizels M *et al.* (1999) Single system ureteral ectopia in boys associated with bladder outlet obstruction. *J Urol* **161**: 1297–300.

Matsuki M, Matsuo M, Kaji Y *et al.* (1998) Ectopic ureter draining into seminal vesical cyst: usefulness of MRI. *Radiat Med* **16**: 309–11.

Meyer R (1946) Normal and abnormal development of the ureter in the human embryo: a mechanistic consideration. *Anat Rec* **96**: 355.

Monfort G, Guys JM, Coquet M *et al.* (1992) Surgical management of duplex ureteroceles. *J Pediatr Surg* **27**: 634.

Mor Y, Goldwasser B, Ben-Chaim J *et al.* (1994) Upper pole heminephrectomy for duplex systems in children: a modified technical approach. *Br J Urol* **73**: 584.

Nussbaum AR, Dorst JP, Jeffs RD *et al.* (1986) Ectopic ureter and ureteroceles: their varied sonographic manifestations. *Radiology* **159**: 227.

O'Brien W, Matsumoto AH, Grant EG *et al.* (1990) Percutaneous nephrostomy in infants. *Urology* **36**: 269.

Parvinen T (1976) Complete ureteral triplication. *J Pediatr Surg* **11**: 1039.

Passerini GG, Calabro A, Aragona F *et al.* (1986) Blind ureterocele. *Eur Urol* **12**: 331.

Patil U, Mathews R (1995) Minimal surgery with renal preservation in anomalous complete duplicated systems: is it feasible? *J Urol* **154**: 727–8.

Pattaras JG, Rushton HG, Majd M (1999) The role of ^{99m}technetium dimercapto-succinic acid renal scans in the evaluation of accult ectopic ureters in girls with paradoxical incontinence. *J Urol* **162**: 821–5.

Pfister C, Ravasse P, Barret E *et al.* (1998) The value of endoscopic treatment for ureteroceles during the neonatal period. *J Urol* **159**: 1006–9.

Plaire JC, Pope JC IV, Kropp BP *et al.* (1997) Management of ectopic ureters: experience with the upper tract approach. *J Urol* **158**: 1245–7.

Pode D, Shapiro A, Lebensart P (1983) Unilateral triplication of the collecting system in a horseshoe kidney. *J Urol* **130**: 533.

Pope JC IV, Brock JW III, Adams MC *et al.* (2001) Congenital anomalies of the kidney and urinary tract – role of the loss of function mutation in the pluripotent angiotensin type 2 receptor gene. *J Urol* **165**: 196–202.

Prewitt LH Jr, Lebowitz RL (1976) The single ectopic ureter. *AJR Am JRoentgenol* **127**: 941–8.

Rassweiler JJ, Henkel TO, Joyce AD *et al.* (1993) The technique of transperitoneal laparoscopic nephrectomy, adrenalectomy and nephroureterectomy. *Eur Urol* **23**: 425.

Rich MA, Keating MA, Snyder HM *et al.* (1990) Low transurethral incision of single system intravesical ureteroceles in children. *J Urol* **144**: 120.

Rickwood AM, Reiner I, Jones M *et al.* (1992) Current management of duplex-system ureteroceles: experience with 4 patients. *Br J Urol* **70**: 196.

Rosenfeld DL, Lis E (1993) Gartner's duct cyst with a single vaginal ectopic ureter and associated renal dysplasia or agenesis. *J Ultrasound Med* **12**: 775–8.

Sariola H, Aufderheide E, Bernhardt H *et al.* (1988) Antibodies to cell surface ganglioside GD3 perturb inductive epithelial–mesenchymal interactions. *Cell* **54**: 235.

Scherz HC, Kaplan GW, Packer MG *et al.* (1989) Renal function and vesicoureteral reflux in children with ureteroceles. *J Urol* **142**: 538.

Schulmann CC (1976) The single ectopic ureter. *Eur Urol* **2**: 64.

Senn S, Beasley SW, Ahmed S *et al.* (1992) Renal function and vesicoureteral reflux in children with ureteroceles. *J Pediatr Surg* **27**: 192.

Share JC, Lebowitz RL (1989) Ectopic ureterocele without ureteral and calyceal dilatation (ureterocele disproportion): findings on urography and sonography. *AJR Am J Roentgenol* **152**: 567–71.

Smith FL, Ritchie EL, Maizels M *et al.* (1989) Surgery for duplex kidneys with ectopic ureters: ipsilateral ureteroureterostomy versus polar nephrectomy. *J Urol* **142**: 532.

Sole GM, Randall J, Arkell DG (1987) Ureteropyelostomy: a simple and effective treatment for symptomatic ureterioureteric reflux. *Br J Urol* **60**: 325.

Spencer JR, Maizel M (1987) Inhibition of protein glycosylation causes renal dysplasia in the chick embryo. *J Urol* **138**: 94.

Stephens FD (1971) Caecoureterocele and concepts on the embryology and aetiology of ureteroceles. *Aust NZ J Surg* **40**: 239.

Stephens FD (1983) *Congenital malformations of the urinary tract*. New York: Praeger, 320–2.

Sumfest JM, Burns MW, Mitchell ME *et al.* (1995) Pseudoureterocele: potential for misdiagnosis of an ectopic ureter as a ureterocele. *Br J Urol* **75**: 401.

Suzuki K, Ihara H, Kurita Y *et al.* (1993) Laparoscopic nephrectomy for atrophic kidney associated with ectopic ureter in a child. *Eur Urol* **23**: 463.

Tanagho EA (1976) Embryologic basis for lower ureteral anomalies: a hypothesis. *Urology* **7**: 451.

Tank ES (1986) Experience with endoscopic incisions and open unroofing of ureteroceles. *J Urol* **136**: 241–2.

Tokunaka S, Goth T, Koyanagi T *et al.* (1981) The morphological study of ureterocele: a possible clue to its embryogenesis as evidenced by a locally arrested myogenesis. *J Urol* **126**: 726.

Unson AC, Lattimer JK, Melicow MM (1961) ureteroceles in infants and children: report based on 44 cases. *Pediatrics* **27**: 971.

Wakhlu A, Dalela D, Tandon RK *et al.* (1998) The single ectopic ureter. *Br J Urol* **82**: 246–51.

Weigert C (1877) Uebeteinige bil dunfehter der uretern. *Virchows Arch* **70**: 490.

Weiss JP, Duckett JW, Snyder HM (1984) Single vaginal ectopic ureter, is it really a rarity? *J Urol* **132**: 1177.

Whitaker J, Danks GN (1966) A study of the inheritance of duplication of the kidneys and ureters. *J Urol* **95**: 176.

Williams DI (1980) The ectopic ureter: diagnostic problems. *Br J Urol* **52**: 257.

Williams DI, Lightwood RG (1972) Bilateral single ectopic ureters. *Br J Urol* **44**: 267.

Wines RD, O'Flynn JD (1972) Transurethral treatment of ureteroceles. *Br J Urol* **44**: 207.

Wyly JB, Lebowitz RL (1984) Refluxing urethral ectopic ureters: recognition by the cyclic voiding cystourethrogram. *AJR AM J Roentgenol* **142**: 1263.

Ureterovesical and other ureteral obstructions

24

David A. Bloom and H.P. Koo

History of ureteral surgery

Claudius Galen, in the second century AD, performed the first known recorded deliberate ureteral operative procedure, this being experimental ureteral ligation in a living dog (Bloom *et al.*, 1999b). It took nearly two millennia, however, for safe and humane surgery with a high expectation of success to become a practical reality in humans and other animals, owing to the synergism of anesthesia, antisepsis/asepsis, and antibiotics. Towards the end of the nineteenth century the main ureteral disorders requiring operative intervention were stone disease and tuberculosis. In the pediatric arena, the upper ureter fell into surgical cross-hairs when Trendelenburg's method of correcting ureteropelvic junction stenosis was described in 1912 in Ramon Guiteras' urology textbook (Bernstein *et al.*, 1999). Young's landmark textbook of urology in 1926 described ureterotomy for stone or stricture, ureterectomy for tuberculosis or cancer, operation for fistula, and management of trauma. Regarding the latter, Young wrote:

> We have never had to carry out the operation for traumatism of the ureter, but have frequently transplanted the lower portion of the ureter after it has been excised with vesical tumors. In such cases we have found that the best procedure is simply to puncture the bladder with a clamp, and draw the ureter well within it, then to fasten it there by sutures behind the bladder and also within the bladder … The probabilities are that it matters little what is done to the ureter within the bladder...It is impossible to produce an artificial sphincter for the ureter, and one has to trust to keeping the bladder free from infection to preserve the kidney in its functional efficiency (Young and Davis, 1926).

Pediatric ureteral pathology

Obstruction and vesicoureteral reflux (VUR) cause most of the ureteral problems in pediatric urology. These pathologic situations tend to deform the ureter and this is usually evidenced by dilatation. The typical scenerio in earlier days of pediatric urology was this: a child had a clinical problem (failure to thrive, infection, pain, or hematuria) and urologic imaging revealed upper tract dilatation (hydroureteronephrosis). The patient's symptoms and the hydronephrosis were usually thought to be related, and a surgical solution was provided. Antenatal and screening studies have changed the scenerio: imaging studies may reveal urinary tract dilatation in the absence of symptoms and if the dilatation is considered likely to cause eventual harm, pre-emptive surgical correction is offered.

Nomenclature and the wide ureter

The language and terminology used to describe ureteral pathology tend to shape the therapeutic response. Thus, an obstructive megaureter demands relief of the obstruction. Precision with nomenclature is imperative. Herein, a few ureteral terms are defined that are sometimes unclear. *Ureteral duplication* requires that each ureter, from a functionally distinct renal subunit, has an individual insertion into the bladder or on the ectopic pathway. A *bifid ureter*, in contrast, consists of two distinct ureters proximally which become conjoint distally such that the terminal portion, even if only a few millimeters in length, enters the bladder at a single ureteric orifice.

The term *wide ureter* implies that a normal standard of ureteral width exists, perhaps based on age or physical size. The term wide ureter is invoked heuristically; one's eyes seem to recognize that subtle difference between normal and wide. It is useful, however, to pick a rough standard, such as a diameter of 5 mm, as the upper limit of normal (Cussen, 1971). Ureteral dilatation is described in the literature by several terms including megaureter, megaloureter, ureterectasis, ureterectasia, or wide ureter. These morphologic terms say nothing about the etiology of the ureteral distortion, which may be obstructive, refluxing, or simply dysmorphic. Terminal ureteral dilatation without involvement of the proximal ureter or renal collecting system is a common observation in children, but tends to be simply dysmorphic rather than of functional significance, and is virtually never progressive (Williams and Hulme-Moir, 1970).

Hendren's description of megaureter is still the most accurate and compact: 'Megaureter is a descriptive term for a ureter that is wide and sometimes very tortuous; it is not a diagnosis. A megaureter can be refluxing or obstructive' (Hendren, 1998). The terms primary and secondary megaureter are of historic interest and some authors have given good operational descriptions (Wilcox and Mouriquand, 1998). The older literature can be misleading when those terms lead to subjective decisions that mandate an operation or non-operative surveillance, in the absence of clinical or investigational evidence of obstruction. It is preferable to abandon the primary and secondary terminology and rely on the adjectives obstructive or refluxing, which are applied when clinical or investigational evidence warrants. This mission, however straightforward when one applies the term refluxing, is not always easy with the obstructive adverb.

Ureteral obstruction as a clinical problem

Obstruction is a problematic word for the genitourinary surgeon. Complete obstruction is easy enough to understand: no urine can pass the point in question. However, transitional regions of the urinary tract, such as the ureteropelvic junction (UPJ) and the ureterovesical junction (UVJ), may offer minor physiologic impediments to flow and some obstruction at these junctions may become important. Generally, urinary tract obstruction is incomplete. Symptoms, progressive dilatation, and deteriorating function make

Table 24.1 Explanations for wide ureters

Unobstructed	Obstructed
Refluxing ureter	Retrocaval ureter
Prune belly syndrome	Ureteral valve
Diuresis-provoked	Ureteral stricture
Simple ureterectasis	Uretrovesical junction
Infection	obstruction:
	Congenital
	Acquired

the diagnosis of true obstruction easy, but more often than not assessments and plans must be made without benefit of prolonged observation and these obvious clinical and investigational markers. A wide ureter in the absence of current reflux or obstruction may have been the result of reflux or obstruction that is long absent (or perhaps intermittent). Some wide ureters are simply unexplained dysmorphic phenomena, whereas wide ureters occasionally develop in relation to prolonged diuresis (Table 24.1).

Evaluation of ureteral obstruction

When ureteral obstruction is suspected, evidence-based diagnosis is the next step and this is usually accomplished by some form of urinary tract imaging. Ultrasonography is a practical first step to ascertain any dilatation of the urinary tract. Genitourinary sonography must always evaluate the entire urinary tract. A renal/upper ureteral sonogram alone is incomplete. Although ultrasonography is an excellent modality to detect hydroureteronephrosis and major structural anomalies, the recognition of dilatation alone is not proof of obstruction. Conversely, the absence of significant visual dilatation is not proof that there is no obstruction, as the following two cases illustrate.

Case 1: a 12-year-old girl complained of weekly episodes of flank pain. Four years previously she had undergone a dismembered pyeloplasty for UPJ obstruction, and postoperative studies including sonography (severe hydronephrosis improved to mild) and diuretic renography (a markedly prolonged half-time improved to equivalence) were normal. These studies were repeated several times after the new complaints surfaced, but without evidence of obstruction. After more than one year of persistent complaints, a percutaneous nephrostomy was placed. The pain episodes disappeared. Fluoroscopic Whitaker pressure perfusions, supine and sitting, were normal, but obstruction was revealed on certain torso rotations. Reoperative pyeloplasty solved the complaints and she has been well for the ensuing 7 years.

Case 2: a 21-year-old woman was well for 3.5 years after her third renal transplantation (for focal glomerulosclerosis). Over a 4 month period she noted vague discomfort and intermittent tenderness in the area of the graft and repeatedly called this to the clinicians' attention. Examinations, however, elicited no pain or tenderness. There was no sign of infection or rejection. Her serum creatinine remained normal and several renal sonograms were stable without evidence of hydronephrosis. Then, after a few days of increased pain, myalgias, and malaise she was admitted in profound shock with an elevated creatinine and mild to moderate hydronephrosis. She was resuscitated and a percutaneous nephrostomy was placed. An antegrade nephrostogram revealed a high ureteral structure. Correction of this is pending.

These cases demonstrate that, while ultrasonography is a useful screening test, one cannot rely on it to disprove obstruction, particularly when the clinical situation does not match the test.

The intravenous pyelogram (IVP), once the diagnostic mainstay for obstructive uropathy, is still a very useful modality, offering many clues to obstruction. Delayed visualization of the renogram or late visualization of the collecting system and ureter can be evidence of a blockage. The IVP may also identify the precise point of obstruction, for example by ureteral columnization on delayed films. As this test receives less use, however, its technical nuances are lost through disuse atrophy and diminished educational exposure. In evaluation of acute ureteral obstruction, usually by a stone, the spiral computed tomographic (CT) scan has become the latest and best diagnostic mainstay. For the non-acute diagnostic evaluation, CT urography combines localization and some functional information, much like the IVP, but the anatomic detail and adjacent structure visualization are far more precise.

Nuclear renography has utility in the evaluation of ureteral obstruction, although it may be less useful than in instances of UPJ obstruction. A diuretic-stimulated (^{99m}Tc) MAG-3 (technetium-99m-mercapto-acetyltriglycine) nuclear renal scan is currently in wide use and affords good anatomic detail. The renal scan will show roughly how well one kidney performs in relation to its contralateral mate. Evidence for obstruction, however, must be gleaned from a delay in collecting system visualization (much as is done with the IVP) or ascertained from prolonged drainage half-times. These half-times are limited by the designation of critical areas of interest, which becomes a rough guess in the area of the distal ureter where bladder and ureter overlap.

The Whitaker pressure perfusion test, although uncommonly indicated, can provide evidence for obstruction in four ways: (1) placement of the percutaneous tube, alone, can resolve symptoms and thereby facilitate diagnosis; (2) infusion of contrast can provoke symptoms; (3) the contrast can visually be held up at the point of obstruction; and (4) a rise in pressure during perfusion can indicate obstruction (see Chapter 20).

Ureteral exposure and surgical principles

The upper ureter may be approached by any of the usual renal exposures. Mid-ureter access requires a flank approach and the lower ureter is found by Gibson, low mid-line, or Pfannenstiel incisions. Hinman (1993, 1998) explains these incisions clearly.

The pediatric ureter is less forgiving than an adult ureter. An infant's ureter is delicate and susceptible to damage from manual pressure, forceps handling, prolonged stretch, or mild thermal injury from electrocautery. Overt damage will result in early ischemia and a poor surgical result. Subclinical damage may result in fibrosis and delayed dysfunction, years or decades later. Once a ureter is dismembered, either proximally at the UPJ, or distally, its blood supply is immediately compromised and even a small additional harm from axial tension or pressure will have some cost. Optical magnification, extraordinary operative finesse, minimal use of electrocautery (with bipolar cautery near the ureter), stay sutures to handle the ureter and fine suture materials are advantageous for the pediatric genitourinary surgeon (Koo and Bloom, 1999).

Uretero-vascular anomalies: retrocaval (circumcaval) and retroiliac ureter

Although these lesions are congenital, they tend to present in later life, typically the fourth decade, with a predilection for males. In the early human embryo the major venous channels are the posterior cardinal veins and minor venous channels (the subcardinal veins). The channels come to lie ventral to the developing ureter. By the 15 mm stage, supracardinal veins, which lie dorsal to the developing ureter, are present. In normal embryologic development the posterior cardinal vein, caudal to the renal vein, regresses, thereby allowing the ureter to assume its normal location ventral to the supracardinal vein (which eventually becomes the vena cava). The subcardinal vein becomes the gonadal vein. (See also Chapter 1.)

Persistence of the right posterior cardinal vein, which is ventral to the definitive ureteral position, results in the typical retrocaval ureter. The right side is affected except in instances of situs inversus. Symptoms are upper tract infection, pain, calculus, and hematuria. Bateson and Akinson (1969) and Kenawi and Williams (1976) recognized two main types of retrocaval ureter. The more common low loop variant (type I) has the typical reverse J configuration on IVP or retrograde pyelography, with the dilated upper ureter lateral to the vena cava at the third to fourth lumbar vertebral level and the distal non-dilated portion medial. A high loop variant (type II) has been described, which can mimic a UPJ obstruction (Fig. 24.1a). Surgical correction is performed only when the retrocaval ureter is symptomatic, and usually consists of a dismembered ureteroureterostomy or dismembered pyeloplasty if the obstructed element is high enough. Goodwin, for many years during his career, advocated division and reanastomosis of the vena cava to restore the normal ureteral position, although it is not known whether he ever accomplished this (Goodwin W, personal communication, 1979). CT urography shows the ureteral–caval relationships precisely (Fig. 24.1b).

The rarity of retrocaval ureter as a clinical entity is apparent in Considine's report that found only two patients operated for this in the Glasgow Royal Infirmary in 30 years. The first, a 30-year-old woman with two episodes of right flank pain nausea and emesis, underwent pelvic resection and reconstruction in 1949 by Mr Arthur Jacobs, a legendary figure in urology. The second patient, a 29-year-old man, had right flank pain and hematuria. A calculus was found in the strictured retrocaval segment which was excised and a ureteroureterostomy was performed. The author's

first two conclusions were: (1) the discovery of this condition is not itself an indication for its operative correction; and (2) the plan of a corrective action cannot be decided until the operative findings are known. One operative option mentioned was section and reanastomosis of the inferior vena cava (IVC) (Considine, 1966). A variant caval-ureteric anomaly is the obstructive periureteric venous ring in which the deviated ureter effectively splits the vena cava and thus may not have the typical radiologic retrocaval appearance (LePage and Baldwin, 1972).

Retroiliac ureter is rare and may occur on either or both sides, typically at the L_5 level. Concurrent problems, particularly of the mesonephric duct, are common. Other vascular obstructions, such as from uterine and hypogastric vessels, may occur, but it is important to distinguish true obstruction from a vascular impression. Hanna (1972) reported on a patient of DI Williams with bilateral retroiliac artery ureters, horseshoe kidney, and VUR. Two related cases were found in the literature. Epididymitis, hematuria, and

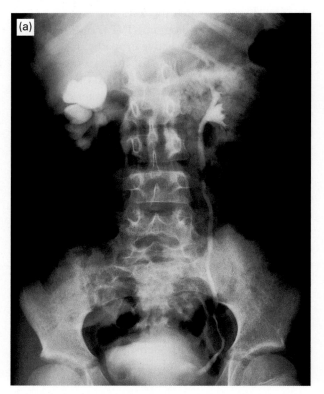

Figure 24.1 (a) IVP: right hydronephrosis secondary to retrocaval ureter in a 12 year old boy with flank pain. (b) *Shown opposite.*

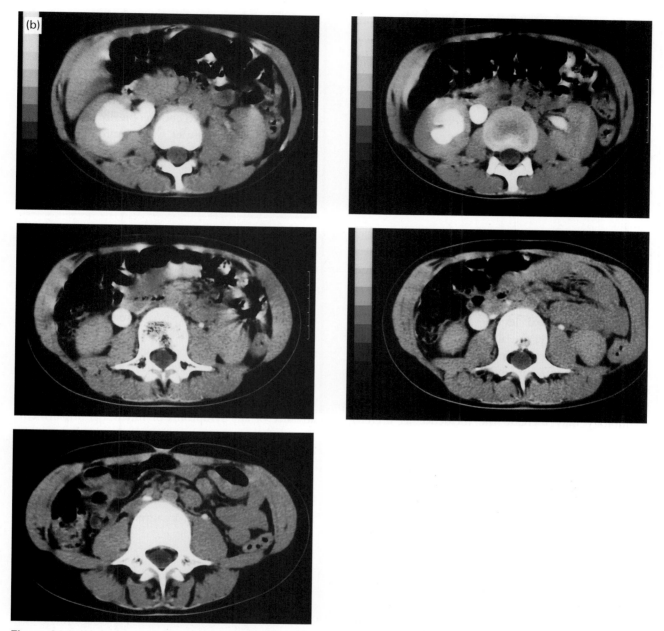

Figure 24.1 (*b*) *Continued.* CT scans of the same patient as (*a*).

urinary infection were the presenting symptoms. Ureteral remodeling and reimplantation were performed in Hanna's case, the others being managed by ureteral division and reanastomosis. A duplicated vena cava with right retrocaval ureter containing a fibroepithelial polyp presented with pyelonephritis in a 15-year-old boy (Clements *et al.*, 1978). Another odd variant was the distal common ensheathment of ureters found in a 2-year-old boy with a high right retrocaval ureter (Salem and Luck, 1976).

Ureteral valves

The literature can be confusing in the realm of ureteral valves owing to the inclusion of lesions at the UPJ and UVJ in some reports (Maizels and Stephens, 1980). The transverse folds observed in newborns and called folds of Östling are non-obstructive lesions that disappear with time as the ureter grows and straightens (Östling, 1942). For all practical purposes such findings may be excluded and ureteral valves defined as those uncommon obstructive lesions occurring in the ureter between its proximal and distal endpoints. Two sorts of ureteral valve seem to exist: the congenital annular transverse folds of epithelium and smooth muscle (Noe and Scaljon, 1979), and the eccentric folds and kinks that occur in dilated ureters, which can become obstructive as peristaltic waves and fibrosis shape and fix them. Obstructive lesions in the ureter need surgical redress, whether by endoscopy, open excision, ureter-oureterostomy, or replacement.

Ureteral stricture

A stricture is a narrowing, and a narrowing becomes significant to the patient and clinician when it becomes obstructive, either clinically or radiologically. Although several lesions have been described under this category, the authors' opinion is that the use of the term stricture implies histologic change secondary to trauma or inflammation. Discounting stenosis at the UPJ and UVJ, ureteral obstruction from stricture is rare (Allen, 1970), although new technology may increase the incidence as ureteroscopy and percutaneous endoscopic adventures proliferate.

Trauma to the ureter is the source of most ureteral strictures in clinical practice. In the past, the trauma was typically received during open surgery for malignancy or gynecologic procedures. In the future endo-scopic procedures are expected to be the primary source. Surgical management has a variety of interventional options. Strictures may be multiple and good surgical judgment mandates complete evaluation of the collecting system proximal and distal to the stricture. Short and recently acquired endoscopic injuries may be repaired endoscopically, but long segment and fibrotic injuries will require exicision and anatomosis, or replacement.

Ureterovesical obstruction

The obstructive label should be applied when clinical or investigational evidence is at hand (Table 24.2). Controversy still abounds regarding that precise fork in the road where the obstructive megaureter diverges from the non-obstructive megaureter. Many dilated ureters, although visually severe, may not represent an obstructive threat to their renal moieties. In former pediatric urologic practice, children with megaureters presented with urinary infection, hematuria, pain, and failure to thrive. At present, most megaureters are discovered by prenatal sonography in advance of any symptoms or functional impairment. Some of these megaureters tend to normalize visually over time and never seem to cause a problem (Elder, 1992; Baskin *et al.*, 1994; Liu *et al.*, 1994).

The cause of congenital distal ureteral obstruction is not known and the histologic and ultrastructural findings vary. Investigators agree that the organization

Table 24.2 Evidence of ureteral obstruction

Symptomatic	Infection
	Pain
Simple imaging	Hydronephrosis: in the absence of UPJ obstruction:
	Calyceal dilatation
	Renal pelvic dilatation: AP diameter > 40 mm
	Ureterectasis
	Progressive dilatation, proximal ureteral dilatation or panureteral dilatation > 5 mm
	Trapping of contrast on delayed IVP or VCUG
	Positive resistive indices on Doppler sonogram
	Calculus proximal to suspected obstruction
Provocative testing	Diuretic renal scan:
	Diminished or declining relative renal contribution
	Increased half-time
	Positive Whitaker pressure perfusion test

The presence of two or more of these findings in a patient is highly suspicious for obstruction.
UPJ = ureteropelvic junction; AP = anteroposterior; IVP = intravenous pyelography; VCUG = voiding cystourethrography.

and relationship of smooth muscle and extracellular matrix are altered (McLaughlin *et al.*, 1973; Tanagho, 1973; Hanna *et al.*, 1976; MacKinnon, 1977; Medel and Quesada, 1985). The most consistent finding seems to be the predominance of circular smooth muscle with increased collagen deposition between the muscle bundles of the obstructing segment. The structural abnormalities lead to disruption in myoelectric propagation and peristalsis, ultimately affecting the free efflux of urine and resulting in functional obstruction. The segment may be short or long (Fig. 24.2). Lee *et al.* (1998) distinguished histologically between wide ureters that were the result of obstruction and wide ureters due to reflux. Refluxing wide ureters had susbstantially less type I and more type III collagen than either normal ureters or obstructed megaureters.

UVJ obstruction may occur without an inherent distal ureteral abnormality (previously this was described as secondary obstructive megaureter). This form of obstruction usually occurs with bladder dysfunction from myelodysplasia or posterior urethral valves (PUV). Although obstruction is not present within the ureters, progressive ureteral dilatation occurs when there is increasing difficulty with the propulsion of urine across the thickened bladder wall at the UVJ. The ureterectasis that occurs in most cases improves once the cause of the vesical dysfunction and elevated bladder pressures has been addressed. Long-standing bladder abnormalities may lead to permanent damage to the intrinsic ureteral peristaltic mechanisms.

Evaluation

Ultrasonography is the best initial study for a child in whom a urinary abnormality is suspected. Complete urologic evaluation includes the bladder and bony pelvic structures in addition to the upper urinary tract. Renal parenchyma, renal pelvis, ureter (including the retrovesical ureter), bladder, and gonadal–müllerian structures in girls comprise a complete report. Hydronephrosis can be graded according to the Society for Fetal Urology scale (Maizels *et al.*, 1994). Longitudinal and transverse sonographic images at the bladder level are sensitive in detecting ureteral dilatation. If dilatation is detected, a voiding cystourethrogram (VCUG) is indicated to evaluate for VUR and to assess the bladder and urethra for likely causes of ureteral dilatation (Fig. 24.3). A renal function study such as the diuretic renal scan (DRS) provides relative renal values and may reveal obstruction. Technetium-99m-diethylenetriaminepentacetic acid ([^{99m}Tc]DTPA) and MAG-3 are the radionuclides currently in wide use. Although the IVP has generally been replaced by the DRS, the IVP will be especially valuable in some clinical situations. For example, calyceal preservation (which is best evaluated

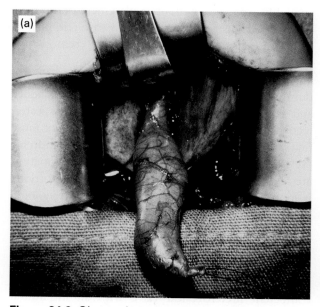
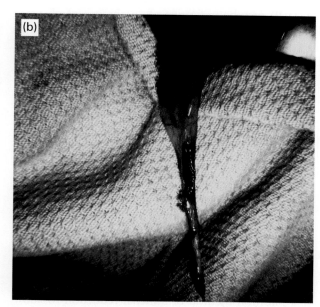

Figure 24.2 Obstructive megaureters. (*a*) Short terminal obstructive element. (*b*) Long, narrowed distal obstructive element.

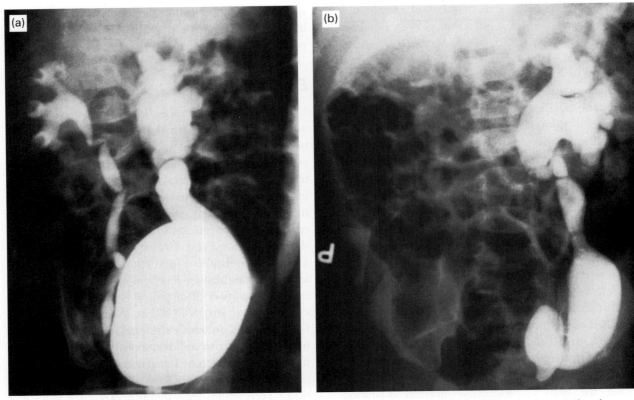

Figure 24.3 (*a*) Child with bilateral reflux and dilated collecting system with significant calycectatic changes. (*b*) Six-hour drainage film of same patient. Note that the right side is completely empty; note also the sharp cut-off on the left at the ureterovesical junction. This left side combined the worst features of two problems, reflux and obstruction.

by IVP) may be indicative of an absence of obstruction in spite of significant ureteral dilation. The Whitaker pressure perfusion test may also help to reveal obstruction, but it is invasive, costly, and only uncommonly necessary to make an accurate clinical decision (Whitaker, 1973).

Treatment

In a crisis, percutaneous nephrostomy is a short-term solution for an obstructive megaureter. The decompression may also allow ureteral distension to decrease enough that a simple ureteroneocystomy will suffice later. The definitive procedure, however, is resection of the obstructive element and ureteroneocystostomy (Vereecken and Proesmans, 1999). A very wide ureter will require a Hendren-type tapering or a plication method of lumenal reduction to allow reconstruction of a functional UVJ. The Great Ormond Street group in London recently reported

favorable experience with open placement of double J stents which delayed or avoided ureteric reimplantation, and usually obviated ureteric remodeling (Koehler *et al.*, 1999).

The surgical principles of wide ureter reconstruction have evolved from direct plug-in to the bladder and cutaneous ureterostomy to more sophisticated reconstruction. The obstructed ureteral element must first be defined and completely excised. Hendren's excisional tapering recognized that form and function are related; thus, a ureter with anatomic proportions is more likely to perform its designated physiologic task (Hendren, 1969a). He defined the less vascular side of the wide ureter, excised it, and closed the reconfigured ureter over a catheter before reimplantation (Fig. 24.4). By reducing the reimplanted segment to a diameter of around 5 mm, he created a competent ureterovesical valve with an intramural tunnel several centimeters in length (see Fig. 25.35). The non-excisional remodeling technique introduced by Kalicinski *et al.* (1977) expanded on Hendren's plan, by tailoring without excision of native tissue or much interruption of the blood supply. This folding method may be used with an absorbable running suture to tailor the wide ureter over an 8–10 Fr catheter, then folding and tacking the excluded segment over the working ureteral moiety (see Figs. 25.36, 25.37). In Ehrlich's modification, the longitudinal suture runs down the center of the dilated ureter so that, when folded, both ureteral lumena are open (Ehrlich, 1985). The running suture, however, is completed shy of the terminal ureter and a few interrupted sutures complete the tailoring. The reason for this is that the traction and manipulation of the ureter may render the terminus less robust than it had started out, after excision of the obstructive element. If excision of a short segment of more distal ureter is necessary after the tailoring and folding process, it can then easily be accomplished without compromising the more proximal running suture. At the ultimate terminal portion of the ureter a few sutures are placed to occlude the access to the excluded moiety and secure it to the new ureteric orifice. Note that a few seconds of unrecognized axial tension on the ureter can severely impair its blood supply. As the ureter is being mobilized and during folding and plication, the surgeon needs to be on the alert for this risk.

The failed reimplant

Ureteroneocystostomy, whether for reflux or renal transplantation, is one of the most successful operative procedures in pediatric urology. Success rates, whether by advancement techniques, cross-trigonal reimplantation, or extravesical detrusorrhaphy, are generally 98% or better when the bladder is normal (Ehrlich, 1982; Ohl *et al.*, 1988; Houle *et al.*, 1992; Keneally *et al.*, 1995). Newer techniques such as trigonal splitting and laparoscopic methods should be taken up only with great caution as the existing standards of practice are so good. Failure of a ureteroneocystomy, although uncommon, is a problem that a busy pediatric urology team must face (Hendren, 1969b; Bloom and Ritchey, 1991). The failure may take the form of obstruction or reflux.

Obstruction is the more dangerous form of failure, leaving the upper tracts at immediate risk. Obstruction may be due to angulation of the distal ureter. This is most commonly seen after Politano–Leadbetter reimplants that position the intramural tunnel too laterally such that the filled bladder kinks the distal ureter. This is best avoided by placing the intramural tunnel in a medial and fairly fixed portion of the posterior aspect of the bladder and by dividing the obliterated umbilical artery when extravesical reimplants are performed. Correction of the malpositioned ureter requires reposition of the intramural tunnel. Obstruction may also result from distal ureteral fibrosis and stricture, which are the result of ureteral injury. These are likely to result from traumatic dissection of a ureter, excessive traction on the ureter, or damage from electrocautery. Obvious injury may produce early stricture, but subclinical damage to the distal ureter may result in late fibrosis. As always, prevention is preferable to correction. Distal ureteral stenosis requires repeat ureteroneocystostomy. The fibrosis is rarely such a discrete lesion that ureterotomy will be curative, and a significant length of narrow and aperistaltic ureter is unlikely to be restored to normal by a longitudinal incision. The abnormal ureter must be excised carefully without axial tension or other impairment to the residual ureter, such that the viability of the new distal segment is absolutely dependable. Ureteroneocystotomy will then require an advancement, Politano–Leadbetter, or cross-trigonal reimplant, or a psoas hitch or Boari flap may be necessary (Fig. 24.5). Occasionally, ureteral replacement with appendix or bowel segment may be necessary to bridge a long gap although transureteroureterostomy may be an easier solution.

Persisting reflux is the other form of failure of a reimplant. When this occurs, the possibility of occult bladder dysfunction must be entertained. Therefore, a precise elimination history, voiding diary, and urodynamic assessment are useful studies before reoperative ureteroneocystostomy is performed. Lower tract dysfunction associated with poor toilet habits, such as infrequent voiding, should be corrected before reoperation. Persisting reflux can be due to an inadequate intramural tunnel or inadequate detrusor backing. The former condition is the more likely scenario in reflux to a transplanted kidney. The latter condition may occur in a well-performed reimplant in a child with an unstable bladder and detrusor-sphincter dyssynergia. In this instance, the intramural tunnel may be more than long enough (well in excess of the desired 4:1 ratio between intramural tunnel and ureteral diameter), but the detrusor backing is lacking.

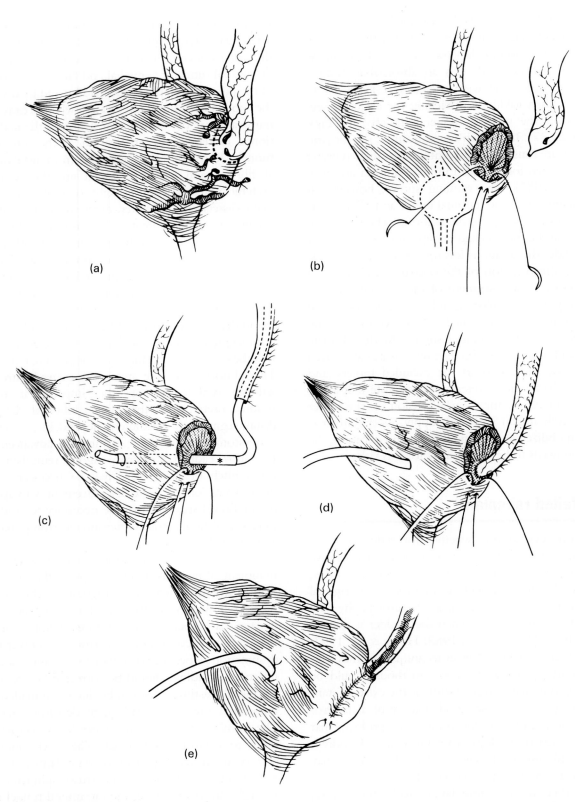

(a)

(b)

(c)

(d)

(e)

Figure 24.4 Detrusorrhaphy for megaureter. (*a*) Exposing the intramurcal ureter. (*b, c*) Advancing the tapered mega-ureter. (*d*) Anastomosing the tapered ureter to the bladder. (*e*) The cut margins of the detrusor flaps are reapproximated creating the tunnel. (Adapted from Chaviano and Maizels, 1987.)

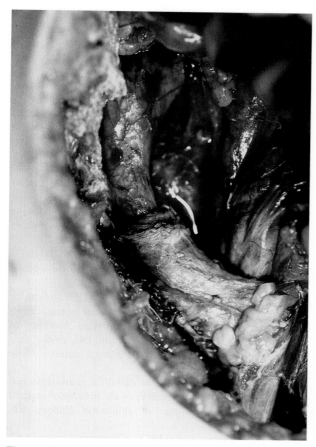

Figure 24.5 Replacement of a long obstructive terminal ureteral element using a Boari flap ureteroneocystostomy.

Reoperative ureteroneocystostomy is technically demanding, with higher stakes than at the first reimplant. Correctable underlying and associated factors, such as detrusor dysfunction and constipation, need to be addressed preoperatively. A dismembered ureteroneocystostomy is almost always the preferred reoperative procedure. The bladder is opened, the ureter mobilized, a stenotic or dysfunctional segment removed, and a cross-trigonal, or Politano–Leadbetter procedure performed. In the latter instance, the new entry point of ureter to bladder must be somewhat medial in a relatively fixed portion of bladder so that obstructive angulation does not occur during bladder filling. The authors generally stent a reoperative reimplant for 3 weeks with a small caliber tube. If the distal ureter is too short for simple reimplantation, a psoas hitch, Boari flap, or ureteral

substitution with bowel or appendix will be necessary, although a more simple solution is to perform a transureteroureterostomy, anastamosing the refluxing ureter into the normal, contralateral ureter. In some instances of clinically significant reflux after renal transplantation the reflux may be corrected by detrussorhaphy, using a conventional extravesical technique (Fig. 24.4).

Other ureteral problems

Ureteral neoplasms are rare in children and tend to be benign. The primary differential diagnosis is stone, and Bergman's radiographic sign may be of use, wherein dilatation below the lesion signals neoplasm, but constriction below is more typical of stone (Faerber and Bloom, 1999).

Replacement of a ureter is a rare necessity in pediatric urology, and the occasion is most likely to be related to a severe congenital atresia or trauma of some sort. The appendix is a useful spare part for a right ureteral deficiency. The ileal ureter is the classic modality for any major ureteral replacement (Tveter *et al.*, 1980). A Yang–Monti tube may be another serviceable method (Yang, 1993; Monti *et al.*, 1997; Bloom *et al.*, 1999a).

Outcome surveillance, and conclusion

It could be claimed that no one is cured of a given disease until that person dies of something else. Perhaps it is naive to expect a lifetime guarantee for any operative procedure, including ureteral reconstructions. The unknown natural histories of the diseases themselves, along with the thousands of tiny injuries imparted surgically, mandate surveillance far beyond federal and insurance carrier global periods. Surveillance, however, need not be complex, invasive, or expensive. Genitourinary history, physical examination, blood pressure, urine analysis, and occasional ultrasonography are usually all that are needed beyond the first postoperative year. Surveillance should extend at least until the child stops growing. For third-party payers who question the value of surveillance, one might counter that one's automobile will undoubtedly need more attention than a lower urinary tract reconstruction. Sequential renal scans or invasive procedures should be resisted unless there is a strong need to know.

Inasmuch as a wide ureter is not necessarily obstructive, some further evidence of harm or threat is generally sought before embarking on surgical management. The authors no longer find the terms primary and secondary megaureter useful, preferring instead to use the term wide ureter alone, appending refluxing or obstructive when evidence is present.

References

Allen TD (1970) Congenital ureteral strictures. *J Urol* **104**: 196–204.

Baskin LS, Zderic SA, Snyder HM *et al.* (1994) Primary dilated megaureter: long-term follow-up. *J Urol* **152**: 618.

Bateson EM, Atkinson D (1969) Circumcaval ureter: a new classification. *Clin Radiol* **20**: 173–7.

Bernstein AM, Koo HP, Bloom DA (1999) Beyond the Trendelenburg position: Friedrich Trendelenburg's life and surgical constrictions. *Surgery* **126**: 78–82.

Bloom DA, Ritchey ML (1991) The failed ureteral reimplantation: postoperative evaluation of the failed reimplant. *Dialog Pediatr Urol* **14**: 2–4

Bloom DA, Koo HP, Manzoni G (1999a) Paul Mitrofanoff and the Mitrofanoff principle. *Contemp Urol* Feb: 15–6.

Bloom DA, Milen MT, Heininger JC (1999b) Claudius Galen: from a 20th century genitourinary perspective. *J Urol* **161**: 12–9.

Chaviano AH, Maizels M (1987) Detrusorrhaphy for megaureter. In: Resmick MI, Kursh E (eds) *Current therapy in genitourinary surgery*. Philadelphia, PA: BC Decker, 203–8.

Clements JC, McLeod DG, Greene WR, Stutzman RE (1978) A case report: duplicated vena cava with right retrocaval ureter and a ureteral tumor. *J Urol* **119**: 284–5.

Considine J (1966) Retrocaval ureter. *Br J Urol* **38**: 412–23.

Cussen LJ (1971) The morphology of congenital dilation of the ureter: intrinsic ureteral lesions. *Aust NZ J Surg* **31**: 185.

Ehrlich RM (1982) Success of the transvesical advancement technique for vesicoureteral reflux. *J Urol* **128**: 554–7.

Ehrlich RM (1985) The ureteral folding technique for megaureter surgery. *J Urol* **134**: 668.

Elder JS (1992) *In utero* ultrasonography – impact on urology. *J Endourol* **6**: 279.

Faerber GJ, Bloom DA (1999) The origin and utility of Bergman's sign. *Contemp Urol* Jan: 16–7.

Hanna MK (1972) Bilateral retroiliac-artery ureters. *Br J Urol* **44**: 339–44.

Hanna MK, Jeffs RD, Sturgess JM *et al.* (1976) Ureteral structure and ultrastructure. Part II. Congenital ureteropelvic junction obstruction and primary obstructive megaureter. *J Urol* **116**: 725.

Hendren WH (1969a) Operative repair of megaureter in childhood. *J Urol* **101**: 491–5.

Hendren WH (1969b) Reoperation of the failed ureteral reimplantation. *J Urol* **101**: 403.

Hendren WH III (1998) Commentary. In Hinman F Jr (ed.) *Atlas of urologic surgery*. 2nd edition. Philadelphia, PA: WB Saunders, 807–8.

Hinman F Jr (1993) *Atlas of urosurgical anatomy*. Philadelphia, PA: WB Saunders, 148–58.

Hinman F Jr (1998) *Atlas of urologic surgery*. 2nd edition. Philadelphia, PA: WB Saunders, 488–98.

Houle AM, McLorie GA, Heritz DM *et al.* (1992) Extravesical nondismembered ureteroplasty with detrusorrhaphy: a renewed technique to correct vesicoureteral reflux in children. *J Urol* **148**: 704–7.

Kalicinski ZM, Kansy K, Kotarginska B *et al.* (1977) Surgery of megaureters: modification of Hendren's operation. *J Pediatr Surg* **12**: 183.

Kenawi MM, Williams DI (1976) Circumcaval ureter: a report of four cases in children with a review of the literature and a new classification system. *Br J Urol* **48**: 183–92.

Keneally MJ, Bloom DA, Ritchey ML, Panzl AC (1995) Outcome analysis of bilateral Cohen cross-trigonal ureteroneocystostomy. *Urology* **46**: 393–5.

Koehler ML, Wilcox DT, Gordon I *et al.* (1999) Primary obstructive megaureter managed by ureteric stenting: experience and long-term outcome. American Academy of Pediatrics Annual Meeting, Washington, DC, 1999.

Koo HP, Bloom DA (1999) Lower ureteral reconstruction. *Urol Clin North Am* **26**: 167–73.

Lee BR, Silver RI, Partin AW *et al.* (1998) A quantitative histologic nalysis of collagen subtypes: the primary obstructed and refluxing megaurter of childhood *Urology*. **51**: 820–3.

LePage JR, Baldwin GN (1972) Obstructive periureteric venous ring. *Radiology* **104**: 313–5.

Liu JYA, Dhillon HK, Yeung CK *et al.* (1994) Clinical outcome and management of prenatally diagnosed primary megaureters. *J Urol* **152**: 614.

MacKinnon KC (1977) Primary megaureter. *Birth Defects* **13**: 15.

McLaughlin AP, Pfister RC, Leadbetter WF *et al.* (1973) The pathophysiology of primary megaureter. *J Urol* **109**: 805–11.

Maizels M, Stephens FD (1980) Valves of the ureter as a cause of primary obstruction of the ureter: anatomic, embryologic and clinical aspects. *J Urol* **123**: 742–7.

Maizels M, Mitchell B, Kass E *et al.* (1994) Outcome of nonspecific hydronephrosis in the infant: a report from the Society of Fetal Urology. *J Urol* **152**: 2324–7.

Medel R, Quesada EM (1985) Ultrastructural characteristics of collagen tissue in normal and congenitally dilated ureter. *Eur Urol* **11**: 324–9.

Monti PR, Lara RC, Dutra MA *et al.* (1997) New techniques for construction of efferent conduits based on the Mitrofanoff principle. *Urology* **49**: 112–5.

Noe HN, Scaljon W (1979) Case profile: ureteral valves. *Urology* **14**: 411–2.

Ohl DA, Konnak JW, Campbell DA *et al.* (1988) Extravesical ureteroneocystostomy in renal transplantation. *J Urol* **139**: 499–502.

Östling K (1942) The genesis of hydronephrosis. *Acta Chir Scand* Suppl **72**: 5–122.

Salem RJ, Luck RJ (1973) Midline ensheathed ureters. *Br J Urol* **48**: 18.

Tanagho EA (1973) Intrauterine fetal ureteral obstruction. *J Urol* **109**: 196.

Tveter KJ, Bloom DA, Goodwin WE (1980) Ileal ureter: current status. *Eur Urol* **6**: 321–7.

Vereecken RL, Proesmans W (1999) A review of ninety-two obstructive megaureters in children. *Eur Urol* **36**: 342–7.

Whitaker RH (1973) Methods of assessing obstruction in the dilated ureter. *Br J Urol* **45**: 15.

Wilcox D, Mouriquand P (1998) Management of megaureter in children. *Eur Urol* **34**: 73–8.

Williams DI, Hulme-Moir I (1970) Primary obstructive megaureter. *Br J Urol* **42**: 140.

Yang WH (1993) Yang needle tunneling technique creating antireflux and continent mechanism. *J Urol* **150**: 830–4.

Young HH, Davis DM (1926) *Young's practice of urology*. Volume II. Philadelphia, PA: WB Saunders, 318–9.

Vesicoureteral reflux

25

Stephen A. Kramer

Historic review

Vesicoureteral reflux (VUR) is the abnormal flow of urine from the bladder into the upper urinary tract. Reflux was recognized as early as medieval times by Galen and Leonardo da Vinci (Polk, 1965; Lines, 1982). Semblino first demonstrated reflux experimentally in 1883 (Levitt and Weiss, 1985). In 1893, Pozzi was the first to observe reflux in humans when he noted urine flow from the cut end of the distal ureter after nephrectomy (Walker, 1987). In 1898, Young and Wesson concluded that patients with a normal ureterovesical junction (UVJ) did not have VUR (Young and Wesson, 1921). Sampson observed in 1903 that the normal obliquity of the ureter through the bladder prevented reflux (Walker, 1921). Hutch's classic studies on the pathophysiology of reflux in paraplegic patients demonstrated the relationship between reflux and chronic pyelonephritis and led the way for the widespread use of voiding cystourethrography (VCUG) in the evaluation of patients with unexplained hydronephrosis or recurrent urinary tract infections (UTIs) or both (Hutch, 1952).

Tanagho *et al.* (1965) performed experiments on the ureteral trigonal complex in dogs and demonstrated that incision of the trigonal musculature distal to the ureteral orifice produced VUR. Ransley and Risdon (1975a) showed that resection of the roof of the submucosal tunnel in piglets consistently resulted in VUR. Kiruluta *et al.* (1986) demonstrated that maturation of the adrenergic fibers in the bladder has a role in the presence or absence of reflux.

Incidence and epidemiology

The prevalence of VUR in healthy children is probably less than 1% and varies depending on race and country of origin. Politano (1960) and Lich *et al.* (1964) found no evidence of reflux in large series of patients undergoing cystography. Ransley (1978) found only seven instances of reflux in a series of 535 VCUGs performed in presumably normal neonates, infants, and children. Iannaccone and Panzironi (1955) reported only one instance of reflux in a series of 50 assessable infants without urologic disease who underwent voiding cystourethrography. Jones and Headstream (1958) found reflux in only 1 of 100 children evaluated.

Manley suggested that reflux occurs more commonly in children with fair skin, blond hair, and blue eyes (Walker, 1987). Conversely, others have found a higher incidence of reflux only in red-headed children. Askari and Belman (1982) noted that reflux occurred ten times more frequently in white girls with UTI than in black girls with infections. Peters *et al.* (1967) found no instances of reflux in 56 black children who underwent cystography.

Diagnosis

Clinical presentation

The widespread use of obstetric ultrasonography and early screening of infants at risk for urinary tract abnormalities has led to detection of a significant number of fetuses with hydronephrosis. Between 10 and 40% of patients with hydronephrosis *in utero* have renal pelvic dilatation from primary VUR. The majority of these babies are boys with high-grade bilateral reflux (Paltiel and Lebowitz, 1989; Elder, 1992). The etiology of this severe reflux may be due to transient bladder outlet obstruction occurring *in utero*, that persists into infancy and childhood (Avni and Schulman, 1996) or simply, high voiding pressures.

Infants and young children frequently present with non-specific symptoms related to UTI. These may include fever, lethargy, anorexia, nausea, vomiting, and failure to thrive. Older children usually present with lower tract symptoms such as dysuria or with flank pain and tenderness and fever secondary to acute pyelonephritis. The symptomatic presentation of VUR is almost always in conjunction with an associated UTI. Sterile reflux is a rare and unusual cause of flank pain.

Fever is the most important symptom to differentiate children with upper tract infections (pyelonephritis) from those with lower tract infections (cystitis) (Govan and Palmer, 1969). Woodard and Holden (1976) evaluated 350 children with UTI and found that 90% of those with reflux had a temperature greater than 38.5°C. Conversely, only 40% of children without reflux had a similar temperature increase.

However, Majd *et al.* (1991), in a prospective analysis of 94 children evaluated with documented febrile UTI, found that, in general, clinical parameters were poor indicators of pyelonephritis. Upon evaluating WBC elevation, ESR >25, temperature >39.4°C, chills, lethargy, flank tenderness and gastrointestinal (GI) symptoms, only temperature >39.4°C, WBC > 17 000 cell/mm, and GI symptoms correlated statistically with scan-proven acute pyelonephritis. And these correlations were weak.

Radiologic evaluation of lower tract

Voiding cystourethrography

The diagnosis of VUR is established accurately by use of VCUG with fluoroscopy. The dynamic VCUG clearly delineates the bladder outline, bladder neck, and urethral anatomy and gives an accurate estimation of bladder capacity. The key to successful VCUG is an experienced pediatric uroradiologist and gentle and confident personnel. It often helps to have the parents with the child when the study is performed.

VUR may occur with bladder filling or during voiding, or both. Conway *et al.* (1972) observed reflux during bladder filling three times more frequently than during voiding. The rate of urinary flow has been shown to have an effect on the presence or absence of VUR. High flow rates are associated with an increase in the frequency and magnitude of ureteral peristalsis, which prevents VUR (Briggs *et al.*, 1972). Conversely, low flow rates due to either dehydration or poor renal function may increase the possi-

bility of detecting VUR. Contrast medium temperature does not appear to affect the incidence of VUR. Zerin (1993) compared the use of room temperature contrast to body temperature medium in a large series of children undergoing VCUG. He found no difference in the prevalence of VUR or in bladder capacity between the two groups.

Reflux may be diagnosed with the patient in either the awake or the anesthetized state (Poznanski and Poznanski, 1969; Woodard and Filardi, 1976; Lyon, 1977; Timmons *et al.*, 1977). Cystography in awake patients may result in artificially increased bladder pressures, because of straining to resist bladder filling (King, 1976). However, the majority do not require anethesia. In fact, most do not need sedation. Anesthesia results in a decrease in glomerular filtration rate (GFR) and, consequently, in urinary flow rates (Mazze *et al.*, 1963). Sleep cystography can be useful in selected persons (Woodard and Filardi, 1976; Timmons *et al.*, 1977) but this technique should be reserved for those who require cystoscopy during the same period of anesthetization.

The optimal hydrostatic pressure for VCU is still controversial. Gravity flow should be used at no greater than 70–100 cmH$_2$O, controlled by the height of the infusion bottle above the bladder (Levitt and Weiss, 1985). Intravesical pressure is an important factor in producing reflux, and minimal degrees of reflux may occur only at high intravesical pressures, as with detrusor contractions.

All patients with a history of prenatal hydronephrosis should have postnatal VCUG to rule out VUR. Any infant or child with a first UTI with or without fever should undergo radiographic assessment of the urinary tract. In a study of 350 children with UTI, 10% of those with documented reflux were afebrile at presentation. The diagnosis of reflux would have been missed if patients without fever had been excluded from VCUG (Woodard and Holden, 1976).

The timing of the VCUG in relation to the presence or absence of UTI is an important consideration. Acute cystitis may result in edema at the UVJ or produce an increase in intravesical pressure and cause transient VUR (Van Gool and Tanagho, 1977). Bacteriuria may produce ureteral atony and decreased peristalsis and may also be responsible for VUR (Jeff and Allen, 1962; Kaveggia *et al.*, 1966). Historically, VCUG was deferred for at least 3–4 weeks after the urine was sterile. However, it has been shown clearly that many children have reflux only during an acute infection (Walker, 1987; Kaplan, 1990). Most pediatric urologists maintain that it is important to document reflux that occurs only during a UTI, because it would justify giving the patient prophylactic antibiotic therapy. There is little risk of performing VCUG in the presence of reflux and recent UTI if the patient has adequate antibiotic coverage for a few days before the study.

Cyclic VCUGs increase the detection of VUR in between 15 and 40% of patients and should be performed routinely (Fettich and Kenda, 1992; Paltiel *et al.*, 1992). Tailored low-dose fluoroscopic VCUG is as accurate as standard or 105 mm images (Diamond *et al.*, 1996a). Substituting digital video fluoroscopic hard copies for 105 mm spot films reduces fluoroscopic time, particularly over the gonads. Digital imaging without spot films definitely decreases the radiation dosage. Pulsed fluoroscopy has the ability to lower the dose even further. If reflux is demonstrated, the study can be converted to standard fluoroscopic imaging to quantitate the grade of reflux.

Radionuclide cystography

Radionuclide cystography is ideal for patients who may require repeated or longitudinal studies annually and for screening siblings (Conway *et al.*, 1972; Nasrallah *et al.*, 1978). This test offers two advantages: it subjects the patient to less radiation exposure and is more sensitive than the standard VCUG. A dose of 0.5 mCi of technetium 99 (^{99}Tm)-pertechnetate in isotonic saline is instilled in the bladder. This provides a gonadal radiation dose of only $4-5 \times 10^{-5}$ Gy, which is significantly less than the exposure with conventional VCUG with fluoroscopy (Blaufox *et al.*, 1971). In addition to minimizing the risk from radiation, this technique allows for prolonged observation under the gamma camera, thereby enhancing the sensitivity of the test by providing a continuous cystogram (Stewart, 1953).

Indirect cystography

The use of indirect cystography by scanning the bladder at the time of a radionuclide renal scan is grossly inaccurate and cannot be recommended to detect VUR (see Chapter 6). Compared with conventional direct radionuclide cystography, this technique is associated with at least a 50% false-negative rate (Levitt and Weiss, 1985) and is particularly unreliable

with milder grades of reflux. Furthermore, gonadal radiation exposure may be higher with indirect radionuclide cystography than with direct radioisotope cystography, because radiation exposure increases further when a prolonged period is required to induce voiding.

Ultrasonography

Ultrasonography has been proposed as an in-office technique for follow-up of patients with reflux or to detect reflux in siblings. Pfister *et al.* (1982) instilled a carbonated solution into the bladder and were able to detect CO_2 bubbles in the upper urinary tract by sonography (Levitt and Weiss, 1985). Atala *et al.* (1993b) studied sonicated albumin injected into the bladder and found echogenicity in the ureters during reflux. Although this is an easy technique and eliminates ionizing radiation, it is associated with a significant incidence of false-negative results, particularly in patients with low-grade reflux. Ultrasonography cannot be recommended as a routine test for the detection of VUR (Blane *et al.*, 1993; Stockland *et al.*, 1994).

Radiologic evaluation of upper tract

Excretory urography

Assessment of upper tract anatomy is performed after VCUG. Excretory urography (IVP) has been the standard for the evaluation of upper tract anatomy in children with febrile UTI. This study can assess the renal parenchyma, calyceal architecture, presence or absence of duplication, and renal atrophy. Excretory urographic signs suggestive of VUR include pyelonephritic scarring, ureteral dilatation (particularly the lower ureter), longitudinal striations or folds of the renal pelvis or upper ureters, and renal growth retardation. Ginalski *et al.* (1985) studied a group of 141 children undergoing surgery for VUR and found that preoperative excretory urography demonstrated signs suggestive of reflux in 68% of refluxing renal units. In 21% of renal units, renal growth retardation was the only radiographic sign; therefore, patients with renal growth retardation should undergo VCUG to rule out reflux. In patients undergoing excretory urography who have evidence of pyelonephritic scarring without obstruction, reflux may be found on VCUG in up to 85% (Scott and Stansfeld, 1968; Filly *et al.*, 1974; Govan *et al.*, 1975; Smellie *et al.*,

1975; Claësson and Lindberg, 1977; Shah *et al.*, 1978). Delayed emptying of the ureter after voiding suggests an abnormal distal ureteral segment and concomitant ureterovesical obstruction, which may occur in up to 10% of ureters with reflux (Weiss and Lytton, 1974).

Excretory urography should be delayed approximately 3–4 weeks after an acute UTI has cleared. Infection with coliform organisms may result in ureteral stasis, and excretory urography performed during infection may show dilated ureters (Teague and Boyarsky, 1968) (Fig. 25.1). However, children with a UTI who have persistent fever and symptoms despite antibiotic therapy should undergo excretory urography emergently to rule out obstruction.

Ultrasonography

Ultrasonography is a safe, accurate, and non-invasive test to study upper tract anatomy. This test can detect hydronephrosis, renal duplication in the presence of an obstructed upper pole segment, and gross renal scars. Renal ultrasonography should be performed in children with UTI and negative results on VCUG.

Isotope renography

Radioisotopic renal scanning is the most accurate test of upper tract function and evaluation of renal scars in patients with VUR. Technetium 99m (^{99m}Tc)-dimercaptosuccinic acid (DMSA) is the best agent for visualizing cortical tissue and evaluating the presence or absence of renal scarring. In large clinical series, DMSA scintigraphy has been shown to be much more sensitive than either excretory urography or ultrasonography in the diagnosis of acute pyelonephritis (Elison *et al.*, 1992). Rushton *et al.* (1988) studied experimentally induced pyelonephritis in piglets and found that DMSA scintigraphy correlated with histopathologic findings in 95% of animals. In

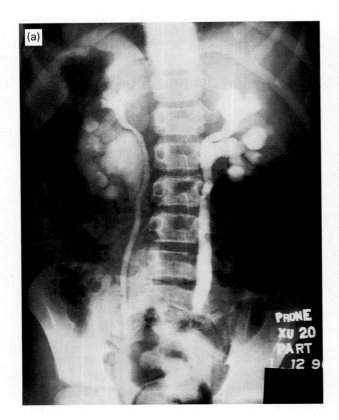

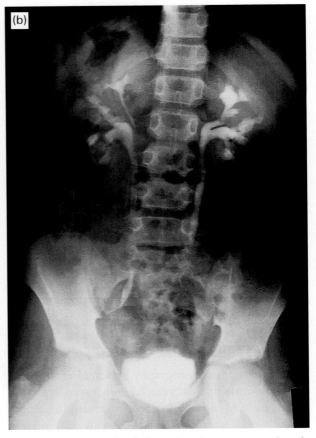

Figure 25.1 (*a*) Excretory urogram performed during acute pyelonephritis showing bilateral hydroureteronephrosis and duplication of the left collecting system. (*b*) Excretory urogram performed 6 weeks after pyelonephritis showing resolution of hydroureteronephrosis bilaterally. (From Kramer, 1992.)

follow-up clinical studies, these authors confirmed the accuracy of DMSA renal scans (Rushton *et al.* 1992) (see Chapter 10).

DMSA renal (single-photon emission computed tomography) SPECT is superior to planar DMSA in the detection of renal scarring due to acute pyelonephritis. These differences are particularly apparent in children younger than 3 years old (Yen *et al.*, 1996).

Classification and grading of reflux

The major etiologic categories of VUR include (1) primary VUR due to congenital malimplantation of the ureter with lateral ectopia; (2) chronic infection with edema and distortion of the ureterovesical angle; (3) bladder outlet obstruction with decompensation of the bladder and UVJ, such as a posterior urethral valve (PUV) and urethral stricture; (4) neuropathic bladder dysfunction with concomitant malfunction of the UVJ, such as myelomeningocele or paraplegia; and (5) traumatic reflux, which may occur after basket extraction of a ureteral calculus or surgical disruption of the UVJ.

The grading system used by the International Reflux Study Group places particular emphasis on the anatomy of the fornices and calyces (Fig. 25.2). Reflux is graded I–V. There are subtle variations within grades III and IV reflux (Fig. 25.3).

Urodynamic evaluation

Urodyamic studies (UDS), including cystometrography, electromyography, urinary flow studies with postvoid residual urines, and occasionally videourodynamics, may be helpful in selected patients with VUR. Preoperative UDS should be performed in patients with urgency, frequency, urge incontinence (uninhibited detrusor contractions), squatting maneuvers, or encopresis, all of which may suggest an occult neuropathic bladder with secondary reflux. These studies are also important in children with a sacral dimple, hairy patch, decreased perineal sensation, or decreased rectal tone. UDS is also indicated in children in whom the radiographic studies show sacral agenesis, dysgenesis, or a thick-walled or vertical bladder with diverticula and in patients with persistent VUR after a technically successful ureteroneocystostomy (Mesrobian *et al.*, 1985).

The results of cystometric studies are difficult to interpret in children with high grades of reflux. In patients with increased bladder pressure, the study is probably accurate, although much of the fluid is dissipated throughout the ureters and collecting system. A bladder with decreased compliance that has transmitted pressure through the UVJ and produces increased pressures with filling and voiding certainly places the upper tracts at risk for damage. Conversely, in patients with low detrusor pressures, reflux may cause false-negative results because of a pop-off mechanism from the incompetent ureteral orifice. Placement of Fogarty catheters into the ureteral orifices to prevent reflux at the time of cystometrography has been suggested (Woodside and Borden, 1982) but is very difficult in practice, and this technique is rarely used.

Patients with abnormal findings on UDS are clearly at higher risk for failure of ureteroneocystostomy.

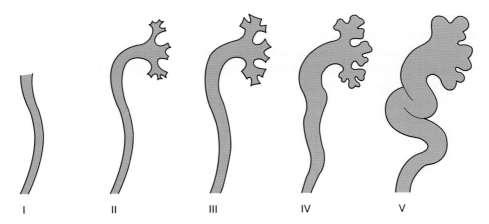

Figure 25.2 International Reflux Classification. (From Walker, 1987, with permission of Year Book Medical Publishers.)

Grade III   Grade IV

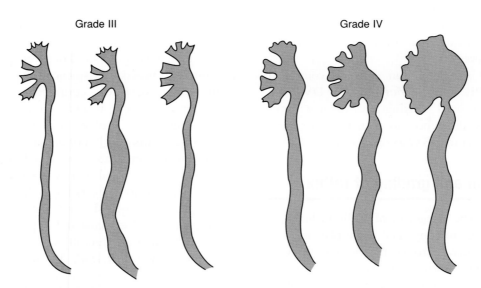

Figure 25.3 Variations with grade III and IV of the International Reflux Classification. (From Walker, 1987, with permission of Year Book Medical Publishers.)

These abnormal bladders should be treated medically before undergoing surgery. Children with detrusor instability or detrusor-sphincter dyssynergia may require frequent or timed voiding, double voiding, anticholinergic therapy, or intermittent catheterization before surgical correction of reflux (Koff and Murtagh, 1983). Patients with high-pressure voiding and decreased detrusor compliance may require pharmacologic therapy, intermittent catheterization, or augmentation cystoplasty in conjunction with ureteral reimplantation. (See discussion of antireflux surgery in the neuropathic bladder.)

Etiology and pathogenesis of primary reflux

The anatomic features that characterize the normal valve mechanism of the UVJ include an oblique entry of the ureter into the bladder (Harrison, 1888), an adequate length of the intramural ureter (especially of its submucosal segment) (Johnston, 1962; King *et al.*, 1974), and support of the detrusor muscle (King, 1976) (Fig. 25.4). The extravesical ureter consists of three muscle layers: an inner longitudinal, a middle circular, and an outer longitudinal layer. The ureteral adventitia and circular muscle layer continue into the bladder wall in the upper part of the ureteral hiatus to form Waldeyer's sheath, which attaches the ureter to the hiatus. This attachment is lax, and during bladder

filling, the hiatus can slide along the extravesical ureter. Within the bladder, the circular layer disappears and the longitudinal muscle fibers continue distally beyond the ureteral orifice into the trigone and intertwine with fibers from the contralateral ureter, forming Bell's muscle of the trigone and the posterior urethra (Mathisen, 1964) (Fig. 25.5). This anatomic complex acts as a single functional unit, and experimental interruption of this unit results in incompetence of the ureterovesical angle and VUR (Tanagho *et al.*, 1965). The well-established continuity between the ureter and the trigone (ureterotrigonal complex) prevents excessive mobility of the orifice by fixing it in position.

With bladder filling, the ureteral lumen is flattened between the bladder mucosa and the detrusor muscle, thereby creating a flap-valve mechanism that prevents VUR. This valve mechanism is probably more passive than active (Young and Wesson, 1921; Tanagho *et al.*, 1965). The passive nature of the mechanism of the ureterovesical angle is well demonstrated by the fact that reflux cannot be produced in a post-mortem specimen (Kelalis, 1985). During micturition, contraction of the detrusor muscle results in an increase in intravesical pressure, which may herniate the ureteral orifice through the wall of the bladder. This herniation does not occur with normal and adequate fixation of the ureterovesical junction, but it is likely to occur with maldevelopment of the trigonal region and lateral displacement of the ureteral orifice. The ureterotrigonal longitudinal muscles close the ureteral meatus

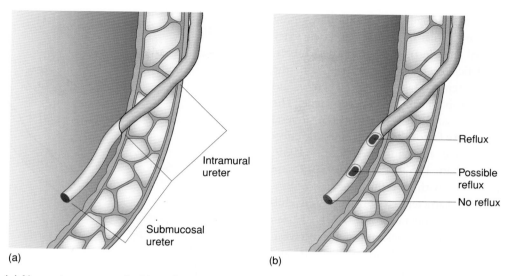

(a)   (b)

Figure 25.4 (*a*) Normal ureterovesical junction: demonstration of the length of the intravesical submucosal ureteral segment. (*b*) Refluxing ureterovesical junction: same anatomic features as non-refluxing orifice, except for an inadequate length of intravesical submucosal ureter, are shown. Some orifices reflux intermittently with borderline submucosal tunnels. (Modified from Politano, 1975, with permission of Lippincott Williams & Wilkins.)

and submucosal tunnel during a detrusor contraction and provide the 'active' component of the UVJ (Stephens and Lenaghan, 1962; Tanagho *et al.*, 1969).

The most important factor in maintaining the one-way characteristic of the UVJ is the occlusion of the ureteral lumen as the increase in intravesical pressure compresses it against the detrusor muscle. The ureteral orifice must be immobile and, thus, must have adequate detrusor support. Paraureteral diverticula tend to enlarge and to obliterate the submucosal tunnel by displacing the intramural ureter extravesically, resulting in incompetence of the ureterovesical junction.

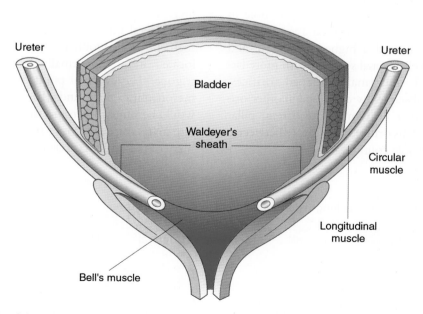

Figure 25.5 Passage of the ureter through the ureteral hiatus in the bladder wall. The drawing illustrates how Bell's muscle is a direct continuation of the longitudinal muscle of the ureter. (Modified from Mathisen, 1964, with permission of *Surgery, Gynecology and Obstetrics*.)

Primary VUR is a congenital condition resulting from an inadequate valvular mechanism and deficiency of the longitudinal muscle of the submucosal ureter. The degree of deficiency usually correlates with the degree of incompetence of the UVJ. There is no obstruction or neuropathic bladder component. The ratio of the submucosal tunnel length to the ureteral diameter is the primary factor that determines the effectiveness of this valve mechanism (Paquin, 1959; Stephens and Lenaghan, 1962). Paquin (1959) found that in normal children without reflux, the ratio of tunnel length to ureteral diameter was 5:1, whereas in children with reflux, the same ratio was 1.4:1. Cussen (1967) documented the relationship among intravesical ureteral length, submucosal ureteral length, and ureteral diameters in normal children (Table 25.1). The length of the intravesical ureter (intramural plus submucosal segments) has been estimated to average 1.3 cm in adults and 0.5 cm in neonates (Hutch, 1961).

Lyon *et al.* (1969) described four basic orifice shapes: cone, stadium, horseshoe, and golf-hole. The position (Fig. 25.6) and shape (Fig. 25.7) of the ureteral orifice correlate well with the length of the intravesical tunnel. Orifices that were placed laterally showed a higher incidence of reflux and probably had shorter submucosal tunnels. Lyon *et al.* (1969) found a 4% prevalence of reflux in patients with a normal orifice configuration, 28% incidence of reflux in those with a stadium orifice, 83% in those with a horseshoe shape, and 100% when the orifice was golf-hole in appearance. Heale (1979) confirmed Lyon's earlier observations and reported a higher prevalence and grade of reflux as well as renal scarring with more laterally placed and abnormally shaped orifices. Stephens (1980) subsequently described another orifice configuration that he termed the 'lateral pillar defect' (Fig. 25.7). This orifice lies midway between a horseshoe and golf-hole configuration.

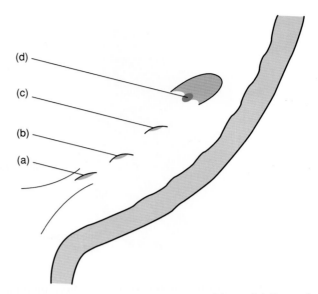

Figure 25.6 Four different orifice positions. (*a*) Normal position; (*b*) moderately lateral; (*c*) very lateral; (*d*) orifice at the mouth of a diverticulum. (From Glassberg *et al.*, 1987, with permission of the authors.)

Abnormal location and configuration of the ureteral orifice may be associated with developmental renal anomalies. The 'ureteral bud theory' proposed by Mackie and Stephens (1975) attempted to correlate renal morphology, based on a quantitative scale of hypoplasia and dysplasia, with the position of the ureteral orifice. These authors postulated that, when the ureteral bud did not arise from the appropriate segment of the wolffian duct, the ureteral orifice was located in an abnormally lateral position on the trigone. The eventual point of contact between the mesonephric duct and the nephrogenic blastema would be similarly ectopic, making it less likely to differentiate normally. More severe degrees of displacement of the orifice correlated well with high scores on

Table 25.1 Mean ureteral tunnel lengths and diameters in normal children

Age (years)	Intravesical ureteral length (mm)	Submucosal ureteral length (mm)	Ureteral diameter at ureterovesical junction (mm)
1–3	7	3	1.4
3–6	7	3	1.7
6–9	9	4	2.0
9–12	12	6	1.9

Adapted from Cussen (1967) with permission of Lippincott Williams & Wilkins.

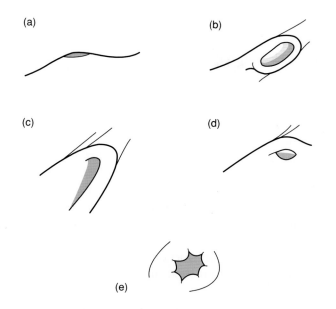

Figure 25.7 Orifice morphology. (a) Normal cone or volcanic orifice; (b) stadium orifice; (c) horseshoe orifice; (d) lateral pillar defect orifice; (e) golf-hole orifice. (From Glassberg et al., 1987, with permission of the authors.)

the hypoplasia/dysplasia scale (Fig. 25.8). Sommer and Stephens (1981) showed a correlation between an abnormal position of the ureteral orifice with reflux and associated renal dysplasia and scarring in children.

Reflux nephropathy can be present at birth without any prior UTI. This has been referred to as primary or congenital reflux nephropathy and corresponds to the abnormal ureteral bud theory of Mackie and Stephens (1975). These changes have been described in patients noted to have prenatal VUR and were proven as newborns on DMSA scan (Najmaldin et al., 1990; Gordon et al., 1990; Anderson and Rickwood, 1991).

Relationship of vesicoureteral reflux and renal scarring

Experimental studies

Although some studies suggest that renal scarring may occur on a congenital basis (Mackie and Stephens, 1975; Sommer and Stephens, 1981), the majority of

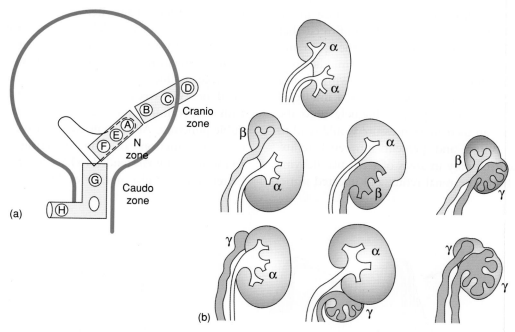

Figure 25.8 (a) Possible sites of ureteral orifices. Dissection of stillborn material reveals that orifices on the trigone in the normal position A or in the E and F positions are associated with normal (α) kidneys. Refluxing orifices in the B, C, or D positions are associated with hypoplastic (β) or dysplastic (γ) kidneys shown in (b). The more lateral the orifice, the worse the renal segment, because development in utero is apparently impaired if the ureteral bud arises from an abnormal position. (b) The renal segment in duplicated systems. A dark blue ureter indicates reflux. (From Mackie et al. (1975), with permission of WB Saunders Company.)

evidence supports the concept that renal scarring is an acquired phenomenon. The importance of intrarenal reflux in the pathogenesis of pyelonephritic scarring has been demonstrated experimentally. Intrarenal reflux is defined as the extension of refluxed urine into the collecting tubules of the nephrons. This theory provides a readily apparent mechanism by which urinary microorganisms may gain access to the renal parenchyma and produce renal scarring.

Ransley and Risdon (1975a) studied the effects of experimentally induced VUR on the papillary anatomy in piglets. Because the pig possesses renal papillary morphology similar to that in humans, this animal model is ideal to study the mechanisms of intrarenal reflux and renal scarring (Ransley and Risdon, 1975b). These authors studied the effect of low-pressure and high-pressure reflux under both sterile and infected conditions (Ransley and Risdon, 1978). The ureters of young Welsh pigs were cannulated and contrast medium was instilled through the catheter into the renal pelvis at a predetermined peak pressure (Ransley, 1978). The areas of renal parenchyma susceptible to intrarenal reflux and subsequent scarring were drained by papillae with flat or concave area cribrosa and large papillary ducts (Fig. 25.9). These concave papillae occurred predominantly in the polar regions of the kidney. VCUG confirmed that intrarenal reflux occurred exclusively at the upper and lower poles. Conversely, papillae in the middle areas of the renal medulla were cone-shaped with slit-like papillary ducts that closed with increased intrarenal pressure. These orifices opened obliquely onto the surface, so that an increase in pressure would tend to occlude the orifice and prevent intrarenal reflux. Scarring occurred only in areas of renal parenchyma exposed to both intrarenal reflux and infected urine.

Scarring did not occur in any animal subjected to either high-pressure or low-pressure sterile reflux. These elegant studies support the hypothesis that the development of new renal scars essentially occurs only in the presence of UTI, VUR, and intrarenal reflux (Edwards *et al.*, 1977; Ransley and Risdon, 1978; Torres *et al.*, 1984).

The only exception to this statement is the study by Hodson *et al.* (1975b) of sterile reflux in Sinclair miniature piglets. They placed a silver wire ring around the urethra to produce high intravesical pressures and promote intrarenal reflux. These experiments documented that sterile VUR could result in renal scarring experimentally, but only in the presence of severe outlet obstruction. Intrarenal reflux was essential for scar formation, and the severity and duration of intrarenal reflux correlated well with the degree of renal scarring (Hodson and Edwards, 1960).

Torres *et al.* (1984) studied the effect of bacterial immunization on experimental reflux nephropathy in piglets. These authors used the experimental model of reflux nephropathy described by Hodson *et al.* (1975b) and modified by Ransley and Risdon (1978). Male piglets underwent surgical creation of VUR at 2 weeks of age. Between the ages of 2 and 6 weeks, one-half of the piglets received subcutaneous injections of formalin-killed alum-precipitated *Escherichia coli* in incomplete Freund's adjuvant and one-half received incomplete Freund's adjuvant and vehicle alone. At 6 weeks of age, all piglets were infected with an identical strain of *E. coli* introduced by suprapubic puncture. All animals were killed 6 weeks after the introduction of the infecting organisms. Immunized animals tended to have less renal scarring, better renal tubular uptake of DMSA, significantly

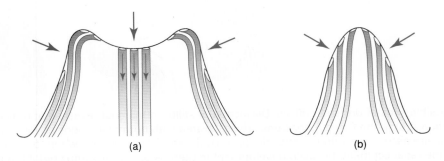

Figure 25.9 Anatomy of confluent and simple papillae. (*a*) Concave; (*b*) cone-shaped. (Modified from Ransley 1977, with permission of Springer-Verlag.)

lower serum creatinine values, and less mesangial cell proliferation in glomeruli than their non-immunized counterparts. The authors concluded that previous exposure to a specific bacterial strain and bacterial immunization had at least a mild protective effect on the development of reflux nephropathy. In a subsequent study, Torres *et al.* (1985) reviewed various pathogenetic factors that were thought to be important in the development of reflux nephropathy. The three independent risk factors studied were (1) radiographic evidence of intrarenal reflux, (2) P-fimbriation of the bacterial strain, and (3) absence of previous immunization. Animals with no or only one risk factor had significantly less scarring, fewer glomerular lesions, and lower serum creatinine values than animals with two or three factors present. The authors concluded that in the experimental animal, several independent pathogenetic factors appear to have a synergistic effect on the development of reflux nephropathy.

The initial immunologic response in acute renal infection and the early formation of renal scars have been studied in rat models by direct inoculation of *E. coli* into the kidneys or into the systemic circulation or bladder in combination with transient ureteral obstruction. Active production of antibodies against the invading organism occurs systemically and in the kidney. During these inoculations, there is a depression of the cell-mediated immunity to non-specific stimulants that is secondary to the generation of a suppressor-lymphocyte population in response to renal infection. Many of the basic observations in the rat and pig models of pyelonephritis have been reproduced, expanded, and brought closer to the human disease in a primate model developed by Roberts *et al.* (1985). They postulated that the final determinant of renal scarring is that intrarenal reflux, in the presence of infection, causes an exudative reaction with the release of oxygen free radicals and proteolytic enzymes that develop in fibrosis and scarring. These investigators injected a bacterial inoculum into the renal pelvis of primates and produced intrarenal reflux, demonstrating that infected urine could produce renal scarring in the absence of VUR or obstruction.

Superoxide, an enzyme toxic to the renal tubular cells, is produced by neutrophils during the process of phagocytosis of bacteria. Roberts *et al.* (1982) postulated that the pathogenesis of renal scarring was the result of the inflammatory response itself and that superoxide was responsible for renal parenchymal damage. Administration of superoxide dismutase, an antagonist of superoxide, prevented tubular cell damage without interfering with phagocytosis of bacteria.

Urinary extravasation in the renal interstitium may provoke renal damage either by directly eliciting fibrosis or by initiating an autoimmune reaction against Tamm–Horsfall protein (THP), even in the absence of urinary infection (Cotran and Pennington, 1981). This mucoprotein, a normal constituent of urine, is produced in high concentration by the tubular epithelial cells of the loop of Henle and distal nephron and is a primary constituent of renal tubular casts. Immunofluorescent techniques have demonstrated extratubular THP in the interstitium of kidneys with VUR and intrarenal reflux. Such deposits of the protein are associated with inflammatory infiltrates and fibrosis. Although extratubular THP may serve as a marker for urinary extravasation, further investigations regarding the role of THP and extratubular urinary extravasation are warranted.

Clinical studies

Hodson (1959) was the first to recognize the frequent occurrence of renal scars in children with recurrent UTI. Of children with renal scars, 97% showed radiographic evidence of VUR. Hodson *et al.* (1975b) proposed that segmental scarring in chronic atrophic pyelonephritis was due to the reflux of urine into the tubules of the kidney, which either carried infection into the parenchyma or damaged the kidney by urodynamic forces. Hodson and Edwards (1960) observed that the scars were most often polar in location and associated with calyceal clubbing.

Bailey (1973) coined the term 'reflux nephropathy' to describe the radiographic abnormality of renal scarring in the presence of VUR. Hinman and Baumann (1973) introduced the terms 'high-pressure reflux' and 'low-pressure reflux' to indicate reflux that occurred during bladder filling (low pressure) and reflux that occurred during voiding (high pressure).

Studies of papillary morphology in human kidneys indicate that at least two-thirds of papillae are concave and allow intrarenal reflux (Ransley and Risdon, 1978). Intrarenal reflux has been observed in 5–15%

of neonates and infants with VUR (Rose *et al.*, 1975). Rolleston *et al.* (1970) detected intrarenal reflux only in children younger than 5 years and only in those with moderate to severe degrees of reflux. Rolleston *et al.* (1970) observed that infants with severe reflux were more likely to have renal damage than children with lesser degrees of reflux. Furthermore, there was a significant correlation between the presence of intrarenal reflux and the subsequent development of renal scarring in the affected area.

The characteristic scarring associated with reflux nephropathy is frequently present at the time of the initial diagnosis. Renal scars usually develop during the first few years of life and rarely after the age of 5 years (Rolleston *et al.*, 1974; Smellie and Normand, 1979). The studies by Ransley and Risdon (1978, 1981), among others (Tamminen and Kaprio, 1977; Funston and Cremin, 1978; Cremin, 1979), provided a possible explanation for this development of scars early in life. Those areas of the kidney that are drained by compound papillae are susceptible to intrarenal reflux and vulnerable to the damaging effects of VUR of infected urine (Ransley and Risdon, 1978, 1981). During the first weeks of life, small amounts of pressure in the renal pelvis can produce intrarenal reflux into these vulnerable areas of the kidney. Thereafter, increasing amounts of pressure are necessary to produce a similar effect (Funston and Cremin, 1978). Scars develop in these areas at the time of the first urinary infection during infancy, whereas the remaining areas drain by non-refluxing papillae and remain unscarred despite persistence of the VUR and recurrent UTI. Marginally refluxing papillae may be transformed into refluxing papillae by (1) high-pressure voiding, (2) hydronephrosis, or (3) scarring and associated contraction from other susceptible areas of the kidney. This sequence of events accounts for the diffusely scarred kidney sometimes seen on excretory urography.

Becu *et al.* (1988) proposed a different mechanism for the pathogenesis of renal scarring. These authors studied 27 kidneys from children with a diagnosis of primary non-obstructive reflux who underwent nephrectomy. They concluded that the decreased size of deformities present in patients with reflux nephropathy was the result of either a dysplastic developmental arrest or a primary dwarfism with focal segmental tubular atrophy and glomerular obsolescence rather than an inflammatory response.

Synopsis of experimental and clinical studies

Experimental evidence and clinical observation suggest that the pathogenesis of reflux nephropathy is multifactorial. An interactive view of the different mechanisms that have been proposed to explain the pathogenesis of reflux nephropathy and the more rare development of progressive renal insufficiency is illustrated in Figure 25.10. Although the clinical relevance of some of the proposed mechanisms remains controversial, the multifactorial concept of the pathogenesis of reflux nephropathy helps us to understand the spectrum of clinical observations.

Vesicoureteral reflux and urinary tract infections

Hodson and Edwards (1960) showed that reflux occurred more commonly in children with UTI than in those with sterile urine. VUR has been documented in 29–50% of children with UTI undergoing VCUG (Kunin *et al.*, 1964; Savage *et al.*, 1969; Shopfner, 1970; Wein and Schoenberg, 1972; Levitt and Weiss, 1985). In children with UTI, the prevalence of VUR is inversely proportional to age (Baker *et al.*, 1966; Smellie *et al.*, 1975). In a group of patients with UTI, reflux occurred in 70% of those younger than 1 year of age, in 25% of children at 4 years of age, in 15% at 12 years of age, and in 5.2% of adults (Baker *et al.*, 1966). Walker (1987) studied a group of young girls with asymptomatic bacteriuria and found that reflux occurred in 29% of preschool-aged children but in only 23% of school-aged children.

Govan and Palmer (1969) showed that children with reflux tended to present with UTI approximately 2 years earlier than children with UTI and no reflux. Conversely, others (Smellie *et al.*, 1981b) found no age difference at presentation among children with UTI with or without VUR. From 30 to 40% of patients investigated for renal insufficiency and found to have radiographic features of reflux nephropathy have no definite history of UTI (Bakshandeh *et al.*, 1976). These observations may be explained in that UTIs in infants and children are underdiagnosed and scarring often occurs early in life when the history is obscure and the presenting symptoms of infection may be mistaken for another febrile illness. Transient febrile illnesses with non-specific symptomatology are

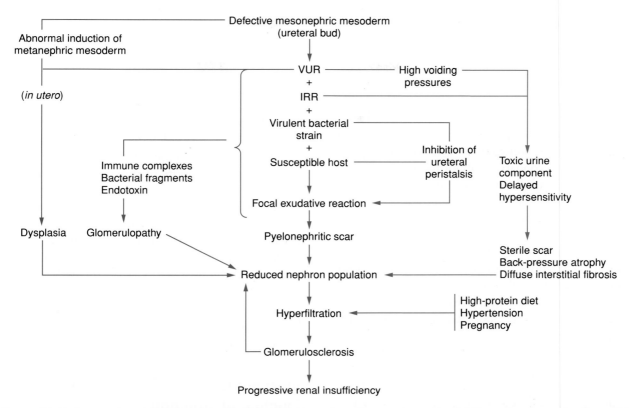

Figure 25.10 Integrative view of pathogenetic mechanisms in reflux nephropathy. VUR, vesicoureteral reflux; IRR, intrarenal reflux. (Modified from Kramer, 1984, with permission of William J. Miller Associates.)

generally not considered indications for urinary culture in the usual pediatric practice.

In 1980 an international prospective randomized clinical trial was initiated among a group of major teaching hospitals in the USA and Europe (Levitt and Weiss, 1985). Patients with primary grade IV (International Classification) reflux were accepted into the trial as well as patients with grade III reflux beyond infancy in the European group. Several important observations were noted after 5 years of study. The incidence of UTIs developing during the first 5 years of follow-up was similar between the medically and surgically treated groups. However, the incidence of pyelonephritis was statistically higher in the medically treated group (Jodal *et al.*, 1992).

Calculi

The occurrence of primary VUR and urinary calculi in infants and children has been reported infrequently (Malek and Kelalis, 1975). The incidence of VUR in patients with calculi is approximately 8%, whereas 0.5% of patients with VUR have calculi (Roberts and Atwell, 1989). VCU should be performed routinely in children with staghorn calculi (Malek, 1976; Lue *et al.*, 1982).

Secondary vesicoureteral reflux

Infectious

UTI can produce VUR (Jeffs and Allen, 1962; Schoenberg *et al.*, 1964; Kaveggia *et al.*, 1966), and infection may delay spontaneous resolution of reflux (Roberts and Riopelle, 1978). Transient reflux may occur in a marginally competent ureterovesical orifice because of bladder inflammation or infection. Reflux secondary to UTI will generally resolve spontaneously with treatment of the infection and disappearance of the inflammatory changes at the UVJ. VUR may predispose children to UTI by contributing to increased residual urine, which acts as a fertile incubation medium for urinary pathogens in susceptible children.

Neuropathic

Neuropathic dysfunction is an important cause of secondary VUR (Hinman and Baumann, 1973; Allen, 1985). Reflux can occur in conjunction with a neuropathic bladder in 15–60% of patients (Woods and Atwell, 1982; Sidi *et al.*, 1986). Dysfunctional voiding due to detrusor-sphincter dyssynergia and uninhibited detrusor contractions can be an acquired phenomenon secondary to abnormal voiding. These abnormal voiding patterns may result in high intravesical pressure and UTIs and produce VUR in patients with a previously normal VCU (Kondo *et al.*, 1983).

The association of infection, reflux, uninhibited bladder contractions, infrequent voiding, and constipation in neurologically normal children has been well documented (Koff and Murtagh, 1983; Nasrallah and Simon, 1984; Seruca, 1989; Koff *et al.*, 1998). The peak incidence of VUR occurs in children between 3 and 5 years of age. This period is also the peak age for dysfunctional voiding (Allen, 1985). The most common urodynamic abnormality in patients with VUR is uninhibited bladder contractions, and this correlates clinically with urgency, frequency, urge incontinence, and nocturnal enuresis (Taylor, 1984; Homsy *et al.*, 1985). Taylor *et al.* (1982) showed that 75% of girls with reflux had evidence of uninhibited bladder contractions. Reflux has been observed in approximately 50% of children with UTI undergoing urodynamic evaluation for an abnormal voiding pattern (Allen 1979; Koff and Murtagh, 1983). The majority of patients with breakthrough UTIs will have dysfunctional voiding or constipation. Furthermore, these patients have delayed reflux resolution, are at increased risk for pyelonephritis and renal scarring, and account for the majority of failed ureteral reimplantations (Naseer and Steinhardt, 1997).

Koff and Murtagh (1983) treated 62 neurologically normal children who had VUR with and without uninhibited bladder contractions. They found that patients with uninhibited contractions treated with anticholinergic therapy showed a statistically significant improvement in resolution of recurrent UTI and reflux when compared with a control group of children with normal cystometric findings. Homsy *et al.* (1985) and Seruca (1989) reported equally good success in treating children with voiding dysfunction with anticholinergic therapy. They observed significant resolution or reduction (or both) in the stage of reflux in the majority of children treated. Clearly, bladder instability can be an important factor in causing and perpetuating reflux, and therapy directed at decreasing intravesical pressures could decrease the incidence of UTI and VUR.

The acceptance and effectiveness of clean intermittent catheterization as a means to drain the bladder and the use of anticholinergic medication to lower bladder pressures have obviated the need for urinary diversion in the majority of children with neuropathic bladder due to meningomyelocele (Bauer *et al.*, 1982). Most low-grade reflux in these patients resolves with intermittent catheterization and pharmacologic therapy (Nasrallah and Simon, 1984; Taylor, 1984). In a large series of children with reflux and neuropathic bladder, 124 of 200 (62%) either ceased to have reflux or the reflux was downgraded while the patient was maintained on intermittent catheterization and antibiotic prophylaxis (Kaplan and Firlit, 1983).

Vesicoureteral reflux and ureteropelvic junction obstruction

The coexistence of VUR and ureteropelvic junction (UPJ) obstruction is well documented (Whitaker, 1976; DeKlerk *et al.*, 1979; Lebowitz and Blickman, 1983; Maizels *et al.*, 1984). The incidence of reflux in large series of patients with UPJ obstruction ranges from 5 to 24% (Lebowitz and Blickman, 1983; Kelalis and Kramer, 1987; Hollowell *et al.*, 1989). Maizels *et al.* (1984) found VUR in 11 of 124 patients (9%) undergoing pyeloplasty. In a retrospective series of 200 children with UPJ obstruction, Lebowitz and Blickman (1983) found that 10% had associated VUR. In a study of 120 patients with UPJ obstruction undergoing VCUG, Hollowell *et al.* (1989) found that 17 (14%) demonstrated VUR. In each of these studies, the majority of patients had incidental reflux that resolved spontaneously over time.

The incidence of UPJ obstruction in patients with VUR ranges from 0.8 to 14% (Lebowitz and Blickman, 1983; Hollowell *et al.*, 1989; Leighton and Mayne, 1989). In a retrospective review of 2800 patients with VUR, Lebowitz and Blickman (1983) found UPJ obstruction in 0.8%. 'Apparent' UPJ obstruction is suggested at VCUG when there is disproportionate ureteral and pelvic dilatation, the pelvis being more dilated than the ureter. A delayed

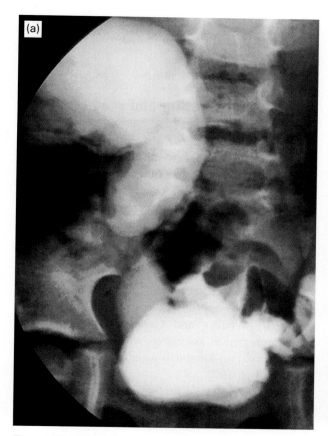 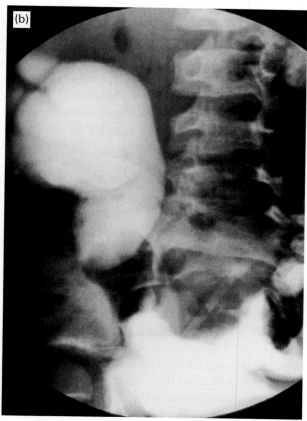

Figure 25.11 Voiding cystourethrography showing (*a*) massive reflux into the right kidney and (*b*) delayed drainage in the lower pole of a duplex kidney consistent with secondary ureteropelvic junction obstruction.

drainage film may resolve the question, but a lasix-stimulated renal scan may be necessary for final determination. Patients with significant VUR and concomitant UPJ obstruction secondary to fixed kinks should undergo primary pyeloplasty (Maizels *et al.*, 1984) (Fig. 25.11). Primary ureteral reimplantation may provoke an acute UPJ decompensation and obstruction that requires subsequent pyeloplasty (Hollowell *et al.*, 1989; Leighton and Mayne, 1989). Ureteral reimplantation should be reserved for patients with persistent high-grade reflux after successful pyeloplasty (Kelalis and Kramer, 1987).

Vesicoureteral reflux in siblings

The familial incidence of VUR among siblings of patients with reflux ranges from 8 to 45% (Tobenkin, 1964; Van den Abbeele *et al.*, 1987). This compares with a prevalence of less than 1% spontaneous VUR cases in the general population. Although the pattern of genetic transmission is undetermined, investigators favor a polygenic or multifactorial mode of inheritance (Burger and Burger, 1974; Levitt and Weiss, 1985). Dwoskin (1976) found 26.5% of siblings to have VUR from 125 families of probands with reflux. Noe (1992) screened 354 siblings of 275 patients who had VUR and found that 119 (34%) had reflux. There was no evidence of either UTI or voiding dysfunction in 75% of these siblings. The highest incidence of reflux was found in the siblings of patients with radiographic evidence of renal scarring. Twenty per cent of siblings of patients with dysfunctional voiding demonstrated reflux. In patients without symptoms of bladder dysfunction, 38% of siblings had reflux. In both groups, reflux in siblings occurred unrelated to grade, scarring, frequency of infections, or age of the index case.

In a large series of patients with VUR, Connolly *et al.* (1997) found reflux in 37% of siblings. However, when siblings older than 6 years were screened, the detection rate decreased to 7%. Puri *et al.* (1998)

screened 624 consecutive patients with reflux and identified 44% of siblings with reflux. Buonomo *et al.* (1993) reviewed 16 symptom-free siblings of children with VUR and found six (38%) to have scarring on DMSA renal scanning. They recommended early screening of siblings in order to detect renal damage.

Most pediatric urologists obtain a radionuclide VCUG in younger siblings of index patients with reflux (Noe, 1995). In those with documented reflux, upper tract evaluation with excretory urography, ultrasonography, or isotope renography is recommended. Noe *et al.* (1992) reported that 66% of the offspring of children with reflux exhibited reflux and recommended screening the offspring of all patients with a history of reflux.

Vesicoureteral reflux in boys

In the first year of life, particularly in infancy, the majority of VUR occurs in boys. Most of these infant boys have increased voiding detrusor pressures and higher grades of reflux than their female counterparts. Throughout the first several months of life, voiding pressures decrease, detrusor hyperreflexia resolves, and postvoid residuals improve (Chandra *et al.*, 1996; Sillen *et al.*, 1996). In these selected patients, the rate of spontaneous resolution is approximately 60% for grade IV reflux and up to 40% for grade V (Fichtner *et al.*, 1993).

There are only a few series of males with primary VUR. Decter *et al.* (1988) reported 86 boys with VUR, two-thirds of whom presented because of UTI, and 15% had symptoms of voiding dysfunction without infection. Approximately 20% of patients had renal scars at diagnosis. Boys with low-grade reflux who presented with UTI were treated initially with antibiotics, but the therapy was discontinued as they grew older. Older boys with low-grade reflux who had not presented with a UTI were only observed. These patients were assumed to be at minimal risk for scarring after urinary infection, and long-term antibiotic therapy and aggressive follow-up were not necessary. Decisions for surgery were based on persistent reflux and the cystoscopic assessment of the orifice position, configuration, and tunnel length, although it is unclear what clinical significance this has. Seventy-three per cent of boys underwent surgery because of high-grade reflux or abnormal location of the orifice on cystoscopy. Thirteen per cent had

reimplantation because of breakthrough UTI, 10% because of age and 3.3% because of progressive scarring.

Vesicoureteral reflux and pregnancy

Physiologic changes in the urinary tract during pregnancy result from the secretion of prostaglandins and progesterone-like hormones and often produce decreased peristalsis, ureteral tortuosity, and hydro-ureteronephrosis. Anatomic changes include lateral displacement of the intravesical ureter, a perpendicular course of the distal ureter, and ureteral obstruction from the gravid uterus. The prevalence of asymptomatic bacteriuria during pregnancy is between 4 and 7%. Pyelonephritis occurs in 20–40% of pregnant women with asymptomatic bacteriuria (Heidrick *et al.*, 1967; Whalley and Cunningham, 1977) and when untreated is associated with premature labor, prematurity, and low-birth-weight babies (Mattingly and Borkowf, 1978).

Heidrick *et al.* (1967) reported a disproportionately high incidence of acute pyelonephritis during pregnancy in women with recurrent bacteriuria and reflux compared with women without reflux (Hutch, 1961). Williams *et al.* (1968) evaluated 100 women with asymptomatic bacteriuria during pregnancy, all of whom were treated with an acute course of antibiotic therapy. Cystography performed 4–6 months postpartum showed VUR in 21 patients. The incidence of bacteriuria after delivery was higher in patients with reflux (63%) than in those without reflux (16%). Furthermore, the incidence of renal scarring was also higher in women with reflux (48%) than in those without reflux (9%). Bacteriuria was more difficult to clear during pregnancy, despite antibiotic therapy, in patients with reflux (33%) compared with those without reflux (67%) ($P < 0.0005$) (Williams *et al.*, 1968).

In a series of 41 women, all with a history of childhood UTIs, the women with persistent reflux developed more pyelonephritis (37%) than those without reflux (6%). All patients with VUR who developed pyelonephritis had renal scars (Martinell *et al.*, 1990). Patients with renal scars were at higher risk for bacteriuria (47%), pyelonephritis (13%), and hypertension (37%) than women without scars.

Austenfeld and Snow (1988) reviewed the records of 67 women who had undergone surgical correction of reflux by ureteroneocystostomy and had a minimum of 15 years of follow-up. Thirty women became pregnant, for a total of 64 pregnancies. During pregnancy, 17 of 30 women (57%) had one or more UTIs and five of 30 (17%) had one or more episodes of pyelonephritis. The incidence of pyelonephritis during pregnancy (17%) was statistically higher than the 4% incidence of pyelonephritis in these women before pregnancy. There were eight spontaneous abortions. These results suggest that women with surgically corrected reflux are at greater risk for pyelonephritis than controls. In a follow-up study from the same institution, Mansfield *et al.* (1995) reviewed the incidence of bacteriuria in women with a history of VUR. In sexually active women who had undergone ureteroneocystostomy, 75% developed bacteriuria and 65% developed bacteriuria during pregnancy. In sexually active women with a history of VUR who did not undergo reimplantation, 62% developed bacteriuria with sexual activity but only 15% had bacteriuria with pregnancy. Fetal loss was 15% among those with a history of ureteroneocystostomy and 18% among those without ureteroneocystostomy. This study suggests that there are pregnant women with a history of childhood UTIs who are at risk for pyelonephritis during pregnancy regardless of whether their VUR was corrected.

Pregnancy has been shown in long-term studies of women with moderate renal failure to have an adverse effect on renal function (Becker *et al.*, 1986). The outcome of pregnancy in women with reflux nephropathy is dependent on the degree of renal impairment and the presence of hypertension and proteinuria (Jungers *et al.*, 1986; Weaver and Craswell, 1987). Women with hypertension and moderate renal insufficiency in the initial stages of pregnancy are at risk for hypertension and accelerated decline in renal function during pregnancy. Kincaid-Smith and Fairley (1987) noted that 36% of women with moderate renal insufficiency developed hypertension and 8% had accelerated decline in renal function throughout pregnancy.

Renal scarring, particularly bilateral, and renal insufficiency are the real threats to maternal complications and fetal loss (Jungers *et al.*, 1996). In a series of 41 women with 77 pregnancies, women with renal scarring or hypertension were at significantly increased risk for pre-eclampsia, premature birth, and acute renal failure (Bukowski *et al.*, 1998). In a series of 345 pregnancies, el-Khatib *et al.* (1994) reported 137 with reflux nephropathy. Of this group, fetal loss

was 12% and maternal complications were 39%. These complications occurred only in patients with bilateral scarring and impaired renal function (creatinine > 1.2 mg/dl). Women with VUR and no scars were not at increased risk for complications.

The critical risk factors for pyelonephritis during pregnancy include (1) the presence of pathogenic bacteria, (2) a history of childhood UTIs, (3) renal scarring with or without reflux, and (4) chronic renal insufficiency. The arguments for repair of VUR prior to pregnancy include attempts to decrease potential pregnancy complications such as pyelonephritis and further renal deterioration in patients with scars. The arguments against repair of VUR include evidence that further development of renal scarring is minimal in adults, ureteroneocystostomy has not been proven to protect pregnant women from pyelonephritis (Austenfeld and Snow, 1988), and ureteroneocystostomy has not been proven to prevent renal deterioration in patients with established scars (Malek *et al.*, 1983b).

The options for the management of the adolescent girl with VUR include (1) discontinuing antibiotic prophylaxis and observation, (2) continuing prophylaxis indefinitely, (3) endoscopic repair of VUR, and (4) ureteroneocystostomy. Most pediatric urologists have traditionally advocated correcting persistent reflux in adolescent girls. The author's recommendation is to (1) correct dysfunctional voiding and constipation, (2) discontinue prophylactic antibiotics at 8–9 years of age in girls with mild VUR and no history of breakthrough UTIs, (3) correct reflux in those with renal scarring because these patients are at increased risk for pyelonephritis during pregnancy, (4) screen for bacteriuria during pregnancy and consider prophylaxis, and (5) consider prophylaxis for pregnant patients with scars and no reflux and follow them indefinitely because of the risk of hypertension.

Medical management of reflux

Natural history

The natural tendency for VUR is to improve or resolve spontaneously over time, and this observation should warrant initial medical management of most patients with low-grade reflux. There is a strong inverse correlation between the severity of reflux at the time of initial diagnosis and the likelihood of spontaneous resolution. The resolution or persistence of reflux is related directly to the location and configuration of the UVJ. Elongation of the submucosal tunnel with growth increases the ratio between the length of the submucosal tunnel and the diameter of the ureter and tends to correct the abnormality of the valve mechanism (Stephens and Lenaghan, 1962; King *et al.*, 1974). Spontaneous cessation of VUR occurs significantly more often in children with unilateral than with bilateral reflux (Tamminen-Mobius *et al.*, 1992).

Several objective criteria can be used to predict the chance of resolution of VUR. The presence of ureteral dilatation, abnormal position and configuration of the ureteral orifice, and a paraureteral diverticulum, particularly when the ureter enters the diverticulum, all suggest the need for surgical intervention. Smellie and Normand (1979) observed spontaneous resolution of VUR in 80% of kidneys with undilated ureters on VCU (grades I and II). Edwards *et al.* (1977) found that reflux ceased spontaneously in 85% of children with ureters of normal caliber. Conversely, only 41% of kidneys with ureteral dilatation and grade III, IV, or V reflux underwent spontaneous resolution of reflux (Smellie and Normand, 1979). In a surveillance study of children with VUR observed for 4–10 years, King *et al.* (1974) reported no cases of spontaneous cure of reflux when the orifice was golf-hole in shape and when there was absence of an intravesical ureter. In a large retrospective series, Skoog *et al.* (1987) showed that reflux resolved in approximately 90% of those with grade I, 80% with grade II, 50% with grade III, 10% with grade IV, and essentially none with grade V. In the series of Duckett (1983), reflux resolved spontaneously in 63% of patients with grade II, 53% of those with grade III, and 33% of those with grade IV reflux. In most series, conservative medical treatment of grade IV VUR has been shown to be less successful than surgery (Scholtmeijer, 1993).

It had been suggested that spontaneous resolution of reflux most often occurs within the first few years after diagnosis and the rate of reflux resolution remains constant throughout childhood, at approximately 10–15% per year (Smellie and Normand, 1979). Puberty has not been associated with an increased rate of spontaneous cessation of reflux (Edwards *et al.*, 1977). In a large series of children with VUR, moderate grades of VUR almost always resolved within a 4-year period of observation and were not likely to resolve after that interval (McLorie *et al.*, 1990). This group included 112 patients (86 female and 26 male) with grade III, IV, or V reflux who were observed non-operatively. Sixty-one patients had grade III, 38 had grade IV, and 13 had grade V reflux. Of the patients with grade III reflux, 21% had resolution of reflux in an average of 2.6 years. Grade IV reflux resolved in only one patient after 2.9 years of follow-up, and 86% of patients with grade IV reflux ultimately had surgical correction. Patients with grade V reflux clearly benefited from early surgical repair.

The Pediatric VUR Guidelines Panel retrospectively reviewed large series of patients treated with continuous antibiotic therapy (Elder *et al.*, 1997). The probability of reflux resolution with continuous prophylaxis is shown in Figure 25.12 and Figure 25.13. Lower grades of reflux correlated with a better chance of spontaneous resolution. In children with grades I and II reflux, there was no difference in patient age at presentation or laterality with respect to resolution of reflux. In patients with grade III reflux, patient age and laterality (unilateral versus bilateral) were important prognostic indicators. Older children and those with bilateral reflux had less chance of undergoing spontaneous resolution of reflux. Patients with bilateral grade IV reflux most often underwent surgical correction.

Vesicoureteral reflux and growth

Renal growth

The effect of reflux on growth of the kidney is related to the presence of a normal or abnormal contralateral kidney, infection of the urinary tract, and the grade of VUR in the affected kidney. Claësson *et al.* (1981) found compensatory hypertrophy in the contralateral normal kidney in patients with unilateral reflux and scarring. Children with VUR and recurrent UTI are clearly at increased risk for renal scars and renal growth retardation (Hannerz *et al.*, 1989). Smellie *et al.* (1981a) studied the effects of VUR on renal growth in a series of 76 children with various degrees of reflux. Renal growth was impaired in only those patients with documented UTI and higher grades of reflux (Tables 25.2, 25.3). Lyon (1973) and Redman *et al.* (1974) used bipolar renal measurements and

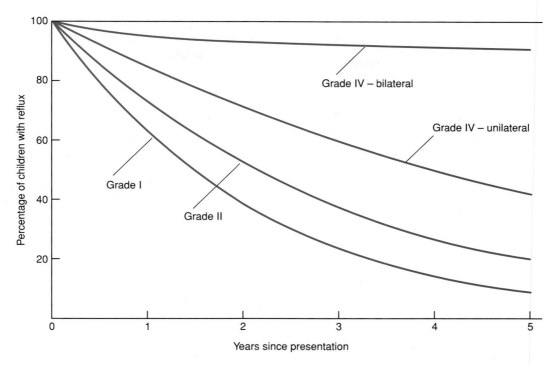

Figure 25.12 Per cent chance of reflux persistence for 1–5 years after presentation for reflux grades I, II, and IV. (Modified from Elder *et al.*, 1997, with permission of Lippincott Williams & Wilkins.)

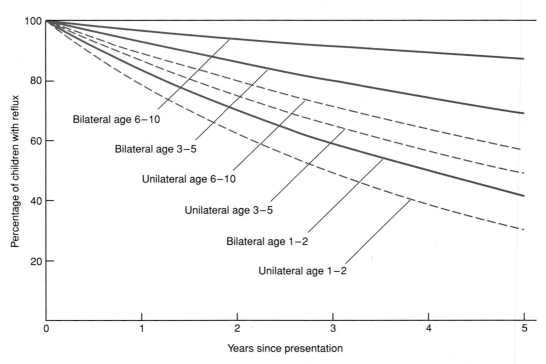

Figure 25.13 Per cent chance of reflux persistence for 1–5 years after presentation for grade III reflux by patient age at presentation. (From Elder *et al.*, 1997, with permission of Lippincott Williams & Wilkins.)

Table 25.2 Renal growth in 111 kidneys with vesicoureteral reflux related to recurrence of infection during 791 kidney-years of observation[a]

Renal growth	Infection	No infection	Total
Normal	20	80	100
Slow	10	1	11

[a] $\xi^2 = 25.3$, df $= 1$, $p = 0.001$.
From Smellie *et al.* (1981a), with permission of the journal.

Table 25.3 Renal growth in 111 kidneys with vesicoureteral reflux related to grade of reflux on first diagnosis[a]

Renal growth	Vesicoureteral reflux[b]		
	Grades I–III	Grade IV	Total
Accelerated or normal	88	12[c]	100
Slow	5	6[d]	11

[a] $\xi^2 = 13.20$, df $= 1$, $p = 0.001$.
[b] Grade I reflux was minimal, grades II and III extended up to the kidney without dilatation, grade II on voiding only. Grade IV included all reflux with dilatation of the ureter or renal pelvis.
[c] Three kidneys were scarred.
[d] Five kidneys were scarred; all six were exposed to infection. From Smellie *et al.* (1981a), with permission of the journal.

observed a subnormal rate of renal growth in the presence of VUR without documented UTI.

Various methods have been used to evaluate renal growth, including determinations of renal length, renal area, and parenchymal thickness (Currarino, 1965; Gatewood *et al.*, 1965; Klare *et al.*, 1980). Sequential measurements of renal length by excretory urography are inaccurate (Redman *et al.*, 1974; Hodson, 1975a; Hodson, 1979). Scar formation occurs predominantly at the renal poles, and this contracture, combined with intervening hypertrophy of normal parenchyma, makes interpretation of renal size by using renal length alone unreliable. Hodson (1979) and Hodson *et al.* (1975a) recommended calculating the ratio of bipolar parenchymal thickness to total renal length. In a study of patients with renal duplication, Hannerz *et al.* (1989) found that parenchymal thickness was a more accurate predictor of renal growth than either renal length or renal area.

Several authors reported accelerated renal growth after successful antireflux surgery (McRae *et al.*, 1974; Willscher *et al.*, 1976b; Atwell and Vijay, 1978; Ginalski *et al.*, 1985). Scott and Stansfeld (1968) reported that successful ureteral reimplantation produced a significant increase in renal growth compared with medical management. In a series of 22 patients with a unilateral atrophic kidney and VUR, significant growth of the atrophic kidney was observed in 15 of 22 patients (68%) after ureteral reimplantation (Carson *et al.*, 1982). In seven of 22 children (32%), the small kidney grew proportionally to its mate, suggesting that preservation of small atrophic kidneys is more appropriate than nephrectomy.

Hagberg *et al.* (1984) studied renal growth after ureteral reimplantation for gross reflux in infancy. In infants in whom the kidneys already had significant parenchymal loss at presentation, an early antireflux operation did not influence renal growth significantly. However, kidneys that had minimal parenchymal reduction at presentation showed normal growth postoperatively but did not 'catch up' to normal kidney size.

Willscher *et al.* (1976b) reported on 94 children who had antireflux surgery and found that reflux in kidneys without radiographic evidence of pyelonephritic scarring had accelerated growth postoperatively. In children with bilateral parenchymal scars, there was also increased growth postoperatively. However, in patients with unilateral renal scarring, renal growth did not increase postoperatively.

Ultimately, there may be no difference in rates of renal growth whether VUR is treated medically or surgically (Claësson *et al.*, 1981; Birmingham Reflux Study Group, 1983; Birmingham Reflux Study Group, 1987; Scott *et al.*, 1986). Although renal growth may be greater in patients with surgical correction than in those treated medically, accelerated renal growth is known to occur during puberty in medically treated patients; therefore, these differences may not be significant in long-term follow-up (Claësson *et al.*, 1981). Both spontaneous resolution of reflux and surgical correction will increase renal blood flow, decrease voiding pressure effects on the kidney, and allow the small kidney to resume growth. Evidence from the Birmingham Reflux Study Group (1983, 1987) showed that when patients were allocated on a random basis to either medical treatment or surgery, there was no significant difference in renal growth or renal parenchymal scarring between the treatment groups.

Somatic growth

Elimination of VUR has been suggested to result in an increase in somatic growth (Merrell and Mowad, 1979; Sutton and Atwell, 1989). Smellie *et al.* (1983) documented normal somatic growth in 51 girls with VUR who were maintained on low-dose prophylactic antibiotic therapy. None of these patients had surgical treatment. Merrell and Mowad (1979) showed that physical growth of prepubertal children with VUR is accelerated after successful antireflux surgery. Sutton and Atwell (1989) studied a series of children with primary VUR. Patients undergoing medical treatment were observed during 1 year of treatment and those undergoing surgical correction were observed for 2 years postoperatively. Patients who had successful surgical correction of reflux showed a moderate but significant increase in height and weight compared with patients who had medical treatment alone.

Renal scarring

Approximately 30–50% of patients with VUR have renal scarring on initial evaluation. Arant (1992) showed that even mild to moderate VUR could be associated with renal injury. In a prospective 5-year follow-up study of infants and children younger than 5 years treated medically, renal scarring was present in about 10% of those with grade I or II reflux and in 28% of those with grade III reflux. In a large series of patients with normal kidneys, Smellie and Normand (1979) reported that new renal scars developed in only 83 of 1720 (5%). Of these 83 children, 80 had a history of reflux and 79 had UTI. Although the majority of patients with reflux in whom renal scars develop show them at an early age, renal scarring is not confined exclusively to young children. Smellie *et al.* (1985) documented newly diagnosed renal scars in 34 of 87 patients (39%) who were older than 5 years when scarring developed. In most of these patients, treatment of UTI was delayed, which may explain the progression of renal scarring documented subsequently.

The onset of new renal scarring is related directly to the successful use of low-dose antibiotic therapy to maintain sterile urine. Children with uncomplicated primary reflux in whom continuous low-dose chemoprophylaxis maintains sterile urine rarely have scars. Smellie and Normand (1979) followed a large group of children with VUR and reported that new scarring

developed in only two patients while receiving continuous low-dose chemoprophylaxis, in a 7–15-year follow-up. Both of these patients had breakthrough UTI and moderate to severe reflux. Lenaghan *et al.* (1976) used intermittent short courses of antibacterial drugs for the treatment of recurrent infections in children with reflux. Of 76 kidneys that were initially normal, renal scarring developed in 16 (21%). Of 44 kidneys with established scars, additional scarring developed in 66%. All patients with new or progressive scarring had intercurrent infections.

Randomized prospective studies have shown no significant difference between medical and surgical treatment with respect to development of new scars or progression of pre-existing scars (Birmingham Reflux Study Group, 1987). The Birmingham Reflux Study Group (1987) found ten new developing scars in a long-term follow-up of more than 5 years. These new scars affected 3.8% of operated renal units and 4.5% of spontaneously resolved VUR. All scars developed within the first 2 years after randomization in the study. Because the complete formation of scars visible on imaging studies can be delayed, the 3.8% incidence of scarring found postoperatively may be causally related to ascending UTI preoperatively (Beetz *et al.*, 1989).

In the International Reflux Study, there was no difference between medical and surgical treatment in terms of renal size and growth, the development of new radiographic scars or areas of parenchymal thinning, or the progression of established scarring (Smellie, 1992). More new scars developed in children with parenchymal thinning at entry than in those with scarred or normal kidneys at entry. Younger patients at entry were found to develop more scars than older children (Olbing *et al.*, 1992). Patients with renal scars should have their blood pressure checked annually throughout their lives.

Long-term follow-up in adults with corrected or uncorrected VUR has been reported (Hawtrey *et al.*, 1983; Torres *et al.*, 1983; Malek *et al.*, 1983a; Malek *et al.*, 1983b; Neves *et al.*, 1984; De Sy *et al.*, 1986; Nativ *et al.*, 1987; Zucchelli and Gaggi, 1988). Malek *et al.* (1983a) studied 67 adults with primary VUR and found a significant correlation between the severity of reflux and the extent of renal scarring. The age of the patients at the time of the first recognized UTI and the frequency and pattern of subsequent infections did not correlate with the severity of renal scarring.

Hypertension

Reflux nephropathy is the most common disorder leading to severe hypertension in children. The variability of hypertension is affected by the degree of parenchymal damage, the involvement of one or both kidneys, the degree of renal insufficiency, and the age of the patient. Inasmuch as hypertension may develop many years after renal damage, blood pressure measurements should be performed once or twice a year in these children for the rest of their lives.

Hypertension may develop in 10–20% of children with VUR and renal scars (Smellie et al., 1975). In a series of 189 patients with VUR observed for a mean of 10.8 years, Beetz et al. (1989) found that 61 patients (32%) had renal scars. In seven of those 61 patients (11.5%), moderate arterial hypertension developed. Wallace et al. (1978) reported hypertension in 11% of patients with unilateral renal scarring and in 19% of children with bilateral renal scars who were observed more than 10 years after ureteroneocystostomy for correction of VUR.

Hypertension is a well-known long-term complication in children and young adults with reflux nephropathy in whom end-stage renal failure develops (Torres et al., 1983). In an analysis of 100 children with severe hypertension, Gill et al. (1976) found 14 children with reflux nephropathy. Holland (1979) reviewed the literature and found 177 patients with hypertension associated with reflux and renal scarring. The overwhelming majority of patients were female and most patients had a history of previous UTI (Table 25.4).

Malek et al. (1983b) reported a 32% incidence of hypertension in long-term follow-up of adults with reflux nephropathy. This incidence of hypertension is approximately twice that expected in a normal white population. Hypertension developed in three of 67 patients (4%) with unilateral scarring and in 19 of 67 (28%) of those with bilateral renal scarring (Torres et al., 1983). Spontaneous resolution of reflux or surgical correction by ureteral reimplantation did not protect against the development of hypertension (Stickler et al., 1971; Stecker et al., 1977; Malek et al., 1983b). Moreau et al. (1979–80) found hypertension in approximately 5% of the 15–25-year-old patients with renal scarring and normal renal function. In older patients, the prevalence increased to 41%. Kincaid-Smith et al. (1984) reported a prevalence of 45% in adult women with renal scarring.

In patients with hypertension in association with a poorly functioning renal unit, unilateral nephrectomy or partial nephrectomy has been used to cure hypertension. In these selected patients, renal vein renin studies should be performed preoperatively. It is often necessary to obtain segmental renal vein renin measurements to determine accurately the source of the affected renal segment. Patients with unilateral renal scarring and localized increased renal vein renin ratios greater than 1.5 most often achieve cure or significant improvement in hypertension after unilateral nephrectomy (Levitt and Weiss, 1985). Conversely, patients with asymmetric bilateral renal scarring and localized increased renal vein renin ratios are less successfully treated by unilateral nephrectomy.

Renal insufficiency

VUR is or has been present in 30–40% of children who have renal failure before the age of 16 years and in 20% of adults who have renal failure before the age of 50 years. Reflux nephropathy and renal

Table 25.4 Hypertension associated with reflux and renal scarring

Diagnosis	No. of cases	Female:male ratio	Prior history of UTI (%)	Prevalence of VUR	
				No. with VUR	No. of VCUs done (%)
Chronic pyelonephritis	99	4:1	66	36/43	(84)
Segmental hypoplasia	49	5:1	8	9/21	(43)
Primary interstitial nephritis	15	4:1	–	10/11	(91)
Reflux nephropathy	8	8:0	75	8/8	(100)
Ask–Upmark kidney	6	6:0	50	2/2	(100)

UTI = urinary tract infection; VUR = vesicoureteral reflux; VCU = voiding cystourethrogram.
Modified from Holland (1979) with permission of Masson Publishing USA.

insufficiency are often detected during the course of diagnostic evaluation for hypertension or proteinuria in older children. Significant proteinuria has been a constant finding in patients with reflux and progressive deterioration of renal function (Torres *et al.*, 1983; Malek *et al.*, 1983b). In long-term follow-up of 67 adults (mean age, 29 years) with primary bilateral VUR who underwent bilateral ureteroneocystostomy, Torres *et al.* (1983) found that renal insufficiency occurred only in those with bilateral renal scarring. The presence or absence of proteinuria was an excellent prognostic indicator, and significant proteinuria was found almost exclusively in patients with renal insufficiency. The glomerular lesions of reflux nephropathy will vary depending on the degree of proteinuria and alteration in renal function (Torres *et al.*, 1980a). In patients with significant proteinuria, segmental sclerotic lesions similar to idiopathic focal sclerosing glomerulonephrosis have been documented.

Genetic markers such as HLA-B12 in female patients, HLA-B8 in combination with HLA-A9 or HLA-Bw15 in male patients, and HLA-Bw15 in patients of both sexes have been found with end-stage renal disease (ESRD) secondary to reflux nephropathy (Torres *et al.*, 1980a). It has been postulated that these markers may be a link to a gene that confers susceptibility to renal damage by VUR.

The role of antireflux surgery in patients with advanced reflux nephropathy and compromised renal function remains controversial (Torres *et al.*, 1980b). In a series of papers from the Mayo Clinic, it has been shown that surgical correction of reflux in adults with severely damaged kidneys and significant proteinuria did not prevent the progression of renal insufficiency (Torres *et al.*, 1980b; Malek *et al.*, 1983b; Neves *et al.*, 1984). Patients with mean serum creatinine values greater than 2.75 mg/dl often had progression to renal failure despite successful surgical correction of reflux (Torres *et al.*, 1980b).

Salvatierra and Tanagho (1977) recommended surgical correction of bilateral reflux even in older children and adolescents with reflux nephropathy and compromised renal function. They believed that successful surgical correction may (1) retard the rate of progression toward end-stage renal failure, (2) prevent the accelerated deterioration that sometimes occurs in patients with reflux nephropathy after an episode of acute pyelonephritis, and (3) maximize somatic growth in this subset of patients. Benefits in correcting reflux in patients with ESRD include (1) less severe anemia in those who retain their native kidneys and are receiving renal dialysis, (2) decreased threat to life from pyelonephritis due to reflux in an immunosuppressed patient, and (3) decreased need for bilateral nephrectomies in preparation for renal transplantation (Salvatierra and Tanagho, 1977).

Antibiotic prophylaxis

The primary goals in the management of VUR are the prevention of ascending pyelonephritis and renal scarring. Prospective studies have shown clearly that long-term continuous chemoprophylaxis can prevent parenchymal damage. Medical management of VUR consists of preventing UTI by frequent voiding, avoidance of constipation, ensuring low-pressure voiding, and continuous low-dose chemoprophylaxis until reflux has resolved. Long-term antibacterial therapy is usually safe and well tolerated by the majority of children. Despite rare side-effects in isolated patients, most children tolerate long-term antibacterial therapy for years without sequelae. Chemoprophylactic agents should achieve high urinary concentrations and have activity against a broad spectrum of urinary pathogens. Antibacterial therapy is usually prescribed in a liquid form and calculated to be one-half of the standard therapeutic dose. The prophylactic medication should be given once daily at bedtime, because that is the time when the dry child will retain urine longest and infection is likely to develop.

Either trimethoprim–sulfamethoxazole (Septra) or nitrofurantoin macrocrystals (Macrodantin) is an excellent initial choice for antibiotic therapy. Trimethoprim–sulfamethoxazole is contraindicated in children younger than 1 month of age. Sulfa and trimethoprim–sulfa combinations have been associated with blood dyscrasias, Stevens–Johnson syndrome, gastrointestinal symptoms, and central nervous system abnormalities. Some suggest that a complete blood cell count should be made at 6-month intervals to rule out leukopenia and thrombocytopenia.

Rare side-effects of nitrofurantoin include interstitial pneumonitis or pulmonary fibrosis, exfoliative dermatitis, hemolytic anemia, and peripheral neuropathies. It may cause gastrointestinal disturbance and is best given in combination with food or milk. This drug is contraindicated in patients with renal insufficiency, because it may result in peripheral neuropathy.

Nitrofurantoin should not be used in children younger than 2 months old. Children allergic to sulfa or nitrofurantoin are candidates for cephalosporins, trimethoprim, nalidixic acid (NegGram), or methenamine mandelate (Mandelamine)–ascorbic acid.

Cefixime (Suprax) is an excellent third-generation cephalosporin, that can be used for patients with recurrent breakthrough infections while taking trimethoprim–sulfamethoxazole or nitrofurantoin macrocrystals. The author has used this antibiotic for years in difficult cases and remains very impressed with its tolerability and effectiveness. Ciprofloxacin is another excellent antibiotic, that can be used selectively in older children with recurrent or resistant UTIs. Pediatric infectious disease colleagues should be consulted before it is used in children.

After reflux has been diagnosed, urine culture may be obtained every few months to rule out occult UTI. Home culture programs allow the parents to culture the urine at frequent intervals (1–3 months) at a fraction of the cost of coming to the clinic. Negative cultures are usually reliable; however, positive cultures should be confirmed in the clinic with a specimen obtained by catheter, and treatment altered accordingly. Children with known reflux who have fever should have urine cultures to rule out UTI, regardless of symptoms.

Inasmuch as resolution of reflux is approximately 10–15% per year, radionuclide cystography should be performed at 12–18-month intervals. The upper tract is evaluated with either a DMSA renal scan or renal ultrasonography as clinically indicated. Antibiotics should be continued until reflux resolves, documented by a cyclic cystogram or until the child with low-grade reflux reaches 7–8 years of age without a breakthrough infection (Belman, 1995). If the child develops febrile infections and becomes symptomatic, additional studies are performed at that time.

Surgical management

The choice of technique should be individualized for the patient and will be biased by the surgeon's preference and experience. Although various surgical procedures have been advocated for the correction of VUR, all successful reimplantations involve the development of an adequate length of submucosal ureter as it courses into the bladder. This maneuver permits physiologic valve-like flattening or closing of the distal ureteral segment during periods of increased intravesical pressure, as encountered with a full bladder and during voiding. Prevention of reflux may also be dependent on shortening of the muscular fibers of the trigone, which in turn elongates and constricts the intramural and intravesical portion of the distal ureter (Tanagho et al., 1965).

Absolute indications for surgical correction of reflux include (1) pyelonephritis despite antibiotic chemoprophylaxis, (2) non-compliance with medical management or breakthrough infections during medical treatment, (3) a refluxing ureter that opens into a bladder diverticulum, (4) ureteral obstruction in association with reflux, and (5) the cystoscopic observation of a golf-hole orifice with no submucosal tunnel. The surgical results of the International Reflux Study documented overall success rates greater than 95% (Duckett et al., 1992; Hjalmas et al., 1992).

Successful surgical correction of reflux decreases the risk of pyelonephritis, eliminates progressive renal scarring, and has been associated with resumption of renal growth. Even though successful antireflux surgery prevents recurrent infections in the majority of children, 20–40% of patients have recurrent cystitis despite correction of reflux (Willscher et al., 1976a,b; Beetz et al., 1989). Postoperative UTI has been noted to occur equally with all grades of reflux (Wacksman et al., 1978). These lower tract infections should not affect renal growth or renal function.

General surgical principles

Endoscopy

Cystoscopic examination is rarely necessary but when done should be accomplished with anesthesia. Although orifice shape and position can be assessed accurately during cystoscopy, the degree of bladder filling must be taken into account in describing the shape of the orifice and its position. Primary VUR is most likely to be associated with some degree of ureterovesical angle incompetence or measurable deficiencies of the submucosal tunnel, or both. Because reflux often occurs with a full bladder at voiding, it is important to assess the configuration and shape of the orifice during moderate bladder distention. Progressive bladder filling displaces the orifice laterally and changes its appearance towards a more abnormal type. Many orifices that appear normal at initial observation clearly become incompetent with progressive bladder filling. Urethral dilation, internal urethrotomy, and urethral meatotomy are not beneficial for children with VUR.

King *et al.* (1974) stated that cystoscopic examination and measurement of submucosal tunnel length is an important prognostic measurement for predicting the likelihood of spontaneous resolution of VUR. Conversely, Duckett and Bellinger (1982) reported inconsistencies with the measurement of submucosal tunnel length and resolution of reflux. They reported that the cystoscopic appearance of the ureteral orifices does not help in predicting whether reflux will resolve. The decision to perform ureteroneocystostomy should be based on the clinical history and severity of reflux.

Preliminary treatment of associated pathology such as persistent UTI or bladder-outlet obstruction should precede ureteral reimplantation. Ureteral reimplantation should be done in the absence of infection and not sooner than several weeks after an acute UTI has been eliminated. Mucosal edema from residual infection will compromise an already delicate operation and increase the chance of surgical failure.

Surgical technique, use of catheters and stents, and pain management

The initial step in successful ureteral reimplantation surgery in children is the administration of excellent anesthesia, preferably by a pediatric anesthesiologist. Preoperative enemas are not necessary in most patients; however, those with neuropathic bladders or a history of constipation may benefit from preoperative bowel cathartics. A rolled towel placed under the buttocks and lower sacrum displaces the pelvis anteriorly and provides better exposure. The hips are abducted and the knees are flexed slightly.

A transverse crease incision is made two fingerbreadths above the pubic symphysis just to the lateral borders of the rectus muscle. This classical Pfannenstiel incision will permit further lateral extension if necessary. The anterior rectus sheath is divided transversely to achieve adequate exposure. The rectus muscles are retracted laterally and the peritoneum is swept superiorly to provide access to the bladder. Extravesical dissection should be limited because extensive bladder mobilization can result in injury to adjacent vessels or produce vesical dysfunction and a secondary neuropathic bladder. The bladder is opened vertically in the midline down to 2 cm above the bladder neck. Manipulation of the interior of the bladder with sponges or suction is avoided to prevent edema and mucosal bleeding. The Dennis–Brown retractor provides excellent exposure. Saline-soaked sponges are placed beneath each blade of the retractor to prevent mucosal hemorrhage and edema.

A successful reimplantation involves straightening any kinks or angulation of the terminal ureter, decreasing the caliber of a dilated ureter to allow an appropriate length-to-width ratio for reimplantation, mobilization of the ureter to release any fibrous attachments, and prevention of injury to the surrounding peritoneal envelope or intraperitoneal viscera. The bladder mucosa should be handled carefully and with atraumatic instruments.

Tagging sutures of fine silk and fine chromic catgut on atraumatic pop-off needles are used to secure the superior and inferior aspects of the ureteral meatus for traction and orientation. The ureter is intubated with a 3 or 5 Fr feeding tube. Mucosal incisions are made around the ureteral meatus with either a knife blade or pinpoint electrocautery. Dissection should continue close to the ureter to preserve the bladder mucosa. A deep, 6 o'clock incision through the bladder wall divides the ureterotrigonal continuity and affords access to the retroperitoneal space. Dissection can then be continued in this plane easily and safely. All muscle bundles should be cut and coagulated well away from the ureter. The ureter should be completely freed from its muscle attachments. Use of a vein retractor placed through the ureteral hiatus allows visualization of the peritoneum so that it can be swept well away from the posterior bladder wall.

Periureteral bleeding should be isolated carefully with fine vascular forceps and gently electrofulgurated or suture ligated. Any portion of the ureter that appears to have a compromised blood supply should be excised back to normal tissue.

Division and spatulation of the ureter should be done with tenotomy scissors. Mucosal flaps should be developed widely to allow the ureter to reside clearly in its submucosal tunnel. Any muscular bleeding encountered during development of the submucosal flaps should be controlled carefully with electrocautery or sutures, or both. The ureteral hiatus should be closed snugly to establish a competent ureterovesical angle.

Urinary diversion in girls is accomplished through a urethral Foley catheter. In boys, a suprapubic cystostomy tube is used by some surgeons to avoid a catheter within the urethra and risking iatrogenic stricture. Suprapubic tubes should be placed high on the dome of the bladder to avoid irritation of the trigone. In patients with a history of neuropathic vesical dysfunction, the suprapubic catheter should be clamped in order to assess bladder function and residual urine volume prior to catheter removal. Drains are not used except in patients who undergo excision and ureteral tapering for megaureter.

Urethral catheters are usually left in place for 2–3 days until the urine becomes clear. Early removal of the catheter shortens hospital stay considerably (McCool and Joseph, 1995) and most patients are sent home by the third or fourth day postoperatively. Brandell and Brock (1993) recommended using neither vesical nor urethral catheters postoperatively. No postoperative complications were reported in their study.

Stents are optional, but if used, they should be soft and non-reactive. Stents are probably indicated when the ureter has been excised and tapered, in children with a solitary kidney, in cases of extensive dissection, particularly with a great deal of edema, and in reoperative cases. Indwelling ureteral stents may be used to avoid possible obstruction by circumventing the edema at the ureteral orifice and to maintain ureteral fixation. Small stents can be troublesome because the lumen of the stent may become occluded with blood, which may then occlude the ureter. When stenting a ureter, Silastic tubing of appropriate size and length, small feeding tubes, or single J catheters may be used. Stents are brought out through separate stab wounds in the bladder and through the skin and removed a few days after the operation. Most series show that morbidity and operative failure are comparable between stented and non-stented groups (Fort et al., 1983). Stents seldom do harm but may lengthen hospitalization and will not in themselves prevent subsequent complications when a suitable, anatomic reconstruction cannot be achieved.

The author's group has eliminated the use of continuous postoperative epidural anesthetic agents in patients undergoing ureteroneocystostomy. In a review of a large series of children who underwent uncomplicated ureteroneocystostomy and received epidural anesthetic agents postoperatively, there was a significant increase in the incidence of postoperative fever and 25% had catheter-related problems that often resulted in early removal of the epidural catheter (Cain et al., 1995). Most importantly, the cost of pain

management was significantly greater than that of a standard narcotic regimen. This modality was replaced with perioperative ketorolac tromethamine (Toradal), which led to a significant improvement in early ambulation and dismissal from the hospital (Anderson and Kevorkian, 1998). Patients continue receiving pediatric belladonna and opium (B&O) suppositories or other analgesics as necessary.

Appropriate antibiotic coverage should be maintained during hospitalization and followed by prolonged chemotherapy for several months postoperatively with sulfonamides, nitrofurantoin, or another form of antibacterial treatment. The initial radiographic studies are performed at 3–4 months and include either cyclic radionuclide cystography or standard VCUG and radiographic imaging of the upper tracts. If initial studies show no obstruction or reflux, subsequent studies include upper tract evaluation with ultrasonography or DMSA scanning at intervals of 12 months, 36 months, and 5 years postoperatively. Although extremely rare, late obstruction or reappearance of reflux may occur several years after an apparently successful operation; therefore, periodic upper tract evaluations have been recommended through puberty (Mesrobian et al., 1985). However, success with modern antireflux procedures is so high, delayed follow-up is being carried out less and less often (see postoperative results)

Surgical options: open surgical procedures

Suprahiatal repairs

Hutch-1

Hutch (1952) popularized antireflux surgery in the early 1950s by introducing the concept of constructing an antireflux valve by elongating the intravesical portion of the ureter. The transvesical approach of the Hutch-1 technique involves incising the mucosa cephalad and lateral to the original hiatus and developing submucosal flaps bilaterally (Hutch, 1963) (Fig. 25.14). The detrusor musculature is closed under the ureter, and the overlying mucosa is closed over the ureter. This technique leaves the orifice in an abnormal lateral position. It is also not possible to correct any ureteral kinks or adhesions or to perform ureteral tapering. The technique should be applied only to the normal or slightly dilated ureter. The dis-

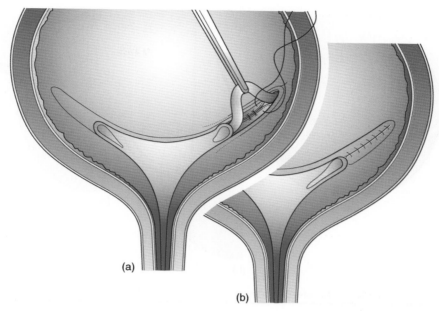

Figure 25.14 Hutch-1 technique of ureteroneocystostomy. (Modified from Kramer 1992.)

tal ureteral continuity and blood supply are not interrupted, and therefore this procedure may be applicable to patients in whom the blood supply of the ureter has been compromised superiorly from a previous pyelostomy or ureterostomy.

Lich–Grégoir

This extravesical antireflux procedure does not require opening the bladder and eliminates the risk of urinary contamination of the wound. Because the ureters are not reimplanted, they do not need stenting (Lich *et al.*, 1961; Grégoir and Van Regemorter, 1964). The operation can be performed in a relatively short time and requires minimal hospitalization.

The ureters are identified and isolated, and the lateral umbilical ligaments are ligated and transected. The posterior aspect of the bladder, where the antirefluxplasty is to be performed, is freed from the peritoneal pouch. The incision of the bladder muscle is performed cephalad and lateral to the ureteral hiatus and along the natural course of the ureter (Fig. 21.15). The incision is made through the serosal and muscular layers down to the mucosal layer. The muscular coat is undermined sufficiently to create an adequate bed for the ureter. The extension of the incision depends on the diameter of the ureter. The ureter is placed into the mucosal bed and the overlying muscle is closed with running absorbable sutures. It is impor-

tant that the tunnel be fashioned vertically on the posterior wall and that the incision does not interfere with the ureterotrigonal continuity (Marberger *et al.*, 1978).

Various authors have used this technique with success rates greater than 90% (Palken, 1970; Grégoir and Schulman, 1977; Arap *et al.*, 1981; Brühl *et al.*, 1988; Beetz *et al.*, 1989). The Lich–Grégoir procedure has particular advantages and applicability in the renal transplant population. Although this operation has been applied successfully in patients with ureteral duplication and paraureteral diverticula, others (Linn *et al.*, 1989) believe that a Hutch diverticulum is a contraindication for this procedure.

Detrusorrhaphy

Extravesical detrusorrhaphy is a modification of the Lich–Grégoir antireflux procedure that incorporates ureteral advancement into the repair (Daines and Hodgson, 1971; Zaontz *et al.*, 1987). The bladder is rotated to expose the involved ureter and its detrusor hiatus. The ureter is dissected circumferentially at the ureteral hiatus so that the ureter is attached only with the bladder mucosa (Fig. 25.16a, b). An incision is made in the bladder muscle both proximally and distally from the ureteral hiatus to create a muscular defect. Submucosal flaps are developed. The ureteral orifice is advanced onto the trigone toward the vesical

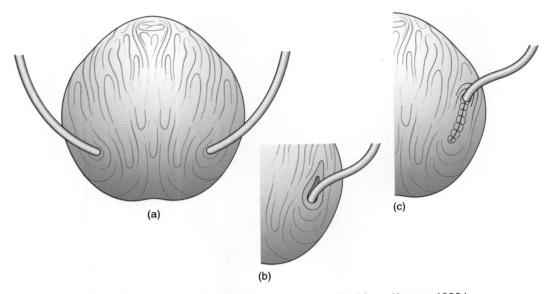

Figure 25.15 Lich–Grégoir technique of ureteroneocystostomy. (Modified from Kramer 1992.)

neck with a pair of Vest-type sutures (Fig. 25.17). Sutures are placed through the distal detrusor and ureteral muscle such that tying the pair of Vest sutures advances and anchors the ureteral orifice distally and creates a new long submucosal tunnel (Fig. 25.18). The procedure has been successful in more than 90% of patients (Zaontz *et al.*, 1987; Burbige *et al.*, 1996; Wacksman and Sheldon, 1999), including patients with megaureters (McLorie *et al.*, 1994).

Between 6 and 15% of patients have experienced transient inadequate bladder emptying after bilateral extravesical detrusorrhaphy (Houle *et al.*, 1992; Lapointe *et al.*, 1998). Transient postoperative urinary retention has been reported, despite attempts to minimize detrusor dissection (Lipski *et al.*, 1998). Postoperative voiding dysfunction is more pronounced in younger children and in those with a history of pre-operative voiding dysfunction (Minevich *et al.*, 1998). Patients may require intermittent self-catheterization

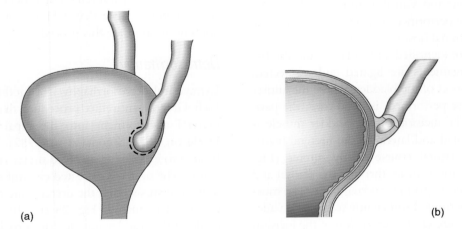

Figure 25.16 Detrusorrhaphy. (*a*) After ureteral mobilization, the detrusor is incised (dotted lines) at the level of the ureteral hiatus; (*b*) sagittal section demonstrating a ureteral hiatus. (From Zaontz *et al.*, 1987, with permission of Lippincott Williams & Wilkins.)

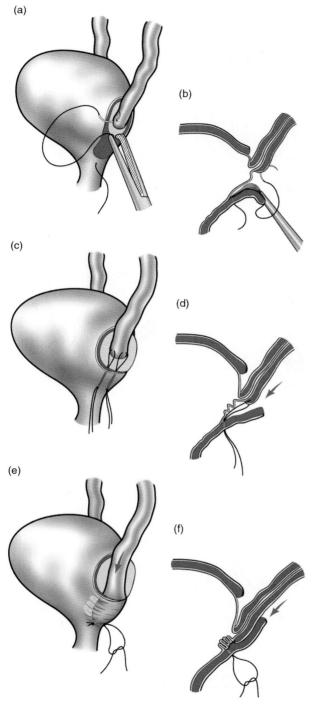

for several weeks, until spontaneous voiding and complete bladder emptying return. Therefore, this procedure is probably not the best choice in children with bilateral VUR (Fung *et al.*, 1995; Steinbrecher and Rangecroft, 1997).

This technique has been used unilaterally, with excellent success, including no problems with voiding dysfunction and a very low incidence (< 4%) of new-onset contralateral reflux (Mevorach *et al.*, 1998). The infrequency of contralateral reflux may be related to minimal trigonal dissection.

Politano–Leadbetter

One of the most widely used surgical techniques for ureteroneocystostomy was described by Politano and Leadbetter (1958). This technique achieves most of the basic objectives of ureteroneocystostomy and can be applied to kinked and dilated ureters in which the caliber of the ureter needs to be reduced. A circumferential incision is made around the ureteral orifice, and the ureter is freed from the ureterotrigonal continuity. The ureter is mobilized intravesically. It is then passed extravesically and brought inside the bladder through a new hiatus that lies superior and lateral to the original ureteral hiatus. It is imperative that the peritoneum be swept superiorly away from the ureter

Figure 25.17 (*a*) Bladder mucosa is elevated off the bladder wall muscle, and Vest-type sutures are placed; (*b*) sagittal section shows a suture passing between the undermined mucosa and detrusor; (*c*) alignment of Vest sutures after placement; (*d*) sagittal section demonstrating appropriate positioning of sutures; (*e*) tying Vest sutures advances and anchors the ureter onto the trigone; (*f*) sagittal section of ureteromeatal advancement. (Modified from Zaontz *et al.*, 1987, with permission of Lippincott Williams & Wilkins.)

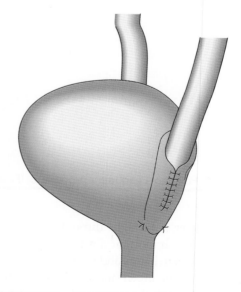

Figure 25.18 Closure of detrusor flaps over the ureter allows for a long submucosal tunnel and completes detrusorrhaphy (Modified from Zaontz *et al.*, 1987, with permission of Lippincott Williams & Wilkins.)

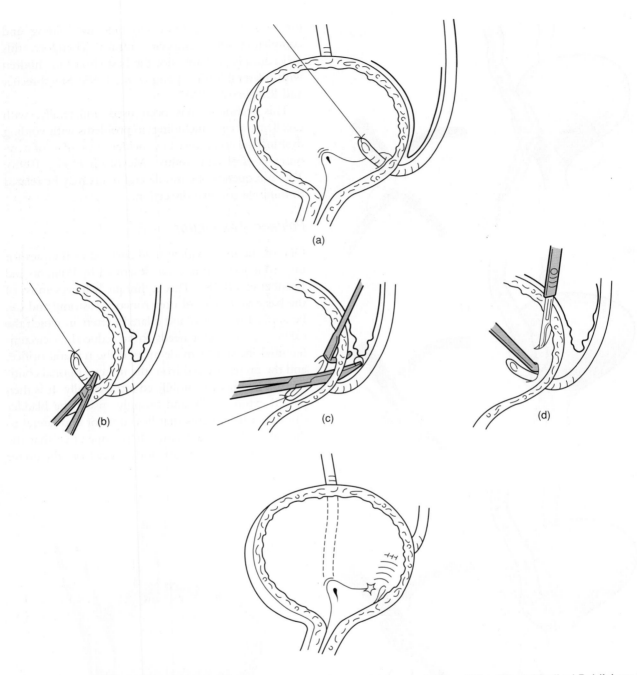

Figure 25.19 Politano–Leadbetter procedure. (From Walker, 1987, with permission of Year Book Medical Publishers.)

before the ureter is brought through its new hiatus (Fig. 25.19). It is important not to kink the ureter at the level of the new hiatus and to prevent inadvertent transposition of the ureter around the lateral umbilical ligament through the peritoneal cavity or perhaps through bowel (Fig. 25.20).

Most surgeons prefer to combine an extravesical approach with the intravesical approach, to ensure that the ureter has a straight course without kinks and that the peritoneal cavity has not been entered. The lateral umbilical ligaments should be transected to prevent kinking of the ureter. After the ureter has been brought through its new superior and lateral hiatus, a submucosal tunnel is developed from the site of the new hiatus inferiorly down to the site of the original ureteral hiatus. The distal terminal ureter is

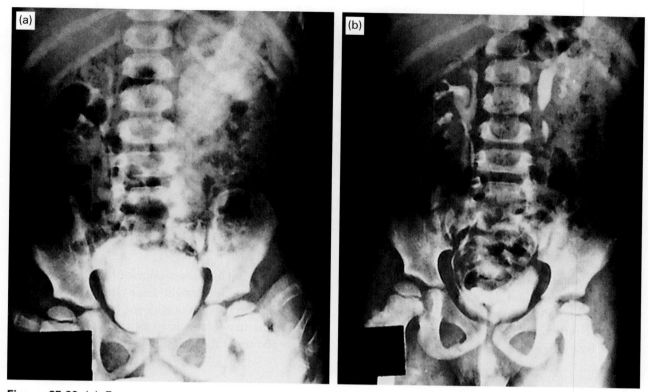

Figure 25.20 (*a*) Excretory urogram 3 months after ureteroneocystostomy; left hydronephrosis. At secondary ureteroneocystostomy the left ureter was found to traverse the lumen of the sigmoid. (*b*) Postoperative urogram.

discarded to remove any obstructive component or mucosa traumatized from placement of tagging sutures. A long intravesical ureteral segment is created in which the ureter lies submucosally and is supported by intact and unincised detrusor muscle.

The results of this procedure compare very favorably to other contemporary operations. In a large series of patients undergoing two different types of ureteroneocystostomy, the Politano–Leadbetter technique was successful in 98% and the Cohen cross-trigonal reimplantation in 97% (Burbige, 1991). Ellsworth and Merguerian (1995) reported similar results between detrusorrhaphy and the Politano–Leadbetter operations.

Kelalis

Kelalis (1985) described a technique in which the ureteral hiatus is created posteromedially on a relatively immobile part of the bladder. Advancing the ureteral orifice distally lengthens the submucosal tunnel. The operation is performed transvesically;

however, if there is any doubt about the proper position of the ureteral hiatus, extravesical dissection should be accomplished. The ureter must be mobilized sufficiently to prevent acute angulation as it enters its new course into the bladder. This technique has the advantage of creating a tunnel that has good support and places the ureter into a position in the bladder that will change little with bladder filling. This prevents intermittent or permanent ureteral obstruction, known as J-hooking of the ureter.

The ureter is intubated with a 5 Fr Stamey feeding tube, and traction sutures of fine silk and chromic catgut are placed inferomedially and superolaterally to the orifice. These tagging sutures allow the operator to apply tension to the ureter without grasping the ureter itself. They also identify the proper anatomic orientation of the orifice and thus avoid twisting the ureter after its transposition into the bladder. The mucosal cuff around the orifice is outlined circumferentially by using electrocautery or scissor dissection. The plane of cleavage is established between the adventitia of the ureter and the fibers of the bladder.

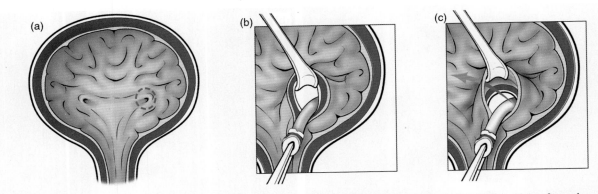

Figure 25.21 Kelalis procedure: the ureter is mobilized using both blunt and sharp dissection. Use of a vein retractor placed through the ureteral hiatus allows visualization of the peritoneum. (Modified from Kramer, 1992.)

Sufficient mobilization of the ureter is easily achieved by using both blunt and sharp dissection. The base of the bladder is elevated with a vein retractor, and the peritoneal reflection is pushed superiorly from the bladder base (Fig. 25.21). This ensures that there is no obstruction in the new course of the ureter as it re-enters the bladder. A right-angle clamp is passed from the old ureteral hiatus outside the bladder to the point where the new hiatus is to be created (Fig. 25.22). Once the tip of the clamp appears in the bladder and

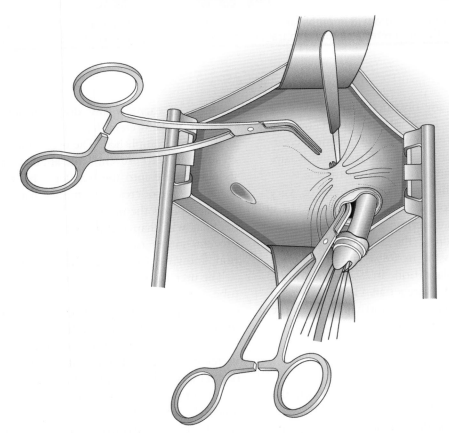

Figure 25.22 A right-angle clamp is passed from the old ureteral hiatus outside the bladder to the point where the new hiatus is to be created. (Modified from Kramer, 1992.)

the new hiatus is stretched to avoid subsequent narrowing, a second clamp is attached to its tip and guided into the bladder to such a position that it can grasp the traction sutures and pull the ureter into the bladder via the new hiatus (Fig. 25.23). The defect in the original hiatus musculature is closed with interrupted Vicryl sutures. Submucosal flaps are developed and a submucosal tunnel is constructed. The ureter is brought through this tunnel into the anteromedial portion of the mucosal defect (Fig. 25.24). It is important to reinsert a ureteral catheter into the reimplanted ureter and advance it all the way to the kidney to exclude any obstruction or angulation of the ureter. The distal end of the ureter is removed routinely inasmuch as this end is often stenotic and aperistaltic or it may be traumatized during dissection.

The mucosal cuff of the ureter is sutured to the mucosa of the bladder with several interrupted sutures of fine Vicryl or chromic catgut. The most distal suture should encompass bladder muscle as well as mucosa because this stitch serves to anchor the ureter into position and re-establish the ureterotrigonal continuity. The remaining ureteral mucosal sutures can be stitched to the bladder mucosa only. The bladder mucosa overlying the original ureteral hiatus is closed in a linear fashion with running absorbable sutures.

Paquin

The Paquin ureteroneocystostomy procedure combines transvesical and extravesical approaches and allows correction of normal-sized ureters or megaureters (Paquin, 1959; Woodard and Keats, 1973) (Fig. 25.25). This technique differs from the Politano–Leadbetter procedure in that the bladder wall is split open posterior and lateral to the chosen site of the new hiatus.

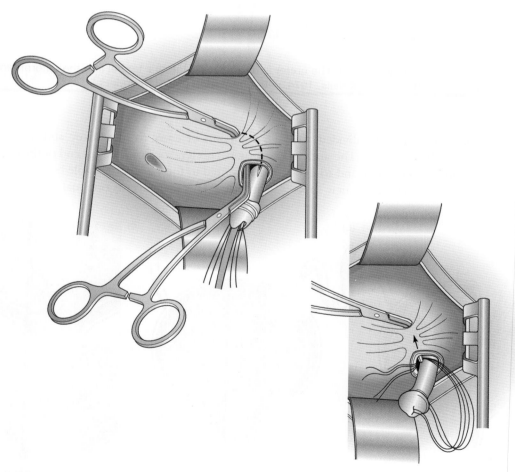

Figure 25.23 The ureter is pulled into the bladder via the new hiatus. (Modified from Kramer, 1992.)

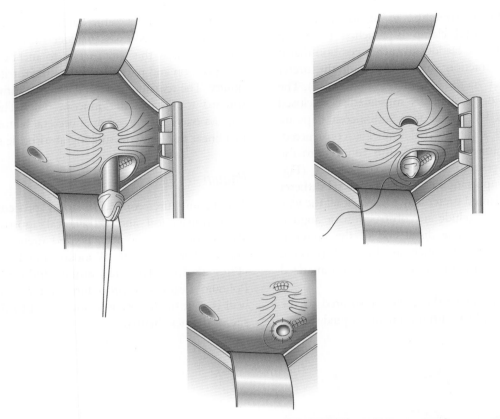

Figure 25.24 Submucosal flaps are developed. The ureter is brought through this tunnel into the anteromedial portion of the mucosal defect. (Modified from Kelalis, 1974, with permission of WB Saunders.)

In his original description, Paquin divided the distal terminal ureter and left it in place. The author prefers to mobilize the ureter completely and to develop a submucosal tunnel from the ureter's new superior point of entry to just below and medial to the original ureteral orifice. The cut end of the ureter may be everted to form a cuff or nipple before it is sutured in place. This maneuver is optional.

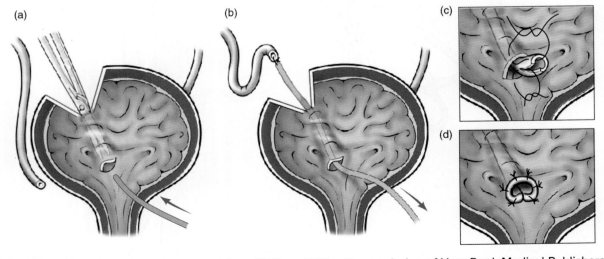

Figure 25.25 Paquin procedure. (Modified from Walker, 1987, with permission of Year Book Medical Publishers.)

A modified Paquin procedure is frequently used for secondary repairs in which extravesical mobilization is necessary and the ureter is short and wide (Mesrobian *et al.*, 1985). A psoas hitch is an important adjunct to this technique. The bladder should be opened obliquely on its anterolateral surface. The corresponding side of the bladder is brought up to the psoas muscle and sutured with Vicryl or polydioxanone sutures lateral to the iliac vessels (Prout and Koontz, 1970). Care should be taken to avoid the genitofemoral nerve. This maneuver allows a long intravesical ureter and maintains the new ureteral hiatus at a fixed point, so that neither kinking nor obstruction may occur.

Infrahiatal repairs

Mathisen

Mathisen (1964) described a combined extravesical and intravesical procedure that advanced the ureter down onto the trigone (Fig. 25.26). This procedure has wide applicability and is associated with minimal complications and excellent success.

Glenn–Anderson

The advantage of the Glenn–Anderson advancement technique is that the ureter enters the bladder through the normal ureteral hiatus and, thus, the chance of kinking or obstruction (J-hooking) of the ureter because of a high ureteral hiatus is virtually eliminated (Glenn and Anderson, 1967). The infrahiatal principle is most applicable to patients in whom the ureteral orifice is superolateral and there is enough space between the original ureteral hiatus and the bladder neck to advance the intravesical ureter. Ureteral length is gained by dissecting and freeing the intravesical ureter. After the ureter has been freed transvesically, a submucosal tunnel is developed from the ureteral hiatus distally towards the bladder neck. Creation of the tunnel distally may be difficult at times, and it may be necessary to incise the bladder mucosa distally and elevate the mucosa laterally and medially to create a trough for the ureter. The underlying detrusor muscle is closed with interrupted sutures of Vicryl, with the knots tied in an inverted

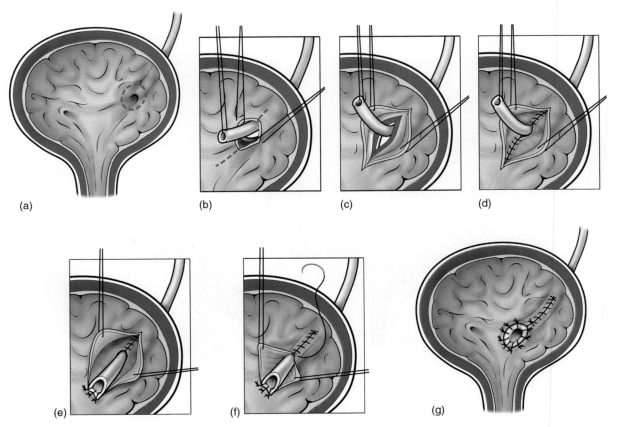

(a)　　　(b)　　　(c)　　　(d)

(e)　　　(f)　　　(g)

Figure 25.26 Mathisen procedure. (Modified from Mathisen, 1964, with permission of *Surgery, Gynecology and Obstetrics*.)

fashion. The ureter is placed onto the bladder musculature, and the mucosa is sutured over it. The technique is simple, can be accomplished rapidly, and avoids extravesical dissection. It places the ureter in its proper physioanatomical position on the trigonal musculature.

Glenn and Anderson (1978) offered a modification of their original technique. Whereas the original procedure described mobilization of only the terminal 2–3 cm of ureter, the modified technique allows extension of the ureteral hiatus superiorly to achieve a longer tunnel (Fig. 25.27). The modified technique involves the development of a larger hiatus that provides visibility of the extravesical and extraperitoneal space, peritoneum, and contiguous structures. The development of this large hiatus permits mobilization of at least 8–10 cm of distal ureter. Subsequent closure of the enlarged hiatus distal to the point of bladder entry of the ureter creates a longer submucosal tunnel and diminishes the necessity of extensive submucosal dissection onto the trigone. Success of the original and modified repairs has been greater than 90% (Gonzales *et al.*, 1972; Glenn and Anderson, 1978).

Cohen

The Cohen technique is simple, safe, and effective for the prevention of VUR (Cohen, 1975). It is the most widely used procedure in Europe and perhaps the USA today. The advantages of this technique include minimal angulation at the ureteral hiatus (Fig. 25.28). The ureters are mobilized transvesically and separate submucosal tunnels are created for each ureter, so that each ureter opens on the opposite side from its hiatus. The ureters can be criss-crossed anywhere on the bladder floor with good results.

In large series of patients with all grades of reflux, successful results have been reported in more than 95% of patients (Wacksman *et al.*, 1992; Kennelly *et al.*, 1995). Kondo and Otani (1987) reported a 100% success rate for correction of primary reflux and 89% for secondary reflux. Ehrlich (1982) described a 98% success rate in 229 ureters reimplanted for primary reflux and a 95% success rate in 109 ureters corrected for secondary reflux or obstructive megaureter. Glassberg *et al.* (1985) recommended a modification of the original technique for patients with dilated ureters and small bladders. This modified technique

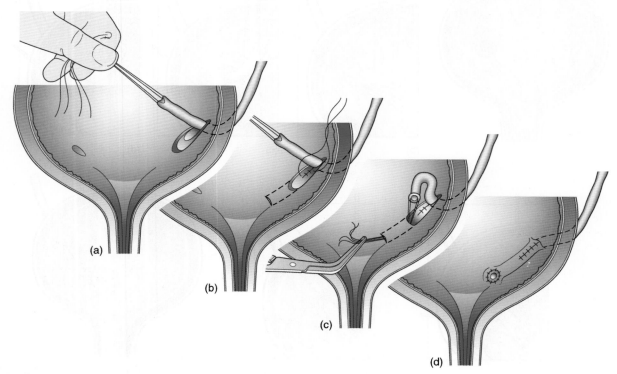

(a)

(b)

(c)

(d)

Figure 25.27 Modification of the Glenn–Anderson technique. (From Kramer, 1992, with permission of the Mayo Foundation.)

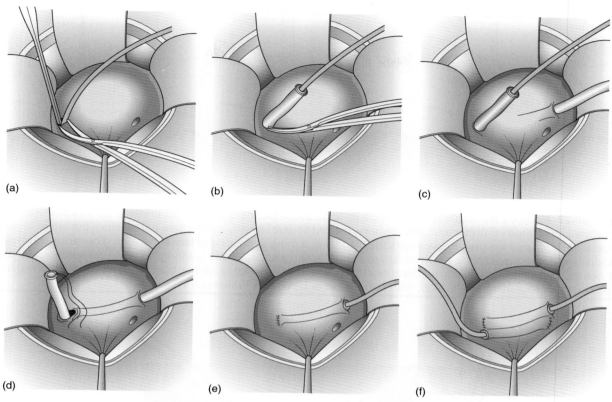

Figure 25.28 Cohen technique. (*a*) A circumferential incision is made around the ureteral orifice. (*b*) The ureter is freed by sharp dissection, always staying close to it and not straying into extraneous planes. (*c*) The site for the new orifice is chosen at a point superior and lateral to contralateral orifice. The mucosa at this site is incised and a sub-mucosal tunnel is fashioned cephalad to the trigone with semipointed scissors. (*d*) The ureter is advanced through the tunnel. (*e*) The ureter is sewn into place, making sure that at least one or two sutures have incorporated a good bite of bladder muscle. Detrusor in previously dissected hiatus is closed inferiorly, with care taken not to compromise the ureter. The mucosa is closed as a separate layer. (*f*) In cases of bilateral reimplantation, a separate sub-mucosal tunnel is fashioned within the trigone. The new orifice for the second ureter is placed either at the inferior aspect of the closed contralateral ureteral hiatus or inferior and lateral to it. (Modified from Glassberg *et al.*, 1985, with permission of Lippincott Williams & Wilkins.)

involves incising the bladder at the superolateral margin of the hiatus and mobilizing the peritoneum superiorly. This incision allows the ureter to enter the bladder in a more superior and lateral position, thus creating a longer tunnel (Figs. 25.29, 25.30).

Because of the criss-cross positioning of the ureteral meatus, problems may arise if retrograde ureteral catheterization becomes necessary (Lamesch, 1981). A Cystocath may be placed within the bladder and simultaneous cystoscopy performed. The ureters are catheterized through the Cystocath trocar, while a second observer directs the catheters cystoscopically. A flexible-tip, manually controllable retrograde catheter (Cook Urological, Spencer, IN, USA) is available. In the author's experience, this maneuver is still challenging and often unsuccessful.

Gil–Vernet

Gil–Vernet (1984) described a technique based on the principle that the intrinsic muscular fibers of the transmural ureter may provide sphincteric action in preventing reflux. This procedure advances the ureters across the trigone and approximates them in the midline, thereby increasing the intramural length of each distal ureter. A non-absorbable mattress suture is placed at the base of each ureter, including the periurethral sheath of Waldeyer and the intrinsic ureteral musculature, and tied in the midline. The original technique has been modified in that absorbable sutures are used to advance the ureters (Carini *et al.*, 1985). Solok *et al.* (1988) reported success in 94% of renal units with grades II, III, or IV

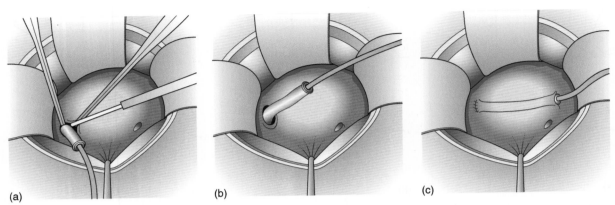

Figure 25.29 Modified technique for difficult cases (e.g., infant bladders and dilated ureters). (*a*) The posterior wall of the bladder is lifted off ureter and, with cautery, incised superolaterally, taking care not to injure the ureter or peritoneum. (*b*) Note that the ureter now enters the bladder at a more superior and lateral position. The retroperitoneum is visualized better through the newly enlarged hiatus, which also facilitates tailoring. (*c*) A longer submucosal tunnel can be fashioned, inasmuch as the tunnel is made in a wider area of the bladder, well above the trigone. (Modified from Glassberg *et al*., 1985, with permission of Lippincott Williams & Wilkins.)

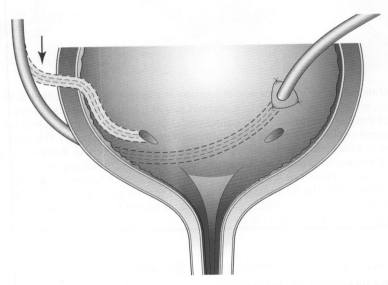

Figure 25.30 Gentle curve of the ureter in the Cohen technique compared with the hitch that can occur when the ureter (*dotted lines*) is passed through the new hiatus (*arrow*) as in the Politano–Leadbetter procedure. (Modified from Glassberg *et al*., 1985, with permission of Lippincott Williams & Wilkins.)

VUR. Carini *et al*. (1985) also stressed the ease and simplicity of the Gil–Vernet technique and reported successful results in 13 of 14 patients undergoing surgical treatment for reflux.

Submucosal injection techniques

The principle of endoscopic injection is identical to that of a formal open ureteroneocystostomy: to create solid support behind the refluxing intravesical ureter. The success of the procedure depends on the ability of the surgeon to place the implant within the lamina propria at a position just proximal to the ureteral orifice. This injection elevates the ureteral orifice on a 'hillock' and causes the orifice to assume an inverted, crescentic appearance. If the needle is not placed correctly, the injection may occur into the ureteral lumen or detrusor musculature and result in an implantation that extrudes superficially into the bladder lumen, deeply into the bladder wall, or perhaps extravesically.

The submucosal injection of any substance for the treatment of VUR should be limited to specific clinical situations, and the risks and unanswered long-term concerns should be discussed thoroughly with the parents. The ideal substance should conserve its volume and be non-migratory and non-antigenic. Endoscopic injection therapy for reflux is a reasonable alternative for correction of reflux after failed ureteral reimplantation in selected patients with neuropathic bladder dysfunction in whom open surgical techniques are less likely to produce a successful result or in those with persistent reflux after complicated augmentation or reconstruction procedures.

Polytetrafluoroethylene

Polytef paste is a sterile mixture of polytetrafluoroethylene (Teflon), glycerin, and polysorbate (Malizia et al., 1984). Injection of this substance has been used for many years to enlarge displaced or deformed vocal cords in patients with dysphonia (Arnold, 1963). The subureteric injection of polytetrafluoroethylene for correction of VUR was first used by Matouschek (1981) and applied to both the bladder neck and ureter by Politano et al. (1974). Subsequently, an experimental study (Puri and O'Donnell, 1984) and its clinical application in children (O'Donnell and Puri, 1984) demonstrated that it was possible to correct VUR by the endoscopic injection of polytetrafluoroethylene under the submucosal ureter. The Polytef particles stimulate an ingrowth of fibroblasts at the site of injection, and this tends to hold the particles within the tissues (O'Donnell and Puri, 1984).

The injection technique is straightforward, can be performed as an outpatient procedure, and requires approximately 5–15 min under anesthesia. The bladder must be nearly empty to keep the ureteral orifice flat rather than displaced laterally, as occurs during bladder filling. The needle is composed of a 5 Fr Nylon catheter onto which is wedged a 21G needle or a rigid needle of the same dimensions. The 13.5 Storz cystoscope or 9.5 or 11 Fr Wolf cystoscope (Richard Wolf Medical Instruments, Rosemont, IL, USA) with offset lens is used. The needle is introduced 3–4 mm distal to the orifice, and as the injection proceeds, the distal ureter flattens and the orifice closes, assuming a slit-like configuration at the conclusion of the procedure (Fig. 25.31). Some authors have advocated the use of a 4 Fr ureteral catheter or Fogarty catheter to elevate the ureteral orifice during injection

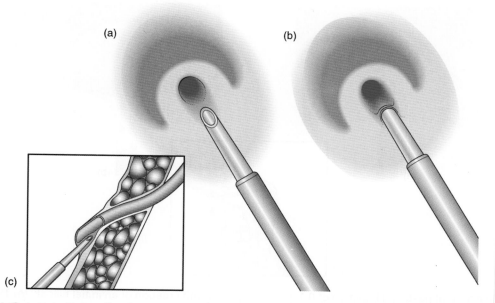

Figure 25.31 Subureteric needle placement. (a) Needle positioned at the 6 o'clock position, bevel up; (b) needle inserted in the subureteric space; lever up on needle to ensure superficial placement; (c) cut-away view to indicate superficial subureteric placement of the needle before injection. (Modified from Kramer, 1992.)

to help to prevent perforation of the ureteral wall while avoiding the detrusor muscle. When the needle is positioned properly, approximately 0.4–0.6 ml of Teflon paste is injected to provide a subureteric buttress (Fig. 25.32).

Dewan and Higgs (1995) retrospectively reviewed videotapes of treatments to assess predictors of treatment failures. The visual mound of paste and meticulous placement of the needle were predictors of success. Conversely, injections into large ureteral orifices usually did not produce a classic 'hillock'; however, successful results were achieved with larger volumes of paste.

Schulman and Sassine (1992) reported their experience with 180 patients with 256 refluxing units treated with the endoscopic injection of Teflon. More than 50% of the patients had grade III, IV, or V VUR. In children with primary VUR, 87% were successfully treated with a single injection and 93% with a second injection. At 5-year follow-up, no morbidity or complications were reported.

Puri (1995) reported his 10-year experience with a large series of patients who underwent Teflon injection for VUR. He noted a 76% overall success with a single injection and 85% with repeated injections. Dessouki *et al.* (1993) reported a series of 38 patients with an 84% success rate with a single injection and

ultimately 100% with two or three injections. Ninety-five per cent of successfully treated patients remained without reflux at 2–5 years postoperatively. Farkas *et al.* (1990) reported their experience with Teflon in 115 ureters with reflux and noted a 96% cure rate after an initial injection in those with primary VUR. Patients with dilated ureters and golf-hole orifices did not respond to endoscopic Teflon injection therapy. Michael *et al.* (1993) used Teflon in 100 refluxing units and reported a 77% success rate with one injection and 90% with a second injection. Dewan and Goh (1994) reviewed their 2-year experience with Teflon in 47 children with 60 refluxing units and reported that 82% were corrected after a single injection and 90% after a second injection.

Some centers have reported less success with subureteric Teflon. Mattar *et al.* (1994) noted only a 43% success rate after a single injection; resolution of reflux improved to 74% after a second injection. Sweeny and Thomas (1987) reported a 65% success rate after Teflon injection. Brown (1989) compared open ureteroneocystostomy to the subureteric injection of Polytef paste for primary treatment of VUR. Surgical reimplantation cured reflux in 98% of 76 ureters, whereas endoscopic procedures were successful in only 70% of 40 ureters. Patients undergoing endoscopic surgery required more hospital admis-

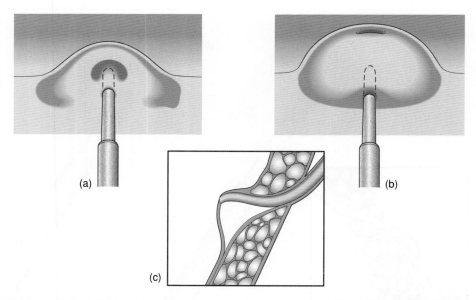

Figure 25.32 Injection of paste. (*a*) Injection of 0.1–0.2 ml of paste, with creation of an initial hillock. (*b*) Then, 0.3–0.4 ml of paste is injected at completion of the procedure. Note the crescentic appearance of the orifice. The final result should look like a volcano. (*c*) Side view of the completed procedure to indicate support and lengthening of the ureter on the bead, with only minor compression of the distal segment. (Modified from Kramer, 1992.)

sions, more anesthetics, and more VCUGs than did those in the surgically reimplanted group. Brown (1989) concluded that open reimplantation remains the procedure of choice if surgery is indicated for patients with VUR.

Engel *et al.* (1997) reviewed the efficiency of subureteric Teflon compared with ureteroneocystostomy in treating VUR in children with neuropathic bladders. In this group of patients, success rates following a Cohen ureteroneocystostomy were significantly greater (84%) than with Teflon (57%). The cumulative success rate after a second Teflon injection was only 61%.

Teflon has been used to correct persistent VUR after failed ureteroneocystostomy (Kumar and Puri, 1998). In a series of 31 children with 40 high-grade refluxing units after failed ureteroneocystostomy, successful results were obtained in 68% of patients after a single injection. Seven ureters required two injections and four ureters required three injections for the correction of VUR. VCUGs were obtained 3 years postoperatively.

Patients with complete ureteral duplication have been more difficult to treat, and success rates have been lower than with single systems. Success rates for reflux into duplex ureters range between 59 and 82% after an initial injection (Farkas *et al.*, 1990; Miyakita *et al.*, 1993). Furthermore, the presence of a paraureteral diverticulum is extremely difficult to correct because of lack of adequate detrusor muscle support.

Ultrasonography, computed tomographic (CT) scanning, and magnetic resonance imaging (MRI) have been used to determine the size and location of the Teflon mass after subureteric injection (Mann *et al.*, 1988; Gore *et al.*, 1989; Kirsch *et al.*, 1990). Sonographically, the Teflon paste at the injection site appears as a hyperechoic locus within the bladder wall, with distal shadowing (Mann *et al.*, 1988). On CT scanning, Teflon was seen in various locations relative to the bladder wall, and the location did not correlate with success or failure of the submucosal injection procedure (Gore *et al.*, 1989). Kaplan (1990) reported that the injected volume of the Teflon bead remained constant at 2 years with follow-up with MRI.

Despite encouraging success rates with this procedure, concern remains regarding the safety of injectable Polytef substance in children. Data from animal experiments demonstrated the development of a giant cell reaction locally at the injection site and migration of small Teflon particles beyond the injec-

tion site. Malizia *et al.* (1984) studied periurethral Polytef injection in animals and found distant migration of Teflon particles in monkeys to the pelvic lymph nodes, lungs, brain, kidneys, and spleen. A similar study performed with smaller injection volumes placed suburethrally in monkeys showed local migration around the bladder and distal migration to the periaortic and pelvic nodes and, in male monkeys, the testicles (Malizia *et al.*, 1988). Furthermore, the subureteric injection sites have been monitored with both CT and MRI, and the granulomas enlarge over time. Longer term follow-up in monkeys demonstrated persistent masses (granulomas) radiographically and at autopsy. Aaronson *et al.* (1993) demonstrated that Teflon injection into an animal bladder resulted in the migration of numerous small particles to the brain and lungs. They hypothesized that following the 'sting' procedure, small particles may lodge in the brain and obstruct the microcirculation.

A Teflon granuloma has been reported after particle migration to the lung in a patient treated with periurethral injection of Polytef paste (Mittleman and Marraccini, 1983). Elder (1988) reported two unusual complications after the injection of Polytef paste. The paste was found inside the corpora cavernosa of a patient with bladder exstrophy who had had periurethral injection in an attempt to attain continence. There was moderate scarring within the spongy tissue, and histologic examination confirmed a marked giant cell reaction. In another patient, a scrotal abscess and a urethrocutaneous fistula developed after periurethral injection of Polytef paste. Elder thought that these two complications were a direct result of injecting into periurethral scar tissue.

The development of local granulomas and distant migration has discouraged most pediatric urologists from using Teflon paste in children. The US Food and Drug Administration has not approved Teflon paste for urologic use. Further research studies are necessary to develop a safe material that is biocompatible and permanent, causes little inflammatory response, and does not migrate from the injection site.

Collagen

Cross-linked bovine collagen has been used widely for years for hemostatic agents, in cardiac valves, and in the injectable form as a soft-tissue substitute. Glutaraldehyde cross-linked bovine collagen preparation (Zyplast; Collagen Corporation, Palo Alto, CA,

USA) is a bovine corium collagen that is solubilized by exposure to pepsin in acetic acid and purified by ultrafiltration and ion-exchange chromatography (Gearhart, 1990). After purification, the collagen is reconstituted in a neutral solution, harvested, and resuspended in saline to provide non-cross-linked collagen. It is important to distinguish the cross-linked agent from the non-cross-linked substance (Zyderm; Collagen Corporation). Zyplast demonstrates 90–100% wet weight persistence as a stable implant in subdermal and suburothelial injection in animals (Gearhart, 1990). Zyplast is less viscous than Polytef paste, which allows for easier injection through a 23 or 25G needle. Zyplast is a safe and effective alternative to Teflon paste for the endoscopic treatment of VUR. The major drawback is the inability of collagen to conserve its volume over time.

In a series of 57 patients (92 ureters) from Johns Hopkins University, subureteric collagen corrected VUR in 75% at 1 month and 65% at 1 year post-injection (Leonard et al., 1991). Thirty-three per cent of patients required two and 5% required three injections. The initial grades of reflux influenced the cure rates. Patients with lower-grade reflux (I, II, or III) had a cure rate of 80% at 1 month. Ureters with higher grade reflux (grade IV or V) had cure rates of only 40% at 1 month. Lipsky and Wurnschimmel (1993) used collagen in 67 children and reported a 61% success rate.

Frey et al. (1992) reported a series of 66 children with 97 refluxing units and noted a 59% cure rate after one injection and a 77% rate after two injections. The mean follow-up was 18.5 months. In a follow-up study, Frey et al. (1997) compared GAX 65 with GAX 35 collagen. GAX 65 is a second-generation glutaraldehyde cross-linked collagen. Sixteen children were treated with GAX 65 and 12 with GAX 35. Short-term success rates for GAX 65 were 88% at 3 months, compared with 59% for GAX 35 at 3 months. These investigators concluded that GAX 65 appears to have significantly better implant volume preservation than GAX 35.

In patients with duplicated ureters, the use of collagen to correct VUR has given discouraging results (Reunanen, 1997). In a series of 24 children with duplication and VUR, success rates at 1 month, 6 months, 2 years, and 4 years were only 46, 25, 22, and 23%, respectively. Eventually, 83% of these children required ureteroneocystostomy. In patients who subsequently require an open procedure, the operative repair does not appear to be compromised (Frey et al., 1992).

Histologic studies have shown that there is no significant foreign body giant cell reaction in response to the implanted collagen. The amount of inflammation, neovascularization, and fibroblastic ingrowth is relatively minimal (Leonard et al., 1991). Histologic analysis of the collagen deposits removed at open ureteroneocystostomy demonstrated that endogenous fibroblasts invade the collagen implant and produce new human collagen, replacing the implant (Frey et al., 1994).

Other products

Various alternative injectable substances have been investigated experimentally and clinically. Polyvinyl alcohol foam (Ivalon) was found to be biocompatible and permanent, and to cause minimal inflammatory responses at the injection site (Merguerian et al., 1990). The endoscopic injection of blood was used with variable success in dogs to correct reflux. The animals' blood was heparinized and injected subureterically and then thrombin and protamine were added to form a clot (Kohri et al., 1988). Smith et al. (1994) studied polydimethysilox (Macroplastique) in mongrel dogs and noted a well-encapsulated foreign body reaction at the injection site, but local and distant migration was noted in two animals. Autologous fat has been used to correct VUR, but the results were poor, owing to presumed reabsorption (Chancellor et al., 1994).

Atala et al. (1992) have described new and novel methods to correct VUR endoscopically. These investigators developed an inflatable, detachable, and self-sealing silicone balloon that was implanted through a cystoscope. More recently, this group used chondrocytes in a biodegradable polymer solution to treat VUR in an animal model (Atala et al., 1994) and clinically (Diamond and Caldamone, 1998). The chondrocytes were grown from a small cartilage specimen harvested from the ear. Success rates of 60% were noted at 3 months and 79% after repeated injections with short follow-up. However, these studies are ongoing and the long-term results are not yet known.

Laparoscopic repairs

Laparoscopic correction of VUR has been described in animal models (Atala et al., 1993a; Schimberg et al., 1994) as well as in clinical trials (Ehrlich et al., 1994). The proposed advantages of this technique include smaller incisions, shorter hospitalizations, and decreased postoperative discomfort. Although technically feasible (and with reasonable success in small series), the prolonged operative time for this procedure outweighs its potential benefits over standard open and/or endoscopic techniques. In two small series of patients, endoscopic trigonoplasty has been performed to correct VUR. Preliminary results with short-term follow-up yielded only moderate success rates with significant complications (Cartwright et al., 1996; Okamura et al., 1996).

Antireflux surgery in the neuropathic bladder

It is important to recognize voiding dysfunction before embarking on surgical treatment of reflux, because voiding dysfunction will ultimately lead to failure and persistent reflux. Patients with urinary urgency, frequency, urge incontinence, or abnormal physical findings should be evaluated preoperatively with urodynamic studies. VCUG may show a thick-walled and trabeculated bladder with increased capacity and large postvoiding residual. Even though intermittent catheterization, anticholinergic agents, and antibiotic prophylaxis should be the first line of treatment for patients with neuropathic bladder and VUR, some children may require ureteroneocystostomy (Kass et al. 1981; Kaplan, 1990). The indications for antireflux surgery in these patients are similar to those for patients with primary reflux and include breakthrough UTI and the development of progressive renal scarring. However, since most of these patients are on CIC, bacteriuria is the rule and the clinical diagnosis of UTI and pyelonephritis may be hard to verify. A DMSA renal scan can be helpful.

Ureteral reimplantation has been shown to be an effective method for correcting reflux in children with neurogenic bladder dysfunction (Bauer et al., 1982; Evans et al., 1986). Ureteroneocystostomy is more difficult, and it is often necessary to inject saline submucosally to facilitate creation of the tunnel. Techniques that involve bringing the ureter through a new hiatus (suprahiatal ureteroneocystostomy) have not been as successful as those involving infrahiatal advancement procedures. In patients with a neuropathic bladder, contralateral reflux after ureteral reim-

plantation may occur in up to 50% (Johnston et al., 1976), particulary if aggressive medical management is not pursued. One of the most important reasons for failure in patients undergoing ureteral reimplantation is undiagnosed occult neuropathic bladder secondary to detrusor-sphincter dyssynergia. These patients must be maintained on anticholinergic medication and intermittent catheterization postoperatively to keep bladder pressures low. Failures may occur late and are often the result of UVJ obstruction due to abnormalities in bladder dynamics with increased intravesical pressures.

A select group of patients with neuropathic bladder and high voiding pressure may require augmentation cystoplasty in addition to ureteroneocystostomy. Enterocystoplasty effectively lowers bladder pressures, and the success of ureteral reimplantation into either the bladder or bowel segment has been well documented. The use of enterocystoplasty alone may normalize detrusor pressure and correct reflux without the necessity of performing ureteral reimplantation (Nasrallah and Aliabadi, 1991) (see Chapter 16).

Vesicoureteral reflux and ureteral duplication

VUR is the most common abnormality associated with complete ureteral duplication. Approximately 10% of children undergoing antireflux surgery have complete or incomplete duplication of the collecting system (Kelalis, 1985). Lower pole reflux most often persists and is unlikely to abate with growth (Kelalis, 1971). Spontaneous resolution of reflux occurred in only 22% of patients with renal duplication followed non-operatively during a 13-year period of observation (Kaplan et al., 1978). Husmann and Allen (1991) compared a series of patients with grade II VUR with and without complete renal duplication. During a 2-year observation period, reflux ceased spontaneously in only 10% with duplication, compared with 35% of patients with a single system ($p < 0.01$).

Conversely, others have shown that reflux into the lower pole of a duplex kidney did not constitute an absolute indication for early surgical intervention. Ben-Ami et al. (1989) compared a series of children with grades I, II, or III reflux into the lower pole of a duplicated collecting system with a control group of children with reflux into a single collecting system. There were no significant differences between the two groups with respect to resolution of reflux or incidence of new parenchymal scars.

Peppas *et al.* (1991) reviewed the records of 56 children with reflux into a duplicated lower pole system. Of the 70 refluxing units, 18% demonstrated resolution of reflux within 42 months, 23% were stable on prophylaxis at the time of the review, and 57% had undergone surgical repair. However, of the patients with grades I–III reflux, 58% had spontaneous resolution. The conclusion reached was that resolution of reflux in the presence of duplication is similar to that for the single system, dependent upon grade at the time of recognition.

In patients with an incomplete ureteral duplication, a single ureteral orifice enters the bladder but reflux affects both components of the duplication. These patients should undergo conventional ureteroneocystostomy. In rare cases, the duplicated ureters adjoin in the juxtavesical region and form a V-type duplication. If operative intervention is indicated, it is preferable that the two ureters be converted into complete duplication by resecting the common stem and reimplanting both ureters as a unit through a single submucosal tunnel. Simple reimplantation without excision of the distal ureter may accentuate the functional obstruction at the union of the two ureters. This may result in ureteroureteral reflux and produce hydroureteronephrosis (Scott, 1963).

When complete ureteral duplication is present, reflux essentially always involves the lower segment orifice. Several surgical alternatives are available for correcting this type of reflux. Reimplanting the ureters via a common submucosal tunnel after the two ureters have been mobilized in their common sheath generally produces excellent results, providing that the lower pole ureter is not greatly dilated relative to the normal upper pole ureter (Ellsworth *et al.*, 1996). This technique eliminates reflux in the lower ureter without disturbing the function of the upper segment. A theoretical disadvantage of this procedure is that the larger ureter may obstruct the smaller one.

In the presence of significant dilatation of the lower pole ureter, distal ureteroureterostomy is an acceptable alternative to common sheath reimplantation (Bracci *et al.*, 1979; Bieri *et al.*, 1998). This operation converts a duplex system into a bifid system and allows removal of the refluxing ureteral stump (Figs. 25.33a, b) (Bockrath *et al.* 1983; Ahmed and Boucaut, 1988). The procedure can be accomplished without opening the bladder; it is simple and associated with a high degree of success even in the presence of a dilated ureter.

Another technique to bypass the UVJ is pyeloureterostomy, in which the renal pelvis is anastomosed end to side into the upper pole ureter (Fig. 25.33c). The anastomosis must be angled correctly and be approximately 2 cm in length, so that the end result is similar to the naturally occurring bifid renal pelvis. This flank approach allows examination and biopsy of the involved renal segment (Belman *et al.*, 1974). Patients undergoing either a ureteroureterostomy or pyeloureterostomy must have one normal draining non-refluxing unit. This anastomosis may be difficult if the caliber of the recipient ureter is small.

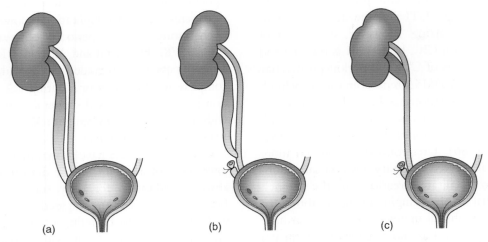

(a)   (b)   (c)

Figure 25.33 (*a*) Complete duplication with reflux in the lower segment; (*b*) ureteroureterostomy; (*c*) pyeloureterostomy. (Modified from Kramer, 1992, with permission of the Mayo Foundation.)

In either case, the anastomotic area is drained and no stents are used. The distal ureter is excised and the stump ligated.

In some patients with lower pole reflux, the involved renal segment may be dysplastic and require lower pole heminephrectomy. The lower pole ureter is dissected as far down as safely possible, taking care to preserve the blood supply to the intact upper pole ureter. The ureteral stump should be ligated, with appropriate paravesical drainage for a few days, or the ureter may be split open down to the bladder. It is unusual for the ureteral stump to be associated with postoperative infection or to act as a vesical diverticulum. Total nephrectomy is almost never justified.

Preliminary drainage

Children with VUR occasionally present with azotemia and acute urinary sepsis. In these patients, it probably is wise to place a urethral catheter temporarily to minimize stasis and to treat the infection appropriately. In small infants with significant ureteral dilatation, megacystis, and UTI, either intermittent catheterization or a cutaneous vesicostomy may be preferable to initial ureteroneocystostomy. Intermittent catheterization or cutaneous vesicostomy may be continued for 1–2 years, at which time ureteral reimplantation can be accomplished more successfully. The author prefers to close the cutaneous vesicostomy initially, allowing the bladder mucosa and muscle to return to normal. A second VCUG is performed a few months later, and if reflux persists, a ureteroneocystostomy is performed.

Postoperative results

The two criteria for judging the success of ureteroneocystostomy are the elimination of VUR and the absence of obstructive hydroureteronephrosis. The literature is replete with series documenting greater than 90% success after various reimplantation techniques (Politano, 1963; Palken, 1970; Gonzales *et al.*, 1972; Woodard and Keats, 1973). Recently, the need for VCUG postoperatively has been questioned. In a series of 332 patients undergoing various repairs for VUR, successful results were reported in 94% and the only risk factor associated with failure was a postoperative UTI (Bomalaski *et al.*, 1997). These authors concluded that no postoperative radiographs are necessary in patients undergoing a non-tapered ureteroneocystostomy without a neuropathic bladder. In a literature review of more than 1000 patients, Bisignani and Decter (1997) found that 98% of patients had an initial successful result. Of the 2% who had failure, 85% had spontaneous resolution with time. They recommended no postoperative VCUG as a significant cost-saving measure. Despite these recent observations, most surgeons continue to recommend postoperative imaging studies to document the success of their efforts.

The incidence of clinical pyelonephritis is markedly decreased after successful ureteroneocystostomy. Govan and Palmer (1969) reported a decrease in pyelonephritis from 50% to less than 10% after successful reimplantation. Willscher *et al.* (1976a) reported that even though UTI recurred postoperatively in approximately 20% of patients, fewer than 2% had clinical pyelonephritis. Bacteriuria may occur in up to 30% of patients postoperatively and does not correlate with either the preoperative urographic appearance or the severity of the reflux (Wacksman *et al.*, 1978). This is approximately the same incidence of bacteriuria in children with no reflux and in those with reflux who are being treated medically.

Complications

Complications after ureteral reimplantation result from either preoperative planning errors or errors in intraoperative technique. UTI should be eliminated before operation. Cystitis and mucosal edema compromise the ability to achieve a sufficient submucosal tunnel and increase the risk of postoperative ureteral obstruction. An occult neuropathic bladder may contribute to failure of ureteral reimplantation. It is important that children with reflux and diurnal enuresis, squatting maneuvers, constipation, or encopresis be evaluated thoroughly with complete urodynamic studies before surgery to rule out detrusor-sphincter dyssynergia. In patients with a neuropathic bladder, it is important to normalize detrusor dynamics as much as possible preoperatively. This may include frequent or timed voiding, intermittent catheterization, and anticholinergic therapy. It is very difficult to make this diagnosis in children who are in diapers. In these infants, the obvious bladder lesion is often discovered intraoperatively, when the bladder is opened or during attempts at creating a submucosal tunnel.

Excessive tissue handling during ureteral mobilization may contribute to postoperative edema or devascularization of the ureter. Technical errors intraoperatively include ureteral perforation, ureteral transection, or avulsion during mobilization. Ureteral obstruction may occur secondary to creation of a too tight detrusor hiatus, passing the ureter through a peritoneal fold or intraperitoneal structure, and placement of the bladder neohiatus too cephalad and lateral.

Early perioperative complications include bleeding, catheter obstruction or dislodgment, sepsis, ureteral obstruction, anuria, and prolonged ileus. Postoperative gross hematuria usually resolves within 36–48 hours, but it may require catheter irrigation. Hematuria beyond 3–4 days may be the result of irritation from the catheter and can often be corrected by its removal. Occasionally, ileus develops postoperatively in children because of anticholinergic and narcotic therapy. These situations respond quite adequately to either glycerin or bisacodyl (Dulcolax) suppositories. Prolonged ileus usually reflects ureteral obstruction, subtle sepsis, retroperitoneal leakage of urine, retroperitoneal hematoma, or passage of a ureter through the peritoneum or a segment of intestine. Ileus that persists for more than 48 hours postoperatively is of concern and should promote a careful review of kidneys, ureters, and bladder, as well as upright studies.

Interval management

Early postoperative ureteral obstruction is most often due to detrusor edema. Ureteral obstruction may present with oliguria, anuria if bilateral, flank pain, nausea and vomiting, sepsis, or prolonged ileus. Hydronephrosis secondary to ureteral obstruction is confirmed by renal ultrasonography. It is suspected when the degree of dilatation on the sonogram is greater than the maximum noted on the preoperative cystogram. The options for interval management for patients with early postoperative UVJ obstruction include observation, placement of percutaneous nephrostomy tubes, or internal ureteral stents. In patients with mild obstruction but with good urine output, observation alone may be indicated. If significant obstruction exists, as evidenced by severe hydronephrosis or delayed visualization on isotope renography, percutaneous nephrostomy tubes can be placed temporarily until the edema resolves. It is best to postpone reoperation for at least 3 months to allow the edema and postsurgical reaction to subside.

Nephrostograms can be obtained periodically during this interval to reassess ureteral patency, and occasionally, an obstructed system will open up. Endoscopic visualization and catheterization of the recently reimplanted ureters in the immediate postoperative period may be difficult, particularly in children who have undergone a cross-trigonal reimplantation.

Obstruction

The incidence of ureterovesical junction obstruction requiring reoperation is between 1 and 4%. Obstruction after ureteral reimplantation may occur as a result of one of three major causes.

Mechanical factors

Mechanical obstruction may result from the presence of paravesical scar tissue, ureteral kinking and angulation, and an intraperitoneal course of the ureter with resultant angulation at the point of entry or exit from the peritoneum. Frequently, this obstruction is intermittent, and it results from angulation of the ureter at its new hiatus (J-hooking), when the entrance has been placed too high and laterally on the bladder wall. In these instances, a film taken with the bladder full will show hydroureteronephrosis; with the bladder empty, it will show regression of hydroureteronephrosis (Fig. 25.34).

Ischemia

Devascularization of the lower ureter can occur with subsequent stricture formation. Avoidance of aggressive dissection of the ureter during intravesical mobilization can prevent distal ureteral ischemia. Ischemia may also develop by creating a ureteral hiatus that is too tight or by twisting of the distal ureteral segment.

Neuropathic bladder

Unrecognized neuropathic bladder may produce obstruction secondary to a thick-walled, trabeculated detrusor. The level of the obstruction may be extravesical, intravesical, or at the bladder wall. Extravesical obstruction can be prevented by avoiding injury to blood vessels contiguous to the ureter (i.e. the uterine artery) that might result in bleeding and hematoma, with subsequent ureteral scarring and compression of the distal ureter. Penetration of the peritoneum may occur during development of a new hiatus and should be avoided by adequate visualization during dissec-

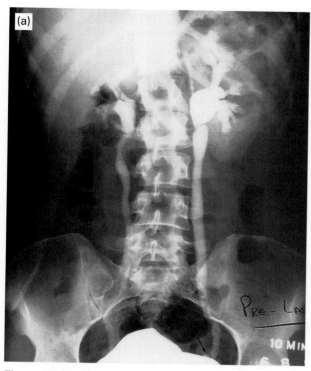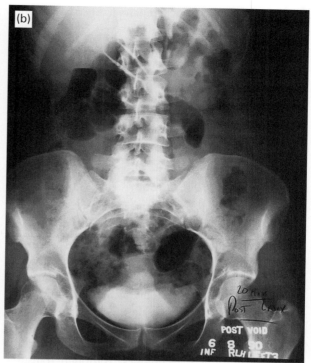

Figure 25.34 J-hooking of the ureter. (*a*) Excretory urogram with the bladder full; (*b*) with the bladder empty. Note regression of dilatation of the ureter and straightening of its course. No reflux was demonstrated. (From Kramer, 1992)

tion. Kinking and J-hooking of the ureter should be prevented by choosing a more medial hiatus in the posterior, less expansile portion of the bladder. When the bladder wall is thick and trabeculated, it is preferable to reimplant the ureter by one of the techniques that does not require creation of a new hiatus.

Reflux

The incidence of persistent VUR requiring reoperation is between 1 and 3%. The mechanisms of failure in patients in whom VUR develops include either a short submucosal tunnel or an unrecognized neuropathic bladder. A short submucosal tunnel is usually due to malposition of the ureteral orifice or to its retraction after inadequate trigonal fixation. Problems associated with an unrecognized neuropathic bladder are described above.

VUR that appears on the initial VCUG within a few months after surgery does not always signify failure. It may take several months for inflammatory changes to resolve and the antireflux flap-valve mechanism to become competent (Willscher *et al.*, 1976a). Rarely, high-grade reflux that persists after a technically satisfactory ureteral reimplantation may resolve

spontaneously several months after reimplantation (Siegelbaum and Rabinovitch, 1987). Voiding dysfunction may also play a role.

Definitive management

The options for definitive management include nonsurgical, endoscopic, and open repairs.

Non-surgical repair

The treatment of failed ureteral reimplantation due to an occult or primary neuropathic bladder should be directed at the bladder alone. This may consist of frequent voiding, double voiding, anticholinergic therapy, or clean intermittent catheterization (or a combination of these). Behavioral modification with the institution of proper voiding habits and treatment of constipation, if present, must be incorporated into the overall treatment plan.

Endoscopic repair

In children with low-grade VUR, collagen is an acceptable alternative to open reoperative ureteroneocystostomy. Balloon dilation may be a reasonable alternative to open surgical repairs for partial obstruction if the obstruction is discovered early and the stricture to be dilated is short (Shore *et al.*, 1986). Early dilation has been associated with better long-term results than dilation carried out after several months (Hulbert *et al.*, 1988; Mesrobian and Kelalis, 1989). However, this technique cannot be expected to be successful if the distal ureter is partially devascularized.

Open surgical procedures

The majority of failed ureteral reimplantations can be salvaged with various well-described techniques. In the author's experience, failure due to UVJ obstruction has been treated most reliably with a Paquin ureteral reimplantation combined with a psoas hitch (Table 25.5) (Mesrobian *et al.*, 1985). This technique allows construction of a long submucosal tunnel and immobilizes the new hiatus. Failed ureteral reimplantation due to VUR can be managed effectively by using various ureteral advancement techniques. Although transureteroureterostomy has not been extensively used in our series, this is an excellent surgical option, especially when bilateral reimplantation becomes necessary into a small and scarred bladder.

Occasionally, the ureter can become atonic, scarred, and shortened after multiple attempts at reimplantation. Selected patients may require an augmentation cystoplasty to alter bladder dynamics or for reimplantation of the refluxing ureter into the bowel segment.

The overall success after reoperation for UVJ obstruction or VUR is approximately 80%. Surgery is more likely to be successful in patients with persistent VUR than for persistent UVJ obstruction (Mesrobian *et al.*, 1985). This finding may be the result of a higher proportion of patients in the obstructed group who have a neuropathic bladder as the primary cause of failure of the original reimplantation.

It is suggested that patients be followed carefully after ureteral reimplantation. Growth spurts and hormonal changes at puberty may alter the configuration of the UVJ. Obstruction rather than reflux is the most significant late serious complication and, therefore, periodic ultrasonographic examinations of the urinary tract are advisable during this interval. Additionally, those with renal scarring require periodic blood pressure measurement.

Contralateral reflux

Contralateral reflux most often resolves with prolonged follow-up, and the incidence of persistent contralateral reflux in patients undergoing unilateral ureteroneocystostomy is only 3–5% (Hanani *et al.*, 1983; Quinlan and O'Donnell, 1985; Burno *et al.*, 1998; Noe, 1998). There are specific patients at higher risk for the development of contralateral reflux, and the additional morbidity of bilateral reimplantation for unilateral reflux in this select group of patients is low.

Contralateral reflux occurs more often in patients with a previous history of reflux on that side, but no

Table 25.5 Results of reoperation for ureterovesical junction obstruction and vesicoureteral reflux

Procedure	Renal units		Success	
	n	%	*n*	%
Ureterovesical junction obstruction				
Modified Paquin	32	65	25	78
Modified Politano–Leadbetter	15	31	8	53
Advancement	2	4	1	50
Total	49	100	34	69
Vesicoureteral reflux				
Modified Paquin	15	31	13	87
Modified Politano–Leadbetter	17	36	17	100
Advancement	14	29	11	79
Transureteroureterostomy	2	4	2	100
Total	48	100	43	90

From Mesrobian *et al.* (1985) with permission of Lippincott Williams & Wilkins.

reflux at the time of ipsilateral reimplantation. This observation supports the concept that contralateral reflux is the result of an incompetent contralateral ureteral orifice that was not reimplanted. Parrott and Woodard (1976) found contralateral reflux in eight of 40 children (20%) undergoing unilateral reimplantation. Fifty per cent of these patients had an abnormal-appearing orifice at the time of cystoscopy before ipsilateral reimplantation. Warren et al. (1972) found an abnormal orifice in four of 11 patients (36%) in whom contralateral reflux developed. In patients with unilateral reflux, bilateral reimplantation should be considered in those who have a history of prior reflux in the now non-refluxing side and an abnormal location and configuration of the non-refluxing orifice (Ross et al., 1995). Caione et al. (1997) proposed a novel method of contralateral ureteral meatal advancement to prevent contralateral reflux. This technique was effective in preventing VUR in all cases, compared with an 11% incidence of contralateral reflux in their control group.

Another proposed cause for contralateral reflux is the disturbance of the ureterotrigonal continuity on the contralateral side during surgical dissection. Kumar and Puri (1997) found only a 7% incidence of contralateral reflux following subureteric Teflon injection in patients with unilateral reflux. This low rate of contralateral reflux was thought to be due to non-interference of the contralateral trigone following the endoscopic injection technique. However, Hoenig et al. (1996) reported no difference in contralateral reflux between patients undergoing a Cohen cross-trigonal repair and those undergoing a Glenn–Anderson advancement. Overall, 19% of patients had contralateral reflux (Cohen, 21%, and Glenn-Anderson, 17%), of whom 61% had spontaneous resolution of that re-acquired reflux. These authors concluded that trigonal distortion was probably not the cause of contralateral reflux, considering the similar incidence of reflux between the two procedures.

Diamond et al. (1996b) identified high-grade reflux and reflux into duplex systems as significant risk factors for the development of contralateral reflux postoperatively. They speculated that loss of a 'pop-off' mechanism was likely to be responsible for the development of contralateral reflux. Conversely, McCool et al. (1997) reported that the preoperative grade of reflux, the presence of a duplicated system, or the endoscopic appearance of the ureteral orifice did not influence the development of contralateral reflux.

Megaureter

Congenital megaureter may occur as a result of primary VUR, primary UVJ obstruction, posterior urethral valves, prune-belly syndrome, neuropathic bladder, ectopic ureterocele, or an iatrogenic cause, often the result of failed ureteroneocystostomy (Kelalis and Kramer, 1983). Patients with obstructive or refluxing megaureter require reduction in the ureteral caliber at the time of ureteral reimplantation. This is done to achieve an adequate length-to-width ratio in the new intravesical ureter, to relieve ureteral dilatation, to allow effective ureteral peristalsis, and to eliminate residual urine within the ureter. Some megaureters show both reflux and obstruction (Whitaker and Flower, 1979).

Refluxing ureters larger than 1 cm in diameter almost always require reduction in ureteral caliber. There is often a relatively aperistaltic distal segment (Tanagho, 1971). Surgical correction for obstructive megaureter responds well to various techniques (Rabinowitz et al., 1979), whereas surgical results in refluxing megaureters have been less satisfactory (Johnston and Farkas, 1975). Overall success rates range from 54% (Coleman and McGovern, 1979) to greater than 90% (Ehrlich, 1982; McLorie et al., 1994) for ureteroneocystostomy of megaureters.

Excision and tapering

Approximately 10–12 cm of distal ureter should be mobilized transvesically. The entire tapering procedure and reimplantation can be performed intravesically without the need to transpose the ureter into the paravesical space. Meticulous attention must be paid to the blood supply of the ureter during dissection. The ureter has a medial mesentery from the kidney to the pelvic brim, but the blood supply is lateral in the true pelvis. The tortuous ureter is straightened, and the lower redundant portion is excised. The lower third of the ureter should be reduced in caliber to encompass not only the submucosal tunnel but also a few centimeters proximal to the ureteral hiatus (Johnston, 1967). Hanna (1979) has advocated a one-stage total remodeling of the dilated and tortuous ureter, but this is rarely necessary in most patients.

The segment of the ureter to be removed can be marked with Babcock or Hendren clamps, which are used to trap the ureteral catheter in the segment of the ureter to be preserved (Fig. 25.35). Caliber

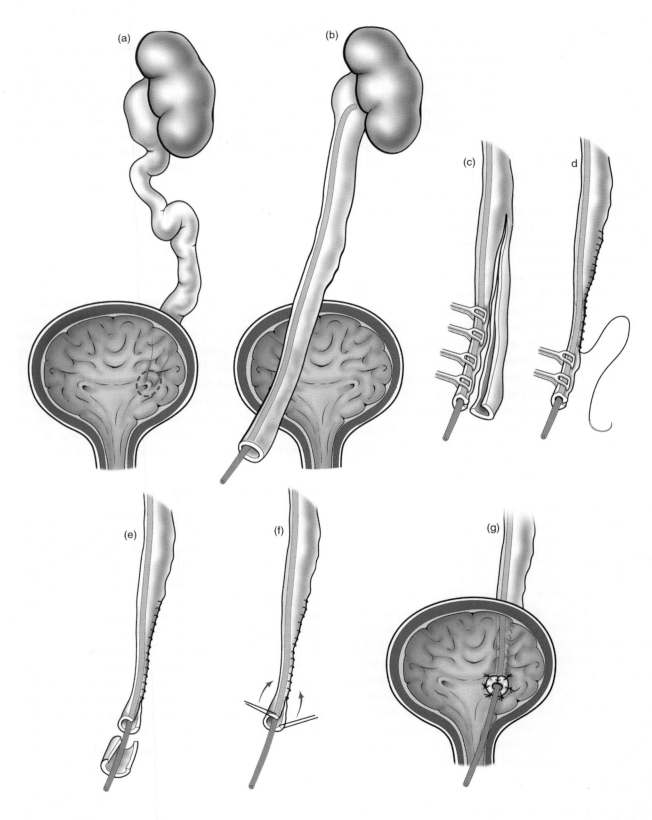

Figure 25.35 Technique of ureteral caliber reduction. (Modified from Kramer, 1992, with permission of Mayo Foundation.)

reduction is achieved by excising the 'antimesenteric' ureter. The intact ureter that is left behind is subsequently closed in two layers with fine continuous and interrupted absorbable sutures. There should be a gradual transition between the reduced ureteral caliber and the dilated proximal ureter. An 8 Fr ureteral catheter should fit loosely within the ureter. A ureteroneocystostomy is accomplished, and any excessive ureteral length after tapering is removed. The remodeled ureter should be stented for 7–10 days.

Diamond and Parulkar (1998) described a technique of ureteral tailoring *in situ* for persistent reflux in the dilated reimplanted ureter. This procedure is useful in selected patients with postoperative reflux in whom tunnel length and muscular backing are adequate but the diameter of the ureter remains wide.

Ureteral folding

The ureteral folding technique, first reported by Kaliciński *et al.* (1977) (Fig. 25.36) and modified by Starr (1979) (Fig. 25.37), involves reduction of ureteral caliber without excision of the ureteral wall. The lateral excluded ureteral lumen is folded either anteriorly or posteriorly with multiple interrupted sutures along the medial wall. The reduction of the ureteral caliber should extend for a few centimeters proximal to the bladder wall. A ureteroneocystostomy by one of the accepted techniques is performed. The bulk of the folded ureter usually does not interfere with placement into the submucosal tunnel. How-

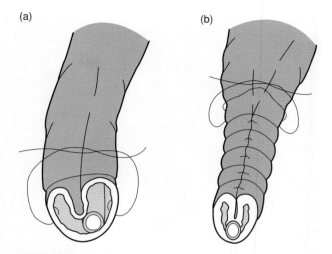

Figure 25.37 Starr technique for ureteral folding.

ever, in some patients, the ureter is too wide and bulky, and formal excision and tapering should be accomplished. This technique has the advantage of preserving blood supply, and it reduces the chance of suture line leakage; therefore, it does not require prolonged ureteral stenting. Stents are optional with this procedure, but if used, they are usually removed within 48–72 hours. This technique has produced excellent results, with a low incidence of complications (Ehrlich, 1985).

The results of ureteral caliber reduction, either excising or folding, should not be based exclusively on the appearance of the excretory urogram (Figs. 25.38, 25.39) but also on the resumption of renal growth and function, that is probably best evaluated by

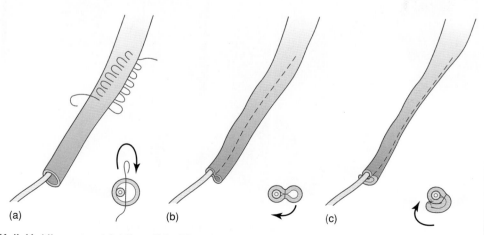

Figure 25.36 Kaliciński's ureteral folding. (Modified from Kramer, 1992.)

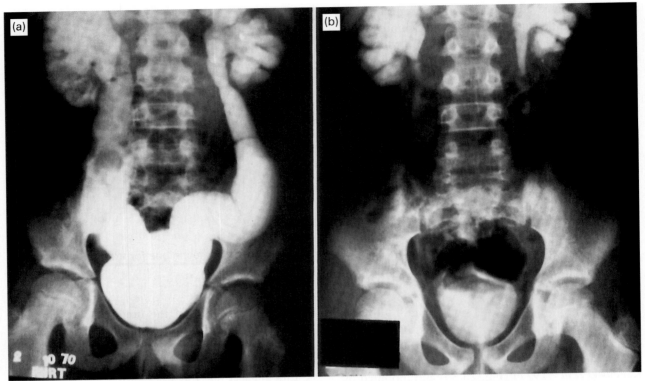

Figure 25.38 Reflux megaureter. Excretory urograms before (*a*) and 1 year after (*b*) ureteral caliber reduction.

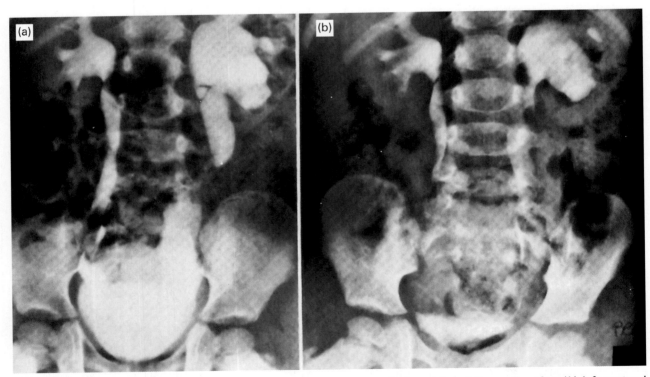

Figure 25.39 Primary obstructive megaureter. Excretory urograms before (*a*) and 5 months after (*b*) left ureteral reduction.

diuretic-stimulated renal scan, and the elimination of pyelonephritis. In neonates with bilateral refluxing megaureters and megacystis, preliminary diversion by cutaneous vesicostomy may be indicated. In neonates and infants with bilateral obstructive megaureters and a small bladder capacity, a unilateral ureteral caliber reduction, which uses up most of the bladder base, and transureteroureterostomy of the contralateral ureter may be technically easier than bilateral ureteral reimplantation with ureteral tapering.

References

Aaronson IA, Rames RA, Greene WB *et al*. (1993) Endoscopic treatment of reflux: migration of Teflon to the lungs and brain. *Eur Urol* **23**: 394–9.

Ahmed S, Boucaut HA (1988) Vesicoureteral reflux in complete ureteral duplication: surgical options. *J Urol* **140**: 1092–4.

Allen TD (1979) Vesicoureteral reflux as a manifestation of dysfunctional voiding. In: Hodson CJ, Kincaid-Smith P (eds) *Reflux nephropathy*. New York: Masson Publishing, 171–80.

Allen TD (1985) Vesicoureteral reflux and the unstable bladder (Letter). *J Urol* **134**: 1180.

Anderson C, Kevorkian T (1998) Perioperative use of Ketoralac in the pediatric patient. *Soc Pediatr Urol Newslett* **1**: 2–5.

Anderson PAM, Rickwood AMK (1991) Features of primary vesicoureteric reflux detected by prenatal sonography. *Br J Urol* **67**: 267.

Arant BS Jr (1992) Medical management of mild and moderate vesicoureteral reflux: followup studies of infants and young children. A preliminary report of the Southwest Pediatric Nephrology Study Group. *J Urol* **148**: 1683–7.

Arap S, Abrão EG, Menezes de Góes G (1981) Treatment and prevention of complications after extravesical antireflux technique. *Eur Urol* **7**: 263–7.

Arnold GE (1963) Alleviation of aphonia or dysphonia through intrachordal injection of Teflon paste. *Ann Otol Rhinol Laryngol* **72**: 384–95.

Askari A, Belman AB (1982) Vesicoureteral reflux in black girls. *J Urol* **127**: 747–8.

Atala A, Peters CA, Retik AB *et al*. (1992) Endoscopic treatment of vesicoureteral reflux with a self-detachable balloon system. *J Urol* **148**: 724–7.

Atala A, Kavoussi LR, Goldstein DS *et al*. (1993a) Laparoscopic correction of vesicoureteral reflux. *J Urol* **150**: 748–51.

Atala A, Wible JH, Share JC *et al*. (1993b) Sonography with sonicated albumin in the detection of vesicoureteral reflux. *J Urol* **150**: 756–8.

Atala A, Kim W, Paige KT *et al*. (1994) Endoscopic treatment of vesicoureteral reflux with a chondrocyte-alginate suspension. *J Urol* **152**: 641–3.

Atwell JD, Vijay MR (1978) Renal growth following reimplantation of the ureters for reflux. *Br J Urol* **50**: 367–79.

Austenfeld MS, Snow BW (1988) Complications of pregnancy in women after reimplantation for vesicoureteral reflux. *J Urol* **140**: 1103–6.

Avni EF, Schulman CC (1996) The origin of vesico-ureteric reflux in male newborns: further evidence in favour of a transient fetal urethral obstruction. *Br J Urol* **78**: 454–9.

Bailey RR (1973) The relationship of vesico-ureteric reflux to urinary tract infection and chronic pyelonephritis – reflux nephropathy. *Clin Nephrol* **1**: 132–41.

Baker R, Maxted W, Maglath J *et al*. (1966) Relation of age, sex and infection to reflux: data indicating high spontaneous cure rate in pediatric patients. *J Urol* **95**: 27–32.

Bakshandeh K, Lynne C, Carrion H (1976) Vesicoureteral reflux and end stage renal disease. *J Urol* **116**: 557–8.

Bauer SB, Colodny AH, Retik AB (1982) The management of vesicoureteral reflux in children with myelodysplasia. *J Urol* **128**: 102–5.

Becker GJ, Ihle BU, Fairley KF *et al*. (1986) Effect of pregnancy on moderate renal failure in reflux nephropathy. *BMJ* **292**: 796–8.

Becu L, Quesada EM, Medel R *et al*. (1988) Small kidney associated with primary vesicoureteral reflux in children: a pathological overhaul. *Eur Urol* **14**: 127–40.

Beetz R, Schulte-Wisserman H, Tröger J *et al*. (1989) Long-term follow-up of children with surgically treated vesicorenal reflux: postoperative incidence of urinary tract infections, renal scars and arterial hypertension. *Eur Urol* **16**: 366–71.

Belman AB (1995) A perspective on vesicoureteral reflux. *Urol Clin North Am* **22**: 139–49.

Belman AB, Filmer RB, King LR (1974) Surgical management of duplication of the collecting system. *J Urol* **112**: 316–21.

Ben-Ami T, Gayer G, Hertz M *et al*. (1989) The natural history of reflux in the lower pole of duplicated collecting systems: a controlled study. *Pediatr Radiol* **19**: 308–10.

Bieri M, Smith CK, Smith AY *et al*. (1998) Ipsilateral uretero-ureterostomy for single ureteral reflux or obstruction in a duplicate system. *J Urol* **159**: 1016–8.

Birmingham Reflux Study Group (1983) Prospective trial of operative versus non-operative treatment of severe vesicoureteric reflux: two years' observation in 96 children. *BMJ* **287**: 171–4.

Birmingham Reflux Study Group (1987) Prospective trial of operative versus non-operative treatment of severe vesicoureteric reflux in children: five years' observation. *BMJ* **295**: 237–41.

Bisignani G, Decter RM (1997) Voiding cystourethrography after uncomplicated ureteral reimplantation in children: is it necessary? *J Urol* **158**: 1229–31.

Blane CE, DiPietro MA, Zerin JM *et al*. (1993) Renal sonography is not a reliable screening examination for vesicoureteral reflux. *J Urol* **150**: 752–5.

Blaufox MD, Gruskin A, Sandler P *et al*. (1971) Radionuclide scintigraphy for detection of vesicoureteral reflux in children. *J Pediatr* **79**: 239–46.

Bockrath JM, Maizels M, Firlit CF (1983) The use of lower ipsilateral ureteroureterostomy to treat vesicoureteral reflux or obstruction in children with duplex ureters. *J Urol* **129**: 543–4.

Bomalaski MD, Ritchey ML, Bloom DA (1997) What imaging studies are necessary to determine outcome after ureteroneocystostomy? *J Urol* **158**: 1226–8.

Bracci U, Miano L, Laurenti C (1979) Ureteroureterostomy in complete ureteral duplication. *Eur Urol* **5**: 347–51.

Brandell RA, Brock JW III (1993) Ureteral reimplantation: postoperative management without catheters. *Urology* **42**: 705–7.

Briggs EM, Constantinou CE, Govan DE (1972) Dynamics of the upper urinary tract: the relationship of urine flow rate and rate of ureteral peristalsis. *Invest Urol* **10**: 56–62.

Brown S (1989) Open versus endoscopic surgery in the treatment of vesicoureteral reflux. *J Urol* **142**: 499–500.

Brühl P, van Ahlen H, Mallmann R (1988) Antireflux procedure by Lich–Grégoir: indications and results. *Eur Urol* **14**: 37–40.

Bukowski TP, Betrus GG, Aquilina JW *et al*. (1998) Urinary tract infections and pregnancy in women who underwent antireflux surgery in childhood. *J Urol* **159**: 1286–9.

Buonomo C, Treves ST, Jones B *et al*. (1993) Silent renal damage in symptom-free siblings of children with vesicoureteral reflux: assessment with technetium Tc 99m dimercaptosuccinic acid scintigraphy. *J Pediatr* **122**: 721–3.

Burbige KA (1991) Ureteral reimplantation: a comparison of results with the cross-trigonal and Politano–Leadbetter techniques in 120 patients. *J Urol* **146**: 1352–3.

Burbige KA, Miller M, Connor JP (1996) Extravesical ureteral reimplantation: results in 128 patients. *J Urol* **155**: 1721–2.

Burger RH, Burger SE (1974) Genetic determinants of urologic disease. *Urol Clin North Am* **1**: 419–40.

Burno DK, Glazier DB, Zaontz MR (1998) Lessons learned about contralateral reflux after unilateral extravesical ureteral advancement in children. *J Urol* **160**: 995–7.

Cain MP, Husmann DA, McLaren RH *et al*. (1995) Continuous epidural anesthesia after ureteroneocystostomy in children. *J Urol* **154**: 791–3.

Caione P, Capozza N, Lais A *et al*. (1997) Contralateral ureteral meatal advancement in unilateral antireflux surgery. *J Urol* **158**: 1216–8.

Carini M, Selli C, Lenzi R *et al*. (1985) Surgical treatment of vesicoureteral reflux with bilateral medialization of the ureteral orifices. *Eur Urol* **11**: 181–3.

Carson CC III, Kelalis PP, Hoffman AD (1982) Renal growth in small kidneys after ureteroneocystostomy. *J Urol* **127**: 1146–8.

Cartwright PC, Snow BW, Mansfield JC *et al*. (1996) Percutaneous endoscopic trigonoplasty: a minimally invasive approach to correct vesicoureteral reflux. *J Urol* **156**: 661–4.

Chancellor MB, Rivas DA, Liberman SN *et al*. (1994) Cystoscopic autogenous fat injection treatment of vesicoureteral reflux in spinal cord injury. *J Am Parapleg Soc* **17**: 50–4.

Chandra M, Maddix H, McVicar M (1996) Transient urodynamic dysfunction of infancy: relationship to urinary tract infections and vesicoureteral reflux. *J Urol* **155**: 673–7.

Claësson I, Lindberg U (1977) Asymptomatic bacteriuria in schoolgirls: VII. A follow-up study of the urinary tract in treated and untreated schoolgirls with asymptomatic bacteriuria. *Radiology* **124**: 179–83.

Claësson I, Jacobsson B, Jodal U *et al*. (1981) Compensatory kidney growth in children with urinary tract infection and unilateral renal scarring: an epidemiologic study. *Kidney Int* **20**: 759–64.

Cohen SJ (1975) Ureterozystoneostomie: eine neue antireflux Technik. *Aktuelle Urol* **6**: 1.

Coleman JW, McGovern JH (1979) A 20-year experience with pediatric ureteral reimplantation: surgical results in 701 children. In: Hodson CJ, Kincaid-Smith P (eds) *Reflux Nephropathy*. New York: Masson Publishing, 299–305.

Connolly LP, Treves ST, Connolly SA *et al*. (1997) Vesicoureteral reflux in children: incidence and severity in siblings. *J Urol* **157**: 2287–90.

Conway JJ, King LR, Belman AB *et al*. (1972) Detection of vesicoureteral reflux with radionuclide cystography: a comparison with roentgenographic cystography. *Am J Roentgenol Radium Ther Nucl Med* **115**: 720–7.

Cotran RS, Pennington JE (1981) Urinary tract infection, pyelonephritis, and reflux nephropathy. In Brenner BM, Rector FC Jr (eds) *The kidney*, Volume 2, 2nd edition. Philadelphia, PA: WB Saunders, 1571–632.

Cremin BJ (1979) Observations on vesico-ureteric reflux and intrarenal reflux: a review and survey of material. *Clin Radiol* **30**: 607–21.

Currarino G (1965) Roentgenographic estimation of kidney size in normal individuals with emphasis on children. *AJR Am J Roentgenol* **93**: 464–6.

Cussen LJ (1967) Dimensions of the normal ureter in infancy and childhood. *Invest Urol* **5**: 164–78.

Daines SL, Hodgson NB (1971) Management of reflux in total duplication anomalies. *J Urol* **105**: 720–4.

Decter RM, Roth DR, Gonzales ET Jr (1988) Vesicoureteral reflux in boys. *J Urol* **140**: 1089–91.

DeKlerk DP, Reiner WG, Jeffs RD (1979) Vesicoureteral reflux and ureteropelvic junction obstruction: late occurrence of ureteropelvic obstruction after successful ureteroneocystostomy. *J Urol* **121**: 816–8.

Dessouki T, Staerman F, Abbar A *et al*. (1993) Treatment of primary vesicoureteric reflux by polytetrafluoroethylene injection: a middle-term follow-up study. *Eur Urol* **23**: 375–8.

De Sy WA, de Meyer JM, Oosterlinck W *et al*. (1986) Antireflux in adults: a long-term follow-up. *Eur Urol* **12**: 395–7.

Dewan PA, Goh DW (1994) Subureteric Polytef injection in the management of vesico-ureteric reflux in children. *J Paediatr Child Health* **30**: 324–7.

Dewan PA, Higgs MJ (1995) Correlation of the endoscopic appearance with clinical outcome for submucous Polytef paste injection in vesico-ureteric reflux. *Aust N Z J Surg* **65**: 642–4.

Diamond DA, Caldamone AA (1998) Endoscopic treatment of vesicoureteral reflux in children using autologous chondrocytes: preliminary results. presented at American Academy of Pediatrics, Section on Urology Annual Meeting. San Francisco, California, October 17–19, 1998.

Diamond DA, Parulkar BG (1998) Ureteral tailoring *in situ*: a practical approach to persistent reflux in the dilated reimplanted ureter. *J Urol* **160**: 998–1000.

Diamond DA, Kleinman PK, Spevak M *et al.* (1996a) The tailored low dose fluoroscopic voiding cystogram for familial reflux screening. *J Urol* **155**: 681–2.

Diamond DA, Rabinowitz R, Hoenig D *et al.* (1996b) The mechanism of new onset contralateral reflux following unilateral ureteroneocystostomy. *J Urol* **156**: 665–7.

Duckett JW (1983) Vesicoureteral reflux: a 'conservative' analysis. *Am J Kidney Dis* **3**: 139–44.

Duckett JW, Bellinger MF (1982) A plea for standardized grading of vesicoureteral reflux. *Eur Urol* **8**: 74–7.

Duckett JW, Walker RD, Weiss R (1992) Surgical results: International Reflux Study in Children – United States branch. *J Urol* **148**: 1674–5.

Dwoskin JY (1976) Sibling uropathy. *J Urol* **115**: 726–7.

Edwards D, Normand ICS, Prescod N *et al.* (1977) Disappearance of vesicoureteric reflux during long-term prophylaxis of urinary tract infection in children. *BMJ* **2**: 285–8.

Ehrlich RM (1982) Success of the transvesical advancement technique for vesicoureteral reflux. *J Urol* **128**: 554–7.

Ehrlich RM (1985) The ureteral folding technique for megaureter surgery. *J Urol* **134**: 668–70.

Ehrlich RM, Gershman A, Fuchs G (1994) Laparoscopic vesicoureteroplasty in children: initial case reports. *Urology* **43**: 255–61.

Elder JS (1988) Complications of periurethral Teflon injection. *Soc Pediatr Urol Newslett* 41–2, August 25.

Elder JS (1992) Commentary: importance of antenatal diagnosis of vesicoureteral reflux. *J Urol* **148**: 1750–4.

Elder JS, Peters CA, Arant BS Jr *et al.* (1997) Pediatric Vesicoureteral Reflux Guidelines Panel summary report on the management of primary vesicoureteral reflux in children. *J Urol* **157**: 1846–51.

Elison BS, Taylor D, Van der Wall H *et al.* (1992) Comparison of DMSA scintigraphy with intravenous urography for the detection of renal scarring and its correlation with vesicoureteric reflux. *Br J Urol* **69**: 294–302.

el-Khatib M, Packham DK, Becker GJ *et al.* (1994) Pregnancy-related complications in women with reflux nephropathy. *Clin Nephrol* **41**: 50–5.

Ellsworth PI, Merguerian PA (1995) Detrusorrhaphy for the repair of vesicoureteral reflux: comparison with the Leadbetter-Politano ureteroneocystostomy. *J Pediatr Surg* **30**: 600–3.

Ellsworth PI, Lim DJ, Walker RD *et al.* (1996) Common sheath reimplantation yields excellent results in the treatment of vesicoureteral reflux in duplicated collecting systems. *J Urol* **155**: 1407–9.

Engel JD, Palmer LS, Cheng EY *et al.* (1997) Surgical versus endoscopic correction of vesicoureteral reflux in children with neurogenic bladder dysfunction. *J Urol* **157**: 2291–4.

Evans RJ, Raezer DM, Shrom SH (1986) Surgical treatment of reflux in neurologically impaired child. *Urology* **28**: 31–5.

Farkas A, Moriel EZ, Lupa S (1990) Endoscopic correction of vesicoureteral reflux: our experience with 115 ureters. *J Urol* **144**: 534–6.

Fettich JJ, Kenda RB (1992) Cyclic direct radionuclide voiding cystography: increasing reliability in detecting vesicoureteral reflux in children. *Pediatr Radiol* **22**: 337–8.

Fichtner J, Iwasaki K, Shrestha G *et al.* (1993) Primary vesicoureteral reflux in children under one year of age: the case for conservative management? *Int Urol Nephrol* **25**: 141–6.

Filly R, Friedland GW, Govan DE *et al.* (1974) Development and progression of clubbing and scarring in children with recurrent urinary tract infections. *Radiology* **113**: 145–53.

Fort KF, Selman SH, Kropp KA (1983) A retrospective analysis of the use of ureteral stents in children undergoing ureteroneocystostomy. *J Urol* **129**: 545–7.

Frey P, Berger D, Jenny P *et al.* (1992) Subureteral collagen injection for the endoscopic treatment of vesicoureteral reflux in children. Followup study of 97 treated ureters and histological analysis of collagen implants. *J Urol* **148**: 718–23.

Frey P, Lutz N, Berger D *et al.* (1994) Histological behavior of glutaraldehyde cross-linked bovine collagen injected into the human bladder for the treatment of vesicoureteral reflux. *J Urol* **152**: 632–5.

Frey P, Gudinchet F, Jenny P (1997) GAX **65**: new injectable cross-linked collagen for the endoscopic treatment of vesicoureteral reflux – a double-blind study evaluating its efficiency in children. *J Urol* **158**: 1210–2.

Fung LC, McLorie GA, Jain U *et al.* (1995) Voiding efficiency after ureteral reimplantation: a comparison of extravesical and intravesical techniques. *J Urol* **153**: 1972–5.

Funston MR, Cremin BJ (1978) Intrarenal reflux – papillary morphology and pressure relationships in children's necropsy kidneys. *Br J Radiol* **51**: 665–70.

Gatewood OMB, Glasser RJ, Vanhoutte JJ (1965) Roentgen evaluation of renal size in pediatric age groups. *Am J Dis Child* **110**: 162–5.

Gearhart JP (1990) Endoscopic management of vesicoureteral reflux. In: Paulson DF (ed.), Kramer SA (Guest ed.) *Problems in urology*. Volume 4, No. 4. Philadelphia, PA: JB Lippincott, 639–47.

Gil-Vernet JM (1984) A new technique for surgical correction of vesicoureteral reflux. *J Urol* **131**: 456–8.

Gill DB, da Costa BM, Cameron JS *et al.* (1976) Analysis of 100 children with severe and persistent hypertension. *Arch Dis Child* **51**: 951–6.

Ginalski J-M, Michaud A, Genton N (1985) Renal growth retardation in children: sign suggestive of vesicoureteral reflux? *AJR Am J Roentgenol* **145**: 617–9.

Glassberg KI, Laungani G, Wasnick RJ *et al.* (1985) Transverse ureteral advancement technique of ureteroneocystostomy (Cohen reimplant) and a modification for difficult cases (experience with 121 ureters). *J Urol* **134**: 304–7.

Glassberg KI, Hackett RE, Waterhouse K (1987) Congenital anomalies of the kidney, ureter, and bladder. In: Kendall AR, Karafin L, Goldsmith HS (eds) *Urology*. Volume 1. Philadelphia, PA: Harper & Row.

Glenn JF, Anderson EE (1967) Distal tunnel ureteral reimplantation. *J Urol* **97**: 623–6.

Glenn JF, Anderson EE (1978) Technical considerations in distant tunnel ureteral reimplantation. *J Urol* **119**: 194–8.

Gonzales ET, Glenn JF, Anderson EE (1972) Results of distal tunnel ureteral reimplantation. *J Urol* **107**: 572–5.

Gordon AC, Thomas DFM, Arthur AJ *et al.* (1990) Prenatally diagnosed reflux: a follow-up study. *Br J Urol* **65**: 407.

Gore MD, Fernbach SK, Donaldson JS *et al.* (1989) Radiographic evaluation of subureteric injection of Teflon to correct vesicoureteral reflux. *AJR Am J Roentgenol* **152**: 115–9.

Govan DE, Palmer JM (1969) Urinary tract infection in children: the influence of successful antireflux operations in morbidity from infection. *Pediatrics* **44**: 677–84.

Govan DE, Fair WR, Friedland GW *et al.* (1975) Management of children with urinary tract infections: the Stanford experience. *Urology* **6**: 273–86.

Grégoir W, Schulman CC (1977) Die extravesikale antireflux-plastik. *Urologe A* **16**: 124–7.

Grégoir W, Van Regemorter G (1964) Le reflux vésico-urétéral congénital. *Urol Int* **18**: 122–36.

Hagberg S, Hjälmå SK, Jacobsson B *et al.* (1984) Renal growth after antireflux surgery in infants. *Z Kinderchir* **39**: 52–4.

Hanani Y, Goldwasser B, Jonas P *et al.* (1983) Management of unilateral reflux by ipsilateral ureteroneocystostomy – is it sufficient? *J Urol* **129**: 1022–3.

Hanna MK (1979) New surgical method for one-stage total remodeling of massively dilated and tortuous ureter: tapering *in situ* technique. *Urology* **14**: 453–64.

Hannerz L, Wikstad I, Celsi G *et al.* (1989) Influence of vesicoureteral reflux and urinary tract infection on renal growth in children with upper urinary tract duplication. *Acta Radiol* **30**: 391–4.

Harrison R (1888) On the possibility and utility of washing out the pelvis of the kidney and the ureters through the bladder. *Lancet* i: 463.

Hawtrey CE, Culp DA, Loening S *et al.* (1983) Ureterovesical reflux in an adolescent and adult population. *J Urol* **130**: 1067–9.

Heale WF (1979) Age of presentation and pathogenesis of reflux nephropathy. In: Hodson CJ, Kincaid-Smith P (eds) *Reflux nephropathy*. New York: Masson Publishing, 140–6.

Heidrick WP, Mattingly RF, Amberg JR (1967) Vesicoureteral reflux in pregnancy. *Obstet Gynecol* **29**: 571–8.

Hinman F, Baumann FW (1973) Vesical and ureteral damage from voiding dysfunction in boys without neurologic or obstructive disease. *J Urol* **109**: 727–32.

Hjalmas K, Lohr G, Tamminen-Mobius T *et al.* (1992) Surgical results in the International Reflux Study in Children (Europe). *J Urol* **148**: 1657–61.

Hodson CJ (1959) The radiological diagnosis of pyelonephritis. *Proc R Soc Med* **52**: 669–72.

Hodson CJ (1979) Reflux nephropathy: scoring the damage. In: Hodson CJ, Kincaid-Smith P (eds) *Reflux nephropathy*. New York: Masson Publishing, 29–38.

Hodson CJ, Edwards D (1960) Chronic pyelonephritis and vesicoureteric reflux. *Clin Radiol* **11**: 219–31.

Hodson CJ, Davies Z, Prescod A (1975a) Renal parenchymal radiographic measurement in infants and children. *Pediatr Radiol* **3**: 16–9.

Hodson CJ, Maling TMJ, McManamon PJ *et al.* (1975b) The pathogenesis of reflux nephropathy (chronic atrophic pyelonephritis). *Br J Radiol* **13** (Suppl): 1–26.

Hoenig DM, Diamond DA, Rabinowitz R *et al.* (1996) Contralateral reflux after unilateral ureteral reimplantation. *J Urol* **156**: 196–7.

Holland NH (1979) Reflux nephropathy and hypertension. In: Hodson CJ, Kincaid-Smith P (eds) *Reflux nephropathy*. New York: Masson Publishing, 257–62.

Hollowell JG, Altman HG, Snyder HM III *et al.* (1989) Co-existing ureteropelvic junction obstruction and vesicoureteral reflux: diagnostic and therapeutic implications. *J Urol* **142**: 490–3.

Homsy YL, Nsouli I, Hamburger B *et al.* (1985) Effects of oxybutynin on vesicoureteral reflux in children. *J Urol* **134**: 1168–71.

Houle AM, McLorie GA, Heritz DM *et al.* (1992) Extravesical nondismembered ureteroplasty with detrusorrhaphy: a renewed technique to correct vesicoureteral reflux in children. *J Urol* **148**: 704–7.

Hulbert JC, Hunter D, Castaneda-Zuniga W (1988) Classification and techniques for the reconstitution of acquired strictures in the region of the ureteropelvic junction. *J Urol* **140**: 468–72.

Husmann DA, Allen TD (1991) Resolution of vesicoureteral reflux in completely duplicated systems: fact or fiction? *J Urol* **145**: 1022–3.

Hutch JA (1952) Vesico-ureteral reflux in the paraplegic: cause and correction. *J Urol* **68**: 457–69.

Hutch JA (1961) Theory of maturation of the intravesical ureter. *J Urol* **86**: 534–8.

Hutch JA (1963) Ureteric advancement operation: anatomy, technique and early results. *J Urol* **89**: 180–4.

Iannaccone G, Panzironi PE (1955) Ureteral reflux in normal infants. *Acta Radiol* **44**: 451–6.

Jeffs RD, Allen MS (1962) The relationship between uretero-vesical reflux and infection. *J Urol* **88**: 691–5.

Jodal U, Koskimies O, Hanson E *et al.* on behalf of The International Reflux Study in Children (1992) Infection pattern in children with vesicoureteral reflux randomly allocated to operation or long-term antibacterial prophylaxis. *J Urol* **148**: 1650–2.

Johnston JH (1962) Vesico-ureteric reflux: its anatomical mechanism, causation, effects and treatment in the child. *Ann R Coll Surg Engl* **30**: 324–41.

Johnston JH (1967) Reconstructive surgery of mega-ureter in childhood. *Br J Urol* **39**: 17–21.

Johnston JH, Farkas A (1975) The congenital refluxing megaureter: experiences with surgical reconstruction. *Br J Urol* **47**: 153–9.

Johnston JH, Shapiro SR, Thomas GG (1976) Anti-reflux surgery in the congenital neuropathic bladder. *Br J Urol* **48**: 639–42.

Jones BW, Headstream JW (1958) Vesicoureteral reflux in children. *J Urol* **80**: 114–5.

Jungers P, Forget D, Henry-Amar M *et al.* (1986) Chronic kidney disease and pregnancy. *Adv Nephrol Necker Hosp* **15**: 103–41.

Jungers P, Houillier P, Chauveau D *et al.* (1996) Pregnancy in women with reflux nephropathy. *Kidney Int* **50**: 593–9.

Kaliciński ZH, Kansy J, Kotarbińska B *et al.* (1977) Surgery of megaureters – modification of Hendren's operation. *J Pediatr Surg* **12**: 183–8.

Kaplan WE (1990) Early evaluation and treatment of children with meningomyelocele. In: Paulson DF (ed.), Kramer SA (Guest ed.) *Problems in urology*, Volume 4, No. 4. Philadelphia, PA: JB Lippincott, 676–89.

Kaplan WE, Firlit CF (1983) Management of reflux in the myelodysplastic child. *J Urol* **129**: 1195–7.

Kaplan WE, Nasrallah P, King LR (1978) Reflux in complete duplication in children. *J Urol* **120**: 220–2.

Kass EJ, Koff SA, Diokno AC (1981) Fate of vesicoureteral reflux in children with neuropathic bladders managed by intermittent catheterization. *J Urol* **125**: 63–4.

Kaveggia L, King LR, Grana L *et al.* (1966) Pyelonephritis: a cause of vesicoureteral reflux? *J Urol* **95**: 158–63.

Kelalis PP (1971) Proper perspective on vesicoureteral reflux. *Mayo Clin Proc* **46**: 807–18.

Kelalis PP (1974) The present status of surgery for vesicoureteral reflux. *Urol Clin North Am* **1**: 457–69.

Kelalis PP (1985) Surgical correction of vesicoureteral reflux. In: Kelalis PP, King LR, Belman AB (eds) *Clinical pediatric urology*. 2nd edition. Philadelphia, PA: WB Saunders, 381–419.

Kelalis PP, Kramer SA (1983) Complications of megaureter surgery. *Urol Clin North Am* **10**: 417–22.

Kelalis PP, Kramer SA (1987) Anomalies of renal ectopy and fusion. In: Libertino JA (ed.) *Pediatric and adult reconstructive urologic surgery*, 2nd edition. Baltimore, MD: Williams & Wilkins, 102–8.

Kennelly MJ, Bloom DA, Ritchey ML *et al.* (1995) Outcome analysis of bilateral Cohen cross-trigonal ureteroneocystostomy. *Urology* **46**: 393–5.

Kincaid-Smith P, Fairley KF (1987) Renal disease in pregnancy. Three controversial areas: mesangial IgA nephropathy, focal glomerular sclerosis (focal and segmental hyalinosis and sclerosis), and reflux nephropathy. *Am J Kidney Dis* **9**: 328–33.

Kincaid-Smith PS, Bastos MG, Becker GJ (1984) Reflux nephropathy in the adult. *Contrib Nephrol* **39**: 94–101.

King LR (1976) Vesicoureteral reflux: history, etiology and conservative management. In: Kelalis PP, King LR, Belman AB (eds) *Clinical pediatric urology*. Volume 1. Philadelphia, PA: WB Saunders, 342–65.

King LR, Kazmi SO, Belman AB (1974) Natural history of vesicoureteral reflux: outcome of a trial of nonoperative therapy. *Urol Clin North Am* **1**: 441–55.

Kirsch MD, Donaldson JS, Kaplan WE (1990) MR appearance of subureteric injection of Teflon to correct vesicoureteral reflux. *J Comput Assist Tomogr* **14**: 673–4.

Kiruluta HG, Fraser K, Owen L (1986) The significance of the adrenergic nerves in the etiology of vesicoureteral reflux. *J Urol* **136**: 232–5.

Klare B, Geiselhardt B, Wesch H *et al.* (1980) Radiological kidney size in childhood. *Pediatr Radiol* **9**: 153–60.

Koff SA, Murtagh DS (1983) The uninhibited bladder in children: effect of treatment on recurrence of urinary infection and on vesicoureteral reflux resolution. *J Urol* **130**: 1138–41.

Koff SA, Wagner TT, Jayanthi VR (1998) The relationship among dysfunctional elimination syndromes, primary vesicoureteral reflux and urinary tract infections in children. *J Urol* **160**: 1019–22.

Kohri K, Kataoka K, Akiyama T *et al.* (1988) Treatment of vesicoureteral reflux by endoscopic injection of blood. *Urol Int* **43**: 324–6.

Kondo A, Kobayashi M, Otani T *et al.* (1983) Children with unstable bladder: clinical and urodynamic observation. *J Urol* **129**: 88–91.

Kondo A, Otani T (1987) Correction of reflux with the ureteric crossover method: clinical experience in 50 patients. *Br J Urol* **60**: 36–8.

Kramer SA (1984) Experimental vesicoureteral reflux. *Dialog Pediatr Urol* **7**: 1–8.

Kramer SA (1992) Vesicoureteral reflux. In: Kelalis PP, King LR, Belman AB (eds) *Clinical pediatric urology*. Volume 1. 3rd edition. Philadelphia, PA: WB Saunders, 441–99.

Kumar R, Puri P (1997) Newly diagnosed contralateral reflux after successful unilateral endoscopic correction: is it due to the pop-off mechanism? *J Urol* **158**: 1213–5.

Kumar R, Puri P (1998) Endoscopic correction of vesicoureteric reflux in failed reimplanted ureters. *Eur Urol* **33**: 98–100.

Kunin CM, Deutscher R, Paquin A Jr (1964) Urinary tract infections in school children: an epidemiologic, clinical and laboratory study. *Medicine (Baltimore)* **43**: 91–130.

Lamesch AJ (1981) Retrograde catheterization of the ureter after antireflux plasty by the Cohen technique of transverse advancement. *J Urol* **125**: 73–4.

Lapointe SP, Barrieras D, Leblanc B *et al.* (1998) Modified Lich–Grégoir ureteral reimplantation: experience of a Canadian center. *J Urol* **159**: 1662–4.

Lebowitz RL, Blickman JG (1983) The coexistence of ureteropelvic junction obstruction and reflux. *AJR Am J Roentgenol* **140**: 231–8.

Leighton DM, Mayne V (1989) Obstruction in the refluxing urinary tract – a common phenomenon. *Clin Radiol* **40**: 271–3.

Lenaghan D, Whitaker JG, Jensen F *et al.* (1976) The natural history of reflux and long-term effects of reflux on the kidney. *J Urol* **115**: 728–30.

Leonard MP, Canning DA, Peters CA *et al.* (1991) Endoscopic injection of glutaraldehyde cross-linked bovine dermal collagen for correction of vesicoureteral reflux. *J Urol* **145**: 115–9.

Levitt SB, Weiss RA (1985) Vesicoureteral reflux. Natural history, classification, and reflux nephropathy. In: Kelalis PP, King LR, Belman AB (eds) *Clinical pediatric urology*. 2nd edition. Philadelphia, PA: WB Saunders Co., 355–80.

Lich R Jr, Howerton LW, Davis LA (1961) Recurrent urosepsis in children. *J Urol* **86**: 554–8.

Lich R Jr, Howerton LW Jr, Goode LS *et al.* (1964) The ureterovesical junction of the newborn. *J Urol* **92**: 436–8.

Lines D (1982) 15th century ureteric reflux. *Lancet* **ii**: 1473.

Linn R, Ginesin Y, Bolkier M *et al.* (1989) Lich–Grégoir antireflux operation: a surgical experience and 5–20 years of follow-up in 149 ureters. *Eur Urol* **16**: 200–3.

Lipsky H, Wurnschimmel E (1993) Endoscopic treatment of vesicoureteric reflux with collagen. Five years' experience. *Br J Urol* **72**: 965–8.

Lipski BA, Mitchell ME, Burns MW (1998) Voiding dysfunction after bilateral extravesical ureteral reimplantation. *J Urol* **159**: 1019–21.

Lue TF, Macchia RJ, Pastore L *et al.* (1982) Vesicoureteral reflux and staghorn calculi. *J Urol* **127**: 247–8.

Lyon RP (1973) Renal arrest. *J Urol* **109**: 707–10.

Lyon RP (1977) What does urethral dilation really do? *Birth Defects* **13**: 439–41.

Lyon RP, Marshall S, Tanagho EA (1969) The ureteral orifice: its configuration and competency. *J Urol* **102**: 504–9.

McCool AC, Joseph DB (1995) Postoperative hospitalization of children undergoing cross-trigonal ureteroneocystostomy. *J Urol* **154**: 794–6.

McCool AC, Perez LM, Joseph DB (1997) Contralateral vesicoureteral reflux after simple and tapered unilateral ureteroneocystostomy revisited. *J Urol* **158**: 1219–20.

McLorie GA, McKenna PH, Jumper BM *et al.* (1990) High grade vesicoureteral reflux: analysis of observational therapy. *J Urol* **144**: 537–40.

McLorie GA, Jayanthi VR, Kinahan TJ *et al.* (1994) A modified extravesical technique for megaureter repair. *Br J Urol* **74**: 715–9.

McRae CU, Shannon FT, Utley WLF (1974) Effect on renal growth of reimplantation of refluxing ureters. *Lancet* **1**: 1310–2.

Mackie GG, Stephens FD (1975) Duplex kidneys: a correlation of renal dysplasia with position of the ureteral orifice. *J Urol* **114**: 274–80.

Mackie GG, Awang H, Stephens FD (1975) The ureteric orifice: the embryologic key to radiologic status of duplex kidneys. *J Pediatr Surg* **10**: 473–81.

Maizels M, Smith CK, Firlit CF (1984) The management of children with vesicoureteral reflux and ureteropelvic junction obstruction. *J Urol* **131**: 722–7.

Majd M, Rushton HG, Jantausch B, Wiedermann B (1991) Relationshop among vesicoureteral reflux, P-fimbriated *Escherichia coli*, and acute pyelonephritis in children with febrile urinary tract infection. *J Ped* **119**: 578–85.

Malek RS (1976) Urolithiasis. In: Kelalis PP, King LR, Belman AB (eds) *Clinical pediatric urology*. Volume 2. Philadelphia, PA: WB Saunders, 870.

Malek RS, Kelalis PP (1975) Pediatric nephrolithiasis. *J Urol* **113**: 545–51.

Malek RS, Svensson JP, Torres VE (1983a) Vesicoureteral reflux in the adult: I. Factors in pathogenesis. *J Urol* **130**: 37–40.

Malek RS, Svensson J, Neves RJ *et al.* (1983b) Vesicoureteral reflux in the adult: III. Surgical correction: risks and benefits. *J Urol* **130**: 882–6.

Malizia AA Jr, Reiman HM, Myers RP *et al.* (1984) Migration and granulomatous reaction after periurethral injection of polytef (Teflon). *JAMA* **251**: 3277–81.

Malizia AA Jr, Woodard JR, Rushton HG *et al.* (1988) Intravesical/subureteric injection of polytef: serial radiologic imaging (abstract). *J Urol* **139**: 185A.

Mann CI, Jequier S, Patriguin H *et al.* (1988) Intramural Teflon injection of the ureter for treatment of vesicoureteral reflux: sonographic appearance. *AJR Am J Roentgenol* **151**: 543–5.

Mansfield JT, Snow BW, Cartwright PC *et al.* (1995) Complications of pregnancy in women after childhood reimplantation for vesicoureteral reflux: an update with 25 years of followup. *J Urol* **154**: 787–90.

Marberger M, Altwein JE, Straub E *et al.* (1978) The Lich–Grégoir antireflux plasty: experiences with 371 children. *J Urol* **120**: 216–9.

Martinell J, Jodal U, Lidin-Janson G (1990) Pregnancies in women with and without renal scarring after urinary infections in childhood. *BMJ* **300**: 840–4.

Mathisen W (1964) Vesicoureteral reflux and its surgical correction. *Surg Gynecol Obstet* **118**: 965–71.

Matouschek E (1981) Die Behandlung des Vesikorenalen refluxes durch transurethrale einspritzung von Teflonpaste. *Urologe A* **20**: 263–4.

Mattar SG, Orr JD, MacKinlay GA (1994) Endoscopic treatment of vesico-ureteric reflux in children by subureteric Teflon injection: the Edinburgh experience. *J R Coll Surg Edin* **39**: 17–9.

Mattingly RF, Borkowf HI (1978) Clinical implications of ureteral reflux in pregnancy. *Clin Obstet Gynecol* **21**: 863–73.

Mazze RI, Schwartz FD, Slocum HC *et al.* (1963) Renal function during anesthesia and surgery: 1. Effects of halothane anesthesia. *Anesthesiology* **24**: 279–84.

Merguerian PA, McLorie GA, Khoury AE *et al.* (1990) Submucosal injection of polyvinyl alcohol foam in rabbit bladder. *J Urol* **144**: 531–3.

Merrell RW, Mowad JJ (1979) Increased physical growth after successful antireflux operation. *J Urol* **122**: 523–7.

Mesrobian H-GJ, Kelalis PP (1989) Ureterocalicostomy: indications and results in 21 patients. *J Urol* **142**: 1285–7.

Mesrobian H-GJ, Kramer SA, Kelalis PP (1985) Reoperative ureteroneocystostomy: review of 69 patients. *J Urol* **133**: 388–90.

Mevorach RA, Merguerian PA, Balcolm AH (1998) Detrusorrhaphy for repair of unilateral vesicoureteral reflux: report of 76 patients using a modified technique. *Urology* **51** (Suppl 5A): 12–4.

Michael V, Davaris P, Arhontakis A *et al.* (1993) Effects of submucosal Teflon paste injection in vesicoureteric reflux: results with 1- and 2-year follow-up data. *Eur Urol* **23**: 379–81.

Minevich E, Aronoff D, Wacksman J *et al.* (1998) Voiding dysfunction after bilateral extravesical detrusorrhaphy. *J Urol* **160**: 1004–6.

Mittleman R, Marraccini JV (1983) Pulmonary Teflon granulomas following periurethral Teflon injection for urinary incontinence (Letter). *Arch Pathol Lab Med* **107**: 611–2.

Miyakita H, Ninan GK, Puri P (1993) Endoscopic correction of vesico-ureteric reflux in duplex systems. *Eur Urol* **24**: 111–5.

Moreau JF, Grenier P, Grünfeld JP *et al.* (1979–80) Renal clubbing and scarring in adults: a retrospective study of 110 cases. *Urol Radiol* **1**: 129–36.

Najmaldin A, Burge DM, Atwell TD (1990) Reflux nephropathy secondary to intraureterine vesicoureteric reflux. *J Pediatr Surg* **25**: 387.

Naseer SR, Steinhardt GF (1997) New renal scars in children with urinary tract infections, vesicoureteral reflux and voiding dysfunction: a prospective evaluation. *J Urol* **158**: 566–8.

Nasrallah PF, Aliabadi HA (1991) Bladder augmentation in patients with neurogenic bladder and vesicoureteral reflux. *J Urol* **146**: 563–6.

Nasrallah PF, Conway JJ, King LR *et al.* (1978) Quantitative nuclear cystogram: aid in determining spontaneous resolution of vesicoureteral reflux. *Urology* **12**: 654–8.

Nasrallah PF, Simon JW (1984) Reflux and voiding abnormalities in children. *Urology* **24**: 243–5.

Nativ O, Hertz M, Hanani Y *et al.* (1987) Vesicoureteral reflux in adults: a review of 95 patients. *Eur Urol* **13**: 229–32.

Neves RJ, Torres VE, Malek RS *et al.* (1984) Vesicoureteral reflux in the adult. IV. Medical versus surgical management. *J Urol* **132**: 882–5.

Noe HN (1992) The long-term results of prospective sibling reflux screening. *J Urol* **148**: 1739–42.

Noe HN (1995) The current status of screening for vesicoureteral reflux. *Pediatr Nephrol* **9**: 638–41.

Noe HN (1998) The risk and risk factors of contralateral reflux following repair of simple unilateral primary reflux. *J Urol* **160**: 849–50.

Noe HN, Wyatt RJ, Peeden JN Jr *et al.* (1992) The transmission of vesicoureteral reflux from parent to child. *J Urol* **148**: 1869–71.

O'Donnell B, Puri P (1984) Treatment of vesicoureteric reflux by endoscopic injection of Teflon. *BMJ* **289**: 7–9.

Okamura K, Yamada Y, Tsuji Y *et al.* (1996) Endoscopic trigonoplasty in pediatric patients with primary vesicoureteral reflux: preliminary report. *J Urol* **156**: 198–200.

Olbing H, Claësson I, Ebel KD *et al.* (1992) Renal scars and parenchymal thinning in children with vesicoureteral reflux: a 5-year report of the International Reflux Study in Children (European branch). *J Urol* **148**: 1653–6.

Palken M (1970) Surgical correction of vesicoureteral reflux in children: results with the use of a single standard technique. *J Urol* **104**: 765–8.

Paltiel HJ, Lebowitz RL (1989) Neonatal hydronephrosis due to primary vesicoureteral reflux: trends in diagnosis and treatment. *Radiology* **170**: 787–9.

Paltiel HJ, Rupich RC, Kiruluta HG (1992) Enhanced detection of vesicoureteral reflux in infants and children with the use of cyclic voiding cystourethrography. *Radiology* **184**: 753–5.

Paquin AJ Jr (1959) Ureterovesical anastomosis: the description and evaluation of a technique. *J Urol* **82**: 573–83.

Parrott TS, Woodard JR (1976) Reflux in opposite ureter after successful correction of unilateral vesicoureteral reflux. *Urology* **7**: 276–8.

Peppas DS, Skoog SJ, Canning DA *et al.* (1991) Nonsurgical management of primary vesicoureteral reflux in complete ureteral duplication: is it justified? *J Urol* 1594–95.

Peters PC, Johnson DE, Jackson JH Jr (1967) The incidence of vesicoureteral reflux in the premature child. *J Urol* **97**: 259–60.

Pfister RR, Biber RJ, Rose JS *et al.* (1982) Monitoring ureteral reflux with ultrasound. Presented at the Urologic Section of the 51st American Academy of Pediatrics meeting, October 6, 1982.

Politano VA (1960) Vesicoureteral reflux in children. *JAMA* **172**: 1252–6.

Politano VA (1963) One hundred reimplantations and five years. *J Urol* **90**: 696–9.

Politano VA (1975) Vesicoureteral reflux. In: Glenn JF (ed.) *Urologic Surgery.* 2nd edition. New York: Harper & Row, 272–93.

Politano VA, Leadbetter WF (1958) An operative technique for the correction of vesicoureteral reflux. *J Urol* **79**: 932–41.

Politano VA, Small MP, Harper JM *et al.* (1974) Periurethral Teflon injection for urinary incontinence. *J Urol* **111**: 180–3.

Polk HC Jr (1965) Notes on Galenic urology. *Urol Surv* **15**: 2–6.

Poznanski E, Poznanski AK (1969) Psychogenic influences on voiding: observations from voiding cystourethrography. *Psychosomatics* **10**: 339–42.

Prout GR Jr, Koontz WW Jr (1970) Partial vesical immobilization: an important adjunct to ureteroneocystostomy. *J Urol* **103**: 147–51.

Puri P (1995) Ten year experience with subureteric Teflon (polytetrafluoroethylene) injection (STING) in the treatment of vesico-ureteric reflux. *Br J Urol* **75**: 126–31.

Puri P, O'Donnell B (1984) Correction of experimentally produced vesicoureteric reflux in the piglet by intravesical injection of Teflon. *BMJ* **289**: 5–7.

Puri P, Cascio S, Lakshmandass G *et al.* (1998) Urinary tract infection and renal damage in sibling vesicoureteral reflux. *J Urol* **160**: 1028–30.

Quinlan D, O'Donnell B (1985) Unilateral ureteric reimplantation for primary vesicoureteric reflux in children. *Br J Urol* **57**: 406–9.

Rabinowitz R, Barkin M, Schillinger JF *et al.* (1979) Surgical treatment of the massively dilated primary megaureter in children. *Br J Urol* **51**: 19–23.

Ransley PG (1977) Intrarenal reflux: anatomical, dynamic and radiological studies – Part I. *Urol Res* **5**: 61–9.

Ransley PG (1978) Vesicoureteric reflux: continuing surgical dilemma. *Urology* **12**: 246–55.

Ransley PG, Risdon RA (1975a) Renal papillary morphology and intrarenal reflux in the young pig. *Urol Res* **3**: 105–9.

Ransley PG, Risdon RA (1975b) Renal papillary morphology in infants and young children. *Urol Res* **3**: 111–3.

Ransley PG, Risdon RA (1978) Reflux and renal scarring. *Br J Radiol* **14** (Suppl): 1–35.

Ransley PG, Risdon RA (1981) Reflux nephropathy: effects of antimicrobial therapy on the evolution of the early pyelonephritic scar. *Kidney Int* **20**: 733–42.

Redman JF, Scriber LJ, Bissada NK (1974) Apparent failure of renal growth secondary to vesicoureteral reflux. *Urology* **3**: 704–7.

Reunanen M (1997) Endoscopic collagen injection: its limits in correcting vesico-ureteral reflux in duplicated ureters. *Eur Urol* **31**: 243–5.

Roberts JA, Riopelle AJ (1978) Vesicoureteral reflux in the primate: III. Effect of urinary tract infection on maturation of the ureterovesical junction. *Pediatrics* **61**: 853–7.

Roberts JA, Roth JK Jr, Domingue G et al. (1982) Immunology of pyelonephritis in the primary model. *J Urol* **128**: 1394–400.

Roberts JA, Suarez GM, Kaack B et al. (1985) Experimental pyelonephritis in the monkey. VII. Ascending pyelonephritis in the absence of vesicoureteral reflux. *J Urol* **133**: 1068–75.

Roberts JP, Atwell JD (1989) Vesicoureteric reflux and urinary calculi in children. *Br J Urol* **64**: 10–2.

Rolleston GL, Shannon FT, Utley WLF (1970) Relationship of infantile vesicoureteric reflux to renal damage. *BMJ* **1**: 460–3.

Rolleston GL, Maling TMJ, Hodson CJ (1974) Intrarenal reflux and the scarred kidney. *Arch Dis Child* **49**: 531–9.

Rose JS, Glassberg KI, Waterhouse K (1975) Intrarenal reflux and its relationship to renal scarring. *J Urol* **113**: 400–3.

Ross JH, Kay R, Nasrallah P (1995) Contralateral reflux after unilateral ureteral reimplantation in patients with a history of resolved contralateral reflux. *J Urol* **154**: 1171–2.

Rushton HG, Majd M, Chandra R et al. (1988) Evaluation of [99m]technetium-dimercapto-succinic acid renal scans in experimental acute pyelonephritis in piglets. *J Urol* **140**: 1169–74.

Rushton HG, Majd M, Jantausch B et al. (1992) Renal scarring following reflux and nonreflux pyelonephritis in children: evaluation with [99m]technetium-dimercaptosuccinic acid scintigraphy. *J Urol* **147**: 1327–32.

Salvatierra O Jr, Tanagho EA (1977) Reflux as a cause of end stage kidney disease: report of 32 cases. *J Urol* **117**: 441–3.

Savage DCL, Wilson MI, Ross EM et al. (1969) Asymptomatic bacteriuria in girl entrants to Dundee Primary Schools. *BMJ* **iii**: 75–80.

Schimberg W, Wacksman J, Rudd R et al. (1994) Laparoscopic correction of vesicoureteral reflux in the pig. *J Urol* **151**: 1664–7.

Schoenberg HW, Beisswanger P, Howard WJ et al. (1964) Effect of lower urinary tract infection upon ureteral function. *J Urol* **92**: 107–8.

Scholtmeijer RJ (1993) Treatment of vesicoureteric reflux. Results of a prospective study. *Br J Urol* **71**: 346–9.

Schulman CC, Sassine AM (1992) Endoscopic treatment of vesicoureteral reflux. *Eur J Pediat Surg* **2**: 32–4.

Scott JE (1963) Ureteric reflux in the duplex kidney. *Acta Urol Belg* **31**: 73–84.

Scott JES, Stansfeld JM (1968) Ureteric reflux and kidney scarring in children. *Arch Dis Child* **43**: 468–70.

Scott JD, Blackford HN, Joyce MRL et al. (1986) Renal function following surgical correction of vesico-ureteric reflux in childhood. *Br J Urol* **58**: 119–24.

Seruca H (1989) Vesicoureteral reflux and voiding dysfunction: a prospective study. *J Urol* **142**: 494–8.

Shah KJ, Robins DG, White RHR (1978) Renal scarring and vesicoureteric reflux. *Arch Dis Child* **53**: 210–7.

Shopfner CE (1970) Vesicoureteral reflux: five-year re-evaluation. *Radiology* **95**: 637–48.

Shore N, Bartone FF, Miller A et al. (1986) Balloon dilation of upper ureteral strictures in primates. *J Urol* **136**: 342–3.

Sidi AA, Peng W, Gonzalez R (1986) Vesicoureteral reflux in children with myelodysplasia: natural history and results of treatment. *J Urol* **136**: 329–31.

Siegelbaum MH, Rabinovitch HH (1987) Delayed spontaneous resolution of high grade vesicoureteral reflux after reimplantation. *J Urol* **138**: 1205–6.

Sillen U, Bachelard M, Hermanson G et al. (1996) Gross bilateral reflux in infants: gradual decrease of initial detrusor hypercontractility. *J Urol* **155**: 668–72.

Skoog SJ, Belman AB, Majd M (1987) A nonsurgical approach to the management of primary vesicoureteral reflux. *J Urol* **138**: 941–6.

Smellie J, Edwards D, Hunter N et al. (1975) Vesico-ureteric reflux and renal scarring. *Kidney Int* **8** (Suppl 4): S65–72.

Smellie JM (1992) Commentary: management of children with severe vesicoureteral reflux. *J Urol* **148**: 1676–8.

Smellie JM, Normand C (1979) Reflux nephropathy in childhood. In: Hodson CJ, Kincaid-Smith P (eds) *Reflux nephropathy*. New York: Masson Publishing, 14–20.

Smellie JM, Edwards D, Normand ICS et al. (1981a) Effect of vesicoureteric reflux on renal growth in children with urinary tract infection. *Arch Dis Child* **56**: 593–600.

Smellie JM, Normand ICS, Katz G (1981b) Children with urinary infection: a comparison of those with and those without vesicoureteric reflux. *Kidney Int* **20**: 717–22.

Smellie JM, Preece MA, Paton AM (1983) Normal somatic growth in children receiving low-dose prophylactic cotrimoxazole. *Eur J Pediatr* **140**: 301–4.

Smellie JM, Ransley PG, Normand ICS et al. (1985) Development of new renal scars: a collaborative study. *BMJ* **290**: 1957–60.

Smith DP, Kaplan WE, Oyasu R (1994) Evaluation of polydimethylsiloxane as an alternative in the endoscopic treatment of vesicoureteral reflux. *J Urol* **152**: 1221–4.

Solok V, Erözenci A, Kural A et al. (1988) Correction of vesicoureteral reflux by the Gil–Vernet procedure. *Eur Urol* **14**: 214–5.

Sommer JT, Stephens FD (1981) Morphogenesis of nephropathy with partial ureteral obstruction and vesicoureteral reflux. *J Urol* **125**: 67–72.

Starr A (1979) Ureteral plication: a new concept in ureteral tailoring for megaureter. *Invest Urol* **17**: 153–8.

Stecker JF Jr, Read BP, Poutasse EF (1977) Pediatric hypertension as a delayed sequela of reflux-induced chronic pyelonephritis. *J Urol* **118**: 644–6.

Steinbrecher HA, Rangecroft L (1997) The use of the detrusorrhaphy for vesico-ureteric reflux: the way forward? *Br J Urol* **79**: 971–4.

Stephens FD (1980) Ureteric configurations and cystoscopy schema. *Soc Pediatr Urol Newslett*, January 23, 2.

Stephens FD, Lenaghan D (1962) The anatomical basis and dynamics of vesicoureteral reflux. *J Urol* **87**: 669–80.

Stewart CM (1953) Delayed cystograms. *J Urol* **70**: 588–93.

Stickler GB, Kelalis PP, Burke EC *et al.* (1971) Primary interstitial nephritis with reflux. *Am J Dis Child* **122**: 144–8.

Stockland E, Hellstrom M, Hansson S *et al.* (1994) Reliability of ultrasonography in identification of reflux nephropathy in children. *BMJ* **309**: 235–9.

Sutton R, Atwell JD (1989) Physical growth velocity during conservative treatment and following subsequent surgical treatment for primary vesicoureteric reflux. *Br J Urol* **63**: 245–50.

Sweeney LE, Thomas PS (1987) Evaluation of sub-ureteric Teflon injection as an antireflux procedure. *Ann Radiol (Paris)* **30**: 478–81.

Tamminen TE, Kaprio EA (1977) The relation of the shape of renal papillae and of collecting duct openings to intrarenal reflux. *Br J Urol* **49**: 345–54.

Tamminen-Mobius T, Brunier E, Ebel KD *et al.* on behalf of The International Reflux Study in Children (1992) Cessation of vesicoureteral reflux for 5 years in infants and children allocated to medical treatment. *J Urol* **148**: 1662–6.

Tanagho EA (1971) Ureteral tailoring. *J Urol* **106**: 194–7.

Tanagho EA, Hutch JA, Meyers FH *et al.* (1965) Primary vesicoureteral reflux: experimental studies of its etiology. *J Urol* **93**: 165–76.

Tanagho EA, Guthrie TH, Lyon RP (1969) The intravesical ureter in primary reflux. *J Urol* **101**: 824–32.

Taylor CM (1984) Unstable bladder activity and the rate of resolution of vesico-ureteric reflux. *Contrib Nephrol* **39**: 238–46.

Taylor CM, Corkery JJ, White RHR (1982) Micturition symptoms and unstable bladder activity in girls with primary vesicoureteric reflux. *Br J Urol* **54**: 494–8.

Teague N, Boyarsky S (1968) The effect of coliform bacilli upon ureteral peristalsis. *Invest Urol* **5**: 423–6.

Timmons JW, Watts FB, Perlmutter AD (1977) A comparison of awake and anesthesia cystography. *Birth Defects* **13**: 363–4.

Tobenkin MI (1964) Hereditary vesicoureteral reflux. *South Med J* **57**: 139–47.

Torres VE, Moore SB, Kurtz SB *et al.* (1980a) In search of a marker for genetic susceptibility to reflux nephropathy. *Clin Nephrol* **14**: 217–22.

Torres VE, Velosa JA, Holley KE *et al.* (1980b) The progression of vesicoureteral reflux nephropathy. *Ann Intern Med* **92**: 776–84.

Torres VE, Kramer SA, Holley KE *et al.* (1984) Effect of bacterial immunization on experimental reflux nephropathy. *J Urol* **131**: 772–6.

Torres VE, Kramer SA, Holley KE *et al.* (1985) Interaction of multiple risk factors in the pathogenesis of experimental reflux nephropathy in the pig. *J Urol* **133**: 131–5.

Torres VE, Malek RS, Svensson JP (1983) Vesicoureteral reflux in the adult. II. Nephropathy, hypertension and stones. *J Urol* **130**: 41–4.

Van den Abbeele AD, Treves ST, Lebowitz RL *et al.* (1987) Vesicoureteral reflux in asymptomatic siblings of patients with known reflux: radionuclide cystography. *Pediatrics* **79**: 147–53.

Van Gool J, Tanagho EA (1977) External sphincter activity and recurrent urinary tract infection in girls. *Urology* **10**: 348–53.

Wacksman J, Anderson EE, Glenn JF (1978) Management of vesicoureteral reflux. *J Urol* **119**: 814–6.

Wacksman J, Gilbert A, Sheldon CA (1992) Results of the renewed extravesical reimplant for surgical correction of vesicoureteral reflux. *J Urol* **148**: 359–61.

Wacksman J, Sheldon C (1999) Results of the 're-newed' extravesical reimplant – a quantum leap forward in the surgical management of vesicoureteral reflux. Abstract No. 350, presented at AUA Meeting, May 13–17, 1990, New Orleans.

Walker RD (1987) Vesicoureteral reflux. In: Gillenwater JY, Grayhack JT, Howards SS *et al.* (eds) *Adult and pediatric urology*. Volume 2. Chicago, IL: Year Book Medical Publishers, 1676–708.

Wallace DMA, Rothwell DL, Williams DI (1978) The long-term follow-up of surgically treated vesicoureteric reflux. *Br J Urol* **50**: 479–84.

Warren MM, Kelalis PP, Stickler GB (1972) Unilateral ureteroneocystostomy: the fate of the contralateral ureter. *J Urol* **107**: 466–8.

Weaver E, Craswell P (1987) Pregnancy outcome in women with reflux nephropathy – a review of experience at the Royal Women's Hospital Brisbane, 1977–1986. *Aust N Z J Obstet Gynaecol* **27**: 106–11.

Wein AJ, Schoenberg HW (1972) A review of 402 girls with recurrent urinary tract infection. *J Urol* **107**: 329–31.

Weiss RM, Lytton B (1974) Vesicoureteral reflux and distal ureteral obstruction. *J Urol* **111**: 245–9.

Whalley PJ, Cunningham FG (1977) Short-term versus continuous antimicrobial therapy for asymptomatic bacteriuria in pregnancy. *Obstet Gynecol* **49**: 262–5.

Whitaker RH (1976) Reflux induced pelvic-ureteric obstruction. *Br J Urol* **48**: 555–60.

Whitaker RH, Flower CDR (1979) Ureters that show both reflux and obstruction. *Br J Urol* **51**: 471–4.

Williams GL, Davies DKL, Evans KT *et al.* (1968) Vesicoureteric reflux in patients with bacteriuria in pregnancy. *Lancet* **ii**: 1202–5.

Willscher MK, Bauer SB, Zammuto PJ *et al.* (1976a) Infection of the urinary tract after anti-reflux surgery. *J Pediatr* **89**: 743–7.

Willscher MK, Bauer SB, Zammuto PJ *et al.* (1976b) Renal growth and urinary infection following antireflux surgery in infants and children. *J Urol* **115**: 722–5.

Woodard JR, Filardi G (1976) The demonstration of vesicoureteral reflux under general anesthesia. *J Urol* **116**: 501–2.

Woodard JR, Holden S (1976) The prognostic significance of fever in childhood urinary infections: observations in 350 consecutive patients. *Clin Pediatr (Philadelphia)* **15**: 1051–4.

Woodard JR, Keats G (1973) Ureteral reimplantation: Paquin's procedure after 12 years. *J Urol* **109**: 891–4.

Woods C, Atwell JD (1982) Vesico-ureteric reflux in the neuropathic bladder with particular reference to the development of renal scarring. *Eur Urol* **8**: 23–8.

Woodside JR, Borden TS (1982) Determination of true intravesical filling pressure in patients with vesicoureteral reflux by Fogarty catheter occlusion of ureters. *J Urol* **127**: 1149–52.

Yen TC, Chen WP, Chang SL *et al.* (1996) Technetium-99m-DMSA renal SPECT in diagnosing and monitoring pediatric acute pyelonephritis. *J Nucl Med* **37**: 1349–53.

Young HH, Wesson MB (1921) The anatomy and surgery of the trigone. *Arch Surg* **3**: 1.

Zaontz MR, Maizels M, Sugar EC *et al.* (1987) Detrusorrhaphy: extravesical ureteral advancement to correct vesicoureteral reflux in children. *J Urol* **138**: 947–9.

Zerin JM (1993) Impact of contrast medium temperature on bladder capacity and cystographic diagnosis of vesicoureteral reflux in children. *Radiology* **187**: 161–4.

Zucchelli P, Gaggi R (1988) Vesicoureteral reflux and reflux nephropathy in adults. *Contrib Nephrol* **61**: 210–9.

Imperforate anus, urogenital sinus, and cloaca

Curtis A. Sheldon

26

Introduction

The management of anorectal malformations (ARMs), including cloacal malformations (CMs) and urogenital sinus malformations (UGSMs), is pertinent to the practice of pediatric urology. ARM and urogenital sinus anomalies are commonly associated with surgically relevant urinary tract and vaginal pathology, the reconstruction for which the pediatric urologist is generally responsible.

The history of imperforate anus management dates back to the seventh century, where the earliest reports of survival with surgery (rupture of an obstructing anal membrane) may be found. In 1835, a perineal proctoplasty was performed by Amusset, and in the 1850s, various authors reported the use of colostomy, which opened the door for successful management of high ARM. An abdominal–perineal pull-through procedure was undertaken in the 1880s (McLeod, 1880; Hadra, 1885) and advanced further by Rhoads et al. (1948). In 1953, Stevens promoted a direct sacral approach to reconstruction, and in 1967, Kiesewetter combined these approaches into a two-stage sacroabdominoperineal pull-through procedure.

The seminal advances that ushered in the modern era of ARM management were those of Peña for imperforate anus and Hendren for CMs and UGSMs. However, other significant contributions have advanced the management of ARMs and UGSMs. These include the creation of the intestinal neovagina (Pratt, 1972; Hensle and Dean, 1992; Hendren and Atala, 1994). Subsequently, intestine was used as an interposition for the short vagina. Skin tube inversion as a complement to difficult vaginal reconstruction has further facilitated care (Passerini-Glazel, 1989; Sheldon et al., 1994a; DiBenedetto et al., 1997).

Of significant impact was the recognition of the high incidence of urologic abnormalities associated

with ARMs (Smith, 1968; Santulli et al., 1971; Belman & King, 1972; Weiner and Kieswetter, 1973; McLorie et al., 1987). Recognition of the high incidence of spinal cord abnormalities, including occult spinal dysraphisms such as tethered cord, lipomas, neurenteric cysts and diastematomyelia, significantly advanced the management of these patients (Carson et al., 1984; Karrer et al., 1988; Sheldon et al., 1991; Boemers et al., 1996). Patients with ARMs frequently require complex urinary reconstruction for which unique concerns must be addressed (Sheldon et al., 1994b).

The development of the Malone antegrade continence enema or continence cecostomy (Malone et al., 1990) has tremendously advanced the management of fecal incontinence and fecal retention in children with neurologic conditions such as myelomeningocele. Subsequently, this procedure has been proven to be highly applicable to the management of children with ARMs (Sheldon et al., 1997b; Malone and Curry, 1999). The use of this procedure has been extended to enable fecal undiversion in children with ARMs who have previously undergone colostomy for refractory fecal incontinence with success (Sheldon et al., 1997b) (se Chaptwe 18).

While relatively uncommon, ARMs and UGSMs are critically important to the reconstructive surgeon owing to their tremendous morbidity and significant mortality. Anorectal malformations occur in 1 in 4000 to 1 in 5000 live births (Brenner, 1925; Trusler and Wilkinson, 1962; Santulli et al., 1971). UGSMs represent a complex array of anomalies for which a true incidence of occurrence is difficult to estimate. Vaginal agenesis occurs in 1 in 4000 to 1 in 5000 live female births (Bryan, 1949) and cloacal anomalies occur in 1 in 50 000 live births (Hendren, 1982).

The incidence of mortality with ARMs and UGSMs has dropped dramatically over time.

However, on occasion, infants will still succumb to renal failure, cardiac anomalies, and sepsis (in particular, urosepsis and aspiration pneumonia). The morbidity associated with these anomalies is extensive and includes psychosocial developmental disorders, fecal incontinence, urinary incontinence, urinary tract infection, impaired intercourse, impaired fertility, as well as other abnormalities such as limb anomalies, vertebral anomalies, neurologic deficits, and tracheoesophageal fistulae.

Spectrum of abnormalities encountered

It is now known that urinary, genital and anorectal development are intimately interconnected. This has been emphasized with the recognition of two important constellations of anomaly patterns. As early as 1829 an association was recognized between vaginal agenesis and other congenital anomalies (Mayer, 1829). This observation was subsequently confirmed (Kuster, 1910; Rokitanski, 1938), following which this pattern of anomalies was referred to as the Mayer–Rokitanski–Kuster syndrome. Hauser and Schreiner (1961) emphasized the association of vaginal agenesis with skeletal and renal anomalies. This association became known as the Rokitanski–Kuster–Hauser syndrome. Upper tract anomalies are encountered in approximately one-third of these patients, mostly consisting of renal agenesis, renal ectopia, and renal fusion anomalies (Fore *et al.*, 1975; Griffin *et al.*, 1976). Frequent skeletal anomalies were also noted, many of which involved abnormal cervical and thoracic somite development. Duncan *et al.* (1975) referred to this as the MURCS association: müllarian duct aplasia, renal aplasia, and cervicothoracic somite association.

Similar to those observations associated with vaginal agenesis, repetitive patterns of anomalies were seen with anorectal anomalies (Say and Gerald, 1968; Quan and Smith, 1973; Barry and Auldist, 1974; Temtamy and Miller, 1974; Wendeken *et al.*, 1977; Weber *et al.*, 1980; Uehling *et al.*, 1983; Muraji and Mahour, 1984; Weaver and Mapstone, 1986; Beals and Rolfe, 1989; Brock *et al.*, 1987). This constellation originally became known as the VATER association: vertebral, anorectal, tracheoesophageal, and radial. Later, it was expanded to the VACTERL association: vertebral, anorectal, cardiac, trachoesophageal, radial/renal, and limb.

The presentation of patients with ARM and UGSM can be quite varied. Some patients present with an abnormal antenatal sonogram demonstrating renal anomalies, associated myelomeningocele, hydrocolpos, or exstrophy. Most frequently, patients present with an abnormal neonatal examination. In general, this consists of an absent perineal orifice, most commonly anus, occasionally vagina, or both. An abdominal mass may be encountered, often secondary to hydrometrocolpos, urinary retention, or hydronephrosis. In addition, an interlabial mass may allow detection of hydrometrocolpos. Patients may present with failure to evacuate either feces or urine, incontinence of urine, and urinary tract infection (UTI). Older children may present with failure to menstruate or with pain and abdominal mass associated with obstructed menstrual flow.

It is not surprising that an anatomic area of such complex anatomy as the perineum, which develops over such a brief duration, would have a high incidence of congenital anomalies. Table 26.1 outlines common female congenital anomalies involving the urethra, vagina, and anorectum. Common anorectal abnormalities include stenosis, ectopic anus, covered anus, imperforate anus (high or low), and atresia. Of note is the fact that many vaginal anomalies may be associated with anorectal malformation in girls, including congenital vaginal obstruction, vaginal agenesis, and duplication anomalies. UGSMs represent anomalies involving both the female urethra and vagina and may occur in the setting of intersex but may also occur in the absence of intersex states. A commonly associated vaginal and anorectal abnormality is that of imperforate anus with fistula to the vestibular or vaginal regions. Rarely, a fistula without imperforate anus may be encountered. Cloacal anomalies and cloacal exstrophy represent anomalies that involve the urethra, vagina, and anorectum.

Similarly, Table 26.2 outlines commonly encountered urethral and anorectal anomalies encountered in the male. As in the female, the spectrum of ARMs, includes anal stenosis, ectopic anus, covered anus, imperforate anus, and anorectal atresia. Of note is the fact that hypospadias, urethral duplication, urethral agenesis, urethral stricture, and valves have all been described in association with ARMs. The urethra and anorectum may be jointly involved in those patients who have imperforate anus with fistula to the bladder, prostatic urethra, or bulbar urethra. Urethral fistula without imperforate anus (White *et al.*, 1978; Hong

Table 26.1 Common female congenital anomalies

Urethra	Vagina	Anorectum

Epispadias
Ectopic ureterocele
	Congenital obstruction[a]
	  Imperforate hymen
	  Transverse septum
	  Obstructive duplications
	  Atresia
	Agenesis[a]
	  With intersex
	  Without intersex
	Duplication anomalies[a]
	Urogenital sinus
	  With intersex
	  Without intersex
		Stenosis
		Ectopic
		Covered
		Imperforate
		  Low
		  High
		Atresia

	Imperforate anus with fistula
	  Vestibular
	  Vaginal	

	Fistula without imperforate anus Cloaca Cloacal exstrophy	

[a]May be associated with anorectal malformations.

et al., 1992) may be encountered but is relatively rare. As with the female, cloacal exstrophy involves a severe anomaly of development involving the urethra and anorectum.

Embryology

The surgeon who has some knowledge of embryology, however imperfect or controversial, will be better prepared to understand the relationship of the anus and rectum to surrounding structures and to the fistulas that so frequently connect the rectum to the genitourinary system (*Raffensperger, 1990*).

The understanding of the embryology of ARM is severely compromised by limited studies of both normal and abnormal human embryos. However, animal studies raise major questions regarding the current theories of ARM embryogenesis (Kluth and Lambrecht, 1997). These studies suggest that the embryonic cloaca never passes through a stage that resembles the 'persistent cloaca' which is recognized clinically. This line of investigation suggests that ARMs may arise from a short cloacal membrane associated with deficient dorsal cloacal anlage. Impaired septation may

not ultimately prove to be etiologic of ARMs, as classically conceptualized.

Nonetheless, the classic embryologic concepts remain useful because they predict human disease patterns (O'Rahilly and Müller, 1992; Skandalakis and Gray, 1994). Figure 26.1 depicts a classical approach

Table 26.2 Common male congenital anomalies

Urethra	Anorectum

Hypospadias[a]
Epispadias
  Isolated
  With Exstrophy
Duplication[a]
Agenesis[a]
Stricture[a]
  Congenital
  Acquired
Valves[a]
	Stenosis
	Ectopic
	Covered
	Imperforate
	  Low
	  High
	Atresia

Imperforate anus with fistula
  Bladder
  Prostatic urethra
  Bulbar urethra
Fistula without imperforate anus
Cloacal exstrophy	

[a]May be associated with anorectal malformations.

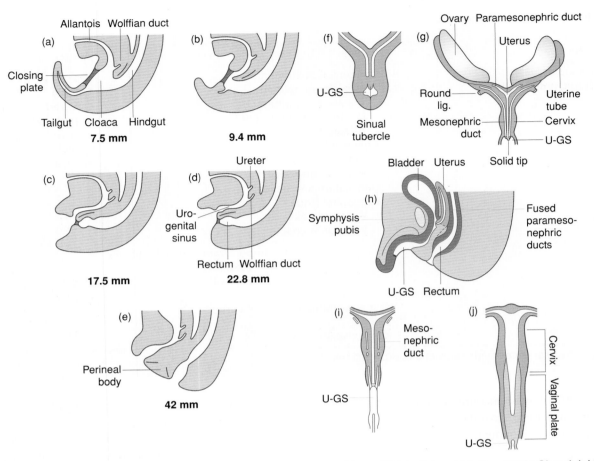

Figure 26.1 Embryology of cloacal and urogenital development. (From O'Raholly and Muller, 1992; Skandalakis *et al.*, 1994.) (U-GS = urogenital sinus.)

to the embryologic derivation of the rectum, anus, vagina, and urethra. The closing plate of the cloaca (the cloacal membrane) is comprised of only two layers, the endoderm and ectoderm, in immediate apposition (Fig. 26.1a). The urorectal septum (Fig. 26.1b) functions as a mesodermal tissue wedge, the medial portion of which (Tourneux fold) is progressively driven caudally toward the cloacal membrane by progressive fusion of the lateral ridges (Rathke folds) which grow inward from the sides of the cloaca. The urorectal septum divides the cloacal membrane into the urogenital membrane and the anal membrane, which subsequently ruptures (Fig. 26.1c, d). Differential growth causes the anal membrane to be displaced caudally and depressed below the surface, forming the anal pit. The pectinate line in the fully developed human represents the level of the anal membrane. Further differential growth separates the urogenital and anal orifices with the formation of the perineal body (Fig. 26.1e).

It follows, then, that one might conceive the origin of the various ARMs as depicted in Figure 26.2, as reviewed by Paidas and Peña (1997). Here, failure of the Rathke fold (RF) development results in the rectoprostatic urethral fistula (RPUF) in males, and the high rectovaginal fistula (RVFH) and common cloaca (CC) in females. Similarly, failure of both Rathke and Tourneux fold (TF) development results in the rectovesical fistula in males and common cloaca in females. Malalignment of Tourneux and Rathke folds causes rectobulbarurethral fistulae (RUF) in males and rectovestibular (RVBF) and low rectovaginal fistulae (RVFL) in females. A mesodermal defect at the level of the perineal body results in perineal fistulae (PF). Partial or complete failure of anal membrane absorption results in anal stenosis (AS) or rectal atresia (RA), respectively. Arrest of anal pit formation results in imperforate anus without fistula, while abnormal fusion of the genital folds gives rise to the covered anus.

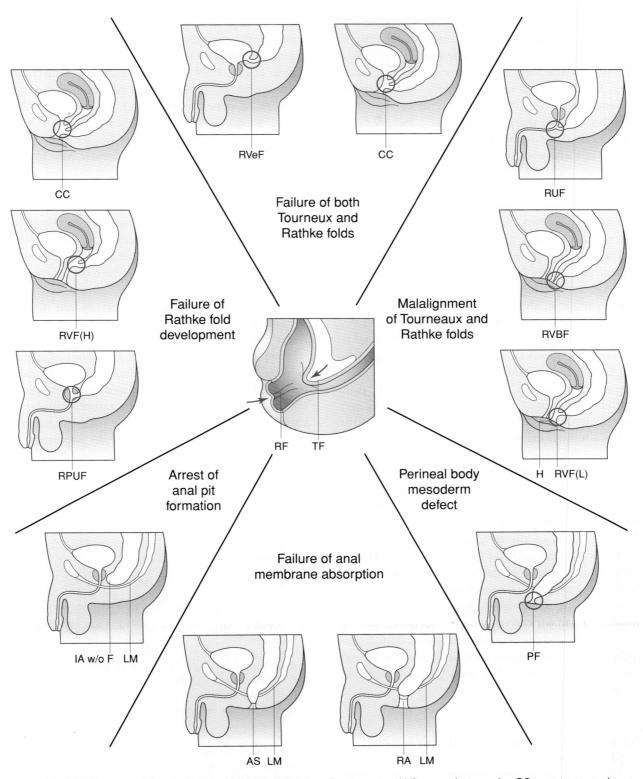

Figure 26.2 Spectrum of anomalies associated with imperforate anus. (AS = anal stenosis; CC = common cloaca; IA w/o F = imperforate anus without fistula; RF = rathic fold; RA = rectal atresia; RPUF = recto-prostatic urethral fistula; RUF = rectourethral fistula; RVF(H) = rectovaginal fistula (high); RVF(L) = rectovaginal fistula (low); RVeF = rectrovesicle fistula; RVBF = rectovestibular fistula; TF = tourneux fold; LM = levator muscle; (Redrawn after Paidas and Peña A, 1997.)

The developing mesonephric duct induces the formation of the paramesonephric ducts which arise as coelomic invaginations (O'Rhailly and Müller, 1992). The paramesonephric ducts grow caudally to insert into the urogenital sinus. Caudally, they fuse to become the uterus, while cranially the unfused portions become the uterine or fallopian tubes. A sinual tubercle develops at the site of insertion of the solid tip of the paramesonephric duct and the urogenital sinus (Fig. 26.1f–h). This intimate embryologic relationship between the mesonephric and paramesonephric ducts explains the high incidence of upper tract urinary anomalies encountered with anomalous vaginal development.

The developing vagina becomes occluded by the vaginal plate (Fig. 26.1i). With differential growth, the vagina elongates and slides caudally down the dorsal surface of the urethra to establish a separate vestibular opening, as the vaginal plate desquamates to create the vaginal lumen. The hymen is believed to represent the junction of the sinual tubercle and the urogenital sinus. Failure of the hymen to rupture (imperforate hymen) and failure of vaginal plate canalization (vaginal atresias and vaginal septa) may cause hydrocolpos (obstructive fluid distension of the vagina) or hydrometrocolpos (obstructive fluid distension of both the vagina and uterus). After menarche, vaginal obstruction may result in hematocolpos or hematometrocolpos (obstructive distension with blood). Müllerian (or uterine) aplasia represents absence of the uterus and results from inadequate caudal progression of the developing paramesonephric ducts. Here, the distal most vagina, ovaries, and external genitalia are normal. An unicornate uterus occurs from developmental failure of one paramesonephric duct, while uterus didelphys (two uteri, two cervices, and two vaginas), uterus duplex bicollis (two uteri, two cervices, and one vagina) and uterus duplex unicollis or bicornuate uterus (two uteri, one cervix, and one vagina) arise from various degrees of failure of paramesonephric duct fusion.

Anomalies of anorectal development: imperforate anus

Imperforate anus exists as a large spectrum of anomalies and, for this reason, classification systems are essential. Stephens and Smith (1986) presented a classification for anal rectal malformations, outlined in

Table 26.3. This classification is quite detailed and anatomically precise and useful for investigation. A recent study of 1992 patients with ARMs from Japan (Endo *et al.*, 1999) demonstrated the incidence of these anomalies (Table 26.4). 'Low' lesions represented 58% of patients, with 'high' and 'intermediate' lesions found in 26% and 11%, respectively. Only 13% of female ARMs were classified as 'high', most of which were cloacal malformations (CM). In contrast, 35% of males had 'high' lesions, 81% of whom had rectourethral fistulae. 'Low' lesions were encountered in 49% and 72% of males and females, respectively, most of which represented anocutaneous or anovestibular fistulae. 'Intermediate' lesions are less common but very important because they are managed as high lesions but may appear to be low lesions on examination. More recently, Brock and Peña (1992) promoted a classification system that is extremely useful clinically (Table 26.5). For both males and females, patients are divided into those for whom no colostomy is required, for whom colostomy is required, and complex malformations. In both males and females, those patients for whom no colostomy is required represent a rather simple spectrum of ARMs. In contrast, those patients requiring colostomy represent a more diverse population of patients with more difficult anatomic problems.

Table 26.3 Wingspread classification of anorectal malformations

Female	Male
High	**High**
Anorectal agenesis	Anorectal agenesis
Rectovaginal fistula	Rectoprostatic fistula
No fistula	Rectovesical fistula
Rectal atresia	No fistula
	Rectal atresia
Intermediate	**Intermediate**
Rectovestibular fistula	Rectobulbar fistula
Rectovaginal fistula	Anal agenesis without
Anal agenesis without	fistula
fistula	
Low	**Low**
Anovestibular fistula	Anocutaneous fistula
Anocutaneous fistula	Anal stenosis
Anal stenosis	Rare malformations
Cloaca	
Rare malformations	

After Stephens and Smith (1986).

Table 26.4 Incidence of anorectal anomalies

Male		Female		Total
High (35%)		High (13%)		High (26%)
Rectourethral fistula	81%	Cloaca	86%	
Rectovesical fistula	10%	Anorectal agenesis without fistula	5%	
Anorectal agenesis without fistula	8%	Rectovaginal fistula	5%	
Rectal atresia	1%	Rectovesical fistula	2%	
		Rectal atresia	2%	
Intermediate (14%)		Intermediate (7%)		Intermediate (11%)
Rectobulbar fistula	56%	Rectovestibular fistula	54%	
Anal agenesis without fistula	38%	Anal agenesis without fistula	21%	
Anorectal stenosis	7%	Rectovaginal fistula	20%	
		Anorectal stenosis	5%	
Low (49%)		Low (72%)		Low (58%)
Anocutaneous fistula	65%	Anovestibular fistula	42%	
Covered anal stenosis	21%	Anocutaneous fistula	30%	
Covered anus	14%	Anovulvar fistula	17%	
		Covered anus	6%	
		Covered anal stenosis	4%	
		Other	1%	
Miscellaneous (2%)		Miscellaneous (8%)		Miscellaneous (5%)

From Endo *et al*. (1999).

Table 26.5 Peña classification of anorectal malformations and fistulae

Female	Male
No colostomy required	No colostomy required
Rectoperineal (cutaneous) fistula	Rectoperineal (cutaneous) fistula
	Anal stenosis
	Anal membrane
Colostomy required	Colostomy required
Vestibular fistula	Rectourethral fistula:
Vaginal fistula	Bulbar
Anorectal agenesis without fistula	Prostatic
Rectal atresia	Rectovesical fistula
Persistent cloaca	Anorectal agenesis without fistula
	Rectal atresia
Complex malformations	Complex malformations

From Brock and Peña (1992).

The management of the patient with imperforate anus is outlined in Figures 26.3 and 26.4. Neonatal evaluation begins with a detailed physical examination followed by a period of observation usually ranging between 18 and 24 hours. This not only enables medical stabilization and exclusion of important associated congenital anomalies, but also helps in determining the level of the imperforate anus. Patients who pass meconium through the urethra or into the bladder may be detected by direct inspection or by urinalysis. This indicates a high imperforate anus. In contrast, those patients who pass meconium through a perineal fistula generally will have a low imperforate anus. In males, the 'bucket handle' abnormality as well as a mid-raphe fistula suggest a low imperforate anus. As noted in Figure 26.3, patients with a 'rocker-bottom' anomaly or females with rectovestibular or rectovaginal fistulae fall, in general, into a high

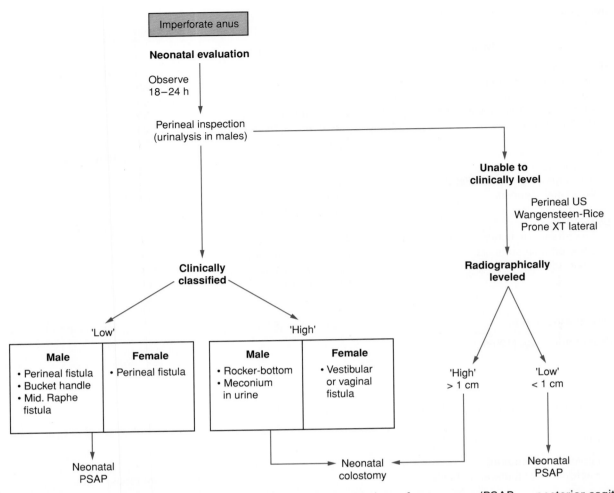

Figure 26.3 Neonatal evaluation and management of patient with imperforate anus. (PSAP = posterior-sagital anoplasty.)

imperforate anus category. Those patients with high lesions require neonatal colostomy, whereas those with a low lesion can be managed with a neonatal posterior sagittal anoplasty.

Some patients are unable to be clinically classified and require radiographic evaluation. This may be done with a perineal ultrasound, a Wangensteen–Rice 'invertogram' or a prone, cross-table, lateral X-ray study. Those infants with a radiographically determined distance between the rectal pouch and perineum exceeding 1 cm have high lesions and those with distances less than 1 cm have low lesions. Occasionally, contrast injected into a cutaneous or vestibular lesion may help to distinguish between an intermediate and a low lesion.

As outlined in Figure 26.4, the goals of management in the first few years of life are to protect the upper urinary tracts, ensure low pressure urinary drainage, normalize anorectal anatomy, and minimize any neurologic deficit that might arise from treatable spinal pathology. All patients are evaluated with an abdominal sonogram to include the kidneys, a contrast voiding cystourethrogram (VCUG), a spinal sonogram and determination of postvoid residual volume of urine (PVR). Depending on these findings, patients occasionally require intermittent catheterization, cutaneous vesicostomy, or even spinal surgery. Those patients who receive colostomy will undergo definitive anorectal reconstruction in the form of posterior-sagittal anorectoplasty (PSAP), usually between 1 and 6 months of age, but occasionally older depending on the presence of other congenital anomalies.

The type of colostomy performed is extremely important. Figure 26.5 outlines the course of an infant who received a partially diverting colostomy for high imperforate anus and who had incomplete bladder emptying. This child suffered severe urosepsis resulting in acute tubular necrosis and significant azotemia which ultimately resolved following creation of a vesi-

costomy and revision of the colostomy to an end colostomy. Accordingly, patients with rectourinary fistulae, particularly, those with incomplete bladder emptying and vesicoureteral reflux (VUR), should be managed with a completely diverting colostomy.

As outlined in Figure 26.4, the goals of management of the preschool and school-aged child with

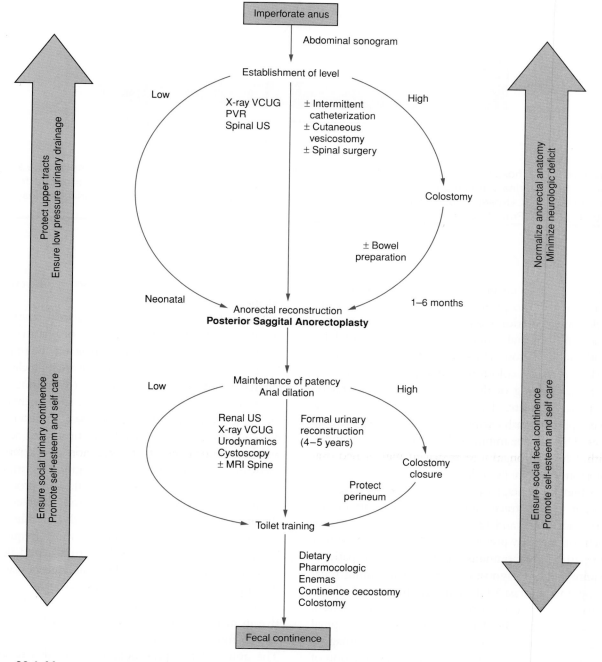

Figure 26.4 Management strategy for imperforate anus (± = possible).

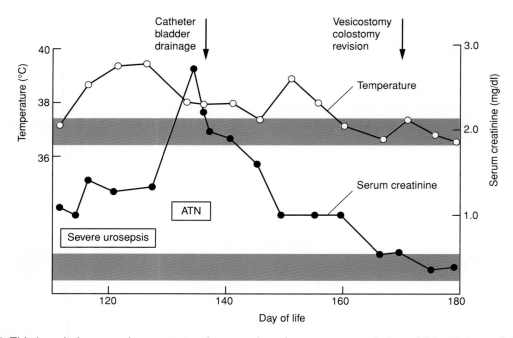

Figure 26.5 This hospital course demonstrates the sequelae of severe urosepsis in a child with imperforate anus in whom chronic urinary retention was unrecognized and a partially diverting colostomy was performed for high imperforate anus. Urosepsis persisted despite antibiotic therapy and resolved only after appropriate drainage had been instituted. (From Sheldon *et al.*, 1991.)

ARMs are to ensure social urinary and fecal continence and to promote self-esteem and self-care. Following posterior sagittal anorectoplasty, maintenance of anorectal patency is generally ensured by gentle anal dilation. Those patients who have previously received a colostomy undergo colostomy closure once healing of the posterior sagittal anorectoplasty is complete. These children often develop a severe perineal rash owing to the sudden exposure to feces. This may be minimized by the aggressive application of antifungal ointment in the early post-colostomy closure period.

A high percentage of children will either have significant urinary tract anomalies or fail to attain urinary continence and require urinary reconstruction. Such patients may present to the urologist for the first time after toilet training has failed. These patients require careful diagnostic evaluation including renal sonogram, contrast VCUG, urodynamics, and often a cystoscopy prior to formal urinary reconstruction. Those patients who have not had previous spinal imaging will require a magnetic resonance imaging (MRI) study of the spine, as ultrasound evaluation of the spine cannot be performed beyond the age of 6 months because of the presence of vertebral calcification.

Those children who fail to attain fecal continence are often readily managed by dietary or pharmacologic intervention. Occasionally, enemas may be required to achieve continence. Most effective are high cleaning enemas administered at night (Shandling and Gilmour, 1987). Not uncommonly, such enemas are incompletely successful or cannot be administered by the child, resulting in their being unable to achieve self-care. In this setting, the creation of a continent cecostomy for purposes of antegrade continence enema has been extremely beneficial. This procedure consists of making a continent and catheterizable channel connecting the cecum and the skin. The appendix is used for this purpose most frequently, however, other channels, such as tubularized ileum, have also been used successfully. This concept was first developed and presented by Malone *et al.* (1990). Subsequently, this procedure was proven to be effective in many children who have extremely deformed and dysfunctional anal canals (Sheldon *et al.*, 1997b). The utility of this procedure was extended to allow fecal undiversion for children who had previously received colostomies for refractory fecal incontinence.

The surgical management of ARMs has been detailed recently (Paidas and Peña, 1997) and is illustrated in Figures 26.6 and 26.7. These procedures are performed with the patient prone, with the pelvis elevated into a 'jack-knife' position and with a Foley catheter indwelling. Figure 26.6 depicts the approach to low lesions, as illustrated by the anoperineal fistula (Fig. 26.6a) and the anal vestibular fistula (Fig.

26.6b–e). The perineal fistula in both males and females is corrected in the newborn period without a diverting colostomy. Electrical stimulation (Fig. 26.7) allows determination of the position of the sphincteric mechanism.

The fistula is mobilized through a circumferential incision. A vertical incision is created posteriorly, directly in the midline through the external sphincter mechanism, enabling the rectum to be transposed

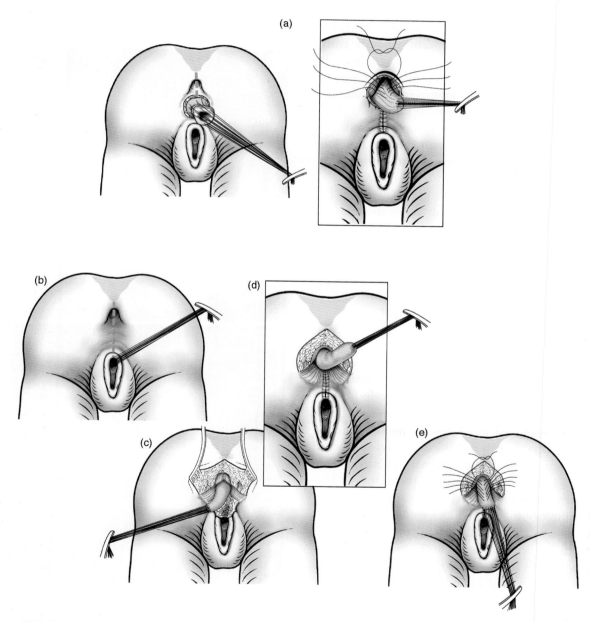

Figure 26.6 Surgical management of anorectal malformations (low lesions). See text. Redrawn from Paidas and Peña A, 1997.)

posteriorly to the site of the external sphincter mechanism. Similarly, the anovestibular fistula may also be corrected through a limited posterior sagittal approach. Many surgeons approach this in the newborn period without a protecting colostomy. Others prefer a colostomy with early definitive correction of the anorectal malformation subsequently. The fistula is circumscribed (Fig. 26.6b) and, again, a vertical midline incision is created extending through the sphincteric mechanism identified by electrical stimulation.

The rectum is gently dissected free from the underlying vagina to which it is, generally, intimately attached (Fig. 26.6c). Once the rectum is sufficiently mobilized to prevent tension, the perineal body is reconstructed in two layers, establishing clear separation between the anus and vagina and the anterior edge of the sphincteric muscle is approximated (Fig. 26.6d). Posteriorly, the muscle complex is approximated and anchored to the rectum (Fig. 26.6e), following which the anocutaneous anastomosis is completed.

Prior to this approach, the only access to these defects was either through the perineum, the abdomen, or a combination of the two. Surgical procedures frequently involved blind maneuvers with the consequent risk of injuring important structures. The rectum was pulled down through a path that was assumed to be the right one (*Peña, 1990*).

High lesions are managed by a similar, but more extensive, approach (Fig. 26.8). This is illustrated in a male with a rectourethral fistula who previously had a diverting colostomy. The patient is prone with an indwelling Foley catheter. A midline incision extends from the coccyx (which is divided distally) to a point through and beyond the external sphincter (Fig. 26.8a), identified by electrical stimulation. The sphincteric muscle complex and levator muscle are divided directly in the midline, guided by electrical stimulation to minimize any resultant nerve injury. The rectum is opened distally in the midline between traction sutures (Fig. 26.8b), enabling the rectourethral fistula to be identified (Fig. 26.8c,d). A series of traction sutures is placed just proximal to the fistula, allowing a plane to be developed between the rectum and the underlying urogenital structures (Fig. 26.8e–g).

Once mobilization is complete, the urethral fistula is sutured closed under direct vision and with the protection of an indwelling Foley catheter, making urethral injury very unlikely. The perineal body is constructed in two layers and the anterior edge of the external muscle complex is approximated. The levator muscle is approximated over the rectum (Fig. 26.8h), following which the posterior edge of the external sphincteric muscle complex is approximated and anchored to the rectum to prevent prolapse (Fig. 26.8i). The anocutaneous anastomosis is completed and the posterior–sagittal incision is closed in layers (Fig. 26.8j–k).

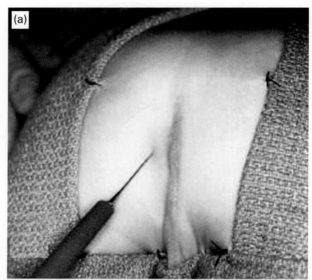

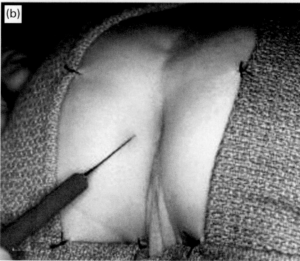

Figure 26.7 Identification of the location of the external striated muscle complex: (*a*) prior to stimulation; (*b*) during stimulation. Dimpling localizes the site of the muscle complex.

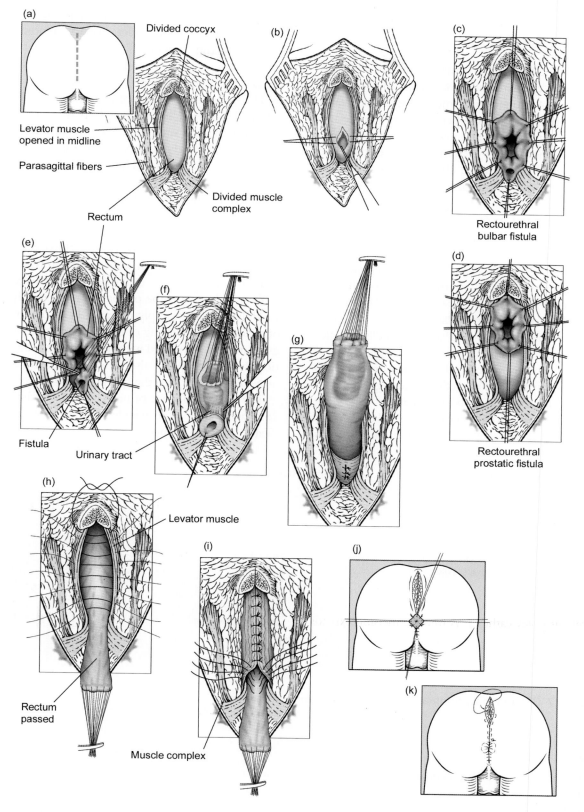

Figure 26.8 Surgical management of anorectal malformations (high lesions). See text. (Redrawn from Paidas and Peña A, 1997.)

Urologic problems associated with imperforate anus

The mean incidence of structural anomalies of the urinary tract is estimated at 35% (Table 26.6). A 1987 review of 484 patients with imperforate anus detailed several critical relationships between imperforate anus and upper tract urinary anomalies (Table 26.7, 26.8). Fistulae connecting the rectum with the urinary tract are frequently encountered abnormalities. Excluding these, structural genitourinary anomalies were seen in 38% of patients. Non-fistula genitourinary anomalies were encountered in 60% of the patients with high lesions and were seen equally in males and females. Such anomalies were encountered in 25% of low lesions (25% for males and 20% for females). Of great significance is the fact that renal mortality was encountered in 3.5% of these patients. Death from renal failure occurred in 6.4% of patients with high anorectal abnormalities (7.2% male, 3.8% female). Renal mortality was encountered in only 1.1% of patients with low anorectal malformations (1.5% male, 0.8% female). This reflects the high incidence of conditions threatening both kidneys.

Table 26.8 reviews the incidence of bilateral upper tract urinary abnormalities threatening renal function which explains the significant renal mortality. Symmetric bilateral upper tract urinary abnormalities occurred in 36 patients (7%) and include bilateral reflux, bilateral agenesis, and bilateral hypoplasia–dysplasia. Asymmetric abnormalities were encountered in 32 (7%) patients. Most of these had reflux on one side and agenesis, hypoplasia–dysplasia, or obstructive pathology on the other. The overall incidence of lesions placing both kidneys at risk was 14%.

The importance of VUR in this population of patients at risk for urinary tract infection and voiding dysfunction cannot be overstated. The true overall incidence of vesicoureteral reflux (i.e. the incidence encountered in patients who received a screening VCUG) was 33%. As in any patient, the development of a UTI in a child with imperforate anus demands prompt and aggressive evaluation and management. Often overlooked is the presentation of epididymitis. Epididymitis may simply reflect UTI in the presence of dysfunctional voiding or urethral stricture pathology or may be associated with intermittent catheterization. It may, however, also be associated with ectopic ureteral insertion into the genital pathway.

The mean incidence of neurovesical dysfunction is 25% and varies quite widely among reported series (Table 26.9). As expected, high anorectal malforma-

Table 26.6 Structural abnormalities of the genitourinary (GU) tract

Series	No.	Gu Anomaly (%)
Smith (1968)	195	60
Santulli et al. (1971)	1166	26
Belman and King (1972)	143	36
Wiener and Kiesewetter (1973)	200	28
Hoekstra (1983)	150	50
McLorie et al. (1987)	484	38
Rich et al. (1988)	244	48
Metts et al. (1977)	105	41
Total	2687	50

Table 26.7 Genitourinary anomalies in patients with imperforate anus

484 patients	High			Low			Overall
	Male	Female	Total	Male	Female	Total	
GU anomalies excluding fistulae	60%	62%	60%	25%	20%	25%	42%
Renal mortality	7.2%	3.8%	6.4%	1.5%	0.8%	1.1%	3.5%

GU = genitourinary.
From McLorie et al. (1987).

Table 26.8 Bilateral upper tract urinary abnormalities threatening renal function

Symmetric		Asymmetric	
Pathology	No.	Pathology	No.
Bilateral reflux	22	Reflux/agenesis	14
Bilateral agenesis	16	Reflux/hypoplasia–dysplasia	6
Bilateral UPJ obstruction	5	Reflux/ectopia	3
Hypoplasia–dysplasia	1	Reflux/UPJ obstruction	3
Bilateral duplication		Reflux/primary obstructing megaureter	1
		Dysplasia/UPJ obstruction	1
		Agenesis/hypoplasia–dysplasia	3
		Agenesis/ectopia	1
Total	36(7%)	Total	32(7%)

Overall incidence of lesions placing both kidneys at risk = 14%.
True overall incidence of vesicoureteral reflux (patients screened by voiding cystourethrography) = 44/133 (33%).
UPJ = ureteropelvic junction.
From McLorie *et al.* (1987).

tions have the greatest incidence. However, the incidence in low lesions is quite significant as well and all patients with ARM should be screened. As previously noted, the recognition of the high incidence of occult spinal dysraphism has had a major impact on the management of these patients (Carson *et al.*, 1984; Karrer *et al.*, 1988; Sheldon *et al.*, 1991; Warf *et al.*, 1993). Such lesions have been demonstrated to have significant implications for the urinary tract, to be potentially progressive and may improve following surgical correction (Cumes, 1977; Al-Mefty *et al.*, 1980; Yoneyama *et al.*, 1985; Hellstrom *et al.*, 1985; Warf *et al.*, 1993). Although the timing of surgical intervention remains controversial, some authors suggest that early surgical intervention results in the best functional neurologic outcome (Sato *et al.*, 1993).

Screening ultrasonography has proven useful in the diagnosis of occult spinal dysraphism in infants (Raghavendra *et al.*, 1983; Scheible *et al.*, 1983).

Table 26.9 Incidence of neuropathic bladder in ARM

Series	No.	NVD (%)
Sheldon *et al.* (1992)	90	24
Kakizaki *et al.* (1994)	21	43
Boemers *et al.* (1996)	90	57
Capitanucci *et al.* (1996)	14	18
Total	215	25

NVD = neurovesical dysfunction.

Older children generally require MRI for diagnosis. The significance of these dysraphic states became apparent in the early 1990s. Table 26.10 outlines an early experience, where dysfunctional voiding was encountered in 31% and 5% high and low ARMs, respectively. Structural spinal cord pathology was encountered in 12% and 4%, respectively. More recent data (Appignani *et al.*, 1994) suggest that screening by MRI for occult dysraphic myelodysplasia yields an even higher incidence of spinal cord pathology. They encountered dysraphic states in 17% of low ARMs, 34% of high ARMs, 46% of cloacal anomalies, and 100% of patients with cloacal exstrophy.

Of great importance to the surgeon is whether or not surgical correction of ARMs is etiologic in the development of the neuropathic bladder. Ralph *et al.* (1993) evaluated 58 patients with imperforate anus who had reached an age of 18 years or greater. Of these, 43 patients had received rectal pull-through procedures while the remainder received cutback procedures. They found evidence for a neuropathic bladder in 32 patients (55%). Ninety-one per cent of these neuropathic bladders were hyperreflexic in nature. Thirty patients (52%) had spinal deformities, 21 (70%) of which had evidence for neurovesical dysfunction. Only three patients (5.2%) had hypotonic bladders, normal spinal anatomy and high ARMs and were felt likely to have iatrogenic neurovesical dysfunction. Boemers *et al.* (1995) evaluated 32 patients with ARMs who underwent posterior-sagittal anorectoplasty (PSARP) employing urodynamic

Table 26.10 Spinal abnormalities in patients with anorectal malformations

Type of anorectal malformation	No. of patients	Dysfunctional voiding		Structural cord lesion[a]	
		No.	%	No.	%
High	25	8	31	3	12
Low	56	3	5	2	4
Anorectal stenosis	2	1	50	1	50
Cloaca	5	3	60	—	—
Cloacal exstrophy	2	1	50	1	50
Total	90	16	18	7	8

[a]Six tethered cords and one lumbar stenosis.
From Sheldon et al. (1991).

investigation. In 27 patients, urodynamic investigation was performed both before and after PSARP. No evidence of somatic nerve injury was encountered in this series. Detrusor failure suggestive of autonomic denervation was encountered in three males, two of whom had combined PSARP with transabdominal dissection. The authors concluded that, in the absence of transabdominal dissection and significant retrovesical dissection, PSARP did not affect lower urinary tract function.

Another important urologic problem which may be extremely problematic is that of hyperchloremic metabolic acidosis (Iwai et al., 1978; Caldemone et al., 1979). This condition usually occurs as the result of urine passing from the bladder, through a rectovesical or rectourethral fistula and into the defunctionalized distal limb of colon following initial diverting colostomy. The resultant absorption of urinary constituents by the bowel results in the metabolic abnormality. The occurrence of this complication requires the presence of a urorectal fistula and is facilitated by a long segment of defunctionalized colon (large absorptive surface) communicating with the fistula. Additionally, the presence of distal urinary obstruction, which may be structural (stricture) or functional (neurovesical dysfunction), facilitates this risk. UTI and renal insufficiency may also potentiate this metabolic abnormality. Hyperchloremic metabolic acidosis may be avoided by the creation of a low, fully diverting colostomy and by ensuring effective bladder drainage. Once established, hyperchloremic metabolic acidosis is treated by the administration of oral alkalinizing agents, intermittent catheterization, vesicostomy, or early anorectal reconstruction with division of the fistula, depending on the clinical setting.

Vaginal problems in patients with imperforate anus

Often overlooked, and underestimated, are the long-term vaginal and reproductive problems that can occur in girls with imperforate anus (Fleming et al., 1986). While most girls experiencing such complications fall into the category of cloacal anomalies, such complications can occur in girls with imperforate anus alone. Problems may occur as a result of scarring from reconstructive vaginal surgery, from primary vaginal anomalies, such as vaginal agenesis, or from the surgical violation of the vagina in the correction of imperforate anus associated with rectovaginal fistula.

Transperitoneal pelvic surgery, needed in many of these children, may result in peritoneal adhesions that may adversely affect tubal function, impairing fertility and promoting ectopic pregnancy. Consequently, it is imperative that the managing physician as well as the patient be aware of the potential of such complications and that long-term follow-up is maintained. Some children will require subsequent introital surgery in order to facilitate intercourse. Such surgery is generally deferred until adolescence.

Anomalies of vaginal development: urogenital sinus and vaginal agenesis

Vaginal anomalies offer a unique challenge for the reconstructive surgeon. They represent a complex constellation of abnormalities with highly variable anatomy. In addition, the vagina may be relatively difficult to expose surgically compared with other organ systems commonly requiring restorative surgery. It is imperative that the surgeon attempt to delineate vaginal anatomy preoperatively but be prepared to alter the planned procedure based on operative findings. Consequently, the surgeon must be familiar with a wide range of surgical options in order to adapt the reconstruction to the patient's unique anatomy.

Vaginal anomalies may be classified as outlined in Figure 26.9. The majority of surgically significant vaginal anomalies encountered are urogenital sinus malformations (UGSMs), cloacal malformations (CMs) and vaginal agenesis. The majority of UGSMs and vaginal agenesis malformations occur in association with intersex states. It is important to realize, however, that a significant number will be encountered in the absence of intersex states.

The presentation of vaginal anomalies can be quite varied. Some congenital vaginal malformations are suggested by antenatal ultrasonography (Geifman-Holtzman *et al.*, 1997; Cacciaguerra *et al.*, 1998), that may demonstrate either hydrocolpos, hydronephrosis, or both. Most vaginal anomalies are diagnosed during the examination of a newborn who has an obvious congenital deformity. The examiner may note ambiguous genitalia or the presence of only one or two orifices on the female perineum. Some anomalies will be diagnosed during the evaluation of UTI, or when urethral catheterization is attempted and the urethral meatus cannot be located. Less commonly, an absent or abnormal vaginal introitus will be noted on a routine examination later in childhood and, rarely, an anomaly will be detected incidentally during abdominal or pelvic imaging for other pathology. Occasionally, vaginal anomalies will present at menarche, with failure to menstruate or pain from sequestration of menstrual fluid.

The newborn presenting with any suggestion of vaginal abnormality should be evaluated immediately by a surgeon familiar with the entire spectrum of diagnostic possibilities. One must exclude intersex states that may be accompanied by the risk of life-threatening electrolyte disorders. The evaluation and management of intersex states have been reviewed recently (Sheldon, 1997). One must also exclude associated renal and bladder pathology that may have high morbidity if not treated promptly. The surgeon must be prepared to undertake prompt diversion of urine and/or stool as indicated by the clinical setting. Hydrocolpos, when present, must often be promptly decompressed in order to alleviate obstructive uropathy and respiratory compromise, and to prevent or relieve infectious complications.

Urogenital sinus malformations

Classification of UGSMs is difficult owing to the tremendous variability of the presenting anatomy. An attempt at classification does, however, provide a framework for the initial selection of appropriate surgical approaches (Table 26.11). Figure 26.10 provides an overview of the management of children with UGSMs. The first phase of management focuses on protecting the upper urinary tracts, ensuring low-pressure urinary drainage and normalizing the perineal anatomy. Urogenital sinus abnormalities are usually primary in nature but may be secondary, as seen with traumatic disruption of the female urethra or patients with cloacas who are referred for vaginal reconstruction after previously undergoing an anorec-

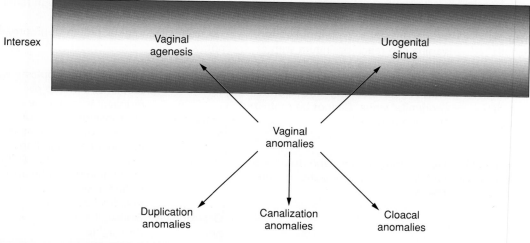

Figure 26.9 Spectrum of vaginal anomalies.

tal reconstructive procedure. It must be emphasized that the most appropriate management of cloacal anomalies is a single-stage reconstruction addressing correction of the ARM, the vaginal malformation, and the urethra in one setting.

Patients with primary urogenital sinus anomalies undergo an immediate neonatal evaluation to delineate their anatomy and to exclude the presence of intersex states. Further, an immediate assessment is made as to whether or not hydrocolpos is present and problematic. Most cases involving hydrocolpos can be managed by intermittent catheterization of the urogenital sinus, vesicostomy, or a combination of the two. Occasionally, vaginostomy will be necessary.

Early anatomic diagnostic procedures may be required in order to facilitate patient management. Abdominal and pelvic ultrasonography is always indicated, as is the determination of postvoid residual volume. Genitoscopy is the preferred method for delineating detail regarding anatomy, while genitography is used only rarely. As will be discussed later, it is important to recognize that many children with vaginal abnormalities will have underlying neuropathic bladders and occult spinal pathology may be present in some. Accordingly, spinal ultrasonography is indicated in selected patients, primarily those without an identifiable intersex state. Definitive anatomic reconstruction is undertaken usually between 3 and 12 months of age. The second stage of management generally begins at the age of 4–5 years as the child prepares to enter school. Here, the focus is ensuring social urinary continence and the promotion of self-esteem. Subsequently, self-care and the insurance of functional vaginal dimensions play a critical role.

Reconstruction of the UGSM begins with careful attention to preparation. Prophylactic antibiotics are routinely administered and all patients with high urogenital malformations undergoing surgery receive a thorough bowel preparation. Preoperative catheter insertion greatly assists in the delineation of anatomy

Table 26.11 Urogenital sinus malformations

Class	Group	Description	Intersex	Common Surgical Options
Low	Wide	Normal or near normal vaginal introitus with urethra 'inserting' into well-developed vagina or 'vaginalized' urogenital sinus	Usually not	Minimal: observation only; urethral meatus obscured: buttock, or alternate, inlay flap over vaginal tube neourethra reconstruction
	Narrow	Confluence of urethra and vagina obscured by midline fusion, usually of labioscrotal folds	Usually	Labioscrotal inlay flap feminizing genitoplasty
High	Wide	Normal or near normal vaginal introitus with urethra 'inserting' into well-developed vagina or 'vaginalized' urogenital sinus	Usually not	Buttock, or alternate, inlay flap over vaginal tube neourethra reconstruction
	Narrow with adequate vaginal length	Usually long, narrow urogenital sinus with vagina 'inserting' into 'urethralized' urogenital sinus. With mobilization, vagina can reach perineum with or without small cutaneous flaps	Usually	Vaginal pull-through feminizing genitoplasty
			Occasionally not	Vaginal pull-through procedure
	Narrow with inadequate vaginal length	Usually long, narrow urogenital sinus with vagina 'inserting' into 'urethralized' urogenital sinus. Cannot be mobilized to reach perineum	Usually	Feminizing genitoplasty with tubularized M-flap or mucocutaneous tube
			Ocassionally not	Interposition procedure such as bowel segment, rotation flaps or pudendal–thigh flaps
	Narrow wtih rudimentary vagina	Usually blind ending and associated with absent or hypoplastic uterine tissue	Usually	Excise, if significant, and create neovagina with tubularized M-flap, mucocutaneous tube or intestinal segment
			Ocassionally not	Excise, if significant, and create neovagina

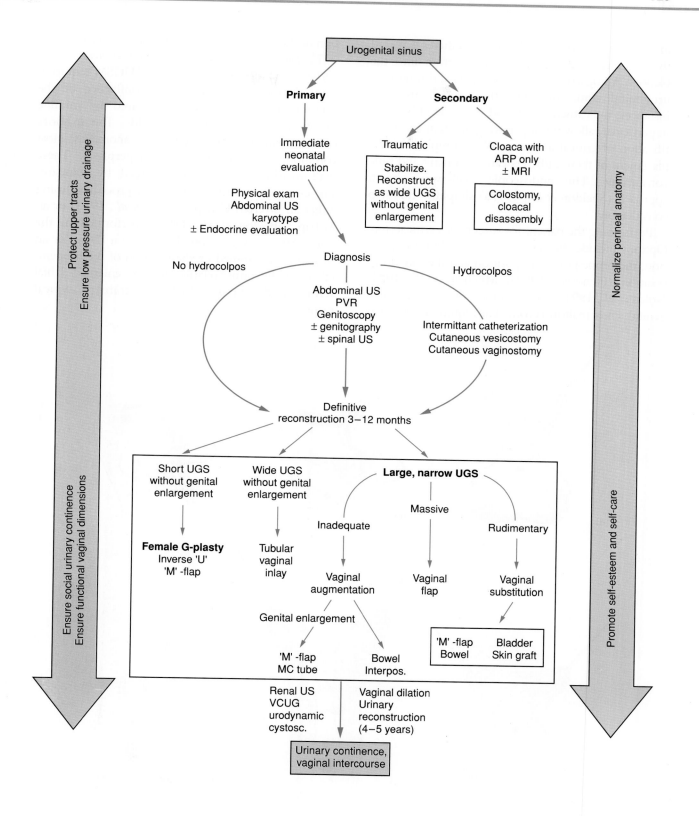

Figure 26.10 Management strategy for urogenital sinus malformations.

intraoperatively. In general, a Foley catheter is placed through the urogenital sinus and urethra into the bladder. A Fogarty catheter is also passed through the urogenital sinus and into the vagina. In both instances, the catheter itself and the inflated balloon, in particular, allow intraoperative palpation and identification of critical anatomy. With complex lesions, placement of these catheters can be difficult and time consuming. The endoscopic peel-away sheath approach (Sheldon *et al.*, 1997a) simplifies this step considerably.

Positioning the patient for surgery is a critical step. Options include the standard dorsal lithotomy position, the prone jack-knife position and the 'sky-diver' position (Hendren, 1980a; Mitchell *et al.*, 1982; Nolan *et al.*, 1991). Not uncommonly, complex urogenital sinus malformations will require a combination of these positions for single-stage reconstruction.

The low urogenital sinus with genital enlargement is, perhaps, the most common type of UGSM requiring surgical restoration. Here, the confluence of the urethra and the vagina is obscured by midline fusion, usually of labioscrotal folds. The majority of these patients represent intersex anomalies, most commonly congenital adrenal hyperplasia. These malformations are readily managed by standard, single-stage feminizing genitoplasty procedures using either an inverted U-flap (Snyder *et al.*, 1983) or an M-flap (Sheldon *et al.*, 1994a) performed in the dorsal lithotomy position. The use of a U-flap or an M-flap is determined by the position of the urogenital sinus introitus relative to the enlarged labial scrotal folds. Figure 26.11 illustrates a typical reconstruction.

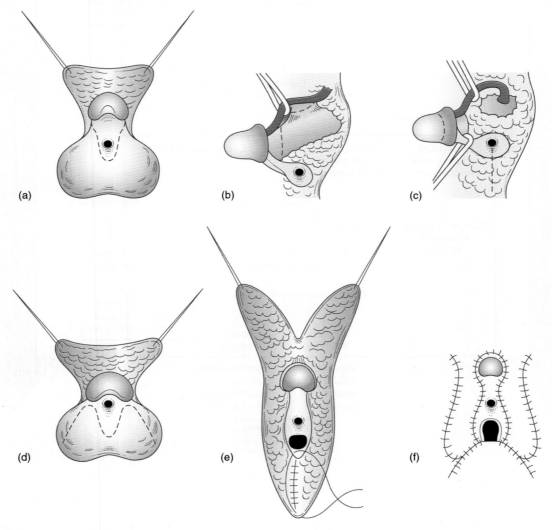

Figure 26.11 Feminizing genitoplasty. See text. (From Sheldon, 1997.)

An incision is made along the lateral edges of the urethral sulcus bilaterally and connected immediately proximal to the urogenital sinus-introitus (Fig. 26.11a). The incision is continued around the dorsum at the hypertrophied clitoris just proximal to the coronal sulcus, allowing the dorsal prepuce to be mobilized (Fig. 26.11b, e). With preservation of the urethral sulcus and the dorsal neurovascular complex, the corpora cavernosa are excised and the remaining ends oversewn with absorbable suture material. A clitoroplasty is undertaken, for which a variety of reconstructive options is available. The clitoris is then recessed and approximated to the tissue immediately adjacent to the symphysis pubis. The urogenital sinus is incised in the midline and an M-flap is developed as shown in Figure 26.11d and reconfigured by midline approximation (Fig. 26.11e). The dorsal prepuce is split in the midline and brought inferiorly on each side of the reduced clitoris to reconstruct the labia minora. This approach has enabled a highly successful outcome from both a cosmetic and functional perspective, as demonstrated in Figure 26.12. Urogenital sinus mobilization and advancement is routinely employed to enable exteriorization of both the urethra and vagina.

The wide UGSM without genital enlargement is an important and distinctive form of the anomaly. Such individuals have a normal or nearly normal vaginal introitus, with the urethra inserting into a well-developed vagina. The majority of these patients do not represent intersex states. The insertion of the urethra into the vagina may occur anywhere from a point just distal to the cervix to a point very near the vaginal introitus. Patients with a very minimal urogenital sinus will often be entirely asymptomatic and generally do not require surgical intervention. With the exception of the most minimal conditions, most patients require urethal lengthening and are readily reconstructed employing the vaginal tube–buttock flap approach (Hendren, 1980a; Mitchell *et al.*, 1982). This procedure is illustrated in Figure 26.13a.

The patient is positioned in the sky-diver position with retractors placed within the vagina to expose the anterior vaginal wall. An inverted U incision is made to outline the tissue used for neourethral reconstruction.

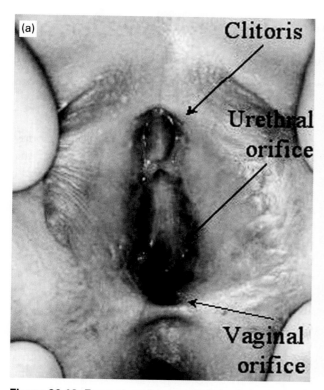 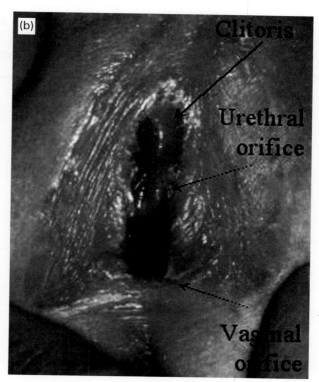

Figure 26.12 Examples of urogenital sinus reconstruction for congenital adrenal hyperplasia, demonstrating normal clitoral size, exteriorized urethral orifice and a vaginal vault of normal caliber and depth for age following M-flap feminizing genoplasty.

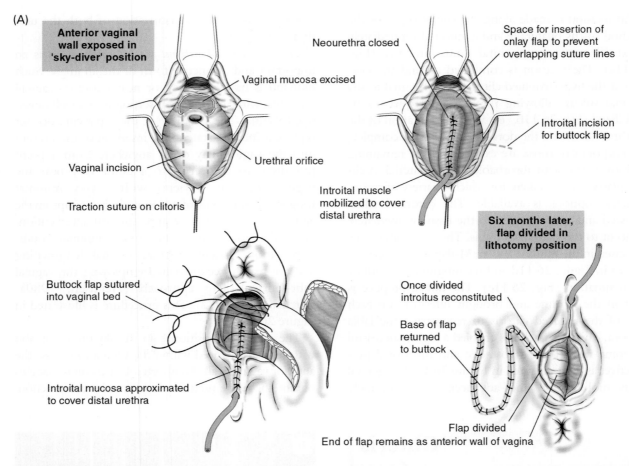

(A)

Anterior vaginal wall exposed in 'sky-diver' position

Vaginal mucosa excised

Vaginal incision

Urethral orifice

Traction suture on clitoris

Neourethra closed

Space for insertion of onlay flap to prevent overlapping suture lines

Introital incision for buttock flap

Introital muscle mobilized to cover distal urethra

Six months later, flap divided in lithotomy position

Buttock flap sutured into vaginal bed

Introital mucosa approximated to cover distal urethra

Once divided introitus reconstituted

Base of flap returned to buttock

Flap divided
End of flap remains as anterior wall of vagina

Figure 26.13 Reconstruction for urogenital sinus with wide vaginal introitus. (*A*) From Hendren (1998b). (*B*) and (*C*) *Shown opposite.* See text.

The resultant midline tongue of tissue should be generous in order to prevent tension upon closure. Importantly, vaginal mucosa should be excised proximally to create an additional bed for the onlay flap to help prevent the occurrence of overlapping suture lines and, thereby, minimize the risk of fistula formation. The neourethra is closed in one or two layers. Introital muscle is mobilized to cover the distal urethra and an introital incision is created to allow the placement of a buttock flap. The distal neourethra is covered by the approximation of introital mucosa and the remainder is covered by the generous buttock flap, which is swung into position and sutured in place. The resultant buttock defect is then closed. After approximately 6 months, the patient is returned to the operating room and, in the lithotomy position, the inlay flap is divided at the level of the introitus, the base of the flap is returned to the buttock and the

once divided introitus is reconstituted. Other reported successful variations on this approach include the posteriorly based buttock flap (Nolan *et al.*, 1991) (Fig. 26.13B) and the preputial inlay flap (Sheldon *et al.*, 1994a) (Fig. 26.13C).

The high, narrow UGSM provides the greatest reconstructive challenge. Here, a labioscrotal inlay flap cannot be used because it will still leave the patient with a urogenital sinus and an obscured urethra, difficult to access. In addition, the cosmetic appearance with this type of approach is completely unacceptable. These patients usually have a long, narrow urogenital sinus. The vagina appears to insert into a rather significantly masculinized urethra, often into a structure resembling a verumontanum. Occasionally, the vaginal insertion will occur at a very high level, even as high as the bladder trigone. These anomalies can be classified as having adequate vaginal length,

(B)

(C)

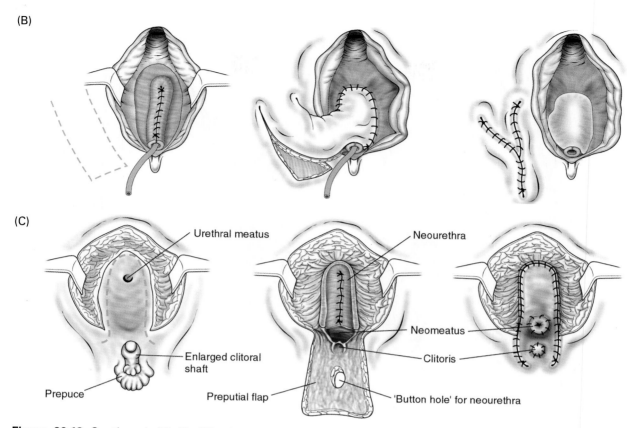

Urethral meatus

Neourethra

Enlarged clitoral shaft

Prepuce

Preputial flap

Neomeatus

Clitoris

'Button hole' for neourethra

Figure 26.13 *Continued.* (*B*) Modification based on posteriorly based buttock flap. (From Nolan *et al.*, 1991.) (*C*) Modification based on preputial flap. (From Sheldon *et al.*, 1994a.)

inadequate vaginal length, or a rudimentary vagina. Most, but certainly not all, will have an identifiable intersex state. Patients with adequate vaginal length are those for whom careful and thorough vaginal mobilization enables the vagina to reach the perineum as a pull-through procedure using simple, local skin flaps for vaginal exteriorization. Multiple reconstructive options for vaginal exteriorization are available (Passerini-Glazel, 1989; Gonzalez and Fernandes, 1990; Donahoe and Gustafson, 1994; Sheldon *et al.*, 1994; Donahoe and Schnitzer, 1998), the selection of which generally depends on the configuration of the external genitalia (Fig. 26.14A–E).

Patients with inadequate vaginal length represent those for whom the vagina cannot be sufficiently mobilized to reach the perineum (Fig. 26.15). Here, the first priority is to ensure that adequate vaginal mobilization has been achieved. Excellent exposure for mobilization can be achieved through a lower abdominal incision. The vagina may be mobilized extravesically (transperitoneally) or transvesically

(Passerini-Glazel, 1989; Parrott and Woodard, 1991), depending on the anatomy encountered, as shown in Figure 26.16. This approach is clearly superior in those uncommon instances where the vagina enters at or above the bladder neck.

The majority of patients achieve adequate exposure through a prone, jack-knife approach. Vaginal exposure is obtained via an incision similar to that used for PSARP, as described previously. Exposure may include midline incision through the urogenital sinus and extending through the anorectum to the coccyx (Peña *et al.*, 1992) or a midline incision ending with the incision of only the anterior anorectal wall (Di Benedetto *et al.*, 1997; Domini *et al.*, 1997). Alternatively, a midline incision ending with a transversely oriented incision allows a skin flap to be developed anterior to the anus, through which the anorectum may be deflected posteriorly without entry of the anorectal canal, yet enabling excellent exposure (Hendren, 1996; Rink *et al.*, 1997).

(A)

(B)

(C)

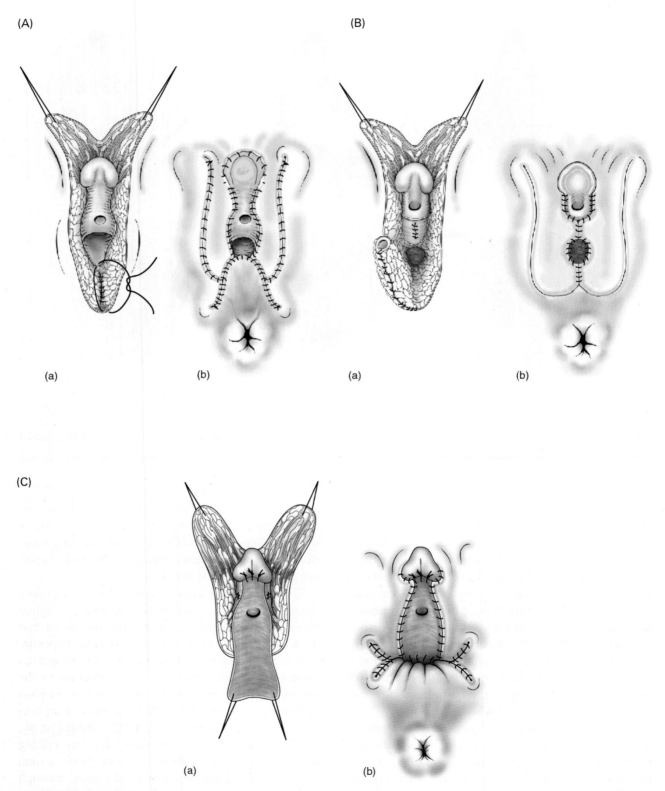

(a)　　(b)　　(a)　　(b)

(a)　　(b)

Figure 26.14 Representative techniques for vaginal exteriorization in the face of abnormally enlarged and masculinized genitalia. (*A*) Prominent labioscrotal folds, short urogenital sinus. (From Sheldon, 1997.) (*B*) Prominent labioscrotal folds, long urogenital sinus. (From 1997.) (*C*) Prominent phallus and urethra, long urogenital sinus. (From Passerini-Glazel, 1989.) (*D*) and (*E*) *Shown opposite.*

(D)

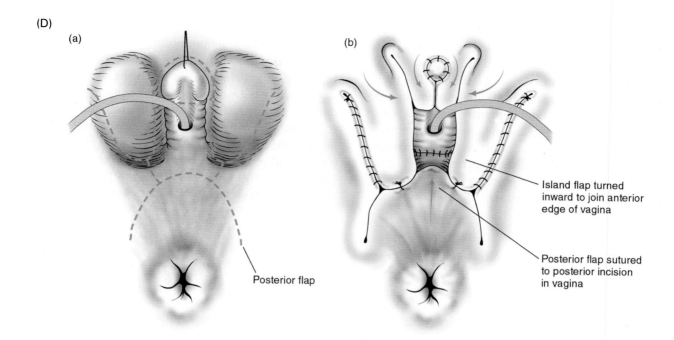

(a)

Posterior flap

(b)

Island flap turned inward to join anterior edge of vagina

Posterior flap sutured to posterior incision in vagina

(E)

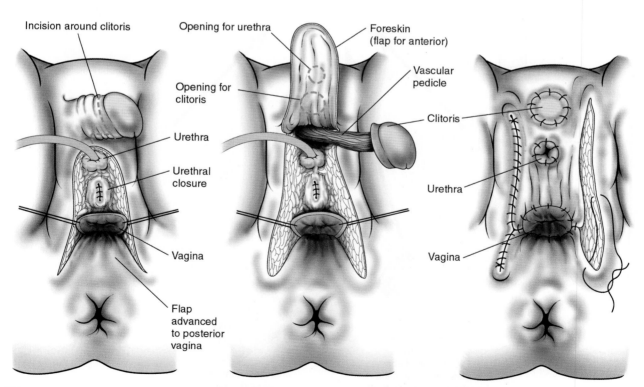

Incision around clitoris

Opening for urethra

Foreskin (flap for anterior)

Opening for clitoris

Vascular pedicle

Urethra

Clitoris

Urethral closure

Vagina

Urethra

Vagina

Flap advanced to posterior vagina

Figure 26.14 *Continued.* (*D*) Labioscrotal transposition, long urogenital sinus. (From Donahoe and Schnitzer, 1998.) (*E*) Prominent phallus, non-prominent urethra, long urogenital sinus. (From Gonzalez and Fernandez, 1990.)

Exposure involving incision of the anorectum may be done with or without a covering colostomy. Those surgeons not using a colostomy must do so in full awareness of the increased risk of infection. The resultant inflammatory changes from such infection may be sufficiently severe not only to destroy the initial repair but also to compromise any subsequent attempts at reconstruction. In general, whenever a single-stage reconstruction combines clitoroplasty and vaginal reconstruction employing a posterior sagittal approach, the procedure is best begun with clitoroplasty in the dorsal lithotomy position and vaginal reconstruction in the prone jack-knife position.

When a significant distance remains between the vagina and the perineum, or when the depth of the vaginal vault is insufficient, an interposition procedure is required. Patients with significant genital enlargement may be reconstructed using a mucocutaneous tube (Paserini-Glazel, 1989) if a prominent phallus and phallic urethra are present, or a tubularized M-flap (Sheldon *et al.*, 1994a) in the setting of prominent labioscrotal folds. Creation of a mucocuta-

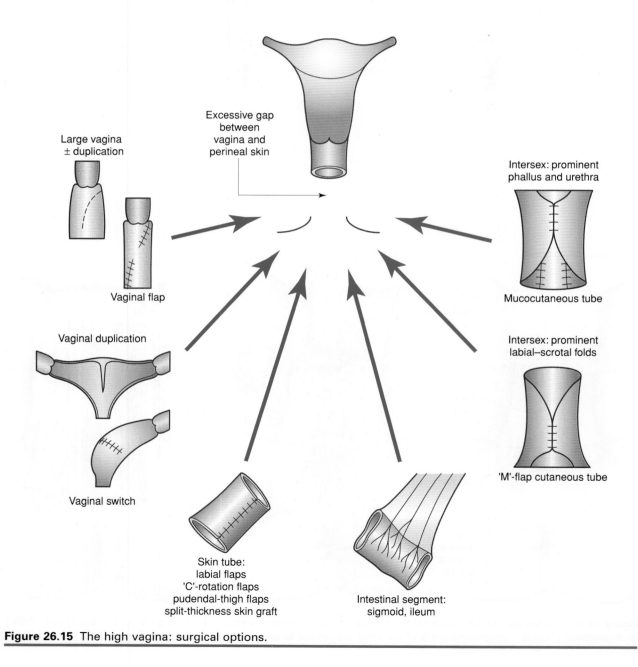

Figure 26.15 The high vagina: surgical options.

neous tube begins with mobilization of the phallic urethra, surgical excision of the corpora cavernosa, and clitoroplasty (Fig. 26.17a–d). The phallic foreskin is split dorsally and ventrally in the midline, and the dorsal surface of the mobilized phallic urethra is divided in the midline, creating a small flap proximally that is approximated to the edge of the clitoris (Fig. 26.17e–g). The foreskin flaps are swung caudally and anastomosed to the detubularized phallic urethra (Fig. 26.17h), following which the mucocutaneous plate is tubularized and swung internally to be anastomosed to the end of the vagina (Fig. 26.17i–k).

The tubularized M-flap (Fig. 26.18) is performed in a similar way to that previously described in the feminizing genitoplasty for short UGSMs. Here, a generous M-flap is developed and ultimately the clitoris is mobilized with excision of the corpora cavernosa and reduced (Fig. 26.18a, b). Dissection is continued in a plane caudal to the urogenital sinus until the vaginal insertion is identified. The vagina is separated from the urogenital sinus and the defect in the urogenital sinus is closed such that the urogenital sinus becomes the urethra (Fig. 26.18c). The M-flap is tubularized (Fig. 26.18d, e) and inverted internally

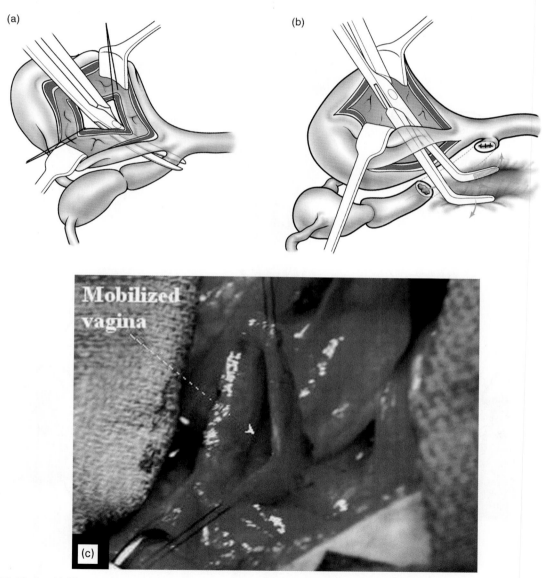

Figure 26.16 (*a*, *b*) Transvesical mobilization of the high inserting vagina. (From Parrott and Woodard, 1991.) (*c*) Intraoperative photograph demonstrating the excellent mobilization of the vagina achievable from an abdominal approach.

to be anastomosed to the vagina, bridging the gap between the vagina and the perineum (Fig. 26.18f). An example of a patient reconstructed with an M-flap cutaneous tube is shown in (Fig. 26.18g, h).

In the absence of genital enlargement, extensive local flaps may be used to exteriorize the vagina (Fig. 26.19) (Hagarty *et al.*, 1988; Wee *et al.*, 1989; Parrot and Woodard, 1991; Joseph, 1997; Rink *et*

Ventral **Dorsal**

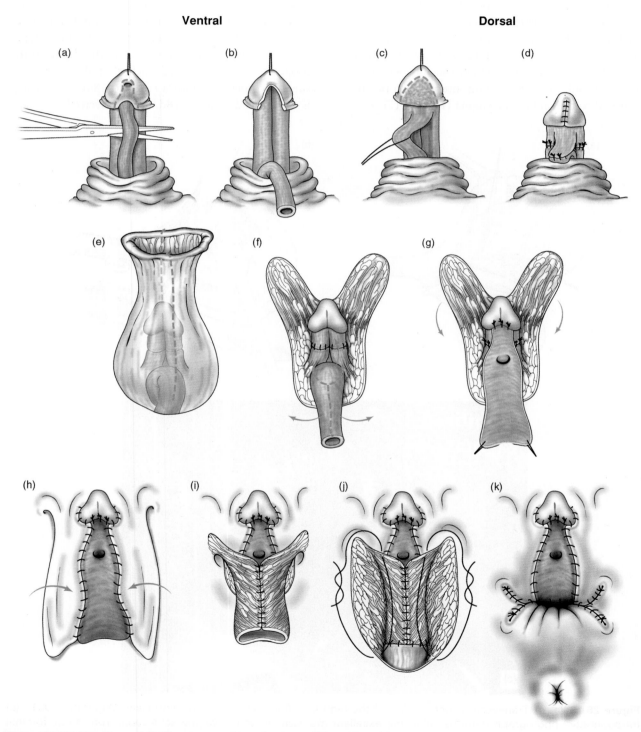

Figure 26.17 The Passerini–Glazel procedure. See text. (From Aaronson, 1992.)

al., 1997). A capacious vagina, when encountered, may allow the creation of a tubularized vaginal flap (Fig. 26.20) (Kiely and Peña, 1998). A favorable duplication anomaly may enable a vaginal-switch procedure (Kiely and Peña, 1998) (Fig. 26.21). The latter two options find their greatest application in the setting of cloacal malformations. A bowel interposition remains an excellent and very versatile alternative (Fig. 26.22). Here, a segment of large or small bowel is mobilized on its mesentery, anastomosed to the vagina on one end and to the perineum on the other.

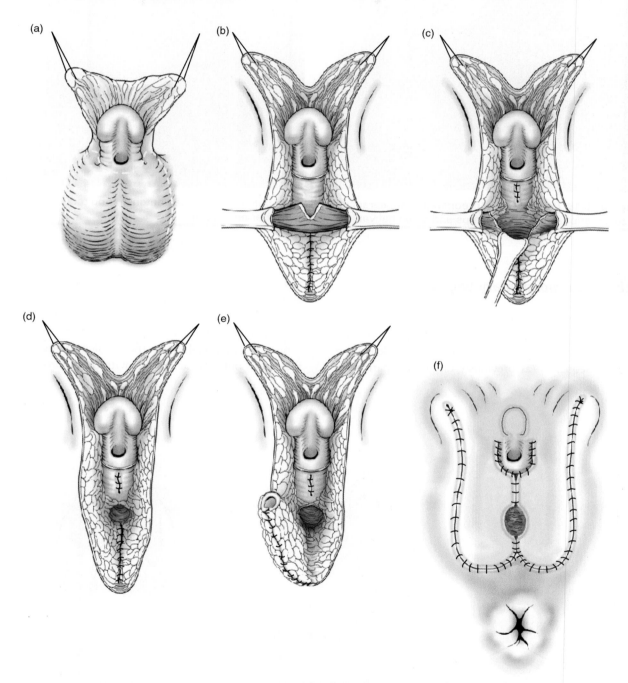

Figure 26.18 (*a–f*) Feminizing genitoplasty, high lesion. (From Sheldon, 1997.) (*g, h*) Feminizing genitoplasty (high lesion) reconstructed employing an M-flap cutaneous tube in a patient with true hermaphroditism: (*g*) and (*h*) *Shown over page.*

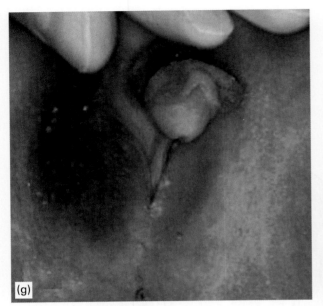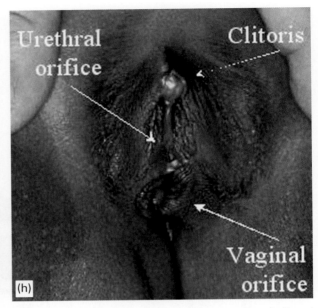

Figure 26.18 *Continued.* (*g*) preoperative appearance; (*h*) postoperative appearance demonstrating reduced clitoral size, exteriorized urethra meatus and a vaginal vault of normal caliber and depth.

Absent or rudimentary vagina

Reconstruction of a rudimentary urogenital sinus vagina or an absent vagina requires an unique approach. Such lesions may be isolated, part of a multiple malformation sequence (as previously discussed), part of an intersex state, or they may accompany imperforate anus. Colonic vaginal substitution offers an excellent approach to the management of these patients (Fig. 26.23) (Hensle and Dean, 1992; Hendren and Atala, 1994). Figure 26.24 shows the excellent cosmetic and functional outcome achievable with this approach.

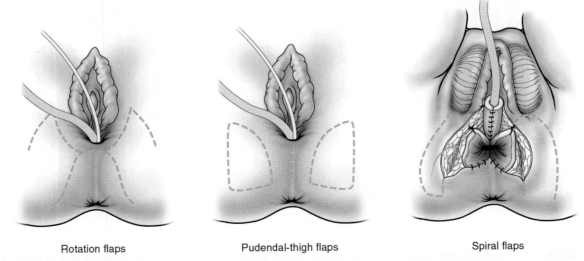

Rotation flaps   Pudendal-thigh flaps   Spiral flaps

Figure 26.19 Local cutaneous flap useful for vaginal reconstruction. (Modified from Parrott and Woodard, 1991; Joseph, 1997; Rink *et al.* 1997.)

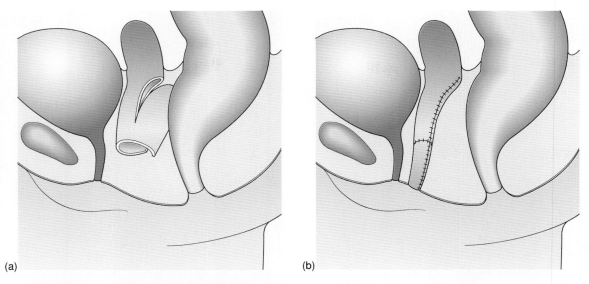

Figure 26.20 Vaginal extension from vaginal flap. (From Peña, 1990.)

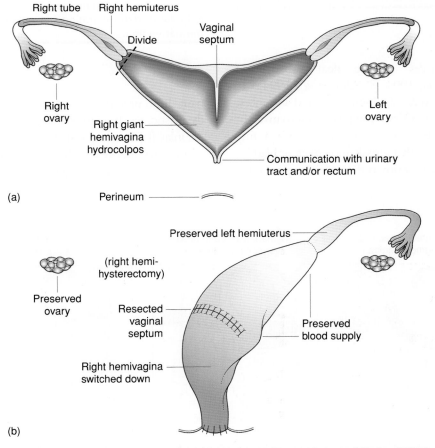

Figure 26.21 Vaginal switch procedure for vaginal externalization. (From Kiely and Peña, 1998.)

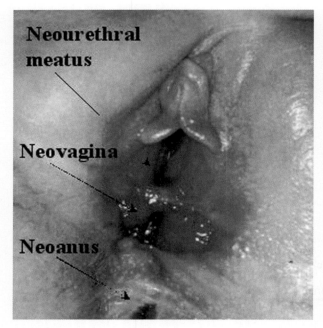

Figure 26.22 Reconstruction of severely dysmorphic child with cloacal anomaly. Extremely high and short vagina reconstructed with an interposed intestinal segment. Vagina of normal depth and caliber for age.

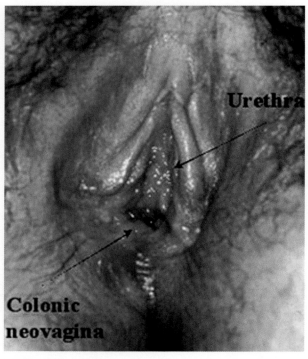

Figure 26.24 Reconstruction for vaginal agenesis employing a colonic neovagina. Vagina accepts a vaginal dilator, demonstrating normal caliber and depth of the neovagina.

Other alternatives include ileal substitution (Hendren and Atala, 1994; Sheldon *et al.*, 1994a) as shown in Figure 26.25. In highly selected instances, bladder substitution offers an excellent alternative. In Figure 26.26a–d, the patient presented with a tiny hypoplastic bladder with a grossly incompetent bladder neck and UGSM with a tiny rudimentary vaginal rem-

nant. Both ureters were ectopic and both kidneys were dysplastic, resulting in end-stage renal disease (ESRD). An inlay flap technique allowed exposure of the bladder as a vagina, following which a portion of the appendix was mobilized and brought anterior to the vagina as an

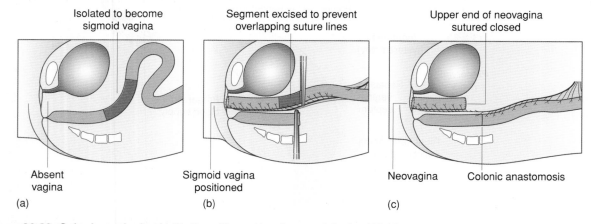

Figure 26.23 Colonic vaginal substitution. (From Hendren and Atala, 1994.)

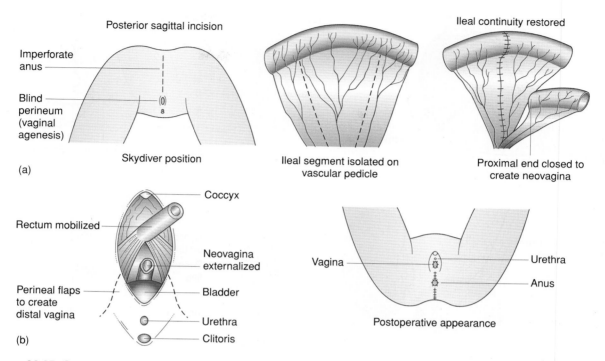

Figure 26.25 Construction of neovagina employing an ileal segment in a patient with vaginal agenesis associated with imperforate anus. (From Sheldon *et al.*, 1994a.)

orthotopic neourethra. The remainder of the appendix was implanted into an orthotopic gastric neobladder in a Mitrofanoff fashion. She subsequently received a living related donor transplant, completing a total anatomic urinary tract replacement (Sheldon and Welch, 1998).

In Figure 26.26e, a tiny hypoplastic bladder was again encountered with a severely incompetent bladder outlet. A solitary kidney drained through an ectopic ureter, resulting in total urinary incontinence, although renal function was well preserved. The bladder was not deemed suitable for reconstruction and was used for vaginal reconstruction, again with a perineal inlay flap. A composite neobladder (stomach and ileum) was created into which her ureter was implanted. Because the appendix had been previously removed, the distal ureter was used to create a catheterizable continence mechanism. She has excellent vaginal dimensions, is continent, and has stable renal function.

In the setting of prominent genital enlargement involving large labioscrotal folds, an extensive tubularized M-flap may be used to create the entire neovagina (Fig. 26.27) (Sheldon *et al.*, 1994a). Other options include, progressive, direct dilation without operation (Frank, 1938), creation of the vagina with split-thickness skin grafting (McIndoe, 1950; Marshall, 1980) and the gracilis musculocutaneous flap (McGraw *et al.*, 1976).

The importance of neurovesical dysfunction accompanying urogenital sinus anomalies and cloacal malformations cannot be over-emphasized. All such patients must be carefully evaluated and followed to ensure that neurovesical dysfunction, if present, is adequately treated (Sheldon *et al.*, 1994a). In addition, long-term gynecologic follow-up is necessary (Mollitt *et al.*, 1981; Levitt *et al.*, 1998). Such patients are at risk not only for vaginal stenosis, which would complicate intercourse, but also for obstructive genital complications resulting in hydrocolpos, pyocolpos, hematocolpos, hematometrocolpos, tubo-ovarian abscess, and endometriosis.

One critically important issue for those patients with a UGSM who have neurovesical dysfunction is reliable access for intermittent catheterization. This has been successfully addressed in several ways. An anterior detrusor tube has been used to create a neourethra that courses orthotopically to exit in a nor-

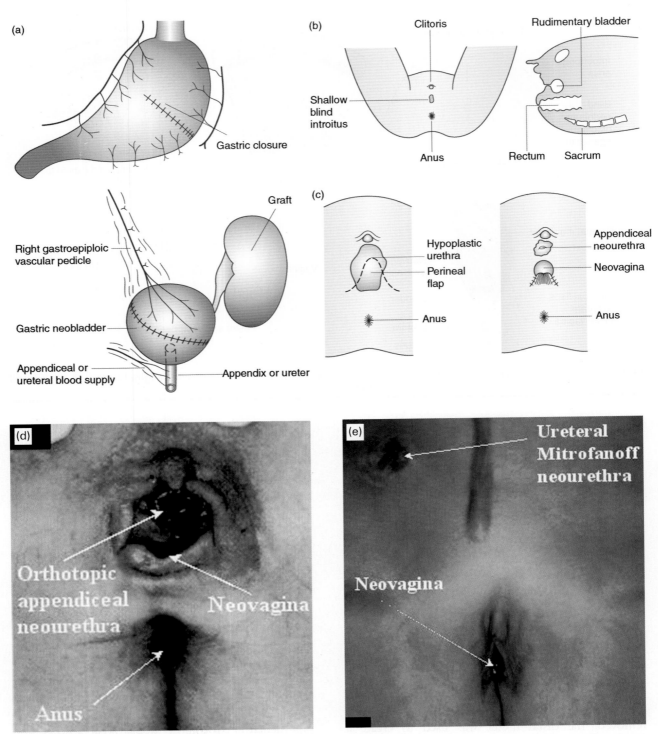

Figure 26.26 (*a–c*) Vaginal reconstruction employing a bladder substitution technique: (a) total anatomic urinary replacement (b) preoperative anatomy; (c) reconstruction employing a perineal inlay flap bladder substitution and an appendiceal neourethra. (From Sheldon *et al.*, 1994a; Sheldon and Welch, 1998.) (*d*) Appearance of perineum of a child with a urogenital sinus malformation, a tiny hypoplastic bladder, and a rudimentary vaginal remnant employing an inlay flap bladder substitution technique. (From Sheldon *et al.*, 1994a.) (*e*) Appearance of a child with a urogenital sinus malformation, a tiny hypoplastic bladder, and a rudimentary vaginal remnant reconstructed employing an inlay flap bladder substitution technique. A composite neobladder (stomach and ileum) was constructed along with an ureteral Mitrofanoff neourethra.

mal perineal position and provide continent cathe-terizable access (Diamond and Ransley, 1987). The vaginal mucosal tube–buttock flap technique to leng-then the urethra can also provide reliable access for intermittent catheterization and, in some instances, creates sufficient bladder outlet resistance to achieve continence (Hendren, 1980a, 1998; Gonzalez, 1985).

The vaginal tube–buttock flap is not capable of achieving continence in all patients, particularly those with a very deficient bladder outlet mechanism. In these instances, a bladder neck reconstruction such as the Young–Dees–Leadbetter procedure will be required. Some of these neourethras may be difficult to catheterize and the use of a Coudé catheter

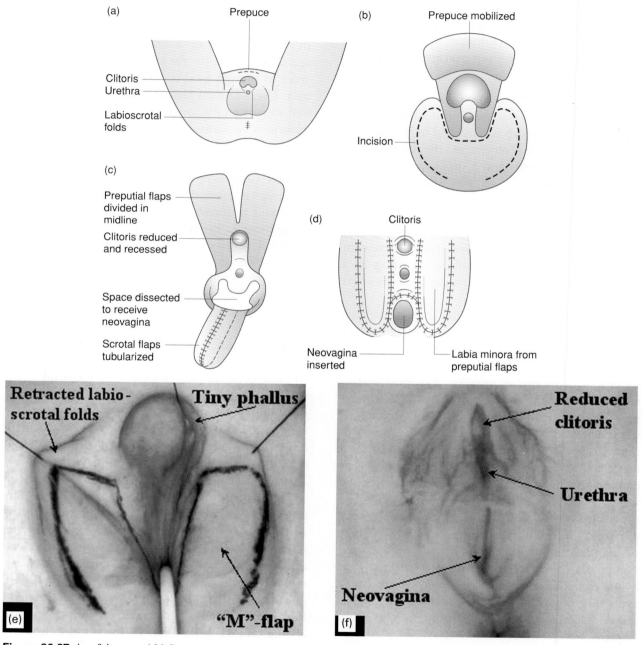

Figure 26.27 (a–d) Inverted M-flap neovagina. (From Sheldon et al., 1994a.) (e, f) Appearance of a patient with incom-plete androgen insensitivity and absent vagina reconstructed employing an M-flap cutaneous tube neovagina tech-nique: (e) preoperative appearance; (f) postoperative appearance. Vagina of normal depth and caliber for age.

or a curved metal catheter may facilitate catheterization. The Mitrofanoff neourethra provides excellent access when other techniques fail or are not applicable.

Anomalies of both anorectal and vaginal development: cloaca

> Cloaca is the Latin word for sewer ... A persisting cloaca is normal in birds, reptiles and some fish. However, a persistent cloaca can be disastrous for the human infant if it is not managed properly (*Hendren, 1997*).

The cloaca is one of the most complex congenital anomalies for which successful restorative surgery is feasible. The approach is simplified by the recognition that the cloaca represents the combination of an imperforate anus and a urogenital sinus malformation. Accordingly, all the principles already discussed in this chapter are applicable to this complex and highly heterogeneous patient population. Cloacal anatomy is sufficiently diverse so as to defy meaningful classification. Rather, it is best thought of as a spectrum of abnormalities occurring as a continuum, one gradually blending into the next (Fig. 26.28).

From a surgical perspective, the level of insertion of the rectum is generally immaterial, as all patients are managed with an initial diverting colostomy. As with the PSARP for imperforate anus, the rectum is divided from its site of insertion and mobilized to reach the perineum. The configuration of the remaining urogenital sinus, however, has tremendous surgical implications. Patients with very short urogenital sinus remnants are readily managed by total urogenital advancement (Peña, 1997), with excellent cosmetic and functional outcome. Otherwise, the vagina is dissected off the urogenital sinus. The urogenital sinus is closed to become the urethra and the vagina is mobilized for exteriorization. A short vagina may require interposition with a tubularized vaginal flap (most appropriate for cloacas with hydrocolpos) or a vaginal switch procedure (most applicable to patients with vaginal and uterine duplication). Occasionally, bowel interposition is necessary (Fig. 26.23).

A rare (and unique) form of cloaca is the posterior cloaca (Peña and Kessler, 1998). Here, the cloaca drains through a posteriorly located orifice rather than the usual anterior orifice. This draining orifice may represent a normally positioned anus. The surgical management of these infants is significantly different from that for other cloacal anomalies.

Figure 26.29 outlines the conceptual approach to the management of cloacal malformations. During the first phase of management, attention is directed towards protection of the upper urinary tracts, the maintenance of low-pressure urinary drainage, normalization of perineal anatomy, and minimalization of any neurologic deficit related to spinal cord anomaly. The presence of a cloacal malformation is an urgent indication for the creation of a colostomy in order to prevent fecal contamination of the urinary tract. The colostomy should be positioned so as to be well away from the lower midline abdomen, where a subsequent vesicostomy may be necessary. Contrast cystography, measurement of postvoid residual volume, and spinal ultrasonography are necessary in all patients. Genitoscopy may be indicated at the time of colostomy in selected patients, particularly those with significant hydrocolpos. Depending on the findings, intermittent catheterization, cutaneous vesicostomy, or spinal surgery may be indicated. Patients with hydrocolpos require prompt and aggressive management, which may involve intermittent catheterization of the urogenital sinus and/or cutaneous vesicostomy. Occasionally, cutaneous vaginostomy will be necessary.

At approximately 6–12 months of age, most patients are able to undergo posterior sagittal anorectal urethrovaginoplasty (PSARUVP) following careful bowel preparation. Those patients with a low urogenital sinus abnormality are managed by an advancement technique (Peña, 1997), while those with a high urogenital sinus anomaly are managed by complete cloacal disassembly and reassembly as described by Paidos and Peña (1997) (Fig. 26.30).

The patient is positioned in the prone jack-knife position as for PSARP. The striated muscle complex is identified by electrical stimulation and a midline incision is created, this time extending from the cloacal orifice to the coccyx. The levator muscles are divided in the midline under electrical stimulation guidance. The cloaca is opened precisely in the midline, exposing the urogenital sinus, urethra, vagina, and rectum (Fig. 26.30a). A row of fine traction sutures facilitates dissection of the rectum off its attachment to the vagina (Fig. 26.30b). The rectum is fully mobilized and traction sutures are placed in the

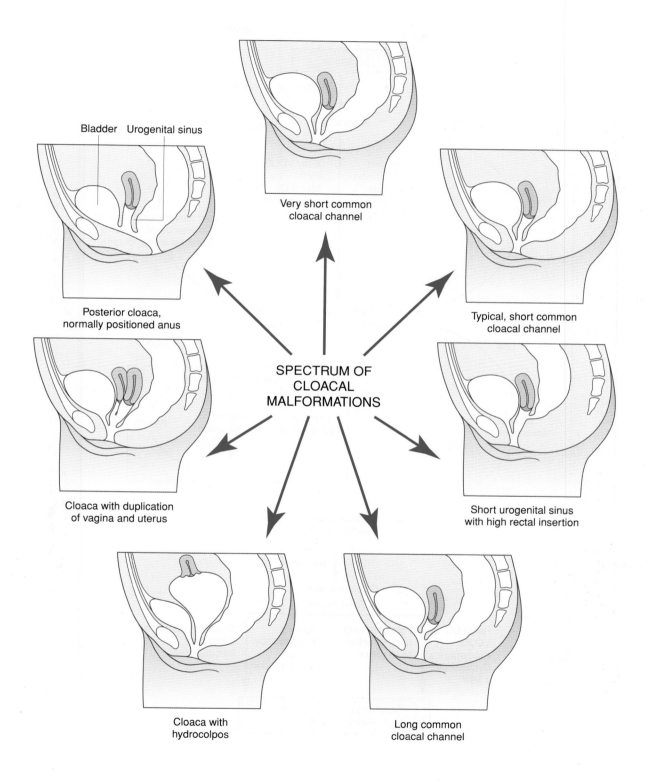

Bladder   Urogenital sinus

Posterior cloaca,
normally positioned anus

Very short common
cloacal channel

Typical, short common
cloacal channel

SPECTRUM OF
CLOACAL
MALFORMATIONS

Cloaca with duplication
of vagina and uterus

Short urogenital sinus
with high rectal insertion

Cloaca with
hydrocolpos

Long common
cloacal channel

Figure 26.28 Spectrum of cloacal malformation. (From Brock and Peña, 1992; Peña and Kessler, 1998.)

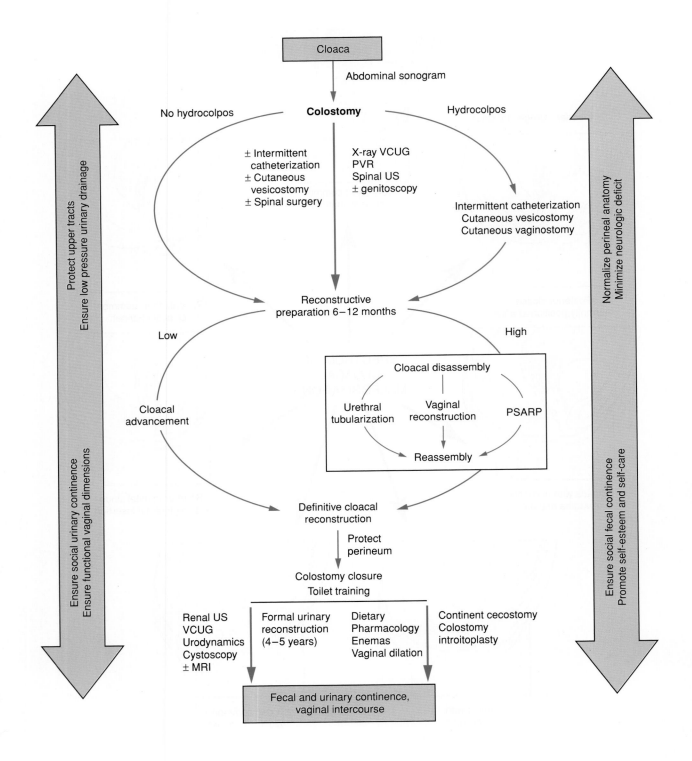

Figure 26.29 Management strategy for cloacal anomaly.

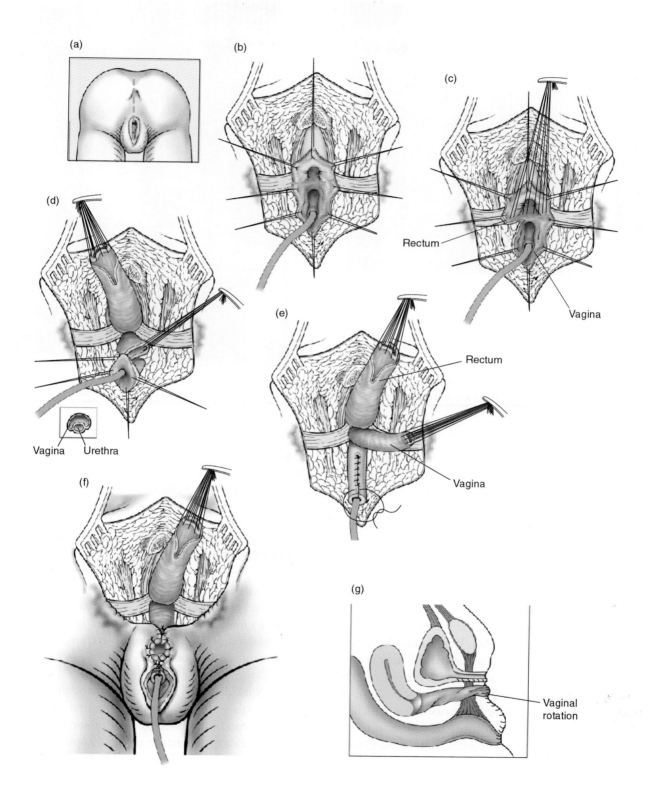

Figure 26.30 Cloacal reconstruction. See text. (Redrawn from Paidas and Peña, 1997.)

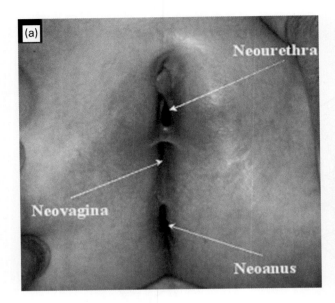

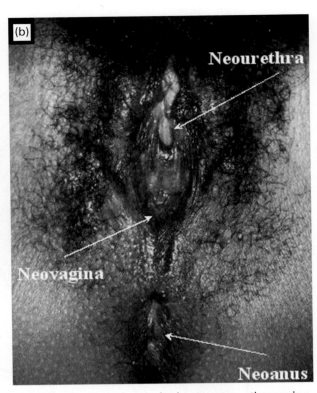

Figure 26.31 (*a*) Appearance of child following cloacal reconstruction by posterior sagittal anorectourethrovaginoplasty (PSARUVP). (*b*) Appearance of more mature patient following reoperative cloacal reconstruction.

vagina. The vagina is carefully dissected off the urethra, which is difficult owing to the intense adherence of these structures, which basically share a common wall, and the fact that the vagina wraps itself around the dorsal half of the urethra (Fig. 26.30c). Often, this dissection leaves a defect on the anterior surface of the vagina, which is sutured closed. The vagina is then mobilized and the urogenital sinus tubularized over a catheter to become the urethra (Fig. 26.30d–e). A two-layer closure of skin allows a small distance between the urethra and the vagina, which is then exteriorized (Fig. 26.30f). When a vaginal suture line is present, the vagina is rotated 90° to prevent overlapping suture lines and minimize the risk of urethrovaginal fistula (Fig. 26.30g). The anorectum is reconstructed as previously described for PSARP. These principles enable reconstruction of most complex anomalies with very successful outcomes. Figure 26.31a shows an infant following PSARUVP, and Figure 26.31b shows a more mature patient who received reoperative cloacal reconstruction. She has a neuropathic bladder managed by bladder neck reconstruction and intermittent catheterization, and a neu-

ropathic rectum managed by continent cecostomy. She is continent of both urine and stool, and has normal vaginal depth and caliber for her age.

Urologic reconstruction in patients with anorectal malformations

Genitourinary reconstruction is best undertaken as an integral part of imperforate anus reconstruction. Failure to do so results in the loss of surgical alternatives, unnecessary reoperative procedures and compromised outcomes (*Sheldon, 1994b*).

The high incidence of significant urinary and genital tract anomalies in patients with imperforate anus, the significant morbidity associated with these anomalies, and the intricate association of these anomalies with those accompanying ARMs mandate that their management be done as an integral part of imperforate anus care. Consequently, it is necessary that the general surgeon have a clear understanding of the implication of genitourinary pathology and that the pediatric urologist be familiar with the management of imperforate anus.

These patients are at risk for both urinary and fecal incontinence. It is certainly inappropriate to treat urinary incontinence without solving the problem of fecal incontinence, because the patient will still require diapers and will not experience a significant change in his or her social integration. These problems should be addressed concomitantly and in a coordinated fashion, as the treatment of one may have

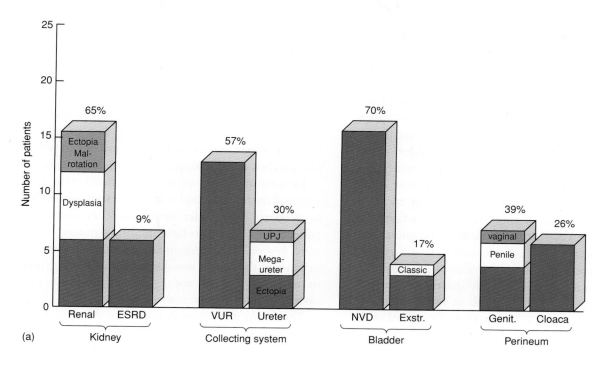

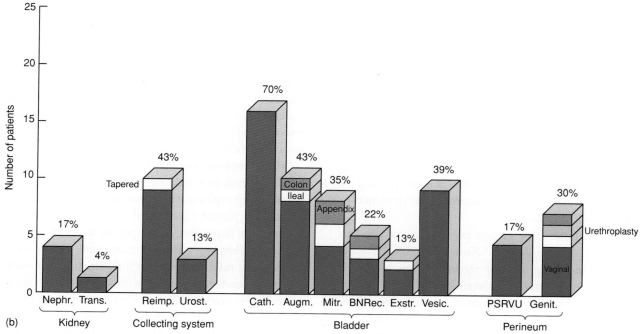

Figure 26.32 (*a*) Genitourinary abnormalities and (*b*) genitourinary surgical procedures in patients with anorectal malformations. (From Sheldon *et al.*, 1994b.) (NVD = neurovesical dysfunction.)

a significant influence on the management of the other. For example, anticholinergic therapy to control uninhibited detrusor contractions may adversely affect anorectal function by causing constipation. Similarly, loss of the ileocecal valve with procedures such as ileocecocystoplasty may exacerbate fecal soilage in patients with ARM by preventing the production of formed stool. Further, sigmoid colocystoplasty in patients with imperforate anus runs the risk of ischemic injury to the anorectum by dividing the descending blood supply.

From the genitourinary perspective, incidental appendectomy should always be avoided, as the appendix may be needed for either antegrade continence enema or Mitrofanoff neourethral bladder access. Imperforate anus surgery should never be undertaken without an indwelling Foley catheter, because of the risk of inadvertent urethral injury. Inability to pass a catheter at the time of anorectal reconstruction is an indication for a cystoscopic evaluation and guidance in catheter placement. All patients with rectourinary fistulae, but especially those with reflux and neurovesical dysfunction, should have a fully diverting colostomy with a short distal colonic limb in order to prevent ongoing fecal urinary contamination. Placement of the colostomy is important. Patients at risk for future vesicostomy (e.g. high-grade VUR, neurovesical dysfunction, and hydrocolpos) should have the colostomy positioned so as not to interfere with a possible subsequent vesicostomy.

The implications of genitourinary surgery in patients with ARMs have been addressed previously (Sheldon *et al.*, 1994b). Figure 26.32a outlines the genitourinary abnormalities encountered in 90 consecutive patients with ARMs managed over a 5-year period. Twenty-three patients had genitourinary anomalies requiring surgical intervention. Of these, 65% had primary renal pathology (9% had ESRD), 87% had collecting system abnormalities placing the kidneys at risk, 70% had neurovesical dysfunction, and 26% had CMs.

The genitourinary surgery procedures required are shown in Figure 26.32b. Note that 70% of those patients requiring urinary reconstruction ultimately required intermittent catheterization. It is important to recognize that the presence of a rectourethral fistula in the male may impair the ability to perform intermittent catheterization even after the fistula has been divided. Usually, intermittent catheterization can be readily performed in this setting employing a Coudé

catheter. Problematic diverticula from the perspective of infection, voiding difficulties, and catheterization problems may occasionally be managed by endoscopic fulguration (Husmann and Allen, 1997). Rarely, surgical excision may be required.

More than 40% of these patients required ureteral reimplantation and bladder augmentation. Twenty-two per cent required bladder neck reconstruction for incontinence and 35% required a Mitrofanoff neourethra for alternate continent catheterizable bladder access. Nine patients required temporary vesicostomy, three for neonatal urosepsis, four for neurovesical dysfunction and hydronephrosis not responding to intermittent catheterization, one to control hyperchloremic metabolic acidosis, and one to relieve hydrocolpos complicating a cloacal malformation.

Importantly, none of the 16 patients with neurovesical dysfunction had evidence to support PSARP as a source of bladder denervation. Further, four patients were found to have urethral stricture. Three were proven to be congenital and not iatrogenic in origin and the fourth was suspected to be congenital in origin but this was not definitively proven by preoperative urethrography or endoscopy.

The 18 surgical complications occurring in 14 of these 23 patients requiring genitourinary reconstruction are particularly instructive. Nine complications occurred secondary to surgery performed before referral to the author's institution. Four patients with cloacas were referred for vaginal reconstruction after previous anorectal pull-through with no effort made to correct the UGSM. Two of these subsequently had urogenital sinus surgery using inlay flap techniques and both of these developed urethrovaginal fistulae. Three patients had ureteral reimplantation before referral which failed as a result of not recognizing an associated neuropathic bladder.

Nine complications occurred following referral. Two patients developed delayed small bowel obstruction necessitating exploratory laparotomy and lysis of adhesions. One patient experienced intraoperative collapse as a result of latex allergy. One patient developed a lymphocele following transplantation, and one patient developed a mild recurrent urethral stricture following urethroplasty for congenital stricture that was simply corrected by urethral dilation. One patient developed a urethral calculus that occurred secondary to urethral erosion of a suture placed for approximation of the pubis for cloacal exstrophy reconstruction. Two patients developed stenosis of their catheterizable channels corrected by stomal revision. Both had previously undergone incidental appendectomy such that one patient had a ureteral 'Mitrofanoff' and the other had a tubularized ileal 'Mitrofanoff'. One patient reconstructed for a cloacal malformation developed late vaginal stenosis.

This experience emphasizes several important principles. (1) Most neurovesical dysfunction and urethral strictures encountered in patients with ARMs are not iatrogenic but congenital in origin. (2) VUR is highly significant in that it often occurs bilaterally or, if unilateral, occurs in conjunction with a disease that threatens the contralateral kidney. In addition, it is often associated with neurovesical dysfunction. (3) Ureteral reimplantation into a dysfunctional bladder is vulnerable to failure unless the underlying bladder dysfunction has been controlled. (4) Prompt and efficient decompression of obstructive hydronephrosis is essential in order to optimize long-term renal function. (5) Patients with ARM have a similar risk for latex allergy as do the myelomeningocele population. (6) The combination of neurovesical dysfunction or urethral stricture and rectourinary fistulae predisposes the patient to critical neonatal illness such as sepsis and hyperchloremic metabolic acidosis. (7) A low, fully diverting colostomy is most protective of the urinary tract. (8) Patients with cloacas should never have their anorectal and urogenital sinus malformations corrected separately. The best results are attained by a single-stage PSARUVP. Those patients who present for correction of a UGSM who have previously undergone an anorectal pull-through procedure are best corrected by reoperative PSARUVP complete with repeat mobilization of the rectum. Both patients managed in this fashion in this series were successfully reconstructed.

Renal transplantation in the setting of ARMs and UGSMs deserves additional comment. ESRD in this setting has very significant implications (Sharma *et al.*, 1993; Sheldon *et al.*, 1994; Sheldon, 1996). Peritoneal dialysis can be seriously compromised by the presence of multiple adhesions secondary to prior transabdominal surgical procedures. Every effort must be made to preserve the peritoneal cavity in the very young, as hemodialysis access is difficult and associated with significant long-term complications such as superior vena caval thrombosis.

Renal transplantation in patients with ARMs and UGSMs is extremely challenging, as the majority of these patients with ESRD have major bladder pathology that must be controlled or corrected prior to

transplantation, in order to optimize outcome. In addition, significant vascular anomalies are not infrequent in these patients (Dykes *et al.*, 1993). It has been clearly demonstrated, however, that successful renal transplantation in the setting of imperforate anus can be achieved (Sharma *et al.*, 1993; Sheldon *et al.*, 1994; Sheldon, 1996). Successful renal transplantation in patients with UGSMs, CMs, and cloacal exstrophy has also been reported (Sheldon *et al.*, 1994; Sheldon, 1996). The complex nature of transplant management in patients with ARMs and UGSMs is highlighted by three cases.

The patient in Fig. 26.26 presented with a UGSM with a tiny hypoplastic bladder, a rudimentary vagina, and ectopic ureters draining dysplastic kidneys. She underwent creation of a neovagina using the hypoplastic bladder and then underwent total anatomic urinary replacement with the creation of an appendiceal orthotopic neourethra and an orthotopic gastric neobladder, followed by living related donor transplantation. The second patient was born with cloacal exstrophy and had the cloacal plate removed as an infant. She was managed with an ileostomy and a cutaneous ureterostomy draining a solitary kidney. This kidney was lost over the ensuing years secondary to hydronephrosis and urosepsis. She presented for renal transplantation and underwent creation of an orthotopic neourethra using a segment of ureter and creation of an orthotopic neobladder using a gastric segment. She subsequently underwent renal transplantation. Both of these patients with total anatomic urinary tract replacement continue to have satisfactory renal function and are continent of urine on intermittent catheterization (Sheldon and Welch, 1998).

The third patient (Fig. 26.33) presented after several decompressive procedures were performed at the referring institution. These included a gastrostomy, a colostomy with mucus fistula for imperforate anus, a vesicostomy for neuropathic bladder, and bilateral cutaneous ureterostomies for bilateral hydronephrosis accompanied by profound renal insufficiency. This child presented with end-stage renal failure for transplantation. His surgical preparation consisted of posterior sagittal anorectoplasty, followed by takedown of colostomy, gastrocystoplasty, creation of a Mitrofanoff neourethra, and native nephrectomy. He subsequently underwent living related transplantation and has excellent renal function and is continent of urine on intermittent catheterization.

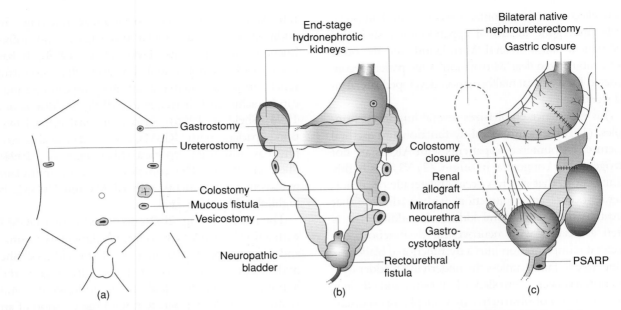

Figure 26.33 Urinary reconstruction and renal transplantation in a patient with the VATER association: (*a*) preoperative appearance; (*b*) preoperative urinary and colonic status; (*c*) postreconstructive status.

The principles outlined in this chapter regarding the management of ARMs and UGSMs, along with the advancements in the science of perioperative surgical management and transplantation, have clearly enabled even those children born with the most devastating congenital anomalies to be restored to health and a functional social status.

References

Aaronson IA (1992) Sexual differentiation and intersexuality. In: Kelalis PP, King LR, Belman AB (eds) *Clinical pediatric urology*. 3rd edition. Philadelphia, PA: WB Saunders, 1011.

Al-Mefty O, Kandzari S, Fox J (1980) Neurogenic bladder and the tethered spinal cord syndrome. *J Urol* **122**: 112–15.

Appignani BA, Jaramillo D, Barnes PD *et al*. (1994) Dysraphic myelodysplasias associated with urogenital and anorectal anomalies: prevalence and types seen with MR imaging. *AJR Am J Roentgenol* **163**: 1199–203.

Barry JE, Auldist AW (1974) The Vater association. One end of a spectrum of anomalies. *Am J Dis Child* **128**: 769–71.

Beals RK, Rolfe B (1989) Current concepts review – VATER association. *J Bone Joint Surg* **71**: 948–50.

Belman AB, King L (1972) Urinary tract abnormalities associated with imperforate anus. *J Urol* **108**: 823.

Boemers TML, Bax KMA, Rovekamp MH *et al*. (1995) The effect of posterior sagittal anorectoplasty PSARP and it variants on lower urinary tract function in children with anorectal malformations. *J Urol* **153**: 191–3.

Boemers TM, de Jong TP, van Gool JD *et al*. (1996) Urologic problems in anorectal malformations. Part **2**: Functional urologic sequelae. *J Pediatr Surg* **31**: 634–7.

Brock WA, Peña A (1992) Cloacal abnormalities and imperforate anus, In: Kelalis PP, King LR, Belman AB (eds) *Clinical pediatric urology*. Volume 2. Philadelphia, PA: WB Saunders, 922.

Cacciaguerra S, Lo presti L, Di Leo L *et al*. (1998) Prenatal diagnosis of cloacal anomaly. *Scand J Urol Nephrol* **32**: 77.

Caldamone AA, Emmens RW, Rabinowitz R (1979) Hyperchloremic acidosis and imperforate anus. *J Urol* **122**: 817–18.

Capitanucci ML, Rivosecchi M, Silveri M *et al*. (1996) Neurovesical dysfunction due to spinal dysraphism in anorectal anomalies. *Eur J Pediatr Surg* **6**: 159–62.

Carson JA, Barnes PD, Tunell WP *et al*. (1984) Imperforate anus: the neurologic implication of sacral abnormalities. *J Pediatr Surg* **19**: 838–42.

Cumes D (1977) Sacral dysgenesis associated with occult spinal dysraphism causing neurogenic bladder dysfunction. *J Urol* **117**: 127–8.

Diamond DA, Ransley PG (1987) Use of the anterior detrusor tube in managing urogenital sinus anomalies. *J Urol* **138**: 1057–9.

Di Benedetto V, Gioviale M, Bagnara V *et al*. (1997) The anterior sagittal transanorectal approach: a modified approach to 1-stage clitoral vaginoplasty in severely masculinized female pseudohermaphrodites – preliminary results. *J Urol* **157**: 330–2.

Domini R, Rossi F, Ceccarelli PL *et al.* (1997) Anterior sagittal transanorectal approach to the urogenital sinus in adrenogenital syndrome: preliminary report. *J Pediatr Surg* **32**: 714–6.

Donahoe PK, Gustafson ML (1994) Early one-stage surgical reconstruction of the extremely high vagina in patients with congenital adrenal hyperplasia. *J Pediatr Surg* **29**: 352–8.

Donahoe PK, Schnitzer JJ (1998) Ambiguous genitalia in the newborn. In: O'Neill JA, Rowe MI, Grosfeld JL *et al.* (eds) *Pediatric surgery*. 5th edition: St Louis, MO: Mosby Year Book, 1810–11.

Duncan PA, Shapiro LR, Stangel JJ *et al.* (1975) The MURCS association: mullerian duct aplasia, renal aplasia, and cervicothoracic somite dysplasia. *J Pediatr* **95**: 399–402.

Dykes EH, Oesch I, Ransley PG, Hendren WH (1993) Abnormal aorta and iliac arteries in children with urogenital abnormalities. *J Pediatr Surg* **28**: 696–700.

Endo M, Hayashi A, Ishihara M *et al.* (1999) Analysis of 1,992 patients with anorectal malformations over the past two decades in Japan. *J Pediatr Surg* **34**: 435–41.

Fleming SE, Hall R, Gysler M *et al.* (1986) Imperforate anus in females: frequency of genital tract involvement, incidence of associated anomalies, and functional outcome. *J Pediatr Surg* **21**: 146–50.

Fore SR, Hammond CB, Parker RT (1975) Urologic and genital anomalies in patients with congenital absence of the vagina. *Obstet Gynecol* **46**: 410–6.

Frank RT (1938) The formation of an artificial vagina without operation. *Am J Obstet Gynecol* **35**: 1053.

Geifman-Holtzman O, Crane SS, Winderl L *et al.* (1997) Persistent urogenital sinus: prenatal diagnosis and pregnancy complications. *Am J Obstet Gynecol* **176**: 709–11.

Gonzalez R (1985) Reconstruction of the female urethra to allow intermittent catheterization for neurogenic bladders and urogenital sinus anomalies. *J Urol* **133**: 478–80.

Gonzalez R, Fernandes ET (1990) Single-stage feminization genitoplasty. *J Urol* **143**: 776–8.

Griffin JE, Edwards C, Madden JD *et al.* (1976) Congenital absence of the vagina. *Ann Intern Med* **85**: 224–36.

Hadra R (1885) Demonstration zweier Fälle von Atresie ani vulvalis. *Berlin Clin Wochenschr* **22**: 340.

Hagerty RC, Vaughn TR, Lutz MH (1988) The perineal artery axial flap in reconstruction of the vagina. *Plast Reconstr Surg* **82**: 344–5.

Hauser GA, Schreiner WE (1961) Das Mayer–Rokitansky–Kuster Syndrome. *Schweiz Med Wochenschr* **91**: 381.

Hellstrom WJ, Edwards MS, Kogan B (1985) Urological aspects of the tethered cord syndrome. *J Urol* **135**: 317–20.

Hendren WH (1980a) Construction of female urethra from vaginal wall and a perineal flap. *J Urol* **123**: 657–64.

Hendren WH (1980b) Urogenital sinus and anorectal malformation: experience with 22 cases. *J Pediatr Surg* **15**: 628–41.

Hendren WH (1982) Further experience in reconstructive surgery for cloacal anomalies. *J Pediatr Surg* **17**: 695–717.

Hendren WH (1996) Urogenital sinus and cloacal malformations. *Semin in Pediatr Surg* **5**: 72–9.

Hendren WH (1997) Management of cloacal malformations. *Sem Pediatr Surg* **6**: 217–27.

Hendren WH (1998a) Cloaca, the most severe degree of imperforate anus – experience with 195 cases. *Ann Surg* **228**: 331–46.

Hendren WH (1998b) Construction of a female urethra using the vaginal wall and a buttock flap: experience with 40 cases. *J Pediatr Surg* **33**: 180–7.

Hendren WH, Atala A (1994) Use of bowel for vaginal reconstruction. *J Urol* **152**: 752–5.

Hensle TW, Dean GE (1992) Vaginal replacement in children. *J Urol* **148**: 677–9.

Hoekstra WJ (1983) Urogenital tract abnormalities associated with congenital anorectal anomalies. *J Urol* **130**: 962–3.

Hong AR, Croitoru DP, Nguyen LT *et al.* (1992) Congenital urethral fistula with normal anus: a report of two cases. *J Pediatr Surg* **27**: 1278–80.

Husmann DA, Allen TD (1997) Endoscopic management of infected enlarged prostatic utricles and remnants of rectourethral fistula tract of high imperforate anus. *J Urol* **157**: 1902–6.

Iwai N, Ogita S, Shirasaka S *et al.* (1978) Hyperchloremic acidosis in an infant with imperforate anus and rectourethral fistula. *J Pediatr Surg* **13**: 437–8.

Joseph VT (1997) Pudendal–thigh flap vaginoplasty in the reconstruction of genital anomalies. *J Pediatr Surg* **32**: 62–5.

Kakizaki H, Nonomura K, Asano Y *et al.* (1994) Preexisting neurogenic voiding dysfunction in children with imperforate anus: problems in management. *J Urol* **151**: 1041–4.

Karrer FM, Flannery AM, Nelson MD *et al.* (1988) Anorectal malformations: evaluation of associated spinal dysraphic syndromes. *J Pediatr Surg* **23**: 45.

Kiely EM, Peña A (1998) Anorectal malformations. In: O'Neill JA, Rowe MI, Grosfeld JL *et al.* (eds) *Pediatric surgery*. 5th edition. St Louis: Mosby Year Book, 1425–48.

Kluth D, Lambrecht W (1997) Current concepts in the embryology of anorectal malformations. *Semin Pediatr Surg* 180–6.

Kuster H (1910) Uterus bipartitus solidus rudimentarius cum vagina solida. *Z Geburtshilfe Perinatol* **67**: 692.

Levitt MA, Stein DM, Peña A (1998) Gynecologic concerns in the treatment of teenagers with cloaca. *J Pediatr Surg* **33**: 188–93.

McCraw J, Massey F, Shanklin K *et al.* (1976) Vaginal reconstruction using gracilis myocutaneous flaps. *Plast & Reconstr Surg* **38**: 176–83.

McIndoe AH (1950) The treatment of congenital absence and obliterative conditions of the vagina. *Br J Plast Surg* **2**: 254.

McLeod N (1880) A case of imperforate anus, with a suggestion for a new method of treatment. *BMJ* **ii**: 657.

McLorie GA, Sheldon CA, Fleisher M *et al.* (1987) The genitourinary system in patients with imperforate anus. *J Pediatr Surg* **22**: 1100–109.

Malone PSJ, Curry JL (1999) The MACE procedure. *Dialog Pediatr Urol* **22**: 2.

Malone PS, Ransley PG, Kiely EM (1990) Preliminary report: the antegrade continence enema. *Lancet* **336**: 1217–18.

Marshall FF (1980) Vaginal agenesis. *Clin Plast Surg* **7**: 175–8.

Mayer CAJ (1829) Uber verdoppelungen des uterus und ihre arten, nebst bemerkungen uber hasenscarte und wolfsrachen. *J Chir Auger* **13**: 525.

Metts JC, Kotkin L, Kasper S *et al.* (1997) Genital malformations and coexistent urinary tract or spinal anomalies in patients with imperforate anus. *J Urol* **158**: 1298–300.

Mitchell ME, Hensle TW, Crooks KK (1982) Urethral reconstruction in the young female using a perineal pedicle flap. *J Pediatr Surg* **17**: 687–94.

Mollitt DL, Schullinger JN, Santulli TV *et al.* (1981) Complications at menarche of urogenital sinus with associated anorectal malformations. *J Pediatr Surg* **16**: 349–52.

Muraji T, Mahour HG (1984) Surgical problems in patients with VATER-associated anomalies. *J Pediatr Surg* **19**: 550–4.

Nolan JF, Stillwell TJ, Barttelbort SW *et al.* (1991) Urethrovaginal reconstruction using a perineal artery axial flap. *J Urol* **146**: 843–9.

O'Rahilly R, Müller F (1992) *Human embryology and teratology.* New York: Wiley-Liss, 216.

Paidas CN, Peña A (1997) Rectum and anus. In: Oldham KT, Colombani PM, Foglia RP (eds) *Surgery of infants and children: scientific principles and practice.* Philadelphia, PA: Lippincott-Raven, 1323–62.

Parrott TS, Woodard JR (1991) Abdominoperitoneal approach to management of the high, short vagina in the adrenogenital syndrome. *J Urol* **146**: 647–8.

Passarini-Glazel G (1989) A new 1-stage procedure for cliterovaginoplasty in severely masuclinized female pseudo-hermaphrodites. *J Urol* **142**: 55–8.

Peña A (ed.) (1990) *Atlas of surgical management of anorectal malformations.* New York: Springer.

Peña A (1997) Total urogenital mobilization: an easier way to repair cloacas. *J Pediatr Surg* **32**: 263–7.

Peña A, Kessler O (1998) Posterior cloaca: a unique defect. *J Pediatr Surg* **33**: 407.

Peña A, Filmer B, Bonilla E *et al.* (1992) Transanorectal approach for the treatment of urogenital sinus: preliminary report. *J Pediatr Surg* **27**: 681–5.

Peña A, Kessler O (1998) Posterior cloaca: a unique defect. *J Pediatr Surg* **33**: 407–12.

Pratt JH (1972) Vaginal atresia corrected by the use of small and large bowel. *Clin Obstet Gynecol* **15**: 639–49.

Quan L, Smith DW (1973) The VATER association. *J Pediatr* **82**: 104–7.

Raffensperger JG (ed.) (1990) *Swenson's pediatric surgery.* 5th edition. Norwalk, CT: Appleton & Lange.

Raghavendra BN, Epstein FJ, Pinto RS *et al.* (1983) The tethered spinal cord: diagnosis by high-resolution real-time ultrasound. *Radiology* **149**: 123–8.

Ralph DJ, Woodhouse CR, Ransley PG (1993) The management of the neuropathic bladder in adolescents with imperforate anus. *J Urol* **148**: 366–8.

Rhoads JE, Pipes RL, Randall JP (1948) A simultaneous abdominal and perineal approach in operations for imperforate anus with atresia of the rectum and rectosigmoid. *Ann Surg* **127**: 552.

Rich MA, Brock WA, Peña A (1988) Spectrum of genitourinary malformations in patients with imperforate anus. *Pediatr Surg Int* **3**: 110.

Rink RC, Pope JC, Kropp BP *et al.* (1997) Reconstruction of the high urogenital sinus: early perineal prone approach without division of the rectum. *J Urol* **158**: 1293–7.

Rokitanski K (1938) Uber die sogenannten verdoppelungen des uterus. *Med Jb Ost Staat* **26**: 39.

Santulli TV, Schullinger JN, Kiesewetter WB, Bill AH (1971) Imperforate anus: a survey from the members of the Surgical Section of the American Academy of Pediatrics. *J Pediatr Surg* **6**: 484–7.

Sato S, Shirane R, Yoshimoto T (1993) Evaluation of tethered cord syndrome associated with anorectal malformations. *Neurosurgery* **32**: 1025–7.

Say P, Gerald PS (1968) A new polydactyly/imperforate anus/vertebral anomalies syndrome? *Lancet* **ii**: 688.

Scheible W, James VE, Leopold GR *et al.* (1983) Occult spinal dysraphism in infants: screening with high-resolution real-time ultrasound. *Radiology* **146**: 743–6.

Shandling B, Gilmour RF (1987) The enema continence catheter in spina bifida: successful bowel management. *J Pediatr Surg* **22**: 271–3.

Sharma AK, Kashtan CE, Nevins TE (1993) The management of end-stage renal disease in infants with imperforate anus. *Pediatr Nephrol* **7**: 721–4.

Sheldon CA (1997) Intersex states. In: Oldham KT, Colombani PM, Foglia RP (eds) *Surgery of infants and children: scientific principles and practice.* Philadelphia, PA: Lippincott-Raven, 1577–616.

Sheldon CA, Welch TR (1998) Total anatomic urinary tract replacement and renal transplantation: a surgical strategy to correct severe genitourinary anomalies. *J Pediatr Surg* **33**: 635–8.

Sheldon C, Cormier M, Crone K *et al.* (1991) Occult neurovesical dysfunction in children with imperforate anus and its variants. *J Pediatr Surg* **26**: 49–54.

Sheldon CA, Gilbert A, Lewis AG (1994a) Vaginal reconstruction: critical technical principles. *J Urol* **152**: 190–5.

Sheldon CA, Gilbert A, Lewis AG *et al.* (1994b) Surgical implications of genitourinary tract anomalies in patients with imperforate anus. *J Urol* **152**: 196–9.

Sheldon CA, Gonzalez R, Burns MW *et al.* (1994c) Renal transplantation into the dysfunctional bladder: the role of adjunctive bladder reconstruction. *J Urol* **152**: 972–5.

Sheldon CA, Minevich E, Wacksman J (1997a) A peel away sheath endoscopic technique for difficult pediatric urethral intubation problems. *J Urol* **157**: 1880–1.

Sheldon CA, Minevich E, Wacksman J *et al.* (1997b) Role of the antegrade continence enema in the management of the most debilitating childhood rectourogenital anomalies. *J Urol* **158**: 1277–9.

Skandalakis JE, Gray SW (eds) (1994) *Embryology for surgeons.* 2nd edition. Baltimore, MD: Williams and Wilkins, 244.

Skandalakis JE, Gray SW, Ricketts R (1994) The colon and rectum. In: Skandalakis JE, Gray S (eds) *Embryology for surgeons.* 2nd edition. Baltimore, MD: Williams and Wilkins, 244.

Smith DE (1968) Urinary anomalies and complications in imperforate anus and rectum. *J Pediatr Surg* **3**: 337–49.

Snyder HM, Retik AB, Bauer SB *et al.* (1983) Feminizing genitoplasty: a synthesis. *J Urol* **129**: 1024–6.

Stephens FD, Smith ED (1986) Classification, identification and assessment of surgical treatment of anorectal anomalies. *Pediatr Surg Int* **1**: 200.

Temtamy SA, Miller JD (1974) Extending the scope of the VATER association: definition of the VATER syndrome. *J Pediatr* **85**: 345–9.

Trusler GA, Wilkinson RH (1962) Imperforate anus: a review of 147 cases. *Can J Surg* **5**: 169.

Uehling DT, Gilbert E, Chesney R (1983) Urologic implications of the VATER association. *J Urol* **129**: 352–4.

Warf BC, Scott RM, Barnes PD *et al.* (1993) Tethered spinal cord in patients with anorectal and urogenital malformations. *Pediatr Neurosurg* **19**: 25–30.

Weaver DD, Mapstone CL (1986) The VATER association: analysis of 46 patients. *Am J Dis Child* **140**: 225–9.

Weber TR, Smith W, Grosfeld JL (1980) Surgical experience in infants with the VATER association. *J Pediatr Surg* **15**: 849–54.

Wee JTK, Joseph VT (1989) A new technique of vaginal reconstruction using neurovascular pedendal-thigh flaps: a preliminary report. *Plast and Reconstr Surg* **83**: 701–9.

Wendelken JR, Sethney HT, Halverstadt DB (1977) Urologic abnormalities associated with imperforate anus. *Urology* **10**: 239.

White JJ, Haller JA, Scott JR *et al.* (1978) N-type anorectal malformations. *J Pediatr Surg* **13**: 631–7.

Wiener ES, Kiesewetter WB (1973) Urologic abnormalities associated with imperforate anus. *J Pediatr Surg* **8**: 151–7.

Yoneyama T, Fukui J, Ohtsuka K *et al.* (1985) Urinary tract dysfunctions in tethered spinal cord syndrome: improvement after surgical untethering. *J Urol* **133**: 999–1001.

Bladder anomalies, exstrophy, and epispadias

27

Richard W. Grady and Michael E. Mitchell

Exstrophy

Formal descriptions of exstrophy date back to at least 1597 with Sherk Von Grafenberg's description of this congenital defect, although possible depictions of exstrophy also exist on Assyrian tablets from 2000 BC. Chaussier first coined the term 'exstrophie' to describe this defect in 1780 following detailed descriptions of it by Mowat in 1748. Because exstrophy is usually a non-lethal defect, its natural history is known and described by various authors. Our understanding of exstrophy has resulted in the synthesis of various diseases into a common group. Since the nineteenth century, various efforts to manage the problem have been described. Because exstrophic conditions are rare, these approaches were empiric and often unsuccessful. More focused efforts in the twentieth century have led to a better understanding of exstrophy. Currently, the exstrophic diseases are considered a spectrum of processes related by certain principle anatomic features. They are referred to as the exstrophy–epispadias complex (Gearhart and Jeffs, 1996). This complex includes:

- epispadias
- classic bladder exstrophy
- cloacal exstrophy
- exstrophy variants.

Anatomic pathology

Bladder exstrophy; classic exstrophy

Brock and O'Neill (1988) described exstrophy as 'if one blade of a pair of scissors were passed through the urethra of a normal person; the other blade were used to cut through the skin, abdominal wall, anterior wall of the bladder and urethra, and the symphysis pubis;

and the cut edges were then folded laterally as if the pages of a book were being opened' (Fig. 27.1).

Anatomic features of exstrophy include the presence of an open defect covered by a layer of urothelium on the anterior abdominal wall representing the bladder and urethra. At birth, the urothelium is usually normal in appearance. However, ectopic bowel mucosa or polypoid lesions consistent with cystitis cystica and/or

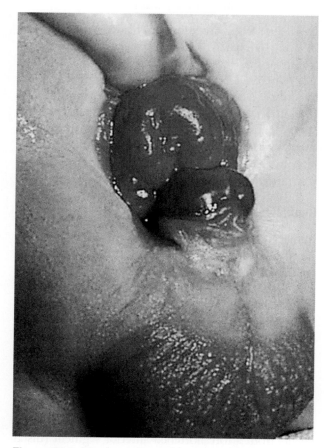

Figure 27.1 Newborn boy with classic bladder exstrophy. Note evidence of anterior placement of the bladder and urethra.

glandularis may be present. If left untreated and without meticulous protection after birth, the exposed urothelium will undergo squamous metaplasia in response to acute and chronic inflammation. Other inflammatory changes such as cystitis cystica and/or glandularis will then be seen. When left chronically exposed to the environment, the areas of squamous metaplasia often undergo malignant degeneration to adenocarcinoma or squamous cell carcinoma (O'Kane and Megaw, 1968; Gupta and Gupta, 1976).

Associated anomalies

Classic exstrophy and epispadias have a relatively low incidence of associated anomalies. In contrast, patients with cloacal exstrophy have associated anomalies more often than not (Beckwith, 1966; Diamond and Jeffs, 1985). These anomalies can affect the upper urinary tract, intestines, skeletal system, and neurologic system.

Kidneys and upper urinary tract

Renal anomalies can occur with bladder exstrophy but they are not characteristic. Associated renal abnormalities include cystic dysplasia, ureteropelvic junction (UPJ) obstruction, pelvic kidney, megaureter, renal hypoplasia, and horseshoe kidney (O'Donnell, 1984). In contrast, vesicoureteral reflux (VUR) does occur almost universally after exstrophy closure due to the lateral placement of the ureteral orifices on the bladder plate in association with the lateral and inferior pathway of the ureters into the bladder.

Genitalia

In males the penis is broad and shortened because the corpora cavernosa are splayed laterally, attached to the separated pubic bones. The penis is deflected dorsally and may have true intrinsic dorsal chordee because of angulated corpora cavernosa. Because of the varying degree of pubic diastasis associated with exstrophy, the penis appears variably foreshortened. Further, magnetic resonance imaging (MRI) evaluation of the penile length of adult male exstrophy and epispadias patients reveals that the total corporeal length is significantly shorter than in a normal control population. This corporeal shortening apparently results from a foreshortened anterior segment (distal to the pelvic attachment); the posterior corporeal segment is unaffected in exstrophy patients (Silver *et al.*, 1997).

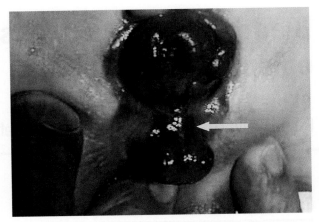

Figure 27.2 Newborn boy with classic bladder exstrophy. The white arrow indicates the posterior urethra and location of verumontanum.

The short urethral plate results in the glans penis lying in close approximation to the prostatic utricle (Fig. 27.2). The ejaculatory ducts empty at the prostatic utricle exposed on the urethral plate. The vas and ejaculatory ducts are probably unaffected in classic exstrophy unless iatrogenically damaged (Hanna and Williams, 1972). Innervation to the penis is also normal. The cavernosal nerves are located on the lateral aspects of the corporeal bodies with exstrophy. Normally these nerves can be found on the dorsal aspect of the penis after they traverse the posterolateral aspects of the prostate and the membranous urethra (Woodhouse and Kellett, 1984). The prostate is also incompletely formed in exstrophy (Hamper *et al.*, 1991; Gearhart *et al.*, 1993a). The scrotum is usually not affected, although most exstrophy patients have an increased distance between the base of the penile shaft and the scrotum and a broadening of the scrotum, dependent on the degree of diastasis. The testes may be undescended. Because of the underlying bladder neck anomalies, exstrophic patients may have impaired fertility. A particular problem is retrograde ejaculation if the bladder neck cannot close completely following bladder reconstruction (Lattimer *et al.*, 1978; Avolio, 1996; Ben-Chaim *et al.*, 1996).

In the female with bladder exstrophy, the mons pubis is absent. In association with a bifid clitoris, the anterior labia are laterally displaced although they fuse in the midline posteriorly. The vagina and introitus are also displaced anteriorly relative to their usual position. The vaginal opening may be stenotic in these patients but this is not a characteristic feature. It may result from improper primary closure. Internal genital structures (uterus, cervix, fallopian tubes, and ovaries) are unaffected in classic exstrophy. Uterine prolapse due to deficient pelvic floor support can occur in the older exstrophy patient and poses particular problems with pregnancy (O'Neill, 1998). Early primary bladder reconstruction may decrease this risk. Uterine suspension procedures, such as sacrocolpopexy, can be employed in these situations as well.

Anorectal and intestinal abnormalities

The anus is often located rather ventrally in the exstrophy complex. Surgical procedures involving these patients should preserve the anal sphincter mechanism. However, some exstrophic patients will have insufficient anal continence due to the underlying abnormalities of the pelvic floor support structures including the levator ani and puborectalis muscles. Anal sphincter weakness not only impacts fecal continence but also limits the use of ureterosigmoidostomy and its variants, for example rectal bladder and ileocecal ureterosigmoidostomy. In untreated patients rectal prolapse can also occur owing to insufficient pelvic floor support. This is usually definitively treated with formal exstrophy repair that corrects the lack of anterior pelvic support. In the interim, most rectal prolapse is intermittent and reducible (Gearhart and Jeffs, 1996)

Skeletal abnormalities

Diastasis of the pubic symphysis occurs as part of the exstrophy complex (Fig. 27.3). This results from outward rotation of the inominate bones along both sacroiliac joints. Outward rotation of the pubic rami at the iliac and ischial junctions is also present.

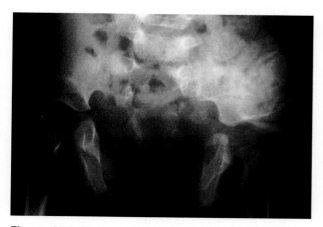

Figure 27.3 Plain abdominal radiograph demonstrating pubic diastasis in a patient with bladder exstrophy.

Sponseller *et al.* (1995) noted other differences in the pelvic anatomy of patients with exstrophy, including (1) increased intertriradiate distance, (2) external rotation and shortening (by 30%) of the anterior segment of the iliac bone, and (3) external rotation of the posterior segment of ileum. These pelvic bone abnormalities contribute to the splaying of the penis associated with exstrophy and epispadias and cause the penis to appear foreshortened. Gait abnormalities in these children arise as a consequence of these bone abnormalities. Many children learn to ambulate with a wide, waddling gait. This gait abnormality resolves as the children grow. Orthopedic procedures to reapproximate the pubis symphyses do not appear to offer any long-term benefits from an orthopedic viewpoint. Osteotomies to reapproximate the pubis symphysis do, however, increase the chance of successful primary bladder closure in selected patients and may play a significant role in securing continence and support of the pelvic diaphragm (Aadalen *et al.*, 1980; Ben-Chaim *et al.*, 1995b).

Fascial abnormalities

Fascial abnormalities include the rectus fascial defect associated with the exposed bladder. Inferiorly, the pelvic floor support structures are also compromised. At the inferior portion of the fascial defect, patients possess an anteriorly located intersymphyseal ligament or band representing the attenuated urogenital diaphragm. The rectus muscles diverge laterally with the widened pubis symphysis. This abdominal wall defect is most severe in cloacal exstrophy.

Inguinal hernias are commonly associated with exstrophy in both male and female patients (Stringer *et al.*, 1994; Connolly *et al.*, 1995) (Fig. 27.4). The majority of these hernias are indirect. They probably occur as a consequence of enlarged internal and external inguinal rings in conjunction with compromised fascial support and lack of obliquity of the inguinal canal (Husmann *et al.*, 1990a). In a review of patients from Toronto Sick Children's Hospital, 56% of classic male exstrophy patients and 15% of classic female exstrophy patients developed inguinal hernias over a 10-year period. The authors recommended that these hernias be repaired at the time of primary bladder closure to prevent incarceration, which could occur in 50% of patients in the first 2 years of life (Churchill *et al.*, 1997). Reinforcement of the transversalis and internal oblique fascia during hernia repair decreases the incidence of later direct inguinal hernias.

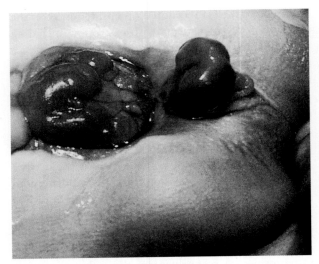

Figure 27.4 Evidence of an inguinal hernia in this newborn male with bladder exstrophy as demonstrated by the inguinal bulge.

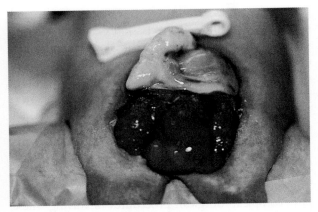

Figure 27.5 Newborn male with cloacal exstrophy.

Umbilical hernias are repaired at the time of the exstrophy closure. An omphalocele may also be associated with bladder exstrophy, although this is rare (Yazbeck *et al.*, 1986).

Neurologic system

Spinal cord abnormalities are the exception rather than the rule in bladder exstrophy. Occult spina bifida and even myelomeningocele can be seen in combination with bladder exstrophy but this is a rare occurrence.

Cloacal exstrophy

The bladder plate associated with cloacal exstrophy is divided in half by the hindgut plate; the hindgut plate represents the cecum, the deformation in the development of the colon that occurs with cloacal exstrophy. Ileum enters and intussuscepts into the middle of the hindgut creating the 'trunk of an elephant's face' appearance with appendiceal appendages located laterally to give the impression of 'tusks on the face of the elephant' (Warren and Ziegler, 1993) (Fig. 27.5).

As with classic bladder exstrophy, the bladder neck (internal urethral sphincter) and external urethral sphincter are not fully developed owing to the open bladder, and urethral remnants located on the anterior and dorsal surfaces of the body wall and penis, respectively. When the innervation to these structures is intact, anatomic closure offers the possibility of

achieving urinary continence, at least theoretically (Toguri *et al.*, 1978; Shapiro *et al.*, 1985). The urethral plate is characteristically short as well.

Associated anomalies

Kidneys and upper urinary tract

Renal anomalies are much more common with cloacal exstrophy. They include anomalies of location such as pelvic kidneys and crossed fused ectopia. Horseshoe kidneys, renal agenesis, and UPJ obstruction may also occur (O'Neill, 1998).

Genitalia

In cloacal exstrophy the penis (may be small) is separated into two hemiphalluses due to the wide pubic diastasis (Fig. 27.6). This can make subsequent reconstructive efforts technically more challenging if a male phenotype is preserved. Cryptorchidism is the rule with cloacal exstrophy.

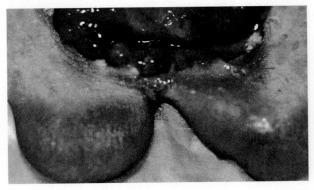

Figure 27.6 Newborn male with cloacal exstrophy. Note the virtual absence of the phallus.

For girls, in addition to the genital pathology described above with bladder exstrophy, uterus didelphys and other fusion anomalies of the müllerian duct structures are commonly seen in up to two-thirds of cloacal exstrophy patients. Vaginal agenesis occurs in one-third of girls with cloacal exstrophy.

Anorectal and intestinal abnormalities

Associated intestinal abnormalities specific to cloacal exstrophy include imperforate anus, foreshortening of the midgut, bowel duplication, malrotation, intestinal atresia, and Meckel's diverticulum (O'Neill, 1998). These are in addition to the exstrophy of hindgut, ileal intussusception, and exposed appendices that are considered part of the primary pathology of cloacal exstrophy. There is no colon internally.

Skeletal abnormalities

In addition to the features seen with bladder exstrophy, patients with cloacal exstrophy can have other skeletal abnormalities. Skeletal anomalies are seen in as many as one-half of patients with cloacal exstrophy. Anomalies include congenital hip dislocation, talipes equinovarus, and a variety of limb deficiencies and spinal anormalies (Sponseller *et al.*, 1995).

Fascial abnormalities

The fascial anomalies associated with cloacal exstrophy include those described in bladder exstrophy, but the defects are more severe. Further, omphaloceles often occur in association with cloacal exstrophy (Hesser *et al.*, 1984; Lund and Hendren, 1993). These can be closed during the initial bladder closure if they are small. If the omphalocele is large, it may require closure as a primary procedure with reapproximated bladder halves acting as a silo to reduce intra-abdominal pressure. Alternatively, omphaloceles may be treated with antiseptic paint to promote skin overgrowth. The authors' preference is to proceed with a staged surgical omphalocele correction with primary reconstruction of the bladder at a later date if the infant is a surgical candidate. Intra-abdominal pressure following omphalocele closure can determine whether the surgeon may proceed with primary bladder closure at the same time as the omphalocele repair. Usually, these operations must be staged. Aggressive, one-stage closure of a cloacal exstrophy can lead to organ ischemia from increased intra-abdominal pressure. Rupture of an omphalocele requires immediate surgery in these babies and takes precedence over other considerations. This is a rare occurrence.

Neurologic abnormalities

Abnormalities of the lower spinal cord in cloacal exstrophy patients are the rule (Howell *et al.*, 1983; Hurwitz *et al.*, 1987; Lund and Hendren, 1993). Most have lumbar or sacral cord involvement, but thoracic level myelodysplasia has been reported (Lund and Hendren, 1993). Management of cloacal exstrophy must then be coordinated with neurosurgical plans to close the neural tube defect, which usually takes precedence.

Epispadias

Isolated epispadias can be considered the least severe problem of the exstrophy–epispadias complex (Fig. 27.7). It does not involve the body of the bladder. However, as in exstrophy, the urethra is represented as a plate of tissue located dorsally on the penis. The genital anomalies described above are also seen in epispadias. These include lateral splaying of the penis and dorsal chordee in boys. In affected girls, the clitoris is bifid, the perineal body is broadened, and the vagina is anterior to its orthotopic or typical position. Widening of the pubic diastasis occurs as well. Importantly, the bladder neck is also frequently involved: it is often wide and incompetent. This directly affects the continence mechanism of these children and impacts the ability to achieve urinary continence. In boys with epispadias, continence exists if the epispadias is distal and

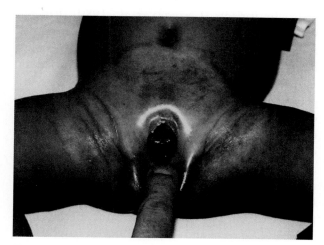

Figure 27.7 Penopubic epispadias in a 3-month-old male. Skin demarcation is due to chronic urine contact dermatitis in this patient.

the bladder neck is normally formed. In girls, however, continence is invariably affected to some degree because of the coexisting urethral and bladder neck ectasia. Because the features of epispadias are shared with bladder exstrophy, clinicians consider these anomalies as part of the exstrophy–epispadias complex.

Exstrophy variants

In the exstrophy–epispadias complex, variations in bladder plate size and compliance are commonplace but no system to quantify these differences has been devised. Phallic size and degree of phallic separation also vary from patient to patient. However, despite these variations the underlying features are consistent for classic forms of the exstrophy complex.

Variants have also been recognized, however, patients with atypical physical findings are referred to as exstrophy variant patients. These patients have some but not all of the typical features of bladder or cloacal exstrophy as well as other features not typically associated with bladder exstrophy. These include 'covered' exstrophy and superior vesical fissure. Patients with exstrophy variants may have anatomically normal genitalia despite their bladder and/or colon anomalies.

Bladder exstrophy variants include those with separated pubes and a lower abdominal fascial defect but which are not associated with any significant anomaly of the urinary tract. These are labeled as pseudo-exstrophy (Marshall and Muecke, 1968; Mitchell et al., 1993; Swana et al., 1997). If such defects also have an isolated ectopic bowel segment in association with these findings they are referred to as 'covered' exstrophy variants (Cerniglia et al., 1989). Patients with superior vesical fissure also have the muscular and skeletal defects associated with bladder exstrophy, but only the upper portion of the bladder is affected, so that the bladder neck and urethra are intact and the genitalia are less significantly affected than in classic exstrophy (Kizilcan et al., 1994). Duplicate exstrophy may occur. Patients with this variation have a superior vesical fissure associated with normal fascial abdominal wall development, so that only components of the bladder are ectopic. Such patients can have genital anomalies consistent with classic exstrophy as well, but this association is variable (Nielsen et al., 1980; Pineschi and Chiella, 1982; Sheldon et al., 1990; Andiran and Tanyel, 1999).

Cloacal exstrophy variants also exist. These patients possess some of the features of cloacal exstrophy, such as an exposed hindgut plate and separated bladder plates, but may not have the typical genital involvement (Manzoni et al., 1987; Stoler et al., 1993; Goldfischer et al., 1997; Radhakrishnan, 1998). Hypospadias has been described in association with cloacal exstrophy, as well as normal genitalia in both male and female patients. These patients may also have other atypical features such as accessory appendages or limb malformation. These findings, in association with prenatal ultrasound examinations that document twin gestations early in some pregnancies, suggest that partial conjoined twinning may be the cause of cloacal exstrophy variants in some cases (Goldfischer et al., 1997; Grady et al., 1997) (Fig. 27.8).

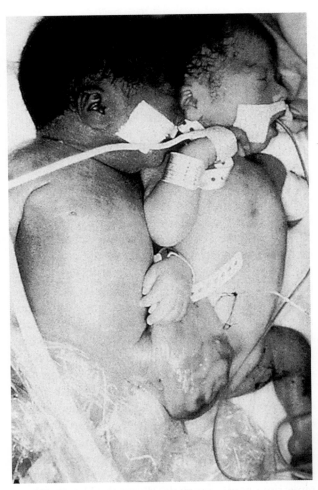

Figure 27.8 Conjoined twins connected by a membranous omphalocele sac containing a shared segment of distal ileum, cecum, and colon draining to a common exstrophic cloaca; an example of an exstrophy variant.

Embryology

Normal bladder development

Normal bladder development results in an organ that functions to store and evacuate urine. This process, known as bladder cycling, requires the bladder to store urine at low intravesical pressures during filling while maintaining continence at the level of the bladder neck. Subsequent evacuation of urine from the bladder requires a coordinated contraction of the detrusor in conjunction with relaxation of the bladder outlet. Coordinated storage and emptying require normal innervation of the bladder and sphincter mechanisms (Klimberg, 1988).

During embryogenesis, the ureteral buds first appear during the 4th week of gestation. At this time the bladder has not completely formed from the anterior urogenital sinus. Before the bladder is closed, mesenchyme grows inwards towards the midline between the bilaminar (ectoderm and endoderm) layers of the cloacal membrane. This mesenchyme later differentiates into the abdominal wall musculature and fascia. Subsequently, the urorectal septum separates the bladder from rectum by growing downwards between them. Abnormalities in the appearance, timing, and function of the cloacal membrane are implicated in the causation of exstrophy. In this fashion, the urinary bladder arises during the 8th week of fetal development when the ventral portion of the urogenital sinus begins to expand (Klimberg, 1988). With bladder filling, the mesenchymal tissue surrounding this structure differentiates into smooth muscle, which will eventually become the detrusor muscle. Ingrowth of neuronal tissue into this smooth muscle to form motor units is critical to the development of a functional bladder (Hoyes *et al.*, 1973). Embryogenesis of the pelvic floor is also important in normal fetal bladder development and function; the pelvic floor acts as a dynamic support for the bladder, which aids in both continence and volitional voiding (Galloway, 1997).

Theories of pathogenesis of exstrophy

Improvements in our understanding of embryogenesis have led to some insight into the cause of exstrophy. In the premodern era, trauma to the unborn child or ulceration of the abdominal wall and bladder between 2 and 3 months of life was felt to be the underlying cause. Current theories implicate an error in embryogenesis rather than an event of arrested development, since the developing human embryo does not normally pass through a stage that corresponds to exstrophy (Muecke, 1964). Animal models suggest that exstrophy results from pathophysiologic events involving the cloacal membrane. This membrane serves to separate the coelomic cavity from the amniotic space in early development. The cloacal membrane can first be identified during development at 2–3 weeks of gestation. By the 4th week of development, it forms the ventral wall of the urogenital sinus with the unfused primordia of the genital tubercles sitting cephalad and lateral to it. With further development, these primordia grow and fuse in the midline, and mesoderm grows towards the midline creating the infraumbilical abdominal wall. Simultaneously, the urorectal septum migrates medially and caudally to separate the cloaca into the urogenital sinus and rectum (Warren and Ziegler, 1993).

Marshall and Muecke (1962) proposed that exstrophy was caused by persistence of the cloacal membrane during early fetal development, based on autopsy studies of fetuses with bladder exstrophy done earlier in the twentieth century. Persistence of the membrane would create a wedge effect that would keep the medially encroaching mesoderm from fusing in the midline. To study this hypothesis further, Muecke (1964) created an animal model of cloacal exstrophy using the developing chick embryo. By placing a plastic triangle in the region of the tail bud, he created cloacal exstrophy and concluded that exstrophy was due to persistence of the cloacal membrane, as Marshall had originally postulated.

Other experimental models implicate the cloacal membrane in the pathophysiology of exstrophy as well. Thomalla *et al.* (1985) developed a model of cloacal exstrophy in the developing chick embryo by using a CO_2 laser to create an early dehiscence in the tail bud caudal to the omphalomesenteric vessels. Their results suggest that exstrophy may be caused by failure of the mesoderm to ingrow between the ectoderm and endoderm of the cloacal membrane, which then ruptures to produce exstrophy (Fig. 27.9). They hypothesize that such an event could be caused by early hypoxic infarction in the region of the tail bud with subsequent cellular loss of the mesoderm, and herniation of the developing bladder or cloaca. This type of ischemic injury has been implicated as the cause of gastroschisis and may explain the spectrum of exstrophy–epispadias complex (Thomalla *et al.*, 1980).

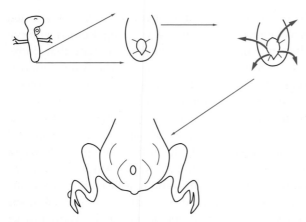

Figure 27.9 Schematic diagram of the chick model of cloacal exstrophy. (Adapted from Thomalla and Rudolph, 1985, with permission.)

Other proposed theories for exstrophy include caudal displacement of the paired primordia of the genital tubercles. Exstrophy occurs, according to this mechanism, when the primordia of the genital tubercles fuse caudal to their usual location relative to where the urorectal fold divides the cloaca into the urogenital sinus and rectum (Patten and Barry, 1952). This theory readily explains the spectrum of variation seen in the exstrophy–epispadias complex. However, it fails to explain the higher incidence of exstrophy compared to epispadias; one would anticipate a higher incidence of epispadias if caudal displacement were the underlying cause of exstrophy–epispadias because it would represent the most minimal example of this phenomena (Warren and Ziegler, 1993).

The underlying cause of exstrophy remains in question because it is a rare birth defect and no naturally occurring animal models exist. The chick model has inherent limitations since chicks normally possess a cloaca and do not form a bladder. Other animal models used to study bladder exstrophy have proven difficult to create. Slaughenhoupt *et al.* (1996) have created an exstrophy model using sheep but have not published any data regarding bladder development.

Incidence

Bladder exstrophy occurs at a rate of one per 10 000 to 50 000 livebirths (Lattimer and Smith, 1966; Engel, 1974). This anomaly has long been recognized to occur more commonly in males than females, with a ratio of 3–6:1 reported in the literature (Ives *et al.*, 1980, 1987). Cloacal exstrophy occurs even more rarely, with an incidence of 1 in 200 000 to 400 000 livebirths (Ziegler *et al.*, 1986).

Genetic factors involved in exstrophy remain incompletely defined. Because of associated anomalies, patients with bladder exstrophy often have to overcome significant obstacles to reproduce. Men may need to resort to artificial insemination because their seminal emissions may reflux into the bladder or the ejaculatory ducts may be secondarily obstructed. Further, sexual intercourse can be difficult for some patients owing to deformity of the phallus. In the 1800s prevailing thought declared males with bladder exstrophy impotent because of the deformities of the penis. Women with exstrophy were (and still are) prone to uterine prolapse and miscarriage. In the mid-nineteenth century, few women with bladder exstrophy successfully delivered (Gross, 1876). Difficulties with conception and pregnancy are still a problem today despite *in vitro* fertilization and careful obstetric care (Burbige *et al.*, 1986). This may explain, in part, why familial patterns of inheritance of exstrophy are infrequent. To date, 18 familial cases of bladder exstrophy have been reported, the most recent of which describes a mother and son with bladder exstrophy (Messelink *et al.*, 1994). In 1984, a survey of pediatric urologists and surgeons turned up nine cases related to 2500 index cases of bladder exstrophy; this same survery also reported twins and noted discordance in both fraternal and identical twinships (Shapiro *et al.*, 1984). In a study population of greater than 6 million births with 208 cases of exstrophy, no patient had a family history for this anomaly (Jeffs, 1987). Current recommendations on counseling about the risk of recurrence in a sibling of a patient with exstrophy estimate about 1% to a 1 in 70 chance of transmission to progeny (Messelink *et al.*, 1994). Based on these findings the occurrence of bladder exstrophy appears to be multifactorial rather than directly genetically based; combined environmental and developmental factors may play a significant role in the cause of the exstrophy–epispadias complex.

Antenatal diagnosis

Prenatal detection of bladder exstrophy is possible. Ultrasonography can reliably detect exstrophy before the 20th week of gestation (McLaughlin *et al.*, 1984;

Langer, 1993; Paidas *et al.*, 1994; Gearhart *et al.*, 1995; Pinette *et al.*, 1996; Austin *et al.*, 1998; Brun *et al.*, 1998; Cacciari *et al.*, 1999) (Fig. 27.10). Absence of bladder filling in the presence of normal kidneys in association with a low-set umbilical cord suggests the diagnosis. Sonographic examination may also reveal a semisolid mass protruding from the abdominal wall, as well as the above findings (Jaffe *et al.*, 1990; Barth *et al.*, 1990). Gearhart *et al.* (1995) reviewed the antenatal ultrasonographic studies of 25 women who delivered live infants with exstrophy and found:

- an absent bladder in 71% of the studies;
- a lower abdominal protrusion in 47% of the studies;
- an anteriorly displaced scrotum with a small phallus in 57% of the male fetuses;
- a low-set umbilical cord in 29% of the studies;
- abnormal iliac crest widening in 18%.

Amniotic fluid levels will be normal since urine production is normal in these fetuses. Prenatal diagnosis is valuable in the management of bladder exstrophy because it allows optimal perinatal management of these infants, including delivery near a pediatric center equipped to treat babies with this unusual anomaly. Unfortunately, many affected fetuses are not detected antenatally (Skari *et al.*, 1998).

Antenatal diagnosis also allows the parents the opportunity to discuss termination of the pregnancy. Such a discussion should include a pediatric urologist experienced in the treatment of bladder exstrophy. The overall prognosis of these children is excellent if they are referred to medical centers with physicians experienced in the treatment of this disorder. Unfortunately, because of the rarity of bladder exstrophy, healthcare providers who lack insight and knowledge of this disorder often counsel prospective parents of these patients. For example, in one recent article, the authors state '... the point of termination [of the pregnancy] may be underlined by the poor long term results in boys, who mostly end up with severe sexual dysfunction' (Messelink *et al.*, 1994). Such

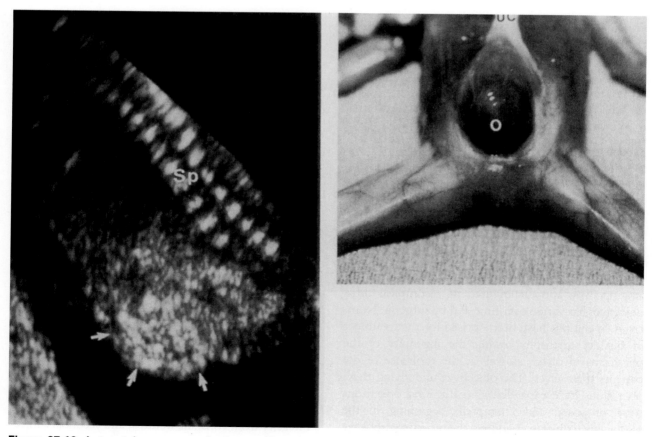

Figure 27.10 Antenatal sonogram of a fetus with exstrophy and a photograph of a fetus with confirmed exstrophy at autopsy. (Adapted from Mirk *et al.*, 1986, with permission.)

recommendations are based on an outdated understanding of bladder exstrophy. The authors believe that counseling recommendations for termination for bladder exstrophy would be akin to recommending therapeutic termination in a child diagnosed antenatally with a cleft lip and palate or ventricular septal defect. Unfortunately, the counseling of these families by healthcare providers who are unaware of the true prognosis of patients with bladder exstrophy has led to an increase in the abortion rate of these fetuses who have an otherwise treatable condition with a satisfactory long-term outcome and life expectancy when appropriately managed (Cacciari *et al.*, 1999).

Treatment philosophies

Goals of reconstruction of exstrophy and epispadias

In the treatment of exstrophy, objectives for reconstruction can be placed broadly in the following categories.

Principal objectives:
- urinary continence;
- reconstruction to allow volitional voiding;
- a low-pressure urine storage reservoir;
- preservation of kidney function;
- functionally and cosmetically acceptable external genitalia.

Secondary objectives:
- minimization of urinary tract infections (UTIs);
- minimization of the risk for urinary calculi;
- minimization of the risk for malignancy associated with the urinary tract;
- reconstruction of the abdominal wall fascia;
- reconstruction of the pelvic floor.

Successful achievement of these goals remains challenging. The approaches used to accomplish these objectives has varied over time and by surgeon. Numerous operations have been devised for the treatment of bladder exstrophy testing the ingenuity of the physicians involved, as well as the resilience of the patients themselves. The objectives underlying these operations have expanded since the first operations were proposed and attempted, beginning in the 1800s. Such objectives address the primary pathology and problems associated with exstrophy and its management. These problems include the following.

Primary pathophysiology (untreated):
- urinary incontinence
- UTI
- urinary calculi
- bladder malignancy
- pelvic floor prolapse
- inguinal herniation
- inadequate phallus in males with subsequent social and psychological sequelae.

Potential complications (associated with management of exstrophy):
- malignancy (related to the use of intestine in bladder reconstruction or for urinary diversion)
- urinary tract infection
- urinary tract obstruction
- uterine prolapse
- severe penile shortening with dorsal chordee
- inadequate bladder emptying
- urinary incontinence
- urinary calculi
- kidney damage

Natural history of exstrophy

Because the bladder exstrophy–epispadias complex is not a lethal anomaly, children with bladder exstrophy or epispadias can survive untreated. Before the modern era of surgery and anesthesia, this was the rule. These children are often quite intelligent, with many achieving postgraduate education degrees. Reports exist of such patients with classic bladder exstrophy living into their eighth decade (O'Kane and Megaw, 1968). In contrast, until recently patients born with cloacal exstrophy died shortly after birth from electrolyte abnormalities and malnutrition due to the short small intestine.

Because bladder exstrophy is a serious anomaly, the morbidity experienced by these patients was often severe and included the problems noted above. Patients left untreated covered the exposed bladder with a variety of undergarments, including linament-soaked rags or cotton and wool bolsters. In addition to the problems listed above, the surrounding skin around the exstrophic bladder was often inflamed secondary to urine contact dermatitis, loss of skin integrity from constant wetness, and secondary infection. These patients were often social pariahs because of the odor and hygiene problems. Up to the nineteenth century, many considered bladder exstrophy irreparable, as evidenced by these comments:

> Exstrophy of the bladder, unless the patient is willing to assume the (often mortal) risk of an autoplastic operation, is utterly irremediable; all that can be done is to palliate the patient's suffering by attention to cleanliness, and by the use of a closely-fitting flexible gutta-percha shield, furnished with a gum-elastic bottle for receiving urine ... When this cannot be obtained, the part must be kept constantly covered with a thick, soft compress, renewed as often as it becomes wet and disagreeable. The skin around may be protected, if necessary, with pomatum, simple cerate, or zinc treatment (Gross, 1876).

Early attempts at surgical reconstruction

The morbidity of exstrophy led surgeons to begin empiric approaches to the operative correction of this anomaly. Surgeons in the nineteenth century attempted urinary reconstructive or diversion procedures to treat these patients. Initial efforts were directed at partial reconstruction of the abdominal wall to allow the application of a urinary receptacle to collect urine. The first successful record of this form of repair is attributed to Dr Pancoast in 1859. He used skin flaps from the abdominal wall:

> In the treatment of exstrophy of the bladder the principal objects aimed at are either to establish a channel for the conveyance of the urine to the rectum or perineum, or to cover its exposed and sensitive mucus membrane with flaps of skin, thereby protecting it from contact of the clothing, and preventing excoriation of the surrounding parts, as well as facilitating the adjustment of an apparatus for receiving the urine (Gross, 1876).
>
> A flap is taken from one side of the abdomen or groin, dissected up, and turned over like the leaf of a book so that the epidermis comes into contact with the mucous membrane. A second flap is then taken from the groin on the opposite side and its raw surface applied to the raw surface of the former flap ... thus a thick bridge is formed over the cleft (Coulson, 1881).

Drs Wood and Maury also described variations on the use of skin flaps to reconstruct the abdominal wall (Wood, 1869; Gross, 1876). Wood used a full-thickness skin graft from the abdominal wall followed by a lateral, pyriform flap from each groin held in place with hare-lip pins, wire sutures, and broad straps of adhesive plaster which were removed 6–8

days after surgery (Fig. 27.11). In contrast, Maury created perineal and scrotal skin flaps to repair bladder exstrophy. These procedures represented early attempts at anatomic closure but did not address the functional reconstruction of these bladders, namely to achieve satisfactory storage and emptying of urine. Van Buren aptly stated the common sentiment of the time:

> The most that can be promised by operative interference is to leave behind a fistula, more or less large, over which a urinal must be constantly worn. The patient's virility is not returned to him, nor is his condition very materially bettered. A less dangerous and equally efficacious mode of treatment seems to be to adapt a suitable urinal to the parts as they are left by Nature, such a one as shall shield them from injury, and keep the patient dry and clean (Van Buren and Keyes, 1874).

Others, such as Simon, approached the surgical treatment by attempting urinary diversion in these patients through the creation of a ureteral sigmoid fistula. Results were poor; one patient died of peritonitis in the immediate postoperative period and the other died of renal failure secondary to chronic pyelonephritis (Gross, 1876).

These early efforts suffered from lack of understanding of the physiology of the urinary tract and bladder and subsequently how these operations would affect urine storage and emptying, kidney function, electrolyte homeostasis, the propensity for urinary tract infection (UTI) or calculus formation, fertility, and sexual

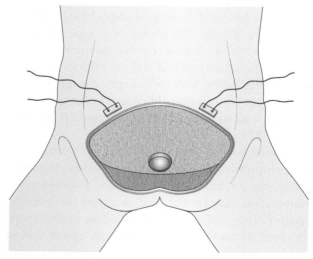

Figure 27.11 Early operation for bladder exstrophy as proposed by Maury in the mid-nineteenth century.

function. Complications from these operations were often life threatening. That patients were willing to assume this risk in the treatment of this anomaly demonstrates the impact that it had on their lives.

The modern era: operative procedures in the management of exstrophy

Despite the innumerable operations that have been applied to the treatment of exstrophy, operations for exstrophy fall largely into two categories. The first group includes operations designed to remove the exstrophic bladder and replace it with a form of urinary diversion. The second group includes reconstructive procedures designed to reconstruct the bladder either in multiple stages or in a single stage.

Perioperative care of the patient with exstrophy

Preoperative care

To prevent trauma to the exposed bladder plate after delivery, the umbilical cord should be ligated with silk suture rather than a plastic or metal clamp. The authors routinely cover the exstrophic bladder with a hydrated gel dressing such as Vigilon. This dressing protects the bladder plate effectively and allows handling of the infant with minimal risk of trauma to the bladder. In some circumstances, this dressing has been used for over 2 months with minimal inflammation of the bladder noted at the time of total primary repair. If a hydrated dressing is unavailable, covering the exposed bladder with plastic wrap, especially during transportation, is an acceptable alternative. Either dressing should be replaced and the bladder irrigated with normal saline with each diaper change. Others advocate the use of a humidified air incubator with no dressing at all to minimize bladder trauma (Churchill et al., 1997).

Routine use of intravenous antibiotic therapy in the preoperative and postoperative period decreases the chance for infection. In addition, a sonographic examination may be obtained to assess the kidneys preoperatively and to establish a baseline examination for later ultrasonographic studies. A spinal sonographic examination should be performed if sacral dimpling or other signs of spina bifida are noted on physical examination.

Operative considerations

In the newborn period, primary exstrophy closure is performed using general inhalation anesthesia. The use of nitrous oxide during primary closure is inadvisable because it may cause bowel and peritoneal distension. This reduces surgical exposure during the operation and increases the risk of primary wound dehiscence due to bowel distension. Gearhart (1999) uses a nasogastric tube to decrease abdominal distension in the postoperative period. The present authors do not use nasogastric suction in most patients but routinely use a one-time caudal block to reduce the anesthetic requirement during the operation.

For patients older than 3 days or with a wide pubic diastasis, osteotomies are used in the majority of cases to facilitate closure and increase the chance of later urinary continence (Aadalen et al., 1980; Ben-Chaim et al., 1995b).

Postoperative considerations

One can apply a variety of methods to stabilize pelvic ring closure following bladder closure. A spica cast may be used for 3 weeks to prevent external hip rotation and optimize pubic apposition (Fig. 27.12). Modified Buck's traction may also be used in the postoperative period for 4 weeks. The newborn is fitted with a 'sled' to be used when the child is out of traction for feeding and bathing in this situation. The authors do not advocate Buck's traction because this makes performing daily activities and routine care difficult. An external fixation device also provides satis-

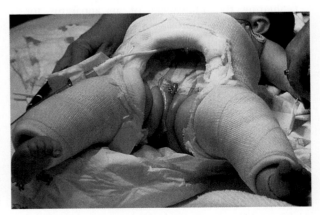

Figure 27.12 Use of a spica cast following complete primary repair for exstrophy to reduce tension on the closure by preventing hip abduction in the postoperative period.

factory immobilization. Fixator pins for these devices should be cleaned several times a day to reduce the risk of infection. If the pins become loose, a cast should be applied, or the patient placed in traction. 'Mummy wrapping' to immobilize the pelvis is unreliable (Gearhart, 1999).

Because of the high incidence of vesicoureteral reflux (VUR), low-dose antibiotic therapy should be prescribed in all babies after bladder closure to prevent pyelonephritis. This is continued until the reflux is corrected or resolves spontaneously.

Postoperative factors recognized to increase the success of the initial reconstruction include:

- use of osteotomies (in selected cases) or non-newborn closure (>24–48 h);
- postoperative immobilization;
- use of postoperative antibiotics;
- ureteral stenting catheters;
- adequate postoperative pain management;
- avoidance of abdominal distension;
- adequate nutritional support;
- secure fixation of urinary drainage catheters.

Anatomic reconstruction of exstrophy

The first efforts at anatomic reconstruction of the exstrophic bladder are usually attributed to Trendelenberg (1906). In 1881 he described an exstrophy closure emphasizing the importance of pubic reapproximation in front of the reconstructed bladder to achieve continence and prevent dehiscence. This effort ultimately proved unsuccessful. Because of discouraging results such as this, bladder reconstruction was largely abandoned and replaced by urinary diversion, most notably ureterosigmoidostomy, in the early part of the twentieth century.

Not all attempts at bladder reconstruction for exstrophy were abandoned. Various surgeons reported occasional successful attempts during this time. However, these results were uncommon and difficult to reproduce. For example, Young (1942) reported the first successful primary bladder closure. He achieved urinary continence in a young girl. Primary reconstructive efforts by others remained inconsistent and largely unsuccessful during this period. Since Young's successful report in 1942, other investigators intermittently achieved a satisfactory result with a one-stage reconstructive effort to repair the exstrophied bladder. Ansell (1971) reported a one-stage

closure with a successful outcome in a newborn female. Ansell (1979) was also one of the early advocates for primary closure of bladder exstrophy in the newborn period and reported 28 babies closed in this fashion. Montagnani (1982) described a one-stage functional bladder reconstruction in two female babies aged 8 and 13 months. His procedure included inominate osteotomy, bladder closure, an antireflux procedure, and narrowing of the bladder outlet followed by pubic reapproximation. Continence was achieved in one of the patients. The second patient required further bladder neck reconstruction to achieve continence. Fuchs et al. (1996) achieved urinary continence in eight of 15 patients whose problem was also approached in a single-stage effort. However, several large series of patients who underwent single-stage reconstruction in the 1960s and 1970s reported continence rates of only 10–30% (Ezell and Carlson, 1970; King and Wendel, 1972; Engel, 1973; Megalli and Lattimer, 1973; Williams and Keeton, 1973; Johnston and Kogan, 1974). Renal damage was as high as 90% in these series, generally because of bladder outlet obstruction (King and Wendel, 1972).

Because of these complications and the low rate of urinary continence, reconstructive surgical efforts were subsequently directed towards staged bladder reconstruction, an approach pioneered and advocated by Jeffs as well as others (Jeffs, 1977; Saltzman et al., 1985). More recently, new techniques of single-stage reconstruction for exstrophy have been advocated by Mitchell, Fuchs, Kelly, and others. Continence rates in these series approach or equal those reported in series of patients whose defect is closed using staged surgical reconstruction (Fuchs et al., 1996; Grady et al., 1999).

Complete primary repair for exstrophy

Complete primary reconstruction of the exstrophied bladder is best done in the newborn period. Primary reconstruction then is technically easier than in an older child. It also offers theoretical advantages as it may maximize the opportunity for 'normal' bladder development and the potential for urinary continence. The bony pelvis remains pliable in the newborn period so that osteotomies may be avoided in some cases, usually if closure can be performed within the first 72 hours of life.

The authors' experience with early ablation of posterior urethral valves (PUV) suggests that early restoration of non-obstructive emptying and filling of the bladder allows the bladder to regain some or all of its normal physiologic and developmental potential (Mitchell and Close, 1996; Close *et al.*, 1997; Close, 1999). This, in turn, implies that the bladder progresses through developmental milestones that occur in the first few months of life and which may be irreversibly lost if missed. Precedence for this form of organ development is noted in the brain with the acquisition of language and visual perception. Finally, early primary bladder reconstruction creates a more normal appearing baby, thus fostering improved bonding between parents and infant.

Grady and Mitchell (1998, 1999) advocated the complete primary repair, or Mitchell technique, in this period. This technique moves the bladder, bladder neck, and urethra posteriorly within the pelvis. This repositions the proximal urethra within the pelvic diaphragm in an anatomically more normal position to maximize the effect of the pelvic muscles and support structures for the achievement of urinary continence. Posterior movement of the bladder neck and urethra also facilitates reapproximation of the pubic symphysis which, in turn, helps to prevent anterior migration of the urethra and bladder neck and provides a more anatomically normal muscular pelvic diaphragm.

By employing total penile disassembly as part of the exstrophy closure, this repair also reduces anterior tension on the urethra because the urethra is separated from its attachments to the underlying corporeal bodies. These attachments otherwise pull the urethral plate anteriorly, preventing posterior placement of the proximal urethra and bladder neck in the pelvis. Tension reduction decreases the risk of bladder dehiscence and also reduces dorsal pull on the corporeal bodies that may contribute to dorsal chordee in males. Combining the epispadias repair with primary closure allows the most important aspect of primary closure, i.e. division of the intersymphyseal ligament or band located posterior to the urethra in these patients. In order to divide this ligament, the urethral plate must be separated from the corpora cavernosa.

Neonatal closure using this technique optimizes the chance for early bladder cycling and consequent normal bladder development. It may also obviate the need for a multistaged repair of the exstrophic bladder including further bladder neck reconstruction, bladder augmentation, and penile reconstructive surgery.

Technique for primary reconstruction

Before starting the dissection, 3.5 Fr umbilical artery catheters are placed into both ureters and sutured in place with 5.0 chromic suture (Fig. 27.13). Initial dissection is directed at separating the bladder plate from the adjacent skin (Fig. 27.14). This dissection is then carried inferiorly. Fine-tip electrocautery (Colorado tip) may be used for this dissection. To aid in dissection, traction sutures are placed into each hemiglans of the penis. These sutures are initially oriented transversely in the hemiglans. They will rotate to a parallel vertical orientation as the corporeal bodies rotate medially after dissection of the corporeal bod-

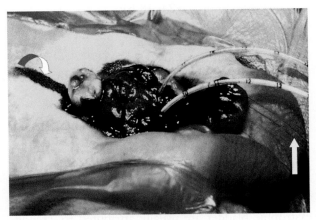

Figure 27.13 Markings indicate lines of initial dissection. The curved arrow indicates where the incision is carried above the vessels of the cord so that the umbilicus can be constructed superiorly. Straight white arrows demonstrate stay sutures in the hemiglans of the penis.

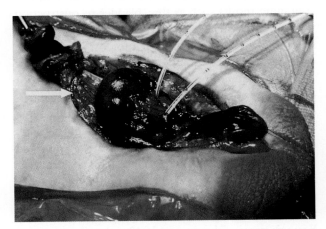

Figure 27.14 Dissection is initiated superiorly and extended inferiorly to circumscribe the bladder plate and urethra completely. The bladder and urethra are considered a single unit.

ies and urethral wedge (urethral plate plus underlying corpora spongiosa) from each other. This repair precludes division of the proximal urethral wedge since this would devascularize the more distal urethra. Fortunately, because the bladder and urethra are moved posteriorly in the pelvis as a unit, division of the urethral wedge is not required. However, in some cases, because the urethra is too short, a male patient will be left with a hypospadias that will require later surgical reconstruction. With the urethral wedge left intact, one can also avoid the use of paraexstrophy skin flaps used to lengthen the urethra, which can result in an irregular tortuous urethra that may make subsequent urethral catheterization and cystoscopy difficult.

The penile dissection begins along the ventral aspect of the penis as a circumcising incision (Fig. 27.15). This should precede dissection of the urethral wedge from the corporeal bodies because it is easier to identify Buck's fascia ventrally. The plane of dissection is between Buck's fascia and the overlying tissue. Staining the plate with methylene blue or brilliant green facilitates dissection of the urethral wedge. Injection of the surrounding tissues with 0.25% lidocaine and 1:200 000 U/ml epinephrine also improves hemostasis and assists the dissection. One should take care not to narrow the urethral wedge as this will be tubularized later. Urethral wedge dissection is carried proximally to the bladder neck. Careful dissection of the lateral penile shaft skin and dartos fascia from the corporeal bodies is paramount since the neurovascular bundles are usually located in this lateral position on the corpora (Woodhouse and Kellett, 1984).

As described by Mitchell and Bagli (1996), the penis is disassembled into three components: the right and left corporeal bodies with their respective hemiglans, and the urethral wedge (urothelium with underlying corpora spongiosa) (Fig. 27.16). This dissection is easiest to initiate proximally and ventrally. The plane of dissection should be at the level of the tunica albuginea on the corpora. Once a plane is created between the urethral wedge and the corporeal bodies, the dissection is extended distally to separate the three components from each other completely. The hemiglans may be completely separated from each other since they depend on a separate blood supply based on the paired, lateral neurovascular bundles. It is important to keep the underlying corpora spongiosum with the urethral plate; the blood supply to the urethral plate is based on this corporeal tissue, which should appear wedge shaped after its dissection from the underlying corpora cavernosa. This urethral/corporeal spongiosal component will later be tubularized and placed *ventral* to the corporeal bodies.

Proximal dissection of the urethral wedge away from the corporeal bodies is critical to the posterior placement of the bladder neck and proximal urethra. Division of the intersymphyseal ligaments posterior to the urethral wedge is absolutely necessary to allow the bladder to achieve a posterior position in the pelvis. Failure to dissect the bladder and urethral wedge adequately from these surrounding structures will cause anterior tension along the urethral plate and prevent posterior movement of the bladder in the pelvis.

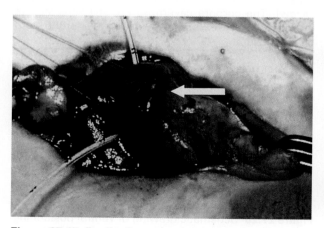

Figure 27.15 Penile dissection begins ventrally. A ventral incision is made at the base of the glans penis as a circumcising incision (*arrow*). This is carried dorsally.

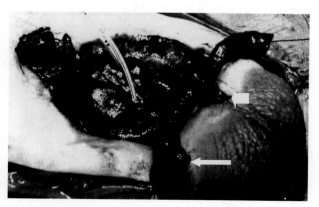

Figure 27.16 Separation of the corporeal bodies (*narrow arrow*) from each other and the urethral wedge (*wide arrow*). This dissection is then carried proximally to separate the proximal corpora from the bulbar urethra.

Once the bladder and urethral wedge are adequately dissected from the surrounding tissues, they can be closed. Prior to reapproximating the bladder, a suprapubic tube is placed and brought out superiorly. A primary closure of the bladder may then be performed using a three-layer closure with monofilament absorbable suture (Monocryl). The urethra is tubularized using a two-layer running closure with monofilament suture (Figs. 27.17, 27.18). The authors have not performed ureteral reimplantation at this time, although this may be considered.

The pubic symphysis is then reapproximated using 0.0 polydiaxonone interrupted sutures (Fig. 27.19). Knots are placed anterior to prevent suture erosion into the bladder neck. Rectus fascia is reapproximated using a running 2.0 polydiaxonone suture. The tubularized urethra is located ventral to the corporeal bodies following pubic reapproximation (Fig. 27.20).

The corporeal bodies will tend to rotate medially; this rotation assists in correcting the dorsal chordee and can be readily appreciated by observing the vertical lie of the previously horizontally placed glans traction sutures. Occasionally, significant discrepancies in the dorsal and ventral lengths of the corpora will require dorsal dermal graft insertion. However, this is rarely needed in newborns. The corpora are reapproximated with fine interrupted sutures along their dorsal aspect.

The urethra can then be brought between each hemiglans ventrally to create an orthotopic meatus. The glans is reconfigured using interrupted mattress sutures of polydiaxonone suture (PDS) followed by horizontal mattress sutures of 7.0 monofilament suture (Maxxon) to reapproximate the glans epithelium. The neourethral meatus is matured with 7.0 braided polyglactin suture (Vicryl) as in a standard hypospadias repair. Some glans tissue is usually removed dorsally to create a conical appearing glans. Occasionally, the urethra is too short to reach the

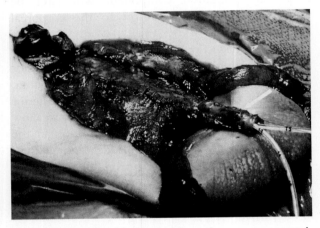

Figure 27.17 The bladder and urethra are reapproximated using running absorbable suture material.

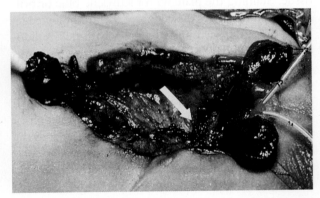

Figure 27.19 Reapproximation of pubis symphysis (*arrow*). The corpora cavernosa are still separated at this point. Penile reassembly takes place after the symphysis closure.

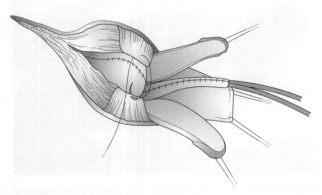

Figure 27.18 Schematic drawing of bladder and urethral closure demonstrating the continuity of these structures.

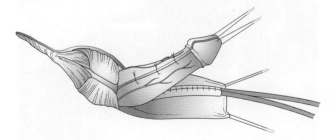

Figure 27.20 Schematic drawing of ventral positioning of the urethra. This allows the bladder and urethra to be positioned posteriorly in an anatomically more normal location.

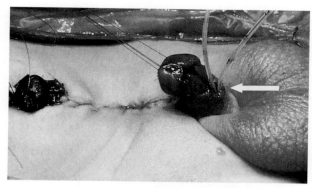

Figure 27.21 White arrow indicates midshaft hypospadias after complete primary exstrophy repair.

glans. In this situation the urethra may be matured along the ventral aspect of the penis to produce a hypospadias (Fig. 27.21). This can be corrected at a later date as a second-stage procedure. Redundant shaft skin may be left ventrally for later penile reconstructive procedures.

The penile shaft skin is reconfigured using either a primary dorsal closure or reversed Byars flaps if needed to provide dorsal skin coverage. The skin covering the abdominal wall is approximated using a two-layer running closure of absorbable monofilament suture.

Staged reconstruction for exstrophy

In contrast to the high rate of renal damage reported from multiple centers using a single-stage reconstructive effort to close bladder exstrophy in the 1970s, results from a staged reconstruction approach appeared significantly better at that time. Jeffs and colleagues reviewed their results with staged reconstruction and noted normal upper urinary tracts in 87% (DeMaria *et al.*, 1980). Later studies from Johns Hopkins also reported low rates of renal damage (12% and 17% respectively) (Lepor and Jeffs, 1983; Oesterling and Jeffs, 1987).

Urinary continence rates after single-stage closure in the 1960s and 1970s were not consistent. Continence ranged from 0 to 45% with an average of 17% (Ezell and Carlson, 1970; Marshall and Muecke, 1970; Cendron, 1971; King and Wendel, 1972; Engel, 1973; Megalli and Lattimer, 1973; Williams and Keeton, 1973; Johnston and Kogan, 1974). In contrast, staged efforts by Jeffs and others resulted in continence rates of 60–88% (Cendron and Mollard, 1971; Jeffs, 1977; Mollard, 1980; Mesrobian *et al.*,

1988; Ritchey *et al.*, 1988; Connor *et al.*, 1989; Gearhart and Jeffs, 1989; Husmann *et al.*, 1989) (Fig. 27.22). These results prompted a shift from single-stage reconstruction to planned multiple-stage reconstruction in the treatment of bladder exstrophy. Planned staged reconstruction (the Jeffs technique) subsequently became the standard approach.

Others using the staged approach for exstrophy reconstruction have generally noted lower rates of urinary continence, as low as 9%, with the need for clean intermittent catheterization (CIC) to achieve continence in as many as 60% of these patients (Hollowell *et al.*, 1993; Jones *et al.*, 1993; Woodhouse and Redgrave, 1996). These series reflect the variable success of staged reconstruction. Conversion rates from such reconstructive efforts to urinary diversion range from 7.4 to 59.4% (Mesrobian *et al.*, 1988; Mollard *et al.*, 1994; Woodhouse and Redgrave, 1996).

As currently employed, the staged approach to bladder exstrophy reconstruction includes:

- initial bladder closure, ideally in the newborn period;
- epispadias repair, usually performed at 12–18 months of age but may be combined with initial bladder closure;
- bladder neck reconstruction, usually performed at 4–5 years of age or when age appropriate for toilet training and bladder capacity adequate (>60 ml).

Factors to consider with staged reconstruction

Initial bladder closure

A number of factors can impact the ability to achieve urinary reconstruction via bladder reconstruction in exstrophy patients. These include:

- primary failure (dehiscence) of the initial bladder closure;
- outlet obstruction;
- bladder prolapse;
- chronic urinary tract infection.

Failure of the initial closure, in particular, significantly decreases the chance for eventual continence with volitional voiding (Lowe and Jeffs, 1983; Gearhart *et al.*, 1996). Gearhart *et al.* (1993c) reported that only 40% of patients after a failed primary closure attempt will ultimately achieve a bladder capacity adequate for

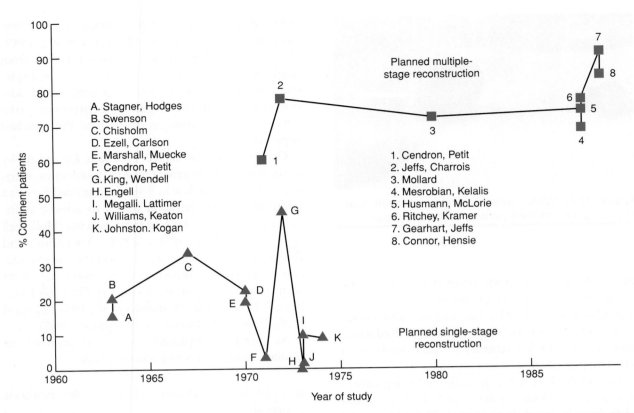

Figure 27.22 Historical data on continence rates in planned multiple-stage versus planned single-stage reconstruction. (Adapted from Churchill *et al.*, 1997, with permission.)

bladder neck reconstruction. If more than two closure attempts are required, chances for continence decrease to below 20% (Gearhart *et al.*, 1996). The initial closure must be performed to prevent bladder prolapse but avoid outlet obstruction. The use of osteotomies and postoperative immobilization improves the success of initial bladder closure as well as the postoperative factors listed above.

Technique for initial bladder closure

Ureteral catheters are placed to aid in ureteral visualization prior to making the initial incision. These may be secured with 5-0 or 6-0 chromic suture. Dissection begins with a circumferential incision around the bladder plate (Fig. 27.23). This can be initiated at the umbilicus. The underlying detrusor muscle is mobilized from the rectus sheath to expose the peritoneum. Extraperitoneal dissection lateral to the bladder exposes the retroperitoneal space and identifies the intersymphyseal band. This band should be transected to allow the bladder and bladder neck to be placed deep into the pelvis. After a suprapubic tube

has been placed, the bladder is closed in the midline in multiple layers with a running 3-0 absorbable suture. The posterior urethra is also closed at the base of the penis over a 14 Fr catheter. To reapproximate the pubis symphysis, 0 PDS or no. 2 Nylon suture may be used. The authors recommend PDS using a figure-of-eight suture with the knot placed anteriorly to prevent erosion into the bladder. The umbilicus may be used as the site to bring the urinary drainage catheters out to the skin.

Osteotomies

Trendelenberg first recognized the importance of osteotomies in exstrophy closure at the turn of the century. Osteotomies optimize pubic symphysis apposition and anatomic positioning of the bladder, bladder neck, and urethra in the pelvis. This also improves the reapproximation of the corporeal and clitoral bodies. Finally, osteotomies may decrease the risk of later uterine prolapse because the anterior closure brings the pelvic diaphragm into a more normal anatomic position to offer more support.

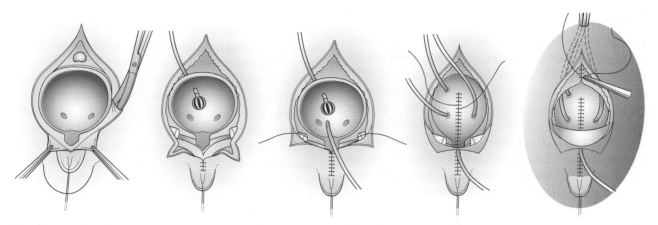

Figure 27.23 Primary bladder closure. These diagrams demonstrate the sequence of initial bladder closure in a staged repair for bladder exstrophy in the male patient. From left to right: (1) completion of dissection around the bladder and urethral plate; (2) placement of a suprapubic drainage tube after corporal reapproximation; (3) tubularization of the urethral plate over the catheter; (4) following two-layer closure of the bladder and urethral plate, the bladder is reduced in the pelvis and fixed with sutures; (5) drainage tubes are brought out superiorly and the fascia, subcutaneous tissue, and skin are reapproximated. (Adapted from Brock and O'Neill, 1998, with permission.)

The need for osteotomy is best determined under general anesthesia. Candidates for osteotomy include those more than 72 hours old, newborns with a wide pubic diastasis, newborns with cloacal exstrophy, and patients who have had a previously failed closure. Osteotomies are usually performed at the same setting as bladder closure to help to secure the closure.

Osteotomies may be performed by an anterior or posterior approach or in combination. Posterior iliac osteotomies are performed with the patient in a prone position, dividing the iliacs about 1 cm lateral to the sacroiliac joints. The patient is then repositioned for the bladder closure. Anterior iliac osteotomies offer the advantage of a single position and sterile field (Figs. 27.24, 27.25). Compared with posterior iliac osteotomies, an anterior approach has also been shown to result in less blood loss and better apposition and mobility of the pubic rami. The group at Johns Hopkins uses combined anterior innominate and vertical iliac osteotomies because of superior initial and long-term results when compared with anterior iliac osteotomies alone (Sponseller *et al.*, 1991). Both osteotomies may be performed through the same anterior skin incisions. McKenna *et al.* (1994) also described the use of a diagonal mid-iliac osteotomy performed through the same incision as the exstrophy closure. Division of the superior pubic ramus has also been described; this is not as effective as the other methods when used alone but may be utilized in newborns (Schmidt *et al.*, 1993; Frey, 1996).

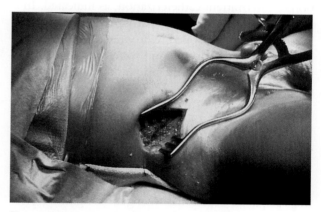

Figure 27.24 Photograph demonstrating exposure of the bony pelvis for anterior iliac osteotomy.

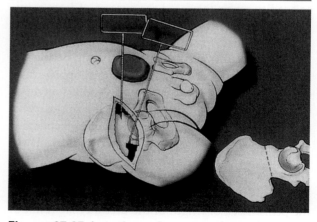

Figure 27.25 Location of an anterior osteotomy, performed here with a Gigli saw. (Adapted from Brock and O'Neill, 1998, with permission.)

Urinary outlet obstruction

Urinary outlet obstruction is diagnosed when post-void residuals are significant, especially when greater than one-half the actual bladder capacity. Outlet obstruction increases the risk of renal damage, especially if unrecognized for several months or more (Husmann *et al.*, 1990b). Obstruction increases the risk of UTI, as well as potentially raising bladder storage pressures to dangerous levels as well as decreasing the chances for urinary continence. The bladder outlet following initial bladder closure should be assessed with sounds or bougies 4–6 weeks after closure to detect obstruction. Routine sonography of the bladder and upper urinary tracts should also be performed 3 months after closure to detect hydronephrosis that may indicate obstruction. Evidence of hydronephrosis in combination with high postvoid residual urine volumes requires further evaluation with cystoscopy and urethral dilation or the institution of intermittent catheterization, as indicated. In a review of 68 patients at Toronto Sick Children's Hospital, 23% developed hydroureteronephrosis following the initial closure and were then successfully treated with dilation of the bladder outlet or the institution of CIC (Husmann *et al.*, 1990b).

Epispadias repair

Since the initial description by Jeffs of the staged reconstructive approach to exstrophy, the timing of the epispadias repair has changed. Originally, Jeffs advocated epispadias repair as the last stage of reconstruction. However, he later recognized that earlier epispadias repair increased the success of later continence procedures by stimulating bladder growth and increasing bladder capacity (Gearhart and Jeffs, 1989). Epispadias repair is now typically performed at 12–18 months of age when a staged approach to extrophy repair has been employed. Various methods can be used. These include Cantwell–Ransley techniques and their modifications or complete penile disassembly (Mitchell technique) or its variants. These procedures are discussed in more detail below. Both employ dissection of the corporeal bodies and transposition of the urethral plate to the ventral aspect of the penis. Lack of length of the urethra may result in hypospadias with either of these techniques. This can be corrected later in a variety of ways using operations described for hypospadias repair.

More recently, Gearhart and colleagues have adopted a single-stage approach and reported on combining bladder closure and epispadias repair in 15 boys. They performed this combined approach as the initial procedure for one boy and used it as a salvage procedure in 14 boys who had previous closure failures. They found that combining a repeat bladder closure with epispadias repair optimized the use of osteotomies and was as successful as staging these operations. Furthermore, two boys who underwent combined repair became continent without further bladder neck reconstruction. They now recommend combined bladder closure and epispadias repair as the preferred management of patients who have had previously failed bladder closure (Gearhart *et al.*, 1998). Some surgeons use topical or intramuscular testosterone to increase the size of the phallus prior to performing the epispadias repair (Gearhart, 1998; Perovic *et al.*, 1999).

Techniques for epispadias repair

The goals of epispadias repair include achieving a straight penis and urethra, easy urethral catheterization, normal erectile function, and a cosmetically satisfactory phallus. These goals allow the patient to stand while voiding and to have intromission during intercourse. Epispadias repair can prove challenging and a variety of surgical procedures have been devised to correct this anomaly. Two of the more successful and popular procedures are described below.

Modified Cantwell–Ransley repair

Cantwell (1895) first described mobilization of the urethra, moving it ventrally for epispadias repair. Ransley subsequently modified this technique and reported on his results in 1988 (Ransley and Woppin, 1988) (Fig. 27.26). To begin this procedure, a stay suture is placed into the glans penis. A reverse MAGPI (meatal advancement-glanuloplasty) or IPGAM procedure at the distal urethral plate allows advancement of the urethral meatus onto the glans. Following this, skin incisions are made on the lateral edges of the urethral plate and around the epispadic meatus. The plate is dissected from the corporeal bodies up to the level of the glans distally and to the prostatic urethra proximally. Glanular wings should be developed distally as well. The corporeal bodies are then separated from each other. This allows them to be rotated medially. The urethra is then tubularized over a 6 or 8 Fr urethral catheter, using running 6-0 absorbable sutures. The corporeal bodies are rotated over and above the urethra and reapproximated using 5-0 absorbable sutures in an interrupted fashion. Cavernocavernosotomies may be performed prior to reappproximating the corporeal bodies to help to correct persistent chordee. These are performed at the point of maximal angulation. The neurovascular bundles may require mobilization to avoid injury if cavernosotomies are performed. The glans wings are then closed over the urethra using interrupted 5-0 absorbable sutures. Penile shaft skin can be trimmed and tailored to cover the penis using interrupted 5-0 or 6-0 absorbable sutures. Z-plasties at the level of the pubis decrease the risk of a dorsal retractile scar at the base of the penis. A recent review of this technique in 40 patients revealed a successful anatomic and functional result in 90% at a mean follow-up period of 3 years (Lottman and Mellin, 1999). Complications requiring further procedure occurred in 45% and were more common in patients who underwent this procedure as part of a staged exstophy closure as compared with isolated epispadias repair.

Complete penile disassembly

The authors have exclusively used the complete penile disassembly or the Mitchell technique for epispadias repair since 1989. Mitchell and Bagli reported their results in 1996. Complete penile disassembly offers several advantages over the modified Cantwell–Ransley technique. The planes of dissection extend anatomically to the bladder neck. This facilitates its use with bladder neck reconstruction. Complete mobilization of the urethral wedge from the corporeal bodies by disassembly also creates a more normal appearance of the penis by allowing ventral placement of the urethra (Figs. 27.27–27.29). A detailed description of the surgical technique is included in the section on complete primary repair of exstrophy above. Zaontz *et al.* (1998) reported on a multicenter experience using this technique and found that 16/17 boys had straight erections following repair. Three patients developed pinpoint fistulae, of which two closed spontaneously. Perovic *et al.* (1999) have described variants of this technique for epispadias that may be used in selected circumstances.

Bladder neck reconstruction

With a staged approach to exstrophy repair, bladder neck reconstruction is performed when the child is at an appropriate age for toilet training. This is typically

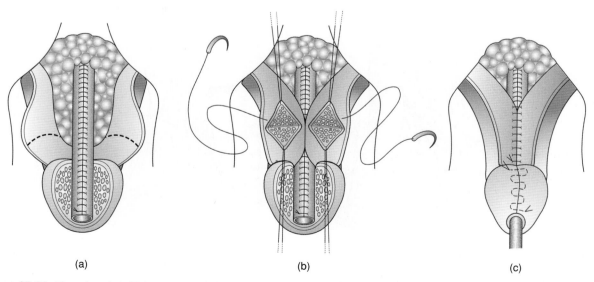

(a) (b) (c)

Figure 27.26 Line drawing illustrating the steps for the Cantwell–Ransley repair for espispadias. (*a*) The tubularized urethral plate is placed in a dorsal groove incision in the glans penis. The dotted lines indicate the site of incision for the cavernosa–cavernosotomies; (*b*) approximation of the corpora cavernosa and performance of cavernosal anastamosis; (*c*) glans closure over urethra and skin closure. (Adapted from Brock and O'Neill, 1998, with permission.)

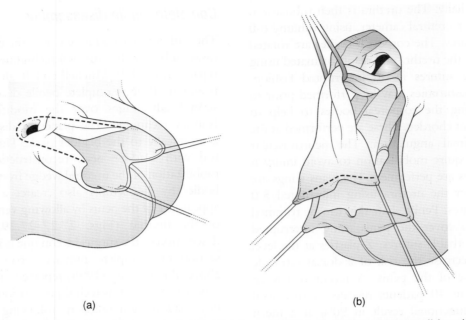

(a)   (b)

Figure 27.27 Complete penile disassembly technique. (*a*) lines of initial dissection circumscribing the urethral plate and bladder neck. (*b*) Careful dissection of the urethra from the underlying corporeal bodies. Dotted line indicates the site of distal incision to free the urethra entirely from the glans. (Adapted from Mitchell and Bagli, 1996, with permission.)

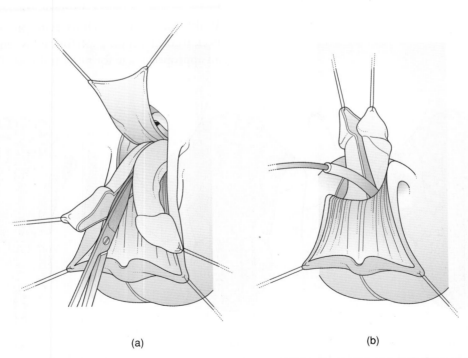

(a)   (b)

Figure 27.28 Complete penile disassembly technique. (*a*) Corporeal bodies and two hemiglans are separated by a longitudinal midline incision. (*b*) The urethra is tubularized and brought to the ventrum. The corpora are reapproximated dorsally. They will rotate medially when adequately dissected from each other. (Adapted from Mitchell and Bagli, 1996, with permission.)

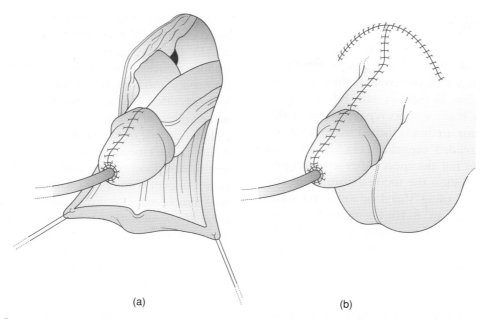

(a) (b)

Figure 27.29 Complete penile disassembly technique. (*a*) Completion of urethral meatus; (*b*) completion of shaft skin coverage. (Adapted from Mitchell and Bagli, 1996, with permission.)

at 4–5 years of age. Advocates of staged reconstruction emphasize the importance of achieving adequate bladder capacity prior to performing bladder neck reconstruction. A bladder capacity less than 60 ml under anesthesia or during urodynamic evaluation decreases the success of bladder neck reconstruction (Jeffs *et al.*, 1982; Lepor and Jeffs, 1983). Factors that increase the potential for the bladder to achieve adequate capacity prior to bladder neck reconstruction include:

- avoidance of UTIs;
- complete bladder emptying with institution of CIC if bladder emptying is incomplete;
- epispadias repair;
- avoidance of bladder prolapse (Churchill *et al.*, 1997).

To reconstruct the bladder neck for exstrophy most surgeons employ a Young–Dees or a Leadbetter approach or a combination of these techniques. They are described in detail below. Neoureterocystostomy may be required at the time of bladder neck reconstruction to correct VUR and to move the ureters from the lower bladder where bladder neck reconstruction will use some of the bladder base to form the new bladder neck. The Cohen technique is often used. However, others have described a cephalotrigonal technique that is particularly applicable because of the angle of ureteral entry into the exstrophic bladder (Canning *et al.*, 1993). The Marshall–Marchetti–Kranz bladder neck suspension or a bladder neck wrap using rectus muscle or fascia or gracilis may be combined with bladder neck reconstruction as well. Bladder neck reconstruction requires adequate bladder capacity because detrusor volume is reduced.

Preoperative assessment

Following a careful history and physical examination, cystourethroscopy is performed before open bladder neck reconstruction. Cystoscopy provides information regarding bladder capacity and the status of any previous repairs, including correction of epispadias.

Urodynamic evaluation should also be considered because it allows preoperative detection of detrusor hyperactivity or atony as well as assessment of functional bladder capacity and leak point pressures. However, the urethra of these patients may be difficult to catheterize. In these situations the cystourethroscopic examination may be combined with suprapubic placement of a urodynamic catheter to be used later that day for the urodynamic evaluation.

Mitchell repair

This repair uses a modification of the Leadbetter procedure (Jones *et al.*, 1993). The authors currently use this modification as their preferred method of bladder neck reconstruction in patients with bladder exstrophy who require bladder outlet repair. In this modification the anterior urethra is incised transversely and the incision extended cephalad (Fig. 27.30). The incision is made full thickness. After cross-trigonal ureteral reimplantation the urethral strip is tubularized in two layers using Vicryl or monocryl suture (4-0 or 5-0) over an 8–10 Fr urethral catheter, depending on the size of the patient. The bladder may be closed in continuity with the urethral closure. This procedure effectively narrows and lengthens the urethra. It also moves fibrotic tissue at the level of the original bladder neck away from the new bladder neck. Following the closure, circumferential dissection around the new bladder neck may be performed if a combined bladder neck wrap or sling will be placed simultaneously.

Postoperatively, urine is drained through a combination of ureteral stents, a suprapubic tube, and a 6 Fr (Kendall) urethral catheter. The urethral catheter is removed 7–10 days after the operation. Ureteral stents are removed 10–14 days after surgery. The suprapubic tube remains for 3 weeks. The tube should be clamped before removal and postvoid residual urine volumes measured to assess for urinary retention before removing the suprapubic tube. As with any bladder neck reconstruction procedure (without augmentation), several months of adjustment will be required before the patient develops adequate bladder awareness, capacity, and control to achieve prolonged intervals of urinary continence.

Occasionally, trigonal tubularization must be combined with bladder augmentation because of small bladder capacity; most bladder neck repairs decrease bladder capacity since bladder is used to create the continence mechanism (Mansi and Ahmed, 1993). Stomach offers the best potential to preserve spontaneous volitional voiding in this group, but places these children at risk of the hematuria–dysuria syndrome, which can be especially troubling in the face of persistent urinary incontinence and intact sensory innervation (Ganesan *et al.*, 1993). Other intestinal segments may also be used according to the surgeon's preference. If augmentation is required, appendicovesicostomy or another form of the Mitrofanoff operation should be performed simultaneously in those children who have difficult urethras to negotiate, because they may require intermittent catheterization to empty the bladder after bladder neck reconstruction.

Young–Dees–Leadbetter procedure

To perform a Young–Dees–Leadbetter (YDL) procedure (Figs. 27.31, 27.32), a strip of posterior bladder mucosa approximately 1–1.5 cm wide and 3–4 cm long is outlined and rolled into a tube over an 8 or 10 Fr urethral catheter using interrupted or running polyglycolic acid sutures (4-0 or 5-0). The use of an epinephrine-soaked sponge during this dissection aids in hemostasis and visualization. Triangular flaps of demucosalized detrusor muscle are developed on either side of the mucosal tube and subsequently wrapped over it in a double-breasted technique using 3-0 polyglycolic acid sutures (Churchill *et al.*, 1997). This reinforces the neobladder, decreases the risk of fistula, and augments the outlet resistance (Ben-Chaim and Gearhart, 1996).

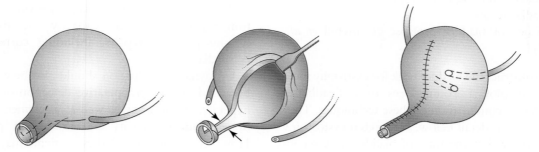

Figure 27.30 Mitchell bladder neck reconstruction. (*a*) Dotted lines represent incisions that will construct posterior bladder strip that will become urethra. (*b*) Retractor pulling inferior most portion of bladder superiorly, effectively enlarging bladder dome. Posterior strip (arrows) is 1.5 cm in width. Ureters detached from bladder. (*c*) Strip and bladder closed, ureters reimplanted into bladder at high level.

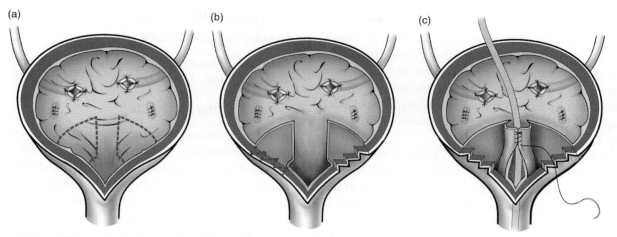

Figure 27.31 Principles of the Young–Dees–Leadbetter procedure. This is performed as the third stage of a staged reconstructive approach to exstrophy. The ureters are reimplanted as shown here to prevent vesicoureteral reflux and move them out of the area of the bladder neck reconstruction. The base of the bladder is reconstructed to lengthen the urethra and reinforce the bladder neck. (Adapted from Brock and O'Neill, 1998, with permission.)

Gearhart advocates the use of intraoperative urodynamic studies. Retrospective studies have shown that intraoperative closure pressures of 70–100 cmH$_2$O will prevent urinary leakage at 50 cmH$_2$O postoperatively (Canning *et al.*, 1993). Postoperative management is similar to that following the Mitchell repair. Some surgeons recommend avoidance of an urethral catheter in the postoperative period because of concerns that it may adversely affect later urinary continence. Urinary drainage is then achieved through ureteral catheters and suprapubic tube drainage (Gearhart and Jeffs, 1996).

Results

Bladder neck reconstruction in YDL procedures and its variants has yielded success rates of 30% to over 80% urinary continence for patients with bladder exstrophy (Mollard, 1980; Jones *et al.*, 1993; Gearhart *et al.*, 1993b). Many factors influence the outcome of surgery. For instance, an initial failed bladder closure or prior failed bladder neck reconstruction reduces the chance of subsequent urinary continence (Gearhart *et al.*, 1996). Use of iliac osteotomies to provide a tension-free anastomosis, and patient immobilization

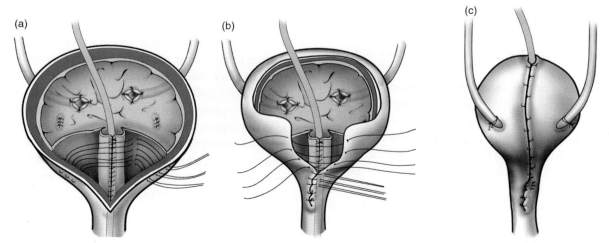

Figure 27.32 Principles of the Young–Dees–Leadbetter procedure. The bladder neck closure is reinforced with a pants-over-vest closure. Drainage catheters are brought out superiorly. (Adapted from Brock and O'Neill, 1998, with permission.)

through the use of spica casting or Bryant's traction in the postoperative period increases the success of bladder closure and subsequent continence (Gearhart et al., 1996; Lottman et al., 1997). Delayed bladder closure increases the likelihood of the eventual need for bladder augmentation due to inadequate bladder capacity that, in turn, reduces the chance of volitional voiding.

Woodhouse and Redgrave (1996) reported that eight of 13 patients with initially successful bladder closures and bladder neck reconstruction required further surgery in their second decade of life because of poorly compliant, low-capacity bladders that caused urinary incontinence. Surgeons who care for these patients must be committed to their long-term follow-up as late complications may develop.

Failed repair

Gearhart and Jeffs (1996) noted that patients who are not initially continent (defined by a dry interval of 3 hours) after bladder neck reconstruction may achieve urinary continence later. However, such patients rarely improve if they remain wet 1–2 years after surgery. Kramer and Kelalis (1982) have also observed some male patients who became continent after puberty and postulated that prostatic enlargement may have created enough additional resistance to achieve urinary continence. While this observation appears valid in patients who have undergone epispadias repair, exstrophy patients do not achieve continence with puberty. Based on magnetic resonance imaging studies in these patients, prostatic volume is equivalent to age-matched controls but the configuration of this gland remains abnormal so that it does not surround the urethra (Gearhart and Jeffs, 1996).

Patients who fail to achieve continence after bladder neck reconstruction should undergo urodynamic evaluation. Some patients will demonstrate uninhibited bladder contractions resulting from increased resistance at the bladder neck after reconstruction and treatment with anticholinergic agents, such as oxybutynin, may significantly improve continence.

If urodynamic evaluation reveals a bladder with adequate capacity but low leak point pressures, a second YDL procedure can be performed. However, this is unusual. More commonly, patients demonstrate an inadequate bladder capacity and require bladder augmentation (Gearhart and Jeffs, 1996).

Alternatives to the Young–Dees–Leadbetter procedure

After failed bladder neck reconstruction using an YDL procedure, several options are available.

Artificial urinary sphincter

An artificial urinary sphincter may be used to achieve urinary continence in patients who have adequate bladder capacity and compliance but an incompetent bladder neck after bladder neck reconstruction (Decter et al., 1988). This device preserves the ability to void volitionally, but because of the requirements for later revision and the dexterity required to use it, is not the first choice for younger patients. Others have described its use in combination with bladder augmentation. In one series of 11 patients who underwent sigmoid augmentation with artificial urinary sphincter placement, nine are continent. However, these patients required multiple operative revisions to achieve this degree of continence (Light and Scott, 1983). Sphincter erosion into the bladder neck or bowel segment can also occur (Gearhart and Jeffs, 1988).

Bladder neck wrap/sling

Bladder neck wraps and slings may also be used. However, series reporting on the use of bladder neck wraps suggest that this procedure does not consistently maintain long-term urinary continence, especially in male patients who constitute the gender majority in exstrophy (Decter, 1993; Kurzrock et al., 1996).

Collagen therapy

Several authors have used collagen injections at the bladder neck to treat patients with stress incontinence after bladder neck reconstruction (Caione et al., 1993; Ben-Chaim et al., 1995a). Ben-Chaim et al. (1995a) reported an improvement in continence in 53% of patients after collagen therapy, although most required multiple injections. It may be used as an adjunctive procedure for those patients who demonstrate slight leakage due to stress incontinence after bladder neck reconstruction.

Bladder neck closure

Bladder neck closure in conjunction with appendicovesicostomy is also an option in those patients who have failed multiple attempts at bladder neck reconstruction. It should be reserved as a last resort because it eliminates the chance to void per urethra and commits the patient to lifelong intermittent catheterization.

Urinary diversion

Proponents of urinary diversion for the treatment of exstrophy argue that the varying continence rates achieved with functional reconstruction demonstrate the unreliability of this approach (Hohenfellner and Stein, 1996). The use of the native bladder will often require later bladder augmentation with intestinal segments to achieve a functional bladder storage capacity. Certainly, some centers report poor rates of continence after primary reconstruction and some urodynamic studies demonstrate low urine flow rates and poor contractility in patients following primary bladder reconstruction (Nisonson and Lattimer, 1972; Hollowell et al., 1992).

Primary urinary diversion avoids many complications associated with functional reconstruction, including urinary retention and subsequent kidney damage, a predisposition to UTI, and later dependence on CIC to empty the bladder, with its own possible complications of urethral stricture formation, epididymitis, and UTI (Hohenfellner and Stein, 1996). Advocates of early urinary diversion also cite a decreased risk of epididymitis and obstruction of the vas deferens by the creation of a receptacle with a suprapubic window at the level of the prostatic urethra (Hohenfellner and Stein, 1996). Diversion can be combined with cosmetic operative procedures for the external genitalia and epispadias repair.

Urinary diversion is used to provide urinary continence in patients who have failed multiple attempts at functional reconstruction. Some also advocate primary urinary diversion for patients with bladder plates deemed too small to close. However, because one cannot accurately predict which bladder plates will increase significantly in size after primary closure, this should not be used as a criterion for primary diversion, and the authors do not divert the urine primarily in exstrophy patients. Arap has described preservation of the very small bladder by tubularizing it as the continence mechanism after anastamosing the ureters to a sigmoid conduit in an antireflux manner. Final reconstruction involves attachment of the sigmoid conduit to the neourethra and reconstruction of the abdominal wall.

Because of the difficulties encountered with functional bladder reconstruction, advocates of early urinary diversion argue that their approach achieves the primary goals of surgical intervention for bladder exstrophy with fewer operations and higher success rates than are achieved with bladder closure and urethral reconstruction. Ureterosigmoidostomy became the treatment of choice for bladder exstrophy patients as a primary and secondary treatment because of the dismal results associated with primary bladder reconstruction in the early twentieth century and well into the 1970s. The long-term complications, including hyperchloremic metabolic acidosis, risk of chronic pyelonephritis, and a 250–500-fold increased risk of colonic adenocarcinoma at the site of ureteral anastomosis, dampened enthusiasm for this procedure despite the reduction in metabolic complications following improvements in ureteral reimplantation (Leadbetter, 1951; Spence et al., 1975; Husmann and Spence, 1990). Ureterosigmoidostomy was subsequently replaced by incontinent urinary diversions such as the colonic and ileal conduits. A significant disadvantage of these forms of urinary diversion is the incontinent abdominal stoma associated with these conduits. The popularization of CIC allowed the development, since the 1980s, of continent urinary diversions such as the Indiana pouch, which was developed for patients with exstrophy and is now the preferred method of urinary diversion to the abdomen in this population (see Chapter 17).

Rectal reservoirs

Various investigators have made significant improvements on the use of the rectum as a urinary reservoir, including the Mainz II pouch and the Sigma pouch (Ghoneim et al., 1981; Hohenfellner, 1992). Use of a rectal reservoir permits urinary continence without the reliance on CIC required with other forms of continent urinary diversion. Hohenfellner and Stein (1996) report a 92% rate of renal preservation in their series of children treated primarily with a urinary rectal reservoir (Mainz II pouch) since 1991. Continence rates of 97% in school-aged children are reported using this technique. The Heitz–Boyer–Hovelaque procedure involves isolation of a rectal segment for ureteral implantation followed by posterior sagittal pull-through of the sigmoid colon through the anal sphincter to achieve both urinary and fecal continence. A small series using this procedure reported continence rates of 95% with acceptable complication rates (Tacciuoli *et al.*, 1977).

Complications of this form of diversion include fecal–urinary incontinence in patients with impaired anorectal sphincter control (Gearhart and Jeffs, 1996). Metabolic electrolyte imbalances can be treated with complete, frequent emptying of the rectal reservoir, which reduces the contact time between urine and the absorptive rectal mucosa, along with oral bicarbonate replacement. Oral bicarbonate replacement is recommended for all patients who have a base deficit of 2.5 mmol/l or greater (Hohenfellner and Stein, 1996). The risk of malignant degeneration remains with use of a rectal urinary reservoir. Various modifications to the rectal reservoir to prevent admixture of feces and urine may theoretically decrease the incidence of adenocarcinoma formation if it is due to conversion of urinary nitrates into carcinogenic nitrites by fecal bacteria (Crissey *et al.*, 1980). Long-term results are not yet available.

Approaches to urinary diversion

Methods to construct urinary diversions include the following (see Chapter 17):

1 Continent diversions:
  (a) external diversions (continent urinary reservoir):
      ■ Indiana pouch
      ■ Mainz pouch
      ■ Penn pouch
      ■ Kock pouch
      ■ others
  (b) internal diversions (rectal sphincter-based continence)
      ■ ureterosigmoidostomy
      ■ Sigma pouch
      ■ Ghoneim reservoir
      ■ Gersuny
      ■ Heitz–Boyer–Hovelacque
      ■ rectal bladder with proximal colostomy
      ■ ileocecal ureterosigmoidostomy.
2 Incontinent diversions:
      ■ ileal conduit
      ■ colon conduit
      ■ ileocecal conduit.

Management of cloacal exstrophy

Although cloacal exstrophy has been recognized as a disease entity for at least several hundred years,

Spencer (1965) became the first surgeon to report the successful repair and survival of an infant with this anomaly. Mortality rates of infants with cloacal exstrophy remained high for years following this initial success. In 1979, the mortality rate of a contemporary series stood at 50% (Welch, 1979). Affected infants routinely died of malnutrition and sepsis. With continuing improvements in total parenteral nutrition and neonatal management, mortality rates are currently less than 10% (Davidoff *et al.*, 1996). Issues of quality of life are now paramount in this patient group.

Perioperative management

Because the care of patients with cloacal exstrophy involves multiple organ systems, these patients are best cared for by a team of experienced physicians. Advances in neonatal care, intravenous nutrition, and the surgical procedures have markedly reduced the mortality and morbidity of this disease. Nonetheless, management remains challenging.

In the neonatal period, the bladder and hindgut plate should be covered with a hydrophilic gel (Vigilon) dressing to protect these structures. The umbilical cord should be ligated with a silk suture to prevent an umbilical clamp from abrading the bladder or hindgut plate. Antibiotic prophylaxis is routinely used in these patients because of the high incidence of renal abnormalities.

Preoperative studies include ultrasonography and karyotyping. Sonographic examination allows the evaluation of the upper urinary tracts, internal genital structures, and spinal cord. Because the genital anomalies associated with cloacal exstrophy may make it difficult to identify the gender of the baby accurately, karyotyping is used to define the chromosomal sex in situations where the gender of the infant is unclear.

Initial closure

As indicated above, closure of a cloacal exstrophy should involve a team of pediatric surgeons and pediatric urologists experienced in the care of these children. If the baby is medically stable, the initial reconstructive procedures should be performed within the first 48 hours of life, thus taking advantage of the pliable bony pelvis if closure of the entire defect is possible. The size of the omphalocele and the size of the hindgut plate and bladder plates largely dictate the extent of the initial closure. A large omphalocele containing liver may preclude any attempt at simultaneous bladder closure (O'Neill, 1998). In this situation, the omphalocele and plates should be appropriately protected until staged reconstructive procedures can be undertaken.

Before the dissection begins, ureteral catheters are placed in the ureteral orifices and secured in place with 5.0 chromic suture. The omphalocele associated with the cloacal exstrophy is approached. The omphalocele should be repaired first. The initial dissection is begun superiorly. The umbilical vessels are ligated and the bladder plates separated from the adjacent skin using sharp dissection, for example Colorado tip electrocautery. The medial hindgut plate is separated from the paired, separated bladder plates during this stage of the closure. The ileum should be detached from the hindgut plate. The hindgut is then tubularized and reattached to the ileum to lengthen the intestine. The distal end of this segment will be used as a colostomy at the end of the procedure.

After the hindgut has been separated from the bladder plates, the bladder halfs are reapproximated. Primary bladder closure may be performed at this time if the intra-abdominal pressure remains low after omphalocele closure. This can be determined clinically by assessing ventilatory effort. Increased abdominal pressure may also result in organ ischemia following closure. When possible, a one-stage closure is performed using the complete primary repair technique described as for bladder exstrophy. The decision to proceed with one-stage closure versus staged reconstruction must be weighed carefully and highlights the importance of involving surgeons experienced in the care of these patients.

Because of the wide pubic diastasis in cloacal exstrophy, pubic reapproximation usually requires iliac osteotomies. This can be determined by assessing the lower extremities and external genitalia for ischemia during the pubic reapproximation before osteotomies are performed.

The high incidence of neurologic abnormalities in this patient population also impacts on the potential for urinary continence (Appignani *et al.*, 1994). This factor must also be considered when counseling patients' families and when choosing the reconstructive technique to use to provide these children with a functional and safe urinary tract.

Genitourinary reconstruction

Gender assignment for patients with cloacal exstrophy is currently under scrutiny both by the medical profession and by the lay public (see Chapter 30). Traditionally, male patients underwent sex conversion in infancy because of concerns that the small, separated hemi-phalluses in these patients were inadequate for reconstruction and later sexual function. This approach was supported by anecdotal data of unsatisfied patients following reconstruction as males (Lund and Hendren, 1993). These observations, in conjunction with the prevailing notion that humans were gender neutral at birth and so could undergo gender conversion safely in infancy, have recently been questioned (Diamond and Sigmundson, 1997). Recent evidence suggests that gender imprinting occurs during fetal development (Gorski, 1999). Gender identity now appears to be a much more complex issue than previously thought.

The authors' institutional experience with external genital reconstruction in this patient population covers a period when patients were both gender converted and later when male gender was maintained. These patients are now routinely reconstructed as males whenever technically possible. Many gender reassigned individuals will later identify themselves in a male gender role in adolescence and adulthood (Mitchell, 1999). Technically, however, reconstruction of external male genitalia in the cloacal exstrophy population can be quite difficult. The wide pubic diastasis and small phallic size add to the complexity because it is difficult to bring the two phallic halves together in the midline.

Gastrointestinal reconstruction

Short-gut syndrome is usually present in patients with cloacal exstrophy at birth. The effects of malabsorption and fluid loss from this are most significant early in life (Husmann *et al.*, 1988). Many such children require parenteral nutritional support in early infancy (Georgeson and Breaux, 1992; Husmann *et al.*, 1988). Therefore, the hindgut should be constructed and placed in continuity with the intestine during initial reconstruction. This may improve nutrition and also preserves intestinal tissue that may be used in later reconstruction of the urinary tract or to form a vagina. Rickham (1960) noted the importance of preservation of the hindgut in the intestine in his report of the first surviving neonate with cloacal exstrophy. Although hindgut can be closed with the bladder to augment bladder capacity, it is preferable to reconstruct these patients with the goal of providing maximal functional bowel length.

At the time of the initial procedure, the bladder plates are separated from the hindgut segment. The hindgut is then tubularized with the terminal portion of the ileum and exteriorized as a colostomy. In the event of colonic duplication, all intestinal segments should be preserved, if possible, and placed end-to-end in series. Appendiceal segments should also be preserved for possible use in later reconstruction of the urinary tract as for a Mitrofanoff procedure.

Long-term concerns in exstrophy

Psychosocial concerns

Children with exstrophy face significant challenges in the development of their psychosocial identity. Reiner *et al.* (1999) have noted that 'in children with exstrophy, psychosocial and psychosexual hurdles are the rule' rather than the exception. Unfortunately, this area of development has been poorly studied to date. A preliminary study of 135 children and adolescents with bladder exstrophy revealed that a detailed sexual and social history was rarely part of the routine evaluation of these children. Other studies have shown that adolescent males with exstrophy were psychosexually delayed by 2–4 years compared with their peers and delayed by 4–6 years in sexual activity. Data on teenage girls with exstrophy are incomplete, but Reiner has noted that these girls struggle with sexual self-esteem issues such as body image, genital perception, and genital appearance. Current recommendations include regular assessment of social development.

Psychiatric input should be initiated at birth with parental education about concerns. Child assessment should then begin as early as 12–18 months of age and periodically after that. Evaluation and intervention are also useful prior to operative procedures. Reiner *et al.* (1999) have found that anxiety and psychosexual disorders are universal in their patients. Routine patient and parental education is critical.

Sexual function

As exstrophy patients age, sexual function, along with urinary continence and physical appearance, become major concerns. Libido for patients with exstrophy is characteristically present with or without surgical correction. Woodhouse noted that many older patients with exstrophy develop stable partnerships. He found 33 of 43 patients married or living with a partner. However, sexual counseling in these patients is paramount because of the difficulties that they face. For male patients, erectile function is usually intact (Woodhouse *et al.*, 1983; Woodhouse, 1986). Variable degrees of chordee can create difficulty in achieving intercourse for some patients (Woodhouse, 1986). In these situations, a female superior position provides closer apposition of the genitalia for intercourse. For female patients, sexual function is often intact (Woodhouse *et al.*, 1983). In Woodhouse's series, 14 of 23 patients had normal intercourse (Woodhouse and Hinsch 1997).

Ejaculation is often present as well, despite the extensive reconstructive procedures that are done for these patients. The seminal emission may be slow and continue for several hours after orgasm. Further, sperm quality and quantity is often impaired. This may be due to partial obstruction or recurrent UTIs. Despite this, some male patients are fertile and successful pregnancies have been recorded (Mesrobian *et al.*, 1988). Fertility is unimpaired in female patients with exstrophy, although uterine prolapse occurs more commonly because of the lack of pelvic floor support structures. This may make bed-rest necessary in the later stages of pregnancy (Woodhouse, 1999).

Other bladder abnormalities

Other anomalies related to bladder development can occur. These are uncommon phenomena and include bladder agenesis, duplication, diverticula formation, and megacystis.

Bladder diverticula

Bladder diverticula occur when bladder mucosa herniates between the muscular fibers of the detrusor. In children, these typically occur just lateral and cephalad to the ureteral orifice (Bjelland and Freudlich, 1975) (Fig. 27.33). Bladder diverticula can also occur at the dome of the bladder. Diverticula in this location are typically seen in association with urinary outlet obstruction or prune belly syndrome (Caldamone, 1987).

In children, bladder diverticula are usually congenital and not due to obstruction (Cendron and Alain, 1972). The bladders of these children are typically

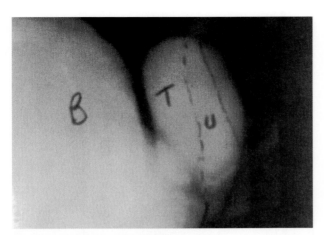

Figure 27.33 Bladder diverticulum. Voiding cysto-urethrography demonstrates filling of a bladder diverticulum (T) and vesicoureteral reflux. U = ureter; B = bladder. (Adapted from Caldamone, 1987, with permission.)

smooth-walled and the diverticula are solitary. They are believed to develop because of an inherent weakness in the detrusor muscle. Post-mortem studies of paraureteral bladder diverticula demonstrated deficiencies in Waldeyer's fascial sheath (Stephens, 1979). Bladder diverticula also occur in association with certain syndromes, including Menke's syndrome and Ehlers–Danlos syndrome (Levard *et al.*, 1989; Proud *et al.*, 1996).

Bladder diverticula may be acquired. Acquired diverticula develop secondary to urinary outlet obstruction such as posterior or anterior urethral valves, urethral stricture disease, or neurogenic or functional (Hinman's syndrome) bladder dysfunction. Acquired diverticula are often multiple and seen in association with bladder trabeculation. They can resolve after the obstruction is relieved (Caldamone, 1987).

The optimum imaging study for diagnosis is a voiding cystourethrogram (VCUG) with a postvoid film. However, bladder diverticula may be seen on sonographic examination as well if the bladder is examined when empty and full (Caldamone, 1987). Excretory urography is a suboptimal radiographic study to diagnose a bladder diverticulum because diverticula can be overshadowed by the bladder during this study. Allen and Atwell (1980) reported 24 children with bladder diverticula, only two of whom were diagnosed by excretory urography.

Small bladder diverticula that empty with voiding are not clinically significant and do not require surgical intervention. However, bladder diverticula can cause outlet obstruction at the bladder neck, VUR, or ureteral obstruction. Paraureteral diverticula can cause VUR or may just be associated with it. Primary VUR has an associated diveticulum with it in 8–13% of cases (Barrett *et al.*, 1976). Ureteral orifices that enter into the diverticulum will persistently reflux because of the lack of submucosal tunnel and detrusor support. In girls these diverticula may resolve spontaneously with spontaneous resolution of the VUR as well. Spontaneous resolution is less common in boys, in whom the diverticula tend to be larger (Amar, 1972). Diverticula may require surgical correction if they are associated with persistent VUR. They are usually excised in this situation at the time of ureteral reimplantation.

Larger diverticula will require operative resection if they cause urinary outlet or ureteral obstruction. Barrett *et al.* (1976) noted diverticulum-related obstruction in 5% of these patients. Diverticulum-associated ureteral obstruction should be confirmed by Lasix renography. If the associated kidney demonstrates minimal function, the kidney, ureter, and diverticulum may be surgically removed. Otherwise, diverticulectomy with ureteral reimplantation is the procedure of choice. Urinary outlet-associated obstruction by diverticula occurs less frequently. These patients may present with abnormal voiding patterns, UTIs, or hydronephrosis (Taylor *et al.*, 1979; Verghese and Belman, 1984). Importantly, if bladder diverticula occur secondary to obstruction, the cause of outlet obstruction must be corrected first before making decisions about the management of the bladder diverticulum.

Bladder agenesis and hypoplasia

Complete agenesis of the bladder occurs rarely and is usually found in association with other severe anomalies. Only eight cases have been reported in viable newborns. These babies had associated urogenital anomalies along with orthopedic and neurologic abnormalities (Graham, 1972). The majority of babies born with this anomaly are female (Caldamone, 1987).

Hypotheses for the development of bladder agenesis include failure of the lower portion of the mesonephric ducts to develop into the bladder (Palmer and Russi, 1969). Bladder agenesis may also occur owing to the loss of the anterior division of the cloaca (Krull *et al.*, 1988). It may also represent the most severe form of ureteral ectopia (Caldamone, 1987).

In female patients with bladder agenesis, the ureters empty into the müllerian structures so they may terminate in the uterus, anterior vaginal wall, or vestibule. This allows preservation of renal function. In the male patient with bladder agenesis, cloacal or urachal persistence is the only means of achieving urinary drainage. Treatment options in these patients include urinary diversion, either internally or externally (Caldamone, 1987).

Bladder hypoplasia typically occurs secondary to urinary outlet failure such as severe epispadias or ectopic ureters, or secondary to oliguria or anuria from renal dysplasia. With these conditions the bladder does not cycle urine, remaining small and poorly compliant. These bladders may attain function after the primary abnormality is corrected. However, bladder augmentation is generally required to achieve adequate capacity (Caldamone, 1987).

Bladder duplication

This abnormality may be complete or incomplete. Only 45 cases of complete duplication have been reported in the literature (Kapoor and Saha, 1987). With complete duplication, the bladders are on either side of the midline and possess separate muscular walls (Fig. 27.34). The associated ipsilateral ureter enters into its respective bladder. Duplication of the genitalia occurs in the majority of these cases as well. In males this is seen as duplication of the penis and in females as duplication of the vagina and uterus (Satler and Mossman, 1968). Hindgut duplication occurs in almost one-half of these cases and duplication of lumbar vertebrae has also been reported (Caldamone, 1987).

With incomplete bladder duplication, the bladder units communicate distally and drain into a common urethra. The wall separating them is full thickness, in contrast to septation of the bladder where the wall may be mucosa alone or muscularis and mucosa. Duplication of other structures and organ systems typically does not occur in association with incomplete bladder duplication. This anomaly is not considered to have serious consequences (Uhlir, 1968).

Congenital megacystis

This rare entity describes a large bladder. When associated with massive VUR the bladder empties poorly during fetal development recycling urine into the upper tracts. Although the bladder is normal, this process leads to its gradual increase in size. Surgical

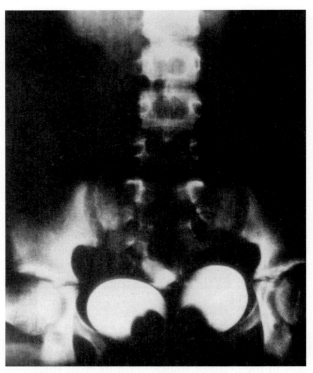

Figure 27.34 Complete duplication of the bladder and urethra. (Adapted from Caldamone, 1987, with permission.)

correction of the VUR can correct megacystis in this situation. This entity is also referred to as megacystis–megaureter syndrome (Williams, 1957).

Megacysytis is also described in association with microcolon. This is known as the megacystis–microcolon–hypoperistalsis syndrome. It probably represents a functional obstruction of the bladder and intestine, although the etiology is not understood at this time. Secondary forms of megacystis may occur secondary to urethral obstruction from urethral valves, extrinsic compression of the bladder outlet, or a neuropathic bladder (Caldamone, 1987). Megacystis due to these causes is optimally managed by correcting the underlying abnormality. Finally, a group of patients exists with large bladders and no apparent etiology. Proposed causes of megacystis in this group include transient bladder obstruction *in utero*, cerebral anoxia, and metabolic abnormalities.

Urachal abnormalities

Congenital urachal anomalies are uncommon. The reported incidence of patent urachus in pediatric autopsy series is 1:761 and 1:5000 for urachal cyst (Rubin, 1967). They typically present in early childhood but may remain unrecognized and clinically silent until adulthood. Urachal anomalies occur when the normal process of urachal involution is interrupted. These anomalies include (Fig. 27.35):

- patent urachus
- urachal cyst or sinus
- alternating urachal sinus
- vesicourachal diverticulum.

Urachal anomalies usually occur in isolation. Males are affected twice as commonly as females (Caldamone, 1987).

Embryology

The urachus develops from the anterior portion of the cloaca. As the bladder enlarges and descends, the urachus becomes apparent as the attachment from the allantois to the dome of the bladder. The urachus progressively narrows and obliterates to become a fibromuscular strand connecting the umbilicus to the dome of the bladder. Failure of the urachus to obliterate results in one of the abnormalities above. The urachus lies between the transversalis fascia and the peritoneum. An umbilicovesical fascial sheath that forms a self-contained space surrounds it. Histologically, the urachus is composed of three layers, an outer smooth muscle layer, a submucosal tissue layer, and an inner layer of cuboidal or transitional epithelium.

Patent urachus

This anomaly is typically recognized in the neonate. The neonate will present with a wet umbilicus. Discharge of urine may be minimal or intermittent. At delivery, a patent urachus should be suspected if the umbilical cord is enlarged or edematous or when it sloughs in a delayed fashion (Fig. 27.36). This diagnosis may be confirmed by sending the discharge fluid for urea nitrogen and creatinine or by intravesical instillation of colored dye. Evaluation should include a VCUG to evaluate for bladder outlet obstruction and may also include a fistulagram if the tract is not well visualized by cystography (Fig. 27.37). A patent urachus may be managed conservatively if no urinary outlet obstruction exists and the patency is small. If drainage persists for several months, the urachus should be excised along with a cuff of bladder to prevent calculus formation in a retained urachal segment (Nix *et al.*, 1958) (Fig. 27.38). Other possible causes of a wet umbilicus include omphalitis, granulation of a healing umbilical stump, infection of an umbilical vessel, external urachal sinus, and a patent vitelline or omphalomesenteric duct (Caldamone, 1987).

Urachal cyst

This lesion occurs when the umbilical end of the urachus is obliterated and the urachus fills with desquamated epithelium. Most urachal cysts develop in the

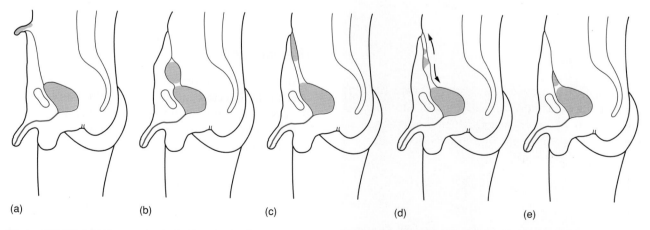

(a)   (b)   (c)   (d)   (e)

Figure 27.35 (*a*) Patent urachus, which communicates between the bladder and umbilicus; (*b*) urachal cyst, loculated section, usually in the lower third of the urachal segment; (*c*) urachal sinus, which drains to the umbilicus in most cases; (*d*) alternating urachal sinus, which drains to the bladder and umbilicus; (*e*) vesicourachal diverticulum, which extend halfway to the umbilicus. This does not need to be removed but may predispose to adenocarcinoma. (Adapted from Bauer and Retik, 1978, with permission.)

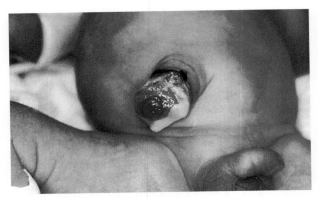

Figure 27.36 Newborn male baby with a patent urachus. Note thickening of the umbilical cord.

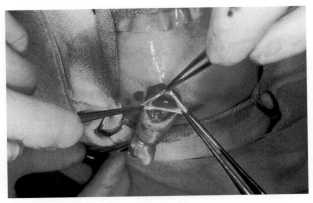

Figure 27.38 Resection of patent urachus in the same patient as in Figure 27.36. Resection includes removal of a cuff of bladder tissue at the dome of the bladder, which is displayed open in this photograph.

distal third of the urachus. Urachal cysts typically present in childhood or early adult life when they become infected. Signs and symptoms of infection include fever, suprapubic pain and tenderness, irritative voiding symptoms, and a palpable supra-

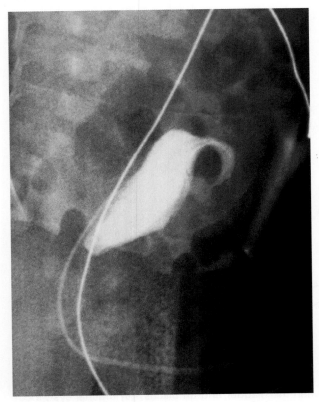

Figure 27.37 Voiding cystourethrogram of the same newborn male baby with patent urachus as in Figure 27.36. Note the curvilinear arc of contrast filling the urachus.

pubic mass. They may drain spontaneously into the bladder, cutaneously, or into the peritoneal cavity. Urachal cysts can also present as an asymptomatic suprapubic mass. Imaging evaluation should include sonographic examination to define the mass and demonstrate its relationship to the bladder and peritoneum. Voiding cystography and cystoscopy may also be performed to assess the degree of bladder involvement. Computed tomographic scans may also be useful. Initial management should involve incision and drainage of the cyst or percutaneous catheter drainage. Definitive cyst excision is performed after inflammation has subsided to minimize the risk of injuring adjacent structures (Caldamone, 1987).

Urachal sinus

A urachal sinus occurs when a urachal cyst becomes chronically infected and drains into the umbilicus. If the cyst intermittently drains into the bladder as well, it may form an alternating sinus to both the bladder and umbilicus. Typically, these patients present in childhood with periumbilical pain and tenderness associated with intermittent drainage of clear or cloudy fluid. Management, as with the urachal cyst, first involves treatment of associated infection followed by definitive excision of the sinus tract. Because of its location, a urachal sinus may involve adjacent intraperitoneal structures. Careful attention should be paid to avoiding injury to these structures at the time of surgical resection of the sinus.

Vesicourachal diverticulum

This anomaly is usually seen in association with prune belly syndrome. It has also been associated with bladder outlet obstruction, but may occur as an isolated finding. These diverticula usually do not predispose to infection or urinary stasis. A vesicourachal diverticulum does not require surgical intervention unless it drains poorly or contracts paradoxically.

References

Aadalen RJ et al. (1980) Exstrophy of the bladder: long-term results of bilateral posterior iliac osteotomies and two-stage anatomic repair. Clin Orthop **151**: 193–200.

Allen NH, Atwell JD (1980) The paraureteric diverticulum in childhood. Br J Urol **52**: 264–8.

Amar AD (1972) Vesicoureteral reflux associated with congenital bladder diverticulum in boys and young men. J Urol **107**: 966–8.

Andiran F, Tanyel FC (1999) Duplicate exstrophy of the bladder. J Pediatr Surg **34**: 626–7.

Ansell JS (1971) Primary closure of exstrophy in the newborn: a preliminary report. Northwest Med **70**: 842–4.

Ansell JS (1979) Surgical treatment of exstrophy of the bladder with emphasis on neonatal primary closure: personal experience with 28 consecutive cases treated at the University of Washington hospitals from 1962 to 1977: techniques and results. J Urol **121**: 650–3.

Appignani BA et al. (1994) Dysraphic myelodysplasias associated with urogenital and anorectal anomalies: prevalence and types seen with MR imaging. AJR Am J Roentgenol **163**: 1199–1203.

Austin PF et al. (1998) The prenatal diagnosis of cloacal exstrophy. J Urol **160**: 1179–81.

Avolio L et al. (1996) The long-term outcome in men with exstrophy/epispadias: sexual function and social integration. J Urol **156**: 822–5.

Barrett DM, Malek RS, Kelalis PP (1976) Observations on vesical diverticulum in childhood. J Urol **116**: 234–6.

Barth RA, Filly RA, Sondheimer FK (1990) Prenatal sonographic findings in bladder exstrophy. J Ultrasound Med **9**: 359–61.

Bauer SB, Retik AB (1978) Urachal anomalies and related umbilical disorders. Urol Clin North Am **5**: 184–95.

Beckwith JB (1966) The congenitally malformed. VII. Exstrophy of the bladder and cloacal exstrophy. Northwest Med **65**: 407–10.

Ben-Chaim J, Jeffs RD, Peppas DS, Gearhart JP (1995a) Submucosal bladder neck injections of glutaraldehyde cross-linked bovine collagen for the treatment of urinary incontinence in patients with the exstrophy/epispadias complex. J Urol **154**: 862–4.

Ben-Chaim J et al. (1995b) Applications of osteotomy in the cloacal exstrophy patient. J Urol **154**: 865–7.

Ben-Chaim J et al. (1996) The outcome of patients with classic bladder exstrophy in adult life. J Urol **155**: 1251–2.

Ben-Chaim J, Gearhart JP (1996) Current management of bladder exstrophy. Tech Urol **2**: 22–33.

Bjelland JC, Freudlich IM (1975) Radiology case of the month. Case no. 4. Hutch diverticulum complicated by a post-operative pelvic hematoma. Ariz Med **32**: 885–7.

Brock III J, O'Neill J Jr (1988) Bladder exstrophy. In: O'Neill JA, Rowe MI, Grosfeld JL et al. (eds) Pediatric surgery. 5th edition. Volume 2. Philadelphia, PA: Mosby Year Book, 1709–32.

Brun M et al. (1998) Diagnostic prenatal ultrasonography of malformations of the fetal anterior abdominal wall. J Radiol **79**: 1461–8.

Burbige KA et al. (1986) Pregnancy and sexual function in women with bladder exstrophy. Urology **28**: 12–14.

Cacciari A et al. (1999) Prenatal diagnosis of bladder exstrophy: what counseling? J Urol **161**: 259–61; discussion 262.

Caione P, Lais A, de Gennaro M, Capozza N (1993) Glutaraldehyde cross-linked bovine collagen in exstrophy/epispadias complex. J Urol **150**: 631–3.

Caldamone A (1987) Anomalies of the bladder and cloaca. In: Gillenwater J, Grayhack J, Howards S, Duckett J (eds) Adult and pediatric urology. Philadelphia, PA: Mosby Year Book 2023–54.

Canning DA et al. (1993) The cephalotrigonal reimplant in bladder neck reconstruction for patients with exstrophy or epispadias. J Urol **150**: 156–8.

Cantwell V (1895) Operative treatment of epispadias by transplantation of the urethra. Ann Surg **22**: 689–701.

Cendron J (1971) Bladder reconstruction. Method derived from that of Trendelenbourg. Ann Chir Infant **12**: 371–81.

Cendron J, Alain JL (1972) Bladder diverticulum in children without obstruction of the lower urinary tract. Apropos of 43 cases. J Urol Nephrol (Paris) **78**: 793–805.

Cendron J, Mollard P (1971) Treatment of bladder exstrophy. Therapeutic indications. Ann Chir Infant **12**: 481–2.

Cerniglia FR Jr, Roth DR, Gonzales ET Jr (1989) Covered exstrophy and visceral sequestration in a male newborn: case report. J Urol **141**: 903–4.

Churchill B, Merguerian PA, Khoury AE et al. (1997) Bladder exstrophy and epispadias. In: BaK, O'Donnell S, (eds) Pediatric urology. 3rd edition. Oxford: Reed Elsevier, 495–508.

Close C (1999) Urethral valves and the potential for healing in very young patients. AUA Update Ser 1–20.

Close C, Carr MC, Burns MW, Mitchell ME (1997) Lower urinary tract changes after early valve ablation: is early diversion warranted? J Urol **157**: 984–8.

Connolly JA et al. (1995) Prevalence and repair of inguinal hernias in children with bladder exstrophy. J Urol **154**: 1900–1.

Connor JP et al. (1989) Long-term followup of 207 patients with bladder exstrophy: an evolution in treatment. J Urol **142**: 793–5; discussion 795–6.

Coulson WJ (1881) The diseases of the bladder and prostate gland. 6th edition. New York: William Wood & Co.

Crissey M, Steel G, Gittes R (1980) Rat model for carcinogenesis in ureterosigmoidostomy. *Science* **207**: 1079–80.

Davidoff AM *et al*. (1996) Management of the gastrointestinal tract and nutrition in patients with cloacal exstrophy. *J Pediatr Surg* **31**: 771–3.

Decter R (1993) Use of the fascial sling for neurogenic incontinence: lessons learned. *J Urol* **150**: 683–6.

Decter R, Roth DR, Fishman IJ *et al*. (1988) Use of the AS800 device in exstrophy and epispadias. *J Urol* **140**: 1202–3.

DeMaria JE *et al*. (1980) Renal function in continent patients after surgical closure of bladder exstrophy. *J Urol* **124**: 85–8.

Diamond DA, Jeffs RD (1985) Cloacal exstrophy: a 22-year experience. *J Urol* **133**: 779–82.

Diamond M, Sigmundson HK (1997) Management of intersexuality. Guidelines for dealing with persons with ambiguous genitalia. *Arch Pediatr Adolesc Med* **151**: 1046–50.

Engel RM (1973) Bladder exstrophy: vesicoplasty or urinary diversion? *Urology* **2**: 20–4.

Engel RM (1974) Exstrophy of the bladder and associated anomalies. *Birth Defects Orig Artic Ser* **10**: 146–9.

Epidemiology of bladder exstrophy and epispadias: a communication from the International Clearinghouse for Birth Defects Monitoring Systems (1987) *Teratology* **36**: 221–7.

Ezell WW, Carlson HE (1970) A realistic look at exstrophy of the bladder. *Br J Urol* **42**: 197–202.

Figueroa-Colon R *et al*. (1996) Impact of intestinal lengthening on the nutritional outcome for children with short bowel syndrome. *J Pediatr Surg* **31**: 912–6.

Frey P (1996) Bilateral anterior pubic osteotomy in bladder exstrophy closure. *J Urol* **156**: 812–15.

Fuchs J, Gluer S, Mildenberger H (1996) One-stage reconstruction of bladder exstrophy. *Eur J Pediatr Surg* **6**: 212–15.

Galloway N (1997) The biology of continence. *Department of Urology*, Seattle, WA: University of Washington, 4.

Ganesan G, Nguyen DH, Adams MC *et al*. (1993) Lower urinary tract reconstruction using stomach and the artifical urinary sphincter. *J Urol* **149**: 1107–9.

Gearhart J (1999) Bladder and cloacal exstrophy. In SB, Gonzales E (eds) *Pediatric urology practice*. Philadelphia, PA: Lippincott Williams & Wilkins. 339–63.

Gearhart JP (1998) Evolution of epispadias repair – timing, techniques and results (Editorial; comment). *J Urol* **160**: 177–8.

Gearhart JP, Jeffs RD (1988) Augmentation cystoplasty in the failed exstrophy reconstruction. *J Urol* **139**: 790–3.

Gearhart J, Jeffs RD (1996) Exstrophy of the bladder, epispadias, and other bladder anomalies. In: Walsh P, Retik A, Stamey T, Vaughan D (eds) *Campbell's urology*. 6th edition. Volume 2. Philadelphia, PA: WB Saunders, 1772–821.

Gearhart J, Jeffs RD (1989) Bladder exstrophy: increase in capacity following epispadias repair. *J Urol* **142**: 525–9; discussion 542–3.

Gearhart JP *et al*. (1993a) Prostate size and configuration in adults with bladder exstrophy. *J Urol* **149**: 308–10.

Gearhart J, Canning DA, Peppas DS, Jeffs RD (1993b) Techniques to create continence in the failed bladder exstrophy closure patient. *J Urol* **150**: 441–3.

Gearhart JP, Peppas DS, Jeffs RD (1993c) The failed exstrophy closure: strategy for management. *Br J Urol* **71**: 217–20.

Gearhart JP *et al*. (1995) Criteria for the prenatal diagnosis of classic bladder exstrophy. *Obstet Gynecol* **85**: 961–4.

Gearhart J, Ben-Chaim J, Sciortino C *et al*. (1996) The multiple reoperative bladder exstrophy closure: what affects the potential of the bladder. *Urology* **47**: 240–3.

Gearhart J, Mathews R, Taylor S, Jeffs RD (1998) Combined bladder closure and epispadias repair in the reconstruction of bladder exstrophy. *J Urol* **160**: 1182–5.

Georgeson KE, Breaux CW Jr (1992) Outcome and intestinal adaptation in neonatal short-bowel syndrome. *J Pediatr Surg* **27**: 344–8; discussion 348–50.

Ghoneim M, Shebab-El-din A, Ashmallah A, Gaballah M (1981) Evolution of the rectal bladder as a method for urinary diversion. *J Urol* **126**: 737–41.

Goldfischer ER *et al*. (1997) Omphalopagus twins with covered cloacal exstrophy. *J Urol* **157**: 1004–5.

Gorski R (1999) Hypothalamic imprinting by steroid hormones – 20 year review. In: *Gender Reassignment Meeting*, 1999, Dallas, TX.

Grady RW, Mitchell ME (1998) Newborn exstrophy closure and epispadias repair. *World J Urol* **16**: 200–4.

Grady RW, Mitchell ME (1999) Complete primary repair of exstrophy. *J Urol* **162**: 1415–20.

Grady R, Carr MC, Mitchell ME (1997) Cloacal exstrophy variants: challenging the current hypothesis. In: Northwest Urology Society Annual Meeting, 1997, Seattle, WA.

Grady RW, Carr MC, Mitchell ME (1999) Complete primary closure of bladder exstrophy. Epispadias and bladder exstrophy repair. *Urol Clin North Am* **26**: 95–109, viii.

Graham SD (1972) Agenesis of bladder. *J Urol* **107**: 660–1.

Gross S (1876) *A practical treatise on the diseases, injuries, and malformations of the urinary bladder, the prostate gland, and the urethra*. 3rd edition. Philadelphia, PA: Henry C. Lea.

Gupta N, G IM (1976) Ectopia vesicae complicated by squamous cell carcinoma. *Br J Urol* **48**: 244.

Hamper UM *et al*. (1991) Bladder exstrophy–epispadias complex: prostatic evaluation by transrectal ultrasonography. *Prostate* **19**: 133–40.

Hanna MK, Williams DI (1972) Genital function in males with vesical exstrophy and epispadias. *Br J Urol* **44**: 169–74.

Hesser JW, Murata Y, Swalwell CI (1984) Exstrophy of cloaca with omphalocele: two cases. *Am J Obstet Gynecol* **150**: 1004–6.

Hohenfellner R (1992) Ureterosigmoidostomy: past, present and future. *Scand J Urol Nephrol* **142** (Suppl): 86–9.

Hohenfellner R, Stein R (1996) Primary urinary diversion in patients with bladder exstrophy (Editorial). *Urology* **48**: 828–30.

Hollowell JG et al. (1992) Lower urinary tract function after exstrophy closure. *Pediatr Nephrol* **6**: 428–32.

Hollowell J, Hill PD, Duffy PG, Ransley PG (1993) Evaluation and and treatment of incontinence after bladder neck reconstruction in exstrophy and epispadias. *Br J Urol* **71**: 743–9.

Howell C et al. (1983) Optimal management of cloacal exstrophy. *J Pediatr Surg* **18**: 365–9.

Hoyes A, Ramus NI, Martin BGH (1973) Ultrastructural aspects of the development of the innervation of the vesical musculature in the early human fetus. *Invest Urol* **10**: 307–11.

Hurwitz RS et al. (1987) Cloacal exstrophy: a report of 34 cases. *J Urol* **138**: 1060–4.

Husmann D, Spence H (1990) Current status of tumor of the bowel following ureterosigmoidostomy: a review. *J Urol* **144**: 607–10.

Husmann DA et al. (1988) Management of the hindgut in cloacal exstrophy: terminal ileostomy versus colostomy. *J Pediatr Surg* **23**: 1107–13.

Husmann DA, McLorie GA, Churchill BM (1989) Closure of the exstrophic bladder: an evaluation of the factors leading to its success and its importance on urinary continence. *J Urol* **142**: 522–4; discussion 542–3.

Husmann DA et al. (1990a) Inguinal pathology and its association with classical bladder exstrophy. *J Pediatr Surg* **25**: 332–4.

Husmann DA, McLorie GA, Churchill BM (1990b) Factors predisposing to renal scarring: following staged reconstruction of classical bladder exstrophy. *J Pediatr Surg* **25**: 500–4.

Ives E, Coffey R, Carter CO (1980) A family study of bladder exstrophy. *J Med Genet* **17**: 139–41.

Jaffe R, Schoenfeld A, Ovadia J (1990) Sonographic findings in the prenatal diagnosis of bladder exstrophy. *Am J Obstet Gynecol* **162**: 675–8.

Jeffs RD (1977) Functional closure of bladder exstrophy. *Birth Defects Orig Artic Ser* **13**: 171–3.

Jeffs RD (1987) Exstrophy, epispadias, and cloacal and urogenital sinus abnormalities. *Pediatr Clin North Am* **34**: 1233–57.

Jeffs RD, Guice SL, Oesch I (1982) The factors in successful exstrophy closure. *J Urol* **127**: 974–6.

Johnston JH, Kogan SJ (1974) The exstrophic anomalies and their surgical reconstruction. *Curr Probl Surg* 1–39.

Jones JA, Mitchell ME, Rink RC (1993) Improved results using a modification of the Young–Dees–Leadbetter bladder neck repair. *Br J Urol* **71**: 555–61.

Kapoor R, Saha MM (1987) Complete duplication of the bladder, urethra and external genitalia in a neonate – a case report. *J Urol* **137**: 1243–4.

King L, Wendel E (1972) Primary cystectomy and permanent urinary diversion in the treatment of exstrophy of the urinary bladder. In: Scott R, Gordon H, Carlton C, Beach P (eds) *Current controversies in urologic management.* Philadelphia, PA: WB Saunders, 242–50.

Kizilcan F et al. (1994) Superior vesical fissure: an exstrophy variant or a distinct clinical entity. *Eur Urol* **26**: 187–8.

Klimberg I (1988) The development of voiding control. *AUA Update Series* **7**: 162–7.

Kramer S, Kelalis PP (1982) Assessment of urinary continence in epispadias: a review of 94 patients. *J Urol* **128**: 290–3.

Krull CL, Heyns CF, de Klerk DP (1988) Agenesis of the bladder and urethra: a case report. *J Urol* **140**: 793–4.

Kurzrock H, Lowe P, Hardy BE (1996) Bladder wall pedicle wraparound sling for neurogenic urinary incontinence in children. *J Urol* **155**: 305–8.

Langer JC (1993) Fetal abdominal wall defects. *Semin Pediatr Surg* **2**: 121–8.

Lattimer JK, Smith MJ (1966) Exstrophy closure: a followup on 70 cases. *J Urol* **95**: 356–9.

Lattimer JK, MacFarlane MT, Puchner PJ (1978) Male exstrophy patients: a preliminary report on the reproductive capability. *Trans Am Assoc Genitourin Surg*, **70**: 42–4.

Leadbetter W (1951) Consideration of problems incident to performance of uretero-enterostomy: report of a technique. *J Urol* **65**: 818–30.

Lepor H, Jeffs RD (1983) Primary bladder closure and bladder neck reconstruction in classical bladder exstrophy. *J Urol* **130**: 1142–5.

Levard G et al. (1989) *Urinary bladder diverticula and the Ehlers–Danlos syndrome in children.* J Pediatr Surg **24**: 1184–6.

Light JK, Scott FB (1983) Treatment of the epispadias–exstrophy complex with the AS792 artificial urinary sphincter. *J Urol* **129**: 738–40.

Lottman HB, Melin Y (1999) Male epispadias repair: surgical and functional results with the Cantwell–Ransley procedure in 40 patients. *J Urol* **162**: 1176–80.

Lottman H, Melin Y, Cendron M et al. (1997) Bladder exstrophy: evaluation of factors leading to continence with spontaneous voiding after staged reconstruction. *J Urol* **158**: 1041–4.

Lowe FC, Jeffs RD (1983) Wound dehiscence in bladder exstrophy: an examination of the etiologies and factors for initial failure and subsequent success. *J Urol* **130**: 312–15.

Lund DP, Hendren WH (1993) Cloacal exstrophy: experience with 20 cases. *J Pediatr Surg* **28**: 1360–8; discussion 1368–9.

McKenna PH et al. (1994) Iliac osteotomy: a model to compare the options in bladder and cloacal exstrophy reconstruction. *J Urol* **151**: 182–6; discussion 186–7.

McLaughlin JF, Marks WM, Jones G (1984) Prospective management of exstrophy of the cloaca and myelocystocele following prenatal ultrasound recognition of neural tube defects in identical twins. *Am J Med Genet* **19**: 721–7.

Mansi M, Ahmed S (1993) Young–Dees–Leadbetter bladder neck reconstruction for sphincteric urinary incontinence: the value of augmentation cystoplasty. *Scand J Urol Nephrol* **27**: 509–17.

Manzoni GA, Ransley PG, Hurwitz RS (1987) Cloacal exstrophy and cloacal exstrophy variants: a proposed system of classification. *J Urol* **138**: 1065–8.

Marshall V, Muecke E (1962) Variations in exstrophy of the bladder. *J Urol* **88**: 766–96.

Marshall V, Muecke EC (1968) Congenital abnormalities of the bladder. In: *Handbuch de Urologie*. New York: Springer, 165.

Marshall VF, Muecke EC (1970) Functional closure of typical exstrophy of the bladder. *J Urol* **104**: 205–12.

Megalli M, Lattimer JK (1973) Review of the management of 140 cases of exstrophy of the bladder. *J Urol* **109**: 246–8.

Mesrobian HG, Kelalis PP, Kramer SA (1988) Long-term followup of 103 patients with bladder exstrophy. *J Urol* **139**: 719–22.

Messelink EJ et al. (1994) Four cases of bladder exstrophy in two families. *J Med Genet* **31**: 490–2.

Mirk P, Calisti A, Fileni A (1986) Prenatal sonographic diagnosis of bladder exstrophy. *J Ultrasound Med* **5**: 291–4.

Mitchell M (1999) The challnege of cloacal exstrophy. In: *Gender Reassignment Meeting*, 1999, Dallas, TX.

Mitchell M, Close C (1996) Early primary valve ablation for posterior urethral valves. *Semin Pediatr Surg* **5**: 66–71.

Mitchell ME, Bagli DJ (1996) Complete penile disassembly for epispadias repair: the Mitchell technique. *J Urol* **155**: 300–4.

Mitchell, W, Venable D, Patel AJ (1993) Pseudoexstrophy. *Urology* **41**: 134–6.

Mollard P (1980) Bladder reconstruction in exstrophy. *J Urol* **124**: 525–9.

Mollard P, Mouriquand PD, Buttin X (1994) Urinary continence after reconstruction of classical bladder exstrophy (73 cases). *Br J Urol* **73**: 298–302.

Montagnani CA (1982) One stage functional reconstruction of exstrophied bladder: report of two cases with six-year follow-up. *Z Kinderchir* **37**: 23–7.

Muecke E (1964) The role of the cloacal membrane in exstrophy: the first successful experimental study. *J Urol* **92**: 659–67.

Nielsen OH, Nielsen R, Parvinen T (1980) Duplicate exstrophy of the bladder. *Ann Chir Gynaecol* **69**: 32–6.

Nisonson I, Lattimer JK (1972) How well can the exstrophied bladder work? *J Urol* **107**: 664–6.

Nix J, Menville JG, Albert M (1958) Congenital patent urachus. *J Urol* **79**: 264–7.

O'Donnell B (1984) The lessons of 40 bladder extrophies in 20 years. *J Pediatr Surg* **19**: 547–9.

O'Kane HO, Megaw JM (1968) Carcinoma in the exstrophic bladder. *Br J Surg* **55**: 631–5.

O'Neill JJ (1998) Cloacal exstrophy. In: O'Neill JJ, Rowe S (eds) *Pediatric surgery*. Philadelphia, PA: Mosby Year Book, 1725–32.

Oesterling JE, Jeffs RD (1987) The importance of a successful initial bladder closure in the surgical management of classical bladder exstrophy: analysis of 144 patients treated at the Johns Hopkins Hospital between 1975 and 1985. *J Urol* **137**: 258–62.

Paidas MJ, Crombleholme TM, Robertson FM (1994) Prenatal diagnosis and management of the fetus with an abdominal wall defect. *Semin Perinatol* **18**: 196–214.

Palmer JM, Russi MF (1969) Persistent urogenital sinus with absence of the bladder and urethra. *J Urol* **102**: 590–4.

Patten B, Barry A (1952) The genesis of exstrophy of the bladder and epispadias. *Am J Anat* **90**: 35–53.

Perovic SV, VV Djordjevic MLJ, Djakovic NG (1999) Penile disassembly technique for epispadias repair: variants of technique. *J Urol* **162**: 1181–4.

Pineschi A, Chiella E (1982) Duplicate exstrophy of the bladder: a case report. *Z Kinderchir* **35**: 35–7.

Pinette MG et al. (1996) Prenatal diagnosis of fetal bladder and cloacal exstrophy by ultrasound. A report of three cases. *J Reprod Med* **41**: 132–4.

Proud VK et al. (1996) Distinctive Menkes disease variant with occipital horns: delineation of natural history and clinical phenotype. *Am J Med Genet* **65**: 44–51.

Radhakrishnan J (1998) Double-barrelled colovaginoplasty in a patient with cloacal exstrophy variant. *J Pediatr Surg* **33**: 1402–3.

Ransley P, Woppin M (1988) Bladder exstrophy closure and epispadias repair. In: Spitz L (ed.) *Operative surgery: pediatric surgery*. London: Butterworths, 620–32.

Reiner WG, Gearhart JP, Jeffs R (1999) Psychosexual dysfunction in males with genital anomalies: late adolescence, Tanner stages IV to VI. *J Am Acad Child Adolesc Psychiatr* **38**: 865–72.

Rickham P (1960) Vesicointestinal fissure. *Arch Dis Child* **35**: 97–101.

Ritchey ML, Kramer SA, Kelalis PP (1988) Vesical neck reconstruction in patients with epispadias-exstrophy. *J Urol* **139**: 1278–81.

Rubin A (1967) *Handbook of congenital malformations*. Philadelphia, PA: WB Saunders, 334.

Saltzman B, Mininberg DT, Muecke EC (1985) Exstrophy of bladder: evolution of management. *Urology* **26**: 383–8.

Satler E, Mossman HW (1968) A case report of a double bladder and double urethra in the female child. *J Urol* **79**: 274–6.

Schmidt AH et al. (1993) Pelvic osteotomy for bladder exstrophy. *J Pediatr Orthop* **13**: 214–19.

Shapiro E, Jeffs RD, Gearhart JP, Lepor H (1985) Muscarinic cholinergic receptors in bladder exstrophy: insights into surgical management. *J Urol* **134**: 308–10.

Shapiro E, Lepor H, Jeffs RD (1984) The inheritance of the exstrophy–epispadias complex. *J Urol* **132**: 308–10.

Sheldon CA et al. (1990) Duplicate bladder exstrophy: a new variant of clinical and embryological significance. *J Urol* **144**: 334–6.

Silver RI et al. (1997) Penile length in adulthood after exstrophy reconstruction. *J Urol* **157**: 999–1003.

Skari H et al. (1998) Consequences of prenatal ultrasound diagnosis: a preliminary report on neonates with congenital malformations. *Acta Obstet Gynecol Scand* **77**: 635–42.

Slaughenhoupt B, Chen CJ, Gearhart JP (1996) Creation of a model of bladder exstrophy in the fetal lamb. *J Urol* **156**: 816–18.

Spence H, Hoffman W, Pate V (1975) Exstrophy of the bladder. Long term results in a series of 37 cases treated by ureterosigmoidostomy. *J Urol* **114**: 131–7.

Spencer R (1965) Exstrophia splanchnica (exstrophy of the cloaca). *Surgery* **57**: 751–5.

Sponseller PD, Gearhart JP, Jeffs RD (1991) Anterior innominate osteotomies for failure or late closure of bladder exstrophy. *J Urol* **146**: 137–40.

Sponseller PD *et al.* (1995) The anatomy of the pelvis in the exstrophy complex. *J Bone Joint Surg Am* **77**: 177–89.

Stephens FD (1979) The vesicoureteral hiatus and paraureteral diverticula. *J Urol* **121**: 786–91.

Stoler JM, Doody DP, Holmes LB (1993) A case of a closed partial cloacal septation defect with a patent urachus. *Teratology* **48**: 97–103.

Stringer MD, Duffy PG, Ransley PG (1994) Inguinal hernias associated with bladder exstrophy. *Br J Urol* **73**: 308–9.

Swana HS, Gallagher PG, Weiss RM (1997) Pseudoexstrophy of the bladder: case report and literature review. *J Pediatr Surg* **32**: 1480–1.

Tacciuoli M, Laurenti C, Racheli T (1977) Sixteen years' experience with the Heitz Boyer–Hovelacque procedure for exstrophy of the bladder. *Br J Urol* **49**: 385–90.

Taylor WN *et al.* (1979) Bladder diverticula causing posterior urethral obstruction in children. *J Urol* **122**: 415.

Thomalla J, Rudolph R, Seal G *et al.* (1980) Gastroschisis induced in the chick embryo with the CO_2 laser. *Surg Forum* **35**: 634–7.

Thomalla JV, Rudolph RA *et al.* (1985) Induction of cloacal exstrophy in the chick embryo using the CO_2 laser. *J Urol* **134**: 991–5.

Toguri A, Churchill BM, Schillinger JF, Jeffs RD (1978) Continence in cases of bladder exstrophy. *J Urol* **119**: 538–40.

Trendelenberg F (1906) The treatment of ectopia vesicae. *Ann Surg* **44**: 981–9.

Uhlir K (1968) Rare malformations of the bladder. *J Urol* **99**: 53–8.

Van Buren W, Keyes ED (1874) *A practical treatise on the surgical diseases of the genito-urinary organs, including syphilis.* New York: Appleton and Company.

Verghese M, Belman AB (1984) Urinary retention secondary to congenital bladder deverticula in infants. *J Urol* **132**: 1186–89.

Warren B, Ziegler M (1993) Exstrophy of the cloaca. In: Ashcraft K, Holden T (eds) *Pediatric surgery*. 2nd edition. Philadelphia, PA: WB Saunders, 402.

Welch K (1979) Cloacal exstrophy. In: Ravitch M (ed.) *Pediatric surgery*. Chicago, IL: Year Book Medical Publishers.

Williams D (1957) Congenital bladder neck obstruction and megaureter. *Br J Urol* **29**: 389.

Williams DI, Keeton JE (1973) Further progress with reconstruction of the exstrophied bladder. *Br J Surg* **60**: 203–7.

Wood J (1869) *Lancet* i: 259.

Woodhouse CR (1986) The management of erectile deformity in adults with exstrophy and epispadias. *J Urol* **135**: 932–5.

Woodhouse CR (1999) The gynaecology of exstrophy. *BJU Int* 83 (Suppl 3): 34–8.

Woodhouse C, Redgrave NG (1996) Late failure of the reconstructed exstrophy bladder. *Br J Urol* **77**: 590–2.

Woodhouse CR, Hinsch R (1997) The anatomy and reconstruction of the adult female genitalia in classical exstrophy. *Br J Urol* **79**: 618–22.

Woodhouse CR, Kellett MJ (1984), Anatomy of the penis and its deformities in exstrophy and epispadias. *J Urol* **132**: 1122–4.

Woodhouse CR, Ransley PG, Williams DI (1983) The patient with exstrophy in adult life. *Br J Urol* **55**: 632–5.

Yazbeck S, Ndoye M, Khan AH (1986) Omphalocele: a 25-year experience. *J Pediatr Surg* **21**: 761–3.

Young H (1942) Exstrophy of the bladder: the first case in which a normal bladder and urinary control have been obtained by plastic operations. *Surg Gynecol Obstet* **74**: 729–37.

Zaontz MR *et al.* (1998) Multicenter experience with the Mitchell technique for epispadias repair. *J Urol* **160**: 172–6.

Ziegler M, Duckett JW, Howell JG (1986) Cloacal exstrophy. In: Welch J (ed.) *Pediatric surgery*. Chicago, IL: Year Book Medical Publishers.

Urethral valve and other anomalies of the male urethra

28

Kenneth I. Glassberg and Mark Horowitz

The male urethra

The male urethra can be divided into anterior and posterior segments. The posterior segment is composed of the prostatic and membranous urethra while the anterior segment includes the bulbous and penile urethra. That area that runs from the bladder neck to the proximal margin of the urogenital membrane, including the urethra within the prostate gland, is referred to as the prostatic urethra. The segment of urethra that lies within the urogenital diaphragm, i.e. the striated muscles of the external sphincter, is referred to as the membranous urethra. The area just distal to the urogenital diaphragm and proximal to the penoscrotal junction is the bulbous urethra. The urethra lying within the penile shaft and glans is referred to as the penile, anterior or pendulous urethra.

Posterior urethral valves

A posterior urethral valve (PUV) is the most common cause of bladder outlet obstruction in boys. It is associated with a dilated posterior urethra, poor urinary stream, incomplete emptying of the bladder, usually bilateral hydroureteronephrosis, frequently vesicoureteral reflux (VUR) and bladder diverticula, sometimes renal failure and poor growth, and occasionally urinary ascites or perirenal urinoma. Classically, the diagnosis is made on a voiding cysto-urethrogram (VCUG).

Embryology and anatomy

Young *et al.* (1919) recognized three distinct types of congenital valvular obstruction of the posterior urethra. They classified PUV as follows: a type I valve is the bicuspid type that usually is seen originating on

the floor of the urethra arising from the distal lateral aspect of the verumontanum extending distally and anteriorly to fuse in the midline (Fig. 28.1a, b). A type II valve runs between the verumontanum and the bladder neck, while type III appears distal to the verumontanum as a circular, non-oblique diaphragm usually just distal to the verumontanum.

Type I valves make up the vast majority of PUV. They are obstructive to the antegrade flow of urine since they fill with urine during micturition (like sails catching the wind) and meet together in the midline, making the aperture between the valves considerably smaller. In some cases, the valves are less rigid and more distendable and may prolapse further down the urethra, simulating the windsock valves previously described by Fields and Stephens (1974). Type II valves probably do not represent an obstructive phenomenon but appear as prominent longitudinal folds in a posterior urethra that is dilated secondary to some other, more distal, obstruction. Type III valves may represent an entirely different entity, as Williams and Eckstein (1965) have suggested, a form of congenital urethral stricture (Fig. 28.2a–h). Since the type III diaphragm is not a rigid stricture and is comprised mostly of mucosa, the latter description may be inappropriate.

In the normal urethra small, distinct, paired lateral folds (plicae colliculi) arise at the lateral distal edge of the verumontanum bilaterally and traverse a short distance distally to attach onto the lateral walls of the urethra. Stephens (1983a) believes that these folds represent the embryologic integration of the wolffian ducts into the urethra. PUV also arise at the distal lateral aspect of the verumontanum but extend more distally in an oblique fashion along the lateral walls of the urethra and continue anteriorly, where they fuse and form a circumferential obstruction. The normal mucosal folds, the plicae colliculi, do not appear in

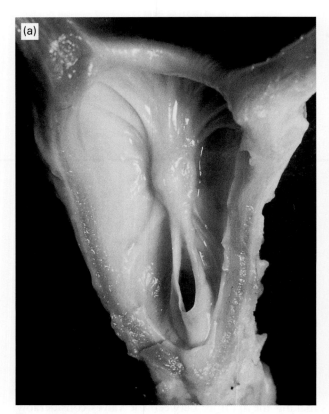 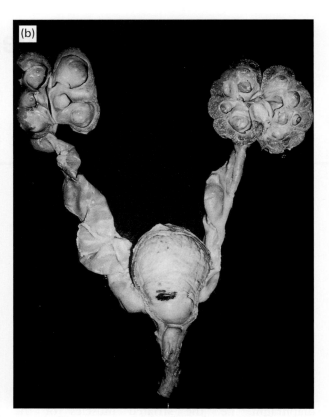

Figure 28.1 (a) Autopsy specimen of type I posterior urethral valve. The ventrum of the posterior urethra has been removed, allowing visualization of the prominent bladder neck, verumontanum, and posterior urethral valve. Note the oblique course of the valve, beginning on the floor at the verumontanum and fusing anteriorly further down the urethra. (b) The bladder is thick walled and severely trabeculated. The ureters are dilated and tortuous. The kidneys are severely hydronephrotic with thin parenchyma. (From Johnston and Kulatilake, 1972, with permission.)

patients with PUV. As a result, it seems logical to assume that PUV actually represent an exaggeration of the normal plica colliculi with distal anterior fusion resulting from an abnormal integration, insertion, or absorption of the wolffian ducts into the posterior urethra, an etiology that is supported by Stephens (1983a). Even as far back as 1870, Tolmatshew proposed that PUV represent enlargement of normal urethral folds (Fig. 28.3a–c).

According to Stephens (1983a), prior to the cloaca separating into the anorectal canal posteriorly and the urogenital sinus anteriorly, the wolffian (mesonephric) ducts insert laterally on the cloaca. As the cloaca divides the opening of each wolffian duct migrates posteriomedially and cranially to open at the verumontanum, leaving remnants just distal and lateral to the verumonantum, i.e. plica colliculi. Stephens believes that PUV result from the wolffian ducts entering the cloaca more anteriorly, not migrating posteriomedially

as in normals and, instead, fusing anteriorly in the midline leaving behind the PUV (Fig. 28.4a–f).

Because PUV simulate the normally appearing mucosal folds, except that they are usually thicker, more prominent, and fused anteriorly, one must consider the existence of a spectrum of PUV, as there is a spectrum of disease in any congenital anomaly. As a result, those valves that have a smaller aperture between the leaflets with a larger area of anterior fusion are generally more obstructive than those with a larger aperture and a less prominent anterior component. Debate exists as to whether prominent folds without anterior fusion can be obstructive. Plica colliculi themselves represent normal non-obstructive folds. Because endoscopically plica colliculi appear much more prominent in prepubertal boys than in adult men, the urologist who does not frequently perform cystoscopy in children may misinterpret the presence of normal urethral folds as PUV. The prob-

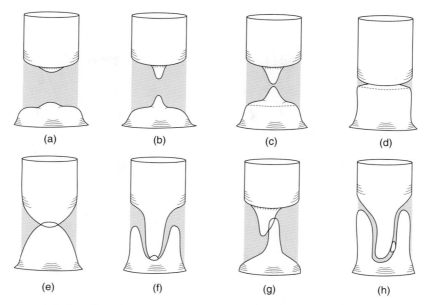

Figure 28.2 Development of type III valves. (*a–d*) Normal canalization of the urogenital membrane. (*d*) Shows normal slight constriction at the level of the perineal membrane. (*e*)Stricture formation. (*f*) Canalization by central downgrowth and circumferencial ingrowth, resulting in a bulging membrane with a central stenotic orifice. (*g, h*) Side openings creating valvular 'windsock' membranes.

lem in diagnosing lesser degrees of valves (what Hendren (1974), refers to as 'mini valves') is determining where the transition is between normal plicae colliculi and obstructive PUV. Some have suggested that milder degrees of obstruction may be associated with dysfunctional voiding symptomatology, nocturnal enuresis, and teenage and adult prostatitis, and

some resect these prominent folds assuming that they represent minivalves (Mahony, 1974; Mahony and Laferte, 1974; Arnold and Ginsburg, 1974). Even before Hendren's drawing attention to the phenomenon of minivalves, Williams and Eckstein (1965) discussed the risks of overdiagnosing normal mucosal folds as obstructive valves. In a recent report

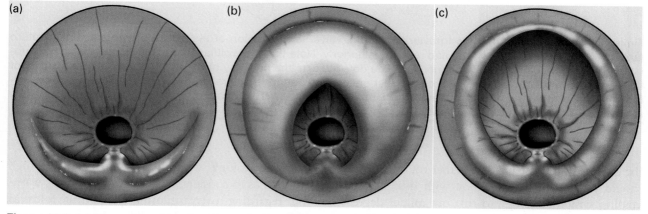

Figure 28.3 (*a*) Normal urethra demonstrating prominent normal folds, i.e. plicae colliculi, arising from the verumontanum and inserting on the lateral wall. These is no evidence of anterior fusion. (*b*) Obstructive posterior urethral valve arising from verumontanum fusing anteriorly and more distally. (*c*) 'Minivalves': less obstructive valves, but pathologic since leaflets fuse anteriorly.

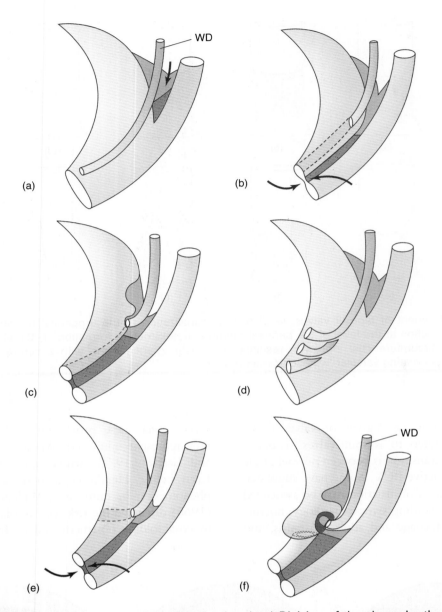

Figure 28.4 Development of type I posterior urethral valve. (*a–c*) Division of the cloaca by the anorectal septum (*arrows*) into the bladder anteriorly and rectum posteriorly. Note that the wolffian ducts (WD) initially insert anterio-laterally and then migrate to a posterior site. The dots indicate the pathway of migration of the receding orifice of the duct. (*d–f*) More anterior location of the duct orifice with abnormal migration giving rise to an oblique circumferential 'valve' structure with its proximal aspect arising from the verumontanum and fusing distally and obliquely in an anterior position. (From Stephens, 1976, with permission.)

the question was raised as to whether routine VCUG should be obtained in any boy with dysfunctional voiding symptomatology to rule out milder degrees of valvular obstruction (Arena *et al.*, 1999). If this advice were followed, radiology suites would be overflowing. In another study, almost one-half the valves reported were in boys with dysfunctional voiding

symptomatology without hydronephrosis, which compels us to consider Williams and Eckstein's warning regarding overdiagnosing prominent folds as PUV (Pieretti, 1993) (Fig. 28.5a–c).

Dewan *et al.* (1992) and Dewan (1993, 1996, 1999), after observing PUV in a number of previously uninstrumented infant urethras, believe that what has

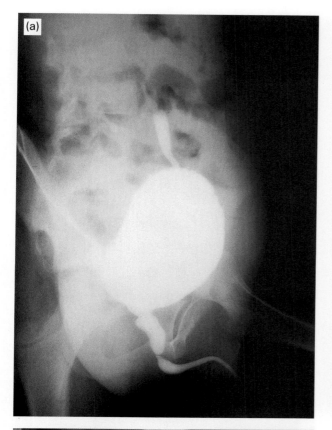

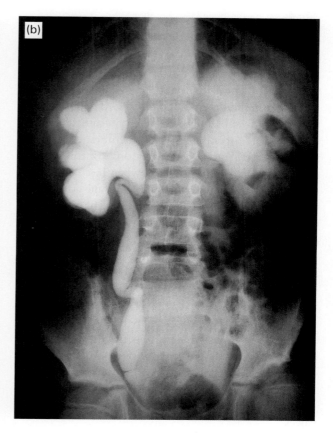

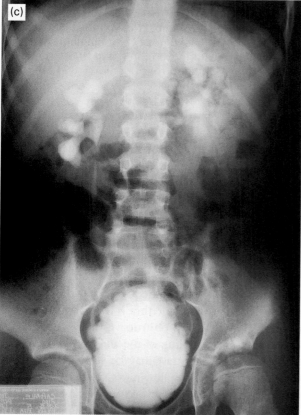

Figure 28.5 An 11-year-old boy with day and night wetting. (*a*) Voiding cystourethrogram demonstrating a dilated posterior urethra. Note that the anterior urethra fills fairly well, indicating a less obstructive valve. Cystoscopy confirmed that this was a type I valve with anterior fusion. (*b*) Intravenous pyelogram demonstrating bilateral hydroureteronephrosis. (*c*) Intravenous pyelogram 1 year after valve ablation demonstrating significantly less dilatation. The patient is asymptomatic.

been referred to as 'posterior urethral valves' actually is a single obstructive membrane with a small defect or opening in the posterior midline of the urethra that allows for the passage of urine. Dewan (1993), therefore, prefers to call the entity 'congenital obstructing posterior urethral membrane (COPUM)'. He believes that, with the subsequent passage of a catheter or cystoscope, the opening in the membrane becomes stretched or enlarged. Depending on how the opening enlarges will cause the surgeon, when performing cystourethroscopy, to perceive the membrane as type I or type III valves. He believes that both represent a COPUM. The membrane that exists with a central opening that sometimes is perceived as a type III PUV occurs more distally, i.e. within the bulbous urethra, and that entity is not a COPUM or valve, but one sometimes referred to as a Cobb's collar or congenital urethral stricture (Dewan et al., 1994, 1995). The present authors agree with Dewan that PUV is not an abnormality represented by two discrete valves, but anatomically is a singular obstructive structure. However, there is probably no need to change the term 'valve' to 'membrane'. The singular term 'posterior urethral valve' is preferable to the plural 'posterior urethral valves'.

Radiologic appearance on voiding cystourethrography

The diagnosis of a PUV is made on the VCUG. The posterior urethra is much more dilated than normal and significantly more dilated than the anterior urethra. It frequently takes on a shield shape or squared-off appearance. Often the distal aspect of the dilated posterior urethra will appear to overlap the urethra beyond the obstruction or, in the words of Williams and Eckstein (1965), 'bulge forward over the bulbar region' (Fig. 28.6). The bladder neck most often is clearly demarcated and may appear as a thick muscular collar (Fig. 28.7) as described by Waterhouse (1964), or as a posterior and/or anterior indentation between the shield-shaped posterior urethra and bladder (Fig. 28.6). The radiologic appearance of a PUV can be summarized as:

- widened posterior urethra (sometimes shield shaped);
- most often anterior urethra only partially filled;
- prominent bladder neck (most often demarcated as a prominent posterior lip and/or anterior lip and sometimes as an annular band);

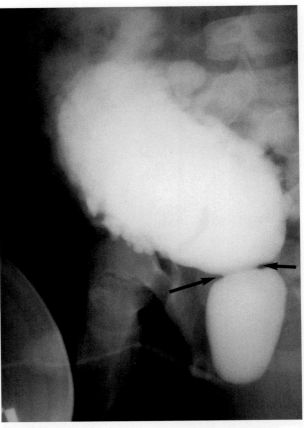

Figure 28.6 Diagnosis of posterior urethral valves on voiding cystourethrogram. Note the shield-shaped posterior urethra that bulges over the bulbous urethra, the collapsed anterior urethra, and the prominent bladder neck outlined by posterior and anterior indentations (*arrows*).

- sometimes the posterior urethra will bulge forward over the bulbous urethra;
- lucencies representing valve leaflets may or may not be visualized.

Normal plica colliculi as well as PUV leaflets may appear as lucencies (Fig. 28.8). Frequently, however, when a PUV is present, lucencies representing the valve leaflets are not seen and the posterior urethral dilatation alone suggests the presence of PUV.

Usually, the anterior urethra is less full than normal during voiding but less obstructive valves can be associated with greater filling of the anterior urethra (Fig. 28.5a). In some, contrast may be seen refluxing into the ejaculatory ducts. Following valve ablation, ejaculatory duct reflux may persist or even become apparent.

Often, pediatric radiologists performing a VCUG

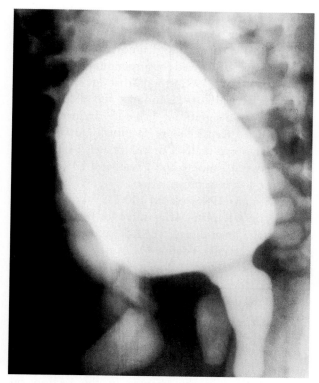

Figure 28.7 Bladder neck represented by an opaque radiographic collar. The bladder neck lumen appears wider than the bladder neck typically seen on a normal voiding cystourethrogram.

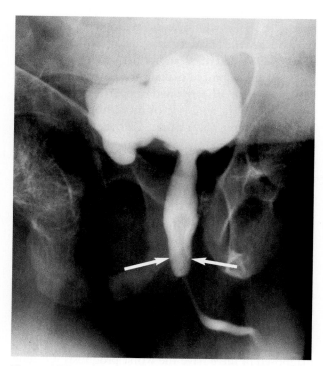

Figure 28.8 Valve leaflets seen as lucencies (*arrows*).

will leave the urethral catheter in place during voiding in case the bladder needs to be refilled. Ditchfield *et al.* (1995) found that the catheter does not obscure the diagnosis. Lebowitz (1996) agrees that the catheter will not obscure the valves. However, he finds the catheter a drawback when the preablation VCUG is needed for comparison with the postablation VCUG to determine the adequacy of surgery. He suggests that if a valve is diagnosed on a VCUG when a catheter is in place, the catheter should be removed after refilling the bladder. Repeat voiding images can then be obtained without a catheter and be used, if needed, for later comparison with postablation images.

The severity of the disease and how successfully the surgeon feels that the valve was ablated will determine how soon after valve resection or ablation a VCUG should be obtained to confirm the absence of residual obstruction. The VCUG can be performed in combination with a urodynamic evaluation (i.e. videourodynamic examination) so that bladder function can be evaluated simultaneously. Often, there is some residual dilatation of the posterior urethra following valve ablation; which may last a lifetime. However, when there is fullness, it is important to rule out any residual obstructing valve tissue or a stricture that might be due to the urethral instrumentation, before concluding that it is residual dilatation only.

Incidence

PUV are the most common cause of congenital urethral obstruction. Although first described by Morgani and Benjamin (1769), again by Langenback (1802), discussed by Young *et al.* (1919), and reported in 55 clinical cases by Campbell (1937), Campbell still had reason to write 14 years later: 'Valvular obstruction of the posterior urethra is not uncommon; it simply fails to be recognized' (Campbell, 1951). In the USA, it was not until the late 1950s and early 1960s that the diagnosis started to be entertained when the VCUG became the means for its diagnosis (Griesbach *et al.*, 1959; Waterhouse, 1961; Hamm and Waterhouse, 1961).

Casale (1999) estimated the incidence of PUV to be 1 in 8000–25 000 live male births. Atwall (1983) suggested a frequency of 1 in 5000–12 500, and King (1985) reported an occurrence of 1 in 5000–8000 live male births. These reports, however, may be somewhat conservative in their estimate. For example, in

Yorkshire, UK, approximately six live male births occur each year with PUV, implying an incidence of 1 in 4000 live male births, and this statistic does not take into account another ten male fetuses with severe *in utero* urethral obstruction that are electively aborted each year (Hutton *et al.*, 1994). In Oman, the calculated incidence of PUV is 1 in 2375 newborn males (Rajab *et al.*, 1996). The incidence in Oman and in Yorkshire seems to correlate more closely with the present authors' experience.

Presentation and prognosis

Fetal urine contributes approximately 90% of the amniotic fluid volume. In the most severely affected PUV fetuses, i.e. those with dysplastic kidneys or hydronephrotic, shell-like kidneys, not enough urine is produced or voided, and oligohydramnios results. Such a fetus may spontaneously abort or, if it survives to delivery, may be stillborn or have respiratory distress secondary to pulmonary hypoplasia. Landers and Hanson (1990) believe that decreased amniotic fluid will not allow chest mobility, lung expansion, or lung development. Oligohydramnios is usually associated with the facial features and limb deformations of Potter's syndrome.

Denes *et al.* (1997) found that 35% (15 of 43) of their PUV cases presented *in utero*. The newborns not detected *in utero* presented with non-specific gastrointestinal symptoms, respiratory distress, or abdominal distension or a mass, the latter representing a distended bladder or hydronephrotic kidney. Older infants in the series presented with urinary tract infection (UTI) or an abdominal mass. In other series, poor urinary stream and other lower tract symptomatology are major presenting signs in older children.

In early reports, perinatal mortality was reported at approximately 50% and usually was secondary to sepsis, respiratory problems, acidosis, and uremia (Williams, 1954; Johnston and Kulatilake, 1972). The higher incidence of prenatal diagnosis, elective termination of pregnancy, and better perinatal care have lowered perinatal mortality to between 0 and 10% (Churchill *et al.*, 1983, 1990; Parkhouse *et al.*, 1988; Reinberg *et al.*, 1992). Those with respiratory difficulties at birth secondary to pulmonary hypoplasia have the worst prognosis. In a group of boys presenting between birth and 10 years of age and diagnosed between 1966 and 1975 (before the widespread use of *in utero* sonograms), Parkhouse *et al.*

(1988) found a 21% renal failure rate during long-term follow-up occurring at a mean of 15 years. When 102 PUV patients, diagnosed between 1969 and 1979, were followed for a minimum of 10 years, Merguerian *et al.* (1992) found that age of presentation (i.e. 1 month, 1–12 months and older than 1 year) was not a significant factor in the incidence of renal failure. Renal failure eventually occurred in 14.7% diagnosed under 1 month of age, 14.3% diagnosed between 1 month and 1 year, and 10% in those aged over 1 year at presentation.

Smith *et al.* (1996) placed 100 PUV boys of varying ages on a Kaplan–Meier curve for both the onset of end-stage renal disease (ESRD) and chronic renal failure. The latter was defined as a sustained creatinine greater than 2.0 mg/dl for at least 1 month. They found the development of ESRD to be 6% before 1 year of age and uncommon between the ages of 1 and 10 years. At 10 years of age, the rate was $10 \pm 3\%$ and, at age 20, $38 \pm 8\%$. The chronic renal failure curve preceded the curve for ESRD by approximately 5 years. The significance of serum creatinine levels is discussed later in the chapter in the section on prognostic indicators.

Prenatal diagnosis and prognosis

The diagnosis of PUV is suspected *in utero* when a male fetus is seen with bilateral hydroureteronephrosis and a thick-walled bladder that does not empty. Cohen *et al.* (1998) described additional sonographic findings that are helpful in making the diagnosis of PUV in fetuses with *in utero* hydronephrosis, i.e. dilated posterior urethra with one or more bright echogenic lines representing valve tissue. This same group previously had identified these echogenic lines in the dilated posterior urethra in three of five PUV neonates using a transperineal sonographic technique (Cohen *et al.*, 1994). Mahoney (1994) has likened the *in utero* sonographic appearance of the bladder and urethra to a 'keyhole' where the dilated, thick-walled bladder takes on the upper appearance of the keyhole and the dilated posterior urethra makes up the lower aspect. Kaefer *et al.* (1997) consider the combination of *in utero* renal hyperechogenecity (sometimes representing dysplasia), oligohydramnios, and bladder distention as strong indicators of outlet obstruction.

Reinberg *et al.* (1992) found that those patients diagnosed *in utero* have the worst prognosis. Of nine such patients, one died of pulmonary hypoplasia one day after birth, five were surviving with renal failure, and three required transplantation. Others have not found such poor prognosis for the *in utero* group, particularly when the diagnosis is made in the third trimester after a normal *in utero* ultrasound had been obtained in the second trimester. For example, when Hutton *et al.* (1994) divided infants into those diagnosed at or before 24 weeks' gestation and those after 24 weeks, those diagnosed at or before 24 weeks had a poorer outcome, i.e. 53% (nine of 17 patients) died or developed renal failure (mean follow-up 3.9 years) compared with only one poor outcome in 14 patients diagnosed after 24 weeks. Making the data even more compelling is that for all 14 patients who were diagnosed after 24 weeks, a normal *in utero* sonogram had been obtained before 24 weeks. El-Ghoniemi *et al.* (1999) reported that renal failure developed in two of five boys diagnosed *in utero* before 24 weeks and in four of 25 diagnosed after 24 weeks, but made no comment as to whether or not a negative ultrasound study had been obtained before 24 weeks.

Dinneen *et al.* (1993) also found the gestational age of 24 weeks to be significant. In a group of 42 patients who had undergone antenatal sonograms, a fetal uropathy was diagnosed in only 19, and in only three of the 19 was it diagnosed before 24 weeks' gestation. Of the remaining 16 cases that were diagnosed *in utero* after 24 weeks, an *in utero* sonographic study had been obtained before 24 weeks and in none was fetal uropathy identifiable. Dinneen *et al.* (1993) suggest that, if routine sonograms were obtained in the third trimester in those babies who had normal renal ultrasounds in the second trimester, more cases of PUV would be diagnosed *in utero*. They speculate that in some PUV fetuses the urachus is patent in the second trimester, as in fetal lambs with infravesical obstruction (Harrison *et al.*, 1983), thus protecting the kidneys from increased bladder pressure. However, once the urachus closes hydronephrosis becomes apparent. Perhaps it is those fetuses with early closure of the urachus, whose kidneys are then no longer protected during a period when the kidney is rapidly developing, that are most vulnerable to the effects of obstruction.

Where the diagnosis is made before 20 weeks, massive dilatation is often seen and the kidneys are likely to be very poorly functioning with cysts and dysplasia present. Intrauterine intervention, such as vesicoamniotic shunting, is unlikely to salvage such kidneys. If untreated, many such fetuses would spontaneously abort.

Those that survive to term are likely to be stillborn with pulmonary hypoplasia (Dinneen *et al.*, 1993).

Early prenatal diagnosis allows in-depth counseling of parents, informing them of a 50% chance of renal failure or death in those diagnosed at 24 weeks or earlier. Likewise, the obstetrician and urologist can advise the parents of the good outcome that is likely when the diagnosis is made after 24 weeks, provided that a normal sonogram had been obtained before 24 weeks. However, the accuracy of *in utero* diagnosis is poor. For example, in one study, only 27 of 51 fetuses with the presumptive *in utero* diagnosis of PUV, made on the basis of bilateral hydronephrosis and a large bladder, actually had PUV (El-Ghoniemi *et al.*, 1999). Severe oligohydramnios is a more ominous sign.

Familial posterior urethral valves

While familial PUV is a rare entity, PUV have been reported in non-twin siblings (Farkas and Skinner, 1976; Borzi *et al.*, 1992), identical twins (Williams and Kapila, 1973; Kroovand *et al.*, 1977; Grajewski and Glassberg, 1983) and in one family in two successive generations (Hanlon-Lundberg *et al.*, 1994). In the latter, the father and paternal uncle had been diagnosed with PUV in childhood. The diagnosis in the reported infant was suspected *in utero* and confirmed postnatally. In the identical twin case reported by Williams and Kapila (1973), each patient had a large bladder diverticulum and ipsilateral hydronephrosis, in one twin on the left and in the other on the right. In the case of identical twins reported by Grajewski and Glassberg (1983), one twin presented at 18 months with urosepsis and was found to have severe bilateral hydronephrosis and compromised renal function. The brother presented at 5 years of age with the chief complaint of straining on urination. That latter sibling was 13 cm taller and 4 kg heavier, and had a normal blood urea nitrogen (BUN) and serum creatinine, grade II unilateral VUR, and no hydronephrosis. These twin boys illustrate the spectrum of disease associated with PUV. Both boys had obstructive valve leaflets meeting anteriorly, not the 'minivalves' without anterior fusion. However, one valve was more obstructive than the other, causing major destruction to the kidneys and a shorter stature because of compromised renal function. In the other, in spite of unilateral reflux the upper tracts were normal (Fig. 28.9a–e).

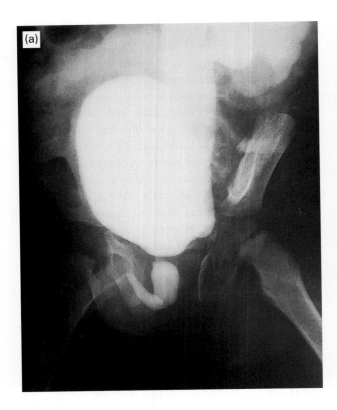

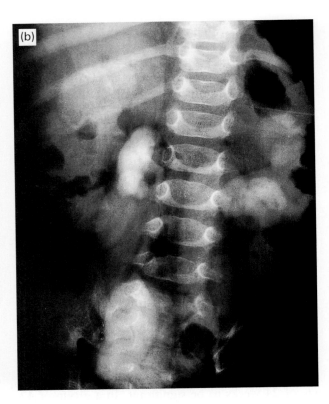

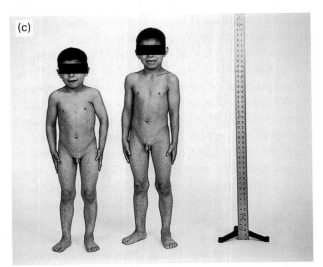

Figure 28.9 Clinical spectrum of posterior urethral valves (PUV) illustrated in identical twin boys. (*a*) Voiding cystourethrogram (VCUG) demonstrating PUV and severe vesicoureteral reflux in a 15-month-old boy presenting with urinary sepsis and renal failure. (*b*) Intravenous pyelogram demonstrating severe hydroureteronephrosis. (*c*) The previously unknown identical twin (right) presented 3 years later with straining to urinate. This twin was 13 cm taller and 4 kg heavier than his brother (left), and represents the more benign end of the spectrum of PUV. (*d*) and (*e*) *Continued opposite.*

Management

In the late 1950s, with the increasing use of the VCUG, the diagnosis of PUV became more frequent. At that time, incandescent bulbs for small cystoscopes offered poor illumination, the field of view was small, and hook electrodes were not available. Fulguration of the valves was often performed after retropubic exposure, even by splitting the pubis to gain exposure, or transvesically (Waterhouse, 1961). Traumatic breaking of the valves with sounds or catheters was another mode of treatment. Johnston (1966) sometimes fulgurated valves via an auroscope inserted through a perineal urethrotomy. RK Waterhouse (personal communication) used a wire stylet in a ureteral catheter, passed through a pediatric cystoscope. By making contact between an electrocautery and the wire stylet, the valve could then be ablated under vision. The approach was later popularized by Hendren (1974).

Today, most valve ablation is accomplished transurethrally. Using a small pediatric resectoscope, the valve leaflets are caught with a right-angle hook or loop electrode and, preferably with the cutting current, incised at the 4 or 5 and 7 or 8 o'clock position. Williams *et al.* (1973) preferred incising at the 12

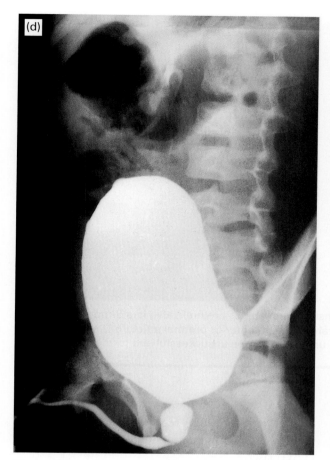 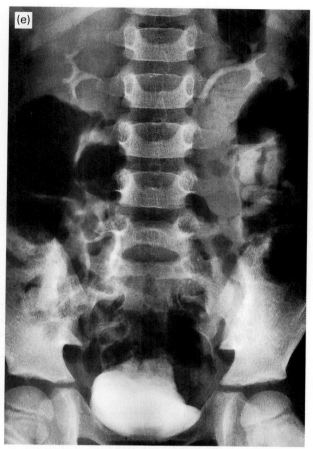

Figure 28.9 *Continued.* (*d*) VCUG of the taller twin demonstrates PUV but with better filling of the anterior urethra and only grade II right vesicoureteral reflux. (*e*) Intravenous urogram of the taller twin demonstrating normal kidneys. (From Grajewski and Glassberg, 1983, with permission.)

o'clock position and Gonzales (1998) at the 4, 8, and 12 o'clock positions. The valve remnants can be left behind. Overaggressive attempts to fulgurate the remaining tissue can cause strictures. Myers and Walker (1981) found a 50% incidence of urethral stricture in infants under 1 year of age following valve ablation. Of the seven strictures, two developed in the membranous area, so they could have developed secondary to the fulguration. Five developed elsewhere, four in the bulbous area and one more distally, suggesting that these five strictures could have occurred secondary to urethral trauma. Because of this experience, they recommended treating young infants with temporary diversion and delaying the valve ablation until the age of 9–12 months. However, as cystoscopes have become smaller, with better optics and better working units, most infant urethras can be negotiated with only a small incidence of urethral

stricture (Fig. 28.10a, b). Crooks (1982) found only three of 36 infants with PUV to have developed a urethral stricture following valve ablation and, in all three, the ablation was done at the time of a vesicostomy. He then hypothesized that a dry urethra caused the stricture and recommended that a valve ablation not be done at a time when no urine is passing through the urethra. He also cautioned against using a loop for the fulguration. Lal *et al.* (1998) evaluated 82 PUV boys. All newborns and infants with small-caliber urethras underwent temporary diversion and valve ablation was delayed until 9 months of age. Even though all underwent transurethral valve ablation with a fulgurating current at the 5, 7, and 12 o'clock positions, only three (3.6%) developed a urethral stricture. In two of the three, ablation was done while a vesicostomy was in place, i.e. a dry urethra. However, a dry fulguration was done in 34 others

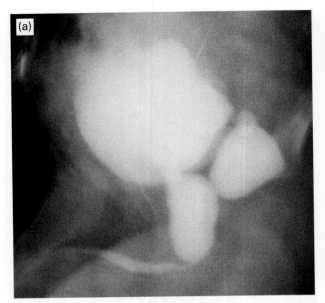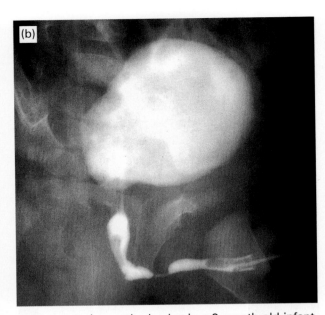

Figure 28.10 (a) Voiding cystourethrogram (VCUG) demonstrating posterior urethral valve in a 3-month-old infant. Note the large bladder diveticulum. (b) Six months after valve ablation anterior urethral stricture is seen, although none was seen on initial postvalve ablation VCUG. Optical urethrotomy was unsuccessful and formal urethroplasty was eventually required to correct the obstruction.

who did not develop strictures. In addition, a loop electrode was used in all patients and did not seem to predispose to stricture formation as had been suggested by Crooks (1982). At Toronto's Hospital for Sick Children, the incidence of stricture following valve ablation alone was 9% (12 of 131 boys). When valve ablation was done through a perineal urethrostomy, the incidence of stricture rose to 21% (nine of 43 boys) (Churchill *et al.*, 1983).

The valve leaflet can also be caught with some form of transurethral hook. The 'Whitaker hook' became the most popular and still is used at some centers, especially in small infants. The Whitaker hook is a small, 6 Fr insulated rod with the metal exposed only on the inside of the hook where contact is made with the valve (Whitaker and Sherwood, 1986). The rod is passed into the urethra and, under fluoroscopic vision, the valve is caught by the hook and obliterated with electrocautery. Zaontz and Gibbons (1984) suggested ablating PUV in an antegrade fashion when a vesicostomy is in place. In a logical extension of this concept, Zaontz and Firlit (1985) reported antegrade ablation through a percutaneous cystostomy for premature and low birthweight infants with a small urethra.

Ehrlich *et al.* (1987) reported ablating the valve with a neodymium: yttrium aluminum garnet (YAG) laser.

As soon as the diagnosis of PUV is suggested, the baby should be placed on a prophylactic antibiotic and the bladder drained. In a newborn, a 5 or 8 Fr feeding tube may be held in place with clear transparent dressing tape. The feeding tube is left in place until a VCUG is obtained to make the diagnosis. In patients with severe hydrouretero-nephrosis or elevated BUN and serum creatinine, the feeding tube is left in place while serum electrolyte abnormalities are corrected, upper tracts decompress, and the BUN and serum creatinine levels fall. On occasion, the catheter can cause severe bladder spasm and the bladder can become palpable as a small fist as it clamps down around the catheter. In such situations, the bladder may also clamp down around the ureteral hiatus, such that urine may not drain into the bladder and creatinine levels may not fall until the catheter has been removed and more definitive treatment initiated (Noe and Jerkins, 1983; Sarkas *et al.*, 1995).

Alternatives to treatment following catheter drainage include valve ablation alone (Mitchell and Close, 1996; Smith *et al.*, 1996) or temporary vesicostomy

(Duckett, 1974a, b). Supravesical temporary diversion in the form of loop ureterostomy (Johnston, 1963), Sober-Y pelvioureterostomy (Sober, 1972), ring ureterostomy (Williams and Cromie, 1976), end ureterostomy, cutaneous pyelostomy, surgically placed tube nephrostomy drainage (Waldbaum and Marshall, 1970), percutaneously placed nephrostomy or cystostomy tube drainage (Holmdahl *et al.*, 1995), and total reconstruction of the urinary tract, including ureteral reimplantation and tailoring, at the time of valve ablation (Hendren, 1970) (Fig. 28.11) are reserved for exceptional circumstances.

If the upper tracts decompress and serum creatinine falls, primary ablation is the best alternative. In patients whose upper tracts fail to decompress significantly, whose serum creatinine does not fall, or whose urethra is small (as in a small premature baby), consideration is given to vesicostomy. Traditionally, those who have the most severe dilatation, poorest renal function and little improvement on catheter drainage have undergone supravesical diversion, an option which is growing progressively less popular. In such situations, the surgeon must realize that the kidneys may be so compromised that there is little potential for improvement following diversion. (Further discussion of the pros and cons of supravesical diversion is included in the primary valve ablation versus temporary diversion section.)

Hendren (1970) recommended urinary tract remodeling and ureteral reimplantation at the time of valve ablation in patients with severe hydroureteronephrosis. Johnston and Kulatilake (1972), however, found that over time the dilatation will decrease spontaneously in many of these boys following relief of obstruction (Fig. 28.12). In those patients with severe dilatation and elevated serum creatinine, Johnston (1963) recommended temporary cutaneous loop ureterostomies and credited F. Douglas Stephens with describing the procedure. The ureterostomy is closed 1–2 years later, or at a time

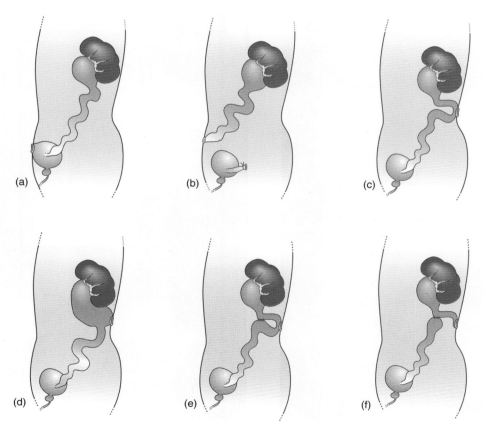

Figure 28.11 Various temporary diversions for posterior urethral valves with some of historical note: (*a*) cutaneous vesicostomy; (*b*) cutaneous ureterostomy; (*c*) cutaneous loop ureterostomy; (*d*) cutaneous pyelostomy; (*e*) ring ureterostomy; (*f*) Sober-Y-ureterostomy.

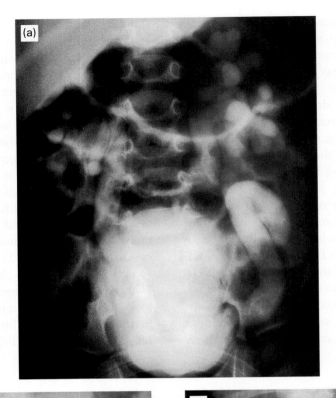

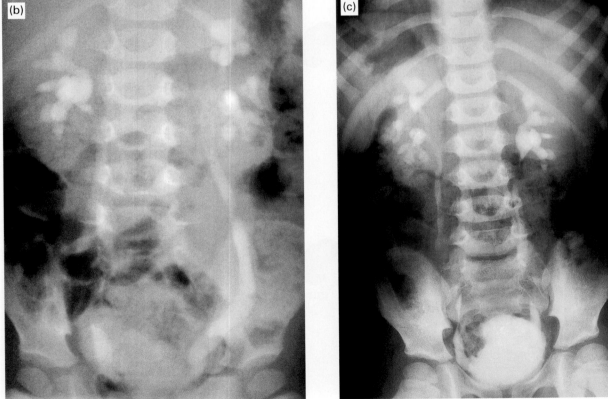

Figure 28.12 (*a*) Intravenous pyelogram in a 1-year-old boy with posterior urethral valves revealing dilated, tortuous ureters. (*b*) Two years after primary valve ablation there is marked improvement. (*c*) Further improvement is seen after another 2 years of follow-up. (From Glassberg *et al.*, 1982, with permission.)

when it is appropriate for the child to come out of diapers. It is no longer clear that high diversion is better than a vesicostomy unless the ureters are obstructed or the upper tracts infected.

Duckett (1974a, b) had suggested a Blocksom vesicostomy in those with severe disease, but later on warned that vesicostomies were being done too often. He became a proponent of primary valve ablation, reserving vesicostomy for those in whom valve ablation is not technically possible (Crooks, 1982). The procedure is simple to perform and does not involve skin flaps. A 2–3 cm horizontal incision is made midway between the pubic symphysis and the umbilicus. The dome of the bladder is identified and the peritoneum stripped away. The dome is then opened and sewn 1 cm from its edge to the rectus fascia with interrupted polyglycolic acid sutures. The bladder edges are sewn to the skin edges with chromic or polyglycolic acid sutures. Stomal stenosis is sometimes seen but less often than prolapse. It is important to externalize the bladder dome, since lower stomas are more prone to prolapse. It is important to be aware that the bladder often contains residual urine in varying amounts following vesicostomy. Residual urine, particularly in patients with VUR, may be associated with urine infections even though the vesicostomy stoma may be open. Clean intermittent catheterization (CIC) in such infants via the abdominal stoma may be required, but vesicostomy closure and valve resection should be considered. In Noe and Jerkins' (1985) series of 35 children with vesicostomy, ten developed prolapse (two of whom required revision), one stomal stenosis that required revision, and another a parastomal hernia. UTI was the most common complication.

Williams favored cutaneous pyelostomy for the most severely affected, but was concerned with the possibility that it could lead to a small, non-compliant bladder (Williams and Cromie, 1976). Therefore, he recommended, as an alternative, the Sober-Y pelvioureterostomy in which the pelvis or proximal ureter is brought to the skin. At the same time, an ipsilateral ureteropyelostomy is done so that some urine can drain into the bladder (Sober, 1972). Williams and Cromie (1976) suggested the ring ureterostomy as an alternative to the Sober-Y ureterostomy; this procedure also allows some urine to pass down the ureter into the bladder. Since in both the Sober-Y and ring ureterostomies the bladder will be allowed to fill, both require transurethral valve ablation at the time of

diversion. In addition, both take longer than cutaneous pyelostomy or loop ureterostomy, a disadvantage in a baby who may be septic or with compromised renal function. At the time of undiversion, however, the Sober-Y and ring ureterostomy are easier to take down than the cutaneous pyelostomy or loop ureterostomy (Fig. 28.11).

In utero *management*

Since pulmonary hypoplasia and renal failure are the major causes of death in neonates with PUV, efforts have been made to treat fetuses with significant disease before birth. However, not all fetuses suspected of having PUV when *in utero* actually have a PUV. Any procedure is also a procedure on the mother as well, and can induce premature labor or sepsis. In addition, if the kidneys already are dysplastic, intervention is unlikely to be of benefit.

A major indication for prenatal shunting is evidence of decreasing amniotic fluid. Shunting in such situations probably decreases the risk of pulmonary disease (Lome *et al.*, 1972). Decreased urine output leads to oligohydramnios but not all cases of oligohydramnios are associated with pulmonary hypoplasia, nor are all cases of pulmonary hypoplasia secondary to oligohydramnios.

Harrison *et al.* (1982) suggested that intervention should be avoided in fetuses with well-functioning kidneys, as well as in fetuses whose kidneys are too damaged to benefit from intervention. *In utero* ultrasound studies demonstrating hyperechogenic kidneys, particularly with cysts, suggest a poor prognosis. The following amniotic fluid values are indicative of good renal function (Glick *et al.*, 1985; Harrison, 1993, 1994):

- total protein   < 20   mg/dl
- β2-microglobulin   < 4.0   mg/dl
- calcium   < 100 mg/dl
- chloride   < 90   mg/dl
- osmolality   < 200 mg/dl.

Intervention is indicated if amniotic fluid volume decreases significantly and renal function is adequate to produce enough urine to increase amniotic fluid volume. If an initial sonogram demonstrates oligohydramnios, there is no way of knowing how long it has been present. In such situations, it becomes difficult to predict the effectiveness of shunting on renal and pulmonary function. If the fetus has developed oligihydramnios on serial ultrasound studies, is near term, and the lungs are mature, early delivery is often indicated. If the lungs are immature, a shunting procedure should be considered. Percutaneously placed vesicoamniotic shunts are usually employed when the diagnosis is made early (second trimester) and there is associated oligohydramnios. Hundreds of such procedures have been performed. The shunts often are displaced and replacement may be required. Open fetal cystostomy has been done and involves a hysterotomy. Estes *et al.* (1992) used a fetoscope endoscopically to place a wire mesh stent between the fetal bladder and amniotic sac. They felt that this approach, under direct vision, insures better initial positioning of the shunt and less chance of harming the fetus. Quintero *et al.* (1995) went a step further and successfully performed percutaneous endoscopic valve ablation, passing the 'scope through

the mother's abdomen and uterus and then through the fetus' abdomen and bladder to do an antegrade fulguration of the valve. The operation was done at 19 weeks gestation. The mother went into preterm labor at 31 weeks. The child was born with a small omental herniation through the abdominal wall and died on day 4 with pulmonary hypoplasia (Fig. 28.13).

In utero placed shunts or surgery to the fetus have not gained general acceptance since it is not clear that intervention does more good than harm. *In utero* procedures should still be pursued at a limited number of institutions and should still be considered experimental. Infants born with pulmonary hypoplasia will require immediate intubation and ventilation. Extracorporeal membrane oxygenation (ECMO) is used at most centers to assist oxygenation for these neonates (Gibbons *et al.*, 1993).

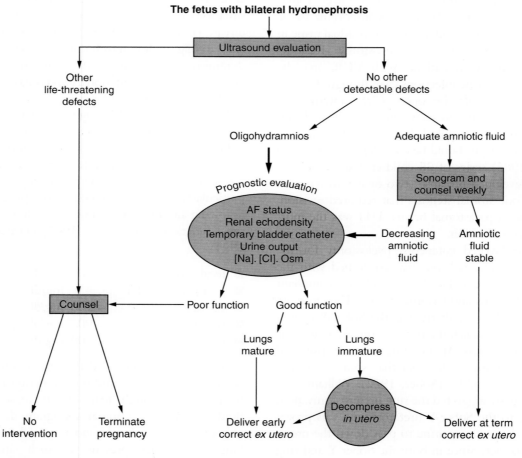

Figure 28.13 Scheme for the management of the fetus with bilateral hydronephrosis. (From Glick *et al.*, 1985, with permission.) (LAF = amniotic fluid.)

Persistent upper tract dilatation and the 'valve bladder'

No matter what treatment is initiated, i.e. valve ablation, temporary diversion and later undiversion with valve ablation, or total urinary tract reconstruction, some patients will have persistent upper tract dilatation while others will dramatically improve (Fig. 28.14). In the mid-1970s, in an effort to determine which systems with persistent dilatation and no VUR were actually obstructed, percutaneous renal pelvic pressure studies with constant perfusion of contrast (Whitaker test) were performed (Whitaker, 1973; Glassberg *et al.*, 1982). One of the boys, with markedly dilated renal pelves, while undergoing sonography to mark the kidneys for needle placement, expressed a need to urinate. After doing so, it was found that his renal pelves had decompressed to the degree that it was considered too risky to attempt the Whitaker study (Fig. 28.15a, b). At this point, it was realized, as did Whitaker (1973), that the bladder had something to do with upper tract dilatation in some patients. Numerous intravenous urograms were retrospectively reanalysed in PUV patients with persistent dilatation. An almost uniform finding was that hydroureteronephrosis was most marked when the bladder had some degree of filling, but when the bladder was empty the dilatation was significantly less.

In order to evaluate the relationship between bladder filling and upper tract dilatation, Whitaker studies were performed on patients at varying levels of bladder filling. Upper tracts without reflux in PUV patients were placed into three categories (Glassberg, 1982, 1985; Glassberg *et al.*, 1982):

- type I: unobstructed with the bladder empty, unobstructed during bladder filling;
- type II: unobstructed with the bladder empty, obstructed with bladder filling;
- type III: obstructed with the bladder empty, obstructed with bladder filling.

The majority of the units tested fell into the type II category, i.e. unobstructed with the bladder empty and obstructed with bladder filling, even when patients had undergone previous ureteral reimplantation and tailoring (Table 28.1). In most systems, the pelvic pressure rose with early bladder filling, well before reaching capacity. Small pressure elevations in the bladder were associated with large pressure elevations in the kidney. Surprisingly, only one of 13 units studied was categorized as type III, i.e. obstructed with the bladder empty and with filling (Glassberg *et*

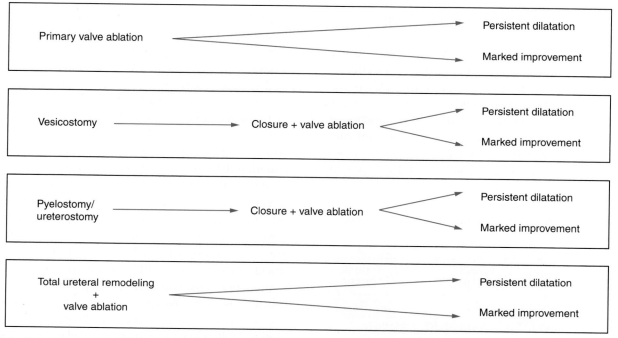

Figure 28.14 Upper tract outcome following four forms of initial management.

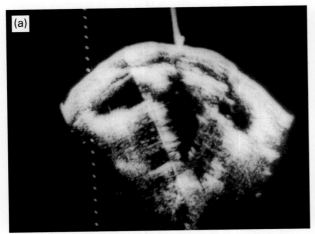
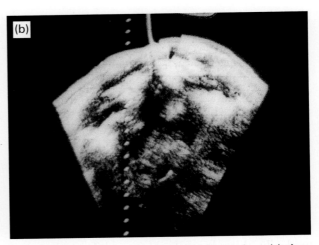

Figure 28.15 Renal sonogram in an 8-year-old boy with persistent hydronephrosis, 6 years after valve ablation. (a) Renal images just before voiding; (b) immediately after voiding, the renal pelvic dilatation has collapsed. (This is the study that opened our eyes to the effect of bladder filling on upper tract dilatation in patients with posterior urethral valves). (From Glassberg *et al.*, 1982, with permission.)

al., 1982; Glassberg, 1985). That patient underwent a ureteral reimplantation for distal ureteric obstruction and did well. Whitaker (1973) had noted previously that reimplantation of dilated ureters into the bladders of PUV patients was often not associated with lessening of the dilatation, and occassionally the dilatation worsened. Cukier (1980) reimplanted eight ureters with persistent dilatation and no reflux and, in five of these, the dilatation remained unchanged following surgery. On the basis of these findings, it was concluded that it is unusual for there to be a fixed or distal ureteric obstruction in PUV patients and that the persistent dilatation is more related to the effect of intravesical pressure on the upper tracts. Others also found distal obstruction to be infrequent. For example, Tietjen *et al.* (1997) found distal obstruction in only two of 52 units in 26 PUV patients evaluated with Whitaker studies and Lal *et al.* (1998) could only document obstruction in one of 16 boys with

severe hydronephrosis by antegrade pyelography. If the thick-walled, poorly compliant bladder is the cause of persistent obstruction and not distal ureteric obstruction, then it becomes understandable why ureteral reimplantation in PUV patients has not been widely successful in decreasing hydronephrosis, since one would still be implanting the ureter through the same thick, non-compliant bladder wall (Glassberg, 1983).

Another major cause of persistent upper tract dilatation in PUV patients is high urine output secondary to a decreased ability to concentrate urine. Patients with a history of PUV may have urine output 2–4 times the normal volume for their age. This phenomenon is particularly found in patients with persistent dilatation (Glassberg *et al.*, 1982; Glassberg, 1985). Of the 15 PUV children with persistent dilatation studied by Glassberg (1985), all had a concentrating defect with an inability to achieve a specific gravity ≥ 1.008 after a 14-hour fast. In five of the patients, pitressin was given as a test dose (10 mg/kg) and all five were unable to achieve urine osmolalities above serum values. This finding supports the diagnosis of nephrogenic diabetes insipidus. In one patient, the diagnosis of PUV had been missed while an endocrinologist had been treating him for central diabetes insipidus. Baum *et al.* (1974) had already reported on a case of permanent nephrogenic diabetes insipidus following valve ablation similar to another patient reported in the literature prior to that. Since it

Table 28.1 Whitaker pressure findings in 12 dilated renal units

Type I ↓BE↓BF	Type II ↓BE↑BF	Type III ↑BE↑BF
4	7	1

↓ = decreased; ↑ = increased; BE = bladder empty; BF = bladder filling.

is not uncommon for patients with primary (central) diabetes insipidus to have large bladders and dilated tortuous ureters, one can imagine the effect of high urinary output in perpetuating continued ureteral dilatation and tortuosity in PUV patients (Shapiro *et al.*, 1978). In patients whose upper tracts are dependent on the bladder being empty, a large urine output does not allow for the bladder to stay empty for more than a few minutes at a time. As a result, type II systems are challenged even more. Nephrogenic diabetes insipidus can be treated with thiazides and salt restriction. However, such a regimen carries the potential risk of depleting valve patients of sodium (Glassberg, 1985). Other treatment options are discussed below.

Dinneen *et al.* (1995), more recently, identified moderately impaired urinary concentrating ability (unable to concentrate > 800 μOsm/kg) in 59% (31 of 51) of boys with previously treated posterior urethral valves and severe impairment (unable to concentrate > 300 μOsm/kg) in 16% (eight of 51). The authors did not indicate whether it was the boys with persistent dilatation who had a poorer concentrating ability. They also were able to correlate glomerular filtration rate (GFR), maximum urinary concentration, and 24-hour urine volumes. They proposed the following formula based on their findings:

$$GFR(ml/min \text{ per } 1.73 \text{ m}^2)^* = \frac{\text{Maximum osmolality}}{8} + 6$$

(*Corrected surface area.)

If urinary osmolality were > 800 μOsm/kg, the GFR was likely to be > 80 ml/min per 1.73 m² surface area. However, if it were < 400 μOsm/kg, it was likely to be < 60 ml/min per 1.73 m² SA.

Incontinence in PUV patients is a well-recognized entity. Whitaker (1973) felt that in the majority of cases it was related to prior bladder neck surgery or to persistent dilatation of the posterior urethra. However, none of the patients in the Glassberg *et al.* (1979) study with persistent upper tract dilatation had previous bladder neck surgery, yet all of the type II patients also had incontinence. This quadrate of findings of persistent upper tract dilatation, nephrogenic diabetes insipidus, non-compliant bladder, and incontinence was reported at the 1979 American Urological Association meeting in New York (Glassberg *et al.*, 1979) and later published (Glassberg *et al.*, 1982). In the same year, Bauer *et al.* (1979) reported that eight

of 62 (13%) PUV boys had varying degrees of incontinence years following valve ablation. All eight boys had an intact external urethral sphincter on urodynamic examination. Three of the eight had a prior YV-plasty, which was thought to have contributed to their incontinence. Seven of the eight boys were found to have a hypertonic bladder, uninhibited contractions, or a small bladder. Duckett and Snow (1986) used the term 'full bladder syndrome' for patients with PUV, but this term is inaccurate because the dilatation also occurs with early bladder filling. A better term, which is used more often, was coined by Mitchell (1980) at the Southeastern Section, AUA, as the 'valve bladder syndrome'.

Urodynamic findings

After Bauer *et al.* (1979) at Boston Children's Hospital identified eight incontinent PUV boys with abnormal urodynamic studies, he along with Peters *et al.* (1990) evaluated 41 PUV patients, 35 with signs and symptoms of incontinence, three with frequency, two with hydronephrosis, and one with infection. Three boys were found to have a normal urodynamic examination: two had high voiding pressure secondary to outlet resistance and one had external sphincter damage from previous surgery. Of the remaining patients, a hyperreflexic bladder was identified in ten, a small, poorly compliant bladder in 11 and myogenic failure with overflow incontinence in 14 patients. They defined myogenic failure as an inability to sustain a voiding detrussor contraction (Fig. 28.16). In another similar investigation, Parkhouse and Woodhouse (1990) evaluated 42 consecutive post-ablation PUV patients at the Hospital for Sick Children, Great Ormond Street, London. They used videourodynamics to determine the incidence of bladder dysfunction in PUV patients. Of the 42 patients, only ten had a normal urodynamic examination. Of the 32 abnormal studies, 20 had detrusor instability, eight had bladder hypocompliance, and four had acontractile bladders. The terms detrusor instability, bladder hypocompliance and acontractile bladder correspond to the terms of hyperreflexic, small, poorly compliant, and myogenic failure used by Peters *et al.* (1990). Their study is important because it demonstrated that despite correction of the distal obstruction, approximately 75% of the boys continue to have abnormal bladder dynamics (Fig. 28.17).

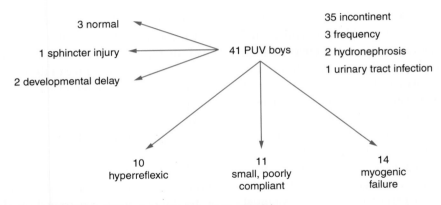

Figure 28.16 Urodynamic findings. (Data from Peters *et al.*, 1990.)

Kim *et al.* (1997a) studied 31 of this author's patients, the majority of whom had voiding symptomatology or persistent hydronephrosis at a mean of 54 months following valve ablation (Fig. 28.18). Only three were found to have a normal urodynamic examination and these patients had no symptomatology. Because the findings of both instability and poor compliance were present in the majority of patients with an abnormal urodynamic examination, the patients were divided differently, i.e. instability alone, decreased compliance alone, or a combination of the two. There was a strong correlation between the degree of compliance loss and the presence of instability. None of the 31 patients had any evidence of an acontractile or myogenic failure bladder. This differs from the report by Peters *et al.* (1990) in which myogenic failure represented the largest number of patients, being present in 14 of 41 patients, and Parkhouse and Woodhouse's (1990) study in which

four of 31 patients had myogenic failure. Of interest, perhaps, is that none of the 31 patients in Kim's group had been on any long-term course of anticholinergic medication prior to the study or at the time of the study. Two patients developed myogenic failure but only after being placed on oxybutynin therapy, in one case for 13 months and in the other for 16 months. This was probably an anticholinergic-induced myogenic failure. Once the authors had made this observation regarding anticholinergic-induced myogenic failure, they approached Woodhouse regarding the Parkhouse and Woodhouse (1990) study in which four patients had myogenic failure, and asked whether any of their four myogenic failure patients had been on or were on anticholinergics at the time of the study. Woodhouse replied that in all likelihood these patients were managed with anticholinergics at some time and possibly around the time of their videourodynamic examination. Bauer, when asked the same question, said that the patients were not on anticholinergics at the time of their developing myogenic failure and that it was the older boys who developed myogenic failure. The urodynamic findings of Jaureguizar *et al.* (1994), after long-term follow-up of 39 PUV patients, must also be included. They too did not find any with a myogenic bladder, but in a subsequent study with a larger series of PUV patients, i.e. 59 patients, Jaureguizar *et al.* (1999) found that three had developed myogenic failure. No mention was made regarding either the age of these three patients or whether or not any of them had been on anticholinergic therapy.

Compliance will significantly improve and instability will disappear in almost all patients following anticholinergic medication. Of the 31 patients in the

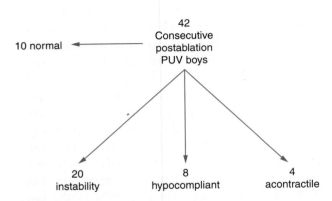

Figure 28.17 Urodynamic findings. (Data from Parkhouse and Woodhouse, 1990.)

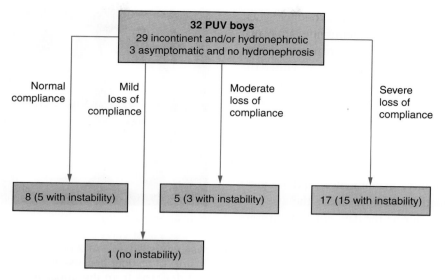

Figure 28.18 Urodynamic findings. (Data from Kim *et al.*, 1997a.)

Kim *et al.* (1997a) series, two underwent bladder augmentation because of severe compliance loss and an inadequate response to anticholinergic medication. A third patient, who did not respond to anticholinergic medication, was placed on CIC in preparation for augmentation and in this patient the augmentation was no longer necessary as bladder dynamics improved dramatically with CIC. This response to CIC is similar to that reported by Campaiola *et al.* (1985) in four PUV patients. Two others in Kim's study, as mentioned above, were maintained on CIC for their oxybutynin-induced myogenic failure. Also of significance is that VUR was present in ten of the 31 boys at the time of the initial urodynamic examination and, in seven, it resolved with anticholinergic medication and in another after CIC was instituted. In general, varying degrees of persistent hydronephrosis demonstrate improvement while on anticholinergic medication. Since fixed obstruction of the ureterovesical junction (UVJ) seems to be rare, the more obstructed patient with more distended upper tracts and higher serum creatinine levels may do well by treating the bladder aggressively after valve ablation with anticholinergics and if necessary CIC. However, to treat all comers with primary valve ablation and to ignore the bladder dynamics as the child grows is, in the authors' opinion, pure bravado and dangerous.

Johnston and Kulajilake (1972) found that incontinence, when present in PUV patients, 'always'

stopped spontaneously at puberty and considered its cessation secondary to the development of the prostate. Egami and Smith (1982) suggested that the wetting is a consequence of prolonged dilatation of the sphincters and posterior urethra and improves as the posterior urethra shrinks. More recent investigations suggest that perhaps it is the changing dynamics of the bladder itself that leads to continence with increasing age (Holmdahl *et al.*, 1996; DeGennaro *et al.*, 1996). For example, Holmdahl *et al.* (1996) found that two-thirds of valve patients (eight of 12) have instability during filling at the age of 5 years and considered the instability the major cause of incontinence. However, with growth, particularly after puberty, they found that instability diminishes, incontinence disappears, and bladder capacity increases on average to twice normal (mean 992 ml, range 610–1274 ml). In some, after puberty, the change may be so extreme that unsustained contractions (i.e. myogenic failure) may occur (three of six patients) (Holmdahl *et al.*, 1996).

DeGennaro *et al.* (1996) also found a tendency towards bladder hypocontractibility in older PUV boys. In a larger investigated group than Holmdahl's, i.e. 48 boys, they also found that younger PUV boys frequently have hypercontractibility and hypocompliance but with age the bladder often becomes larger, more compliant, and even hypocontractile. They considered that this evolution to hypocontractibility might represent bladder decompensation secondary to chronically elevated pressures when younger. Their findings support attempts at identifying abnormal urodynamic parameters early and correcting them when they are identified. No mention in either the Holmdahl *et al*. (1996) study or the DeGennaro *et al*. (1996) study was made as to whether or not these patients were on long-term anticholinergic medication and whether or not the hypocontractibility could have been anticholinergic induced.

In another study, Holmdahl *et al*. (1997) found that bladder instability, incontinence, and frequent small-volume urinations in boys under the age of 6 years were common during the day, but at night boys were dry, with higher bladder capacity and less instability. Perhaps increased urine output and high bladder volumes during sleep eventually lead to decompensated high volume bladders that cannot sustain a detrusor contraction. Holmdahl *et al*. (1996) found that myogenic failure occurs in older valve boys who had dysfunctional bladders when younger. If that is the case, it is our job to see whether this can be prevented. Therefore, poor compliance and instability must be treated with anticholinergic medication or CIC. Holmdahl (1997) warns that bladder augmentation should be avoided in young children since their bladders dilate with time anyway. She also warns against augmentation as a treatment for incontinence since incontinence lessens with time as well. Holmdahl recommends CIC for the non-compliant and unstable bladder early on, especially since these bladders turn out to have improved capacities and less instability following a period of CIC than if left alone. However, since these boys are sensate, it is often difficult to keep them on CIC.

One must be careful of studies that determine postvoid residuals by catheterization, particularly in valve patients, since the filling bladder can obstruct the upper tracts. As the catheter empties the bladder, it also decompresses and unobstructs the upper tracts. Urine from the upper tracts now rushes into the bladder, increasing the amount of urine drained by the catheter (Fig. 28.19). This leads to false calculations of actual residual urine volumes and can increase the number of patients diagnosed with myogenic failure. The presence of residual urine can only be determined by immediate postvoid X-ray images of contrast-filled bladders or by sonography. For example, Holmdahl *et al*. (1998) found that residual urine volumes determined by ultrasound during free voiding were

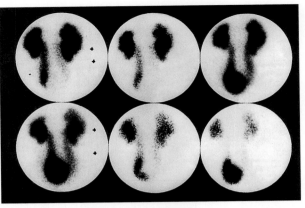

Figure 28.19 DTPA renal scan in a 12-year-old boy, 11 years after valve ablation and in the pre-furosemide washout scan era. At 2 hours, the isotope is not seen in area of bladder because the full bladder has obstructed drainage from the upper tracts. Immediately after voiding and complete emptying, the bladder refills and reobstructs the upper tracts. The same phenomenon is seen at 3 hours when voiding is repeated. (From Glassberg *et al*., 1982, with permission.)

smaller than those determined by catheter drainage whether the urodynamic catheter was a suprapubic or transurethral one. They attributed the higher urine residuals to the fact that the bladder was maximally filled via the catheter. It is more likely, however, that the volumes were high because the catheter drained not only residual bladder urine but also urine that drained from the upper tracts.

Following valve ablation some bladders will improve on their own and some will not. Consideration should be given as to whether or not all patients should be placed on empiric anticholinergic medication following valve ablation, rather than taking the 'wait and see' approach. Certainly, the vast majority of infants will have elevated pressures in the early months following ablation, and starting the majority of PUV patients on anticholinergic medication with subsequent titration or discontinuation after re-evaluation may be the more reasonable approach. If this is not done, then certainly, a proactive approach must be taken as regards urodynamic studies, and these studies obtained soon after valve ablation.

It is important that any patient with incontinence or persistent hydroureteronephrosis be investigated urodynamically, preferably with videourodynamics. Incontinence is a sign of bladder instability and poor compliance and usually is associated with persistent hydronephrosis. Bladder instability and hypocompliance usually improve with anticholinergic medication. Improving compliance often results in improvement in hydronephrosis. If anticholinergic medication does not solve the problem, CIC should be undertaken. If the latter does not improve bladder dynamics, augmentation or urinary diversion must be seriously considered (Kim *et al.*, 1997a).

Kajbafizadeh *et al.* (1995) found that in PUV patients with an augmented valve bladder, in contradistinction to patients with an augmented, neuropathic bladder or exstrophy bladder, the majority can void spontaneously without a large postvoid residual. They found gastrocystoplasty to be associated with the highest incidence of postoperative problems: five of seven patients with gastrocystoplasty had prolonged dysuria despite taking histamine antagonists and two had the hematuria–dysuria syndrome. However, use of intestine may result in azotemia. A segment of bowel that is too large may be floppy and not allow efficient emptying of the bladder. In such patients, CIC is required. Dilated ureters associated with non-functioning kidneys should not be removed at the time of a nephrectomy if the possibility exists that an augmentation might be necessary in the future. The ureter is an excellent alternative to bowel.

Tanagho (1982) pointed out that the entire bladder, bladder neck, and trigone hypertrophy *in utero* secondary to the outlet obstruction. He felt that extensive trigonal stretch and hypertrophy create resistance at the UVJ and cause persistent upper tract dilatation. He suggested that if anticholinergic drugs were ineffective in diminishing upper tract dilatation, one might consider resecting the interureteric ridge in order to weaken the trigonal hold on the lower end of the ureter. Conceivably, since trigonal tone is largely dependent on α-sympathomatic stimulation, one might achieve the same theoretical result of lessening hydroureteronephrosis by using an α-blocking drug. For example, when McGuire (1975) and Weiss (1982) used phenoxybenzamine in two boys with persistent upper tract dilatation and bladder neck obstruction, the dilatation markedly diminished. In one boy, when the phenoxybenzamine was stopped the dilatation returned, and it diminished once again after it was reinstituted. Was the response secondary to the effects of phenoxybenzamine on the trigone, the bladder neck, or both?

Histologic studies

Bladder wall changes that occur *in utero* secondary to partial outlet obstruction have drawn a great deal of attention to animal experimentation and the bladder wall histology of PUV boys. Classically, bladder obstruction has been thought to induce bladder muscle hypertrophy followed by replacement of muscle tissue with connective tissue, the latter event leading to decreased compliance (Keating, 1994). However, it seems that more is involved, including diminished blood perfusion (Gosling *et al.*, 1986), a reduction in nerve density with a decrease in autonomic detrusor innervation (Speakman *et al.*, 1987; Hsu *et al.*, 1994), and diminished mitochondrial enzyme activity (Gosling *et al.*, 1986).

Urethral obstruction causes significant changes in bladder histology and compliance. Two components of the bladder wall, i.e. muscle and matrix, are most responsible for the bladder's compliance. The cellular components of the bladder wall are muscle cells and fibroblasts, while collagen and elastin make up the structural components. The developing *in utero* bladder will respond differently in the relative proportion of its components than does the adult with acquired obstruction. Ultimately, compliance is dependent on tonus, that is the state of tension in muscles contractile elements, and elasticity, that is its ability to stretch and recoil, which is a reflection of the passive elements collagen and elastin (Keating, 1994).

Peters *et al.* (1992) demonstrated in the obstructed fetal sheep bladder a 4.6-fold increase in bladder weight reflecting a 5.8-fold increase in smooth muscle mass. The latter is mostly secondary to hypertrophy rather than hyperplasia. Urothelial cell growth also occurs and may result from stimulation by heparin-binding epidermal growth factor (HB-EGF), a chemical that Borer *et al.* (1999) have demonstrated to be increased in obstructed mice bladders.

There are 15 different types of collagen in humans. The two principal ones specific for the bladder are type I and type III. Type I collagen has been found to be stiffer and thicker than type III. Thus, when Kim *et al.* (1991) found more of the stiff type I than the more compliant and thinner type III collagen in biopsies of 'valve bladders', they suggested that *in utero* outlet obstruction leads to a small hypocompliant bladder because of its predilection to induce type I collagen formation. A problem in their interpretation is that Ewalt *et al.* (1992) found more type III than type I in their bladder biopsies.

Primary valve ablation versus temporary diversion

Comparing the outcome of supravesical diversion to primary transurethral valve ablation is a fruitless argument. Showing similar outcomes for the two groups implies that supravesical diversion is of benefit since it usually is the thicker walled-bladder with the more grossly dilated system that ends up with diversion.

At Toronto's Hospital for Sick Children, Krueger *et al.* (1980b) found that long-term follow-up demonstrated that infants treated with temporary supravesical diversion, especially under the age of 1 year, ended up with lower serum creatinine levels and were taller than children treated with valve ablation alone. The results become even more impressive when one considers that it was the sicker infants with higher serum creatinine levels who were the ones more likely to be diverted.

In a similar study, Jaureguizar *et al.* (1994) compared the outcome of 35 boys who were managed initially with either temporary cutaneous pyelostomy/ureterostomy or primary valve ablation. The chosen treatment was based on the preference of two individual senior surgeons. Since one preferred primary ablation and the other temporary supravesical diversion, the two groups, more or less, were equal before therapy. Those in the temporarily diverted group ended up with better creatinine clearances, better bladder function, and ultimately were taller. Poor renal function had a high association with non-compliant bladders and the majority of non-compliant bladders were seen in the primary valve ablation group.

In a very significant study comparing valve ablation alone and diversion, Lyon *et al.* (1992) evaluated 25 PUV patients initially treated with valve ablation alone. Eight patients subsequently were diverted. They found better growth in the diverted patients than in the non-diverted patients, with decompression of the upper tracts. Even though diversion initially was intended to be for 2–6 years, six patients were left diverted for 10 or more years with end cutaneous ureterostomies because of the good results, the

remaining two were left diverted for 7 and 4 years. Six of 18 (35%) non-diverted patients went into renal failure, while five of eight (63%) diverted patients went into renal failure. Since the diverted group represented the more severely affected patients, the higher incidence of renal failure is not surprising. What is more significant is that linear growth was normal in the diverted renal failure patients and impaired in the non-diverted renal failure patients.

Lyon *et al.* (1992) suggested that diversion and decompression of the upper tracts allow for better growth and recommended that diversion be used more frequently in PUV children. In a subsequent study, Lyon (2000) felt that it was not the bladder causing the problem but rather the very large amounts of hypotonic urine that these patients produced and the inefficiency of the already large ureters to transport the increased load. Now that we have a better understanding of the 'valve bladder', similar results can be achieved with a less invasive approach by aggressively treating abnormal dynamics with anticholinergic medication and, if ineffective, CIC or even bladder augmentation.

Tietjen *et al.* (1997) prefer vesicostomy to supravesical diversion in the patient whose creatinine has not fallen or whose dilatation has not lessened while on catheter drainage. It is their view that most supravesical diversions have been done in patients whose dilatation and serum creatinine levels would have come down with time or in patients whose kidneys have been so badly damaged that proximal diversion is too late. They found that of 26 boys who had undergone proximal diversion, 22 (85%) had dysplasia on biopsy. They also believe that ureteral obstruction in most cases is only temporary and found that anatomic obstruction of the distal ureter is rare (see section on Persistent ureteral dilatation) Whitaker (1973) believed that some wide ureters may not drain with an indwelling bladder catheter because they may have become overstretched and atonic secondary to prolonged outlet obstruction and high bladder pressures; it may take some time before effective peristaltic waves establish themselves and the dilatation can lessen. Tietjen *et al.* (1997) reserve supravesical diversion for the patient whose dilatation and creatinine have not lessened following vesicostomy and in whom an actual obstruction has been proven. They do not recommend its use for primary treatment, except for sepsis. If vesicostomy, instead of supravesical diversion, is employed as the primary treatment for infants whose serum creatinine has not fallen significantly with catheter drainage, and/or for infants whose upper tract dilatation has not diminished significantly with catheter drainage, fewer supravesical diversions will subsequently be required, along with their obligatory and sometimes complex undiversions.

In a report on their experience with vesicostomy, Noe and Jerkins (1985) initially feared that, in valve patients, vesicostomy may not adequately decompress the upper urinary system, especially if any supravesical obstruction was present. However, in actuality, any suspected ureteral obstruction was almost always found to be temporary. For example, of their 35 children who underwent vesicostomy (21 with PUV), only one patient had inadequate upper tract drainage and that patient had a duplication anomaly, not PUV.

Walker and Padron (1990) compared their series of infants managed with vesicostomy with other series managed initially with valve ablation and found no apparent difference in outcomes and complications.

Rounding out the debate, regarding diversion and primary ablation, Reinberg *et al.* (1992) found that the type of primary surgical treatment (transurethral valve ablation, vesicostomy, or high urinary diversion) did not influence progression to renal failure or body growth. This study differs from that of Lyon *et al.* (1992) in which initial, temporary diversions were prolonged for many years; in the study by Reinberg *et al.* (1992), temporary diversions really were temporary.

Some observers fear vesicostomy less than temporary supravesical diversion since in the former urine still flows into the bladder. In addition, vesicostomy is simpler to perform than supravesical diversion and is simpler to reverse. Bilateral cutaneous pyelostomies or ureterostomies require bilateral surgery. Depending on the status of the bladder and presence or absence of reflux, one can close one side first, perhaps that which is more poorly functioning, in order to cycle the bladder. Once it is clear that bladder dynamics are reasonable, the contralateral side can be safely closed. In patients with a vesicostomy and reflux, if the bladder is small at the time of vesicostomy closure, it would be imprudent to perform a bilateral reimplantation at the same time. In such patients it is best to close the vesicostomy and ablate the valves. Once the bladder has gained good capacity and good dynamics, if reflux persists, reimplantation can be done later. Patients can be started on anticholinergic medication just before vesicostomy closure (Fig. 28.20).

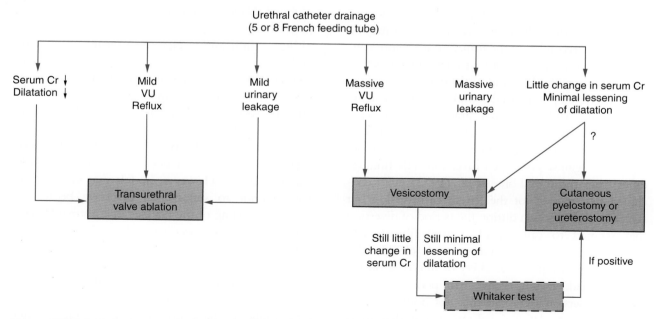

Figure 28.20 Initial management of the infant with a posterior urethral valve.

The defunctionalized bladder

Much has been written regarding the outcome of the temporarily diverted bladder in PUV patients. However, it is important first to understand what happens to a normal bladder when defunctionalized, in order to understand the diverted bladder in PUV patients. In dogs with a normal bladder, for example, Chun et al. (1989) demonstrated that bladder compliance and capacity following supravesical diversion decrease significantly. When they studied isolated biopsied muscle strips of diverted bladders, there was a decrease in contractility to muscarinic stimulation along with a decrease in muscarinic receptor density. However, once the urinary tract was reconstructed, the bladders recovered to prediverted status with normal compliance and the biopsied muscle strips had normal ability to respond to muscarinic agents. Bladder capacity not only returned to normal, but often returned to above-normal values. Studies that report decreased bladder compliance following supravesical diversion in PUV patients, therefore, may only be reporting a normal physiologic response. Even though the bladder in PUV patients will become smaller while diverted, following reconstitution of the urinary tract most such bladders will expand and, according to Kim et al. (1996) and Lome et al. (1972), sometimes even become larger. However, in a few PUV patients, the bladder will stay contracted following undiversion.

Cycling a still diverted bladder, in order to increase its capacity, is difficult. Therefore, in some, it may be necessary to reconstitute the urinary tract before considering augmentation in order to determine whether the bladder, with time and anticholinergic medication, will develop improved compliance and capacity.

Tanagho (1974) felt that previously obstructed bladders diverted the longest have the greatest risk of failing to expand following undiversion and therefore cautioned against prolonged diversion. His findings differ from those of Lome et al. (1972), who concluded that it was not the length of diversion but rather vesical infection during the period of diversion that seemed to cause bladder wall fibrosis and decreased compliance. Khoury et al. (1990) also acknowledge the potential effect of infection on the diverted bladder, but believe that poor storage in some bladders in PUV patients has nothing to do with temporary defunctionalization and that these bladders would have been non-compliant regardless of the initial form of management. They believe instead that it is the pathologic changes that occur before treatment that determine which bladders will remain non-compliant.

Close et al. (1997) compared 23 PUV patients who underwent primary valve ablation with eight who had undergone temporary diversion. The diverted group included two diverted by vesicostomy, three by ureterostomy, and three by vesicostomy and ureterostomy. Each patient was evaluated urodynamically and by bladder sonography employing a grading system. They found compliance and the bladder sonogram score, in general, to be better in the primary ablation group. In addition, they found that the diverted children were far less likely to be continent by the age of 4 years after reconstruction. Six of the 23 primary valve ablation patients and six of eight of the diverted group had a serum creatinine greater than 1.2 mg/dl before valve ablation and after stabilization with a draining urethral catheter. These six patients in each group were selected in an effort to compare near-equal patients from each group. They found that there was no significant difference in serum creatinine during follow-up in the two groups, but also found that the bladders in the diverted group had poorer compliance and a poorer grade on the sonogram scale, and that the children were more often incontinent at the age of 4 years. They theorized that the bladders were worse in the diverted group because the absence of normal bladder cycling inhibited bladder recovery. However, some parameters (e.g. massive hydroureteronephrosis, massive VUR, significantly elevated serum creatinine levels) that led to some boys being diverted were parameters that also were associated with poor bladder recovery. Perhaps, these two groups of six patients were not equivalent after all, making comparisons difficult.

Duckett supported Close et al's (1997) conclusions regarding diversion (Duckett and Snow, 1986; Duckett, 1997). However, he felt that vesicostomy was superior to supravesical diversion because it allows for cycling of the bladder in a normal fashion but with voiding occurring through the stoma. Furthermore, he suggested that a 'valve bladder' does not occur after primary ablation (Duckett and Snow, 1986; Duckett, 1997). Conflicting data were reported by Campaiola et al. (1985) in four patients who were found to have non-compliant bladders after being treated with primary valve ablation alone.

In Noe and Jerkins (1985) series of 35 children with vesicostomy (21 with PUV), 19 had undergone closure and all but one had good capacity after closure. In the exception, a contracted bladder was attributed to a prolonged period of infections and suprapubic tube drainage prior to referral and the vesicostomy. In a previous paper, Noe and Jerkins (1983) acknowledged the existence of temporary upper tract obstruction in PUV patients following decompression of the bladder. They suggested that, if a supravesical diversion is being considered, a temporary type of intubated drainage should be tried first.

Because so many fear a negative effect of diversion on the bladder, Kim et al. (1996) did a comparative urodynamic evaluation in a group of 32 PUV patients at a mean of 71 months following valve ablation. Patients were separated into three groups: (1) primary transurethral valve ablation (20 boys); (2) vesicostomy followed by vesicostomy closure and valve ablation (eight boys); and (3) cutaneous pyelostomy followed by undiversion and valve ablation (four boys). Surprisingly, patients who underwent vesicostomy or pyelostomy had bladders with larger functional capacity, better compliance, and less instability (Tables 28.2, 28.3). The mean length of time of diversion was 25 months. The findings are significant in that the sicker infants, who were more likely to have poorer bladders and underwent primary temporary diversion, in general, were the ones eventually to have the better bladders. These results are not meant to imply that temporary diversion should be used more often, but rather that one should not hesitate to employ temporary diversion, when appropriate, because of the fear that it might harm the bladder. The authors agree with Khoury et al. (1990) that those bladders that are poorly compliant following temporary diversion and subsequent undiversion are probably poor bladders to begin with, whether divert-

Table 28.2 Percentage of expected bladder capacity for age[a] following three forms of initial therapy

Type of initial therapy	Expected bladder capacity for age following therapy (%)
Valve ablation (20 boys)	90
Vesicostomy (five boys)	196
Pyelostomy (four boys)	123

[a]Based on Koff's formula [expected volume for age (in ounces) = age + 2 (in ounces)]. From Kim et al. (1996).

ed or not diverted. Temporary diversion probably does not or rarely harms the bladder and if it does have an effect on the bladder, it is more often a positive one. Putting the bladder at rest may ultimately improve capacity and compliance. Perhaps just as temporary diversion can improve bladder dynamics, CIC also, by not allowing the bladder to overfill, represents another way of putting the bladder to rest.

One more recent study must also be commented upon. Jaureguizar et al. (1999) also compared long-term bladder function in 59 patients initially treated by either primary valve ablation or temporary cutaneous pyelostomy/ureterostomy. They found no significant differences in bladder function between the two treatment groups and also concluded that neonatal supravesical urinary diversion has no adverse effects on bladder function and that poor bladder function is probably a consequence of detrusor muscle damage in utero.

Clearly, a non-compliant bladder can be seen after valve ablation alone, after temporary vesicostomy, and after temporary supravesical diversion. It still is not clear how often, if ever, supravesical diversion

Table 28.3 Bladder compliance[a] following three forms of initial therapy

Initial management	Moderately impaired	Severely impaired	Percent with impairment
Valve ablation	8	4	67% (12/18)
Vesicostomy	1	0	20% (1/5)
Pyelostomy	0	1	25% (1/4)

[a]Compliance = $\Delta V/\Delta P$; severely impaired < 10 ml/cm; moderately impaired 10–20 ml/cm; mildly impaired 21–30 ml/cm (none had mildly impaired compliance).

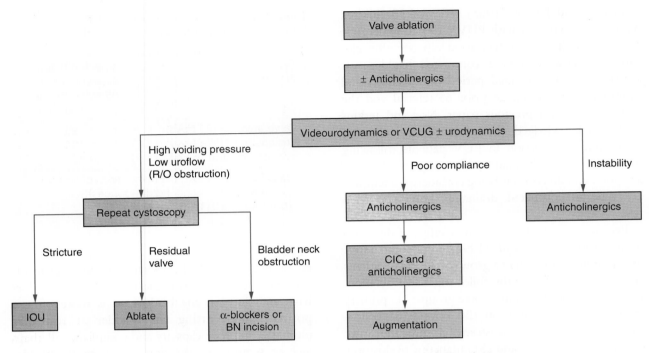

VCUG: voiding cystourethrogram; CIC: clean intermittent catheterization; IOU: internal optical urethrotomy.

Figure 28.21 Management following valve ablation.

causes a non-compliant bladder and to what degree the status of the bladder before treatment determines ultimate bladder function (Fig. 28.21).

The bladder neck

In the 1950s and 1960s, the diagnosis of bladder neck obstruction was too often made in 'valve' patients on the basis of the bladder neck's prominence on VCUG and patients were too often treated by Y-V-plasties to the bladder neck. This procedure can contribute to future incontinence or retrograde ejaculation. Waterhouse (1964) pointed out that the bladder neck usually is not narrow and the 'pseudonarrow' appearance is only relative in comparison to an adjacent dilated posterior urethra. Often what appears as a narrow lumen at the bladder neck on VCUG in the boy with a PUV may, in fact, be a lumen that is wider or the same size as the bladder neck lumen in a normal boy (Fig. 28.22). Waterhouse (1964), therefore, cautioned against overdiagnosing associated bladder neck obstruction. However, it is important, when evaluating patients' postvalve ablation that a flow rate, radiographic voiding study, and voiding pressure be obtained when there is any question regarding blad-

der function. Outlet obstruction, whether due to persistent residual valve tissue, stricture, or bladder neck obstruction, can be associated with a normal voiding flow rate because an abnormally elevated voiding pressure can overcome the obstruction. If there is no obvious obstruction distal to the bladder neck in patients with a high voiding pressure, the bladder neck must not be overlooked as a cause (Kim *et al.*, 1997a). If the bladder neck does not open during voiding on an imaging study, preferably a videourodynamic exam, secondary bladder neck obstruction may be the cause and treatment options include a transurethral bladder neck incision at 12 o'clock or α-blockers. McGuire and Weiss (1975) and Weiss (1982) treated PUV patients with persistent upper tract dilatation and bladder neck hypertrophy with phenoxybenzamine, an α-blocker, with good results in two patients. Therapy with newer α-blocking agents is gaining popularity. In those patients in whom the diagnosis of bladder neck obstruction is documented on videourodynamic studies, α-blockers often will dramatically increase voiding flow rates and improve continence. Pharmacotherapy of this type should precede any consideration of bladder neck incision.

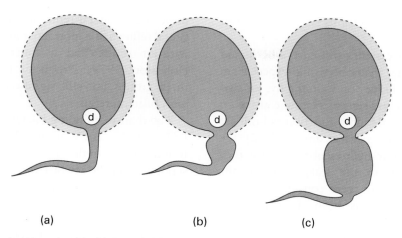

(a)　　　　　　　(b)　　　　　　　(c)

Figure 28.22 Sketch showing the bladder neck lumen with the same diameter (*d*) in three hypothetical patients: (a) normal; (b) mildly obstructed posterior urethral valves (PUV) and (c) severely obstructed PUV. Note the illusion of bladder neck obstruction in the two valve examples, even though the lumen is the same size in each sketch. (From Waterhouse, 1964, with permission.)

Perirenal urinomas and urinary ascites

Urinary extravasation from the kidney or the bladder can occur perinatally when there is bladder outlet obstruction. More commonly, it occurs from the kidney and is manifested as a subcapsular or perirenal urinoma or finds its way into the peritoneal cavity, causing urinary ascites. In the latter, on a plain X-ray of the abdomen, the intestines will be situated centrally and the abdomen will have a ground-glass appearance (Fig. 28.23). When a neonate is identified with urinary ascites, 70% are secondary to PUV (Scott, 1976). The first surviving case of urinary ascites secondary to PUV was reported by Davis and James (1952).

Debate exits regarding the mechanism of urine entry into the peritoneal cavity. One mechanism that has been considered proposes a direct communication between the fornices and the peritoneal cavity. Alternatively, leakage of urine into the perirenal space with subsequent transudation of the urine into the peritoneal cavity has been suggested. The latter is the more likely mechanism.

Mitchell and Garrett (1980) reviewed the literature and found 22 cases of urinary leakage in PUV patients where the site of rupture was determined to be the kidney and added seven of their own. Leakage occurred from the right kidney in 17 patients, from the left in 11, and in one, the extravasation was bilateral. When a VCUG was done, reflux to the ipsilateral leaking kidney was identified 71% of the time. When reflux is identified, active

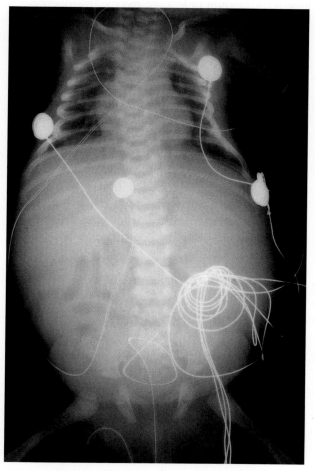

Figure 28.23 Flat plate of the distended abdomen of a newborn with a posterior urethral valve and urinary ascites. Note the 'ground-glass' appearance of the abdomen and the centrally located bowel gas.

extravasation of urine from a fornix is sometimes seen on fluoroscopy.

Patients with urinary ascites will have a BUN and serum creatinine higher than one would expect from the appearance of the kidney on sonography, for two reasons: (1) the BUN and serum creatinine are often elevated relative to actual kidney function as both are reabsorbed through the peritoneum; and (2) the kidneys may not appear hydronephrotic since they decompress secondary to the leakage. Originally urinary leakage and ascites were considered a poor prognostic sign, but it has been determined by Rittenberg *et al*. (1988) to act as a pop-off mechanism, preserving kidneys from excessive pressure (Fig. 28.24a–f).

Mitchell and Garrett (1980) found bladder drainage alone to be adequate treatment in 19% of PUV patients with urinary leakage. If catheter drainage lessens the amount of leakage and the hydronephrosis decreases, transurethral ablation of the valves is appropriate. However, when the extravasation is major, the urethral catheter ineffective in draining the upper tracts, and the BUN and serum creatinine do not fall significantly, a vesicostomy is preferable. If supravesical diversion is considered, cutaneous pyelostomy is not usually feasible since the pelvis may be collapsed secondary to the urinary leakage, making it difficult to bring it to the skin.

Urinomas can be confused with large renal cysts. If the urinomas are large or the urinary ascites very tense, respiratory compromise can result, with elevation of the diaphragm. If that is the case, the urinoma or ascites should be drained percutaneously.

Vesicoureteral reflux and the pop-off mechanisms

Over 50% of patients with PUV have VUR (Johnston, 1979; Egami and Smith, 1982; Scott, 1985). Scott (1985) found that reflux was present in 53% of ureters and in 72% of children. Approximately one-third of boys with PUV have bilateral VUR at presentation, one-third unilateral reflux, and one-third no reflux (Scott, 1985; Rittenberg *et al*., 1988). At a time when perinatal mortality was high in valve patients, Johnston (1979) reviewed his valve patients from the two previous decades. He found that the prognosis for bilateral reflux was worse than that for unilateral reflux and that those without reflux had the best prognosis. He found that the mortality rate in those with bilateral reflux was 57%, those with unilateral reflux had a mortality rate of 17.4%, and those without reflux had a mortality rate of 9.1% (Johnston, 1979). Prognosis is better now for all three groups but still significantly worse for those with bilateral reflux.

The chance of finding bilateral VUR seems to decline with age. For example, Parkhouse *et al*. (1988) found bilateral reflux in 37% (23 of 62 boys) presenting under the age of 1 year, statistics similar to the incidence of bilateral reflux in the Johnston (1979) and the Scott (1985) series. However, in those who presented later than 1 year of age, bilateral reflux was found in only one of 29 (3%). In agreement with Johnston, they found that bilateral reflux was associated with a higher rate of mortality and renal failure. Parkhouse *et al*. (1988) found that the incidence of unilateral reflux did not vary as much with age. Unilateral reflux was present in 30% of those who presented under 1 year of age and also in 30% who presented after 1 year of age (Parkhouse *et al*., 1988).

Unilateral reflux is more frequently seen on the left, particularly when the reflux is severe. For example, in boys with severe unilateral reflux, the reflux was on the left in 14 of 18 patients in Hoover and Duckett's (1982) series, in seven of eight in the study by Greenfield *et al*. (1983), and in eight of 12 of those reported by Cuckow *et al*. (1997). When reflux is on the right it is more often associated with a better kidney and has a better chance of spontaneous cessation.

Lal *et al*. (1998) found, at presentation, reflux in 44 of 84 boys (52%) who ranged in age from birth to 50 years. The reflux resolved in 24 of the 62 (38.7%) renal units with reflux of grade III or more and in all four units with unilateral grade II reflux. Kim *et al*. (1997) identified abnormal bladder urodynamic parameters in those with persistent reflux following valve ablation and, furthermore, found that correcting abnormal dynamics then led to reflux disappearance in the majority.

In 1982, Hoover and Duckett (1982) reported the association of severe unilateral VUR and ipsilateral renal dysplasia in boys with valves and found dysplasia in ten of 12 kidneys. They also observed that the unilateral reflux in association with a non-functioning kidney occurred predominantly on the left side (11 of the 12 cases; 92%). They recommended early nephroureterectomy both because the kidney was not functioning and in order to improve voiding

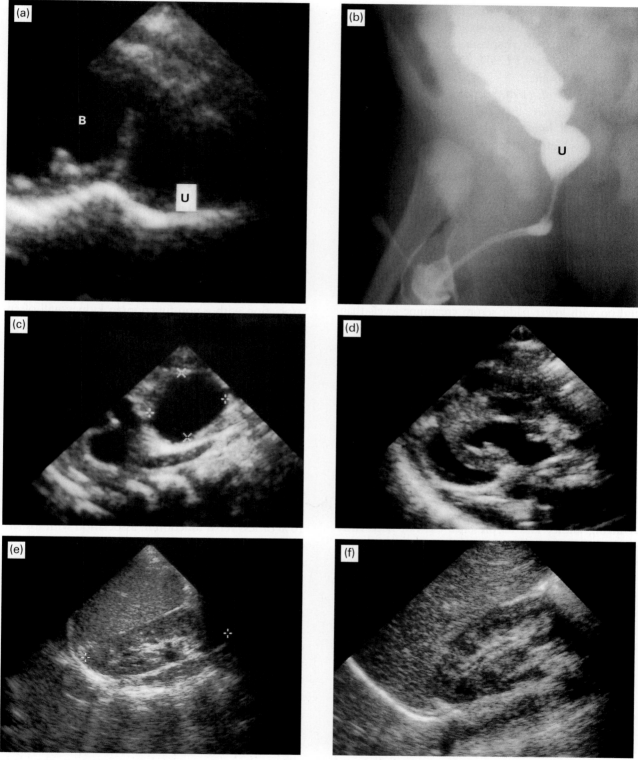

Figure 28.24 (*a*) Sonogram of bladder (B) and dilated posterior urethra (U) in an infant with a posterior urethral valve. (*b*) Voiding cystourethrogram demonstrating valve. (*c*) Urinoma in the left renal fossa inferior to the kidney on sonogram. (*d*) Urinoma superior to the right kidney. (*e, f*) Left and right non-hydronephrotic kidneys following valve ablation. Note that the good outcome might have been secondary to the urinary leak acting as a pop-off mechanism.

dynamics so that there no longer would be a pool of urine in the refluxing ureter on voiding. This combination of VUR, renal dysplasia, and PUV has been referred to as the VURD (vesicoureteral reflux-dysplasia) syndrome.

Greenfield *et al*. (1983) reported in 1983 that the contralateral kidney, in VURD syndrome boys, had good function and concluded that it had been protected from high bladder pressures by the severely refluxing unit acting as a 'pop-off' mechanism. Five years later, Rittenberg *et al*. (1988) proposed that a unilateral refluxing ureter was one of three possible pop-off mechanisms preserving renal function. The other two are a large congenital bladder diverticulum and, as described above, urinary leakage from the kidney manifested either as urinary ascites or as a perirenal urinoma. Overall, they found that patients with one of these pop-off mechanisms were more likely to end up with lower nadir serum creatinine levels than patients with no pop-off phenomenon. Unfortunately, Rittenberg *et al*. (1988) did not examine each pop-off mechanism separately but grouped all three together. Contradicting the theory regarding the beneficial effect of unilateral reflux as a pop off mechanism is Johnston's (1979) earlier finding that mortality was greater with unilateral reflux than with no reflux, as well as the finding of Parkhouse *et al*. (1988) that boys with unilateral VUR have a similar outcome to those without reflux. Cuckow *et al*. (1997) questioned the theory in 1997 and concluded that the VURD syndrome is not protective of the contralateral non-refluxing kidney and its presence did not necessarily mean that the prognosis was better. They found that with long-term follow-up the percentage of patients with VURD syndrome who have normal serum creatinine levels dramatically falls with age, leading them to conclude that patients in other studies may not have been followed sufficiently long. For example, in the Greenfield *et al*. (1983) study, patients were followed for only 6 years, and in the Rittenberg *et al*. (1988) study, the length of follow-up was not stated.

The correlation of severe VUR and renal dysplasia or hypodysplasia in valve patients also was analysed by Henneberry and Stephens (1980) and Schwarz *et al*. (1981). They concluded that it was not the reflux that caused the hypodysplasia, but instead abnormal ureteric budding caused a triad of anomalies: renal dysplasia, lateral ureteric orifice ectopia, and reflux. According to their theory, if the ureteric bud forms too early or too distal on the wolffian duct, it will lay down a laterally placed ureteric orifice and reach a peripheral area of the differentiating blastema, resulting in abnormal renal differentiation, i.e. hypodysplasia. They also found that lateral ectopia alone, even without reflux, was associated with dysplasia. In order for the diagnosis of dysplasia to be met, one must have at least primitive ducts present. Loose mesenchymal tissue and cartilage are usually present as well (Fig. 28.25a–d). The pathologic findings in one series of eight patients with severe unilateral VUR and non-functioning kidneys (Greenfield *et al*., 1983), however, were not supportive of true dysplasia as in other series. Instead, their pathologic findings consisted predominantly of hydronephrosis, interstitial inflammation, and diffuse atrophy.

Antireflux surgery considerations

Johnston (1979) found that even massive reflux in association with a non-functioning kidney will often resolve spontaneously. He also found, before anticholinergic medication was typically prescribed for valve patients, that reimplanting dilated reflux ureters into thick-walled bladders did not provide uniform good results. Kim *et al*. (1997a, b) found that reflux can disappear in either situation. Reimplanting ureters into thick-walled bladders can also provide good results, provided that abnormal urodynamics are corrected before surgery. Correcting abnormal bladder dynamics not only provides a better medium for reimplanting the ureter, but may also result in spontaneous resolution of the reflux. Of 11 boys with 10% or less renal function in association with ipsilateral reflux, the reflux was on the left in six and on the right in five. Three nephroureterectomies were done, five ureters were reimplanted without removing the poorly functioning ipsilateral kidney, and in four, the reflux spontaneously resolved. All four whose reflux stopped without surgery did so after being treated for abnormal urodynamic parameters. Of the five reimplanted ureters, four reimplantations were done at the time of implanting a contralateral reflux ureter, rather than performing another operation through a flank incision to remove the poorly functioning kidney. In the fifth patient, the reimplantation was done to preserve a kidney with 10% renal function. In the five who underwent successful reimplantation, the bladder was improved with anticholinergic medication in four and with augmentation in one. It is important to recognize the significance of providing an optimum environment in order to achieve a successful reim-

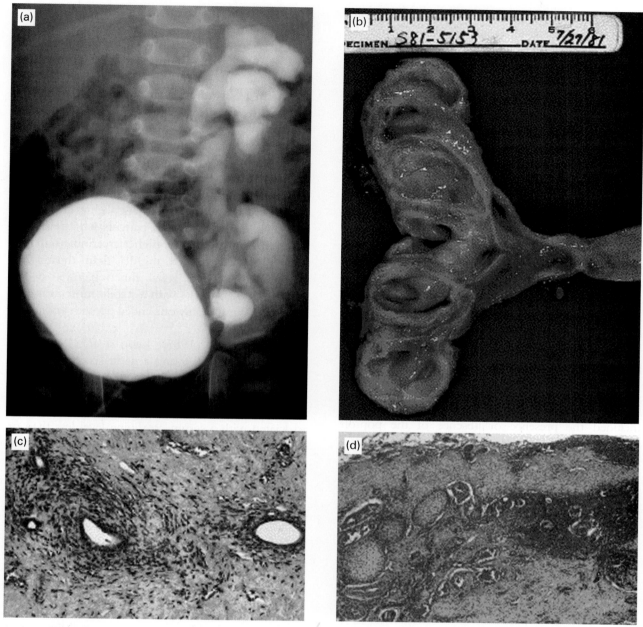

Figure 28.25 (*a*) Cystogram of a child with a posterior urethral valve and grade V left reflux, a large paraureteric diverticulum, and a non-functioning left kidney. (*b*) Sagittal section through the nephrectomy specimen showing dilated calyces and thin cortex. (*c*) Primitive ducts, the sine qua non of dysplasia, and loose parenchymal tissue are seen in one area (× 100). (*d*) Cartilage is identified in another area (× 40). (From Glassberg and Filmer, 1985, with permission.)

plant. These patients did not have the VURD syndrome since four of the 11 patients had bilateral reflux. No negative clinical sequella resulted from failure to remove a poorly functioning kidney in eight patients. If the contralateral kidney is not optimal, it is preferable to preserve as much function as possible

and to perform a reimplantation rather than a nephroureterectomy, particularly if there is greater than 10% function remaining. This may help to prevent hyperfiltration glomerulopathy. In the setting of bilateral reflux, bilateral reimplantation should be considered instead of unilateral nephroureterectomy and contralateral reimplantation. This approach preserves as much renal tissue as possible and limits the patient to one surgical incision. Subsequent nephroureterectomy has not been necessary, at least in the present authors' experience. The other reason to preserve a large, dilated ureter is its potential use for bladder augmentation if that becomes necessary in the future (Kim *et al.*, 1997b).

Before reimplantation or nephroureterectomy is done for a reflux ureter, abnormal urodynamic parameters should be corrected, in part for a successful reimplant but also to avoid the high pressure to the contralateral kidney once a possible pop-off release has been eliminated. Both Johnston (1960, 1979) and Rittenberg *et al.* (1988) felt that this philosophy applies especially when operating on large bladder diverticula. As a final note, Puri and Kumar (1996) have achieved excellent antireflux results in PUV patients with endoscopic subureteric injection of polytetrafluoroethylene (Teflon).

Prognostic indicators

Several investigators have tried to identify prognostic indicators of patients with PUV. Studies have included the presence or absence of the pop-off phenomenon, the laterality of reflux, the age at presentation after birth, the age of presentation *in utero* (all discussed above), the presence or absence of incontinence, serum creatinine level after catheter drainage or at 1 year of age, and the presence or absence of pyramids visualized by renal sonography.

Incontinence

Incontinence implies a poorly compliant and unstable bladder and associated persistent hydronephrosis. Churchill *et al.* (1983) found the incidence of incontinence to be 29% (51/178), while Conner and Burbige (1990) identified a 19% incidence of incontinence at a mean of 6.8 years after diagnosis. Merguerian *et al.* (1992) found that incontinence was not a risk factor for developing renal failure. Parkhouse *et al.* (1988), however, found incontinence at the age of 5 years to be associated with a 46% incidence of renal failure, while continence at 5 years carried only a 5% risk. If incontinence implies a poor prognosis, as the latter study suggests, it then behooves us to answer the question: if abnormal urodynamic parameters and incontinence are corrected early on, will prognosis improve? In many, the likely answer is 'yes'.

Serum creatinine

Numerous studies have tried to determine what nadir level of serum creatinine is of prognostic value. Conner and Burbige (1990) found that, of 31 PUV boys with a serum creatinine level of less than 1.0 mg/dl at 1 year of age, none developed progressive renal failure. However, when the serum creatinine was greater than 1.0 mg/dl at 1 year, seven of 19 developed progressive renal disease (mean follow-up 7 years). Merguerian *et al.* (1992) used the term stabilization creatinine, defined as the lowest serum creatinine measurement achieved during follow-up. They found that patients who developed poor renal function had a higher creatinine stabilization level (2.0 ± 0.8 mg/dl) than those with maintained adequate renal function (0.5 ± 0.2 mg/dl). Of 54 patients with a stabilization creatinine less than 1.0 mg% only one ended up with poor renal function.

Warshaw *et al.* (1985), Lyon *et al.* (1992), and Denes *et al.* (1997) found a nadir serum creatinine level of 0.8 mg/dl or less in the first year of life to be of significant prognostic value. In Warshaw's series, nadir serum creatinine of 0.8 mg/dl or less was associated with a serum creatinine level less than or equal to 1.1 mg/dl at the time of final evaluation (mean follow-up 5.8 years). In those with nadir creatinine levels greater than 0.8 mg/dl the follow-up mean serum creatinine value was 1.6 mg/dl. Lyon *et al.* (1992) found that of 12 boys whose creatinine was 0.8 mg/dl or less following treatment, two developed renal failure. However, when the serum creatinine was greater than 0.8 mg/dl, nine of 13 boys went on to renal failure. The average age for developing renal failure was 13 years.

Denes *et al.* (1997) studied the most recent creatinine clearance in 43 patients at a mean follow-up of 8.5 years (range 50–219 months) and divided them into two groups: group I, those with a recent creatinine clearance of 69 ml/min or less per 1.73 m²; and group II, those with clearances greater than 70 ml/min. In group I, mean serum creatinine was 3.60 mg/dl at presentation and 1.7 mg/dl after at least 4 days of catheter drainage; mean nadir serum creatinine during the first year of life was 1.7 mg/dl. In group II patients, mean serum creatinine was 2.4 mg/dl at presentation and 0.6 mg/dl after drainage; mean nadir creatinine during the first year of life was 0.6 mg/dl. Only one patient in group II had a serum creatinine as high as 0.8 mg/dl. They concluded that having a serum creatinine of 0.8 mg/dl or less both after at least 4 days of catheter drainage and during the first year of life correlates with an excellent prognosis.

Sonographic findings

Hulbert *et al.* (1992) suggested that it was helpful to determine whether there were definable medullary pyramids in at least one kidney on sonography. If definable pyramids were present, serum creatinine levels remained lower than 0.8 mg% over a mean of 4 years. Of 11 boys in whom the medullary pyramids were not identifiable, seven ended up with serum creatinine levels greater than 0.8 mg%, five of whom later developed renal insufficiency. It was of interest that in nine of the 11 with absent medullary pyramids there was also either unilateral or bilateral VUR. Duel *et al.* (1998) found that loss of corticomedullary differentiation, i.e. definable medullary pyramids, and increased renal echogenicity on sonography, were less sensitive and less specific markers for predicting outcome when compared with nadir serum creatinine and creatinine clearance in the first year of life. However, in the face of normal echogenicity and normal corticomedullary differentiation, poor renal function was unlikely. Prognostic signs are listed below.

Favorable prognostic signs:

■ *in utero* presentation after 24 weeks, provided a normal sonogram before 24 weeks;
■ sonographic appearance of pyramids in at least one kidney;
■ nadir serum creatinine < 0.8 m%;
■ no reflux;
■ continence at the age of 5 years;
■ presence of pop-off phenomenon
   (a) urinary leak (urinary ascites or urinoma)
   (b) large bladder diverticulum
   (c) unilateral VUR (?)

Unfavourable prognostic signs:

■ *in utero* presentation before 24 weeks;
■ hyperechogenic kidneys, no pyramids seen;
■ lowest serum creatinine > 0.8 m%;
■ bilateral VUR;
■ incontinence;
■ absence of pop-off phenomenon.

Fertility and cryptochordism

Cryptorchidism occurs in 12% of PUV patients and in 5% it is bilateral. In comparision, the general population has a 0.7–0.8% incidence of cryptorchidism and 10% incidence of bilaterality (Krueger *et al.*, 1980a).

PUV can present in adulthood with almost-dry orgasms secondary to semen pooling in the posterior urethra (Páramo *et al.*, 1983). Even after valve ablation in childhood, adult patients may have a widened posterior urethra resulting in poor ejaculatory expulsion force.

Woodhouse *et al.* (1989) undertook the only thorough study of sexual function and fertility in PUV adults. They interviewed 21 men, 19–37 years old, who were treated in childhood for PUV. Two men had a history of epididymoorchitis and two had undergone orchiopexy. Three men were on dialysis, including the only man in the group who was impotent. Almost 50% of the men complained of slow or dry ejaculation, although they seemed to have the normal sensation of orgasm. Ejaculates were obtained from nine men. Total sperm count, motility, and percentage of abnormal forms were unremarkable. Unique for this group of men was that five of the nine specimens were so viscous that they had to be cut with a knife to divide them; the viscous specimens had exceptionally high pH values. Another unique finding was a shaking motion of the sperm in almost all specimens, the type of motion sometimes associated with the presence of sperm antibodies, although none was found. There was no difference in the semen analysis of those with a propulsive ejaculation compared with those with a slow flow. Urine samples following ejaculation did not demonstrate retrograde ejaculation. Conclusions regarding fertility in PUV patients are difficult to make based on a series with a mean age of only 24.6 years.

Renal transplantation

It is often commented that long-term follow-up is necessary to determine outcome in patients with PUV. This statement is made because some 'valve patients' seem to go into renal failure in their teenage years and it is not always easy to predict by serum creatinine (SC) values those for whom dialysis or transplantation will be required, and when. In order to predict patient outcome more accurately, Arbus and Bacheyle (1981) addressed this shortcoming in management and showed that the rate of deterioration of renal function can best be determined by using the fraction 1/SC and plotting linear regression with multiple SC values. The more values obtained and plotted, the more precisely one can determine when dialysis or renal transplantation will be warranted. They found from the regressions that predictions using at least six 1/SC values over time would predict a fairly accurate outcome. Thus, an elevated serum creatinine level could help in defining definitive outcome (i.e. the need for dialysis or transplantation) as opposed to palliative therapy. In a patient with a serum creatinine level of 5 mg%, by using the linear regression graph of 1/SC, one could then predict which patients with a SC of 5 mg% might require definitive therapy in the next year and which might require definitive therapy in a few years (Arbus and Bacheyle, 1981).

The majority of transplant patients with a history of a PUV valve ultimately have abnormal urodynamic findings. It is important to correct bladder dynamics prior to renal transplantation. However, long-term follow-up studies have yielded contradicting results when comparing the outcome of transplantation in valve patients with controls.

Churchill et al. (1988) found poorer graft survival in patients who had had PUV than in other groups. They theorized that the ureters in such patients had difficulty delivering urine to a bladder that, in retrospect, was likely to have had higher pressures during the storage phase. When comparing children with a history of isolated VUR as controls and children with a history of PUV, Reinberg et al. (1988) found that graft survival was 73% in the reflux group and 75% in the valve group at 5 years. Renal function, however, was significantly better in those with VUR alone than in those with a history of PUV. Groenewegen et al. (1993) found graft survival after 5 years to be less in patients with PUV than in a matched control group (50% vs 65%). They also found serum creatinine levels to be higher in the PUV patients. However, the findings were not statistically significant.

Two studies from the University of Alabama (Bryant et al., 1991; Indudhara et al., 1998), evaluated valve patients following renal transplantation, after 5 years in one and after 10 years in the other. The graft survival was slightly higher but not significantly so in the valve patients after 5 years when compared with a control group (62.3% vs 48%). Serum creatinine levels, however, as in the Reinberg et al. (1988) study, were significantly increased (1.2 mg% in controls vs 2.2 mg% in the valve group). They suspected that abnormal bladder dynamics played a role in their elevation.

While serum creatinine remained relatively unchanged over the next 5 years in the Alabama valve group, it continued to increase in the control group and, while mean serum creatinine levels remained higher in the valve group, there was no longer a statistical difference in the serum creatinine levels between the two groups (Indudhara et al., 1998). In another study, Rajagopalan et al. (1994) found no significant difference in graft survival, mean serum creatinine levels, or adjusted serum creatinine levels in valve patients when compared with controls at the end of 5 years.

While the evidence may not be strong that renal function may be worse with time following transplantation in patients with a history of PUV, based on the current literature one must not underestimate the 'valve bladder' and the possible detrimental role that it can play on the transplanted ureter and its associated kidney.

In a more definitive approach to determine whether a valve bladder is associated with poorer long-term graft function, Salomon et al. (2000) split PUV transplant patients into two groups, those with and those without dysfunctional voiding symptoms, the latter representing the more typical valve bladder. They found a difference between the two groups, in that graft survival was significantly better in the non-valve bladder group. In the future, when comparing PUV transplant patients and their graft outcome to controls, the PUV patients should be separated into two groups, those with normal bladders and those with abnormal bladders, and each subgroup should be compared with the control group. Separately, the present authors strongly agree with Thomalla et al. (1989) that it is necessary to evaluate bladder dynamics before transplantation, especially in those who have a history of voiding symptoms. Abnormal parameters must be corrected, even if bladder augmentation is required. Transplantation can be successful even when the transplant ureter is implanted into the augmented bladder.

Anterior urethral valves

Anterior urethral valves are rare, with the largest series reporting 17 patients (Williams and Retik, 1969). They are important causes of obstruction in children (Firlit *et al.*, 1978). They occur about ten times less frequently than PUV. Most anterior urethral valves are congenital in nature, but valves may be acquired after trauma or surgery. They can be located anywhere in the urethra: approximately 40% occur in the bulbar urethra, 30% at the penoscrotal junction, and the remaining 30% in the penile urethra. There is a dispute in the literature as to whether or not anterior urethral valves can exist without an associated diverticulum. Both lesions are characterized by a ventral outpouching of the anterior urethra and as urine distends the outpouching, the distal lip is elevated and pressed against the dorsal wall of the urethra, creating an obstruction. Patients present in a similar manner to those with PUV. The clinical spectrum ranges from mild urethral dilatation to bilateral hydronephrosis with renal insufficiency, both representing different degrees of urinary tract obstruction. They too can cause histologic and dynamic bladder changes. Today, most patients present with antenatal hydronephrosis. Other means of presentation include urethral ballooning, UTI, hematuria, and obstructive voiding symptoms. One-third of patients present with a visible urethral diverticulum on the ventral shaft or bulb of the penis and therefore the role the valve plays may be missed. Compression of the urethra after voiding causes some urine to dribble out from the meatus. Fewer than 5% of patients with anterior valves progress to chronic renal failure. Patients with significant upper tract deterioration often present at a younger age. All patients should be evaluated with VCUG and renal sonography or excretory urography. Cystoscopy and retrograde urethrography may fail to demonstrate the valve as it remains open with retrograde flow. Baseline serum creatinine should be assessed, especially in cases with bilateral hydronephrosis.

The age of the patient, degree of upper tract involvement, and the type of valve dictate the appropriate treatment. Approximately one-half of all patients can be treated with simple transurethral fulguration. Van Savage *et al.* (1997) proposed an algorithm of treatment based on the severity of disease. Transurethral fulguration of anterior urethral valves is the preferred treatment for patients with a normal serum creatinine and only mild to moderate hydronephrosis. The aim of endoscopic treatment is to cut the distal lip of the valve to allow the urethral lumen to open. Attempts are not made to resect the valve completely. Patients must have an adequate sized urethra for cystoscopy. Insufficient corpus spongiosum tissue puts these patients at increased risk for postoperative subcutaneous extravasation and an iatrogenic urethrocutaneous fistula. A urethroplasty and open resection of the valve are recommended for patients with an associated massive urethral diverticulum. The urethral diverticulum should be widely laid open and the excess mucosa excised. A double-breasted closure is then performed. Patients with persistent high serum creatinine despite catheter drainage of their bladders may benefit from vesicostomy.

Congenital anterior urethral diverticula

Urethral diverticula in the male is a rare condition that is usually diagnosed as part of an investigation of patients with lower urinary tact symptoms such as dysuria, frequency, and postvoid dribbling.

Ventral midline diverticula arising from cystic dilatations of the Cowper's gland ducts (syringoceles) and dorsal urethral diverticula of the fossa navicularis (lacuna magna) are the most common congenital diverticula of the male anterior urethra.

Syringoceles

The cystic dilatations and diverticula arising from the main duct of Cowper's bulbourethral gland were named Cowper's syringoceles by Maizels *et al.* (1983), who divided them into four groups depending on their radiographic appearance (Fig. 28.26): (1) simple syringocele, a minimally dilated duct; (2) perforate syringocele, a bulbous duct draining into the urethra by a spatulous ostium; (3) imperforate syringocele, a duct resembling a submucosal cyst appearing as a radiolucent mass protruding into the urethra on VCUG; and (4) ruptured syringocele, a membrane remaining after the rupture of a dilated duct (Maizels *et al.*, 1983). The perforate and ruptured syringoceles have the urethroscopic appearance of a diverticulum and cause urethral infections, hematuria, dysuria, and urinary dribbling (Sant and Kaleli, 1985). The imperforate and simple syringoceles can cause compression of the urethra resulting in voiding difficulties.

(a) 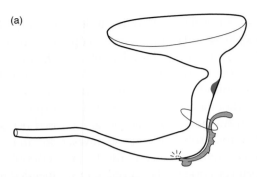   (b)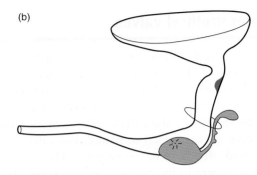

Figure 28.26 Cowper's gland and duct abnormalities: (a) normal anatomy. (b, c) Cowper's syringoceles; (d) abnormal entry site of the duct into the bulbous urethra.

These patients can also present with a mass in the perineum and hydronephrosis. Cystic dilatations of the duct of Cowper's gland can be acquired or congenital. Cystourethroscopy or retrograde urethrography confirms the diagnosis. The treatment of choice is unroofing of the diverticulum by transurethral incision, thereby marsupializing it into the urethra.

Recently, Bevers *et al.*, (2000) proposed a simplified and clinically useful classification which differentiates between open and closed syringoceles. Open syringoceles may cause postvoid incontinence, while the closed type may cause an infravesical obstruction. The closed syringocele is the equivalent of what Maizels labeled the imperforate syringocele.

Lacuna magna

Morgani (1719) was the first to describe this entity. Guérin (1950) referred to the flap of tissue overlying the lacunae or diverticulum as a valve, i.e. the valve of Guérin. Sommer and Stephens (1980) suggested that the valve of Guérin is a remnant of an embryologic septum that persists between the canalized glanular ingrowth of ectodermal tissue and the distally advancing urethra. They are lined by squamous epithelium (Fig. 28.27).

Sommer and Stephens (1980) first associated this previously described anomaly with specific urologic complaints in boys in 1980. A lacuna magna usually causes no symptoms and may be present in 30% of boys (Bellinger *et al.*, 1983). Symptoms include postvoid dribbling of blood or bloody urine, blood spotting, and pain on urination. Friedman and King (1992) reported on six boys with dysuria and blood spotting. The diagnosis can be made on cystoscopy when the actual diverticulum can be seen on the roof of the distal urethra or on VCUG when it fills with con-

trast. The contrast-filled diverticulum can be mistaken for a drop of urine on the penile skin. Sommer and Stephens (1980) discussed blindly probing the diverticulum with a lacrimal duct probe and incising the valve of Guérin with blunt-tipped scissors passed through the meatus. Bellinger *et al.* (1983) suggested grasping the valve with forceps and pulling it to the meatus, where it could then be incised under direct vision. Seskin and Glassberg (1994) reported on six patients who presented with blood spotting and/or pain and had negative urinalysis and cultures. All patients had a VCUG and a cystoscopy, both studies showing the lacuna magna. All patients were treated endoscopically using a pediatric resectoscope and right-angle wire electrode. The valves were incised with cutting current and the base of the diverticulum was fulgurated.

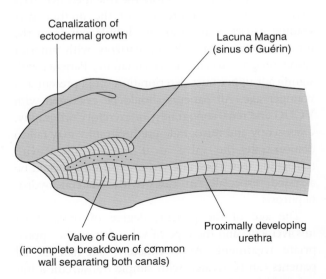

Figure 28.27 Embryologic formation of fossa navicularis and lacuna magna. (From Seskin and Glassberg, 1994, with permission, and adapted from Stephens, 1983b.)

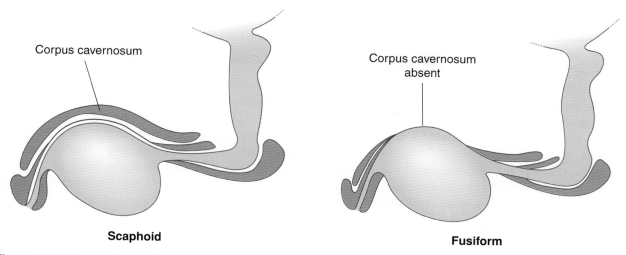

Scaphoid

Fusiform

Figure 28.28 Types of megalourethra (left) scaphoid; (right) fusiform.

Megalourethra and large diverticula

Megalourethra is a rare congenital disorder most commonly associated with the prune belly disorder. It is divided into the scaphoid and fusiform types (Fig. 28.28).

Narrow-mouthed saccular diverticula, wide-mouthed saccular diverticula, and scaphoid diverticula are three types of diverticula of the floor of the anterior urethra. All three are due to defects in the corpus spongiosum, with the scaphoid megalourethra also having a defect in the corpus spongiosum. Although rare, the wide-mouthed saccular diverticulum is the most common congenital lesion obstructing the anterior urethra during voiding. The distal lip of the diverticulum is elevated during voiding, forcing it against the roof of the urethra. Patients present in an almost identical manner to those with anterior urethral valves. They have a poor stream with a palpable or visible swelling on the ventral surface of the penis. On VCUG the urethra is usually dilated proximal to the diverticulum, and the urethra distal to the diverticulum may be narrow or invisible.

Patients with scaphoid megalourethra have no corpus spongiosum along the ventral surface of the penis. During voiding the anterior urethra swells through this defect and the penis elongates (Fig. 28.29). There is no bulge on the dorsal surface of the penis because both corpora cavernosa are present. These patients are very susceptible to infection and therefore should not be catheterized. Anomalies associated with scaphoid megalourethra include prune belly syndrome, hypo-

spadias, hypoplastic or dysplastic kidneys, and supernumerary digits. Management is primarily cosmetic if the upper tracts are not at risk for infection or deterioration.

The fusiform megalourethra is a congenital anomaly involving the distal. Large defects are present in the corpus spongiosum and in both corpora cavernosa, leaving the urethra poorly supported only by fibrous tissue and penile skin. When patients void, the entire penis elongates and swells in a fusiform manner. Since there are no corporeal bodies, the penis is soft and flabby, consisting primarily of skin. Most often these patients have other associated, often fatal conditions such as covered exstrophy of the bladder and congenital rectovesical fistula. The prognosis for patients with fusiform megalourethra is very poor.

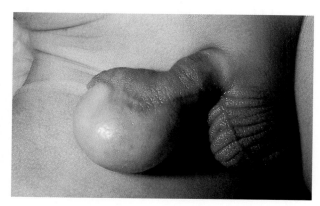

Figure 28.29 Scaphoid megalourethra. Note how the penis bulges and elongates in this anomaly lacking corpus spongiosum.

Congenital urethral polyps

Usually arising from the verumontanum, urethral polyps are benign congenital lesions. The stalks of urethral polyps consist of vascular fibrous tissue and smooth muscle covered by transitional epithelium. Possible etiologies include abnormal protrusion of the urethral wall and metaplastic changes secondary to maternal estrogens. Presenting symptoms include hematuria, dysuria, and incontinence. Most patients present with hesitancy, diminished stream, incomplete emptying, and urinary retention. Physical examination is usually not helpful except in cases where the polyp is so large that it can be felt on rectal examination. A filling defect located between the bladder and anterior urethra on VCUG is seen with voiding. After voiding, the polyp retracts and its tip occupies the region of the bladder neck or trigone. This 'flip-flop' appearance is pathognomonic for posterior urethral polyps. Polyps that prolapse into the bladder are often seen on sonogram.

Traditionally, urethral polyps were approached suprapubically. Most lesions are now managed by transurethral resection with fulguration of the base. With resection there is a potential risk of urethral injury and damage to the nearby sphincter, and the polyp may recur if the base is not destroyed.

Gleason and Kramer (1994) reviewed the symptoms, radiographic findings, treatment, and natural history of children with genitourinary polyps seen between 1957 and 1992. The mean age at presentation was 8.9 years and one-half of all patients presented with obstructive lower urinary tract voiding complaints. None of the patients had hydronephrosis.

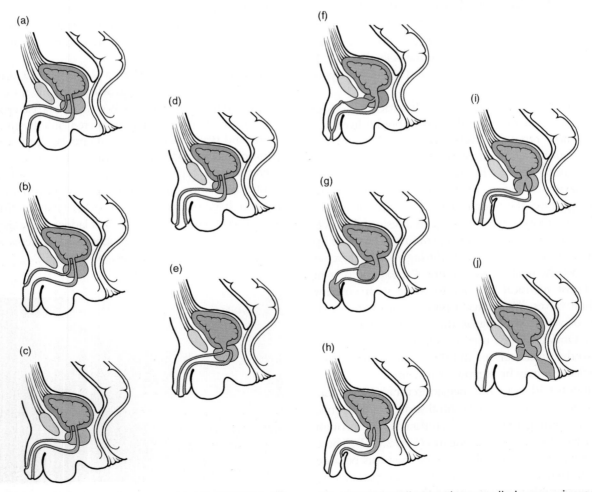

Figure 28.30 Ten variations of urethral duplications. Those with one epispadiac urethra usually have an increased separation of the pubic symphysis. The normal distance between the ends of the pubes is 10 mm or less. (From Colodny, 1990, with permission.)

Anterior urethral polyps are extremely rare. These polyps arise from the ventral wall of the urethra and patients present with hematuria, dysuria, weak stream, and occasionally postvoid dribbling. They are benign lesions and treatment consists of transurethral excision or fulguration.

Urethral duplication

Partial or complete, patients with this anomaly have two urethras, one of which is normal, and the other an accessory urethra. It is an extremely rare congenital anomaly. The two urethras are usually aligned in a sagittal plane, one above the other, with the ventral urethra having a lumen that is closer to normal than the often stenotic or hypoplastic dorsal urethra. The minority of duplications are collateral, the two channels lying side by side. Patients can present with incontinence, UTI, outflow obstruction, double or split stream, or can be asymptomatic with the duplication being found on routine physical examination. The symptoms will depend on the type of duplication.

Many hypotheses have been proposed for the embryologic explanation of duplication anomalies. The dorsal, epispadiac channel types can be explained by a partial failure of the ingrowth of the lateral mesoderm between the ectodermal and endodermal layers of the cloacal membrane in the midline. Abnormal canalization of the urethral plate explains the distal hypospadiac duplication variant.

Several classifications exist but the one offered by Woodhouse and Williams (1979) is based on the final destination of the accessory urethra, sex, completeness, and the relationship of the two urethras to each other. In the complete type, each urethra has a separate origin from a different bladder openings and the urethras terminate separately. In the dorsal (hypospadiac) variety, the accessory urethra terminates on the ventral aspect of the penis. In the more common ventral (epispadiac) variety the accessory urethra terminates on the dorsum anywhere from the glans penis to the penopubic junction. In the incomplete type there is only one urethra originating from the bladder. The accessory urethra arises from the dorsum (incomplete epispadiac sagittal duplication) or ventrum (incomplete hypospadiac sagittal duplication) of the bulbous urethra. Both accessory urethras terminate anywhere from the subglanular to the penoscrotal location (Fig. 28.30).

The most widely used classification by Effman *et al.*, (1976) classified duplication of the urethra into three types, as summarized below:

Type I: blind incomplete urethral duplication (accessory urethra):
(A) distal: opening on the dorsal or ventral surface of the penis but not communicating with the urethra or bladder (most common type);
(B) proximal; opening from urethral channel but ending blindly in the periurethral tissue; may be difficult to differentiate from urethral diverticula or Cowper's ducts (rare).

Type II: completely patent urethral duplication:
(A) two meati: (1) two non-communicating urethras arising independently from the bladder; (2) second channel arising from the first and coursing independently into a second meatus;
(B) one meatus; two urethras arising from the bladder or posterior urethra and uniting into a common channel distally.

Type III: urethral duplication as a component of partial or complete caudal duplication.

Using Effman's classification, type I (incomplete) is the most common type, is almost always asymptomatic, and requires no treatment. Of the complete types, the most common are two non-communicating channels arising independently from the bladder and coursing separately through the penis and then exiting as two separate meati. The ventral urethra is normal in caliber and has its meatus in a normal glanular position. The meatus of the dorsal channel has an epispadiac location and its lumen is quite narrow and sometimes hypoplastic. In a few instances the meatus of the dorsal (accessory) channel is positioned normally and the meatus of the ventral channel is located in a hypospadiac location. In type IIA2, one urethra arises from the other and has a second meatal opening. In most cases the accessory urethra originates at the level of the prostatic urethra and the normal urethra is located ventrally as in type IIA1. The most serious form of type IIA2 duplication occurs when the ventral meatus is located at the anterior anal margin. The dorsal urethra is hypoplastic and most of the urine passes through the ventral channel and exits in the perineum. The rarest of complete patent duplication anomalies is type IIB. In this situation the urethras unite to form a single channel, that ends in a normally positioned meatus.

The exception to the rule of the ventral urethra being the more normal and functional one is congenital posterior urethroperineal fistula, the so-called 'Y-fistula'. This represents a variant of duplication where the accessory urethra extends from the posterior urethra to the perineum. In this subset of urethral duplication, the ventral urethra is less functional and tends to be lined with transitional cell epithelium. Patients usually present with perineal leakage of urine and may present at any age. The diagnosis is made with VCUG or retrograde urethrography and treatment involves excision of the ventral urethra. Brown *et al.* (1990) reported a case of urethroperineal fistula that originated from the posterior urethra between the bladder neck and verumontanum and terminated in the perineum. The patient had a normal dorsal urethra and leaked from the rectum after voiding. Glassberg *et al.* (1978) reported on two patients with an accessory urethra that terminated in the perineum and originated from the bladder passing just anterior to the bladder neck, passing anterior to the prostate, and crossing the normal urethra.

Double stream is the most common complaint. The extent of patients' complaints depends on how much urine comes from each opening, the location of the openings, and how parallel the two streams are to each other. Incontinence, usually stress related, is secondary to inadequate development of the sphincter mechanism of the accessory urethra. The incomplete distal crypt associated with hypospadias is often confused with urethral duplication by inexperienced examiners.

Narrowing or obstruction of the distal dorsal channel leads to proximal dilatation with secondary compression and obstruction of the more normal, ventral urethra. These patients present with complaints of decreased force of stream, straining, and infection.

VCUG usually demonstrates both channels, assuming that both channels are patent and carry enough urine to be visualized. Occasionally, all or part of the dorsal urethra is so small that it is not visualized on the VCUG. Retrograde urethrograms of each channel (separately and together) help to delineate the anatomy in this situation. It is usually easy to catheterize the ventral urethra and quite difficult to catheterize the dorsal, accessory urethra. Cystoscopy can be performed to locate the site of a urethroperineal fistula.

Treatment of duplication anomalies depends on the anatomy of the duplication and its clinical manifestations. Double stream and incontinence are the symptoms that most often lead to surgical correction. A combination of surgical techniques is required to correct this malformation. A posterior sagittal trans-anorectal approach based on splitting the anterior rectal wall has been suggested for the difficult-to-reach posterior urethra. A protective colostomy is recommended for this approach. This technique provides excellent exposure of the retrourethral region, permitting simple and safe surgery. Complete excision of the accessory urethra should always be attempted. Other options include excision of a distal common septum to create a single channel, and reconstruction and anastomosis of two urethras into one in instances where the glanular urethra is adequate in caliber.

Occasionally, the urethroperineal fistula can be managed endoscopically. The fistulous tract can be cannulated with a 4 Fr ureteral catheter passed through the perineal opening. Cystoscopy then allows for visualization of the communication with the urethra, which can then be fulgurated with a bugbee electrode.

Williams and Bloomberg (1975) reported on nine patients with a form of incomplete urethral duplication where the urethra bifurcates just below the bladder neck and the ventral limb opens at the anal verge. The dorsal limb follows the normal anatomic course but is usually severely stenotic. The aim of surgery in this group was to create a second complete urethral channel to the tip of the penis. Options in the treatment of these Y-type fistulae include mobilization of the perineal limb with distal urethroplasty, as advocated by Belman (1977), or marsupialization of the atretic urethra with a secondary urethroplasty at a later date, as suggested by Stephens and Donnellan (1977). This secondary procedure can be performed using preputial island flap technique. If the dorsal urethra can be catheterized, Passerini *et al.* (1988) have shown that gentle, gradual prolonged dilation *in situ* may allow eventual use of this, often very narrow, urethral channel.

References

Arbus GS, Bacheyle GS (1981) Method for predicting when children with progressive renal disease may reach high serum creatinine levels. *Pediatrics* **67**: 871–3.

Arena JG, Bomalaski MD, Coplen DE *et al.* (1999) Delayed presentation of posterior urethral valves. Read at the Annual meeting of the American Urologic Association, Dallas, TX, 2 May 1999.

Arnold SJ, Ginsberg A (1974) Radiographic and photoendoscopic studies in posterior urethral vales in enuretic boys. *Urology* **4**: 145–54.

Atwell JD (1983) Posterior urethral valves in the British Isles: a multicenter BAPS review. *J Pediatr Surg* **18**: 70–4.

Bauer SB, Dieppa RA, Libib KK, Retik AB (1979) The bladder in boys with posterior urethral valves: a urodynamic assessment. *J Urol* **121**: 769–73.

Baum NA, Burger R, Catlon CE (1974) Nephrogenic diabetes insipidus associated with posterior urethral valves. *Urology* **4**: 581–3.

Bellinger MF, Purohit GS, Duckett JW, Cromie WJ (1983) Lacuna magna: a hidden case of dysuria and bloody spotting in boys. *J Pediatr Surg* **18**: 163–6.

Belman AB (1977) The repair of the H-type urethrorectal fistula using a scrotal flap urethroplasty. *J Urol* **118**: 659–61.

Bevers RFM, Abberberk EM, Boon TA (2000) Cowper's syringocele: symptoms, classification and treatment of an unappreciated problem. *J Urol* **163**: 782–4.

Borer JG, Park JM, Atala A *et al.* (1999) Heparin binding EGF-like growth factor expression increases selectivity in bladder smooth muscle in response to lower urinary tract obstruction. *Lab Invest* **79**: 1335–45.

Borzi PA, Beasley SW, Fowler R (1992) Posterior urethral valves in non-twin siblings. *Br J Urol* **70**: 201.

Brown WI, Dillon PW, Hensle TW (1990) Congenital urethral–perineal fistula: diagnosis and new surgical management. *Urology* **36**: 157–9.

Bryant JE, Joseph DB, Kohaut EC, Diethelm AG (1991) Renal transplantation in children with posterior urethral valves. *J Urol* **146**: 1585–7.

Campaiola JM, Perlmutter AD, Steinhardt GF (1985) Non-compliant bladder resulting from posterior urethral valves. *J Urol* **134**: 708–10.

Campbell M (1937) *Pediatric urology*. Volume 1. New York: Macmillan Corporation, 52.

Campbell M (1951) *Clinical pediatric urology*. Philadelphia, PA: WB Saunders, 336.

Casale AJ (1999) Posterior urethral valves and other obstructions of the urethra. In: Gonzales ET, Bauer SB (eds) *Pediatric urology practice*. Philadelphia, PA: Lippincott, Williams and Wilkins, 223–44.

Chun AL, Ruzich JV, Wein AJ, Levin RM (1989) Functional and pharmacological effects of ureteral diversion. *J Urol* **141**: 403–7.

Churchill BM, Krueger RP, Fleischer MH, Hardy BE (1983) Complications of posterior urethral valve surgery and their prevention. *Urol Clin North Am* **10**: 519–30.

Churchill BM, Sheldon CA, McLorie GA, Arbus GS (1988) Factors influencing patients and graft survival in 300 cadaveric renal transplants. *J Urol* **140**: 1129–33.

Churchill BM, McLorie GA, Khoury AE *et al.* (1990) Emergency treatment and long-term follow-up of posterior urethral valves. *Urol Clin North Am* **17**: 125–6.

Close CE, Carr MC, Burns MW, Mitchell ME (1997) Lower urinary tract changes after early valve ablation in neonates and infants: is early diversion warranted? *J Urol* **157**: 984–8.

Cohen HL, Susman M, Haller JO (1994) Posterior urethral valves: transperineal ultrasound for imaging and diagnosis in male infants. *Radiology* **192**: 261–4.

Cohen HL, Zinn HL, Patel A *et al.* (1998) Prenatal sonographic diagnosis of posterior urethral valves: identification of valves and thickening of the posterior wall. *J Clin Ultrasound* **26**: 366–70.

Colodny AH (1990) Urethral lesions in infants and children. In: Gillenwater JY, Grayhack JT, Howards SS, Duckett JW (eds) *Adult and pediatric urology*. Volume 2. Chicago, IL: Year Book Medical Publishers, 1799.

Connor JP, Burbige KA (1990) Long-term urinary continence and renal function in neonates with posterior urethral valves. *J Urol* **144**: 1209–11.

Crooks KK (1982) Urethral structures following transurethral resection of posterior urethral valves. *J Urol* **127**: 1153–4.

Cuckow PM, Dinneen MD, Risdon RA *et al.* (1997) Long-term renal function in the posterior urethral valves, unilateral reflux and renal dysplasia syndrome. *J Urol* **158**: 1004–7.

Cukier J (1980) Treatment of posterior urethral valves. Presented at the International Assembly for Pediatric Urology, Pinehurst, N C, 5–8 November 1980.

Davis JA, James U (1952) Congenital urethral obstruction presenting in the neonatal period. *Proc R Soc Med* **45**: 401.

DeGennaro M, Mosiello G, Capitanucci ML *et al.* (1996) Early detection of bladder dysfunction following posterior urethral valves. *Eur J Pediatr Surg* **6**: 163–5.

Denes ED, Barthold JS, Gonzalez R (1997) Early prognostic valves of serum creatinine levels in children with posterior urethral valves. *J Urol* **157**: 1441–3.

Dewan PA (1993) Congenital obstructing posterior urethral membrane (COPUM): further evidence for a common morphological diagnosis. *Pediatr Surg Int* **8**: 45–50.

Dewan PA (1996) Letter to the Editor. *J Pediatr Surg* **31**: 867.

Dewan PA (1999) Urethral valves or COPUM? Changing the nomenclature. *Contemp Urol* **11**: 15–27.

Dewan PA, Goh DG, Crameri J (1995) Cobb's collar. *Pediatr Surg Int* **10**: 243–6.

Dewan PA, Zappata SM, Ransky PG, Duffy PG (1992) Endoscopic reappraisal of the morphology of congenital obstruction of the posterior urethra. *Br J Urol* **70**: 439–44.

Dewan PA, Keenan RJ, Morris LL *et al.* (1994) Congenital urethral obstruction: Cobb's collar or prolapsed congenital obstruction posterior urethral membrane (COPUM). *Br J Urol* **73**: 91–5.

Dinneen M, Dhillon HK, Ward HC *et al.* (1993) Antenatal diagnosis of posterior urethral valves. *Br J Urol* **72**: 364–9.

Dinneen MD, Duffy PG, Barratt TM, Ransley PG (1995) Persistent polyuria after posterior urethral valves. *Br J Urol* **75**: 236–40.

Ditchfield MR, Grattan-Smith JD, deCampo JF, Hutson JM (1995) Voiding cystourethrography in boys: does the presence of the catheter obscure the diagnosis of posterior urethral valves? *AJR Am J Roentgenol* **164**: 1233–5.

Duckett JW Jr (1974a) Current management of posterior urethral valves. *Urol Clin North Am* **1**: 471–83.

Duckett JW Jr (1974b) Cutaneous vesicostomy in childhood. The Blocksom technique. *Urol Clin North Am* **1**: 484–95.

Duckett JW Jr (1997) Editorial comment. *J Urol* **157**: 988.

Duckett JW, Snow BW (1986) Disorders of the urethra. In: Walsh PC, Gittes RF, Perlmutter AD *et al.* (eds) *Campbell's urology*. 5th edition. Philadelphia, PA: WB Saunders, 2000.

Duel BP, Mogbo K, Barthold JS, Gonzalez R (1998) Prognostic valve of initial real ultrasound in patients with posterior urethral valves. *J Urol* **160**: 1198–200.

Effman EL, Lebowitz RL, Colodny AH (1976) Duplication of the urethra. *Radiology* **119**: 179–85.

Egami K, Smith ED (1982) A study of the sequelae of posterior urethral valves. *J Urol* **127**: 84–7.

Ehrlich RM, Shamberg A, Fine RN (1987) Neodynium:YAG laser ablation of posterior urethra valves. *J Urol* **138**: 959–62.

El-Ghoniemi A, Desgrippes A, Luton D *et al.* (1999) Outcome of posterior urethral valves: to what extent is it improved by prenatal diagnosis? *J Urol* **162**: 846–8.

Estes JM, MacGilliuray TE, Hedrick MH *et al.* (1992) Fetoscopic surgery for the treatment of congenital anomalies. *J Pediatr Surg* **27**: 950–4.

Ewalt DH, Howard PS, Blyth B *et al.* (1992) Is lamina propria matrix responsible for normal bladder compliance? *J Urol* **148**: 544–9.

Farkas A, Skinner DG (1976) Posterior urethral valves in siblings. *Br J Urol* **48**: 76.

Field PL, Stephens FD (1974) Congenital urethral membranes causing urethral obstruction. *J Urol* **111**: 250–5.

Firlit RS, Firlit CF, King LR (1978) Obstructing anterior urethral valves in children. *J Urol* **119**: 819–21.

Friedman RM, King LR (1992) Valve of Guerin – an elusive cause of dysuria and hematuria in young boys. *J Urol* **147**: 385A (Abstract 691).

Gibbons MD, Horan JJ, Dejter SW Jr, Keszler M (1993) Extracorporeal membrane oxygenation: an adjunct in the management of the neonate urinary tract anomalies. *J Urol* **150**: 434–7.

Glassberg KI (1982) Persistent ureteral dilatation following valve ablation (Editorial comments). *Dialog Pediatr Urol* **5**: 2.

Glassberg KI (1983) Comments. In: Churchill BN (ed.) *Posterior urethral valves management. Dialog Pediatr Urol* **6**: 7.

Glassberg KI (1985) Current issues regarding posterior urethral valves. *Urol Clin North Am* **12**: 175–85.

Glassberg KI, Filmer RB (1985) Renal dysplasia, renal hypoplasia and cystic disease of the kidney. In: Kelalis P, King LR, Belman AB (eds) *Clinical pediatric urology*. 2nd edition.l Philadelphia, PA: WB Saunders.

Glassberg KI, Schwartz R, Haller JO (1978) Vesicoperineal accessory urethra. *J Urol* **120**: 255–6.

Glassberg KI, Schneider M, Waterhouse RK (1979) Observations of the dilated ureter following posterior urethral valve ablation. Read at the Annual Meeting of the American Urologic Association, New York, 13 May 1979.

Glassberg KI, Schneider M, Haller JO *et al.* (1982) Observations on persistently dilated ureter after posterior urethral valve ablation. *Urology* **20**: 20–8.

Gleason PE, Kramer SA (1994) Genitourinary polyps in children. *Urology* **144**: 106–9.

Glick PL, Harrison MR, Globus MS *et al.* (1985) Management of the fetus with hydronephrosis II. Prognostic criteria and selection for treatment. *J Pediatr Surg* **20**: 376–87.

Gonzales ET Jr (1998) Posterior urethral valves and other anomalies. In: Walsh PC, Retik AB, Vaughan ED Jr, Wein AJ (eds) *Campbell's urology*. 7th edition. Philadelphia, PA: WB Saunders, 2069–91.

Gosling JA, Gilpin SA, Dixon JS, Gilpin CJ (1986) Decrease in autonomic innervation of human detrusor muscle in outflow obstruction. *J Urol* **136**: 501–4.

Grajewski RS, Glassberg KI (1983) The variable effect posterior urethral valves as illustrated in identical twins. *J Urol* **130**: 1188–90.

Greenfield SP, Hensle TW, Berdon WE, Wigger HJ (1983) Unilateral vesicoureteral reflux and unilateral nonfunctioning kidney associated with posterior urethral valves – a syndrome? *J Urol* **130**: 733–8.

Griesbach WA, Waterhouse RK, Mellins HZ (1959) Voiding cystourethrography in the diagnosis of congenital posterior urethral valves. *Am J Roentgenol* **82**: 521–9.

Groenewegen AA, Sukhai RN, Nauta J, Sholtmeyer RJ, Nijman RJM (1993) Results of renal transplantation in boys treated for posterior urethral valves. *J Urol* **149**: 1517–20.

Guérin A (1950) In: Chamerot C (ed.) *Elements de chirugie operatiore*. Paris, **60**: 749.

Hamm FC, Waterhouse RK (1961) Changing concepts in lower urinary tract obstruction in children. *JAMA* **175**: 854–7.

Hanlon-Lundberg KM, Verp MS, Loy G (1994) Posterior urethral valves in successive generations. *Am J Perinatol* **11**: 37–9.

Harrison MR (1993) Fetal surgery. In: *Fetal Medicine* (Special Issue). *West J Med* **159**: 341–9.

Harrison MR (1994) Fetal surgical therapy. *Lancet* **343**: 897–902.

Harrison MR, Golbys MS, Filly RA (1982) Fetal surgery for congenital hydronephrosis. *N Engl J Med* **306**: 591–3.

Harrison MR, Ross N, Noall R (1983) Correction of congenital hydronephrosis *in-utero*. I. The model: fetal urethral obstruction produces hydronephrosis and pulmonary hypoplasia in fetal lambs. *J Pediatr Surg* **18**: 247–56.

Hendren WH (1970) A new approach to infants with severe obstructive uropathy: early complete reconstruction. *J Pediatr Surg* **5**: 184–99.

Hendren WH (1974) Posterior urethral valves in boys: a broad clinical spectrum. *J Urol* **106**: 298–307.

Henneberry MO, Stephens FD (1980) Renal hypoplasia and dysplasia in infants with posterior urethral valves. *J Urol* **123**: 912–15.

Holmdahl G (1997) Bladder dysfunction in boys with posterior urethral valves. *Scand J Urol Nephrol* **188** (Suppl): 1–36.

Holmdahl G, Sillen U, Bachelara M *et al.* (1995) The changing urodynamic pattern in valve bladders during infancy. *J Urol* **153**: 463–7.

Holmdahl G, Sillen U, Hanson E *et al.* (1996) Bladder dysfunction in boys with posterior urethral valves before and after puberty. *J Urol* **155**: 694–8.

Holmdahl G, Sillen U, Bertilsson M *et al.* (1997) Natural filling cystometry in small boys with posterior urethral valves: unstable valve bladders become stable during sleep. *J Urol* **158**: 1017–21.

Holmdahl G, Hanson E, Hanson M *et al.* (1998) Four-hour voiding observations in young boys with posterior urethral valves. *J Urol* **160**: 1477–81.

Hoover DL, Duckett JW Jr (1982) Posterior urethral valves, unilateral reflux and renal dysplasia: a syndrome. *J Urol* **128**: 994–7.

Hsu TH, Levin RM, Wein AJ, Haugaard N (1994) Alterations of mitochondrial oxidative metabolism in rabbit urinary bladder after partial outlet obstruction. *Molec Cell Biochem* **141**: 21–6.

Hulbert WC, Rosenberg HK, Cartwright PC *et al.* (1992) The predictive valve of ultrasonography in evaluation of infants with posterior urethral valves. *J Urol* **148**: 122–4.

Hutton KAR, Thomas DFM, Arthur RJ *et al.* (1994) Prenatally detected posterior urethral valves: is gestational age at detection a predictor of outcome? *J Urol* **152**: 698–701.

Indudhara R, Joseph DB, Perez LM, Diethelm AG (1998) Renal transplantation in children with posterior urethral valves revisited: a ten-year follow up. *J Urol* **160**: 1201–3.

Jaureguizar E, Lopez Pereira P, Bueno J, Espinosa y Navarro L (1994) Pronóstico de los pacientes con válvulas de uretra posterior según tratamiento inicial y su comportamiento urodinámico. *Cir Pediatr* **7**: 128–31.

Jaureguizar E, Lopez Pereira P, Martinez Urrutia MJ *et al.* (1999) Does neonatal pyelo-ureterostomy worsen bladder function in children with posterior urethral valves. *Pediatrics* **104**: 820 (40A).

Johnston JH (1960) Vesical diverticula without urinary obstruction in childhood. *J Urol* **84**: 535–8.

Johnston JH (1963) Temporary cutaneous urethrostomy in the management of advanced congenital urethral obstruction. *Arch Dis Child* **38**: 161–6.

Johnston JH (1966) Posterior urethral valves: an operative technique using an electric auriscope. *J Pediatr Surg* **1**: 583–4.

Johnston JH (1979) Vesicoureteral reflux with urethral valves. *Br J Urol* **51**: 100–4.

Johnston JH (1984) Reflux secondary to severe urethral obstruction. In: *Management of vesicoureteral reflux*. Baltimore, MD: Williams and Wilkins.

Johnston JH, Kulatilake AE (1972) Posterior urethral valves: results and sequelae. In: Johnston JH, Sholtmeijer (eds) *Problems in paediatric urology*. Amsterdam: Excerpta Medica, 161–79.

Kaefer M, Peters M, Retik AB (1997) Increased renal echogenecity: a sonographic sign in differentiating between obstructive and non-obstructive etiologies of *in-utero* bladder distention. *J Urol* **158**: 1026–9.

Kajbafizadeh AM, Quinn FM, Duffy DG, Ransley PG (1995) Augmentation cystoplasty in boys with posterior urethral valves. *J Urol* **154**: 874–7.

Keating MA (1994) The noncompliant bladder: principles in pathogenesis and pathophysiology. *Prob Urol* **8**: 348–60.

Khoury AE, Houle AM, McLorie GA, Churchill BM (1990) Cutaneous vesicostomy effect on bladder's eventual function. In: Hussman D, McConnell J (eds) *Subject of controversy: bladder dysfunction. Dialog Pediatr Urol* **13**: 4.

Kim KM, Kogan BA, Massad CA, Huang Y-C (1991) Collagen and elastin in the obstructed fetal bladder. *J Urol* **146**: 528–31.

Kim YH, Horowitz M, Combs AJ, Nitti VW, Libretti D, Glassberg KI (1996) Comparative urodynamic findings after valve ablation, vesicostomy or proximal diversion. *J Urol* **156**: 673–6.

Kim YH, Horowitz M, Combs AJ, Nitti VW, Borer J, Glassberg KI (1997a) Management of posterior urethral valves on the basis of urodynamic findings. *J Urol* **158**: 1011–16.

Kim YH, Horowitz M, Combs AJ, Nitti VW, Glassberg KI (1997b) The management of unilaterally poorly functioning kidneys in patients with posterior urethral valves. *J Urol* **158**: 1001–3.

King LR (1985) Posterior urethra. In: Kelalis PP, King LR, Belman AB (eds) *Urology* 2nd edition. Philadelphia, PA: WB Saunders, 527–58.

Kroovand RL, Weinberg N, Emani A (1977) Posterior urethral valves in identical twins. *Pediatrics* **60**: 748.

Krueger RP, Hardy BE, Churchill BM (1980a) Cryptorchidism in boys with posterior urethral valves. *J Urol* **124**: 101–2.

Krueger RP, Hardy BE, Churchill BM (1980b) Growth in boys with posterior urethral valves, primary valve resection versus upper tract diversion. *Urol Clin North Am* **7**: 265–72.

Lal R, Bhatnagar V, Mitra DK (1998) Urethral strictures after fulguration of posterior urethral valves. *J Pediatr Surg* **33**: 518–19.

Lal R, Bhatnagar V, Mitra DK (1998) Upper-tract changes insipidus associated with posterior urethral valves. *Pediatr Surg Int* **13**: 396–9.

Landers S, Hanson TN (1990) Pulmonary problems associated with congenital malformations. In: Gonzales ET, Roth DR (eds) *Common problems in pediatric urology*. St Louis, MO: Mosby Year Book, 85.

Langenback CJ (1802) Ueber eine ein fache und sichere methode des St e in schnittes. Stahel: Würzberg. (Cited in Dewan, 1999.)

Lebowitz RL (1996) Voiding cystourethrography in boys: the presence of the catheter does not obscure the diagnosis of posterior urethral valves but prevents estimation of the adequacy of transurethral fulguration (Letter to the Editor). *AJR Am J Roentgenol* **166**: 724.

Lome LG, Howat JM, Williams DI (1972) The temporarily defunctionalized bladder in children. *J Urol* **107**: 469–72.

Lyon RP (2000) Urine specific gravity – neglected and resurrected. Presented at the American Association of Genitourinary Surgeons, Annual Meeting, San Antonio, TX 5–8 April 2000.

Lyon RP, Marshall S, Baskin LS (1992) Normal growth with renal insufficiency owing to posterior urethral valves: valve of long-term diversion, a twenty-year follow-up. *Urol Int* **48**: 125–9.

McGuire EJ, Weiss RM (1975) Secondary bladder neck obstruction in patients with urethral valves: treatment with phenoxybenzamine. *Urology* **5**: 756–8.

Mahoney BS (1994) Ultrasound evaluation of the fetal genitourinary system. In: Callen PW (ed.) *Ultrasonography in obstetrics and gynecology*. 3rd edition. Philadelphia, PA: WB Saunders, 400–10.

Mahony DT (1974) Studies of enuresis I. Incidence of obstructive lesions and pathopathology of enuresis. *J Urol* **4**: 145.

Mahony DT, Laferte RO (1974) Congenital posterior urethral valves in adult males. *Urology* **3**: 724–34.

Maizels M, Stephens FD, King LR, Firlit CF (1983) Cowper's syringocele: a classification of dilatations of Cowper's gland duct based upon clinical characteristics of 8 boys. *J Urol* **129**: 111–14.

Merguerian PA, McLorie GA, Churchill BM *et al.* (1992) Radiographic and serologic correlates of azotemia in patients with posterior urethral valves. *J Urol* **148**: 1499–503.

Mininberg DT (1999) Genitourinary anomalies. In: Petrikovsky BM (eds) *Fetal disorders: diagnosis and management*. New York: Wiley-Liss, 123–9.

Mitchell ME (1980) Valve bladder syndrome. Read at the Annual Meeting of the North Central Section, American Urologic Association, Hamilton, Bermuda, 1980.

Mitchell MM, Close CE (1996) Early primary valve ablation for posterior urethral valves. *Semin Pediatr Surg* **5**: 66–71.

Mitchell ME, Garrett RA (1980) Perirenal urinary extravasation associated with urethral valves in infants. *J Urol* **124**: 68.

Morgani GB (1719) Adversaria anatomica omina. *Padua Journal Comius* Part 1, Article **10**: 5.

Morgani G, Benjamin A (1769) The seats and causes of diseases investigated by anatomy; in five books, containing a great variety of dissections, with remarks, to which are added very accurate and copious indexes of the principal things and names therein contained. In: Millar A, Cadell T (eds); trans. Alexander B. London, 540–56. (Cited in Arnold and Ginsberg, 1974.)

Myers DA, Walker RD II (1981) Prevention of urethral structures in the management of posterior urethral valves. *J Urol* **126**: 655–7.

Noe HN, Jerkins GR (1983) Oliguria and renal failure following decompression of the bladder in children with posterior urethral valves. *J Urol* **129**: 595–7.

Noe HN, Jerkins GR (1985) Cutaneous vesicostomy experience in infants and children. *J Urol* **134**: 301–2.

Páramo PG, Martinez-Piñeiro JA, dela Peña J, Páramo PS Jr (1983) Andrological implications of congenital posterior urethral valves in adults. *Eur Urol* **9**: 359–61.

Parkhouse HF, Barratt TM, Dillon MJ *et al.* (1988) Long-term outcome of boys with posterior urethral valves. *Br J Urol* **62**: 59–62.

Parkhouse HF, Woodhouse CRJ (1990) Long-term status of patients with posterior urethral valves. *Urol Clin North Am* **17**: 373–8.

Passerini-Glazel G, Araguna F, Chiozza L (1988) The PADUA (progressive augmentation by dilating the urethra anterior) procedure for the treatment of severe urethral hypoplasia. *J Urol* **140**: 1247–9.

Peters CA, Bolkier M, Bauer SB *et al.* (1990) The urodynamic consequences of posterior urethral valves. *J Urol* **144**: 122–6.

Peters CA, Vasavada DS, Dator D *et al.* (1992) The effect of obstruction on the developing bladder. *J Urol* **148**: 491–6.

Pieretti RV (1993) The mild end of the clinical spectrum of posterior urethral valves. *J Pediatr Surg* **28**: 701–6.

Puri P, Kumar R (1996) Endoscopic correction of vesicoureteral reflux secondary to posterior urethral valves. *J Urol* **156** (Suppl): 680–2.

Quintero RA, Hume R, Smith C *et al.* (1995) Percutaneous fetal cystoscopy and endoscopic fulguration of posterior urethral valves. *Am J Obstet Gynecol* **172**: 206–9.

Rajab A, Freeman NV, Patton M (1996) The frequency of posterior urethral valves in Oman. *Br J Urol* **77**: 900–4.

Rajagopala PR, Hanevold JD, Orak JB *et al.* (1994) Valve bladder does not affect the outcome of renal transplants in children with renal failure due to posterior urethral valves. *Transplant Proc* **26**: 115–16.

Reinberg Y, Gonzalez R, Fryd D *et al.* (1988) The outcome of renal transplantation in children with posterior urethral valves. *J Urol* **140**: 1491–3.

Reinberg T, de Castano I, Gonzalez R (1992) Influence of initial therapy on progression of renal failure and body growth in children with posterior urethral valves. *J Urol* **148**: 532–3.

Reinberg Y, deCastano I, Gonzales R (1992) Prognosis for patients with prenatally diagnosed posterior urethral valves. *J Urol* **148**: 125–6.

Rittenberg MH, Hulbert WC, Snyder HM III, Duckett JW Jr (1988) Protective factors in posterior urethral valves. *J Urol* **140**: 1993–6.

Salomon L, Fontaine E, Guest G *et al.* (2000) Role of the bladder in delayed failure of kidney transplants in boys with posterior urethral valves. *J Urol* **163**: 1282–5.

Sant GR, Kaleli A (1985) Cowpers syringocele causing incontinence in an adult. *J Urol* **133**: 279–80.

Sarkas, P, Robert M, Lopez C *et al.* (1995) Obstructive anuria following fulguration of posterior urethral valves and foley catheter drainage bladder. *Br J Urol* **76**: 664–5.

Schwarz RD, Stephens FD, Cussen LJ (1981) The pathogenesis of renal dysplasia. Part II: The significance of lateral and medial ectopy of the ureteric orifice. *Invest Urol* **19**: 97–100.

Scott JES (1985) Management of congenital posterior urethral valves. *Br J Urol* **57**: 71–7.

Scott TW (1976) Urinary ascites secondary to posterior urethral valves. *J Urol* **116**: 87–91.

Seskin FE, Glassberg KI (1994) Lacuna magna in 6 boys with post-void bleeding and dysuria: alternative approach to treatment. *J Urol* **152**: 980–2.

Shapiro SR, Woerner S, Adelman RD, Palmer JM (1978) Diabetes insipidus and hydronephrosis. *J Urol* **119**: 715–19.

Smith GHH, Canning DA, Schulman SL *et al.* (1996) The long-term outcome of posterior urethral valves treated with primary valve ablation and observation. *J Urol* **155**: 1730–4.

Sober I (1972) Pelviourethrostomy-en-Y. *J Urol* **107**: 473–5.

Sommer JT, Stephens FD (1980) Dorsal diverticulum of the fossa navicularis. *J Urol* **124**: 94–7.

Speakman MJ, Brading AF, Gilpin CJ *et al.* (1987) Bladder outflow obstruction: a cause of denervation supersensitivity. *J Urol* **138**: 1461–6.

Stephens FD (1976) In: Kelalis PB, King LR (eds) *Clinical pediatric urology*. Philadelphia, PA: WB Saunders.

Stephens FD (1983a) Congenital intrinsic lesions of the posterior urethra. In: Stephens FD (ed.) *Congenital malformations of the urinary tract*. New York: Praeger, 95–125.

Stephens FD (1983b) Congenital malformations of the urinary tract. In: Stephens FD (ed.) *Congenital malformations of the urinary tract*. New York: Praeger Scientific, 142.

Stephens FD, Donnellan WL (1977) H-type urethroanal fistula. *J Pediatr Surg* **12**: 95–102.

Tanagho EA (1974) Consequently Congenitally obstructed bladders: fate after prolonged defunctionalization. *J Urol* **111**: 102–9.

Tanagho EA (1982) Comments. In: Glassberg KI (ed.) *Persistent upper tract dilatation following valve ablation. Dialog Pediatr Urol* **5**: 4, 5.

Thomalla JV, Mitchell ME, Leapman SB, Filo RS (1989) Renal transplantation into the reconstructed bladder. *J Urol* **14**: 265–8.

Tietjen DN, Gloor JM, Hussman DA (1997) Proximal urinary diversion in the management of posterior urethral valves: is it necessary? *J Urol* **158**: 1008–10.

Tolmathshew N (1870) Ein Fall con semilunaren Klappen der Hurröhre und von vergrösserte vesicular prostatica. *Virch Arch (Pathol Anat)* **49**: 348.

uretra posterior según tratamiento inicial y su comportamiento urodinámico. *Cir Pediatr* **7**: 128–31.

Van Savage JG, Khoury AE, McLorie GA, Bagli DJ (1997) An algorithm for the management of anterior urethral valves. *J Urol* **158**: 1030–2.

Waldbaum RS, Marshall VF (1970) Posterior urethral valves: evaluation and management. *J Urol* **103**: 801–9.

Walker RD, Padron M (1990) The management of posterior urethral valves by initial vesicostomy and delayed valve ablation. *J Urol* **144**: 1212–14.

Warshaw BL, Hymes LC, Trulock TS, Woodard JR (1985) Prognostic features in infants with obstructive uropathy due to posterior urethral valves. *J Urol* **133**: 240–3.

Waterhouse RK (1961) Voiding cystourethrography: a simple technique. *J Urol* **85**: 103–4.

Waterhouse RK (1964) The dilated posterior urethra I. Male. *J Urol* **91**: 71–5.

Weiss RM (1982) Comments. In: Glassberg KI (ed.) *Persistent ureteral dilatation following valve ablation. Dialog Pediatr Urol* **5**: 4, 5.

Whitaker RA, Keeton JE, Williams DI (1972) Posterior urethral valves: a study of urinary control after operation. *J Urol* **108**: 167–71.

Whitaker RH (1973) The ureter in posterior urethral valves. *Br J Urol* **45**: 395–403.

Whitaker RH, Sherwood T (1986) An improved hook for destroying posterior urethral valves. *J Urol* **135**: 531–2.

Williams DI (1954) Congenital valves in the posterior urethra. *Br J Urol* **26**: 623–7.

Williams DI, Bloomberg S (1975) Bifid urethra with pre-anal accessory track (Y duplication). *Br J Urol* **47**: 882.

Williams DI, Cromie WJ (1976) Ring ureterostomy. *Br J Urol* **47**: 789–92.

Williams DI, Eckstein HB (1965) Obstructive valves in the posterior urethra. *J Urol* **93**: 236.

Williams DI, Retik AB (1969) Congenital valves and diverticula of the anterior urethra. *Br J Urol* **41**: 228–34.

Williams DI, Whitaker RA, Barratt TM, Keeton JE (1973) Urethral valves. *Br J Urol* **45**: 200–10.

Williams N, Kapila L (1973) Posterior urethral valves in twins with mirror image abnormalities. *Br J Urol* **71**: 615–16.

Woodhouse CR, Williams DI (1979) Duplication of the lower urinary tract in children. *Br J Urol* **51**: 481–7.

Woodhouse CRJ, Reilly JM, Bahadur G (1989) Sexual function and fertility in patients treated for posterior urethral valves. *J Urol* **142**: 586–8.

Young HH, Frontz WA, Baldwin JC (1919) Congenital obstruction of the posterior urethra. *J Urol* **3**: 289–354.

Zaontz MR, Firlit CF (1985) Percutaneous antegrade ablation of posterior urethral valves in premature underweight term neonates: an alternative to primary vesicostomy. *J Urol* **134**: 139–41.

Zaontz MR, Gibbons MD (1984) An antegrade technique for ablation of posterior urethral valves. *J Urol* **132**: 982–4.

Prune belly syndrome

29

Steven J. Skoog

Introduction

Prune belly syndrome is classically defined by three abnormalities: deficiency of the abdominal wall musculature, bilateral cryptorchidism, and a dilated dysmorphic urinary tract. The scope of involvement of the genitourinary system, combined with the visible appearance of the abdominal wall in the male child with the prune belly syndrome, sets the stage for the intense interest and controversy which surrounds this developmental anomaly (Fig. 29.1). The name of the syndrome itself has been a point of contention because of its harsh portrayal of the patient (Stephens, 1983).

A rich history surrounds the recognition of the essential components of the prune belly syndrome (Table 29.1). The abdominal wall 'tumidity' was noted by Frolich (1839). Parker (1895) reported the autopsy findings of a male infant with absent abdominal muscles. He recognized the essential elements of the syndrome to include: (1) the large flaccid abdominal wall with absent musculature; (2) the undescended testes; and (3) the hypertrophied and dilated renal collecting system and bladder without urethral obstruction. Osler (1901) is credited with giving the syndrome its name 'prune belly'. He described the distended and deficient abdominal wall in a 6-year-old male, who presented with difficulty in passing urine. Upon review of this reference, however, the term 'prune belly' is not specifically mentioned. Nonetheless, prune belly syndrome is, at present, the most widely accepted appellation (Duckett, 1986). Other popular synonyms, such as urethral obstruction malformation complex, the triad syndrome, abdominal muscle deficiency syndrome, and mesenchymal dysplasia syndrome, reflect the etiologic biases of the respective authors (Nunn and Stephens, 1961; Ives, 1974; Welsh and Kearney, 1974; Pagon et al., 1979).

The criterion of cryptorchidism effectively eliminates the syndrome in female patients, but the descriptive term 'prune belly' is applicable and has been recognized in females, who constitute about 3–5% of recorded cases (Rabinowitz and Schillinger, 1977) (Fig. 29.1c). In females with a prune belly there is a strong association with omphalocele and bladder outlet obstructive lesions (Guvenc et al., 1995). In a review by Reinberg et al. (1991), 40% of female patients had anorectal anomalies and the perinatal mortality was 40%. The principles of management are essentially the same as in the male patient.

The incidence of prune belly syndrome is 1 in 29 000 to 1 in 40 000 livebirths (Garlinger and Ott, 1974; Greskovich and Nyberg, 1988). An increased incidence of this syndrome has been reported in Nigeria (Adeyokunnu and Familuse, 1982) as well as in Saskatchewan, Canada (Ives, 1974). In a population-based study from New York State the livebirth prevalence was 3.2 per 100 000. Twins, blacks, and children born to younger mothers appear to be at higher risk (Druschel, 1995). Maternal cocaine abuse during pregnancy has also been associated with prune belly syndrome (Greenfield et al., 1991). The terminology of 'pseudoprune' has been suggested to define females and males who do not have the complete triad of prune belly syndrome (Duckett, 1986). It is possible in males to have urinary tract dilatation, without obstruction, not associated with the abdominal wall deficiency or undescended testes. Isolated dilatation of the posterior urethra, without obstruction, the urologic hallmark of the pseudoprune, has been suggested as a limited form of the syndrome, a manifestation of mesenchymal dysplasia (King, 1969). However, the underlying uropathy and clinical course in patients with pseudoprune belly syndrome are unpredictable and in one series 63% went on to renal failure (Bellah et al., 1996).

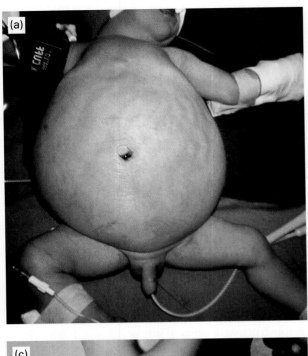

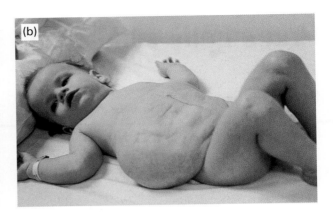

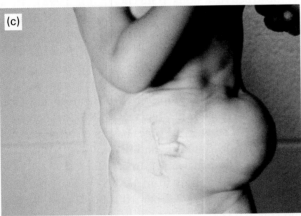

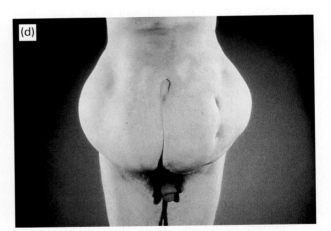

Figure 29.1 (*a*) Newborn with prune belly syndrome, urinary ascites, and pulmonary hypoplasia. Outline of the bowel is visible through the abdominal wall. (*b*) Six-month-old child with prune belly syndrome before comprehensive reconstruction. (*c*) Four-year-old female with hemiprune belly. (*d*) Adult with prune belly syndrome exhibiting pot belly configuration.

The prognosis for infants and children with the prune belly syndrome has dramatically improved from a mortality rate in the preantibiotic era of 70%, to 20% today. The latter infants are usually stillborn or die in the neonatal period, secondary to renal failure and pulmonary hypoplasia (Eagle and Barrett, 1950; Fallat *et al.*, 1989).

One of the major areas of controversy is the role of surgical reconstruction in the management of prune belly syndrome. Early series stressed the importance of relief of obstruction and stasis by high ureteros-

tomies or catheter drainage. The latter often met with disastrous infectious complications and an additional 30% mortality reported in the first 2 years of life (Eagle and Barrett, 1950; Waldbaum and Marshall, 1970). Later reports of successful, early urinary reconstruction professed improved urinary drainage and improved radiographic configuration of the urinary tract. Long-term follow-up demonstrated stabilization of renal function (Welsh and Kearney, 1974; Jeffs *et al.*, 1977; Rabinowitz and Barkin, 1978; Woodard and Parrott, 1978a; Randolph *et al.*,

Table 29.1 History of prune belly syndrome

Year	Author	Discovery
1839	Frolich	Described abdominal wall abnormality
1895	Parker	Recognized all three components to the syndrome
1901	Osler	Coined the name prune belly syndrome
1903	Strumme	Proposed obstructive theory of prune belly syndrome
1961	Nunn and Stephens	Proposed theory of mesenchymal dysplasia as etiology of syndrome

1981a). However, with improved antibiotics available for prophylaxis and better means to test the urodynamic and functional aspects of the upper and lower urinary tracts, the need for extensive tailoring of the urinary tract has been questioned. Prevention of urinary infection and preservation of renal function may be equally obtainable with 'watchful waiting' (Williams and Burkholder, 1967; Burke et al., 1969; Duckett, 1976; Tank and McCoy, 1983). Woodhouse et al. (1979) reported a normal serum creatinine in 27 patients with prune belly syndrome who had limited surgical intervention over a 29 year period. Patients living as long as 70 years have been reported (Eagle and Barrett, 1950). More recent experience advocates the importance of watchful waiting in regards to the urinary tract but, mindful of psychological and fertility considerations, current practice stresses a more active, early surgical role in correction of the abdominal wall defect and the cryptorchid testes (Burbidge et al., 1987; Fallat et al., 1989; Woodard, 1998; Woodard and Smith, 1998).

Antenatal diagnosis of the prune belly syndrome by ultrasound is not reliable. Unfortunately, other causes of prenatal hydronephrosis, such as posterior urethral valves (PUV) and primary vesicoureteral reflux (VUR), cannot be differentiated as a result of their common sonographic features (Glazer et al., 1982). This, coupled with the facts that fetal renal function is difficult to assess and fetal intervention has not been documented to benefit subsequent development of the kidneys, has resulted in recommendations against fetal intervention in prune belly syndrome (Kramer, 1983; Snow and Duckett, 1987; Woodard and Smith, 1998).

The etiology and pathophysiology of prune belly syndrome remain in question. The report of an animal model based on early urethral ligation resulting in all the features of the syndrome has not yet provided much-needed answers (Gonzales et al., 1990). The proposed theories of pathogenesis and supporting arguments will be discussed later in this chapter.

A further improvement in the treatment of prune belly syndrome has been the application of dialysis and renal transplantation. The assessment of lower urinary tract function and elimination of urinary stasis is critical prior to transplant (Shenasky and Whelchel, 1976). Transplantation offers hope to those patients with initial poor renal function due to renal dysplasia and to those patients who gradually develop renal failure, despite appropriate urologic intervention.

Theories of etiology and embryogenesis

Inheritance

A variety of genetic inheritance patterns has been suggested as etiologic in prune belly syndrome to explain its familiar occurrence. One must remember, however, that most cases are sporadic and have a normal karyotype (Garlinger and Ott 1974; Woodard and Trulock, 1996). Prune belly syndrome has been reported in male siblings, cousins, and twins (Sladezyk, 1967; Petersen et al., 1972; Riccardi and Grum, 1977; Adeyokunnu and Familuse, 1982). The majority of twins described in the literature, however, are discordant for prune belly syndrome, which speaks strongly against a genetic etiology. Ives (1974), in her analysis of twinning and its relationship to prune belly syndrome, noted 11 pairs of twins discordant for the syndrome. Six were monozygous and five were of unknown zygosity. Of the 250 cases of prune belly syndrome reviewed, 11 cases or 4% occurred in twins, compared with the 1.25% incidence of twinning in the general population. Unequal division of mesodermal cells, occurring at the primitive streak formation, may explain the discordant monozygotic twinning phenomenon.

Williams was one of the first to suggest that prune belly syndrome was due to a sex-linked recessive trait. This would explain the male predominance of the syndrome, and its occurrence in male siblings, in concordant twins, and in association with Turner syndrome (Williams and Burkholder, 1967; Lubinsky et al., 1980). The vast majority of twins, however, are discordant for the syndrome and its presence in three females with documented 46 XX karyotypes speaks strongly against a sex-linked pattern of inheritance (Rabinowitz and Shillinger, 1977).

Autosomal dominant and autosomal recessive inheritance have also been reported (Adeyokunnu and Familuse, 1982). Male predominance, lack of consanguinity, and lack of extensive pedigrees in new cases due to associated infertility, make any association with single gene inheritance uncertain at this time (Garlinger and Ott, 1974). Riccardi and Grum (1977) have proposed an interesting hypothesis of the genetic inheritance of prune belly syndrome. They suggest a two-step autosomal dominant mutation with sex-limited expression that partially mimics X-linkage. This pattern would explain male predominance, as well as the small number of affected family members.

Specific chromosomal abnormalities are rare. Trisomy 18 has been demonstrated in prune belly syndrome in seven documented cases (Hoagland et al., 1988). Trisomy 18 is also associated with other genitourinary abnormalities, including renal dysplasia and hypoplasia, horseshoe kidney, duplication anomalies, and persistent nodular renal blastema (Moerman et al., 1982). A cause-and-effect relationship is only speculative. Trisomy 21 and prune belly syndrome have been reported in three patients (Curry et al., 1984; Amacker et al., 1986). A careful analysis of incidence rates and birth rates suggests, however, that these are independent events, occurring together by chance alone (Baird and Sadovnick, 1987).

An association with Turner syndrome has been reported on four occasions. This suggests that the gene responsible for the syndrome may be located on the X chromosome and is recessively transmitted. However, it is more likely to represent the occurrence of the prune belly phenotype in the female as a result of other causes of abdominal distension such as impaired lymphatic development with chylous ascites (Pagon et al., 1979; Lubinsky et al., 1980; Adeyokunnu and Familuse, 1982). Although mosaicism for a monosome of chromosome number 16 in two male siblings with prune belly syndrome has been documented, its importance etiologically cannot be determined (Harley et al., 1972). An extracentric chromosomal fragment was reported in association with prune belly syndrome. The same aberration, however, was present in two phenotypically normal male family members (Halbrecht et al., 1972).

Fetal development

Three major theories have been proposed to explain the clinical features of the prune belly syndrome. As with most theories, none completely explains the entire constellation of findings in the syndrome, and all are marred by conjecture and speculation.

Fetal outlet obstruction

Strumme (1903) proposed that the syndrome was the final expression of any obstructive lesion producing significant back pressure at a critical time during development. The dilatation of the urinary tract and secondary pressure atrophy of the abdominal wall produced the clinical features common to prune belly syndrome (Fig. 29.2). Subsequent clinical reviews reflected this belief and called attention to the need to alleviate the obstructing lesions commonly found in the posterior urethra (Eagle and Barrett, 1950; Lattimer, 1958; Rogers and Ostrow, 1973; Berdon et al., 1977). However, improved methods of radiographic diagnosis of obstruction with the voiding cystourethrogram (VCUG), post-mortem anatomic enbloc dissections, and the application of urodynamics cast doubt on the anatomic presence of obstructions (Nunn and Stephens, 1961; Williams and Burkholder, 1967; Burke et al., 1969; Straub and Spranger, 1981). Sebsequent clinical reports found obstructing lesions in 10–20% of patients, in contrast to up to 80% thought to be present as reported in earlier series (Lattimer, 1958; Tank and McCoy, 1983). It has been proposed that those infants with the most severe manifestations of the syndrome have the 'lethal variant' (an anatomic obstructing lesion) leading to pulmonary hypoplasia, renal dysplasia, and death (Rogers and Ostrow, 1973). This distinction is particularly important when studying the theories of pathogenesis, inasmuch as most articles that indicate obstruction as the primary cause are based on autopsy information (Berdon et al., 1977; Wigger and Blanc, 1977; Hoagland and Hutchins, 1987).

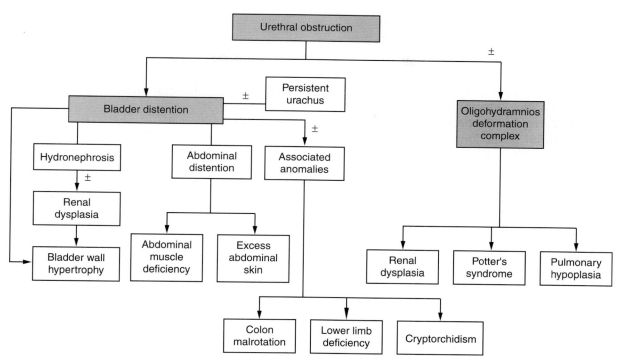

Figure 29.2 Urethral obstruction, whether anatomic or functional, is the proposed etiology of prune belly syndrome and its associated anomalies.

The source of the obstruction may be true areas of stenosis, atresia, valves, or pinpoint diaphragms at the junction of the posterior and membranous urethra. Recent theories have suggested a 'functional obstruction' present *in utero*, secondary to prostatic hypoplasia, as the specific etiology of the syndrome. This 'obstruction' is thought to be the result of conformational changes in the prostatic urethra during voiding, creating a valve-like mechanism (Moerman *et al.*, 1984; Hoagland and Hutchins, 1987). The most recent lesion suggested as the etiology of prune belly syndrome is a transient obstruction at the junction of the glanular and penile urethra. This was based on evidence of anterior, urethral dilatation in patients with prune belly syndrome, as measured on radiographs from a VCUG, and comparison made with children with urinary tract infections (UTIs) and children with PUV (Beasley *et al.*, 1988). This theory is supported by the high incidence of megalourethra seen with prune belly syndrome (Sellers *et al.*, 1976; Kroovand *et al.*, 1982).

The obstructive theory contends that the abdominal wall findings are secondary to the pressure effects of the distended bladder on the developing myotomes of the abdominal wall. This is supported by the extent of muscular involvement being greatest in the transversus abdominis, obliques, and lower rectus muscles, i.e. those directly over the bladder. Histologic studies and electron microscopy of the abdominal wall, however, have failed to demonstrate a pattern of atrophy, but rather one of developmental arrest (O'Kell, 1969; Mininberg *et al.*, 1974; Stephens, 1983). In addition, the absence histologically of any aponeurotic layer of the affected muscles opposes an atrophic cause (Stephens, 1983).

More recent evidence from prenatal sonography in patients with prune belly syndrome and other disease processes that cause the prune belly phenotype suggests that the abdominal wall laxity may be a secondary effect of abdominal distension. Transient ascitic distension may produce the finding in those patients with the syndrome who have no urethral obstruction (Monie and Monie, 1979; Pagon *et al.*, 1979; Smythe, 1981; Nakayama *et al.*, 1984; Cazorla *et al.*, 1997). Urinary ascites has been demonstrated *in utero* in patients with prune belly syndrome. The urine is theorized to leak into the abdomen via the distended urinary tract and spontaneously reabsorbs at the end of gestation, which explains its clinical absence at birth (Symonds and Driscoll, 1974; Monie and Monie, 1979; Smythe, 1981; Golbus *et al.*, 1982; Fitzsimmons *et al.*, 1985). Other causes of *in utero* abdominal wall distension and the prune belly phenotype include non-immune ascites, intestinal duplication, PUV, amniotic band syndrome, visceromegaly, polycystic kidneys, impaired lymphatic drainage in Turner syndrome, and cystic adenomatoid malformation of the lung (Pagon *et al.*, 1979; Nakayama *et al.*, 1984; Kuruvilla *et al.*, 1987; Chen *et al.*, 1997).

The 'urethral obstruction malformation complex' is the terminology now applied to the theory of fetal outlet obstruction as the etiology of prune belly syndrome (Fig. 29.2). The timing and severity of the obstructive phenomena are critical. Distension of the urinary tract at 13–15 weeks of gestation could produce the degenerative changes in the abdominal wall and urinary tract, preventing gut rotation and prostatic development (Wheatley *et al.*, 1996). This broader application of Strumme's original hypothesis, however, fails to explain (1) the lack of hypertrophy and hyperplasia normally present in the obstructed urinary tract, (2) the diffuse replacement of smooth and skeletal muscle by fibrous and collagenous tissue, (3) normal or low intravesical pressures assessed urodynamically, (4) absent obstruction but presence of renal dysgenesis in the majority of patients, (5) other causes of *in utero* outlet obstruction not associated with abdominal wall laxity, and (6) the excessively high incidence of cryptorchid testes. All these factors are common in prune belly syndrome and cannot be completely explained on the basis of obstruction alone

(Nunn and Stephens, 1961; Osathanondh and Potter, 1964; Williams and Burkholder, 1967; Palmer and Tesluck, 1974; Straub and Spranger, 1981).

Theory of mesodermal arrest

The theory of mesodermal arrest is based on an embryologic aberration of mesenchymal development as the etiology of prune belly syndrome (Fig. 29.3) (Nunn and Stephens, 1961). Urinary tract obstruction occurs in some patients as a consequence of the primary defect and may increase the pathological severity (Wheatley *et al.*, 1996). Stephens and Gupta (1994) proposed that all three systems, the genitourinary tract, the testes, and the abdominal wall, would be vulnerable to a mesodermal defect occurring between 6 and 10 weeks of gestation. A noxious insult occurring when the lateral plate mesoderm has already extended to the midline, with failure of myoblast differentiation and migration ventrally and caudally, would explain the abdominal wall findings (Wigger and Blanc, 1977). At the same time, the urinary tract is developing from the visceral layer of the lateral plate mesoderm. The same insult would impair differentiation of the mesoderm, which forms the smooth muscle of the urinary tract, resulting in the characteristic dilatation and dysmorphic features common to the syndrome. The kidneys are concurrently differentiating from the para-axial mesoderm. A defect in induction by the ureteral bud or an abnormality in the metanephric blastema, with or without subsequent urinary tract obstruction, would account

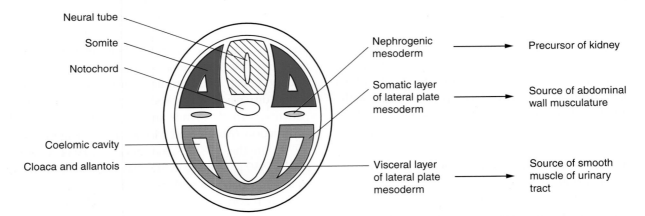

Figure 29.3 Cross-section of fetus at 6–10 weeks of gestation. An embryologic insult to both layers of the lateral plate mesoderm and the nephrogenic mesoderm could explain the majority of findings seen in the prune belly syndrome.

for the renal dysplasia commonly associated with prune belly syndrome (Wigger and Blanc, 1977; Greskovich and Nyberg, 1988; Stephens and Gupta, 1994).

Some authors have suggested that this insult must occur early in the 3rd week of embryogenesis, at the primitive streak stage of development. At the division of the embryonic disk an unequal distribution of mesoderm could explain the discordant occurrence in monozygotic twins (Ives, 1974). This localized defect in mesodermal development would also explain the abnormalities seen in the prostate and urethra, and in testicular descent. According to this theory, the prostatic hypoplasia with poor glandular development, and abnormalities in the mesenchyme of the testicular gubernaculum, result in unresponsiveness of these tissues to hormonal stimulation (Wigger and Blanc, 1977; Deklerk and Scott, 1978; Elder et al., 1982; Fallon et al., 1982). This unresponsiveness of the gubernaculum to hormonal stimulation, the diminished intra-abdominal pressure, and potential mechanical obstruction by an enlarged bladder all contribute to the maldescent of the testes in the prune belly syndrome.

The mesodermal arrest theory is further supported by the histologic findings in the abdominal wall, the urinary tract, and the male genital tract. The abundance of fibrous tissue, collagen, and connective tissue, with sparsely placed smooth muscle throughout the urinary tract, point more to an inherent problem with mesodermal differentiation than to one of obstruction. Bladder outlet obstruction, as seen in PUV, results in hypertrophy and hyperplasia in the urinary tract, with normally developed seminal ducts and seminal vesicles and prostate glands proximal to the obstruction. These features are noticeably absent in the prune belly syndrome (Nunn and Stephens, 1961; Cussen, 1971; Mininberg et al., 1974; Deklerk and Scott, 1978; Straub and Spranger, 1981; Stephens and Gupta, 1994). Other arguments that support the mesodermal arrest theory include the absence of anatomic obstruction in the majority of patients and the demonstration of urodynamically unobstructed urinary tracts. This theory also provides an adequate explanation for the high association with megalourethra (Nunn and Stephens, 1961; Snyder et al., 1976; Kroovand et al., 1982).

Nevertheless, the mesodermal arrest theory does not explain the male predominance of the syndrome. It also fails to explain the myriad of associated anomalies and the presence of the abdominal wall abnormalities with a normal urinary tract. In addition, obstructive urethral lesions, whether anatomic or functional, are associated with the syndrome. The development of an animal model, with all the features of the syndrome after fetal urethral ligation, has been reported (Moerman et al., 1984; Hoagland and Hutchins, 1987; Gonzales et al., 1990).

The yolk sac theory

Stephens has recently proposed a new theory to explain the features of the prune belly syndrome. It is based on an error in embryogenesis of the yolk sac and allantois. Inherent in this theory is the contention that the bladder and prostatic urethra are derived, to a greater degree than customarily accepted, from the allantois. If an abnormally large amount of the yolk sac is retained inside the embryo, owing to overgrowth of the lateral folds of the discoid embryo, it could affect the development of the abdominal wall, resulting in the prune belly phenotype. A critical aspect of this theory is the overdevelopment of the allantoic diverticulum. This structure grows out from the yolk sac contiguous with the body stalk. If it becomes excessively large owing to the oversized intra-abdominal yolk sac, it would become incorporated into the urinary tract as the redundant enlarged urachus, bladder, and prostatic urethra that characterize the prune belly syndrome (Stephens, 1983; Stephens and Gupta, 1994). Unfortunately, this theory does not explain the errors in development of the upper urinary tract or male genital tract.

Spectrum of disease

As is true with many diseases and syndromes in medicine, prune belly syndrome represents a spectrum of severity of disease (Table 29.2). Three major categories can be broadly defined.

A review of most series demonstrates that approximately 20% of newborns will die in the perinatal period as a consequence of pulmonary hypoplasia and pulmonary complications (Woodard and Parrott, 1978a; Burbidge et al., 1987; Fallat et al., 1989). Their births are often associated with oligohydramnios, and when these infants are stillborn, the classic features of Potter's syndrome are observed (Potter, 1972; Perlman and Levin, 1974). In this subset (category I), severe renal dysplasia is present,

Table 29.2 Spectrum of prune belly syndrome

Category classification	Distinguishing characteristics
I	Oligohydramnios, pulmonary hypoplasia, or pneumothorax. May have urethral obstruction or patent urachus and clubfoot
II	Typical external features and uropathy of the full-blown syndrome but no immediate problem with survival. May have mild or unilateral renal dysplasia. May or may not develop urosepsis or gradual azotemia
III	External features may be mild or incomplete. Uropathy is less severe and renal function stable

and high urinary diversion, which is often performed, is generally to no avail (Welsh and Kearney, 1974). Initial normal serum creatinine progressively rises in spite of urinary diversion. These patients may also have urethral obstruction or atresia, the 'lethal variant' of the syndrome, unless associated with a patent urachus (Rogers and Ostrow, 1973).

The next group (category II) includes those infants who do not have severe pulmonary hypoplasia but have severe involvement of the urinary tract. This involvement may manifest itself as moderate to severe renal failure with azotemia and failure to thrive. The clinical course is one of either stabilization of renal function or progressive azotemia. Surgical intervention to tailor the urinary tract, in order to provide unimpeded drainage and decrease stasis, has been successfully performed, although its impact on long-term renal function continues to be debated (Waldbaum and Marshall, 1970; Randolph, 1977; Woodard and Parrott, 1978a).

The last category of patients with prune belly syndrome (category III) comprises those with the external abdominal features and undescended testes but in whom neither pulmonary nor renal function is severely impaired. They constitute the majority of patients with prune belly syndrome (Woodhouse *et al.*, 1982; Woodard, 1998). Although these infants may have severe dilatation of the urinary tract, they have stable renal function. General agreement exists that patients in this category require little if any urologic reconstructive surgery (Woodard and Smith, 1998).

Classifications of the syndrome based on the clinical spectrum of the disease have been formulated by numerous authors; all take into consideration initial and subsequent renal function (Welsh and Kearney, 1974; Berdon *et al.*, 1977; Woodhouse *et al.*, 1982; Woodard and Smith, 1998). The classifications have similar, clinically distinctive parameters to segregate the patients prognostically. The clinical classification of prune belly syndrome provides a framework for a more rational approach to overall management, which is determined on an individual basis (Greskovich and Nyberg, 1988). Woodard's classification is shown in Table 29.2.

Clinical features

Abdominal wall

The wrinkled, floppy abdominal wall (see Fig. 29.1) that characterizes the syndrome results from a deficiency of the underlying musculature. Autopsy studies have shown that the muscles most severely affected are those ventral and lateral in location. The epaxial and hypaxial trunk muscles develop normally. The order of severity of involvement from most to least involved is: transversus abdominis, rectus abdominis below the umbilicus, internal oblique, external oblique, and rectus abdominis above the umbilicis (Parker, 1895; Eagle and Barrett, 1950). There is cephalic displacement of the umbilicus due to unopposed contraction of the upper rectus abdominis muscle. The diminished muscle mass, if severe, allows one to observe spontaneous contraction of the underlying bowel and easily palpate the abdominal organs and kidneys (Fig. 29.1a). Because the muscular deficiency may not be symmetric, a more dominant flank bulge on one side of the abdomen is often present and coincides with the dilated distal ureter (Fig. 29.1b).

Electromyographic studies of the abdominal wall have confirmed the anatomic findings. The lower, midline musculature demonstrates the least amount of electrical activity. Recruitment of voluntary motor units is greatest in the upper lateral musculature (Randolph *et al.*, 1981b).

Autopsy studies of the abdominal wall have demonstrated normal segmental nerve distribution and normal blood supply (Wigger and Blanc, 1977; Stephens, 1983). The distribution of muscle fibers is haphazard and, in the most severe cases, the entire thickness of the abdominal wall consists only of skin, connective tissue, superficial fascia, and the peritoneum (Fig. 29.4). In the infant there is no aponeurotic layer that might represent atrophied muscle (Williams and Burkholder, 1967) Fortunately, the poorly developed abdominal wall heals well despite the limited layers for suturing.

Microscopic examination demonstrates fatty infiltration interdigitated with muscle fibers. These fibers have been characterized as hypoplastic, atrophic, and hypertrophic, adding further confusion to an apparent etiology (Afifi *et al.*, 1972; Mininberg *et al.*, 1974). Others have found the muscle cells to be clear and normal in appearance and at times associated with myotubular embryonic cells similar to those seen in the fetus of about 10 weeks' gestation (O'Kell, 1969; Stephens, 1983). Ultrastructural abnormalities, demonstrated by electron microscopy, include loss of coherence and orientation of the Z-bands,

mitochondrial disruption, and clumping of glycogen granules. These changes are non-specific, but are consistent with the hypoplastic histologic changes (Mininberg *et al.*, 1974).

The functionally impaired abdominal wall can result in significant morbidity. These infants are unable to sit up directly from the supine position and this delays the onset of walking (Duckett, 1986). The lack of mechanical assistance from the abdominal wall contributes to the noted difficulties with respiratory infections and chronic constipation (Geary *et al.*, 1986).

Kidneys

Renal dysmorphism is the common denominator of the upper urinary tract in prune belly syndrome. Both grossly and radiologically, cystic dilatation of the calyces and renal pelvis is present (Fig. 29.5). Infundibular narrowing, without obstruction, is common and occasional ureteropelvic junction (UPJ)

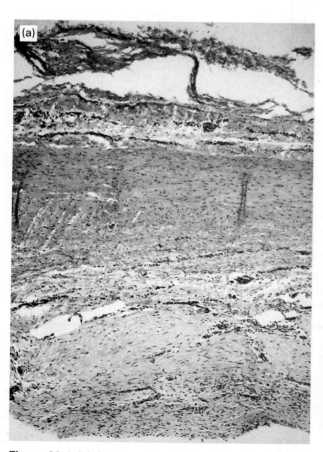
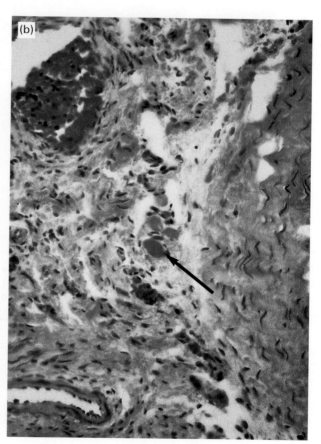

Figure 29.4 (*a*) Cross-section of the abdominal wall of a infant with prune belly syndrome. Note the scant and haphazard arrangement of muscle fibers. (*b*) High-power view of abdominal wall composed largely of collagen and fibrous tissue. The arrow points to scant skeletal muscle fibers.

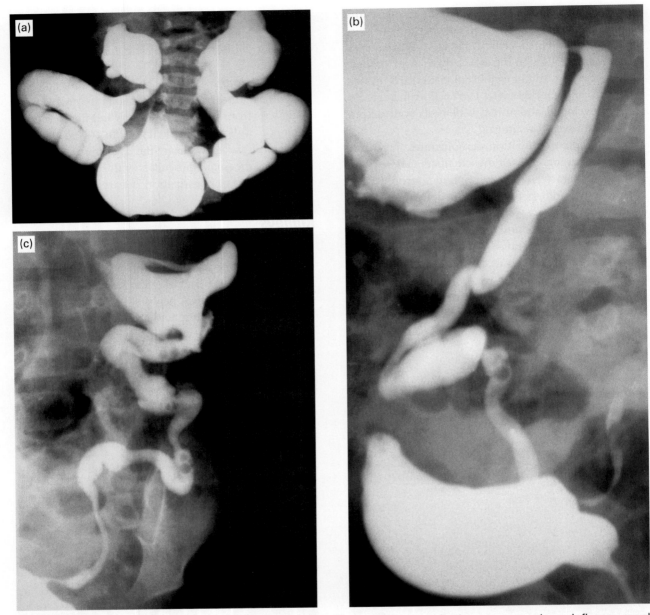

Figure 29.5 (*a*) Retrograde cystogram demonstrates the dilated, tortuous, refluxing ureters; enlarged, floppy, renal pelvis, and distended bladder with urachal remnant. (*b*) Retrograde cystogram demonstrates vesicoureteral reflux into a dysmorphic ureter and renal pelvis with pseudoureteropelvic junction obstruction. (*c*) Same patient as in (*b*) but left ureter and pelvis visualized.

obstruction may be present (Woodard and Parrott, 1978a). There may be wide individual variations in each renal unit in terms of appearance and function as well as location and rotation (Wigger and Blanc, 1977).

Prognosis is directly related to renal function and the degree of renal dysplasia. Stephens (1983) proposed pathogenic mechanisms to explain the develop-

ment of dysplasia. These include (1) defects of the ureteric bud or its branches, (2) qualitative or quantitative deficiencies of the nephrogenic mesenchyme, and (3) vascular ischemic insults with resultant ureteric obstruction and renal cystic dysplasia. He suggested that the dysplasia of the prune belly syndrome is due to a combination of a ureteric bud and metanephric defect.

The most severe degree of dysplasia is recognized from autopsy studies and associated with both Potter's type II and IV renal cystic changes (Osathanondh and Potter, 1964; Wigger and Blanc, 1977). These patients have associated distal outlet obstruction (urethral atresia) with a non-patent urachus, and they are usually stillborn. The kidneys are small, with disorganizational features of dysplasia and probably become impaired before significant nephron formation at the stage of ampullary development (Berdon *et al.*, 1977).

In contrast, some patients have hydronephrosis but adequate renal function. The degree of hydronephrosis may not correlate with ureteral dilatation or the abdominal wall deficiency. The thinned out renal parenchyma, often seen with congenital UPJ obstruction, is absent and the parenchyma is often well preserved (Fig. 29.6). The dilatation is attributed to the mesenchymal defect and deficient smooth muscle, not to obstruction. Consequently, some resolution in the degree of dilatation can occur spontaneously in follow-up (Fig. 29.7). Urinary infection rather than obstruction represents the greatest threat to the kidneys.

Ureters

The ureters are elongated, tortuous, and dilated. The abnormal ureters are the radiographic hallmark of the syndrome (Snow and Duckett, 1987). The lower one-third of the ureter is more profoundly affected than the proximal portion, an important consideration at the time of reconstructive surgery. The lower ureteral segments occupy the flared out flanks of the abdomen. Although fluoroscopic studies demonstrate ineffective peristalsis over its entire length, true obstructive lesions of the ureter are exceptional. However, pleat-like valves at the ureterovesical junction (UVJ) have been documented in two cases. These were created by a common wall valve at the junction of a dilated and non-dilated ureteral segment (Maizels and Stephens, 1980).

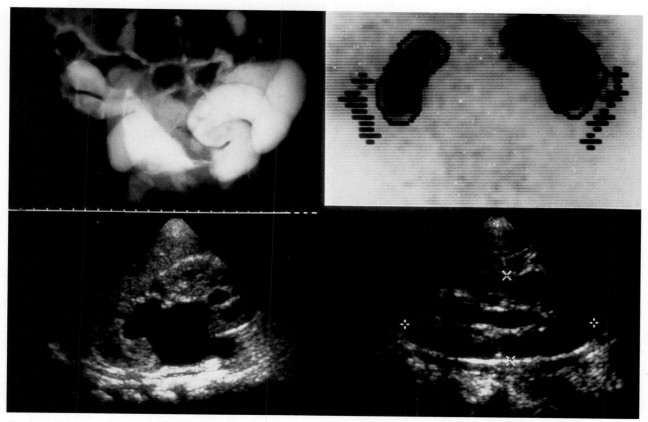

Figure 29.6 Intravenous pyelogram, DMSA renal scan, and renal sonogram of a 1-year-old child with prune belly syndrome. Despite gross dilatation and dysmorphic features of the renal pelvis and ureters, the renal scan and sonogram are remarkably normal. Renal function was normal.

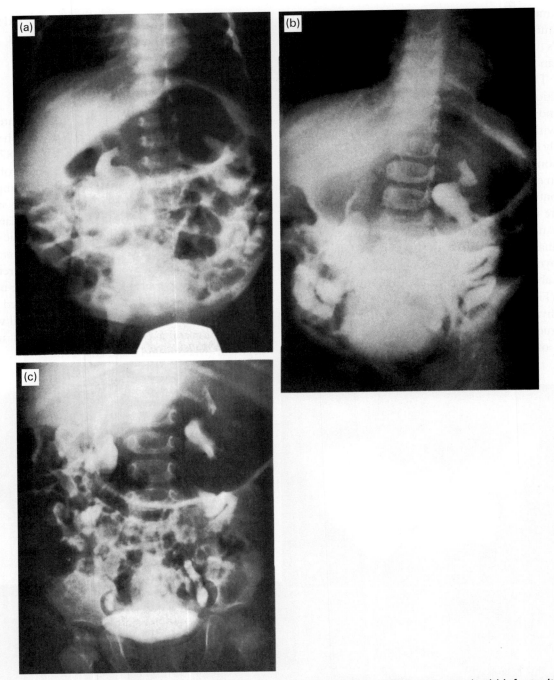

Figure 29.7 Progressive improvement with growth. (*a*) excretory urogram (IVP) in a 1-month-old infant with prune belly syndrome. (*b*) IVP at 1 year. (*c*) IVP at the age of 2 years and 6 months. This child takes prophylactic antibiotics and has had no infections and no surgical procedures. Serum creatinine is 0.5 mg/dl.

VUR is seen in greater than 70% of patients (Fig. 29.5). The conventional system of grading reflux is difficult to apply because of the dysmorphic features of the ureter, renal pelvis, and calyces (Fallat *et al.*, 1989).

Histologic examination of the ureter demonstrates a profound alteration in the content and architecture of the ureteral wall. The hypertrophy and hyperplasia of the smooth muscle cells, which characterize the dilated ureters due to obstruction or VUR, are absent in the prune belly syndrome. Instead, a diffuse increase in the connective tissue with replacement of the smooth muscle is present. The ratio of collagen to smooth muscle, especially in refluxing ureters, is markedly elevated in patients with prune belly syndrome (Gearhart *et al.*, 1995). There is no differentiation into longitudinal and circular muscle layers. The patchy distribution of smooth muscle is present in both the dilated and narrowed ureteral segments. The upper ureter has more smooth muscle cells than the lower portion (Nunn and Stephens, 1961; Palmer and Tesluck, 1974). A marked decrease in the number of nerve plexuses, with degeneration of non-myelinated Schwann fibers, has also been reported. This may contribute to poor ureteral peristalsis even after corrective surgery (Ehrlich and Brown, 1977). Ultrastructural examination of the smooth muscle cells of the ureter reveals a decrease in the number of thick and thin myofilaments, obviously contributing to poor muscle cell performance (Palmer and Tesluck, 1974; Hanna *et al.*, 1977). These histologic and pathologic features are important to remember during reconstructive efforts. Because the upper ureter is potentially the best, its future should not be risked by using it for temporary cutaneous diversion. The dilatation and ineffective peristalsis of the ureters in prune belly syndrome result in urinary stasis and a heightened risk of infection, which can generally be prevented with long term, continuous antibacterial prophylaxis.

Bladder

The bladder is thick walled and grossly enlarged but trabeculations are usually absent (Fig. 29.8). Its normal contour is deviated by a pseudodiverticulum which consists of the urachal remnant, giving the bladder an hour-glass configuration. A patent urachus may be present, especially in association with urethral atresia or microurethra. The trigone is splayed and the ureteric orifices are located laterally, explaining the common association with VUR (Stephens, 1983). The bladder neck is characteristically quite wide at its junction with the prostatic urethra (Fig. 29.9).

Histologic evaluation of the bladder, like that of the ureter, demonstrates an alteration in the ratio of connective tissue to smooth muscle. The extent of involvement, however, is less, and smooth muscle hypertrophy can be present (Perlmutter, 1976; Wigger and Blanc, 1977). The increased bladder thickness is largely due to fibrocytes and collagen. The anatomic innervation of the bladder is normal. No abnormality in the distribution of ganglion cells is present (Nunn and Stephens, 1961; Burke *et al.*, 1969).

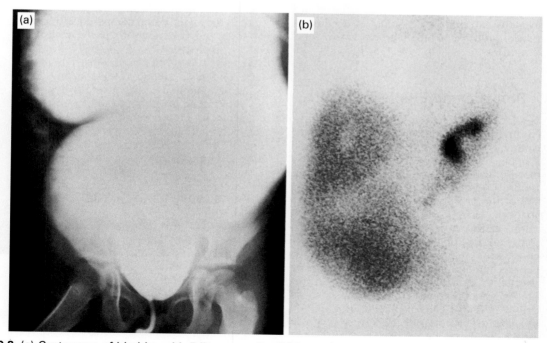

Figure 29.8 (*a*) Cystogram of bladder with 5 liter capacity. (*b*) Lateral view of renal scan demonstrating the urinary bladder (left) higher than the upper pole of the solitary functioning kidney (right).

The bladder in prune belly syndrome has efficient low-pressure storage; however, its ability to empty is compromised by VUR and poor contractility. Urodynamic assessment of the bladder has demonstrated normal balanced voiding in some patients regardless of the gross anatomic and radiologic features (Nunn and Stephens, 1961). Three distinct patterns of voiding have been observed: normal, prolonged voiding with a low peak velocity, and an intermittent pattern. The voiding pattern does not correlate with residual urine volume (Kinahan *et al.*, 1992). Maximum urinary flow rates and voiding pressures may be within normal limits for age; however, the filling phase of the cystometrogram is shifted to the right, with a markedly delayed first sensation to void. Bladder instability with uninhibited contractions is present infrequently and usually does not explain the urinary incontinence often present (Williams and Burkholder, 1967; Snyder *et al.*, 1976; Kinahan *et al.*, 1992). In those patients with unbalanced voiding manifested by urinary incontinence, an increase in residual urine and a decrease in flow rates may be noted. Spontaneous improvement as well as deterioration in voiding efficiency is not unusual and

mandates the need for regular urodynamic assessment and possible surgical intervention or intermittent self-catheterization.

Prostate and posterior urethra

The radiographic appearance of the prostatic urethra is quite distinctive. The bladder neck is open and the posterior urethra is dilated and elongated, and tapers at the membranous urethra (Figs. 29.9, 29.10). The anterior wall of the prostate is shorter than the posterior wall. It frequently has a localized sacculation which represents a utricular diverticulum (Fig. 29.10a). At times, reflux into the vas deferens may be present (Fig. 29.10b). The verumontanum is small or absent. True obstructive lesions at the junction of the prostatic and membranous urethra have been described in 20% of infants, usually those with the worst prognosis. These obstructions have been described as stenosis, true valves, atresia, diaphragms, and diverticula (Lattimer, 1958; Bourne and Cerny, 1967; Berdon *et al.*, 1977; Wigger and Blanc, 1977). A kinking of the prostatic urethra during voiding, as a result of asymmetry of its anterior and posterior walls,

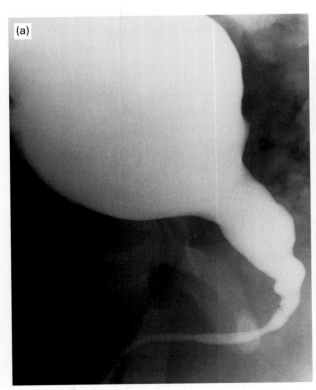

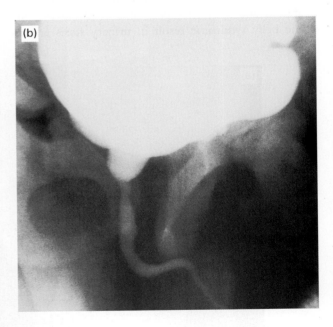

Figure 29.9 (*a, b*) The voiding cystourethrograms detail the grossly enlarged, but non-trabeculated bladder. The bladder neck is widely patent, with dilatation of the posterior urethra. No valve or stenosis is present.

has been suggested as a functional obstruction in prune belly syndrome. Stephens assigned a type IV valve classification to these lesions (Stephens, 1983; Hoagland and Hutchins, 1987).

Lack of development of the epithelial portion of the prostate is a constant component of the syndrome. Compared with normal children and children with PUV, patients with prune belly syndrome have either absent or sparsely distributed prostatic epithelial glands (Nunn and Stephens, 1961; Deklerk and Scott, 1978; Stephens and Gupta, 1994). The prostatic hypoplasia results from an inability of the urogenital mesenchyme to induce epithelial differentiation (Deklerk and Scott, 1978). Prostatic hypoplasia is one of the etiologies of infertility in this syndrome (Hinman, 1980).

Accessory male sexual organs

As with the other mesenchyme derived genitourinary organs in the prune belly syndrome, abnormalities of the epididymis, seminal vesicles, and vas deferens have also been noted. Autopsy findings demonstrate lack of continuity between the ductuli efferentes and rete testes. The body of the epididymis is frequently detached from the testis; a common finding with abdominal undescended testes. The vas deferens is abnormally thickened and may drain ectopically (Cabral et al., 1988). The seminal vesicles may be dilated with diverticular formation but usually are atretic or absent, another diagnostic feature of prune belly syndrome (Stephens and Gupta, 1994). All of

these findings have significance with regard to the known infertility associated with prune belly syndrome (Stephens, 1983).

Anterior urethra

The recognized abnormalities of the anterior urethra in prune belly syndrome range from urethral atresia to fusiform megalourethra (Fig. 29.11, 29.12a). Surviving patients with urethral atresia or microurethra have a patent urachus. It has been suggested that the microurethra in prune belly is normally formed but unused and can be progressively dilated to a functional caliber (Passerini-Glazel et al., 1988).

Bulbous urethral dilatation has been demonstrated in 68% of patients with prune belly syndrome by Kroovand et al. (1982). Two of their patients had a fusiform megalourethra. Comparative measurements of anterior urethral diameters in patients with prune belly syndrome with normal patients have confirmed a dilated anterior urethra in patients with prune belly syndrome (Hutson and Beasley, 1987). A transient obstruction during fetal development at the junction of the glanular and penile urethra may explain this common radiographic finding, as well as the known association of prune belly syndrome with megalourethra (Sellers et al., 1976).

Both types of megalourethra, scaphoid and fusiform, are associated with prune belly syndrome. The fusiform megalourethra, accompanied by deficient corpora cavernosa, is a more severe defect frequently associated with renal dysplasia and lethal

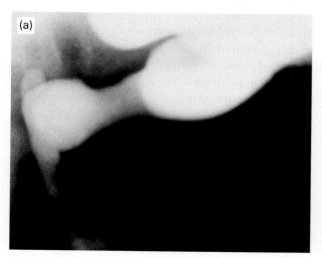 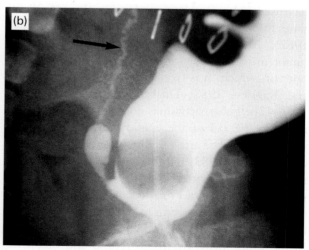

Figure 29.10 (*a*) Voiding cystourethrogram outlines the dilated posterior urethra with a utricular diverticulum. (*b*) Same as in (*a*), but reflux of contrast into the vas deferens (*arrow*), which drained into the prostatic utricle.

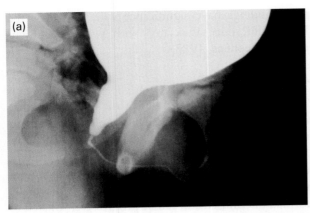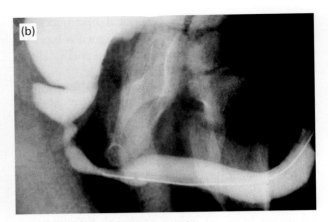

Figure 29.11 (*a*) Atretic or microurethra of prune belly syndrome. (*b*) Scaphoid megalourethra.

anomalies (Fig. 29.12). Scaphoid megalourethra is characterized as a deficiency of the corpus spongiosum only with normal glans and fossa navicularis (Fig. 29.11). In a series of 26 patients with this anomaly, ten had prune belly syndrome (Shrom *et al.*, 1981). It has been suggested that the mesenchymal developmental arrest that accounts for the major features of the syndrome could also explain the urethral malformations (Kroovand *et al.*, 1982).

Testis

Bilateral cryptorchidism is an essential component of the prune belly syndrome. In the majority of patients the testes are intra-abdominal, overlying the ectatic ureters at the pelvic inlet. The intra-abdominal position of the testes predisposes these patients to increased risk of malignant degeneration of 30–50 times that of a normally descended testis (Batata *et al.*, 1982). At least three documented cases of testis tumor in prune belly syndrome have been reported, one of which was retroperitoneal (Woodhouse and Ransley, 1983; Duckett, 1986; Sayre *et al.*, 1986). The gubernaculum is normally attached proximally to the tail of the epididymis, travels via the inguinal canal, and attaches distally at the pubic tubercle (Stephens, 1983). No testicular histologic abnormality has been noted, and the nerve supply of the gubernaculum is intact (Tayakkanontak, 1963).

Histologically, the germinal epithelium of the fetal and neonatal testes is indistinguishable from normal in the prune belly syndrome (Nunn and Stephens, 1961). However, comparative, quantitative analysis of spermatogonia in fetuses with prune belly syn-

drome has demonstrated a significantly decreased number of spermatogonia and marked Leydig cell hyperplasia, well before expected testicular descent, thus implying some intrinsic testicular abnormality (Orvis *et al.*, 1988). Absent spermatogenesis due to prolonged intra-abdominal location has been histologically documented (Uehling *et al.*, 1984). Azoospermia was present in adults when a semen sample was analysed (Woodhouse and Snyder, 1985). No patient with prune belly syndrome has been reported to have fathered a child. Nevertheless, early orchidopexy is advocated for these patients to optimize potential spermatogenesis, to improve evaluation for possible malignancy, and to promote better psychological health (Woodard and Parrott, 1978b; Fallat *et al.*, 1989).

The etiology of maldescent in prune belly syndrome is multifactorial. Mechanical obstruction by the enlarged bladder is contributory, as the incidence of cryptorchidism is also increased in other diseases associated with a enlarged bladder, such as PUV (Krueger *et al.*, 1980). The mechanical effects of the intermuscular pressure of the abdominal muscles pushing the testis toward the scrotum are deficient in the prune belly syndrome. In addition, given the mesenchymal abnormalities of the syndrome, the ability of the gubernaculum to respond hormonally to guide the testes to the scrotum may be impaired (Elder *et al.*, 1982).

Sexual function and fertility

Woodhouse and Snyder (1985) studied sexual function in nine adult patients with prune belly syndrome.

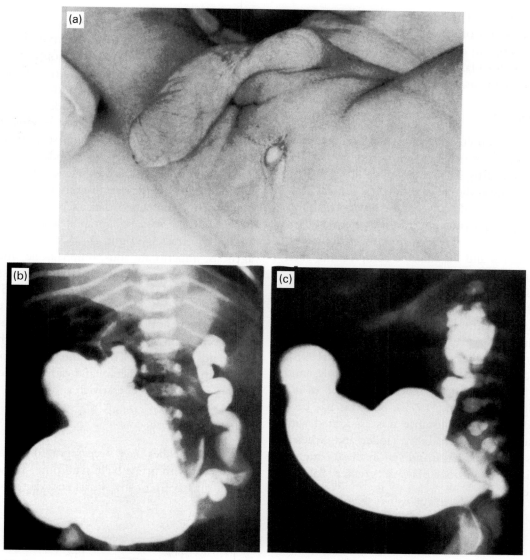

Figure 29.12 Severe manifestation of prune belly syndrome. (*a*) This newborn with prune belly syndrome also has megalourethra and imperforate anus. At autopsy, severe renal dysplasia and pulmonary hypoplasia were apparent. (*b*) Cystogram. (*c*) Voiding cystourethrogram: note urethral stenosis and urachal diverticulum.

All had normal libido, with normal erections and orgasm. Seven had retrograde ejaculation. All patients studied to date are azoospermic (Woodhouse and Snyder, 1985; Burbidge *et al.*, 1987). These patients all had orchidopexy performed late in childhood. Earlier orchidopexy may improve spermatogenesis (Woodard and Parrott, 1978b).

Patients with prune belly syndrome have multiple factors, other than spermatogenesis, that contribute to infertility. An open bladder neck and poorly developed prostate result in retrograde ejaculation. Associated abnormalities of the prostatic epithelium

and seminal vesicles affect the amount and content of the seminal fluid. Vas deferens obstruction and epididymal abnormalities associated with maldescent affect sperm delivery and maturation.

Associated anomalies

Abnormalities of other organ systems result in long-term morbidity for as many as 75% of patients with prune belly syndrome (Fig. 29.13) (Geary *et al.*, 1986). Growth was impaired in 32% of surviving patients in one large series and was poorly correlated with renal function. This impairment was most manifest in the first year of life, with subsequent stabilization but incomplete catch-up growth (Geary *et al.*, 1986). Developmental delay has also been documented in selected patients.

Orthopedic

In most series musculoskeletal anomalies predominate in frequency of non-urologic pathology. Of the patients reviewed by Tuck and Smith (1978), 50% had one or more orthopedic anomalies. Lateral dimples of the elbows and knees are the mildest manifestation of the compression effect of intrauterine oligohydramnios. More severe deformities, attributed to oligohydramnios and intrauterine compression, such as lower limb deficiencies and arthrogryposis, are recognized usually at autopsy (Pagon *et al.*, 1979; Carey *et al.*, 1982). Congenital dislocation of the hips, the most frequent musculoskeletal finding, requires early institution of treatment and may be resistant to conventional therapy (Brinker *et al.*, 1995). Talipes equinovarus, polydactyly, syndactyly, and torticollis have also been reported (Burke *et al.*, 1969; Wigger and Blanc, 1977). Scoliosis has been recognized and in one instance was associated with thoracic segmental insensibility (Joller and Scheier, 1986). As prognosis has improved in these patients, orthopedic intervention plays a greater role in management.

Gastrointestinal

Gastrointestinal anomalies are observed in over 30% of autopsied patients and are commonly recognized in the postnatal period. The majority of anomalies, such as malrotation, atresia, stenosis, and volvulus, are due to persistence of the embryonic wide mesentery, with absent fixation to the posterior abdominal wall (Wright *et al.*, 1986). This same suspension abnormality allows the spleen to wander freely in the abdominal cavity, and acute splenic torsion has been reported on two occasions (Teramoto *et al.*, 1981). It has been recommended that all patients with prune belly syndrome have radiographic assessment of their alimentary tract (Wright *et al.*, 1986). Anorectal agenesis, imperforate anus, omphalocele, and gastroschisis have occasionally been reported in association with prune belly syndrome (Short *et al.*, 1985; Wright *et al.*, 1986; Walker *et al.*, 1987). Chronic constipation is a frequent problem in these children, attributed to a decrease in abdominal wall pressure, which normally aids evacuation. This requires continuous attention with long-term dietary and cathartic intervention (Geary *et al.*, 1986; Greskovich and Nyberg, 1988).

Cardiac

Cardiac anomalies have been reported in up to 10% of patients with prune belly syndrome. These include patent ductus arteriosus, artrial and ventricular septal

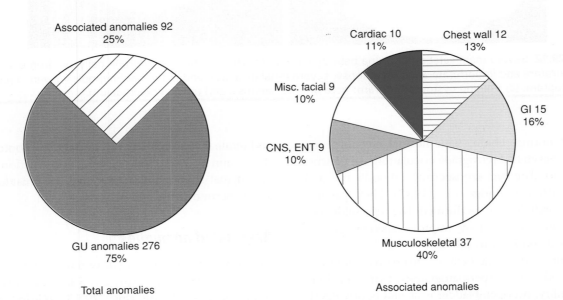

Figure 29.13 Associated anomalies constitute 25% of all anomalies from a large series of patients with prune belly syndrome. CNS: central nervous system; GI: gastrointestinal; GU: genitourinary. (Adapted from Welsh, 1979).

defects, and tetralogy of Fallot (Adebonojo, 1973; Welsh, 1979). The severity of the cardiac involvement will dictate initial care of the infant, as the urologic anomalies rarely demand immediate treatment.

Pulmonary

Pulmonary and respiratory difficulties pervade the lives of these patients from birth to adulthood. Clinically significant pulmonary problems were noted in 55% of survivors (Geary et al., 1986). In the most severe form, pulmonary hypoplasia is associated with oligohydramnios and renal dysplasia, and is incompatible with life. Initial prognosis is dependent on pulmonary development. Pneumothorax and pneumomediastinum may be present at birth, with or without pulmonary hypoplasia, and an early chest X-ray is advised. Chest-wall deformities and abdominal muscle deficiency impair mechanical ventilation, resulting in ventilitory limitation and a high incidence of lobar atelectasis and pneumonia (Alford et al., 1978; Ewig et al., 1996). Chronic bronchitis and the development of respiratory insufficiency following upper respiratory infections or anesthetics are well recognized, and appropriate pulmonary support must be provided (Alford et al., 1978; Geary et al., 1986).

The non-urologic associated anomalies in patients with prune belly syndrome are a major source of morbidity and mortality. Close cooperation with all physicians involved with the patients' care allows an individualized approach. Urologic anomalies rarely require emergency treatment.

Patient management

Prenatal

Fetal hydronephrosis can be accurately recognized by ultrasonography, and when present, is usually diagnosed prior to 20 weeks' gestation. The ability to diagnosis the etiology of the hydronephrosis, however, is questionable. The accuracy varies from 30 to 85% (Elder, 1990). The majority of patients with prune belly syndrome have no demonstrable obstruction, regardless of the hydronephrosis. In addition, renal function does not correlate with the amount of dilatation present in the urinary tract. Thus, intervention to relieve obstruction in a fetus with a specific diagnosis of prune belly syndrome is difficult to justify. Even in instances of true obstruction, reviews

have failed to document a beneficial effect of fetal intervention on subsequent renal function or pulmonary development (Kramer, 1983; Elder, 1990).

Although there are reports in the literature of antenatal intervention and even termination of pregnancy based on the ultrasonic findings of prune belly syndrome, one should carefully weigh the decision to perform these invasive procedures (Gadziala et al., 1982; Golbus et al., 1982; Prescia et al., 1982). Fetal intervention in prune belly syndrome is not warranted except in the rare instance of dystocia secondary to fetal bladder distension. Decompression at the time of labor and delivery may be necessary (Gadziala et al., 1982; Meizner et al., 1985).

Newborn

The appearance of the abdominal wall leaves little doubt as to the diagnosis in the newborn. Fortunately, this is not a true urologic emergency, thus allowing a thorough multisystem evaluation to rule out significant cardiac, pulmonary, or other associated malformations (Alford et al., 1978). An immediate chest X-ray is necessary to exclude associated pneumothorax and pneumomediastinum. The presence of severe pulmonary hypoplasia with progressive inability to oxygenate the infant immediately affects prognosis. This is usually associated with the antenatal demonstration of oligohydramnios a product of severely impaired renal function (Perlman and Levin, 1974).

The evaluation of renal function is tempered by the knowledge of developmental renal physiology. Because initial creatinine measurements reflect maternal renal function, repetitive sampling is necessary. If after 48–72 hours the serum creatinine is greater than 1.0 mg/dl in the term infant or 1.5 mg/dl in the preterm infant, a degree of renal insufficiency is present. A progressive rise in serum creatinine over the first few weeks of life portends a poor prognosis. If initial nadir creatinine is less than 0.7 mg/dl then subsequent renal failure is unlikely (Noh et al., 1999). Urine is sent for baseline culture and antibiotic prophylaxis is initiated. Measurement of serum and urinary electrolytes at birth can be helpful in assessing sodium conservation, implying adequate renal function (Appleman and Golbus, 1986). In the premature and full-term infant the glomerular filtration rate (GFR) is initially low, then rapidly increases (Arant, 1978). This must be remembered in relation to the administration of intravenous contrast agents, which may rapidly elevate plasma osmolality, causing intraventricular hemorrhage as well as further impairment of renal function (Chevalier, 1989).

Radiologic assessment in the newborn is tempered by the known risks of intravenous contrast and the introduction of infection with retrograde studies. Initial sonographic and nuclear medicine scans, which give both anatomic and functional information, are preferred (Fig. 29.6). Renal sonograms provide information on cortical thickness, presence of cystic changes, and renal size. Examinations before and after voiding give a clue to the presence of VUR, and postvoid residual urine. The diethylene triamine-pentaacetic acid (DTPA) renal scan and the mercaptoacetyltriglycine (MAG-3) renal scan provide both functional and anatomic information. Blood flow, differential renal function, and drainage in response to furosemide (Lasix) can be assessed and compared with subsequent studies (Fig. 29.14). The limitations of diuresis renography in demon-strating obstruction in patients with prune belly syndrome have been noted. A Whitaker test may be necessary on occasion as the definitive study to rule out significant obstruction (Snow and Duckett, 1987). Dimercaptosuccinic acid (DMSA) renal scan is performed rather than intravenous pyelography IVP to evaluate renal size, tubular mass, and differential function. Comparative studies are invaluable to assess renal growth and scarring as these patients are observed in the future (Rushton et al., 1988).

Initially, a VCUG is performed in those infants with abnormal renal function to ensure that a true anatomic, urethral obstruction is not present (Figs. 29.5, 29.11). This 'lethal variant' and the potential confusion with PUV 'masquerading' as prune belly syndrome must be diagnosed, as treatment changes dramatically (Rogers and Ostrow, 1973; Krueger, 1981; Aaronson, 1983). The VCUG also demon-strates VUR in up to 70% of patients and bladder

(a)

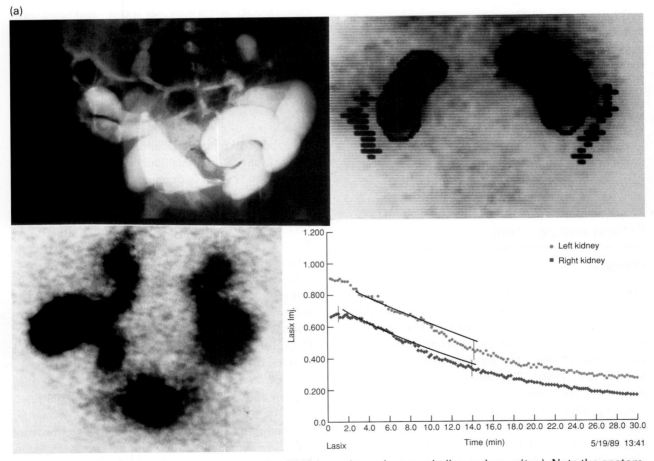

Figure 29.14 (*a*) Intravenous pyelogram and lasix DMSA renal scan in prune belly syndrome (*top*). Note the anatomic definition of the renal scan (*bottom*) and adequate drainage of upper collecting system (*diagram*). Renal function was normal. (*Continued on the next page.*)

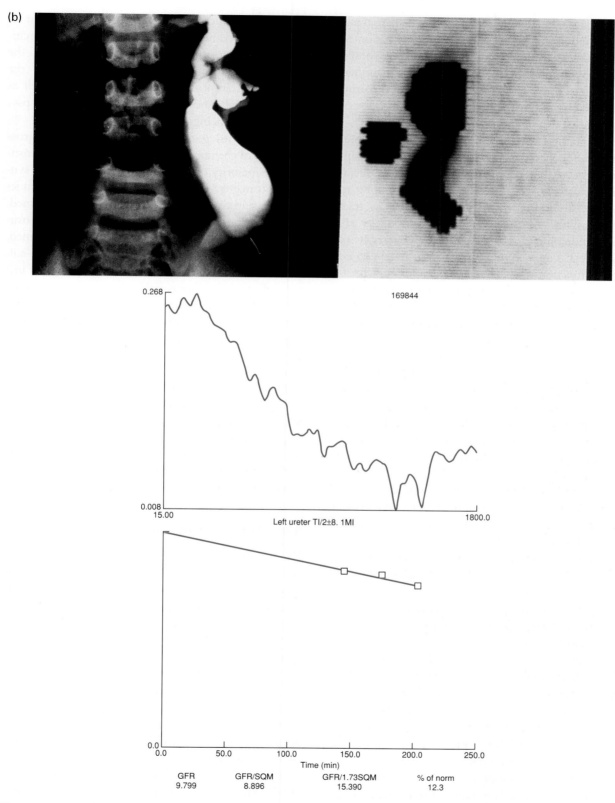

Figure 29.14 *Continued.* (*b*) Cystogram and Lasix renal scan with glomerular filtration rate (GFR) in a patient with poor renal function. The scan demonstrates adequate drainage but the solitary kidney functions poorly (GFR = 15.3 ml/min per 1.73 m²).

emptying is assessed (Fig. 29.5). All infants are treated with antibiotics prior to sterile catheterization to decrease the risk of infection. Instrumentation should be kept to a minimum to avoid bacterial contamination. In general, the radiologic assessment of the urinary tract is tailored by the management philosophy of the individual urologic surgeon.

The overall goals of initial management are to preserve renal function and prevent infection. The attainment of these goals is possible via a variety of therapeutic approaches, ranging from watchful waiting to immediate surgical reconstruction of the urinary tract (Waldbaum and Marshall, 1970; Woodhouse et al., 1979; Randolph et al., 1981a). When a philosophy of management is applied to a classification system based on renal function (Table 29.2), individualized treatment is accomplished. Early surgical intervention in the neonate is avoided, unless a rising creatinine or infection intervenes, requiring early vesicostomy. Unless salvaged by extraordinary means (extracorporeal membrane oxygenation with or without dialysis), patients with category I disease associated with prenatal oligohydramnios and postnatal pulmonary hypoplasia usually die in the immediate postnatal period as a result of pulmonary complications. In those few infants surviving the pulmonary insult, high urinary diversion by cutaneous pyelostomy has been attempted to provide optimal urinary drainage (Randolph, 1977). Unfortunately, recovery of renal function is not usually possible because of the severe underlying renal dysplasia.

Patients with category II involvement are serially monitored for infection and a decrease in renal function. All such infants and children are placed on long-term prophylactic antibiotics. With documentation of infection, failure of adequate renal growth, or decreasing renal function, aggressive reconstruction of the urinary tract is pursued. The authors' approach, like Woodard's (Figs. 29.15, 29.16), involves surgical remodeling to eliminate stasis and VUR and optimize drainage (Randolph et al., 1981a). If renal insufficiency is severe or infection is initially present, a period of urinary diversion by means of cutaneous vesicostomy is recommended (Fig. 29.17) (Duckett, 1974). Cutaneous ureterostomies probably do little to improve drainage. In addition, the upper ureter is anatomically and histologically the most normal and should be preserved if later tailored reconstruction is elected (Palmer and Tesluck, 1974; Hanna et al., 1977). The authors' approach has been aggressive with children who have significant abdominal wall pathology, including operation usually at 1 year of age. At that time, the abdominoplasty and orchidopexy are performed along with tailoring of the urinary tract when indicated. This optimizes the potential for improved urinary drainage, as well as addressing the issues of subsequent fertility and psychological wellbeing (Fallat et al., 1989).

Patients with good renal function, despite gross dilatation of the upper and lower urinary tract, constitute the majority of individuals with prune belly syndrome (category III). Serial assessment of renal function by selective imaging techniques is performed. Surgical reconstruction of the urinary tract is not usually necessary. Antibiotic prophylaxis is maintained, for example a daily single dose of trimethoprim–sulfamethoxazole or nitrofurantoin. Development of urinary infections or a measurable decrease in renal function mandates urodynamic assessment of the urinary tract. The demonstration of significant residual urine with unbalanced voiding warrants surgical intervention to promote emptying (Snyder et al., 1976; Woodhouse et al., 1982). Upper tract stasis should be evaluated and a Whitaker test performed, if necessary, to rule out obstruction (Whitaker, 1973). The results of these specific tests will help to determine the type of surgical intervention. All such patients will benefit from early orchidopexy and abdominoplasty. Correction of the abdominal wall may improve defecation and voiding efficiency (Smith et al., 1998).

Anesthetic considerations

The patient with prune belly syndrome presents unique problems to the anesthesiologist. Previous reports have commented on respiratory difficulties due to the abnormal mechanics of pulmonary ventilation. The deficient abdominal musculature weakens the ability to cough effectively and predisposes to postoperative atelectasis and infection (Hannington-Kiff, 1970). In one case, prolonged, postoperative ventilation was necessary to clear secretions effectively and oxygenate the patient adequately (Karamanian et al., 1974). In a review of 36 patients with prune belly syndrome, postoperative respiratory infection developed following eight of 133 anesthetics, all of which resolved with antibiotics and physiotherapy (Henderson et al., 1987). There were no intraoperative respiratory difficulties. Three deaths occurred in the postoperative period, one of which was partially contributed to by pneumonia, as a result of ineffective cough.

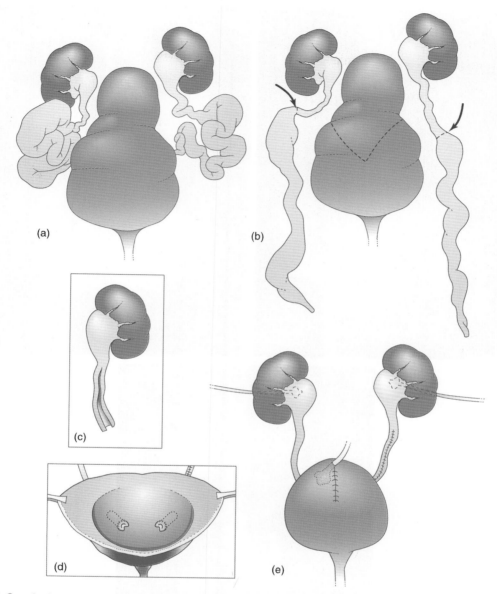

Figure 29.15 Surgical technique used for extensive reconstruction of prune belly uropathy. The operation is performed transperitoneally. No attempt is made to straighten the lower ureter, inasmuch as only the upper portion of the ureter is needed for the reimplantation. The ureter may or may not require tapering. The dome of the bladder is excised (*b*; *dotted line*) in most patients. Ureteral stents (not shown) are used; nephrostomy tubes are rarely used.

All these patients require careful preoperative pulmonary assessment. An antecedent history of recurrent respiratory infections warrants aggressive physiotherapy, postural drainage, and intermittent positive-pressure breathing treatments. Specific antibiotic therapy should be given (Karamanian *et al.*, 1974). Judicious use of postoperative analgesics, which may produce respiratory depression, is advised.

Operative interventions in prune belly syndrome

Vesicourethral dysfunction

Internal urethrotomy

In a small percentage of patients a true obstruction, at the junction of the prostatic and membranous ure-

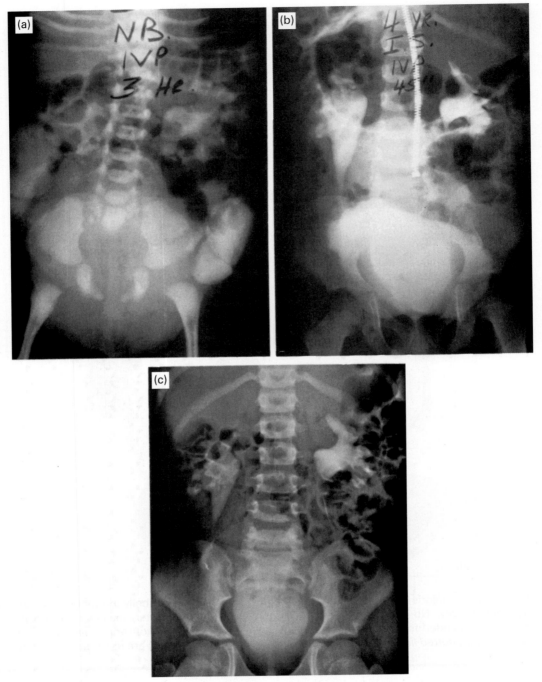

Figure 29.16 Results of neonatal reconstruction. Excretory urograms prior to surgery (*a*), and at 3 years (*b*) and 10 years (*c*) following a single primary reconstruction.

thra, is present. This has been called a 'type 4' valve by Stephens. This redundancy partially obstructs the membranous urethra, and transurethral incision at the 12 o'clock position has been advised to improve voiding and decrease residual urine (King, 1969).

Urodynamic assessment in patients with prune belly syndrome, although infrequently reported, may prove valuable (Nunn and Stephens, 1961; Williams and Burkholder, 1967; Snyder *et al.*, 1976). The demonstration of residual urine with infection indicates the need for further testing. If a low flow rate is associated with significant residual urine and normal voiding pressure, then intervention to lower urethral resistance is warranted (Snyder *et al.*, 1976). Endoscopic incision of the external urinary sphincter by hot or cold knife, to decrease outlet resistance, was successful in ten of 11 cases, improving emptying (Cukier, 1977). Most authors who advocate minimal surgical intervention stress the need to assess carefully lower tract dynamics and demand routine urine flow rates and assessment of residual urine, preferably by ultrasound, in follow-up. Transurethral external sphincterotomy may be the first step to balanced voiding, but clean intermittent catheterization (CIC) should be considered as an alternative if the urodynamic criteria for outlet obstruction

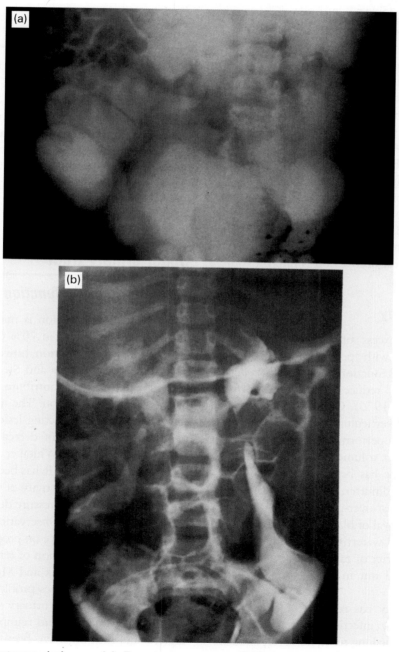

Figure 29.17 Vesicostomy drainage. (*a*) Excretory urogram (IVP) in an 18-month-old boy with prune belly syndrome; (*b*) IVP 10 years later with cutaneous vesicostomy alone.

are absent (Snyder *et al.*, 1976; Cukier, 1977; Woodhouse *et al.*, 1979; Kinahan *et al.*, 1992).

Vesicostomy

When the patient's condition is complicated by urinary infection or deteriorating renal function in the perinatal period, a cutaneous vesicostomy is the drainage procedure of choice (Duckett *et al.*, 1980; Duckett, 1986). This provides a vent that decompresses the entire urinary tract (Fig. 29.17). The procedure is performed by making a small transverse incision midway between the umbilicus and the pubic symphysis. The rectus fascia is incised and a small amount of it and the skin removed. The dome of the bladder is mobilized and brought to the skin. The wall of the bladder is sewn to the fascia and matured to the skin. A generous stoma is advocated to prevent stomal stenosis (Snow and Duckett, 1987). A urachal diverticulum, if present, can be excised. The vesicostomy serves as an initial temporary drainage procedure prior to more extensive reconstruction (Woodard, 1985). The only potential disadvantage of vesicostomy is ineffective drainage of the redundant, tortuous, ureters or associated UPJ obstruction. This is unlikely, however, because true supravesical obstruction is rarely a component of this syndrome.

Reduction cystoplasty

Bladder volumes in excess of 3 liters have been recorded in children with prune belly syndrome (Snyder *et al.*, 1976). Reduction cystoplasty has been suggested as a means to reduce volume and improve emptying (Perlmutter, 1976). Concomitant removal of a dilated urachal diverticulum, which contributes to inefficient voiding, is performed. A variety of techniques to reduce bladder volume and produce a more efficient spherical shape has been proposed (Binard and Zoedler, 1968; Perlmutter, 1976; Woodard and Trulock, 1996). A 'vest-over-pants' closure of the bladder wall after removal of bladder epithelial strips, or simple resection and watertight closure have been performed in the majority of cases. Reduction cystoplasty has been carried out in many patients, with clinical improvement.

Reduction cystoplasty has resulted in fewer hospitalizations for urinary infections and has initially improved voiding. In the long term, however, bladder capacity and voiding efficiency have not been demonstrated to be improved (Bukowski and Perlmutter,

1994). Comparison of urodynamic voiding parameters between patients who underwent reconstruction, as compared to those who did not has demonstrated no significant difference. Consequently, some authors do not recommend reduction cystoplasty in light of the effective and safe application of CIC, although removal of a urachal pseudodiverticulum may be advantageous (Snow and Duckett, 1987; Kinahan *et al.*, 1992).

Anterior urethra

Prune belly syndrome is associated with microurethra and megalourethra (Fig. 29.11). Utilization of the unused 'micro' anterior urethra is advocated. Successful progressive soft dilatation of the urethra with normal voiding has been reported (Passerini-Glazel *et al.*, 1988). If the anterior urethra is not usable, urethroplasty techniques combining skin flaps and grafts may be necessary to bridge the anterior urethral defect. Megalourethra can be repaired using hypospadias operative techniques.

Upper urinary tract

Vesicoureteral dysfunction

Vesicoureteral dysfunction is manifested most commonly as VUR, found in 70% of patients. Ureteral valves and UVJ obstruction, however, have also rarely been described (Maizels and Stephens, 1980). Both conditions potentially contribute to urinary stasis and increased risk of infection. The indications for surgical correction of obstructing lesions should be based on the demonstration of decreasing renal function, infection, or a positive Whitaker test.

Surgery to repair VUR has been contested because of the poor peristaltic activity of the ureters and their dissipation of voiding pressure due to increased capacity (Duckett, 1986). Observation of those patients, who remain infection free on prophylactic antibiotics, has confirmed preservation of renal function (Woodhouse *et al.*, 1982; Tank and McCoy, 1983). When urinary infection becomes problematic, correction of reflux and reduction of urinary stasis become necessary. Formal tapering and reimplantation, as well as ureteral imbrication, have been used as part of the comprehensive approach to management (Fig. 29.18) (Fallat *et al.*, 1989). The authors found no difference in the complication rate with either procedure, and nine of 13 patients had successful elimination of their reflux. Ureteral imbrication, rather than excisional ureteroplasty may produce fewer problems with stenosis (Duckett, 1986). Because the imbricated ureter is very bulky, a very long and wide subepithelial tunnel is required for successful reimplantation.

Comprehensive reconstruction

Total urinary reconstruction, including reduction cystoplasty with bilateral ureteral tapering and reimplantation with resection of the distal ureter, is applied to a selected population of patients (Fig. 29.15). Reconstruction may be combined with abdominoplasty and bilateral orchidopexy, usually before 2 years of age (Randolph *et al.*, 1981a; Woodard, 1998). This aggressive approach was used in 15 patients in one series. Serial measurements of creatinine up to 13 years later documented preservation of renal function (Fallat *et al.*, 1989). VUR was corrected in nine of 13 patients and improved in three. Because of the known urinary stasis that occurs in these patients, all are maintained on lifelong antibiotic prophylaxis. Therefore, the decrease in urinary infection cannot be totally attributed to the surgical result.

Urinary reconstruction is similar to that proposed by Woodward (Figs. 29.15). One approach is to make a wide lower abdominal incision that extends from the tip of the 12th rib, along the anterior superior iliac spine to the pubis and then curves upward to the opposite 12th rib, as introduced by Randolph *et*

al. (1981b). This tends to spare the segmental nerve and vascular supply of the abdominal wall for reconstruction. In addition, at the time of excision of the redundant abdominal wall, that portion with the most muscle fibers is preserved. The exposure of the urinary tract provided with this incision is exceptional and plays a role in the decision to reconstruct the urinary tract. Alternatively, a midline approach can be utilized, as proposed by Chilich *et al.* (1986) or Monfort *et al.* (1991) (see 'Abdominoplasty').

The posterior peritoneum is incised along the length of the ureters. The spermatic vessels are mobilized distally, care being taken not to compromise the peritoneal attachments of the vas deferens if a Fowler–Stephens orchidopexy is required. The bladder is opened in the midline with cautery. The laterally placed ureteral orifices are recognized and each ureter is mobilized. The extreme length of the mobilized ureters allows for resection of their distal third, usually the most abnormal portion. Formal tapering or imbrication is performed (Fig. 29.18) (Hendren, 1970; Ehrlich, 1985). The ureters are then reimplanted, using a transtrigonal or Politano–Leadbetter technique. The operated ureters are stented and the stents are brought out through the bladder and separate abdominal incisions.

Prior to reduction cystoplasty, the testes are mobilized with a wide apron of posterior peritoneum (Fig. 29.19). Fortunately, if the reconstruction is performed before 2 years of age, a standard orchidopexy with intact spermatic vessels can be performed in 80% of cases (Woodard and Parrott, 1978b; Fallat *et al.*, 1989). Otherwise, a delayed or formal Fowler–Stephens orchidopexy will be necessary (Ransley *et al.*, 1984).

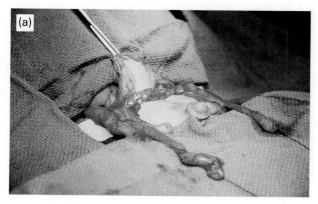
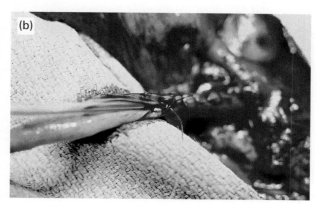

Figure 29.18 (*a*) Both ureters have been mobilized prior to reimplantation and tapering. (*b*) The ureter is closed in two layers with a running, locking suture.

The bladder is reduced in size by resection of the urachal remnant and the huge bladder dome. A strip of bladder epithelium can be removed from one of the lateral walls and closed by the vest-over-pants technique. The bladder is drained transabdominally with a Malecot catheter. The previously mobilized testes are brought up through the distal abdominal wall at the pubic tubercle. A dartos pouch is created in the scrotum and each testis is secured in the pouch with permanent sutures.

The redundant abdominal wall is then held taut and marked in the midline and laterally at the costo-vertebral angles to outline the tissue to be excised (Fig. 29.20) (Randolph *et al.*, 1981b). Avoidance of removal of excessive amounts of abdominal wall is critical. The second line of incision parallels the previous incision. A large wedge of full-thickness abdominal wall is removed (Fig. 29.19). The closure of the abdominal wall starts with placement of key sutures of 0 or 1–0 non-absorbable sutures at the anterior iliac spines and at each pubic tubercle. These sutures should include the periosteum of the bone and a full thickness of the proximal opposing tissue edge. The tension created occasionally allows for removal of additional lateral redundant abdominal wall. Each section between the key sutures is closed with interrupted sutures opposing the full thickness of the abdominal tissue. The subcutaneous tissue is closed to prevent dead space and the skin is approximated with a subcuticular absorbable suture.

All patients undergo preoperative enemas to clear the colon, and require good bowel decompression postoperatively. Postoperative abdominal distension must be avoided and a rectal tube placed during surgery is often valuable.

Cryptorchidism

The early correction of the cryptorchid intra-abdominal testes by a transabdominal approach is recommended to optimize spermatogenesis, facilitate examination for testicular malignancy, and improve testicular salvage. This can be performed at the time of comprehensive reconstruction, with a high success rate (Woodard and Parrott, 1978b; Randolph *et al.*, 1981a; Fallat *et al.*, 1989). If orchidopexy is performed in the first a years of life, a standard technique with preservation of the spermatic vessels is often possible. Orchidopexy in older children frequently requires division of the spermatic vessels, with an increased risk for atrophy (Docimo, 1995). To avoid atrophy, a broad, peritoneal pedicle mobilized with the long-looping vas, combined with early ligation of the spermatic vessels above the point of confluence of the vas and spermatic artery, is recommended (Fowler and Stephens, 1959). An 80% success rate for intra-abdominal testes has been attained with this premeditated approach (Gibbons *et al.*, 1979). Overall, successful orchidopexy can be expected in the majority of patients.

A recent consideration is the laparoscopic orchiopexy and laparoscopic staged Fowler–Stephens orchiopexy. Laparoscopic orchiopexy can be applied unilaterally or bilaterally in the older child with insufficient spermatic vessel length. Frequently, the testes can be positioned in the scrotum with the sper-

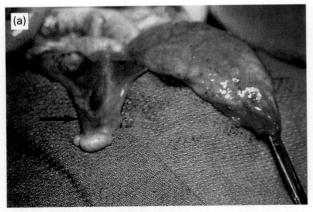
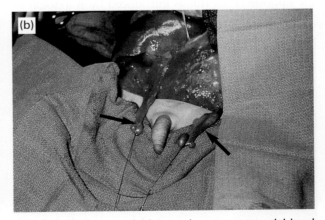

Figure 29.19 (*a*) The widely mobilized peritoneum with intact spermatic vessels (*arrows*) ensures good blood supply to the testis. (*b*) Achieving adequate length to secure the testes in the scrotum is not difficult in the child less than 2 years of age.

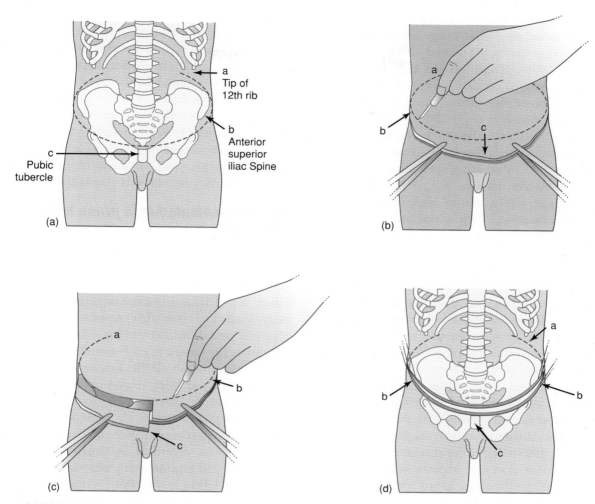

Figure 29.20 Technique of Randolph abdominoplasty. (*a*) A curvilinear incision extends from the tip of the twelfth rib, along the anterior superior iliac spine to the pubic tubercle and onto the opposite 12th rib. (*b*) A parallel incision is made, avoiding removal of too much abdominal wall. (*c*) Rhomboid-like pieces of abdominal wall are removed. (*d*) Critical non-absorbable sutures are placed at both anterior superior iliac spines and at the pubic tubercle. These are placed through the full thickness of the abdominal wall and include the periosteum.

matic vessels intact (Docimo *et al.*, 1995). This technique is particularly useful in the older child or in the patient requiring no other surgery. The staged technique involves laparoscopic ligation of the spermatic vessels *in situ*, without mobilization of the testis or cord structures. This optimizes the subsequent development of collateral circulation, via the vasal and spermatic vascular arcade (Ransley *et al.*, 1984; Bloom, 1991; Yu *et al.*, 1995). The second-stage repair is performed 6 months later, either through open surgery or laparoscopically.

Microvascular testicular autotransplantation has been used in patients with prune belly syndrome. The spermatic vessels are anastomosed to the inferior epigastric vessels, with microsurgical vascular techniques (Wacksman *et al.*, 1980). This is generally reserved for older patients as a last salvage effort (Woodard, 1985). Recent advances in male factor infertility and assisted reproductive techniques may improve the chances for fertility in patients with prune belly syndrome. Consequently, all efforts to repair the cryptorchid testis should be performed early.

Abdominoplasty

Abdominal wall reconstruction plays a significant role in the treatment of patients with prune belly syndrome. Abdominoplasty had previously been performed to improve body image, self-esteem, and psychological wellbeing (Woodard, 1998; Woodard and Smith, 1998). Recent studies suggest that the improved abdominal contour, with repositioning of the most functional musculature, also improves voiding efficiency (Smith *et al.*, 1998). The decrease in residual urine has obvious benefit in the prevention of urinary infection. In addition, abdominoplasty was subjectively felt to improve defecation and the sensation of bladder fullness.

The surgical approaches to abdominoplasty are based on preservation of the lateral and upper parts of the abdominal wall, the sites of the most normal musculature. The authors have achieved good cosmetic and functional results using the abdominoplasty as described by Randolph *et al.* (1981b). This technique (Figs. 29.20, 29.21) excises the most abnormal segment of redundant abdominal wall, provides excellent exposure for urinary reconstruction and orchidopexy, and preserves segmental motor nerves to the retained abdominal musculature. In 16 patients in whom this technique was used, nine had an excellent cosmetic improvement in abdominal contour, while in seven a slight protuberance remained. There were no serious complications related to the abdominoplasty procedure (Fallat *et al.*, 1989). The major criticisms of this technique are that it does not improve abdominal wall thickness, and lateral bulging is not completely eliminated. This technique has been favored by a number of surgeons (Duckett, 1986; Snow and Duckett, 1987).

Surgical approaches to abdominal wall reconstruction that use a midline incision with extensive subcutaneous dissection and a pants-over-vest closure have also been described (Ehrlich *et al.*, 1986; Monfort *et al.*, 1991). These techniques preserve the umbilicus, uses the full thickness of the abdominal wall, and provide narrowing at the waist. Excellent cosmetic results with a high degree of patient satisfaction have been reported with both the Ehrlich and Monfort techniques (Figs. 29.22, 29.23) (Ehrlich *et al.*, 1986; Monfort *et al.*, 1991; Parrott and Woodard, 1992; Woodard and Smith, 1998). A new adaptation using an extraperitoneal plication of the abdominal wall through a midline incision decreases the extent of fascial dissection, avoids entering the peritoneal cavity, and decreases postoperative recovery time (Furness *et al.*, 1998). This simplification seems most appropriate for patients not requiring other concomitant intra-abdominal surgical procedures.

Non-operative treatments include the use of abdominal binders and elasticized corsets (Fig. 29.24). These aids do not address the psychological implications of the abdominal disfigurement, which have generally been ignored in the past (Ehrlich *et al.*, 1986). The importance of body image during the formative years of childhood cannot be overestimated. The abdominoplasty provides these males with freedom from abdominal binders, a more natural waisted physique, and the ability to wear normal pants and participate in sports (Fallat *et al.*, 1989).

Renal transplantation in prune belly syndrome

Progressive renal insufficiency resulting from renal dysplasia, reflux nephropathy, and recurrent pyelonephritis can be successfully treated by transplantation. Renal transplantation in patients with prune belly syndrome was first reported in 1976 by Shenasky and Whelchel (1976). The age at transplantation has ranged from 8 months to 21 years of age (Dreikorn *et al.*, 1978; Reinberg *et al.*, 1989). Both cadaver and living-related donor kidneys have been successfully transplanted. In a retrospective review of eight patients with prune belly syndrome who underwent transplantation, there was no statistically significant difference in patient deaths, graft survival, or graft function compared with age-matched controls (Reinberg *et al.*, 1989). A more recent retrospective analysis of graft survival at 10 years of 47% was not statistically significantly different from age-matched control patients (Fontaine *et al.*, 1997). The success of renal transplantation was in part attributed to the low-pressure urine storage provided by the bladder in prune belly syndrome (Gonzalez, 1997).

Prior to transplantation, bilateral nephroureterectomies were performed in all reported cases. Radiographic and urodynamic assessment of the lower urinary tract is recommended to ensure absence of obstruction and balanced voiding (Messing *et al.*, 1985). The use of CIC to empty the decompensated bladder is not a contraindication to renal transplantation (Kogan *et al.*, 1986; Reinberg *et al.*, 1989). All patients should be kept on antibiotic prophylaxis. An unusual complication of transplantation in prune belly syndrome is allograft torsion (Marvin *et al.*, 1995). The torsion, with resultant graft loss, was thought to be the result of a lack of abdominal wall tone. Nephropexy has been recommended to avoid this disastrous complication.

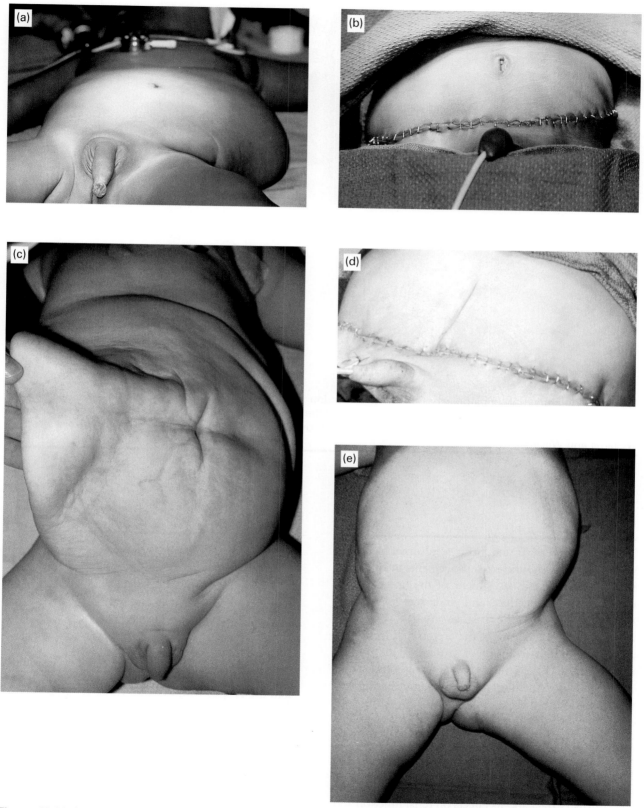

Figure 29.21 (*a, b*) Preoperative and immediate postoperative results of abdominoplasty. (*c–e*) Preoperative and postoperative, and 18 months following abdominoplasty in a 9-month-old child.

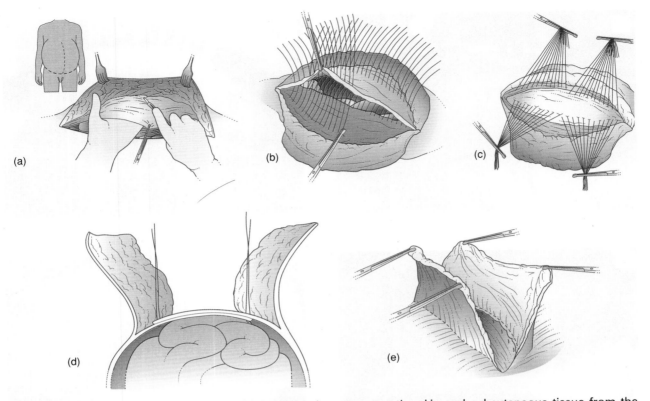

Figure 29.22 Ehrlich abdominoplasty. (*a*) Sharp dissection separates the skin and subcutaneous tissue from the musculofascial layer. (*b–d*) A 'vest-over-pants' closure of the musculofascial layers. The umbilicus can be saved on a separate pedicle. (*e*) The excess abdominal skin is removed. (From Ehrlich *et al.*, 1986, with permission from Williams and Wilkins.)

Conclusions

The treatment of prune belly syndrome has been refined through significant improvements in antibiotic therapy, urodynamic assessment of the urinary tract, diagnosis of obstruction, and understanding of the natural history of the disease. A less extensive approach to the tailoring of the ureters and bladder is advocated in the majority of patients with normal renal function. When infection and stasis compromise renal growth or function, aggressive surgical intervention to promote drainage is advised. All infants with adequate renal function will benefit from abdominoplasty and orchidopexy performed at 12–24 months of age. The long-term psychological benefits and the potential for improved fertility await further study. Because of the changing urodynamic condition of the lower urinary tract and its effects on renal function and infections, all of these patients require careful lifelong antibacterial prophylaxis and urologic surveillance.

References

Aaronson IA (1983) Posterior urethral valve masquerading as the prune belly syndrome. *Br J Urol* **55**: 508–12.

Adebonojo FO (1973) Dysplasia of the abdominal musculature with multiple congenital anomalies: prune belly or triad syndrome. *J Nat Med Assoc* **65**: 327–9.

Adeyokunnu AA, Familuse JB (1982) Prune belly syndrome in two siblings and a first cousin: possible genetic implications. *Am J Dis Child* **136**: 23–5.

Afifi AK, Rebeiz JM, Adonia SJ *et al.* (1972) The myopathy of prune belly syndrome. *J Neurol Sci* **15**: 153–65.

Alford BA, Peoples WM, Resnick JS *et al.* (1978) Pulmonary complications associated with the prune-belly syndrome. *Radiology* **129**: 401–7.

Amacker EA, Grass FS, Hickey DE *et al.* (1986) An association of prune belly anomaly with trisomy 21. *Am J Med Genet* **23**: 919–23.

Appleman Z, Golbus MS (1986) The management of fetal urinary tract obstruction. *Clin Obstet Gynecol* **29**: 483–6.

Arant BS Jr (1978) Development patterns of renal functional maturation compared in the human neonate. *J Pediatr* **92**: 705–12.

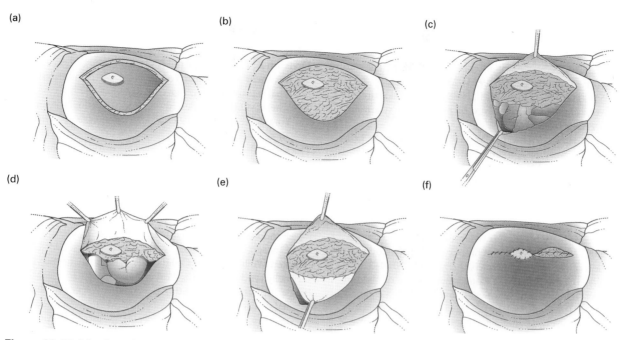

Figure 29.23 Monfort abdominoplasty. (*a*) An almond-shaped incision is made on the abdomen from the xiphoid to the pubic symphysis. (*b*) The full thickness of skin is removed, sparing the umbilicus. (*c*) The peritoneum is opened lateral to the musculofascial layer. Intra-abdominal surgery can be easily performed through these incisions. (*d*) The parietal peritoneum is incised at a level to achieve a normal-appearing waistline. (*e*) The edges of the musculofascial plate are sewn to the peritoneal incisions. (*f*) The lateral skin flaps are trimmed and sutured together in the midline. (From Monfort *et al.*, 1991, with permission from Williams and Wilkins.)

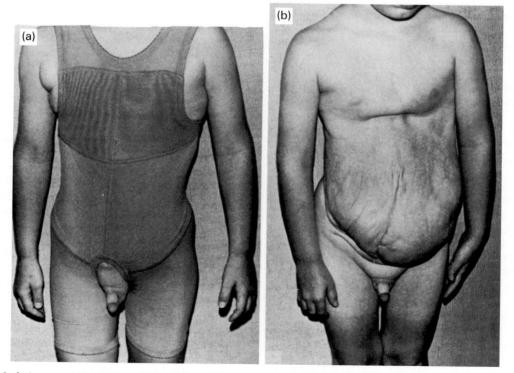

Figure 29.24 A 4-year-old boy, (*a*) with and (*b*) without his elasticized corset.

Baird PA, Sadovnick AD (1987) Letter to the editor: prune belly anomaly in Down syndrome. *Am J Med Genet* **26**: 747–8.

Batata MS, Chu FCH, Hilaris BI *et al.* (1982) Testicular cancer in cryptorchids. *Cancer* **49**: 1023–30.

Beasley SW, Henay F, Hutson JM (1988) The anterior urethra provides clues to the aetiology of prune belly syndrome. *Pediatr Surg Int* **3**: 169.

Bellah RD, States LJ, Duckett JW (1996) Pseudoprune belly syndrome: imaging, findings and outcome. *AJR Am J Roentgenol* **167**: 1389–93.

Berdon WE, Baker DH, Wigger HJ *et al.* (1977) The radiologic and pathologic spectrum of prune belly syndrome. *Radiol Clin North Am* **15**: 83–92.

Binard JE, Zoedler D (1968) Treatment of hypotonic decompensated urinary bladder. *Int Surg* **50**: 502–7.

Bloom DA (1991) Two step orchiopexy with pelviscopic clip ligation of the spermatic vessels. *J Urol* **145**: 1030–3.

Bourne CW, Cerny JC (1967) Congenital absence of abdominal muscles: report of six cases. *J Urol* **98**: 252–5.

Brinker MR, Palutis RS, Sarwark JF (1995) The orthopedic manifestations of prune belly (Eagle–Barrett) syndrome. *J Bone Joint Surg* **77**: 251–7.

Bukowski TP, Perlmutter AD (1994) Reduction cystoplasty in the prune belly syndrome: a long-term follow-up. *J Urol* **152**: 2113–16.

Burbidge KA, Amodio J, Berdon WE *et al.* (1987) Prune belly syndrome: 35 years of experience. *J Urol* **137**: 86–90.

Burke EC, Shin MH, Kelalis PP (1969) Prune belly syndrome: clinical findings and survival. *Am J Dis Child* **117**: 668–71.

Cabral B, Majidi A, Gonzales R (1988) Ectopic vasa deferentia in an infant with the prune belly syndrome. *J Urol (Paris)* **94**: 223–6.

Carey JC, Eggert L, Curry CJR (1982) Lower limb deficiency and the urethral obstruction sequence. *Birth Defects* **18**: 19–28.

Cazorla E, Ruiz F, Abad A *et al.* (1997) Prune belly syndrome: early antenatal diagnosis. *Eur J Obstet Gynecol Reprod Biol* **72**: 31–3.

Chen CP, Liu FF, Jan SW *et al.* (1997) First report of distal obstructive uropathy and prune belly syndrome in an infant with amniotic band syndrome. *Am J Perinatol* **14**: 31–3.

Chevalier RL (1989) Perinatal renal development and physiology. *AUA Update Ser* **8**: 58–60.

Cukier J (1977) Resection of the urethra with the prune belly syndrome. *Birth Defects* **13**: 95–6.

Curry CJR, Jensen K, Holland J *et al.* (1984) The Potter sequence: a clinical analysis of 80 cases. *Am J Med Genet* **19**: 679–702.

Cussen LJ (1971) The morphology of congenital dilatation of the ureter: intrinsic ureteral lesions. *Aust N Z J Surg* **41**: 185–94.

Deklerk DP, Scott WW (1978) Prostatic maldevelopment in the prune belly syndrome: a defect in prostatic stromal–epithelial interaction. *J Urol* **120**: 341–4.

Docimo SG (1995) The results of surgical therapy for cryptorchidism: a literature review and analysis. *J Urol* **154**: 1148–52.

Docimo SG, Moore RG, Kavoussi LR (1995) Laparoscopic orchidopexy in the prune belly syndrome: a case report and review of the literature. *Urology* **45**: 679–81.

Dreikorn K, Palmtag H, Rohl L (1978) Prune belly syndrome: treatment of terminal renal failure by hemodialysis and renal transplantation. *Eur Urol* **3**: 245–7.

Druschel CM (1995) A descriptive study of prune belly in New York State 1983 to 1989. *Arch Pediatr Adolesc Med* **149**: 70–6.

Duckett JW Jr (1974) Cutaneous vesicostomy in childhood. *Urol Clin North Am* **1**: 485–92.

Duckett JW Jr (1976) The prune belly syndrome. In: Kelalis PP, King LR, Belman AB (eds) *Clinical pediatric urology*. Philadelphia, PA: WB Saunders, 615–35.

Duckett JW (1986) Prune belly syndrome. In: Welsh KJ, Randolph JG, Ravich MM *et al.* (eds) *Pediatric surgery*. Chicago, IL: Year Book Medical Publishers, 1193–1203.

Duckett JW Jr, Knutrud O, Hohenfellner R *et al.* (1980) Prune belly syndrome. *Dialog Pediatr Urol* **3**: 1–7.

Eagle JF, Barrett GS (1950) Congenital deficiency of abdominal musculature with associated genitourinary abnormalities. A syndrome: report of 9 cases. *Pediatrics* **6**: 721–36.

Ehrlich RM (1985) The ureteral folding technique for megaureter surgery. *J Urol* **134**: 668–70.

Ehrlich RM, Brown WJ (1977) Ultrastructural anatomic observations of the ureter in prune belly syndrome. *Birth Defects* **13**: 101–3.

Ehrlich RM, Lesavoy MA, Fine RN (1986) Total abdominal wall reconstruction in the prune belly syndrome. *J Urol* **136**: 282–5.

Elder JS (1990) Intrauterine intervention for obstructive uropathy. *Kidney* **22**: 19–24.

Elder JS, Isaacs JT, Walsh PC (1982) Androgenic sensitivity of the gubernaculum testis: evidence for hormonal/mechanical interactions in testicular descent. *J Urol* **127**: 170–6.

Ewig JM, Grissom NT, Wohl ME (1996) The effect of the absence of abdominal muscles on pulmonary function and exercise. *Am J Respir Crit Care Med* **153**: 1314–21.

Fallat ME, Skoog SJ, Belman AT *et al.* (1989) The prune belly syndrome: a comprehensive approach to management. *J Urol* **142**: 802–5.

Fallon B, Welton M, Hawtrey C (1982) Congenital anomalies associated with cryptorchidism. *J Urol* **127**: 91–3.

Fitzsimmons RB, Keohane C, Galvin J (1985) Prune belly syndrome with ultrasound demonstration of reduced megacystis *in utero*. *Br J Radiol* **58**: 374–6.

Fontaine E, Salomon L, Gaganadoux MF *et al.* (1997) Long term results of renal transplantation in children with the prune belly syndrome. *J Urol* **158**: 892–4.

Fowler R, Stephens FD (1959) The role of testicular vascular anatomy in the salvage of high undescended testes. *Aust NZ J Surg* **29**: 92–6.

Frolich F (1839) Der Mangel der Muskeln, insbesondere der Seitenbauch muskeln. Dissertation. Wurzburg: C.A. Zurn.

Furness PD III, Cheng EY, Franco I *et al.* (1998) The prune belly syndrome: a new and simplified technique for abdominal wall reconstruction. *J Urol* **160**: 1195–7.

Gadziala NA, Kavade CY, Doherty FJ et al. (1982) Intrauterine decompression of megalocystis during the second trimester of pregnancy. *Am J Obstet Gynecol* **144**: 355–6.

Garlinger P, Ott J (1974) Prune belly syndrome: possible genetic implications. *Birth Defects* **10**: 173–80.

Gearhart JP, Lee BR, Partin AW et al. (1995) The quantitative histological evaluation of the dilated ureter of childhood. II: Ectopia, posterior urethral valves and the prune belly syndrome. *J Urol* **153**: 172–6.

Geary DF, MacLusky IB, Churchill BM et al. (1986) A broader spectrum of abnormalities in the prune belly syndrome. *J Urol* **135**: 324–6.

Gibbons DM, Cromie WJ, Duckett JW (1979) Management of the abdominal undescended testicle. *J Urol* **122**: 76–9.

Glazer GM, Filly RA, Callen PW (1982) The varied sonographic appearance of the urinary tract in the fetus and newborn with urethral obstruction. *Radiology* **144**: 563–8.

Golbus MS, Harrison MR, Filly RA et al. (1982) *In utero* treatment of urinary tract obstruction. *Am J Obstet Gynecol* **142**: 383–8.

Gonzalez R (1997) Editorial: Renal transplantation into abnormal bladders. *J Urol* **158**: 895.

Gonzalez R, Reinberg Y, Burke B et al. (1990) Early bladder outlet obstruction in fetal lambs induces renal dysplasia and the prune belly syndrome. *J Pediatr Surg* **25**: 342–5.

Greenfield SP, Rutigliano E, Steinhardt G et al. (1991) Genitourinary tract malformations and maternal cocaine abuse. *Urology* **37**: 455–9.

Greskovich FJ, Nyberg LM (1988) The prune belly syndrome: a review of its etiology, defects, treatment and prognosis. *J Urol* **140**: 707–12.

Guvenc M, Guvenc H, Aygun AD et al. (1995) Prune-belly syndrome associated with omphalocele in a female newborn. *J Pediatr Surg* **30**: 896–7.

Halbrecht I, Komulus L, Shabtai F (1972) Prune belly syndrome with chromosomal fragment. *Am J Dis Child* **123**: 518.

Hanna MK, Jeffs RD, Sturgess JM et al. (1977) Ureteral structure and ultrastructure. Part III. The congenitally dilated ureter (megaureter). *J Urol* **117**: 24–7.

Hannington-Kiff JG (1970) Prune belly syndrome and general anesthesia. *Br J Anesth* **42**: 649–52.

Harley LM, Chen Y, Rattner WH (1972) Prune belly syndrome. *J Urol* **108**: 174–6.

Henderson AM, Vallis CJ, Sumner E (1987) Anesthesia in the prune belly syndrome: a review of 36 cases. *Anesthesia* **42**: 54–60.

Hendren WH (1970) Functional restoration of decompensated ureters in children. *Am J Surg* **119**: 477–82.

Hinman F (1980) Alternatives to orchiectomy. *J Urol* **123**: 548–51.

Hoagland MH, Hutchins GM (1987) Obstructive lesions of the lower urinary tract in the prune belly syndrome. *Arch Pathol Lab Med* **111**: 154–6.

Hoagland MH, Frank KA, Hutchins GM (1988) Prune belly syndrome with prostatic hypoplasia, bladder wall rupture, and massive ascites in a fetus with trisomy 18. *Arch Pathol Lab Med* **112**: 1126–8.

Hutson JM, Beasley SW (1987) Aetiology of the prune belly syndrome. *Aust Paediatr J* **23**: 309–10.

Ives EJ (1974) The abdominal muscle deficiency triad syndrome – experience with ten cases. *Birth Defects* **10**: 127–35.

Jeffs RD, Comisarow RH, Hanna MK (1977) The early assessment for individualized treatment in the prune belly syndrome. *Birth Defects* **13**: 97–9.

Joller R, Scheier H (1986) Complete thoracic segmental insensibility accompanying prune belly syndrome with scoliosis. *Spine* **11**: 496–8.

Karamanian A, Kravath R, Nagashima H et al. (1974) Anesthetic management of prune belly syndrome: a case report. *Br J Anesth* **46**: 897–9.

Kinahan TJ, Churchill BM, McLorie GA et al. (1992) The efficiency of bladder emptying in prune belly syndrome. *J Urol* **148**: 600–3.

King LR (1969) Idiopathic dilatation of the posterior urethra in boys without bladder outlet obstruction. *J Urol* **102**: 783–7.

Kogan SJ, Weiss R, Hanna M et al. (1986) Successful renal transplantation into a patient with neurogenic bladder managed by clean intermittent catheterization. *J Urol* **135**: 563–5.

Kramer SA (1983) Current status of fetal intervention for hydronephrosis. *J Urol* **130**: 641.

Kroovand RL, Al-Ansari RM, Perlmutter AD (1982) Urethral and genital malformations in prune belly syndrome. *J Urol* **127**: 94–6.

Krueger RP (1981) Posterior urethral valves masquerading as prune belly syndrome. *Urology* **18**: 182–4.

Krueger RP, Hardy BE, Churchill BM (1980) Cryptorchidism in boys with posterior urethral valves. *J Urol* **124**: 101–2.

Kuruvilla AC, Kesler KR, Williams JW et al. (1987) Congenital cystic adenomatoid malformation of the lungs associated with prune belly syndrome. *J Pediatr Surg* **22**: 370–1.

Lattimer JK (1958) Congenital deficiency of the abdominal musculature and associated genitourinary anomalies: a report of 22 cases. *J Urol* **79**: 343–52.

Lubinsky M, Doyle K, Trunca C (1980) The association of prune belly with Turner's syndrome. *Am J Dis Child* **134**: 1171–2.

Maizels M, Stephens FD (1980) Valves of the ureter as a cause of primary obstruction of the ureter: anatomic, embryologic and clinical aspects. *J Urol* **123**: 742–7.

Marvin RG, Halff GA, Elshihabi I (1995) Renal allograft torsion associated with prune belly syndrome. *Pediatr Nephrol* **9**: 81–2.

Messing EM, Dibbell DG, Belzer FO (1985) Bilateral rectus femoris pedicle flaps for detrusor augmentation in the prune belly syndrome. *J Urol* **134**: 1202–4.

Meizner I, Bar-Zui J, Katz M (1985) Prenatal ultrasound diagnosis of the extreme form of prune belly syndrome. *J Clin Ultrasound* **13**: 581–3.

Mininberg DT, Montoya F, Okada K et al. (1974) Subcellular muscle studies in the prune belly syndrome. *J Urol* **109**: 524–6.

Moerman P, Fryns KP, Godderis PI (1982) Spectrum of clinical and autopsy findings in trisomy 18 syndrome. *J Genet Hum* **30**: 17–38.

Moerman P, Fryns JP, Goddeeris P *et al*. (1984) Pathogenesis of the prune-belly syndrome: a functional urethral obstruction caused by prostatic hypoplasia. *Pediatrics* **73**: 470–5.

Monfort G, Guys JM, Bocciardi A *et al*. (1991) A novel technique for reconstruction of the abdominal wall in prune belly syndrome. *J Urol* **146**: 639–40.

Monie IW, Monie BJ (1979) Prune belly and fetal ascites. *Teratology* **19**: 111–17.

Nakayama DK, Harrison MR, Chinn DH *et al*. (1984) Pathogenesis of prune belly. *Am J Dis Child* **138**: 834–6.

Noh PH, Cooper CS, Zderic SA *et al*. (1999) Prognostic factors in patients with prune belly syndrome. *J Urol* **162**: 1399–401.

Nunn IN, Stephens FD (1961) The triad syndrome: a composite anomaly of the abdominal wall, urinary system and testes. *J Urol* **86**: 782–94.

O'Kell RT (1969) Embryonic abdominal musculature associated with anomalies of the genitourinary and gastrointestinal system. *Am J Obstet Gynecol* **105**: 1283–4.

Orvis BR, Bottles K, Kogan BA (1988) Testicular histology in fetuses with prune belly syndrome and posterior urethral valves. *J Urol* **139**: 335–7.

Osathanondh V, Potter EL (1964) Pathogenesis of polycystic kidneys. *Arch Pathol* **77**: 510–12.

Osler WO (1901) Absence of the abdominal muscles, with distended and hypertrophied urinary bladder. *Bull Johns Hopkins Hosp* **12**: 331–3.

Pagon RA, Smith DW, Shepard TH (1979) Urethral obstruction malformation complex: a cause of abdominal muscle deficiency and the 'prune belly'. *J Pediatr* **94**: 900–6.

Palmer JM, Tesluck H (1974) Ureteral pathology in the prune belly syndrome. *J Urol* **111**: 701–7.

Parker RW (1895) Case of an infant in whom some of the abdominal muscles were absent. *Trans Clin Soc Lond* **28**: 201–3.

Parrott TS, Woodard JRR (1992) The Monfort operation for the abdominal wall reconstruction in the prune belly syndrome. *J Urol* **148**: 688–90.

Passerini-Glazel G, Araguna F, Chiozza L *et al*. (1988) The P.A.D.U.A. (progressive augmentation by dilating the urethral anterior) procedure for the treatment of severe urethral hypoplasia. *J Urol* **140**: 1247–9.

Perlman M, Levin M (1974) Fetal pulmonary hypoplasia, anuria, and oligohydramnios: clinicopathologic observations and review of the literature. *Am J Obstet Gynecol* **118**: 1119–22.

Perlmutter AD (1976) Reduction cystoplasty in prune belly syndrome. *J Urol* **116**: 356–62.

Petersen DS, Fish L, Cass AS (1972) Twins with congenital deficiency of abdominal musculature. *J Urol* **107**: 670–2.

Potter EL (1972) Abnormal development of the kidney. In: Potter EL (ed.) *Normal and abnormal development of the kidney*. Chicago, IL Year Book Medical Publishers 154–220.

Prescia G, Cruz JM, Weeks D (1982) Prenatal diagnosis of prune belly syndrome by means of raised maternal alpha-fetoprotein level. *J Genet Hum* **30**: 271–3.

Rabinowitz R, Barkin M (1978) Urinary tract reconstruction in the prune belly syndrome. *Urology* **12**: 333–5.

Rabinowitz R, Schillinger JF (1977) Prune belly syndrome in the female subject. *J Urol* **115**: 454–6.

Randolph JG (1977) Total surgical reconstruction for patients with abdominal muscular deficiency ('prune belly') syndrome. *J Pediatr Surg* **12**: 1033–43.

Randolph JG, Cavett C, Eng G (1981a) Surgical correction and rehabilitation for children with 'prune belly syndrome'. *Ann Surg* **193**: 757–62.

Randolph JG, Cavett C, Eng G (1981b) Abdominal wall reconstruction in the prune belly syndrome. *J Pediatr Surg* **16**: 960–4.

Ransley PG, Vordermark JS, Caldamone AA, Bellinger MF (1984) Preliminary ligation of the gonadal vessels prior to orchidopexy for the intra-abdominal testicle: a staged Fowler–Stephens procedure. *World J Urol* **2**: 266–9.

Reinberg Y, Manivel JC, Fryd P *et al*. (1989) The outcome of renal transplantation in children with the prune belly syndrome. *J Urol* **142**: 1541–2.

Reinberg Y, Shapiro E, Manivel JC (1991) Prune belly syndrome in females: a triad of abdominal musculature deficiency and anomalies of the urinary and genital systems. *J Pediatr* **118**: 395–8.

Riccardi VM, Grum CM (1977) The prune belly syndrome: heterogeneity and superficial X-linkage mimicry. *J Med Genet* **14**: 266–70.

Rogers LW, Ostrow PT (1973) The prune belly syndrome: report of 20 cases and description of a lethal variant. *J Pediatr* **83**: 786–93.

Rushton HG, Majd M, Chandra R, Yim D (1988) Evaluation of 99m technetium dimercaptosuccinic acid renal scans in experimental acute pyelonephritis in piglets. *J Urol* **140**: 1169–74.

Sayre R, Stephens R, Chonko AM (1986) Prune belly syndrome and retroperitoneal germ cell tumor. *Am J Med* **81**: 895–7.

Sellers BB, McNeal R, Smith RV *et al*. (1976) Congenital megalourethra associated with prune belly syndrome. *J Urol* **116**: 814–15.

Shenasky JH, Whelchel JD (1976) Renal transplantation in prune belly syndrome. *J Urol* **115**: 112–13.

Short KL, Groff DB, Cook L (1985) The concomitant presence of gastrochesis and prune belly syndrome in a twin. *J Pediatr Surg* **20**: 186–7.

Shrom SH, Cromie WJ, Duckett JW (1981) Megalourethra. *Urology* **17**: 152–6.

Sladezyk VE (1967) Das gehaufte familiare Duftreten des angeborenen Bauchmuskel-wanddefektes. *Zbl Chir* **92**: 426–8.

Smith CA, Smith EA, Parrott TS *et al*. (1998) Voiding function in patients with the prune belly syndrome after Monfort abdominoplasty. *J Urol* **159**: 1675–9.

Smythe AR (1981) Ultrasonic detection of fetal ascites and bladder dilatation with resulting prune belly. *J Pediatr* **98**: 978–80.

Snow BS, Duckett JW (1987) Prune belly syndrome. In: Gillenwater JY, Grayhack JT, Howards SS, Duckett JW (eds) *Adult and pediatric urology*. Chicago, IL: Year Book Medical Publishers, 1709–25.

Snyder HM, Harrison NW, Whitfield HN *et al*. (1976) Urodynamics in the prune belly syndrome. *Br J Urol* **48**: 663–70.

Stephens FD (1983) Triad (prune belly) syndrome. In: Stephens FD (ed.) *Congenital malformations of the urinary tract*. New York: Praeger, 485–511.

Stephens FD, Gupta D (1994) Pathogenesis of the prune belly syndrome. *J Urol* 152: 2328–31.

Straub E, Spranger J (1981) Etiology and pathogenesis of the prune belly syndrome. *Kidney Int* 20: 695–9.

Strumme EG (1903) Über die symmetrischen krongenitalen Bauchmuskeldefekte unt Über die Kombination derselben mit anderen Bildungsanomalien des Rumpfres. *Mitt Grenzigeb Med Chir* 11: 548–51.

Symonds DA, Driscoll SG (1974) Massive fetal ascites, urethral atresia and cytomegalic inclusion disease. *Am J Dis Child* 127: 895–7.

Tank ES, McCoy GB (1983) Limited surgical intervention in the prune belly syndrome. *J Pediatr Surg* 18: 688–91.

Tayakkanontak K (1963) The gubernaculum and its nerve supply. *Aust N Z J Surg* 33: 61–3.

Teramoto R, Opas LM, Andrassy R (1981) Splenic torsion with prune belly syndrome. *J Pediatr* 98: 91–2.

Tuch BA, Smith TK (1978) Prune belly syndrome: a report of twelve cases and review of the literature. *J Bone Joint Surg* 60: 109–11.

Uehling DT, Zadina SP, Gilbert E (1984) Testicular histology in triad syndrome. *Urology* 23: 364–6.

Wacksman J, Dinner M, Staffon RA (1980) Technique of testicular autotransplantation using a microvascular anastomosis. *Surg Obstet Gynecol* 150: 399–401.

Waldbaum RS, Marshall VS (1970) The prune belly syndrome: a diagnostic therapeutic plan. *J Urol* 103: 668–74.

Walker J, Prokurat AI, Irving IM (1987) Prune belly syndrome associated with exomphalos and anorectal agenesis. *J Pediatr Surg* 22: 215–17.

Welsh K, Kearney GP (1974) Abdominal musculature deficiency syndrome: prune belly. *J Urol* 111: 693–7.

Welsh KJ (1979) Abdominal musculature deficiency syndrome. In: Ravich MM, Welch KJ, Benson CD *et al.* (eds) *Pediatric surgery*. 3rd edition. Chicago, IL: Year Book Medical Publishers, 1220–32.

Wheatley JM, Stephens FD, Hutson JM (1996) Prune belly syndrome: ongoing controversies regarding pathogenesis and management. *Semin Pediatr Surg* 5: 95–106.

Whitaker RH (1973) Methods of assessing obstruction in dilated ureters. *Br J Urol* 45: 15–22.

Wigger JH, Blanc WA (1977) The prune belly syndrome. *Pathol Ann* 12: 17–39.

Williams DI, Burkholder GV (1967) The prune belly syndrome. *J Urol* 98: 244–9.

Woodard JR (1985) Prune-belly syndrome. In: Kelalis PP, King LR, Belman AB (eds) *Clinical pediatric urology*. Philadelphia, PA: WB Saunders, 805–24.

Woodard JR (1998) Editorial: Lessons learned in 3 decades of managing the prune belly syndrome. *J Urol* 159: 1680.

Woodard JR, Parrott TS (1978a) Reconstruction of the urinary tract in prune belly uropathy. *J Urol* 119: 824–8.

Woodard JR, Parrott TS (1978b) Orchidopexy in the prune belly syndrome. *Br J Urol* 50: 348–51.

Woodard JR, Trulock TS (1996) Prune belly syndrome. In: Walsh PC, Retik AB, Vaughan ED Jr, Wein AJ (eds) *Campbell's urology*. Philadelphia, PA: WB Saunders, 2159–2167.

Woodard JR, Smith EA (1998) Prune belly syndrome. In: Walsh PC, Retik AB, Vaughan ED Jr, Wein AJ (eds) *Campbell's urology*. Philadelphia, PA: WB Saunders, 1917–1938.

Woodhouse CRJ, Kellett MJ, Williams DI (1979) Minimal surgical interference in the prune belly syndrome. *Br J Urol* 51: 475–80.

Woodhouse CRJ, Ransley PG (1983) Teratoma of the testis in the prune belly syndrome. *Br J Urol* 55: 580–1.

Woodhouse CRJ, Ransley PG, Williams DI (1982) Prune belly syndrome – report of 47 cases. *Arch Dis Child* 57: 856–9.

Woodhouse CRJ, Snyder HM III (1985) Testicular and sexual function in adults with prune belly syndrome. *J Urol* 133: 607–9.

Wright JR, Barth RF, Neff JC *et al.* (1986) Gastrointestinal malformations associated with prune belly syndrome: three cases and a review of the literature. *Pediatr Pathol* 5: 421–48.

Yu TJ, Lai MK, Chen WF *et al.* (1995) Two stage orchiopexy with laparoscopic clip ligation of the spermatic vessels in prune belly syndrome. *J Pediatr Surg* 30: 870–2.

Gender identity and sex assignment

30

William G. Reiner

Introduction

For as the physician considers that the body will receive no benefit from taking food until the internal obstacles have been removed, so the purifier of the soul is conscious that his patient will receive no benefit from the application of knowledge until he is refuted, and from refutation learns modesty; he must be purged of his prejudices first and made to think that he knows only what he knows, and no more

[Plato, *Sophist*, 230 BC (tr. Jowettt)].

The decision-making process about sex assignment in the newborn with ambiguous genitalia is in a state of transition (Wilson and Reiner, 1998). Diagnoses and etiologies of disorders of sexual differentiation can be carefully delineated using appropriate biochemical, radiographic, and chromosomal studies. Yet few descriptive outcome data are available and it is not at all clear that a definitive diagnosis will dictate the choice of sex of rearing (Reiner, 1997a, 1999). It *is* clear that errors of sexual differentiation create an unusual and unique matrix for the development of psychosexual and psychosocial vulnerabilities and disorders in such children.

From a psychosexual vantage point it is important that the precise diagnosis be identified as quickly as possible in order to correlate the available clinical and research data with a prudent assignment of sex of rearing. Nevertheless, the sense of urgency must be tempered by the lack of diagnosis-specific outcome data for sex of rearing assignment. Prudence would dictate an assignment offering the least likelihood of the appearance of inappropriate secondary sexual changes at puberty or of a later self-declaration by a child or adolescent of inappropriate assignment of gender. An inappropriate choice of sex assignment can be disastrous, for a child reared in the wrong gender is likely to suffer from severe emotional difficulties, including gender confusion (Reiner, 1997a,

1999; Wilson and Reiner, 1998). However, deficient or inadequate genitalia can create novel and complex psychosexual developmental problems. What is the proper approach?

It is imperative that the multidisciplinary team comprehend the full ambiguity of any given clinical situation. Both the causes and effects of ambiguous genitalia infuse global ramifications for child development. A definitive diagnosis may not dispel the ambiguity. On the contrary, with numerous diagnoses the child's own recognition of gender identity may be difficult to predict and may only become apparent as the child develops and behaviors are observed or the child declares a gender identity. Contrary to the traditional paradigm of sex assignment in the neonate with ambiguous genitalia, current clinical and research data demand a variety of paradigms and a distinct flexibility in the clinical approach in order to provide the child with the best possible clinical outcome (Reiner, 1997a, b, 1999; Wilson and Reiner, 1998).

Clinical outcome data must transcend purely medical and surgical results. The child's developmental trajectory may well supersede structural and physiologic considerations. In other words, psychological health is paramount in child development. Mind and body cannot be separated any more than can mind and brain. Sexual function or fertility may be less important than the child's perception of gender identity. For example, if a 46 XX genetic female with congenital adrenal hyperplasia (CAH) perceives gender identity as male, is sexually attracted to females, and is uninterested in bearing children, then that child's potential fertility may not be relevant.

Ambiguity is foreign to neither parenting processes nor experiences. Quite the contrary, child rearing and parenting are often marked by ambiguity and ambivalence. While it is true that some tolerate ambiguity better than others, most parents can accept complex circumstances and move forward in child rearing if they are prepared and counseled about the nature of the ambiguity and offered supportive interventions during the child's development. Sophisticated psychiatric intervention can and should begin at the time of birth. The child psychiatrist, familiar with the basic science and clinical applications of medicine and surgery as well as being well versed in child development and parent effectiveness training, is the ideal member of the team to provide or direct such interventions. Not only can the psychiatrist educate the parents during open discussions, but he or she can also initiate an early outline for parenting skills that will incorporate potential child needs, parental needs, observational skills, and methods of coping with social requirements in the face of the ambiguity.

Thus, the ambiguity of the genitalia reflects and implies a potentially greater ambiguity in the child's development and portends vulnerabilities for the parents (Wilson and Reiner, 1998). The distinct genetic, physiologic, and anatomic incongruity of any given phenotype provides the material for psychiatric interventions tailored to each specific and unique clinical situation and to the parents' personalities and parenting styles. The ambiguity itself can be used as a positive reinforcement for parent effectiveness training. This early intervention should initiate the integration of the medical, surgical, and psychiatric team approaches to the developing infant and child.

Let us first evaluate the past and the present clinical and research data before addressing a new paradigm for the care of neonates with ambiguous genitalia.

The traditional paradigm

As it has evolved since the 1950s, four stipulations are generally embodied by the traditional paradigm for the approach to the neonate with ambiguous genitalia (Bradley et al., 1998; Glassberg, 1998):

- urgency of diagnosis and sex assignment;
- adequacy of the phallus;
- fertility, especially in the 46 XX neonate with CAH;
- potential cosmetic appearance of the reconstructed genitalia.

In the past, the treatment team argued for urgency and early gender assignment so that early surgical reconstruction would obviate the trauma of the parents or others seeing the intersex nature of the child with each diaper change. If a 46 XY male were born with an inadequate phallus, the child would be sex reassigned at birth, castrated, and reconstructed shortly thereafter. A 46 XX female born with an enlarged clitoris and fused labioscrotal folds would be sex assigned female and reconstructed shortly thereafter. In general, 46 XX female newborns with CAH were sex assigned female because of potential fertility, regardless of the degree of external virilization. Finally, the potential cosmetic appearance of the reconstructed genitalia was integrated into the first three criteria, recognizing that external female genitalia are generally easier to construct than male. In addition, it was felt in the past that gender identity is firmly established by about 18–24 months of age.

The treatment team generally counseled the parents not to discuss gender assignment or gender issues with other family members or friends (Bradley et al., 1998; Glassberg, 1998). Most importantly, they argued, the child was never to learn about the issues surrounding sex assignment. A sense of secrecy was thus advertently or inadvertently created.

In the last few years numerous data have challenged the traditional paradigm. Case reports have variously supported or refuted the paradigm (Reiner, 1996; Diamond and Sigmundson, 1997; Bradley et al., 1998; Schobur, 1998; Woodhouse, 1998). Lay support groups have challenged medical decision making. Preliminary clinical research data (Reiner, 2000b) from outcome studies cast doubt on prior assumptions and imply that the etiology of gender identity may be more biologically based than has been accepted over the last four decades. This combination of limited research and anecdotal data serves to emphasize a central and paramount question: is it ethical to subscribe to a specific medical and surgical approach when outcome data are lacking both for intervention and for no intervention? A related and important question arises: is it ethical to withhold important personal and medical data from a patient? The child's sex of rearing, after all, and a child's gender identity have profound lifelong implications for that child. This analytic climate, then, has led to a vigorous reappraisal of the approach to the neonate with ambiguous genitalia.

Sex assignment in the neonate with ambiguous genitalia: a reappraisal

Ultimately, an appropriate goal of the investigation of the newborn with ambiguous genitalia is to reveal those data concerning its genetic and steroid metabolism, internal ductal anatomy, gonadal histology, and degree of masculinization of the brain. The assessment and integration of these data should provide a rational decision for the appropriate sex of rearing. In other words, any decision will hopefully match the child's long-term sense of self. It is important to note that there are no data characterizing the psychological impact of early versus later surgery on the parents, let alone the child. In the normal genetic male with hypospadias or cryptorchidism, however, it may be wise to complete surgical correction quite early, to avoid significant memory for hypospadias surgery and to maximize gonadal function for cryptorchidism.

How do we measure virilization? How do we assess masculinization of the brain? What do we know and how do we know it? What is important in clinical outcomes and to whom is it important? Answers to these questions should provide the foundation for any paradigm or paradigms that may be needed in decision making for sex assignment in these children. Answers to these questions, however, are neither obvious nor facile.

In the first place there is a myriad of clinical diagnoses and neonatal presentations. It is not even clear whether two children with identical diagnoses will necessarily have the same or similar outcomes. Thus, each diagnosis and conceivably even each child could possibly suffer divergent outcomes. In order to comprehend how to approach children with ambiguous genitalia it will be necessary to understand how the child develops, responds, and perceives its identity. These are all functions determined by or dependent on the brain.

The brain

Developmentally, the central nervous system is defined by a set of probability patterns of neuronal development and synaptic interconnections. These patterns are critical for both brain development and function. Sexual dimorphism is one such pattern (Giedd *et al.*, 1997; De Courten-Myers, 1999) and is an integral facet of the integrated systems of brain activity and function. It is expressed in the developing brain at least as early as the end of the first or the beginning of the second trimester. Gender differences are found in cortical regions, deeper nuclei and ganglia, hemispheric interconnections, and in neuronal processes and synapses (Raisman and Field, 1971; Swaab *et al.*, 1995; Gorski, 1998; Kirn and Lombroso, 1998; Young and Chang, 1998). The full extent of such sexual dimorphism is not entirely known. Nevertheless, in view of such dimorphism it is little wonder that sexually dimorphic behaviors, performance, and even psychiatric disease patterns are both obvious and subtle as well as discernible (Zucker *et al.*, 1996; Giedd *et al.*, 1997; De Courten-Myers, 1999), often at remarkably young ages (Hines and Kaufman, 1994; Giedd *et al.*, 1997; Berenbaum, 1999), and cross-culturally (Slijper, 1984; Sato and Koizumi, 1991; Dittmann *et al.*, 1992), and may potentially be detectable in infancy or perhaps even in utero (DiPietro, 1981; 1996; McFadden, 1998). These findings raise fascinating possibilities for the future. It is also increasingly clear that children can come to recognize their gender identity when it differs from their infancy-assigned identity without major psychological collapse or psychiatric illness, although supportive, educational, and cognitive-based interventions are extremely important. Clinical and preliminary research data imply that gender identity may be established well before 18 months of age (Reiner, 1997a, 1999; Wilson and Reiner, 1998; Reiner *et al.*, 2000).

Like the cascade of events of embryonic sex determination, the complex interaction of events leading to sexual dimorphism of the brain has not yet been fully delineated. Nevertheless, critical periods for androgen brain imprinting, and possibly estrogen imprinting in the female, almost surely exist in human development as in other animals (Raisman and Field, 1971; Swaab *et al.*, 1995; Fitch and Denenberg, 1998; Gorski, 1998; Kirn and Lombroso, 1998; Young and Chang, 1998). Sexually dimorphic effects or coeffects of müllerian inhibiting substance (MIS), growth hormone, and other important circulating embryonic hormones are conceivable but unknown. The effects of the postnatal surge of testosterone in male infants as well as the correlation between the degree of external genital virilization and masculinization of the brain are also not clear. However, such a correlation may exist (Slijper, 1984; Sato and Koizumi, 1991; Dittmann *et al.*, 1992; Swaab *et al.*, 1995; Reiner, 1999).

Sexual dimorphism and sex assignment guidelines

Methodologies for studying sexually dimorphic behaviors and interests and for assessing gender identity continue to be refined. This is important because gender confusion may well be common throughout preadolescence, adolescence, and adulthood in many of the sex assigned and sex reassigned patients (Meyer-Bahlburg *et al.*, 1994; Reiner, 1999). Newer methodological techniques have improved the correlation between research findings and apparent gender identity outcomes, or perhaps what can be termed 'appropriate' outcomes, that is, outcomes consistent with what a child would perceive without external pressures to the contrary (Hines and Kaufman, 1994; Meyer-Bahlburg *et al.*, 1994; Berenbaum, 1999; Reiner *et al.*, 2000). In an appropriate outcome the child would be devoid or nearly devoid of gender confusion. If more technical data can be shown to provide a similar correlation, then future sex assignment decision-making processes may be rendered less controversial (DiPietro, 1996). The sexual dimorphism of click-evoked otoacoustic emissions (CEOAEs) may be such an example (McFadden, 1998). These are echo-like waveforms emitted by normal-hearing cochleas in response to a brief transient click sound. These CEOAEs are known to be differentially stronger in females than in males. The technology is easily performed at the bedside. In the meantime, clinical and research data are limited, yet clinical realities demand guidelines for decision making.

Sex assignment

Guidelines must take into account clinical situations, social demands, basic science and clinical research data, and medical and surgical potential. A dearth of information requires that guidelines must necessarily be general and perhaps even ambiguous. That is, ethical standards preclude specific recommendations when the outcome is unclear, regardless of the approach. Guidelines need to specify diagnostic and therapeutic options available to the patients and thus to the parents. Because of our incomplete knowledge, doctrinaire decisions or marked variation in clinical practice is probably unwise and imprudent. Non-specific guidelines are likely to become more specific as

clinical research outcome data accrues (Shaneyfelt *et al.*, 1999). Any guidelines should be questioned if they are not evidentiary in form (Cook and Giacomini, 1999).

It is in this light that generalized guidelines to sex assignment are offered in the spirit of assisting the treatment team as well as the parents in admittedly ambiguous circumstances. Two important caveats must be emphasized: (1) remove nothing that the child might later desire, and (2) be flexible. Surgical reconstructions are by nature traumatic. More importantly, tissue removed cannot be replaced. This rather obvious concept begets the second theme: flexibility. Flexibility in decision making will discourage surgical reconstructions that might later be regretted. It also allows for changes in clinical decisions if a child's individual and specific outcome appears to diverge from what was expected or predicted. Rather than emphasizing good reproductive function, sexual function, or normal looking genitalia (Bradley *et al.*, 1998; Glassberg, 1998), present guidelines should be predicated upon clinical outcome. A successful outcome ultimately is determined by the patient, not by preconceived notions. Again, without the luxury of prognosis the treatment team must be wary of irreversible surgical interventions until the child is sure of gender.

For example, gonadectomy can generally be postponed, as long as puberty is not approaching, until the child's declaration of identity, thus determining the fate of the gonad. Similarly, genital reconstruction can await such recognition of a child's perception of gender identity. The argument that the child's genitalia must have a good cosmetic appearance begs the question: a good appearance for whom? Experience with children with major reconstruction of the genitalia has shown that they spontaneously undress in front of virtually no one, whereas normal children explore nudity with apparent glee from about 2–6 years of age. Psychosexual anxiety in the group with genital abnormalities generally precludes their own genital self-exploration and often even genital awareness (Reiner *et al.*, 1999, 2000; Reiner, 2000). Thus, a good cosmetic appearance of the genitalia can await the child's recognition of gender identity, at which time he or she will nearly always desire reconstruction in line with that recognized identity. At that time, the child is likely to desire a good cosmetic appearance, even though their fervent genital modesty will probably remain.

Realizing that malformations in a newborn virtually always create psychological vulnerabilities in the parents, one must avoid the notion that emotional trauma can be obviated with medical or surgical approaches. Rather, continued psychological interventions are necessary for the parents and cannot be ignored. In addition, repeated assessments of the child throughout development encourage maximum understanding of the child's psychosexual and psychosocial directions and vulnerabilities, and thus determine an appropriate evolution of clinical decisions. It is this flexibility, with regular surgical, endocrinologic, pediatric, and psychiatric assessments, that can provide the child with the best potential clinical outcome. Surgical reconstruction can await, and can be directed by, an understanding of the child's perception of self, including gender identity, whenever that perception becomes clear. Children are highly likely to desire surgical reconstruction before adolescence and their involvement in decision making is likely to enhance their clinical outcome (Wilson and Reiner, 1998).

Psychosocial and psychosexual ramifications of sex assignment decisions are by nature complex and profound (Reiner *et al.*, 1999, 2000; Reiner, 2000). Longitudinal follow-up studies of homogeneous target populations are only now underway (Reiner, 1997a, 1999, 2000, unpublished data; Reiner *et al.*, 1999, 2000). It is sufficient to note that sex assignment decisions will have lifelong effects on the child.

No algorithm for sex assignment is likely to be entirely satisfactory. However, it is becoming increasingly clear that to determine sex assignment based on a child's genetic sex, the appearance of the external genitalia, potential fertility, or even social norms or parental desires is unsatisfactory. Given that the most important data for a specific child, its own sense of gender identity, may not be available until techniques of assessment are further refined, the following guidelines, carefully delineated and discussed with the parents, can assist in clinical decision making when combined with the available data.

General guidelines

When the phenotypic appearance of the genitalia is ambiguous, appropriate biochemical, radiographic, and chromosomal studies should be completed. The degree of external virilization should be carefully noted and recorded. Careful photographs are helpful. The parents should be informed of the ambiguity and that clinical investigation is underway. They should be advised that a sex assignment decision will be based on the appropriate data. The child psychiatrist can begin to assess the psychological effects of such ambiguity on the parents and initiate appropriate interventions. These may be supportive, educational, cognitive, or a combination of these.

Because of the likelihood of androgen imprinting, the quantity, timing, and duration of androgen exposure will all play a role in determining the degree of masculinization of the brain. Such variables are also pivotal for external virilization. Therefore, questions of potential sexual function, genital appearance, or even fertility may be subsumed by the intensity of *in utero* androgen effects on the brain. The intensity of androgen exposure that decrees a male gender identity may be below those androgen levels found in the typical male (Reiner, 1996). Thus, external virilization could potentially be a sensitive marker for masculine gender identity. It is probably wise to obtain neonatal serum androgen and perhaps MIS levels in any infant with external virilization. Otoacoustic emissions, which are simple to obtain, might also be of benefit (McFadden, 1998) and should be performed whenever possible. All data should be recorded and reported in any case series.

It must be emphasized that once any true medical emergency is diagnosed and medical intervention initiated, sex assignment should be determined quickly but not urgently. The treatment team must perform a rational and comprehensive evaluation. The parents must be provided with all of the investigational data and the options, and educated about the available clinical research data. They should understand normal genital variations. The team should gradually reassure the parents that, although the clinical situation appears ambiguous, it is very likely that their child will ultimately recognize its sense of gender identity. Thus, by being flexible the treatment team encourages flexibility in the parents, while reassuring them that they will receive support throughout their child's development. The parents must be given ample time before reaching a decision. Repetitive education is vital because initially their recall and comprehension are likely to be poor.

The parents may comprehend that phallic size and even potential for fertility, for example, may not affect gender identity. Gender identity does need to be assigned, but the parents can recognize the importance of flexibility. They can deduce the significance of an appropriate assignment of sex and that surgical correction will inevitably be indicated in the future. The parents will require interventions and support for their sense of loss, grief, or guilt. They also need to recognize their central role in the sex assignment decision. Referral to a support group may be helpful.

Early surgical and medical interventions should be directed at the child's physical health. Gonadectomy should be performed in those cases and at such time that malignant degeneration of the gonads is a significant risk. As reproductive technology improves, delaying gonadectomy in other cases permits the maximum chance for fertility as well as better recognition of the child's gender identity. Furthermore, in those cases in which the child's gender identity is congruent with the gonads, the requirement for exogenous hormones after puberty may be avoided.

Understanding and accepting the child's ultimate sense of gender identity not only decreases the possibility of gender confusion but also enables the child to play some role and have some control in his or her medical treatment. There are no data to show that postnatal feminizing hormones affect the evolution of gender identity. Thus, although steroid hormones have powerful behavioral implications at and after puberty, it would appear that imprinting during critical periods of early brain development may determine the intensity and even the possibility of those effects at puberty.

Because the child's psychosexual development is at least partly biologically determined, and because of ethical considerations in an open society, the treatment team should advise open communication between parent and child regarding the medical history. This is not to say that the child should be inundated with the realities of ambiguity. Rather, it is to argue for the ongoing involvement of the child psychiatrist with the parents and with the child in order to help the parents to assist the child's development within the context of that ambiguity. The child's questions should be answered simply and directly. Again, recurrent psychiatric assessments, including gender identity assessments, during the child's development are critical. Experience with complex gender identity issues in children with a myriad of diagnoses has shown that gender assessments may be fairly accurate after the age of 5 years and sometimes even younger (DiPietro, 1981, 1996; Berenbaum, 1999; Reiner et al., 2000). Indeed, children can often reassign their sex as young as 5 or 6 years of age (Reiner et al., 2000), well before the development of abstract reasoning.

Surgical genital reconstruction should be performed only after gender identity has been established, usually between the ages of 6 and 8 years. Although there are certain psychological disadvantages to surgical procedures on the genitalia once long-term memory has developed, the tragedy of a surgery later regretted is obvious.

These children are likely to endure psychosexual dysfunctions regardless of the approach taken (Reiner et al., 1999; Reiner, 2000). Gender confusion in a child with inappropriate assignment of sex accentuates the psychosexual vulnerabilities. Therefore, these children require frequent psychiatric assessment and intervention. It is very likely that genital reconstruction will be completed before puberty. Nevertheless, it is conceivable that some children may not come to clinical attention until an age more typical of adolescence. Limited case reports imply that these patients can do reasonably well (Reiner, 1996; Diamond and Sigmundson, 1997).

Knowing that sex assignment can be made independent of surgical reconstruction, attention surrounding the issue of an unequivocal sex-of-rearing approach becomes moot. Sex of rearing can be decided by the parents over the first few days or 1–2 weeks of the baby's life, after the treatment team has provided maximum data and the most likely gender outcome has been predicted by the data. Parents no longer will need to be bound by the tension and anxiety of attempting to maintain a sex of rearing that they fear may be incorrect or that may be discoverable by their child. Rather, they can pay attention to more typical child-rearing problems while they are learning to observe their child's behaviors and to discuss these regularly with the treatment team. If the child's developmental trajectory deviates from the assigned gender, interventions can gradually prepare the parents and child for a reassignment. Children seem to be quite tolerant of such interventions, whereas parents will probably experience a more difficult transition and acceptance.

This is not to argue that this transitional approach to sex assignment and sex of rearing will be without its own complexities and parent and child vulnerabilities. No approach to these children is without risk.

Rather, this transitional approach should increase the opportunity for children with ambiguous genitalia to achieve psychosocial and psychosexual development with a minimum of confusion until such time that outcome data can better enhance our predictive skills. In the absence of empirical data to support the traditional paradigm, such a transitional approach appears to be most reasonable from parental, social, psychological, and even legal perspectives.

The central element of this transitional paradigm is the following: a living system, although dependent on its environment, is not determined by it. The pattern of organization remains the same. The systems pattern of organization of the brain that leads to gender identity formation appears to be strongly biological. Once the brain has been organized under the influence of steroid hormones, be it female development or male development, and once the critical periods of that development have elapsed, the pattern of gender identity may not be able to change very much. That environment influences its appearance, that social norms play a part in gender roles, that hormones impact its expression do not detract from the realization that the pattern of gender identity remains. The gender interconnections of the brain interact with and relate to other interconnections within the brain and within the environment, and the essence of the child's existence lies in those relationships. These neuronal systems determine our capacity for reacting to and being influenced by the environment.

With these points in mind, let us proceed to a set of outcome-based guidelines.

Specific guidelines

1 *Significant* or *moderate* virilization of the external genitalia: regardless of the genotype, serious consideration should be given to a sex assignment of male.

   (a) 46 XY or 46 XY/45 X0 mosaic genotype: gender identity is most likely to be male. Often these 46 XY children demonstrate male gender identity by the age of 3 or 4 years and can be surgically reconstructed at a fairly young age.

   (b) 46 XX genotype (CAH): in 46 XX females with CAH (or significant exogenous androgen exposure) the ovaries can be ignored well into the prepubertal years while careful assessments slowly delineate the unfolding of the child's gender identity. At the very least, the treatment

team must educate the parents that their child's behaviors may be more male typical than female typical. Female gender identity may be associated with homosexual or bisexual behaviors. Pregnancy after adolescence may be avoided.

2 *Mild* virilization of the external genitalia: the genotype may be only a fair predictor of future gender identity.

   (a) 46 XY or 46 XY/45 X0 mosaic genotype: the testes have probably failed to develop properly. If serum androgen levels at birth are very low or if MIS is low or absent, female sex assignment must be seriously considered. However, other than for prevention of gonadal malignant degeneration surgical reconstruction should await the child's determination of gender identity. Patients with micropenis have scrotal fusion and generally will have male gender identity. They should be reared as male.

   (b) 46 XX genotype: in many cases of simple virilizing CAH, gender identity is likely to be female (Berenbaun, 1999). Fertility issues may therefore be very important. With low neonatal serum androgen levels and absent MIS, gender identity is most likely to be female. Therefore, sex assignment as female is indicated. Female gender identity may be associated with homosexual or bisexual behaviors. Some such children may recognize themselves as male. Appropriate surgical reconstruction based on a child's gender identity should be performed before the onset of puberty.

3 *Feminine* external genitalia or *clitoral hypertrophy* only: regardless of the genotype gender identity is likely to be female. Sex assignment as female is indicated. Vaginal reconstruction should be conducted at an appropriate age for surgical success. Gonads can be treated based on medical or developmental considerations (e.g. malignancy potential and breast development).

Within intersex conditions, the degree of androgen responsiveness or activity may vary and the timing of exposure may differ for brain and genitalia. Thus, for example, 46 XY children with 5a-reductase deficiency are best assigned male. Accentuated virilization will generally occur with puberty, but the brain is probably already imprinted. Incomplete androgen insensitivity syndrome children should be assigned according to the above guidelines but with the caveat that brain imprinting will be very difficult to predict. These children may have a female gender identity or a male gender identity, and the children may even virilize further at puberty as a result of residual receptor or hormonal activity. True hermaphrodites with their variable chromosomal and phenotypic pictures also fall within the above guidelines, with gender assignment based on predicted gender identity. Similarly, Klinefelter and Turner syndromes fall within the guidelines and should be sex assigned male and female, respectively.

Conclusions

Thus, with our present knowledge external genital appearance can be used to estimate the degree and timing of androgen exposure of the brain and therefore can *estimate* an appropriate sex of rearing. Nevertheless, the critical awareness is that surgical reconstruction should be reserved for those patients whose gender identity is solidly established. This will probably occur by about the age of 6–8 years. In 46 XX CAH females who present a mixed behavioral picture through their early school years, ample time should be allotted for full gender identity assessment because of potential fertility. Thus, these children may have to be reassessed regularly until they are 9 or 10 years of age, although surgical decisions can probably be made before the onset of puberty. This approach can also be used for other children with a mixed behavioral picture during development. Psychosexual and psychosocial ramifications for all of these children warrant the continued involvement of the experienced child psychiatrist.

References

Berenbaum SA (1999) Effects of early androgens on sex-typed activities and interests in adolescents with congenital adrenal hyperplasia. *Horm Behav* **35**: 102–10.

Bradley SJ, Oliver GD, Chernick AB, Zucker KJ (1998) Experiment of nurture: ablatio penis at 2 months, sex reassignment at 7 months, and a psychosexual follow-up in young adulthood. *Pediatrics* **102**: 132–3.

Cook D, Giacomini M (1999) The trials and tribulations of clinical practice guidelines. *JAMA* **281**: 1950–1.

De Courten-Myers GM (1999) The human cerebral cortex: gender differences in structure and function. *J Neuropathol Exp Neurol* **58**: 217–26.

Diamond M, Sigmundson HK (1997) Sex reassignment at birth: Long-term review and clinical implications. *Arch Pediatr Adolesc Med* **151**: 298–304.

DiPietro JA (1981) Rough and tumble play: a function of gender. *Dev Psychol* **17**: 50–8.

DiPietro JA (1996) Fetal neurobehavioral development. *Child Dev* **67**: 2553–67.

Dittmann RW, Kappes ME, Kappes MH (1992) Sexual behavior in adolescent and adult females with congenital adrenal hyperplasia. *Psychoneuroendocrinology* **17**: 153–70.

Fitch RH, Denenberg VH (1998) A role for ovarian hormones in sexual differentiation of the brain. *Behav Brain Sci* **21**: 311–52.

Giedd JN, Castellanos FX, Rajapakse JC et al. (1997) Sexual dimorphism of the developing human brain. *Prog Neuropsychopharmacol Biol Psychiatry* **21**: 1185–201.

Glassberg KI (1998) The intersex infant: early gender assignment and surgical reconstruction. *J Pediatr Adolesc Gynecol* **11**: 151–4.

Gorski RA (1998) Sexual differentiation of the brain. In: Bittar EE, Bittar N (eds) *Principles of medical biology: reproductive endocrinology and biology*. Stamford, CT: JAI Press, 1–23.

Hines M, Kaufman FR (1994) Androgen and the development of human sex-typical behavior: rough-and-tumble play and sex of preferred playmates in children with congenital adrenal hyperplasia (CAH). *Child Dev* **65**: 1042–53.

Kirn J, Lombroso PJ (1998) Development of the cerebral cortex: XI. Sexual dimorphism in the brain. *J Am Acad Child Adolesc Psychiatry* **37**: 1228–30.

McFadden D (1998) Sex differences in the auditory system. *Dev Neuropsychol* **14**: 261–98.

Meyer-Bahlburg HFL, Sandberg DE, Yager TJ et al. (1994) Questionnaire scales for the assessment of atypical gender development in girls and boys. *J Psychol Hum Sexuality* **6**: 19–39.

Raisman G, Field PM (1971) Sexual dimorphism in the preoptic area of the rat. *Science* **173**: 731–3.

Reiner WG (1996) Case study: sex reassignment in a teenage girl. *J Am Acad Child Adolesc Psychiatry* **35**: 799–803.

Reiner WG (1997a) Sex assignment in the neonate with intersex or inadequate genitalia. *Arch Pediatr Adolesc Med* **151**: 1044–5.

Reiner WG (1997b) To be male or female – that is the question (editorial). *Arch Pediatr Adolesc Med* **151**: 224–5.

Reiner WG (1999) Assignment of sex in neonates with ambiguous genitalia. *Curr Opin Pediatr* **11**: 363–5.

Reiner WG (2000) Psychosexual dysfunction in males with genital anomalies: pre- and early adolescence, Tanner stages I–III (in press).

Reiner WG, Meyer-Bahlburg HFL, Gearhart JP (2000) Female-assigned genetic males: androgens and male gender identity (in press).

Reiner WG, Gearhart JP, Jeffs R (1999) Psychosexual dysfunction in males with genital anomalies: late adolescence, Tanner stages IV–VI. *J Am Acad Child Adolesc Psychiatry* **38**: 865–72.

Sato T, Koizumi S (1991) Effects of fetal androgen on childhood behavior. *Acta Paediatr Jpn* **33**: 639–44.

Schobur JM (1998) Early feminizing genitoplasty or watchful waiting. *J Pediatr Adolesc Gynecol* **11**: 154–6.

Shaneyfelt TM, Mayo-Smith MF, Rothwangl J (1999) Are guidelines following guidelines? The methodological quality of clinical practice guidelines in the peer-reviewed medical literature. *JAMA* **281**: 1900–5.

Slijper FM (1984) Androgens and gender role behaviour in girls with congenital adrenal hyperplasia (CAH). *Prog Brain Res* **61**: 417–22.

Swaab DF, Gooren LJ, Hoffman MA (1995) Brain research, gender and sexual orientation. *J Homosex* **28**: 283–301.

Wilson BE, Reiner WG (1998) Management of intersex: a shifting paradigm. *J Clin Ethics* **9**: 360–9.

Woodhouse CR (1998) Sexual function in boys born with exstrophy, myelomeningocele, and micropenis. *Urology* **52**: 3–11.

Young WJ, Chang C (1998) Ontogeny and autoregulation of androgen receptor mRNA expression in the nervous system. *Endocrine* **9**: 79–88.

Zucker KJ, Bradley SJ, Oliver G *et al*. (1996) Psychosexual development of women with congenital adrenal hyperplasia. *Horm Behav* **30**: 300–18.

Sexual differentiation and intersexuality　31

Ian A. Aaronson

Introduction

Intersexuality represents a rare but important group of disorders which usually present at birth with ambiguity of the external genitalia. It is imperative that these conditions are recognized early and steps taken to identify the underlying cause as, in some cases, a delay may result in sudden collapse and death from an underlying metabolic disorder. Deciding the appropriate sex of rearing is often problematic. Although a provisional assignment, based on the appearance of the external genitalia, can often be made, this is generally best delayed until the definitive diagnosis is determined.

The investigation of these cases is best managed by a team comprising a pediatric urologist, a pediatric endocrinologist, a geneticist, a radiologist, a pathologist, and a clinical psychologist or pediatric psychiatrist, all of whom should have a special interest in intersexuality. The object of investigation is not to reveal the true sex of the child, for this concept is of little practical value. Instead, it is to provide information concerning the chromosomes, internal duct anatomy, gonadal histology and steroid metabolism upon which to base a rational recommendation as to the appropriate sex of rearing.

Normal sexual differentiation

Ambiguity of the external genitalia results from either virilization of otherwise normal female external genitalia or an arrest of the process of masculinization which normally occurs between 7 and 14 weeks gestation. An understanding of intersex disorders depends, therefore, on an appreciation of the basic steps that lead to normal sexual differentiation.

During the first 6 weeks after conception, the internal and external genitalia of the male and female embryo are identical (Fig. 31.1). The gonads comprise a condensation of cells on the caudal aspect of the urogenital ridge alongside which lie the developing wolffian and müllerian ducts. These are destined to form, respectively, the male and female internal ducts. The external genitalia are represented by a genital tubercle, urethral folds, and labioscrotal swellings that surround the urogenital groove (Fig. 31.2).

The external genitalia

In the female the external genitalia require little adaptation to assume their definitive form. The genital tubercle becomes the glans of the clitoris and the urogenital groove the vestibule. The urethral folds remain small and separate, forming the labia minora, and the genital swellings the labia majora.

The external genitalia of the male, in contrast, undergo a rapid and profound modification. Beginning in the 8th week, the genital tubercle begins to enlarge and elongate. Growth, however, is initially disproportionate so that in the early stages there is some ventral curvature of the developing penis. In parallel with this growth the urogenital groove begins to close over, commencing proximally, as a result of

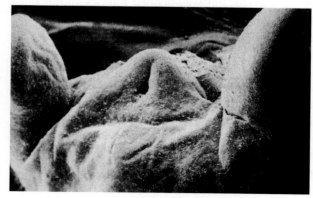

Figure 31.1 External genitalia at the indifferent stage in a 7-week embryo. Scanning electron micrograph. (From Rowsell and Morgan, 1987, *Br J Plast Surg* **40**: 201–5, with permission.)

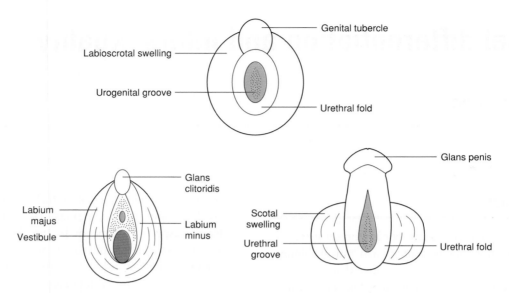

Figure 31.2 Differentiation of the external genitalia. Diagram illustrating the fate of the anlagen in the female (bottom left) and male (bottom right).

the migration of mesenchyme which sweeps around to build up tissue ventrally between the newly formed urethra and the skin, thus correcting the chordee. The genital swellings expand and migrate caudally to form the scrotum. Development of the external genitalia is thus almost entirely complete by the end of the 3rd month (Fig. 31.3).

The internal genitalia

The gonads in the early embryo are identical in both sexes and appear as swellings in the central portion of the urogenital ridges on either side of the midline on the dorsal aspect of the coelomic cavity. The earliest manifestation of ovarian differentiation is meiosis of the germ cells, but well-defined follicles appear only late in fetal life when steroid production can be demonstrated for the first time. By the 9th week, the wolffian ducts have begun to regress, sometimes leaving vestiges in the form of the epoophoron of the ovary at one end and Gartner's duct distally. From this point onwards, the müllerian ducts differentiate into the fallopian tubes and, after fusion of their caudal ends, form the body and cervix of the uterus together with the upper third of the vagina, which establishes continuity with the urogenital sinus (Fig. 31.4).

The first signs of testicular organization can be recognized at 42 days when cells in the medial portion of the mesonephros aggregate as cords of primordial Sertoli cells. These envelope inflowing germ cells,

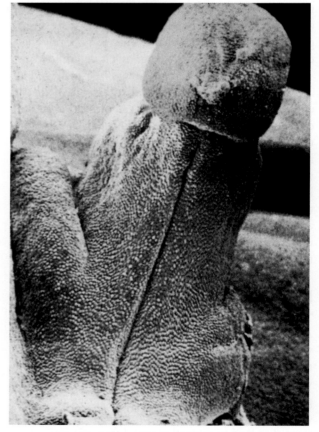

Figure 31.3 Phallus of a male fetus at 12 weeks' gestation. The ventral raphe marks the site of fusion of the urethral folds. Scanning electron micrograph. (From Rowsell and Morgan, 1987, *Br J Plast Surg* **40**: 201–5, with permission.)

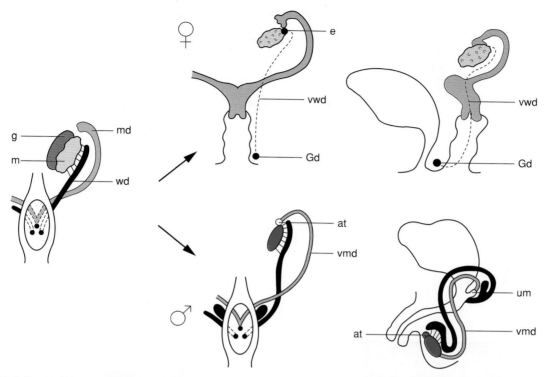

Figure 31.4 Fate of the wolffian and müllerian ducts. In the male, the wolffian duct forms the epididymis, vas, and seminal vesicle. Note the remnants of the müllerian duct. In the female, the müllerian ducts form the fallopian tubes, uterus, and upper third of the vagina. Note the remnants of the wolffian duct. g=gonad; m=mesonephros; md=müllerian duct; wd=wolffian duct; at=appendix testis; vmd=vestigial müllerian duct; um=utriculus masculinus; e=epoophoron; vwd=vestigial wolffian duct; Gd=Gartner's duct.

thus forming primordial tubules. Leydig cells migrate into the developing testicular interstitium where they come to rest in clusters between the tubules. Differentiation of the testis precedes that of the ovary and occurs primarily in the central, medullary portion of the indifferent gonad.

The wolffian or mesonephric duct, which first appeared during the 3rd week of fetal life as solid cords adjacent to the nephrogenic ridge, grows to form the epididymis, vas, ejaculatory duct, and seminal vesicle. The rudimentary prostate also forms at this stage. A vestige of the müllerian duct is frequently encountered as an appendix testis at one end and a small utriculus masculinus at the other.

The sexual differentiation cascade

The foundations of our understanding of mammalian sexual differentiation are the pioneering experiments of Alfred Jost carried out in rabbit embryos in wartime France in the 1940s. He showed that excising the primordial gonads in the early embryo result-

ed in rabbits with internal and external genitalia that were entirely female irrespective of their genetic sex. He concluded firstly, that the chromosomes did not directly determine phenotypic sex and, secondly, that female differentiation did not depend on the presence of gonads and was, therefore, the pathway of default (Jost, 1947).

In a second series of experiments, Jost replaced the primordial gonads with a crystal of testosterone prioprionate. He observed that the external genitalia subsequently masculinized and the wolffian ducts developed but the müllerian ducts also persisted and went on to form fallopian tubes and a uterus. He concluded that, for normal masculinization to occur, the testes must secrete not only testosterone, but another substance which was responsible for suppression of the müllerian ducts which he called 'l'hormone inhibitrice' (Jost, 1970). This was eventually confirmed by Blanchard and Josso (1974) and it is now known in the European literature as anti-müllerian hormone and the North American literature as müllerian inhibiting substance (MIS) (Fig. 31.5).

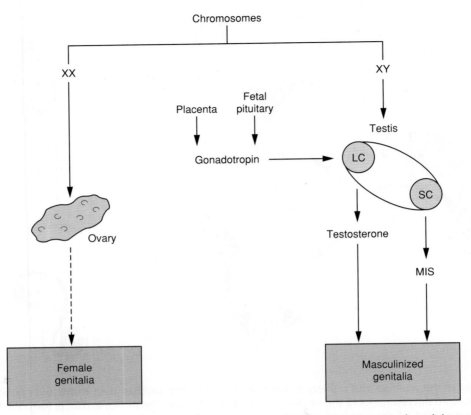

Figure 31.5 Pathways of normal sexual differentiation. The role of the chromosomes is solely to determine the nature of the gonads. Gonadotropin stimulation of the testes releases testosterone. This, together with müllerian inhibiting substance (MIS), determines the nature of the internal ducts and external genitalia. SC=Sertoli cells; LC=Leydig cells.

Molecular basis of testis development

The differentiation of the internal and external genitalia along male lines is a response to a signal from the Y chromosome directing the indifferent gonad to form a testis. Thus, embryos with either a 46,XY or a 47,XXY karyotype will develop testes, whereas among those without a Y chromosome, for example a 46,XX or 45,XO karyotype, the gonad will differentiate in the direction of an ovary. It was not long after the importance of the Y chromosome in testicular development was appreciated that the quest for what came to be known as the testis determining factor was underway.

SRY gene

The search for the precise locus on the Y chromosome responsible for testicular differentiation ended, after several false leads. In 1990 Sinclair *et al.*, examining translocated material in XX males, identified a 35 kb sequence in the 11.3 band of the short arm of the Y chromosome, adjacent to the pseudoautosomal boundary, which was identical to that found in normal males. This was designated the sex-determining region of the Y chromosome (SRY). Support for its role in testis determination came from mouse embryos, where it was found to be expressed exclusively in the caudal urogenital ridge at the earliest stages of development. Conclusive evidence came from elegant experiments in which a 14 kb DNA fragment from the SRY region was inserted in the genome of female mouse embryos. They subsequently developed testes and a male phenotype (Koopman *et al.*, 1991). The SRY gene is now known to comprise a single exon within which lie 237 base pairs (bp) that encode an evolutionarily highly conserved group of 79 amino acids known as the HMG box, so called because of their homology to the widely distributed highly mobile group of proteins. The gene acts as a transcription factor, the protein product of which binds to specific sequences causing partial unraveling of the DNA double helix. This spatial rearrangement exposes adjacent regions of DNA which are potential binding sites for the products of other genes.

The realization that genes other than SRY are involved in the formation of a testis came from the study of 46,XY individuals raised as females because their testes had failed to develop. In 85% of these cases, the SRY gene appeared to be entirely normal. Furthermore, failure of testicular development is a feature of several other clinical syndromes in which specific chromosomal mutations and deletions have been identified. The genes which are presently recognized as being essential for testicular development and their presumed site of action are recorded in Fig. 31.6.

WT-1 gene

Among patients with the WAGR (**W**ilms' tumor, **a**niridia, **g**igantism, and **r**enogenital) syndrome and the related Denys–Drash syndrome, in which the testes may be dysgenetic, defects in the WT-1 tumor suppressor gene have now been identified. Study of human embryos has revealed that the WT-1 gene is expressed not only, as expected, in the developing kidney but also in the primitive gonad, confirming its role early on in the testicular developmental cascade (Pritchard-Jones *et al.*, 1990).

SF-1

Steroidogenic factor-1 (SF-1) is a nuclear receptor protein that regulates the production of hydroxylase

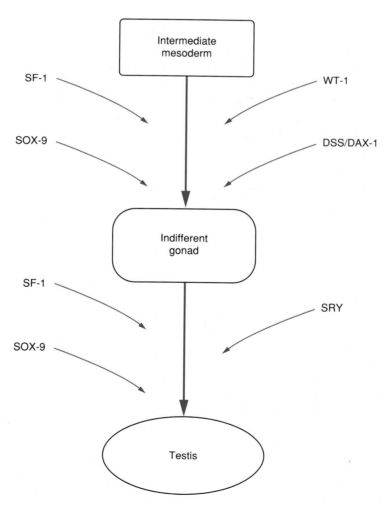

Figure 31.6 Diagram showing genes believed to be involved in testicular development and their presumed site of action.

enzymes essential for steroid synthesis. In addition to its expression in the adrenal glands, ovaries, and Leydig cells of the testes, transcripts of the SF-1 gene have been detected in the mouse urogenital ridge at the stage of the indifferent gonad before Leydig cells become apparent, suggesting an early role in testicular development. This was confirmed when mice bred for a deletion for the structurally very similar Ftz-F1 gene died shortly after birth and were found at autopsy to have not only adrenal agenesis but also absent gonads (Luo *et al.*, 1994).

SOX-9

Mutations of the SOX-9 gene are routinely found in patients with campomelic dysplasia, a dominantly inherited and usually fatal osteochondrodysplasia. Among those with an XY karyotype approximately 75% also have dysgenetic gonads, which give rise to the ambiguous genitalia that are a characteristic feature of this condition.

In the human fetus SOX-9 has been found to be abundantly expressed in chondrocytes but also in the differentiating testis, indicating that it has a role, although relatively late, in testicular development (Wagner *et al.*, 1994). In the mouse embryo, SOX-9 was found to be expressed in the genital ridge before any gonadal differentiation had occurred (Kent *et al.*, 1996), suggesting that the gene may act at two distinct sites. Its precise action is presently unclear but may be primarily concerned with the formation of a connective tissue framework upon which the integrated architecture of both bones and testes depend.

DAX-1 gene

Bernstein *et al.* (1980) reported a pair of female siblings with dysgenetic gonads who had a 46,XY karyotype in which a portion of the short arm of the X chromosome was duplicated. This raised the question of whether suppression of their testes was the result of a double dose of X material, reminiscent of the sex-determining mechanism in more primitive life forms. Other patients were subsequently identified in whom it was shown their SRY gene was intact. Analysis of the X fragment confirmed it to be a duplication of part of the Xp21 band (Bardoni *et al.*, 1994). This was designated the dosage-sensitive sex reversal region of the X (DSS) that overlaps a locus where deletions are known to occur in patients with congenital adrenal hypoplasia (CAH). The gene responsible for sex reversal in these cases was therefore designated DAX-1 (for Dss-Ahc critical region of X).

In the mouse embryo DAX-1 is expressed in the urogenital ridge (Swain *et al.*, 1996), suggesting that this gene is concerned with the early stages of testicular development. Curiously, males with CAH, who would be expected to have a defective DAX-1 gene, are found to have normal testes, indicating that we do not yet fully understand the interaction of this gene with others involved in the formation of the testis.

Other autosomal genes

Evidence for the involvement of other genes in the development and differentiation of the testes comes from several case reports. Bennett *et al.* (1993) described a 46,XY female with gonadal dysgenesis in whom a terminal deletion was found in the short arm of chromosome 9. Another XY patient with ambiguous genitalia and testicular dysgenesis was reported by Wilkie *et al.* (1993) in whom a deletion was noted in the long arm of chromosome 10. Gonadal dysgenesis with subsequent phenotypic ambiguity is also a feature of a number of multiple defect syndromes, including the Smith–Lemli–Opitz, the genito-palato-cardiac, and the α-thalassemia mental retardation syndromes.

Until recently, it was assumed that the genes involved in testicular development function positively as transcription activators triggering the next step along the developmental cascade. However, several paradoxes remained. Most notable was the observation that some XX males seemed to be totally lacking the SRY gene yet had apparently normal testes. To explain this, McElreavey *et al.* (1993) proposed that the SRY gene product acts to suppress another hitherto unidentified gene, which they called 'gene Z', the role of which is to inhibit testis formation. Although much progress has been made, we are still far from finally understanding the molecular complexities of testicular development.

Testosterone

Although it has been suggested there is some autonomous testosterone synthesis by the Leydig cells, it is generally accepted that production is initially dependent on stimulation by placental gonadotropin. This triggers the conversion of cholesterol via five sequential enzymic steps to testosterone which can first be detected in the 8-week embryo, reaching a peak concentration at 12 weeks. At this stage, the circulation is only just established so that its early action of stimulating the development of the adjacent wolffian duct is by local diffusion. The concentration of testosterone reaching the external genitalia is relatively low and is augmented by the enzyme 5α-reductase, which converts testosterone to dihydrotestosterone, a substance that is approximately 2.5 times more potent. The action of both hormones, however, depends on the presence in the target cells of functioning androgen receptors.

By 14 weeks, the genitalia are complete but testosterone continues to be secreted for the remainder of gestation under the influence of fetal pituitary gonadotropin and results in continuing growth of the penis (Aaronson, 1994).

Müllerian inhibiting substance

This hormone is produced by the immature Sertoli cells, of which the early tubules are largely composed. It is active only during a very brief window between 7 and 8 weeks of gestation. It has been identified as a glycoprotein polymer consisting of two subunits linked by disulfide bonds (Picard and Josso, 1984). MIS is a member of the transforming growth factor-β (TGF-β) 'superfamily' of growth factors, that regulate cell growth and differentiation. It is secreted as a prohormone that undergoes protease cleavage to expose its active carboxyl terminus (Nachtigal and Ingraham, 1996). This hormone then binds to an MIS receptor on the mesenchymal cells that surround the müllerian duct (Lane and Donahoe, 1998). The nature of the interaction between these cells and duct epithelium is presently not clear but the consequence is reabsorption of the müllerian duct system.

It is now appreciated that MIS has actions other than related to müllerian duct inhibition. MIS receptors are also expressed in Leydig cells, where the hormone appears to act as a negative-feedback regulator of testosterone production (Racine et al., 1998). Evidence for this comes from the study of two sets of male transgenic mice. The testes of those unable to produce MIS showed Leydig cell hyperplasia, whereas those which overexpressed MIS appeared to be testosterone deficient and had internal and external genitalia that were feminized (Behringer, 1995). The inhibitory action of MIS on testosterone production appears to be both at the level of Leydig cell differentiation and on intracellular steroid synthesis.

In spite of much progress, MIS in many respects remains a mystery hormone. It continues to be secreted throughout gestation long after the brief window of müllerian inhibition has passed. Hutson (1985) has suggested that its role at this stage is in inducing testicular descent. The hormone, however, goes on being produced in high concentrations throughout childhood, falling only at puberty. It is also secreted in trace amounts by the ovary in girls in whom levels markedly rise at puberty where it appears to regulate aromatase activity. Furthermore, its receptors have been identified in many other tissues throughout the body but its role in these situations remains obscure.

Ovarian development

The mechanisms governing the transformation of the indifferent gonad into an ovary are poorly understood. There is some evidence that DSS/DAX-1 may play a role but what other genes are involved is presently a matter of speculation.

Sexual differentiation of the brain

There is little doubt that boys are psychologically quite different from girls. For many years, it was generally assumed that this was largely the result of the way in which the child was reared rather than because of any intrinsic differences. It was argued, therefore, largely because of the teaching of Money et al. (1955), that if a sex change were carried out prior to about 18 months of age, when sexual identity begins to be established, a satisfactory outcome could be anticipated.

During the 1990s, however, it has become apparent that testosterone imprinting of the fetal brain may play a role in determining an ultimately male gender identity. The evidence for this comes from both clinical and experimental studies. Several clinical reviews have confirmed a widely held impression that girls with CAH are more tomboyish in their behavior than controls. Furthermore, as adolescents and adults, they are less likely then their peers to form lasting heterosexual relationships, marry, or have children (Zucker et al., 1996). Money et al. (1984) reported that as women, these patients showed a significantly increased incidence of bisexuality and homosexuality, although this has not been confirmed by others (Kuhnle et al., 1995).

It is not certain, however, that these behavioral differences can be attributed solely to testosterone imprinting of the brain, either antenatally or in the immediate postnatal period. Many of these patients had been poorly controlled medically and had often undergone genital surgery late in childhood and were left with external genitalia which were, both cosmetically and functionally, unsatisfactory. Furthermore, when these patients were compared with a group of controls who had other chronic medical conditions or had undergone genital surgery but had not been exposed to testosterone, the differences were less striking (Hurtig and Rosenthal, 1987).

There is experimental evidence, derived mainly from rats, indicating that a period exists in early life during which androgens can produce irreversible effects on the brain (Goiski, 1985). For example, the administration of androgens to female rats during a critical phase of perinatal development results in enlargement of several groups of sexually dimorphic nuclei in the hypothalamus which become as prominent as in the male. Upon reaching sexual maturity, these females exhibit male-type mating behavior (Gorski, 1998).

Anatomic studies of the human brain have revealed some differences between males and females, notably in the region of the hypothalamus, but these seem likely to be concerned more with pituitary than higher functions. Morphologic changes in other regions of the brain, for example the corpus callosum and cerebral hemispheres, have also been described but these are, in the main, subtle and inconsistent. Attempts to define male type brain anatomy in females exposed to testosterone in early life are handicapped by the rarity of such material. Several studies have claimed to identify changes in the brains of homosexuals and transsexuals (Zhou *et al.*, 1995), but these have been criticized on the grounds of methodology (Breedlove, 1995).

The most fruitful avenue for detecting the role of androgen exposure on the developing human brain probably lies in careful long-term clinical studies of intersex patients and other males reassigned as females because of a hopelessly inadequate penis. These are presently being undertaken.

Causes of intersexuality

The underlying principles governing the causes of genital ambiguity are straightforward. Because the development of a female phenotype is an autonomous process, ambiguity in a genetically female fetus having normal ovaries can only arise as a result of a hormonal milieu in which there is an excess of androgens at a critical phase of development. These may originate either from the fetus itself, because of CAH or, much more rarely, from a placental enzyme defect, or alternatively, from the mother, reaching the fetus via the placental circulation (Fig. 31.7).

As masculinization of the genitalia is an active process, ambiguity can only arise in the presence of a 46,XY karyotype when there is failure of one of the steps along the male developmental pathway resulting in an arrest of the masculinizing process (Fig. 31.8). This may occur very early because of a gene defect that prevents the formation of a normal testis. In other cases, the testes may have formed normally, but either the Leydig cells may be unresponsive to gonadotropin stimulation or the enzymes they contain may fail to elaborate sufficient testosterone to permit adequate masculinization of the genitalia. Among fetuses in which there is adequate testosterone production, the problem may lie in the peripheral tissues, where either the 5-α-reductase enzyme fails to convert testosterone to dihydrotestosterone or androgen receptor function is impaired. MIS production or action may also be defective. The genes responsible for each of the above steps have now been identified and cloned, giving rise to the possibility of precise diagnosis at the molecular level (Table 31.1).

Classification of the intersex disorders

The intersex disorders are most conveniently classified under four main headings, based on gonadal histology (Fig. 31.9). This is both conceptually simple and clinically relevant, as the histology of the gonads will largely determine the future of the infant with regard to fertility potential, the risk for malignant degeneration, endocrine function and possible gender identity.

1. *Female pseudohermaphroditism*: two histologically normal ovaries are present. The karyotype is invariably 46,XX, but the external genitalia show a variable degree of virilization. By far the most common example of this group is CAH.

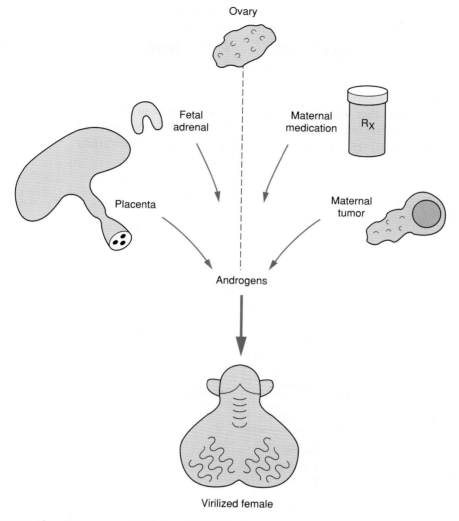

Ovary

Fetal
adrenal

Maternal
medication

R~x~

Placenta

Maternal
tumor

Androgens

Virilized female

Figure 31.7 Causes of ambiguous genitalia in a 46,XX female.

2. *True hermaphroditism*: both ovarian and testicular tissue are found in the same patient. The karyotype is variable but the appearance of the external genitalia reflects the amount of testicular tissue in the gonads.

3. *Male pseudohermaphroditism*: two histologically normal testes are present. The karyotype is invariably 46,XY, and the external genitalia show either partial or complete failure of masculinization. The most frequent underlying cause is androgen insensitivity.

4. *Conditions with dysgenetic gonads*: the gonads are histologically disordered, and usually contain abundant fibrous stroma. The appearance of the external genitalia is variable, but the karyotype frequently shows both XY and XO cell lines.

Criteria for investigation

Infants whose genitalia are clearly ambiguous will be referred for investigation at birth because of the difficulty of sex assignment. In many cases, however, the appearance may be deceptive. For example, an infant may be assumed to be a boy because the penis is fully developed and urine is passed from its tip, but may in fact be a severely virilized girl with CAH. Similarly, an apparently female infant with only slight clitoral hypertrophy may be a male with severe androgen insensitivity whose intra-abdominal testes will need to be removed to prevent malignant degeneration.

It is necessary, therefore, to have well-defined clinical criteria for investigating intersexuality. These must to some extent be arbitrary in as much as even the mildest degree of hypospadias can be regarded as a form of incomplete masculinization. However, the incidence of an identifiable form of intersexuality increases with severity of hypospadias or if one gonad is also incompletely descended (Kaefer *et al.*, 1999).

The phenotypic appearances that warrant investigation for intersexuality are tabulated in Table 31.2 and illustrated in Figures 31.10–15. Among these examples, three occur in apparent girls, whereas in three the patient looks like a boy. The remaining group comprises those in whom the external genitalia are clearly ambiguous so that the sex cannot immediately be decided. In spite of these comprehensive criteria, an additional small number of children will only come to light in adolescence because of amenorrhea, virilization, inappropriate breast development, or the onset of cyclical 'hematuria'.

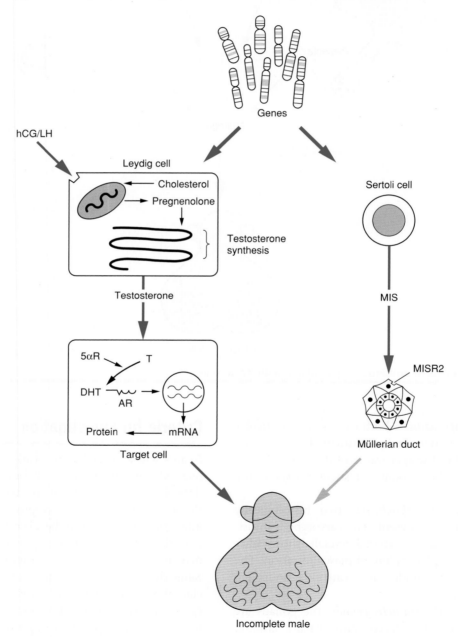

Figure 31.8 Causes of ambiguous genitalia in 46,XY male. A block may occur at any stage in the pathway of male differentiation, resulting in incomplete masculinization. T=testosterone; 5αR=5α-reductase; DHT=dihydrotestosterone; AR=androgen receptor; MISR2=MIS receptor-2.

Table 31.1 Loci of genes involved in the male developmental cascade

Gene	Chromosome	Locus
Testis development		
SRY	Y chromosome	p11.3
DSS/DAX-1	X chromosome	p21–22
SF-1	Chromosome 9	q33
WT-1	Chromosome 11	p13
SOX-9	Chromosome 17	q24–25
Testosterone biosynthesis		
hCG receptor	Chromosome 2	p21
StAR protein	Chromosome 8	p11.2
3β HSD-2	Chromosome 1	p13.1
17α OH	Chromosome 10	q24.3
17-20 lyase	Chromosome 10	q24.3
17β HSD-3	Chromosome 9	q22
Target tissues		
5α reductase-2	Chromosome 2	p23
T/DHT receptor	X chromosome	q11–12
Müllerian duct regression		
MIS	Chromosome 19	p13.2
MIS receptor-2	Chromosome 12	q12–13

Investigation of the intersex patient

Talking with the family

Intersex disorders are one of the most distressing problems to be encountered at birth because of the uncertainty that clouds the newborn's most basic identity. The first interview, therefore, is of critical importance in order to put the problem in its correct perspective. This is best carried out by the member of the intersex team who will be responsible for long-term follow-up so that a personal relationship with the family can be established.

At the outset, it is usually best to offer the simple explanation that nature either did not complete the differentiation of the genitalia or there has been some overstimulation, and that tests will need to be conducted to determine the cause of the problem. Reassurance should be given that surgery can be offered so that the genitalia will look appropriate and have the potential to function adequately. While investigations are being carried out, speculation as to the likely outcome should be avoided so that what has been said does not have to be retracted. It is best, therefore, to refer to the newborn at this stage as 'baby' rather than he or she.

Once the definitive diagnosis has been established and a consensus reached among the intersex team as to the recommended sex of rearing, a second interview takes place with the parents at which time the nature of the underlying problem is explained and its implications, particularly with regard to the need for long-term hormone therapy and fertility, are discussed. As much detail as seems appropriate for each individual family is given. Among infants whom it is proposed should be raised as girls and who were exposed to androgens *in utero*, the possibility should be raised that this may have an effect on psychosexual development. It should also be explained that the spectrum of normal psychosexual development is very wide and that even among children born without any overt problem with their genitalia or hormones, their eventual sexual orientation and gender identity can never be assumed. Nevertheless, parents should be reassured that, although published follow-up studies are presently few, it is the experience of most physicians familiar with these disorders that the majority of children raised as girls, particularly with CAH, seem to do well.

With such a step-by-step approach the parents will almost invariably gain confidence in both their physician and their own ability to raise their child in a positive manner.

Taking a history

Clinical evaluation begins with the taking of a family history. Most intersex states are recessively inherited disorders, so that careful inquiry may reveal a neonatal death among siblings or cousins, abnormalities of the genitalia, an unusual course at puberty, or a family history of infertility. Inquiries should also be made concerning any medication that may have been taken during pregnancy, particularly treatment for recurrent spontaneous abortion or other steroids, including the casual use of hormonal contraceptives.

Examining the baby

A general examination should first be carried out looking for an abnormal facial appearance or other dysmorphic features suggesting a multiple malformation syndrome. In particular, Turner syndrome, featuring a short broad neck and widely spaced nipples suggests the presence of a 45,XO cell line. Abnormal skin pigmentation from high levels of adrenocorticotrophic hormone (ACTH) will suggest the diagnosis of CAH.

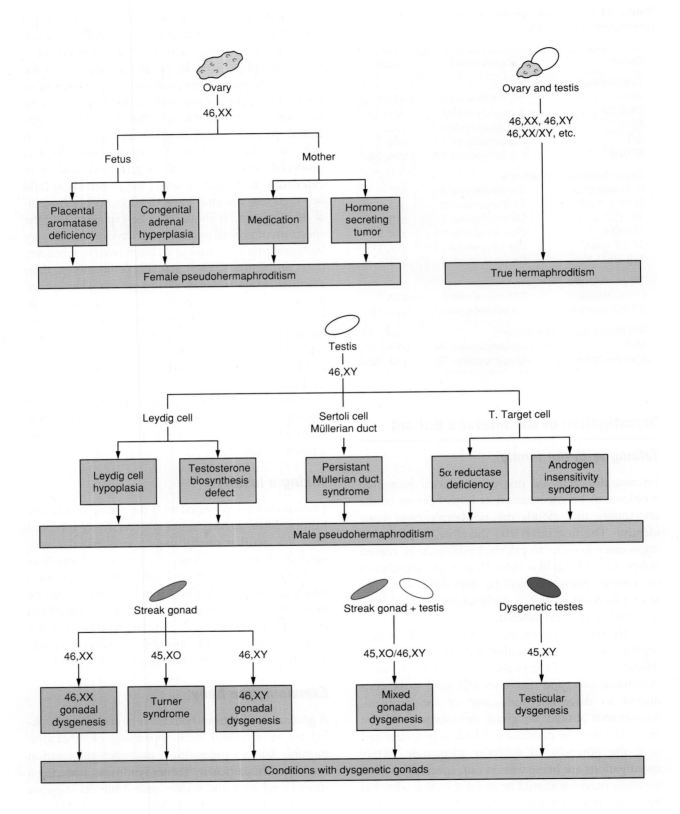

Figure 31.9 Classification of intersex disorders: a scheme based on the histology of the gonads.

Table 31.2 Clinical criteria for the investigation of intersexuality

'Female'	'Unsure'	'Male'
Clitoral hypertrophy	Ambiguous	Impalpable testes
Skin-fused labia		Severe hypospadias
Palpable gonad		Hypospadias and UDT

Occasionally, the mother may have a virilized or cushingoid appearance, betraying placental aromatase deficiency or a functioning ovarian or adrenal tumor.

The size of the phallus should now be assessed. As chordee is usually present, the initial impression is often that it is much smaller than it actually is. Stretched length measurements are rarely possible, but the distance from the pubis to the tip of the glans

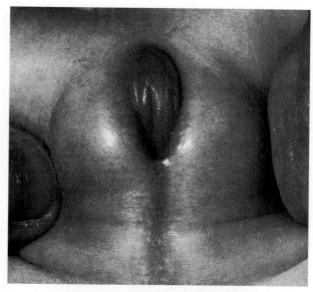

Figure 31.11 Intersexuality: an apparent female with almost complete skin fusion of the labia.

along the dorsum of the phallus should be recorded while holding back the prepubic fat. The girth of the corpora should also be determined by rolling them between the fingers. The position of the urethral meatus is now noted. This is sometimes difficult to determine unless the infant actually voids during the examination, but even when it seems small, it is almost always wide enough to allow adequate urination. The labioscrotal folds are then inspected for asymmetry and the degree of rugosity of the skin.

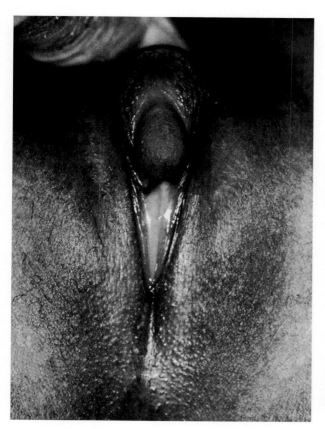

Figure 31.10 Intersexuality: an apparent female with moderate clitoral hypertrophy.

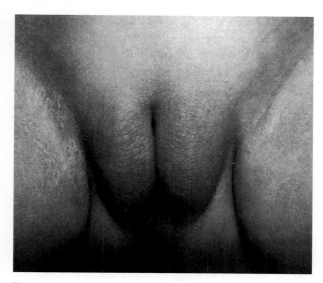

Figure 31.12 Intersexuality: an apparent female with a left inguinal hernia containing a gonad.

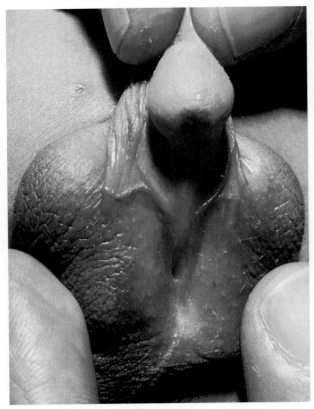

Figure 31.13 Intersexuality: ambiguous genitalia. This infant displays an enlarged clitoris, urethral folds, a single urogenital sinus opening, and empty, fused labioscrotal folds.

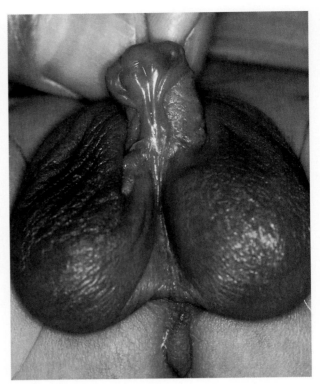

Figure 31.14 Intersexuality: an apparent male with hypospadias and a cleft scrotum. Both gonads are fully descended.

A careful attempt is now made to feel a gonad. With an assistant holding the infant's thighs abducted, and with warm hands, the fingers are swept down along the line of the inguinal canal on each side beginning well above the site of the internal inguinal ring. Any gonad brought down towards the scrotum by this maneuver is gently grasped by the other hand and its size and consistency are noted.

The appearance of the external genitalia varies so widely among patients who have the same condition that it is generally unwise to attempt a definitive diagnosis from the physical findings alone. There is only one deduction that can be safely made. If a gonad is palpable, the condition is not female pseudohermaphroditism, in which the gonads invariably comprise normal ovaries lying within the abdominal cavity. Nevertheless, some tentative conclusions can be drawn. For example, the presence of a well-developed phallus indicates that significant levels of testosterone were present *in utero*. Asymmetric development of the scrotum suggests an abnormality of the gonads with

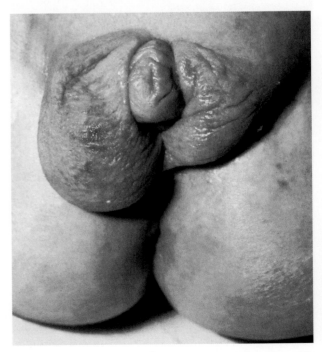

Figure 31.15 Intersexuality: an apparent male with hypospadias and left cryptorchidism.

production of testosterone by that on the better developed side.

Cytogenetic investigations

There are currently a number of methods available to help in the cytogenetic diagnosis of intersex disorders. The choice will depend on the suspicion as to the nature of the underlying condition and the laboratory facilities available.

Buccal smear

This time-honored method still has a place in those parts of the world where more sophisticated cytogenetic studies are not readily available. It depends on the identification of a dense dot, or Barr body, in the periphery of the nucleus of buccal mucosal epithelium which represents the second X chromosome. The technique is straightforward and depends simply on obtaining a scraping from the lining of the cheek, staining with hemotoxolin and eosin and examining it under ordinary light microscopy. The Barr bodies, however, are only identified in approximately 30% of the cells examine. As it offers no other genetic information, the usefulness of the technique is limited to confirming a female genotype among patients in whom a laboratory diagnosis of CAH has been made.

Fluorescent in situ hybridization

Many cytogenetic laboratories are now able to carry out fluorescent *in situ* hybridization (FISH) staining of lymphocytes, which rapidly identifies the X and Y chromosomes. The technique is faster and less expensive than karyotyping. It depends on the binding of a fluorescent labeled X or Y chromosome antibody probe to its target which, when examined under ultraviolet light microscopy, appears as a bright red or green dot (Fig. 31.16). Like the buccal smear, however, its role is mainly confined to demonstrating the presence of a second X chromosome in patients with confirmed CAH. In laboratories which provide this test as a routine service, the results can be available within a few hours.

Karyotype

Nowadays, G-banded karyotyping is the standard method of examining chromosomes in intersex patients. Lymphocytes are obtained from a small sample of venous blood or, in the case of a premature baby, from the bone marrow. These are incubated for 24 hours, at which time the culture is inoculated with colchicine to arrest mitosis in metaphase. The chromosomes are then seen to best advantage, photographed and displayed in sequence. A minimum of 30 lymphocytes should be examined to exclude mosaicism with a 95% probability. The method, however, is time consuming, so that the results are rarely available before 2 or 3 days.

Among patients with ambiguous genitalia, a 46,XX karyotype is usually indicative of female pseudohermaphroditism or, less often, true hermaphroditism. The finding of a 46,XY karyotype is less specific and will be found in all male pseudohermaphrodites, in the XY form of gonadal dysgenesis and also in some cases of true hermaphroditism (Fig. 31.17). A 46,XY/46,XX line or other combinations may be found in true hermaphroditism, whereas a mixture of 46,XY and 45,XO cell lines is the rule in mixed gonadal dysgenesis. The identification of a few 45,XO cells in a predominantly 46,XY karyotype obtained from peripheral blood will suggest the diagnosis of testicular dysgenesis.

Gene probe studies

These sophisticated genetic techniques hold out the promise of being able to make a definitive diagnosis by identifying mutations and deletions in genes specific to individual intersex conditions. Most of the genes in the complex pathway of normal sexual development have now been identified and cloned, and commercial kits are becoming available for automated analysis.

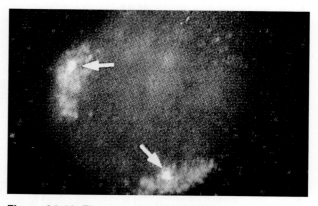

Figure 31.16 Flourescent *in situ* hybridization probe of a lymphocyte showing bright signals from the two X chromosomes (*arrows*).

Gene probe studies depend on the amplification by polymerase chain reaction of short, single-chain DNA sequences suspected of being abnormal and comparing these on an electrophoretic strip to a control sample. Presently, however, few laboratories can carry out these studies on a routine basis. There are also several limitations to the technique. Large and complex genes require very lengthy analysis, although the recognition of mutation 'hot spots' allows better targeting. The identification of a mutation, however, does not necessarily mean that it is clinically significant. Furthermore, when mutations are not found this could simply be the result of a laboratory error, or that the appropriate part of the gene was not screened. Nonetheless, among conditions in which the relevant gene is small and therefore amenable to thorough analysis, the most frequent site of the mutation is known, and there is a very low incidence of inconsequential mutations, the technique can be very valuable, particularly for conditions in which the diagnosis by other means is difficult.

Imaging studies

Ultrasonography

An ultrasound scan using a 15 mHz transducer should be carried out of the pelvis in all infants suspected of having an intersex condition in an effort to identify a uterus. Among infants with female pseudohermaphroditism, it appears as a moderately echogenic oval struc-

ture with a central cavity. In transverse images the uterus lies in or slightly to one side of the midline between the rectum and the posterior wall of the bladder, which may appear indented (Fig. 31.18). In longitudinal images, the central endometrial stripe is usually well seen, as is the cervix which indents the vault of the vagina (Fig. 31.19). When the vagina is distended with urine, a high insertion into the urogenital sinus above the pelvic floor should be suspected.

In most other intersex states, the uterus is often a rudimentary structure and more difficult to identify, particularly if the bladder is overdistended or empty. However, with patience and moderate bladder filling, which can be achieved by feeding the baby during the examination, it is sometimes possible to recognize the unicornuate uterus frequently associated with mixed gonadal dysgenesis or true hermaphroditism (Wright et al., 1995; Kutteh et al., 1995).

Intra-abdominal gonads are difficult to locate or characterize by ultrasound scanning. Ovaries can sometimes be seen behind the bladder lying close to its posterior wall lateral to the position of the ureters. This is often easier in the newborn when they may contain follicular cysts (Fig. 31.20). It should be noted, however, that even among normal infant girls both ovaries are routinely seen in only a minority of cases (Cohen et al., 1993).

A gonad that is palpable in the groin or fully descended should always be scanned by ultrasound. A

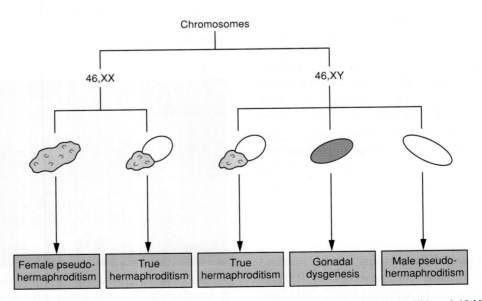

Figure 31.17 Diagram showing possible causes of genital ambiguity associated with 46,XX and 46,XY karyotypes.

testis can usually be recognized by its size, shape, and homogeneous low-intensity echo pattern. Dysgenetic testes are usually smaller than normal and may show mixed echogenicity. The very bright echoes of calcification will suggest the development of a gonadoblastoma. The presence of a cyst within a palpable gonad suggests the diagnosis of an ovotestis (Sohaib *et al.*, 1997). It must also be remembered that the sonographic findings may be confusing because of an associated inguinal hernia that may contain a uterus, fallopian tube, contralateral gonad, omentum, or a loop of bowel.

The adrenal glands should also be routinely examined to exclude a tumor or the massive enlargement characteristic of congenital lipoid hyperplasia (Takaya

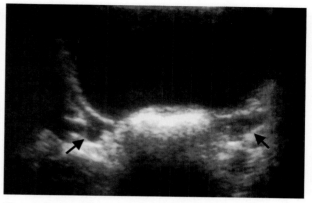

Figure 31.20 Transverse sonogram through the bladder in a neonate showing both ovaries (*arrows*). The uterus is enlarged.

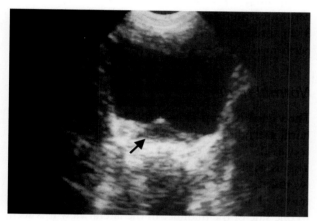

Figure 31.18 Sonogram scan of an infant with congenital adrenal hyperplasia showing a uterus indenting the posterior wall of the bladder (*arrow*) (transverse scan).

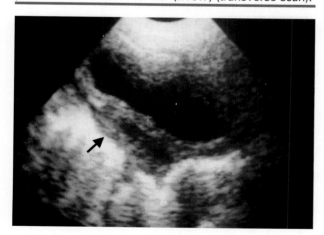

Figure 31.19 Sonogram of an infant with congenital adrenal hyperplasia showing a thick-walled uterus (*arrow*). The endometrial cavity is well seen (longitudinal scan).

et al., 1998). Although there have been claims that the diagnosis of the more common forms of congenital adrenal hyperplasia can be made by measuring adrenal size, this is unreliable. At birth, the normal adrenal gland is a very large structure measuring approximately one-half the length of the kidney. However, during the first few weeks this rapidly shrinks down as the fetal zone, which initially makes up 80% of the gland, involutes (Menzel and Hauffa, 1990). Furthermore, the shape of the gland resembles a Salvador Dali 'soft watch' rather than a pyramid, and its low echogenicity make its margins difficult to define. Although techniques have been described for accurately measuring the dimensions of the glands (Sivit *et al.*, 1991), these have not attracted much support because of significant observer error. The presence of two normal kidneys, however, should be routinely verified.

In addition to the initial diagnostic work-up, ultrasonography has an important role in long-term follow-up. Among boys with gonadal dysgenesis the retained testis should be scanned regularly because of the possible development of a tumor. Similarly, among boys being followed with the Denys–Drash syndrome, the kidneys should be kept under periodic review because of the risk of Wilms' tumor.

The routine use of antenatal ultrasound scanning has, on occasion, led to the diagnosis of ambiguous genitalia being made *in utero*. The penis and clitoris are initially indistinguishable but from 20 weeks onwards the penis progressively enlarges and the anatomy becomes clearer (Shapiro, 1999). At about this time the scrotum can also be recognized, initially as a hillock, posteriorly. The diagnosis of ambiguous genitalia will be suggested by the continuing apparent small size of the penis, which is tethered down with chordee, in conjunction with clefting or asymmetry of the developing scrotum. Fortuitous micturition by the fetus during the examination may allow the position of the urethral meatus to be determined by a Doppler flow study.

Genitography

A genitogram should be obtained in all cases of intersexuality, although the technique used should be tailored according to the specific information sought. It is therefore advantageous to defer this examination until the results of other investigations are known.

Among infants with CAH, the purpose of the study is solely to identify the level at which the vagina opens into the urogenital sinus with particular reference to the pelvic floor. This information is essential in planning the surgical approach for vaginoplasty. In other cases, its value lies in confirming the presence of a vagina, identifying a cervical impression, and outlining a uterine canal and fallopian tubes. Alternatively, one or both vasa may be filled in a retrograde manner from the vaginal vault.

These radiologic findings contribute towards the diagnosis but are not themselves diagnostic because, they may not only be identical in a number of different conditions, but also vary within each condition. It can be inferred, however, that on the side of a fallopian tube, the ipsilateral gonad failed during intra-uterine life to produce an adequate amount of MIS. The presence of a vagina is less helpful diagnostically because it is formed mainly from the urogenital sinus.

Techniques

The radiologist should first be given a working differential diagnosis based on the results of other investigations. Undiluted water-soluble contrast medium is preferred, which should be injected by hand under fluoroscopy, using either a single-catheter or a double-catheter technique (Aaronson and Cremin, 1984). Often the catheter preferentially enters the vagina (Fig. 31.21). When, instead, it passes up into the bladder, cystography should be carried out, which will often show the vagina during the voiding phase (Fig. 31.22).

In order to identify the uterine canal and fallopian tubes, a tapered nozzle is fitted to the syringe or a 6 Fr Foley catheter used and the balloon inflated with a small volume of sterile water to occlude the distal urogenital sinus channel (Fig. 31.23). Care should be taken when injecting contrast medium not to overfill the system as extravasation or intraperitoneal spill can easily occur. Spot films are taken both in the frontal and lateral projections, which need to be of high quality if the vasa are to be identified.

When the genitogram fails to demonstrate any ducts, the position of the verumontanum, which appears as a shallow filling defect on the posterior urethral wall, should be noted. When this is lying in a lower position than normal, urethroscopy may be carried out with the patient under general anesthesia. An opening will usually be found in the center of the verumontanum that can be cannulated with a 3 Fr ureteral catheter and a direct genitogram performed.

Normal findings

The vagina is a capacious structure, even in the newborn, extending to the superior pubic ramus with a convex filling defect in its apex formed by the cervix. This is easily obscured, however, if the fornices are overfilled. The uterine canal appears as a streak of contrast medium which, in the anterior projection, may lie to one side of the midline. In the lateral view it is seen to arch over the back of the bladder (Fig. 31.24). Contrast material often fills the fallopian tubes, sometimes spilling into the peritoneal cavity.

Although a vagina will be demonstrated in most intersex disorders, its size and configuration vary widely. In the syndromes of androgen insensitivity, it is usually short with a rounded vault that only reaches to the level of the mid pubis. In syndromes associated with dysgenetic gonads and in true hermaphroditism, a uterine canal is often outlined but the cervix is usually too rudimentary to be apparent. In CAH, the length and size of the vagina are generally inversely proportional to the degree of virilization but the cervix, body of the uterus, and tubes are invariably normal.

In some cases of penoscrotal or perineal hypospadias in which no other evidence of intersexuality can be demonstrated, an enlarged utriculus masculinus may sometimes be seen. This is also a common finding in the prune belly syndrome.

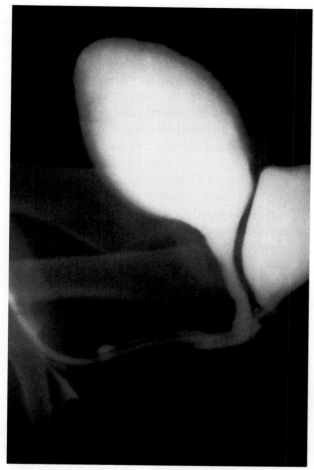

Figure 31.21 Technique of genitography: the vagina has been catheterized via the urogenital sinus opening.

Other imaging studies

The role of magnetic resonance imaging in the diagnosis of intersex conditions is currently being explored. Good definition of the pelvic tissue planes can usually be obtained using T_1-weighted images allowing paired structures and the relationship of the vagina to the pelvic floor to be clearly seen. Gonads are better seen with T_2-weighted images but they are frequently elusive (Secaf *et al.*, 1994). However, because of the long acquisition time for multiple 3 mm sections, infants need to be either heavily sedated or put under general anesthesia to avoid movement artifact. Computed tomography also has these limitations as well as the added disadvantage of ionizing radiation. The high quality of the images currently obtainable with ultrasound, as well as cost considerations, therefore, make this the preferred imaging modality in the intersex patient.

Endocrine studies

Biochemical investigations are the primary means of identifying CAH and placental aromatase deficiency in virilized girls. Among boys, they identify defects of testosterone biosynthesis and 5α-reductase deficiency. In all of these conditions, the diagnosis will be unequivocally established when the assay of hormones above and below a suspected enzyme block reveals either a greatly elevated concentration of the substrate or an elevated substrate to product ratio. Endocrine studies can also be helpful in suspected cases of androgen insensitivity. The specific hormones that need to be measured in the various intersex disorders are discussed in the relevant sections of this chapter.

Hormone studies are a valuable means of determining the presence of functioning testicular tissue. There are two windows of opportunity during which the measurement of basal testosterone concentration alone will suffice. The first is immediately after birth

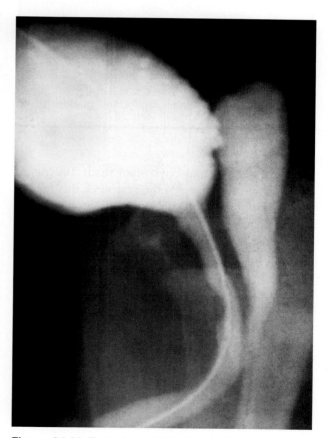

Figure 31.22 Technique of genitography: the vagina has been filled during the voiding phase of a cysto-urethrogram.

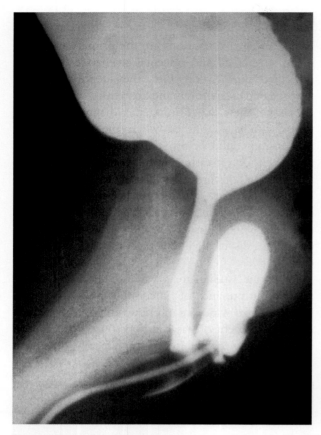

Figure 31.23 Technique of genitography: a balloon catheter has occluded the distal urogenital sinus channel, allowing both the vagina and bladder to be filled.

when levels in normal boys often reach 100 ng/dl. However, in the course of the first week this rapidly falls to below 50 ng/dl. Beginning about 4 weeks of age, a second opportunity arises as a result of the post-natal surge in luteinizing hormone (LH) secretion. This peaks by 2 months of age when serum testosterone concentration reaches adult levels, but there-after it progressively declines so that by 6 months of age it is barely detectable (Fig. 31.25). Between these two periods, and for the remainder of infancy and childhood, detection of testosterone from functioning testicular tissue will require human chorionic gonado-tropin (hCG) stimulation. A commonly employed regime is to give this in the dose of 1500 IU on alter-nate days for 2–3 doses measuring serum testosterone concentration 48 hours after the last dose.

The measurement of MIS is also a sensitive marker of functioning testicular tissue (Gustafson *et al.*, 1993). However, because of its inverse relationship to

serum testosterone concentration, levels remain low for the first few months of life. Once the postnatal testosterone peak has passed, serum MIS levels rise to a mean of 50 ng/ml and remain elevated until puberty (Fig. 31.26). Absolute MIS concentrations vary from child to child and can range from 10 to over 500 ng/ml. Even the lower value is still ten times higher than that found in normal girls (Lee *et al.*, 1996). Beyond the first few months of age, the mea-surement of MIS has a clear advantage over testos-terone in that hCG stimulation is not necessary. Furthermore, unlike testosterone, which is also pro-duced by the adrenal glands, MIS is secreted only by the Sertoli cells and is therefore testis specific.

Rey *et al.* (1999) found that the absolute serum concentration of MIS could be correlated with gonadal histology. Thus, among children having only ovarian tissue or gonadal dysgenesis, levels were either undetectable or very low. Those with testicular

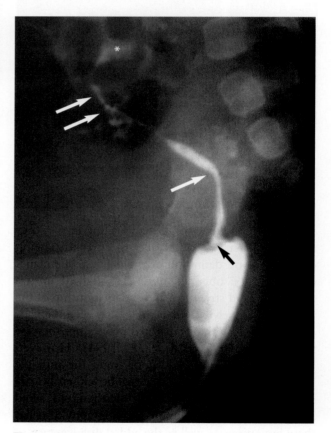

Figure 31.24 Normal vaginogram, lateral projection. Note the cervical impression in the vault of the vagina (*black arrow*), and contrast medium in the uterine canal (*white arrow*) and a fallopian tube (*double arrow*). There is spillage into the peritoneal cavity (*).

dysgenesis or true hermaphroditism had levels that were somewhat reduced, whereas those with defective testosterone biosynthesis had concentrations that were generally above the normal range.

Commercial kits are now available for the assay of MIS and an increasing number of laboratories provides this test on a routine basis. The combination of serum MIS and hCG-stimulated testosterone levels provides a confident predictor of the presence of functioning testicular tissue.

Gonadal histology

Biopsy of the gonads is unnecessary when a definitive diagnosis has been unequivocally established biochemically, but in all other situations is essential. Palpable gonads are best exposed via an inguinal incision so that a commonly associated hernial sac can be dealt with at the same time. The skin incision can then be extended, if necessary, for a minilaparotomy to identify internal duct structures.

When the gonads are impalpable they should be inspected either by laparoscopy using additional ports for biopsy or by a minilaparotomy carried out through a small Pfannenstiel or lower midline inci-

sion. Provided the same precautions are taken as for laparoscopy and there is minimal handling of the bowel, patients can usually be discharged home on the following day.

The gonad must first be fully exposed by delivering it from its coverings. Its color and consistency should be noted, paying particular attention to any nodules lying in the hilum of the gland. The adjacent tissues are then carefully examined to identify a fallopian tube which can be distinguished from a dissociated epididymis by the presence of fimbria surrounding a central os. A vas is also sought alongside the vessels. If the gonad appears homogeneous, it should first be bivalved to expose its central portion and a deep but thin wedge excised. In some dysgenetic gonads or ovotestes the histologic picture may not be uniform. A running 6-0 absorbable suture is used to close the fibrous capsule, taking care to avoid including deep tissue in which important vessels may run.

Although the diagnosis is often apparent by the gross appearance of the gonad, one should always obtain histologic confirmation before proceeding any further. If the surgeon and pathologist have considerable experience with intersex disorders and the thera-

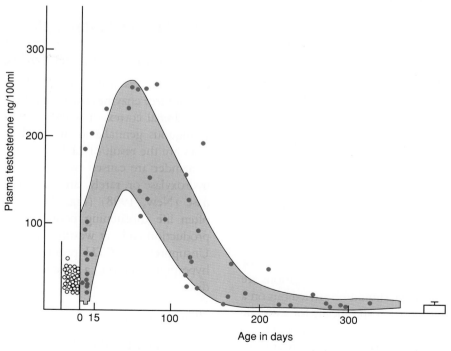

Figure 31.25 Plasma testosterone concentrations in normal male infants during the first year of life. Note the postnatal surge which peaks at around 2 months of age. (Data from Forest MG.)

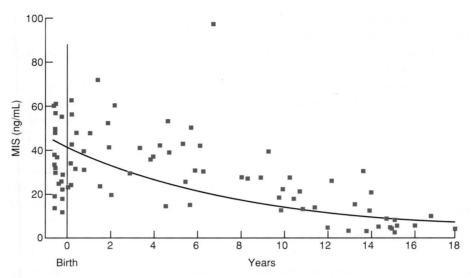

Figure 31.26 Plasma müllerian inhibiting substance concentrations in normal boys from birth to adolescence. (Data from Josso, N.V. (1995) *Hormone Res* **43**: 243–48.)

peutic options have been fully discussed with the family beforehand, a frozen section may suffice and definitive surgery carried out at the same sitting. In most situations, however, it is wiser to confine the first procedure to a biopsy in order to establish the diagnosis.

Sequence of investigations

As CAH is the most common single cause of intersexuality, it is most productive to begin with the appropriate endocrine studies in infants in whom a gonad cannot be felt (Fig. 31.27). When the diagnosis of 21-hydroxylase or 11β-hydroxylase deficiency is unequivocally established, no further investigation is necessary other than a urogenital sinogram. This determines the level of the confluence of the vagina with the urogenital sinus. The parents, however, will be reassured if they know for certain that their child has two X chromosomes, which can be convincingly shown by a rapid FISH study. They will also be reassured by having a normal uterus pointed out to them on an ultrasound scan.

Among patients in whom a gonad is palpable or the CAH screen is negative, further investigations are necessary. A full karyotype should be carried out on a minimum of 30 cells, looking specifically for a mosaic pattern. A pelvic ultrasound scan and genitogram are also carried out, the latter directed specifically at identifying internal duct structures. Further hormonal investigations are also appropriate, looking specifi-

cally for evidence of testicular tissue and, if confirmed, for defects in testosterone biosynthesis or 5α-reductase activity. Unless the definitive diagnosis has at this stage been clearly established, it will be necessary to inspect and biopsy the gonads. According to the biopsy findings, analysis of specific genes may be warranted.

Female pseudohermaphroditism

Congenital adrenal hyperplasia

CAH is the result of a recessively inherited defect of one of three enzymes essential for cortisol synthesis in the adrenal cortex. It is the most common cause of ambiguous genitalia in the newborn. Over 90% of cases are the result of 21-hydroxylase deficiency. The remainder are caused by a deficiency of either 11β-hydroxylase or, rarely, 3β-hydroxysteroid dehydrogenase (New, 1998) (Fig. 31.28). The condition is often life threatening because of impaired cortisol production and salt wasting, leading to hypotension. Unsuppressed ACTH production gives rise to skin hyperpigmentation, a characteristic marker of the disease.

Clinical features

Girls with 21-hydroxylase deficiency show a wide spectrum of virilization, ranging from mild clitoral hypertrophy to what appears to be a normal penis

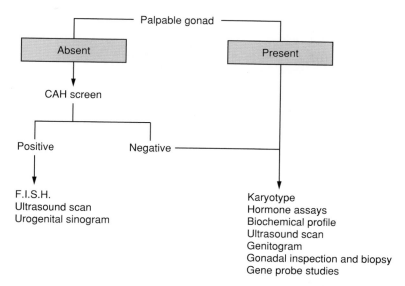

Figure 31.27 Recommended sequence of investigation of intersex disorders based on the clinical findings. FISH=fluorescent *in situ* hybridization probe.

with a well-developed but empty scrotum. Most will have moderate enlargement of a clitoris that is tethered down by chordee, at the base of which urine is passed through a single urogenital sinus opening. The labia majora are usually prominent and often rugose (Fig. 31.29). Irrespective of the degree of virilization, however, genital symmetry is always preserved and the gonads are impalpable. Internally, the uterus and fallopian tubes are normal but during childhood the ovaries may become polycystic. No male structures are present as these have regressed by the time androgen levels become elevated.

About two-thirds of these infants have evidence of salt loss as a result of impaired aldosterone production. If this is severe and unrecognized, the presentation will be with lethargy, vomiting, and diarrhea, leading to dehydration and circulatory collapse. Death is then usually rapid from hyperkalemia and a severe metabolic acidosis.

Unrecognized survivors tend to grow rapidly and develop a muscular build. Bone age is advanced, but the epiphyses fuse early so that these children ultimately remain short. There is precocious growth of pubic and axillary hair, acne is common, and maturation of sweat glands gives these children a characteristically adult odor. Menstruation is scanty or absent and breast development is suppressed. Prostatic tissue may also form which, over many years, may hypertrophy or even become neoplastic (Winter *et al.*, 1996).

Diagnosis

The diagnosis of CAH will be foremost in the mind when an infant is encountered with symmetrical virilization of the genitalia and whose gonads are impalpable, especially when there is a family history of the disease. Plasma cortisol, glucose, and electrolyte concentrations should be urgently checked and the blood pressure monitored, while awaiting the results of confirmatory hormone assays.

The diagnosis is established by finding elevated plasma concentrations of 17-hydroxyprogesterone and androstenedione. The former is a particularly sensitive marker, as it accumulates in concentrations that are often several hundred times higher than normal. Although the production of deoxycorticosterone (DOC) and deoxycortisol is relatively suppressed, these assays are less diagnostically useful as they frequently reach the low normal range. In salt wasters hyponatremia and hyperkalemia may be manifest but their onset is often delayed. The diagnosis of salt wasting, however, can be made by finding a raised serum renin concentration or an altered serum renin to aldosterone ratio. It should be noted that among severe salt losers, the renin concentration may actually be low as a result of depletion of its substrate. In suspected mild cases an ACTH stimulation test should be carried out measuring the ratio of 17-hydroxyprogesterone to deoxycortisol 1 hour after injection.

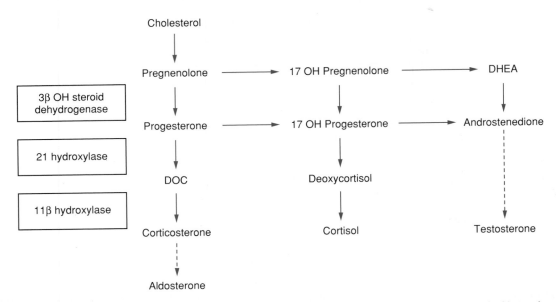

Figure 31.28 The three enzymes causing congenital adrenal hyperplasia in girls (in boxes). Note the specific pathways they regulate.

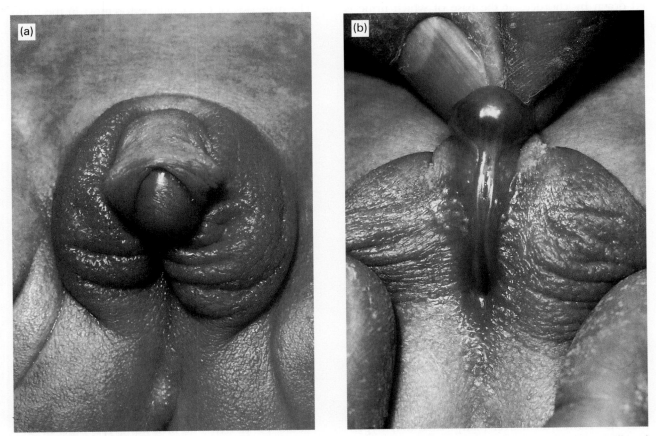

Figure 31.29 External genitalia of a newborn girl with congenital adrenal hyperplasia. Note the significant clitoral hypertrophy, urogenital sinus opening and the redundant, rugose labia majora: (*a*) dorsal, and (*b*) ventral views.

Most laboratories can provide a rapid assay of plasma 17-hydroxyprogesterone, but when this is not available, the urinary concentration of its principal metabolites, namely pregnanetriol and 17 ketosteroids, can be assayed. Ideally, this determination should be from a 24-hour urine specimen, but because of the difficulty in ensuring a complete collection in infants, this can be extrapolated from urine collected over a shorter period by simultaneously measuring creatinine excretion. However, as steroid excretion varies over 24 hours, the diagnosis may be missed.

An ultrasound scan of the pelvis using the full bladder as an acoustic window will confirm the presence of a well-developed uterus. A urogenital sinogram will usually demonstrate a capacious vagina with a cervical impression within its vault. The uterine cavity and fallopian tubes may also be filled. The radiologist should be asked to pay particular attention to demonstrating clearly the site at which the vagina joins with the urethra with respect to the level of the pelvic floor (Figs 31.30, 31.31).

21-Hydroxylase deficiency

The reported incidence of classical 21-hydroxylase deficiency is about 1 in 15 000 births. Increasingly, however, a non-classical, late-onset variety is being recognized which suggests that CAH may well be the most common of all inherited metabolic disorders.

11b-Hydroxylase deficiency

This enzyme defect accounts for fewer than 10% of cases of CAH. Biochemically, there is an accumulation of 17-hydroxyprogesterone, as is the case with 21-hydroxylase deficiency, but unlike the latter, there is also a build-up of deoxycorticosterone, which causes salt retention. Consequently, about two-thirds of these patients become hypertensive, although often not until childhood. In general, the more severely virilized the external genitalia, the more likely hypertension is to develop.

The diagnosis is established by finding elevated serum 17-hydroxyprogesterone and deoxycorticosterone levels and also an increase in 11-deoxycortisol production. The latter is usually identified by measuring the concentration of its tetrahydro metabolites which appear in urine. Serum sodium concentration is usually normal as excess sodium is excreted in the urine, but serum potassium levels may be raised. Serum renin concentration is low.

3β-Hydroxysteroid dehydrogenase deficiency

In this rare disorder there is a block early in the pathway of cortisol metabolism leading to an accumulation of 17-hydroxypregnenolone and dehydroepiandrosterone (DHEA). The latter, however, is only weakly androgenic, so that the resulting virilization is usually mild with modest clitoral hypertrophy and slight rugosity of the labia majora. There is usually a single urogenital sinus opening, but in some cases the vagina and urethra may open separately in the vulva.

The mild virilization of the genitalia in these cases is deceptive, as the metabolic consequences of this condition are often profound with salt wasting and circulatory collapse. However, mild cases are now being recognized in which aldosterone is produced in sufficient quantity for sodium homeostasis. The diagnosis is established by finding elevated serum DHEA and 17-hydroxypregnenolone concentrations associated with low serum levels of aldosterone and cortisol. Among the three enzyme defects responsible for

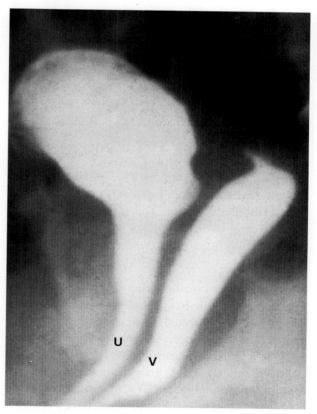

Figure 31.30 Urogenital sinogram of a girl with congenital adrenal hyperplasia showing a low confluence of the vagina (V) and urethra (U).

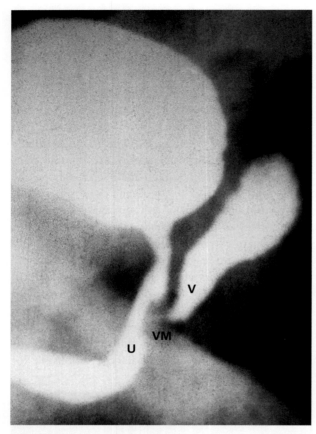

Figure 31.31 Urogenital sinogram of a girl with congenital adrenal hyperplasia. The vagina (V) enters the urethra (U) above the pelvic floor. The verumontanum (VM) is well seen, but the cervix is obscured by overfilling of the fornices.

ambiguous genitalia in girls, 3β-hydroxysteroid dehydrogenase deficiency is the only one also to cause genital ambiguity in boys. This is discussed below.

Genetic diagnosis of congenital adrenal hyperplasia

Progress has been made during the 1990s in understanding the genetic basis for CAH in order to identify carriers and affected fetuses. The gene for 21-hydroxylase deficiency, assigned to chromosome 6p21.3, is a large structure secluded in the human leukocyte antigen (HLA) gene cluster region. It comprises a functioning gene (CYP 21) and a non-functioning pseudogene (CYP 21p) which have a complex interaction (Wedell, 1996). Over 36 mutations have hitherto been described. Approximately 20% of patients have a large deletion, all of whom have severe

clinical manifestations of the disease. The remaining 80% have mostly point mutations that cluster in several hot spots, thus facilitating the diagnosis by gene probes. However, in some cases no mutations have been found (Nimkarn et al., 1999). Presently, there does not seem to be any clear correlation between specific mutations and the clinical patterns of simple virilizing, salt wasting, and late-onset types of the disease (Wilson et al., 1995).

The genes responsible for encoding 11β-hydroxylase and 3β-hydroxysteroid dehydrogenase have been cloned. However, reports of specific mutations are not well documented.

Medical treatment

Patients with CAH require lifelong steroid therapy to replace the deficient cortisol as well as suppress the ACTH drive to the adrenal cortex. This should be under the long-term supervision of a pediatric endocrinologist. Dose adjustments are frequently needed based on 17-hydroxyprogesterone concentration, somatic growth and appearance, and bone maturation as determined by radiographs of the hands and wrists. In salt-losing patients, fludrocortisone and often sodium chloride supplements will be needed and their doses adjusted to maintain plasma renin levels and the plasma renin to aldosterone ratios in the normal range. This steroid is also sometimes given to non-salt-losing patients in order to reduce their cortisol requirements. The dose of both of these medications may need to be increased in times of illness or severe injury, or to cover surgery. As children get older, many compensate for salt loss by dietary means and no longer need fludrocortisone. However, it may have to be reintroduced in times of metabolic stress.

Although medical treatment is generally satisfactory, adequate suppression of ACTH drive is difficult to achieve in about 25% of cases. These children show poor growth, re-enlargement of the clitoris and increasing rugosity of the labia, hirsutism, acne, and a deepening voice. Increasing the dose of steroids to achieve better control often results in a cushingoid appearance as well as psychological and behavioral problems. In such cases, alternative medications such as ketoconazole, which blocks steroid synthesis, may be helpful. The efficacy of new ACTH blockers and androgen antagonists is presently being explored in clinical trials.

An alternative approach to the treatment of the most difficult and refractory cases of CAH is total adrenalectomy (van Wyk *et al.*, 1996). This produces a surgical Addisonian state which, however, is generally easier to manage. The sympathetic nervous system appears to fully compensate for the missing adrenal glands so that catecholamine replacement is not necessary. Although initially recommended as a treatment of last resort, advocates of the operation argue that it is best carried out during the first year of life to prevent the irreversible somatic changes that can result from poor medical control. Such patients may be predicted from the family history and by finding a null mutation for the 21-hydroxylase gene which is known to correlate with severe clinical manifestations.

Genital surgery

Patients with mild virilization may be watched as it can be anticipated that with good medical control the clitoris will become proportionately smaller and the labia less prominent. A small cutback to expose the vagina may be all that is required. In most patients, however, the clitoris is markedly enlarged and the labia redundant and rugose, an appearance which, for most parents, is clearly abnormal and distressing (see Chapter 30).

Antenatal diagnosis and treatment

21-Hydroxylase and 11β-hydroxylase deficiencies can be discovered when the fetal adrenal cortex begins to function during the second trimester. Elevated 17-hydroxyprogesterone concentration is found in the amniotic fluid. However, by this time, the external genitalia of affected fetuses are already masculinized. In order to prevent this, a strong case can be made for offering high-dose dexamethasone treatment to suppress the fetal ACTH drive in mothers known to be at risk.

To be effective, treatment must be started by the 8th week of gestation, before the diagnosis can be confirmed. Consequently, many unaffected fetuses will also be treated. Being a recessively inherited disorder, only one in four will have the disease, of whom one-half will be boys. Thus, only 1 in 8 fetuses is likely to benefit. Nonetheless, treatment is effective and will result in genitalia that look externally normal or show only mild clitoral hypertrophy (Mercado *et al.*, 1995). However, the vagina usually remains concealed and will need to be exteriorized.

The risk of exposing a developing fetus to high-dose steroids during the period of organogenesis raised concerns that other congenital defects, particularly cleft palate, would be induced. But this does not seem to be the case, allaying ethical concerns that unaffected fetuses may be harmed. However, about 10% of mothers will develop fluid retention, edema, and hypertension during the first trimester, the incidence rising to 50% if treatment is prolonged beyond this period. Whether there is any benefit in continuing treatment throughout pregnancy, in order to protect the developing fetal brain from the effects of androgens, is presently unknown.

Long-term outcome

In spite of the difficulties of adequate medical control in some patients, the long-term outcome for the majority of women with CAH with regard to their general health and psychological wellbeing is good. However, the majority remain below the mean for height (Premawardhana *et al.*, 1997). The reason for short stature is not entirely clear but appears to be related to both inadequate suppression of testosterone and an excess of replacement cortisol (Girgis and Winter, 1997). Menstrual irregularity is also common and fertility somewhat reduced. In some cases this can be attributed to a lack of interest in forming heterosexual relationships or sexual activity, but in many it appears to be related to the inadequacy of the reconstruction of their genitalia giving rise to both psychological stress and physical pain (Meyer-Bahlburg, 1999).

The rare, severely virilized 46,XX patients with CAH raised as boys require hysterosalpingoophorectomy and resection of as much of the vagina as can be conveniently reached from an intraperitoneal approach. They will also require lifelong testosterone as well as cortisol and, often, fludrocortisone replacement therapy. Long-term follow-up data on this rare group of patients are sparse but short stature appears to be the rule and psychological problems are apparently common (Nihoul-Fékété C., personal communication, 1999).

Surgery in boys with congenital adrenal hyperplasia

Although CAH affects boys with the same frequency as girls, those with 21-hydroxylase and 11β-hydroxylase deficiencies do not have any ambiguity of their genitalia. They do, however, need to take cortisol to correct the metabolic defect but are frequently not motivated to do so and are therefore poorly controlled. Continuing ACTH drive may then result in Leydig cell adenomas which usually present as bilateral testicular enlargement. Although mostly seen in adult life, these have been reported in adolescents and children. They are benign, multifocal, and poorly encapsulated lesions which can be difficult to distinguish histologically from Leydig cell tumors (Walker et al., 1997). Most regress with the resumption of steroid treatment. For those that persist, surgical enucleation can be carried out with preservation of the remaining testicular tissue.

Placental aromatase deficiency

Female fetuses may become virilized as a result of a recessively inherited deficiency of aromatase, an enzyme particularly abundant in the placenta that converts androgens to estrogen. Since the first description by Shozu et al. (1991), fewer than a dozen cases have been reported (Ludwig et al., 1998).

The specific action of the enzyme is the synthesis of estrone, estradiole, and estriol from dehydroepandrosterone sulfate (DHEA-S). This substance is derived from the androstenedione and testosterone secreted by both the fetal and maternal adrenal glands. From the 8th week onwards, when placental syncitial trophoblast aromatase normally becomes active, all three of these androgens accumulate above the block, causing masculinization not only of the fetal external genitalia but also of the mother (Harada et al., 1992).

At birth the majority of infants have been severely virilized with a large phallus and fusion of rugose labioscrotal folds. However, postnatally these appearances tend to improve. Although the internal genitalia are developmentally normal, the ovaries undergo progressive polycystic changes during childhood also reflecting a deficiency of aromatase in this organ (Ito et al., 1993). At puberty, in response to the rise in LH and follicle-stimulating hormone (FSH) levels and the reaccumulation of androgens, virilization reappears, manifest by clitoral hypertrophy, hirsutism, acne, a deepening voice, and amenorrhea. Postpartum, the maternal signs of virilization resolve.

The diagnosis of aromatase deficiency presently depends on finding high serum concentrations of androstenedione, testosterone, and DHEA-S in conjunction with very low or undetectable levels of estrogen. Serum LH and FSH levels are also usually raised. In equivocal cases the diagnosis may be revealed by a DHEA-S loading test. The cloning of the aromatase gene has allowed mutations to be recognized, thus potentially opening the way for genetic diagnosis of both affected individuals and heterozygous carriers (Bulun, 1996).

Treatment with estrogen is effective in reducing androgen levels by inhibiting gonadotropin production. This had been started at puberty, but a case can be made for giving regular low doses of estrogen during childhood to prevent cystic changes in the ovaries and normalize bone density and growth (Mullis et al., 1997). It may also be beneficial in affected male siblings to prevent the excessive bone growth and osteoporosis to which they are prone.

Exogenous virilization
Maternal medication

Occasionally, a female neonate is encountered with a slightly enlarged clitoris and normal ovaries in whom no biochemical abnormality can be demonstrated (Fig. 31.32). In the past, many such cases were encountered that were the result of mothers being given progestational agents in the first trimester of pregnancy as treatment for recurrent spontaneous abortion. This cause is now rare, but a detailed history should nonetheless be taken of any medications that may have been taken by the mother, particularly oral contraceptives which may have been initiated after pregnancy had become established.

Luteoma of pregnancy

In this condition, the maternal ovaries contain small, benign, fleshy nodules that histologically resemble the luteinized thecal cells seen in mature follicles. They appear to be the result of overstimulation of the ovarian stroma by gonadotropins in early pregnancy. The lesions are hormonally active producing androgens that may mildly virilize a female fetus as well as the mother. Their incidence is uncertain, but it seems likely that the majority are asymptomatic. Among mothers who developed signs of virilization, about 70% of their fetuses will be affected (McClamrock and Adashi, 1992).

Postpartum, the luteomas regress and the signs of virilization in the mother resolve. The genitalia of the baby also improve in appearance so that surgery is rarely necessary.

Theca–lutein cysts

These maternal ovarian lesions are sometimes encountered incidentally on an antenatal ultrasound scan. Like luteomas of pregnancy, they appear to be a response to gonadotropin stimulation, but the lesions are cystic rather than solid. Diabetic mothers and those with a multiple pregnancy seem particularly susceptible. However, only 30% of mothers with identified lesions show signs of virilization. Most babies are unaffected and when clitoral hypertrophy is present it is usually mild.

Other maternal tumors

Isolated reports appear from time to time of fetal virilization resulting from androgen-secreting Sertoli–Leydig cell tumors of the ovary, a hormonally active

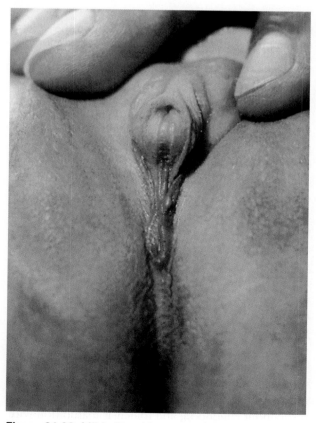

Figure 31.32 Mild clitoral hypertrophy.

Krukenberg tumor, or maternal adrenal cortical adenomas. Such occurrences are very rare, not only because of the infrequency of these tumors but also because of the critical timing necessary to cause ambiguity without impairing fertility.

Virilizing childhood tumors

Very occasionally a female infant is born with normal external genitalia who, in childhood, shows progressive hirsutism and enlargement of the clitoris. The diagnosis of late-onset CAH will be suspected, but when this has been excluded the possibility of a hormonally active ovarian or adrenal tumor must be considered (Masiakos *et al.*, 1997).

True hermaphroditism

Although true hermaphroditism is a rare form of intersexuality in Europe and North America, in central and southern Africa it is among the most common forms (Aaronson, 1985). Most cases are sporadic, but among families with the condition autosomal recessive and dominant forms of transmission have been described.

Clinical features

The appearance of the external genitalia in true hermaphroditism varies widely, ranging from unambiguously female with only mild clitoral hypertrophy to obviously male. Most lie towards the male end of the spectrum, having a large phallus with chordee and a single urogenital sinus opening in the hypospadiac position. Both gonads may be fully descended but when one remains high there is usually a corresponding asymmetry of the scrotum (Fig. 31.33). Late presentation is common, particularly in Africa, where those raised as boys may first be seen at puberty because of breast enlargement, cyclic hematuria or the sudden onset of a painful swelling in the scrotum as a result of a ruptured follicular cyst. The diagnosis may also be delayed in girls until the onset of virilization at puberty, or only come to light in adult life when investigations are carried out for infertility.

Karyotype

There is a marked geographic variation in the karyotypic findings in true hermaphroditism. In Africa, where the condition is common, the vast majority are

46,XX with no obvious mosaicism in the lympho-cytes, pudendal skin, or gonads. By contrast, in Europe and North America, mosaicism is the rule, with 46,XX/46,XY and 47,XXX/46,XY lines being the most common. A 46,XY karyotype is seen in about 7% of patients and is evenly distributed throughout Asia, Europe, and North America (Krob *et al.*, 1994)

The presence of testicular tissue with what appears to be a pure 46,XX karyotype has long been a puzzle. Translocation of the SRY gene to an X chromosome or autosome has been suspected, but this seems to be the case in only 10% of patients (McElreavey *et al.*, 1992). For the remainder, it has been postulated that there is either mosaicism which eludes detection, or possibly, that testicular tissue has developed as the result of a chromosomal mutation in the absence of SRY material (Berkovitz *et al.*, 1992). Several families have also been reported among whom both true her-maphroditism and 46,XX males have occurred, indi-cating that these conditions are genetically related (Slaney *et al.*, 1998).

The development of ovarian tissue in patients with a pure 46,XY karyotype is also puzzling. In some cases, this may be the result of an inactivating muta-tion of the SRY gene (Hiort and Klauber, 1995), but in others the cause must remain speculative until the genetic basis for normal ovarian development is bet-ter understood.

The coexistence of ovarian and testicular tissue in patients with a 46,XX/46,XY karyotype is less myster-ious although the reason for this chromosomal picture has been a source of speculation. Some are mosaics but others appear to be chimeras resulting from either double fertilization or the fusion of two zygotes of the opposite sex (Giltay *et al.*, 1998).

The gonads

The gonads in true hermaphroditism contain, by definition, both testicular and ovarian elements. The latter is distinguished from streak tissue by the pres-ence of at least one well-formed ovarian follicle. The most common distribution is in the form of bilateral ovotestes, but any combination may be found (Table 31.3). Curiously, testicular tissue tends to predominate on the right, perhaps related to the normally delayed differentiation of the gonad on this side.

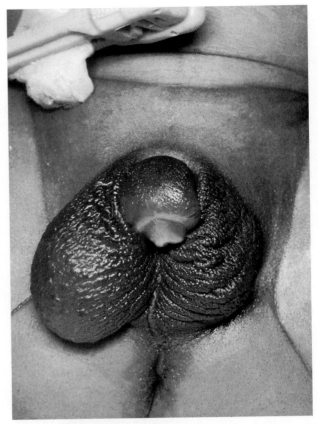

Figure 31.33 True hermaphroditism: note the scrotal asymmetry. The left gonad was an intra-abdominal ovotestis.

Most ovotestes are intra-abdominal, but some are scrotal in position, particularly when the ovarian com-ponent is small (Figs 31.34, 31.35). About 80% of ovotestes show an obvious polar distribution with a clear demarcation between the two components. The ovarian portion is yellow and firm with a granular surface which, in the newborn, may be expanded by a follicular cyst. The testicular portion is soft and pink as the tunica albuginea is often lacking. Rarely, the gonad may comprise an outer ovarian cortex conceal-ing a medullary zone of testicular tissue, reflecting the developmental potential of the outer and inner zones of the primordial gonad. In other cases there is a uni-form admixture of the two components. One gonad is occasionally absent.

Histologically, ovarian tissue is generally well dev-eloped, although the follicles are often fewer than normal. The appearance tends to remain stable throughout childhood, and follicular maturation with ovulation occurs at puberty. Testicular tissue, in contrast, although often appearing normal at birth, tends to degenerate during childhood with the progressive deposition of interstitial fibrous tissue and tubular atrophy (Fig. 31.36). Spermatogenesis is rare.

The endocrine function of the gonads appears to parallel the histologic findings. Ovarian tissue is capable of producing estrogen and progesterone and this seems to be sustained throughout the reproductive phase of adult life. By contrast, testosterone production by testicular tissue may be normal in early infancy, but thereafter tends to decline progressively (Aaronson, 1990).

Tumors have been reported in both components of the gonad. In the testis these have usually been seminomas, but gonadoblastomas and dysgerminomas are also described. Tumors arise less commonly in ovarian tissue, where they may take the form of dysgerminomas or other ovarian cell types commonly seen in women.

The prevalence of tumors is difficult to determine. Based on an extensive review of the literature, van Niekerk (1981) found an incidence of about 2.6%, but this may exaggerate the true figure inasmuch as those cases complicated by malignancy are more likely to be reported. Furthermore, most of these tumors arose in patients in whom the underlying condition was not initially recognized and testicular tissue was, consequently, retained in the abdominal cavity. For the individual who is correctly diagnosed and appropriately managed, the incidence of subsequent tumor formation is probably very low.

Internal ducts

The internal ductal anatomy parallels the histology of the ipsilateral gonad. Thus, on the side of an ovary, there is usually a well-developed fallopian tube and complete regression of the wolffian duct. A partially

Table 31.3 Gonadal findings among 47 patients with true hermaphroditism (from Aaronson, 1990)

Right gonad	Number	Left gonad
Ovotestis	19	Ovotestis
Ovotestis	13	Ovary
Testis	6	Ovary
Testis	6	Ovotestis
Ovary	2	Ovotestis
Ovary	1	Testis

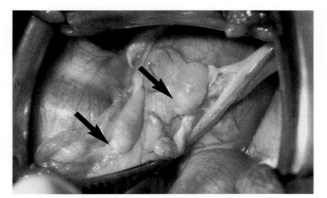

Figure 31.34 True hermaphroditism with bilateral intra-abdominal ovotestes. Note the smaller, ovarian portions (*arrows*).

or fully descended testis is usually accompanied by an epididymis and a well-formed vas with complete suppression of the müllerian ducts, indicating adequate antenatal secretion of both testosterone and MIS. In the presence of ovotestes, both duct systems are usually represented, although their degree of

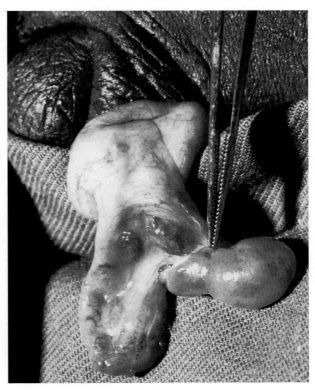

Figure 31.35 True hermaphroditism: a fully descended ovotestis showing a clear demarcation between the ovarian (left) and testicular (right) portions.

development is proportional to the volume of testicular tissue present. The uterus, however, is often rudimentary and the cervix rarely well defined. It is characteristic of true hermaphroditism that, even in the well-virilized patient, the vagina is usually capacious and opens into the urogenital sinus below the pelvic floor.

Diagnosis

The diagnosis of true hermaphroditism will be determined by gonadal biopsy but will be suspected when the karyotype reveals a 46,XX/46,XY or more complex picture. It should also be suspected in a 46,XX patient in whom the CAH screen is negative. The phenotypic appearance, however, is too variable to be helpful.

An ultrasound scan of the pelvis will sometime delineate the vagina and a small uterus behind the bladder. Determining the nature of intra-abdominal gonads is difficult but, when palpable and imaged directly, ovarian tissue may be distinguished from the homogeneous, low-intensity echo pattern of a testis, particularly if follicular cysts are present (Eberenz *et al.*, 1991).

Genitography should be tailored to delineate not only the vagina but also the uterine canal and any fallopian tube that may be present (Fig. 31.37). The demonstration of the confluence of the vagina with the urethra is essential for planning surgery.

Endocrine studies are valuable in suspected true hermaphrodites to confirm the presence of function-ing testicular tissue. The serum testosterone concentration will reflect its volume and can be measured directly immediately after birth and during the first few months postnatally when LH levels are elevated. At other times an hCG stimulation test will be necessary. MIS levels should also be measured but are particularly useful after the first few months of age when the serum testosterone concentration has fallen to very low levels. There is no ready marker for the presence of ovarian tissue in childhood, although Mendez *et al.* (1998) found that an hMG (human menopausal gonadotropin) stimulation test may be helpful in this regard, although this requires a prolonged course of injections.

Biopsy of a palpable gonad can be carried out through the scrotum if it is fully descended, but in most cases it is best approached through an inguinal incision which can be extended to inspect the internal genitalia. When the gonads are impalpable they may be biopsied and the internal genitalia inspected either laparoscopically or by a minilaparotomy. Because of the difficulty in some cases of distinguishing an ovotestis from a dysgenetic gonad on frozen section, it is generally best to defer definitive surgery until paraffin sections have been reviewed and a definitive surgical plan formulated.

Sex assignment

Among all the intersex disorders, true hermaphroditism offers the most freedom of choice with regard to the sex of rearing. Factors that favor rearing as a male are the presence of a good-sized phallus and a substantial volume of testicular tissue and subsequent testosterone production that may have encoded a male gender identity. It should be remembered, however, that a fall-off in endocrine function of testicular tissue that has been brought down into the scrotum must be anticipated and that testosterone replacement may be needed at puberty. Infants in whom the gonads are predominantly ovarian are generally raised as girls inasmuch as testosterone imprinting is unlikely to have been significant, the phallus is usually inadequate, the uterus is often fairly well developed and the vagina can be exteriorized without difficulty. Fertility among patients with true hermaphroditism raised as males has been alleged but is poorly documented. However, it is well recognized among women, some of whom have gone on to bear many children (Tiltman and Sweerts, 1982).

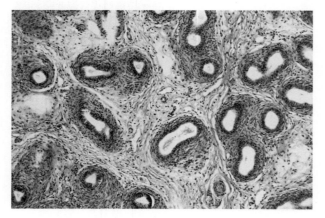

Figure 31.36 True hermaphroditism: testicular biopsy from a 4-year-old boy showing tubular atrophy. Hematoxylin and eosin. Original magnification × 80.

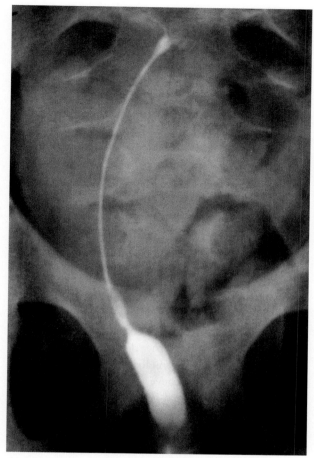

Figure 31.37 True hermaphroditism: genitogram showing a capacious vagina, uterine canal, and single fallopian tube.

Surgical management

The surgical management of true hermaphroditism consists initially of excising all inappropriate gonadal and duct tissues. When the sex of rearing is to be female, an intact ovary together with its adjacent tube is left *in situ* together with the uterus. A predominantly ovarian ovotestis may also be conserved as there is usually a sharp plane of demarcation (Fig. 31.38), provided that all testicular tissue can be safely removed without compromising the blood supply to the ovarian portion. The vas should be left *in situ* to further safeguard vascularity. Feminizing genitoplasty is then completed. Postoperatively, the presence of any residual testicular tissue should be determined by measuring serum MIS levels. However, this should be delayed for several weeks after the gonad was handled to allow any potential function to return.

When the sex of rearing is to be male, a predominantly testicular ovotestes is managed in a similar fashion, which will be straightforward when the ovarian component consists of a small overlying cap that can be easily trimmed away. All testicular tissue, however, must be brought down into the scrotum, using the Fowler–Stephens technique, if necessary, in which the principal gonadal vessels are ligated. In such cases, the ipsilateral fallopian tube should be left undisturbed to avoid damage to the collateral blood supply, upon which the survival of the gonad will depend. Ovotestes that do not lend themselves to partial conservation should be removed together with the fallopian tubes, uterus, and vagina as far as can be conveniently reached. Repair of the hypospadias is usually performed between 6 and 18 months of age.

Male pseudohermaphroditism

These patients have histologically normal testes but external genitalia which are either incongruous with their male genotype or ambiguous. The underlying cause is either defective synthesis of testosterone by the Leydig cells or, more frequently, an inadequate response to this hormone by the peripheral tissues.

Leydig cell hypoplasia

This condition was first described by Schwartz *et al.* (1981). Subsequently, only several dozen cases have been reported. The underlying cause is a defect in the hCG/LH receptor of the Leydig cells, the function of which is to trigger testosterone biosynthesis. Family studies have indicated an autosomal recessive inheritance pattern (Kremer *et al.*, 1995).

The classical, severe form of the disease causes a phenotype indistinguishable from complete androgen insensitivity in which the external genitalia are female and the vagina is short and blind ending. The testes may be palpable in the groin or intra-abdominal. An incomplete form of the condition is now recognized presenting with a small penis with hypospadias and incomplete descent of the testicles. A few cases of micropenis have also been attributed to this condition.

Histologically, Leydig cells are sparse or unidentifiable. Development of the müllerian ducts is completely suppressed but a rudimentary vas or epididymis may be present. This suggests that these

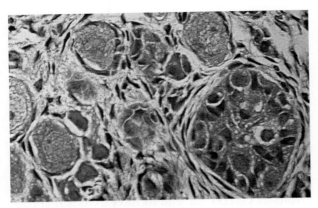

Figure 31.38 True hermaphroditism: ovotestis sectioned to show the sharp demarcation between the ovarian (left) and testicular (right) portions. Hematoxylin and eosin. Original magnification × 200.

structures can respond to very low levels of testosterone or, alternatively, that this hormone is produced autonomously by the Leydig cells independent of hCG and LH stimulation. At puberty, unlike in the androgen insensitivity syndrome, there is no breast development (Toledo, 1992).

Leydig cell hypoplasia can be distinguished from androgen insensitivity immediately postnatally by finding a very low serum testosterone concentration in the presence of normal or high LH levels. Thereafter, it will be necessary to carry out a gonadotropin-releasing hormone stimulation test which will demonstrate a normal LH response by the anterior pituitary, but no corresponding rise in serum testosterone or its precursors. This should be confirmed by an hCG stimulation test. The gene which encodes the Leydig cell hCG/LH receptor has been cloned, permitting study of mutations (Martens *et al.*, 1998). Because these patients will respond to exogenous testosterone, whenever possible they should be raised as males.

Girls who have inherited the condition also have defective LH receptors but their genitalia are normal. They usually come to light at puberty because of primary amenorrhea, but their breast development is normal (Stavrou *et al.*, 1998).

Testosterone biosynthesis defects

The Leydig cells are the main source of testosterone synthesis in boys and their normal function in early fetal life is essential for masculinization to occur (Fig. 31.39). The five enzymic steps necessary for the con-

version of intracellular cholesterol to testosterone are illustrated in Fig. 31.40. It will be seen that the first four of these replicate the pathways in the adrenal gland, although the contribution of this organ to testosterone synthesis is normally small.

Deficiency of each of these enzymes has been well described, although reports in the literature are few, suggesting that some patients may go unrecognized. The diagnosis can be established by identifying an increased concentration of the enzyme substrate or, in mild cases, an increase in substrate to product ratio, although an hCG stimulation test may be necessary to bring this out (Aaronson *et al.*, 1997). The genes encoding these enzymes have been cloned, permitting mutations to be identified.

Clinically, the external genitalia of patients with defects of testosterone synthesis show a wide spectrum. The vasa are usually present in spite of low serum testosterone levels, and the müllerian ducts are fully suppressed. At puberty the gonadotropin drive may partially overcome the defect with increasing masculinization of the genitalia, so that a male sex of rearing is desirable whenever possible. In addition to testosterone, which may be required at puberty, cortisol and fludrocortisone may be needed if the pathways in the adrenal glands are also significantly affected.

Congenital lipoid adrenal hyperplasia

Congenital lipoid adrenal hyperplasia has long been regarded as a rare and usually fatal defect of 20-22 desmolase function in the adrenal glands and testes. As this enzyme, which mediates the conversion of cholesterol to pregnenolone, lies at the head of the steroid cascade, impaired function will reduce the production of aldosterone and cortisol as well as testosterone. Classically, these babies look like normal girls but rapidly collapse and at autopsy are found to have adrenal glands that are massively distended with cholesterol and cholesterol esters (Prader and Gurtner, 1955).

The recent cloning of the 20-22 desmolase gene led to the surprising discovery that it, and the enzyme that it encodes, were both structurally normal (Lin *et al.*, 1991). The true underlying defect was eventually traced to a small but metabolically crucial protein now known as steroid acute reaction protein (StAR) which controls the access of substrate to 20-22 desmolase (Lin *et al.*, 1995).

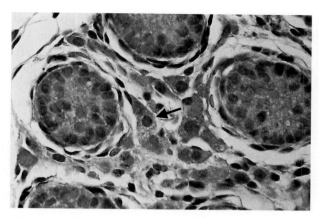

Figure 31.39 Leydig cells (*arrow*) appear prominent in this biopsy of a neonatal testis. Hematoxylin and eosin. Original magnification × 200.

StAR protein

StAR is a short, 285 amino acid polypeptide which is expressed in both the Leydig cells and the adrenal gland. It is physiologically important in the latter, where it is rapidly synthesized in response to ACTH, and triggers the immediate production of adrenal cortical steroids. It is believed to function by opening cholesterol transport channels in the mitochondrial membrane and thus acts as gatekeeper for the acute adrenocortical stress response (Bose *et al.*, 1998). In the Leydig cells, deficiency of the protein blocks testosterone biosynthesis.

Although congenital lipoid adrenal hyperplasia is undoubtedly an uncommon condition, more cases are now coming to light, particularly among Palestinians, Koreans, and Japanese. From these reports, it is becoming apparent that the condition shows a spectrum of severity with some patients surviving until adolescence. The classical presentation, seen in 50% of patients, is of a phenotypic girl who develops vomiting, diarrhea, severe salt loss and hypovolemic collapse, in whom the entire adrenal cortex is replaced by lipid. The remainder, however, show some degree of masculinization of their genitalia (Nakae *et al.*, 1997), and may be entirely asymptomatic for many weeks. In this group of patients, the cells of the definitive cortex are initially intact, allowing some steroid synthesis to take place. In time, however, these too become distended and disrupted by lipid accumulation so that the function of enzymes beyond 20-22 desmolase on the steroid cascade becomes secondarily impaired and symptoms appear (Miller, 1997).

The diagnosis of congenital lipoid adrenal hyperplasia should be suspected when there is hyperpigmentation of the skin in an apparent girl in whom the karyotype is found to be 46,XY. Biochemical investigations will reveal severe salt loss and hyperkalemia and very low levels of all adrenal steroids. Among virilized, milder cases, the diagnosis is difficult to establish biochemically as serum cortisol and testosterone concentrations may initially be in the low normal range. An abdominal ultrasound scan may be helpful by demonstrating adrenal enlargement.

Because of the predominantly female phenotype, all surviving patients have been raised as girls and given hormone replacement therapy. Histologic

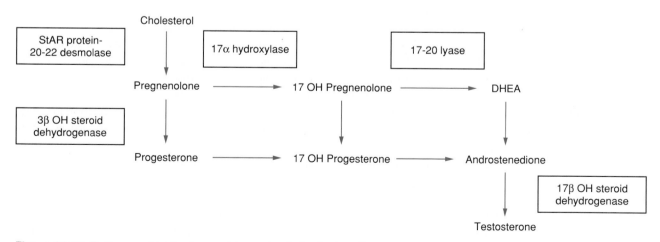

Figure 31.40 Pathway of testosterone biosynthesis in the Leydig cell, showing the five enzymes (in boxes) and the steps they regulate. Compare with the cortisol pathway in the adrenal gland (Fig. 31.28). (StAR = steroid acute reaction protein.)

examination of their testes, which will need to be removed, shows the Leydig cells to have a foamy appearance similar to, although less striking than, that found in the adrenal glands (Aya *et al.*, 1997).

As the inheritance pattern of congenital lipoid adrenal hyperplasia is autosomal recessive, it is assumed that the incidence among genetic females is the same as boys but, surprisingly, only a few such cases have been reported. The ovaries appear to be spared throughout childhood, and at puberty the breasts develop and menstruation occurs. Secondary amenorrhea, however, appears to be the rule as lipids accumulate in the ovaries and progressively inhibit function.

3β-Hydroxysteroid dehydrogenase type 2 deficiency

Deficiency of this enzyme, which was first described by Bongiovanni in 1961, causes ambiguity of the external genitalia in both boys and girls. The production of androstenedione, the immediate precursor of testosterone, is impaired and there is an accumulation above the block of 17-hydroxypregnenolone and DHEA. Because the latter is a weak androgen, masculinization of boys is incomplete but girls become mildly virilized.

3β-Hydroxysteroid dehydrogenase is a widely distributed enzyme which exists in two isoforms. Type 1 is found in the placenta as well as other tissues, but defects are not recognized clinically (Morel *et al.*, 1997). Type 2 is found in the adrenal glands, where it mediates mineralocorticoid, glucocorticoid, and testosterone synthesis, as well as in the testes and ovaries.

3β-Hydroxysteroid dehydrogenase deficiency seems to be a rare condition but is probably underdiagnosed as the relevant biochemical studies are rarely performed. In the classical case, boys present at birth with penoscrotal or perineal hypospadias and, usually, fully descended testes. Cortisol deficiency and salt wasting become apparent early, leading to collapse in the neonatal period. A non-salt-losing variety is now recognized, raising the possibility that the adrenal and testicular enzymes may be under independent genetic control. Mild cases with a later onset have also been described (Mebarki *et al.*, 1995).

The diagnosis of 3β-hydroxysteroid dehydrogenase deficiency can readily be made in the florid case by measuring the concentration of steroids above and below the suspected block. Thus, pregnenolone, 17-hydroxypregnenolone, and DHEA concentrations are raised, whereas progesterone, 17-hydroxyprogesterone, and androstenedione levels are low. Deoxycortisol and corticosterone concentrations are also usually low.

In less severe cases the diagnosis can be more difficult to establish, particularly in early infancy, when the enzyme is normally relatively inefficient. Interpretation of the biochemical results may also be confused by the action of the type 1 isoenzyme in peripheral tissues. Genetic diagnosis may prove helpful in these cases, particularly as the gene is small and therefore accessible to thorough examination.

Cortisol replacement is necessary in most cases, which corrects the biochemical deficiencies, and the hypospadias is repaired at the appropriate time. Fertility in these patients has not been well documented.

17α-Hydroxylase and 17-20 lyase deficiency

The enzyme mediating both 17α-hydroxylase and 17-20 lyase activity is a single polypeptide which is expressed in both the adrenal glands and gonads. Deficiency of the enzyme was first reported by Biglieri *et al.* (1966), although it was only several years later that its association with ambiguous genitalia was recognized (New, 1970). Affected boys are usually well masculinized with a variable degree of hypospadias. Hypertension is common because of the accumulation of steroids on the aldosterone pathway. The association of hypospadias and hypertension should therefore lead to a suspicion of the diagnosis. Gynecomastia may develop at puberty.

When the defect is severe the external genitalia of these babies will look predominantly female with mild clitoral hypertrophy (Monno *et al.*, 1997). However, there does not appear to be any correlation between the severity of the hypertension and the phenotype, suggesting that either the adrenal and testicular enzymes are affected differently, or the impairment may only affect the 17α-hydroylase or the 17-20 lyase function. Girls with this enzyme defect are also hypertensive, but the underlying cause is not usually appreciated until they are investigated for primary amenorrhea.

The biochemical diagnosis is established by finding raised progesterone, DOC, and corticosterone, and reduced DHEA and androstenedione concentrations in the serum. The ratio of pregnenolone to 17-hydroxypregnenolone and progesterone to 17-hydroxyprogesterone will also be elevated. Serum sodium levels may also be raised, with corresponding hypokalemia.

The enzyme is encoded by a small gene spanning 6.6 kb. A mutation hot spot has been identified on exon 8 which may facilitate genetic diagnosis (Hermans *et al.*, 1996).

17β-Hydroxysteroid dehydrogenase type 3 deficiency

This recessively inherited enzyme defect, also known as 17-ketosteroid reductase deficiency, was first described by Saez *et al.* (1971). The enzyme appears to be expressed exclusively in the testes, where it catalyses the conversion of androstenedione to testosterone. Its distribution is presently unknown but it is common among the Palestinian population of the Gaza region, where it has been estimated that 1 in 100 males are affected (Rösler *et al.*, 1996).

Clinically, most patients present as phenotypic females with clitoral hypertrophy and a urogenital sinus, although one or both testes are often palpable in the groin. Most are therefore raised as girls, but at puberty marked virilization occurs with the development of a muscular build, hirsutism, enlargement of the phallus, and partial descent of the testes. Many of these patients, as is the case with 5α-reductase deficiency, reassign themselves as males. The underlying biochemical change responsible for this virilization is believed to be the rapid accumulation of androstenedione in response to the pubertal LH drive, which is converted by a 17β-hydroxysteroid dehydrogenase isoenzyme in peripheral tissues to testosterone.

At least four isoenzymes of 17β-hydroxysteroid dehydrogenase, which are essential for androgen and estrogen synthesis, have been identified and numbered according to the order in which their DNA was cloned. Type 1 is found in the placenta and ovary, whereas type 2 is abundant in extraglandular tissues such as the liver, skin, and fat. Type 3 is found exclusively in the testes (Andersson and Moghrabi, 1997). All three isoenzymes are the product of separate genes. Girls who are homozygous for 17β-hydroxysteroid dehydrogenase deficiency are clinically unaffected.

Diagnosis

The biochemical diagnosis is made by finding an elevated androstenedione concentration in the serum in the presence of low testosterone levels. Beyond the first few months of age, an hCG stimulation test will be necessary to demonstrate an increase in the ratio of these hormones. The enzyme also mediates the conversion of DHEA to androstenediol, and estrone to estradiol. Assays of these substances are therefore helpful in making the diagnosis.

Management

Because of the responsiveness of these patients to exogenous testosterone, preference should always be given to raising these children as boys. A test course of parenteral testosterone is given to observe phallic growth. Because of the spontaneous improvement that occurs in this condition, exogenous testosterone may not be necessary at puberty.

5α-Reductase deficiency

Epidemiology

This condition, in which the conversion of testosterone to dihydrotestosterone is impaired, was first recognized independently by Imperato-McGinley *et al.* (1974) among inbred villagers in the Dominican Republic, and by Walsh *et al.* (1974) who described affected siblings in an African–American family. Clusters of cases have since been reported in Papua New Guinea, the Middle East, and Central and South America among communities where consanguinity is common. Presently, approximately 100 cases have been well documented among 50 families, only a few of whom are from Europe or North America. A striking feature of the condition is the progressive masculinization that occurs towards puberty, so that those raised as girls often develop a male gender identity (Mendonca *et al.*, 1996). In communities where such patients are well known, they are often given a special designation. For example, among the Sambians of Papua New Guinea, the term 'kwoluaatmwol' or 'turnim man' is applied. Because of the difficulty in making the diagnosis, particularly in mild cases, it is likely that 5α-reductase deficiency is more prevalent then is presently recognized.

The enzyme

5α-Reductase exists as two separate isoenzymes. Type 1, distinguished by its optimal *in vitro* function at an alkaline pH, is found in many tissues of the body but, hitherto, no deficiency disease has been described.

Type 2, responsible for genital ambiguity, was the second of the two isoenzymes to be identified. It is a 254 amino acid protein that is expressed mainly in the prostate gland and external genitalia, although some activity has also been found in the liver and brain (Aumuller *et al.*, 1996). The substrate for the enzyme is testosterone, which it converts to dihydrotestosterone, a compound that binds more avidly to the androgen receptors of target cells.

The gene that encodes the enzyme is relatively small, but over 30 distinct point mutations have now been identified in patients and their families, mostly of the missense or nonsense type. These usually result in a single amino acid change in the enzyme, which alters its efficacy (Thigpen *et al.*, 1992).

Clinical features

Among the early cases described were boys who had severe hypospadias with a small vagina opening separately on the perineum. Consequently, the condition was originally known as pseudovaginal perineoscrotal hypospadias. It is now recognized that the phenotypic appearance embraces a wide spectrum. However, at birth most babies look more female then male, having an enlarged clitoris and a single urogenital sinus opening that conceals a blind-ending vagina. The testes, however, although undescended, are frequently palpable in the groin. Less often, the phenotype is predominantly male, presenting as hypospadias together with an undescended testis.

If unrecognized, these children virilize at puberty with marked enlargement of the phallus, progressive descent of one or both testes, and the development of a strikingly muscular build. Breast development, however, does not occur, and axillary and pubic hair are sparse or absent. These patients do not develop acne, which is common among their peers at this age, and the prostate remains small. These changes appear to be brought about by the rapid rise in serum testosterone at puberty, confirming the diminishing importance of 5α-reductase during childhood.

Diagnosis

Every effort should be made to make the diagnosis of 5α-reductase deficiency whenever male pseudohermaphroditism is diagnosed, as the predictable slide towards masculinization would favor male as the sex of rearing. In the classical case, this will be confirmed by finding an elevated serum testosterone to dihydrotestosterone ratio, frequently in the order of 50:1, compared with the normal ratio of approximately 5–10:1. An early-morning serum sample may suffice during the first few months of life, but at other times an hCG stimulation test will be necessary. Initially, 5000 IU hCG can be given and serum levels of testosterone and dihydrotestosterone measured in a sample drawn 48 hours later. If the ratios remain within the normal range, 1500 IU is given on alternate days for five doses, and the levels are remeasured 24 hours after the last dose.

Among less florid cases, the diagnosis of 5α-reductase deficiency is difficult. This is due in part to the normally wide range of testosterone to dihydrotestosterone ratios. Additionally, among patients with the androgen insensitivity syndrome, there may be a secondary inhibition of 5α-reductase activity brought about by the interaction of the enzyme with the androgen receptor in peripheral tissues (Imperato-McGinley *et al.*, 1982). The situation is further complicated by the fact that LH secretion may also be stimulated. Thus, the finding of elevated LH and testosterone levels may suggest the diagnosis of androgen insensitivity syndrome. To overcome these problems, Imperato-McGinley *et al.* (1986) have proposed that, in addition to the serum testosterone to dihydrotestosterone ratios, the ratio of 5β-tetrahydrocortisol to 5α-tetrahydrocortisol in the urine should be measured. These values reflect 5α-reductase activity in the liver and will be elevated only in primary 5α-reductase deficiency.

These biochemical methods have now largely replaced the traditional *in vitro* measurement of testosterone conversion to dihydrotestosterone in cultured pudendal skin fibroblasts. Presently, the possibility of genetic diagnosis looks encouraging because of the small size of the gene, a low incidence of polymorphism, and the availability of a rapid screening method (Hiort *et al.*, 1996).

Management

Among communities where 5α-reductase deficiency is endemic and well recognized, approximately 75% of those raised as girls spontaneously change their gender identity, with alterations in their sexual behavior becoming apparent from as early as 8 years of age. In cases where the diagnosis is firmly established, male should therefore be the sex of rearing whenever this is practical. The extent to which these psychological changes are the result of testosterone imprinting of the brain rather than a reaction to evident virilization is presently unclear. There is no doubt that cultural pressures may also play a role for, in many parts of the developing world, there is a strong bias towards raising children as males, particularly because of the stigma attached to a female who is certain to be infertile. Among those to be raised as boys, dihydrotestosterone cream or, alternatively, high doses of parenteral testosterone will often improve the size of the penis. Hypospadias repair is then carried out 6 months later when maximum benefit will be seen, and the testes are brought down into the scrotum.

Among infants in whom the phallus is extremely small or where androgen treatment has been disappointing, a feminizing genitoplasty and bilateral orchiectomies should be considered. The parents, however, should be cautioned that the ultimate gender identify of the child cannot be confidently predicted.

Fertility

Fertility among patients raised as boys is usually impaired as a result of the small size of the prostate and correspondingly low seminal fluid volume. Sperm counts, however, are variable and in some cases have been within the normal range. Ivarsson (1996) has reported two brothers with 5α-reductase deficiency who have fathered children.

Complete androgen insensitivity syndrome

The first detailed clinical description of this syndrome was given in a classic paper by Morris (1953). He thought that the testes of these women produced a feminizing hormone and therefore called the condition 'testicular feminization'. It was over 20 years later, however, that the underlying cause was recognized as a defect in the androgen receptors (Keenen *et al.*, 1974). Complete androgen insensitivity syndrome (CAIS) is probably the most common cause of male pseudohermaphroditism, with an estimated incidence of 1 in 20 000 male births (Quigley *et al.*, 1995). It also occurs in many other mammals and is the best studied of all receptor deficiency diseases.

Clinical features

The external genitalia of babies with complete androgen insensitivity look entirely female and the diagnosis will not be suspected unless there is a fami-

ly history of the condition. Sometimes, however, the presentation is with an inguinal hernia when a testis is found in the sac. It has been estimated that between 1 and 2% of all girls with an inguinal hernia will have the condition and it has, therefore, been recommended they should be routinely karyotyped. However, the diagnosis can be ruled-out by simply identifying the gonad at the time of surgical repair, either directly or by laparoscopy through the peritoneal defect. When there is no family history, the majority of patients come to light only at puberty when they are investigated for primary amenorrhea.

When unrecognized, puberty follows a male pattern, occurring a little later than expected, with a pronounced growth spurt so that these women are taller than their peers. The breasts are usually well developed, although the nipples remain small. Axillary and pubic hair, which are testosterone dependent, is usually scanty or absent, giving rise to the descriptive term 'hairless women'. Similarly, facial hair is absent and as adolescents they do not develop acne. The labia and clitoris remain infantile but the vagina, which opens in the normal position in the vulva, is usually adequate in caliber although short and blind ending. A testis is palpable in the groin on one or both sides in the majority of cases (Viner *et al.*, 1997).

Female internal genitalia are usually absent, although in up to one-third a rudimentary uterus and fallopian tubes will be found (Rutgers and Scully, 1991). MIS appears to be produced in normal concentration by the testes, suggesting that some interaction with functioning androgen receptors is necessary for it to be effective. Rudimentary vasa and epididymides may also be present, indicating the exquisite sensitivity of these structures to androgens.

Histologically, the testes are initially normal, although the Leydig cells are prominent. During childhood, however, they undergo progressive tubular atrophy similar to that seen in boys with cryptorchidism. Testes that are retained in the abdominal cavity are susceptible to malignant degeneration, usually in the form of seminomas. The overall risk has been calculated to be 3% at the age of 20 years, rising to 30% by 50 years of age. Hamartomatous nodules comprising Leydig cells, Sertoli cells, spermatogonia, and fibrous tissue also develop as a result of the high levels of circulating LH (Scully, 1991).

The androgen receptor

The androgen receptor is encoded by a single-copy X chromosome gene assigned to Xq11-12 and is transmitted by the mother to male infants in a recessive fashion. Over 200 mutations have hitherto been described, making these the most diverse of all reported gene defects.

The androgen receptor protein can be identified as early as 8 weeks' gestation in many tissues throughout the body. It is thought to reside in the cell cytoplasm and binds both testosterone and dihydrotestosterone. The bound receptor then migrates into the nucleus, where it triggers a series of steps culminating in the production of mRNA (Fig. 31.41). The androgen receptor is modulated by a complex mechanism in which testosterone appears, overall, to downregulate its activity.

Diagnosis

The diagnosis of CAIS is straightforward when, among families known to have the condition, a newborn baby girl is found to have a 46 XY karyotype. Among sporadic cases the diagnosis is more difficult.

Classically, the diagnosis is made at puberty by finding the concentration of both LH and testosterone to be well above normal, a consequence of the impaired feedback of testosterone on the anterior pituitary gland in which the androgen receptors are also thought to be defective. Elevation of LH and testosterone concentrations may also be seen in the first few months postnatally, although often they are normal. In some cases, the serum level of MIS during the first year of life may be raised but in others this is also normal. Because of these difficulties, the diagnosis of complete androgen insensitivity is usually assumed in a phenotypic female if the testes are histologically normal and defects in testosterone biosynthesis and 5α-reductase activity have been excluded.

Patients with complete androgen insensitivity are invariably raised as girls and, provided follow-up can be assured, intra-abdominal testes may be left in place until puberty to allow their estrogen production to enhance breast development. However, they must be removed immediately afterwards as malignant degeneration has been described in an adolescent as young as 14 years. When palpable, it is best to remove them early through separate inguinal incisions because of the risk of bowel strangulation in the associated hernia (Fig. 31.42). Estrogen is begun at puberty to induce breast development, and thereafter should be continued to maintain bone density, but patient compliance is often poor (Soule et al., 1995). A gynecologic examination should also be carried out at puberty to determine the caliber and length of the vagina; however, surgical intervention is rarely necessary.

Girls with complete androgen insensitivity should be told that they will be unable to conceive but can have children by adoption. It is also preferable that they are told that they have a 46,XY karyotype, although it should be explained that this has no relevance to their female status.

Partial androgen insensitivity syndrome

The incidence of this condition is presently uncertain because of the difficulty in firmly establishing the diagnosis. It probably accounts, however, for a substantial portion of patients with male pseudohermaphroditism in whom no other cause can be found. The syndromes described by Reifenstein (1947), Gilbert-Dreyfus et al. (1957), Lubs et al. (1959) and Rosewater et al. (1965) are now believed to be examples of this condition.

Clinical features

Partial androgen insensitivity syndrome (PAIS) embraces a wide phenotypic spectrum ranging from slight clitoral hypertrophy with the vagina opening in the normal position to mild hypospadias (Table 31.4). Most recognized cases fall somewhere between these extremes with some degree of genital ambiguity. It is thought that some infertile males represent the mildest form of this condition (Aiman et al., 1979). At puberty, virilization is frequently disappointing so that an initial decision to assign these patients as males may be regretted. Consequently, PAIS presents one of the most difficult management problems among all intersex disorders.

Imaging studies

The findings on genitography will parallel the degree of ambiguity of the genitalia. A blind-ending vagina will usually be identified entering the urogenital sinus below the level of the pelvic floor. The vault is often rounded and smooth, from which filling of slender vasa may sometimes be seen (Fig. 31.43). Ultrasonography of palpable testes will reveal a normal, homogeneous echo pattern.

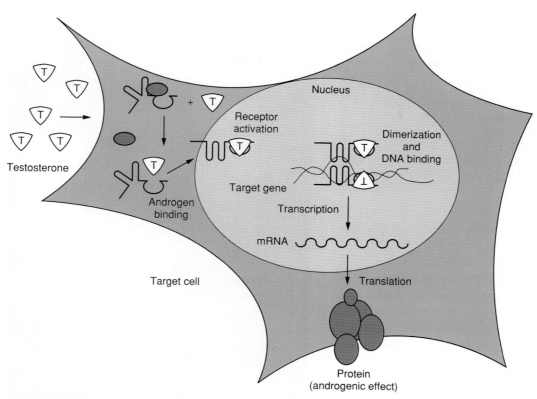

Figure 31.41 Androgen receptor binding in the target cell: the molecular events involved in induction of an androgen effect within the target cell. The initial step is the binding of androgen 'T' to the intracellular androgen receptor. This results in removal of inhibitory proteins (oval) and activation of the receptor to its DNA-binding state. Within the cell nucleus, the receptor complex undergoes dimerization and binding to a hormone response element, regulatory DNA sequence in or near a target gene. This interaction of the receptor dimer with its target gene regulates gene transcription. The same sequence of events occurs in the presence of dihydrotestosterone. (From Quigley *et al*. 1995, with permission.)

Diagnosis

In clinical practice a firm diagnosis of partial androgen insensitivity is rarely made but is often inferred from the clinical and biochemical findings.

Biochemical studies

Although an elevated serum testosterone level is suggestive of the diagnosis of partial androgen insensitivity, this may be difficult to discern because of the wide range normally seen immediately after birth. However, unlike in the complete form of the disease, high levels may be found during the first few months associated with an unusually high level of LH. The testosterone to dihydrotestosterone ratio may be slightly raised, reflecting a secondary insensitivity to 5α-reductase, but this does not

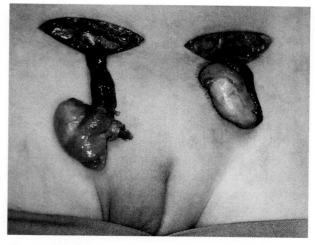

Figure 31.42 Complete androgen insensitivity syndrome: bilateral inguinal explorations revealed apparently normal testes.

Table 31.4 Clinical grading of androgen insensitivity (after Quigley *et al.*, 1995)

Classification	Phenotype
Grade 1	Normal male, infertile
Grade 2	Mild or moderate hypospadias
Grade 3	Severe hypospadias
Grade 4	Ambiguous
Grade 5	Clitoral hypertrophy
Grade 6	Normal female, pubic hair
Grade 7	Normal female, no pubic hair

usually reach the ratios commonly seen in true 5α-reductase deficiency.

For many years, the mainstay of diagnosis of partial androgen insensitivity was the measurement of the *in vitro* binding of testosterone by genital skin fibroblasts. In about one-third of cases, however, no defect in binding could be demonstrated and these patients were, therefore, thought to have a 'post-receptor defect'. It is now appreciated that the androgen-receptor has not only an androgen-binding domain, which this technique quantifies, but also a domain that binds the receptor to nuclear DNA, which it does not measure. In spite of this limitation the method is still sometimes used for diagnosis.

The measurement of free serum sex hormone binding globulin has been proposed by Sinnecker *et al.* (1997) as an alternative test for androgen insensitivity. It depends on the fact that, in complete androgen insensitivity, the globulin is unable to bind androgens so that its concentration in the free form remains high, as is the case in women. Patients with partial androgen insensitivity have free globulin levels that lie somewhere between the normal range for males and females. In children an oral load of Stanozolol, a synthetic androgen, must first be given because of their relatively low serum testosterone levels. Although useful in childhood, the test has proved disappointing in the first few months of life.

Because of the inconclusive nature of all of these diagnostic tests, attention is presently focused on the detection of mutations and deletions in the androgen receptor gene.

Gene probe studies

The androgen receptor gene is a large structure spanning between 75 and 90 kb comprising eight exons and seven introns (Fig. 31.44). It is made up of an

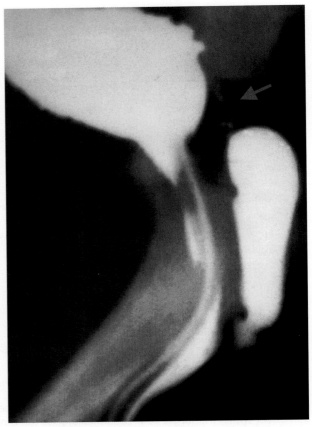

Figure 31.43 Partial androgen insensitivity syndrome: genitogram showing a rounded vaginal vault and faint filling of the vasa (*arrow*).

NH$_2$ transcription activation terminal, a highly conserved DNA binding domain encoded by exons 2 and 3, a hinge region that appears to target androgen receptor protein to the nucleus, and a COOH steroid binding domain encoded by exons 4–8. Eighty-five per cent of the defects hitherto described occur in the steroid binding domain, with the remaining 15% occurring in the DNA binding domain. In over 90% of cases, the mutations are confined to a few base pairs. 'Hot spots' have been identified in exons 5, 6, and 7, and kits are now available for automated sequencing to screen these regions. However, because of its large size, screening of the entire gene is presently not practical.

Analysis of the several hundred mutations and deletions that have been identified thus far reveals that there is little correlation with the phenotypic findings. An exception is the complete deletion of the gene which, although very rare, is invariably associated with complete androgen insensitivity. The much more common point mutations are associated with a wide phenotypic spectrum, with variations occurring even among siblings who have the same mutation. Cases of androgen insensitivity have also been reported in which no gene defect could be identified. This may have been the result of a laboratory error or mosaicism with only certain cells being affected. Alternatively, mutations may have been present in parts of exons not screened or even within introns (Brüggenwirth *et al.*, 1997). It is also possible that these cases may represent defects, not of the androgen receptor gene itself, but of other genes that may lie upstream or downstream.

In spite of these difficulties, gene analysis has proved useful in screening families with known mutations to detect carriers. It has also been used for antenatal diagnosis by chorionic villae sampling. However, about 25% of all cases of androgen insensitivity are not familial but arise as a *de novo* mutation (Boehmer *et al.*, 1997), thus limiting its value.

Management

The management of patients with partial androgen insensitivity is difficult because, unlike individuals with 5α-reductase or 17β-hydroxysteroid dehydrogenase deficiencies, those with receptor defects are unlikely to develop a satisfactory sized penis at puberty (Fig. 31.45). When the phallus is small most clinicians prefer to give a prolonged course of testosterone to see what growth can be obtained. Gene studies may have some predictive value insofar as those in whom the mutation occurs in the DNA binding domain are likely to have a particularly poor response (Tincello *et al.*, 1997).

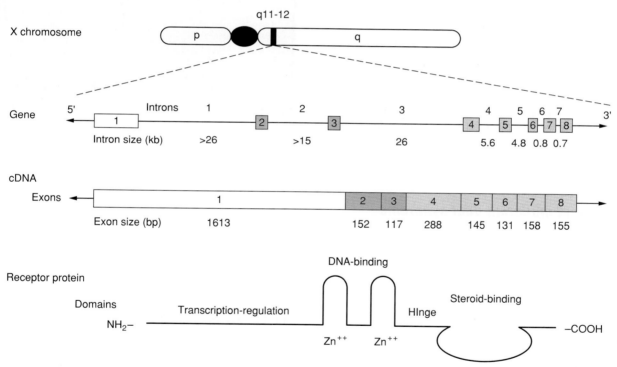

Figure 31.44 The X-chromosomal locus of the AR gene and structural organization of the gene and protein. (Top) The AR gene is located in the pericentromeric region of the long arm of the X-chromosome at Xq11-12. (Middle), The AR gene spans 75–90 kb of genomic DNA, the eight coding exons (numbered within boxes) being separated by introns (numbered above the diagram) ranging from 0.7 kb to more than 26 kb in size. Intron sizes are given beneath the diagram. The AR complementary DNA comprises a coding region of approximately 2760 bp. The base pair sizes of the eight exons are given below the diagram. Exon 1 encodes the amino-terminal domain; exons 2 and 3 encode the DNA-binding domain; the 5′-region of exon 4 encodes the hinge region including the nuclear targeting signal; the 3′-portion of exon 4 and exons 5–8 encode the steroid-binding domain. (Bottom) Schematic representation of the AR protein (not intended to represent the actual 3D structure). The main functional domains of the AR are, from left to right: the amino-terminal, transcription-regulation domain; the DNA-binding domain, comprising a pair of zinc-binding motifs (zinc fingers); the hinge region, containing the nuclear-targeting sequence; the steroid-binding domain. (From Quigley *et al.* 1995, with permission).

The testes should be removed when female is to be the sex of rearing as soon as this decision is made because of the risk that some virilization, which may include irreversible deepening of the voice, will occur at puberty. Breast development can be satisfactorily induced with estrogen.

When the size of the penis is adequate, or shows a good response to testosterone administration, male will usually be the sex of rearing. The hypospadias is repaired and both testes are brought down into the scrotum. The testes should, however, remain under long-term surveillance, both clinically and by ultrasound scanning, because of an increased risk of tumors. Fertility among men with partial androgen insensitivity is poorly documented.

Kennedy disease

This X-linked condition is a variant of motor neurone disease in which there is progressive androgen resistance that first becomes apparent in adult life (MacLean *et al.*, 1995). The latter is manifest by testicular atrophy, declining production of testosterone and the development of gynecomastia. These patients have a unique mutation in their androgen receptor gene comprising 20 CAG trinucleotide repeat sequences. The association of these two conditions suggests that androgens may be required for the integrity of anterior horn cells.

Persistent müllerian duct syndrome

This uncommon condition is usually classified as a variety of male pseudohermaphroditism, although it does not cause any ambiguity of the external genitalia. It is the result of a defect in either the production or the peripheral action of MIS (Guerrier *et al.*, 1989), and usually only comes to light in adult life when a fallopian tube or uterus is encountered during the repair of an inguinal hernia, hence the descriptive name of 'hernia uteri inguinalis'. The condition is only rarely encountered in childhood (Karnak *et al.*, 1997).

The patients often present with an inguinal hernia and a non-palpable contralateral testis. At exploration, both testes are found in the hernia sac because the testes are unusually mobile, so that one is frequently drawn across to the opposite side. Additionally, the fallopian tubes and often the uterus, may also be delivered into the wound. In about 20% of cases the presentation is with bilateral cryptorchidism. Because

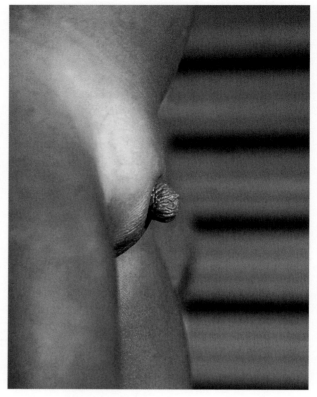

Figure 31.45 Partial androgen insensitivity syndrome in an 11 year old raised as a boy. Note the very small penis.

of their extreme mobility testis torsion is common, so that at surgery only blind-ending spermatic vessels may be found (Imbeaud *et al.*, 1995). In such cases, the penis is also likely to be small.

Histologically, the testes appear normal, but in time undergo the atrophic changes usually seen with cryptorchidism. The epididymides are well developed but the vasa are short and run down towards the urethra in the wall of the uterus. The uterus is otherwise normal but at puberty remains infantile because of the lack of estrogen stimulation. The vagina is short and opens via a narrow communication into the mid-prostatic urethra at the center of the verumontanum.

The underlying cause in 50% of cases of persistent müllerian duct syndrome is a severe defect of Sertoli cell MIS production. Most of the patients reported in this group, who come from inbred communities bordering the Mediterranean Sea or the Middle East, have a diverse range of mutations in their MIS gene. The remaining 50% of patients have a defect in the MISR-2 receptor where the mutations tend to be more homogeneous, comprised often of a 27 bp deletion in exon 10 (Imbeaud *et al.*, 1996). Biochemically, the two varieties are easily distinguished by finding very low or unrecordable MIS levels in the group with a Sertoli cell defect, whereas levels are normal or elevated when the defect lies in the receptor.

Patients with persistent müllerian duct syndrome are assumed to be potentially fertile, although this has not been well documented. The surgical challenge in these patients, therefore, is to move both testes down to the scrotum, retaining both their blood supply and continuity of the vasa. This is best achieved by dividing the fallopian tubes and bringing the distal portion down with the testes. The proximal ends of the tubes are then removed together with the central portion of the uterus, but preserving a strip of the lateral uterine wall to protect the vasa.

Disorders with dysgenetic gonads

In this group of disorders the gonads fail to differentiate completely into either an ovary or a testis. Histologically, they form a spectrum ranging from streaks of fibrous tissue to testicular dysgenesis in which the gonads may be recognizable as testes but show a variable degree of disorganization. Mixed gonadal dysgenesis is the most common of these disorders, in which one gonad is represented by a fibrous streak and the other a well-formed testicle. The karyotypic findings are variable but frequently include a 46,XO cell line. Clinically, external genitalia range from entirely female to obviously male with hypospadias and cryptorchidism. Some of the features of Turner syndrome may be seen in those harboring a 45,XO cell line, whereas others may exhibit the dysmorphic features of a multiple malformation syndrome.

Gonadal dysgenesis

In this group of patients, whose gonads consist of bilateral undifferentiated streak tissue, the external genitalia are unambiguously female. Their importance lies, among those whose karyotype contains Y chromosome material, in the risk that their gonads will undergo malignant degeneration. Among those whose dysgenetic gonads are part of a broader syndrome, manifestations of the latter may also pose a threat to life.

Turner syndrome

This syndrome, first described by Henry Turner in 1938, remains a purely descriptive term for a constellation of somatic abnormalities in infertile women with streak gonads who typically have a 45,XO karyotype.

The outward features of the syndrome are easily recognizable, although not all are necessarily present in any given patient (Hall and Gilchrist, 1990). They include a webbed neck deformity with low hairline, low-set ears, a shield-like chest with widely spaced nipples, and an increased carrying angle at the elbows. Lymphodema of the hands and feet is common in infants and children, in whom pigmented skin lesions may also be found. Older children are of short stature.

Coarctation of the aorta is present in 30% of cases and such a finding should, therefore, always alert the physician to the possibility of Turner syndrome. Renal anomalies are also found in about 30% of patients, particularly a horseshoe kidney, other fusion anomalies, and unilateral renal agenesis. At puberty, secondary sexual features are poorly developed or absent and primary amenorrhea is the rule.

The external genitalia are unambiguously female. The ovaries are histologically normal at birth but within a few months become atretic with the eventual disappearance of the ova. They are hormonally sluggish and, by the time the diagnosis is usually made, consist of bilateral streaks in the broad ligaments which histologically resemble ovarian type stroma but are devoid of follicles. The risk for malignant degeneration is generally regarded as very low. The vagina, uterus, and fallopian tubes develop normally but remain infantile.

Although classically Turner patients have a pure 45,XO karyotype, sophisticated techniques have revealed that some harbor Y chromosome material. Turner syndrome should therefore be regarded not as a unique entity but, rather, as part of the broad spectrum of gonadal dysgenesis.

Because of the known risk of malignancy developing in dysgenetic gonads containing Y material, this should be diligently looked for, particularly if there is any virilization of the external genitalia. Lo *et al.* (1996) recommend that 100 rather than 30 cells should be examined when karyotyping patients with any somatic features of Turner syndrome. However, as Y material may be confined to the gonads, a case can be made that these should be routinely biopsied and karyotyped using, if available, an SRY probe (Lopez *et al.*, 1998). Those found to be positive should be removed. They can otherwise be left *in situ* so that the patient may benefit from any potential hormonal function.

Noonan syndrome

The condition is a common disorder seen in both males and females who show some of the phenotypic features of Turner syndrome (Noonan, 1994). Males often have undescended testes. It is inherited as an autosomal dominant disorder with many patients representing spontaneous mutation. Females are fertile and have normal internal genitalia.

46,XX gonadal dysgenesis

In this rare condition the patients appear to be normal girls but harbor streak gonads indistinguishable from those in Turner syndrome. The diagnosis usually only comes to light at puberty when the investigation of primary amenorrhea reveals high gonadotropin but low estrogen levels and laparoscopy identifies two streak gonads. The importance of the condition lies in the possibility that these patients, like those with Turner syndrome, may harbor latent Y material. The gonads should therefore be biopsied (Letterie and Page, 1995).

46,XY gonadal dysgenesis

Patients with this condition, known as Swyer's syndrome, have streak gonads that are indistinguishable from those found in the 46,XX variety of gonadal dysgenesis (Swyer, 1955). The external genitalia are those of a normal female and there is a well-formed uterus with fallopian tubes (Fig. 31.46). Its importance lies in the strong tendency of the gonads to develop tumors. The incidence rises with increasing age, reaching about 50% by 30 years, by far the most common type being a gonadoblastoma.

Gene defects

It has for long been suspected that the underlying cause of the failure of the gonads to develop into normal testes lies in a defect in the genes involved in testicular development and differentiation. The SRY gene was the obvious candidate, but mutations are found in only 15% of cases (Fuqua *et al.*, 1996). Other genes in the testicular developmental cascade

have also been studied for defects, but, so far, no consistent pattern has emerged.

Why the presence of a Y chromosome in these patients should pose a risk for tumor formation has long been a puzzle. Page (1987) suggested that they may have a disabled gene on the Y chromosome, which he called the 'gonadoblastoma-Y' gene, that allows malignant degeneration to occur. Although the SRY gene appears to be intact, among some patients with 46,XY gonadal dysgenesis a deletion has been found on the short arm of the Y chromosome near the centromere (Tsuchiya *et al.*, 1995), thus supporting Page's hypothesis.

Tumors associated with gonadal dysgenesis

Gonadoblastoma

This tumor is specific to dysgenetic gonads and its development may be heralded by the sudden appearance of virilization or breast development. To the naked eye it appears as a discrete, firm, pale, nodule that, if large, may replace the gonad. Histologically, the tumor forms nests of germ cells between which Sertoli cells and stromal tissue may be partially organized to form primitive sex cords (Fig. 31.47). In some cases there is attempted tubule formation, emphasizing that the various varieties of dysgenetic gonads form a continuous spectrum. The tumors frequently calcify, are bilateral in about one-third of cases, and have been described at all ages, including in a fetus. Although the lesion is non-invasive and does not metastasize there is increasing evidence, based on the morphology of the nuclei, their DNA content, and biochemical studies, that it is premalignant (Jorgensen *et al.*, 1997). Fifty per cent of gonadoblastomas will have undergone transformation into dysgerminomas at the time of diagnosis.

Dysgerminoma

Dysgerminomas are the female equivalent of a seminoma and are usually seen in normal girls in whom it is a fairly common malignancy. Those arising in dysgenetic gonads are assumed to have had their origin in a gonadoblastoma, although by the time of diagnosis this element may be overgrown. The behavior of dysgerminomas arising in dysgenetic gonads is assumed to be similar to the more common variety which, although frankly malignant, are usually slow

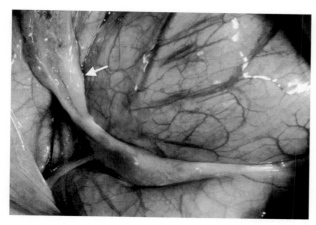

Figure 31.46 XY gonadal dysgenesis: the streak gonad on the left broad ligament (*arrow*) showed a few testicular elements on microscopy.

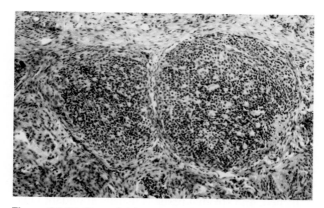

Figure 31.47 Gonadoblastoma: photomicrograph showing two nests of dark staining tumor cells in a background of dysgenetic gonadal tissue. Hematoxylin and eosin. Original magnification × 60.

growing and are sensitive to both chemotherapy and radiotherapy. However, in about 10% of cases the tumor contains yolk sac, embryonal, choriocarcinoma, or tertomatous elements, and behaves in a very aggressive manner. Although unusual at so young an age, a locally invasive dysgerminoma was reported by Muller *et al*. (1992) in a 9-year-old girl. The overall 10 year survival for dysgerminomas is about 80% (Casey *et al*., 1996).

Mixed gonadal dysgenesis

This condition, first described by Sohval in 1963, can be regarded as lying at the midpoint of a spectrum between Turner syndrome and testicular dysgenesis (Davidoff and Federman, 1973). The condition is aptly named inasmuch as the gonads comprise, in the classical case, a testicle on one side and a streak gonad on the other.

Patients typically present at birth with ambiguous genitalia. The phallus varies in size but is often modest, with the urethra opening at some point along its ventral aspect. The labioscrotal folds are characteristically asymmetric, with a gonad frequently being palpable or fully descended on the better developed side (Fig. 31.48).

The testis shows considerable histologic variation. In some cases it is clearly disordered with irregularly branched or sparse tubules and an abundance of interstitial tissue. Those that are descended may have normal architecture, but with increasing age this often shows atrophy with a corresponding decline in Leydig cell function.

The contralateral streak gonad is nearly always located intra-abdominally, lying in the position of an ovary on the broad ligament. In the classic case, it is histologically indistinguishable from other streak gonads but sometimes there are a few rudimentary tubules or even an ovarian follicle. Distinguishing this condition from true hermaphroditism can, therefore, be difficult, particularly when these components are found in the same gonad rather then showing the usual lateral segregation.

The internal duct structures largely parallel the gonadal findings. Thus, on the side of the streak gonad a well-developed fallopian tube and unicornuate uterus will be found; on the opposite side, the vas and epididymis are often well formed and the müllerian system is rudimentary or absent. The vagina generally opens into the urethra below the pelvic floor and tends to be capacious.

The karyotype in mixed gonadal dysgenesis is typically 46,XX/45,XO with both cell lines evenly distributed throughout the body. However, some variants have 47,XXY or 47,XYY cell lines, whereas in others, only a 46,XY or 45,XO line can be demonstrated.

Biochemically, serum testosterone levels at birth are frequently in the normal male range and subsequently show a brisk response to hCG stimulation. Similarly, MIS levels are also in the male range. However, at puberty the rise in serum testosterone is frequently disappointing in spite of high LH and FSH levels.

Tumors, mainly gonadoblastomas and dysgerminomas, may arise either in the streak gonad or in the testis. Embryonal cell tumors have also occurred in the testicle in childhood, while seminomas may be seen after puberty, the majority having arisen in gonads that were retained in the abdominal cavity. The risk for tumors in histologically normal descended testes is probably low but has not been accurately determined.

The management of mixed gonadal dysgenesis has historically been influenced by the generally small size of the phallus, the malignant potential of the gonads, and the ultimately poor Leydig cell function of the testes. Consequently, most infants have hitherto been raised as girls, the gonads removed early, and a feminizing genitoplasty carried out.

Among those showing a moderate degree of masculinization strong consideration should be given to raising the child as a boy, particularly if the testicle has fully descended into the scrotum. A biopsy,

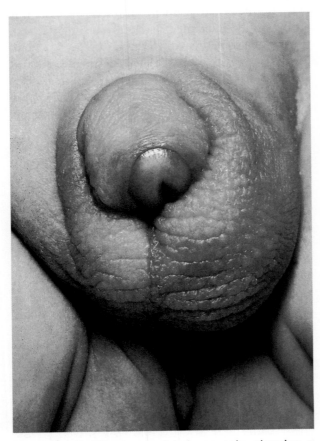

Figure 31.48 Mixed gonadal dysgenesis, showing a flat and empty right hemiscrotum in a boy with hypospadias.

however, must first be taken looking for evidence of dysgenesis or carcinoma *in situ*, which has been described in both adolescents and children (Ramani *et al.*, 1993), retaining the testis only if it is histologically normal. The contralateral streak gonad is removed together with the ipsilateral fallopian tube and hemiuterus, and the vagina resected as far as can be conveniently reached. Long-term observation is important because of the risk of possible tumor formation in a retained testis and the need to monitor Leydig cell function. When the testis has been removed testosterone replacement therapy is initiated at puberty.

Testicular dysgenesis

In this condition, described by Rajfer *et al.* (1978) as dysgenetic male pseudohermaphroditism, both testes comprise a mixture of disordered tubules and an excess of stromal tissue. These produce little testosterone or MIS, so that the external genitalia are incompletely masculinized and some müllerian duct structures are preserved.

At birth, the external genitalia show a variable degree of ambiguity and often asymmetry corresponding to the degree of testicular differentiation. The testes are usually small and devoid of covering and frequently lie within an inguinal hernial sac which also contains a fallopian tube (Fig. 31.49). Histologically, the tubules are hypoplastic, disordered and frequently branched, and stromal tissue is usually abundant (Fig. 31.50). The Sertoli cells, although capable of MIS synthesis, are reduced in number (Rey *et al.*, 1996). As gonadoblastomas and dysgerminomas have been described in this condition as early as in the newborn period, all dysgenetic tissue should be removed upon diagnosis.

Patients with testicular dysgenesis classically have a pure 46,XY karyotype, although a diligent search of many tissues may reveal a latent 45,XO cell line, especially among those showing some features of Turner syndrome.

Syndromes with gonadal dysgenesis

It has long been recognized that dysgenetic gonads are a frequent finding in several multiple malformation syndromes. The recent availability of gene probes has allowed several specific mutations to be recognized, particularly of the Wilms' tumor suppressor (WT-1) gene assigned to chromosome 11p13.

Denys–Drash syndrome

This condition was first described by Denys *et al.* (1967) in a child with 46,XX/46,XY karyotype and subsequently by Drash *et al.* (1970) in a boy in whom the karyotype was 46,XY. It is characterized by the triad of Wilms' tumor, pseudohermaphroditism, and a rapidly progressive nephropathy. Over 95% of cases show missense point mutations of the WT-1 gene, usually in exons 8 and 9 (Pelletier *et al.*, 1991). The renal lesion often starts as foci of nodular renal blastema in both kidneys that progresses to Wilms' tumor, although characteristically this shows prognostically favorable histology. The genitalia have a variable degree of ambiguity ranging from apparent simple hypospadias to predominantly female with clitoral hypertrophy, the appearance corresponding to the degree of testicular differentiation in the dysgenetic gonads. The nephropathy, which rapidly leads to nephrotic syndrome, usually has its onset in early infancy and, histologically, shows a characteristic diffuse mesangial sclerosis. Such a histological finding in an infant with apparently isolated nephrotic syndrome should lead to a search for a mutation in the WT-1 gene (Schumacher *et al.*, 1998).

Variations of the Denys–Drash syndrome are now well recognized. In some cases the genitalia are normal (Schmitt *et al.*, 1995), whereas in others the onset of nephropathy may be delayed by several years.

Frasier syndrome

The association of male pseudohermaphroditism and nephrotic syndrome was first described by Frasier *et al.* (1964). The nephropathy is slowly progressive with end-stage renal failure occurring in the teens. Renal biopsy reveals a non-specific focal glomerulosclerosis but Wilms' tumors do not occur. The gonads show a variable degree of testicular differentiation but are frequently streak-like with a corresponding female phenotype.

The Denys–Drash and Frasier syndromes are now viewed as being part of a broad spectrum of conditions in which mutations or deletions may be found in the WT-1 gene (Barbaux *et al.*, 1997). This covers isolated Wilms' tumor in which the testes and the genitalia are normal, the WAGR syndrome (**W**ilms' tumor, **a**niridia, **g**igantism, and **r**enogenital syndrome) in which hypospadias and cryptorchidism are commonly seen, as well as the Denys–Drash and Frasier syndromes. It has recently been suggested that

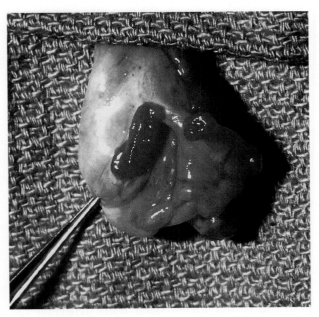

Figure 31.49 Testicular dysgenesis: a fallopian tube lies adjacent to the small testis. Both were found in an inguinal hernial sac.

isolated diffuse mesangial sclerosis, presenting as early-onset nephrotic syndrome, is also part of this spectrum (Jeanpierre *et al.*, 1998).

Chromosome 9p deletion syndrome

Dysgenetic testes are also a feature of a syndrome with a characteristic facies comprising upward slanting palpable fissures, inner epicanthic folds, a flat nasal bridge, and a short, webbed neck (Alfi *et al.*, 1973), in which there is a deletion in chromosome

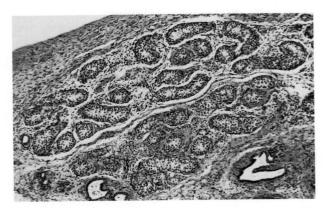

Figure 31.50 Testicular dysgenesis: photomicrograph of a cluster of fairly orderly tubules on a background of dysgenetic stromal tissue. Hematoxylin and eosin. Original magnification × 80.

9p24. Histologically, the testes may be small with disordered architecture, but they have some endocrine function so the genitalia are partially masculinized (Veitia *et al.*, 1997). In others the gonads are predominantly fibrous streaks (Flejter *et al.*, 1998). Tracheoesophageal fistula, choanal atresia, congenital heart disease, and mental retardation have also been described in this syndrome.

α-Thalassemia–Mental Retardation (ATR-X) syndrome

This X-linked recessive mental retardation syndrome is also associated with ambiguous genitalia (Wilkie *et al.*, 1990). These patients have a characteristic facial appearance which includes microcephaly and also have a short stature. The external genitalia show a spectrum ranging from mild clitoral hypertrophy to hypospadias and undescended testes reflecting the degree of testicular differentiation in the dysgenetic gonads (Reardon *et al.*, 1995). The thalassemia is caused by the presence of hemoglobin H in the red corpuscles, which can be identified by electrophoresis. The underlying mutation has been localized to Xq12.2, but a variant of the syndrome without thalassemia has been described in which the mutation occurred in Xq13.3 (Ion *et al.*, 1996).

Campomelic dysplasia

Patients with this rare osteochondrodysplasia are recognized by a Robin-like facies, bowed, short limbs, and a narrow thorax. Tracheomalacia is often present, which can lead to respiratory distress. The gonads are usually represented by bilateral fibrous streaks in both 46,XX and 46,XY cases (Houston *et al.*, 1983). Because of the failure of the external genitalia to masculinize, those with 46,XY karyotype are usually assumed at birth to be girls. Karyotyping is therefore required as those carrying a Y chromosome are at risk for developing gonadal tumors (Hong *et al.*, 1995).

The underlying gene defect in campomelic dysplasia is a mutation of the SOX-9 gene on the long arm of chromosome 17, which is known to be involved in the testicular developmental cascade. So far, 24 different mutations have been described in this gene, but there does not presently seem to be any clear correlation between these and the phenotype (Meyer *et al.*, 1997). The inheritance pattern of the condition is unclear.

Dysgenetic gonads have also been described from time to time in patients with a wide variety of chromosomal defects associated with other multiple malformation syndromes. From these, further insights into the genetic control of gonadal development have been gained.

Sex assignment

All infants whose genitalia are suggestive of an underlying intersex disorder should be investigated expeditiously. The results of the biochemical, radiographic, and basic chromosomal studies will become available within a few days, when the need for gonadal biopsy can be determined. The provisional sex of rearing is often decided by the appearance of the external genitalia, but this may have to be modified in the light of the definitive diagnosis and future development. In coming to a final recommendation, the following criteria must be carefully considered.

Age of presentation

The age of presentation has traditionally been regarded as one of the most important criteria in determining the sex of rearing, in the belief that by the third year sexual identity becomes fixed. However, this must be reconsidered as it is now apparent that the development of gender identity is a gradual process demonstrating considerable plasticity. In cases where, in retrospect, an inappropriate decision was made at birth, skilled psychiatric help may permit a relative smooth transition to the opposite sex during childhood or even beyond (see Chapter 30).

Fertility potential

All female infants with pseudohermaphroditism are potentially fertile, regardless of how severely they may have been virilized, so that most have been raised as girls. However, it is now recognized that among salt losing patients with CAH, heterosexual interest and a desire for motherhood are often reduced. The primacy of fertility therefore needs to be reconsidered.

Severely virilized females with CAH who have been raised as boys, usually because of a missed diagnosis, are probably best left in that role and surgery recommended for the removal of the internal genitalia. For the newborn infant correctly diagnosed with 46,XX CAH who has a near normal looking penis and a small, very high vagina, the decision as to the appropriate sex of rearing is currently problematic, because of the sparcity of follow-up data of such individuals.

Among other intersex conditions, pregnancies have been recorded among true hermaphrodites raised as girls and, rather less often, among men with defects of testosterone biosynthesis and 5α-reductase activity.

Assisted reproductive techniques have altered the traditional view as to what constitutes infertility. Among males with a rudimentary prostate and severely reduced sperm count, intracytoplasmic injection of spermatozoa into an oocyte and subsequent implantation of the embryo into the partner's uterus has produced successful pregnancies. Women with gonadal dysgenesis in whom the uterus is usually normal can receive an embryo conceived by *in vitro* techniques using donor oocytes. A unicornuate uterus may also sustain a pregnancy, but the risk of spontaneous abortion and preterm labor is high, with less than one-third going to term (Raga *et al.*, 1997). Such uteri generally do not respond well to oxytocins, so that elective cesarean section is necessary.

Nevertheless, assisted reproductive techniques presently have a low success rate and also carry the risk of transmitting defective genes to the embryo. Among male embryos there is also an increased incidence of hypospadias, which appears to be related to the progestins given to the mother to aid implantation (Silver *et al.*, 1999). Anomalies of sex chromosomes have also been described, including a 46,XX/46,XY chiamera with true hermaphroditism, apparently the result of fusion of two of the embryos that had been implanted into the uterus (Strain *et al.*, 1998).

Size of the penis

The size of the phallus and its potential to develop at puberty into a sexually functional penis are of major importance when one is considering male as the sex of rearing. Although a large penile size is certainly not a prerequisite for a satisfactory sexual relationship (Reilly and Woodhouse, 1989), it must be anticipated that boys who emerge from puberty with a very small penis are likely to have significant psychological problems. Careful assessment of penile size by palpation rather than appearance is therefore essential. In equivocal cases, when male is being considered as the sex of rearing, the response to androgen stimulation should be determined before coming to a final decision. The severity of the hypospadias should not be a consideration, for the results of hypospadias repair using current surgical techniques are generally, from both the cosmetic and functional points of view, very satisfactory.

The vagina

The presence of a capacious, low-lying vagina is advantageous if assignment as a female is being considered, but this is not of critical importance. A vagina that enters the urogenital sinus at or above the pelvic floor presents a major surgical challenge, but current techniques allow a satisfactory vaginoplasty to be carried out even in these cases.

Endocrine function

Because of the ease with which exogenous estrogen or testosterone can be given, the ability of the gonads to produce these hormones is not a major factor in sex assignment. Nevertheless, there is clearly an advantage in retaining a gonad of the appropriate sex if it is likely to function adequately.

Among the intersex disorders, the ovaries in most cases of female pseudohermaphroditism will be normal. Ovarian tissue in true hermaphroditism, if present in sufficient volume, is likely to produce an adequate amount of estrogen throughout the reproductive phase of adult life. However, testicular tissue in this condition and in mixed gonadal dysgenesis may initially produce an adequate amount of testosterone but this often declines, so that supplements may eventually become necessary.

Malignant change

Histologically abnormal gonads should always be removed with the exception of girls with streak gonads who do not harbor any Y chromosomal material. When female is the sex of rearing, the uterus, even if unicornuate, should be left *in situ* for potential embryo implantation even though the gonad may have been excised.

Histologically abnormal testes carry a risk for malignant degeneration, but their removal does not preclude male as the sex of rearing if this is thought desirable because of the degree of masculinization. The parents can be reassured that, with replacement therapy, normal pubertal development can be anticipated and that testicular prostheses can be inserted into the scrotum in due course. The risk of malignant degeneration in retained müllerian structures appears to be very low.

Antenatal testosterone exposure

Recent publicity surrounding several boys who suffered traumatic penile amputation in early infancy and were raised initially as girls only subsequently to reassign themselves as boys has resulted in a re-evaluation of the significance of antenatal exposure of the brain to testosterone with regard to ultimate sexual identity (Diamond and Sigmundson, 1997). However, long-term follow-up studies among women with CAH exposed to testosterone *in utero* indicate that, although there are some exceptions (Meyer-Bahlburg *et al.*, 1996), the majority do not seem to have problems in this regard.

Human sexuality is a highly complex matter (Pillard and Bailey, 1995), and antenatal testosterone exposure is but one possible influence among many that may impact on ultimate gender identity. Others include the possible influence of unidentified genes on the Y chromosome, familial and cultural pressures and, doubtless, factors intrinsic to each individual that are not yet understood. Nonetheless, the potential effects that androgens may have had on the developing brain must be seriously considered in recommending gender assignment. Although these cannot be accurately assessed, it is reasonable, in the absence of any other guide, to assume that they parallel the degree to which the external genitalia have masculinized. However, how much weight should be given to this consideration will remain uncertain until the results of long-term, multicenter follow-up studies become available (see Chapter 30).

Feminizing surgery

Indications and timing of surgery

Infants who are to be raised as girls have hitherto generally undergone clitoral reduction and vulvo-vaginoplasty in early infancy, often in the immediate postnatal period. Those with congenital adrenal hyperplasia, however, were first stabilized on replacement therapy. However, the point of view has recently been put forward that the preservation of clitoral function should take precedence over appearance and, as the functional results of surgical techniques are presently not well documented (Alizia *et al.*, 1999), there should be a reluctance to recommend surgery which may prove to be harmful. Furthermore, among those infants with severe virilization, the possibility of

an eventual male sexual identity becoming established may mean that any irreversible feminizing procedure carried out in infancy may, in the fullness of time, be regretted. Such children, it has been argued, should be left to assign themselves.

There is, however, a counterargument that most parents prefer to have their infant's genitalia looking appropriate to their sex of rearing as soon as possible and that current surgical techniques have the potential to leave the sensory and erectile functions of the clitoris intact. Furthermore, there is the anxiety that allowing children to grow up with genitalia that, in most people's estimation, are clearly abnormal, may bring its own harvest of adverse psychological sequelae. Until long-term follow-up studies become available this debate is bound to continue.

Nowadays, there is general agreement that those with only mild clitoral hypertrophy should not undergo early surgery in anticipation that, as the adverse hormonal milieu abates, there will be a relative reduction in the size of the clitoris and a corresponding improvement in the appearance of the labia. In such cases the only surgery necessary will be a limited procedure to bring the vagina out onto the surface of the perineum.

Among infants with more severe virilization whose parents request feminizing genitoplasty, the author believes it is appropriate to offer surgery to reduce the size of the clitoris, fashion labia minora from the prepuce, trim the labia majora to an appropriate size and exteriorize the vagina. Such surgery can usually be carried out during the first few months after birth. However, the parents should understand, and the surgical consent form should specify that the long term outcome of feminizing genitoplasty has not been fully evaluated and that no guarantee can be given as to the ultimate gender identity of their child.

Clitoral recession

Currently, the indications for this relatively simple procedure are few. It should be strictly reserved for cases in which surgery is requested by the parents and the clitoris is only slightly enlarged, for if it is too bulky, the procedure is very likely to be followed by painful erections. The initial steps of the operation are common to both clitoral recession and the more frequently performed clitoral reduction.

The infant is placed in the frog-leg position. After the skin has been prepared, a drape is sutured in front of the anus to exclude it from the field. A catheter is inserted into the bladder, and the urogenital sinus laid open in the midline using cutting electrocautery as far back as necessary to expose the urethral orifice. The lateral margins of the mucosal strip are then sutured to the adjacent skin with a short, running, 6-0 absorbable suture.

The adherent prepuce is now freed to fully expose the coronal sulcus, and a traction suture is placed well back on the glans. A transverse incision is then made just proximal to the coronal sulcus through the dorsal skin and subcutaneous tissue, and extended on either side for three-quarters of the clitoral circumference so as to leave a ventral midline strip intact. Using fine curved scissors, the surgeon then develops a plane just above Buck's fascia, and the skin of the prepuce and clitoral shaft, together with a generous covering of subcutaneous tissue, are allowed to fall back. This is then cut back to the midline in the manner of Byar's flaps in order to expose the prepubic fascia. The suspensory ligament of the clitoris is now divided and the fat swept away, revealing the perichondrium covering the inferior aspect of the symphysis pubis. Superficial dorsal veins may need to be divided at this point.

In the technique of clitoral recession described by Randolph and Hung (1970), the corpora are now gathered in two 4-0 non-absorbable sutures placed lateral to the neurovascular bundles and hitched to the undersurface of the symphysis, taking a good bite of the perichondrium to ensure firm fixation. A superficial wedge of tissue is then excised from the dorsum of the glans, and, after coagulation of any bleeding points, the sutures are tied and the clitoris is snugged down beneath the pubis.

A vulvoplasty is then carried out by extending the incisions on either side of the preserved midline strip further caudally to the level of the vaginal orifice. Any redundant labioscrotal skin is excised as a long ellipse, and after the preputial flaps are trimmed to a suitable length, these are brought down to form labia minora. Interrupted 6-0 absorbable sutures are then placed to bring the skin edges together, starting with the glans. If the initial dorsal incision was not extended back too far, the glans remains partially covered by a pleasing hood.

Reduction clitoroplasty

This will be the operation of choice for most infants with clitoromegaly (Fig. 31.51). The initial steps of this procedure are the same as for clitoral recession,

but here the central portions of the corporeal bodies are excised. The surgeon first mobilizes and preserves the dorsal neurovascular bundles by incising Buck's fascia laterally in the 3 o'clock and 9 o'clock positions, thereby preserving bundles of the dorsal nerves that fan out laterally as they approach the glans (Baskin, 1999) (Fig. 31.52). The exposure of the corporeal bodies needs to be carried well back beyond their bifurcation to the inferior pubic rami where, after bulldog clamps are placed for hemostasis, they are transected. The remaining proximal and distal portions of the corporeal bodies are then reapproximated using interrupted 5-0 absorbable sutures placed in the investing fascia, thereby optimizing the potential for erectile function (Mollard *et al.*, 1981).

The glans is reduced by excision of a superficial triangle of dorsal tissue, leaving the ventral and lateral two-thirds of sensate epithelium intact. It is then attached to the inferior surface of the symphysis pubis using two 4-0 non-absorbable sutures, with care being taken not to entrap the broad fascial band containing the neurovascular bundles as the sutures are snugged down. The vulvoplasty is then completed as described above (Fig. 31.53).

Low vaginoplasty

Before any vaginal surgery is undertaken, the position of the vagina with respects to both the pelvic floor and perineal skin must be accurately determined from the genitogram, supplemented if necessary by endoscopy. In most cases, low vaginoplasty can be carried out at the same time as the clitoroplasty. Early surgery is advantageous because, in the immediate postnatal period, the vaginal wall is more substantial than in later childhood as a result of maternal estrogen stimulation. This facilitites handling of the tissues.

When the vagina opens very low, it may be laid open by a simple cutback, suturing the vaginal wall to the perineal skin with 6-0 absorbable sutures. In most cases, however, a posteriorly based U-flap will be necessary to ensure a tension-free anastomosis, reducing the risk of postoperative stenosis.

A urethral catheter is first inserted into the bladder by means of a fine curved sound as a guide. If any difficulty is encountered the skin is cut back in the midline to expose the urethral meatus. The posterior flap, which must be sufficiently long to reach the vagina without tension and wide enough to ensure a good blood supply, is elevated together with a generous cov-

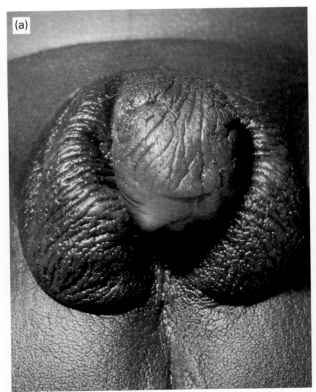 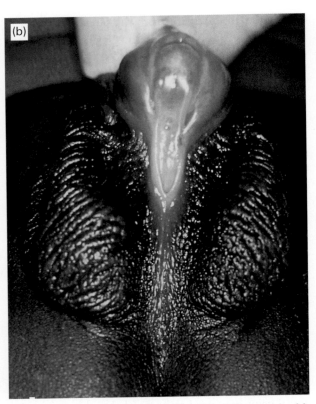

Figure 31.51 Reduction clitoroplasty. The preoperative appearance of the external genitalia of a virilized girl with congenital adrenal hyperplasia: (*a*) dorsal, and (*b*) ventral views.

ering of subcutaneous tissue (Fig. 31.54). A plane is then developed in the midline immediately behind the urethra to expose the vagina. The posterior wall of the vagina is now widely opened in the same plane to expose its cavity and the tip of the skin flap sutured down. The remainder of the flap is brought down using multiple 6-0 absorbable sutures. The vulvoplasty, if not previously carried out, is now completed. The urethral catheter is removed after 24 hours. Ten days postoperatively, the vagina is inspected under general anesthesia and its caliber determined, separating any filmy adhesions that may have formed in the interim.

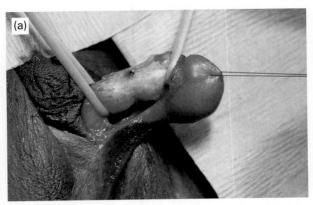 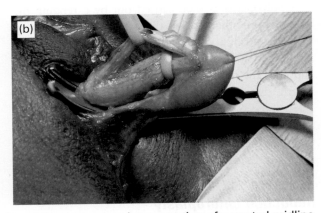

Figure 31.52 Operative photographs showing (*a*) mobilization of the corpora and preservation of a ventral midline strip of skin and urethral mucosa. The preputial and shaft skin have been allowed to fall back. (*b*) Lateral incisions are made in Buck's fascia and the dorsal neurovascular bundles are elevated. A bulldog clamp is placed for hemostasis and the central portion of the corporeal bodies is resected.

Exposure of the high vagina

Perineal approach

Reconstruction of the genitalia in severely virilized CAH presents particular difficulties because of the high position and often small size of the vagina. In such cases it may be approached from below, but exposure is limited and great care is needed to safeguard the external urethral sphincter, the nerves and muscles of the pelvic floor, and the urethra and rectum.

Hendren operation

A Fogarty catheter is first introduced endoscopically into the vagina to facilitate its identification during the dissection, and the balloon inflated. A second catheter is then placed in the bladder. The rectum is then cleaned by insertion of a Betadine swab, which is retained for the duration of the procedure. The operation begins by the creation of two U-shaped perineal skin flaps, one based posteriorly and the other anteri-

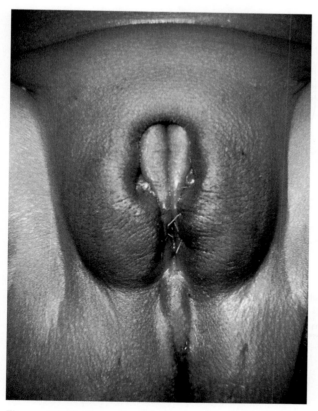

Figure 31.53 Operative photograph: the clitoris has been sutured to the inferior aspect of the pubis, the labia majora have been reduced and labia minora fashioned by Byar's flaps from the preputial skin.

orly. These are elevated and the dissection continued, keeping strictly to the midline until, with gentle traction on the Fogarty catheter, the vagina can be felt in the depths of the field. A nerve stimulator is used at this point to identify the levator muscles and external urethral sphincter. The former is divided in the sagittal plane and the vaginal wall is stabilized with a series of 6-0 silk stay sutures. The Fogarty catheter is withdrawn. The vagina is then detached from the urethra and opened as widely as possible. The urethral defect is carefully closed transversely with interrupted 6-0 polyglycolic acid sutures. Using cautious blunt dissection, the surgeon mobilizes the vagina from the back of the bladder and rectum, which must be constantly safeguarded, reaching as far as the peritoneal reflection to obtain as much length as possible. The anterior and posterior skin flaps are then brought down and sutured to the vaginal margins.

The mobilization of a high vagina is sometimes very difficult, particularly when there has been prior infection in a hydrocolpos. It may then be necessary to turn the child and free the vagina via a laparotomy from the back of the bladder, safeguarding the ureters to which it may be adherent. It is then brought down through the pelvic floor and, after closing the abdomen, is anastomosed to the previously prepared perineal skin flaps without tension. With experience the operation can be safely carried out in children between 6 months and 1 year of age (Hendren and Atala, 1995).

Passerini–Glazel operation

For the severely virilized infant whose phallus resembles a normal penis, a satisfactory total reconstruction can be carried out using the technique described by Passerini-Glazel (1989). This takes advantage of the sheath of penile skin, which is tubularized and brought up through the perineum to form the lower portion of the vagina, and also provides a cosmetically pleasing midline strip of mucosa in the vulva (Fig. 31.55).

The patient is positioned and prepared for both a perineal and an abdominal dissection, although the procedure can usually be carried out entirely from below. A circumferential incision is first made around the coronal sulcus, and the skin and subcutaneous tissue are peeled back to the base of the penis. The corpus spongiosum is then separated from the corpora cavernosa and laid open. The skin sleeve is split dorsally and ventrally in the midline, and the corpora cavernosa are transected close to the inferior pubic

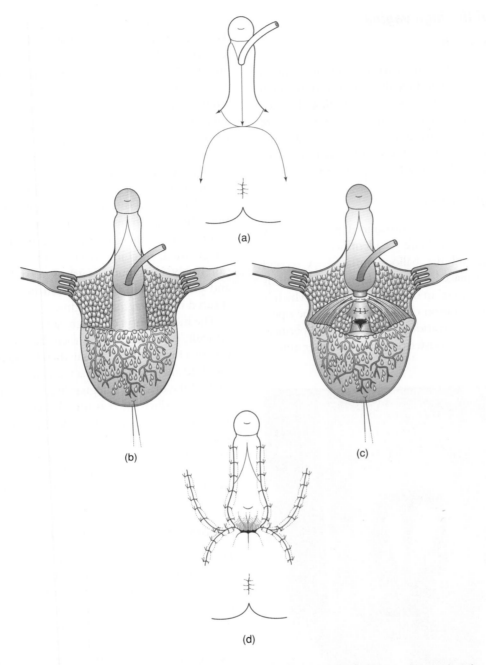

Figure 31.54 Vaginoplasty: (*a*) lines of incision. Note that when a clitoroplasty has been previously performed, the labia minora are remobilized; (*b*) invented U flap to expose vagina; (*c*) deep exposure of a high-lying vagina. The external urethral sphincter, pelvic floor muscles, and rectum must be safeguarded; (*d*) the completed vaginoplasty.

rami after careful preservation of the dorsal neurovascular bundles. A wedge resection of the glans is carried out, and the corporeal stumps are brought together by fine interrupted circumferential sutures. The split penile skin is then brought down on either side and sutured to the opened spongiosum. The resulting rectangular flap is rolled in with a running suture to form a composite tube that will serve as the lower portion of the vagina. The upper vagina is then exposed as in Hendren's operation and the anastomosis completed. Finally, the skin margins are brought together to complete the vulvoplasty.

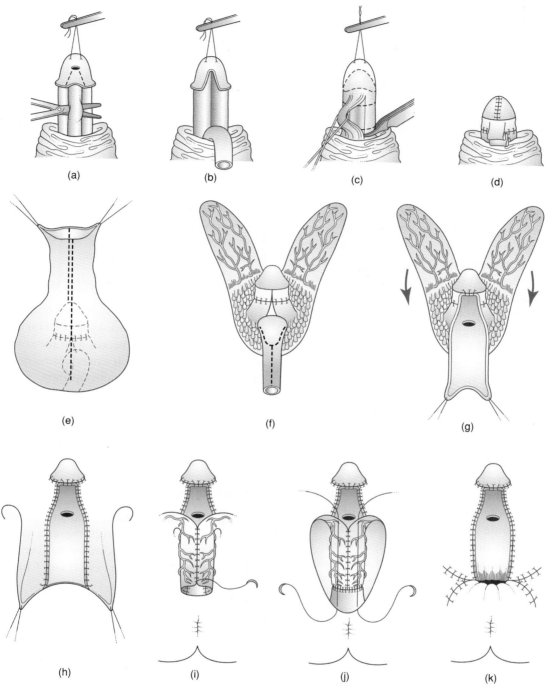

Figure 31.55 The Passerini–Glazel operation for one-stage correction of total virilization. (*a*) The penis is degloved and the urethra and corpus spongiosum separated from the corpora cavernosa. (*b*) The corpus spongiosum is detached from the glans. (*c*) The dorsal neurovascular bundles are mobilized on a generous strip of investing fascia and the bulk of the corpora cavernosa resected. A deep wedge is excised from the ventral glans. (*d*) The glans is closed and the corporeal stumps are reapproximated. (*e*) The penile skin tube is cut back dorsally and ventrally. (*f*) The skin flaps are elevated and the urethra and corpus spongiosum are incised as indicated. (*g*) They are laid open. The dorsal flap is sutured to the base of the glans. (*h*) The skin flaps are brought down and sutured to the lateral edges of the urethra. (*i*) The composite flap is rolled into a tube with a running stitch. (*j*) The upper portion of the vagina is now exposed and prepared as in Fig. 35.54(c). The skin tube is sutured to the vagina and its now distal end drawn down to the perineal skin. (*k*) The final appearance of the vulva.

Posterior sagittal vaginoplasty

This approach was originally described for the total reconstruction of a cloacal anomaly but is adapted for repair of a urogenital sinus by opening the posterior and anterior walls of the intervening rectum (Peña et al., 1992). This provides excellent exposure of the vagina and its insertion into the urethra and, provided the dissection is carried out strictly in the midline, safeguards the pelvic nerves and the integrity of the pelvic floor musculature. Unless a perfect bowel preparation can be assured a preliminary colostomy will be necessary.

A Fogarty catheter is first inserted into the vagina endoscopically and the balloon inflated. A Foley catheter is inserted into the bladder and the rectum cleaned with Betadine solution. With the patient in the prone, jack-knife position, an incision is made extending from the tip of coccyx anteriorly to the urogenital sinus opening. The dissection proceeds through the perineal body and fat until the muscle bundles of the levator ani are encountered. These are carefully identified by electrical stimulation and marked with multiple, long, 6-0 silk sutures to facilitate accurate realignment at the end of the procedure. The posterior and anterior rectal walls are then opened in the midline, and the position of the vagina and its junction with the urethra determined by feeling for the presence of the Fogarty balloon and urethral catheter. The inferior aspect of the posterior vaginal wall is now marked with a series of 6-0 silk stay sutures, gentle traction upon which allows the junction with the urethra to be clearly defined. The vagina is then detached, the urethral defect closed with fine polyglycolic sutures, and the vagina widely opened. Continuing gentle traction and blunt dissection in the surrounding connective tissues allow the vagina to be progressively mobilized towards the perineum to which it is sutured.

Because of the difficulty which is sometimes encountered in separating the vagina from the urethral wall, to which it may be fused for some distance above the confluence, it is often easier to carry out a total urogenital sinus mobilization in which the sinus, urethra, and vagina are freed as a single unit, sweeping around these structures by blunt dissection up as far as the peritoneal reflection posteriorly while anteriorly reaching as high as the anterior bladder wall (Peña, 1997). These structures are progressively mobilized together down towards the perineum, where the redundant portion of the urogenital sinus is excised. When the confluence of the vagina and urethra is at the level of the pelvic floor, both structures can be anastomosed separately to the perineal skin, leaving them attached at their common wall. When the confluence is higher, the maneuver is still very useful in order to allow formal separation to take place in the center of the operative field. After completion of the perineal anastomoses the anterior and posterior rectal walls are closed in layers and the pelvic floor musculature is then accurately reapproximated prior to closing the superficial tissues. The colostomy is retained for 6 weeks postoperatively when, after satisfactory healing of the rectum has been confirmed, it is closed. Posterior sagittal vaginoplasty is best carried out between 6 and 12 months of age.

Anterior sagittal transanorectal vaginoplasty

This operation, described by Domini et al. (1997), is carried out in the prone, jack-knife position but, unlike the Peña approach, commences with the anterior wall of the anal sphincter and is extended anteriorly in the midline to the urogenital sinus opening. The incision is then extended up the anterior rectal wall, allowing exposure of the vagina up to the level of the pelvic floor. This variation on the Peña procedure minimizes the risk of a rectal stricture but provides more limited access to a vagina that is very high.

Vaginal replacement

When the vagina is very high and small, replacement with a segment of bowel, usually sigmoid colon, will be necessary. The operative technique has been well described by Hensle and Dean (1992) (see Chapter 26).

Surgical outcomes

Long-term follow-up studies of feminizing genitoplasty are sparse. Those that have been published describe the outcomes of techniques which have now largely been abandoned.

The assessment of clitoral function after surgery has generally been confined to the demonstration of nerve conduction. Among a group of patients who underwent reduction clitoroplasty with preservation of the dorsal neurovascular bundles, sensation and the elicitation of evoked potentials were well preserved (Gearhart et al., 1995). Although these observations do not directly measure erogenous sensation, they do confirm that the neurologic pathways are intact. The objective assessment of a erectile function, although widely used for men, has not hitherto been applied to women who have undergone genitoplasty. Sexual fulfillment is a complex matter involving not only clitoral but also vaginal sensation as well as critical psychological factors that act via mechanisms that are not fully understood. This is illustrated by the observations that some women who had undergone clitorodectomy as infants many years previously have been capable of orgasm, whereas it is estimated that fully 20% of adult women who have never had any genital surgery are anorgasmic.

Vaginal stenosis remains a common problem after all types of vaginoplasty, particularly if there has been tension on the anastomosis with the perineal skin. Examination under anesthesia is therefore advisable prior to the onset of puberty to ensure that menstruation can occur unimpeded. Unless stenosis is severe, an adequate caliber for intercourse can usually be obtained by serial dilations begun in the late teens (Costa *et al.*, 1997).

Revirilization of the reduced clitoris and labia is sometimes seen among patients with CAH who are poorly controlled medically. Any revision surgery should be postponed until the patients are brought fully under medical control.

Surgery in boys

The external genitalia

All infants raised as boys need chordee correction and hypospadias repair. Currently, even in severe cases this is usually carried out as a one-stage procedure by one of the standard techniques (see Chapter 32). The preferred age is 6 months and in most case the infant can be discharged home on the same day with an indwelling catheter draining between double diapers.

Orchidopexy, if required, is carried out at the same time. However, if the hypospadias repair has been particularly complex, it may be deferred for 6 months.

The internal genitalia

Removal of the fallopian tubes and uterus is usually straightforward, as they are often rudimentary structures in these children. The intraperitoneal dissection begins laterally, and after the fallopian branches of the gonadal vessels are ligated, the tubes are freed from the peritoneum of the broad ligament on either side. The dissection continues close to the uterus as far as the peritoneal reflection, which is opened widely to allow identification of the ureters. Here, small uterine vessels may be encountered that are coagulated. With traction on the uterus, the upper vagina is progressively mobilized by blunt dissection and, safeguarding the ureters, is cross-clamped as low as can be safely reached. The stump is then transfixed with a 2-0 absorbable suture. The vaginal remnant does not, as a rule, give rise to any problems.

Excision of a utriculus masculinus

Excision of an isolated utriculus is not usually necessary unless there have been recurrent episodes of urinary infection or epididymitis. The most satisfactory surgical approach is through the trigone of the bladder, which gives direct access to the anterior wall of the utriculus and allows careful separation of this from the bladder and the ureters (di Benedetto *et al.*, 1997). The vasa sometimes run down laterally on the utricular wall to enter the verumontanum, but more often open into its dome. Their continuity can be preserved by retaining lateral strips of utricular wall which are then tubularized. Alternatively, the vasa may be transected when they enter the utriculus and reimplanted in an antirefluxing manner into the bladder for seminal fluid harvesting. Current assisted reproductive techniques also offer an alternative approach to fertility. At the end of the procedure the posterior bladder wall is closed in a watertight manner in layers and the anterior wall closed with temporary suprapubic catheter drainage.

Total penile construction

These techniques, which are a surgical *tour de force*, are mainly used in adults who have sustained the accidental loss of their penis. Their application to children has generally been confined to cases of accidental circumcision injury, but also to a few cases of aphallia and micropenis (Gilbert *et al.*, 1993). Among intersex patients their potential application is confined to those very rare individuals raised as girls but who ask for the construction of a penis because of a change in their gender identity.

The technique with which there is most experience employs a composite flap comprising skin, fat, and the superficial lamina of fascia, together with arteries, veins, and nerves, that is raised from the forearm. This leaves a large defect that is covered by a full-thickness skin graft. Although the resulting penis, which has protective sensation, can be cosmetically satisfactory, complications are common. These include stricture and fistulae related to the construction of the urethra in up to 50% of cases and, rather less often, loss of the entire graft as the result of arterial or venous thrombosis (Jordan *et al.*, 1994). Successful grafts subsequently require a prosthesis to be inserted for erectile function.

In order to avoid the unsightly scarring of the forearm and the need for a prosthesis inherent with the forearm flap technique, Sadove *et al.* (1993) have described a lower limb composite fibula flap in which the lower portion of this bone serves as a stiffening rod. Postoperatively, however, a prolonged period of rehabilitation is necessary and unaided walking is achieved only after 3 months. Because of the adult dimensions of the constructed organ this technique has not yet been applied to children.

Although the availability of such formidable techniques is advantageous for adults suffering penile trauma, the complexity of the procedure, suboptimal cosmesis and function, and significant postoperative morbidity confine their potential applications among children to a few, highly selected individuals.

References

Aaronson IA (1985) True hermaphroditism: a review of 41 cases with observations on testicular histology and function. *Br J Urol* **57**: 775–9.

Aaronson IA (1990) Les hermaphrodites vrais. In: Cukier J (ed.) *Journees urologiques de necker: ambiguités sexuelles.* Paris: Masson, 41–7.

Aaronson IA (1994) Micropenis: medical and surgical implications. *J Urol* **152**: 4–14.

Aaronson IA, Cremin BJ (1984) *Clinical pediatric uroradiology.* Edinburgh: Churchill Livingstone, 385.

Aaronson IA, Cakmak MA, Key LL (1997) Defects of the testosterone biosynthetic pathway in boys with hypospadias. *J Urol* **157**: 1884–8.

Aiman J, Griffin JE, Gazak SM *et al.* (1979) Androgen insensitivity as a cause of infertility in otherwise normal men. *N Engl J Med* **300**: 223–7.

Alfi O, Donnell GN, Crandall BF *et al.* (1973) Deletion of the short arm of chromosome 9 (46, 9p-): a new deletion syndrome. *Ann Genet* **16**: 17–22.

Alizai NK, Thomas DF, Lilford RT (1999) Feminizing genitoplasty for congenital adrenal hyperplasia: what happens at puberty? *J Urol* **161**: 1588–91.

Andersson S, Moghrabi N (1997) Physiology and molecular genetics of 17β-hydroxysteroid dehydrogenases. *Steroids* **62**: 143–7.

Aumuller G, Eicheler W, Renneberg H *et al.* (1996) Immunocytochemical evidence for different subcellular localization of 5α-reductase isoenzymes in human tissues. *Acta Anat* **156**: 241–52.

Aya M, Ogata T, Sakaguchi A *et al.* (1997) Testicular histopathology in congenital lipoid adrenal hyperplasia: a light and electron microscopy study. *Horm Res* **47**: 121–5.

Barbaux S, Niaudet P, Gubler M-C *et al.* (1997) Donor splice-site mutations in WT-1 are responsible for Frazier syndrome. *Nature Genet* **17**: 467–70.

Bardoni B, Zanaria E, Guioli S *et al.* (1994) A dose sensitive locus at chromosome Xp21 is involved in male to female sex reversal. *Nature Genet* **7**: 497–501.

Baskin LS (1999) Fetal genital anatomy reconstructive implications. *J Urol* **162**: 527–9.

Behringer RR (1995) The müllerian inhibitor and mammalian sexual development. *Phil Trans R Soc Lond B* **350**: 285–8.

Bennett CP, Docherty Z, Robb SA (1993) Deletion 9p and sex reversal. *J Med Genet* **30**: 518–20.

Berkovitz GD, Fechner PY, Marcantonio SM *et al.* (1992) The role of the sex determining region of the Y chromosome (SRY) in the etiology of 46XX true hermaphroditism. *Hum Genet* **88**: 411–16.

Bernstein R, Koo GU, Wachtel SS (1980) Abnormality of the X chromosome in human 46XY female siblings and dysgenetic ovaries. *Science* **207**: 768–9.

Biglieri EG, Herron MA, Brust N (1966) 17 hydroxylation deficiency in man. *J Clin Invest* **45**: 1946–54, 1966.

Blanchard MG, Josso N (1974) Source of the anti-müllerian hormone synthesized by the fetal testis: müllerian inhibiting activity of fetal bovine Sertoli cells in tissue culture. *Pediatr Res* **8**: 968–71.

Boehmer AL, Brinkmann AO, Niermeijer MF *et al.* (1997) Germ line and somatic mosaicism in the androgen insensitivity syndrome: implications for genetic counseling. *Am J Hum Genet* **60**: 1003–6.

Bongiovanni AM (1961) Unusual steroid pattern in congenital adrenal hyperplasia: deficiency of 3β-hydroxysteroid dehydrogenase. *J Clin Endocrinol Metab* **21**: 860–2.

Bose HS, Baldwin MA, Miller WL (1998) Incorrect folding of steroidogenic acute regulatory protein (StAR) in congenital lipoid adrenal hyperplasia. *Biochemistry* **37**: 9768–75.

Breedlove, SM (1995) Another important organ. *Nature* **378**: 15–16.

Brüggenwirth MT, Boehmer AL, Ramnarain S. *et al.* (1997) Molecular analysis of the androgen receptor gene in a family with receptor positive partial androgen insensitivity. An unusual type of intronic mutation. *Am J Hum Genet* **61**: 1067–77.

Bulun SE (1996) Aromatase deficiency in women and men. Would you have predicted the phenotypes? *J Clin Endocr Metab* **81**: 867–71.

Casey AC, Bhodauria S, Shapter A. *et al.* (1996) Dysgerminoma: the role of conservative surgery. *Gynecol Oncol* **63**: 352–7.

Cohen HL, Shapiro MA, Mandel FS. *et al.* (1993) Normal ovaries in neonates and infants: a sonographic study of 77 patients one day to 24 months old. *AJR Am J Roentgenol* **160**: 583–6.

Costa EM, Mendonca BB, Inacio M. *et al.* (1997) Management of ambiguous genitalia in pseudohermaphrodites: new perspectives on vaginal dilatation. *Fertil Steril* **67**: 229–32.

Davidoff F, Federman DD (1973) Mixed gonadal dysgenesis. *Pediatrics* **52**: 725–42.

Denys P, Malvaus P, van der Berghe H *et al.* (1967) Association d'un syndrome anatomo-pathologique de pseudohermaphrodisme masculin, d'une tumeur de Wilms, d'une nephropathie parenchymateuse et d'un mosaicisme XX/XY. *Arch Franc Pediatr* **24**: 729–39.

Diamond M, Sigmundson HK (1997) Management of intersexuality: guidelines for dealing with persons with ambiguous genitalia. *Arch Pediatr Adolesc Med* **151**: 1046–50.

di Benedetto V, Bagnara V, Guys JM *et al.* (1997) A transvesical approach to müllerian duct remnants. *Pediatr Surg Int* **12**: 151–4.

Domini R, Rossi F, Caccarelli PL *et al.* (1997) Anterior sagittal transrectal approach to the urogenital sinus in adrenogenital syndrome: preliminary report. *J Pediatr Surg* **32**: 714–16.

Drash A, Sherman F, Hartmann W *et al.* (1970) A syndrome of pseudohermaphroditism, Wilms' tumor, hypertension and degenerative renal disease. *J Pediatr* **76**: 585–93.

Eberenz W, Rosenberg HK, Moshang T *et al.* (1991) True hermaphroditism: sonographic demonstration of ovotestes. *Radiology* **179**: 429–31.

Flejter WL, Fergestad J, Gorski J *et al.* (1998) A gene involved in XY sex reversal is located on chromosome 9, distal to marker D9S1779. *Am J Hum Genet* **63**: 794–802.

Frasier S, Bashore RA, Mosier HD (1964) Gonadoblastoma associated with pure gonadal dysgenesis in monozygotic twins. *J Pediatr* **64**: 740–5.

Fuqua JS, Sher ES, Fechner PY *et al.* (1996) Linkage analysis of a kindred with inherited 46XY partial gonadal dysgenesis. *J Clin Endocrinol Metab* **81**: 4479–83.

Gearhart JP, Burnett A, Owen JH (1995) Measurement of pudendal evoked potentials during feminizing genitoplasty: technique and applications. *J Urol* **153**: 481–7.

Gilbert DA, Jordan GH, Devine CJ *et al.* (1993) Phallic reconstruction in prepubertal and adolescent boys. *J Urol* **149**: 1521–6.

Gilbert-Dreyfus S, Sabaoun CA, Balausch J (1957) Etude d'un cas familial d'androgynoidisme avec hypospadie grave, gynecomastie et hyperestrogenie. *Ann Endocrinol Paris* **18**: 93–101.

Giltay JC, Brunt T, Beemer FA *et al.* (1998) Polymorphic detection of the parthenogenetic maternal and double paternal contribution to a 46XX/46XY hermaphrodite. *Am J Hum Genet* **62**: 937–40.

Girgis R, Winter JS (1997) The effect of glucocorticoid replacement therapy on growth, bone mineral density, and bone turnover makers in children with congenital adrenal hyperplasia. J Clin Endocrinol Metab **82**: 3926–9.

Gorski RA (1985) Sexual dimorphisms of the brain. *J Anim Sci* **61**: 38–61.

Gorski RA (1998) Sexual differentiation of the brain. In: Bittar EE, Bittar N (eds) *Principles of medical biology: reproductive endocrinology and biology.* Stamford, CT: JAI Press, 1–23.

Guerrier D, Tran D, van der Winden JM *et al.* (1989) The persistent müllerian duct syndrome: a molecular approach. *J Clin Endocrinol Metab* **68**: 46–52, 1989.

Gustafson ML, Lee MM, Asmundson L *et al.* (1993) Müllerian inhibiting substance in the diagnosis and management of intersex and gonadal abnormalities. *J Pediatr Surg* **28**: 439–44.

Hall JG, Gilchrist DM (1990) Turner syndrome and its variants. *Pediatr Clin North Am* **37**: 1421–40.

Harada N, Ogawa H, Shozu M *et al.* (1992) Biochemical and molecular genetic analyses on placental aromatase (P-450arom) deficiency. *J Biol Chem* **267**: 4781–5.

Hendren WH, Atala A (1995) Repair of high vagina in girls with severely masculinized anatomy from the adrenogenital syndrome. *J Pediatr Surg* **30**: 91–4.

Hensle TW, Dean GE (1992) Vaginal replacement in children. *J Urol* **148**: 677–9.

Hermans C, de Plaen J-F, de Nayer P *et al.* (1996) Case report: 17 alpha hydroxylase/17-20 lyase deficiency: a rare cause of endocrine hypertension. *Am J Med Sci* **312**: 126–9.

Hiort O, Klauber GT (1995) True hermaphroditism with 46XY karyotype and a point mutation in the SRY gene. *J Pediatr* **126**: 1022.

Hiort O, Sinnecker GH, Willenbring H *et al.* (1996) Nonisotopic single strand conformation analysis of the 5α-reductase type 2 gene for the diagnosis of 5α-reductase deficiency. *J Clin Endocrinol Metab* **81**: 3415–18.

Hong JR, Barber M, Scott CI *et al.* (1995) 3-year old phenotypic female with campomelic dysplasia and bilateral gonadoblastoma. *J Pediatr Surg* **30**: 1735–7.

Houston CS, Opitz JM, Spranger JW *et al.* (1983) The campomelic syndrome: review, report of 17 cases and follow-up in the currently 17 year old boy first reported by Maroteaux *et al.* in 1971. *Am J Med Genet* **15**: 3–38.

Hurtig AL, Rosenthal IM (1987) Psychological findings in early treated cases of female pseudohermaphroditism caused by virilizing congenital adrenal hyperplasia. *Arch Sexual Behav* **16**: 209–23.

Hutson JM (1985) A biphasic model for hormonal control of testicular descent. *Lancet* **ii**: 419–21.

Imbeaud S, Rey R, Berta P *et al.* (1995) Testicular degeneration in three patients with the persistent müllerian duct syndrome. *Eur J Pediatr* **154**: 187–90.

Imbeaud S, Belville C, Messika-Zeitoun L *et al.* (1996) A 27 base-pair deletion of the anti-müllerian type II receptor gene is the most common cause of the persistent müllerian duct syndrome. *Hum Molec Genet* **5**: 1269–77.

Imperato-McGinley J, Guerrero L, Gautier T *et al.* (1974) Steroid 5-alpha-reductase deficiency in man: an inherited form of male pseudohermaphroditism. *Science* **186**: 1213–15.

Imperato-McGinley J, Peterson RE, Gautier T *et al.* (1982) Hormonal evaluation of a large kindred with complete androgen insensitivity: evidence for secondary 5α-reductase deficiency. *J Clin Endocrinol Metab* **54**: 931–41.

Imperato-McGinley J, Gautier T, Pichard OM et al. (1986) The diagnosis of 5α-reductase deficiency in infancy. *J Clin Endocrinol Metab* **63**: 1313–18.

Ion A, Telvi L, Chaussain JL et al. (1996) A novel mutation in the putative DNA helicase XH2 is responsible for male to female sex reversal associated with an atypical form of the ATR-X syndrome. *Am J Med Genet* **58**: 1185–91.

Ito Y, Fisher CR, Conte FA et al. (1993) Molecular basis of aromatase deficiency in adult female with sexual infantilism and polycystic ovaries. *Proc Natl Acad Sci USA* **90**: 11673–7.

Ivarsson S-A: 5α-Reductase deficient men are fertile. *Euro J Pediatr* **155**: 425.

Jeanpierre C, Denamur E, Henry I et al. (1998) Identification of constitutional WT-1 mutations in patients with isolated diffuse mesangial sclerosis, and analysis of genotype/phenotype correlations by use of a computerized mutation database. *Am J Med Genet* **62**: 824–33.

Jordan GH, Alter GJ, Gilbert GA (1994) Penile prosthesis implantation in total phalloplasty. *J Urol* **152**: 410–14.

Jorgensen N, Muller J, Jaubert F et al. (1997) Heterogeneity of gonadoblastoma germ cells: similarities with immature germ cells, spermatogonia and testicular carcinoma in situ cells. *Histopathology* **30**: 177–86.

Jost A (1947) Recherches sur la differenciation sexuelle de l'embryon du lapin. *Arch d'Anat Microsc Morphol Exp* **26**: 271–2.

Jost A (1970) Hormonal factors in the sex differentiation of the mammalian foetus. *Phil Trans R Soc Lond B* **259**: 119–30.

Kaefer M, Diamond D, Hendren WH et al. (1999) The incidence of intersex in children with cryptorchidism and hypospadias: stratification based on gonadal palpability and meatal position. *J Urol* **162**: 1003–6.

Karnak I, Tanyel FC, Akcoren Z (1997) Transverse testicular ectopia with persistent müllerian duct syndrome. *J Pediatr Surg* **32**: 1362–4.

Keenan BS, Meyer WJ, Hadjian AJ et al. (1974) Syndrome of androgen insensitivity in man: absence of 5α-dihydrotestosterone binding protein in skin fibroblasts. *J Clin Endocrinol Metab* **38**: 1143–6.

Kent J, Wheatley SC, Andrews JE et al. (1996) A male-specific role for SOX-9 in vertebrate sex determination. *Development* **122**: 2813–22.

Koopman P, Gubbay J, Vivian N et al. (1991) Male development of chromosomally female mice transgenic for SRY. *Nature* **351**: 117–21.

Kremer H, Kraaij R, Toledo JP et al. (1995) Male pseudohermaphroditism due to homozygous missense mutation of the luteinizing hormone receptor gene. *Nature Genet* **9**: 160–4.

Krob G, Braun A, Kuhnle U (1994) True hermaphroditism: geographical distribution, clinical findings, chromosomes and gonadal histology. *Eur J Pediatr* **153**: 2–10.

Kuhnle U, Bullinger M, Schwarz HP (1995) The quality of life in adult female patients with congenital adrenal hyperplasia: a comprehensive study of the impact of genital malformations and chronic disease on female patients life. *Eur J Pediatr* **154**: 708–16.

Kutteh WH, Santos-Ramos R, Ermel LD (1995) Accuracy of ultrasonic detection of the uterus in newborn infants: implications for infants with ambiguous genitalia. *Ultrasound Obstet Gynecol* **5**: 109–13.

Lane AH, Donahoe PK (1998) New insights into müllerian inhibiting substance and its mechanism of action. *J Endocrinol* **158**: 1–6.

Lee MM, Donahoe PK, Hasegawa T et al. (1996) Müllerian inhibiting substance in humans: normal levels from infancy to adulthood. *J Clin Endocrinol Metab* **81**: 571–6.

Letterie GS, Page DC (1995) Dysgerminoma and gonadal dysgenesis in a 46XX female with no evidence of Y chromosomal DNA. *Gynecol Oncol* **57**: 423–5.

Lin D, Gitelman SE, Saenger P et al. (1991) Normal genes for the cholesterol side chain cleavage enzyme P450scc in congenital lipoid adrenal hyperplasia. *J Clin Invest* **88**: 1955–62.

Lin D, Sugawara T, Strauss JF et al. (1995) Role of steroidogenic acute regulatory protein in adrenal and gonadal steriodogenesis. *Science* **267**: 1828–31.

Lo KW, Lam SK, Cheung TH et al. (1996) Gonadoblastoma in patient with Turner's syndrome. *J Obstet Gynecol Res* **22**: 35–41.

Lopez M, Canto P, Aguinaga M et al. (1998) Frequency of Y chromosomal material in Mexican patients with Ullrich–Turner syndrome. *Am J Med Genet* **76**: 120–4.

Lubs HA, Vilar O, Bergenstal DM (1959) Familial male pseudohermaphroditism with labial testes and partial feminization: endocrine studies and genetic aspects. *J Clin Endocrinol* **19**: 1110–20.

Ludwig M, Beck A, Wickert L et al. (1998) Female pseudohermaphroditism associated with a novel homozygous G-to-A (V370-To-M) substitution in the P450 aromatase gene. *J Pediatr Endocrinol Metab* **11**: 657–64.

Luo X, Ikeda Y, Parker KL (1994) A cell specific nuclear receptor is essential for adrenal and gonadal development and sexual differentiation. *Cell* **77**: 481–90.

McClamrock HD, Adashi EY (1992) Gestational hyperandrogenism. *Fertil Steril* **57**: 257–74.

McElreavey K, Rappoport R, Vilain E et al. (1992) A minority of 46XX true hermaphrodites are positive for the Y-DNA sequence including SRY. *Hum Genet* **90**: 121–5.

McElreavey K, Vilain E, Abbas N et al. (1993) A regulatory cascade hypothesis for mammalian sex determination: SRY represses a negative regulator of male development. *Proc Natl Acad Sci USA* **90**: 3368–72.

MacLean HE, Choi W-T, Rekaris G et al. (1995) Abnormal androgen receptor binding affinity in subjects with Kennedy's disease (spinal and bulbar muscular atrophy). *J Clin Endocrinol Metab* **80**: 508–16.

Martens JW, Verhoef-Post M, Abelin N et al. (1998) A homozygous mutation in the luteinizing hormone receptor causes partial Leydig cell hypoplasia: correlation between receptor activity and phenotype. *Molec Endocrinol* **12**: 775–84.

Masiakos PT, Flynn CE, Donahoe PK (1997) Masculinizing and feminizing syndromes caused by functioning tumors. *Semin Pediatr Surg* **5**:147–55.

Mebarki F, Sanchez R, Rheaume E *et al.* (1995) Nonsalt-losing male pseudohermaphroditism due to the novel homozygous N200S mutation in the type II 3β-hydroxysteroid dehydrogenase gene. *J Clin Endocrinol Metab* **80**: 2127–34.

Mendez JP, Schiavon R, Diaz-Cueto L *et al.* (1998) A reliable endocrine test with human menopausal gonadotropins for diagnosis of true hermaphroditism in early infancy. *J Clin Endocrinol Metab* **83**: 3523–6.

Mendonca BB, Inacio M, Costa EM *et al.* (1996) Male pseudo-hermaphroditism due to steroid 5α-reductase 2 deficiency. *Medicine* **75**: 64–76.

Menzel D, Hauffa BP (1990) Changes in size and sonographic characteristics of the adrenal glands during the first year of life and the sonographic diagnosis of adrenal hyperplasia in infants with 21-hydroxylase deficiency. *J Clin Ultrasound* **18**: 619–25.

Mercado AB, Wilson RC, Cheng KL *et al.* (1995) Prenatal treatment and diagnosis of congenital adrenal hyperplasia owing to steroid 21-hydroxylase deficiency. *J Clin Endocrinol Metab* **80**: 2014–20.

Meyer J, Sudbeck P, Held M *et al.* (1997) Mutation analysis of the SOX9 gene in campomelic dysplasia and autosomal sex reversal: Lack of genotype/phenotype correlations. *Hum Molec Genet* **6**: 91–8.

Meyer-Bahlburg HF (1999) What causes low rates of child-bearing in congenital adrenal hyperplasia? *J Clin Endocrinol Lab Med* **84**: 1844–7.

Meyer-Bahlburg HF, Gruen RS, New MI *et al.* (1996) Gender change from female to male in classical congenital adrenal hyperplasia. *Horm Behav* **30**: 319–32.

Miller WL (1997) Congenital lipoid adrenal hyperplasia: the human gene knockout for the steroidogenic acute regulatory protein. *J Molec Endocrinol* **19**: 227–40.

Mollard P, Juskiewenski S, Sarkissian J (1981) Clitoroplasty in intersex: a new technique. *Br J Urol* **53**: 371–3.

Money J, Hampson JG, Hampson JL (1955) Herma-phroditism: recommendations concerning assignment of sex, change of sex and psychologic management. *Bull Johns Hopkins Hosp* **97**: 284–300.

Money J, Schwartz M, Lewis VG (1984) Adult erotosexual status and fetal hormonal masculinization and demasculinization: 46XX congenital virilizing adrenal hyperplasia and 46XY androgen insensitivity syndrome compared. *Psychoneuroendocrinology* **9**: 405–14.

Monno S, Mizushima Y, Toyoda W *et al.* (1997) A new variant of the cytochrome P450c17 (CYP17) gene mutation in three patients with 17α-hydroxylase deficiency. *Ann Hum Genet* **61**: 275–9.

Morel Y, Mebarki F, Rhéaume E *et al.* (1997) Structure-function relationships of 3β-hydroxysteroid dehydro-genase: contribution made by molecular genetics of 3β-hydroxysteroid dehydrogenase deficiency. *Steroids* **62**: 176–84.

Morris JM (1953) The syndrome of testicular feminization in male pseudohermaphrodites. *Am J Obstet Gynecol* **65**: 1192–211.

Muller J, Visfeldt J, Philip J *et al.* (1992) Carcinoma *in situ*, gonadoblastoma, and early invasive neoplasia in a nine year old girl with 46XY gonadal dysgenesis. *APMIS* **100**: 170–4.

Mullis PE, Yoshimura N, Kuhlmann B *et al.* (1997) Aromatase deficiency in a female who is compound heterozygous for two new point mutations in the P450 arom gene: impact of estrogens on hypergonadotropic hypogonadism, multi-cystic ovaries and bone densitometry in childhood. *J Clin Endocrinol Metab* **82**: 1739–45.

Nachtigal M, Ingraham HA (1996) Bioactivation of müllerian inhibiting substance during gonadal development by a Kex2/subtilisin-like endoprotease. *Proc Natl Acad Sci USA* **93**: 7711–16.

Nakae J, Tajima T, Sugawara T *et al.* (1997) Analysis of the steroidogenic acute regulatory protein (StAR) gene in Japanese patients with congenital adrenal hyperplasia. *Hum Molec Genet* **6**: 571–6.

New MI (1970) Male pseudohermaphroditism due to 17 alpha hydroxylase deficiency. *J Clin Invest* **49**: 1930–41.

New MI (1998) Diagnosis and management of congenital adrenal hyperplasia. *Ann Rev Med* **49**: 311–28.

Nimkarn S, Cerame BI, Wei J-Q *et al.* (1999) Congenital adrenal hyperplasia (21-hydroxylase deficiency) without demonstrable genetic mutations. *J Clin Endocrinol Metab* **84**: 378–81.

Noonan JA (1994) Noonan syndrome. An update and review for the primary pediatrician. *Clin Pediatr* **33**: 548–56.

Page DC (1987) Hypothesis: a Y-chromosome gene causes gonadoblastoma in dysgenetic gonads. *Development* **101**: 151–5.

Passerini-Glazel G (1989) A new one-stage procedure for cli-torovaginoplasty in severely masculinized female pseudo-hermaphrodites. *J Urol* **142**: 565–8.

Pelletier J, Bruening W, Kashtan CE *et al.* (1991) Germ line mutations in the Wilms' tumor suppressor gene are associated with abnormal urogenital development in Denys–Drash syndrome. *Cell* **67**: 437–47.

Peña A (1997) Total urogenital mobilization: an easier way to repair cloacas. *J Pediatr Surg* **32**: 263–8.

Peña A, Filmer B, Bonilla E *et al.* (1992) Transanorectal approach for the treatment of urogenital sinus: preliminary report. *J Pediatr Surg* **27**: 681–5.

Picard JY, Josso N (1984) Purification of testicular anti-müllerian hormone allowing direct visualization of the pure glycoprotein and determination of yield and purification factor. *Molec Cell Endocrinol* **34**: 23–9.

Pillard R, Bailey JM (1995) Biological perspectives in sexual orientation. *Psychiatr Clin North Am* **18**: 71–84.

Prader A, Gurtner HP (1955) Das Syndrom des Pseudo-hermaphroditismus masculinus bei kongenitaler Neben-nierenrindenhyperplasie ohne Androgenuberproduktion (Adrenaler Pseudohermaphroditismus masculinis). *Helv Paediatr Acta* **10**: 397–412.

Premawardhana LD, Hughes IA, Read GF *et al.* (1997) Longer term outcomes in females with congenital adrenal hyperplasia (CAH): the Cardiff experience. *Clin Endocrinol* **46**: 327–32.

Pritchard-Jones K, Fleming S, Davidson D *et al.* (1990) The candidate Wilms' tumour gene is involved in genitourinary development. *Nature* **346**: 194–7.

Quigley CA, de Bellis A, Marschke KB *et al.* (1995) Androgen receptor defects: historical, clinical and molecular perspec-tives. *Endocr Rev* **16**: 271–321.

Racine C, Rey R, Forest MG et al. (1998) Receptors for anti-müllerian hormone on Leydig cells are responsible for its effects on steroidogenesis and cell differentiation. *Proc Natl Acad Sci USA* **95**: 594–9.

Raga F, Bauset C, Remohi J et al. (1997) Reproductive impact of congenital müllerian anomalies. *Hum Reprod* **12**: 2277–81.

Rajfer J, Mendelson G, Arnheim J et al. (1978) Dysgenetic male pseudohermaphroditism. *J Urol* **119**: 525–7.

Ramani P, Yeung CK, Habeebu SS (1993): Testicular intratubular germ cell neoplasia in children and adolescents with intersex. *Am J Surg Pathol* **17**: 1124–33.

Randolph JG, Hung W (1970) Reduction clitoroplasty in females with hypertrophied clitoris. *J Pediatr Surg* **105**: 224–31.

Reardon W, Gibbons RJ, Winter RM et al. (1995) Male pseudohermaphroditism in sibs with the α-thalassemia/mental retardation (ATR-X) syndrome. *Am J Med Genet* **55**: 285–7.

Reifenstein EC (1947) Hereditary familial hypogonadism. *Proc Am Fed Clin Res* **3**: 86.

Reilly JM, Woodhouse CR (1989) Small penis and the male sexual role. *J Urol* **142**: 569–71.

Rey R, Al-Attar L, Louis F et al. (1996) Testicular dysgenesis does not effect suppression of anti müllerian hormone by Sertoli cells in premeiotic seminiferous tubules. *Am J Pathol* **148**: 1689–98.

Rey RA, Belville C, Nihoul-Fékété C et al. (1999) Evaluation of gonadal function in 107 intersex patients by means of serum antimüllerian hormone measurement. *J Clin Endocrinol Metab* **84**: 627–31.

Rosewater S, Gwinup G, Hamwi JG (1965) Familial gynecomastia. *Ann Intern Med* **63**: 377–85.

Rösler A, Silverstein S, Abeliovich D (1996) A (R80Q) mutation in 17β-hydroxysteroid dehydrogenase type 3 gene among Arabs of Israel is associated with pseudohermaphroditism in males and normal asymptomatic females. *J Clin Endocrinol Metab* **81**: 1827–31.

Rutgers JL, Scully RE (1991) The androgen insensitivity syndrome (testicular feminization): a clinicopathologic study of 43 cases. *Int J Gynecol Pathol* **10**: 126–44.

Sadove CR, Sengezer M, McRoberts W et al. (1993) One stage total reconstruction with a full sensate osteocutaneous fibular flap. *Plast Reconstruct Surg* **92**: 1314–25.

Saez JM, de Peretti E, Morera AM et al. (1971) Familial male pseudohermaphroditism with gynecomastia due to testicular 17-ketosteroid reductase defect: I. Studies *in vivo*. *J Clin Endocrinol Metab* **32**: 604–10.

Schmitt K, Zabel B, Tulzer G et al. (1995) Nephropathy with Wilms' tumor or gonadal dysgenesis: incomplete Denys–Drash syndrome or separate disease? *Eur J Pediatr* **154**: 577–81.

Schumacher V, Scharer K, Wuhl E et al. (1998) Spectrum of early onset nephrotic syndrome associated with WT-1 missense mutations. *Kidney Int* **53**: 1594–600.

Schwartz M, Imperato-McGinley J, Peterson RE et al. (1981) Male pseudohermaphroditism secondary to an abnormality in Leydig cell differentiation. *J Clin Endocrinol Metab* **53**: 123–7.

Scully RF (1991) Gonadal pathology and genetically determined diseases. *Monogr Pathol* **88**: 257–85.

Secaf E, Hricak H, Gooding CA et al. (1994) Role of MRI in the evaluation of ambiguous genitalia. *Pediatr Radiol* **24**: 231–5.

Shapiro E (1999) The sonographic appearance of the normal and abnormal fetal genitalia. *J Urol* **162**: 530–3.

Shozu M, Akasofu K, Marada T et al. (1991) The new cause of female pseudohermaphroditism: placental aromatase deficiency. *J Clin Endocrinol Metab* **72**: 560–6.

Silver RI, Rodriguez R, Chang TS et al. (1999) *In vitro* fertilization is associated with an increased risk of hypospadias. *J Urol* **161**: 1954–7.

Sinclair, AH, Berta P, Palmer MS (1990) A gene from the human sex determining region encodes a protein with homology to a conserved DNA binding motif. *Nature* **346**: 240–4.

Sinnecker GH, Hiort O, Nitsche GM et al. (1997) Functional assessment and clinical classification of androgen sensitivity in patients with mutations of the androgen receptor gene. *Eur J Pediatr* **156**: 7–14.

Sivit CJ, Hung W, Taylor GA et al. (1991) Sonography in neonatal congenital adrenal hyperplasia. *AJR Am J Roentgenol* **156**: 141–3.

Slaney SF, Chalmers IJ, Affara NA et al. (1998) An autosomal or X linked mutation results in true hermaphrodites and 46XX males in the same family. *J Med Genet* **35**: 17–22.

Sohaib SA, Webb JA, Rees MC et al. (1997) Case report: ultrasonographic appearance of ovotestes in a true hermaphrodite. *Clin Radiol* **52**: 312–14.

Sohval AR (1963) 'Mixed' gonadal dysgenesis: a variety of hermaphroditism. *Am J Hum Genet* **15**: 155–57.

Soule JG, Conway G, Prelevic GM et al. (1995) Osteopenia as a feature of the androgen insensitivity syndrome. *Clin Endocrinol* **43**: 671–5.

Stavrou SS, Zhu Y-S, Cai L-Q et al. (1998) A novel mutation of the human luteinizing hormone receptor in 46XY and 46XX sisters. *J Clin Endocrinol Metab* **83**: 2091–8.

Strain L, Dean JC, Hamilton MP et al. (1998) A true hermaphrodite chimera resulting from embryo amalgamation after *in vitro* fertilization. *N Engl J Med* **338**: 166–9.

Swain A, Zanaria E, Hacker A et al. (1996) DAX-1 expression is consistent with a role in sex determination as well as in adrenal and hypothalamus function. *Nature Genet* **12**: 404–9.

Swyer GI (1955) Male pseudohermaphroditism: a hitherto undescribed form. *BMJ* **2**: 709–12.

Takaya J, Ishihara R, Kino M et al. (1998) A patient with congenital lipoid adrenal hyperplasia evaluated by serial abdominal ultrasonography. *Eur J Pediatr* **157**: 544–6.

Thigpen AE, Davis DL, Milatovich A et al. (1992) Molecular genetics of 5α-reductase deficiency. *J Clin Invest* **90**: 799–809.

Tiltman AJ, Sweerts M (1982) Multiparity in a covert true hermaphrodite. *Obstet Gynecol* **60**: 752–4.

Tincello DG, Saunders PT, Hodgins MB et al. (1997) Correlation of clinical, endocrine and molecular abnormalities with *in vitro* responses to high dose testosterone in patients with partial androgen insensitivity syndrome. *Clin Endocrinol* **46**: 497–506.

Toledo SP (1992) Leydig cell hypoplasia leading to two different phenotypes: male pseudohermaphroditism and primary hypogonadism not associated with this. *Clin Endocrinol* **36**: 521–2.

Tsuchiya K, Reijo R, Page DC *et al.* (1995) Gonadoblastoma: molecular definition of the susceptibility region on the Y chromosome. *Am J Hum Genet* **57**: 1400–7.

Turner HH (1938) A syndrome of infantilism, congenital webbed neck and cubitus valgus. *Endocrinology* **23**: 566–74.

van Niekerk WA (1981) True hermaphroditism. In: *The intersex child. pediatric and adolescent endocrinology*. Volume 8. Basel: Karger, 80–99.

van Wyk JJ, Gunther DF, Ritzen EM *et al.* (1996) The use of adrenalectomy as a treatment for congenital adrenal hyperplasia. *J Clin Endocrinol Metab* **81**: 3180–9.

Veitia R, Nunes M, Brauner R *et al.* (1997) Deletion of distal 9p associated with 46XY male to female sex reversal: Definition of the break points at 9p23.3-p24.1. *Genomics* **41**: 271–4.

Viner RM, Teoh Y, Williams DM *et al.* (1997) Androgen insensitivity syndrome: a survey of diagnostic procedure and management in the U.K. *Arch Dis Child* **77**: 305–9.

Wagner T, Wirth J, Meyer J *et al.* (1994) Autosomal sex reversal and campomelic dysplasia are caused by mutations in and around the SRY-related gene SOX9. *Cell* **79**: 1111–20.

Walker BR, Skoog SJ, Winslow BH *et al.* (1997) Testis sparing surgery for steroid unresponsive testicular tumors of the adrenogenital syndrome. *J Urol* **157**:1460–3.

Walsh PC, Madden JD, Harrod MJ *et al.* (1974) Familial incomplete male pseudohermaphroditism, type 2. Decreased dihydrotestosterone formation in pseudovaginal perineoscrotal hypospadias. *N Engl J Med* **291**: 944–9.

Wedell A (1996) Molecular approaches for the diagnosis of 21-hydroxylase deficiency and congenital adrenal hyperplasia. *Clin Lab Med* **16**: 125–37.

Wilkie AO, Zeitlin HL, Lindenbaum RH *et al.* (1990) Clinical features and molecular analysis of the α thalassemia/mental retardation syndrome: II Cases without detectable abnormality of the α globulin complex. *Am J Hum Genet* **46**: 1127–40.

Wilkie AO, Campbell FM, Daubeney P *et al.* (1993) Complete and partial XY sex reversal associated with terminal deletion of 10q: report of 2 cases and literature review. *Am J Med Genet* **46**: 597–600.

Wilson RC, Mercado AB, Cheng KC *et al.* (1995) Steroid 21-hydroxylase deficiency: genotype may not predict phenotype. *J Clin Endocrinol Metab* **80**: 2322–9.

Winter JL, Chapman PH, Powell DE *et al.* (1996) Female pseudohermaphroditism due to congenital adrenal hyperplasia complicated by adenocarcinoma of the prostate and clear cell carcinoma of the endometrium. *Am J Clin Pathol* **106**: 660–4.

Wright NB, Smith C, Rickwood AM. *et al.* (1995) Imaging children with ambiguous genitalia and intersex states. *Clin Radiol* **50**: 823–9.

Zhou J-N, Hofman MA, Gooren LJ *et al.* (1995) A sex difference in the human brain and its relation to transsexuality. *Nature* **378**: 68–70.

Zucker KJ, Bradley ST, Oliver G *et al.* (1996) Psychosexual development of women with congenital adrenal hyperplasia. *Horm Behav* **30**: 300–18.

Hypospadias and chordee

32

A. Barry Belman

Introduction

As in the third edition of *Clinical Pediatric Urology*, this chapter will not review the historical aspects of the subject unless they have direct applicability. The interested reader is referred to the first two editions or to other treatises on the subject.

Hypospadias is one of the most common congenital urogenital problems. It also continues to be one of our most challenging and gratifying problems. Over the past several years significant advances have occurred which have raised the bar of expectations for success. The current challenge is to create a normal appearing penis in a single operation with only a small risk of a complication. Duckett (1981a) aptly applied the name hypospadiology to the study of this subject.

Etiology

In most cases hypospadias is a spontaneous occurrence without an obvious underlying cause. However, inheritance plays a role in approximately 20–25% of cases (Bauer *et al.*, 1981). The exact mode of inheritance remains unclear. In siblings there appears to be about a 10-fold risk for hypospadias (Kallen *et al.*, 1986).

Penile development is a product of the effects of the stimulus of testosterone produced by the fetal testes on androgen-sensitive structures. These include the wolffian structures as well as the genital tubercle and labioscrotal folds. It has been postulated that a reduced response to gonadotrophin may be responsible for inadequate testosterone production. However, no difference in maternal serum gonadotrophin levels during early pregnancy was noted between a control group and those who had children with hypospadias (or cryptorchidism) (Kiely *et al.*, 1995). Walsh, *et al.*

(1976) found no difference in testosterone response to human chorionic gonadotropin (hCG) in 11 boys with hypospadias, but there have also been several reports of diminished testosterone production in boys with hypospadias (Knorr *et al.*, 1979; Allen and Griffin, 1984; Nonomura *et al.*, 1984; Shima *et al.*, 1986). Since penile development is a product of testosterone stimulation, androgen-binding capability has been studied extensively (Evans Ball *et al.*, 1991; Bentvelsen *et al.*, 1995; Sutherland *et al.*, 1996). No specific factor has been isolated as a consistent cause. Aaronson *et al.* (1997) reported a 50% incidence of a testosterone biosynthetic defect in a group of boys with penoscrotal and proximal shaft hypospadias. They concluded that there may be a deficiency in the structure or rate of maturation of enzymes that lead to testosterone production. The impact on testosterone production influences penile development in the early weeks of gestation.

No relationship has been identified between the use of oral contraceptives and hypsopadias (Kallen *et al.*, 1991; Ramen-Wilms *et al.*, 1995). Macnab and Zouves (1991) reported two boys with hypospadias in a group of 53 males born as a result of *in vitro* fertilization, suggesting that excessive early hormonal levels can play a role. Use of progestational hormones in early pregnancy has previously been thought to be a causal factor (Aarskog, 1979).

Kallen *et al.* (1986) reported other factors that appear to play a role. These included maternal age, with an increased incidence in older mothers. The risk was particularly great for those having their first child. Twin births also increased the risk, particularly in male–male twinning, with a lower incidence in male–female twins. However, Weidner *et al.* (1999), reported no relationship to maternal age in a review of hypospadias incidence in Denmark but found a correlation with decreasing birth weight. In addition, not all monozygotic twins will both have hypospadias. Fredell *et al.* (1998) evaluated 18 monozygotic twins discordant for hypospadias and in 16 the twin with the lower birth weight had hypospadias, suggesting that some environmental factor affecting overall development played a role. Stoll *et al.* (1990) found no etiologic factors in a total of 176 boys with hypospadias other than low placental weight.

Embryology and associated abnormalities

At about 6 weeks' gestation the genital tubercle becomes evident. Under the stimulation of fetal testosterone it enlarges. Parallel folds form along the undersurface of this tubercle between which lies the urethral groove that ultimately becomes the urethral plate. The scrotum forms from swellings on either side of the urethral groove. With growth of the phallus the urethral folds unite over the urethral groove from proximal to distal, forming the urethra. Any arrest in development will cause hypospadias (Fig. 32.1). However, the glanular urethra distal to the fossa navicularis is formed by an ingrowth of tissue that cores through the glans to meet the more proximal urethra. Failed attempts to form this most distal part of the urethra are evident by the blind-ending pits noted in the distal urethral plate in some boys with hypospadias.

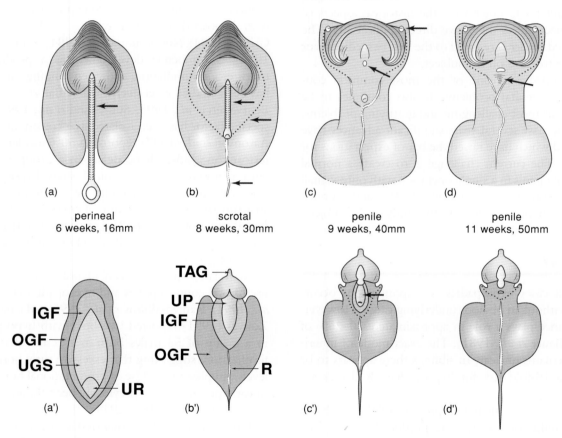

Figure 32.1 Diagrams of clinical forms of hypospadias and corresponding embryologic stages of development of the urethra with approximate gestational times of occurrence and corresponding crown–rump lengths. (*a*) Perineal, rudimentary urethral plate (*arrow*); separated scrota. (*a'*) Roof of urogenital sinus remains uncanalized (IGF, OGF = inner and outer genital folds; UGS = urogenital sinus; UR = urethral orifice). (*b*) Scrotal orifice of clitoral hypospadias; perineal raphe (*lowest arrow*); bifurcation at orifice and branches (*middle arrow*); and rudimentary plate (*top arrow*). (*b'*) Roof of UGS partly canalized; partly uncanalized urethral plate (UP), scrotal raphe (R), and epithelial glanular tag (TAG). (*c*) Mid-penile orifice. Orifice of Littre gland (*arrow*); dog-ear (*top arrow*). (*c'*) Uncanalized plate in urethral groove (*arrow*); prepuce begins. (*d*) Distal penile orifice, raphe bifurcation mid-penile; posterior extended triangle (*arrow*). (*d'*) Urethral plate uncanalized anterior to orifice. (*e*) – (*h'*) *Shown opposite.* (From Stephens, Smith and Hudson *et al.*, 1996, with permission.)

Foreskin development is related to urethral development and hypospadias is almost always associated with a hooded prepuce. The exception is the megameatal variant (Kumar, 1986). Because the foreskin is complete, hypospadias is often not recognized until circumcision is carried out in this group or, in the uncircumcised boy, until the foreskin retracts.

One should think of hypospadias as an isolated abnormality, although it may be found to coexist with other malformations in patients with complex congenital syndromes and chromosomal defects (see Chapters 3 and 31). In a review of 700 cases, associated extragenital abnormalities were noted in 6.7% with no particular organ system affected more than any other (Latifoglu *et al.*, 1998). There are reports of

an increased incidence of undescended testes and hernias in boys with hypospadias variably reported as from 7 to 10% (Khuri *et al.*, 1981; Kulkarni *et al.*, 1991; Weidner *et al.*, 1999). There have also been reports of increased urinary abnormalities in boys with hypospadias, which has led to the recommendation for routine visualization of the urinary tract (Fallon *et al.*, 1976; Ikoma *et al.*, 1979; Shafir *et al.*, 1982; Moore, 1990). Nevertheless, in the absence of other congenital anomalies which might suggest additional problems screening of the upper urinary tract is hard to justify since it is unlikely that a clinically significant abnormality will be found.

One abnormality that can be anticipated in patients with severe hypospadias is an enlarged utricle

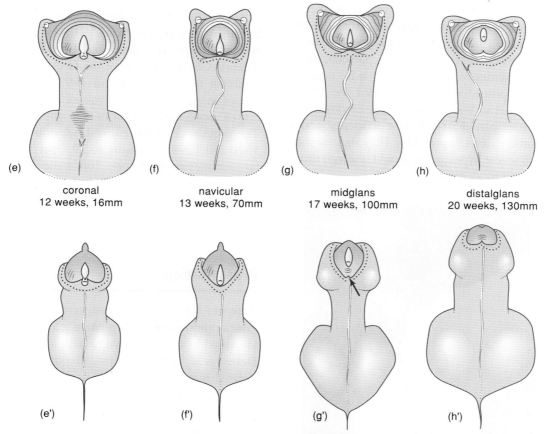

Figure 32.1 *Continued.* Diagrams of clinical forms of hypospadias and corresponding embryologic stages of development of the urethra with approximate gestational times of occurrence and corresponding crown–rump lengths. (*e*) Coronal orifice confluent with navicular groove; prepuce deficient ventrally. (*e′*) Branches of raphe extending to dorsal fringe of prepuce; primitive ostium open. (*f*) Glanular navicular orifice projected onto base of glans; inner and outer layers of prepuce converge on posterior lip of orifice. (*f′*) Ventral component of prepuce developing; coronal orifice closes. (*g*) Mid-glanular orifice with lip rudimentary frenulum. (*g′*) Normal frenular attachments to glans (*arrow*). (*h*) Subapical distal glanular orifice mildly stenotic; deviated penile raphe; false prepuce formed chiefly from G-skin; skewed mini-triangle. (*h′*) Normal orifice on summit; prepuce, frenulum, and raphe normal. (From Stephens, Smith and Hudson *et al.*, 1996, with permission.)

(Fig. 32.2). Devine *et al.* (1980) reported enlargement of the utriculus masculinus in 57% of boys with perineal hypospadias and 10% in those with a penoscrotal meatus. Ikoma *et al.* (1986) reported utricular enlargement in 27.5% of 280 boys with hypospadias. An enlarged utricle does not generally have any clinical significance, although it may complicate catheterization. Placing some type of stylet or guide in the catheter or feeding tube directing it anteriorly will assist its passage. Stasis in the utricle may be a rare cause of urinary tract infection (UTI) or, over the years, result in stone formation (Ritchey *et al.*, 1988). Under the rare circumstances when surgical excision of the utricle is required, it should be approached with caution since the vasa may be located along its lateral walls. At exploration a uterus and tubes may be noted, suggesting that more boys with severe hypospadias than is commonly appreciated have a degree of intersex (Ikoma *et al.*, 1986). In fact, in a report by Albers *et al.* (1997), when full evaluation was pursued, identifiable abnormalities were noted in 12 of 33 patients with severe hypospadias. These included the Drash syndrome, partial androgen insensitivity, chromosomal abnormalities, partial 5α reductase deficiency, and a variety of others (see Chapter 31). They suggest that all boys with severe hypospadias should undergo thorough evaluation to identify a cause.

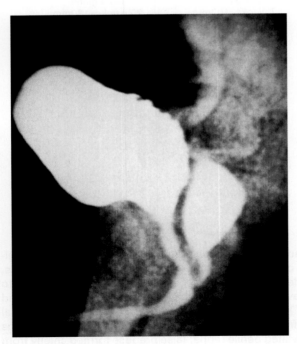

Figure 32.2 Voiding cystourethogram in a boy with hypospadias and significant utricular enlargement.

Editorial note: Practically speaking, it is safe to assume that the child with hypospadias and two palpable gonads can be considered a male and genital reconstruction may be pursued without further evaluation.

Incidence

The incidence of hypospadias varies geographically. Kallen (1988) reported a prevalence ranging from 0.26 per 1000 births (both male and female) in Mexico to 2.11 in Hungary. In the same report it was cited that there were 2.6 per 1000 livebirths in Scandinavia. More recently an incidence of 4 in 1000 male (0.4 in 100) births was found in Denmark between 1983 and 1992 (Weidner *et al.*, 1999). Sweet *et al.* (1974) reported the highest incidence, 4.1 per 1000 livebirths in a review from 1940–1970. In 1997 a review of the prevalence of hypospadias in the Atlanta, Georgia, region of the USA reported a near doubling between 1968 and 1993, with an annual rate of increase of 2.9% (Paulozzi *et al.*, 1997). The rate of increase was higher in non-whites than whites. The prevalence in the entire USA doubled between 1970 and 1993, increasing to 39.7 per 10 000 births (approximately 0.78 per 100 male births). This increase cannot be attributed to better recognition or reporting since the cases of severe hypospadias increased at an even higher rate, from three- to fivefold. The cause for this increase is unknown.

Presentation

Antenatal sonography may suggest the possibility of a genital abnormality when male genitalia cannot be identified in a fetus known to have a Y chromosome. Devesa *et al.* (1998) reported identifying ten cases of isolated hypospadias on antenatal sonography, six in the second trimester. In most instances hypospadias is recognized in the newborn nursery. However, occasionally mild forms are missed in spite of the fact that incomplete formation of the foreskin serves as a marker. The exception is the child with megameatal hypospadias accompanied by a complete foreskin. For this reason, the foreskin should be retracted completely and the meatus inspected prior to incision or removal of the prepuce.

Upon examination, the penis should be described anatomically, noting both the meatal location and

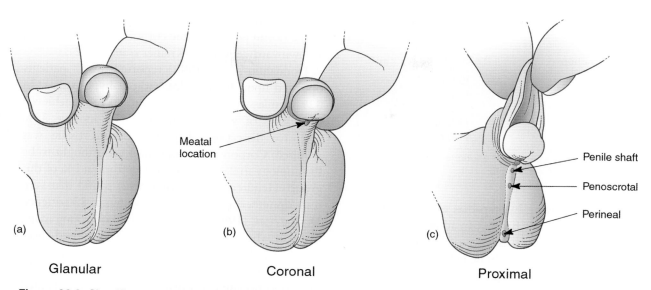

(a) Glanular
(b) Coronal
(c) Proximal

Meatal location

Penile shaft
Penoscrotal
Perineal

Figure 32.3 Classification of hypospadias based on anatomic location of the urethral meatus. Associated chordee is best described in terms of severity: mild, moderate, or severe.

severity of chordee (Fig. 32.3). For example, a boy may have a midshaft hypospadias without chordee or penoscrotal hypospadias with mild, moderate or severe chordee. Meatal position can best be identified by lifting the ventral skin away from the shaft, exaggerating the meatal opening (Fig. 32.4). The child with hypospadias who does not have two gonads clearly palpable is considered as having ambiguous genitalia and intersex evaluation should be pursued prior to hospital discharge (see Chapter 31).

The newborn with an abnormally small penis should undergo early determination as to the capability for penile growth in the future. The normal penile stretched length (base to tip) is 3.5 ± 0.7 cm (Feldman and Smith, 1975). Those below the third percentile are tested further to determine responsiveness to testosterone. Parenteral testosterone, 25 mg given intramuscularly, will demonstrate responsiveness in a few weeks in those capable of responding. Unfortunately, those children with a small penis are less likely to have a normal sized penis when adults (Table 32.1). Ultimate penile length appears to be predetermined and may be dictated by the same developmental abnormality that caused the hypospadias. At this point it does not appear that prepubertal treatment with testosterone alone affects ultimate penile length; however, there is some indication that a combination of testosterone and growth hormone together in early childhood may be a positive stimulus (personal experience).

At the time of initial consultation it may be worthwhile determining both family history and maternal history regarding medications taken during pregnancy. Counseling regarding the risk factors for

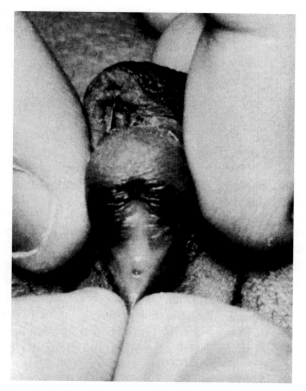

Figure 32.4 Demonstration of hypospadic meatus by pulling outwards on the ventral shaft skin.

Table 32.1 Penile length versus severity of hypospadias

Meatal location	Erect penile length
Glanular	15.0 cm
Coronal	14.5 cm
Distal shaft	13.5 cm
Mid shaft	13.0 cm
Proximal shaft	11.0 cm

Modified from Bracka A (1989) A long term view of hypospadias. *Br J Plast Surg* **42**: 250.

future children having hypospadias can be helpful if there is a known family history. In addition, since the cause of the increasing incidence of hypospadias has not been determined, it might be helpful to start gathering information regarding prenatal factors, including environmental.

Chordee

Chordee is the ventral curvature that accompanies hypospadias in some patients. It occurs more frequently in those with more severe hypospadias but can also be found independent of hypospadias. In those who have chordee without hypospadias the clue on newborn examination is absence of the ventral foreskin. Chordee without hypospadias may simply be a consequence of short ventral skin. However, abnormal development of the distal urethra or ventral corporeal fascia may also play a role.

Ventral curvature of the penis may be a normal phase in fetal phallic development. Kaplan and Lamm (1975), in studies of abortus specimens, found that ventral penile curvature was present in 44% of fetuses through the 6th gestational month (Fig. 32.5).

The cause and treatment of ventral curvature remain controversial in the management of the boy with hypospadias. Devine and Horton (1973) described three pathologic causes of chordee. The first is a consequence of failure of development of the spongiosum in the distal penis. An abnormal, fibrous layer prevents the penis from being straight. If the distal urethra has formed, it is often only a few cell layers in thickness (Fig. 32.6). In their second type the urethra is more normal and the Buck's and dartos fascia are abnormal. The third type, defined by Allen and Spence (1984) as skin chordee, is the result of abnormal superficial (dartos) fascia alone. Finally,

chordee may be the result of disproportionate growth of the dorsal portion of the corporeal bodies, causing a downward deflection (Kramer *et al.*, 1982).

Donnahoo *et al.* (1998) reported on 87 patients operated upon for chordee without hypospadias. In 32% penile straightening (orthoplasty) was achieved by release of ventral skin alone. In another 33% extensive dissection of ventral fibrous tissue was required. Corporeal disproportion was thought to be the etiology in 28% and a short urethra in 7% of this group. Hendren and Caesar (1992) found that ventral skin tethering was the cause in ten of 33 patients. Devine *et al.* (1991) describe a group of 'young men', many of whom were thought to have acquired chordee after puberty. In only one of 26 was ventral dissection alone successful in achieving a straight penis. Disproportionate corporeal growth may be assumed to be the underlying cause.

Chordee correction

The historic method of correcting penile chordee was based on the observation that abnormally developed fibrous tissue on the ventral corporeal fascia was the cause. Therefore, the initial step for repair of hypospadias, after dissection of the ventral skin off the shaft, was to free all the 'abnormal' tissue from the corporeal fascia. Although this concept has become unpopular in recent years, this author generally accepts it. Therefore, when correcting true (not skin) chordee my approach is to aggressively excise that tissue over-

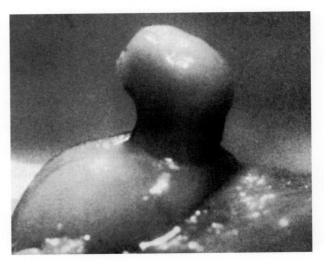

Figure 32.5 Fetal penis demonstrating chordee as part of phallic development. (Courtesy of Dr George W. Kaplan.)

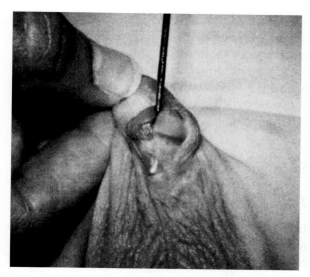

Figure 32.6 Probe in a normally located urethral meatus demonstrating abnormal distal urethra. Spongiosum distal to the penoscrotal junction is absent.

lying the ventral corporeal fascia. Extensive dissection is required, often extending proximal to the hypospadiac meatus, separating the urethra from the deep penile fascia. If release is not achieved by excision of this tissue alone, as demonstrated by an artificial erection (Fig. 32.7), multiple transverse incisions are made in the corporeal fascia, as described by Devine (1983). Some hypospadiologists make a single transverse relaxing incision through the ventral fascia to achieve a straight penis and then apply a graft to cover the resultant fascial defect. Dermal tissue (Devine and Horton, 1975; Kogan et al., 1983; Pope et al., 1996; Lindgren et al., 1998) as well as tunica vaginalis (Perlmutter et al., 1985) have been used to cover the defect. When a graft is applied the repair is generally carried out in two stages, with the urethroplasty performed at a later date. This author has not found it necessary to resort to this maneuver. Chordee is corrected by the method of Devine and the pedicle flap, which has been used to form the urethra, is applied directly over the incised corpora. Devine (1983) also found that an incision along the ventral midline between the corporeal bodies may contribute further to chordee correction. Snow (1989) modified this approach of chordee correction by both incising along the ventral midline and placing dorsal plicating sutures over the neurovascular bundle to rotate the corpora medially. Kass (1993) reported success with simple dorsal rotation without ventral dissection.

Perhaps the most popular method of correcting chordee at the time of writing is by dorsal plication. Nesbit (1965) described the excision of wedges of corporeal fascia as a means of correcting penile bend. The fascial edges are then reapproximated with buried suture. A modification of this technique, tunica albuginia plication, does not require excision of fascia but instead parallel transverse incisions are approximated with non-absorbable 5-0 Prolene (polypropelene) over a buried strip of fascia (Baskin and Duckett, 1994). Although non-absorbable suture is being used, the knots may be felt under the thin penile skin, causing a focus of irritation in some men. Suture that is slowly absorbed, such as (polydiaxanone (PDS), may be preferable.

It has long been taught that the neurovascular bundle is in the midline, splaying laterally as it approaches the coronal sulcus. Based on this observation, either dorsal plication has been carried out lateral to the midline or the neurovascular bundle has been undermined and elevated to avoid injury. Baskin et al. (1998) reported extensive studies of the fetal penis in which nerves were not found at the 12 o'clock position. Instead, they were noted to splay out laterally from the 11 and 1 o'clock position ventrally to the spongiosum. They recommend placing a row of dorsal plicating sutures exclusively along the 12 o'clock position to correct ventral curvature.

Perovic et al. (1998) have a more radical approach to the correction of this problem. They propose complete 'disassembly' of the penis, separating it into its components of the glans with its neurovascular

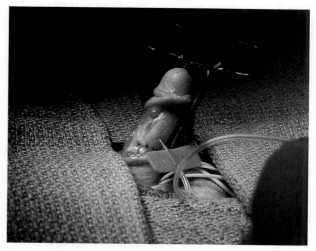

Figure 32.7 Artificial erection test following dorsal plication to correct chordee.

bundle dorsally, the urethra, or urethral plate if hypospadias coexists, and the corpora cavernosa, which may be separated in the midline to some extent. In total, 87 patients were treated by disassembly with complications reported in only four, and all those relating to the urethroplasty.

A persisting question remains: what degree of chordee requires correction? A survey of the members of the Section on Urology of the American Academy of Pediatrics demonstrated a wide perspective in both appreciation of the problem and treatment approaches (Balogna *et al.*, 1999). In spite of the long-standing dogma that urethroplasty should not be attempted until the surgeon is convinced that the penis is straight, it is interesting to note that chordee correction was not the primary concern of 54% of the respondents. The surveyors quantified chordee from 10 to 50°. Surprisingly, 8% of respondents would attempt correction of as little as 10° of chordee, although this author does not believe that represents a functional abnormality (Belman, 1999). Most (75%) of the pediatric urologists who responded would consider intervention for 20° of chordee or greater and virtually all when there is 30° or more. For a defect of 30°, 84% would correct chordee by dorsal plication: 49% would achieve this by incising and suturing the dorsal fascia and 22% would apply plicating sutures alone. Only 13% would excise fascial wedges as described by Nesbit.

Does a mild degree of persisting chordee present a functional problem after pubertal development? Vandersteen and Husmann (1998) reported a retrospective review of older patients who had had earlier correction of hypospadias and chordee. Over a 10 year interval only 34 patients were evaluated at the Mayo Clinic for what was termed 'recurrent chordee'. Of 22 who fit the criteria for their review, 19 had undergone the procedure at another center, so the success of the original surgery cannot be documented. All had been operated upon for severe hypospadias. Since the numbers are so small one must conclude that we are either highly successful in correcting chordee in most patients, or slight, residual chordee has little clinical significance.

Dorsal curvature

Dorsal penile curvature also occurs and surgical correction has been reported (Spiro *et al.*, 1992; Adams *et al.*, 1999). This author does not agree that treatment in childhood is indicated since future problems cannot be predicted. In the unlikely event that sexual dysfunction occurs after pubertal development ventral correction in the same manner as performed for lateral penile bend may be carried out by dissection and plication ventrally.

Surgical correction of hypospadias

Timing of surgery

It has become well accepted that early hypospadias repair is desirable. Manley and Epstein (1981) reported reduced patient anxiety when repairs were carried out before 18 months of age. Belman and Kass (1982) found no increased incidence of surgical complications when surgery is performed at 2–11 months of age. Schultz *et al.* (1983) concluded that the ideal age for genital surgery is between 6 weeks and 12 months of age, after reviewing the psychological ramifications of childhood surgery. Six months of age is ideal for the otherwise healthy child, although surgery may be carried out at either a younger or an older age if supervening medical indications so dictate.

Hormonal stimulation

Preoperative treatment with exogenous testosterone may improve surgical results in boys with a small glans and/or severe chordee and short dorsal skin. The most reliable and simple route is parenteral injection, although testosterone cream may be applied to the penis directly (Sakakibara *et al.*, 1991). Davits *et al.* (1993) found that a dose of 2 mg/kg given 5 and 2 weeks before surgery was effective. The author uses 25 mg testosterone enanthate 6 and 3 weeks before definitive repair. Occasionally three doses are necessary, the first then being given 9 weeks prior to the procedure. Koff *et al.* (1999) have used hCG stimulation 6–8 weeks prior to hypospadias surgery in a group of 12 boys ages 6–12 months. One-half had proximal hypospadias. After a 5-week course of treatment they found a significant reduction in penile chordee and an increase in penile length, that they interpreted as involving primarily the proximal corpora. They suggest that this growth results in a relative decrease in the severity of the hypospadias.

Optical magnification

The use of some form of optical magnification has become the rule, particularly with the acceptance of early repair and the use of fine suture material. Although the operating microscope has been advocated by some (Wesson and Mandell, 1985; Wacksman, 1987; Shapiro, 1989), loupes, with magnification of 2.5 × and higher, are adequate.

Instruments and suture material

Reconstructive surgical techniques should be applied to the repair of hypospadias. These include the use of fine instruments that are non-tissue crushing. Whenever possible traction sutures should be applied to retract skin edges. The reduced complication rates observed during the 1990s are, in part, due to the application of these principles.

Studies evaluating suture material suggest that chromic catgut is the best choice. Bartone *et al.* (1987) compared tissue reaction, granuloma formation, and abscess using baboon foreskin. They recommended against polyglycolic acid (Dexon) and PDS. DiSandro and Palmer (1996) compared results in groups of patients and also concluded that more rapidly absorbed suture, Dexon, or chromic catgut was preferable to PDS. They found a higher incidence of stricture formation but not of urethrocutaneous fistulae when slowly absorbed suture material was used. Ulman *et al.* (1997) compared polyglactine (Vicryl) with PDS in patients undergoing meatal-based (Mathieu) hypospadias repairs. They found a higher incidence of fistulae when Vicryl was used. However, they also refined their technique when using PDS, carrying out running subcuticular (and presumably inverting) anastomoses in that group compared with simple running suture when Vicryl was used.

In spite of these studies, this author has used 6-0 and 7-0 polyglactin suture (Vicryl) exclusively for the past 15 years. I am convinced that surgical technique and the vascularity of the tissues is more important than the specific type of suture material used. Strictures as a complication are almost non-existent in my experience (I believe they are the result of devascularization) and our fistula rates are comparable to those of other successful series. However, owing to its slow dissolution, suture tracts do result when polyglactin larger than 7-0 is used on the skin directly. On that basis 7-0 Vicryl is now being used almost exclusively by me in young boys, even on skin. When 6-0 is used it is only applied subcutaneously.

Control of bleeding

Minimizing blood loss is important since the penis is a highly vascular organ and blood loss in the small child requires strict control. This author prefers the use of needlepoint spot electrocoagulation as the primary means of controlling blood loss. However, coagulation alone is insufficient when incisions are made in the glans or extensive dissection is carried out ventrally to correct chordee. Intermittent application of a rubber band as a tourniquet to the penile base works well, particularly for glanular bleeding. It is released every 10–15 min to allow the tissues to breathe. Alternatively, many use epinephrine, diluted 1:100 000 with 1% lidocaine, which is injected directly into the tissue. Since both of these methods have been used for many years without any evidence of problems one can conclude that both are safe and reliable.

Avoiding complications

Aside from improvement in technical factors such as suture material, instrumentation, and optics, the current success of hypospadias repair can be attributed to the contributions of many of our predecessors. Today's surgeons have been taught fine tissue handling by Charles Devine and Charles Horton, improved use of vascular flaps by Norman Hodgson and John Duckett, and better coverage of suture lines by Durham Smith. Smith (1980) proposed a two-stage hypospadias repair for all patients, using a de-epithelialized flap of ventral tissue at the second stage to cover the urethra and prevent crossing suture lines. Subsequently, this application was applied to single-stage repairs (Belman, 1988; Retik *et al.*, 1988; Ross and Kay, 1997). Modifications include the use of tunica vaginalis (Snow *et al.*, 1995) (Fig. 32.8) and scrotal dartos as a second layer to achieve the same purpose (Churchill *et al.*, 1996).

Urinary diversion

It is rarely necessary to perform suprapubic urinary diversion when repairing hypospadias, no matter how severe the abnormality or how complex the repair. A simple feeding tube inserted into the urinary bladder and draining into a diaper is all that is required. A landmark prospective study by Montagnino *et al.* (1988) compared the rate of urinary infection in a group of children with a closed urinary drainage system with those with an open system, the urine draining into the outer of two diapers. There was no difference in infection rates between the two groups. The use of low-dose oral antibiotics given while the tube is in place has been demonstrated to prevent bacilliuria (Sugar and Firlit, 1988). By using a feeding tube the urine can be directed to the outer diaper, allowing the child to remain dry, reducing skin problems and potential fungal infections during the healing interval. Unfortunately, the feeding tube rubbing against the bladder mucosa and trigone tends to create bladder spasms in some of these children. In most it is of little consequence, but occasionally may be severe. Low-dose oxybutinin given every 6 hours has been effective in minimizing these spasms. Parents must be warned, however, that anticholinergic medication may cause facial flushing and, if given in too high a dose, fever. Rarely, hallucinations may occur.

There is a large experience in correcting distal hypospadias without any type of urinary diversion. Comparative prospective studies have demonstrated no difference in postoperative results when the modified Mathieu and Thiersch-Duplay repair with the Snodgrass modification are done without diversion (McCormack *et al.*, 1993; Hakim *et al.*, 1996; Stecker and Zaontz, 1997). Buson *et al.* (1994), however, found a higher incidence of postoperative complications (4.6% vs. 18.9%) when stents were not used. One of the advantages of the tubeless repair is elimination of bladder spasms associated with the intravesical stent. However, because of painful voiding, older children may occasionally refuse to urinate postoperatively. They may then require secondary catheterization.

Postoperative dressing

A bio-occlusive dressing (Tegoderm) applied directly to the penis is simple and most satisfactory (Gilbert *et al.*, 1986; Ellis and Patil, 1989; Burbige, 1994) (Fig. 32.9). Some prefer to apply a Telfa pad directly to the skin with the bio-occlusive dressing over that (Ellis and Patil, 1989; Duckett, 1996).

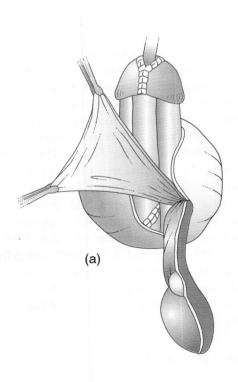
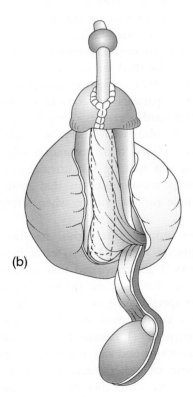

(a)   (b)

Figure 32.8 (*a*) Creation of the tunica vaginalis flap. (*b*) Tunica vaginalis flap covering the neourethra prior to skin closure.

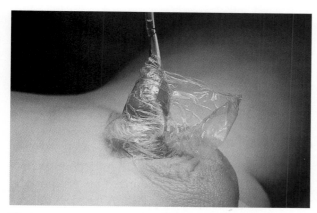

Figure 32.9 Double layer of Tegoderm applied directly to the penis as a postoperative dressing.

For those undergoing more extensive repair, with dissection into the perineum, it is helpful to apply some form of perineal compression. The dressing described by Falkowsky and Firlit (1980) (Fig. 32.10), in addition to the bio-occlusive dressing, is very useful in this situation. The compression dressing remains for 24–48 hours and the bio-occlusive dressing is removed 2–3 days later.

In a prospective, randomized study, van Savage *et al.* (2000) compared the use of a postoperative dressing to no dressing in 100 patients. Efforts were used to compare like groups regarding severity of hypospadias and other technical factors. In a mean follow-up of 1 year no difference in results was reported between the two groups. However, postoperative phone calls were more frequent in the group in which a dressing was not used.

Pain control

Two direct methods are available for controlling intraoperative and postoperative pain: penile block and caudal block (Lau, 1984; Broadman, 1987). Both offer up to 4–6 hours of pain relief. The long-acting analgesic agent bupivacaine 0.25–0.5% is recommended. Penile block can produce a hematoma at the base of the penis and it has been suggested that children with caudal analgesia have difficulty in urinating postoperatively. However, the author has routinely used caudal blocks for postoperative pain relief for circumcision, hernia repair, and orchidopexy for over 15 years with no instances of urinary retention. Chhibber *et al.* (1997) found that a penile block administered at both the onset and termination of

surgery provided better postoperative pain relief than a single injection. Gunter *et al.* (1990) found that preoperative caudal analgesia in conjunction with the inhalant anesthetic agent halothane not only reduced the halothane requirements but also reduced operative blood loss. At the very least, children who are given some measure of intraoperative local analgesia awaken more peacefully and are less restless after surgery. This reduces straining and secondary bleeding, thereby diminishing acute hematoma formation.

Since almost all patients are discharged on the day of surgery, it is important to offer some sort of pain medication to be given at home. Oral acetaminophen given every 4 hours supplemented by ibuprophen every 6 hours usually suffices. Parents must be advised to give food or milk with ibuprofen. Narcotic analgesia is not given to the younger child after hospital discharge.

Cosmesis

Efforts to make the boy with hypospadias appear as normal as possible after surgical correction continue. It has become generally accepted that the urethral meatus belongs in the normal glanular position, in spite of the fact that this may not impact significantly on function compared with having the meatus in the coronal sulcus or proximal glans. The goal is no longer simply to enable the boy to urinate standing up; he should now be able to be indistinguishable

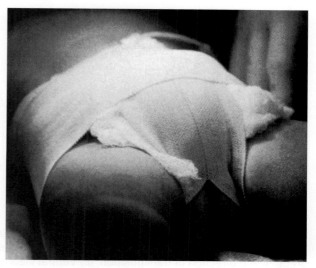

Figure 32.10 Modification of the Falkowski–Firlit compression dressing.

from his congenitally normal (circumcised) counter-parts. The neomeatus has become a recent focus of attention, with efforts to create a slit-like rather than an oval appearance (Snodgrass, 1994).

In most instances correction requires use of the foreskin and results in a circumcised penile appearance. That does not create a problem in the USA and other areas where circumcision is commonly practised, but in other geographic and cultural regions concerns regarding penile appearance and dissatisfaction with the surgical result may center on the absence of the foreskin (Mureau *et al.*, 1995). Unless non-penile tissue is used, successful repair of complex hypospadias requires use of the foreskin, for urethral construction, skin coverage, or both. Efforts have been made not only to preserve but also to reconstruct the foreskin in patients with distal hypospadias (Gilpin *et al.*, 1993; De Jong and Boemers, 1993; Dewan, 1993). For those in whom the foreskin is used or removed, creation of a collar of skin on the ventral surface proximal to the coronal sulcus, as described by Firlit (1987), helps to normalize the appearance of the circumcised penis. The initial incision must be planned to achieve this result (Fig. 32.11).

Length of hospital stay

Most hypospadias repairs are currently done as outpatient or day-surgery procedures. One exception is when a free graft repair is applied. A few days of bed-rest and relative immobilization may facilitate graft inosculation. Another exception is the child with severe hypospadias who requires aggressive proximal dissection between the dorsal urethral plate and ventral corporeal fascia to produce a straight penis. This tends to be bloody, and compression postoperatively for 24–48 hours minimizes postoperative bleeding.

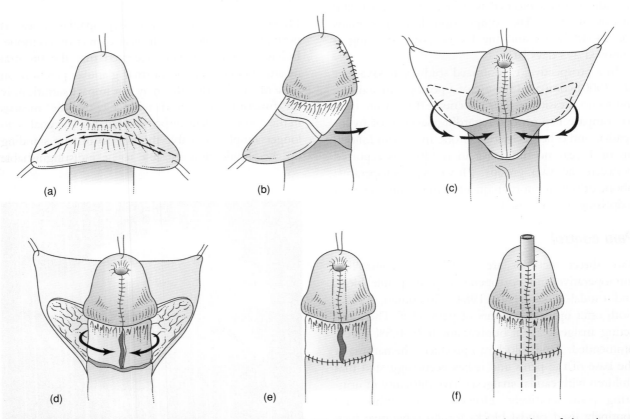

Figure 32.11 Steps used to form the mucosal collar. (*a*) Retracted foreskin indicates the location of the chevron incision and formation of lateral darts (*arrows*). (*b*) Lateral view shows the appearance of the inner surface of the prepuce and direction of transposition. (*c*) Ventral view of phallus before inferomedial migration of the preputial dart. (*d*) Mucosal collar formed from transposed darts. (*e, f*) Completed repair and mucosal collar. (Modified from Firlit, 1987.)

Surgical procedures

Glanular hypospadias
MAGPI

The MAGPI (meatal advancement, glanuloplasty) procedure (Duckett, 1981b), which changed the attitude regarding the goal of ultimate meatal position, has stood the test of time and remains applicable to a very specific group of patients. It requires mobility of the distal urethra and a rounded, not flat, glans. In a review of 1111 patients only 1.2% required a second procedure (Duckett *et al.*, 1991). Park *et al.* (1995) surveyed 90 parents of boys who underwent this procedure and found a 99% satisfaction rate. However, meatal regression can occur (Hastie *et al.*, 1989; Issa and Gearhart, 1989). Originally described as applicable to the subcoronal meatus (Duckett *et al.*, 1991), when applied to coronal hypospadias a 35% failure rate was reported by Unluer *et al.* (1991) Variants of this procedure have been described (Decter, 1991).

A dorsal meatotomy is performed proceeding distal from the meatus incising any skin bridges associated with distal urethral pits. The urethral mucosa is then advanced to the apex of that incision using two or three 7-0 absorbable sutures. A subcoronal incision is then made, preserving the lateral aspects of the hooded prepuce to form Firlit's collar. The lateral aspects of the ventral glans are brought together in the midline, giving the meatus a more normally situated appearance (Fig. 32.12). It is helpful to excise some of the midline ventral epithelium to improve the appearance of the glans. This then allows approximation of ventral glanular tissue proximal to the meatus which, when combined with formation of the subcoronal collar, normalizes the penile appearance.

GAP

GAP (glans approximation procedure) (Dimler *et al.*, 1984; Zaontz, 1989) is best applied when the glans is flat and has a deep and/or wide urethral plate. An ellipse of glans on both sides of the urethral plate is de-epithelialized (Fig. 32.13). The inner epithelial margins are approximated to form the urethra. The outer margins are brought together in the midline to both cover the lengthened urethra and to normalize the appearance of the glans. However, this results in apposing suture lines and risks fistula formation.

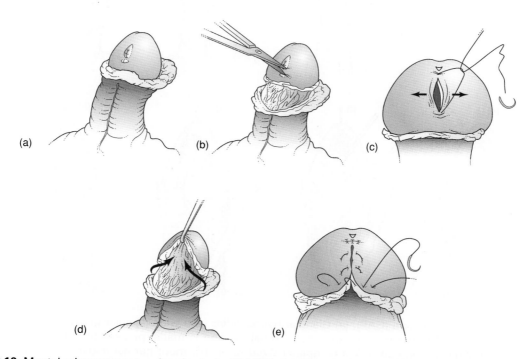

Figure 32.12 Meatal advancement – glanuloplasty (MAGPI). (*a*) Glanular hypospadias without chordee. (*b*) Division of the septum distal to the meatus. (*c*) Advancement of dorsal epithelium distally. (*d, e*) Advancement of the ventral glans and approximation in the midline.

Zaontz (personal communication) has resolved this problem by swinging a de-epithelialized flap over the urethral suture line (Fig. 32.13F, G). Success with this procedure is high (Gittes *et al.*, 1998) and produces a normal appearing penis. The appearance of the penis is further improved by both excising midline submeatal epithelium to bring the ventral glans wings together and creating a subcoronal collar. Compared with the MAGPI procedure, the urethra is lengthened with this operation.

Coronal hypospadias

A number of procedures can be applied successfully to the patient with distal, non-glanular hypospadias. The choice becomes one of personal preference and surgi-

cal experience. The results, in the hands of those with experience, seem to vary little.

Urethral advancement

Introduced by Beck (1898), this procedure requires proximal urethral dissection and mobilization distally to create the meatus in the ideal location (Fig. 32.14). Generally used for distal hypospadias (Spencer and Perlmutter, 1990; Haberlik *et al.*, 1997), long-term follow-up into puberty has demonstrated this to be a durable procedure (Caione *et al.*, 1997). Turner-Warwick *et al.* (1997) recommend that, to avoid utilization of the terminal, atretic portion of the urethra, mobilization all the way to the urethral bulb is required. They refer to this as the BEAM (bulbar

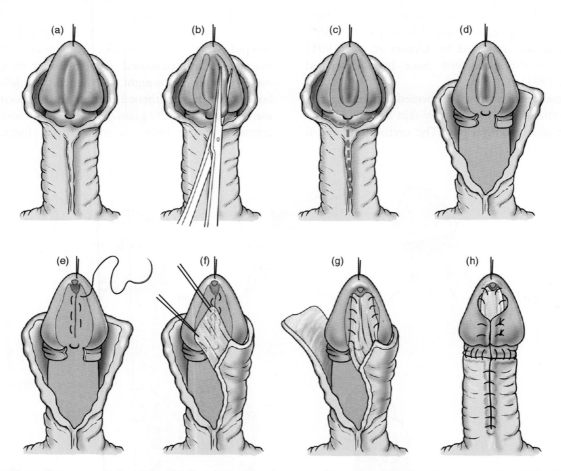

Figure 32.13 Glans approximation (GAP). (*a*) Glanular hypospadias with wide glanular groove. (*b, c*) De-epithelialization of the glans lateral to the groove. (*d*) A subcoronal incision is made, preserving skin for the Firlit collar. Skin in the ventral midline at the corona is de-epithelialized to enable more normal midline closure of the glans. (*e*) Urethral closed in the midline by approximating the inner aspects of the glanular epithelial edges. (*f, g*) The prepuce is split, and the outer edge of one of the halves de-epithelialized and brought ventral to cover midline urethral closure. (*h*) Completed repair.

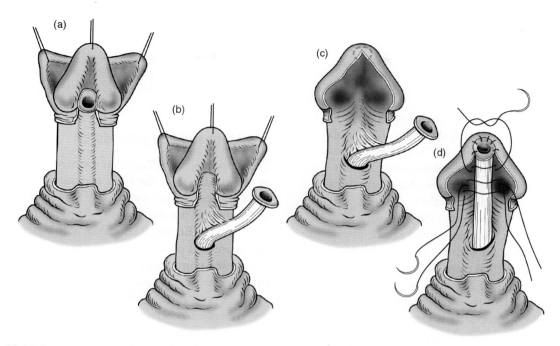

Figure 32.14 Urethral advancement procedure for distal hypospadias. (*a*) A subcoronal incision is made distal to the hypospadiac meatus. (*b*) Urethral dissection from the corpora sufficiently proximal to allow the advance of the normal urethra to the tip of the glans without tension. (*c*) The glans is split and dissected to allow the urethra to lie in the glanular bed without compression. (*d*) The meatus is sutured to the glans and glans closure carried out. (Modified from Spencer and Perlmutter, 1990.)

elongation anastomotic meatoplasty) procedure and suggest that aggressive proximal mobilization is necessary to prevent penile chordee, although that has not been demonstrated to be a problem in other series (Caione *et al.*, 1997). Scrotal hematoma as a complication was reported in five of 76 patients in de Sy and Hoebeke's (1994) experience. They had an opportunity to follow 40 of these patients into adulthood with no late complications noted. Koff *et al.* (1994) combined this procedure with a meatal-based flap-Barcat procedure with a 3.5% reoperation rate.

I tried this operation in the 1970s (Belman, 1997) without having been aware of Beck's prior description but abandoned it shortly thereafter. The amount of dissection required to bring normal urethral tissue into the glans produced significant bleeding and penile edema necessitating an indwelling catheter and compression dressing for a few days. However, the experience reported above suggests that it should be reconsidered as an option, especially when the distal urethra is of good quality. With the availability of the bio-occlusive dressing postoperative care may well be more simplified now.

Megameatal hypospadias repair

As previously described, a variant of hypospadias with an intact foreskin exists. This has been termed megameatal hypospadias based on the appearance of the meatus. Although the meatus may be glanular in location, it is often found at the corona or subcorona. The distal urethra tends to be extremely wide. Because of the width of the urethral plate, the broad flat glans, and abundant ventral skin, repair of this abnormality tends to be quite easy and can be readily accomplished even if the patient has been circumcised. With a tourniquet at the penile base for hemostasis, incisions are made on either side of the urethral plate into the distal glans and the subsequent repair is similar to that of the GAP (Fig. 32.13). However, as described by Duckett and Keating (1989), the dilated, distal urethra may be incised proximally, removing a wedge of urethral tissue to reduce its caliber to a more normal configuration. The urethral plate is then rolled together and closed in the midline, preferably with a running, inverting subcuticular stitch, to create the urethral extension. Then, to avoid crossing suture lines, subcutaneous tissue from the ventral penile shaft is advanced over the urethra, sutured to the depths of the glanular incisions, and the glans closed.

Rolled midline tube

Based on the historic contributions of Duplay (1874), with modifications, the rolled midline tube has gained renewed popularity. King (1970) applied this maneuver to distal hypospadias. Subsequently, results have improved with the application of a de-epithelialized flap covering the midline urethral closure (van Horn and Kass, 1995). Snodgrass (1994) introduced a further modification that has gained recent popularity. In this procedure an incision is made in the dorsal midline of the urethral plate, disrupting its continuity and allowing the two halves to hinge together upon closure (Fig. 32.15). In a multi-institutional review of 148 cases a 7% complication rate was reported, only three of which were meatal stenosis (Snodgrass et al., 1996). To increase the success rate, a de-epithelialized flap was also applied to this procedure (Ross and Kay, 1997). The Snodgrass technique has been applied to reoperative hypospadias surgery as well as to more proximal repairs with reported success (Retik and Borer, 1998; Snodgrass et al., 1998). When applied to complex hypospadias the proximal urethra may

have to be constructed with a pedicle tube while the distal urethra is formed by tubularizing the incised urethral plate (Snodgrass et al., 1998). For those in whom the urethral plate is left intact, incised and rolled into a tube, dorsal plication is necessary for chordee correction.

Meatal-based flap procedures

These operations are based on the method introduced by Ombredanne in the early twentieth century. The Mustardé procedure entails rolling a tube based on skin proximal to the meatus, flipping the resultant tube distally. Because this repair requires transection of the urethral plate distal to the hypospadiac meatus it was used more frequently when it was thought that true chordee accompanied most hypospadias (Belman, 1982). Transection of the tissue distal to the meatus was thought to correct ventral curvature. This procedure has become less popular with greater appreciation that chordee, when it coexists with mild hypospadias, can be corrected by the release of ventral skin alone in most patients. Horton and Devine (1966) introduced a variation of this concept by using a triangular flap of submeatal skin that is anastomosed to a triangularized glanular urethral plate (flip-flap procedure). Perhaps the most popular and enduring

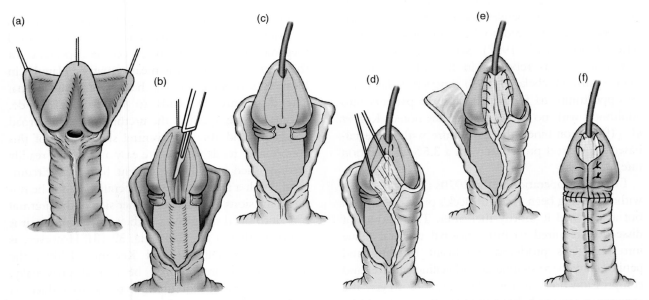

Figure 32.15 Tubularized incised plate urethroplasty (Snodgrass procedure). (*b*) Subcoronal incision proximal to the meatus, with incisions carried along either side of the urethral plate into the glans. Urethral plate incised in midline (dorsal) to allow hinging rolled tube. (*c*) Midline closure of the urethral plate over stent. (*d, e*) A second layer is brought over the neourethra. (*f*) Closure of the skin and glans in the midline. (Modified from Snodgrass *et al.*, 1996).

meatal based flap repair was introduced by Mathieu (1932) and popularized by Wacksman (1981).

The Mathieu procedure

A rectangle of ventral urethral skin proximal to the hypospadiac meatus is outlined, the length determined by the distance from the meatus to the end of the glans. The width should be adequate to form a 10 Fr urethra after anastomotic completion (Fig. 32.16). A subcoronal circumferential incision is carried to the lateral edges of the outlined flap and the flap dissected from the remainder of the ventral skin. Subcutaneous tissue should be maintained with the flap. With adequate hemostasis using epinephrine or a tourniquet, incisions are carried distally on either side of the urethral plate into the glans. These incisions must penetrate to the deep corporeal fascia to allow the glans wings to close over the neourethra without tension. The lateral anastomoses of the flap to the urethral plate are carried out with a running 7-0 subcuticular stitch that inverts the skin edges. Ideally, a second layer of subcutaneous tissue can be closed directly over this suture line; however, fistulae are best prevented by bringing a second layer of tissue over the urethra before closing the glans (Belman, 1988; Retik et al., 1994b) (Fig. 32.17). One or two buried mattressed 6-0 Vicryl is used to approximate the glans and interrupted 7-0 closes the glanular skin edges. Penile skin is ideally closed in the midline with the excess excised to give a normal, circumcised appearance.

The success rate for this operation is excellent. Hakim et al. (1996) reported a complication rate of

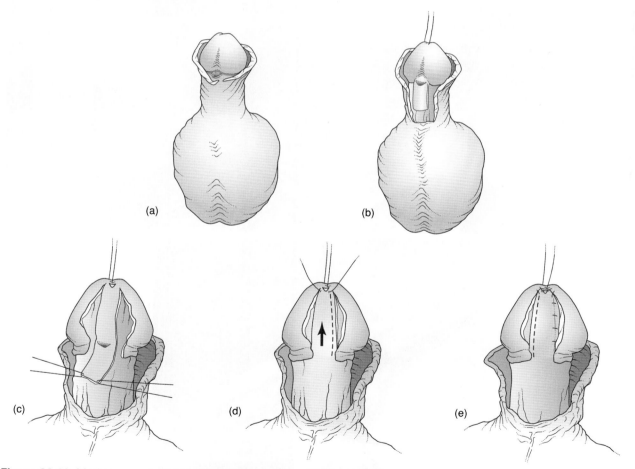

Figure 32.16 Mathieu repair. (*a*) Coronal hypospadias. (*b*) Flap outlined proximal to the meatus. (*c*) Deep incisions in the glans to form the urethral roof (dorsal aspect). (*d*) Left side of anastomosis completed with running subcuticular suture. (*e*) Second layer bringing a subcutaneous tissue of flap over the first suture line on the left and completion of right-sided anastomosis. The final three steps are as per steps (*d–f*) in Figure 32.15.

2.63% in a group of 114 boys when a urethral stent was used postoperatively compared with a complication rate of 3.6% in a group of 222 boys in whom a stent was not used.

Minevich *et al.* (1999) reported a reoperative rate of only 1.5% in a series of 202 patients, 197 of whom had primary repairs. Follow-up was up to 54 months. None in this group had stricture as a complication.

Although it has been suggested that meatal-based flaps can be used to create the urethra in more proximal hypospadias, care must be taken not to incorporate skin which has the future potential to be hair-bearing. Therefore, the Mathieu procedure should be reserved for coronal or subcoronal hypospadias only.

Barcat modification

To bury the urethra more deeply in the glans the urethral plate is mobilized and an incision made into the midline of the glans into which the new urethra is placed. Barthold *et al.* (1996) reported a 5% fistula rate for distal hypospadias when a second layer is placed over the new urethra before glans closure. As noted previously (Koff *et al.*, 1994), this procedure has been combined with urethral mobilization and applied to more proximal hypospadias.

Onlay hypospadias repairs

Hodgson (1978) introduced the concept of using the urethral plate as a base for an onlay of dorsal skin. His procedure involved swinging dorsal skin ventrally

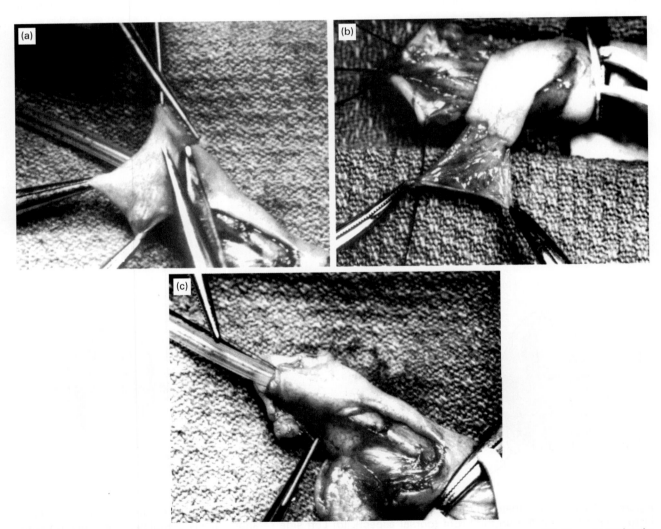

Figure 32.17 (*a*) Left half of a hooded prepuce de-epithelialized using tenotomy scissors. (*b*) Flap completely de-epithelialized. (*c*) De-epithelialized segment placed into the glans covering urethroplasty.

using the buttonhole technique. That not only produced a bulky appearance of the glans but also did not insure that non-hair-bearing skin would be used. Elder *et al.* (1987) modified this concept by swinging the inner layer of the prepuce around the shaft on a vascular pedicle. This allowed tailoring of the anastamosis and precise closure of the glans. Onlay flap repairs have become very popular and can be applied to all patients without penile chordee. Some use this technique for virtually all repairs, even those requiring chordee correction (see below).

The tissue lateral to the urethral plate is sharply incised down to the penile fascia. A subcoronal incision is then made circumferentially to the urethral plate. Skin is dissected proximally to correct any ventral tethering. The procedure as originally described used a transverse pedicle flap of inner preputial skin that was separated from the remainder of the dorsal foreskin. An alternative is to split the foreskin, de-epithelialize the outer skin and apply the inner foreskin as an island pedicle onlay (Belman, 1994) (Fig. 32.18). A tourniquet is applied to the penile base (or dilute epinephrine is injected) for hemostatic control and the incisions are carried into the glans. Instead of separating the inner foreskin of the hooded prepuce the prepuce is split, one half brought ventral, and the outer layer of skin removed (Fig. 32.17). This results in the island flap being served by the blood supply of one-half of the prepuce. The lateral anastomoses are done with inverting 7-0 Vicryl sutures over a no. 8 feeding tube. Because the vascular pedicle is so broad it is sutured to the depths of the glanular incisions to cover the new urethra completely. This procedure is called the split-prepuce *in situ* onlay repair and, in a series of 100 consecutive cases reported by Rushton and Belman (1998), fistulae occurred in only 4%.

Hypospadias with chordee

Several groups have refined the use of vascular-based preputial pedicle flaps for hypospadias repair (Asopa *et al.*, 1971; Hodgson, 1981; Duckett, 1981c; Standoli, 1982; Harris and Jeffrey, 1989). This helped in transforming both the performance and success of this procedure. Although single-stage repairs using free grafts had been carried out prior to this (Horton and Devine, 1973), success rates were less satisfactory. Nevertheless, some still recommend and use preputial free grafts routinely (Stock *et al.*, 1994).

Transverse island tube urethroplasty

Historically, chordee is first released by transection of the urethral plate and ventral dissection. However, when freeing the ventral skin alone does not produce a straight penis, many hypospadiologists use dorsal plication as their primary means for chordee release (Balogna *et al.*, 1999). This has also led to the greater use of onlay flaps rather than pedicle tubes for more proximal hypospadias (Baskin *et al.*, 1994) and, as mentioned previously, an extension of the use of the incised tubularized urethral plate approach (Retik and Borer, 1998).

After the surgeon is satisfied that the penis is straight the undersurface of the hooded foreskin is separated from the remainder of the prepuce. To be certain that adequate tissue is obtained it is ideal to measure both the width and length of skin required and mark the tissue appropriately. Then the foreskin is superficially incised and the flap carefully teased away from the remainder of the dorsal skin (Fig. 32.19). The error made by the novice is to preserve as much pedicle to the flap as possible, endangering the blood supply to the remainder of the dorsal skin. In fact, it takes amazingly little vascularity to maintain viability of the flap. Adequate length of the flap is required to swing the skin ventral without tension. If a complete tube is being constructed, most surgeons first form this over a catheter, carrying out the proximal anastomosis secondarily (Duckett, 1981c). However, by making the spatulated anastomosis first, a running subcuticular inverting 7-0 suture can be used to form the neourethra over the stent (Fig. 32.20). The glans is split and dissected laterally from the deep penile fascia to allow closure over the new urethra without tension. This is very important as glanular disruption is the result of failure to provide a tension-free closure. A second layer of de-epithelialized skin or tunica vaginalis is brought over the entire neourethra to reduce the risk of fistula formation and to add vasculature to the distal urethra. In the past this author used transverse mattressed 6-0 Vicryl to approximate the glans. Although this served its purpose in maintaining the glans closure without disruption, suture tracts in the glans were noted in some patients on delayed follow-up. More recently a buried 6-0 Vicryl vertical mattress suture has been used. This does not incorporate skin. The skin edges are then approximated with 7-0 Vicryl, which does not leave suture tracts. Excess skin is excised to give the penis a normal, circumcised appearance.

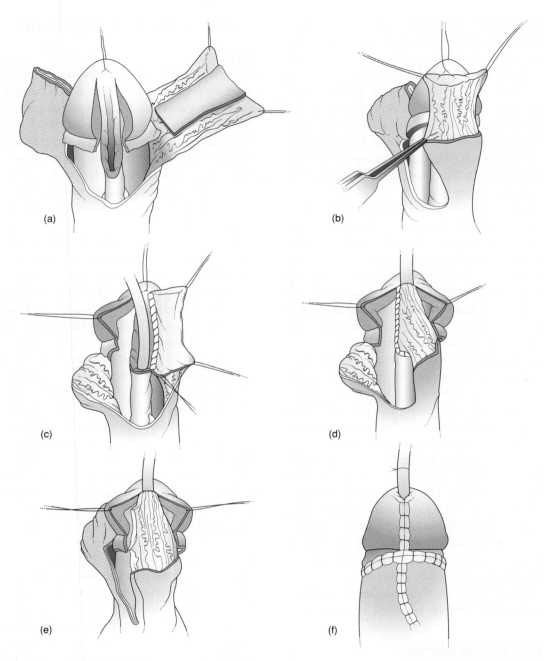

Figure 32.18 (*a*) Skin has been dissected from the penile shaft and freed proximal to the meatus. The foreskin has been split in the midline and deep incisions have been made along the urethral plate to the tunica albuginea. Half of the split prepuce is used for an island flap. An island flap from the inner layer of foreskin was isolated by de-epithelializing adjacent inner foreskin with tenotomy scissors. (*b*) The outer skin of half of the foreskin was de-epithelialized in strips using tenotomy scissors, leaving all of its subcutaneous tissue to serve as a vascular pedicle. No attempt is made to separate the blood supply of the inner and outer layers of the foreskin. (*c*) The onlay island flap is sutured to the urethral plate using running 7-0 polyglactin on the inner surface to invert the skin edges. (*d*) The neourethra is completed using running 7-0 polyglactin inverting subcuticular stitches. The entire blood supply of half of the foreskin is maintained intact to the island flap. (*e*) The vascular pedicle is spread to cover the neourethra completely, and the edges are stitched down beyond the neourethra suture lines to the deep penile fascia with 7-0 polyglactin. (*f*) Completed repair. Redundant skin has been excised. A no. 8 feeding tube remains as an intravesical drip stent, secured in place with 3/0 silk glans traction suture. A double-layer bio-occlusive dressing is used for dressing. (Modified from Rushton and Belman, 1998.)

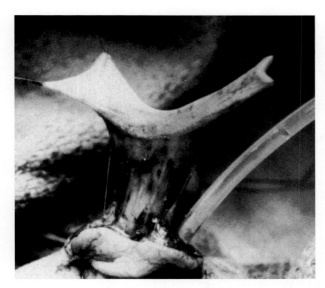

Figure 32.19 Transverse island pedicle flap as seen from the patient's head. Silk sutures are used as traction. Redundant dorsal penile skin is bunched up at base of pedicle. A silicone stent (right) exits the meatus (not visible).

It has also been demonstrated that even in patients with severe hypospadias, chordee can occasionally be released without transecting the urethral plate. Instead, while maintaining its proximal and distal attachments, the plate is elevated from the deep penile fascia and the abnormal tissue beneath it, causing chordee, is excised. This then allows further application of the onlay flap for urethroplasty (Perovic and Vukadinovic, 1994). Although there has been skepticism regarding the vascularity of the plate when this maneuver is carried out (Duckett, 1999a), Mollard and Castagnola (1994) reported a series of patients with hypospadias in whom this approach was attempted. In their experience with 71 boys with proximal penile hypospadias two required dorsal plication to achieve a straight penis. Of 18 perineal hypospadias repairs 61% were corrected without dividing the urethral plate. Only one required dorsal plication to achieve a straight penis.

Scrotal and perineal hypospadias

There is rarely sufficient preputial skin to form the entire urethra in the boy with severe, proximal hypospadias, although preoperative use of testosterone may be helpful. In some, particularly those with penoscrotal transposition (Fig. 32.21), a planned two-stage repair should be considered (Retik et al., 1994a; Greenfield et al., 1994) (Fig. 32.22). When that is done the penis is straightened and skin brought to the ventral surface during the first stage. Urethral construction, generally achieved by rolling a midline tube, is accomplished at the second stage 4–6 months later.

Devine (1983) introduced a single-stage approach to perineal hypospadias. After chordee release he rolled the shiny, presumably hairless, parameatal scrotal skin into a tube extending the meatus to the penoscrotal junction. He then applied a free graft to form the distal urethra. Glassberg (1987) did the same, but formed the penile urethra with a preputial pedicle tube (Fig. 32.23). Following transection of the mid-urethral plate to correct chordee in boys with proximal hypospadias, Flack and Walker (1995) used the proximal and distal ends of the urethral plate as the base for an onlay. They then tubularized the central portion of the island flap to form the mid-urethra. The Koyanagi–Nonomura one-stage procedure applies parameatal foreskin flaps to form the urethra from distal to proximal, rather than from proximal to distal as carried out in the other procedures (Koyanagi et al., 1994). They believe that this somewhat complex procedure can be applied to all forms of hypospadias. Glassberg et al. (1998) reported a series using this procedure, including eight with penoscrotal transposition. Urethrocutaneous fistulae occurred in 50%.

Perovic and Djordjevic (1998) have introduced the most radical method to repair hypospadias, similar to the disassembly technique that has been applied to epispadias (Fig. 32.24). They propose 'separating the penis into its component parts: the glans cap with neurovascular bundle (dorsally) together with the nondivided or divided urethra and urethral plate (ventrally) and the corpora cavernosa'. They performed this procedure in 112 patients, reporting only nine complications. In addition, they believed that they achieved some degree of lengthening for those with small penises. It is unlikely that actual corporeal size is significantly increased by this procedure, but total straightening would optimize penile length.

Free graft repairs

As mentioned previously, urethroplasty using a free graft of tissue from the foreskin was popular until pedicle flaps became so successful. When skin from

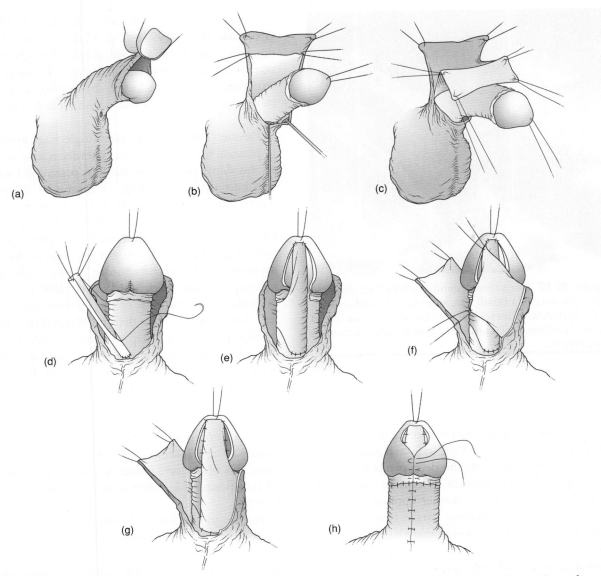

Figure 32.20 Transverse preputial island flap repair. (*a–c*) Release of chordee and dissection of the undersurface of the dorsal prepuce. (*d*) Anastomosis and tubularization of the island flap. (*e*) Creation of meatus (glans split). (*f*) De-epithelialization of the one half of the remaining hooded prepuce used to cover the neourethra. (*g,h*) Completion of ventral skin closure using a midline technique for better cosmesis.

non-penile sites was used results were often complicated by hair growth with full-thickness grafts and contraction of split-thickness grafts. Memmelaar (1947) introduced the bladder mucosa graft. It became popular in the 1980s in cases in which penile skin was not available. Its use was particularly applicable for those patients with complex problems, such as failed hypospadias repair when penile skin is particularly lacking. However, bladder mucosa tolerates surface exposure poorly. Meatal stenosis and meatal pro-

lapse were reported in 68% of a group when the urethra was constructed to the tip of the glans (Kinkead *et al.*, 1994). Reportedly, the meatal problems resolve after 2 years (Li *et al.*, 1995). In addition, in a review of 117 patients who had urethroplasty with bladder mucosa, nephrogenic adenomas were found in six (Weingartner *et al.*, 1997).

Buccal mucosa appears to be better adapted to penile use as it does tolerate exposure to air. The risk of meatal stenosis is low. In a report by Fichtner *et al.*

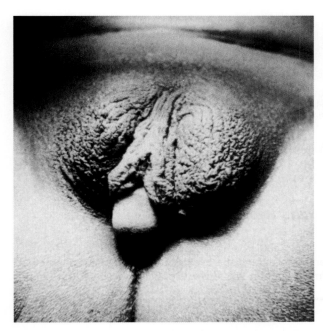

Figure 32.21 Severe penoscrotal transposition requiring multistage repair.

(1998) stenosis occurred in only one of 62 patients when the urethra was constructed from mucosa harvested from the lower lip. The sub-basement membrane vascularity appears to be more abundant in buccal than in bladder mucosa and the epithelial layer is thicker (Duckett, 1996). These qualities appear to enhance its success. Buccal mucosa can be applied as either an onlay or a tube (Kropfl *et al.*, 1998).

In a interesting retrospective analysis, Powell *et al.* (2000) compared a group of children with proximal hypospadias who had either a free graft repair using penile skin to a group having skin flap repairs. Two-thirds of the 142 patients had free graft repairs, applied either as an onlay or a tube. There was no difference in results other than stricture formation. Eight proximal strictures occurred in the free-tube group. Of importance, many of the complications did not become evident for one year, some presenting as late as 4 years post-repair.

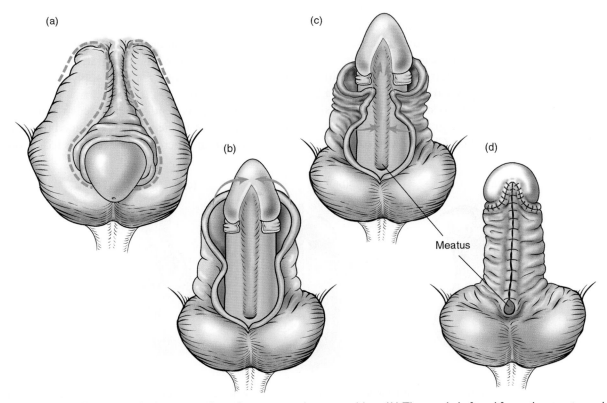

Figure 32.22 (*a*) First stage in the correction of penoscrotal transposition. (*b*) The penis is freed from the scrotum along an incision marked out by the dotted line. This extends around superior aspects of scrotum to enable these to be swung inferiomedially below the penis at closure. (*c*) Chordee released completely by aggressive ventral dissection. The urethral meatus retracts even further proximally. The glans is split. (*d, e*) The prepuce is split and brought ventral to cover the defect. Skin brought into the glans to allow the creation of a distal urethra at the second stage.

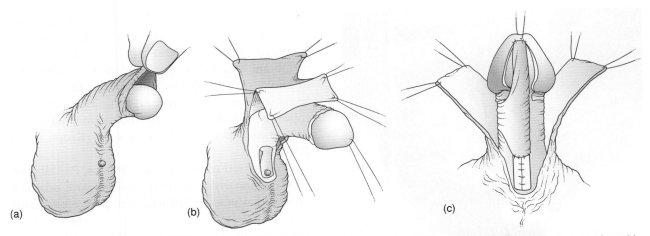

(a)

(b)

(c)

Figure 32.23 (*a*) Midscrotal hypospadias. (*b*) Release of chordee and freeing of the undersurface of the foreskin as a pedicle flap. Note: tissue distal to the meatus is preserved to extend the urethra to the penoscrotal junction. (*c*) Completion of urethroplasty using a midline tube proximally and an island pedicle distally to create the entire urethra in a single stage.

Surgical technique

Aside from site of tissue harvesting there are several steps required to achieve success with free grafts. The tissue must be applied to a well-vascularized bed of healthy tissue and cannot be expected to survive if applied over scar. Therefore, all scar must be removed. Some authorities perform these complex repairs in multiple steps, particularly when they first apply a corporeal patch graft ventrally to straighten the penis and are reluctant to add a free graft over that at the same operation (see section on Chordee correction).

Editorial note: Although I rarely find it necessary to use a free graft to form the urethra, I have applied free grafts of tubularized bladder or buccal mucosa to the ventral corpora even after vigorously incising the fascia to achieve orthoplasty. This graft then serves not only as the urethra but also as the covering of the corpora, acting similarly to the free grafts of tunica vaginalis or dermis that others might apply to the corpora in this situation.

Since free grafts tend to contract, a longer and wider segment of tissue must be obtained to prevent this complication. Therefore, the tissue is rolled loose-

(a)   (b)   (c)

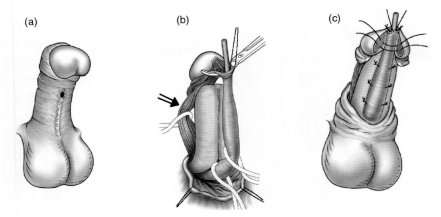

Figure 32.24 Penile disassembly: (*a*) Chordee with distal hypospadias. (*b*) Dorsal neurovascular bundle (*arrow*) and entire glans dissected free from corpus. Entire urethra and its spongiosum freed from ventral corporeal fascia (vessel loops) while urethral plate beyond hypospadiac meatus remains in continuity with urethra and attached to glans. (*c*) Glans split to advance urethra to its end. (*d*) Corpora reattached to glans, urethra advanced into glans and closure carried out to complete repair. For corporeal disproportion causing chordee, corporeal plication can be added. (Modified from Perovic SV *et al*. (1998) A new approach to the treatment of penile curvature. *J Urol* **160**, 1126.)

ly over the appropriate sized stent to prevent stricture formation, in contrast to the pedicle flap tube, which is tailored to the desired size. Finally, the non-mucosal surface requires careful dissection to remove fat, muscle, and appendages (if skin is applied). This is best achieved by pinning the graft to a moist, flat surface and excising the unwanted tissue in strips with fine scissors. Only a thin layer of mucosa and submucosa should remain, which is then applied as either a tube or an onlay.

Although the use of bladder mucosa is no longer recommended, this can easily be harvested by approaching the bladder suprapubically after it is filled. The muscle can be dissected off the mucosa before opening the bladder, allowing one to determine how much is to be harvested while the mucosa is on stretch.

Buccal mucosa can be obtained from the lower lip, but the amount is limited and scar contraction of the lip can lead to later problems. Mucosa from the inner aspect of the cheek is more abundant and healing does not appear to be a problem (Fig. 32.25). However, Stenson's (parotid) duct must be visualized and avoided and only mucosa should be removed. This is facilitated by undermining and elevating the mucosa with a dilute solution of epinephrine (1:100 000). The tissue to be harvested is marked out and sharply outlined with a knife. Then, using tenotomy scissors only mucosa is excised. Aside from avoiding Stenson's duct and the underlying tissue, a margin of tissue should be left at both the corner of the mouth and the tonsillar pillar. The wound is closed with catgut suture and causes very little postoperative morbidity. However, to avoid contracture, graft sites from the lip should not be approximated. If more tissue is required than can be obtained from one cheek, tissue can be obtained from the opposite cheek in a similar manner and the two grafts sutured together to gain either more length or more width. Harvesting may include tissue from the lip and the cheek to gain length (Brock, 1994). It has been recommended that both preoperative and postoperative antibiotics be used when buccal mucosa grafts are harvested (Payne *et al.*, 1998). The graft may also be soaked in a penicillin solution prior to application.

Postoperative complications

Urethrocutaneous fistula

Fistula continues to be the most common postoperative problem following hypospadias repair. However, the incidence is quite low, particularly with the increasing popularity of applying a second complete covering over the neourethra (Snow *et al.*, 1995). In

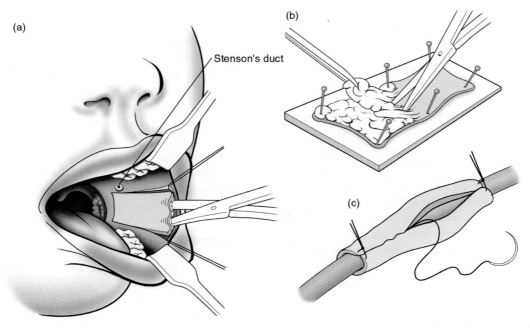

Figure 32.25 (*a*) Buccal mucosa harvest site. The limits of dissection are the anterior tonsillar pillars posteriorly, the corner of the lip anteriorly, and Stensen's duct superiorly. (*b*) Defatting the buccal mucosal graft. (*c*) Tubularizing the graft over a 16 Fr red rubber catheter.

the author's experience the risk of fistula for a distal onlay repair when applying complete coverage between the urethra and skin is less than 5% (Rushton and Belman, 1998). In more complex repairs the risk is between 10 and 20% (Asopa, 1998). With correction of hypospadias being carried out in young children, fistulae, especially those that are very tiny, may not be recognized until the child is toilet trained and voiding in the upright position.

Repair of small urethrocutaneous fistulae is a simple matter done most often as an outpatient procedure. It rarely requires a postoperative urethral stent. The urethra should be calibrated to confirm the absence of distal stenosis. Location of the fistula site is achieved by the retrograde injection of a dilute povidone-iodine (Betadine) solution while the bulbous urethra is being compressed to prevent instillation into the bladder. The secret to successful closure is similar to achieving success with the original repair: optical magnification, the use of fine sutures, careful technique, and covering the suture line completely with a second layer best obtained by de-epithilializing adjacent tissue (Geltzeiler and Belman, 1984; Retik *et al.*, 1988). The fistulous tract is traced to the urethra and excised. An inverting closure is preferred over an intraurethral catheter to prevent urethral narrowing. Larger fistulae may require an onlay flap, which can almost always be obtained from adjacent skin.

Urethral meatal stenosis

Meatal stenosis is a consequence of loss of blood supply to the distal urethra. This is more easily prevented than repaired. The importance of maintaining well-vascularized flaps during initial repair cannot be overemphasized. The addition of vascularized, de-epithelialized tissue over the distal portion of the neourethra may help to prevent this complication (see section on Avoiding complications). If the problem is simply that of a web of scar at the meatus, dilation or a simple ventral incision may resolve the problem. Occasionally a parent is sent home with a urethral dilator which, if inserted on a daily basis, may resolve mild problems.

One of the most frustrating complications is the occurrence of balanitis xerotica obliterans. This can occur years after the repair and its cause is unknown. Uemura *et al.* (2000) reported an incidence of three cases in a series of 796 repairs. Topical steroid applications may initially be tried, however complete exci-

sion with injection of triamcinalone under the involved area may be necessary before attempts at secondary surgery. Recurrence is common.

Stricture formation

Loss of vascularity to the new urethra is the usual cause of strictures. However, contraction of a circular anastamosis may be the etiology. This narrowing can be avoided by spatulation of the anastomosis between the original meatus and the newly constructed urethra. The meatus is incised proximally for a few millimeters to create a fish-mouth appearance prior to attaching the new urethra.

Acute stricture formation may manifest itself with urinary retention after removal of the diverting stent. This requires urgent suprapubic urinary diversion or a proximal urethrotomy. Attempts at catheterization of this newly constructed urethra may disrupt the successfully constructed urethra distal to the troubled area, causing even more problems. If one chooses to perform a proximal urethrotomy, one should be aware that it is often very difficult to find the normal urethra in this circumstance, since a catheter will not be present. Compression of a full bladder with the child under anesthesia may distend that portion proximal to the stenosis, facilitating the effort.

Treatment of strictures generally requires an open procedure; however, a trial of either dilation or visual urethrotomy may be worthwhile. Scherz *et al.* (1989) had success with one or the other of these methods in 46% of patients when the attempt was carried out within the first 3 months following the hypospadias repair. However, cure was achieved in only 16% when treatment was initiated 3 months after the original procedure. Duel *et al.* (1998) reported a 21% resolution with direct vision urethrotomy in a group of 29 patients. In the older patient daily self-dilation with a soft catheter for 6–12 weeks may be successful, but in the young child failure after a single dilation under anesthesia mandates open repair.

Urethral diverticula

Diverticula may be secondary to either distal narrowing or poor support and distensibility of the newly constructed urethra. Indications for surgical excision are recurrent UTIs or significant postvoid urinary dribbling. As is true for fistulae, the urethra should first be calibrated to rule out distal stenosis. Irrigation with Betadine may be used both as an antiseptic solution and to rule out any coincidental fistulae. If a small diverticulum that is not adherent to the overlying skin is present, the repair may be facilitated by retracting the penile skin (degloving), rather than incising over the diverticulum. After diverticular resection and urethral closure, the skin is brought back over the repair, diminishing the chances of complications (Zaontz *et al.*, 1989). If stenosis of the urethra either proximal or distal to the diverticulum coexists, the stenotic area is incised and a portion of the redundant tissue making up the diverticulum brought across the narrowed area. Occasionally, following a tubularized urethroplasty, a large saccular dilatation results, even in the absence of infection or distal narrowing. This may be a consequence of poor tissue support over the urethra or having tubularized too wide a pedicle flap at the time of initial repair. These saccules are best approached by incising down the midline and excising the redundant mucosa. If the submucosa is preserved this redundant tissue is brought together in overlapping layers after closure of the urethra both to prevent leak and to offer tissue support. Recurrence has not been a problem when large diverticula have been dealt with in this manner (Aigen *et al.*, 1987).

Recurrent chordee

In general, if chordee is completely resolved at initial repair it does not re-present as a problem. As previously noted, Vandersteen and Husmann (1998) reviewed a series of patients from the Mayo Clinic and found only 22 who presented with symptomatic chordee as adults. All had had proximal hypospadias repairs. Although the authors interpreted this as recurrent chordee, in many it may have been persisting chordee that was not brought to attention until the onset of sexual activity.

Redo hypospadias repairs

Occasionally hypospadias repairs will disrupt. This may be the result of infection, urinary extravasation, loss of vascularity of a flap, or may be totally unexplainable. Reoperation for complications should be delayed until there is good tissue healing. This generally takes 4–6 months. Ideally, adequate penile skin exists upon which the re-repair can be based.

For distal re-repairs there have been reports of success with incision and hinging of the residual urethral plate (the Snodgrass procedure) (Snodgrass, 1994).

Meatal-based flaps have also been applied in this situation (Wheeler and Malone, 1993; Teague *et al.*, 1994). If a meatal-based flap is used, its base must exist on scar proximal to the meatus. It seems unlikely to this author that the vascularity of a flap which has its base on scar from a previously failed hypospadias repair would be adequate to give a predictably reliable result. Both Hodgson (1983) and Duckett (1994b) expressed the same concern. Secrest *et al.* (1993) report a 53% success rate (47% failure) with a meatal-base flip-flap to repair distal disruption. However, they reported an 88.6% success using an offset pedicle flap of hairless penile skin in the same situation. In general, excellent success can be achieved using ventrolateral penile skin as a pedicle onlay to re-repair failed hypospadias. By incising around the penis along the previous subcoronal incision and freeing dorsally, adequate skin can usually be brought ventral both to create the pedicle flap and to cover the repair. However, Jayanthi *et al.* (1994) had a 53% complication rate using an island pedicle flap in this manner but concluded, nevertheless, that this was a reasonable method of approaching this problem.

Use of a free graft of buccal mucosa to form the urethra is reserved for cases where there is inadequate skin both to create the urethra and to cover the repair. When there is a paucity of skin as well as persistent chordee, a free graft of meshed skin can be applied to the ventral aspect of the penis after correcting chordee as the first stage. The urethra is then tubularized from this skin after complete healing (Secrest *et al.*, 1993; Ehrlich and Alter, 1996). Fortunately, severe complications requiring these types of maneuvers are becoming increasingly rare as hypospadiologists perform more and more primary corrections.

Hensle *et al.* (2001) reviewed the records of 42 men, ages 18–47 years, who had either primary (eight) or redo hypospadias repairs. As anticipated, results were poorest in those who had the most severe problems and who had the least amount of penile skin available for reconstruction. Almost one-third in that group had a complication. However, even those adults who had local tissue available for reconstruction had a 42% complication rate. Most interesting, however, was the 38% complication rate in the eight patients who had had no prior attempts at repair. A higher incidence of wound infections and problems with postoperative erections probably play a role. Adult patients should be made aware of these higher than anticipated risks.

Long-term follow-up

The functional results of hypospadias repair as based on uroflowmetry appear to be satisfactory. Garibay et al. (1995) reported normal flow rates in nine of 11 boys with meatal-based flap distal repairs and in 69% of boys with tubularized repairs. Jayanthi et al. (1995) found that 73% of boys who did not have any postoperative complications had normal urine flow rates.

The long-term psychological aspects of hypospadias appear to be positive. Gender development, identification, and behavior have not been found to be abnormal in most men with previous hypospadias repair (Sandberg et al., 1995). They may have a more negative genital self-concept, but this does not appear to interfere with sexual activity. In societies that do not practise circumcision lack of the foreskin may impact negatively upon self-image (Mureau et al., 1995). Those who had the fewest postoperative complications appeared to have the best self-concept. (Aho et al., 1997).

The future

Tissue from many body sites has been used for urethral replacement, generally with poor success. When adequate penile skin exists it is unnecessary to use other tissue to achieve satisfactory results. The use of tissue expanders under penile skin offers the opportunity to produce more local tissue for that purpose. Cultured urethral epithelium has been used to create tissue ex vitro and used for repair with some success (Romangnoli et al., 1993). Atala et al. (1999) used an onlay of collagen matrix harvested from human cadaver bladders allowing native epithelial ongrowth with good success. Chen et al. (2000) used preserved acellular collagen matrix obtained from porcine bladders to repair experimentally created urethral defects in rabbits. They found host cell infiltration and angiogenesis at 2 weeks, while the implant diameter remained stable. All animals had successful repairs.

Laser soldering has been applied clinically to expedite urethral closure both as an adjunct to the use of sutures and independently (Kirsch et al., 1997). Results suggest that laser soldering may become competitive with the success rates of standard methods of suture anastomosis while shortening operative time.

Conclusions

Hypospadias repair has become one of the most common operative procedures during the 1990s for those surgeons who confine their care to the urologic problems of children. For reasons not clear at this time the incidence of hypospadias appears to be rising. With greater surgical experience and the advances that new approaches have brought, the complication rate has dropped dramatically and cosmesis has improved. Most boys can be expected to appear normal and, unless their families tell them, some will never know that they had genital surgery. This is ideal.

As the responsibility for the care of children with urogenital problems becomes more confined to those with special training and interest we can anticipate further progress in our efforts. However, in the future surgical correction of congenital abnormalities will be an uncommon event with the anticipated explosion of knowledge in genetics and genetic engineering. At the end of this new century a chapter such as this will evoke a smile similar to that one might express in response to a treatise on blood letting. To the future!

References

Aaronson IA, Cakmak MA, Key LL (1997) Defects of the testosterone biosynthetic pathway in boys with hypospadias. *J Urol* **157**: 1884.

Aarskog D (1979) Maternal progestins as a possible cause of hypospadias. *N Engl J Med* **300**: 75.

Adams MC, Chalian VS, Rink RC (1999) Congenital dorsal penile curvature: a potential problem of the long phallus. *J Urol* **161**: 1304.

Aho MO, Tammela OK, Tammela TL (1997) Aspects of adult satisfaction with the results of surgery for hypospadias performed in childhood. *Eur Urol* **32**: 218.

Aigen AB, Khawand N, Skoog SJ et al. (1987) Acquired megalourethra: an uncommon complication of the transverse preputial island flap urethroplasty. *J Urol* **37**: 172.

Albers N, Ulrichs C, Gluer S et al. (1997) Etiologic classification of severe hypospadias: implications for prognosis and management. *J Pediatr* **131**: 386.

Allen TD, Griffin JE (1984) Endocrine studies in patients with advanced hypospadias. *J Urol* **131**: 310.

Allen TD, Spence HM (1984) The surgical treatment of coronal hypospadias and related problems. *J Urol* **100**: 504.

Asopa HS (1998) New concepts in the management of hypospadias and its complications. *Ann R Coll Surg Engl* **80**: 161.

Asopa HS, Elhence EP, Atria SP *et al.* (1971) One stage correction of penile hypospadias using a foreskin tube: a preliminary report. *Int Surg* **55**: 435.

Atala A, Guzman L, Retik AB (1999) A novel inert collagen matrix for hypospadias repair. *J Urol* **162**: 1148.

Balogna RA, Noah TA, Nasrallah PF *et al.* (1999) Chordee: varied opinions and treatments as documented in a survey of the American Academy of Pediatrics, Section on Urology. *Urology* **53**: 608.

Barthold JS, Teer TL, Redman JF (1996) Modified Barcat balanic groove technique for hypospadias repair: experience with 195 cases. *J Urol* **55**: 1735.

Bartone F, Shore N, Newland J *et al.* (1987) The best suture for hypospadias? *Urology* **29**: 517.

Baskin L, Duckett JW (1994) Dorsal tunica albuginea plication (TAP) for hypospadias curvature. *J Urol* **151**: 1668.

Baskin LS, Duckett JW, Ueoka K *et al.* (1994) Changing concepts of hypospadias curvature lead to more onlay island flap procedures. *J Urol* **151**: 191.

Baskin LS, Erol A, Li YW, Cunha GR (1998) Anatomical studies of hypospadias. *J Urol* **160**: 1108.

Bauer SB, Retik AB, Colodny AH (1981) Genetic aspects of hypospadias. *Urol Clin North Am* **8**: 559.

Beck C (1898) A new operation for balanic hypospadias. *NY Med J* **67**: 147.

Belman AB (1982) The modified Mustarde hypospadias repair. *J Urol* **127**: 88.

Belman AB (1988) De-epithelialized skin flap coverage in hypospadias repair. *J Urol* **140**: 1273.

Belman AB (1994) The de-epithelialized flap and its influence on hypospadias repair. *J Urol* **152**: 2332.

Belman AB (1997) Urethroplasty. *Soc Pediatr Urol Newslett* Dec.

Belman AB (1999) Editorial comment. *Urology* **53**: 612.

Belman AB, Kass EJ (1982) Hypospadias repair in children under one year of age. *J Urol* **128**: 1273.

Bentvelsen FM, Brinkmann AO, van der Linden JE *et al.* (1995) Decreased immunoreactive androgen receptor levels are not the cause of isolated hypospadias. *Br J Urol* **76**: 384.

Broadman LM (1987) Regional anesthesia for the pediatric outpatient. *Urol Clin North Am* **5**: 53.

Brock JW III (1994) Autologous buccal mucosal graft for urethral reconstruction. *Urology* **44**: 753.

Burbige KA (1994) Simplified postoperative management of hypospadias repair. *Urology* **43**: 719.

Buson H, Smiley D, Reinberg Y *et al.* (1994) Distal hypospadias repair without stents: is it better? *J Urol* **151**: 1059.

Caione P, Capozza N, Lais A *et al.* (1997) Long-term results of distal urethral advancement glanuloplasty for distal hypospadias. *J Urol* **158**: 1168.

Chen F, Yoo JJ, Atala A (2000) Experimental and clinical experience using tissue regeneration for urethral reconstruction. *Wold J Urol* **18**(1): 67.

Chhibber AK, Perkins FM, Rabinowitz R *et al.* (1997) Penile block timing for postoperative analgesia of hypospadias repair in children. *J Urol* **158**: 1156.

Churchill BM, van Savage JG, Khoury AE *et al.* (1996) The dartos flap as an adjunct in preventing urethrocutaneous fistulas in repeat hypospadias surgery. *J Urol* **156**: 2047.

Davits RJ, van den Aker ES, Scholmeijer RJ *et al.* (1993) Effect of parenteral testosterone therapy on penile development in boys with hypospadias. *Br J Urol* **71**: 593.

Decter RM (1991) M inverted V glansplasty: a procedure for distal hypospadias. *J Urol* **146**: 641.

De Jong TP, Boemers TM (1993) Improved Mathieu repair for coronal and distal shaft hypospadias with moderate chordee. *Br J Urol* **72**: 972.

de Sy WA, Hoebeke P (1994) Urethral advancement for distal hypospadias: 14 years' experience. *Eur Urol* **26**: 90.

Devesa R, Munoz A, Torrents M *et al.* (1998) Prenatal diagnosis of isolated hypospadias. *Prenat Diag* **18**: 779.

Devine CJ Jr (1983) Chordee in hypospadias. In: Glenn JF (ed.) *Urologic surgery.* 3rd edition. Philadelphia, PA: JB Lippincott Co., 775–98.

Devine CJ Jr, Horton CE (1973) Chordee without hypospadias. *J Urol* **110**: 264.

Devine CJ Jr, Horton CE (1975) Use of dermal graft to correct chordee. *J Urol* **113**: 56.

Devine CJ Jr, Gonzales-Serva L, Stecker JF Jr *et al.* (1980) Utricular configuration in hypospadias and intersex. *J Urol* **123**: 407.

Devine CJ Jr, Blackley SK, Horton CE *et al.* (1991) The surgical treatment of chordee without hypospadias in men. *J Urol* **146**: 325.

Dewan PA (1993) Distal hypospadias repair with preputial reconsruction. *J Paediatr Child Health* **29**: 183.

Dimler M, Gibbons MD, Haley A (1984) A modification of the MAGPI procedure. *J Pediatr Surg* **19**: 627.

DiSandro M, Palmer JM (1996) Stricture incidence related to suture material in hypospadias. *J Pediatr Surg* **31**: 881.

Donnahoo KK, Cain MP, Pope JC *et al.* (1998) Etiology, management and surgical complications of congenital chordee without hypospadias. *J Urol* **160**: 1120.

Duckett JW (1996) Hypospadias. *In Adult pediatric urology.* Gillonwater JY, Grayhack JT, Howards SS, Duckett JW (eds), St Louis, Mosby, 2549–90.

Duckett JW (1981a) Foreword: Symposium on Hypospadias. *Urol Clin North Am* **8**: 371.

Duckett JW (1981b) MAGPI (meatoplasty and glanuloplasty): a procedure for subcoronal hypospadias. *Urol Clin North Am* **8**: 513.

Duckett JW (1981c) The island flap technique for hypospadias repair. *Urol Clin North Am* **8**: 503.

Duckett JW (1994a) Editorial comment. *J Urol* **151**: 714.

Duckett JW (1994b) Editorial comment. *J Urol* **152**: 743.

Duckett JW, Keating MA (1989) Technical challenge of the megameatus intact prepuce hypospadias variant: the pyramid procedure. *J Urol* **41**: 1407.

Duckett JW, Snyder HM III (1991) The MAGPI hypospadias repair in 1111 patients. *Ann Surg* **213**: 620.

Duel BP, Barthold JS, Gonzalez R (1998) Management of urethral stricture after hypospadias repair. *J Urol* **160**: 170.

Duplay S (1874) De l'hypspadias perineo-scrotal et de son traitement chirurgical. *Arch Gen Med* **1**: 513.

Ehrlich RM, Alter G (1996) Split-thickness skin graft urethroplasty and tunica vaginalis flaps for failed hypospadias repairs. *J Urol* **155**: 131.

Elder JS, Duckett JW, Snyder HM (1987) Onlay island flap in the repair of mid and distal penile hypospadias without chordee. *J Urol* **138**: 376.

Ellis GF, Patil U (1989) Urologist's perspectives of single-stage hypospadias repair in the 1980s; experience of 100 patients. *Urology* **34**: 262.

Evans BA, Williams DM, Hughes IA (1991) Normal postnatal androgen production and action in isolated micropenis and isolated hypospadias. *Arch Dis Child* **66**: 1033.

Falkowski WS, Firlit CF (1980) Hypospadias surgery: the X-shaped elastic dressing. *J Urol* **123**: 904.

Fallon B, Devine CJ Jr, Horton CE (1976) Congenital anomalies associated with hypospadias. *Urology* **16**: 585.

Feldman KW, Smith DW (1975) Fetal phallic growth and penile standards for newborn male infants. *J Pediatr* **86**: 395.

Fichtner J, Fisch M, Filipas D *et al.* (1998) Refinements in buccal mucosa graft urethroplasty for hypospadias repair. *World J Urol* **16**: 192.

Firlit CF (1987) The mucosal collar in hypospadias surgery. *J Urol* **137**: 80.

Flack CE, Walker RD III (1995) Onlay-tube-onlay urethroplasty technique in primary perineal hypospadias surgery. *J Urol* **154**: 837.

Fredel IL, Lichtenstein P, Pedersen NL *et al.* (1998) Hypospadias is related to birth weight in discordant monozygotic twins. *J Urol* **160**: 2197.

Garibay JT, Reid C, Gonzalez R (1995) Functional evaluation of the results of hypospadias surgery with uroflowmetry. *J Urol* **54**: 835.

Geltzeiler J, Belman AB (1984) Results of closure of urethrocutaneous fistulas in children. *J Urol* **132**: 734.

Gilbert DA, Devine CJ Jr, Winslow BH *et al.* (1986) Microsurgical hypospadias repair. *Plast Reconstr Surg* **77**: 460.

Gilpin D, Clements WD, Boston VE (1993) GRAP repair: single-stage reconstruction of hypospadias as an out-patient procedure. *Br J Urol* **71**: 226.

Gittes GK, Snyder CL, Murphy JP (1998) Glans approximation procedure urethroplasty for the wide, deep meatus. *Urology* **52**: 499.

Glassberg KI (1987) Augmented Duckett repair for severe hypospadias. *J Urol* **138**: 380.

Glassberg KI, Hansbrough F, Horowitz M (1998) The Koyanagi–Nonomura 1-stage buckett repair of severe hypospadias with and without penoscrotal transposition. *J Urol* **160**: 1104.

Greenfield SP, Sadler BT, Wan J (1994) Two-stage repair for severe hypospadias. *J Urol* **152**: 498.

Gunter JB, Forestner JE, Manley CB (1990) Caudal epidural anesthesia reduces blood loss during hypospadias repair. *J Urol* **144**: 517.

Haberlik A, Schmnidt B, Uray E *et al.* (1997) Hypospadias repair using a modification of Beck's procedure: followup. *J Urol* **57**: 2308.

Hakim S, Merguerian PA, Rabinowitz R *et al.* (1996) Outcome analysis of the modified Mathieu hypospadias repair: comparison of stented and unstented repairs. *J Urol* **156**: 836.

Harris DL, Jeffrey RS (1989) One stage repair of hypospadias using split preputial flaps (Harris): the first 100 patients treated. *Br J Urol* **63**: 401.

Hastie KJ, Deshpande SS, Moisey CU (1989) Long-term follow-up of the MAGPI operation for distal hypospadias. *Br J Urol* **63**: 320.

Hendren WH, Caesar RE (1992) Chordee without hypospadias: experience with 33 cases. *J Urol* **147**: 107.

Hensle TW, Tennenbaum SY, Reiley EA, Pollard J (2001) Hypospadias repair in adults: adventures and misadventures. *J Urol* **165**: 77.

Hodgson NB (1978) Hypospadias and urethral duplications. In: Harrison JH, Gittes RF, Perlmutter AD *et al.* (eds) *Campbell's Urology.* 4th edition. Philadelphia, PA: WB Saunders, 1556–95.

Hodgson NB (1981) Use of vascularized flaps in hypospadias repairs. *Urol Clin North Am* **8**: 471.

Hodgson NB (1983) Editorial comment. *J Urol* **130**: 741.

Horton CE, Devine CJ Jr (1966) Hypospadias. In: Gibson T (ed.) *Modern trends in plastic surgery*. London: Butterworth, 268.

Horton CE, Devine CJ Jr (1973) One-stage repairs. In: Horton CE (ed.) *Plastic and reconstructive surgery of the genital area*. Boston, MA: Little Brown and Co, 278.

Ikoma F, Shima H, Yabumoto H *et al.* (1986) Surgical treatment of enlarged prostatic utricle and vagina masculina in patients with hypospadias. *Br J Urol* **58**: 423.

Ikoma HS, Terakawa T, Satoh Y *et al.* (1979) Development anomalies associated with hypospadias. *J Urol* **122**: 619.

Issa MM, Gearhart JP (1989) The failed MAGPI: management and prevention. *Br J Urol* **64**: 169.

Jayanthi VR, McLorie GA, Khoury AE *et al.* (1994) Can previously relocated penile skin be successfully used for salvage hypospadias repair? *J Urol* **152**: 740.

Jayanthi VR, McClorie GA, Khoury AE *et al.* (1995) Functional characteristics of the reconstructed neourethra after island flap urethroplasty. *J Urol* **153**: 1657.

Kallen B (1988) Case control study of hypospadias, based on registry information. *Teratology* **38**: 45.

Kallen B, Bertollini R, Castilla E *et al.* (1986) A joint international study on the epidemiology of hypospadias. *Acta Paediatr Scand* **324** (Suppl): 1–52.

Kallen B, Mastroiacovo P, Lancaster PA *et al.* (1991) Oral contraceptives in the etiology of isolated hypospadias. *Contraception* **44**: 173.

Kaplan GW, Lamm DL (1975) Embryogenesis of chordee. *J Urol* **114**: 769.

Kass EJ (1993) Dorsal corporeal rotation: an alternative technique for the management of severe chordee. *J Urol* **150**: 635.

Khuri F, Hardy BE, Churchill BM (1981) Urologic anomalies associated with hypospadias. *Urol Clin N Am* **8**: 565.

Kiely EA, Chapman RS, Bakproa SL *et al.* (1995) Maternal serum human chorionic gonadotrophin during early pregnancy resulting in boys with hypospadias or cryptorchidism. *Br J Urol* **76**: 389.

King LR (1970) Hypospadias – a one stage repair without skin graft based on a new principle: chordee is sometimes produced by skin alone. *J Urol* **103**: 660.

Kinkead TM, Borzi PA, Duffy PG *et al.* (1994) Long-term follow-up of bladder mucosa graft for male urethral reconstruction. *J Urol* **151**: 1056.

Kirsch AJ, Canning DA, Zderic SA *et al.* (1997) Laser soldering technique for sutureless urethral surgery. *Tech Urol* **3**: 108.

Knorr D, Beckman D, Bidlingmaier F *et al.* (1979) Plasma testosterone in male puberty: II. HCG stimulation test in boys with hypospadias. *Acta Endocrinol (Copenh)* **90**: 365.

Koff SA, Brinkman J, Ulrich J *et al.* (1994) Extensive mobilization of the urethral plate and urethra for repair of hypospadias: the modified Barcat technique. *J Urol* **151**: 466.

Koff SA, Jayanthi VR (1999) Preoperative treatment with human chorionic gonadotropin in infancy decreases the severity of proximal hypospadias and chordee. *J Urol* **162**: 1435.

Kogan SJ, Reda EF, Smey PL *et al.* (1983) Dermal graft correction of extraordinary chordee. *J Urol* **130**: 952.

Koyanagi T, Nonomura K, Yamashita T *et al.* (1994) One-stage repair of hypospadias: is there no simple method universally applicable to all types of hypospadias? *J Urol* **152**: 1232.

Kramer SA, Aydin G, Kelalis PP (1982) Chordee without hypospadias in children. *J Urol* **128**: 539.

Kropfl D, Tucak A, Prlic D, Verweyen A (1998) Using buccal mucosa for urethral reconstruction in primary and reoperative surgery. *Eur Urol* **34**: 216.

Kulkarni BK, Oak SN, Patel MP (1991) Developmental anomalies associated with hypospadias. *J Postgrad Med* **37**: 140.

Kumar S (1986) Hypospadias with normal prepuce. *J Urol* **136**: 1056.

Latifoglu O, Yavuzer R, Demirciler N *et al.* (1998) Extraurogenital congenital anomalies associated with hypospadias: retrospective review of 700 patients. *Ann Plast Surg* **41**: 570.

Lau JTK (1984) Penile block for pain relief after circumcision in children. *Am J Surg* **147**: 797.

Li LC, Zhang X, Zhou SW *et al.* (1995) Experience with repair of hypospadias using bladder mucosa in adolescents and adults. *J Urol* **153**: 1117.

Lindgren BW, Reda EF, Levitt SB *et al.* (1998) Single and multiple dermal grafts for the management of severe penile curvature. *J Urol* **160**: 1128.

McCormack M, Homsy Y, Laberge Y (1993) 'No stent, no diversion' Mathieu hypospadias repair. *Can J Surg* **36**: 152.

Macnab AJ, Zouves C (1991) Hypospadias after assisted reproduction incorporating *in vitro* fertilization and gamete intrafallopian transfer. *Fertil Steril* **56**: 918.

Manley CB, Epstein ES (1981) Early hypospadias repair. *J Urol* **125**: 698.

Mathieu P (1932) Traitement en un temps de l'hypopadias balanique et juxta-balanique. *J Chir* **39**: 481.

Memmelaar J (1947) Use of bladder mucosa in a one-stage repair of hypospadias. *J Urol* **58**: 66.

Minevich E, Pecha BR, Wacksman J, Sheldon CA (1999) Mathieu hypospadias repair: experience in 202 patients. *J Urol* **162**: 2141.

Mollard P, Castagnola C (1994) Hypospadias: the release of chordee without dividing the urethral plate and onlay island flap (92 cases). *J Urol* **152**: 1238.

Montagnino B, Gonzales ET Jr, Roth DR (1988) Open catheter drainage after urethral surgery. *J Urol* **140**: 1250.

Moore CC (1990) The role of routine radiographic screening of boys with hypospadias: a prospective study. *J Pediatr Surg* **25**: 339.

Mureau MA, Slijper FM, Nijman RJ *et al.* (1995) Psychosexual adjustment of children and adolescents after different types of hypospadias surgery: a norm-related study. *J Urol* **54**: 1902.

Nesbit RM (1965) Congenital curvature of the phallus: report of three cases with description of corrective operation. *J Urol* **93**: 230.

Nonomura K, Fujieda K, Sakakibara N *et al.* (1984) Pituitary and gonadal function in prepubertal boys with hypospadias. *J Urol* **132**: 595.

Park JM, Faerber GJ, Bloom DA (1995) Long-term outcome evaluation of patients undergoing the meatal advancement and glanuloplasty procedure. *J Urol* **153**: 1655.

Paulozzi LJ, Erickson JD, Jackson RJ (1997) Hypospadias trends in two US surveillance systems. *Pediatrics* **100**: 831.

Payne CE, Sumfest JM, Deshon GE Jr (1998) Buccal mucosal graft for hypospadias repairs. *Techniques Urol* **4**: 173.

Perlmutter AD, Montgomery BT, Steinhardt GF (1985) Tunica vaginalis free graft for the correction of chordee. *J Urol* **134**: 311.

Perovic S, Vukadinovic F (1994) Onlay island flap urethroplasty for severe hypospadias: a variant of the technique. *J Urol* **151**: 711.

Perovic SV, Djordjevic ML (1998) A new approach in hypospadias repair. *World J Urol* **16**: 195.

Perovic SV, Miroslav LJ, Djordjevic ML, Djakovic NG (1998) A new approach to the treatment of penile curvature. *J Urol* **160**: 1123.

Pope JC IV, Kropp BP, McLaughlin KP *et al.* (1996) Penile orthoplasty using dermal grafts in the outpatient setting. *Urology* **48**: 124.

Powell CR, McAleer I, Alagiri M, Kaplan GW (2000) Comparison of flaps versus grafts in proximal hypospadias surgery. *J Urol* **163**, 1286.

Ramen-Wilms L, Lin-in Tsens A, Wizhardt S *et al.* (1995) Fetal genital effects of first trimester sex hormone exposure: a metaanalysis. *Obstet Gynecol* **85**: 141.

Retik AB, Bauer SB, Mandell J *et al.* (1994a) Management of severe hypospadias with a 2-stage repair. *J Urol* **152**: 749.

Retik AB, Borer JG (1998) Primary and reoperative hypospadias repair with the Snodgrass technique. *World J Urol* **16**: 186.

Retik AB, Keating M, Mandell J (1988) Complications of hypospadias repair. *Urol Clin North Am* **15**: 223.

Retik AB, Mandell J, Bauer SB *et al.* (1994b) Meatal based hypospadias repair with the use of a dorsal subcutaneous flap to prevent urethrocutaneous fistula. *J Urol* **152**: 1229.

Ritchey ML, Benson RC Jr, Kramer SA *et al.* (1988) Management of muellerian duct remnants in the male patient. *J Urol* **140**: 795.

Romangnoli G, De Luca M, Faranda F *et al.* (1993) One-step treatment of proximal hypospadias by the autologous graft of cultured urethral epithelium. *J Urol* **150**: 1204.

Ross JH, Kay R (1997) Use of de-epithelialized local skin flap in hypospadias repairs accomplished by tubularization of the incised urethral plate. *Urology* **50**: 110.

Rushton HG, Belman AB (1998) The split prepuce *in situ* onlay hypospadias repair. *J Urol* **160**: 1334.

Sakakibara N, Nonomura K, Koyanagi T *et al.* (1991) Use of testosterone ointment before hypospadias repair. *Urol Int* **47**: 40.

Sandberg DE, Meyer-Bahlburg HF, Yager TJ *et al.* (1995) Gender development in boys born with hypospadias. *Psychoneuroendocrinoloy* **20**: 693.

Scherz HC, Kaplan GW, Packer MG *et al.* (1989) Urethral strictures after hypospadias repair. *J Urol (Paris)* **95**: 23.

Schultz JR, Klykylo WM, Wacksman J (1983) Timing of elective hypospadias repair in children. *Pediatrics* **71**: 349.

Secrest CL, Jordan GH, Winslow BH *et al.* (1993) Repair of the complications of hypospadias surgery. *J Urol* **150**: 1415.

Shafir R, Hertz M, Boichis H (1982) Vesicoureteral reflux in boys with hypospadias. *Urology* **20**: 29.

Shapiro SR (1989) Hypospadias repair: optical magnification versus Zeiss recontruction microscope. *Urology* **33**: 43.

Shima H, Ikoma F, Yabumoto H *et al.* (1986) Gonadotrophin and testosterone response in prepubertal boys with hypospadias. *J Urol* **135**: 539.

Smith ED (1980) Malformations of the bladder and urethra, and hypospadias. In: Holder TM, Ashcraft KW (eds) *Pediatric surgery*. Philadelphia, PA: WB Saunders, 785.

Snodgrass W (1994) Tubularized, incised plate urethroplasty for distal hypospadias. *J Urol* **151**: 464.

Snodgrass W, Koyle M, Manzoni G *et al.* (1996) Tubularized incised plate hypospadias repair: results of a multicenter experience. *J Urol* **156**: 839.

Snodgrass W, Koyle M, Manzoni G *et al.* (1998) Tubularized incised plate hypospadias repair for proximal hypospadias. *J Urol* **159**: 2129.

Snow BW (1989) Transverse corporeal plication for persistent chordee. *Urology* **34**: 360.

Snow BW, Cartwright PC, Unger K (1995) Tunica vaginalis blanket wrap to prevent urethrocutaneous fistula: an 8-year experience. *J Urol* **153**: 472.

Spencer JR, Perlmutter AD (1990) Sleeve advancement distal hypospadias repair. *J Urol* **144**: 523.

Spiro SA, Seitzinger JW, Hanna MK (1992) Hypospadias with dorsal chordee. *Urology* **39**: 389l.

Standoli L (1982) One stage repair of hypospadias: preputial island flap technique. *Ann Plast Surg* **9**: 81.

Stecker RE, Zaontz MR (1997) Stent free Thiersch–Duplay hypospadias repair with the Snodgrass modification. *J Urol* **158**: 1178.

Stock JA, Cortez J, Scherz HC *et al.* (1994) The management of proximal hypospadias using a 1-stage hypospadias repair with preputial free graft for neourethral construction and a preputial pedicle flap for ventral skin coverage. *J Urol* **152**: 2335.

Stoll C, Alembik Y, Roth MP, Dott B (1990) Genetic and environmental factors in hypospadias. *J Med Genet* **27**: 559.

Sugar EC, Firlit CF (1988) Urinary prophylaxis and postoperative care of children at home with an indwelling catheter after hypospadias repair. *Urology* **32**: 48.

Sutherland RW, Wiener JS, Hicks JP *et al* (1996). Androgen receptor gene mutations are rarely associated with isolated penile hypospadias. *J Urol* **156**: 828.

Sweet RA, Schrott HG, Kurland R *et al.* (1974) Study of the incidence of hypospadias in Rochester, Minnesota, 1940–1970, and a case-controlled comparison of possible etiologic factors. *Mayo Clin Proc* **49**: 52.

Teague JL, Roth DR, Gonzales ET (1994) Repair of hypospadias complications using the meatal based flap urethroplasty. *J Urol* **151**: 470.

Turner-Warwick R, Parkhouse H, Chapple CR (1997) Bulbar elongation anastomotic meatoplasty (BEAM) for subterminal and hypospadias urethroplasty. *J Urol* **158**: 1160.

Uemura S, Hutson JM, Woodward AA, Kelly JH, Chow CW (2000) Balanitis xerotica obliterans with urethral stricture after hypospadias repair. *Pediatr Surg Int* **16**: 144.

Ulman I, Erikei V, Avanoglu A *et al.* (1997) The effect of suturing technique and material on complication rate following hypospadias repair. *Eur J Pediatr Surg* **7**: 156.

Unluer ES, Miroglu C, Ozdiler E *et al.* (1991) Long term follow-up of the MAGPI (meatal advancement and glanuloplasty) operations in distal hypospadias. *Urol Nephrol* **23**: 581.

Vandersteen DR, Husmann DA (1998) Late onset recurrent penile chordee after successful correction at hypospadias repair. *J Urol* **160**: 1131.

van Horn AC, Kass EJ (1995) Glanuloplasty and *in-situ* tubularization of the urethral plate: a simple reliable technique for the majority of boys with hypospadias. *J Urol* **154**: 1505.

van Savage JG, Palanca LG, Slaughenhoupt BL (2000) A prospective randomized trial of dressings versus no dressings for hypospadias repair. *J Urol* **164**: 981.

Wacksman J (1981) Modification of the one stage flip flap procedure to repair distal penile hypospadias. *Urol Clin North Am* **8**: 527.

Wacksman J (1987) Repair of hypospadias using new mouth-controlled microscope. *Urology* **29**: 276.

Walsh PC, Curry N, Mills RC *et al.* (1976) Plasma androgen response to HCG stimulation in prepubertal boys with hypospadias and cryporchidism. *J Clin Endocrinol Metab* **42**: 52.

Weidner IS, Moller H, Jensen TK, Skakkebaek NE (1999) Risk factors for cryptorchidism and hypospadias. *J Urol* **161**: 1606.

Weingartner K, Kozakewich HP, Hendren WH (1997) Nephrogenic adenoma after urethral reconstruction using bladder mucosa: report of 6 cases and review of the literature. *J Urol* **158**: 1175.

Wesson L, Mandell J (1985) Single stage hypospadias repair using the operating microscope. *Microsurgery* **6**: 182.

Wheeler R, Malone P (1993) The role of the Mathieu repair as a salvage procedure. *Br J Urol* **72**: 52.

Zaontz MR, Kaplan WE, Maizels M (1989) Surgical correction of anterior urethral diverticula after hypospadias repair in children. *Urology* **33**: 40.

Zaontz MR (1989) The GAP (glans approximation procedure) for glanular/coronal hypospadias. *J Urol* **141**: 359.

Abnormalities of the penis and scrotum   33

Julia Spencer Barthold and Evan J. Kass

Introduction

Anomalies of the genitalia are common and as a group comprise the most frequent cause of birth defects in males. However, the majority of congenital malformations of the testis and scrotum other than cryptorchidism and hypospadias are extremely rare and often associated with anomalies of other organ systems. Many other developmental abnormalities affecting the genitalia, such as patency of the processus vaginalis (hernia and/or hydrocele), varicocele, and the bell clapper deformity of testicular suspension may not be apparent for many years but are common and have the potential for significant long-term morbidity. Some defects have known etiologies including defined endocrine deficiencies or genetic defects, but for most genital defects the etiology remains unknown. Congenital and acquired abnormalities of male genitalia observed in the pediatric population excluding intersex disorders, hypospadias, and cryptorchidism will be reviewed here.

Normal development of the penis and scrotum

The external genitalia, including the genital tubercle and labioscrotal swellings, are indistinguishable in male and female before the 9th week of human gestation (Ammini *et al.*, 1997). Subsequent development in males proceeds in a proximal to distal fashion. The urethral groove deepens and the urethral folds become distinct and then fuse in the midline. Recent work suggests that creation of the glanular urethra also occurs by fusion of the urethral plate and not by the longstanding concept of ingrowth of surface glanular epithelium (Glenister, 1921; Ammini *et al.*, 1997). The paired labioscrotal swellings attain a more ventral position, either by actual migration or by relative change in position due to lengthening, and are anterior to the genital tubercle by 11 weeks of gestation. Fusion of the urethra up to the coronal sulcus is complete by 12 weeks. Developmental penile curvature is lost and scrotal positioning complete by 13 weeks. Fusion of the urethral folds within the glans proceeds as described for urethral closure in the shaft, and is accompanied by distal growth of the prepuce. By 24 weeks, the meatus is at the glans tip and the prepuce completely covers the glans, to which it is largely adherent.

Penile abnormalities

Prepuce

Normal development

At birth, the normal prepuce is usually partially or completely unretractable because of physiologic adherence between the glans and inner preputial skin and/or tightness of the preputial ring. Ease of retractability of the prepuce increases with age, with complete retraction possible in at least two-thirds of 11–15-year-old and 95% of 16–17-year-old uncircumcised males (Oster, 1968; Herzog and Alvarez, 1986; Kayaba *et al.*, 1996). Therefore, true phimosis is present in childhood only in cases of secondary fibrosis or balanitis xerotica obliterans of the prepuce, which occur in 0.8–1.5% of uncircumcised boys (Rickwood, 1999).

Circumcision

The prevalence of routine neonatal circumcision in the USA has dropped from close to 90% in the mid-1960s to an estimated 64% in 1995 (Laumann *et al.*, 1997; American Academy of Pediatrics, 1999).

Epidemiologic data indicate that there are marked differences in circumcision rates based on socioeconomic class, ethnicity, and religious affiliation. The most recent American Academy of Pediatrics (AAP) Task Force on Circumcision report (1999) supports a growing trend away from neonatal circumcision. However, the degree of controversy surrounding this issue is made clear by the shifts in AAP policy over the last 25 years. In the most recent report, the AAP Task Force acknowledges potential medical benefits to neonatal circumcision but concludes that these do not warrant its routine use. Benefits include reduction in the risk of urinary tract infection (UTI) in infant males and development of penile cancer as an adult. For example, uncircumcised infant boys are three to ten times more likely to develop UTI than circumcised male infants, probably because of an increased rate of periurethral and inner preputial bacterial colonization (American Academy of Pediatrics, 1999). Similarly, penile cancer occurs almost exclusively in uncircumcised males. However, penile hygiene, including foreskin retraction with periodic cleansing, may also play a role. Nevertheless, both of these conditions are rare and their prevention by routine circumcision may not be justified. The argument that the risk of sexually transmitted disease is reduced by circumcision is not supported by available data (Laumann et al., 1997; Van Howe, 1999).

Similarly, the risk of penile problems of sufficient severity to require circumcision is low (Herzog and Alvarez, 1986; American Academy of Pediatrics: Task Force on Circumcision, 1999; Rickwood, 1999). Balanitis and balanoposthitis, characterized by erythema, edema, and purulent preputial discharge involving the glans and/or prepuce, occurs in 3–10% of uncircumcised boys. Paraphimosis, or retraction of a tight preputial ring with consequent severe glanular edema, is rare. Circumcision may be necessary only when these problems are severe or recurrent. Since circumcision in older boys requires general anesthesia and may be associated with morbidity (Griffiths et al., 1985) it should not be performed without a clear medical indication.

Newborn circumcision is performed with the Mogen or Gomco clamp or the Plastibell device (Baskin et al., 1996). Contraindications include hypospadias, chordee, penoscrotal fusion, buried penis, micropenis, and bleeding disorders. Complete separation of the prepuce from the glans with circumferential visualization of the corona is essential for adequate and safe newborn circumcision. Since significant physiologic response to pain has been documented in neonates undergoing circumcision, local anesthetic should be used (American Academy of Pediatric: Task Force on Circumcision, 1999). Choice of anesthetic technique depends on the skills and experience of the surgeon, although penile ring block may be the easiest and most effective alternative (Lander et al., 1997). Older infants and children are circumcised under general anesthesia using a free-hand sleeve resection technique.

Complications of circumcision

The risk of complications after circumcision is 0.2–5% (Baskin et al., 1996). Bleeding is most common, occurring in 0.1% and more often in older boys, but is usually self-limited. Infection typically responds to local care but in rare cases may be associated with sepsis, necrotizing fasciitis, or death. Other complications of varying severity may occur, some of which may require further surgical intervention. Partial denudation of the penile shaft is consequent to removal of an excess amount of skin, but healing takes place uneventfully with local wound care alone. Further intervention is required only to correct secondary chordee or phimosis. Conversely, excess or 'redundant' preputial skin remaining after circumcision is often a source of concern for parents but surgical intervention is rarely required. Resolution of physiologic adherence between the remaining skin and the glans will occur spontaneously after puberty, as in uncircumcised boys. Contracture of the healing edges of skin over the glans may produce secondary phimosis, also known as a trapped penis (Fig. 33.1a). Correction requires excision of scar and in some cases penile skin flaps or Z-plasty for closure. Skin bridges (Fig. 33.1b) between the shaft and glans may cause chordee and should be sharply incised. Inclusion cysts (Fig. 33.1c) comprised of retained subcutaneous epithelium should be completely excised. More severe injuries include glans amputation (Fig. 33.1d), which can often be repaired acutely with success. However, subsequent meatal stenosis may require delayed urethroplasty (Baskin et al., 1997). Total penile necrosis (Fig. 33.1e) is a rare but devastating complication for which gender reassignment has been recommended (Gearhart and Rock, 1989). However, long-term follow-up of such a patient gender reassigned in infancy indicates that this approach is not

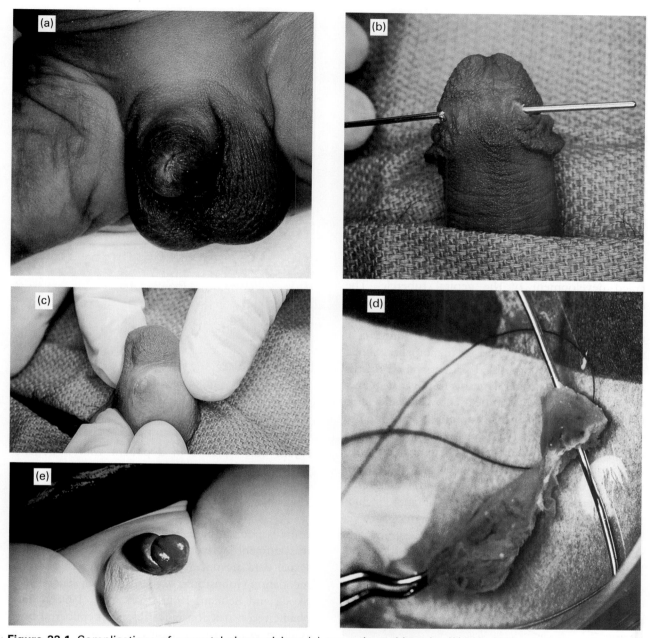

Figure 33.1 Complications of neonatal circumcision: (*a*) secondary phimosis; (*b*) skin bridge between glans and penile skin; (*c*) penile cyst; (*d*) glans amputation; (*e*) penile necrosis.

necessarily appropriate since male gender identity as a consequence of testosterone imprinting may already be well established very early in life (Diamond, 1996).

Meatal stenosis occurs almost exclusively in circumcised boys. The proposed etiologies include frenular devascularization or chronic meatitis from exposure of the unprotected meatus to diaper irritation (Persad *et al.*, 1995; Hensle, 1996). The inci-

dence of symptomatic meatal stenosis after neonatal circumcision appears to be ≤ 10% based on limited available data (Stenham *et al.*, 1986; Persad *et al.*, 1995). Non-specific symptoms such as urethral bleeding, dysuria, or other voiding complaints may be present, but the pathognomonic finding is upward deflection of the urinary stream as a consequence of an acquired ventral web (Fig. 33.2) (American Academy of Pediatrics Urology Section, 1978).

Urinary tract imaging is unlikely to disclose significant pathology in the absence of incontinence or UTI. Meatoplasty or meatotomy can be performed under a brief general anesthetic or, preferably, in the office after a generous application of EMLA cream (Cartwright *et al.*, 1996) (see Chapter 8).

Defects of number or position

Penile agenesis

Penile agenesis, or aphallia, is complete absence of the penis in an otherwise normal phenotypic and genotypic male (Fig. 33.3) (Oesch *et al.*, 1987; Skoog and Belman, 1989). Rudimentary erectile tissue is occasionally present. The estimated incidence is 1 in 10–30 million and the presumed etiology absence or failed development of the genital tubercle. The majority (54%) of patients have other genitourinary anomalies (e.g. cryptorchidism, renal and/or ureteral malformations) with or without gastrointestinal, musculoskeletal, and cardiovascular anomalies. Skoog and Belman (1989) classified patients based on the relationship of the urethral meatus to the anal sphincter, noting increased additional anomalies and mortality with more proximal location of the meatus. The three variations that they described, in decreasing order of frequency, include postsphincteric with anterior perianal urethra, presphincteric with urethrorectal fistula, and urethral atresia with vesicorectal fistula. Surgical intervention during infancy, including urethral transposition and bowel vaginoplasty via a posterior sagittal approach plus orchiectomy and scrotoplasty, is advocated (Stolar *et al.*, 1987; Hendren, 1997). Available data indicate that out-

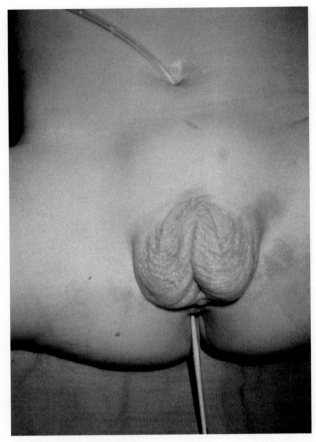

Figure 33.3 Aphallia in a patient with a perianal urethral opening identified by sound.

come is poor in patients raised as males and gender reassignment is advocated; however, detailed psychosexual data are not available to support this recommendation (Johnston *et al.*, 1977; Oesch *et al.*, 1987; Skoog and Belman, 1989; Cifti *et al.*, 1995). Since phallic reconstruction is feasible in prepubertal boys (Gilbert *et al.*, 1993), maintenance of male gender should be considered an option in discussions with the patient's family (see Chapters 30 and 31).

Diphallia

Penile duplication or diphallia occurs in an estimated 1 in 5–6 million births (Marti-Bonmati *et al.*, 1989; Zolfaghari *et al.*, 1995; Hollowell *et al.*, 1997). The proposed etiology is branching or splitting of the genital tubercle soon after the 5th week of gestation. A balanced genetic translocation involving chromosomes 1 and 14 has been reported in one case (Karna and

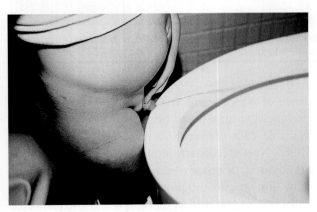

Figure 33.2 Upwardly deflected urinary stream in a boy with significant meatal web.

Kapur, 1994). Variants include partial and complete forms of true diphallia and bifid phallus. In the bifid variant, which is more common, the penis is branched at any point along its length, with each shaft containing a single corpus cavernosum. The designation of true diphallia is reserved for cases in which an accessory tricorporal penis (both cavernosa and spongiosum present), which may be hypoplastic, is present. The accessory organ may be located in the perineum or upper thigh. Ultrasound may be useful to characterize corporal anatomy (Marti-Bonmati *et al.*, 1989). Associated malformations are usually present and may include urethral duplication or agenesis, bladder duplication or exstrophy, hypospadias, epispadias, widened symphysis, cryptorchidism, and/or anorectal, renal, or scrotal anomalies. Surgical repair involves excision of one completely duplicated penis or fusion of the bifid penes with urethral reconstruction.

Abnormal development

Penile torsion

Rotational deformity of the penis, usually in a counterclockwise direction, is most often associated with hypospadias and chordee but may occur as an isolated abnormality (Pomerantz *et al.*, 1978). The incidence in a cohort of normal newborn males was 1.5%, with curvature of at least 90° seen in 0.7% (Ben-Ari *et al.*, 1985). Deviation of the median raphe without torsion was noted in 10% of newborns. Although a functional abnormality is absent if the penis is straight, penile torsion can be corrected in most cases by penile skin degloving and realignment.

Penoscrotal fusion

Foreshortening of an otherwise normal ventral penile shaft occurs when the ventral penoscrotal junction is located distal to its normal position (Fig. 33.4) (Perlmutter and Chamberlain, 1972; Redman 1985a). This abnormality is called penoscrotal fusion or webbed penis, and may be congenital, due to removal of excess ventral skin during circumcision, or associated with hypospadias. Large, bilateral hydroceles in infancy may cause apparent penoscrotal fusion, which disappears with resolution of the hydroceles (Perlmutter and Chamberlain, 1972). Lengthening of the ventral shaft is most simply accomplished by preputial unfurling with or without ventral transfer of dorsal preputial skin. If the foreskin

is not tight, use of the inner preputial skin for ventral shaft coverage during circumcision may be all that is necessary to correct the defect.

Concealed penis

An otherwise normal penis that appears to be small is called a concealed, buried, or inconspicuous penis (Fig. 33.5) (Cromie *et al.*, 1998). Measurements of stretched penile length and penile diameter are normal. Etiologic factors include a prominent prepubic fat pad, generalized obesity, and/or poor fixation of the subcutaneous tissue of the penis to Buck's fascia. Most commonly the patient is asymptomatic and spontaneous resolution can be anticipated with change in body habitus at puberty (Bergeson *et al.*, 1993; Little, 1994). The extent of psychological distress in the untreated patient is unclear and when surgical intervention is elected results are poorly documented. Only Cromie *et al.* (1998) report prolonged (median 5 years) follow-up, with durable improvement in most cases using a preputial unfurling and degloving procedure similar to techniques used to correct penoscrotal fusion. The use of more complex procedures, such as prepubic liposuction or lipectomy, and closure with Z-plasties or skin flaps not only is rarely indicated but may also cause unnecessary scarring. Early failure is reported in as many as 35% of cases and long-term results are unknown (Maizels *et al.*, 1986; Bergeson *et al.*, 1993; Chuang, 1995).

Micropenis

A penis that measures more than 2 or 2.5 standard deviations below the mean in stretched length for age but is otherwise normally formed is called a

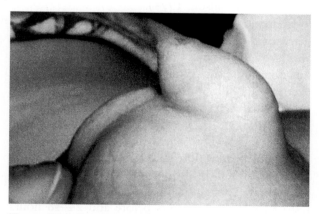

Figure 33.4 Penoscrotal fusion.

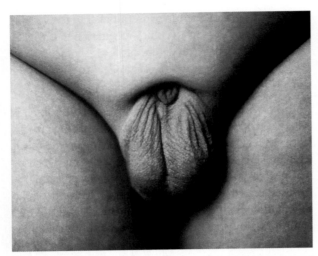

Figure 33.5 Concealed penis in an obese prepubertal boy with normal stretched penile length.

micropenis (Lee *et al.*, 1980b; Aaronson, 1994). In newborns, a stretched length of less than 2.0 cm is considered abnormal. Normal development of the urethra and prepuce implies normal first trimester development, with impaired penile growth occurring in the second and third trimesters. Cryptorchidism may also be present. The most common etiology is gonadotropin deficiency with or without panhypopituitarism (Lee *et al.*, 1980b). Other endocrine causes include growth hormone deficiency, testicular dysgenesis or regression and, rarely, 5α-reductase deficiency (Sinnecker *et al.*, 1996) or partial androgen insensitivity (Quigley *et al.*, 1995). Micropenis may be present in gonadal determination disorders, such as Kleinfelter's syndrome and XX sex reversal, and in Prader–Willi, Lawrence–Moon–Biedl, Robinow, and other rare syndromes, or it may be idiopathic (Lee *et al.*, 1980b; Aaronson, 1994).

Evaluation of patients generally includes karyotype, determination of serum glucose, electrolyte, cortisol, and growth hormone levels, as well as thyroid function tests and pituitary imaging, as indicated (Lee *et al.*, 1980b; Aaronson, 1994). Testicular function can be determined by measuring serum luteinizing hormone (LH), follicle-stimulating hormone (FSH), and testosterone before and after human chorionic gonadotropin (hCG) stimulation. The dose of hCG is 500–1500 International units (approx. 3000 IU/m^2) every other day for 5–7 days with serum testosterone measurements before and 24–48 hours after the last dose. Newborns can be evaluated for the

normal spontaneous surge in serum gonadotropins and testosterone within the first few weeks of life; absence suggests a central (pituitary or hypothalamic) defect.

After diagnostic studies are complete, androgen stimulation therapy using intramuscular depot testosterone, 25 mg every 3–4 weeks for several months in infants, has been recommended to assess penile growth potential (Lee *et al.*, 1980b; Aaronson, 1994). Unfortunately, response to testosterone does not always correlate with adequate penile size in adulthood, and may vary with the etiology of micropenis (Lee *et al.*, 1980a; Money *et al.*, 1985). In this regard, patients with palpable testes (Kogan and Williams, 1977) and significant response to gonadotropin-releasing hormone (GnRH) and hCG stimulation tests (Okuyama *et al.*, 1980) appear more likely to have adequate long-term penile growth, although some do not (Money *et al.*, 1985). Limited data suggest that treatment with dihydrotestosterone cream may be an effective alternative to parenteral testosterone, particularly in peripubertal males and in some patients who have failed testosterone therapy (Choi *et al.*, 1993). In patients with isolated growth hormone deficiency, growth hormone replacement appears to be sufficient for adequate penile growth (Levy and Husmann, 1996). Concerns that early androgen therapy might itself limit long-term penile growth potential are not supported by observations of males with early androgen excess syndromes (Sutherland *et al.*, 1996).

Until recently, routine gender reassignment was recommended for patients who show no penile growth response to testosterone (Lee *et al.*, 1980b; Aaronson, 1994). However, the advisibility of routine gender reassignment in genetic males with functioning testes has been questioned in other contexts (Diamond, 1996), and the long-term results of reassignment for micropenis are not known. Adequate sexual functioning and clear male gender identity in adulthood have been reported in some patients raised as males with persistent small penile size in adulthood (Reilly and Woodhouse, 1989), but not in others (Money *et al.*, 1985). Additional long-term follow-up data are critically needed to facilitate clinical decision making in these patients. Therefore, gender reassignment should be performed with caution and should be accompanied by expert, ongoing patient and family counseling, including a discussion of the risks and benefits of penile reconstruction (see Chapter 30).

Priapism

Priapism is defined as a prolonged, frequently painful penile erection not sustained by sexual activity. The most common pediatric cause is homozygous sickle cell (SS) disease, but other possible etiologies include other hemoglobinopathies, leukemia, local malignancy, viral infections, pelvic infections or appendicitis, trauma, diabetes, amyloidosis, and Fabry's disease (Dewan *et al.*, 1989; Friedman, 1998). Low-flow priapism is usually present in affected boys with sickle cell disease, while a high-flow state is typically present in trauma-induced priapism, but may rarely also be present in sicklers (Ramos *et al.*, 1995; Callewaert *et al.*, 1998). The incidence of priapism in males with sickle cell disease is 2–12% (Tarry *et al.*, 1987; Hamre *et al.*, 1991; Fowler *et al.*, 1991; Sharpsteen *et al.*, 1993; Miller *et al.*, 1995). Stuttering episodes usually lasting less than 24 hours are common in both pediatric and adult patients. Initial episodes may occur in early childhood.

Priapism can be characterized by the site and degree of blood flow or stasis in the erectile tissues. Tumescence is usually limited to the corpora cavernosa but in some cases may also involve the corpus spongiosum, a situation termed tricorporeal priapism (Sharpsteen *et al.*, 1993). Spongiosal involvement, described in postpubertal individuals, is characterized by a firm, tender, engorged glans. Voiding difficulty may occur in some patients. Studies used to characterize degree of blood flow include analysis of aspirated penile blood, technetium-99m (^{99m}Tc) penile flow studies, and color Doppler ultrasonography. Low-flow priapism is characterized by acidosis, hypercarbia, and hypoxemia on penile blood gas analysis. The usefulness and reliability of penile nuclear scans and Doppler studies in children remain unclear. Miller *et al.* (1995) reported that nuclear scans did not predict outcome in a series of pediatric patients with sickle cell-associated priapism.

The initial treatment of patients with priapism due to sickle cell disease is hydration, analgesia, and transfusion to achieve a target hemoglobin S concentration of 30% or less (Seeler, 1973; Tarry *et al.*, 1987; Hamre, 1991; Miller *et al.*, 1995). Prepubertal boys appear to respond more commonly to medical therapy than older patients (Fowler *et al.*, 1991). Exchange transfusion has been associated with acute neurologic events characterized by reversible or irreversible cerebral ischemia, termed the ASPEN syndrome (asso-ciation of sickle cell disease, priapism, exchange transfusion, and neurologic events) (Siegel *et al.*, 1993). Morbidity from this complication may be reduced by gradual or partial exchange transfusion, recognition of prodromal headache, and close monitoring.

Total lack of response to medical therapy after 24–48 hours indicates that the patient may benefit from surgical intervention (Tarry *et al.*, 1987; Miller *et al.*, 1995; Chakrabarty *et al.*, 1996). The older view that surgical intervention in prepubertal patients with sickle cell priapism is unnecessary if not contraindicated (Seeler, 1973) appears unjustified based on documented erectile dysfunction in boys following prolonged episodes of priapism (Mykulak and Glassberg, 1990; Chakrabarty *et al.*, 1996). The patient with high-flow priapism diagnosed by corporeal aspiration and blood gas analysis who does not respond to cavernosum–spongiosum shunting may be a candidate for superselective embolization of dorsal penile and cavernous arteries (Callewaert *et al.*, 1998). For low-flow states, shunting may be performed by bilateral placement of a percutaneous catheter through the glans and corpus cavernosum, as in a modification of Winter's procedure (Ulman *et al.*, 1996) or by formal cavernosum–spongiosum anastomosis in the glans or perineum. These usually produce detumescence. Available long-term follow-up data suggest that potency is more commonly preserved in prepubertal patients, after episodes of shorter duration and when successful intervention occurs early (Emond *et al.*, 1980; Noe *et al.*, 1981; Chakrabarty *et al.*, 1996).

A variety of other treatments is also recommended for patients with sickle cell disease and priapism; however, data are anecdotal or limited. α-Adrenergic agents such as etilefrine (Virag *et al.*, 1996) have been given orally or intracavernosally with some success. This is such a benign therapeutic alternative its use should be considered as the first treatment step. Detumescence with hydroxyurea has been reported (Al Jam'a and Al Dabbous, 1998) but not confirmed in a large series. Other options include treatment with gonadotropin-releasing hormone analogues (Levine and Guss, 1993).

Persistent, apparently painless penile erection has also been observed in newborns (Walker and Casale, 1997). This condition resolves spontaneously in 2–6 days with no adverse sequelae. Associated, possibly contributing factors include polycythemia and birth trauma, although many reported cases are idiopathic.

Scrotal abnormalities

Two main types of scrotal pathology occur in the pediatric population: the commonly observed acute swelling of a normal scrotum (discussed under Inguinoscrotal disease) and the rare abnormalities of scrotal development.

Defects of number or position

Scrotal agenesis

Complete absence of the scrotum is an extremely rare anomaly, reported only twice in the modern literature (Wright, 1993; Verga and Avolio, 1994). The penis was normal in both cases, the perineum was smooth with a median raphe present, and both testes were superior to the expected scrotal site. Successful repair using preputial skin was performed.

Accessory scrotum

Ectopic scrotal tissue in addition to a normally developed scrotum is designated accessory scrotum or, in females, accessory labioscrotal fold. This anomaly is very rare, with 25 cases identified in a recent literature review (Sule et al., 1994). The accessory tissue is located on the perineum in the majority of cases and associated with a perineal lipoma and no other genitourinary anomalies. A case of isolated penile accessory scrotum has also been reported (Coplen et al., 1995). In the absence of a perineal lipoma, accessory perineal scrota are usually associated with other anomalies, including hypospadias, diphallia, defects of scrotal position, anorectal anomalies, and the VACTERL (vertebral, anal, cardiac, tracheoesophageal renal and limb anomalies) association (Spears et al., 1992). Sule et al. (1994) hypothesize that when present, the lipoma disrupts the continuity of the developing labioscrotal fold and the etiology in other cases is generalized perineal maldevelopment.

Ectopic scrotum

Ectopic positioning of the scrotum is usually unilateral, with the ectopic tissue usually suprainguinal but in some cases infrainguinal (femoral) or on the thigh (Lamm and Kaplan, 1977; Elder and Jeffs, 1982; Hoar et al., 1998). The ipsilateral testis is usually present within the ectopic hemiscrotum, although associated cryptorchidism has been reported. Ipsilateral renal and ureteral anomalies are common, so patients should be evaluated for upper tract anomalies. Associated skeletal defects, penile torsion or chordee, and cleft palate have also been reported. The etiology is uncertain, but may be related to a gubernacular defect failure of migration of the labioscrotal fold, or fetal deformation secondary to limb compression (foot). Treatment is generally simply achieved by flap scrotoplasty and orchidopexy.

Bifid scrotum

Incomplete fusion of the labioscrotal folds may produce a partial or complete separation of otherwise normally positioned hemiscrota in patients with severe hypospadias or chordee. The defect may be corrected by excision of the abnormal tissue and creation of a new scrotal raphe with reapproximation of the hemiscrota in the midline.

Penoscrotal transposition

In cases of penoscrotal transposition, part or all of the scrotum is located superior to the penile shaft. The spectrum of findings ranges from a normal sized penis with confluent scrotal tissue both anterior and posterior (shawl or doughnut scrotum) to complete transposition of a rudimentary penis to the perineum behind an intact scrotum, a phenotype similar to that of penile agenesis (Parida et al., 1995). The posterior aspect of the scrotum may be bifid and/or hypoplastic, and hypospadias and chordee are frequently present (Fig. 33.6). However, multiple other anomalies of diverse organ systems have also been identified. These include renal, central nervous system, developmental, gastrointestinal, respiratory, limb, vertebral,

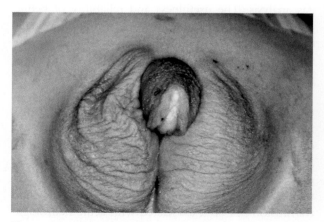

Figure 33.6 Partial penoscrotal transposition and bifid scrotum in patient with proximal hypospadias.

cardiovascular, facial, and ocular anomalies (Parida *et al.*, 1995). Three types of chromosomal defect have been identified: trisomies 8 and 18, and distal deletions of the long arm of chromosome 13 (Bartsch *et al.*, 1996). Correction of the defect may be performed during or subsequent to hypospadias repair by mobilization of the anteriorly placed scrotal skin with ventral transposition and closure, as described by Glenn and Anderson (1973) (see Chapter 32). In some cases ventral penile tethering may occur postoperatively that may be corrected by interposition of thigh-based neurovascular flaps (Levy *et al.*, 1997).

Median raphe cysts

Midline cysts may arise anywhere along the median raphe between the urethral meatus and anus (Sadler *et al.*, 1995; LeVasseur and Perry, 1997; Rattan *et al.*, 1997). Their origin is believed to be epithelial or endothelial rests trapped in an aberrant subcutaneous location during developmental approximation of the urethral and genital folds. They may be large and elongated and appear translucent. Histologically, they are lined with cuboidal or squamous epithelium and contain sebacious material. Rarely, the proximal portion of the cyst may traverse the urogenital diaphragm and extend into the pelvis. Magnetic resonance imaging may be useful to define the extent of the lesion preoperatively if pelvic extension appears likely. Treatment is complete excision of the cysts with midline closure.

Inguinoscrotal disease

Varicocele

Population studies have confirmed the observation that a varicocele first becomes clinically evident between the ages of 10 and 15 years (Steeno *et al.*, 1976) and once a varicocele is present it will normally persist for the remainder of that individual's life (Oster, 1971). The varicocele which has its origin in adolescence may be a major cause of infertility in adults. However, if one waits until adulthood to treat varicocele-induced infertility, success is unlikely for the majority of men (Dubin and Amelar, 1975). Because of this experience, recent efforts have focused on identifying teenagers with an asymptomatic varicocele in an attempt to identify individuals at risk, intervene earlier, and hopefully improve results. Although this approach seems reasonable, the problem for the

clinician has been establishing uniform criteria for treatment. The observation that a varicocele occurs in 15% of men adds to the difficulties in deciding when treatment is indicated. Do we treat all men with a varicocele or just selected ones?

The vast majority of teenagers with a varicocele are discovered during a routine school physical, are asymptomatic, and are unaware of the presence of the varicocele. As a consequence most of the teenagers identified with a varicocele have a grade II (mass or veins 1–2 cm in diameter) or grade III (large mass or veins easily visible and greater than 2 cm in diameter) varicocele. A child with a small varicocele (veins 1 cm or less in diameter) can only be detected by a skilled examiner, and most will escape early detection. No investigators have reported using color Doppler ultrasound to detect a subclinical varicocele in a teenager and therefore this entity appears to have no clinical significance in the teenage population at the current time.

Since most teenagers with a varicocele are detected during a routine physical examination by a primary care physician, it is reasonable to assume that a teenager with a large varicocele is more likely to be diagnosed than one with a small varicocele. Dubin and Amelar (1970) concluded that the size of a varicocele was not a significant fertility variable. However, Fariss *et al.* (1981) and co-workers demonstrated that in adult men found to have a varicocele on routine physical examination there was a greater chance of a man with a large varicocele having a sperm count less than 20 million/ml than a man with a small varicocele. Several other studies have reported that in men with a large varicocele there is greater impairment in semen parameters than in men with a small varicocele (Szabo and Kessler, 1984; Tinga *et al.*, 1984; Steckel *et al.*, 1993). Steeno *et al.* (1976) noted that, with increasing varicocele size, there was progressively more volume loss of the testis ipsilateral to the varicocele. Other studies (Sigman and Jarow, 1997) have also demonstrated lower testicular volumes in men with a large varicocele than those with a small one. This loss of testicular volume may be significant because the seminiferous tubules comprise greater than 50% of the testicular mass, and in adult men total sperm count correlates with testicular volume (Johnson *et al.*, 1980; Rey *et al.*, 1993). Therefore, it is reasonable to conclude that an individual with a large varicocele may be at greater risk for testicular injury than someone with a small varicocele (Haans *et al.*, 1991).

The mechanism by which a varicocele induces testicular injury is still unresolved, although many theories have been proposed. Investigators have noted that a varicocele, both clinically and experimentally, results in an increase in scrotal and testicular temperature (Zorgniotti and MacLeod, 1973). An increase in testicular temperature has been shown to be toxic to the testis in humans as well as other mammals with scrotal testes (Robinson et al., 1968; Amelar and Dubin, 1987; Levine et al., 1990). Aggar (1971) reported that following varicocele correction there was a good correlation between the fall in left testicular temperature and the improvement in spermatogenesis. Kass and Salisz (1991) measured scrotal temperatures in adolescents with grade II and III varicoceles and reported that there was a significant bilateral elevation in scrotal temperature when compared with control subjects without a varicocele. They also noted that the higher the left scrotal temperature the greater the volume loss of the left testis. Following successful varicocele correction scrotal temperature normalized.

In an infertile adult male with a unilateral left varicocele, abnormal testicular histology can be demonstrated in both testes and involves all cell types, although the changes are typically more pronounced in the left testis (Fig. 33.7) (Charney, 1962; Ibrahim et al., 1977; Wang et al., 1991). Similar histopathology has been demonstrated bilaterally in the adolescent with a unilateral varicocele but the abnormalities are less severe (Hienz et al., 1980; Kass et al., 1987).

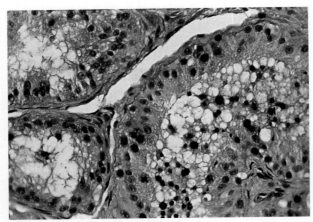

Figure 33.7 Testicular histology in a patient with a varicocele showing Sertoli only tubules and severe maturation arrest. Only 25% of tubules were normal in this patient (× 250).

It is important to note that, while the pathologic changes in the seminiferous tubules, blood vessels, and Sertoli cells are present to varying degrees in infertile men with a varicocele, the relative severity of the abnormality in these cell types is not the key prognostic variable. Investigators have reported that it is the severity of the Leydig cell pathology that is most significant in determining the potential for reversibility of the varicocele-induced testicular injury (Hadziselimovic et al., 1986). Individuals with Leydig cell hyperplasia have a very poor prognosis, while those with Leydig cell atrophy have a better prognosis for fertility following varicocele correction. The prognosis for return of fertility is independent of the degree of tubular pathology and ultimately it is the degree of the pathologic changes in the Leydig–Sertoli cell interrelationship that ultimately decides whether surgery will be successful with regard to fertility (Hadziselimovic et al., 1995). Hadziselimovic et al. (1989) reported that Leydig cell atrophy was the predominant pathologic finding on testicular biopsy in teenagers undergoing varicocele surgery (74%) when compared with adults in whom Leydig cell hyperplasia was more common with atrophy was found in only 22%. These various histologic studies taken as a whole suggest that varicocele-induced histologic abnormalities occur in adolescents and are progressive. The pathology is potentially reversible early on but once Leydig cell hyperplasia is present surgical correction of the varicocele will be unlikely to have beneficial effects.

Varicoceles also induce endocrinologic abnormalities that parallel the histopathology. Weiss et al. (1978) measured the in vitro synthesis in testosterone from testicular biopsy material and noted that there was a significant reduction in testosterone formation in 90% of infertile men with a varicocele. In these same individuals peripheral levels of testosterone and LH were normal. Other investigators have also reported significant varicocele-induced Leydig cell dysfunction and noted that the abnormalities are progressive (Ando et al., 1982; Spera et al., 1983; Su et al., 1995).

An exaggerated gonadotropin response to the administration of GnRH has been demonstrated in infertile men with a varicocele and is thought to be the result of a primary testicular injury. The excessive release of LH following GnRH stimulation is an indicator of Leydig cell dysfunction and the exaggerated FSH response an indicator of an abnormality of the seminiferous tubules. Nagao *et al.* (1986) measured the response to GnRH stimulation and noted that semen and hormonal abnormalities can be observed in both fertile and infertile men with a varicocele, suggesting that there may be some degree of testicular dysfunction in all men with a varicocele, regardless of their fertility status. They suggested that perhaps with increasing age the varicocele-induced testicular injury could become clinically evident in more men. Several investigators (Hudson *et al.*, 1985; Bickel and Dickstein, 1989; Fujisawa *et al.*, 1994; Atikeler *et al.*, 1996; Bablok *et al.*, 1997) demonstrated that the excessive gonadotropin response to GnRH stimulation in infertile men was reversible after varicocele correction only in those individuals whose spermiograms also improved. Individuals who did not demonstrate an improved postoperative gonadotropin response pattern did not show any improvement in their spermiogram.

The gonadotropin response to GnRH stimulation has been shown to be a useful diagnostic tool for evaluating testicular function in teenagers (Lipshultz *et al.*, 1976; Dickerman *et al.*, 1978). Kass *et al.* (1993a) measured the gonadotropin response pattern to GnRH stimulation in adolescent males with a varicocele and compared it with a group of normal teenagers without a varicocele. They noted that an abnormal gonadotropin response was present in almost one-third of teenagers with a varicocele, and that this test may be useful in identifying those varicocele patients with early evidence of testicular injury.

Barwell (1885) was the first to report volume loss of the testis ipsilateral to a varicocele in a teenager, and noted the testis 'became harder and regained some of its dimensions' following surgical correction. In adult men with infertility both testes tend to be smaller than in aged-matched control groups without a varicocele. Kass and Belman (1987) performed varicocele ligation on adolescent males with grade II–III left-sided varicocele and volume loss of the left testis. Significant catch-up growth of the left testis was noted in 80% of patients. Subsequent studies have confirmed their findings and indicate that a varicocele can be responsible for testicular growth retardation, and early successful correction can reverse this process (Laven *et al.*, 1992; Yamamoto *et al.*, 1995; Vasavada *et al.*, 1997). In the majority of adolescents with a varicocele, testicular volume loss is the most common indication of testicular injury and therefore the most significant indication for interven-

tion. Normal testicular size correlates with stage of sexual maturity (Zachmann *et al.*, 1974; Daniel *et al.*, 1982). Testicular volume progressively increases from approximately 4 to 25 ml during pubertal development, making it difficult to calculate a normal testis volume in any individual before adulthood. Most investigators have used the right testis as the 'normal control'. If the left testis is 3 ml or more smaller, then significant testicular volume loss is considered to be present (Fig. 33.8). Accurate testicular volume measurements are possible with a standard Prader orchiometer (Fig. 33.9) and correlate well with volume measurement by ultrasonography; however, the degree of correlation is dependent on the investigator's clinical experience (Behre *et al.*, 1989).

In adults with a varicocele the assessment of a semen sample is a reasonable first step in the evaluation process since there are established normal parameters. Unfortunately, in adolescents it is often difficult to obtain such samples, and even when available, normal adult values for semen volume, spermatozoa concentration, and morphology are not achieved until 2–3 years after the onset of puberty (Janczewski and Bablok, 1985). It is important to remember that a single normal semen analysis does not predict future normality, since the effect of a varicocele may increase with time (Charney, 1962). It is recommended that every adult with a palpable varicocele should have a semen analysis on an annual basis until the completion of his family in order to ensure that abnormalities do not develop.

Current data indicate that it is important to identify and evaluate all teenagers with a varicocele. Certainly no one can predict with absolute certainty whether any adolescent with a varicocele will be fer-

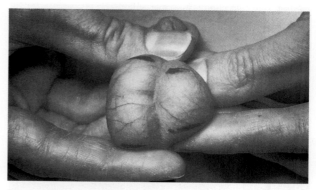

Figure 33.8 Left testicular volume loss in a patient with a left varicocele.

tile or infertile; however, based on existing information it can be expected that many will develop a fertility problem that becomes progressive if left untreated (Okuyama *et al.*, 1988; Paduch and Niedzielski, 1997; Lenzi *et al.*, 1998). Individuals with volume loss of the testis ipsilateral to the varicocele appear to have a greater likelihood of having a normal semen analysis if treated as a teenager than if left untreated (Hosli, 1988; Belloli *et al.*, 1995; Sayfan *et al.*, 1997). Similarly, individuals with large varicoceles may be at future risk for developing testicular volume loss and abnormal semen parameters. Although there are concerns that an abnormal GnRH stimulation test may be associated with similar long-term risks (Kass *et al.*, 1989), that hypothesis is not generally accepted as an indicator for intervention when other parameters are normal. Similarly, it is unclear whether intervention in otherwise normal individuals with bilaterally palpable varicoceles or scrotal discomfort is reasonable, and should not be considered routine. Persistently abnormal semen parameters in older teenagers and adults are of significant concern and should be considered an indication for intervention.

Multiple techniques have been proposed for correction of a varicocele in a teenager (Mandressi *et al.*, 1996; Abdulmaaboud *et al.*, 1998). Selective transvenous embolization of the internal spermatic vein (Lenz *et al.*, 1996; Punekar *et al.*, 1996; Perala *et al.*, 1998) is a complex, invasive procedure with a significant recurrence and non-occlusion rate. Laparoscopic venous ligation (Miersch *et al.*, 1995; Belloli *et al.*, 1996; Humphrey and Najmaldin, 1997; Kattan, 1998) requires intubation and bladder catheterization, and has the potential for significant intra-abdominal complications. Conventional inguinal (Ivanissevich,

1918) and retroperitoneal approaches with attempted preservation of the testicular artery are simple and relatively complication-free procedures but have an unacceptably high risk for failure (Atassi *et al.*, 1995). Current data suggest that the above techniques are not the best choice for varicocele correction in teenagers. The Palomo technique (Palomo, 1949) with mass ligation of the internal spermatic vessels (Ivanissevich, 1918; Hsu *et al.*, 1993; Parrott and Hewatt, 1994; Stern *et al.*, 1998), or the inguinal (Minevich *et al.*, 1998) or subinguinal approach (Marmar and Kim, 1994) with microscopic ligation (Goldstein *et al.*, 1992; Lima *et al.*, 1997; Lemack *et al.*, 1998) of all venous channels are the procedures with the highest success rate and fewest complications, and are the procedures of choice for varicocele correction in teenagers. However, secondary hydrocele is common with mass ligation of the internal spermatic vessels and the potential risk for testicular atrophy, should vasectomy be carried out in the future, must be considered. However, preservation of a single lymphatic vessel may prevent hydrocele.

Acute scrotal disease

Testicular torsion must be considered in any patient who complains of acute scrotal pain and swelling. Torsion of the testis is a surgical emergency because the likelihood of testicular salvage decreases as the duration of torsion increases. Conditions that may mimic testicular torsion, such as torsion of a testicular or epididymal appendage, epididymitis, trauma, hernia, hydrocele, varicocele, and Schönlein–Henoch purpura, generally do not require immediate surgical intervention. The cause of an acute scrotum can usually be established based on a careful history, a thorough physical examination, and appropriate diagnostic tests. The onset, character, and severity of symptoms must be determined. The physical examination includes inspection and palpation of the abdomen, testis, epididymis, scrotum, and inguinal region. Urinalysis should always be performed, but scrotal imaging is necessary only when the diagnosis remains unclear.

History

The history and physical examination can significantly narrow the differential diagnosis of an acute scrotum. Testicular torsion is most common in neonates and postpubertal boys, although it can occur in males of any age. Schönlein–Henoch purpura and torsion of

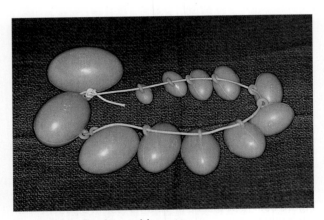

Figure 33.9 Prader orchiometer.

a testicular appendage typically occur in prepubertal boys, whereas epididymitis most often develops in postpubertal boys.

Testicular torsion usually begins abruptly in the early morning and the pain is often severe from the onset. Moderate pain developing gradually over several hours or days is more suggestive of epididymitis or appendiceal torsion.

A history of scrotal trauma is common and does not exclude the diagnosis of testicular torsion. Minor scrotal trauma incurred during sports activities or rough, boisterous play typically causes severe pain of short duration. Pain that persists for more than 1 hour after scrotal trauma is not normal and merits investigation to rule out testicular rupture or acute torsion. Pain that resolves promptly after scrotal trauma only to recur gradually a few days later suggests traumatic epididymitis.

Many patients with testis torsion describe previous episodes of similar pain that lasted for only a short time and resolved spontaneously. Acute on-and-off pain associated with scrotal swelling suggests intermittent torsion with spontaneous detorsion. Voiding dysfunction, congenital genitourinary anomalies, and urethral instrumentation can predispose patients to bacterial UTIs and secondary epididymitis.

Physical examination

A general abdominal examination should be performed, with particular attention given to flank tenderness and bladder distention. The inguinal regions should be examined for obvious hernias and any swelling or erythema. The spermatic cord in the groin may be tender in a patient with epididymitis but typically is not tender in a patient with testicular torsion.

The scrotum should be assessed for discrepancies in size, degree of swelling, presence and location of erythema, thickening of the skin, and position of the testis. Unilateral swelling without skin changes suggests the presence of a hernia or hydrocele. A high-riding testis with an abnormal (transverse) lie may suggest torsion (Fig. 33.10), but this diagnosis is unlikely if the pain has been present for over 12 hours and the scrotum has a normal appearance. In both epididymitis and testicular torsion, the affected hemiscrotum typically displays significant erythema and swelling after 24 hours.

The cremasteric reflex should always be assessed. One study (Caeser and Kaplan, 1994) found that the cremasteric reflex was intact in 100% of boys aged 30 months to 12 years but was not consistently normal in infants and teenagers. The cremasteric reflex is rarely intact in patients with testicular torsion but is usually present in patients with torsion of a testicular or epididymal appendage (Rabinowitz, 1984).

In early torsion, the entire testis is swollen and tender, and is larger than the unaffected testis. Tenderness limited to the upper pole suggests torsion of a testicular appendage, especially when a hard, tender nodule is palpable in this region. A small bluish discoloration representing the necrotic torsed appendage, known as the 'blue dot sign,' may be visible through the skin at the upper pole. This sign is virtually pathognomonic for appendiceal torsion when tenderness is also present. In early epididymitis, the epididymis exhibits tenderness and induration, but the testis itself is not tender. Swelling to the degree that the epididymis is no longer palpable can indicate testis torsion if the symptoms have been present for only a few hours. With both appendiceal torsion and epididymitis, loss of testicular landmarks occurs later in the clinical course. The testis may be elevated to elicit Prehn's sign. Lack of pain relief (negative sign) may contribute to the diagnosis of testicular torsion. If torsion is suspected, manual detorsion can be attempted by rotating the testis away from the midline.

Diagnostic studies

Urinalysis is performed to rule out UTI in any patient with an acute scrotum. Pyuria with or without bacteruria suggests infection and is consistent with epididymitis.

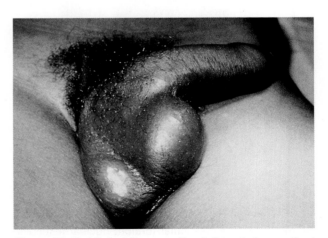

Figure 33.10 High-riding, swollen left testis in a patient with acute spermatic cord torsion.

Historically, it was thought that no imaging studies were useful in confirming the cause of an acute scrotum. Immediate surgical exploration was thus the standard approach when torsion was suspected. However, studies conducted in the past few years have shown that only 16–42% of boys with an acute scrotum have testicular torsion (al Mufti *et al.*, 1995; Lewis *et al.*, 1995; Watkin *et al.*, 1996). Therefore, routine exploration of all children is not reasonable if tests are available to improve diagnostic accuracy.

Initially, Doppler stethoscopes and conventional gray-scale ultrasonography were used to diagnose or exclude the presence of torsion, but these tests lack sensitivity and specificity (Deeg and Wild, 1990). Nuclear testicular flow studies are helpful, and when performed by experienced personnel can reliably identify children with torsion (Fig. 33.11), epididymitis (Fig. 33.12), and late torsion (Fig. 33.13). However, since it is strictly a blood-flow study a testicular scan is not helpful when a hydrocele or hematoma is present because these conditions may mimic the findings of torsion. In addition, it is of critical importance to localize the exact position of the testis, otherwise no reliable test is possible. However, most centers do not have personnel experienced in the performance or interpretation of nuclear medicine scrotal scans.

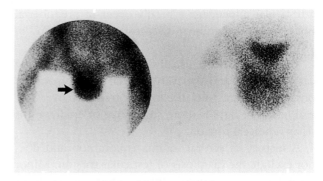

Figure 33.12 Epididymitis: nuclear testicular scan showing flow in both testes and increased activity in the right hemiscrotum (*arrow*).

Color Doppler sonography has become the most popular diagnostic modality to evaluate a child with an acute scrotum because it is non-invasive and has a diagnostic accuracy at least equal to that of nuclear scanning. It can semiquantitatively characterize blood flow, distinguish intratesticular and scrotal wall flow, and also be used to assess other pathologic conditions involving the scrotum (Figs. 33.14–33.16) (Dewire *et al.*, 1992; Wilbert *et al.*, 1993; Brown *et al.*, 1995). Proper technique is essential. When color Doppler examinations are not performed correctly,

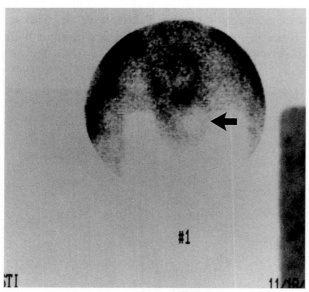

Figure 33.11 Early testicular torsion: nuclear testicular scan showing absence of tracer (*arrow*) in the left testis.

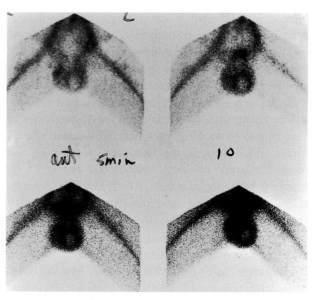

Figure 33.13 Late testicular torsion: nuclear testicular scan showing a 'halo' sign, or increased flow around the avascular left testis.

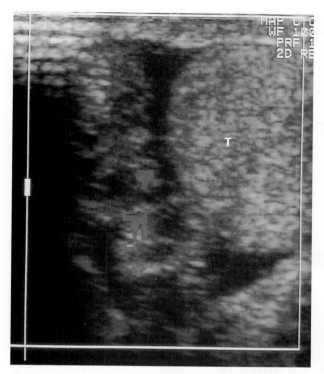

Figure 33.14 Testicular torsion: color Doppler ultrasound showing lack of flow in the testis (T).

studies can be false positive or false negative. Certain caveats are important to remember. It may not be possible to demonstrate a Doppler signal in the small testes of very young boys. Just seeing color dots does not mean that flow is present; one must see a wave

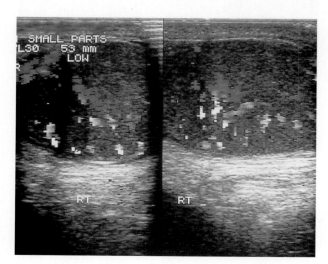

Figure 33.15 Orchitis: color Doppler ultrasound showing increased flow to the right testis.

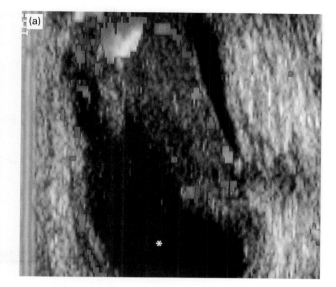

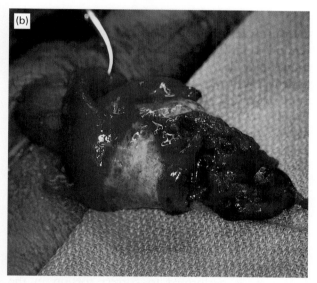

Figure 33.16 Testicular trauma: (*a*) color Doppler ultrasound showing discontinuity of testis and anechoic area at site of hematoma (*asterisk*); (*b*) intraoperative photograph showing disrupted testis with hematoma.

form within the substance of the testis. Reduced flow in a painful testis relative to the normal testis may indicate torsion and exploration is indicated.

Spermatic cord torsion

The suggested protocol for the evaluation of a child with an acute scrotum (Fig. 33.17) states that when the history and physical examination strongly suggest that testicular torsion is present and the duration of

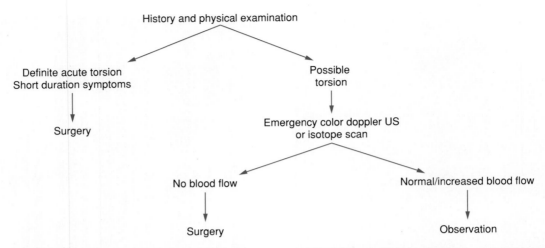

Figure 33.17 Algorithm for evaluation and treatment of patients with acute scrotal pain. (US = ultrasonography.)

the pain is less than 12 hours, urgent surgical intervention is indicated (Kass *et al.*, 1993b). Imaging studies may delay treatment and thereby jeopardize testicular survival. When pain has been present for more than 12 hours or the diagnosis is unclear, color Doppler ultrasound examination can be helpful in making clinical decisions. It is important to remember that most patients with an acute scrotum do not have testicular torsion.

The 'bell clapper' deformity is the underlying cause of testicular torsion in older children. In this deformity, the testicle lacks a normal attachment to the tunica vaginalis and therefore hangs freely. As a result, the spermatic cord can twist within the tunica vaginalis (intravaginal torsion).

Surgery is performed to correct torsion in the affected testis and to anchor the other testis to prevent future torsion. Surgical exploration can usually be accomplished through a single, small, midline incision in the scrotal raphe. Testes that are unequivocally necrotic should be removed. Viable testes should be fixed to the scrotal wall with multiple non-absorbable sutures.

Testicular torsion can also occur perinatally before the entire testis complex has fused to the scrotum. In this type of torsion the testis, spermatic cord, and tunica vaginalis twist *en bloc* (extravaginal torsion) (Fig. 33.18). Clinically, extravaginal torsion generally appears as a hard asymptomatic intrascrotal swelling in the newborn. Erythema or a bluish discoloration of the scrotum is also frequently seen and may be confused with a hydrocele.

The management of perinatal torsion remains controversial. Some surgeons advocate a non-operative approach because of the poor potential for testicular salvage. Others argue that leaving a neonatal

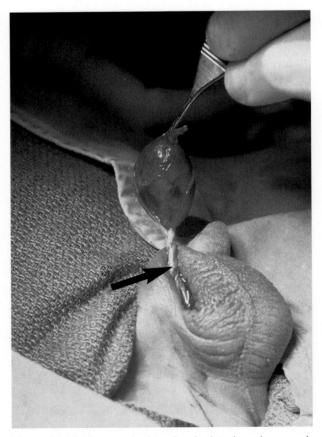

Figure 33.18 Extravaginal torsion (twisted cord – *arrow*).

testis in place may have adverse effects on the contralateral testis and note that cases of bilateral neonatal torsion have been reported (Stone *et al.*, 1995). Also controversial is the question as to whether or not the remaining solitary testis should be fixed in place, although risk of torsion of that testis is no greater than for the general (adult) population.

Torsion of an appendix of the testis or epididymis

The appendix testis, a müllerian duct remnant located at the superior pole of the testicle, is the most common appendage to undergo torsion (Fig. 33.19). The epididymal appendix, located on the head of the epididymis, is a wolffian duct remnant and may also become twisted. Torsion of either appendage produces pain similar to that experienced with testicular torsion, but the onset is more gradual. The cremasteric reflex is not lost with torsion of an appendage. Color Doppler ultrasonography often demonstrates increased blood flow that may be indistinguishable from epididymitis. Occasionally a hypoechoic mass near the upper pole of the testis, the torsed appendage, may be visualized.

Torsion of a testicular appendage may be misinterpreted as epididymitis. However, if the urinalysis is normal, no antibiotic therapy is required. Management entails symptomatic treatment to minimize inflammation and edema. Normal activity may both

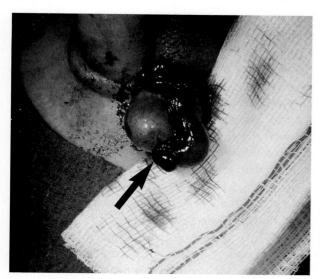

Figure 33.19 Torsion of appendix testis (*arrow*). Note accompanying enlargement and hyperemia of the epididymis.

worsen and prolong the symptoms. Non-steroidal anti-inflammatory drugs (NSAIDs) may offer symptometic relief to some patients. The inflammation usually resolves within 1 week, although the testicular examination may not be completely normal for several weeks with induration in the region of the head of the epididymis persisting for that interval.

Epididymitis or orchitis

Epididymitis in adolescents and young adults is often unrelated to sexual activity and does not present with a UTI. In prepubertal boys, however, bacterial epididymitis is often associated with a urinary tract anomaly (Siegel *et al.*, 1987). Any episode of epididymitis and UTI should be investigated with a renal/bladder sonogram and a voiding cystourethrogram (VCUG) to rule out structural problems. The cause of epididymitis in the majority of young men can often not be determined, however.

Treatment includes empiric antibiotic therapy until the results of a urine culture are known. If the culture is negative, the symptoms are most likely to be due to abacterial chemical epididymitis caused by the retrograde reflux of urine into the vas deferens. Bed-rest and scrotal elevation are often helpful. Symptoms may be alleviated with NSAIDs and analgesics. As with appendiceal torsion, the pain and swelling generally resolve within 1 week. Resolution of epididymal induration may require several weeks.

Scrotal trauma

Severe testicular injury is uncommon and usually results from either a direct blow to the scrotum or a straddle injury. Damage generally occurs when the testis is forcefully compressed against the pubic bones. A spectrum of injuries may occur. Traumatic epididymitis is a non-infectious inflammatory condition that usually occurs within a few days after a blow to the testis (Gordon *et al.*, 1996). Treatment is similar to that of non-traumatic abacterial epididymitis. Scrotal trauma can also result in intratesticular hematoma, hematocele, or laceration of the tunica albuginea (testicular rupture). Color Doppler ultrasonography is the imaging technique of choice (Fig. 33.16). Testicular rupture is a surgical emergency requiring débridement of devascularized tissue and closure of the tunica albuginea. Isolated hematomas and hematoceles are managed on an individual basis.

Lacerations of the scrotum itself are a fairly common occurrence in active boys, usually the consequence of bicycle accidents or getting caught on a fence. Most are superficial and do not involve the tunica vaginalis, requiring only minor suturing with sedation and local anesthesia. Deeper injuries may require a trip to the operating room.

Other acute scrotal disease

Acute idiopathic scrotal edema is another cause of an acute scrotum (Fig. 33.20). This condition is characterized by the rapid onset of significant edema without tenderness. Erythema may be present. The patient is usually afebrile and all diagnostic tests are negative. The etiology of this condition remains unclear. Treatment consists of bed-rest and scrotal elevation. Analgesics are rarely needed.

Schönlein–Henoch purpura, a systemic vasculitic syndrome of uncertain etiology, is characterized by non-thrombocytopenic purpura, arthralgia, renal disease, abdominal pain, gastrointestinal bleeding and, occasionally, scrotal pain and swelling (Wara and Emery, 1991). The onset can be acute or insidious. Hematuria may be present. The syndrome has no specific treatment.

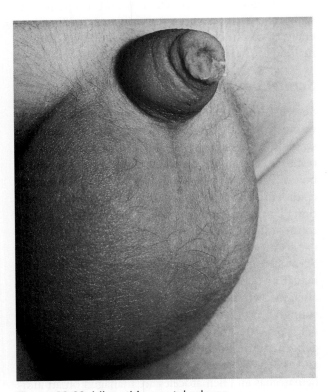

Figure 33.20 Idiopathic scrotal edema.

The overriding need in the child with scrotal edema is to rule out testicular pathology. Color Doppler sonography may be helpful, but it may also be possible to make this determination clinically. If the testes can be manipulated gently into the superficial inguinal pouches and palpated, their non-involvement in the inflammatory process may be proven and no further diagnostic studies need be carried out.

Hernia and hydrocele

Inguinal hernia and hydrocele in childhood is most commonly due to patency of the processus vaginalis, an extension of peritoneum that forms in the first trimester in proximity to the gubernaculum of both sexes (Heyn, 1987). In males, the processus vaginalis migrates distally through the inguinal canal with the masculinized gubernaculum, facilitates descent of the testis, persists distally as the tunica vaginalis, and normally becomes obliterated proximally. In females, the processus vaginalis develops but does not enlarge substantially. In both sexes, failure of closure of the processus creates a potential site for clinical hernia formation, characterized by passage of fluid or intra-abdominal viscera into the persisting sac.

The timing of closure of the processus vaginalis and its relationship to clinical hernia formation can be inferred from data obtained at autopsy, inguinal exploration, intraoperative laparoscopy, and studies of patients requiring ventriculoperitoneal shunts. These studies suggest that the processus is open in more than 80% of individuals at birth, and closure is most common in the first year of life but may occur much later. Patency persists in 15–30% of adults (Rowe et al., 1969; Bronsther et al., 1972). However, clinical hernias develop in fewer than 30% of newborns and 10% of 1 year olds after placement of a ventriculoperitoneal shunt (Clarnette et al., 1998). Similarly, contralateral patency of the processus vaginalis has been reported to be as high as 40–50% of children with unilateral inguinal hernias (Miltenburg et al., 1998). However, only 7% of children who undergo unilateral hernia repair subsequently develop a clinical hernia on the opposite side (Miltenburg et al., 1997). Therefore, not all potential hernias manifest themselves clinically, even in the presence of increased intra-abdominal pressure.

The incidence of pediatric hernia is 10–20 per 1000 and is greater in premature infants (7%), in males (85% of total), and in the first 6 months of life

(30% of total) (Bronsther *et al.*, 1972; Skoog and Conlin, 1995). Clinical hernias are more frequent on the right side and are bilateral in approximately 10% of both male and female children. Incarceration occurs most frequently in the first year of life. Patients may present with an inguinal bulge and/or enlarged scrotum or labium, irritability, vomiting, and obstipation. In the absence of incarceration, a hernia may be diagnosed during the Valsalva maneuver (crying or blowing up a balloon) or by observation of inguinal asymmetry and palpable thickening of the spermatic cord distal to the external ring. These findings may be facilitated by examining the patient in the upright position. The spectrum of anatomic findings is shown in Figure 33.21.

Surgical repair is indicated when the clinical history and physical findings suggest visceral involvement or when fluctuation in size is observed. Prompt repair is also advised in infancy to reduce the risk of incarceration. If an incarcerated hernia requires reduction surgical repair should be urgent, or emergent if peritoneal signs suggest that bowel strangulation is present. The question of contralateral inguinal exploration at the time of repair of the symptomatic hernia is controversial. Some surgeons base their decision on laparoscopic evaluation of the contralateral internal ring (Miltenburg *et al.*, 1998). However, while this may reduce the incidence of routine inguinal exploration, the data cited above suggest that the majority of patent processes vaginales will remain asymptomatic. Routine contralateral exploration may be reasonably limited to situations associated with a higher risk for metachronous hernia and/or morbidity, such as age less than 1 year, history of prematurity,

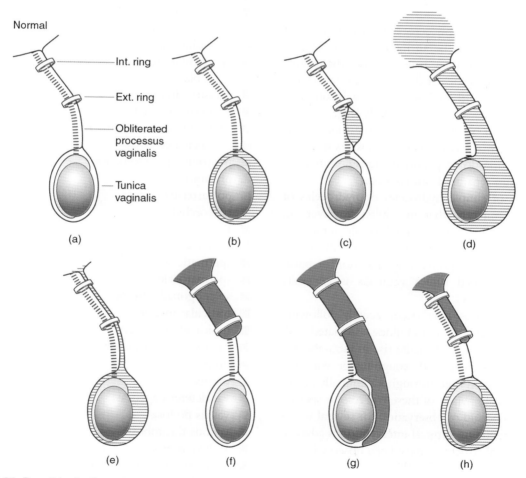

Figure 33.21 Possible findings in patients with hernia and/or hydrocele. Hatched black areas represent fluid and dark blue areas represent intra-abdominal contents: (*a*) normal findings; (*b*) scrotal hydrocele without hernia; (*c*) hydrocele of the cord; (*d*) abdominoscrotal hydrocele; (*e*) communicating hydrocele; (*f*) inguinal hernia; (*g*) inguinolscrotal hernia; (*h*) inguinal hernia and scrotal hydrocele.

and increased abdominal pressure from shunts, dialysis, or ascites.

Principles of repair include a small, transverse incision over the inguinal canal, isolation of the sac with minimal handling of cord structures, reduction of any abdominal viscera, and high ligation of the hernia sac. Formal repair of the internal ring or floor of the canal is rarely needed in children. Generous windowing of an undrained hydrocele, which may be loculated, should be performed after transection and ligation of the hernia sac. The testis should be replaced in its normal position in the scrotum.

Scrotal hydroceles without associated patency of the processus vaginalis are common in newborns and may be quite large. Diagnosis is made by transillumination, and the inability to reduce the mass, forcing the fluid back into the peritoneal cavity, rules out hernia. Most resolve spontaneously and treatment is not recommended.

Persistence of a simple scrotal hydrocele beyond 18 months of age may be an indication for surgical correction. However, there is no evidence that a simple hydrocele risks testicular damage and treatment is generally cosmetic, although some boys will complain of discomfort if the mass is particularly large.

Fluid may also be trapped within the tunica vaginalis of the spermatic cord. The diagnosis is made by identifying a non-decompressible, transilluminatable mass above and separate from the testis.

Treatment of simple hydroceles or hydroceles of the cord is similar to that in adults; however, an inguinal approach is recommended to rule out associated patency of the proximal tunica vaginalis at the level of the internal inguinal ring. Excision or plication of the enlarged tunica vaginalis is generally effective (Lord, 1964).

Finally, hydroceles may occur acutely following minor scrotal trauma or a viral illness associated with coughing or vomiting. The acute rise in intra-abdominal pressure associated with coughing or vomiting may force peritoneal fluid through a minimally patent processus vaginalis. Many of these will resolve spontaneously and a period of observation for several weeks before recommending surgical intervention is advised.

Many unusual structures have been observed within hernia sacs (Bloom *et al.*, 1992):

- abscess
- adrenal hemorrhage
- adrenal tissue, adrenal tumor
- appendix
- bladder
- cystic dysplasia of testis
- dermoid cyst
- ectopic renal tissue
- ectopic testis
- epidermoid cyst of testis
- epididymal cysts, nodules, structural anomalies, tumors
- fat necrosis of scrotum
- fibrous adnexal pseudotumor
- free nodules, calculi
- funniculitis (thrombosis of pampiniform plexus)
- gonad or genital structure of opposite sex
- granulomas (talc, etc.)
- granulomatous disease (sarcoidosis, etc.)
- hemangioma
- intussuscepted processus vaginalis
- lymphangioma
- Meckles (Littre's hernia)
- meconium granuloma
- mesenchymoma
- neuroblastoma
- parasitic disease
- paratesticular cyst
- paratesticular rhabdomyosarcoma
- pedunculated body
- peritonitis pseudotorsion
- pneumoscrotum
- polyarteritis nodosa
- polyorchidism
- Richter's hernia
- scrotal calculi
- spermatic cord tumors
- spermatocele
- splenogonadal fusion
- testicular infarct
- tunica albuginea cyst
- tunica vaginalis tumor
- ureter
- uterus
- vas deferens agenesis
- vasitis nodosa
- venous thrombosis
- Wilms' tumor
- xanthogranuloma (juvenile)

Preoperative clinical findings will suggest the presence of some of these structures, such as spermatic cord tumors. Previously unsuspected discoveries in the inguinal canal become clinically significant in the context of hernia repair if they suggest an additional diagnosis that requires treatment, are confused with normal tissue or are removed inadvertently, producing morbidity. Additional diagnoses of significance include persistent müllerian duct syndrome (usually associated with cryptorchidism), Meckel's diverticulum, intersex abnormalities in phenotypic females, and testicular, vasal, or epididymal anomalies (see below). Since androgen insensitivity syndrome is present in about 1% of girls undergoing hernia repair (Atwell, 1962), routine exposure of the ovary and/or vaginal examination under anesthesia is warranted in these cases.

Incompletely developed portions of vas or epididymis have been identified by microscopic analysis of excised hernia sac tissue in 1.5–4% of cases and may cause concern of vasal injury. These can be differentiated from normal vas and epididymis by their small mean diameter of 0.17–0.26 mm, versus >0.7 mm for normal ducts (Popek, 1990; Gill *et al.*, 1992). Serious injury to the normal vas, bladder, ureter, or testis during hernia/hydrocele repair is uncommon (<2%) (Bronsther *et al.*, 1972; Redman, 1985b; Morecroft *et al.*, 1993). Even in the subset of boys requiring hernia repair in infancy for incarceration, the rate of testicular atrophy is low (2%) (Puri *et al.*, 1984). Hernia recurrence is also rare (<0.5%). Postoperative (new or persistent) hydrocele may be found in 1.5–3.5% of cases but the majority resolve spontaneously within 1 year.

A more severe and unusual form of hydrocele is the abdominoscrotal hydrocele (ASH), which extends from scrotum to retroperitoneum but has no demonstrable communication with the peritoneal cavity (Serels and Kogan, 1996; Gentile *et al.*, 1998; Mohamed *et al.*, 1998). Presentation is usually unilateral but may be bilateral. Bimanual examination confirms an abdominoscrotal mass which transmits a fluid wave; ultrasound may be useful to confirm the diagnosis in some cases. Often present at birth, the ASH may become quite large, extending laterally to the level of the umbilicus or higher. They often do not regress and may enlarge with time. They may rarely cause pain, lower extremity edema, hydronephrosis, and testicular atrophy (Chamberlain *et al.*, 1995; Mohamed *et al.*, 1998).

Proposed etiologies include isolated closure of the processus vaginalis at the internal ring with gradual upward extension of the hydrocele retroperitoneally, or incomplete proximal obliteration of the processus producing a one-way valve mechanism with continued accumulation of fluid (Serels and Kogan, 1996; Gentile *et al.*, 1998). Associated undescended testis may be present. ASH repair is generally performed through a standard inguinal incision, although inbrication of the wall transcrotally may be safer (Belman, 2001). The sac is transected, the distal portion opened widely, and the retroperitoneal portion excised completely to prevent recurrence. Extreme care must be taken to avoid injury to local retroperitoneal structures, such as the vas or ureter, which may be difficult to identify in the folds of the large hydrocele wall (Serels and Kogan, 1996). For this reason the scrotal approach may be preferable. Concomitant orchidopexy is performed, if indicated.

Testicular abnormalities

Congenital testicular anomalies other than cryptorchidism are rare but are often found in association with abnormal testicular descent. Those associated with intersex disorders are reviewed elsewhere (see Chapter 31).

Defects of number and position
Anorchism and monorchism

Absence of one or both testes in otherwise normal phenotypic males is identified in as many as 35% of patients evaluated for non-palpable testes (Turek *et al.*, 1994a; Merry *et al.*, 1997; Cendron *et al.*, 1998). In the majority, the vas and spermatic vessels are present but end blindly distal to the internal inguinal ring, a condition called vanishing testis. Several observations indicate that the likely cause of vanishing testis is antenatal torsion. These include presence of hemosiderin or calcification in 15–85% of specimens examined histologically (Turek *et al.*, 1994a; Merry *et al.*, 1997; Cendron *et al.*, 1998), absence of developmental abnormalities in the contralateral testis (Huff *et al.*, 1991), and sonographic confirmation of prenatal testicular disappearance in a patient with extravaginal torsion (Gong *et al.*, 1996). The diagnosis of anorchism can be made after the first 3 months of age if both elevation of plasma gonadotropins and lack of testosterone response to hCG stimulation are present (Lustig *et al.*, 1987). However, testosterone levels are elevated until about 2 months of age in the normal male. Therefore, absence of measurable levels in this age group suggests anorchia. During mid-childhood, gonadotropin levels may be normal in anorchid boys, but a GnRH stimulation test will reveal an exaggerated gonadotropin response. Contralateral testicular enlargement and elevated FSH levels are present in some, but not all, patients with monorchism (Huff *et al.*, 1992; Palmer *et al.*, 1997). Therefore, diagnosis must be based on laparoscopic and/or surgical findings of blind-ending spermatic vessels. Reduced levels of serum müllerian inhibiting substance may also prove useful in the diagnosis of anorchism (Lee *et al.*, 1997).

Polyorchidism

Supernumerary testis is a rare entity, with fewer than 100 case reports in the literature (Thum, 1991; Merida *et al.*, 1992). The proposed etiology is complete duplication of the genital ridge or separation of the ridge into two or more parts. The extra testis is most commonly located in the scrotum (75%), but may be inguinal (20%) or retroperitoneal (5%). The condition is rarely bilateral (5%). Associated ductal structures on the affected side may be single or duplicated. The anatomic variants described in the literature include shared epididymis and vas (47%), duplicated epididymis and common vas (33%), duplicated epididymis and vas (11%), and absence of both adjacent to the accessory testis (5%). Associated genital anomalies are common and in decreasing order of frequency include inguinal hernia, undescended orthotopic testis, spermatic cord torsion, hydrocele,

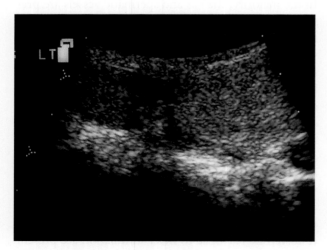

Figure 33.22 Polyorchidism: ultrasound image showing two normal testes on the left side.

testicular tumor, and varicocele. The diagnosis is suspected by physical findings and can often be confirmed sonographically (Fig. 33.22). Surgical intervention is indicated for torsion, hernia/hydrocele, suspected tumor, or cryptorchidism.

Testicular exstrophy

Congenital extrusion of one or both testes outside the scrotum is one of the rarest testicular anomalies (Heyns, 1990; Gupta *et al.*, 1997). There are inadequate data to support any specific etiology, but theories include gubernacular malfunction, scrotal ischemia, or local mesodermal abnormality. No associated anomalies are reported. Treatment is simple scrotal orchidopexy and closure.

Transverse testicular ectopia

The presence of both testes on the same side, each with an intact ipsilateral blood supply, epididymis, and vas, is an uncommon malformation (Golladay and Redman, 1982; Gauderer *et al.*, 1982). The most frequent associated anomalies include inguinal hernia (98%) and persistent müllerian duct syndrome (30%). The absence of a normal attachment of the gubernacular remnant suggests that anomalous development of this structure may predispose to transverse ectopy. Laparoscopy may be useful for both diagnosis and management (Gornall and Pender, 1987; Balaji and Diamond, 1995). Depending on presentation, orchiectomy or orchidopexy is performed with partial excision of müllerian remnants as required to facilitate scrotal placement of the testis.

Other testicular anomalies

Gonadal fusion anomalies

Splenogonadal fusion is a rare anomaly characterized by an abnormal attachment between the left gonad or its internal ductal system and the spleen or accessory splenic tissue (Karaman and Gonzales, 1996; Balaji *et al.*, 1996; Cortes *et al.*, 1996). Almost 150 cases have been reported, with the majority occurring in males. Patients most commonly present with a scrotal mass, inguinal hernia, or undescended testis. Rare presentations include bowel obstruction, ambiguous genitalia, and acute enlargement or traumatic rupture of the scrotal spleen. Two variants are described: a continuous form characterized by a fibrous connection between gonad and spleen which may contain accessory 'spleenlets', and a discontinuous form, with no connection between the gonad and the orthotopic spleen. These subtypes occur with similar frequency. Other congenital anomalies are present in about one-third of cases, including limb, skull or cardiac defects, micrognathia, diaphragmatic hernia, imperforate anus, spina bifida, and hypospadias. Proposed etiologies include adhesion between splenic and gonadal tissue at 5–9 weeks' gestation due to simple fusion or inflammation (Karaman and Gonzales, 1996) and migration of splenic cells into a persistent diaphragmatic gonadal ligament (Cortes *et al.*, 1996). Treatment is based on associated findings, but care should be taken to avoid injury to the associated normal testis (Karaman and Gonzales, 1996).

A single case of hepatogonadal fusion has appeared in the relatively recent literature (Ferro *et al.*, 1996). This patient presented with a right inguinal hernia, and had a histologically proven liver nodule attached to the upper testicular pole and a fibrous attachment to the porta hepatis. No other anomalies were present.

Testicular hypertrophy and macroorchidism

Testicular volume is usually less than 2 ml prior to puberty (Schonfeld, 1943; Fujieda and Matsuura, 1987). After the age of 9–10 years, testicular size is markedly variable but correlates with Tanner stage (Schonfeld, 1943). Unilateral or bilateral enlargement of the testis has many etiologies. Malignant lesions, including primary testicular tumors and leukemia, are rare but should be ruled out initially. Benign causes of increased testicular size include: asymmetric pubertal enlargement (Nisula *et al.*, 1974; Lee *et al.*, 1982), compensatory hypertrophy in some cases of monorchism or cryptorchidism (Laron *et al.*, 1980), macroorchidism associated with fragile X and other mental retardation syndromes (Simko *et al.*, 1989; Lindsay *et al.*, 1996), nodular enlargement in patients with congenital adrenal hyperplasia (Rutgers *et al.*, 1988) and isosexual precocity due to central nervous system (CNS) lesions, excess gonadotropins, testotoxicosis, hypothroidism, and other syndromes (Kletter and Kelch, 1993).

Testicular size discrepancy at puberty in otherwise normal boys is an uncommon finding. If a history of previous inguinal surgery or testicular injury is absent, the proposed cause is asymmetric response of the testis to normal maturational stimulation (Lee *et al.*,

1982). Exaggerated bilateral, benign testicular enlargement is also reported (Nisula *et al.*, 1974). These patients should be evaluated with testicular sonography and, if a tumor is not identified, no further steps are indicated. Over time, the size discrepancy in unilateral cases may persist or resolve (Lee *et al.*, 1982).

Microlithiasis

Microlithiasis is a condition usually reported in adult men, but also found in children (Furness *et al.*, 1998). It is characterized by ultrasonic and/or histologic evidence of multiple calcifications within the testicular parenchyma (Fig. 33.23) (Renshaw, 1998). Adult men with microlithiasis often present with other testicular disease and associated germ cell tumors have been reported in as many as 40% (Backus *et al.*, 1994). By contrast, the prevalence of microlithiasis in men who have had testicular sonography for other reasons is 0.6%. The incidence in the general population is unknown. Microlithiasis identified by pathological examination is not always evident by sonography. However, the histologic type may be helpful in determining the significance of the lesion (Renshaw, 1998). Hematoxylin bodies are associated with germ cell tumors, while laminated calcifications may be present in association with testis tumors, but also

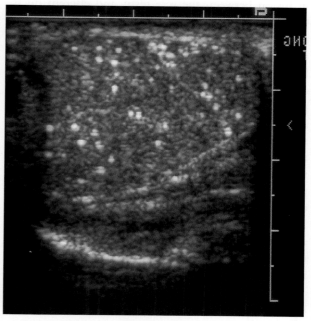

Figure 33.23 Testicular microlithiasis: typical appearance on ultrasound image.

occur in normal boys and in other diseases affecting the testis including cryptorchidism, epididymitis, inguinal hernia, and Klinefelter syndrome.

Histological microlithiasis is even rarer in the pediatric population, identified in only 1 of 2100 autopsies and 1 of 600 testicular biopsies (Nistal *et al.*, 1979). In a multi-institutional series, Furness *et al.* (1998) studied 26 patients aged 6 months to 21 years (mean 12 years) in whom microlithiasis was diagnosed incidentally by sonogram. Reasons for evaluation included hydrocele, epididymitis, varicocele, trauma, testicular or appendix torsion, testicular mass, and unilateral testicular enlargement. There were no cases of clinically evident tumor during a mean follow-up period of slightly more than 2 years. Additional long-term data are required to identify the clinical significance, if any, of testicular microlithiasis in children. For the present, self-examination, yearly ultrasound imaging, and selected biopsy should be used in the surveillance of these patients.

Abnormalities of accessory organs

Cystic dysplasia of rete testis

Cystic dysplasia of the rete testes (also called cystic dysplasia of the testis) has been reported only 15 times in the literature (Bonnet *et al.*, 1997; Wojcik *et al.*, 1997). This lesion is believed to be due to a defect in fusion between the rete testis and efferent ducts. Cystic dysplasia is usually unilateral but may be bilateral, and patients often present in childhood with a testicular or scrotal mass. The diagnosis may be made by identifying multiple small cysts on the medial aspect of the testis, although most of the testicular parenchyma may be compressed by the mass. Associated genitourinary anomalies are common, suggesting that an associated wolffian duct anomaly may be present. Almost all cases are associated with renal anomalies. The most common are agenesis, dysplasia or hypoplasia, and hydronephrosis. Abdominal cryptorchidism is seen in one-third of patients. Preferred treatment is local excision, but an inguinal approach with control of the cord vessels is recommended to rule out tumor. Orchiectomy is performed if testis sparing is not possible.

Wolffian duct system

Since the mesonephric or wolffian duct is the precursor of both ureteral bud and the internal genital ducts, including vas, epididymis, and seminal vesicles, anomalous development frequently affects both the kidney and reproductive tract (Vohra and Morgentaler, 1997). The caudal segment of the wolffian duct, or common mesonephric duct, is the site of origin of the ureteral bud. The middle segment, or common vas precursor, becomes the vas and seminal vesicles, and the upper mesonephric duct become the distal vas and epididymis (Gibbons *et al.*, 1978). It is proposed that defects that appear before the 7th week of gestation (onset of ureteral bud differentiation) may interfere with normal renal and reproductive tract development and after that time the reproductive tract alone is affected (Vohra and Morgentaler, 1997). The timing and extent of the developmental defect probably influence the eventual phenotype.

Agenesis

Absence of the vas deferens is the most common finding in patients with agenesis of wolffian duct derivatives (Charny and Gillenwater, 1965; Donahue and Fauver, 1989; Anguiano *et al.*, 1992; Vohra and Morgentaler, 1997). The lesion may be bilateral or unilateral and in either form occurs in fewer than 1% of males. Vasal agenesis is usually discovered in adult patients with infertility or at the time of planned vasectomy, but may also present during inguinal exploration at any age. Both the unilateral and bilateral forms are associated with agenesis of the epididymis, seminal vesical and/or kidney, but the association is more frequent in unilateral cases. The caput epididymis almost always persists. This observation supports other clinical data indicating similarities between the caput epididymis and the efferent ducts, with the implication that the caput arises from the gonadal ridge rather than the wolffian duct. Mutation of the transmembrane conductance regulator (CFTR) gene is the only known genetic etiology of vasal agenesis. CFTR gene mutations are more common in bilateral (64%) than unilateral (25%) disease and have not been found in patients with bilateral vasal agenesis in association with renal anomalies (Vohra and Morgentaler, 1997). When vasal agenesis is diagnosed in childhood, renal and pelvic sonography and, if abnormal, VCUG should be performed. Vasal agenesis may also be found in patients with cystic fibrosis, even when clinical evidence of the disease is absent.

Anomalies of epididymal attachment

Abnormalities of fusion or suspension of the epididymis are known to be common in patients with cryptorchidism. Turek *et al.* (1994) studied epididymal anatomy in a group of boys undergoing inguinal or scrotal exploration primarily for hydrocele and reported normal anatomy in 96%. However, two other studies have shown a higher incidence (31–39%) of mild suspension or fusion anomalies of the epididymis in boys with hernia/hydrocele, with a greater frequency in those patients with a patent processus vaginalis (Elder, 1992; Barthold and Redman, 1996). The clinical significance of partial epididymal detachment or a long looping epididymis in patients with a normally positioned testis is unclear.

Epididymal cysts

Cysts of the epididymis (spermatocele) (Fig. 33.24) usually appear during puberty or adulthood and are asymptomatic. The etiology is unknown but proposed to be dilated efferent ducts that have failed to fuse with the epididymis (Comiter *et al.*, 1995; Vohra and Morgentaler, 1997). Conditions associated with a higher incidence of epididymal cysts include Von Hippel–Lindau disease and fetal exposure to diethylstilbestrol. Intervention is not usually required, but both excision (Padmore *et al.*, 1996) and sclerotherapy (Daehlin *et al.*, 1997) have been used successfully in symptomatic patients.

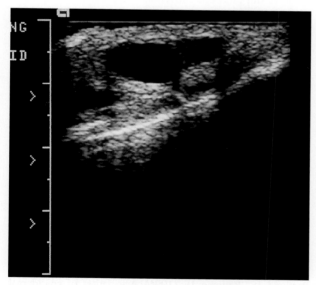

Figure 33.24 Epididymal cysts in a patient with polyorchidism.

Other vasal anomalies

Ectopy of the vas deferens (Gibbons *et al.*, 1978; Nesbitt and King, 1990; Kriss *et al.*, 1995), also called persisting mesonephric duct (Schwartz and Stephens, 1978), is characterized by ectopic insertion of the vas into the urinary tract. Most commonly, fusion of the vas and ureter occurs proximal to the bladder (Borger and Belman, 1975) (vasoureteric insertion), but direct entry of the vas into the bladder (vasovesical insertion) may occur. Approximately 30 cases are reported in the English literature. Proposed mechanisms include ectopic insertion of the ureteral bud and/or aberrant development of the proximal vas precursor (Gibbons *et al.*, 1978; Schwartz and Stephens, 1978). Patients are asymptomatic or present with UTIs and/or epididymitis. Other congenital anomalies are common, including agenesis of the seminal vesicles, imperforate anus, hypospadias, ureteral reflux and/or ectopy, and renal anomalies. The triad of imperforate anus, hypospadias, and ectopic vas was reported in 21% of cases (Hicks *et al.*, 1989). The diagnosis may be made by cystourethrography, retrograde ureterography, or at the time of ureteroneocystostomy. Treatment is based on anatomic findings and clinical indications.

True duplication of the vas deferens is extremely rare. Binderow *et al.* (1993) reported a single case found at the time of inguinal hernia repair in a boy with a normal urinary tract. The authors proposed wolffian duct duplication or ductal bifurcation in the region of the proximal vas precursor as the etiology.

Seminal vesicle cysts

Seminal vesicle cysts are another manifestation of anomalous wolffian duct development (Fuselier and Peters, 1976; Roehrborn *et al.*, 1986; Zaontz and Kass, 1987). Most are associated with renal agenesis with or without ureteral ectopy. Presentation is predominantly in adulthood with pain during micturition, defecation or ejaculation, UTI, or infertility. A palpable mass is appreciated on rectal examination. The diagnosis may be confirmed by abdominal or transrectal sonogram. A computed tomographic scan may be useful to visualize the seminal vesicle and confirm renal agenesis (Fig. 33.25). Excision is indicated in symptomatic patients and is facilitated by a transtrigonal approach (Zaontz and Kass, 1987).

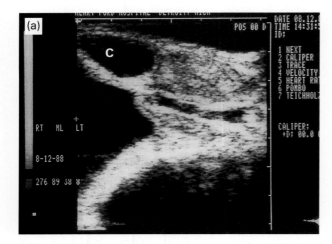

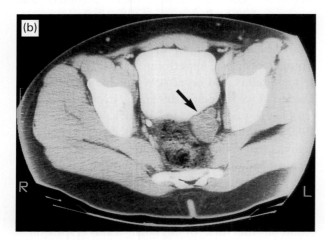

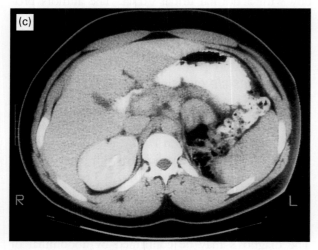

Figure 33.25 Seminal vesical cyst in an adolescent presenting with voiding symptoms and urinary tract infection: (*a*) sonogram showing a cystic structure posterior to the bladder in the left sagital view (C); (*b*) computed tomographic (CT) scan confirming a fluid-filled structure (*arrow*) in the region of the left seminal vesicle. (*c*) Absence of the left kidney on CT scan.

References

Aaronson IA (1994) Micropenis: medical and surgical implications. *J Urol* **152**: 4–14.

Abdulmaaboud MR, Shokeir AA, Farage Y *et al*. (1998) Treatment of varicocele: a comparative study of conventional open surgery, percutaneous retrograde sclerotherapy, and laparoscopy. *Urology* **52**: 294–300.

Agger P (1971) Scrotal and testicular temperature: its relation to sperm count before and after operation for varicocele. *Fertil Steril* **22**: 286–97.

Al Jam'a AH, Al Dabbous IA (1998) Hydroxyurea in the treatment of sickle cell associated priapism. *J Urol* **159**: 1642.

al Mufti RA, Ogedegbe AK, Lafferty K (1995) The use of Doppler ultrasound in the clinical management of acute testicular pain. *Br J Urol* **76**: 625–7.

Amelar RD, Dubin L (1987) Right varicocelectomy in selected infertile patients who have failed to improve after previous left varicocelectomy. *Fertil Steril* **47**: 833–7.

American Academy of Pediatrics Urology Section (1978) Urethral meatal stenosis in males. *Pediatrics* **61**: 778–80.

American Academy of Pediatrics: Task Force on Circumcision (1999) Circumcision policy statement. *Pediatrics* **103**: 686–93.

Ammini AC, Sabherwal U, Mukhopadhyay C *et al*. (1997) Morphogenesis of the human external male genitalia. *Pediatr Surg Int* **12**: 401–6.

Ando S, Giacchetto C, Bealdi E *et al*. (1982) The influence of age on Leydig cell function in patients with varicocele. *Int J Androl* **7**: 104–18.

Anguiano A, Oates RD, Amos JA *et al*. (1992) Congenital bilateral absence of the vas deferens. a primarily genital form of cystic fibrosis. *JAMA* **267**: 1794–7.

Atassi O, Kass EJ, Steinert BW (1995) Testicular growth after successful varicocele correction in adolescents: comparison of artery-sparing techniques with the Palomo procedure. *J Urol* **153**: 482–3.

Atikeler K, Yeni E, Semercioz A *et al*. (1996) The value of the gonadotropin-releasing hormone test as a prognostic factor in infertile patients with varicocele. *Br J Urol* **78**: 632–4.

Atwell JD (1962) Inguinal hernia in female infants and children. *Br J Surg* **50**: 294–7.

Bablok L, Czaplicki M, Fracki S *et al*. (1997) Relationship between semen quality improvement after varicocelectomy and preoperative levels of hypophyseal and gonadal hormones. *Int Urol Nephrol* **29**: 345–9.

Backus ML, Mack LA, Middleton WD *et al*. (1994) Testicular microlithiasis: imaging appearances and pathologic correlation. *Radiology* **192**: 781–5.

Balaji KC, Diamond DA (1995) Laparoscopic diagnosis and management of transverse testicular ectopia. *Urology* **46**: 879–80.

Balaji KC, Caldamone AA, Rabinowitz R *et al*. (1996) Splenogonadal fusion. *J Urol* **156**: 854–6.

Barthold JS, Redman JF (1996) Association of epididymal anomalies with patent processus vaginalis in hernia, hydrocele and cryptorchidism. *J Urol* **156**: 2054–6.

Bartsch O, Kuhnle U, Wu LL *et al.* (1996) Evidence for a critical region for penoscrotal inversion, hypospadias, and imperforate anus within chromosomal region 13q32.2q34. *Am J Med Genet* **65**: 218–21.

Barwell R (1885) One hundred cases of varicocele treated by the subcutaneous wire loop. *Lancet* 1978.

Baskin LS, Canning DA, Snyder HM, Duckett J (1996) Treating complications of circumcision. *Pediatr Emerg Care* **12**: 62–8.

Baskin LS, Canning DA, Snyder HM, Duckett JW (1997) Surgical repair of urethral circumcision injuries. *J Urol* **158**: 2269–71.

Behre HM, Nashan D, Nieschlag E (1989) Objective measurement of testicular volume by ultrasonography: evaluation of the technique and comparison with orchidometer estimates. *Int J Androl* **12**: 395–403.

Belloli G, D'Agostino S, Zen F, Ioverno E (1995) Fertility rates after successful correction of varicocele in adolescence and adulthood. *Eur J Pediatr Surg* **5**: 216–8.

Belloli G, Musi L, D'Agostino S (1996) Laparoscopic surgery for adolescent varicocele: preliminary report on 80 patients. *J Pediatr Surg* **31**: 1488–90.

Belman AB (2001) Abdomenoscrotal hydrocele in infancy. Review and presentation of scrotal approach for correction. *J Urol* **165**: 225.

Ben-Ari J, Merlob P, Mimouni F, Reisner SH (1985) Characteristics of the male genitalia in the newborn: penis. *J Urol* **134**: 521–2.

Bergeson PS, Hopkin RJ, Bailey RB *et al.* (1993) The inconspicuous penis. *Pediatrics* **92**: 794–9.

Bickel A, Dickstein G (1989) Factors predicting the outcome of varicocele repair for subfertility: the value of the luteinizing hormone-releasing hormone test. *J Urol* **142**: 1230–4.

Binderow SR, Shah KD, Dolgin SE (1993) True duplication of the vas deferens. *J Pediatr Surg* **28**: 269–70.

Bloom DA, Wan J, Key D (1992) Disorders of the male external genitalia and inguinal canal. In: Kelalis PP, King LR, Belman AB (eds.) *Clinical pediatric urology.* 3rd edition. Philadelphia, PA: WB Saunders, 1015–49.

Bonnet JP, Aigrain Y, Ferkadji L (1997) Cystic dysplasia of the testis with ipsilateral renal agenesis. A case report and review of the literature. *Eur J Pediatr Surg* **7**: 57–9.

Borger JA, Belman AB (1975) Ureterovas deferens anastamosis associated with imperforate anus: An embryologically predictable occurrence. *J Ped Surg* **10**: 255–7.

Bronsther B, Abrams MW, Elboim C (1972) Inguinal hernias in children – a study of 1000 cases and a review of the literature. *J Am Med Women's Assoc* **27**: 522–35.

Brown JM, Hammers LW, Barton JW *et al.* (1995) Quantitative Doppler assessment of acute scrotal inflammation. *Radiology* **197**: 427–31.

Caesar RE, Kaplan GW (1994) The incidence of the cremasteric reflex in normal boys. *J Urol* **152**: 779–80.

Callewaert P, Stockx L, Bogaert G, Baert L (1998) Post-traumatic high-flow priapism in a 6-year-old boy: management by percutaneous placement of bilateral vascular coils. *Urology* **52**: 134–7.

Cartwright PC, Snow BW, McNees DC (1996) Urethral meatotomy in the office using topical EMLA cream for anesthesia. *J Urol* **156**: 857–9.

Cendron M, Schned AR, Ellsworth PI (1998) Hisological evaluation of the testicular nubbin in the vanishing testis syndrome. *J Urol* **160**: 1161-3.

Chakrabarty A, Upadhyay J, Dhabuwala CB *et al.* (1996) Priapism associated with sickle cell hemoglobinopathy in children: long-term effects on potency. *J Urol* **155**: 1419–23.

Chamberlain SA, Kirsch AJ, Thall EH *et al.* (1995) Testicular dysmorphism associated with abdominoscrotal hydroceles during infancy. *Urology* **46**: 881–2.

Charney CW (1962) Effect of varicocele on fertility. *Fertil Steril* **13**: 47.

Charney CW, Gillenwater JY (1965) Congenital absence of the vas deferens. *J Urol* **93**: 399–401.

Choi SK, Han SW, Kim DH, de Lignieres B (1993) Transdermal dihydrotestosterone therapy and its effects on patients with microphallus. *J Urol* **150**: 657–60.

Chuang J-H (1995) Penoplasty for buried penis. *J Pediatr Surg* **30**: 1256–7.

Cifti AO, Senocak ME, Büyükpamukçu N (1995) Male gender assignment in penile agenesis: a case report and review of the literature. *J Pediatr Surg* **30**: 1358–60.

Clarnette TD, Lam SKL, Hutson JM (1998) Ventriculo-peritoneal shunts in children reveal the natural history of closure of the processus vaginalis. *J Pediatr Surg* **33**: 413–6.

Comiter CV, Bruning CO III, Morgentaler A (1995) Detached ciliary tufts in the epididymis: a lesson in applied anatomy. *Urology* **46**: 740–2.

Coplen DE, Mikkelsen D, Manley CB (1995) Accessory scrotum located on the distal penile shaft. *J Urol* **154**: 1908.

Cortes D, Thorup JM, Visfeldt J (1996) The pathogenesis of cryptorchidism and splenogonadal fusion: a new hypothesis. *Br J Urol* **77**: 285–90.

Cromie WJ, Ritchey ML, Smith RC, Zagaja GP (1998) Anatomical alignment for the correction of buried penis. *J Urol* **160**: 1482–4.

Daehlin L, Tonder B, Kapstad L (1997) Comparison of polidocanol and tetracycline in the sclerotherapy of testicular hydrocele and epididymal cyst. *Br J Urol* **80**: 468–71.

Daniel WA, Feinstein RA, Howard-Peebles P, Baxley WD (1982) Testicular volumes of adolescents. *J Pediatr* **101**: 1009–12.

Deeg KH, Wild F (1990) Colour Doppler imaging – a new method to differentiate torsion of the spermatic cord and epididymo-orchitis. *Eur J Pediatr* **149**: 253–5.

Dewan PA, Tan HL, Auldist AW, Moss DIMcL (1989) Priapism in childhood. *Br J Urol* **64**: 541–5.

Dewire DM, Begun FP, Lawson RK *et al.* (1992) Color Doppler ultrasonography in the evaluation of the acute scrotum. *J Urol* **147**: 89–91.

Diamond M (1996) Prenatal predisposition and the clinical management of some pediatric conditions. *J Sex Marital Ther* **22**: 139–74.

Dickerman Z, Landman J, Prager-Lewin R, Laron Z (1978) Evaluation of testicular function in prepubertal boys by means of the luteinizing hormone-releasing hormone test. *Fertil Steril* **29**: 655.

Donahue RE, Fauver HE (1989) Unilateral absence of the vas deferens. A useful clinical sign. *JAMA* **261**: 1180–2.

Dubin L, Amelar RD (1970) Varicocele size and results of varicocelectomy in selected subfertile men with varicocele. *Fertil Steril* **21**: 606–9.

Dubin L, Amelar RD (1975) Varicocelectomy as therapy in male infertility: a study of 504 cases. *J Urol* **113**: 640–1.

Elder J (1992) Epididymal anomalies associated with hydrocele/hernia and cryptorchidism: Implications regarding testicular descent. *J Urol* **148**: 624–6.

Elder JS, Jeffs RD (1982) Suprainguinal ectopic scrotum and associated anomalies. *J Urol* **127**: 336–8.

Emond AM, Holman R, Hayes RJ, Serjeant GR (1980) Priapism and impotence in homozygous sickle cell disease. *Arch Intern Med* **140**: 1434–7.

Fariss BL, Fenner DK, Plymate SR, *et al*. (1981) Seminal characteristics in the presence of a varicocele as compared with those of expectant fathers and prevasectomy men. *Fertil Steril* **35**: 325–7.

Ferro F, Lais A, Boldrini R *et al*. (1996) Hepatogonadal fusion. *J Pediatr Surg* **31**: 435–6.

Fowler JE Jr, Koshy M, Strub M, Chinn SK (1991) Priapism associated with the sickle cell hemoglobinopathies: prevalence, natural history and sequelae. *J Urol* **145**: 65–8.

Friedman J (1998) Priapism: an unusual presentation of appendicitis. *Pediatr Emerg Care* **14**:143–4.

Fujieda K, Matsuura N (1987) Growth and maturation in the male genitalia from birth to adolescence. I. Change of testicular volume. *Acta Paediatr Jpn* **29**: 214–9.

Fujisawa M, Hayashi A, Imanishi O *et al*. (1994) The significance of gonadotropin-releasing hormone test for predicting fertility after varicocelectomy. *Fertil Steril* **61**: 779–82.

Furness PD, Husmann DA, Brock JW (1998) Mult-institutional study of testicular microlithiasis in childhood: a benign or premalignant condition? *J Urol* **160**: 1151–4.

Fuselier HA, Peters DH (1976) Cyst of seminal vesicle with ipsilateral renal agenesis and ectopic ureter: case report. *J Urol* **116**: 833–5.

Gauderer MWL, Grisoni ER, Stellato TA *et al*. (1982) Transverse testicular ectopia. *J Pediatr Surg* **17**: 43–7.

Gearhart JP, Rock JA (1989) Total ablation of the penis after circumcision with electrocautery. a method of management and long-term followup. *J Urol* **142**: 799–801.

Gentile DP, Rabinowitz R, Hulbert WC (1998) Abdominoscrotal hydrocele in infancy. *Urology* **51** (Suppl 5A): 20–2.

Gibbons MD, Cromie WJ, Duckett JW (1978) Ectopic vas deferens. *J Urol* **120**: 597–604.

Gilbert DA, Jordan GH, Devine CG Jr *et al*. (1993) Phallic construction in prepubertal and adolescent boys. *J Urol* **149**: 1521–6.

Gill B, Favale D, Kogan SJ *et al*. (1992) Significance of accessory ductal structures in hernia sacs. *J Urol* **148**: 697–8.

Glenister TW (1921) The origin and fate of the urethral plate in man. *J Anat (London)* **88**: 413–23.

Glenn JF, Anderson EE (1973) Surgical correction of incomplete penoscrotal transposition. *J Urol* **110**: 603–5.

Goldstein M, Gilbert BR, Dicker AP *et al*. (1992) Microsurgical inguinal varicocelectomy with delivery of the testis: an artery and lymphatic sparing technique. *J Urol* **148**: 1808–11.

Golladay ES, Redman JF (1982) Transverse testicular ectopia. *Urology* **14**: 181–6.

Gong M, Geary ES, Shortliffe LMD (1996) Testicular torsion with contralateral vanishing testis. *Urology* **48**: 306–7.

Gordon LM, Stein SM, Ralls PW (1996) Traumatic epididymitis: evaluation with color Doppler sonography. *AJR Am J Roentgenol* **166**: 1323–5.

Gornall PG, Pender DJ (1987) Crossed testicular ectopia detected by laparoscopy. *Br J Urol* **59**: 283.

Griffiths DM, Atwell JD, Freeman NV (1985) A prospective survey of the indications and morbidity of circumcision in children. *Eur Urol* **11**: 184–7.

Gupta DK, Bajpai M, Rattan S (1997) Testicular exstrophy: bilateral presentation in a newborn. *J Urol* **158**: 599.

Haans LCF, Laven JSE, Mali WPTM *et al*. (1991) Testis volumes, semen quality and hormonal patterns in adolescents with and without a varicocele. *Fertil Steril* **56**: 731–6.

Hadziselimovic F, Leibundgut B, Da Rugna D, Buser MW (1986) The value of testicular biopsy in patients with varicocele. *J Urol* **135**: 707–10.

Hadziselimovic F, Herzog B, Jenny P (1995) The chance for fertility in adolescent boys after corrective surgery for varicocele. *J Urol* **154**: 731–3.

Hadziselimovic F, Herzog B, Liebundgut B *et al*. (1989) Testicular and vascular changes in children and adults with varicocele. *J Urol* **142**: 583–5.

Hamre MR, Harmon EP, Kirkpatrick DV *et al*. (1991) Priapism as a complication of sickle cell disease. *J Urol* **145**: 1–5.

Hendren WH (1997) The genetic male with absent penis and urethrorectal communication: experience with 5 patients. *J Urol* **157**: 1469–74.

Hensle TW (1996) Editorial comment. *J Urol* **156**: 858–9.

Herzog LW, Alvarez SR (1986) The frequency of foreskin problems in uncircumcised children. *Am J Dis Child* **140**: 254–6.

Heyns CF (1987) The gubernaculum during testicular descent in the human fetus. *J Anat* **153**: 93–112.

Heyns CF (1990) Exstrophy of the testis. *J Urol* **144**: 724–5.

Hicks CM, Skoog SJ, Done S (1989) Ectopic vas deferens, imperforate anus and hypospadias: a new triad. *J Urol* **141**: 586–8.

Hienz HA, Voggenthaler J, Weissbach L (1980) Histological findings in testes with varicocele during childhood and their therapeutic consequences. *Eur J Pediatr* **133**: 139–46.

Hoar RM, Calvano CJ, Reddy PP *et al*. (1998) Unilateral suprainguinal ectopic scrotum: the role of the gubernaculum in the formation of an ectopic scrotum. *Teratology* **57**: 64–9.

Hollowell JG Jr, Witherington R, Balagas AJ, Burt JN (1997) Embryologic considerations of diphallus and associated anomalies. *J Urol* **117**: 728–32.

Hosli PO (1988) Varicocele – results after early treatment in children and adolescents. *Z Kinderchir* **43**: 213–5.

Hsu TH, Huang JK, Ho DM *et al*. (1993) Role of the spermatic artery in spermatogenesis and sex hormone synthesis. *Arch Androl* **31**: 191–7.

Hudson RW, Perez-Marrero RA, Crawford VA, McKay DE (1985) Hormonal parameters of men with varicoceles before and after varicocelectomy. *Fertil Steril* **43**: 905–10.

Huff DS, Wu H-Y, Snyder HM *et al.* (1991) Evidence in favor of the mechanical (intrauterine torsion) theory over the endocrinopathy (cryptorchidism) theory in the pathogenesis of testicular agenesis. *J Urol* **146**: 630–1.

Huff DS, Snyder HM, Hadziselimovic F *et al.* (1992) An absent testis is associated with contralateral testicular hypertrophy. *J Urol* **148**: 627–8.

Humphrey GME, Najmaldin AS (1997) Laparoscopy in the management of pediatric varicoceles. *J Pediatr Surg* **32**: 1470–2.

Ibrahim AA, Awad HA, El-Haggar S, Mitawi BA (1977) Bilateral testicular biopsy in men with varicocele. *Fertil Steril* **28**: 663–7.

Ivanissevich O (1918) Left varicocele due to reflux; experience with 4,470 operative cases in forty-two years. *J Int Coll Surg* **34**: 742.

Janczewski Z, Bablok L (1985) Semen characteristics in pubertal boys. I. Semen quality after first ejaculation. *Arch Androl* **15**: 199–205.

Johnston WG Jr, Yeatman GW, Weigel JW (1977) Congenital absence of the penis. *J Urol* **117**: 508–12.

Johnson L, Petty CS, Neaves WB (1980) A comparative study of daily sperm production and testicular composition in humans and rats. *Biol Reprod* **22**: 1233–43.

Karaman MI, Gonzales ET (1996) Splenogonadal fusion: report of 2 cases and review of the literature. *J Urol* **155**: 309–11.

Karna P, Kapur S (1994) Diphallus and associated anomalies with balanced autosomal chromosomal translocation. *Clin Genet* **46**: 209–11.

Kass EJ, Belman AB (1987) Reversal of testicular growth failure by varicocele ligation. *J Urol* **137**: 475–6.

Kass EJ, Chandra RS, Belman AB (1987) Testicular histology in the adolescent with a varicocele. *Pediatrics* **79**: 996–8.

Kass EJ, Freitas JE, Bour JB (1989) Adolescent varicocele: objective indications for treatment. *J Urol* **142**: 579–82.

Kass EJ, Salisz JA (1991) The significance of scrotal temperature elevation in an adolescent with a varicocele. In: Zorgniotti AW (Ed) *Temperature and environmental effects on the testis*. New York: Plenum Press, 245–51.

Kass EJ, Freitas JE, Salisz JA, Steinert BW (1993a) Pituitary gonadal dysfunction in adolescents with varicocele. *Urology* **42**: 179–81.

Kass EJ, Stone KT, Cacciarelli AA, Mitchell B (1993b) Do all children with an acute scrotum require exploration? *J Urol* **150**: 667–9.

Kattan S (1998) Incidence and pattern of varicocele recurrence after laparoscopic ligation of the internal spermatic vein with preservation of the testicular artery. *Scand J Urol Nephrol* **32**: 335–40.

Kayaba H, Tamura H, Kitajima S *et al.* (1996) Analysis of shape and retractability of the prepuce in 603 Japanese boys. *J Urol* **156**: 1813–5.

Kletter GB, Kelch RP (1993) Disorders of puberty in boys. *Endocrinol Metab Clinics North Am* **22**: 455–77.

Kogan SJ, Williams DI (1977) The micropenis syndrome: clinical observations and expectations for growth. *J Urol* **118**: 311–3.

Kriss VM, Miller SD, McRoberts WJ (1995) Ectopia of the vas deferens. *Pediatr Radiol* **25**: 381–2.

Lamm DL, Kaplan GW (1977) Accessory and ectopic scrota. *Urology* **9**: 149–53.

Lander J, Brady-Fryer B, Metcalfe JB *et al.* (1997) Comparison of ring block, dorsal penile nerve block, and topical anesthesia for neonatal circumcision. A randomized clinical trial. *JAMA* **278**: 2157–62.

Laron Z, Dickerman Z, Ritterman I, Kaufman H (1980) Follow-up of boys with unilateral compensatory testicular hypertrophy. *Fertil Steril* **33**: 297–301.

Laumann EO, Mai CM, Zuckerman EW (1997) Circumcision in the United States: prevalence, prophylactic effects, and sexual practice. *JAMA* **277**: 1052–7.

Laven JD, Haans LCF, Mali WPTh *et al.* (1992) Effects of varicocele treatment in adolescents: a randomised study. *Fertil Steril* **58**: 756–62.

Lee MM, Donahoe PK, Silverman BL *et al.* (1997) Measurements of serum mullerian inhibiting substance in the evaluation of children with nonpalpable gonads. *N Engl J Med* **336**: 1480–6.

Lee PA, Danish RK, Mazur T, Migeon CJ (1980a) Micropenis. II. Primary hypogonadism, partial androgen insensitivity syndrome, and idiopathic disorders. *Johns Hopkins Med J* **147**: 175–81.

Lee PA, Mzur T, Danish R *et al.* (1980b) Micropenis. I. Criteria, etiologies and classification. *Johns Hopkins Med J* **146**: 156–63.

Lee PE, Marshall FF, Greco JM, Jeffs RD (1982) Unilateral testicular hypertrophy: an apparently benign occurrence without cryptorchidism. *J Urol* **127**: 329–31.

Lemack GE, Uzzo RG, Schlegel PN, Goldstein M (1998) Microsurgical repair of the adolescent varicocele. *J Urol* **160**: 179–81.

Lenz M, Hof N, Kersting-Sommerhoff B, Bauer W (1996) Anatomic variants of the spermatic vein: importance for percutaneous sclerotherapy of idiopathic varicocele. *Radiology* **198**: 425–31.

Lenzi A, Gandini L, Bagolan P *et al.* (1998) Sperm parameters after early left varicocele treatment. *Fertil Steril* **69**: 347–9.

LeVasseur JG, Perry VE (1997) Perineal median raphe cyst. *Pediatr Dermatol* **14**: 391–2.

Levine LA, Guss SP (1993) Gonadotropin-releasing hormone analogues in the treatment of sickle cell anemia-associated priapism. *J Urol* **150**: 475–7.

Levine RJ, Mathew RM, Chenault CB *et al.* (1990) Differences in the quality of semen in outdoor workers during summer and winter. *N Engl J Med* **323**: 12–6.

Levy JB, Husmann DA (1996) Micr openis secondary to growth hormone deficiency: does treatment with growth hormone alone result in adequate penile growth? *J Urol* **156**: 214–6.

Levy JB, Darson MF, Bite U, Kramer SA (1997) Modified pudendal–thigh flap for correction of penoscrotal transposition. *Urology* **50**: 597–600.

Lewis AG, Bukowski TP, Jarvis PD *et al.* (1995) Evaluation of acute scrotum in the emergency department. *J Pediatr Surg* **30**: 277–82.

Lima M, Domini M, Libri M (1997) The varicocele in pediatric age: 207 cases treated with microsurgical technique. *Eur J Pediatr Surg* **7**: 30–3.

Lindsay S, Splitt M, Edney S *et al.* (1996) PPM-X: a new X-linked mental retardation syndrome with psychosis, pyramidal signs, and macroorchidism maps to Xq28. *Am J Hum Genet* **58**: 1120–6.

Lipshultz LI, Caminos-Torres R, Greenspan CS, Snyder PJ (1976) Testicular function after orchiopexy for unilaterally undescended testis. *N Engl J Med* **295**: 15–8.

Little JR (1994) The inconspicuous or 'disappearing' penis. *Pediatrics* **94**: 240–2.

Lord PH (1964) A bloodless operation for the radical cure of idiopathic hydrocele. *Br J Surg* **51**: 914.

Lustig RH, Conte FA, Kogan BA, Grumbach MM (1987) Ontogeny of gonadotropin secretion in congenital anorchism: sexual dimorphism versus syndrome of gonadal dysgenesis and diagnostic considerations. *J Urol* **138**: 587–91.

Maizels M, Zaontz M, Donovan J *et al.* (1986) Surgical correction of the buried penis: description of a classification system and a technique to correct the disorder. *J Urol* **136**: 268–71.

Mandressi A, Buizza C, Antonelli D, Chisnea S (1996) Is laparoscopy a worthy method to treat varicocele? Comparison between 160 cases of two-port laparoscopic and 120 cases of open inguinal spermatic vein ligation. *J Endourol* **10**: 435–41.

Marmar JL, Kim Y (1994) Subinguinal microsurgical varicocelectomy: a technical critique and statistical analysis of semen and pregnancy data. *J Urol* **152**: 1127–32.

Marti-Bonmati L, Menor F, Gonez J, *et al.* (1989) Value of sonography in true complete diphallia. *J Urol* **142**: 356–7.

Merida MG, Miguelez C, Galiano E, Lopez Perez GA (1992) Polyorchidism: an exceptional case of three homolateral testes. *Eur Urol* **21**: 338–9.

Merry C, Sweeney B, Puri P (1997) The vanishing testis: anatomical and histological findings. *Eur Urol* **31**: 65–7.

Miersch WDE, Schoeneich G, Winter P, Buszello H (1995) Laparoscopic varicocelectomy: indication, technique and surgical results. *Br J Urol* **76**: 636–8.

Miller ST, Rao SP, Dunn EK, Glassberg KI (1995) Priapism in children with sickle cell disease. *J Urol* **154**: 844–7.

Miltenburg DM, Nuchtern JG, Jaksic T *et al.* (1997) Meta-analysis of the risk of metachronous hernia in infants and children. *Am J Surg* **174**: 741–4.

Miltenburg DM, Nuchtern JG, Jaksic T *et al.* (1998) Laparoscopic evaluation of the pediatric inguinal hernia – a meta-analysis. *J Pediatr Surg* **33**: 874–9.

Minevich E, Wacksman J, Lewis AG, Sheldon CA (1998) Inguinal microsurgical varicocelectomy in the adolescent: technique and preliminary results. *J Urol* **159**: 1022–4.

Mohamed AA, Stockdale EJ, Varghese J, Youngson GG (1998) Abdominoscrotal hydrocoeles: little place for conservatism. *Pediatr Surg Int* **13**: 186–8.

Money J, Lehne GK, Pierre-Jerome F (1985) Micropenis: gender, erotosecual coping strategy, and behavioral health in nie pediatric cases followed to adulthood. *Compr Psychiatry* **26**: 29–42.

Morecroft JA, Stringer MD, Higgins M *et al.* (1993) Follow-up after inguinal herniotomy or surgery for hydrocele in boys. *Br J Surg* **80**: 1613–4.

Mykulak DJ, Glassberg KI (1990) Impotence following childhood priapism. *J Urol* **144**: 134–5.

Nagao RR, Plymate SR, Berger RE *et al.* (1986) Comparison of gonadal function between fertile and infertile men with varicoceles. *Fertil Steril* **46**: 930–3.

Nesbitt JA, King LR (1990) Ectopia of the vas deferens. *J Pediatr Surg* **25**: 335–8.

Nistal M, Paniagua R, Díez-Pardo JA (1979) Testicular microlithiasis in 2 children with bilateral cryptorchidism. *J Urol* **121**: 535–7.

Nisula BC, Loriaux DL, Sherins RJ, Kulin HE (1974) Benign bilateral testicular enlargement. *J Clin Endocrinol Metab* **38**: 440–5.

Noe HN, Wilimas J, Jerkins GR (1981) Surgical management of priapism in children with sickle cell anemia. *J Urol* **126**: 770–1.

Oesch IL, Pinter A, Ransley PG (1987) Penile agenesis: a report of six cases. *J Pediatr Surg* **22**: 172–4.

Okuyama A, Nakamura M, Namiki M *et al.* (1988) Surgical repair of varicocele at puberty: preventive treatment for fertility improvement. *J Urol* **139**: 562–4.

Okuyama A, Itatani H, Aono T *et al.* (1980) Prognosis of sexual maturation in prepubertal boys with micropenis. *Arch Androl* **5**: 265–9.

Oster J (1968) Further fate of the foreskin: incidence of preputial adhesions, phimosis, and smegma among Danish schoolboys. *Arch Dis Child* **43**: 200–3.

Oster J (1971) Varicocele in children and adolescents. An investigation of the incidence among Danish school children. *Scand J Urol Nephrol* **5**: 27–32.

Padmore DE, Norman RW, Millard OH (1996) Analyses of indications for and outcomes of epididymectomy. *J Urol* **156**: 95–6.

Paduch DA, Niedzielski J (1997) Repair versus observation in adolescent varicocele: a prospective study. *J Urol* **158**: 1128–32.

Palmer LS, Gill B, Kogan SJ (1997) Endocrine analysis of childhood monorchism. *J Urol* **158**: 594–6.

Palomo A (1949) Radical cure of varicocele by a new technique: preliminary report. *J Urol* **61**: 604.

Parida SK, Hall BD, Barton L, Fujimoto A (1995) Penoscrotal transposition and associated anomalies: report of five new cases and review of the literature. *Am J Med Genet* **59**: 68–75.

Parrott TS, Hewatt L (1994) Ligation of the testicular artery and vein in adolescent varicocele. *J Urol* **152**: 791–3.

Perala JM, Leinonen SAS, Suramo IJI *et al.* (1998) Comparison of early deflation rate of detachable latex and silicone balloons and observations on persistent varicocele. *J Vasc Interv Radiol* **9**: 761–5.

Perlmutter AD, Chamberlain JW (1972) Webbed penis without chordee. *J Urol* **107**: 320–1.

Persad R, Sharma S, McTavish J, *et al.* (1995) Clinical presentation and pathophysiology of meatal stenosis following circumcision. *Br J Urol* **75**: 91–3.

Pomerantz P, Hanna M, Levitt S, Kogan S (1978) Isolated torsion of penis. *Urology* **11**: 37–9.

Popek EJ (1990) Embryonal remnants in inguinal hernia sacs. *Hum Pathol* **21**: 339–49.

Punekar SV, Prem AR, Ridhorkar VR *et al.* (1996) Post-surgical recurrent varicocele: efficacy of internal spermatic venography and steel-coil embolization. *Br J Urol* **77**: 124–8.

Puri P, Guiney EJ, O'Donnell B (1984) Inguinal hernia in infants: the fate of the testis following incarceration. *J Pediatr Surg* **19**: 44–6.

Quigley CA, DeBellis A, Marschke KB *et al.* (1995) Androgen receptor defects: historical, clinical, and molecular perspectives. *Endocrine Rev* **16**: 271–321.

Rabinowitz R (1984) The importance of the cremasteric reflex in acute scrotal swelling in children. *J Urol* **132**: 89–90.

Ramos CE, Park JS, Ritchey ML, Benson GS (1995) High flow priapism associated with sickle cell disease. *J Urol* **153**: 1619–21.

Rattan J, Rattan S, Gupta DK (1997) Epidermoid cyst of the penis with extension into the pelvis. *J Urol* **158**: 593.

Redman JF (1985a) A technique for the correction of penoscrotal fusion. *J Urol* **133**: 432–3.

Redman JF (1985b) Cystectomy: a catastrophic complication of herniorrhaphy. *J Urol* **133**: 97–8.

Reilly JM, Woodhouse CRJ (1989) Small penis and the male sexual role. *J Urol* **142**: 569–71.

Renshaw AA (1998) Testicular calcifications: incidence, histology and proposed pathological criteria for testicular microlithiasis. *J Urol* **160**: 1625–8.

Rey RA, Campo SM, Bedecarras P *et al.* (1993) Is infancy a quiescent period of testicular development? Histological, morphometric, and functional study of the seminiferous tubules of the cebus monkey from birth to the end of puberty. *J Clin Endocrinol Metab* **76**: 1325–31.

Rickwood AMK (1999) Medical indications for circumcision. *BJU Int* **83** (Suppl 1): 45–51.

Robinson P, Rock J, Menkin MF (1968) Control of human spermatogenesis by induced changes of intrascrotal temperature. *JAMA* **204**: 290–7.

Roehrborn CG, Schneider H-J, Rugendorff EW, Hamann W (1986) Embryological and diagnostic aspects of seminal vesicle cysts associated with upper urinary tract malformation. *J Urol* **135**: 1029–32.

Rowe MI, Copelson LW, Clatworthy HW (1969) The patent processus vaginalis and the inguinal hernia. *J Pediatr Surg* **4**: 102–7.

Rutgers JL, Young RH, Scully RE (1988) The testicular 'tumor' of the adrenogenital syndrome: a report of six cases and review of the literature on testicular masses in patients with adrenocortical disorders. *Am J Surg Pathol* **12**: 503–13.

Sadler BT, Greenfield SP, Wan J, Glick PL (1995) Intrascrotal epidermoid cyst with extension into the pelvis. *J Urol* **153**: 1265–6.

Sayfan J, Siplovich L, Koltun L, Benyamin N (1997) Varicocele treatment in pubertal boys prevents testicular growth arrest. *J Urol* **157**: 1456–7.

Schonfeld WA (1943) Primary and secondary sexual characteristics. Study of their development in males from birth through maturity, with biometric study of penis and testes. *Am J Dis Child* **65**: 535–49.

Schwartz R, Stephens FD (1978) The persisting mesonephric duct: high junction of vas deferens and ureter. *J Urol* **120**: 592–6.

Seeler RA (1973) Intensive transfusion therapy for priapism in boys with sickle cell anemia. *J Urol* **110**: 360–1.

Serels S and Kogan S (1996) Bilateral giant abdominoscrotal hydroceles in childhood. *Urology* **47**: 763–5.

Sharpsteen JR Jr, Powars D, Johnson C, *et al.* (1993) Multisystem damage associated with tricorporal priapism in sickle cell disease. *Am J Med* **94**: 289–95.

Siegel A, Snyder H, Duckett JW (1987) Epididymitis in infants and boys: underlying urogenital anomalies and efficacy of imaging modalities. *J Urol* **138**: 1100–3.

Siegel JF, Rich MA, Brock WA (1993) Association of sickle cell disease, priapism, exchange transfusion and neurological events: ASPEN syndrome. *J Urol* **150**: 1480–2.

Sigman M, Jarow JP (1997) Ipsilateral testicular hypotrophy is associated with decreased sperm counts in infertile men with varicoceles. *J Urol* **158**: 605–7.

Simko A, Hornstein L, Soukup S, Bagamery N (1989) Fragile X syndrome: recognition in young children. *Pediatrics* **83**: 547–52.

Sinnecker GH, Hiort O, Dibbelt L *et al.* (1996) Phenotypic classification of male pseudohermaphroditism due to steroid 5a-reductase deficiency. *Am J Med Genet* **63**: 223–30.

Skoog SJ, Belman AB (1989) Aphallia: its classification and management. *J Urol* **141**: 589–92.

Skoog SJ, Conlin MJ (1995) Pediatric hernias and hydroceles. *Urol Clin North Am* **22**: 119–30.

Spears T, Franco I, Reda EF *et al.* (1992) Accessory and ectopic scrotum with VATER association. *Urology* **40**: 343–5.

Spera G, Medolago-Albani L, Coia L *et al.* (1983) Histological, histochemical, and ultrastructural aspects of interstitial tissue from the contralateral testis in infertile men with monolateral varicocele. *Arch Androl* **10**: 73–8.

Steckel J, Dicker AP, Goldstein M (1993) Relationship between varicocele size and response to varicocelectomy. *J Urol* **149**: 769–71.

Steeno O, Knops J, DeClerk L *et al.* (1976) Prevention of fertility disorders by detection and treatment of varicocele at school and college age. *Andrologia* **8**: 47–53.

Stenham A, Malmfors G, Okmian L (1986) Circumcision for phimosis: a follow-up study. *Scand J Urol Nephrol* **20**: 89–92.

Stern R, Kistler W, Scharli AF (1998) The Palomo procedure in the treatment of boys with varicocele: a restrospective study of testicular growth and fertility. *Pediatr Surg Int* **14**: 74–8.

Stolar CJH, Wiener ES, Hensle TW *et al.* (1987) Reconstruction of penile agenesis by a posterior sagittal approach. *J Pediatr Surg* **22**: 1076–80.

Stone KT, Kass EJ, Cacciarelli AA, Gibson DP (1995) Management of suspected antenatal torsion: what is the best strategy? *J Urol* **153**: 782–4.

Su L, Goldstein M, Schlegel PN (1995) The effect of varico-celectomy on serum testosterone levels in infertile men with varicoceles. *J Urol* **154**: 1752–5.

Sule JD, Skoog SJ, Tank ES (1994) Perineal lipoma and the accessory labioscrotal fold: an etiological relationship. *J Urol* **151**: 475–7.

Sutherland RS, Kogan BA, Baskin LS *et al.* (1996) The effect of prepubertal androgen exposure on adult penile length. *J Urol* **156**: 783–7.

Szabo R, Kessler R (1984) Hydrocele following internal spermatic vein ligation: a retroperitoneal study and review of the literature. *J Urol* **132**: 924–5.

Tarry WF, Duckett JW, Snyder HMcC (1987) Urological complications of sickle cell disease in a pediatric population. *J Urol* **138**: 592–4.

Thum G (1991) Polyorchidism: case report and review of the literature. *J Urol* **145**: 370–2.

Tinga DJ, Siemen J, Bruijnen CLAH *et al.* (1984) Factors related to semen improvement and fertility after varicocele operation. *Fertil Steril* **41**: 404–10.

Turek PJ, Ewalt DH, Snyder HM *et al.* (1994a) The absent cryptorchid testis: surgical findings and their implications for diagnosis and etiology. *J Urol* **151**: 718–21.

Turek PJ, Ewalt DH, Snyder HM, Duckett JW (1994b) Normal epididymal anatomy in boys. *J Urol* **151**: 726–7.

Ulman I, Avanoğlu A, Herek Ö *et al.* (1996) A simple method of treating priapism in children. *Br J Urol* **77**: 460–1.

Van Howe RS (1999) Does circumcision influence sexually transmitted diseases? A literature review. *BJU Int* **83** (Suppl 1): 52–62.

Vasavada S, Ross J, Nasrallah P, Kay R (1997) Prepubertal varicoceles. *Urology* **50**: 774–7.

Verga G, Avolio L (1996) Agenesis of the scrotum: an extremely rare anomaly. *J Urol* **156**: 1467.

Virag R, Bachir D, Lee K, Galacteros F (1996) Preventive treatment of priapism in sickle cell disease with oral and self-administered intracavernous injection of etilefrine. *Urology* **47**: 777–81.

Vohra S, Morgentaler A (1997) Congenital anomalies of the vas deferens, epididymis and seminal vesicles. *Urology* **49**: 313–21.

Walker JR, Casale AJ (1997) Prolonged penile erection in the newborn. *Urology* **50**: 796–9.

Wang Y-X, Lei C, Dong S-G *et al.* (1991) Study of bilateral histology and meiotic analysis in men undergoing varicocele ligation. *Fertil Steril* **55**: 152–5.

Wara DW, Emery HM (1991) Collagen vascular diseases. In: Rudolph AM (ed.) *Rudolph's pediatrics*. 19th edition. Norwalk, CT: Appleton & Lange, 490–1.

Watkin NA, Reiger NA, Moisey CU (1996) Is the conservative management of the acute scrotum justified on clinical grounds? *Br J Urol* **78**: 623–7.

Weiss DB, Rodriguez-Rigau LJ, Smith KD, Steinberger E (1978) Leydig cell function in oligospermatic men with varicocele. *J Urol* **120**: 427–30.

Wilbert DM, Schaerfe CW, Stren WD *et al.* (1993) Evaluation of the acute scrotum by color-coded Doppler ultrasonography. *J Urol* **149**: 1475–7.

Wojcik LJ, Hansen K, Diamond DA *et al.* (1997) Cystic dysplasia of the rete testis: a benign congenital lesion associated with ipsilateral urological abnormalities. *J Urol* **158**: 600–4.

Wright JE (1993) Congenital absence of the scrotum: case report and description of an original technique of construction of a scrotum. *J Pediatr Surg* **28**: 264–6.

Yamamoto M, Katsuno S, Yokoi K *et al.* (1995) The effect of varicocelectomy on testicular volume in infertile patients with varicoceles. *Nagoya J Med Sci* **58**: 47–50.

Zachmann M, Prader A, Kind HP *et al.* (1974) Testicular volume during adolescence: cross-sectional and longitudinal studies. *Helv Paediatr Acta* **29**: 61–72.

Zaontz MR, Kass EJ (1987) Ectopic ureter opening into seminal vesicle cyst associated with ipsilateral renal agenesis. *Urology* **24**: 523–5.

Zolfaghari A, Pourissa M, Hajialilou Sh, Amjadi M (1995) True complete diphallia. A case report. *Scand J Urol Nephrol* **29**: 233–5.

Zorgniotti AW, MacLeod J (1973) Studies in temperature, human semen quality and varicocele. *Fertil Steril* **24**: 854–63.

Cryptorchidism

34a

Douglas A. Husmann

Introduction

The optimal goals for treatment of the undescended testicle are to improve fertility, decrease the potential for malignancy, repair the associated hernia, decrease the incidence of spontaneous torsion, and minimize the psychological trauma of an empty scrotum. This chapter will review the current success of pediatric urology to fulfill these objectives (Gill and Kogan, 1997).

Terminology of cryptorchidism

Spontaneously descending testis: a testicle that was not within the scrotum at birth but descends into the scrotum with maturation unaided by hormonal or surgical manipulations.

Ascended testis: a testicle documented to be within the scrotum during the first years of life; however, with time the testis ascends and is unable to be relocated to the scrotum. An ascended testicle can be *primary*, with no antecedent inguinal surgery, or *secondary*, ascensus of the testicle following inguinal cord manipulation after a hernia or hydrocele repair. In this latter situation the testicle becomes entrapped in the inguinal region secondary to scarring, i.e. iatrogenic cryptorchidism.

Gliding testis: a testicle that can be manipulated into the upper scrotum with tension, however, when the tension is released from the testicle it immediately retracts into the inguinal region. Most authors believe that a gliding testicle represents an undescended testicle that is located just distal to the external ring, and should not be confused with a retractile testicle. The importance in determining gliding from a truly retractile testis is the difference in histologic findings. Histologic evaluations of gliding testes have revealed that these testes are at risk of developing pathologic

changes similar to undescended testes, while retractile testes have been routinely noted to be free from pathologic alterations (Puri and Nixon, 1977; Hadziselimovic, 1983b; Wylie, 1984; Hadziselimovic *et al.*, 1987a).

Retractile testis: a testicle that is palpable in the inguinal canal but can be manipulated into the scrotum where it will remain for some time. It is believed that the cremasteric reflex, a function of the genitofemoral nerve, is the physiologic background for the retractile testis. The cremasteric reflex is most active between the ages of 3 and 9 years. Its activity is inversely proportional to testicular weight and/or the level of serum testosterone. Since human chorionic gonadotropin (hCG) or gonadotropin-releasing hormone (GnRH) will increase both testicular weight and testosterone, a retractile testis will invariably descend into the scrotum in response to these agents. Complete relaxation of the cremasteric muscle by general anesthesia and or muscular relaxants has also been helpful in determining a retractile from an undescended or gliding testis. The importance in accurately diagnosing a retractile from a gliding testicle is based on the absence of pathologic alterations in the retractile testis (Farrington, 1968; Puri and Nixon, 1977; Hadziselimov, 1983b; Wylie, 1984; Goh and Hutson, 1992, 1993; Gill and Kogan, 1997; Walker, 1997; Cortes, 1998).

Ectopic testis: classically, a testicle that is distal to the external ring but fails to descend into the scrotum. In most instances the ectopic testis is found in the superficial inguinal pouch, an epifasical location distal to the external ring. Hadziselmovic states that the testicle found in the superficial inguinal pouch is a true undescended testicle, not an ectopic one. In this chapter, a testicle is listed as being ectopic if it is located in the perineum, contralateral scrotum, or femoral region (Hadziselimovic, 1983b; Hadziselimovic *et al.*, 1987a).

True undescended testicle: it is helpful, for investigative and possibly prognostic reasons, to list the location of the undescended testicle found at the time of orchiopexy. The sites of location are listed as intra-abdominal, proximal intracanalicular, distal intracanalicular, or prescrotal, i.e. superficial inguinal pouch.

Normal anatomy of the testis, epididymis, and vas deferens

The arterial supply to the testicle comes primarily from the testicular arteries arising from the aorta just caudal to the renal arteries. Collateral arterial circulation to the testis is supplied by the artery to the vas deferens, a branch of the inferior vesical artery, and the cremasteric artery, a branch of the inferior epigastric artery. The venous drainage of the testicle is via the veins of the pampiniform plexus. These veins eventually coalesce to form a single retroperitoneal vein entering the vena cava on the right or the renal vein on the left (Fowler and Stephens, 1959; Stephens, 1988).

The epididymis serves as a site for sperm maturation and storage. Normally the head of the epididymis (globus major) and the tail of the epididymis (globus minor) are attached to the tunica albuginea of the posterior wall of the testis. The communication between the testicle and the epididymis occurs through the efferent ductules that exit from the mediastinum of the testis to the globus major. The tail of the epididymis turns cranial and becomes the vas deferens.

The tunica vaginalis covers the testicle in its anterior and lateral aspects. It has a peritoneal origin and has both a parietal and visceral component. In the fetus, the tunica vaginalis communicates with the abdominal cavity via the patent processus vaginalis.

Embryology of testicular and germ cell development

Testicular development

Testicular development is under the influence of the sex-determining gene on the short arm of the Y chromosome (SRY). Primordial germ cells are first located in the caudal portion of the yolk sac during the 4th week of gestation. During the 5th week the germ cells migrate along the dorsal mesentery of the hindgut, reaching the urogenital ridge during the 6th week. The urogenital ridge is located in the mesentery (medial side) of the mesonephros, it is originally cigar shaped and stretches alongside the mesonephros from the diaphragm to the first sacral segment. During the 7th week of gestation the SRY gene induces the SRY protein to initiate development of the bipotential gonad into a testis. As differentiation of the testicle occurs, the Sertoli cells appear and begin secreting müllerian inhibitory substance (MIS) by week 8. Leydig cells appear and testosterone secretion begin by week 10. During the 8th week of development, the testis becomes ovoid in configuration and a marked proliferation of germ cells occurs between weeks 8 and 14. As the testis assumes a rounded shape, the cranial and caudal portions of the urogenital ridge become ligamentous in nature. The diaphragmatic gonadal ligament (also known as the cranial gonadal ligament) involutes and is barely discernable by the 13th week of gestation. The caudal connection of the urogenital ridge along with mesonephric inguinal folds join together and run from the testis to the internal inguinal ring. The caudal connection of the testis to the internal ring becomes known as the gubernacular testis (Whitehorn, 1954; Rajfer and Walsh, 1978; Backhouse, 1981; Hutson and Beasley, 1992; Hinman, 1993; Wilson *et al.*, 1993; Cortes, 1998; Silver and Docimo, 1999).

Germ cell development

Under the influence of fetal pituitary gonadotropins, the neonate undergoes a testosterone surge that peaks at 30–90 days and resolves by 6 months of age. During this period gonocytes, under the influence of testosterone, are induced to both multiply and transform to adult dark spermatogonia. Gonocytes that have not been transformed to adult dark spermatogonia after six months of age degenerate. Of interest is the finding that testicular biopsies of descended testes during the first 6 months of life reveal a decreasing number of germ cells per tubular transverse section. The apparent discrepancy between increasing germ cell numbers but decreasing numbers of germ cells per tubular transverse section can be explained by the rapid increase in testicular volume that is also occurring during this timespan. The rapid proliferation of both germ cells and testicular volume results in considerable heterogeneity in germ cell counts between various locations in the testicle, i.e. spermatogonia are not evenly distributed throughout the testis. This fact is extremely important to the physician who is using testicular biopsies to assess fertility potential of the cryptorchid testicle. It is currently recommended that the pathologist needs to evaluate at least 100 tubular transverse sections to prevent inaccurate assessment of fertility potential (Hedinger, 1982; Muller and Skakkebaek, 1983; Muller and Skakkebaek, 1984a; Hadziselimovic, 1986; Huff *et al.*, 1987; Huff *et al.*, 1989; Hadziselimovic *et al.*, 1991; Hinman, 1993; Cortes, 1998; Husmann *et al.*, 1998).

Alterations in testicular and germ cell development in undescended testes

Considerable controversy exists regarding whether or not the cryptorchid testicle has a number of germ cells equal to the descended testicle at the time of birth. The answer to this dispute, although still unknown, is crucial to our understanding of fertility and how it relates to orchiopexy. For example, if the cryptorchid testicle has diminished germ cell counts at birth it is probable that the testicle will continue to have abnormal germ cell counts irrespective of the age of orchiopexy.

Regardless of whether or not the cryptorchid testicle has hypoplasia of germ cells at birth, all authorities have found that there is an additional loss of germ cells that occur if the testicle remains in a non-scrotal position after 1 year of age. It is currently unknown whether the acquired loss of germ cells is due to increased heat from an abnormal testicular position or to an abnormality in gonadotropin and subsequently testosterone secretion that occurs during the first 6 months of life (Hadziselimovic *et al.*, 1984a; Walker, 1997; Hadziselmovic and Herzog, 1997).

Although germ cell hypoplasia may exist within the cryptorchid testicle at birth, the complete lack of germ cells, i.e. germ cell aplasia, appears to be an acquired condition. Necropsy evaluations of fetal cryptorchid testes (age 22–40 weeks of gestation) have routinely found germ cells to be present in all of the testes evaluated. As maturation of the infant occurs, a slow but progressive loss of germ cells in the cryptorchid testicle becomes apparent. Specifically, routine testicular biopsies on infants undergoing orchiopexy at less than 1 year of age reveal a 0.5% incidence of germ cell aplasia. In contrast, 2% of 1 year-old boys undergoing testicular biopsy at the time of orchiopexy had germ cell aplasia. Careful pathologic evaluation of children undergoing orchiopexy between 1 and 2 years of age reveals that a significant increase in the frequency of germ cell aplasia appears to begin at 15 months of age. As the patient with cryptorchidism matures, the number of individuals found to have germ cell aplasia at the time of orchiopexy increases. Specifically, 20% of 2 year olds, up to 40% of 6 year olds and 45% of boys at the age of 10–11 years will have germ cell aplasia (Fig. 34a.1). In contrast to the cryptorchid testicle, testicular biopsies performed on descended testes in children between 1 and 12 years of age reveal a 1% incidence of germ cell aplasia (Fig. 34a.2). The timing for surgical intervention on

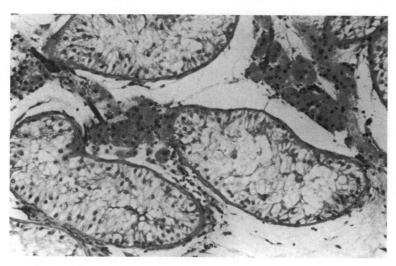

Figure 34a.1 Biopsy specimen of cryptorchid intra-abdominal testis in an 18-year-old boy showing germinal absence, Leydig hyperplasia, and 'Sertoli cell-only' appearance (x 250).

the cryptorchid testicle is currently based on these biopsy results, with routine orchiopexy being recommended by 1 year of age (Sohval, 1954; Hecker and Heinz, 1967; Farrington, 1969; Mengel *et al.*, 1974; Baker and Scrimgeour, 1980; Nistal *et al.*, 1980; Gaudio *et al.*, 1984; Muller and Skakkebaek, 1984a; Coerdt *et al.*, 1985; Hadziselimovic *et al.*, 1986; Schindler *et al.*, 1987; Hadziselimovic *et al.*, 1987a; Kogan, 1988; Orvis *et al.*, 1988; Kogan *et al.*, 1990; Hadziselimovic *et al.*, 1991; Huff *et al.*, 1991; Thorup *et al.*, 1993; McAleer *et al.*, 1995; Cortes, 1998).

Fibrosis around the seminiferous tubules (peritubular fibrosis) occurs as a consequence of testicular undescent. This pathologic entity begins to occur in the undescended testicle by the second year of life and becomes more pronounced with age. Peritubular fibrosis is associated with increased peritubular mucopolysaccharide deposition. The increased deposition of the mucopolysaccharides hinders the exchange of nutrients within the seminiferous tubules and subsequently interferes with spermatogenesis. Diminished sperm count due to testicular undescent is subsequently believed to be due to both the impaired nutrition and diminished number of the remaining germ cells (Hadziselimovic, 1983a).

Testicular descent: the current hypothesis

Following degeneration of the mesonephros at 7–8 weeks of gestation, the testicle is in close proximity to

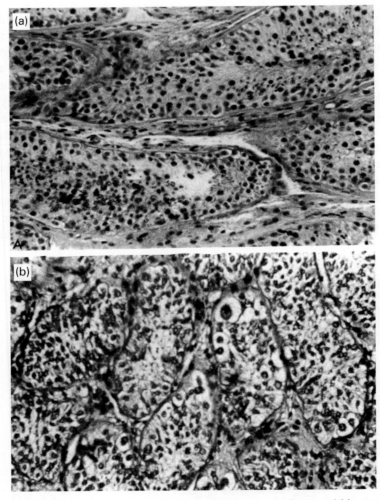

Figure 34a.2 Bilateral biopsy specimens in unilateral cryptorchidism in a 13-year-old boy undergoing orchiectomy. (a) Descended testis with numerous germ cells and active spermatogenesis. (b) Undescended testis with decreased number of germ cells, maturation arrest, and absence of spermatogenesis (a, b, × 200).

the inguinal ring but is highly mobile. In its cephalic portion, the testicle is connected to the kidney and diaphragm via the cranial gonadal ligament. Caudally, the gubernaculum attaches the testis and epididymis to the genital swelling, the precursor of the scrotum. Descent of the testis from its position near the internal inguinal ring into the scrotum can be broken down into two major phases: masculinization of the inguinal canal (gubernacular outgrowth and regression) and transinguinal descent.

Masculinization of the inguinal canal (gubernacular outgrowth and regression)

In the early human embryo the gubernaculum is a jelly-like mass that consists primarily of embryonic mesenchyme. It lies within the developing inguinal canal connecting the testis and epididymis to the scrotum. At 15 weeks of gestation the androgen-independent growth factor descendin, secreted by the testis, stimulates gubernacular outgrowth. The gubernaculum swells due to the combination of hyperplasia of the mesenchymal cells and increased synthesis of the gubernacular extracellular matrix. The extracellular matrix primarily contains hydrophilic acid mucopolysaccharides, such as hyaluronic acid. The hydrophilic nature of this substance results in significant water uptake and enlargement of the gubernaculum, and, by 24 weeks of gestation, the gubernaculum approximates or surpasses the size of the testis. In the human fetus, the testis will eventually herniate through and derives its coverings from the various layers of the abdominal wall. It is noteworthy that the entire inguinal canal is formed around the mesenchymal tissue of the gubernaculum before testicular descent. Indeed, in the developing human fetus prior to the descent of the testis, the inguinal canal will contain the processus vaginalis, the gubernaculum, and the cremasteric muscle. It is currently believed that failure of the gubernaculum to swell results in a constricted or feminized inguinal canal that will prevent testicular descent (Hart, 1910; Wyndham, 1943; Person, 1956; Baumans et al., 1983; Hutson, 1986; Hutson and Donhoe, 1986; Heyns, 1987; Fentener et al., 1988; Spencer et al., 1991; Spencer, 1994; Heyns and Hutson, 1995; Husmann and Levy, 1995; Levy and Husmann, 1995; McMahon et al., 1995).

Gubernacular regression is associated with a decrease in cellular proliferation, a reduction in hyaluronic acid content, and an increase in the cata-bolic enzyme acid phosphatase. In the human fetus, gubernacular regression and testicular descent occur between 24 and 32 weeks of gestation. Although common sense may dictate that the enlarged gubernaculum should regress in front of the descending testicle, scientific investigations have failed to reveal evidence of paratesticular degeneration. Indeed, in some species (swine) the testicle descends alongside the enlarged gubernaculum (Heyns et al., 1990; Heyns and Huston, 1995; Levy and Husmann, 1995; McMahon et al., 1995).

The relationship between gubernacular regression and testicular descent may be integral to our understanding of how androgens control testicular descent. In particular, recent studies have documented that inadequate androgen function is associated with both testicular non-descent and failed gubernacular regression. Although it is unknown how gubernacular regression affects testicular descent, it is hypothesized that androgens control the catabolic enzymes and/or paracrine factors that alter the viscoelastic properties of the gubernaculum. If the catabolic enzymes or paracrine factors are not activated, the gubernaculum would remain more turgid than normal. Under these circumstances, the gubernaculum would serve as an anatomic roadblock to descent of the testis (Husmann, 1991; Spencer et al., 1991; Heyns and Hutson, 1995; Husmann and Levy, 1995; Levy and Husmann, 1995; McMahon et al., 1995).

Transinguinal descent

Transinguinal descent of the testis appears to be predominantly directed by intra-abdominal pressure and occurs between the 24th and 28th weeks of gestation. It is currently believed that the transmission of intra-abdominal pressure to the gonad includes three key components; the patent processus vaginalis, the gubernaculum, and androgen secretion. The patent processus vaginalis is a peritoneal pouch that surrounds and penetrates into the gubernaculum on all but its dorsal side. Elongation and growth of the patent processus appear to be under androgenic control, with androgen blockade resulting in a foreshortened patent processus. It is believed that intra-abdominal pressure is transmitted via the patent processus vaginalis to the tip of the gubernaculum. In turn, the gubernaculum puts traction on the epididymis and testis and initially pulls the testicle into the internal inguinal ring. Once the testicle is within the inguinal canal, intra-abdominal pressure may both push and pull the testis into the scrotum. The patent processus will descend through the canal with the testicle and will eventually reach the scrotum. After the testis has reached the bottom of the scrotum, the gubernaculum regresses and the connection between the processus vaginalis and the peritoneum involutes, leaving the tunica vaginalis to cover the anterior and lateral sides of the testis (Backhouse, 1981; Frey *et al.*, 1983; Frey and Rajfer, 1984; Heyns, 1987; Fentener *et al.*, 1988; Hutson and Beasley, 1992; Shono *et al.*, 1994; Heyns and Hutson, 1995; Husmann and Levy, 1995; Levy and Husmann, 1995; Hutson *et al.*, 1997; Cortes, 1998).

Etiology of cryptorchidism

A complex interplay among the testis, androgens, gubernaculum, patent processus vaginalis, and intra-abdominal pressure is necessary for descent of the testicle. Cryptorchidism can be due to any one of a variety of congenital abnormalities, for example, abnormal or poorly timed androgen secretion (i.e. hypothalamic–testicular malfunction), malformation or anatomic obstruction of the inguinal canal (posterior urethral valves), abnormal development of the gubernaculum, processus vaginalis, abdominal wall (prune belly syndrome) or caudal field defects (imperforate anus, myelodysplasia, gastroschisis, cloacal exstrophy) (Engle, 1932; Fallon *et al.*, 1982; Cortada and Kousseff, 1984; Kaplan *et al.*, 1986; Husmann, 1991; Hutson and Beasley, 1992; Husmann and Levy, 1995; Levy and Husmann, 1995; Walker, 1997; Cortes, 1998; Silver and Docimo, 1999).

Testicular descent: prior hypotheses currently in disfavor

Epididymal and vasal abnormalities: as an etiology of testicular undescent

It has been hypothesized that alterations in mesonephric (wolffian) ductal development are the etiologic cause of cryptorchidism. In fact, the incidence of epididymal–vasal abnormalities in cryptorchid testicles have been reported to range between 15 and 85%, with the more proximal cryptorchid testicles having the higher incidence of abnormalities. The epididymal–vasal abnormalities found to coexist with cryptorchidism are usually divided into one of three categories: agenesis or partial agenesis of the epididymis, vasal atresia, and an elongated vas deferens (Whitehorn, 1954; Lemeh, 1960; Bedford, 1978; Hadziselimovic and Kruslin, 1979; Marshall and Shermata, 1979; Priebe *et al.*, 1979; Backhouse, 1981; Gill *et al.*, 1989; Hinman, 1993; Hadziselimovic and Herzog, 1993).

According to this hypothesis, primary epididymal and vasal maldevelopment may lead to testicular undescent in one of two ways. First, an abnormal epididymis may result in an anomalous attachment of the gubernaculum to the epididymal–testicular complex. Since the gubernacular–epididymal complex leads the testicle into the scrotum, an aberrant gubernacular–epididymal attachment may result in an inappropriate spatial relationship between the testis and the internal inguinal ring. The testicular malposition could theoretically result in the ineffective transfer of intra-abdominal pressure and, subsequently, cryptorchidism. Alternatively, an epididymal abnormality could cause testicular undescent owing to its impact on diffusion of testosterone from the testis. Specifically, according to the Jostarian hypothesis for sexual development, testosterone acts as a paracrine factor, that is it acts locally, not systemically, for sexual development of the internal genitalia and possibly for descent of the testis. Since androgens are aided in their diffusion from the testis via flow down the lumen of the mesonephric ducts, insufficient levels of local testosterone would occur if there were embryologic abnormalities of the wolffian ductal system. Inadequate local levels of testosterone would interfere with both gubernacular regression and elongation of the processus vaginalis. In essence, it is the congenitally abnormal epididymis that interferes with both androgen diffusion and the transmission of intra-abdominal pressure. The argument that an abnormal epididymis could cause abnormal local levels of testosterone is somewhat circuitous, since androgens are necessary to provide normal development of the wolffian ducts. In essence, did abnormal levels of androgens cause the epididymal abnormality or did the epididymal abnormality result in abnormally low levels of local testosterone? (Schultz and Wilson, 1974; Shono *et al.*, 1994; Husmann and Levy, 1995; Levy and Husmann, 1995; McMahon *et al.*, 1995; Spencer-Barthold, 1996; Tong *et al.*, 1996).

The chief argument against this hypothesis is the finding that both epididymal abnormalities and complete absence of the epididymis can be found in descended testes. At present, most authorities believe that it is very unlikely that the epididymal malformations are the etiology of testicular undescent (Scorer and Farrington, 1971; Baikie and Hutson, 1990; Husmann, 1991; Elder, 1992d; Levy and Husmann, 1995; McMahon *et al.*, 1995).

Dual hormonal hypothesis: müllerian inhibitory substance and testosterone

The hypothesis that MIS is responsible for regulating intra-abdominal testicular migration, whereas androgens are responsible for regulating transinguinal testicular migration, arose from two separate findings. First, the majority of patients (70%) with persistent müllerian ductal structures had intra-abdominal testes. Second, 90% of patients with complete testicular feminization had testes that had descended distal to the internal inguinal ring (Hutson, 1986; Hutson and Donahoe, 1986).

This hypothesis has fallen into disfavor because of several contradictory facts. First, the presence of intra-abdominal testes in patients with persistent müllerian ductal syndrome is believed to be due to anatomic blockade caused by the persistence of the müllerian structures. In particular, the persistent fallopian tubes intertwine with the gonadal vasculature and physically block testicular descent. Second, the vast majority of patients with intra-abdominal cryptorchidism do not have persistent müllerian structures. Third, experimental evaluations using female rabbits immunized against MIS revealed that their male offspring had persistent or partial persistence of their müllerian ductal system but still had testicular descent. The arguments against MIS having a role in testicular descent are sufficient enough to discredit this hypothesis (Guerrier *et al.*, 1989; Josso *et al.*, 1993; Husmann and Levy, 1995; Levy and Husmann, 1995; Spencer-Barthold, 1998).

Androgenic control of the genitofemoral nuclei: neuronal control of testicular descent via calcitonin gene-related peptide

According to this hypothesis androgens masculinize the genitofemoral spinal nucleus located at L_1–L_2 and subsequently the genitofemoral nerve. Masculinization of the nuclei and nerve results in an increased number of motor neurons and subsequently an increase in the release of calcitonin gene-related peptide (CGRP). CGRP is a 37 amino acid peptide that induces, maintains, and intensifies the activity of acetylcholine receptors at neuromuscular junctions. Its presumed role in testicular descent is to increase rhythmic contractions of the gubernaculum. It is believed that the increased rhythmic contractions of the gubernaculum aid in the migration of both the gubernaculum and the testicle into the scrotum (Park and Hutson, 1991; Cain *et al.*, 1994; Goh *et al.*, 1994; Husmann *et al.*, 1994; Levy and Husmann, 1995).

Several scientific findings currently exist either to discredit this hypothesis completely or, at a minimum, to suggest that this hypothesis is not applicable to the human. First, it is highly controversial whether or not androgens masculinize the genitofemoral nucleus. Several laboratories have produced contradictory findings (Goh *et al.*, 1994; Cain *et al.*, 1994; Husmann *et al.*, 1994; Spencer-Barthold *et al.*, 1994; Spencer-Barthold *et al.*, 1996). Second, CGRP expression in the sexually dimorphic spinal cord is indeed androgen sensitive; however, androgens decrease and castration increases CGRP expression within the sexually dimorphic neurons. (Popper and Micevych, 1989; Popper and Micevych, 1990; Popper *et al.*, 1992). Third, and perhaps more importantly, CGRP is a neuromuscular transmitter, acting on the muscular component of the rodent's gubernaculum, the cremasteric muscle. In contrast, there is no activity in the mucopolysaccharide or mesenchymal component of the rodent's gubernaculum. Unlike rodents, humans, primates, and ungulates have their gubernaculum almost exclusively made out of mucopolysaccharides. In essence, the human gubernaculum is almost completely lacking the muscle cells that are the very site of CGRP activity. It is therefore possible that CGRP may play some role in the migration of the gubernaculum in the rodent, but highly unlikely that it plays a major role in human testicular descent (Heyns, 1990; Yamanaka *et al.*, 1992; Terada, 1994; Heyns and Hutson, 1995; Husmann and Levy, 1995; Levy and Husmann, 1995; McMahon *et al.*, 1995).

Persistence of the cranial gonadal ligament

It has been hypothesized that the position of the gonad is determined primarily from the sum of the forces elicited by its cephalic (the cranial gonadal ligament) and caudal (the gubernaculum) attachments.

According to this premise, androgens induce lengthening of the craniogonadal ligament, subsequently resulting in descent of the testis. Inadequate androgen exposure results in a thickened cranial gonadal ligament, which tethers the gonad superiorly, thereby preventing its descent. This hypothesis is supported by the finding that antiandrogens in the rodent are associated with foreshortened cranial gonadal ligaments. It is also aided by the presence of cryptorchidism in splenogonadal fusion. In splenogonadal fusion, splenic cells have migrated into the cranial gonadal ligament, resulting in a persistently thickened cranial gonadal ligament that tethers the gonad superiorly (van der Schoot and Elger, 1992; Cain et al., 1995; Spencer-Barthold et al., 1996; Cortes, 1998).

It is this author's opinion that persistence of the cranial gonadal ligament is not a strong etiologic cause of cryptorchidism. Indeed, if it were, one would expect to find cryptorchidism in 100% of children with splenogonadal fusion. Instead, the incidence is at most 44%. Furthermore, only rarely will a thickened craniogonadal ligament be found to be attached to the cryptorchid testicle at the time of orchiopexy (Husmann and Levy, 1995; Cortes, 1998).

Incidence of cryptorchidism

Three major historic and physical findings are associated with an increased risk for cryptorchidism: low birth weight, prematurity, and hypospadias. The relationship between birth weight and testicular undescent is well established, with infants of 900 g or less having approximately a 100% incidence of cryptorchidism. As the birth weight of the infant increases, the incidence of cryptorchidism steadily decreases. The average incidence of testicular undescent in infants of 900–1800 g is 60%, in infants of 1800–2000 g is 25%, in infants of 2000–2700 g is 15%, in infants of 2700–3600 g is 3.3%, and in infants of 3600–5200 g is 0.7%. If gestational age of the infant at birth is less than or equal to 36 weeks, there is a 30% incidence of cryptorchidism, while full-term infants (37–40 weeks of gestation) have a 3.4% incidence of testicular undescent (Cortes, 1998; Walker, 1997; Silver and Docimo, 1999) (Table 34a.1).

The relationship among hypospadias, cryptorchidism, and androgen physiology is recognized. Although the physician must always rule out intersex

when faced with this constellation of findings, it is the rare patient that is found to have a definable intersex disorder. A number of patients coming to the pediatric urologist for treatment of cryptorchidism will have coexisting hypospadias. The incidence of cryptorchidism with hypospadias is directly related to the position of the urethral meatus. Up to 30% of patients with the hypospadiac meatus located proximal to or in the proximal third of the penile shaft will have coexisting cryptorchidism. Patients with a hypospadiac meatus in the middle third, distal third or glanular location have approximately a 10%, 5%, and 2.5% incidence of cryptorchidism, respectively (Ross et al., 1959; Khuri et al., 1981; Cearasco et al., 1986; Walker, 1997; Cortes, 1998; Silver and Docimo, 1999).

Spontaneous descent of the cryptorchid testicle is a frequent occurrence. The incidence of cryptorchidism decreases from 3.4% in full-term infants to approximately 1% at 3 months of age. Similar to the full-term infant, the incidence of cryptorchidism in the premature infant decreases from 30% to 10% from birth to 3 months after the expected date of delivery. It is the rare testicle that will descend into the scrotum after 3 months of age in a full-term infant or after 3 months following the expected date of delivery in a premature infant. In infants with persistent undescended testes, two-thirds will be unilateral and one-third will be bilateral. In those with a unilateral abnormality, the right testicle is affected twice as often as the left (Walker, 1997; Cortes, 1998; Silver and Docimo, 1999).

Table 34a.1 Prevalence of cryptorchidism at various ages

Age	Weight (g)	Incidence (%)
Premature	451–910	100.0
	911–1810	62.0
	1811–2040	25.0
	2041–2490	17.0
	Total	30.3
Full term	2491–2720	12.0
	2721–3630	3.3
	3631–5210	0.7
	Total	3.4
One year		0.7–0.8
School age		0.76–0.95
Adulthood		0.7–1.0

Data from Scorer and Farrington (1971).

It is noteworthy that longitudinal long-term follow-up studies in full-term infants reveal that the incidence of cryptorchidism increases from 1% at 1 year of age to as much as 7% at 7 years of age. The increased incidence of cryptorchidism in the prepubertal child is believed to be related to a misdiagnosis of retractile testis and or testicular ascensus. (See discussion of hCG treatment to differentiate retractile from primary testicular ascensus.) Spontaneous redescent of the testis will occur in the vast majority of these children at puberty, with the incidence of cryptorchidism in the untreated male population at the age of 16 years averaging 1.5% (Johnson, 1939; Smith, 1941; Ward and Hunter, 1960; Buemann et al., 1961; Scorer, 1964; Villumsen and Zachau-Christianson, 1966; Group, 1992; Berkowitz et al., 1993; Gill and Kogan, 1997; Cortes, 1998).

Recent studies have alluded to the fact that there appears to have been an increase in the incidence of cryptorchidism over the past three decades. These reports primarily base their assessment on the increased number of orchiopexies performed during this period. Currently, depending on the locality evaluated and the years reviewed, 2–4% of the males under the age of 40 years will have undergone an orchiopexy. This 2–4% incidence of orchiopexy occurs in the presence of a 1% incidence of cryptorchidism in infants at 1 year of age and 1.5% incidence of testicular undescent in postpubertal untreated males at the age of 16 years. The increased incidence of orchiopexy beyond that of cryptorchidism has resulted in the hypothesis that as many as 50% of the operations performed for testicular undescent may be done in patients with either testicular ascensus or a failure to recognize retractile testes (Browne, 1949; Atwell, 1985; Rajfer et al., 1986; Wilson-Stoney et al., 1990; Berkowitz et al., 1993; Mayr et al., 1995; Gill and Kogan, 1997; Rabinowitz and Hulbert, 1997; Cortes, 1998).

Familial and genetic aspects of cryptorchidism

Over 3000 suspected or proven genetic defects are associated with testicular undescent. If an infant with cryptorchidism presents for evaluation, a review of the family history will reveal that 4–5% of the fathers and 10–15% of the child's male siblings have had a cryptorchid testicle. This is in contrast to the expected incidence of 1% in parents and siblings that could occur by chance alone. The increased paternal and sibling frequency for cryptorchidism satisfies the criteria for a multifactorial (polygenetic) chromosomal defect as the etiology for cryptorchidism (Perrett and O'Rouke, 1969; Rezvani et al., 1976; Jones and Young, 1982).

Diagnosis of cryptorchidism

Historic findings

The patient's history regarding cryptorchidism is frequently unreliable, with the parents often stating that they did not notice whether the testes had been down in the scrotum at birth. In addition, the routine birth and/or well-child examination may fail to record the presence or absence of intrascrotal testes. Without documentation that the testicles were once within the scrotum, it is difficult to ascertain whether the testicles are ascended or cryptorchid.

Physical examination

Examination for testicular undescent should be performed in a warm room with the child naked, lying supine with the legs placed in a frog-like position. The presence or absence of genital abnormalities should be the first item evaluated. The presence of hypospadias indicates the need to rule out an intersex disorder, particularly if neither or only one gonad is palpable. The configuration of the scrotum should be observed. Visualization of the scrotum may reveal an atrophic and empty scrotum or a descended retractile testis. Prior to palpation of the scrotum, the presence of a cremasteric reflex is determined. Close observation of the scrotum or inguinal region during this maneuver will frequently result in an indication of the location of the testicle. Palpation of the abdomen for location of the testis with the fingertips can then be performed by gently rolling the fingertips from the abdominal and inguinal region to the scrotum. If the testicle cannot be palpated it is often beneficial to lubricate the fingertips with K-Y jelly or liquid soap. This decreases the friction between the fingertips and the patient's body and allows the physician to feel a testicle that was not palpable previously.

Inability to palpate the testicle may be due to the patient's obesity, an intra-abdominal location of the testis, an ectopic testis in the perineal or femoral regions, or testicular absence. If the testis is not palpable in the inguinal scrotal region, careful evaluation of the femoral canal and perineum is performed. Retractile testes can often be differentiated from those that are undescended by examining the child with him sitting, cross-legged and leaning forward. This relaxes the abdominal and, subsequently, the cremasteric muscles.

If a unilateral or bilateral undescended testicle is found to coexist with hypospadias, or if bilateral non-palpable undescended testes are found, a karyotype must be performed and the internal pelvic structures evaluated by radiographic methods. Individuals found to have a 46,XY karyotype with bilateral non-palpable testes are further evaluated by a hCG stimulation test unless the testosterone level had been determined during the first weeks of life.

Evaluation of the 46,XY patient with bilateral impalpable gonads: human chorionic gonadotropin hormonal stimulation and measurement of serum müllerian inhibitory substance

In cryptorchidism approximately 20% of the undescended testes are impalpable on the original examination. Surgical findings in these patients reveal the testicle to be present in approximately 60% and absent or associated with a nubbin of fibrous tissue and hemosiderin in approximately 40%. In patients with bilaterally impalpable gonads, initial evaluation should include karyotype and abdominal and pelvic ultrasonography or pelvic magnetic resonance imaging (MRI) to evaluate for the presence of müllerian structures and intersex disorders. If the karyotype is 46,XY and no müllerian structures are identified, an attempt to document bilateral anorchia versus bilateral impalpable gonads is usually performed prior to surgical or laparoscopic exploration. Two diagnostic tests may have some merit, the hCG hormonal stimulation test and the measurement of serum MIS. (Cendron, 1989; Lawson et al., 1991; Diamond and Caldamone, 1992; Cortes, 1998).

Human chorionic gonadotropin hormonal stimulation

To perform this test baseline follicle-stimulating hormone (FSH), luteinizing hormone (LH) and serum testosterone levels are obtained before hCG stimula-

tion. Administration of 1500 units of hCG is performed on alternate days for three injections. LH, FSH, and serum testosterone levels are again obtained within a 24–72 hours timespan after the last hCG injection. If the baseline FSH levels or baseline FSH and LH levels are elevated and there is failure of the serum testosterone to increase following hCG injection, no testicular tissue is present and further evaluation is unnecessary. (A positive response would be an increase in serum testosterone of > 3 times the baseline value.) If, however, baseline FSH and LH are not elevated and no elevation in serum testosterone is noted after hCG injections, the physician cannot rule out the presence of functioning testicular tissue. Approximately 15% of these latter patients will be found to have testicular tissue present upon surgical exploration or laparoscopy. Failure of the testosterone to elevate in response to the initial hCG trial is thought to be due to either a state of chronically depleted substrate and/or a temporal delay in the upregulation of the necessary testicular steroidogenic enzymes (Levitt et al., 1978; Bartone et al., 1984; Jaron et al., 1986; Walker, 1997; Husmann et al., 1998).

Because of the 15% false-positive rate (diagnosed anorchia when testes present) in patients with normal or immeasurable baseline FSH/LH values, some authors have stated that the hCG stimulation test can be bypassed. These authorities recommend obtaining baseline gonadotropin and testosterone levels only. If FSH/LH are elevated and testosterone levels low (<40 ng/ml) they believe that sufficient laboratory proof exists to make the diagnosis of anorchia. If, however, baseline LH and FSH levels are normal or immeasurable, they believe surgical exploration is mandatory (Jarow, 1986).

To prevent the need for surgical exploration and laparoscopy in patients with normal or immeasurable baseline LH and FSH levels, it is necessary to perform a long-term hCG challenge test. In the long-term stimulation test, 1500 units of hCG are administered three times weekly for three weeks. Serum testosterone levels are measured 24–72 hours after the last injection. Failure of serum testosterone to rise to >3 times the initial baseline level confirms the absence of testicular tissue (Riverola et al., 1970; Walker, 1997). However, in most instances hCG stimulation tests can be avoided if serum testosterone measurement is done during the testosterone surge that occurs in the first weeks of life.

Measurement of serum müllerian inhibitory substance

The Sertoli cells secrete MIS in a sexually dimorphic pattern beginning in the 8th week of gestation until puberty. With puberty, secretion of this hormone by the testis decreases and ovarian production increases, eventually resulting in MIS values that overlap between the two sexes. In infants and prepubertal boys, MIS is a highly specific marker of testicular tissue. In prepubertal boys with bilateral impalpable testes, determination of MIS can aid in the determination of bilateral anorchia from cryptorchidism. Specifically, serum MIS values that are normal (> 5 ng/ml) are indicative of testicular function, and laparoscopy or surgical exploration is indicated. Low or undetectable levels of MIS would suggest either anorchia or a dysgenetic gonad. Unfortunately, low or undetectable levels of MIS alone are not conclusive enough to diagnose anorchia. In these situations the physician must proceed with either an hCG test or alternatively laparoscopy to confirm testicular absence. Because of the continued need to confirm anorchia by either an hCG stimulation or laparoscopy, measurement of MIS values normally does not significantly save the patient from additional diagnostic investigations (Josso *et al.*, 1990; Gustafson *et al.*, 1993; Lee *et al.*, 1997).

Localization of the impalpable testicle

It is hoped that an accurate radiologic method to diagnose absent gonadal tissue would prevent the need for additional diagnostic tests (hCG injections) and/or surgery in the patient with non-palpable testis or testes. A variety of radiologic methods has been evaluated, including ultrasonography, abdominal and pelvic computed tomographic (CT) scans, and MRI. A brief review of the sensitivity and specificity of these radiologic methods in the diagnosis of cryptorchidism is provided.

Ultrasonography

Although clinically appealing, ultrasonography is not reliable in its ability to diagnose an absent gonad accurately. Indeed, in one study where the radiologist was blinded to the requesting physician's clinical findings, the ultrasonographer was able to identify only 70% of the palpable testes (Rosenfield *et al.*, 1989; Walker, 1997). In essence, careful physical examination by an experienced clinician was better than ultrasonography alone in the diagnosis of a palpable testis. In this author's clinical experience with the evaluation of 100 impalpable testes, sonography accurately identified the location of the testicle in 15%; 5% of patients had the testicle diagnosed on ultrasonography but surgical exploration revealed that the gubernaculum had been misidentified as the testis, i.e. false positive. Preoperative ultrasound evaluation revealed an absent testis in 80% of the patients. Surgical exploration, however, revealed 40% of these testicles to be present, i.e. false negative (testicular locations, 25% intra-abdominal, and 15% inguinal). Forty per cent of the testes were absent by both ultrasonography and surgical exploration. In our personal experience, the high incidence of false-positive examinations (5%) coupled with the high incidence of false-negative examinations (40%) make ultrasound evaluations of limited value in both the diagnosis of anorchia and the localization of the undescended testis. Use of sonography as a diagnostic tool should be confined to the obese patient.

Computed axial tomography and magnetic resonance imaging

CT and MRI scans can both be effective in localizing the impalpable testicle. Although it is notable that some studies using these modalities have had 100% success in diagnosing anorchia and/or identifying the site of the undescended testis, most studies have a extremely low to zero false-positive rate but a 15% false-negative rate (diagnosing anorchia, usually with an intra-abdominal testicle present). The drawbacks of these two studies are that the CT scan exposes the child to radiation and the MRI requires significant sedation and/or anesthesia in the young infant to perform the test accurately. The information obtained via these tests is not conclusive enough to prevent the need for either laparoscopy or surgical exploration. The performance of these tests outside clinical experimental studies therefore results in an unnecessary cost and should not be performed if surgical exploration is anticipated (Wolverson *et al.*, 1983; Gome-Leon *et al.*, 1986; Sieme *et al.*, 1986; Friedland and Chang, 1988; Hrebinko and Bellinger, 1993; Lan *et al.*, 1998).

Laparoscopy

Short of open surgical exploration, laparoscopy is the most widely used diagnostic modality for the diagnosis and localization of an impalpable testis. Under most circumstances the vas deferens is identified and traced to the internal ring where the gonadal vessels are identified. The intra-abdominal testis can be easily identified via this method. If laparoscopy identifies an atretic vas associated with blind-ending vessels cephalad to the internal ring (a finding consistent with the vanishing testis syndrome) no further exploration or surgery is necessary. If however, the vas and vassal structures are seen entering into the ring, this author believes that surgical exploration of the inguinal region should be performed. The reader should be aware that this latter recommendation is controversial. Some laparoscopists note that they have never found viable testicular tissue in patients with vas and vessels entering into a closed internal ring, i.e. patent processus occluded. They believe that in this circumstance, laparoscopy alone is sufficient to identify testicular absence and no further inguinal exploration is necessary. It can be argued that in these circumstances, a nubbin of testicular tissue can be present and that a risk of developing testicular carcinoma in this nubbin does exist. Factual data to support this latter assumption are, however lacking (Sieme *et al.*, 1986; King, 1996; Godbole *et al.*, 1997; Walker, 1997; Bakr and Kotb, 1998; Baille *et al.*, 1998; Grady *et al.*, 1998; Humphrey *et al.*, 1998; Sieme *et al.*, 1998).

Anorchia (vanishing testis)

The term vanishing testis is given to the intraoperative findings of blind-ending testicular vessels and vas deferens associated with an absent testis. If both testes are lost, the vanishing testes syndrome, the infant is a 46,XY karyotypic male with a fully formed phallus but without testicular tissue via diagnostic tests or surgical exploration (Perman, 1961; Abeyaratne *et al.*, 1969).

If the diagnosis of unilateral monorchia is made, two intraoperative decisions need to be accomplished: (1) should a testicular prosthesis be placed; and (2) should the contralateral testicle be pexed? Although this author does not recommend placement of a testicular prosthesis until the child is postpubertal, some authors will routinely place a juvenile testicular prosthesis to develop the scrotal space and to prevent any psychological trauma of having a vacant scrotum during the formative childhood years. If the testicular prosthesis is placed at this age, placement of another prosthesis will be necessary in the postpubertal period

(Smith and Lattimer, 1975; Pidutti and Morales, 1993).

One of the primary questions regarding the vanishing testis is whether absence of the testicle was due to failure of organogenesis or secondary to a vascular catastrophe, i.e. fetal or neonatal torsion. The contralateral testicle is unlikely to be at any increased risk of torsion over the normal patient population. In addition, the solitary testis could be damaged by the fixation suture, and therefore this author does not pex the remaining testicle. This decision is controversial and adequate scientific information regarding the risk of contralateral intravaginal torsion of the remaining solitary testicle is lacking. Surgeons who believe that the contralateral testicle is at an increased risk of torsion will proceed with its fixation (Walker, 1997).

Long-term follow-up of boys with bilateral anorchia (vanishing testis syndrome) is necessary. Beginning at 10 years of age, FSH and LH measurements are taken at 6 monthly intervals. When the levels begin to rise, indicating the onset of puberty, testosterone replacement therapy is initiated.

Renal abnormalities: the relationship between anorchia and partial or complete vasal agenesis

The relationship among renal, testicular, epididymal, and vasal abnormalities is based on the embryologic development of these structures. In the 4th to 5th week of gestation, the ureteral bud sprouts from the caudal part of the mesonephric duct and grows into the metanephric blastema, where it is responsible for the development of the ureter, renal calyces, and the renal collecting ducts. The testis differentiates on the ventromedial side of the mesonephros during the 7th to 14th week of gestation. Under the stabilizing influence of testosterone, the middle part of the mesonephric duct differentiates into the vas deferens, the seminal vesicle and the ejaculatory duct between 8 and 13 weeks of gestation. If a combination of renal and mesonephric ductal abnormalities exists, the embryologic defect must arise before or during the development of the ureteral bud from the shared mesonephric duct, i.e. before or during the 4th to 5th week of gestation (Whitehorn, 1954; Lemeh, 1960; Backhouse, 1981; Hinman, 1993).

In most circumstances the incidence of coexisting renal abnormalities with cryptorchidism is minimally above the normal frequency and investigation for their presence in a child with cryptorchidism is not warranted. Of note, however, is the high incidence of coexisting renal agenesis when either vasal (partial or complete) or true testicular agenesis/monorchia (as compared to a vanished testis) is found during surgical exploration. In this circumstance ipsilateral renal agenesis will be found to coexist in approximately 20% of the patients. Owing to the high incidence of renal agenesis in this select patient population, a screening renal sonogram should be obtained when either one of these two anomalies is found during surgical exploration (Mercer, 1979; Schlegel, 1996).

Primary and secondary ascended testes

Primary ascensus of the testicle is a relatively new concept, first described by Villumsen and Zachau-Christianson (1966), but more recently brought to attention by Atwell (1985). Once attributed to inadequate physical examinations or inept documentation by the examining physician, longitudinal studies of large patient populations have documented the presence of this phenomenon (Robertson et al., 1988; Group, 1992).

It is currently believed that primary ascent of the testis is related to one of two etiologies. In one group of patients with documented ascensus, proximal retraction of the testis into the inguinal canal or prescrotal space appears to be related to a patent processus vaginalis. In the newborn infant, the inguinal canal is short (approximately 2 cm in length) and associated with a patent processus. With maturity, the proximal processus should close, i.e. fibrose with the distal portion going on to form the tunica vaginalis. In patients with a patent processus, the patent proximal processus is absorbed into the peritoneum, resulting in retraction of the testicle into the inguinal canal or prescrotal space (Atwell, 1985; Robertson et al., 1988). The second group of patients with testicular ascensus comprises individuals with progressive muscle spasticity disorders such as cerebral palsy. Long-term follow-up of children with cerebral palsy has revealed a progressive increase in the incidence of cryptorchidism with maturation. Testicular ascensus in this patient population appears to be due to the increased spasticity of the cremasteric muscle that occurs as a consequence of the neurologic impairment (Smith et al., 1989). The fact that ascensus of the testicle is currently a well-described phenomenon gives impetus to the need for long-term surveillance in children with retractile testis. Children with retractile testis should be examined annually, until documented descent of the testis into the scrotum occurs (Group, 1986).

Secondary testicular ascensus or iatrogenic cryptorchidism is a well-described surgical complication of infantile hydrocele or hernia repairs. Occurring in < 1% of cases, it is assumed that this entity develops after the surgeon pulls the testicle out of the scrotum at the time of the inguinal cord dissection. Failure to replace the testicle into the scrotum upon completion of the operation results in its becoming entrapped by scar tissue in a prescrotal position.

Torsion of the cryptorchid testicle

Testicular torsion of the cryptorchid testis is reported to occur more frequently than torsion of a descended testis. The increased incidence of torsion in cryptorchid testes is presumably due to abnormalities in the testicular–epididymal–tunica vaginalis complex. Torsion of the undescended testis is frequently difficult to diagnose, but should be considered in any male with groin or abdominal pain and an empty scrotum (O'Riordan and Sherman, 1977; Mowad and Konvolinka, 1978; Elder, 1992d; Hutson et al., 1997).

Timing of surgical and hormonal therapy

Orchiopexy is usually performed between 6 and 15 months of age. The minimal age for treatment is based on the fact that delayed descent of the testis is unlikely to occur after 6 months of age. The maximal age is chosen because germ cell aplasia increases significantly after 15 months of age (Hadziselimovic et al., 1984a; Cortes, 1998).

The role of hormonal therapy in the cryptorchid testicle

It is argued that hormonal therapy should be the initial treatment modality for cryptorchidism, based on two major suppositions: (1) it may enhance fertility; and (2) it could prevent the need for a surgical procedure. The concept that hormonal therapy may improve fertility is based on the findings that the cryptorchid testicle has acquired germ cell hypoplasia. Since the transformation of gonocytes to spermatogonia is hypothesized to be both gonadotropin and age dependent, Hadziselimovic postulated that treatment of the cryptorchid testicle, with biopsy-proven germ cell hypoplasia, with long-term GnRH would increase the number of prepubertal spermatogonia and subsequently improve the spermogram in adulthood. He recommended that the following protocol be instituted for the cryptorchid testicle: testicular biopsies should be performed at the time of orchiopexy and individuals with abnormal biopsies (less than 0.2 germ cells per tubular cross-section) should receive GnRH adjunctive treatment (10 μg intranasally every other day for 6 months) postorchiopexy (Hadziselimovic et al., 1984a; Hadziselimovic et al., 1987b; Cortes et al., 1996). Clinical trials using this treatment regimen have revealed significant improvement in germ cell number, as determined by repeat testicular biopsy, provided the boys were younger than 7 years of age at the time of orchiopexy (Hadziselimovic et al., 1984b). Only one laboratory has provided long-term follow-up data. This single study evaluated the spermograms of adults, who were treated as per the recommended protocol, and compared them with a control population with similar testicular biopsy findings at the time of orchiopexy who were managed by orchiopexy alone. This study did document improved spermograms in the GnRH adjuvant-treated population (Hadziselimovic et al., 1987b). Several carefully controlled clinical investigations, from a variety of institutions, are necessary before the routine use of testicular biopsy and adjuvant postoperative GnRH become adopted as the standard of medical care.

Whether or not hormonal therapy can successfully treat the truly cryptorchid testicle is highly controversial, with successful results varying from a high of 75% to as low as 6% (Job et al., 1982; Rajfer et al., 1986; de Munick Keizer Schrama et al., 1986; Waldschmidt et al., 1987; Muller and Skakkebaek, 1997; Walker, 1997). Owing to the great variation in reported success, a variety of hormonal therapies has been recommended: hCG alone (100 IU/kg, maximum single injection of 1500 IU, given twice weekly for 3 weeks, total dose not to exceed 15 000 IU because of possible early closure of the epiphyseal junctions); GnRH alone (200 μg in each nostril three times per day, total of six daily doses, given for 4 weeks), or a combination of hCG followed by GnRH. This author's opinion and experience mirrors that of Rajfer et al. (1986), in that

hormonal therapy does not appear to be very effective in treating a truly undescended testicle, but may be very helpful in determining a retractile versus an undescended testicle.

Polaschik et al. (1996) reviewed retrospectively the use of hCG in boys with non-palpable testes. Of 94 patients (99 testes) identified who received 1500 IU two times weekly preoperatively for four weeks, 39 testes became palpable. Two completely descended. The authors concluded that preoperative hCG stimulation is efficacious in making the non-palpable testis palpable and simplifying orchidopexy poststimulation.

Personal recommendations regarding hormonal therapy

Hormonal therapy for cryptorchidism merits strong consideration in two select circumstances. The strongest indication for its use is in the differentiation between a retractile and a gliding testis. Its application in this situation is strengthened significantly by the recent documentation that the number of orchiopexies performed is greater than the true incidence of cryptorchidism. Since the assumption is that unnecessary operations are being performed on a number of patients with retractile testes, the routine use of hCG or GnRH is recommended prior to orchiopexy in children with a working diagnosis of a gliding testis. The trial of hormonal therapy would either confirm or refute the surgeon's initial clinical impression and save a number of children with retractile testes the morbidity and expense of surgery. However, even if the testicle is found to be in the dependent scrotum following a trial of hormonal therapy, yearly follow-up examinations should be recommended until the child goes through puberty. In rare circumstances, testes that descended into the scrotum in response to gonadotropins ascend with prolonged follow-up, eventually becoming entrapped in the inguinal region and requiring surgery (Aaronson et al., 1989; Walker, 1997).

A weaker indication for the use of hormonal therapy is in the patient with an impalpable testicle who the physician believes may require a Fowler–Stephens maneuver, i.e. dividing the restrictive gonadal vessels and basing the testicular blood supply on the vasal artery (Fowler and Stephens, 1959). The use of hCG therapy in this patient population relies on the scientific findings that gonadotropins increase collateral testicular blood flow and improve testicular survival following testicular artery ligation in the rodent (Levy *et al.*, 1995). It is this author's unsubstantiated belief that pretreatment of this human population, with hCG prior to a Fowler–Stephens maneuver, improves testicular survival.

Cryptorchidism and infertility

Testicular undescent has a known but poorly defined risk of infertility. Currently 2–4% of men in modernized countries will undergo orchiopexy for presumed cryptorchidism. Routine evaluation of the male population presenting to infertility clinics for evaluation reveals that approximately 6% will have a history of orchiopexy or untreated cryptorchidism, i.e. a 1.5–3 fold higher incidence in the patient population than what should be expected (Hargreave *et al.*, 1984).

Owing to the variety of ways in which infertility is reported in cryptorchidism, it is difficult to assess the impact of testicular undescent on fertility. Reviews of this subject report fertility potential via sperm count, testicular biopsy, hormone analysis, and pregnancy rates. The patient attaches the greatest importance to paternity; however, the use of paternity involves several difficulties from a scientific point of view, i.e. biologic paternity, the issue of the women's fertility, the number of patients attempting to achieve paternity, and the time that they have been attempting to acquire paternity.

To compare studies on cryptorchidism and infertility, the physician must be aware of a number of facts that must be equal between the two investigations that they are evaluating: where was the site of the patient's entry into the study, i.e. is it from a infertility clinic? Did the physicians exclude any patients with an abnormal karyotype? Did they note the presence of testicular atrophy or the position of the 'pexed testicle? Did they note the age at the time of orchiopexy? How was the patient treated; hormonally, surgically, or with a combination of the two? What was the position of the testicle at the time of surgery? Is the histology of the testicle known at the time of the orchiopexy? Were there wolffian ductal abnormalities? Did the authors define patient non-participation? In general, fertile patients do not care to deliver semen for analysis and the number of fertile patients after orchiopexy may not be adequately reflected in the data if a large segment of the study group was not evaluated (Mandant *et al.*, 1994).

What methods were used to assess fertility: hormonal studies, testicular biopsies, semen analysis, or pregnancy rates? Comparing and contrasting studies that used different ways to assess fertility is difficult, since investigations comparing testicular biopsy with hormonal studies, semen analysis, and pregnancy rates are extremely rare (Hadziselimovic *et al.*, 1984a; Hadziselimovic *et al.*, 1987b; Cendron *et al.*, 1989; Cortes, 1998). The studies evaluating fertility by semen analysis are also frequently hampered because of the definition of infertility. The World Health Organization defines infertility in men as those having fewer than 20 million sperm cells per milliliter of ejaculate. However, a man can achieve pregnancy with sperm counts of 5 million, if their motility is normal. Indeed, in cryptorchid men paternity has been reported with semen counts ranging from 5 to 60 million sperm/ml of ejaculate (Smith, 1941).

Testicular biopsy at the time of orchiopexy and fertility

Most studies in the scientific literature usually rely on the results of a testicular biopsy obtained at the time of orchiopexy. Although a paucity of data regarding pre-pubertal testicular biopsies and semen analysis at adulthood is available, the following information appears to be reliable. If bilateral testicular biopsies reveal <1% spermatogonia per tubular transverse section (minimum of 100 sections counted), semen analysis at maturity routinely reveals fewer than 1 million sperm/ml of ejaculate. If <1% spermatogonia per tubular transverse section is found unilaterally, approximately 70% of the men will have semen counts of <2 million/ml ejaculate at maturity. In unilateral cryptorchidism, the number of spermatogonia per tubular transverse section is lower in the undescended testicle than in its descended mate; however, counts in both the descended and undescended testicle will be lower than normal (Hecker and Heinz, 1967; Mengel *et al.*, 1974; Lipshultz *et al.*, 1976; Hedinger, 1982; Cendron *et al.*, 1989; Huff *et al.*, 1989).

The physician who chooses to use testicular biopsies to assess the fertility potential of patients must be aware of several factors that limit their prognostic value. First, the biopsy specimen may not reflect the patient's total testicular parenchyma; this may be particularly true in patients undergoing a biopsy for unilateral cryptorchidism. Second, fertility potential may be affected by the postoperative position of the testis. At the time of orchiopexy, biopsies are obtained and the testicle is pexed into position. Long-term follow-up studies of infants undergoing orchiopexy reveal that approximately 30% of the pexed testicles are in the low scrotal position, 66% in the mid and high scrotal position and approximately 4% in the low inguinal position. It is currently unknown what effects postorchiopexy position has on fertility; however, it is hypothesized that the higher the postorchiopexy testicular position, the more likely it is to result in a decrease in semen production (Scorer and Farrington, 1971; Hadziselimovic et al., 1984a; Cortes, 1998). Third, postorchiopexy testicular atrophy (testicular volume < 5 ml) is found in 1.5% of patients. If the atrophy was a result of the surgical procedure, the intraoperative biopsy will not have taken this into account (Kogan et al., 1990). Fourth, and finally, congenital and/or surgically acquired obstruction of the male genital ductal system is not taken into account by the testicular biopsy (Hargreave et al., 1984; Gill and Kogan, 1997).

Fertility potential: bilateral undescended testicles

In general, in individuals with bilateral undescended testes undergoing delayed bilateral orchiopexy, i.e. after 2 years but before 12 years of age, approximately 20% will have normal spermograms (i.e. sperm counts >20 million, normal morphology and motility) at adulthood. Forty per cent of the men will have sperm counts of 5–20 million and approximately 40% will have sperm counts <5 million (Hohenfeller and Eisenhut, 1964; Werder et al., 1976; Bierich, 1982; Hutson and Beasley, 1992; Walker, 1997; Cortes, 1998).

In the child with bilateral cryptorchidism, initial testicular location may play a significant role in fertility. Current studies suggest that if both testes are found in the prescrotal space, patients will usually have normal or near normal semen analysis. In contrast, patients with bilateral impalpable or intra-abdominal testes will usually either be azoospermic or have poor semen quality at adulthood. It is the hope of the urologic community that these latter individuals may have their fertility improved with early surgery (Hargreave, 1997; Walker, 1997).

Fertility potential: unilateral undescended testicles

Clinical studies reporting the sperm concentration for adult men following delayed unilateral orchiopexy vary widely, with the incidence of normal spermograms ranging from 29 to 89%. When several large studies are combined, the overall percentage of men with normal spermograms is approximately 75%. Clinical studies using spermograms to assess fertility suggest that a significant difference exists in the semen analysis between normal and unilateral cryptorchid men. In contrast, studies using paternity to compare the unilateral cryptorchid to the normal male fail to document that paternity is affected. Although testicular biopsies, hormonal analysis, and sperm counts suggest a diminished fertility potential in children undergoing delayed unilateral orchiopexy, no documentation of diminished paternity potential can be proven (Hohenfeller and Eisenhut, 1964; Werder et al., 1976; Bierich, 1982; Gilhooly et al., 1984; Hutson and Beasley, 1992; Lee et al., 1995; Hargreave, 1997; Walker, 1997).

General comments regarding fertility and cryptorchidism

The answer to three major questions can usually assess fertility in men with undescended testes. Is the condition unilateral or bilateral? In the child with bilateral cryptorchidism, what was the initial position of the testes? In the child with bilateral cryptorchidism, at what age was orchiopexy performed? All current studies suggest that the incidence of paternity is similar between the normal patient and the patient with unilateral cryptorchidism irrespective of the age of the orchiopexy. In the child with bilateral cryptorchidism, patients with testes found in the prescrotal space will usually have normal or near normal semen analysis, while individuals with bilateral intra-abdominal testes will usually either be azoospermic or have poor semen quality (Walker, 1997; Hargreave, 1997).

Cryptorchidism and testicular malignancy

Risk of testicular neoplasia

The lifetime risk of developing testicular cancer in men from the general population is approximately 0.3–0.7%, depending on the individual's race and nationality. In contrast to the normal population, the risk of a man with a history of cryptorchidism developing testicular cancer is 3–5%, i.e. a 4–7-fold increased risk (Martin, 1982; Muller et al., 1984;

Giwercman *et al.*, 1987; Whitaker, 1988; Giwercmanl *et al.*, 1989; Haughey *et al.*, 1989; Pinczowski *et al.*, 1991; Forman *et al.*, 1994; Prener *et al.*, 1995; Moller *et al.*, 1996; Moller and Skakkebaek, 1997; Muller and Skakkebaek, 1997; Swerdlow *et al.*, 1997a; Walker, 1997; Cortes, 1998; Sabroe and Olsen, 1998; Silver and Docimo, 1999).

Historically, it was believed that the risk of malignancy within the cryptorchid testicle was increased the more proximally the testicle was located, with intra-abdominal testes having a 20-fold higher risk of developing malignancy than the general population (Hinman and Benteen, 1936; Campbell, 1942; Campbell, 1959; Johnson *et al.*, 1968; Martin, 1982). Unfortunately, studies reporting the increased incidence of testicular malignancies in intra-abdominal testes were flawed. Specifically, patients with an abnormal karyotype and boys with a normal karyotype but abnormal genitalia are at an increased risk of developing a testicular malignancy, irrespective of the presence of cryptorchidism. Since these studies failed to exclude these patients, it is impossible to determine whether the increased risk of malignancy in the intra-abdominal testis was due to its position or to the abnormal phenotype and genotype (Verp and Simpson, 1987; Prener *et al.*, 1995; Moller *et al.*, 1996; Moller and Skakkebaek, 1997; Satge *et al.*, 1997). In current studies, when only patients with bilateral intra-abdominal testes are evaluated, the child with intra-abdominal undescended testis is at only a slightly higher risk of developing a testicular malignancy than the child with inguinal cryptorchidism (Batata *et al.*, 1982; Andrews and Malek, 1992; Swerdlow *et al.*, 1997a).

Why is cryptorchidism associated with testicular malignancy?

Two different explanations exist regarding the association of cryptorchidism with testicular cancer. One hypothesis is based on the assumption that testicular cancer occurs as a consequence of the abnormal position of the testicle (position theory). The other hypothesis is based on the assumption that a common etiologic factor exists that causes both cryptorchidism and testicular neoplasia (common cause theory), (Moller *et al.*, 1996; Prener *et al.*, 1995; Henderson *et al.*, 1979).

If testicular carcinoma is due to testicular position, one would expect to see two pertinent findings on clinical studies. First, in unilateral cryptorchidism, the contralateral descended testicle should be at no higher risk of developing a tumor than the normal patient population. Second, early orchiopexy should decrease the risk of malignancy. Neither of the findings that could substantiate the position theory can be documented to be true. Indeed, in patients with a unilateral undescended testicle, the risk of malignancy developing in the contralateral descended testicle is less than the cryptorchid testicle but is still increased over normal by approximately 2–3 fold. This finding suggests that either an intrinsic testicular abnormality or a common cause, or both, could be responsible for the initiation of both cryptorchidism and testicular neoplasia (Henderson *et al.*, 1979; Prener *et al.*, 1995; Swerdlow *et al.*, 1997a; Cortes, 1998; Silver and Docimo, 1999).

Regarding the ability of early orchiopexy (surgery performed before 2 years of age) to prevent the onset of testicular tumors, current epidemiologic studies are controversial. Although some authors have noted a decrease in the incidence of testicular tumors following early orchiopexy (Chilvers and Pike, 1992; Moller *et al.*, 1996; Moller and Skakkebaek, 1997), others are unable to confirm this finding (Prener *et al.*, 1995; Sabroe and Olsen, 1998). Further fueling the controversy is the fact that even the authors who have seen a decrease in the incidence of cancer following early orchiopexy caution that their data may be spurious owing to the increased number of orchiopexies being performed presumably for retractile testicles (Moller *et al.*, 1996). Over the past few decades, the incidence of orchiopexy has increased significantly, which may be based on the misdiagnosis of retractile testicles being cryptorchid. Since retractile testes are at little or no increased risk of developing cancer, their inclusion in the current database will significantly improve the effect of orchiopexy on the incidence of testicular cancer (Moller *et al.*, 1996; Cortes, 1998).

When large epidemiologic studies are performed to look for common factors found in both cryptorchidism and testicular cancer, three common associations are repetitively found: prematurity, low birth weight, and high maternal age (Swerdlow *et al.*, 1983; Depue, 1984; Moller and Skakkebaek, 1997; Sabroe and Olsen, 1998). The relationship between prematurity and low birth weight has resulted in the hypothesis that an abnormal gene expression for growth may lead to both cryptorchidism and testicular carcinoma (Jones *et al.*, 1997). There are few hard scientific data to support this claim. Regarding increased maternal age as a cause of cryptorchidism and testicular malignancies, it is known that higher concentrations of maternal estrogens are found with increasing maternal age. It is also known that cryptorchidism, testicular atrophy, and testicular neoplasia can be caused by exposure of the fetus to elevated levels of maternal estrogens (Henderson *et al.*, 1979; Depue, 1984; Husmann and Levy, 1995; Levy and Husmann, 1995; Moller and Skakkebaek, 1997; Sabroe and Olsen, 1998). Although still not definitively proven, most of the hard scientific evidence is tilting towards the concept that a common causal factor or factors will lead to both cryptorchidism and testicular neoplasia (Swerdlow *et al.*, 1987; Swerdlow *et al.*, 1997b).

Does orchiopexy result in earlier detection of testicular carcinoma?

It was hoped that orchiopexy of the undescended testicle would result in earlier detection and improved prognosis of testicular carcinoma. Unfortunately, long-term follow-up studies have failed to establish this theory. Approximately 25% of the patients with surgically corrected cryptorchidism and 25% of those with uncorrected cryptorchidism present with metastasis at the time of diagnosis. Disease-free survival of the two groups is dependent on the stage at diagnosis and is essentially equal between the two. The only remarkable difference between the patients with surgically corrected cryptorchidism and the uncorrected cryptorchid patients was the increased incidence of inguinal lymph-node metastasis in the surgically corrected group. Specifically, 10% of the patients who developed cancer following orchiopexy had metastasis to the inguinal lymph-nodes at the time of diagnosis. In contrast, none of the persistent cryptorchid patients who developed cancer had inguinal lymph-node metastasis at the time of diagnosis (Batata *et al.*, 1980; Jones *et al.*, 1991; Raina *et al.*, 1995). Orchiopexy of the cryptorchid testicle has not changed the stage of the tumor at diagnosis, nor has it improved the prognosis. It has, however, changed the lymphatic drainage pathway for the pexed testicle.

Does testicular biopsy, performed at the time of orchiopexy, result in earlier detection of testicular carcinoma?

Carcinoma *in situ* (CIS) of the testis is described as a precursor to testicular germ cell tumors. CIS has been found in up to 8% of infertile patients undergoing testicular biopsy with a history of orchiopexy in childhood (Walker, 1997). Testicular biopsy, to rule out the presence of CIS, has been recommended in the child older than 3 years of age at the time of orchiopexy (Reinberg *et al.*, 1989). Several large studies have, however, failed to show a high yield of CIS when undescended testes were biopsied. The overall incidence of CIS in children (aged 2–18 years) undergoing orchiopexy is approximately 0.4% (Muffly *et al.*, 1984; Hadziselimovic *et al.*, 1984a; Muller and Skakkebaek, 1984b; Bannwart, 1987; Parkinson *et al.*, 1994; Cortes, 1998). This finding is approximately 6-fold lower than the 2–3% lifetime risk of developing testicular neoplasia in the cryptorchid population. The lower incidence than expected may be due to one of a multitude of reasons, including biopsying only one testicle in patients with unilaterally undescended testicle, an inadequate biopsy specimen, or heterogeneity in the location of CIS. In any event, at least three cases of malignant germ cell tumor have developed in patients between the ages of 10 and 32 years who had normal testicular biopsies obtained at the time of orchiopexy (Parkinson *et al.*, 1994). Consequently, most authorities believe that cryptorchid boys are at a significant risk of developing a neoplasia, even in the presence of a normal testicular biopsy (Parkinson *et al.*, 1994; Cortes, 1998).

On reviewing the current literature and combining this with my own experience, the author found 28 boys who had CIS diagnosed following a testicular biopsy at the time of orchiopexy. Age at the time of orchiopexy ranged from 5 months to 16 years. Fifty per cent of the patients reported to have CIS had an underlying abnormality that should have warranted testicular biopsy: four with prune belly syndrome, and ten with either a karyotype abnormality and/or ambiguous genitalia without a karyotype being ascertained (Manuel *et al.*, 1976; Scully, 1981; Verp and Simpson, 1987; Savage and Lowe, 1990; Cortes, 1998). As a result of this information it is recommended that a testicular biopsy be obtained in any cryptorchid male undergoing orchiopexy with a history of prune belly syndrome, or ambiguous genitalia, or abnormal karyotype, or in a postpubertal male (>12 years of age). If CIS is found, re-exploration and orchiectomy are recommended. Alternatively, close self-inspection and interval testicular sonography could be performed; however, the exact incidence of invasive cancer developing in these patients is unknown.

Standard inguinal approach for the repair of the cryptorchid testicle

This author believes that the optimal age for orchiopexy is 6–15 months of age. It should be remembered, however, that conclusive proof that early orchiopexy is better than delayed orchiopexy is lacking.

To perform a routine orchiopexy, the incision is initiated just medial and cephalad to the pubic tubercle and extends laterally 2–3 cm (Fig. 34a.3). The incision through the dermis is performed with the knife and the residual dissection through the subcutaneous tissue is performed with electrocoagulation to prevent hematoma formation. Care must be taken during the dissection down to the external oblique aponeurosis and external ring to avoid injury to a testicle lying in the superficial inguinal pouch. The external oblique fascia is cleaned of fat by blunt dissection and the external ring identified. A small incision is made into the external ring. The ilioinguinal nerve is identified and the external oblique fascia divided over

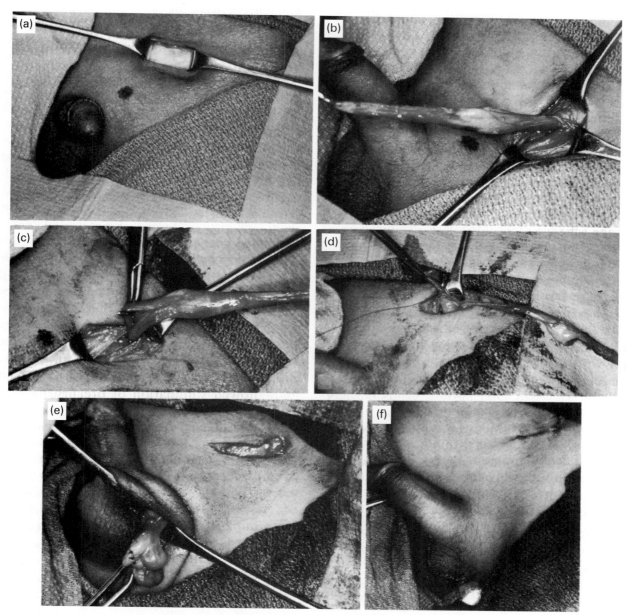

Figure 34a.3 Orchidopexy: technique for palpable undescended testes (see text).

the inguinal canal. The dissection is carried in a cephalad direction until approximately 1 cm of internal oblique muscle is visualized. The external oblique fascia and the ilioinguinal nerve are retracted with stay sutures to the borders of the surgical field.

If the operation is a redo orchiopexy or is performed in a patient who had previously undergone inguinal surgery, it is helpful to preserve the external oblique fascia directly over the inguinal cord. The external oblique fascia is then divided on the medial and lateral borders of the inguinal canal. The two incisions are made parallel to each, extended in a cephalad direction until approximately 1 cm of internal oblique muscle is identified. Cephalad to the internal ring the two incisions are connected by a short horizontal incision through the external oblique fascia, and a small rectangular piece of external oblique fascial is left intact on the spermatic cord to prevent damage to the inguinal structures.

Following incision of the external oblique fascia, the testicular cord and testis are usually visible. Using a Kittner dissector the cord is mobilized from the floor of the inguinal canal and a vessel loop passed around the inguinal structures. The caudal attachments of the testis to the pars gubernacula are divided by electrocoagulation. Meticulous attention is necessary at this point to avoid injury to a looping vas deferens. Once the testicle and cord are freed from the adherent connective tissue and subcutaneous fat, the external spermatic fascia is opened by a combination of sharp dissection and electrocoagulation. The processus vaginalis or hernia sac is usually identifiable at this point on the medial and anterior surface of the spermatic cord. Using non-crushing forceps, the patent processus is unwrapped from the vas deferens and testicular vessels. Once the vessels and vas deferens have been separated from the hernia sac, a vessel loop is passed around these structures and they are identified as being free from the hernia sac throughout the length of the dissection. The hernia sac is then dissected free from the cord for several centimeters cephalad to the internal ring. This maneuver is extremely important in allowing for adequate mobility of the spermatic cord. Indeed, in redo orchiopexies, either failure to divide the patent processus or inadequate cephalad dissection of the patent processus is the most common technical problem resulting in a persistent undescended testicle. If it is necessary to visualize more of the spermatic cord, a small 1–2 cm incision of the internal oblique muscle superior to

the internal ring greatly enhances visualization and mobilization of the spermatic cord. It must be stressed that it is not just the dissection of the peritoneum off the vessels that results in increased spermatic cord length. Indeed, peritoneal mobilization allows visualization of the lateral fascial attachments to the spermatic cord. It is division of these fascial attachments that straightens the vessels to gain length. Mobilization of the peritoneum only allows for improved visualization of the lateral fascial attachments (Browne, 1949).

If after completing the cephalic dissection the testis will still not reach the scrotum, the floor of the inguinal canal can be divided, i.e. the Prentis maneuver (Prentis et al., 1962). This maneuver will add approximately 5–10 mm in length, predominantly by straightening the access of the testicle to the scrotum. Dividing of the inguinal floor does carry some risk and forethought is necessary before proceeding with this maneuver. Division of the floor may be accomplished either by dividing and ligating the deep inferior epigastric arteries or by preserving the vessels and passing the testis and cord under them. Before dividing the epigastric vessels, the surgeon should reflect on whether or not the patient may need testicular autotransplantation for completion of the orchiopexy. Ligation of the epigastric vessels may destroy this option. Although testicular autotransplantation is only rarely performed, consideration regarding whether this procedure will be necessary should be given prior to ligation and destruction of the epigastric vessels. The surgeon should also take great care during the division of the caudal portion of the inguinal floor. During this portion of the procedure, a distended bladder is frequently encountered and inadvertent injury to the bladder may occur unless the surgeon is aware of this possibility.

Once adequate spermatic cord length has been obtained, attention is paid to the fixation of the testicle into the scrotum. The subdartos pouch technique, may be used to pex the testicle in the scrotum. A small 1.0–1.5 cm incision is made in the upper scrotum and a pocket of adequate size to accept the testicle and epididymis is then developed between the skin and the dartos muscle using tenotomy scissors. The index finger is then placed in the inguinal incision and delivered into the scrotal incision. A clamp is passed on the fingertip into the inguinal region, a small attachment of the cauda gubernaculum is grasped, and the testicle delivered into the scrotum. Fixation of the testicle is accomplished by closure of the dartos muscle around the neck of the cord. The testicle and epididymis are placed into the scrotal pouch. Although the present author dislikes fixing the testicle to the scrotum with a stitch, others prefer this method (Walker, 1997).

Surgical options for the impalpable testis or the cryptorchid testis with inadequate cord length

Experience dictates that the vast majority of impalpable or intra-abdominal testes can be manipulated into the scrotum through the inguinal incision described above (Kirsch *et al.*, 1998). Although laparoscopy prior to open surgical exploration is an option, laparoscopy rarely if ever prevents the need for further exploration, increases operative time, and does not in most cases allow the surgeon to determine whether the testicle will reach the lower scrotum. It is therefore this author's preference, in the child with a unilateral non-palpable testis, to proceed with inguinal exploration (see Chapter 34b). In a child with a known intersex disorder or an infant with bilateral impalpable testes, laparoscopy is the best way to proceed. The following section outlines the management of testicles with inadequate spermatic cord length.

Inadequate spermatic cord length found at the time of routine orchiopexy

At the time of orchiopexy the surgeon may be faced with the discovery of inadequate spermatic cord length. In this situation the first maneuver is to verify that all of the routine dissection has been performed: is the patent processus dissected completely free of the cord? Has the internal ring been incised and the retroperitoneal cord mobilized? Are all of the lateral peritoneal attachments divided? Should the inguinal floor or transversalis fascia have been divided? If the inguinal floor or transversalis fascia has been divided, were the deep epigastric vessels preserved or divided? Is the opposite testicle normal?

If the other testicle is normal or if the contralateral undescended testicle has already been successfully pexed, one would normally proceed with a single-stage Fowler–Stephens orchiopexy. If the opposite testicle is still undescended, considerable thought needs to be given before proceeding with the next surgical maneuver. In children with bilateral unde-

scended testicles, the surgical procedure begins on the side where the testicle is most caudally placed. If adequate cord length of the most caudally placed testicle cannot be obtained, it is most likely that the contralateral testicle will be even more difficult to bring down successfully. In this scenario, options should include a staged orchiopexy, or a unilateral Fowler–tevens procedure with plans for a delayed orchiopexy on the contralateral side. If both testes are high and bilateral Fowler–Stevens orchiopexies are being considered, these procedures should be staged because of the chance that a testicle could be lost during the operation. This leaves the surgeon the option of proceeding with an autotransplant procedure of the remaining testicle if the testicle undergoing a Fowler–Stephens orchiopexy should become atrophic.

One-stage Fowler–Stephens orchiopexy

Division of the testicular vessels is necessary when they are too short to allow successful placement of the testes into the scrotum. If the gonadal vessels are divided, preservation of the testis is based on the collateral circulation, the vas deferens, a branch of the inferior vesical artery, and the cremasteric artery, a branch of the inferior epigastric (Fowler and Stephens, 1959; Stephens, 1988). When routinely performing orchiopexies, great care must be taken to preserve the web of vessels that exists between the gonadal vessels and the vas deferens (Fig. 34a.4). By routinely performing a meticulous dissection of the spermatic cord, a single-stage Fowler–Stephens

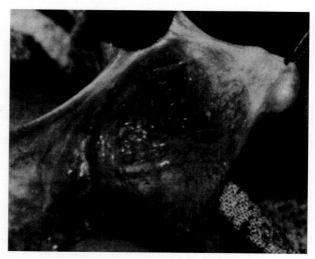

Figure 34a.4 Collateral circulation between vasal and spermatic vessels in an intra-abdominal testis.

orchiopexy can be performed without necessarily preserving the pedicle of peritoneum around the vas. If the routine dissection as described above has been performed and the testicle is still unable to reach the scrotum, the cord is evaluated to verify that it has not been skeletonized. If the cord is skeletonized, one should abandon any thought of proceeding with a Fowler–Stephens orchiopexy and proceed to a staged orchiopexy. If the cord has been preserved, the vas deferens and epididymis are visualized to rule out any segmental vasal atresia or epididymal detachments. If these latter abnormalities are present, a Fowler–Stephens orchiopexy is abandoned (Redman and Mooney, 1993). Then, Doppler is applied to the vasal artery to verify patency. If good Doppler pulses are found, an atraumatic vascular bulldog is used to clamp the gonadal vessels for 5 min. If no Doppler vasal pulses are present or if the testicle becomes cyanotic during the trial clamping of the gonadal vessels, the procedure is abandoned. Fowler and Stephens originally recommended ligation of the testicular artery as high as possible in the retroperitoneum to preserve blood supply. Although this author has performed the operation as described by Fowler and Stephens, I have recently modified my technique as per Koff's recommendations (Koff and Sethi, 1996), leaving the proximal collateral vessels intact and dividing the distal testicular artery close to the testis. In essence, the proximal rather than the distal collaterals preserve testicular blood flow. This incision allows the surgeon to gain another 1–2 cm in spermatic cord length. In my experience, testicular atrophy following a one-stage Fowler–Stephens orchiopexy occurs in approximately 20% of cases.

Besides the possible loss of the testicle, an additional word of caution is advisable for a one-stage Fowler–Stephens orchiopexy. In an attempt to have the testicle reach the scrotum, stretching the testicle into the scrotum with a shortened vas has been reported to result in ureteral obstruction. Care should therefore be given to verify that undo tension of the vas on the ureter does not exist following completion of the orchiopexy (Nguyen and Mitchell, 1993).

Two-stage Fowler–Stephens

A planned two-stage Fowler–Stephens orchiopexy may be considered in patients with prune belly syndrome, intersex disorders, and bilateral impalpable testes. The initial procedure is laparoscopy to assess the testicular location and length of spermatic cord. If the testes are located at or just above the internal inguinal ring, the vast majority of these testes will reach the scrotum either with a standard dissection or via a high extraperitoneal dissection. If, in the surgeon's opinion, the length of the spermatic cord would limit the ability to perform an orchiopexy, a planned two-stage Fowler–Stephens maneuver is performed. Although this procedure can be performed as an open operation, preliminary clipping of the gonadal vessels at the time of laparoscopy is preferable. The second open procedure is delayed for 6–12 months allowing collateral blood flow to the testicle to become established. At the time of the planned second stage, a traditional Fowler–Stevens orchiopexy is performed, taking great care to preserve a broad pedicle of peritoneum over the vas deferens. Testicular atrophy following a planned two-stage Fowler–Stephens technique ranges from 10 to 20% (Ransley, 1984; Elder, 1989; Pascual et al., 1989; Elder, 1992b; Caldamone and Amaral, 1994; Joseph et al., 1996; Baille et al., 1998; Humphrey et al., 1998).

Microvascular anastomosis

It is the rare patient who will need a microvascular testicular autotransplantation. This technique is reserved for use in individuals with a high, solitary, intra-abdominal testis that will not reach the scrotum using standard techniques. This procedure requires the anastomosis of the testicular vessels to the ipsilateral deep inferior epigastric vessels. Success is dependent on the expertise of the operating surgeon in performing the microvascular anastomosis. The average urologist should not attempt this maneuver unless he or she is routinely performing microvascular surgery. Because most urologists do not fit within this category, this procedure should be performed in conjunction with a well-trained and experienced microvascular surgeon.

This procedure may be performed through a Gibson incision. The testicular vessels and vas deferens are mobilized on a wide flap of peritoneum similar to a planned Fowler–Stephens procedure. The subdartos pouch is then formed to prevent excessive movement in the operative field after the microvascular anastomosis is complete. Once the subdartos pouch is formed, the testicular vessels are ligated at their origin. A spatulated end-to-end anastomosis is performed with the inferior epigastric vessels and the testis pexed into the scrotum. Success rates mimic the planned two-stage Fowler–Stephens maneuver, with testicular atrophy found in 10–20% of patients (Silber and Kelly, 1976; Wacksman *et al.*, 1980; Harrison *et al.*, 1990; Burkowski *et al.*, 1995).

Since the rate of testicular atrophy following micro-vascular testicular autotransplant mirrors the testicular atrophy rate following a planned two-stage Fowler–Stephens orchiopexy, considerable controversy exists regarding the indications for autotransplantation (Walker, 1997). In the author's opinion this procedure is rarely indicated and should be pursued only in individuals with a solitary, high intra-abdominal testis.

Staged orchiopexy

When the undescended testicle cannot be brought down into the scrotum with the vessels intact, another option is to perform a staged orchiopexy, pexing the testicle to its lowest possible site, usually in the region of the pubic bone. At the time of the initial operation, the surgeon may opt to wrap the testis in a silastic sheet, both to protect the testis and to facilitate the dissection during the second procedure. The concept of a staged orchiopexy is based on the hypothesis that the gonadal vessels will lengthen given enough time and tension. Although this author has performed numerous successful secondary orchiopexies, I was rarely the initial surgeon. When performing the second procedure it was usually found that little, if any, additional length to the cord had developed. The success of a staged orchiopexy is thus probably directly related to the adequacy of the initial dissection (Firor, 1971; Persky and Albert, 1971; Redman, 1977; Kiesewetter *et al.*, 1981; Steinhardt *et al.*, 1985).

Editorial comment: I have used this method rather than the Fowler–Stephens technique when testes do not easily reach the inferior scrotum. After a delay of 6 months the testes do reach the proper position without tension on the vessels. Viability is excellent (ABB).

Orchiopexy in persistent müllerian ductal syndrome

Persistent müllerian duct syndrome is a rare form of male pseudohermaphroditism caused by failure of the testes to secret MIS during the 8th week of gestation. The affected males have a 46,XY genotype, a fully formed phallus, and undescended testes. Herniation of the müllerian structures through the internal ring (hernia uterine inguinale) and transverse testicular ectopia are encountered frequently in this disorder. The gonadal function of patients with persistent müllerian ductal syndrome may be impaired, with testosterone secretion being normal but infertility a frequent occurrence. It is controversial whether the infertility is due to primary gonadal dysfunction or a consequence of testicular undescent. Since fertility has on occasion been reported within affected individuals, every attempt should be made to place the testicles into the scrotum. Orchiopexy in children with persistent müllerian duct syndrome is no small feat, and the problem is usually encountered when least expected. Indeed, the surgeon is not usually aware of the diagnosis until the gonad is found to be attached to a fallopian tube at the time of surgical exploration. When this phenomenon is encountered in the operative room, a blood sample should be obtained for both karyotype analysis and serum MIS levels. The gonad should be biopsied and replaced along with the herniated müllerian ducts into the pelvis, and the hernia closed. Full evaluation of the patient for an intersex disorder should be performed subsequently (Fernades *et al.*, 1990; Loef *et al.*, 1994; Vandersteen *et al.*, 1997; Rizk *et al.*, 1998).

After confirming a 46,XY karyotype and a normal testicular histology, a second operative procedure is performed. Experience dictates that if the testicle was palpable before the first operation then the gonadal vessels are usually long enough to allow for a successful orchiopexy using standard techniques. If, however, the testicle was impalpable, the testicle may be unable to reach the pelvis, owing, to either a shortened gonadal artery or, in most circumstances, entanglement of the vas deferens with the uterus and tubes. If the gonadal vessels are found to be limiting the dissection, a Fowler–Stephens orchiopexy, ligating the gonadal vessels and leaving the fallopian tubes and vasal structures intact, is performed. Hypothetically, it is tempting to excise the persistent müllerian structures, since leaving the müllerian structures *in situ* could predispose to endometrial malignancies, hematuria, and voiding dysfunctions. Surprisingly, long-term follow-up of patients with müllerian structures left *in situ* reveals these risks to be extremely rare (Fernades *et al.*, 1990; Loef *et al.*, 1994; Vandersteen *et al.*, 1997; Rizk *et al.*, 1998).

If the uterus and fallopian tubes are limiting the dissection, the fimbrae and distal fallopian tube are left intact and severed from the proximal tube. The distal fallopian tube intricately shares blood supply with the gonadal vessels. Injury to the gonadal vessels will frequently occur if complete salpingectomy is performed. Unfortunately, in most cases, this maneuver is still not enough to allow the gonad to reach the scrotum. Excision of the uterine fundus is then necessary. During this dissection, the surgeon must be aware that an extreme risk of vasal injury exists. Strong consideration for partial hysterectomy, leaving the myometrium behind, where it is attached to the vas, should be given (Fernades *et al.*, 1990; Loef *et al.*, 1994; Vandersteen *et al.*, 1997; Rizk *et al.*, 1998).

The true risk of malignancy in testes associated with persistent müllerian duct syndrome is unknown, with reported ranges varying from 2 to 15%. Because of the unknown risk of neoplasia within these gonads, any testicle that cannot be lowered into a palpable position should be excised (Loef *et al.*, 1994; Eastham *et al.*, 1992; Kazim, 1985).

Orchiectomy versus non-surgical management

Although the first consideration in the patient presenting with an undescended testicle is to perform an orchiopexy, there are times when orchiectomy and/or non-surgical management may have considerable merit. One should strongly consider proceeding with an orchiectomy when the descended testis is normal and an abnormal testis is found on exploration, and in the patient with unilateral cryptorchidism greater than 12 years of age.

On rare occasions in patients with profound developmental delay, coupled with significant coexisting physical disabilities, the risks of testicular malignancy should be weighed against the risk of surgery. In the end, the parents and/or legal guardian should to allowed to make an informed decision regarding whether or not they want to proceed with surgery.

Testicular prosthesis

Some authors believe that normal psychosocial development can be hampered by the absence of one testis from the scrotum. Consequently, when one testicle is either removed or congenitally absent, placement of a testicular prosthesis may be of some benefit (Bell, 1974; Smith and Lattimer, 1975).

The main problem in placement of the testicular prosthesis is to find a material that feels natural and is without significant medical legal concerns. The commonly placed silicone-filled testicular prostheses used throughout the 1980s were recalled in the 1990s because of unsubstantiated concerns that the silicone gel may leak out of the prosthesis and cause neoplasia, connective tissue disease, and autoimmune disorders (Pidutti and Morales, 1993; Lakshmanan and Docimo, 1997). Currently, solid silicone polymer testicular prostheses and saline-filled testicular prostheses are available. These new options make placement of the testicular prosthesis more attractive; however, the prosthetic scare of the 1990s has had a significantly negative impact on the placement of these devices.

References

Aaronson I, Hadziselimovic F, Lee P, Rajfer J, Molenaar J, Duckett J (1989) Hormonal therapy in cryptorchidism: Yes? No? *Dialog in Pediatr Urol* 12.

Abeyaratne M, Aherne W, Scott J (1969) The vanishing testis. *Lancet* ii: 822–4.

Andrews P, Malek R (1992) Unilateral cryptorchidism in adults. In: Kursh I, Resnick M (eds) *Current therapy in genitourinary surgery*. New York: Mosby Year Book, 339–44.

Atwell J (1985) Ascent of the testis: fact or fiction. *Br J Urol* 57: 474–7.

Backhouse K (1981) Embryology of the normal and cryptorchid testis. In: Fonkalsrud E, Mengel W (eds). *The undescended testis*. Chicago, IL: Year Book Medical Publishers, 458–62.

Baikie G, Hutson J (1990) Wolffian duct and epididymal agenesis fails to prevent testicular descent. *Pediatr Surg Int* 5: 458–62.

Baille C, Fearns G, Kitteringham L, Turnock R (1998) Management of the impalpable testis: the role of laparoscopy. *Arch Dis Child* 79: 419–22.

Baker T, Scrimgeour J (1980) Development of the gonad in normal and anencephalic human fetuses. *J Reprod Fertil* 60: 193–9.

Bakr A, Kotb M (1998) Laparoscopic orchiopexy: the treatment of choice for the impalpable testis. *Soc Laparosc Surg* 2: 259–62.

Bannwart F (1987) General discussion on CIS. *Int J Androl* 10: 221–4.

Bartone F, Husemann CA, Maizels M, Firlit C (1984) Pitfalls in using human chorionic gondaotropin stimulation test to diagnose anorchia. *J Urol* 132: 563–7.

Batata M, Whitmore W, Chu F, Hilaris B, Grabstald H, Golbey R (1980) Cryptorchidism and testicular cancer. *J Urol* 124: 382–7.

Batata M, Chu F, Hilaris B (1982) Testicular cancer in cryptorchids. *Cancer* 49: 1023–30.

Baumans V, Dijkstra G, Wensing C (1983) The role of a nonandrogenic testicular factor in the process of testicular descent in the dog. *Int J Androl* **6**: 541–52.

Bedford J (1978) Anatomical evidence for the epididymis as the prime mover in the evolution of the scrotum. *Am J Anat* **152**: 483–508.

Bell A (1974) Psychologic implications of scrotal sac and testes for the male child. *Clin Pediatr* **13**: 838–842.

Berkowitz G, Lapinski R, Dolgin S, Gazella J, Bodian C, Holzman I (1993) Prevalence and natural history of cryptorchidism. *Pediatrics* **92**: 44–9.

Berthelsen J, Skakkebaek N, Mogenson P, Sorensen B (1979) Incidence of carcinoma *in situ* of germ cells in contralateral testis of men with testicular tumors. *BMJ* **2**: 363–4.

Bierich J (1982) Undescended testes: treatment with gonadotropin. *Eur J Pediatr* **139**: 275–9.

Browne D (1949) Treatment of the undescended testicle. *Proc R Soc Med* **42**: 643–6.

Buemann B, Henriksen H, Villlumsen A, West A, Zachau-Christiansen B (1961) Incidence of undescended testis in the newborn. *Acta Chir Scand* **283**: 289–93.

Burkowski T, Wacksman J, Billmire D, Sheldon C (1995) Testicular autotransplantation for the intra-abdominal testis. *Microsurgery* **16**: 290–293.

Cain M, Kramer S, Tinall D, Husmann D (1994) Expression of androgen receptor protein within the lumbar spinal cord during ontologic development and following antiandrogen induced cryptorchidism. *J Urol* **152**: 766–9.

Cain M, Kramer S, Tinall D, Husmann D (1995) Flutamide induced cryptorchidism in the rat is associated with altered gubernacular morphology. *Urology* **46**: 553–8.

Caldamone A, Amaral J (1994) Laparoscopic stage 2 Fowler–Stephens orchiopexy. *J Urol* **152**: 1253–6.

Campbell H (1942) Incidence of malignant growth of the undescended testicle. *Arch Surg* **44**: 353–7.

Campbell H (1959) The incidence of malignant growth of the undescended testicle: a reply and re-evaluation. *J Urol* **81**: 663–7.

Cearasco T, Brock W, Kaplan G (1986) Upper urinary tract anomalies with congenital hypospadias: is screening necessary? *J Urol* **135**: 537–42.

Cendron M, Huff D, Keating M, Snyder HMI, Duckett J (1989) Anatomical, morphological and volumetric analysis: a review of 759 cases of testicular maldescent. *J Urol* **142**: 559–62.

Chilvers C, Pike M (1992) Cancer risk in the undescended testicle. *Eur Urol Update Ser* **1**: 74–9.

Coerdt W, Rehder H, Gausmann I, Johannisson R, Gropp A (1985) Quantitative histology of human fetal testes in chromosomal disease. *Pediatr Pathol* **3**: 245–59.

Cortada X, Kousseff B (1984) Cryptorchidism in mental retardation. *J Urol* **131**: 674–6.

Cortes D (1998) Cryptorchidism: aspects of pathogenesis, histology and treatment. *Scand J Urol and Nephrol* **32**: 9–54.

Cortes D, Thorup J, Lindenberg S (1996) Fertility potential after unilateral orchiopexy: an age independent risk of subsequent infertility when biopsies at surgery lack germ cells. *J Urol* **156**: 217–19.

de Munick Keizer Schrama S, Hazebrock F, Drop S, Molenaar J, Visser H (1986) A double-blind placebo controlled study of LHRH treatment of uni and bilateral cryptorchidism. *Lancet* i: 876–82.

Depue R (1984) Maternal and gestational factors affecting the risk of cryptorchidism and inguinal hernia. *Int J Epidemiol* **13**: 311–18.

Diamond DA, Caldamone A (1992) The value of laparoscopy for 106 impalpable testes relative to clinical presentation. *J Urol* **148**: 632–4.

Eastham J, McEvoy K, Sullivan R, Chandrasoma P (1992) A case of simultaneous bilateral nonseminomatous testicular tumors in persisten mullerian duct syndrome. *J Urol* **148**: 1262–4.

Elder J (1989) Laparoscopy and Fowler–Stephens orchiopexy in the management of impalpable testis. *Urol Clin North Am* **16**: 399.

Elder J (1992) Epididymal anomalies associated with hydrocele/hernia and cryptorchidism: implications regarding testicular descent. *J Urol* **148**: 624–6.

Elder J (1992b) Two-stage Fowler–Stephens orchiopexy in the management of intra-abdominal testes. *J Urol* **148**: 1239.

Engle E (1932) Experimentally induced descent of the testis in the Macaus monkey by hormones from the anterior pituitary and pregnancy urine. The role of gonadokinetic hormones in pregnancy blood in the normal descent of the testes in man. *Endocrinology* **16**: 513–20.

Fallon B, Welton M, Hawtrey C (1982) Congenital anomalies asssociated with cryptorchidism. *J Urol* **127**: 91–3.

Farrington G (1968) The position and retractability of the normal testis in childhood with reference to the diagnosis and treatment of cryptorchidism. *J Pediatr Surg* **4**: 606–13.

Farrington G (1969) Histologic observations in cryptorchidism: the congenital germ-cell deficiency of the undescended testis. *J Pediatr Surg* **4**: 606–13.

Fentener vV, JM, van Zolen E, Ursem P, Wensing C (1988) *In vitro* model of the first phase of testicular descent: identification of a low molecular weight factor from fetal testis involved in proliferation of gubernaculum testis cells and distinct from specified polypeptide growth factors and fetal gonadal hormones. *Endocrinology* **123**: 2868–77.

Fernades E, Hollabaugh R, Young J, Wilroy S, Schrock E (1990) Persistent mullerian duct syndrome. *Urology* **36**: 516–18.

Firor H (1971) Two-stage orchiopexy. *Arch Surg* **102**: 598–602.

Forman D, Pike M, Davey G, Dawson S, Baker K, Chilvers C (1994) Aetiology of testicular cancer: association with congenital abnormalities, age at puberty, infertility and exercise. *BMJ* **308**: 1393–9.

Fowler R, Stephens F (1959) The role of testicular vascular anatomy in the salvage of high undescended testes. *Aust N Z J Surg* **29**: 92–106.

Frey H, Peng S, Rajfer J (1983) Synergy of abdominal pressure and androgens in testicular descent. *Biol Reprod* **29**: 1233–9.

Frey H, Rajfer J (1984) Role of the gubernaculum and intrabdominal pressure in the process of testicular descent. *J Urol* **574**–8.

Friedland G, Chang P (1988) The role of imaging in the management of the impalpable undescended testis. *AJR Am J Roentgenol* **151**: 1107–11.

Gaudio E, Paggarino D, Carpino F (1984) Structural and ultrastructural modifications of cryptorchid human testes. *J Urol* **131**: 292–6.

Gilhooly P, Meyers F, Lattimer J (1984) Fertility prospects for children with cryptorchidism. *Am J Dis Child* **138**: 940–3.

Gill B, Kogan S, Starr S, Reda E, Levitt S (1989) Significance of epididymal and ductal anomalies associated with testicular maldescent. *J Urol* **142**: 556–8.

Gill B, Kogan S (1997) Cryptorchidism: current concepts. *Pediatr Clini North Am* **44**: 211–27.

Giwercman A, Grindsted J, Hansen B, Jensen O, Skakkebaek N (1987) Testicular cancer risk in boys with maldescended testis: a cohort study. *J Urol* **138**: 1214–16.

Giwercman A, Bruun E, Frimodt-Moller C, Skakkebaek N (1989) Prevalence of carcinoma *in situ* and other histopathological abnormalities in testes of men with a history of cryptorchidism. *J Urol* **142**: 998–1002.

Godbole P, Morecroft J, MacKinnon A (1997) Laparoscopy for the impalpable testis. *Br J Surg* **84**: 1430–2.

Goh D, Hutson J (1992) Is the retractile testis a normal physiological variant or an anomaly that requires active treatment. *Pediatr Surg Int* **7**: 249–52.

Goh D, Hutson J (1993) The retractile testis: time for reappraisal. *J Pediatr Child Health* **29**: 407–8.

Goh D, Middlesworth W, Farmer P, Hutson J (1994) Prenatal androgen blockade with flutamide inhibits masculinization of the genitofemoral nerve and testicular descent. *J Pediatr Surg* **29**: 836–8.

Gome-Leon M, Ferrios J, Casanova R, Roduguez R, Pedrosa C (1986) The value of computed tomography in the localization of the undescended testis. *Eur J Radiol* **6**: 283–7.

Grady R, Mitchell M, Carr M (1998) Laparoscopic and histologic evaluation of the inguinal vanishing testis. *Urology* **52**: 866–9.

Group JRHCS (1986) Boys with late descending testis: the source of patients with retractile testes undergoing orchiopexy? *BMJ* **293**: 798–9.

Group JRHCS (1992) Cryptorchidism: a prospective study of 7500 consecutive male births, 1984–88. *Arch Dis Child* **67**: 892–9.

Guerrier D *et al.* (1989) The persistent mullerian duct syndrome: a molecular approach. *J Clin Endocrinol Metab* **68**: 46–52.

Gustafson M, Lee M, Asmundson L, MacLaughlin D, Donahoe P (1993) Mullerian inhibiting substance in the diagnosis and managment of intersex and gonadal abnormalities. *J Pediatr Surg* **28**: 439–44.

Hadziselimovic F (1983a) Cryptorchidism: management and implications. Berlin: Springer.

Hadziselimovic F (1983b) Examinations and clinical findings in cryptorchid boys. In: Hadziselimovic F (ed.) *Cryptorchidism: management and implications*. Berlin: Springer 95–98.

Hadziselimovic F, Herzog B (1993) The development and descent of the epididymis. *Eur J Pediatr Surg* **152**: S6–9.

Hadziselmovic F, Herzog B (1997) Treatment with leuteinzing hormone-releasing hormone analogues after successful orchiopexy markedly improves the chance of fertility later in life. *J Urol* **158**: 1193–5.

Hadziselimovic F, Kruslin E (1979) The role of the epididymis in descensus testis and the topographical relationship between the testis and epididymis from the sixth month of pregnancy until immediately after birth. *Anat Embryol* **155**: 191–6.

Hadziselimovic F, Hecker E, Herzog B (1984a) The value of testicular biopsy in cryptorchidism. *Urol Res* **12**: 171–4.

Hadziselimovic F, Hoecht B, Herzog B, Girad J (1984b) Does long-term treatment with buserelin improve the fertility chances of cryptorchid testes? In: Labrie F, Belanger A, Duport A (eds) *Lh-Rh and its analogues* New York: Academic Press 488–506.

Hadziselimovic F, Thommen L, Girad J, Herzog B (1986) The significance of postnantal gonadotropin surge for testicular development in normal and cryptorchid testes. *J Urol* **136**: 274–6.

Hadziselimovic F, Herzog B, Buser M (1987a) Development of cryptorchid testes. *Eur J Pediatr* **146** (Supp 2): S8–12.

Hadziselimovic F, Herzog B, Hocht B, Hecker E, Miescher E, Buser M (1987b) Screening for cryptorchid boys risking sterility and results of long-term buserelin treatment after successful ochiopexy. *Eur J Pediatr* **146** (Supp 2): S59–62.

Hadziselimovic F, Herzog B, Huff D, Manardi G (1991) The morphometric histopathology of undescended testes and testes assoicated with incarcerated inguinal hernia: a comparative study. *J Urol* **146**: 627–9.

Hargreave T (1997) Testis maldescent and male fertility problems. In: O'Donnell B, Koff S (eds) *Pediatric Urology*. 3rd edition. Oxford: Butterworth-Heinemann, 605–7.

Hargreave T, Elton R, Ja W, Busuttil A, Chislom G (1984) Maldescended testis and fertility: a review of 68 cases. *Br J Urol* 734–9.

Harrison C, Kaplan G, Scherz h, Packer M, Jones J (1990) Microvascular autotransplanatation of the intraabdominal testis. *J Urol* **146**: 506–7.

Hart D (1910) The nature and cause of physiological descent of the testes. Part II: Descent in man. *J Anat Physiol* **43**: 4–10.

Haughey B *et al.* (1989) The epidemiology of testicular cancer in upstate New York. *Am J Epidemiol* **130**: 25–36.

Hecker W, Heinz H (1967) Cryptorchidism and fertility. *J Pediatr Surg* **2**: 513–17.

Hedinger C (1982) Histopathology of undescended testes. *Eur J Pediatr* **139**: 266–71.

Henderson B, Bentron B, Jing J, Yu M, Pike M (1979) Risk factors for cancer of the testis in young men. *Int J Cancer* **23**: 598–602.

Heyns C (1987) The gubernaculum during testicular descent. *J Anat* **153**: 93–112.

Heyns C, Human H, Werely C, DP D (1990) The glycosaminoglycan of the gubernaculum during testicular descent in the fetus. *J Urol* **143**: 612–17.

Heyns C, Hutson J (1995) Historical review of theories on testicular descent. *J Urol* **153**: 754–67.

Hinman F Jr (1993) Development of the testis. In: Hinman F Jr (ed.) *Atlas of urosurgical anatomy*. Philadelphia, PA: WB Saunders, 472–83.

Hinman F, Benteen F (1936) The relationship of cryptorchidism to tumor of the testis. *J Urol* **35**: 378–81.

Hohenfeller R, Eisenhut I (1964) Evaluation of fertility in cryptorchidism. *Int J Fertil* **9**: 575–7.

Hrebinko R, Bellinger M (1993) The limited role of imaging techniques in managing children with undescended testes. *J Urol* **150**: 458–60.

Huff D, Hadziselmovic F, Duckett J, Elder J, Snyder H (1987) Germ cell counts in semithin sections of biopsies of 115 unilaterally cryptorchid testes. *Eur J Pediatr* **146** (Suppl 2): S25–7.

Huff D, Hadziselimovic F, McC Snyder HI, Duckett J, Keating M (1989) Postnatal testicular maldevelopment in unilateral cryptorchidism. *J Urol* **142**: 546–8.

Huff D, Hadziselimovic F, McC Snyder HI, Blyth B, Duckett J (1991) Early postnatal testicular maldevelopment in cryptorchidism. *J Urol* **146**: 624–6.

Humphrey G, Najmaldin A, Thomas D (1998) Laparoscopy in the managament of the impalpable undescended testis. *Br J Surg* **85**: 983–5.

Husmann D, Levy J (1995) Current concepts in the pathophysiology of testicular descent. *Urology* **46**: 267–76.

Husmann DM, MJ (1991) Time specific androgen blockade with flutamide is associated with alterations in the genitofemoral nerve morphology. *Endocrinology* **129**: 1409–16.

Husmann D, Boone T, McPhaul M (1994) Flutamide induced testicular undescent in the rat is assocated with alterations in genitofemoral nerve morphology. *J Urol* **151**: 1409–16.

Husmann D, Levy J, Cain M, Tietjen D, Uramoto G (1998) Micropenis: current concepts and controversies. *AUA Update Ser* **17**: 74–9.

Hutson J (1986) Testicular feminization: a model for testicular descent in mice and man. **21**: 195–8.

Hutson J, Beasley S (eds) (1992) *Descent of the testis*. London: Edward Arnold.

Hutson J, Donhoe P (1986) The hormonal control of testicular descent. *Endocrinol Rev* **7**: 270–83.

Hutson J, Hasthorpe S, Heyns C (1997) Anatomical and functional aspects of testicular descent and cryptorchidism. *Endocrine Rev* **18**: 259–80.

Jarow J, Berkovitz G. Migeon C, Gearhart J, Walsh P (1986) Elevation of serum gonadotropins establishes the diagnosis of anorchisim in prepubertal boys with bilateral cryptorchdism. *J Urol* **136**: 277–81.

Job J, Canloebe P, Garagorri J (1982) Hormonal therapy of cryptorchidism with human chorionic gonadotropin (hCG). *Urol Clini North Am* **9**: 405–11.

Johnson D, Woodhead D, Pohl D, Robison J (1968) Cryptorchidism and testicular tumorigenesis. *Surgery* **63**: 919–22.

Johnson W (1939) Cryptorchidism. *JAMA* **113**: 25–7.

Jones B *et al.* (1991) Influence of prior orchiopexy on stage and prognosis of testicular cancer. *Eur Urol* **19**: 201–3.

Jones I, Young I (1982) Familial incidence of cryptorchidism. *J Urol* **127**: 508–11.

Jones M *et al.* (1997) Prenatal risk factors for cryptorchidism, a record linkage. *Paediatr Perinatal Epidemiol* **124**: 383–6.

Joseph D, Law S, Perez L (1996) Two-stage Fowler–Stephens orchidopexy with laparoscopic clipping of the spermatic vessels. *Pediatrics* **98**: 646–8.

Josso N, Legeai L, Forest M, Chaussain J, Brauner R (1990) An enzyme linked immunoassay for anti-mullerian hormone: a new tool for the evaluation of testicular function in infants and children. *J Clin Endocrinol Metab* **20**: 23–7.

Josso N, Picard J, Imbeaus S, Carre-Eusebe D, Zeller J, Adamsbaum C (1993) The persistent mullerian duct syndrome: a rare cause of cryptorchidism. *Eur J Pediatr* **152** (Suppl 2): S76–8.

Kaplan L, Koyle M, Farrer J, Rajfer J (1986) Association between abdominal wall defects and cryptorchidism. *J Urol* **136**: 645–7.

Kazim E (1985) Intraabdominal seminomas in persistent mullerian duct syndrome. *Urology* **26**: 290–2.

Khuri F, Hardy B, Churchill B (1981) Urologic anomalies associated with hypospadias. *Urol Clin* **8**: 565–71.

Kiesewetter W, Mammen K, Kalyglou M (1981) The rationale and results in two stage orchiopexies. *J Pediatr Surg* **16**: 631.

King L (1996) Undescended testis. *JAMA* **276**: 856.

Kirsch A, Escala J, Duckett J *et al.* (1998) Surgical management of the nonpalpable testis: the Children's Hospital of Philadelphia Experience. *J Urol* **159**: 1340–43.

Koff S, Sethi P (1996) Treatment of high undescended testes by low spermatic vessel ligation: an alternative to the Fowler–Stephens technique. *J Urol* **156**: 799.

Kogan S (1988) The case for early orchiopexy. In: King L (ed.) *Urologic surgery in neonates and young infants*. Philadelphia, PA: WB Saunders, 396–416.

Kogan S, Tennenbaum S, Gill B, Reda E, Levitt S (1990) Efficacy of orchiopexy by age 1 year for cryptorchidism. *J Urol* **144**: 508–9.

Lakshmanan Y, Docimo S (1997) Testicular implants. *J Long Term Effects Med Implants* **7**: 65–8.

Lan W, Tan P, Avi V *et al.* (1998) Gadolinium infusion magnetic resonance angiogram: a new noninvasive and accurate method of preoperative localization of the impalpable undescended testis. *J Pediatr Surg* **33**: 123–6.

Lawson A, Gornall P, Buick R, Corkey J (1991) Impalpable testis: testicular vessel division in treatment. *Br J Surg* **78**: 1111–12.

Lee M, Donhoe P, Silverman B *et al.* (1997) Measurements of serum mullerian inhibitory substance in the evaluation of children with nonpalpable gonads. *N Engl J Med* **336**: 1480–6.

Lee P, O'Leary L, Songer N, Bellinger M, Laporte R (1995) Paternity after cryptorchidism; lack of corrleation with age at orchiopexy. *Br J Urol* **75**: 704–7.

Lemeh C (1960) A study of the development and structural relationships of the testis and gubernaculum. *Surg Gynecol Obstet* **110**: 164–72.

Levitt S, Kogan S, Engel R, Weiss R, Martin D, Ehrich R (1978) The impalpable testis: a rational approach to management. *J Urol* **120**: 515–20.

Levy D, Husmann D (1995) The hormonal control of testicular descent. *J Androl* **16**: 459–63.

Levy D, Abdul-Karim F, Miraldi F, Elder J (1995) Effect of human chorionic gonadotropin before spermatic vessel ligation in the prepubertal rat. *J Urol* **154**: 466–9.

Levy J, Husmann D (1995) The hormonal control of testicular descent. *J Androl* **16**: 459–63.

Lipshultz L, Caminos-Torres R, Greenspan C, PJ S (1976) Testicular function after orchiopexy for unilaterally undescended testis. *N Engl J Med* **295**: 15–18.

Loef D et al. (1994) Surgical and genetic aspects of persistent mullerian duct syndrome. *J Pediatr Surg* **29**: 61–5.

McAleer I et al. (1995) Fertility index anlyasis in cryptorchidism. *J Urol* **153**: 1255–8.

McMahon D, Kramer S, Husmann D (1995) Anti-androgen induced cryptorchidism in the pig is associated with failed gubernacular regression and epididymal malformations. *J Urol* **154**: 553–7.

Mandant K et al. (1994) Semen anlalysis of patients who had orchiopexy in childhood. *Eur J Pediatr Surg* **4**: 94–7.

Manuel M, Katyama K, Jones H (1976) The age of gonadal tumors in intersex patients with a Y chromosome. *Am J Obstet Gynecol* **124**: 293–300.

Marshall F, Shermata D (1979) Epididymal abnormalities associated with undescended testis. *J Urol* **121**: 341–2.

Martin D (1982) Malignancy in the cryptorchid testis. *Urol Clin North Am* **9**: 371–6.

Mayr J, Rune G, Holas A, Schimpl G, Schmidt H, Haberlik A (1995) Ascent of the testis in children. *Eur J Pediatr* **154**: 893–5.

McAleer I, Packer M, Kaplan G, Scherz H, Krous H, Billman G (1995) Fertility index analysis in cryptorchidism. *J Urol* **153**: 1255–8.

Mengel W, Heinz H, Sippe WI, Hecker W (1974) Studies on cryptorchidism: a comparison of histological findings in the germinative epithelium before and after the second year of life. *J Pediatr Surg* **9**: 445–50.

Mercer S (1979) Agenesis or atrophy of the testis and vas deferens. *Can J Surg* **22**: 245–6.

Moller H, Prener A, Skakkebaek N (1996) Testicular cancer, cryptorchidism, inguinal hernia, testicular atrophy and genital malformations: case controlled studies in Denmark. *Cancer Cause Control* **7**: 264–74.

Moller H, Skakkebaek N (1997) Testicular cancer and cryptorchidism in relation to prenatal factors: case control studies in Denmark. *Cancer Causes Control* **8**: 904–412.

Mowad J, Konvolinka C (1978) Torsion of the undescended testicle. *Urology* **12**: 567–9.

Muffly K, McWhorter C, Bartone F, Gardner P (1984) The absence of premalignant changes in the cryptorchid testis before adulthood. *J Urol* **131**: 523–5.

Muller J, Skakkebaek N (1983) Quantification of germ cells and seminiferous tubules by sereological examination of testicles from 50 boys who suffered from sudden death. *Int J Androl* **6**: 143–56.

Muller J, Skakkebaek N (1984a) Cryptorchidism and testis cancer: Atypical infantile germ cells followed by carcinoma in situ and invasive carcinoma in adulthood. *Cancer* **54**: 629–634.

Muller J, Skakkebaek N (1984b) Abnormal germ cells in maldescended testes: a study of cell density, nuclear size, deoxyribonucleic acid content in testicular biopsies from 50 boys. *J Urol* **131**: 730–3.

Muller J et al. (1984) Cryptorchidism and testis cancer: atypical infantile germ cells followed by carcinoma in situ and invasive carcinoma in adulthood. *Cancer* **54**: 629–34.

Muller J, Skakkebaek N (1997) Cryptorchidism. *Curr Ther Endocrinol Metab* **6**: 363–6.

Nguyen D, Mitchell M (1993) Ureteral obstruction due to compression by the vas deferens following Fowler–Stephens orchiopexy. *J Urol* **149**: 94–5.

Nistal M, Abaurrea R, Diez-Pardo J (1980) Histological classification of undescended testes. *Hum Pathol* **11**: 666–74.

O'Riordan W, Sherman N (1977) Cryptorchidism and abdominal pain. *J Am Coll Emerg Phys* **6**: 196–9.

Orvis B, Bottles K, Kogan B (1988) Testicular histology in fetuses with prune belly syndrome and posterior urethral valves. *J Urol* **139**: 335–7.

Park W, Hutson J (1991) The gubernaculum shows rhythmic contractility and active movement during testicular descent. *J Pediatr Surg* **26**: 615–17.

Parkinson M, Swerdlow A, Pike M (1994) Carcinoma in situ in boys with cryptorchidism: when can it be detected? *Br J Urol* **73**: 431–5.

Pascual J, Villanueva-Meyer M, Saldio E, Mena I, Rajfer J (1989) Recovery of testicular blood flow following ligation of testicular arteries. *J Urol* **142**: 549–52.

Perman R (1961) Congenital absence of the testicle: monorchism. *J Urol* **85**: 599–601.

Perrett L, O'Rouke D (1969) Hereditary cryptorchidism. *Med J Aust* **1**: 1289–91.

Persky L, Albert D (1971) Staged orchiopexy. *Surg Gynecol Obstet* **132**: 43.

Person A (1956) The relationship of the gubernaculum to the development of the inguinal canal in man. *Anat Rec* **124**: 345–50.

Pidutti R, Morales A (1993) Silicone gel filled testicular prosthesis and systemic disease. *Urology* **42**: 155–8.

Pinczowski D, McLaughlin J, Lackgren G, Adami H, Persson I (1991) Occurrence of testicular cancer in patients operated on for cryptorchidism and inguinal hernia. *J Urol* **146**: 1291–4.

Polascik TJ, Chan-Tack KM, Jeffs RD et al. (1996) Reappraisal of the role of human chorionic gonadotropin in the diagnosis and treatment of the nonpalpable testis: a 10 year experience. *J Urol* **156**: 804–6.

Popper P, Miceyvych P (1989) The effect of castration on calcitonin gene-related peptide in spinal motor neurons. *Neuroendocrinology* **50**: 338–43.

Popper P, Micevych P (1990) Steroid regulation of calcitonin gene-related peptide MRNA expression in motorneuron of the bulbocavernosus. *Molec Brain Res* **8**: 159–66.

Popper P, Ulbarri C, Miceyvych P (1992) The role of target muscles in the expression of calcitonin gene-related peptide mRNA in the spinal nucleus of the bulbocavernosus. *Molec Brain Res* **13**: 43–51.

Prener A, Engholm G, Jensen O (1995) Genital anomalies and risk for testicular cancer in Danish men. *Epidemiology* **7**: 14–17.

Prentis R, Weickgenant C, Moses J, Frazier D (1962) Surgical repair of the undescended testis. *Calif Med* **96**: 401–5.

Priebe C, Holahan J, Ziring P (1979) Abnormalities of the vas deferens and epididymis in cryptrochid boys with congenital rubella. *J Pediatr Surg* **14**: 834–9.

Puri P, Nixon M (1977) Bilateral retractile testes – subsequent effects on fertility. *J Pediatr Surg* **12**: 563–6.

Rabinowitz R, Hulbert W (1997) Late presentation of cryptorchidism: the etiology of testicular re-ascent. **157**: 1892–4.

Raina V, Shukla N, Chen C, Qi Y, Gu D, Gu X (1995) Germ cell tumors in uncorrected cryptorchid testis at Institute Rotary, Cancer Hospital, New Delhi. *Br J Cancer* **71**: 380–2.

Rajfer J, Walsh P (1978) Testicular descent. normal and abnormal. *Urol Clin North Am* **5**: 223–35.

Rajfer J, Handelsman D, Swerdloff R (1986) Hormonal therapy of cryptorchidism. *N Engl J Med* **314**: 466–70.

Ransley P (1984) Preliminary ligation of the gonadal vessels prior to orchiopexy for the intra-abdominal testicle: a staged Fowler Stevens procedure. *World J Urol* **2**: 266–70.

Redman J (1977) The staged orchiopexy: a critical review of the literature. *J Urol* **117**: 113–16.

Redman J, Mooney D (1983) Fowler–Stephens orchiopexy in a patient with prune belly syndrome and segmental atretic vas deferens. *Urology* **41**: 130–3.

Reinberg Y, Manivel J, Fraley E (1989) Carcinoma *in situ* of the testis. *J Urol* **142**: 243–7.

Rezvani I, Rettig K, DiGeorge A (1976) Inheritance of cryptorchidism. *Pediatrics* **58**: 774–6.

Riverola M, Bergada C, Cullen M (1970) hCG stimulation test in prepubertal boys with cryptorchidism, in bilateral anorchia and in male pseudohermaphroditism. *J Clin Endocrinol Metab* **31**: 526–8.

Rizk D *et al.* (1998) Persistent mullerian ductal syndrome. *Arch Gynecol Obstet* **261**: 105–7.

Robertson J, Azmy A, Cochran W (1988) Ascent to ascent of the testis. *Br J Urol* **61**: 146–7.

Rosenfield A, Blair D, Rosenfield N, McCarthy S, Glickman M, Weiss R (1989) The pars infravaginalis gubernaculi and associated structures: an imaging pitfall in the identification of the undescended testis. *Am J Roentgenol* **153**: 775–80.

Ross F, Farmer A, Lindsay W (1959) Hypospadias: a review of 230 cases. *Plast Reconstruct Surg* **24**: 357–68.

Sabroe S, Olsen J (1998) Perinatal correlates of specific histological types of testicular cancer in patients below 35 years of age: a case-cohort study based on midwives records in Denmark. *Int J Cancer* **78**: 140–3.

Satge D, AJ S, Cure H, Leduc B, Sommelet D, Vekemans M (1997) An excess of testicular germ cell tumors in Down's syndrome. *Cancer* **80**: 929–35.

Savage M, Lowe D (1990) Gonadal neoplasia and abnormal sexual differentiation. *Clin Endocrinol* **32**: 519–33.

Schindler A, Diaz P, Cuendet A, Sizonenko P (1987) Cryptorchidism, a morphological study of 670 biopsies. *Helv Pediatr Acta* **42**: 145–58.

Schlegel P (1996) Urogenital anomalies in men with congenital absence of the vas deferens. *J Urol* **155**: 164–8.

Schultz F, Wilson J (1974) Virilization of the wolffian duct in the rat fetus by various androgens. *Endocrinology* **94**: 979–86.

Scorer C (1964) The descent of the testis. *Arch Dis Child* **39**: 605–9.

Scorer C, Farrington G (eds) (1971) *Congenital deformities of the testis and epididymis*. London: Butterworths.

Scully R (1981) Neoplasia associated with anomalous sexual development and abnormal sex chromosomes. *Pediatr Adolesc Endocrinol* **8**: 203–17.

Shono T, Ramm-Anderson S, Goh D, Hutson J (1994) The effect of flutamide on testicular descent in rats examined by scanning electron microscopy. *J Pediatr Surg* **29**: 839–942.

Siemer S, Hunke W, Under M, Kreisser-Haag D (1986) Diagnosis of non palpable testis: value of laparoscopy. *Lagenbecks Arch Chir* **115**: 116–19.

Siemer S, Uder M, Humk U, Bonnet L, Zielger M (1998) Diagnosis of non-palpable testis in childhood: laparoscopic or magnetic resonance imaging. *Urologe-Ausgabe A* **37**: 647–52.

Silber S, Kelly J (1976) Successful autotransplantation of an intra-abdominal testis to the scrotum by microvascular technique. *J Urol* **115**: 452–5.

Silver R, Docimo S (1999) Cryptorchidism. In: Gonzales E, Bauer S (eds) *Pediatric urology practice*. Philadelphia, PA; Lippincott Williams & Wilkins, 499–522.

Smith A, Lattimer J (1975) Psychosexual impact of undescended testes and implanatation of prosthesis. *Med Aspects Hum Sex* **9**: 62.

Smith J *et al.* (1989) The relationship between cerebral palsy and cryptorchidism. *J Pediatr Surg* **24**: 1303–5.

Smith R (1941) The undescended testes. *Lancet* **240**: 747–50.

Sohval A (1954) Testicular dygenesis as an etiologic factor in cryptorchidism. *J Urol* **72**: 693–702.

Spencer J (1994) The endocrinology of testicular descent. *AUA Update Ser* **13**: 94–9.

Spencer J, Torrado T, Sanchez R, Vaugn E, JI-M (1991) Effects of flutamide and finasteride on rat testicular descent. *Endocrinology* **129**: 741–8.

Spencer-Barthold J, Mahler H, Sziszak T, Newton B (1996) Lack of feminization of cremasteric nucleus by prenatal flutamide administration in the rat and pig *J Urol* **156**: 767–71.

Spencer-Barthold J (1998) Letter to the Editor. Re: Testicular descent: a proposed interaction between mullerian inhibitory substance and epidermal growth factor. *J Urol* **160**: 1438–9.

Spencer-Barthold J *et al.* (1996) Lack of feminization of cremasteric nucleus by prenatal flutamide administration in the rat and pig. *J Urol* **156**: 767–71.

Spencer-Barthold J, Mahler N, Newton B (1994) Lack of feminization of the cremasteric nucleus in cryptorchid androgen insensitive rats. *J Urol* **152**: 2280–6.

Steinhardt G, Kroovand R, P. AD (1985) Orchiopexy: planned 2-stage technique. *J Urol* **133**: 434.

Stephens F (1988) Fowler-Stephens orchiopexy. *Semin Urol* **6**: 103.

Swerdlow A, Wood K, Smith P (1983) A case–control study of the etiology of cryptorchidism. *J Epidemiol Commun Health* **37**: 238–44.

Swerdlow A, Huttley S, Smith P (1987) Prenatal and familial associations of testicular cancer. *Br J Cancer* **55**: 571–7.

Swerdlow A, Higgins C, Pike M (1997a) Risk of testicular cancer in cohort of boys with cryptorchidism. *BMJ* **314**: 1507–11.

Swerdlow A, Desavola B, Swanwich M, Mancomchie N (1997b) Risk of breast and testicular cancers in young adult twins in England and Wales: evidence of prenatal and genetic etiology. *Lancet* **350**: 1723–8.

Terada M, Goh D, Farmer P, Hutson J (1994) Calcitonin gene related peptide receptors in the gubernaculum of normal rat and two models of cryptorchidism. *J Urol* **152**: 759–62.

Thorup J, Cortes D, Nielsen O (1993) Clinical and histopathological evaluation of operated maldescended testes after lueteinizing hormone-releasing hormone treatment. *Pediatr Surg Int* **8**: 419–22.

Tong S, Hutson J Watts C (1996) Does testosterone diffuse down the wolffian duct during sexual differentation? *J Urol* **155**: 2057–9.

van der Schoot P, Elger W (1992) Androgen induced prevention of the outgrowth of cranial gonadal suspensory ligaments in fetal rats. *J Androl* **13**: 2280–6.

Vandersteen D, Chaueton A, Ireland K, Tank E (1997) Surgical management of persistent mullerian duct syndrome. *Urology* **49**: 941–5.

Verp M, Simpson J (1987) Abnormal sexual differentiation and neoplasia. *Cancer Genet Cytogenet* **25**: 191–218.

Villumsen A, Zachau-Christianseon B (1966) Spontaneous alterations in postion of the testes. *Arch Dis Child* **41**: 198–200.

Wacksman J, Dinner M, Staffon R (1980) Technique of testicular autotransplantation using a microvascular anastomosis. *Gynecol Obstet* **150**: 399–402.

Waldschmidt J, El Dessouky M, Priefer A (1987) Therapeutic results in cryptorchidism after combination therapy with LHRH nasal spray and hCG. *Eur J Pediatr* **146**: 31–5.

Walker R (1997) Cryptorchidism. In: O'Donnell B, Koff S (eds) *Pediatric Urology*. 3rd edition. Oxford: Butterworth-Heinemann; 569–603.

Ward B, Hunter W (1960) The absent testicle: a report on a survey carried out in Nottingham. *BMJ* i: 1110–11.

Werder E, Illig R, Torresani T *et al.* (1976) Gonadal function in young adults after surgical treatment of cryptorchidism. *BMJ* ii: 1357–9.

Whitaker R (1988) Neoplasia in cryptorchid men. *Semin Urol* **6**: 107–9.

Whitehorn C (1954) Complete unilateral Wolffian duct agensis with homolateral cryptorchidism: a case report, its explanation and treatment; and the mechanism of testicular descent. *J Urol* **72**: 685–92.

Wilson J, Griffin J, Russell D (1993) Steroid 5 alpha reductase 2 deficiency. *Endocrine Rev* **14**: 577–89.

Wilson-Stoney D, McGenity K, Dickson J (1990) Orchiopexy: the younger the better? *J R Coll Surg Edin* **35**: 362–4.

Wolverson M, Houtton E, Heiberg E, Sundara M, Shields J (1983) Comparison of computed tomography with high resolution real time ultrasound in the localization of the impalpable testis. *Radiology* **146**: 133–6.

Wylie G (1984) The retractile testis. *Med J Aust* **140**: 403–5.

Wyndham M (1943) A morphologic study of testicular descent. *J Anat* **77**: 179–85.

Yamanaka J, Metcalf S, Hutson J (1992) Demonstration of calcitonin gene-related peptide in the gubernaculum by computerized densitometry. *J Pediatr Surg* **27**: 876–8.

Evaluation and management of impalpable testes

34b

Israel Franco

Introduction

The impalpable testis accounts for 20% of all cryptorchidism. Testes are considered impalpable when they are intracanalicular and never emerge via the external ring, or are intra-abdominal. They also could be atrophic, dysgenetic, or absent (Table 34b.1) (Levitt et al., 1978). The best time to make the diagnosis of an impalpable testis is in the newborn since the cremasteric reflex is absent or significantly diminished early in life. The absence of large amounts of fat makes it easier to feel a testis at this age. The vast majority of testes that have not descended by 6 months of age are unlikely to descend spontaneously, especially in full-term infants. Spontaneous descent is possible in the premature infant up to the first year of life, so final judgment in premature infants should be postponed accordingly.

Location of the impalpable testis varies widely from series to series, with as many as 45–80% found intracanalicular (Levitt et al., 1978) The variability in these numbers is so great because of the mobility of the testis within the canal.

Table 34b.1 Impalpable testes: compilation of six series

References	No. patients	Testes impalpable	
		n	(%)
Campbell	176	33	(19)
Tibbs	99	19	(19)
Jones	500	102	(21)
Scorer and Farrington	224	21	(9)
Flach	2319	499	(21.5)
Illig et al	112	20	(18)
Totals	3430	694	(20)

Data from Levitt et al. (1978) J Urol **120**: 515–520.

Of greater significance is the child who is monorchid. They account for 33–45% (Franco, 2000) of all children with impalpable testes. Proper diagnosis of this condition is essential for parent and child to ensure that adequate protection is afforded to the remaining testis. Monorchidism is most frequently due to in utero torsion or vascular accidents that occur during development and descent of the testis. True testicular agenesis is rare, representing a small proportion of all monorchid boys. Bilateral in utero torsions or anorchia is also extremely rare. It was reported to occur in 0.6% of 5815 children and has been estimated to occur in 1 of every 20 000 boys (Table 34b.2) (Borbrow and Gough, 1970; Levitt et al., 1978).

Evaluation of the non-palpable testis

The best tool to evaluate the impalpable testis is a good set of hands and a thorough examination in a calm child. Many children have been sent with sonograms indicating an absent testis however, a good examination will generally reveal clues to the presence or absence of the testis. Evaluation of the impalpable testis is best performed by an experienced surgeon who follows the basic guidelines for physical examination. The urologist has an advantage over the pediatrician when evaluating the child with a undescended testis. The pediatrician usually starts the examination at the head and works down to the groin, by which time the child has been prodded and poked by several instruments, making the child cry or tense up, and making palpation of the testis very difficult. The urologist has the benefit of a directed examination. It is best to disrobe the child just before the examination and limit the undressing to the pelvic or lower abdominal area. The appearance of the scrotum is critical to the evaluation of these patients. The testis

Table 34b.2 Incidence of monorchism and anorchism among cryptorchid children

References	No. patients operated	Monorchism	Anorchism		Monorchism or anorchism	
			n	(%)	n	(%)
Gross and Jewett	988	27	6	(0.6)	33	(3)
Curtis and Staggers	93	10	0		10	(10.8)
Tibbs	108	12	1	(0.9)	13	(12)
Bill and Shanahan	100	8	0		8	(8)
Jones	500	13	1	(0.2)	14	(3)
Abeyaratne et al	304	12	4	(1.3)	16	(5)
	2093					
Aynsley-Green et al	3722	Not stated	21	(0.56)		
Totals	5815	82/2093(4)	33/5815	(0.6)	94/2093	(4.5)

Data from Levitt *et al.* (1978) *J Urol* **120**: 515–520.

may be seen to retract upwards as the urologist elicits, a cremasteric reflex. The size and shape of the scrotum provide a clue as to whether a testis ever resided in the scrotum. In some instances, the testis resides in the canal or superficial inguinal pouch, but its gubernacular fibers may tug the scrotum when a cremasteric reflex is elicited. These are clues that help determine whether a testis is present and is intracanalicular or located ectopically (Levitt *et al.*, 1978).

Palpation of the area is the next step to evaluation of the impalpable testis. The clinician starts by stroking the hands from the internal ring to the external ring; this maneuver helps to milk out an intracanalicular testis (Levitt *et al.*, 1978) It is not unusual to be unable to palpate a testis in the superficial inguinal pouch of an obese boy. If nothing is palpable, the examiner should feel over the pubic tubercle; at times, cord structures or a vas-like structure are palpable. Examination of the scrotum is critical in that almost all atrophied testes lie either in the scrotum or in its upper recesses. These nubbins are generally firm and pea sized. When explored, the majority of these nubbins will have a greenish–brown color in the center (hemosiderium). Since all *in utero* torsions are associated with closed internal rings, further laparoscopic exploration is not indicated (Fig. 34b.1a–c) (Tennenbaum *et al.*, 1994).

The decision to remove the nubbins becomes a personal choice in most cases. This author's preference is to remove the nubbin if it can be easily accessed through a scrotal incision, and the majority can be removed in this simple fashion.

If laparoscopy reveals hypoplastic vessels and vas and a closed internal inguinal ring we prefer not to explore the groin to avoid the additional incision. However, if scrotal exploration is carried out primarily and a 'nubbin' found, the tissue should be carefully inspected prior to excision. If tunica vaginalis is present it should be incised and, if patent, is pathognomotic for testicular presence proximally. Further exploration should be pursued to identify that testicle.

The size of the palpable testis is a useful adjunct to the evaluation of the non-palpable testis. Koff (1991) noted that hypertrophy of the palpable testis frequently accompanies unilateral absence. The palpable testis can measure up to 3 cm^3 in volume, however, testes greater than 2 cm^3 are considered hypertrophied. Hypoplastic, rather than atrophic testes, will not result in compensatory hypertrophy of the remaining palpable testis. The hypoplastic remnants may be predicted laparoscopically by the presence of more prominent vessels entering the canal (Fig. 34b.1g)

In all cases that have a testis that measures about 2 ml in volume, one should be prepared for either orchidopexy or removal of the nubbin. Huff *et al.* (1992) noted a wide range in standard deviations from 27 to 74% in testis size, even though there was a statistically significant difference in size between the groups. Their conclusion was that the volume of the contralateral testis is not a reliable criterion for differentiating an absent testis from an intra-abdominal testis.

Radiologic evaluation of the impalpable testes

Urologists prefer to have a 'road map' prior to any surgical procedure to allow us to plan for all possible contingencies that may be encountered. Pneumoperito-

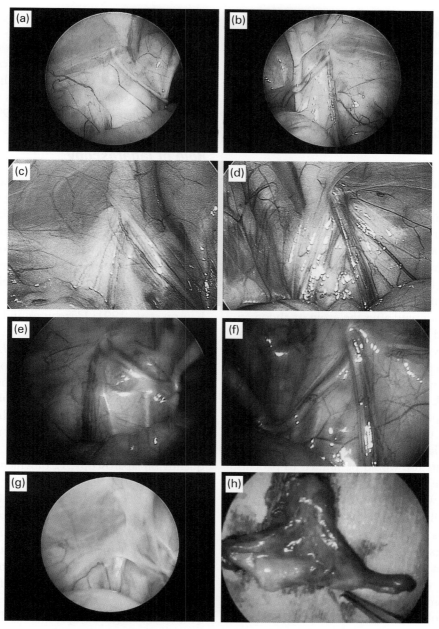

Figure 34b.1 Different appearances of internal ring in suspected *in utero* torsion. (*a*) Classical *in utero* torsion with complete atrophy of vessels and resultant absent or small testicular remnant. (*b*) Normal appearance of the contralateral ring. (*c*) *In utero* torsion with thin vessels. (*d*) Normal contralateral side. (*e*) *In utero* torsion typically seen with larger remnants. (*f*) Normal contralateral side of (*e*). (*g*) Ring of suspected atrophic testis found on examination. The ring was closed but dimpling of the ring by invagination of the processus vaginalis is indicative that this is not atrophy. (*h*) A small dysmorphic testis was found in the groin.

neography using nitrous oxide (andrography) was described by Lunderquist and Rafstedt (1967). This involved filling the abdomen with gas and visualizing the patent inguinal canal. However, failure of the gas to pass into the canal did not preclude an intra-abdominal, dysgenetic, atrophic or absent testis. White *et al*.

(1970) used contrast peritoneography (herniography) in an attempt to localize the testis. This test was fraught with the same drawbacks as Lunderquist's technique, rendering the procedure obsolete.

The desire to locate the testis both preoperatively and postoperatively led to the use of aortography, selective angiography, and spermatic venography. Their most common application today includes cases of autotransplantation to develop a road map of the venous and arterial anatomy before the procedure. Aortography generally does not allow for adequate visualization of gonadal arteries in adults, and even less so in children. Selective gonadal angiography is necessary to visualize the vessels. However, the origin of gonadal arteries is so variable and selective catheterization of these arteries in children is so difficult that this test has had limited success (Notkovich, 1956; Weiss *et al.*, 1977; Khadmin *et al.*, 1980) The need for anesthesia and the risk of arterial injury or thrombosis with transfemoral angiography essentially eliminates this procedure from use today.

Gonadal venography is a safe alternative to angiography and can be performed more readily. The original recommendations for the use of venography were that it was indicated after the groin or abdomen had been explored and no testis was identified. Left-sided venography is generally easier to perform because of the reproducible anatomy. Weiss *et al.* (1977) and Rubin and Gershater (1981) found no false positives with venography when a gonadal vessel terminated in a pampiniform plexus. When vessels terminate blindly or intra-abdominally, or when no vessels are identified, an open operation was recommended. Today, its use would be limited to patients who had extensive abdominal surgery and formation of adhesions that would preclude laparoscopy.

The value of ultrasonography for identifying the undescended testis is questionable. False positive and false negative rates are high, suggesting limited usefulness. Testes that are canalicular are located 70–97% of the time. In a well-designed study by Cain *et al.* (1996) intraabdominal and atrophic testes were correctly identified only 9% and 33% of the time, respectively. Other studies involving intraabdominal testis have localized the testis only 17% of the time. This poor rate of localization underscores the major drawbacks of ultrasonography for evaluation of the intraabdominal testis.

CT scanning for impalpable testes fairs no better than sonography in side-by-side testing, 94% versus 96% sensitivity for CT vs. sonography, respectively. The fact that any false negative studies can occur regardless of the 100% specificity achieved in some studies forces one to consider other evaluation modalities.

Magnetic resonance imaging (MRI) is unable to identify all impalpable testes. False-negative rates range from 7 to 13% for MRI (Lenda *et al.*, 1987; Fritzsch *et al.*, 1987; Tripathi *et al.*, 1992; Sarihan *et al.*, 1998). Gadolinium infusion magnetic resonance angiography has had reported success rates of 100% in a small study involving 17 impalpable testes. This is an encouraging result but studies will be necessary to verify its accuracy (Lam *et al.*, 1998).

Role of laparoscopy

As compared to the various imaging modalities, laparoscopy is capable of providing near 100% accuracy in experienced hands with minimal morbidity. Open exploration at times can be an extensive procedure with subsequent complications that can be avoided with laparoscopy. Furthermore, in multiple studies, 22–58% of patients (Lel-Gohary, 1979; Boddy *et al.*, 1985; Oesch and Ransley, 1987; Lauson *et al.*, 1991; Hazebroek and Molenaar, 1992; Rappe *et al.*, 1992; Gulanikar *et al.*, 1996; Mark and Davidson, 1997; Humphrey *et al.*, 1998) had no testis present, because of agenesis or vanishing testis syndrome. Therefore, it behooves the surgeon to consider laparoscopy before open groin exploration in patients with an impalpable testis. In a very sobering study from England, 59% (13 of 22) of testes deemed absent by groin exploration were identified subsequently on laparoscopy, 12 of which were intra-abdominal (Lakhoo *et al.*, 1996) Similar results have been reported by Perovic and Janic (1994), who identified six testes laparoscopically in 12 patients previously undergoing open surgery. Boddy *et al.* (1985) reported ten of 13 patients with previous negative explorations who were found to have testes at laparoscopy. In some of these series, testes were found to be intra-canalicular or as nubbins that were originally missed on the formal groin explorations. These testes rarely would have been missed if laparoscopy had been performed before groin exploration.

Laparoscopy allows the surgeon to choose the operative technique that will give the patient the best result, without the constraints that are placed on the surgeon given the type of incision originally chosen. If spermatic vessel ligation is necessary, it can be done either laparoscopically or open. Orchidopexy can be done open, laparoscopically assisted, and/or laparoscopically. The issue of whether to remove a nubbin or to leave it *in situ* is controversial. Plotzker *et al.* (1992) reported viable tubular tissue in three of 23 (13%) nubbins removed at surgery. In the author's own series, six of

50 nubbins (12%) had viable testicular tissue in some of the remnants (Franco *et al.*, 2000). Cendron *et al.* (1998) calculated a risk of 0–1.1% of cancer developing based on their finding no viable testicular tissue in these nubbins in a small series of 29 specimens. In this author's experience, 70% of nubbins were located in the scrotum. Therefore, if by inference these testes are descended, theoretically whatever tubules remain are normal with no greater risk for malignancy than the contralateral side. In many of these cases, a groin exploration could have been omitted if laparoscopy had been performed. The flexibility and superior diagnostic reliability of laparoscopy make this technique an integral part of the evaluation and treatment of the child with an impalpable testis.

On the other hand, Belman and Rushton (2001) recently suggested primary scrotal exploration based on their observation that testicular torsion is almost exclusively a scrotal event. Abdominal exploration is reserved by them for those in whom the classic 'nubbin' is not found in the scrotum or in those with a long looping vas and an associated patent processus vaginalis.

Surgical approach to the impalpable testis

Inguinal explorations

Many surgeons perform groin exploration as their procedure of choice for the impalpable testis. During exploration, a thorough dissection to the internal ring should be carried out. If a hernia sac is encountered, tugging on it can often deliver the testis out of its abdominal position. If the testis is still not evident, a limited local exploration of the retroperitoneum should be performed. This is done by incising the internal ring and mobilizing the retroperitoneum. The vas deferens may be identified on the posterior peritoneum and can be traced to its juncture with the spermatic vessels. If this exploration is unsuccessful, the peritoneum must be opened and formal laparotomy performed. Inspection behind the posterior wall of the bladder will usually lead to prompt identification of the vas, which can be traced distally, until the juncture with the spermatic vessels is encountered. If the testis cannot be brought down the inguinal canal, the epigastric vessels can be ligated (Prentiss maneuver) and the testis delivered via a more medial location out of the abdomen. Care should be taken to preserve the peritoneum around the vas, in case the need to perform a Fowler–Stephens orchidopexy arises. While exploring for the impalpable testis, structures resembling a blind-ending spermatic cord, vas deferens, or vessels, should be traced to the internal ring. They should be followed to the point of their divergence proximal to the internal ring. If separation between the vas and vessels is not seen, a blind-ending cord cannot be definitively diagnosed. Occasionally, the vasal vessels are prominent and mistaken for the spermatic vessels, leading to a misdiagnosis of vanishing testis, when in reality what is identified is a long looping vas. The identification of spermatic vessels coursing up the retroperitoneum, diverging from the vas, signals the end of the search. A blind-ending vas and vessels is the sine qua none of testicular absence (Levitt *et al.*, 1978).

Recent advances in laparoscopic technique and technology, combined with the continued refinement and improvement of surgeons' laparoscopic skills, may render routine exploration via an inguinal incision for an impalpable testis an outmoded treatment modality. The arguments are compelling in these patients, with almost 50% of all cases of impalpable testis resulting in nubbins being identified within the inguinal canal or scrotum. Cisek *et al.* (1998) reported a series of 263 impalpable testes, in which a typical groin incision would have left the surgeon compromised 66% of the time compared with the approach optimized as a result of laparoscopic testicular localization. Contrary to these findings, O'Hali *et al.* (1997) concluded that groin exploration is the ideal means for exploring for the impalpable testis. They concluded that the presence of a hernia sac was associated with a testis in all cases and should lead to abdominal exploration. These findings should be enough to obviate laparoscopy. Of 19 cases without a hernia sac, testicular agenesis was documented in five patients. However, in 14 of 19, an intra-abdominal testis was identified. What can be garnered from this study is that the presence of a hernia sac is associated with an undescended testis in all cases (155 impalpable testes), but absence of a hernia sac does not imply absence of an intra-abdominal testis (Fig. 34b.2). Given the present state of the art, there should be very few reasons not to consider laparoscopy as the primary choice in the initial management of the impalpable testis. Only in cases where the examiner has mistakenly thought that he or she palpated a testis or was misled by radiologic imaging should routine groin exploration be performed.

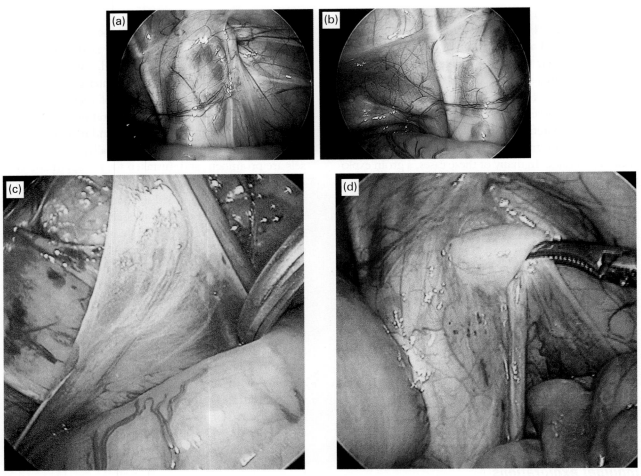

Figure 34b.2 (*a, b*) Closed internal rings with absence of vas. In both the testis was out of sight. (*c*) Note the absent vas in the peritoneal triangle. (*d*) Note the testis with absence of epididymal structures.

The Jones incision for the impalpable testis

When the testis is impalpable and is subsequently found to be a high canalicular testis, either by physical examination or laparoscopy, the Jones approach (Jones and Bagley, 1979) is a good alternative to routine inguinal orchidopexy or laparoscopic orchidopexy. The technique was combined with laparoscopy by Gheiler *et al.* (1997), with 18 out of 19 (95%) testes achieving satisfactory scrotal positioning. The one failure was in a patient who underwent simultaneous Fowler–Stephens orchidopexy. The technique involves making an incision medial to the anterior superior iliac spine (ASIS) (Fig. 34b.3a). The musculature is split and the retroperitoneum entered (Fig. 34b.3b). The peritoneum is mobilized medially and the internal inguinal ring identified (Fig. 34b.3c). The sac is identified and opened, and the testis brought into the field

(Fig. 34b.3d). The hernia sac is ligated and the spermatic vessels are mobilized by incising the lateral spermatic fascia superiorly (Fig. 34b.3e). The subcutaneous tissue is mobilized off the external oblique fascia to the level of the pubic tubercle (Fig. 34b.3f). A small opening, large enough to allow for the testis to pass through the abdominal wall at the pubic tubercle, is made and the testis is brought through this incision (Fig. 34b.3h). The testis is fixed in the scrotum in a subdartos pouch. This technique is the predecessor of the laparoscopic orchidopexy and the basic surgical maneuvers are exactly the same as for laparoscopic orchidopexy.

Orchidopexy by spermatic vessel transection

Orchidopexy by spermatic vessel transection was first

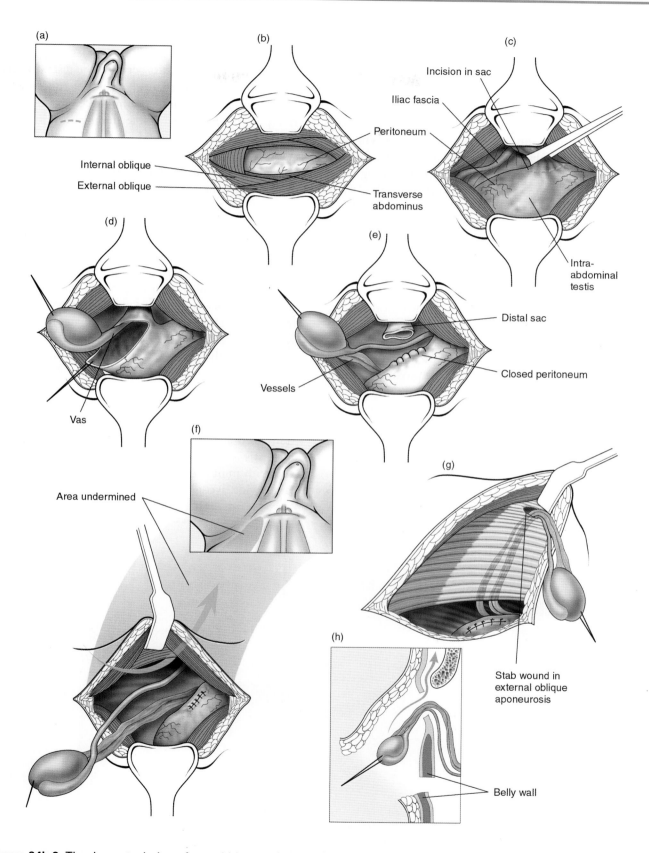

(a)

(b)

Internal oblique

External oblique

Peritoneum

Transverse
abdominus

(c)

Incision in sac

Iliac fascia

Peritoneum

Intra-
abdominal
testis

(d)

Vas

(e)

Vessels

Distal sac

Closed peritoneum

(f)

Area undermined

(g)

Stab wound in
external oblique
aponeurosis

(h)

Belly wall

Figure 34b.3 The Jones technique for orchidopexy (see text).

described by Bevan (1903). It was not popularized until Fowler and Stephens (1959) better characterized the vascular supply of the testis. They advocated temporarily occluding the internal spermatic vessels to test the capacity of its collateral blood supply. Johnston (1977) advocated leaving a medial broad strip of peritoneum, along with the vas to enhance further collateralization of the blood supply. Success rates as high as 89% have been reported using their technique (Kogan *et al.*, 1989) Koff and Seth (1996) recently modified the procedure by making the transections as close to the testis as possible (Fig. 34b.5). They achieved a success rate of 93% in a series of 39 low spermatic transections. The principles of both procedures are similar in that avoidance of manipulation of the vas and cord should be of the highest priority, to prevent damaging the delicate blood supply. Preservation of a strip of peritoneum is essential to the success of the procedure.

The Fowler–Stephens analysis of testicular anatomy and blood flow revealed that the proximal testicular artery is a non-collateralized end artery. However, before it reaches the testis it receives constant collateral communication from the vasal and cremasteric arteries. Fowler and Stephens believe that transection of the main artery too close to the testis would interfere with this collateral blood supply and lead to atrophy. This conclusion led to their recommendation to divide the vessels high to prevent damage to the deli-

cate collateral blood flow. Studies of the vascular anatomy by Jarow (1990) indicate that large-caliber anastomotic channels exist between the testicular and vasal arteries. These channels typically run beneath the tunica albuginea and communicate with the inferior pole of the testes. These findings are in direct contradiction to Fowler and Stephens' findings. Koff states that high ligation may contribute to testicular ischemia during an attempt to preserve the collateral vessels from the vasal artery to the distal testicular artery. High vascular ligation limits or prevents incision and dissection between the ascending and descending loop, which are necessary to unfold the testis. Koff proposes that additional collateral blood flow can be derived from the spermatic vessels that are left intact much higher up than with the typical Fowler–Stephens orchidopexy. In either procedure, it may be that strict adherence to not manipulating the vas and the early decision to perform vessel transection, lead to the good results achieved by several surgeons. Laparoscopic Fowler–Stephens orchidopexy as performed by the present author consists of the high ligation technique. This technique provides a high success rate due to several factors. The vessels are transected as high as possible, and the dissection of the testis is carried out without ever touching the vas and with minimal manipulation of the epididymis. A large, wide, wedge-shaped strip of peritoneum is preserved (Fig. 34b.4a, b). Placement of the testis is

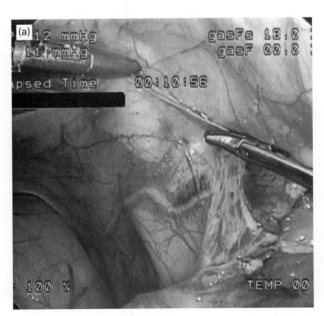 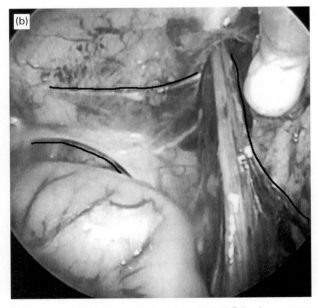

Figure 34b.4 (*a*) Peritoneal tongue in a Fowler–Stephens orchidopexy. (*b*) Peritoneal triangle with VAS in the center

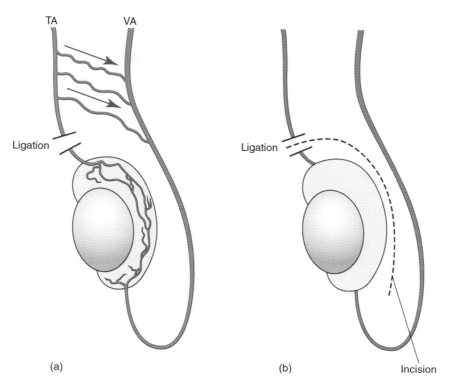

TA   VA

Ligation

Ligation

Incision

(a)   (b)

Figure 34b.5 Low spermatic vessel ligation as advocated by Koff. (Reproduced from Koff and Seth, 1996, with permission.)

done through a medially located anterior abdominal neoinguinal ring, in a fashion similar to Jones, near the pubic tubercle. There is no tension on the testis, even without uncoiling the looped vas or epididymis. Numerous collaterals are seen in the peritoneal strip emanating from sites other then the spermatic vessels. The author has encountered only one-failed Fowler–Stephens orchidopexy to date using the laparoscopic one-stage technique in a virgin case. Two atrophic testes resulted in cases where prior surgery had been performed and extensive dissection of the testis was necessary. In one series of laparoscopic Fowler–Stephens orchidopexies (Lindgren *et al.*, 1999) an overall success rate of 85% was achieved. When patients who had prior inguinal surgery or manipulations of the cord were eliminated, the success rate was 96%. In cases of prior surgery, vessel transection should be avoided and the testis should be approached through either a staged procedure, Jones technique or a microvascular approach. The staged Fowler–Stephens was thought to be a better alternative to one-stage vessel transection. The theory was that the collateral blood supply could mature and

tolerate transplantation of the testis more readily. This concept was supported by work done by Pascual *et al.* (1989) in rats using a xenon washout technique to measure blood flow at 1 hour and 30 days after ligation. Results demonstrated an 80% reduction in blood flow an hour after ligation. However, 30 days later, blood flow returned to normal pretreatment values. Several series have reported very high success rates with this technique (Elder, 1992; Caldamone and Moral, 1994). However, a review of the literature by Docimo (1995) revealed no statistically significant difference between one-stage and two-stage vessel transections. He found that staged Fowler–Stephens orchidopexy had an overall success rate of 76.8% (43/56 testis), compared with the one stage Fowler–Stephens success rate of 68.5% (76/111). These results tend to prove that meticulous preservation of the vasal blood supply is the most important factor in cases of spermatic vessel transection. Variability in surgical technique and tissue handling may account for the wide-ranging differences seen in results achieved with vessel transections.

Microvascular transplantation of the testis

With the advent of microvascular surgery in the 1970s, the first cases of microvascular transplantation were reported by Silber and Kelly (1976). Bukowski and Wacksman (1995) performed 27 autotransplantations with a success rate of 96%. Docimo (1995) reviewed the literature and reported a combined success rate of 83.7% in a total of 86 cases (Table 34b.3). The procedure involves a higher than normal inguinal incision to avoid injuring the inferior epigastric vessels. Dissection is carried down to the level of the inferior epigastric vessels, the retroperitoneum is entered, and the colon is mobilized. The testicle is identified, and the testicular vessels are isolated and divided as high as possible using microvascular hemoclips. The testis is mobilized in a similar fashion to the Fowler–Stephens mobilization, maintaining a wide strip of peritoneum with the vas deferens. The testis is brought through an anterior abdominal incision and placed in the scrotum in a subdartos pouch. Care is taken to make sure that there is no tension on the vas deferens and if necessary the vas is mobilized back to the bladder. The inferior epigastric vessels are isolated. Small branches are ligated as necessary until 8–9 cm of pedicle has been freed up beneath the rectus muscle towards the umbilicus. The inferior epigastric vessels are ligated distally and clips are placed proximally. The edges of the vessels are freshened and flushed with heparinized saline. The testicular artery is anastomosed to the inferior epigastric artery. The testicular artery typically measures 0.5–1 mm in diameter while the epigastric artery is 1–1.5 mm in diameter. The veins are usually equal in size, measuring 1 mm in diameter. The ideal anastomosis is end to end, but occasionally an end-to-side anastomosis is done. Patients are typically immobilized for 24 hours. Recently some groups have mobilized the testis laparoscopically before performing the microvascular anastomosis, thereby minimizing the intra-abdominal dissection. While success rates with this procedure are impressive, they are no different than the success rates obtained by vessel transections as described previously. In the present author's experience and that of Kogan *et al.* (1989) and Koff and Seth (1996), similar results were obtained without using microvascular anastomosis. The only absolute indication for performing a microvascular orchidopexy would be for the patient with a solitary impalpable testis or where there had been prior surgery on the testis, thereby possibly interfering with its collateral blood supply.

Laparoscopic orchidopexy

Laparoscopic orchidopexy seemed to be the logical extension of early attempts at vessel ligation by Bloom (1991) and routine diagnostic laparoscopy. The procedure allows the surgeon to transit from a diagnostic mode to an operative procedure. Laparoscopic orchidopexy was first described by Jordan *et al.* (1992). Subsequently there have been numerous reports using this technique (Caldamone and Amaral, 1994; Jordan and Winslow, 1994; Docimo *et al.*, 1995; Poppas *et al.*, 1996; Lindgren *et al.*, 1998). The original series by Lindgren *et al.*, 1998) was the largest experience of laparoscopic orchidopexies to date. Additional cases have been added to the original report and more than 90 laparoscopic orchidopexies have now been performed. This author's success rate in bringing the testis into a scrotal position without atrophy is 95% in those cases not involving vessel transections.

The original description by Jordan *et al.* (1992) remains relatively unchanged, except for minor variations in delivering the testis out of the abdomen. Routine laparoscopy is performed via an infraumbilical or supraumbilical incision. The supraumbilical incision is preferred by some because it avoids the umbilical vessels during open trocar placement. Open trocar placement is seen as the safest means of entering the abdomen in small children and minimizes complications (Fig. 34b.6). The abdominal space is very small in young children and bowel or vessel injury can occur quite easily with a blind insertion of a sharp instrument. The bladder should be emptied by catheterization to avoid injury during trocar placement. In the prune belly patient, extra caution is necessary when placing the initial trocar, since urachal attachments may extend to the umbilicus. In these patients a supraumbilical incision should be used.

Upon entry into the abdomen (Fig. 34b.7), inspection of the internal ring should be performed. In most cases with an intra-abdominal testis the ring is open. The testis will be found within 1 cm of the ring. Peeping testes can be pushed into the abdomen by pressing on the canal and milking the testis into the abdomen. If the ring is closed on the ipsilateral side of

Table 34b.3 Success of orchiopexy by anatomic position of testis and procedure

	Preoperative position of testes No. successes/total no.(%)					Type of orchiopexy No. successes/total no.(%)				
	Abdominal	Peeping	Canalicular	Distal	Inguinal	Fowler–Stephens	Staged Fowler–Stephens	Transabdominal	Two-stage	Microvascular
Overall	623/842 (74.0)	242/294 (82.3)	593/681 (87.1)	624/674 (92.6)	1388/1566 (88.6)	214/321 (66.7)		65/80 (81.3)	180/248 (72.6)	72/86 (83.7)
After 6 months	420/564 (74.5)	229/279 (82.1)	397/473 (83.9)	603/653 (92.3)	1110/1285 (86.4)	109/174 (62.6)	43/56 (76.8)	44/57 (77.2)	106/149 (71.1)	71/85 (83.5)
To age 6 years	148/211 (70.1)	7/7 (100)	245/257 (95.3) P < 0.05	Not available	535/588 (91.0) p < 0.05	9/19 (47.4)	43/56 (76.8)	11/15 (73.3)	67/84 (79.8)	35/43 (81.4)
							32/43 (74.4) p < 0.05		p < 0.05	
Older than 6 years	107/166 (64.5)	229/279 (82.1)	143/199 (71.9)	159/197 (80.7)	364/428 (85.0) p < 0.05	31/58 (53.4)	9/11 (81.8)	33/42 (78.6)	43/69 (62.3)	37/43 (86.0)
Through 1985	239/345 (69.4)	235/287 (81.9)	263/336 (78.3)	605/655 (92.4)	8 11/889 (91.2)	138/210 (65.7)	Not available	44/57 (77.2)	138/183 (75.4)	23/25 (91.7)
After 1985	384/497 (77.3) p < 0.05	7/7 (100)	330/345 (96.7) p < 0.05	19/19 (100)	577/677 (85.3)	76/111 (68.5)	43/56 (76.8)	21/23 (91.3)	42/65 (64.6)	49/61 (80.3) p < 0.05

Data from Docimo et al., *J Urol* **154**: 1148–52.

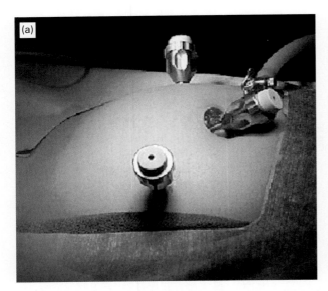
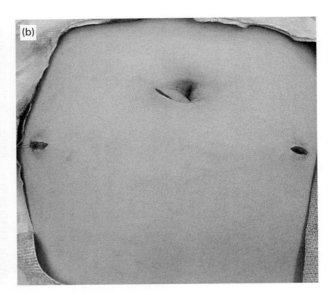

Figure 34b.6 (*a, b*) Trocar placement.

the impalpable testis, it is most likely that the testis has 'vanished'. The vas and vessels will be seen approaching the internal ring and the vessels are generally hypoplastic (Fig. 34b.2). However, a closed ring does not necessarily mean that the testis is absent. Very high abdominal testes may not have any attachments to the internal ring and could reside behind the bowel (Figs. 34b.2a, b, 34b.8a). If neither vessels nor vas are seen approaching the ring, additional trocars should be inserted to explore for the testis. The surgeon has the luxury that the contralateral side can be used as a reference in patients with a unilateral undescended testis (Fig. 34b.8b).

Once the decision to perform a laparoscopic orchidopexy has been made, the working trocars are placed under direct vision (Fig. 34b.6a, b). Trocars are placed at the level of the umbilicus and along the midclavicular line. The size of the working trocars depends on the expectation of whether a vessel transection will be required. The smallest clip applicator available is 5 mm, requiring the use of at least one 5 mm port. Inspection of the placement site will help to avoid injury to the epigastric vessels. In very young children placement of the trocars above the level of the umbilicus is helpful in avoiding the 'crossing sword' phenomenon. This occurs when trocars are bunched close together and either obstruct or interfere with each other. Once the trocars are in place, two grasping forceps are used to pull on the gubernacular attachment and bring as much of it as possible into the abdomen.

Care should be taken to make sure that the vas is not incorporated in this tissue. This tissue is transected using an electrified scissor with a minimal amount of cautery, to prevent transmission of heat to the vas. The dissection is carried medially over the bladder, incising the peritoneum above the vas and continuing towards the contralateral median umbilical ligament (Fig.

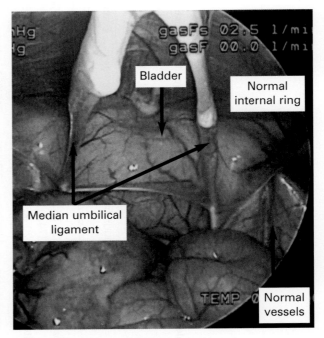

Figure 34b.7 Normal anatomic landmarks.

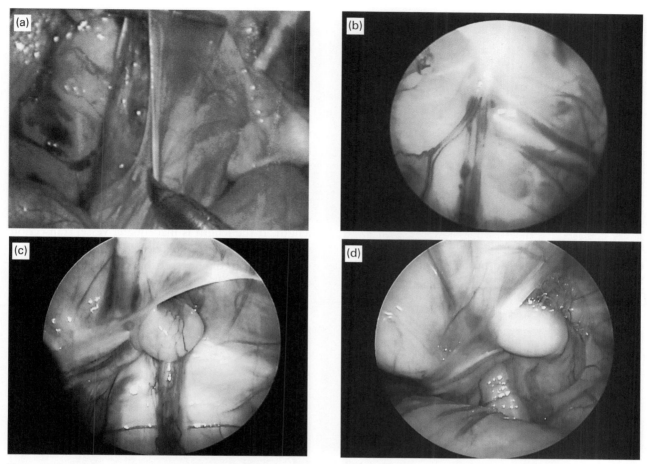

Figure 34b.8 (*a*) Intra-abdominal testis. (*b*) Normal contralateral internal ring. (*c, d*) Peeping testis.

34b.9). A generous piece of peritoneum should be maintained between the cut edge and the vas. The dissection is then carried down the lateral pelvic wall along the spermatic vessels, as high as possible without mobilizing the colon (Fig. 34b.10). The peritoneum is then incised over the spermatic vessels medially towards the root of the mesentery. This maneuver is critical in providing additional length for proper mobilization of the testis into the scrotum (Fig. 34b.11a). This also leaves a generous triangle of peritoneum in case a vessel transection becomes necessary (Fig. 34b.11b, c). The testis is brought out of the abdomen via a neo-ring created in the anterior abdominal wall near the pubic tubercle. The testis is medial to the median umbilical ligament and the bladder (Fig. 34b.12a). The scrotum is invaginated by the index finger and the endodissector is driven over the pubis, into the scrotum, while being guided by the index finger. A small scrotal incision is made and the trocar is brought

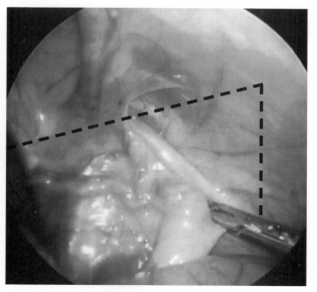

Figure 34b.9 Gubernacular fibers. Dashed lines are incision lines of the peritoneum.

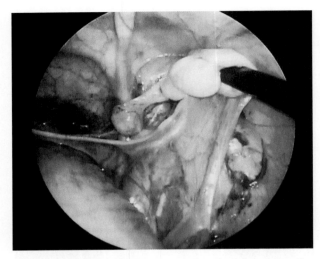

Figure 34b.10 Testis freed up after incising over the bladder and lateral pelvic wall.

out into the field (Fig. 34b.12b). A subdartos pouch is created and a 5 mm trocar is placed over the dissector and guided into the abdomen (Fig. 34b.12c). This trocar can be used to apply clips if vessel transection is necessary while using microinstrumentation. This is a good alternative to using a large center port. The gubernacular attachments of the testis are grasped with an endoallis clamp and the testis is delivered into the field. The testis is fixed in the scrotum in the usual fashion (Fig. 34b.13a).

If testicular positioning is inadequate, further dissection is done while holding the testis to judge the adequacy of the dissection in providing additional length. If the length is inadequate, vessel transection with a clip applier can be elected at this point. Since the vas and feeding vessels have not been dissected, this affords the opportunity for a successful

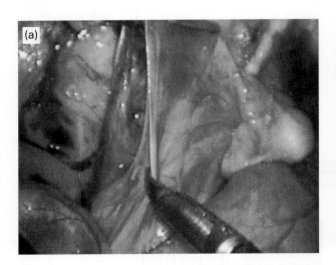

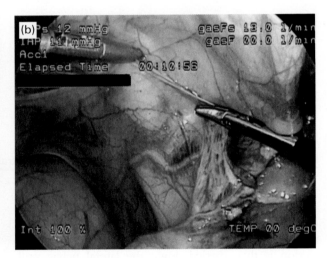

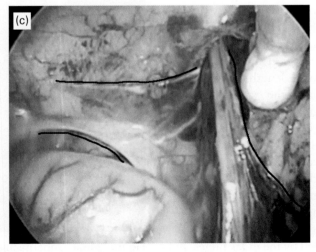

Figure 34b.11 Peritoneum overlying vessels is to be incised.

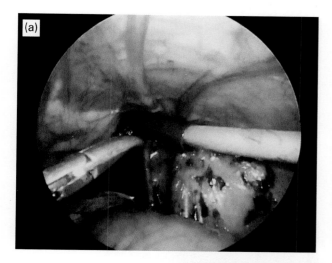

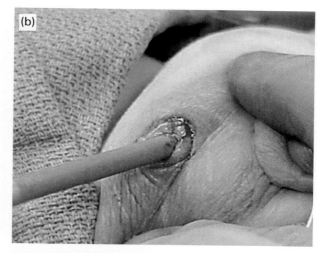

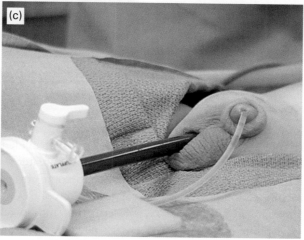

Figure 34b.12 (*a*) Neoinguinal ring between bladder and medium umbilical ligament. (*b*) Subdartos pouch has been created. (*c*) 5 mm trocar back loaded over instrument.

Fowler–Stephens orchidopexy. In 20 virgin laparoscopic Fowler–Stephens orchidopexies, in the author's experience, a 95% success rate was achieved. Two other patients who had had prior surgery on the affected testis failed laparoscopic Fowler–Stephens orchidopexy. The additional dissection to mobilize the testis from the surrounding scar tissue probably accounts for the failure in these cases. Concerns regarding the possible development of a hernia at the internal ring and along the inguinal canal have been unfounded. Initially, laparoscopists stapled or sutured the internal ring, but there is no evidence to suggest that is necessary. The experience of several groups has indicated that the ring scars down and reperitonealizes. No hernias have been seen by the author's group in laparoscopic orchidopexy, even in peeping testes that were removed from deep within the canal.

Complications associated with laparoscopic orchidopexy are the same as with any other procedure. Bowel injuries from cautery or trocar placement can occur. Injury to the iliac vessels during dissection is possible. Avulsion of the gonadal vessels is another complication and usually occurs when additional length is needed to bring the testis into the scrotum. This has occurred when the assistant pulls vigorously on the testis during dissection. The operating surgeon should hold the testis while freeing up additional length to avoid this complication. Identification of the proximal end of the gonadal vessels is the most difficult part of the recovery process from this complication. The vessels retract and go into spasm. These

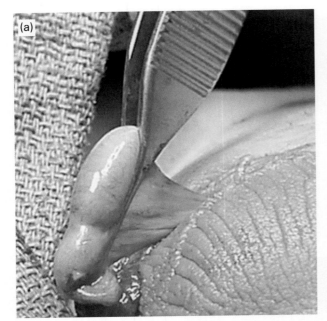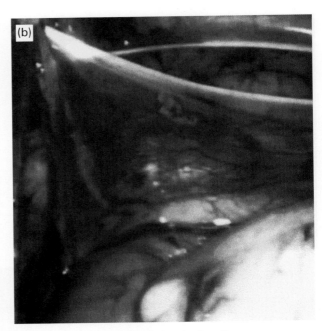

Figure 34b.13 (*a*) The testis is pulled into the scrotum, (*b*) Testis delivered through abdominal wall.

vessels need to be found and clipped. The vessels from the testis generally can be pulled into the scrotum and tied with a silk suture. Another potential catastrophic complication is injury to the femoral vessels. This can be avoided by making sure that the endodissector is passed from the ipsilateral port and aimed medially at all times. Dissecting down to the pubic bone in the window between the bladder and the median umbilical ligament will also prevent injuries to the femoral vessels and the bladder.

In experienced hands, success rates and operative times with laparoscopic orchidopexy are no different than with open surgery. Results with vessel transections are equivalent to open surgery. Laparoscopy affords the surgeon the luxury of proceeding with definitive surgery at the time of diagnostic evaluation. If transition to vessel transection becomes necessary, it can be done even after the testis has been dissected and brought down into the scrotum, without fear of loss of the testis.

Much controversy exists in the literature regarding the risks of postlaparoscopic adhesions. This author has not encountered adhesions in any patients who have had multiple laparoscopic procedures nor have I encountered any episodes of bowel obstruction post-laparoscopy secondary to adhesions. Bowel obstruction at the trocar site is a potential complication of laparoscopy in the immediate postoperative period.

This is due to herniation of bowel into a trocar site that was closed inadequately. Closure of all trocar sites 5 mm or greater is recommended. The advent of microendoscopic equipment, includng endogrip trocar technology introduced by Storz, reduces the risk of herniation and bowel obstruction.

As new modalities become available, surgeons must avail themselves of them and judiciously decide the true indications for their use. A 97% combined satisfactory scrotal placement was achieved in one series (Lindgren *et al.*, 1998) and similar results in other large series confirm that laparoscopic orchidopexy is capable of achieving excellent results. Although laparoscopic surgery is expensive, each year overall costs have decreased with improvements in reusable instruments and a decreased need for disposable instruments.

References

Belman AB and Rushton HG (2001) Is the vanishing testis always a scrotal event? *BJU International* **87**: 480.

Bevin AD (1903) The surgical treatment of undescended testicle: a further contribution. *JAMA* **41**: 718.

Bloom DA (1991) Two-step orchidopexy with pelviscopic clip ligation of the spermatic vessels. *J Urol* **145**: 1030–1.

Boddy SA, Corkery JJ, Gornall P (1985) The place of laparoscopy in the management of the impalpable testis. *Br J Surg* **72**: 918–19.

Borbrow M, Gough MH (1970) Bilateral absence of testes. *Lancet* i: 366.

Bukowski TP, Wacksman FJ, Billmire DA *et al.* (1995). Testicular autotransplantation: a seventeen year review of an effective approach to the management of the intraabdominal testes. *J Urol* **154**: 558–61.

Cain MP, Garra B, Gibbons MD (1996) Scrotal–inguinal ultrasonography: a technique for identifying the nonpalpable inguinal testis without laparoscopy. *J Urol* **33**: 791–4.

Caldamone AA, Maral JF (1994) Laparoscopic stage II Fowler–Stephens orchidopexy. *J Urol* **152**: 1253–6.

Cendron M, Schened AR, Ellsworth PI (1998) Histological evaluation of the testicular nubbin in the vanishing testis syndrome. *J Urol* **160**: 1161–3.

Cisek, LJ, Peters CA, Atala A *et al.* (1998) Current findings in diagnostic laparoscopic evaluation of the nonpalpable testis. *J Urol* **160**: 1145–9.

Docimo SG (1995) The results of surgical therapy for cryptorchidism; a literature review and analysis. *J Urol* **154**: 1148–52.

Docimo SG, Moore RG, Adams J *et al.* (1995) Laparoscopic orchidopexy for the high palpable undescended testis: preliminary experience. *J Urol* **154**: 1513–15.

Elder JS (1992) Two stage Fowler–Stephens orchidopexy in the management of intraabdominal testes. *J Urol* **148**: 1239–41.

Fowler R, Stephens FO (1959) The role of testicular vascular anatomy in the high undescended testes. *Aust NZ J Surg* **29**: 92.

Franco I, Palmer LS, Kolligian MC *et al.* (2000) *JSLS* **4**: 338.

Fritzsch PJ, Hricak H, Kogan BA *et al.* (1987) Undescended testis: value of MR imaging. *Radiology* **164**: 169–73.

Gheiler EL, Spencer-Barthold J, Gonzalez R (1997) Benefits of laparoscopy and the Jones technique for the nonpalpable testis. *J Urol* **158**: 1948–51.

Graif M, Czerniak A, Avigad I, *et al.* (1990) High resolution sonography of the undescended testis in childhood: in analysis of 45 cases. *Isr J Med Sci* **33**: 382–5.

Gulanikar AC, Anderson PA, Schwarz R, Giacomantonio M (1996) Impact of diagnostic laparoscopy in the management of unilateral impalpable testis. *Br J Urol* **77**: 455–7.

Hazebroek FW, Molenaar JC (1992) The management of the impalpable testis by surgery alone. *J Urol* **148**: 620–31.

Huff DS, Snyder, HM Haziselimovic F *et al.* (1992) An absent testis is associated with contralateral testicular hypertrophy. *J Urol* **148**: 627–9.

Humphrey GM, Najmaldin AS, Thomas DF (1998) Laparoscopy in the management of the impalpable undescended testis *Br Jr Surg* **60**: 983–5.

Jarow JP (1990) Intratesticular arterial anatomy. *J Androl* **11**: 255–9.

Johnston JH (1977) Prune belly syndrome. In: Eckstein HB, Henfellner R, Williams DJ (eds) *Surgical pediatric urology*. Philadelphia, PA: WB Saunders, 240.

Jones PF, Bagley FH (1979) An abdominal extraperitoneal approach for the difficult orchidopexy. *Br J Surg* **56**: 14.

Jordan GH, Robey EL, Winslow BH (1992) Laparoendoscopic surgical management of the abdominal/transinguinal undescended testicle. *J Endourol* **6**: 159.

Jordan GH, Winslow BH (1994) Laparoscopic single and staged orchidopexy. *J Urol* **152**: 1249–52.

Khadmim, Seebode JJ, Falla AA (1980) Selective spermatic arteriography for localization for an impalpable undescended testis. *Radiology* **136**: 627–34.

Koff FA, Seth PS (1996) Treatment of high undescended testes by lower spermatic vessel ligation: an alternative to the Fowler–Stephens technique *J Urol* **156**: 799–803.

Koff SA (1991) Does compensatory testicular enlargement predict monorchidism? *J Urol* **146**: 632–4.

Kogan SJ, Houman BZ, Reda EF, Levitt SB (1989) Orchidopexy of the high undescended testis by division of the spermatic vessels: a critical review of 38 selected transections. *J Urol* **141**: 1416–19.

Lakhoo K, Thomas DF, Najmaldin AS (1996) Is inguinal exploration for impalpable an outdated operation. *Br J Urol* **77**: 452–4.

Lam WW, Tam PK, Ai VH *et al.* (1998) Gadolinium-infusion magnetic resonance angiogram: a new, noninvasive, and accurate method of preoperative localization of impalpable undescended testis. *J Pediatr Surg* **33**: 123–6.

Landa HM, Gylys-Morin V, Mattrey RF *et al.* (1987) The magnetic resonance imaging of the cryptorchid testis. *Eur J Pediatr* **29**: S16–17.

Lawson A, Gornall P, Buick RG, Corkery JJ (1991) Impalpable testis: testicular vessel division in treatment *Br J Urol* **78**: 1011–12.

Lel-Gohary MA (1979) The role of laparoscopy in the management of impalpable testis. *Pediatr Surg Int* **33**: 463–5.

Levitt SB, Kogan SJ, Engel RM *et al.* (1978) The impalpable testis: a rational approach to management. *J Urol* **120**: 515–20.

Lindgren BW, Darby EC, Faiella L *et al.* (1998) Laparoscopic orchidopexy: procedure of choice for the nonpalpable testis? *J Urol* **159**: 2132–5.

Lindgren, BW, Franco I, Blick S *et al.* (1999) Laparoscopic Fowler–Stephens orchidopexy for the high abdominal testis. *J Urol* **162**: 990–4.

Lunderquist A, Rafstedt S (1967) Roentgenologic diagnosis of cryptorchidism. *J Urol* **98**: 219–23.

Malone PS, Quiney EJ (1985) A comparison between ultrasonography and laparoscopy in localizing the impalpable undescended testis. *Br J Urol* **57**: 185–6.

Mark SD, Davidson PJ (1997) The role of laparoscopy in evaluation of the impalpable undescended testis. *Aust NZ J Surg* **67**: 332–4.

Notkovich H (1956) Variations of the testicular and ovarian arteries in relation to the renal pedicle. *Surg Gynecol Obstet* **103**: 487.

Oesch I, Ransley PG (1987) Unilaterally impalpable testis. *Eur Urol* **13**: 324–6.

O'Hali W, Anderson P, Giacomantonio M (1997) Management of impalpable testis. Indications for abdominal exploration. *J Pediatr Surg* **148**: 918–20.

Pascual JA, Villanueva-Meyer JS, Salido E *et al.* (1989) Recovery of testicular blood flow following ligation of testicular vessels. *J Urol* **142**: 549–52.

Perovic S, Janic N (1994) Laparoscopy in the diagnosis of nonpalpable testis. *Br J Urol* **73**: 310–13.

Plotzker ED, Rushton HG, Belman AB *et al.* (1992) Laparoscopy for nonpalpable testis in childhood: is inguinal exploration also necessary when vas and vessels exit the internal ring? *J Urol* **148**: 635–8.

Poppas DP, Lemack GE, Mininberg DT (1996) Laparascopic orchidopexy: clinical experience and description of technique. *J Urol* **155**: 708–11.

Rappe BJ, Za De Vries JD, Froeling FM, Debruyne FM (1992) The value of laparoscopy in the management of impalpable cryptorchid testis. *Eur Urol* **21**: 164–7.

Rubin SZ, Gershater (1981) Testicular venography as an accurate indicator of true cryptorchidism. *Can J Surg* **33**: 360–2.

Rubin SZ, Mueller DL, Amundson GM, Wesenberg RL (1986) Ultrasonography and the impalpable testis journal. *Aust N Z J Surg* **56**: 609–11.

Sarihan H, Sari A, Abes M, Dinc H (1998) The nonpalpable undescended testis. Value of magnetic resonance imaging. *Minerva Urol Nefrol* **29**: 233–6.

Silber SJ, Kelly J (1976) Successful autotransplantation of an intraabdominal testis to the scrotum by microvascular technique. *J Urol* **115**: 452–4.

Tennenbaum SY, Lerner SE, McAleer I *et al.* (1994) Preoperative laparoscopic localization of the nonpalpable testis: a critical analysis of a 10 year experience. *J Urol* **151**: 732–4.

Tripathi RP, Jena AN, Gulati P *et al.* (1992) Undescended testis: evaluation by magnetic resonance imaging. *Indian Pediatr* **29**: 433–8.

Weiss RM, Carter AR, Rosenfield AT (1986) High resolution real time ultrasonography in the localization of the undescended testis. *J Urol* **135**: 936–8.

Weiss RM, Glickman MG *et al.* (1977) Preoperative localization of nonpalpable undescended testis. In: *Birth defects, Original Article Series* XIII. Volume 5. New York: Alan R Liss, 273–4.

White JJ, Haller JA, Dorst JP (1970) Congenital inguinal hernia and inguinal herniography. *Surg Clin North Am* **50**: 823–37.

Wolberson MK, Houttuin E, Heiberg E *et al.* (1983) Comparison of computed tomography with high resolution real time ultrasound in the localization of the impalpable undescended testis. *Radiology* **146**: 133–6.

Acute and chronic renal failure

35

Kanwal K. Kher and Marva Moxey-Mims

Introduction

Discovery of renal failure in children, especially in those who are critically ill, brings forth significant diagnostic and management concerns among physicians taking care of these patients. While in many patients renal failure encountered in a hospital environment is transient in nature, in others it may represent the initial detection of previously undiagnosed renal disease. Often, these patients come to medical attention because of one or more complications of chronic renal failure (CRF), such as hypertensive encephalopathy, or congestive cardiac failure resulting from fluid overload. Comprehensive medical care and effective management of these children is best provided by a team of medical personnel composed of a nephrologist, a urologist, a vascular access surgeon, dialysis nursing staff, a nutritionist, and a social worker.

This chapter discusses acute and chronic renal failure in children and approaches the subjects from clinical and patient management perspectives. The pathophysiology of both acute and chronic renal failure is also discussed in detail so as to provide adequate background for understanding the principles of management.

Acute renal failure

Definition

Acute renal failure (ARF) is a clinical disorder characterized by a sudden decline in glomerular filtration rate (GFR). In clinical terms, this represents an elevation of serum creatinine with symptoms of oliguria or anuria. In many cases, especially those associated with mild ischemic insult or nephrotoxic injury, ARF can occur in the absence of oliguria or anuria.

Incidence

The true incidence of ARF in children is unknown. In a recent review of 227 children requiring acute dialysis therapy in a referral hospital, Moghal et al. (1998) reported an incidence of 0.8 cases per 100 000 population, or 3.9 cases per 100 000 children. Since many patients who have ARF may not need dialysis therapy, the reported incidence probably underestimates the true incidence of the disorder.

Classification

ARF is often a secondary disorder that develops in the course of other clinical events or diseases. The underlying causes are usually renal hypoperfusion, intrinsic renal diseases, or urinary outflow obstruction. Accordingly, acute renal failure is classified into three clinical categories: prerenal azotemia, acute intrinsic renal failure, and postrenal failure. Some overlap between these three categories is, however, to be expected. The value of such a classification rests in its utility for both evaluation and management.

Prerenal azotemia

In its strictest sense, prerenal azotemia is not to be regarded as 'failure' of renal function but an appropriate renal response to dehydration and renal hypoperfusion. In all patients with prerenal azotemia, once renal perfusion is re-established recovery of renal function occurs without any residual sequelae. It is, however, important to note that if not treated in time, severe prerenal azotemia has the potential to lead to intrinsic renal damage and progression of ARF.

Renal adaptations to dehydration and renal hypoperfusion are characterized by enhanced tubular sodium and water reabsorption in both the proximal and distal renal tubules. Active reabsorption of sodium followed by passive transport of water in the proximal tubule is promoted by the increased concentration of protein in the peritubular capillaries, while distal tubular sodium absorption is mediated by the renin–angiotensin–aldosterone hormone system (Fig. 35.1) (Ott *et al.*, 1975). Increased water reabsorption in the distal renal tubule is promoted by antidiuretic hormone (ADH) secretion from the posterior pituitary in response to increased plasma osmolality. The net clinical impact of these physiologic alterations is a reduction in urinary volume and an increased renal sodium and water reabsorption in an attempt to preserve intravascular volume.

The clinical hallmarks of prerenal azotemia are oliguria, minimal urinary sodium excretion (<10–15 mEq/l), and an increase in the plasma concentration of blood urea nitrogen (BUN) and creatinine. One of the diagnostic features of prerenal azotemia is a significantly higher rise of BUN than serum creatinine, the resultant BUN:serum creatinine ratio being greater than 20:1 (Thadhani *et al.*, 1996). These alterations result from the enhanced passive tubular reabsorption of urea that follows tubular sodium and water uptake in prerenal azotemia. This contrasts with almost no tubular reabsorption of creatinine from the glomerular ultrafiltrate as it traverses the nephron. Increased BUN:creatinine ratio is a hallmark of prerenal azotemia. However, this characteristic feature may not exist if other compounding conditions are present in addition to azotemia (Table 35.1).

Intrinsic renal failure

Intrinsic renal diseases are the most frequent causes of ARF in children (Bourquina and Zahid, 1993; Arora *et al.*, 1994; Wong *et al.*, 1996). Although the spectrum of intrinsic renal diseases that causes ARF in developing and the developed Western countries is similar, the incidence of each disorder in any given geographic region varies greatly. The referral pattern and the nature of services provided in any given institution additionally influence the reported incidence of various causes. For example, complex cardiovascular surgery and multiorgan failure may predominate as the causes of ARF in a tertiary care unit or an urban teaching hospital, while the hemolytic–uremic syndrome (HUS) may be the dominant cause of ARF in a community-based institution.

In general, four broad categories of intrinsic renal disorders lead to ARF: acute tubular necrosis, glomerulonephritis, tubulointerstitial nephritis, and microangiopathies. The pathogenesis of ARF in each of these disorders varies. For example, in glomerular diseases and microangiopathies, GFR is diminished as a result of structural damage to the glomeruli. In contrast, failure of glomerular filtration develops secondarily in tubulointerstitial disorders, while both glomerular and tubular dysfunctions contribute to the pathogenesis of ARF in ischemic and nephrotoxic renal injury.

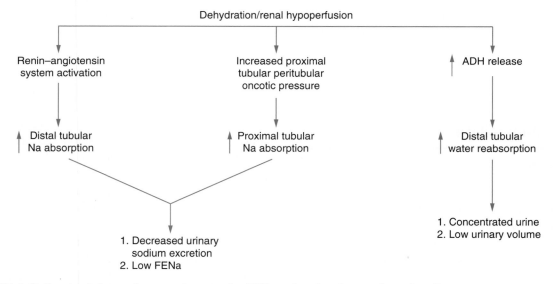

Figure 35.1 Pathophysiology of prerenal azotemia. FENa = fractional excretion of sodium.

Table 35.1 Conditions that alter the blood urea nitrogen: serum creatinine ratio in acute renal failure

High ratio (> 20:1)	Low ratio (< 20:1)
Prerenal azotemia	Malnutrition
Catabolic drug use, e.g. corticosteroids	Hepatic failure
Catabolic states, e.g. sepsis and burns	Volume expansion
Use of hyperalimentation with high amino acid load, high protein intake	Interference in creatinine estimation by ketone bodies and cefotaxime
Gastrointestinal hemorrhage	Following dialysis
Intraperitoneal leak of urine	

Postrenal

ARF due to urinary tract obstruction is encontered less commonly in children than in adults (Bourquina and Zahid, 1993; Arora *et al.*, 1994; Wong *et al.*, 1996). In order to cause ARF, the obstructive lesion in the urinary tract must be located at or below the level of the urinary bladder, except when the patient has a solitary kidney. Apart from the fact that urinary flow is suddenly interrupted, acute urinary tract obstruction also reduces GFR by diminishing renal blood flow, most likely resulting from increased vascular resistance in the preglomerular or afferent arterioles (Havistendahl *et al.*, 1996).

Etiology

In general, dehydration or other forms of prerenal azotemia are responsible for about 20% of cases of ARF in children, while postrenal causes or urinary obstruction account for another 3–20% of cases (Yoshiya *et al.*, 1973; Bourquina and Zahid, 1993; Arora *et al.*, 1994; Kondoth, 1994; Wong *et al.*, 1996; Moghal *et al.*, 1998). Intrinsic renal failure comprises the bulk of patients seen with ARF in tertiary-care pediatric units. Of the intrinsic renal disorders, HUS is the single most common etiology of ARF (Yoshiya *et al.*, 1973; Bourquina and Zahid, 1993; Arora *et al.*, 1994; Wong *et al.*, 1996; Havistendahl *et al.*, 1996; Moghal *et al.*, 1998). Table 35.2 lists the causes of ARF in children, while Table 35.3 compares the distribution of causes of ARF in various geographic regions.

Clinical manifestations

When ARF superimposes on an underlying systemic illness, its presentation overlaps the clinical course of the primary disorder. While the onset of ARF can be slow and subtle in some patients, a dramatic and severe clinical course predominates in other patients. Intrinsic renal diseases, such as glomerulonephritis and tubulointerstitial disorders, are commonly associated with a sudden and symptomatic onset of ARF. An imperceptibly gradual rise in serum creatinine without evidence of oliguria, in contrast, is the usual feature of patients with nephrotoxic ARF induced by drugs, such as aminoglycosides and radiocontrast agents.

During the onset of ARF, serum creatinine usually rises at a rate of 0.5–1.0 mg/day, until a steady state is reached. An accelerated rate of increase of serum creatinine may, however, be encountered in patients with crush injury and other forms of acute renal failure associated with muscle injury or disease (Grossman *et al.*, 1974). In well-established ARF, the rise in BUN parallels the rise of serum creatinine and the normal ratio of BUN:creatinine (10–15:1) is generally maintained.

The manifestations of ARF can take the form of two distinct clinical syndromes: oliguric ARF and non-oliguric ARF.

Oliguric acute renal failure

The characteristic feature of the oliguric ARF is a sudden onset of oliguria, or urine output less than 0.5 ml/kg per hour. Anuria may be present in severe cases. Oliguric ARF is common in glomerular diseases, such as glomerulonephritis, and in severe hypotensive or nephrotoxic injury. Occasionally, acute pyelonephritis and other tubulointerstitial diseases may also manifest oliguric ARF.

Once oliguria is established, the clinical concerns in these patients relate to fluid overload, derangements in electrolyte balance, and metabolic acidosis. Apart from clinical edema, fluid overload may also lead to dilutional hyponatremia and hyponatremic seizures in these patients. Congestive cardiac failure and hyper-

Table 35.2 Etiology of acute renal failure

Prerenal azotemia	Intravascular volume depletion
	Poor cardiac pump function
	Severely raised intra-abdominal pressure
	Burns
Intrinsic renal failure	Hypotension/shock
	Postcardiac surgery
	Sepsis
	Multiorgan failure
	Severe ascites and liver failure
	Nephrotoxic
	Aminoglycosides
	Amphotericin
	Gancyclovir
	Acyclovir
	Non-steroidal anti-inflamatory drugs
	Radiocontrast agents
	Organic solvents
	Carbon tetrachloride
	Methanol
	Toluene
	Ethylene glycol
	Cisplatin
	Bee stings
	Snake bites
	Toxic mushrooms
	Herbal toxin
	Intratubular obstruction
	Pigment nepropathies
	Hemoglobinuria
	Myoglobinuria
	Tumor lysis syndrome
	Crystaluria
	Uric acid
	Sulfonamides
	Acyclovir
	Methotrexate
	Indinavir
	Triamtrene
	Glomerulonephritis
	Postinfections glomerulonephritis
	Membranoproliferative glomerulonephritis
	Rapidly progressive glomerulonephritis
	Interstitial nephritis
	Idiopathic
	Drug induced
	Acute pyelonephritis

Table 35.2 *Continued.*

	Microangiopathic syndromes
	Hemolytic uremic sydrome
	Enterohemorrhagic *E. coli*
	Bone marrow transplant
	Drug induced
	Pregnancy and toxemia
	Malignant hypertension
Postrenal	Bilateral ureteral obstruction
	Stones
	Tumor (retroperitoneal)
	Bladder outlet obstruction
	Obstructed urinary catheter
	Urinary stone
	Bladder clots
	Fungus ball
	Tumor
	Acute-on-chronic obstruction

tension due to intravascular volume expansion can be the consequences of fluid overload resulting from oliguria. Appropriate limitation of fluid intake to prevent secondary complications is, therefore, one of the goals of effective management of an oliguric patient.

Since urinary excretion is the primary source of potassium disposal, the development of oliguria results in an inability to handle effectively the daily intake of potassium, with the resultant risk of hyperkalemia. This risk is further amplified in patients in whom tissue damage, rhabdomyolysis, hemorrhage within body cavities, tumor lysis syndrome, or other forms of catabolic states are additionally present. Since metabolic acidosis promotes exit of potassium from the intracellular sites into the extracellular compartment, it aggravates any existing hyperkalemia and enhances the potential for cardiotoxicity. The risk of cardiotoxicity from hyperkalemia rises as the serum potassium level increases beyond 6.0 mEq/l, eventually leading to arrythmia and cardiac standstill.

Metabolic acidosis in ARF is of the high anion gap variety, and results from retention of the organic acids produced as a result of metabolic activity. Metabolic acidosis impacts many essential cellular functions and makes the clinical management of these patients more challenging.

Recovery in most patients with hypotensive or nephrotoxic injury-associated oliguric ARF usually begins about 2 weeks after onset. Such a recovery is heralded by an increasing urine output, followed by normalization of serum creatinine and the GFR.

Table 35.3 Distribution of the causes of acute renal failure in various parts of the world

	North Africa (Bourquina and Zahid, 1993)	India (Arora *et al.*, 1994)	England (Moghal *et al.*, 1998)
Number of patients	89	52	227
Prerenal (%)	0	0	0
Intrinsic renal disease (%)			
Hemolytic uremic syndrome	13.4	30.8	45
Acute tubular necrosis	12.3	28.8	40
Acute glomerulonephritis	51.6	19.3	7.5
Acute interstitial nephritis	10.1	0	0
Unknown	6.7	0	4
Postrenal (urinary obstruction) (%)	5.6	21.4	3.5

Tubular dysfunction characterized by an inadequate urinary concentrating capacity may, however, persist for a variable period.

Non-oliguric acute renal failure

An elevated serum creatinine and retention of nitrogenous waste products, such as BUN, in face of a normal urinary volume or even polyuria characterize non-oliguric ARF. This form of ARF is commonly seen in patients with mild ischemic or toxic renal injury (Anderson *et al.*, 1977). Non-oliguric ARF can occur in all age groups, including neonates. Non-oliguric ARF is often short-lived and mild in severity, and can be easily overlooked. A high degree of suspicion on the part of treating physicians and the monitoring of renal function while treating patients with potentially nephrotoxic drugs are necessary in order to detect milder variants of non-oliguric ARF.

Despite adequate urine output and a relatively well-preserved fluid balance, patients with non-oliguric ARF may develop severe hyperkalemia. The ease with which fluid balance is maintained in these patients makes the overall management of patients with non-oliguric renal failure easier than those with the oliguric variety. Glomerular ultrastructural changes in experimental models of oliguric and non-oliguric ARF are, however, strikingly similar (Kato *et al.*, 1993).

Specific clinical disorders

Acute tubular necrosis

Acute tubular necrosis (ATN) is a specific term that denotes ARF resulting from renal ischemia or nephrotoxic injury. All other forms of glomerular and tubulointerstitial disorders as causes of ARF are excluded from this definition.

The work of Oliver in the 1950s documented that the predominat morphologic change from both ischemic and nephrotoxic renal injury was that of tubular cell necrosis in the region of medullary thick ascending limb (mTAL) of the loop of Henle (Oliver *et al.*, 1951). He coined the term lower nephron nephrosis to describe these pathologic changes observed in renal ischemia and nephrotoxic injury. While experimental models of ATN generally demonstrate substantial tubular cell damage in the region of proximal tubule and the mTAL, morphologic findings in renal biopsies from patients with clinical ATN are generally minor and patchy in distribution (Solez *et al.*, 1979; Olsen and Hansen, 1990). This discrepancy probably reflects the fact that experimental models of ATN are generated by severe ischemic or nephrotoxic injury with pervasive damage while clinical biopsy samples may not always include deep medullary tissue. Apart from tubular cell damage, the presence of casts within the tubular lumen is also a common finding in ATN. Glomeruli are generally normal when examined by light microscopy, but electron microscopy demonstrates fusion of the foot processes and a narrowing of the diameter of the endothelial fenestrae (Kato *et al.*, 1993).

Pathogenesis

It is best to regard the pathogenesis of ATN as three blended but identifiable phases: initiation, maintenance, and recovery. The initiation phase begins with the onset of renal ischemia or nephrotoxic damage, while the maintenance phase of ATN is to be regarded as the secondary event that results from the ischemic or nephrotoxic insult. Even after renal blood flow is re-established or the nephrotoxic insult ceases, several pathways of tubular cell dysfunction and damage set in motion by the initiating event lead to a decreased GFR during the maintenance phase of ATN. During the recovery phase, tissue repair and re-establishment of GFR allow functional recovery.

Extensive experimental studies of ATN have generated a wealth of information regarding the mechanisms involved in tissue injury and manifestations of ATN. The four key factors that play a role in the pathogenesis are: decreased glomerular blood flow, changes in the glomerular permeability, intratubular obstruction, and tubular backleak (Fig. 35.2). The role played by each of these factors in the pathogenesis of ATN is discussed below.

Renal and glomerular blood flow

While the kidney receives approximately 20–25% of cardiac output, it is uniquely susceptible to tissue injury from hypoperfusion. This susceptibility of the kidney to ischemic injury stems from the fact that the vascular supply and oxygen delivery to the renal tissues are not uniform. While cortical blood flow and oxygen delivery are profuse, the medulla is provided with a low-flow vascular supply with significantly lower oxygen tension in the arterial blood. The metabolic workload and the demand for oxygen delivery in this region, however, are extraordinarily high (Brezis and Rosen, 1995). Consequently, medullary tissue

has a uniquely low tolerance for hypoperfusion and decreased oxygen delivery, rendering it susceptible to ischemic injury and resultant ATN.

Apart from medullary renal tubular cell damage, hypotension and ischemia also induce an immediate and sustained reduction of total renal blood flow as well as glomerular blood flow. The net impact of these vascular flow events is a reduction in GFR. These abnormalities in renal and glomerular blood flow persist even after the renal circulation is restored and blood pressure has returned to normal (Daugharty et al., 1974). Renal arteriolar vasoconstriction, predominantly in the preglomerular or afferent arterioles, is believed to be the cause of decreased total renal blood flow and glomerular blood flow, and a decrease in GFR during ATN (Anderndshorst et al., 1975; Patak et al., 1979).

Enhanced renal synthesis of the potent vasoconstrictor 'endothelin' and a diminished tissue production of the vasodilator 'endothelin-derived nitrous oxide' (EDNO) are considered to play a central role in the renal vasoconstriction and pathogenesis of ATN (Ruschitzka et al., 1999; Goligorsky and Nori, 1999). Other hormones that may also play a significant role in the development of renal vasoconstriction and the pathogenesis of ATN include the renin–angiotensin and prostaglandin–thromboxane systems (Gavras et al., 1971; Swain et al., 1975; Cirino et al., 1990). Exogenous administration of angiotensin II and thromboxane in experimental models causes renal vasoconstriction and ATN, whereas prostaglandins are important renal vasodilatory agents and are believed to protect against ATN. Inhibition of prostagland-

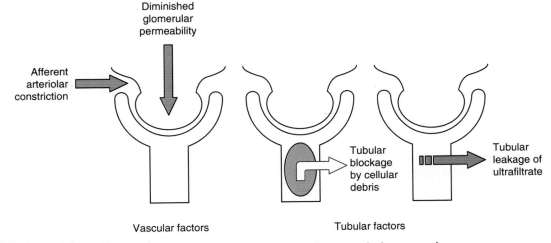

Figure 35.2 Factors that may be involved in the pathogenesis of acute tubular necrosis.

in synthesis by the therapeutic use of non-steroidal anti-inflammatory drugs (NSAIDS) is a well-known cause of ATN (Schaller and Kaplan, 1998).

The significance of renal vasoconstriction and the above-mentioned hormones in the pathogenesis of nephrotoxic ATN is less well defined than in ischemic ATN. Increasing evidence, however, indicates that renal vasoconstriction also plays a significant role in the pathogenesis of nephrotoxic ATN (Yangisawa *et al.*, 1998).

Glomerular permeability

Among other factors, GFR is modulated by the coefficient of filtration (K_f), which is a product of the hydraulic permeability of glomerular capillaries and the filtration surface area. It has been proposed that alterations in K_f may account for a decrease in GFR in ATN (Parekh and Veith, 1981). While some studies have determined an important downward trend in K_f during the course of ATN, most consider the role of diminished K_f as ancillary in determining GFR in this condition (Daugherty *et al.*, 1974; Williams *et al.*, 1981).

Tubular obstruction

The presence of proteinaceous casts and cellular debris in the tubular lumina has been long noted in the experimental models and clinical biopsy samples of ATN (Solez *et al.*, 1979). The matrix of these tubular casts is formed by the Tamm–Horsfall protein, an anionic protein produced by the medullary thick ascending limb (mTAL) of the loop of Henle, in which tubular cell debris may also be trapped. Increased intratubular pressure, presumably due to the nephron obstruction by the casts, has been documented in experimental models of ATN (Tanner and Steinhouse, 1976). Secondary glomerular filtration failure as a result of elevated intratubular pressure is believed by many investigators to contribute towards decreased GFR in ATN.

Tubular backleak

Leaking of the glomerular ultrafiltrate through microscopic breaks in the tubular epithelium and the basement membrane is considered to be another significant reason for low GFR in ATN (Yagil *et al.*, 1988). As a consequence of tubular backleak, the glomerular ultrafiltrate reaches the interstitium, from which it is returned to the systemic circulation, leading to a reduction in GFR. Disruption in the integrity of tight junctions and cell–cell adhesion in the proximal tubules allows a pathway for the passage of glomerular ultrafiltrate to leak from the tubules into the renal interstitium (Kwon *et al.*, 1998).

Preventing acute tubular necrosis

A better understanding of the cellular events involved in ATN has provided an opportunity for minimizing the risks of a prolonged clinical course and reducing the morbidity and mortality associated with this disorder. Some of the clinically applicable therapies currently in use for preventing or minimizing the risk of ATN are discussed below.

Diuretics

Diuretics have long been used in preventing and treating ATN, especially in the context of cardiovascular surgery and renal transplantation. Mannitol, furosemide, and bumetanide are the diuretic agents that have been most used for this purpose. The protective influence of the loop diuretics is mediated by blocking the uptake of sodium and chloride in the thick ascending limb of the loop of Henle. This reduces the metabolic workload for this segment of the renal tubule that is highly susceptible to hypoxic injury. These diuretics may also exert their preventive role hydrodynamically by maintaining a high urine flow rate and flushing the intratubular casts.

The evidence indicating a useful role for loop diuretics in the prevention of ATN is controversial. In some experimental models of ARF, furosemide pretreatment has been found to protect against ATN as well as ameliorte the decline in GFR (Kramer *et al.*, 1980). In other ischemic and nephrotoxic models of ATN, however, the results have been equivocal (Ufferman *et al.*, 1975). In human studies the protective role of loop diuretics in ATN has not been convincingly demonstrated (Shilliday and Allison, 1994; Conger, 1995). Owing to its own toxic effects, including interstitial nephritis and ototoxicity, furosemide should be used judiciously in ATN. Loop diuretics are contraindicated in ATN caused by contrast agents, where they aggravate the toxicity of these nephrotoxic agents (Soloman *et al.*, 1994).

Mannitol, like loop diuretics, has also been used as a renoprotective agent in clinical circumstances and experimental models of ATN. The rationale behind the use of mannitol in ATN is that it prevents tubular cell swelling and maintains an increased tubular flow, thereby preventing intratubular cast formation and intratubular obstruction (Flores *et al.*, 1972). The use of mannitol is recommended for the prevention and treatment of pigment nephropathy (hemoglobinuria and myoglobinuria). Mannitol should be used with caution in conditions where ATN is associated with fluid overload, since its administration may precipitate congestive cardiac failure.

When used early in the course of ATN, both mannitol and loop diuretics can convert oliguric ATN to the non-oliguric type, which is somewhat easier to manage. As a general guide, if an initial trial of loop diuretics or mannitol is not successful in establishing urinary flow in oliguric patients, their use should be curtailed. Loop diuretics are of little use in the treatment of established oliguric or non-oliguric ATN, or in promoting recovery from ATN.

Dopamine

Dopamine, when used in low dose (1 μg/kg per hour) acts as a renal vasodilator and also enhances GFR (McDonald *et al.*, 1964). Despite its salutary impact on renal blood flow and GFR, clinical studies have not confirmed its utility in improving the course or mortality associated with ATN. In a recent randomized, controlled trial, dopamine was not found to improve the outcome or delay the start of dialysis in patients with ATN (Chertow *et al.*, 1996; Anonymous 2000). The consensus among nephrologists at this time is that the use of dopamine in attenuating ATN should be discouraged until further evidence of its impact on the outcome of ATN is determined (Star, 1998).

Calcium channel blockers

Calcium ions are involved in maintaining vascular tone and help in vasoconstriction. Accordingly, calcium channel blockers have been used in clinical practice as vasodilators and antihypertensive agents. Pretreatment with calcium channel blockers has been shown to be protective in experimental models of ATN, where they attenuate the decline in GFR and minimize tubular cell damage (Alvarez *et al.*, 1994). This class of therapeutic agents is particularly useful in the prevention of ATN in renal transplants (Venkat-Raman *et al.*, 1998). Because calcium channel blockers can also induce hypotension and thus compromise renal perfusion, their use in the prevention of ATN in most clinical situations must be carefully monitored.

Natriuretic peptides

Atrial natriuretic peptides (ANP) given after the ischemic event are able to improve the course of ATN, but have not yet been determined to play a role in prevention (Rahman *et al.*, 1994; Allgren *et al.*, 1997). ANP, like diuretics, also may be able to convert oliguric ATN into the non-oliguric type. In contrast to diuretics, the use of ANP also decreases the need for dialysis and improves outcome in ATN. ANP produces these clinically discernible effects by inducing vasodilation in the afferent arteriole while causing efferent arteriolar constriction. The effect is an elevation of intraglomerular filtration pressure and an enhancement of GFR. The future role of ANP in the treatment of ATN appears to be promising but needs to be evaluated critically.

Insulin-like growth factors

Early studies in rats suggested that growth-promoting factors, such as insulin-like growth factor-1 (IGF-1), promote recovery of renal function and decrease the catabolism that is associated with ATN (Miller *et al.*, 1992). Despite early enthusiasm, more recent human trials have not been able show any beneficial effect of IGF-1 in promoting recovery in ATN (Hirschberg *et al.*, 1999). Further studies in this field are necessary to settle the issue.

Toxic nephropathies

The number of drugs and therapeutic agents that can cause ARF is large and ever growing. While a detailed discussion of each of these nephrotoxic agents is beyond the scope of this chapter, three of the common therapeutic agents that may assume significance in the practice of pediatric urology are discussed below.

Contrast nephropathy

The use of contrast agents for diagnostic radiologic studies is a well-known cause of ARF. In most patients (70–90%), contrast-induced ARF is of the non-oliguric variety, but oligura can also occur in severe cases (Porter, 1990). An asymptomatic increase in serum creatinine within 48 hours of intravenous contrast use is a characteristic feature of contrast nephropathy. Demonstration of a persistent nephrogram on delayed images is also a well-described radiographic finding in these patients.

Upon exposure to the contrast agent in a susceptible patient, initial transient renal vasodilation is followed by prolonged vasoconstriction. This interval of vasoconstruction is considered to be the cause of the decline in GFR seen in contrast nephropathy. Proximal tubular damage, as well as tubular obstruction resulting from precipitation of the contrast agent and Tamm–Horsfall protein, also play a contributing role in contrast-induced ARF (Mareau *et al.*, 1975; Dawnay *et al.*, 1985).

Conditions in which the risk for contrast nephropathy is high include diabetes mellitus, intravascular volume depletion and pre-existing renal insufficiency. Clinical states characterized by impaired renal perfusion, such as the nephrotic syndrome, congestive cardiac failure, and cirrhosis are also risk factors (Parfrey *et al.*, 1989). The dose of the contrast agent used is also a relevant determinant of the severity of nephrotoxicity of contrast agents.

Although experimental data suggest that non-ionic contrast agents are less nephrotoxic than ionic contrast agents, a large, randomized, controlled clinical trial in humans was not able to substantiate this claim (Schwab *et al.*, 1989). The strategy for minimizing the risk of contrast agent-associated nephrotoxicity includes adequate hydration, using a lower dose of the contrast agent, and a judicious use of diuretics. Mannitol should be avoided in radiocontrast nephropathy, since it is well known to enhance the nephrotoxicity of these agents (Soloman *et al.*, 1994).

Aminoglycoside nephrotoxicity

Because many patients develop non-oliguric ARF after exposure to aminoglycosides, nephrotoxicity associated with the use of these antibiotics can be easily overlooked. Apart from a rising serum creatinine level, polyuria can be an early indicator of aminoglycoside-induced nephrotoxicity. Although aminoglycoside-associated ARF usually occurs after exposure to these antibiotics for 7–10 days, cases of ARF following a single intravenous dose have also been described (Weir and Mazumdar, 1994).

Aminoglycosides exert their nephrotoxic effects by causing renal vasoconstriction, proximal tubular damage, and necrosis (Hishida *et al.*, 1994). The morphologic hallmark of gentamicin nephrotoxicity is the swelling of proximal tubular lysosomes with accumulation of phospholipids that produce characteristic 'onion-ring' or whorl-shaped images on electron microscopy. Lysosomal phospholipidosis begins early (day 1) after toxic exposure to aminoglycosides, followed by tubular necrosis (day 4), while the process of repair begins around day 7 (Nondereq *et al.*, 1992). It has been suggested that lysosomal dysfunction induced by aminoglycosides leads to proximal tubular cell death and causes ATN.

Risk factors for aminoglycoside nephrotoxicity include a high serum trough level of the antibiotic, intravascular volume depletion, potassium and magnesium depletion, concurrent use of other nephrotoxins, and an increased frequency of aminoglycoside dosing.

Treatment of aminoglycoside-induced ATN should include withdrawal of the drug, if possible. Alternately, the dose and frequency of aminoglycoside administration should be reduced, and intravascular volume expansion considered. Attention should also be paid to preserving a positive potassium and magnesium balance. Recovery from ATN usually occurs within 7–10 days after the last dose of aminoglycoside.

Nephropathy of non-steroidal anti-inflammatory drugs

NSAIDs are increasingly being used as antipyretics and analgesics in children. Despite several studies on the safety of these agents in children, many reports have pointed to the potential for ARF in children treated with NSAIDs (Lesko and Mitchell, 1997; Schaller and Kaplan, 1998). Renal failure resulting from NSAIDs is usually of the non-oliguric type but oliguria can occur, especially if intravascular volume depletion co-exists (Schaller and Kaplan, 1998).

The mechanism of renal failure caused by NSAIDs is the inhibition of vasodilator prostaglandin synthesis in the kidney with resultant intrarenal vasoconstriction. Unless oliguria or other metabolic disturbances are present, renal failure recovers spontaneously and dialysis therapy is generally not necessary.

Hemolytic–uremic syndrome

The HUS is the single most common cause of ARF in children worldwide. The clinical triad of microangiopathic hemolytic anemia, thrombocytopenia, and renal failure characterizes HUS. The typical diarrhea-associated (D$^+$) HUS is usually caused by enterohemorrhagic *Escherichia coli* (O157 H7) infection, while the atypical non-diarrhea-associated HUS (D$^-$) is caused by a wide variety of infective agents and drugs (Remuzzi and Ruggenenti, 1998). Immunosuppressive agents, such as cyclosporine and tacrolimus, infection with Streptococcus pneumoniae, human immunodeficiency virus-1 (HIV-1), and bone marrow transplantation are some of the common causes of D⁻ HUS (Neuhaus et al., 1997; Turner et al., 1997; Bren et al., 1998; Gilbert and Argent, 1998; Kondo et al., 1998). A familial form of D⁻ HUS that is associated with hypocomplementemia and a high mortality rate has also been recognized (Petermann et al., 1998).

The abrupt onset of oliguria, a pale appearance, and the development of petechiae and other bleeding manifestations due to thrombocytopenia mark the onset of HUS. Encephalopathy, cardiomyopthy, colitis, and diabetes mellitus have also been reported in some patients with HUS. Although a renal biopsy is not indicated for establishing the diagnosis of HUS in most cases, it may be considered in patients with atypical clinical characteristics, or in whom diagnostic uncertainty exists.

Treatment of HUS involves manangement of fluid and electrolyte balance, dialysis for treatment of uremia and fluid overload, and the use of supportive therapies, such as blood transfusion. When dialysis treatment is indicated, peritoneal dialysis is generally preferred over hemodialysis, since peritoneal dialysis does not mandate the use of heparin.

The overall prognosis of HUS depends on the severity of the clinical disease and its complications in a given patient. Immediate mortality after onset of HUS is 3–10% , and is usually due to extrarenal complications (Spizzirri et al., 1997; Remuzzi and Ruggenenti, 1998). The incidence of end-stage renal disease (ESRD) following HUS is 3–5%, while chronic renal insufficiency and hypertension occur in about 15% cases (Spizzirri et al., 1997).

Diagnostic evaluation

The goals of diagnostic evaluation in the patient with ARF are: (1) to exclude prerenal azotemia; (2) to exclude acute obstruction as a cause of ARF; and (3) if intrinsic renal disease is suspected, to develop an investigative and treatment plan for it. A carefully taken history and physical examination can provide

Table 35.4 Historic data helpful in distinguishing clinical subgroups of acute renal failure

Prerenal azotemia	Intrinsic renal failure	Urinary obstruction

Intravascular volume depletion
  Diarrhea
  Vomiting
  Removal of fluid via chest-tube or
    other body cavity drains
  Diuretic abuse
	Acute tubular necrosis
	  Significant hypotension
	  Cardiovascular surgery
	  Being on extracorporeal
	    membrane oxygenator (ECMO)
	  Use of nephrotoxic therapies,
	    including over-the-counter drugs
		Sudden onset of anuria
		Abdominal pain
		History of hemorrhage in urinary
		  tract
		History of abdominal mass, tumor
		History of urinary tract surgery

History of poor renal perfusion
  Congestive cardiac failure
  Nephrotic syndrome
  Cirrhosis
	Glomerulonephritis
	  Gross hematuria
	  Edema
	  Skin rash (Henoch–Schönlein
	    purpura, vasculitis syndromes)
	  History of disorders associated
	    with renal disease, systemic
	    erythematosus, scleroderma	

Inadequate fluid intake
  Intentional
  Therapeutic
	Tubulointerstitial diseases
	  Use of drugs: NSAIDS
	  Acute pyelonephritis: dysuria,
	    fever, abdominal or flank pain	

	Glomerular microangiopathy
	  Pale appearance (due to anemia)
	  Petechiae (thrombocytopenia)
	  Edema (oliguria and fluid overload)	

numerous clues to the underlying cause of ARF. Historical data that aid in the diagnosis of ARF are summarized in Table 35.4.

Laboratory studies needed to establish the etiology of ARF in a given patient should be based on the clinical suspicions of its possible etiology. Therefore, not all of the available tests may be necessary in every patient. Figure 35.3 provides pathways for the evaluation of non-surgical (non-obstructive) ATN and oliguria in children. The array of diagnostic tests helpful in distinguishng well-established intrinsic ARF from prerenal azotemia and acute urinary obstruction are listed in Table 35.5. These tests are discussed below in detail.

Urinalysis

Information provided by urinalysis is immensely helpful in the diagnosis of intrinsic renal diseases. A highly concentrated urine favors the diagnosis of prerenal azotemia, while established ARF is usually associated with a low specific gravity. Proteinuria, hematuria, and red cell casts suggest glomerulonephritis, but mild proteinuria and even transient hematuria may also be seen in prerenal azotemia. An abundance of renal tubular cells and tubular cell casts in the urinary sediment aids in the diagnosis of ATN. The presence of white blood cells and casts made of the same cell line may indicate acute pyelonephritis.

Urinary indices

Several tests designed to distinguish oliguria due to prerenal azotemia and ATN are available to clinicians. In general, these tests determine the integrity of tubular function and thus aid in distinguishing prerenal azotemia (where tubular functions are intact) from patients with established ATN (where tubular dysfunction has set in). In order to provide accurate and interpretable results, it is essential that the urine sample obtained for studying urinary indices be collected prior to giving the patient a diuretic or fluid bolus.

Urine and serum osmolality

In patients with oliguria due to prerenal azotemia, urine is expected to be maximally concentrated. In general, a urine osmolality of greater than 500 mOsm/l is suggestive but not diagnostic of prerenal azotemia. A ratio of urine to serum osmolality greater than

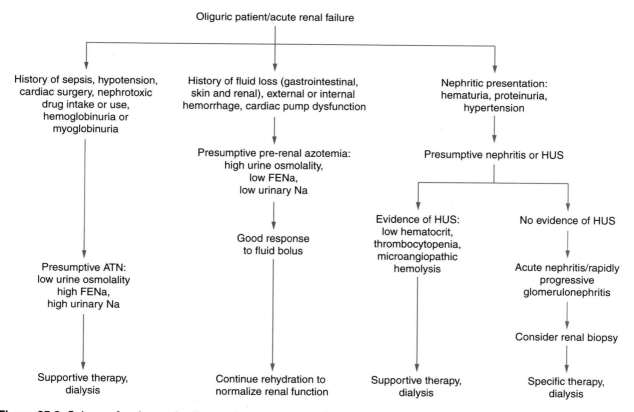

Figure 35.3 Schema for the evaluation and management of non-surgical acute renal failure/oliguria.

Table 35.5 Laboratory findings helpful in differentiating the clinical subgroups of acute renal failure

Laboratory finding	Prerenal azotemia	Established intrinsic renal failure (ATN)	Obstructive ARF
Urine specific gravity	Elevated	Low	Usually low
Urine osmolality	Elevated	Low	Usually low
Urine sodium	< 20 mEq/l	> 20 mEq/l	Usually > 20 mEq/l
FENa	≤ 1.0%	> 3.0%	Usually 1–3% but can be more
BUN: serum creatinine ratio	> 20:1	15–20:1	15–20:1
Renal sonogram	Non-diagnostic	Non-diagnostic	Diagnostic for obstructive lesions
Urinalysis	Mild proteinuria, may have minimal hematuria and granular casts	Diagnostic findings are presence of renal tubular epithelial cells	Non-diagnostic findings

ATN = acute tubular necrosis; ARF = acute renal failure; FENa = fractional excretion of sodium; BUN = blood urea nitrogen.

1.5 is also supportive of the diagnosis of prerenal azotemia. As ATN develops and tubular dysfunction sets in, urinary osmolality resembles that of the glomerular filtrate and the ratio of the urine to serum osmolality decreases below 1.5.

Fractional excretion of sodium

This test determines the fraction of filtered sodium that is excreted in urine and is based on the ability of the tubules to reabsorb sodium. Simultaneously collected samples of urine and serum are obtained. The index is calculated using the following formula:

$$\text{FENa} = \frac{\text{Urine sodium} \times \text{Plasma creatinine}}{\text{Plasma sodium} \times \text{Urine creatinine}} \times 100.$$

Fractional excretion of sodium (FENa) in patients beyond the neonatal period with prerenal azotemia is 1% or less, while in established ATN it can be 3% or more. FENa is not helpful in patients with glomerulonephritis, since values similar to those seen in prerenal azotemia are frequently encountered. Similarly, in patients with obstructive uropathy, FENa can range from an indeterminate range (1.5%) to frankly elevated values (3% or more).

Imaging studies

Renal sonography

Ultrasonographic evaluation of the kidneys, bladder, and vascular tree is important in the search for an etiology of ARF and oliguria. Apart from identifying obstructive lesions of the urinary tract, renal sonography provides essential information regarding the size and echogenicity of the kidney. A variable degree of increase in renal contour and echogenicity due to edema and the inflammatory response can be seen in ATN, acute glomerulonephritis, and acute interstitial diseases. Sonography can also be helpful in detecting thrombi in the main renal vessels. When combined with Doppler imaging of the vascular structures in the renal hilum, aorta, and inferior vena cava it can provide valuable dynamic information regarding the integrity of these vascular structures.

Radionuclide imaging

Imaging of the urinary tract using radioisotopes provides helpful information related to the blood flow, renal excretory function, and integrity of the urinary tract. This imaging technology has replaced intravenous pyelography in the diagnosis of renal diseases. However, once renal function declines significantly, the usefulness of this diagnostic modality becomes less certain. Therefore, radionuclide imaging is useful only in patients with early ARF, especially when obstructive uropathy is considered as the diagnosis. Radionuclide imaging is of little diagnostic value in patients with glomerulonephritis, tubulointerstitial disorders, and ATN.

Renal biopsy

A renal biopsy is not necessary in establishing the diagnosis of ATN in most patients. However, if acute glomerulonephritis or interstitial nephritis is suspected, renal biopsy remains the only definitive test for confirming the diagnosis.

Management of acute renal failure

Non-invasive treatment of ARF consists of providing appropriate management of fluid, electrolyte, and acid–base balance. Dialysis and other forms of renal replacement therapy may be necessary when metabolic decompensation, electrolyte disturbances, or fluid overload create the additional need for such therapeutic support.

Fluid balance

Management of fluid balance requires careful and detailed attention to total fluid intake and output. Euvolemia is maintained in such patients by providing replacement for insensible fluid losses, urine output, and any other measurable losses. While in older patients insensible fluid losses range from 400 to 600 ml/m² per day, in the neonate the insensible losses may be as high as 40 ml/kg per day. Beyond the neonatal period, insensible fluid requirements are 25–30 ml/kg per day.

In non-oliguric acute renal failure, adequate fluid replacement is necessary for the high urine output. Dehydration must be avoided in such patients, as it may lead to further renal hypoperfusion and delay the recovery from ARF. Similarly, as glomerular filtration begins to recover in oliguric ARF, urinary output can increase significantly (diuretic phase), which may also necessitate provision of additional fluid therapy to avoid dehydration. Careful monitoring of urine output becomes mandatory in these patients.

Electrolyte disorders

Prevention of hyperkalemia in patients with ARF is also an important aspect of clinical management. Although serious cardiotoxicity from hyperkalemia usually occurs when serum potassium concentration is greater than 6–7 mEq/l, acidosis and other electrolyte disorders, such as hypocalcemia, can potentiate the risk for sudden cardiac arrythmias (Fig. 35.4). The threat of hyperkalemia is significantly higher in patients with sepsis, burns, rhabdomyolysis, tumor lysis syndrome, and other catabolic or tissue-destructive syndromes. While definitive therapy aims at removal of potassium by dialysis, palliation

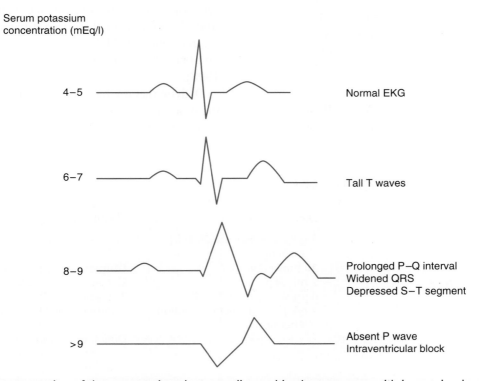

Figure 35.4 Representation of the progressive electrocardiographic changes seen with increasing hyperkalemia.

of hyperkalemia can be achieved by several therapies (Table 35.6). Emergency treatment of patients with hyperkalemic cardiotoxicity consists of administering intravenous calcium and correction of acidosis.

Hyponatremia in ARF is often of dilutional origin and results from fluid overload. Management of hyponatremia under these circumstances requires fluid restriction. Patients developing seizures due to hyponatremia require a rapid correction of the disorder to achieve a serum sodium concentration of 127 mEq/l. This can be accomplished by using a 3% saline solution (513 mEq sodium/l). The total dose of sodium to correct hyponatremia in such emergency situations can be derived from the following formula:

Sodium chloride dose (mEq) = (127 − Present serum concentration) × body weight (kg) × 0.6.

Acidosis

Apart from enhancing the mobilization of potassium from the intracellular stores and increasing the risk for hyperkalemia, metabolic acidosis also contributes to cardiovascular instability, especially the maintenance of blood pressure. In a critically sick patient, treatment of metabolic acidosis requires intravenous sodium bicarbonate supplementation. The dose of intravenous sodium bicarbonate required to correct acidosis can be calculated from the following formula:

Bicarbonate dose (mEq) = (Desired bicarbonate concentration − Present serum bicarbonate concentration) × body weight (kg) × 0.6.

Renal replacement therapies

Dialysis or other forms of renal replacement therapies may be required in patients in whom fluid overload, or other complications of uremia, cannot be addressed by non-invasive means. Three possible forms of renal replacement therapies are available for the treatment of ARF: peritoneal dialysis, hemodialysis, and continuous venovenous hemofiltration (CVVH) or arteriovenous hemofiltration (CAVH). Both CVVH and CAVH are primarily helpful in ameliorating fluid overload, while hemodialysis or peritoneal dialysis can provide an efficient therapy for hyperkalemia, uremia, and fluid overload.

Prognosis

The prognosis for ARF depends on the underlying etiology. Sepsis and multiorgan failure in association with ARF carry a significantly higher mortality than isolated ARF. Fargason and Langman (1993) evaluated the pediatric risk of mortality (PRISM) score in 31 children admitted to the intensive care unit with ARF. The PRISM score of patients who died was significantly higher on the day of dialysis than that of survivors. However, the ability to discriminate survivors from non-survivors was hampered in this study by overlap in these two categories. In adults, the mortality of ARF increases with the increasing number of non-respiratory organ failures (Star, 1998).

Dialytic therapy has had only a modest impact on the mortality of ARF in adult studies. The reduction in the mortality from approximately 91% during

Table 35.6 Emergency treatment of hyperkalemia

Therapy	Dose and route	Comment
Insulin and glucose	1 g/kg glucose + 0.25 U/kg insulin	Transient effect
Calcium	15 mg/kg i.v.	Drug of choice in cardiotoxicity
Sodium bicarbonate	2 mEq/kg	Use as an adjunct to calcium
Albuterol i.v.	4 µg/kg i.v. over 20 min	Transcient effect
Kayexalate	1 g/kg oral or rectal retention enema	Cumbersome and slow to work
Dialysis		Definitive therapy, need vascular access or peritoneal cavity access

World War II to 67% in the Vietnam War may be attributed to preemptive interventions, such as early and appropriate volume replacement, rather than the use of dialysis (Star, 1998).

Chronic renal failure

Definition

The term chronic renal failure (CRF) denotes an irreversible decrement of renal function resulting from loss of more than 50% of the nephron mass. If renal damage or surgical removal affects less than 50% of renal mass, compensatory hypertrophy in the surviving nephron population is able to preserve renal function within a normal range. Accordingly, unless additional complicating issues develop, CRF does not ensue in patients with a solitary kidney.

Incidence

The incidence of CRF in children in the USA has been reported to be 1.5–3 per million of the population (Fogo and Kon, 1994). European data suggest an incidence of around seven patients per million children (Esbjorner *et al.*, 1997). In the USA, pediatric patients with ESRD account for only 1.4% of the total ESRD population (Anonymous, 1999).

Etiology

The North American Pediatric Renal Transplant Cooperative Study (NAPRTCS) data indicate that the most common cause of CRF is obstructive uropathy, followed by renal aplasia, hypoplasia, and dysplasia (Fivush *et al.*, 1998). Overall, about two-thirds of the patients in the registry are reported to have some type of structural anomaly of the urinary tract as the cause of CRF. In contrast, the most common cause of CRF in adults is diabetes mellitus, followed by hypertension and glomerulonephritis. Table 35.7 lists the most common etiologies of CRF in children and adults.

Clinical manifestations

Growth failure

The growth failure associated with CRF is a multifactorial disorder that involves both endocrine and non-endocrine factors:

- younger age of onset of CRF
- primary renal disease
- severity of renal insufficiency
- metabolic acidosis
- salt wasting
- renal osteodystrophy
- protein and caloric malnutrition
- disruption of GH–IGF axis
- anemia
- hypertension
- infection
- prednisone treatment.

Growth failure and resultant short stature is one of the more commonly recognized clinical features of CRF, an association that was first described in the late nineteenth century (Guthrie and Oxon, 1897). Indeed, short stature can be the presenting feature leading to the initial evaluation of a child and discovery of CRF. The height deficits are greatest for younger patients and the risk for growth failure is highest in patients developing CRF at birth or in early infancy (Betts and Magrath, 1974; Abitbol *et al.*, 1990; Fivush *et al.*, 1998). The characteristic growth pattern of children developing renal insufficiency as infants is shown in Figure 35.5.

Table 35.7 Primary disease in pediatric[a] versus adult[b] chronic renal failure

Pediatric	Frequency (%)	Adult	Frequency (%)
Obstructive uropathy	26.1	Diabetes mellitus	41.8
Aplasia/hypoplasia/dysplasia	19.9	Hypertension	25.4
Reflux nephropathy	9.0	Glomerulonephritis	9.3
Focal segmental glomerulosclerosis	6.0	Cystic renal disease	2.2

[a]Adapted from NAPRTCS data (Fivush *et al.*, 1998).
[b]Adapted from USRDS 1999 Annual Report (Anonymous, 1999).

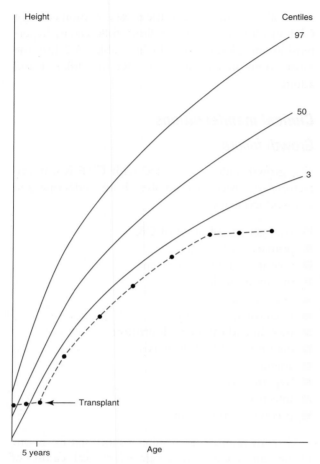

Figure 35.5 Growth impairement in a patient with chronic renal failure due to congenital obstructive uropathy. Flattening of the linear growth as a result of chronic renal failure is evident during the first five years of life. Renal transplantation resulted in only a transient restoration of the linear growth in this patient.

Pathophysiology

Poor nutrition in patients with CRF is a contributor to the development of growth failure. Deficient caloric intake in these patients is caused by dietary restrictions of sodium, potassium, protein, fluid, and possibly alteration in taste (Uauy *et al.*, 1994). Although evident in all age groups, the impact of nutrition on growth is particularly severe and observable in infants (Karlberg, 1990).

Levels of growth hormone (GH) are well documented to be normal in children with CRF, but a state of insensitivity to endogenous GH appears to be present in these patients (Schaefer *et al.*, 1991). GH exerts its action on bone growth by promoting the synthesis of insulin growth factor (IGF) in the liver. Disruption of the GH–IGF axis is considered to be of primary significance in the pathogenesis of growth failure in CRF (Tönshoff *et al.*, 1990). Numerous studies indicate that the levels of IGF-binding proteins 1, 2, 3, 4, and 6 are increased in patients with CRF (Tönshoff *et al.*, 1995; Powell *et al.*, 1997, 1999). It is proposed that this results in an increased binding of IGF, reducing free, biologically active IGF, with resultant failure of linear growth.

Renal osteodystrophy

The combined effects of secondary hyperparathyroidism and derangements in vitamin D metabolism lead to renal osteodystrophy (ROD) in patients with CRF. Apart from severe bone deformities, fractures of long bones, and slipped epiphyses, ROD can also contribute to growth failure in children with CRF. Clinical features include:

- skeletal deformities
- growth retardation
- bone pain
- slipped epiphyses
- pathologic fractures
- genu valgum
- extraskeletal calcifications
- myopathy.

Development of ROD occurs slowly (months) in most older children with CRF, but its onset in neonates and younger children may be rapid. As with growth retardation, ROD is more common in children who develop CRF early in life.

The early indicators of ROD are increased serum alkaline phosphatase and parathyroid hormone levels. Hypocalcemia is usually a late finding in patients with CRF and is not an accurate predictor of ROD. Although X-ray evaluation of long bones can detect the radiologic manifestations of rickets, osteomalacia, and hyperparathyroidism, bone biopsy remains the definitive diagnostic test for assessing the type and severity of ROD.

Radiographic features of ROD include evidence of hyperparathyroidism as well as changes of rickets or osteomalacia. Subperiosteal bone resorption is the radiographic hallmark of hyperparathyroidism and is best seen in the radial aspect of middle and proximal phalanges, clavicles, the femoral neck, and the medial aspect of the proximal tibia (Fig. 35.6) (Kirks,

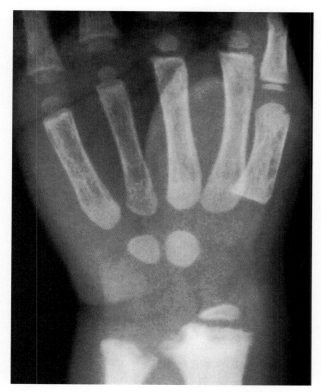

Figure 35.6 Characteristic radiographic changes of renal osteodystrophy seen in the wrist of a patient with chronic renal failure.

1984). Osteosclerosis can also be seen as a distinct feature of ROD in patients with longstanding chronic renal failure. Sclerosis affecting the upper and lower ends of the vertebrae with osteopenia of the intervening vertebral bodies results in a characteristic radiologic appearance known as 'rugger-jersey spine'.

Widening of the epiphyseal ends of the long bones, which results from lack of mineralization of osteoid, along with evidence of 'fraying' and 'cupping', are indicative of rickets. More chronic changes include curvature deformities of long bones manifested as bowing of the legs and ulnar deviation of the hands. Delayed bone age is also a common radiographic finding in patients with CRF. In one study bone age trailed chronologic age by a mean of 2.6 years (Cundall *et al.*, 1988).

Defects in dentition may also be found in children with CRF, particularly those who develop deranged mineral metabolism early in life. The structural dental defects include hypoplasia of the enamel and malformations of the teeth (Koch *et al.*, 1999).

Pathophysiology

Renal osteodystrophy is triggered by phosphate retention, hyperparathyroidism, impaired vitamin D metabolism, and skeletal resistance to the calcemic action of parathyroid hormone (Slatopolsky *et al.*, 1999b). While some independent actions occur, the influences of the aforementioned factors are interrelated and additive.

The kidney plays a pivotal role in vitamin D metabolism. Both provitamin D_3 in the skin (7-dehydrocholesterol) and dietary vitamin D (cholecalciferol) undergo two hydroxylation steps to become bioactive. The first hydroxylation step occurs in the liver, leading to the synthesis of 25-hydroxyvitamin D_3, followed by hydroxylation in the kidney to form the bioactive metabolite, 1,25-dihydroxyvitamin D_3 (calcitriol) (Brunette *et al.*, 1978). Calcitriol regulates mineral metabolism by enhancing gastrointestinal absorption of calcium and phosphorus. This, combined with the action of calcitriol on bone, where it causes resorption, aids in the maintenance of a normal serum calcium concentration.

When GFR falls below 50 ml/min per 1.73 m², serum 1,25-dihydroxyvitamin D_3 levels decrease, leading to hypocalcemia (Portale *et al.*, 1982; Ishimura *et al.*, 1999). Hypocalcemia and the absence of 1,25-dihydroxyvitamin D_3 cause poor mineralization of the osteoid and development of the characteristic features of rickets or osteomalacia. This is the first factor in the development of ROD.

The second factor that promotes the development of ROD is hyperparathyroidism. As GFR declines to about 25 ml/min per 1.73 m², renal excretion of phosphorus is adversely impacted and hyperphosphatemia ensues. In combination with hypocalcemia, hyperphosphatemia stimulates parathyroid hormone secretion and results in a persistent hyperparathyroid state. The pathologic changes in the bones resulting from hyperparathyroidism are collectively termed osteitis fibrosa. These consist of an increased number of osteoclasts and osteoblasts, excess osteoid (mostly woven collagen instead of lamellar collagen seen in healthy bones), and fibrosis of the marrow cavity. This is the most common high-turnover bone lesion of ROD in children (Salusky and Goodman, 1995).

Other factors that contribute to the development of ROD include metabolic acidosis and severe phosphate restriction. Aluminum overload was a significant contributor to the development of ROD in the past (Andreoli *et al.*, 1984) from the use of aluminum-containing phosphate binders. In the USA, aluminum-containing phosphate binders are now very rarely used in the treatment of pediatric CRF (Fivush *et al.*, 1998).

Anemia

A normocytic, normochromic anemia is seen universally in patients with CRF, especially when GFR reaches 20–35 ml/min per 1.73 m² (Chandra *et al.*, 1988). The severity of anemia tends to correlate with the degree of renal dysfunction (Chandra *et al.*, 1988). NAPRTCS data indicate that significant anemia (defined as hematocrit < 30%), is present in 62.9% of pediatric patients with GFR < 10 ml/min per 1.73 m², and in 13.1% of those with GFR between 50 and 75 ml/min per 1.73 m² (Fivush *et al.*, 1998).

The normal kidney synthesizes about 90% of the erythropoietin produced in humans, with the remainder being synthesized in the liver. Erythropoietin acts on erythroid colony-forming cells in the bone marrow via a specific receptor, and promotes the terminal differentiation of erythroid progenitor cells, increasing cellular hemoglobin synthesis and enhancing the rate of release of reticulocytes from the marrow (Sawada *et al.*, 1990). Lack of erythropoietin production by the failing kidneys is the cause of anemia in CRF.

Metabolic acidosis

High anion gap metabolic acidosis is a regular feature of CRF, particularly once GFR decreases to around 25 ml/min per 1.73 m² (Warnock, 1988). Metabolic acidosis in CRF develops because of a diminished ability to excrete hydrogen ions, or endogenous acid load, as well as bicarbonate loss resulting from the inability of the damaged tubules to reabsorb filtered bicarbonate (Warnock, 1988). The high anion gap results from retention of sulfates, phosphates, urates, and hippurates. In early severe CRF a hyperchloremic, normal anion gap metabolic acidosis may be present instead of the high anion gap type of metabolic acidosis (Wallia *et al.*, 1986). Acidosis adversely impacts growth, aggravates hyperkalemia, and induces a protein catabolic state (Jenkins *et al.*, 1989). Its treatment is an essential component of managing ROD.

Electrolyte disorders

Patients with CRF are often in a state of obligatory salt wasting. This is particularly true for patients with interstitial diseases, renal dysplasia, cystic renal diseases, and obstructive uropathy (Terzi *et al.*, 1990). Therefore, sudden and profound sodium restriction may cause hyponatremia, decreasing extracellular volume and renal perfusion, and provoke further deterioration in renal function. Increased sodium loss is mediated by increased sodium excretion in the surviving nephrons by the magnification phenomenon (Bricker *et al.*, 1978). This may result from increased atrial natriuretic factor (Suda *et al.*, 1988). In addition, the natriuretic response to an acute sodium load is blunted in CRF patients, resulting in increased extracellular volume (Kahn *et al.*, 1972).

Renal excretion is the primary route for elimination of potassium. As is the case with the handling of sodium ions, enhanced fractional excretion of potassium in the surviving nephrons attempts to maintain a normal potassium balance (Schultze *et al.*, 1971). Increased fecal potassium excretion also occurs in CRF (Hayes *et al.*, 1967). However, as renal function deteriorates even these adaptive mechanisms are unable to maintain a normal potassium balance unless dietary intake is curtailed.

Patients with renal dysplasia, obstructive uropathy, or tubulointerstitial diseases are particularly at risk for developing hyperkalemia, even when renal function is only modestly compromised. Patients with CRF from other causes usually do not develop hyperkalemia until GFR falls to 10 ml/min per 1.73 m². However, patients with CRF being treated with angiotensin-converting enzyme (ACE) inhibitors are at a higher risk for developing hyperkalemia.

Fluid balance

Patients with CRF have a urinary concentrating defect, producing urine with a fixed osmolality of 300 mOsm/l (isosthenuria). The isosthenuria of CRF is resistant to exogenous vasopressin administration (Holliday *et al.*, 1967). Onset of polyuria or secondary enuresis may be one of the initial manifestations of CRF, especially in those with renal dysplasia, cystic renal diseases, and tubulointerstitial disorders. Providing supplemental water to avoid dehydration should be considered as a part of their therapy.

Patients with CRF are also unable to handle effectively sudden large loads of water. This is especially true when GRF falls below 10 ml/min per 1.73 m^2 and in those with glomerulonephritis as the underlying etiology of CRF.

Metabolic disturbances

Uremia creates an insulin-resistant state (McCaleb *et al.*, 1985). Elevated levels of glucagon (Bilbrey *et al.*, 1975), (El-Bishti *et al.*, 1978), and hyperparathyroidism (Mak, 1998a) may also affect glucose tolerance.

Protein and amino acid metabolism are abnormal in renal failure. Serum concentrations of many amino acids in children with CRF are significantly deranged. The levels of the branched-chain amino acids leucine, valine, and isoleucine, are below normal in CRF (Mak, 1998b). Leucine, in particular, has an anabolic effect on muscle metabolism, and this may be a factor in the abnormal muscle formation and function found in CRF patients who are otherwise well nourished (Sedman *et al.*, 1996). The use of specialized amino acid supplements has proven ineffective (Jones *et al.*, 1980).

Hyperlipidemia is a common finding in patients with CRF, occurring in up to 70% (Attman and Alaupovic, 1991). Hypertriglyceridemia is the prominent abnormality of lipid metabolism in CRF and is thought to be caused by defective catabolism of triglyceride-rich lipoproteins. Metabolic acidosis, hyperinsulinemia, and hyperparathyroidism also impair lipoprotein lipase activity in CRF (Vaziri *et al.*, 1997).

Cardiovascular disorders

The incidence of hypertension in children with renal disease is reported to be 38–78% (Drukker, 1991). As a general rule, hypertension is infrequent in congenital renal disease, but is almost universal in CRF due to primary glomerular disease and renal injury caused by systemic disease (Feld *et al.*, 1996). Irrespective of the etiology of CRF, hypertension accelerates the decline in renal function (Brazy *et al.*, 1989). Hypertension in CRF results from intravascular volume expansion and activation of the renin–angiotensin system (Drukker, 1991; Rosenberg *et al.*, 1994).

Exercise tolerance is lower in children with CRF, is related to the severity of renal failure, and is believed to be due to anemia. Improvement in exercise toler-

ance with correction of anemia with exogenous erythropoitin (rHuEPO) has been documented (Baraldi *et al.*, 1990).

Neurologic impact of chronic renal failure

The onset of CRF in the neonatal period or in early infancy is often associated with significant concerns regarding neurodevelopment. Growth in head circumference is uniformly subnormal in these patients (McGraw and Haka-Ikse, 1985). Gross motor delay, along with global developmental retardation and a lack of maturation on electroencephalography, are common findings in this group (Bock *et al.*, 1989). Progressive encephalopathy characterized by myoclonic seizures, delay in reaching developmental milestones, cerebellar dysfunction, and motor retardation has also been described in non-dialysed infants with CRF (El-Bishti *et al.*, 1978). The etiology of the neurologic dysfunction in these patients is unclear but may include diverse factors, such as malnutrition, uremic toxins, and possible lack of neurotransmitters resulting from deficiency of amino acid precursors.

Medical management of chronic renal failure

The aim of medical therapy is to minimize the clinical impact of metabolic derangements that accompany CRF. Once GFR falls to around 10 ml/min per 1.73 m^2, the patient needs dialysis therapy or renal transplantation.

Treatment of growth failure

Mehls and Ritz (1983) demonstrated that recombinant growth hormone (rhGH) improved growth velocity in uremic growth-retarded rats. Subsequently, numerous studies in children using GH have confirmed these results in humans (Hokken-Koelega *et al.*, 1991; Mehls and Broyer, 1994; Ito *et al.*, 1995; Fine, 1997).

When rhGH treatment is started before bone maturation is complete, final adult height is improved, while discontinuation of rhGH therapy causes a marked reduction in growth velocity (Fine *et al.*, 1996). It is recommended that treatment continue until transplantation or epiphyseal closure.

The presence of ROD may blunt the effects of rhGH and predispose to the development of bone deformities, slipped capital femoral epiphyses, and/or avascular necrosis in children with CRF (Watkins, 1996). It is recommended that ROD is be corrected before initiation of rhGH (Fine, 1997). Complications of rhGH treatment include accelerated glomerulosclerosis, hypercalciuria, pseudotumor cerebri, and potential risk of malignancy (Blethen, 1995).

Supplemental sodium and water in children with dysplasia and/or obstructive uropathy who have polyuria and intravascular volume depletion may prevent growth failure (Sedman *et al.*, 1996). Feeding via a nasogastric tube or gastrostomy may become necessary for supplemental nutritional intake.

Renal osteodystrophy

Since phosphate retention is an important component in the pathogenesis of ROD, restricting dietary phosphorus content is a prudent beginning in the management of ROD. However, such a diet tends to be bland and unpalatable. As a more practical strategy, phosphate binders taken with meals and snacks are used to render phosphorus non-absorbable and promote its excretion in stools.

Aluminum hydroxide is an effective phosphate binder which was used extensively in the past. However, aluminum deposition in the bones leads to the development of anemia and aluminum-induced bone disease. Consequently, it is now rarely recommended as a phosphate binder for patients with CRF. At present, calcium acetate and calcium carbonate are the alternatives most extensively used as phosphate binders in pediatric CRF. The dose of calcium compounds as phosphate binders is empiric and is based on the control of serum phosphorus concentration. Hypercalcemia is a potential side-effect of calcium-containing phosphate binders. Recently, a non-calcium-containing phosphate binder (Renagel) has been approved for use in CRF. The advantage of this compund is its ability to bind phosphorus effectively without causing hypercalcemia (Slatoplosky *et al.*, 1999a). In order to be effective, all phosphate binders need to be taken with meals and snacks.

Bioactive analogs of vitamin D are used to prevent hyperparathyroidism, promote healing of bones, and improve serum calcium concentration. Calcitriol (Rocaltrol) and dihydrotachysterol (DHT) are two commonly used vitamin D compounds. Although both are effective in treating ROD, calcitriol has the advantage of a quick onset and short duration of action (Chan *et al.*, 1994).

Anemia

Administration of rHuEPO is now an accepted and an effective treatment for the anemia of CRF (Eschbach *et al.*, 1989). It can be given intravenously, subcutaneously, or intraperitoneally. The initial starting dose is 100 units/kg per dose, given on three alternating days of the week. In severe cases, a higher dose or more frequent administration may be necessary. After about 4–6 weeks, when the target hematocrit of 36% is reached, the dose can then be adjusted to maintain the hematocrit at that level. Younger children appear to require a higher dose of rHuEPO for effective therapy than older children. The reason for this is unclear since the pharmacokinetics in children is comparable to that seen in adults (Kling *et al.*, 1992).

The benefits of maintaining a higher hematocrit with rHuEPO in CRF are: increased exercise tolerance, improved quality of life, and decreased transfusion requirements, which results in the lower levels of antibodies to histocompatibility antigents. This is of critical advantage for renal transplantation candidates (Brandt *et al.*, 1999). Regression of ventricular hypertrophy, without adversely impacting cardiac function, has also been reported in patients receiving rHuEPO therapy (Portoles *et al.*, 1997).

Suboptimal response to rHuEPO may be secondary to acute and chronic inflammation, infection, aluminum toxicity, and hyperparathyroidism. Iron deficiency causes less effective erythropoiesis (Van Wyck, 1989). Most children receiving rHuEPO therapy require supplemental iron therapy. If the response to iron taken orally is inadequate, intravenous iron therapy may become necessary to achieve the full benefits of rHuEPO therapy (Silverberg *et al.*, 1999).

Adverse effects of rHuEPO therapy include hypertension, hyperkalemia, iron deficiency, and thrombosis of hemodialysis vascular access. Fifty per cent of children with CRF require an escalation of their antihypertensive therapy during rHuEPO treatment (Schaärer *et al.*, 1993). The pathogenesis of hypertension in patients being treated with rHuEPO is not clear, but volume expansion and increased peripheral vascular resistance have been implicated (Vaziri, 1999). Seizures have also been described in some patients undergoing rHuEPO treatment, but most appear to be a result of hypertensive encephalopathy.

Metabolic acidosis

Alkali supplementation is usually required to correct acidosis in patients with CRF. To optimize growth, serum bicarbonate concentration should be maintained between 23 and 25 mEq/l. Sodium bicarbonate can be used as an alkali supplement in older children who can swallow a tablet. In younger children Schol's solution (sodium citrate and citric acid) or Bicitra offer appropriate replacement. The usual dose for alkali therapy is 1–2 mEq/kg of bicarbonate equivalent. Each milliliter of Bicitra provides 1 mEq of bicarbonate equivalent, while a 325 mg tablet of sodium bicarbonate provides 4 mEq of bicarbonate equivalent.

Fluid and electrolyte balance

Sodium and water supplementation is usually necessary in those patients who have polyuria associated with CRF. Fluid restriction is generally unnecessary until GFR is < 10%. In contrast, patients with CRF due to chronic glomerulonephritis generally have low urine output, hypertension, and poor sodium tolerance with even a mild to moderate decrease in GFR. Sodium and water replacement also help to control the hyperkalemia that is exacerbated by volume contraction (Sedman et al., 1996).

Hypertension

The blood pressure in those with hypertension needs to be gradually lowered to prevent decreased renal perfusion and a further reduction in renal function. Diuretics are an effective first-line treatment when volume is an issue, with the stepwise addition of other agents as necessary (Feld et al., 1996). Owing to their renoprotective effect, ACE inhibitors are considered the drug class of choice, (Marcantoni et al., 1999). Also important is the incorporation of non-pharmacologic treatments such as diet and exercise.

Metabolic considerations

Use of lipid-lowering drugs is not recommended for use in children with CRF because of concerns about long-term liver and muscle toxicities. However, dietary maneuvers, such as decreasing the intake of saturated fat while increasing polyunsaturated or monounsaturated fat content in the diet, are helpful and should be undertaken. In addition, correction of secondary hyperparathyroidism can ameliorate the hyperlipidemia of CRF (Vaziri et al., 1997; Slatoplosky et al.,

1999a). In patients who are nephrotic, the use of ACE inhibitors may be helpful by decreasing urinary protein loss, affording renoprotection from hyperfiltration, and thus resulting in improvement in hyperlipidemia (Gansevoort et al., 1994).

Preventing progressive renal damage: role of hyperfiltration

As CRF approaches ESRD the histologic appearance on renal biopsy is similar, regardless of the primary insult, seemingly indicative of an undefined final common pathway for renal tissue damage. Hostetter et al. (1981) and Brenner et al. (1982) proposed that the response to a decrease in functional nephron number leads to an increase in both glomerular capillary plasma flow and glomerular capillary hydraulic pressure. This causes increased single-nephron GFR and glomerular hyperfiltration and the further loss of glomeruli with the resultant cycle of hyperfiltration, glomerular hypertension, and glomerulosclerosis (Fig. 35.7) (Brenner et al., 1996). Hyperfiltration and glomerulosclerosis may also result from massive obesity, chronic obstruction, diabetes mellitus, or congenital or acquired deficits in nephron number causing renal mass reduction (Brenner et al., 1996; Karlen et al., 1996; Brenner and Mackenzie, 1997; Pascual et al., 1998). Glomerular hypertension seems to correlate more closely with glomerular sclerosis than hyperperfusion/hyperfiltration (Brenner et al., 1996). Unilateral nephrectomy for renal donation or secondary to unilateral renal disease does not appear to have this same adverse effect on renal function (Goldfarb, 1995). However, Provoost and Brenner (1993) caution that this conclusion may be premature owing to the relatively short follow-up time of these patients.

The availability of extensive experimental and human data on the correlation of the development of glomerular hypertension to proteinuria and glomerulosclerosis has made it possible to develop therapies aimed at decreasing glomerular hypertension and hyperfiltration processes. This may slow the progression of CRF. Such therapies in current use include a low protein diet (Fouque et al., 1992) and the use of ACE inhibitors or angiotensin II receptor antagonists (Anonymous, 1992; Brenner et al., 1996). The fact that these agents are more efficacious than other non-specific antihypertensives in protecting against progressive glomerulosclerosis is

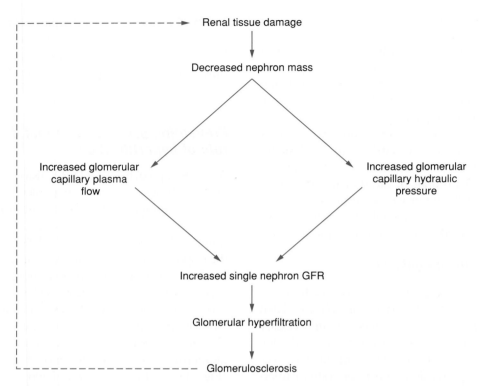

Figure 35.7 Mechanisms involved in hyperfiltration and progressive renal damage. (Adapted from Brenner *et al.*, 1996.)

attributed to their ability to decrease glomerular capillary pressure by preferential dilation of the efferent arteriole, thereby counteracting hyperfiltration.

Non-hemodynamic processes also seem to contribute to progressive renal disease and addressing these may also limit glomerular injury. These include treatment of hyperlipidemia (Samuelsson *et al.*, 1997) and dietary sodium restriction (Bernstein *et al.*, 1990).

References

Abitbol CL, Warady BA, Massie MD *et al.* (1990) Linear growth and anthropometric and nutritional measurements in children with mild to moderate renal insufficiency: a report for the Growth Failure in Children with Renal Diseases Study. *J Pediatr* **116**: S46–S54.

Allgren RL, Marbury TC, Rahman SN *et al.* (1997) Anaritide in acute tubular necrosis. *N Engl J Med* **336**: 828.

Alvarez A, Martul E, Veiga F, Fortez J (1994) Functional, histologic and ultrastructural study of the protective effects of verapamil in experimental ischemic acute renal failure in the rabbit. *Ren Fail* **16**: 193.

Anderndshorst WJ, Finn WF, Gottschalk CW (1975) Pathogenesis of acute renal failure following renal ischemia in the rat. *Circ Res* **37**: 558.

Anderson RJ, Linas SL, Berns AS *et al.* (1977) Nonoliguric acute renal failure. *N Engl J Med* **296**: 1134.

Andreoli SP, Bergstein JM, Sherrard DJ (1984) Aluminum intoxication from aluminum-containing phosphate binders in children with azotemia not undergoing dialysis. *N Engl J Med* **310**: 1079–84.

Anonymous (1992) The Modification of Diet in Renal Disease Study: design, methods, and results from the Feasibility Study. *Am J Kidney Dis* **20**: 18–33.

Anonymous (1999) Incidence and prevalence of ESRD. USRDS 1999. *Am J Kidney Dis* **34** (Suppl. 1): S40–S50.

Anonymous (2000) Low dose dopamine in patients with early renal dysfunction: a placebo controlled randomized trial. *Lancet* **356**: 2139.

Arora P, Kher V, Kohli HS *et al.* (1994) Pattern of acute renal failure at a referral hospital. *Indian Pediatr* **31**: 1047.

Attman PO, Alaupovic P (1991) Lipid abnormalities in chronic renal insufficiency. *Kidney Int* **31** (Suppl): S16–S23.

Baraldi E, Montini G, Zanconato S *et al.* (1990) Exercise tolerance after anemia correction with recombinant human erythropoietin in end-stage renal disease. *Pediatr Nephrol* **4**: 623–6.

Bernstein JA, Feiner HD, Parker M, Dworkin LD (1990) Superiority of salt restriction over diuretics in reducing renal hypertrophy and injury in uninephrectomized SHR. *Am J Physiol* **258**: F1675–81.

Betts PR, Magrath G (1974) Growth pattern and dietary intake of children with chronic renal insufficiency. *BMJ* **2**: 189–93.

Bilbrey GL, Faloona GR, White MC *et al.* (1975) Hyperglucagonemia in uremia reversal by transplantation. *Ann Intern Med* **82**: 525–8.

Blethen SL (1995) Complications of growth hormone therapy in children. *Curr Opin Pediatr* **7**: 466–71.

Bock GH, Conners K, Ruley J *et al.* (1989) Disturbances of brain maturation and neurodevelopment during chronic renal failure in infancy. *J Pediatr* **114**: 231–8.

Bourquina A, Zahid D (1993) Acute renal insufficiency in children, restrospective study of 89 cases. *Ann Pediatr (Paris)* **40**: 603.

Brandt JR, Avner ED, Hickman RO, Watkins SL (1999) Safety and efficacy of erythropoietin in children with chronic renal failure. *Pediatr Nephrol* **13**: 143–7.

Brazy PC, Stead WW, Fitzwilliam JF (1989) Progression of renal insufficiency: role of blood pressure. *Kidney Int* **35**: 670–4.

Bren AF, Kandus A, Buturovic J *et al.* (1998) Cyclosporine-related hemolytic-uremic syndrome in kidney graft recipients: clinical and histomorphologic evaluation. *Transplant Proc* **30**: 1201.

Brenner BM, Lawler EV, Mackenzie HS (1996) The hyperfiltration theory: a paradigm shift in nephrology. *Kidney Int* **49**: 1774–7.

Brenner BM, Mackenzie HS (1997) Nephron mass as a risk factor for progression of renal disease. *Kidney Int* **63** (Suppl): S124–S127.

Brenner BM, Meyer TW, Hostetter TH (1982) Dietary protein intake and the progressive nature of kidney disease: the role of hemodymanically mediated glomerular injury in the pathogenesis of progressive glomerular sclerosis in aging, renal ablation and intrinsic renall disease. *N Engl J Med* **307**: 652–9.

Brezis M, Rosen S (1995) Hypoxia of the renal medulla – its implications for disease. *N Engl J Med* **332**: 647.

Bricker NS, Fine LG, Kaplan M *et al.* (1978) 'Magnification phenomenon' in chronic renal disease. *N Engl J Med* **299**: 1287–93.

Brunette MG, Chan M, Ferriere C *et al.* (1978) Site of 1,25-(OH)$_2$ vitamin D$_3$ synthesis in the kidney. *Nature* **276**: 287–9.

Chan JCM, McEnery PT, Chinchilli VW *et al.* (1994) A prospective, double-blind study of growth failure in children with chronic renal insufficiency and the effectiveness of treatment calcitriol versus dihydrotachysterol. The Growth Failure in Children with Renal Diseases Investigators. *J Pediatr* **124**: 520–8.

Chandra M, Clemons GK, McVicar MI (1988) Relation of serum erythropoietin levels to renal excretory function: evidence for a lowered set point for erythropoietin production in chromic renal failure. *J Pediatr* **113**: 1015–21.

Chertow GM, Sayegh MH, Allgren RL, Lazarus JM (1996) Is the administration of dopamine associated with adverse or favorable outcome in acute renal failure. *Am J Med* **101**: 49.

Cirino M, Morton H, McDonald *et al.* (1990) Thromboxane A$_2$ and prostaglandin endoperoxide analogue effects on porcine renal blood flow. *Am J Physiol* **258**: F109.

Conger JD (1995) Interventions in clinical acute renal failure: where are the data? *Am J Kidney Dis* **26**: 565.

Cundall DR, Brocklebank JT, Buckler JM (1988) Which bone age in chronic renal insufficiency and end-stage renal disease? *Pediatr Nephrol* **2**: 200–4.

Daugharty TM, Ueki IF, Mercer PF, Brenner BM (1974) Dynamics of glomerular ultrafiltration in the rat. V. Response to ischemic injury. *J Clin Invest* **53**: 105.

Dawnay AB, Thornby C, Nockler I *et al.* (1985) Tamm-Horsfall glycoprotein excretion and aggregation during intravenous miography: relevance to ARF. *Invest Radiol* **20**: 53.

Drukker A (1991) Hypertension in children and adolescents with chronic renal failure and end-stage renal disease. *Clin Nephrol Urol* **11**: 152–8.

El-Bishti MM, Counahan RC, Bloom SR *et al.* (1978) Hormonal and metabolic responses to intravenous glucose in children on regular hemodialysis. *Am J Clin Nutr* **31**: 1865–9.

Esbjorner E, Berg U, Hansson S (1997) Epidemiology of chronic renal failure in children: a report from Sweden 1986–1994. Swedish Pediatric Nephrology Association. *Pediatr Nephrol* **11**: 438–42.

Eschbach JW, Kelly MR, Haley NR *et al.* (1989) Treatment of the anemia of progressive renal failure with recombinant human erythropoietin. *N Engl J Med* **321**: 158–63.

Fargason CA, Langman CL (1993) Limitations of the pediatric risk of mortality score in assessing children with acute renal failure. *Pediatr Nephrol* **7**: 703.

Feld LG, Liberman E, Mendoza SA, Springate JE (1996) Management of hypertension in the child with chronic renal disease. *J Pediatr* **129**: S18–S26.

Fine RN (1997) Growth hormone treatment of children with chronic renal insufficiency, end-stage renal disease and following renal transplantation – update 1997. *J Pediatr Endocrinol Metab* **10**: 361–70.

Fine RN, Brown DF, Kuntze J *et al.* (1996) Growth after discontinuation of recombinant human growth hormone therapy in children with chronic renal insufficiency. The Genentech Cooperative Study Group. *J Pediatr* **129**: 883–91.

Fivush BA, Jabs K, Neu AM *et al.* (1998) Chronic renal insufficiency in children and adolescents: the 1996 annual report of NAPRTCS. North American Pediatric Renal Transplant Cooperative Study. *Pediatr Nephrol* **12**: 328–37.

Flores J, DiBona DR, Beck CH, Leaf A (1972) The role of cell swelling in ischemic renal damage and the protective effect of hypertonic solute. *J Clin Invest* **51**: 118.

Fogo A, Kon V (1994) Pathophysiology of progressive renal disease. In: Holliday MA, Barratt TM, Avner ED (eds) *Pediatric nephrology*. Baltimore, MD: Williams & Wilkins, 1228.

Fouque D, Laville M, Boissel J *et al.* (1992) Controlled low protein diets in chronic renal insufficiency: meta-analysis. *BMJ* **304**: 216–20.

Gansevoort RT, Heeg JE, Dikkeschei FD *et al.* (1994) Symptomatic antiproteinuria treatment decreases serum lipoprotein (a) concentration in patients with glomerular proteinuria. *Nephrol Dial Transplant* 9: 244–50.

Gavras H, Lever AF, Brown JJ *et al.* (1971) Acute renal failure, tubular necrosis and myocardial infarction induced in the rabbit by intravenous angiotensin II. *Lancet* ii: 19.

Gilbert RD, Argent AC (1998) Streptococcus pneumoniae-associated hemolytic uremic syndrome. *Pediatr Infect Dis* 17: 530.

Goldfarb DA (1995) Preservation of renal function and the risk of hyperfiltration nephropathy. *Semin Urol Oncol* 13: 292–5.

Goligorsky MS, Nori E (1999) Duality of nitric oxide in acute renal injury. *Semin Nephrol* 19: 263.

Grossman RA, Hamilton RW, Morse BM *et al.* (1974) Nontraumatic rhabdomyolysis and acute renal failure. *N Engl J Med* 291: 807.

Guthrie LG, Oxon MD (1897) Chronic interstitial nephritis in childhood. *Lancet* ii: 585.

Havistendahl JJ, Pedersen TS, Jorgensen HH *et al.* (1996) Renal hemodynamic response to graduated uretor obstruction in the pig. *Nephron* 74: 168.

Hayes CP, McLeod MC, Robinson RR *et al.* (1967) An extrarenal mechanism for the maintenance of potassium balance in severe chronic renal failure. *Trans Assoc Am Phys* 80: 207–16.

Hirschberg R, Kopple J, Lipsett P *et al.* (1999) Multicenter clinical trial of recombinant human insulin-like growth factor-I in patients with acute renal failure. *Kidney Int* 55: 2423.

Hishida A, Nakajima T, Yamada M *et al.* (1994) Roles of hemodynamic and tubular factors in gentamycin-mediated nephropathy. *Ren Fail* 16: 109.

Hokken-Koelega ACS, Stijren T, De Muinck Keizer-Schrama SMPF *et al.* (1991) Placebo-controlled, double-blind, crossover trial of growth hormone treatment in prepubertal children with chronic renal failure. *Lancet* 338: 585–90.

Holliday MA, Egan TJ, Morris CR *et al.* (1967) Pitressin-resistant hyposthenuria in chronic renal disease. *Am J Med* 42: 378–87.

Hostetter TH, Olson JL, Rennke HG *et al.* (1981) Hyperfiltration in remnant nephrons: a potentially adverse response to renal ablation. *Am J Physiol* 241: F85–F93.

Ishimura E, Nishizawa Y, Inaba M *et al.* (1999) Serum levels of 1,25-dihydroxyvitamin D, 24,25-dihydroxyvitamin D, and 25-hydroxyvitamin D in nondialyzed patients with chronic renal failure. *Kidney Int* 55: 1019–27.

Ito K, Kawaguchi H, Shizume K, Hibi I (1995) The effects of recombinant growth hormone (r-hGH, SM-9500, genotropin) on growth failure in children with uremia. Japanese Multi-Center Study (Genotropin) Group on Children with Renal Disease. *Nippon Jinzo Gakkai Shi* 37: 186–93.

Jenkins D, Burton PR, Bennett SE *et al.* (1989) The metabolic consequences of the correction of acidosis in uraemia. *Nephrol Dial Transplant* 4: 92–5.

Jones RW, Dalton N, Start K *et al.* (1980) Oral essential amino acid supplements in children with advanced renal failure. *Am J Clin Nutr* 33: 1696–702.

Kahn T, Mohammad G, Stein RM (1972) Alterations in renal tubular sodium and water reabsorption in chronic renal disease in man. *Kidney Int* 2: 164–74.

Kandoth PW, Agarwal GJ, Dharnidharka MR (1994) Acute renal failure in children requiring dialysis therapy. *Indian Pediatr* 31: 305.

Karlberg J (1990) The infancy–childhood growth spurt. *Acta Pediatr Scand* 367 (Suppl): 111–18.

Karlen J, Linne T, Wikstad I, Aperia A (1996) Incidence of microalbuminuria in children with pyelonephritic scarring. *Pediatr Nephrol* 10: 705–8.

Kato A, Hishida A, Kobayashi S, Honda N (1993) Glomerular alterations in experimental oliguric and nonoliguric acute renal failure. *Ren Fail* 15: 215.

Kirks DR (1984) Skeletal system. In: *Pratical pediatric imaging*. Boston, MA: Little Brown, 314.

Kling PJ, Widness JA, Guillery EN *et al.* (1992) Pharmacokinetics and pharmacodynamics of erythropoietin during therapy in an infant with renal failure. *J Pediatr* 121: 822–5.

Koch MJ, Buhrer R, Pioch T, Scharer K (1999) Enamel hypoplasia of primary teeth in chronic renal failure. *Pediatr Nephrol* 13: 68–72.

Kondo M, Kojima S, Horibe K *et al.* (1998) Hemolytic uremic syndrome after allogeneic or autologous hemopoietic stem cell transplantation for childhood malignancies. *Bone Marrow Transplant* 21: 281.

Kramer HJ, Schuurman J, Wasserman C, Dusing R (1980) Prostaglandin-independent protection by furosemide from oliguric ischemic renal failure in concious rats. *Kidney Int* 17: 455.

Kwon O, Nelson WJ, Sibley R *et al.* (1998) Backleak, tight junctions and cell–cell adhesion in postischemic injury to the renal allograft. *J Clin Invest* 101: 2054.

Lesko SM, Mitchell AA (1997) Renal function after short-term ibuprofen use in children. *Pediatrics* 100: 954.

McCaleb ML, Izzo MS, Lockwood DH (1985) Characterization and partial purification of a factor in human uremic serum that induces insulin resistance. *J Clin Invest* 75: 391–6.

McDonald RH, Goldberg LI, McNay JL, Tuttle EP Jr (1964) Effects of dopamine in man: augmentation of sodium excretion, glomerular filtration rate and renal plasma flow. *J Clin Invest* 43: 1116.

McGraw ME, Haka-Ikse K (1985) Neurologic-developmental sequelae of chronic renal failure in infancy. *J Pediatr* 106: 579–83.

Mak RH (1998a) 1,25-Dihydroxyvitamin D_3 corrects insulin and lipid abnormalities in uremia. *Kidney Int* 53: 1353–7.

Mak RH (1998b) Insulin, branched-chain amino acids, and growth failure in uremia. *Pediatr Nephrol* 12: 637–42.

Marcantoni C, Oldrizzi L, Rugiu C *et al.* (1999) Management of hypertension in renal disease. *Miner Electrolyte Metab* 25: 80–3.

Mareau JM, Drug D, Sabato J *et al.* (1975) Osmotic nephroxix induced by water soluble tri-iodinated contrast media in man. *Radiology* 115: 329.

Mehls O, Broyer M, on behalf of the European/Australian Study Group (1994) Growth response to recombinant human growth hormone in short prepubertal children with chronic renal failure with or without dialysis. *Acta Paediatr Scand* **399** (Suppl): 81–7.

Mehls O, Ritz E (1983) Skeletal growth in experimental uremia. *Kidney Int* **21** (Suppl): S53–S62.

Miller SB, Martin DR, Kissane J *et al.* (1992) Insulin-like growth factor I accelerates recovery from ischemic acute renal failure. *Proc Natl Acad Sci USA* **89**: 11876.

Moghal NE, Brocklebank JT, Meadow SR (1998) A review of acute renal failure in children: incidence, etiology and outcome. *Clin Nephrol* **49**: 91.

Neuhaus TJ, Calonder S, Leumann EP (1997) Heterogeneity of atypical hemolytic uremic syndromes. *Arch Dis Child* **76**: 518.

Nonclercq D, Wrona S, Toubea G *et al.* (1992) Tubular injury and regeneration in the rat kidney following acute exposure to gentamycin: a time-couse study. *Ren Fail* **14**: 507.

Oliver J, MacDowell M, Tracy (1951) The pathogenesis of acute renal failure associated with traumatic and toxic injury. Renal ischemia, nephrotoxic damage and the ischemic episode. *J Clin Invest* **30**: 1307.

Olsen TS, Hansen HE (1990) Ultrastructure of medullary tubules in ischemic acute tubular necrosis and acute interstitial nephritis in man. *APMIS* **98**: 1139.

Ott CE, Hass JA, Cuche L, Knox FG (1975) Effect of increased peritubular protein concentration on proximal tubule reabsorption in the presence and absence of extracellular volume expansion. *J Clin Invest* **55**: 612.

Parekh N, Veith U (1981) Renal hemodynamics and oxygen consumption during postischemic acute renal failure in the rat. *Kidney Int* **19**: 306.

Parfrey PS, Griffiths SM, Barrett BJ *et al.* (1989) Contrast-material induced renal failure in patients with diabetes mellitus, renal insufficiency or both. *N Engl J Med* **320**: 143.

Pascual L, Oliva J, Vega PJ *et al.* (1998) Renal histology in ureteropelvic junction obstruction: are histological changes a consequence of hyperfiltration? *J Urol* **160**: 976–9.

Patak RV, Fadem SZ, Lifshitz MD, Stein JH (1979) Study of the factors which modify the development of norepinephrine-induced acute renal failure in the dog. *Kidney Int* **15**: 227.

Petermann A, Offermann G, Distler A, Sharma AM (1998) Familial hemolytic–uremic syndrome in three generations. *Am J Kidney Dis* **32**: 1063.

Portale AA, Booth BE, Tsai HC *et al.* (1982) Reduced plasma concentration of 1,25-dihydroxyvitamin D in children with moderate renal insufficiency. *Kidney Int* **21**: 627–32.

Porter GA (1990) Experimental contrast-associated nephropathy and its clinical implications. *Am J Cardiol* **66**: 18F.

Portoles J, Torralbo A, Martin P *et al.* (1997) Cardiovascular effects of recombinant human erythropoietin in predialysis patients. *Am J Kidney Dis* **29**: 541–8.

Powell DR, Liu F, Baker BK *et al.* (1997) Insulin-like growth factor binding protein-6 levels are elevated in serum of children with chronic renal failure. *J Clin Endocrinol Metab* **82**: 2978–84.

Powell DR, Durham SK, Brewer ED *et al.* (1999) Effects of chronic renal failure and growth hormone on serum levels of insulin-like growth factor-binding protein-4 (IGFBP-4) and IGFBP-5 in children: a report of the Southwest

Pediatric Nephrology Study Group. *J Clin Endocrinol Metab* **84**: 596–601.

Provoost AP, Brenner BM (1993) Long-term follow-up of humans with single kidneys: the need for longitudinal studies to assess true changes in renal function. *Curr Opin Nephrol Hypertens* **2**: 521–6.

Rahman SN, Kim GE, Mathew AS *et al.* (1994) Effects of atrial natriuretic peptide in clinical acute renal failure. *Kidney Int* **45**: 1731.

Remuzzi G, Ruggenenti P (1998) The hemolytic iremic syndrome. *Kidney Int* **66** (Suppl): S54.

Rosenberg ME, Smith LJ, Correa-Rotter R, Hostetter TH (1994) The paradox of the renin–angiotensin system in chromic renal disease. *Kidney Int* **45**: 403–10.

Ruschitzka F, Shaw S, Gygi D *et al.* (1999) Endothelial dysfunction in acute renal failure: role of circulating and tissue endothelin-1. *J Am Soc Nephrol* **10**: 953.

Salusky IB, Goodman WG (1995) Growth hormone and calcitriol as modifiers of bone formation in renal osteodystrophy. *Kidney Int* **48**: 657–65.

Samuelsson O, Mulec H, Knight-Gibson C *et al.* (1997) Lipoprotein abnormalities are associated with increased rate of progression of human chronic renal insufficiency. *Nephrol Dial Transplant* **12**: 1908–15.

Sawada K, Krantz SB, Dai CH *et al.* (1990) Purification of human blood burst-forming units – erythroid and demonstration of the evolution of erythropoietin receptors. *J Cell Physiol* **142**: 219–30.

Schaärer K, Klare B, Braun A *et al.* (1993) Treatment of renal anemia by subcutaneous erythropoietin in children with preterminal chronic renal failure. *Acta Paediatr* **82**: 953–8.

Schaefer F, Hamill G, Stanhope R *et al.* (1991) Pulsatile growth hormone secretion in prepubertal patients with chronic renal failure. *J Pediatr* **119**: 568–77.

Schaller S, Kaplan B (1998) Acute nonoliguric renal failure in children associated with nonsteroidal antiinflamatory agents. *Pediatr Emerg Care* **14**: 416.

Schultze RG, Taggart DD, Shapiro H *et al.* (1971) On the adaptation of potassium excretion associated with nephron reduction in the dog. *J Clin Invest* **50**: 1061–8.

Schwab SJ, Hlatky MA, Pieper KS *et al.* (1989) Contrast nephrotoxicity: a randomized controlled trial of nonionic and an ionic radiographic contrast agent. *N Engl J Med* **320**: 149.

Sedman A, Friedman A, Boineau F *et al.* (1996) Nutritional management of the child with mild to moderate chronic renal failure. *J Pediatr* **129**: S13–S18.

Shilliday I, Allison ME (1994) Diuretics in acute renal failure. *Ren Fail* **16**: 3.

Silverberg DS, Blum M, Agbaria Z *et al.* (1999) Intravenous iron for the treatment of predialysis anemia. *Kidney Int* **69** (Suppl): S79–S85.

Slatoplosky EA, Burke SK, Dillon MA *et al.* (1999a) RenaGel®, a nonabsorbed calcium- and aluminum-free phosphate binder, lowers serum phosphorus and parathyroid hormone. *Kidney Int* **55**: 299–307.

Slatopolsky E, Dusso A, Brown AJ (1999b) The role of phosphorus in the development of secondary hyperparathyroidism and parathyroid cell proliferation in chronic renal failure. *Am J Med Sci* **317**: 370–6.

Solez K, Morel-Maroger L, Sraer JD (1979) The morphology of 'acute tubular necrosis' in man: analysis in 57 renal biopsies and comparison with glycerol model. *Medicine* **58**: 362.

Solomon R, Werner C, Mann D *et al*. (1994) Effects of saline, mannitol, and furosemide in acute decrease in renal function induced by radiocontrast agents. *N Engl J Med* **331**: 1416.

Spizzirri FD, Rahman RC, Bibloni N *et al*. (1997) Childhood hemolytic uremic syndrome in Argentina: long-term follow-up and prognostic features. *Pediatr Nephrol* **11**: 156.

Star RA (1998) Treatment of acute renal failure. *Kidney Int* **54**: 1817.

Suda S, Weidmann P, Saxenhofer H *et al*. (1988) Atrial natriuretic factor in mild to moderate chronic renal failure. *Hypertension* **11**: 483–90.

Swain JA, Heyndricks GR, Boettcher DH, Vatner SF (1975) Prostaglandin control of renal circulation in the unanesthetized dog and baboon. *Am J Physiol* **229**: 826.

Tanner GA, Steinhause M (1976) Tubular obstruction in ischemia-induced acute renal failure in the rat. *Kidney Int* **10**: 565.

Terzi F, Assael BM, Claris-Appiani A *et al*. (1990) Increased sodium requirement following early postnatal surgical correction of congenital uropathies in infants. *Pediatr Nephrol* **4**: 581–4.

Thadhani R, Pascual M, Bonventre J (1996) Acute renal failure. *N Engl J Med* **334**: 1448.

Tönshoff B, Blum WF, Wingen A-M, Mehls O (1995) Serum insulin-like growth factors (IGFs) and IGF binding proteins 1,2 and 3 in children with chronic renal failure: relationship to height and glomerular filtration rate. The European Study Group for Nutritional Treatment of Chronic Renal Failure in Childhood. *J Clin Endocrinol Metab* **80**: 2684–91.

Tönshoff B, Schaefer F, Mehls O (1990) Disturbance of growth hormone-insulin-like growth factor axis in uremia. *Pediatr Nephrol* **4**: 654–62.

Turner ME, Kher K, Rakusan T *et al*. (1997) Atypical hemolytic uremic syndrome in human immunodeficiency virus-1 infected children. *Pediatr Nephrol* **11**: 161.

Uauy RD, Hogg RJ, Brewer ED *et al*. (1994) Dietary protein and growth in infants with chronic renal insufficiency: a report from the Southwest Pediatric Nephrology Study Group and the University of California. *Pediatr Nephrol* **8**: 45–50.

Ufferman RC, Jaenike JR, Freeman RB, Pabico RC (1975) Effects of furosemide on low-dose mercuric chloride acute renal failure in rats. *Kidney Int* **8**: 362.

Van Wyck DB (1989) Iron management during recombinant human erythropoietin therapy. *Am J Kidney Dis* **14** (Suppl 1): 9–13.

Vaziri ND (1999) Mechanism of erythropoietin-induced hypertension. *Am J Kidney Dis* **33**: 821–8.

Vaziri ND, Wang XQ, Liang K (1997) Secondary hyperparathyroidism downregulates lipoprotein lipase expression in chronic renal failure. *Am J Physiol* **273**: F925–F930.

Venkat-Raman G, Feehaly J, Elliott HL *et al*. (1998) Renal and hemodynamic effects of amlodipine and nifedipine in the hypertensive renal transplant recipients. *Nephrol Dial Transplant* **13**: 261.

Wallia R, Greenberg A, Piraino B *et al* (1986) Serum electrolyte patterns in end stage renal disease. *Am J Kidney Dis* **8**: 98–104.

Warnock DG (1988) Uremic acidosis. *Kidney Int* **34**: 278–87.

Watkins SL (1996) Bone disease in patients receiving growth hormone. *Kidney Int* **53** (Suppl): S126–S127.

Weir BA, Mazumdar DC (1994) Aminoglycoside nephrotoxicity following single-dose cystoscopy prophylaxis. *Ann Pharmacother* **28**: 199.

Williams RH, Thomas CE, Neva LG, Evans AP (1981) Hemodynamic and single nephron function during the maintenence phase of acute renal failure in the dog. *Kidney Int* **19**: 503.

Wong W, McCall E, Anderson B *et al*. (1996) Acute renal failure in the pediatric intensive care unit. *NZ Med J* **109**: 459.

Yagil Y, Myers BD, Jamison RL (1988) Course and pathogenesis of postischemic acute renal failure in the rat. *Am J Physiol* **255**: F257.

Yangisawa H, Nodera M, Umemori Y *et al*. (1998) Role of angiotensin II, endothelin-1, and nitric oxide in $HgCl_2$ induced acute renal failure. *Toxicol Appl Pharmacol* **152**: 315.

Yoshiya K, Ijima K, Yoshikawa N (1973) A clinicopathologic study of 90 children with acute renal failure. *Nippon Jinzo Gakkai Shi* **9**: 483.

Renal transplantation

36

John M. Barry

Introduction

The United States Renal Data System (1999) considers pediatric patients to be those with end-stage renal disease (ESRD) between the ages of 0 and 19 years. The adjusted ESRD rate is about 13 per million US population for this age group, and this is significantly less than the incidence rate for adults. Boys have ESRD more commonly than girls because boys have a higher incidence of congenital disorders such as obstructive uropathy, renal dysplasia, and the triad syndrome. The most common causes of ESRD in children and adults are compared in Table 36.1.

Compared with adults with ESRD, children are more likely to receive chronic peritoneal dialysis than hemodialysis, and they are more likely to undergo renal transplantation. There are fewer constraints on diet and fluid intake with peritoneal dialysis than with hemodialysis, and vascular access for dialysis in small children is problematic. Children with ESRD often suffer growth failure, poor nutrition, depression, anxiety, and loss of self-esteem, and this results in significant family stress (NIH, 1993). Recombinant growth hormone therapy can be used successfully to treat short stature (Yadin and Fine, 1997) and nutritional supplementation can be provided via a nasogastric tube or button gastrostomy. There is a greater availability of parental kidney donors for children than for adults, and children receive preferential points when they are listed for cadaver kidney transplantation (Table 36.2)(UNOS, 1995; Tejani et al., 1998). This has resulted in a greater proportion of living donor kidney transplants than cadaver kidney transplants in children when compared with adults, and a rate of cadaver kidney transplantation that is approximately twice that for young adult ESRD patients 20–24 years of age (US Renal Data System, 1999). The death rate is lower for children who undergo renal transplantation than for those who remain on dialysis; however, sicker children may remain on dialysis and not be offered a transplant.

Kidney transplant survival rates by donor source are presented in Table 36.3 (Tejani et al., 1998). Five-year patient survival rates were 91% and 94% for recipients of cadaver and living donor kidney transplants, respectively. Significant risk factors for kidney transplant failure in children have been shown to be: recipient age under 2 years, cadaver donor age under 6 years, prior transplantation, no antilymphocyte antibody induction, more than five lifetime blood transfusions, no human leukocyte antigen (HLA)-B

Table 36.1 Rank order incidence of end-stage renal disease in children and adults

Rank	Children	Frequency (%)	Adults	Frequency (%)
1	Primary glomerulonephritis	30	Diabetes mellitus	40
2	Cystic/hereditary/congenital diseases	26	Hypertension	27
3	Interstitial nephritis/pyelonephritis	9	Primary glomerulonephritis	10
4	Secondary glomerulonephritis	9	Interstitial nephritis/pyelonephritis	4

Percentages are approximate.
Data from US Renal Data System (1999).

Table 36.2 Point system for cadaver kidney allocation

Variable	Points
Waiting time	1/year
Longest wait	Fraction of 1
PRA > 80%	4
Renal donor	4
Histocompatibility	0–7 (zero A,B,DR mismatch is mandatory share)
Children	
0–10 years old	4
11–17 years old	3

Adapted from UNOS (1995).
PRA: panel reactive antibody. A transplant candidate's serum is tested against a panel of lymphocytes from HLA-typed individuals. If they have a high PRA percentage, it means that they have antibodies to many HLA antigens, and that it will be difficult to get a cross-match negative kidney for them.

or HLA-DR match, and African–American race. The risk of kidney graft loss due to rejection is highest among adolescents because of difficulty adhering to a demanding follow-up regimen.

Selection and preparation of kidney transplant recipients

The pretransplant evaluation is a multidisciplinary process that occurs well in advance of renal transplantation and immunosuppression (Fig. 36.1) (Lemmers and Barry, 1993; Barry, 1998). The purposes of the evaluation are to diagnose the primary renal disease and its risk of recurrence in the kidney transplant and to exclude active invasive infection, obvious operative risk factors, significant risk of post-transplant non-compliance, active malignancy, and anatomy unsuitable for technical success.

Recurrence of original disease as a cause of graft failure is greatest for oxalosis, and then for type II membranoproliferative glomerulonephritis, focal segmental glomerulosclerosis, and hemolytic uremic syndrome, in descending order (Tejani *et al.*, 1998). Type 1 hyperoxaluria is probably best treated with combined liver and kidney transplantation (Watts *et al.*, 1991).

Infection is a major cause of morbidity and the most common cause of death in children after renal transplantation (Tejani *et al.*, 1998; US Renal Data System, 1999). The recommended pretransplant US immunization schedule for children includes immunizations against hepatitis B, diphtheria, tetanus, pertussis, *Haemophilus influenza* type b, polio, mumps, measles, rubella, varicella, and *Pneumococcus* (American Academy of Pediatrics, 1998). Chest radiographs and tuberculin skin tests are used to screen for pulmonary infection. Nephrectomy is done for persistent or recurrent pyelonephritis, persistent nephrolithiasis, or significant hydronephrosis.

The risk of perioperative mortality is very low in children.

The parents and the child must be able to follow a chronic multidrug post-transplant regimen, and pretransplant financial and social evaluations are necessary to identify and correct problems that could result in non-compliance.

If the child has undergone treatment for malignancy, for example bilateral Wilms' tumor, a minimal waiting time of 2 cancer-free years from the time of last cancer treatment is recommended (Kasiske *et al.*, 1995).

Unsuitable anatomy for technical success is usually due to vascular abnormalities or urinary tract dysfunction. If vascular abnormalities are suspected because of other congenital anomalies or prior renal transplantation, Doppler flow studies can be used to screen the potential sites for renal revascularization. Arteriography and venography are reserved for cases with significantly abnormal or unclear findings. The

Table 36.3 Kidney transplant graft survival rates in children

Donor	No.	1 year	2 years	5 years
Cadaver	2502	80%	73%	60%
Living	2213	90%	86%	76%

Data from Tejani *et al.* (1998).

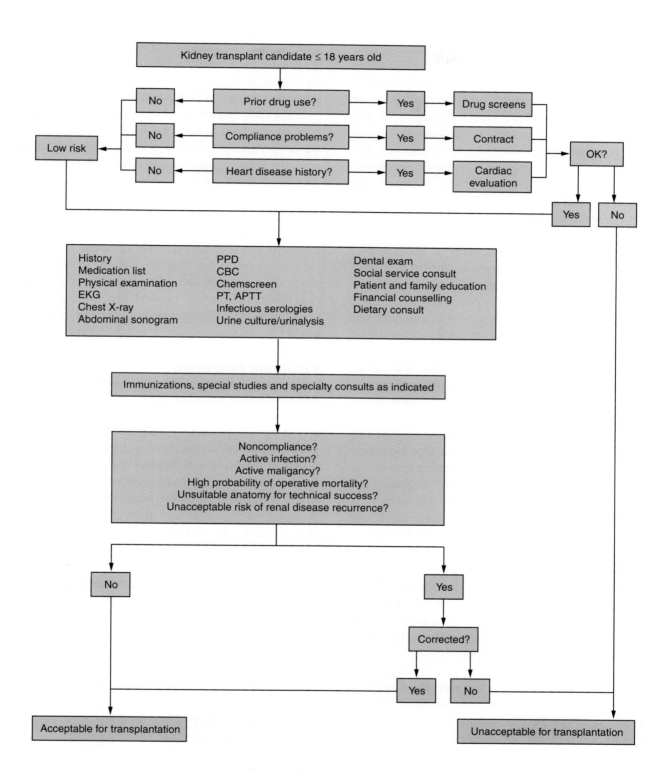

Figure 36.1 Algorithm for the evaluation of pediatric renal transplant candidates. Circumstances may change the order in which data are obtained. EKG, electrocardiogram; CBC, complete blood count; PPD, tuberculin test; PT, prothrombin time; APTT, activate partial prothromboplastin time. (Modified from Lemmers and Barry, 1993; Barry, 1998.)

pretransplant urologic evaluation consists of a history for urologic disease (voiding dysfunction, urinary tract surgeries, infection, obstruction, reflux, stones, and tumors), physical examination (location of scars, stomas and abdominal catheters that could interfere with renal transplantation), urinalysis, bladder or urinary reservoir culture, and sonography of the abdomen and pelvis to include the kidneys, ureters and a postvoid bladder image. In the absence of a history suggestive of urologic abnormalities, hematuria, bacteriuria, calculi, hydronephrosis, or significant bladder residual urine, further imaging of the urinary tract is unnecessary. Patients with suspected voiding dysfunction with or without a history of pyelonephritis are commonly screened with a voiding cystourethrogram and, if necessary, are further evaluated with urodynamics and cystourethroscopy. If a urinary diversion or continent urinary pouch is present, a retrograde contrast study with antibiotic coverage and drainage films will determine its suitability for use or for urinary tract reconstruction during renal transplantation. The urinary reservoir, whether it is a bladder, augmented bladder, or gastrointestinal pouch, must accommodate a reasonable urine volume at low pressure and allow the patient to be dry (Gonzalez, 1997). Bladder augmentation should be restricted to the treatment of urinary incontinence or decreased bladder compliance with proven adverse effects on the upper urinary tract. Urothelial-lined augmentation should be used whenever possible. The care of a patient with a bladder augmentation from stomach or intestine is problematic when the patient has oligoanuria. In the case of the former, peptic perforation is a risk; in the case of the latter, mucus often needs to be irrigated from the bladder on a daily basis. If the bladder has been defunctionalized for a long period, bladder cycling can be done before transplantation in an attempt to determine its compliance. However, transplantation into a small bladder is sometimes necessary because clinical circumstances do not allow a trial of bladder cycling. If, a few months after transplantation, the functionally compromised urinary bladder does not have a reasonable capacity at low pressure and does not allow urinary continence with anticholinergic therapy, augmentation cystoplasty may be necessary to protect the new kidney.

The indications for bilateral nephrectomy in children are the same as in adults. These include uncontrolled hypertension, persistent or recurrent renal infection, renal calculi, renal obstruction, severe proteinuria, persistent antiglomerular basement membrane antibody levels, acquired renal cystic disease with tumors, and kidneys that are so large that there is no room for a renal transplant. It is more common for nephrectomies to be performed at the time of renal transplantation in children than it is in adults.

In the cyclosporine era, donor-specific transfusions have largely been abandoned because of the risk of donor-specific sensitization and the exclusion of a potential kidney donor (Kasiske *et al.*, 1995). They may be of benefit if the process allows reduction in immunosuppression or the exclusion of an ambivalent donor (Barry *et al.*, 1998).

When the patient is admitted for kidney transplantation, donor-specific cytotoxic cross-match results are confirmed to be negative and the history and physical examination focus on a search for acute invasive infections, interval medical problems, and the need for additional cross-matching because of recent blood transfusions.

Recipient operation

After the induction of anesthesia and placement of a central catheter for venous pressure monitoring, fluid and drug administration, and blood sampling, the genitalia and skin are prepared and a Foley catheter is placed in the bladder or bladder substitute. Catheter size is determined by calibration of the urethra or stoma with bougies and the bladder or its substitute is rinsed and then gravity filled to a pressure of approximately 30 cmH$_2$O with a broad-spectrum antibiotic solution (Barry *et al.*, 1998; Lashley *et al.*, 1999). This is facilitated by using a Y-connector so that the bladder can be filled and drained during the transplantation procedure. Abdominal tubes, such as chronic peritoneal dialysis catheters and gastrostomy buttons, can be cleaned with adhesive remover and alcohol, and simply prepped into the operative field. Unless an abdominal stoma can be securely excluded from the operative site, it is irrigated with a broad-spectrum antibiotic solution, the contents are drained, and the stoma is prepped into the surgical site or covered with a sterile antiseptic adhesive barrier.

For children who weigh more than 20 kg, it is usually possible to use an extraperitoneal approach through a modified Gibson incision, much as one would in an adult (Lashley *et al.*, 1999; Barry, 1999b). The sites for renovascular reconstruction are best chosen by placing the kidney graft into the

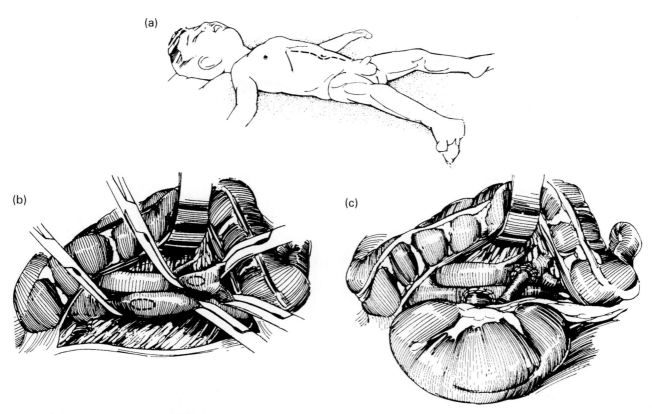

Figure 36.2 Transplantation of adult kidney into small child. (*a*) A transperitoneal vertical midline incision is the most common approach. (*b*) The usual venous anastomotic site is the inferior vena cava. The usual arterial anastomotic sites are the distal aorta or right common iliac artery. (*c*) Revascularization of the adult kidney transplant has been completed. Interrupted vascular suture lines are unnecessary because the anastomoses are the same diameter as if they were in an adult recipient. (From Hinman, 1998a.)

wound and determining the best fit. The renal artery anastomosis is usually completed first because it is the smaller of the two vascular anstomoses and the kidney can be more easily moved about for exposure of the suture line when it has not been tethered by a previously completed venous anastomosis. Whenever possible, the right kidney is transplanted into the left iliac fossa, and the left kidney into the right iliac fossa. This facilitates access for any future open urinary tract repairs because the renal pelvis and proximal ureter are placed anterior and medial to the renal vessels. When a very small child is to receive a large kidney transplant, it is common to use a vertical midline transperitoneal approach, mobilize and retract the right colon and cecum medially, place the kidney in the right retroperitoneum, and anastomose the spatulated renal artery to the aorta or right common iliac artery and the renal vein to the inferior vena cava or common iliac vein (Fig. 36.2) (Hinman,

1998a; Barry *et al.*, 1998; Barry, 1999b; Lashley *et al.*, 1999). It is often necessary to shorten the renal vein when transplanting an adult left kidney into a small child to prevent a kink in the renal vein after revascularization. Since the anastomoses are the same circumference as they would be in an adult, it is not necessary to use an interrupted suture technique (Lashley *et al.*, 1999).

Donor kidneys are usually preserved by simple cold storage after flushing them with an ice-cold high concentration potassium solution. Acute hyperkalemia with renal revascularization can be prevented in children who weigh less than 10 kg by reflushing the kidneys with ice-cold, extracellular potassium-concentration Ringer's lactate solution just prior to transplantation (Barry *et al.*, 1998).

Heparin, 30 units/kg, is administered intravenously before the application of arterial clamps, and low dose heparin, 5–10 units per kg/h i.v., is continued

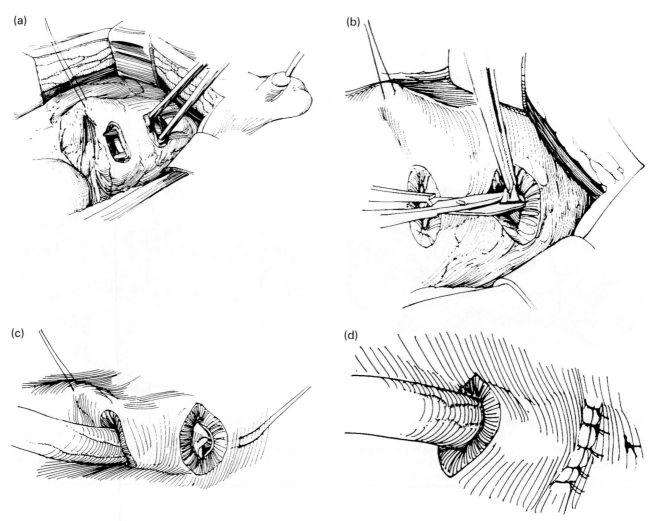

Figure 36.3 Parallel incision extravesical ureteroneocystostomy. (*a*) A submucosal tunnel is created between transverse parallel incisions 2 cm apart after the bladder has been filled with an antibiotic solution through a Y-connector. (*b*) A cystotomy is made after the bladder has been drained. (*c*) The ureter is led through the submucosal tunnel and anastomosed to the bladder mucosa with fine absorbable sutures. A distal mattress suture through all thicknesses of the ureter and bladder anchors the toe of the ureter to the bladder and prevents sliding in the submucosal tunnel. (*d*) Completed extravesical ureteroneocystostomy with closure of the distal seromuscular incision. (From Hinman, 1998b.)

for 3–5 days until the results of a postoperative hypercoagulation profile are known and a determination has been made about long-term anticoagulation. This is because one of the common causes of early graft loss in pediatric kidney transplantation is vascular thrombosis (Tejani *et al.*, 1998). The heparin is not reversed. At the time of renal revascularization, goals for mean arterial pressure, systolic blood pressure, and central venous pressure are ≥ 60 mmHg, ≥ 90 mmHg, and about 10 cmH$_2$O, respectively.

This is usually achieved by the intravenous administration of crystalloid, 15 ml/kg per hour with or without albumin, 0.5 g/kg per hour. Intraoperative blood loss is replaced ml for ml, and sometimes an additional 100 ml of packed red blood cells is administered to replace anticipated acute blood loss into the kidney graft with vascular clamp release in a small child. If the blood pressure goals are not met with intravenous fluid, but the central venous pressure goal has been achieved, up to 5 μg/kg per minute of dopamine is administered. In an attempt to assure a diuresis, mannitol 0.5 g/kg is infused over 1 hour during the vascular anastomoses, and furosemide 1 mg/kg is administered intravenously just before removal of the vascular clamps. The usual sequence for vascular clamp removal is from the proximal vein, then from the artery or arteries, and finally from the distal vein.

Ureteroneocystostomy is the most common form of urinary tract reconstruction. Many surgeons prefer an extravesical technique rather than a transvesical technique because a separate cystotomy is not required, and less ureteral length is necessary (Fig. 36.3) (Hinman, 1998b). It is important to anchor the toe of the spatulated ureter to the muscularis of the bladder to prevent sliding of the ureter in the submucosal tunnel and loss of the antireflux mechanism. Ureteroureterostomy and ureteropyelostomy are optional methods of urinary tract reconstruction. Double-pigtail ureteral stents are used routinely by some surgeons and selectively by others. The generally accepted indications for stent use are premature bladder entry, thickened bladder muscularis, a scarred urinary bladder, and reconstruction by ureteroureterostomy, ureteropyelostomy, or ureteroenterostomy. A closed suction drain is commonly placed in the operative site, and the wound closed by surgeon preference. A subcuticular skin closure with absorbable suture will eliminate the morbidity of suture or clip removal.

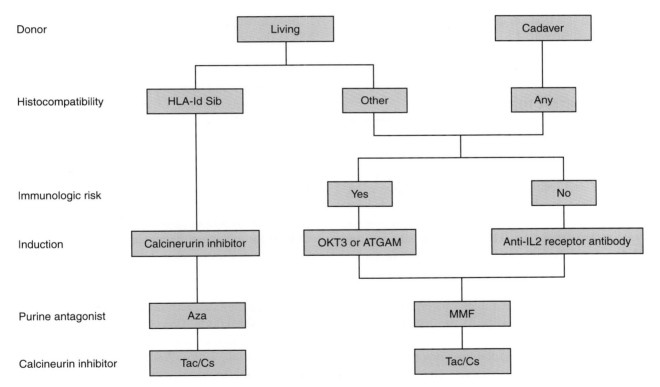

Figure 36.4 Kidney transplant immunosuppression protocol for a child. This algorithm is an example of immunosuppression individuation based on histocompatibility, immunologic risk factors, effectiveness, cost, and toxicity. All recipients receive glucocorticoids. Antibody induction therapy has been shown to prevent, delay, or abrogate rejection crises within the first few months after transplantation. In cadaver kidney transplantation, it allows the kidney to recover from preservation injury before the administration of a nephrotoxic calcineruin inhibitor. Anti-interleukin-2 receptor antibodies (diclizumab and basiliximab) are commonly used for induction therapy. Muromonab-CD3 (OKT3) and antithymocyte gamma globulin (ATGAM) are sometimes used for induction therapy in immunologic high-risk recipients. Immunologic risk factors are high panel reactive antibody levels, African–American recipient, positive flow cross-match, ABO blood group A2 kidney into O or B recipient, and repeat transplantation. Less immunosuppression is necessary in recipients of human leukocyte antigen-identical sibling kidney transplants. (Modified from Barry, 1999a.)

Postoperative care

Insensible fluid loss is replaced with 5% dextrose in 0.45 normal saline. Urinary output is replaced, milliliter for milliliter, with 0.45 normal saline. If a dextrose-containing solution is used for urinary replacement in a diuresing patient, the diuresis can be prolonged because of glucosuria. Pain control is with patient-controlled analgesia with or without epidural analgesia. Perioperative antibiotics are continued until the results of intraoperative bladder and cadaver kidney transplant cultures indicate discontinuance or a change. The bladder catheter is removed on the 5th postoperative day, and a single dose of a broad-spectrum antibiotic is administered. If there is concern about the integrity of the ureteroneocystostomy, a cystogram is done and absence of extravasation is confirmed prior to catheter removal. The closed suction drain is removed when the drainage is ≤ 50 ml/24 h. If a ureteral stent has been placed, it is removed 6–12 weeks later.

Renal allograft rejection

The most common cause of kidney transplant failure in children is rejection (Tejani et al., 1998). The risk of rejection is reduced by histocompatibility between the donor and recipient and by immunosuppression (Barry, 1998). In descending order, the best kidney transplant survival rates are when the kidney is from a monozygotic twin, an HLA-identical sibling, an HLA-half-matched relative, an HLA-mismatched relative, an unrelated living donor, or a cadaver donor.

Hyperacute rejection is very rare. It occurs within days of transplantation and is due to preformed circulating cytotoxic antibodies in the recipient. This type of kidney transplant rejection is prevented by avoidance of renal transplantation when the lymphocytotoxic cross-matches between the donor and recipient are positive. Acute rejection is primarily due to cytotoxic T-lymphocytes, and it is usually reversed with a short course of high-dose glucocorticoids. If this treatment fails and a biopsy indicates persistent acute rejection, an antilymphocyte antibody, such as muromonab CD3 or antilymphocyte gamma-globulin, is usually administered. Chronic transplant nephropathy is due to chronic, antibody-mediated rejection, or to nephrotoxicity from calcineurin inhibitors, such as cyclosporine and tacrolimus.

Prophylactic immunosuppression and infection prophylaxis are outlined as follows (Barry, 1998; Barry et al., 1998) and in Figure 36.4 (Barry, 1999a):

- broad-spectrum i.v. antibiotic perioperatively for skin and urinary tract organisms;
- antibiotic into bladder after anesthesia induction;
- antibiotic wound irrigation intraoperatively;
- trimethoprim–sulfamethoxazole for 6 months to prevent urinary tract infection (UTI) and Pneumocystis pneumonia;
- acyclovir or ganciclovir as necessary to prevent herpes simplex virus-1 (HSV-1), HSV-2, varicella zoster virus (VZV), Epstein–Barr virus (EBV), and cytomegalovirus (CMV) infection;
- CMV immune globulin for 4 months as necessary for risk of primary CMV disease.

Immunosuppression, except in HLA-identical sibling donor kidney transplants, is usually with antilymphocyte antibody induction plus a glucocorticoid, a purine antagonist, and a calceinurin inhibitor. Muromonab CD3 and antilymphocyte gamma-globulin prevent the recognition of donor antigens by the recipient's T-lymphocytes (Burk and Matuszewski, 1997). Muromonab CD3 is associated with the cytokine release syndrome, and acute pulmonary edema occurs in recipients who are fluid overloaded. Because of the need to fill the vascular space of small children who receive adult kidneys to prevent vascular thrombosis and acute kidney graft loss, this agent is usually not used for induction therapy in this group (Barry et al., 1998). Anti-interleukin 2 (IL-2) receptor monoclonal antibodies such as diclizumab (Charpentier and Thurvet, 1998) and basiliximab (Nashan et al., 1997) prevent lymphocyte activation by IL-2 and have almost no side-effects. Glucocorticoids inhibit proinflammatory cytokines and reduce lymphocyte counts (DeMattos et al., 1996). Azathioprine and mycophenolate mofetil interfere with purine synthesis and inhibit proliferation of T- and B-lymphocytes in response to antigens (DeMattos et al., 1996). The calceinurin inhibitors, cyclosporine and tacrolimus, suppress the transcription of IL-2 and other lymphokines (DeMattos et al., 1996). The immunosuppressive protocols used in pediatric and adult renal transplant recipients are similar. However, there are differences in drug dosing because children have less intestinal surface area, increased rates of metabolism, and the need for growth (Ettinger, 1992).

Problems

An algorithm for the management of fluid collections is presented in Figure 36.5 (Barry, 1994). Lymphoceles have been successfully managed by sclerosis (Gilliland *et al.*, 1989) or by drainage into the peritoneal cavity with laparoscopic or open surgical procedures (Gill *et al.*, 1995).

An algorithm for the diagnosis of ureteral obstruction is presented in Figure 36.6 (Barry,

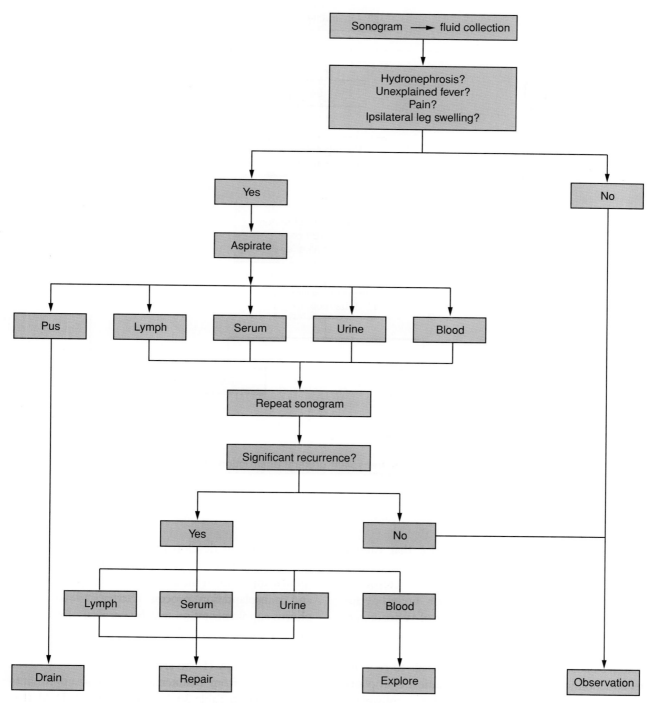

Figure 36.5 Algorithm for evaluation and treatment of perigraft fluid collection. (Modified from Barry, 1994.)

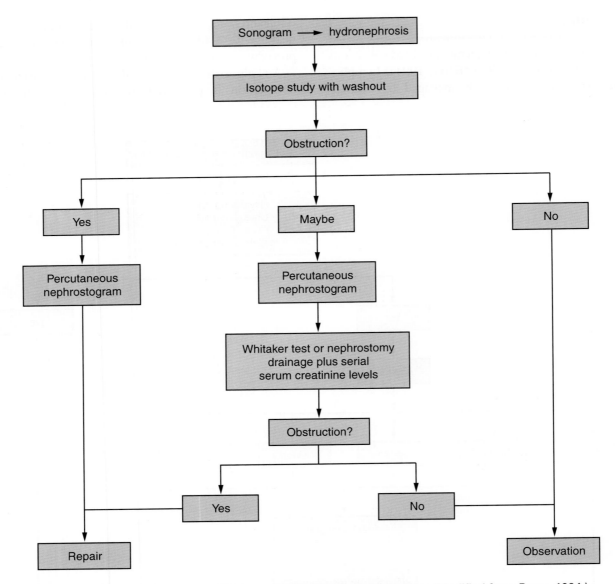

Figure 36.6 Algorithm for evaluation of kidney transplant ureteral obstruction. (Modified from Barry, 1994.)

1994). Ureteral strictures and fistulae that cannot be managed by minimally invasive techniques require urinary tract reconstruction by ureteroneocystostomy, ureteroureterostomy, or ureteropyelostomy. The indications for the repair of vesicoureteral reflux are the same as in non-transplant patients.

If a previously compromised but adequate urinary bladder becomes non-compliant and fails to respond to anticholinergic therapy, augmentation cystoplasty is necessary to protect the kidney transplant (Gonzalez, 1997).

Children can develop marked hypophosphatemia due to secondary hyperparathyroidism or due to tubular injury from the kidney retrieval, preservation, and transplantation process (Better, 1980). Phosphorus supplementation may be necessary for days to months following renal transplantation. Mild hyperparathyroidism usually responds favorably to oral calcitriol therapy (Lobo *et al*., 1995).

Toxicities from maintenance immunosuppressants are outlined in Table 36.4 (Ettinger, 1992; DeMattos *et al*., 1996; Barry *et al*., 1998; Lashley *et al*., 1999).

Table 36.4 Toxicity of maintenance immunosuppressants

Immunosuppressant	Toxicity
Glucocorticoids	Growth failure, abnormal fat distribution, impaired wound healing, dyslipidemia, glucose intolerance, acne
Cyclosporine	Nephrotoxicity, neurotoxicity, hirsutism, gingival hyperplasia, dyslipidemia
Tacrolimus	Nephrotoxicity, neurotoxicity, gastrointestinal upset, glucose intolerance
Azathioprine	Leukopenia
Mycophenolate mofetil	Leukopenia, gastrointestinal upset

Data from Ettinger (1992), DeMattos *et al.* (1996), Barry *et al.* (1998) and Lashley *et al.* (1999).

Growth failure is more common if the child is more than 6 years old at the time of transplantation (Tejani *et al.*, 1998). Following transplantation, growth failure can be managed by conversion of the daily steroid dose to every other day (Jabs *et al.*, 1996), and, in some cases, by tapering the child completely off glucocorticoids (Ingulli *et al.*, 1993). If those maneuvers fail, and if graft function is normal, growth hormone has been administered and resulted in significant growth (Fine *et al.*, 1992). The main concerns about treatment with growth hormone are the risks of malignancy and kidney transplant rejection. A controlled study by the North American Pediatric Renal Transplant Cooperative Study group is currently underway. Hypertension is a common problem. If it is difficult to manage after transplantation, native nephrectomy may facilitate blood pressure control. Tacrolimus and cyclosporine are both nephrotoxic, and both can contribute to post-transplant hypertension (DeMattos *et al.*, 1996). The choice of initial calcineurin inhibitor is often based on the side-effect profile. Although unusual, new-onset diabetes mellitus has been associated with tacrolimus immunosuppression in children (Moxey-Mimms *et al.*, 1998). The pattern of *de novo* malignancies in pediatric organ transplant recipients is different from the general pediatric population, and the predominant neoplasm is lymphoproliferative disease, followed by skin cancer (Penn, 1998).

Conclusions

The preferred treatment for children with ESRD is renal transplantation. Kidney transplantation into small children is a remarkable technical achievement. Renal transplantation should not be considered a cure for ESRD but simply another form of therapy that requires chronic daily drug administration and careful monitoring for compliance, kidney graft dysfunction, and complications. When the transplant is successful, the child is almost completely rehabilitated.

References

American Academy of Pediatrics, Committee on Infectious Diseases (1998) Recommended Childhood Immunization Schedule – United States, January–December, 1998. *Pediatrics* 1998; **101**: 155–6.

Barry JM (1994) Renal transplantation. In: Krane RJ, Siroky MB, Fitzpatrick JM (eds) *Clinical urology*. Philadelphia, PA: J.B. Lippincott, 335–7.

Barry JM (1998) Renal transplantation. In: Walsh PC, Retik AB, Vaughan ED, Wein AJ (eds) *Campbell's urology*. 7th edition. Philadelphia, PA: WB Saunders, 523.

Barry JM (1999a) Renal transplantation. *Curr Opin Urol* **9**: 121–7.

Barry JM (1999b) Technical aspects of renal transplantation. In: Schrier RW, Bennett WM, Henrich WL (eds) *Atlas of diseases of the kidney*. volume 5, Section 2. *Transplantation as treatment of end-stage renal disease 1999*. Philadelphia, PA: Current Medicine, 14.1–12.

Barry JM, Reller KS, Lande MB *et al.* (1998) Transplantation von Spendernieren Erwachsener auf Kinder. *Aktuelle Urol* **29**: 239–45.

Better OS (1980) Tubular dysfunction following kidney transplantation. *Nephron* **25**: 209–13.

Burk ML, Matuszewski KA (1997) Muromonab-CD3 and antithymocyte globulin in renal transplantation. *Ann Pharmacother* **31**: 1370–7.

Charpentier B, Thurvet E (1998) Placebo-controlled study of humanized anti-TAC monoclonal antibody in dual therapy for the prevention of acute rejection after renal transplantation. *Transplant Proc* **30**: 1331–2.

DeMattos AM, Olyaei AJ, Bennett WM (1996) Pharmacology of immunosuppressive medications used in renal diseases and transplantation. *Am J Kidney Dis* **28**: 631–67.

Ettinger RB (1992) Children are different: the challenges of pediatric renal transplantation. *Am J Kidney Dis* **20**: 668–72.

Fine RN, Yadin O, Moultem L *et al.* (1992) Extended recombinant human growth hormone treatment after renal transplantation in children. *J Am Soc Nephrol* **2**: S274–83.

Gill IS, Hodge EE, Munch LC *et al.* (1995) Transperitoneal marsupialization of lymphoceles: a comparison of laparoscopic and open techniques. *J Urol* **153**: 706–11.

Gilliland JD, Spies JB, Brown SB *et al.* (1989) Lymphoceles: percutaneous treatment with povidone-iodine sclerosis. *Radiology* **171**: 227–9.

Gonzalez R (1997) Renal transplantation into abnormal bladders. *J Urol* **158**: 895–6.

Hinman F Jr (1998a) Renal reconstruction: renal transplantation in children. In: Hinman F Jr (ed.) *Atlas of urologic surgery*. 2nd edition. Philadelphia, PA: WB Saunders, 962–3.

Hinman F Jr (1998b) Ureteral reconstruction and excision: ureteroneocystostomy, external tunnel technique. In: Hinman F Jr (ed.) *Atlas of urologic surgery*. 2nd edition. Philadelphia, PA: WB Saunders, 797–8.

Ingulli E, Sharma B, Saing HA *et al.* (1993) Steroid withdrawal, rejection, and mixed lymphocyte reaction in children after renal transplantation. *Kidney Int* **43**: S36–9.

Jabs K, Sullivan EK, Avner ED *et al.* (1996) Alternate-day steroid dosing improves growth without adversely affecting graft survival or long-term graft function: a report of the North American Pediatric Renal Transplant Cooperative Study. *Transplantation* **61**: 31–6.

Kasiske BL, Ramos EL, Gaston RS *et al.* (1995) The evaluation of renal transplant candidates: clinical practice guidelines. *J Am Soci Nephrol* **6**: 1–34.

Lashley DB, Barry JM, DeMattos AM *et al.* (1999) Kidney transplantation in children: a single-center experience. *J Urol* **161**: 1920–5.

Lemmers MJ, Barry JM (1993) Dialysis as compared with transplantation as replacement therapy for end-stage renal disease. *Curr Opin Urol* **3**: 110–5.

Lobo PT, Cortez MS, Stevenson W *et al.* (1995) Normal calcemic hyperparathyroidism associated with relatively low 1,25 vitamin D levels post-renal transplantation can be successfully treated with oral calcitriol. *Clin Transplant* **9**: 277–81.

Moxey-Mimms MM, Kay C, Light JA *et al.* (1998) Increased incidence of insulin-dependent diabetes mellitus in pediatric renal transplant patients receiving tacrolimus (FK506), *Transplantation* **65**: 617–9.

Nashan B, Moor ER, Amlot P *et al.* (1997) Randomized trial of basiliximab versus placebo for control of acute cellular rejection in renal allograft recipients. *Lancet* **350**: 1193–8.

NIH (1993) NIH Consensus Development Conference: Morbidity and Mortality of Dialysis. *NIH Consensus Statement* **11(2)**: 1–31.

Penn I (1998) *De novo* malignancies in pediatric organ transplant recipients. *Pediatr Transplant* **2**: 56–63.

Tejani AH, Sullivan EK, Harmon WE *et al.* (1998) Pediatric renal transplantation – the NAPRTCS experience. In: Cecka JM, Terasaki PI (eds), *Clinical transplants 1997*. Los Angeles, CA: UCLA Tissue Typing Laboratory, 87–100.

United Network for Organ Sharing (UNOS) (1995) *Articles of Incorporation, By-Laws, and Policies:* Policy 3.5, Allocation of Cadaveric Kidneys. Richmond, VA: UNOS, 28 June 1995.

US Renal Data System (1999) *USRDS: 1999 Annual Data Report*. Bethesda, MD: National Institutes of Health, National Institute of Diabetes and Digestive and Kidney Diseases, Division of Kidney, Urologic, and Hematologic Diseases, April 1999.

Watts RWE, Morgan SH, Danpure CJ *et al.* (1991) Combined hepatic and renal transplantation in primary hyperoxaluria type 1: clinical report of nine cases. *Am J Med* 179–88.

Yadin O, Fine RN (1997) Long-term use of recombinant human growth hormone in children with chronic renal insufficiency. *Kidney Int* **58**: S114–117.

Cadaveric kidney: pediatric renal organ donation

37

Lawrence Gibel

Introduction

The need for cadaveric kidneys for transplantation has expanded greatly. The number of patients in the USA with end-stage renal disease has doubled during the 1990s and criteria for candidacy for renal transplantation have also been liberalized. One year cadaveric kidney graft survival improved from 75.7% nationally in 1994 to 84.4% in 1998, with patient survival rates improving from 92.2% to 94.7% (UNOS, 1996). Meanwhile, the number of patients registered on the US national waiting list increased from 13 943 in 1988 to 31 149 in 1995. New annual patient waiting list registrations increased from 11 909 in 1995 to 17 635 in 1998, and median waiting times for transplantation have more than doubled from 400 days in 1988 to 842 days in 1994 (UNOS, 1996). In 1995, the new registrant waiting list accrued at over twice the rate of cadaveric transplants performed (UNOS, 1996). The disparity between need and availability for transplantation of cadaveric hearts and livers is similar, with the impact on patient mortality being far greater among new registrants. Waiting patients are subject to a mortality of 432 and 287 deaths per 1000 patients for hearts and livers, respectively (UNOS, 1996). The paucity of organs for transplantation is a serious and significant healthcare crisis.

Given the dire need for transplantable organs, the transplant community has always attempted to expand the criteria for acceptable donors. Efforts between 1988 and 1995 to use older donors (age > 65 years) and young donors (age < 10 years) were met with reduced graft survival (Fig. 37.1). Donors aged 10 years and younger result in reduced 1 year

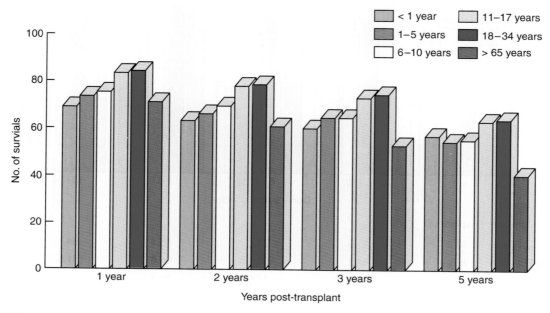

Figure 37.1 Graft survival by donor age (1988–95).

graft survival but no increase in subsequent long-term graft loss compared with donor ages with optimal outcomes. Pediatric donors result in identical transplant recipient survival when compared to optimally aged donors (Fig. 37.2). Strategies using young donors with a reduction in early graft loss due to vascular complications and early rejection have been successful in several single-center series. Comparing 1995 to 1988 UNOS data (Fig. 37.3), the number of pediatric organ donors aged less than 11 years has diminished while the number of donors age 11–17 has increased. The percentage of possible pediatric organ donors who actually undergo kidney donation has increased for donors less than 6 years of age. This increase in donors is particularly striking in infants under 1 year of age (Fig. 37.4).

The use of pediatric cadaveric renal allografts, and whether to use single-unit or dual-unit grafts transplanted *en bloc* remain highly controversial subjects. Often cited observations regarding very young kidney donors include: young donor kidneys do not tolerate the higher arterial pressures seen in adult recipients, they do not tolerate rejection well, they are susceptible to hyperfiltration injury, and they experience an increased risk of vascular thrombosis and increased ureteral complications. However, individual series demonstrate that young donor kidneys can function well after transplantation, and therefore they should be used to increase the availability of cadaveric kidneys for transplantation.

Selection criteria

Most transplant centers restrict the use of kidneys to donors older than 10 years because of national data demonstrating reduced graft survival from younger donors. A minority of centers use younger donors weighing approximately 9–20 kg, usually using both kidneys engrafted *en bloc* to a single recipient. The results have been excellent (Amante and Kahan, 1996; Portoles *et al.*, 1996; Bretan *et al.*, 1997; Lledo-Garcia *et al.*, 1997; Ratner *et al.*, 1997; Burrows *et al.*, 1996; Satterwaiter *et al.*, 1997). Anecdotal experience exists for even younger donors. To date no data are available to establish the minimum acceptable size criteria for either *en bloc* or single allograft donors.

Medical exclusionary criteria are similar to those for adult donors and include disseminated infection, malignancy, and significant renal impairment.

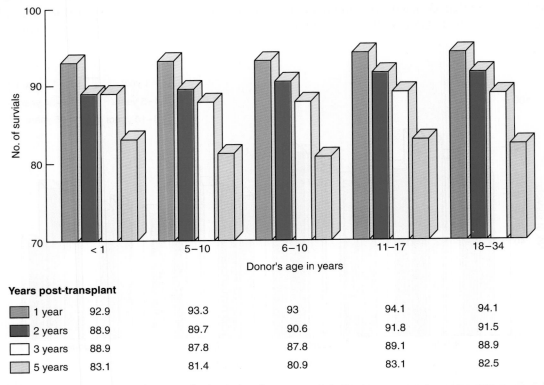

Years post-transplant

	< 1	5–10	6–10	11–17	18–34
1 year	92.9	93.3	93	94.1	94.1
2 years	88.9	89.7	90.6	91.8	91.5
3 years	88.9	87.8	87.8	89.1	88.9
5 years	83.1	81.4	80.9	83.1	82.5

Figure 37.2 Cadaveric kidney patient survival rate by donor age.

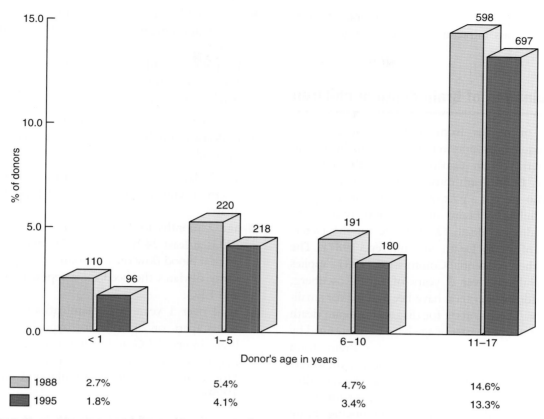

	1988	5.4%	4.7%	14.6%
	1988	2.7%		
	1995	1.8%	4.1%	3.4%	13.3%

Figure 37.3 Percentage of pediatric donors by age. Actual number of donors are shown above bars.

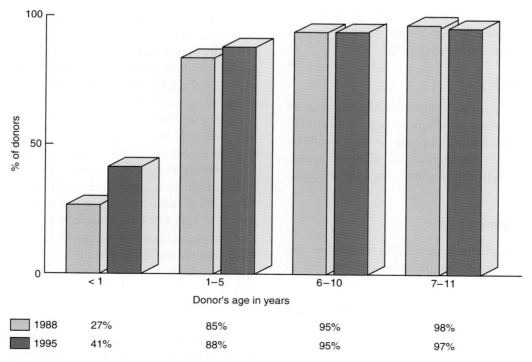

	1988	27%	85%	95%	98%
	1995	41%	88%	95%	97%

Figure 37.4 Percentage of pediatric donors with kidney donation.

Patients with primary, non-malignant brain tumors without previous intracranial surgery are acceptable donors.

Determination of brain death in children

Retrieval of organs from heart-beating cadaveric donors requires pronouncement of death by neurologic criteria (brain death) prior to the retrieval procedure. Brain death must be determined by physicians who are not a part of the donor or transplant service. Children's brains may be more resistant to insults leading to death (Task Force for the Determination of Brain Death in Children, 1987). The report of the Presidential Commission (1981) applies only to children over 5 years of age (Rosenberg, 1995). Additional criteria have been added for smaller children. These criteria for diagnosing brain death in children under 5 years of age have been outlined by the Task Force for the Determination of Brain Death in Children (1987). For term newborns, these recommendations require a waiting period of 7 days during which the patient's status is consistent with apparent neurologic death, before pronouncing brain death. The approach to the pronouncement of brain death can be made more uniform and criteria more specific by incorporating a form that specifies required examinations and their results (Appendix 1) (University of New Mexico Health Sciences Center, Staff Policies and Procedures, 1997).

Medical history

The treating physicians should determine the cause of coma. It is especially important to rule out potentially reversible insults including toxic and metabolic disorders, sedative hypnotic drugs, paralytic agents, hypothermia, hypotension, and surgically treatable conditions.

Physical examination

The criteria for physical examination required for the pronouncement of brain death in children are as follows:

- coma: no spontaneous movement, flaccid tone, no response to stimuli including deep pain (temperature $\geq 32°C$);
- absence of brain stem function (temperature $\geq 32°C$);

- apnea with formal apnea testing confirmed by CO_2 tension greater than 60 mmHg (temperature $\geq 36°C$);
- the patient should not be hypotensive or acidotic, and should not be treated with sedative or paralysing agents.

The examination must remain consistent with brain death throughout the entire specified examination period:

- age 7 days to 2 months: two examinations and electroencephalograms (EEGs) at least 48 hours apart;
- age 2 months to 1 year: two examinations and EEGs at least 24 hours apart. Absence of cerebral arterial blood flow on a radionuclide angiographic study obviates the need for a repeat examination and EEG;
- aged over 1 year: two examinations at least 12 hours apart, or 24 hours for hypoxic or ischemic brain injury. EEG and radionuclide angiography may be used to reduce the observation period (Ad Hoc Committee, 1987; Aboulgound and Levy, 1999).

Determination of brain death in the anencephalic infant and potential for organ donation

Anencephalic infants openly exhibit spontaneous movement and startle reflexes, and have most brainstem functions intact. They usually do not experience neurologic death prior to developing sepsis. Peabody *et al.* (1989). Ashwai *et al.* (1990) studied 12 liveborn anencephalic infants, six receiving intensive care including intubation at birth and six receiving intensive care only at imminent death. Two infants progressed to brainstem death, possibly as a result of birth trauma. Owing to the severe malformation associated with anencephaly neither EEG nor cerebral blood flow estimations are accurate or reliable (Medical Task Force on Anencephaly, 1990).

The natural course of anencephalic infants and the legal requirement for brainstem death in determining death prohibit the vast majority of anencephalic infants from being declared dead by neurologic criteria and becoming organ donors. Furthermore, the generally held reluctance to use kidneys from donors weighing less than approximately 9 kg makes anencephalic infants unlikely candidates for kidney donation.

Counseling the family and approaching permission for organ donation

The death of a child, including determination of brain death, the anticipated discontinuation of life support, and counseling of the family enduring these events, is one of the most difficult and emotionally intense responsibilities with which medical and nursing staff deal in the final care of the child (Peabody *et al.*, 1989). These responsibilities include: (1) educating the family as to the nature of the child's medical problems, what brain death is, and why it occurred; (2) providing emotional support to the family and to other children; and (3) contacting the family's religious liaisons, grief counselor, and/or social worker. It can be expected that educating the family about the patient's medical problems and explaining brain death requires repeated contacts. These are complex issues and the magnitude of the family's grief interferes with the intellectualization of simple facts. Physicians and nurses representing donor retrieval programs should anticipate that, despite completion of the death declaration and excellent counseling by healthcare professionals, families often continue to have difficulty in understanding and accepting the brain death state of their loved one. One frequently encounters families verbalizing the magnitude of these feelings years after death and donation.

The decision to donate organs has provided substantial emotional support and acceptance of the child's death to most families proceeding with organ donation. In order to provide the family with adequate opportunity to consider donation, it is necessary for the family to intellectually accept the death. Grief must progress to the point that the decision makers' emotional state is such that they are able to consider the donation without overwhelming negativity. The progress of the donor family to this state is often referred to as 'decoupling'. It can be expected that for some donor families decoupling may take several hours or days. A basic principle in the psychology of the approach for organ donation is that decoupling must occur before the family is approached about organ donation. Often decoupling is lengthy, and approaching the family about organ donation involves a gradual and repeated educational process blended with the decoupling process, before asking the family for donation. This methodology involves careful observation of the family's grief process and may take many hours. Experience has shown that the request is more successful when it involves healthcare professionals, usually from the local donor organization, who are trained and experienced in the diagnosis of brain death, family grief counseling, and medical and legal issues related to organ donation and transplantation.

The battered child

Brain death is not an unusual occurrence in the battered child. The parents or guardians may be suspected or admit to the injuries leading to the child's death. Unless the state has taken formal steps to remove custody the parents or guardians are still legally the next of kin and responsible for deciding about organ donation. In the author's experience, in this situation the parents or guardians often decide in favor of organ donation.

Medical management of the brain-dead child

The principles of management of the brain-dead child are identical to those of the brain-dead adult. Management includes maintaining hemodynamic and metabolic stability. A complete discussion is beyond the scope of this chapter. However, important points should be recapitulated.

Hemodynamic monitoring and support

Unstable donors are best managed with central venous and arterial line monitoring. Frequently, at the time of and/or shortly after brainstem herniation, the patient experiences a sympathetic storm marked by hypertension as well as tachycardia and pronounced vasoconstriction. This may be treated with the short-acting β-blocker esmolol (Breviblock), which effectively reduces both hypertension and tachycardia (Roza and Johnson, 1999). Alternatively, sodium nitroprusside may be used to treat the hypertension, but may exacerbate the donor's tachycardia.

Management of hypotension requires aggressive fluid resuscitation with resultant central venous pressures in the range of 5–8 cmH_2O, urine output greater than 1 ml/kg per hour, and systolic blood pressure appropriate for age. If, despite adequate fluid replacement urine, output remains low, mannitol or furosemide should be given. Fluid solutions should be warmed to prevent exacerbation of hypothermia. Dopamine at low doses (0.5–2.0 μg/kg/per minute) acts as an ionotrope and vasodilates the renovascular bed system. Higher doses may be needed to maintain adequate perfusion pressure. Advantages of the drug are lost at doses greater than 10 μg/kg/per minute. If the response is inadequate, additional supplemental α-agonists should then be considered (Boyd *et al.*, 1991). Dopamine dosage and α-agonists can often be tapered and discontinued with the addition of thyroxine therapy. Thyroxine (T_4) replacement combined with glucose and insulin loading can improve myocardial glycogen stores (Novitsky *et al.*, 1987; Roza and Johnson, 1999).

Hypothermia

Children are more susceptible than adults to hypothermia, owing to their low body mass and high surface area. Hypothermia may delay the declaration of brain death as it results in significant myocardial depression, decreases oxygen delivery by shifting the oxyhemoglobin dissociation curve to the left, and causes coagulopathy at temperatures lower than 32°C (Roza and Johnson, 1999). Prevention and treatment of hypothermia are essential.

Neurogenic diabetes insipidus

Neurogenic diabetes insipidus is very common in brain-dead donors. However, other causes of polyuria exist, including hyperglycemia, fluid overload, and renal tubular injury. Neurogenic diabetes insipidus is characterized by polyuria, hyperosmolality with serum osmolarity greater than 295 mOsm/l, urine osmolarity less than 300 mOsm/l, and a urine specific gravity less than 1.005. Arginine vasopressin (DDAVP) is generally preferred as replacement therapy owing to its decreased splanchnic vasoconstriction compared with anti-diuretic hormone (ADH).

Frequently used medications for donor management

(1) Hypertension with tachycardia
   ■ esmolol:
   – loading dose 500 μg/kg over 1 min;
   – maintenance dose at 50 μg/kg/ minture;
   – repeat loading dose and increase maintenance dose by 50 μg/kg/per minture until a therapeutic effect is achieved or maximal rate of 300 μg/kg/minute is reached.
(2) Neurogenic diabetes insipidus
   ■ DDAVP:
   – 0.1–0.4 μg/kg i.v. over 30 min;

   – repeat dose in 1 hour if urine output is not adequately controlled;
   – maximum dose 1.2 μg/kg over 4 hours.
(3) Hypotension:
   – dopamine 1–10 μg/kg/per minute;
   – dobutamine 5–10 μg/kg/per minute;
   – epinephrine 0.1 μg/kg (starting dose);
   – thyroxine (T_4); 0.3 μg/kg i.v. followed by 0.15 mg/kg/h i.v. starting dose.

Surgical technique for pediatric cadaveric kidney retrieval and special techniques for engraftment

The surgical technique for the retrieval of cadaveric pediatric kidneys for both isolated and *en bloc* transplants is similar to that for adult donors, with modification of the cannulation technique (Fig. 37.5). Surgical technique must be meticulous because of the smaller and more delicate structures. Cooled (~7°C) preservation fluid using Viaspan (Dupont), 50 ml/kg

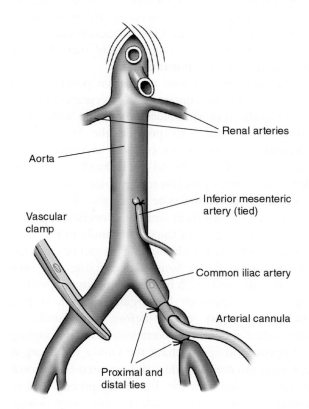

Figure 37.5 Aortic canula placement technique for pediatric cadareric renal donors.

body weight is flushed intraarterially. For retrieval procedures resulting in possible *en bloc* transplantation, modification of the arterial cannula placement, to avoid cannula contact with the aortic lumen, is necessary to prevent intimal injury and increased risk of arterial thrombosis. Cannula placement into the common iliac artery with occlusion of the contralateral iliac system is standard in most centers. Similarly, the use of inferior vena cava cannulae should be avoided. Kidneys that may be transplanted *en bloc* with the usual end-to-side vascular anastomotic technique should be retrieved with the entire length of distal aorta and vena cava, including the bifurcation of the great vessels (Fig. 37.6). When suitably trimmed, the resultant flared distal end is ideally suited to accommodate an appropriately large Carrel patch that will allow for the anticipated growth of the donor kidneys and vasculature (Fig. 37.6b, c). *En bloc* kidneys that are to be transplanted with the standard end-to-side anastomoses require sufficient abdominal aorta to

close the proximal aortic end without comprising the renal arterial orifices. Techniques for achieving this closure are shown in Figure 37.7.

Surgery to minimize ureteral complications recognizes the small ureteral size and delicate ureteral vasculature. Dissection around the renal hilum is minimized. The right ureter may be resected in continuity with the overlying peritoneum and anterior layer of the retroperitoneum. One technique (Fig. 37.8) for the left ureter involves separating the left colon and sigmoid from its mesentery and resecting a small portion of the adjacent sigmoid mesentery *en bloc* with the left ureter. Dissection of both ureters involves dissecting along the iliac arteries and veins, freeing all adjacent tissue, and then retrieving the ureters with all of the tissue anterior to these blood vessels attached. The ureters and their accompanying tissue should also include adjacent segments of the gonadal vessels. The ureters are removed with the overlying anterior and available posterior retroperitoneal tissue. The ureters should be resected close to the bladder. *En bloc* transplantation and its attendant

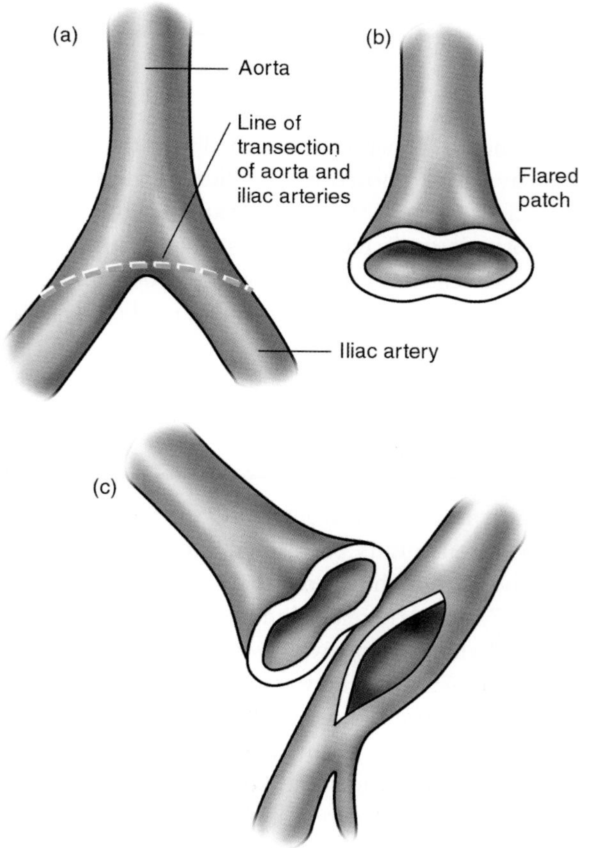

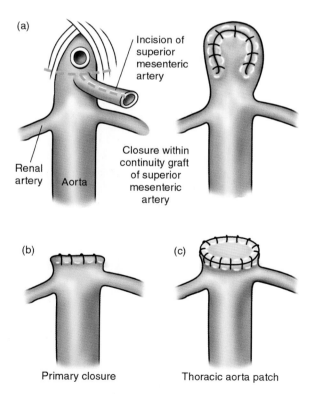

Figure 37.6 (*a*) Technique for trimming distal aorta and (*b*) resultant *en bloc* transplant arterial anastomosis.

Figure 37.7 Closure of proximal aorta in *en bloc* pediatric renal transplantation. (*a*) Using incontinuity superior mestertoric artery. (*b*) Primary closure. (*c*) Patch.

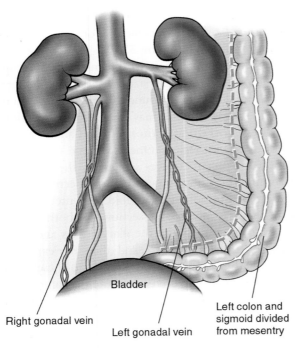

Figure 37.8 Sigmoid messentery taken *en bloc* with the left ureter.

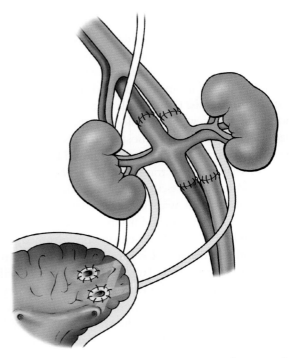

Figure 37.10 Pediatric renal donor engraftment with modified incontinuity vascular techniques. (From Amante and Kahan, 1996, with permission.)

preservation of aortic branches to the ureter is likely to reduce ureteral complications in small donors.

Single allograft pediatric kidneys are transplanted with the same technique as adult kidneys. *En bloc*

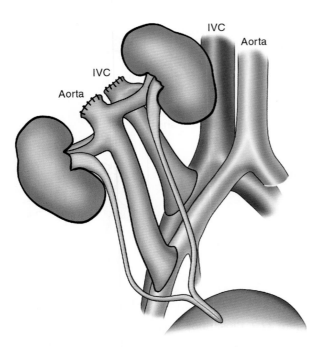

Figure 37.9 *En bloc* graft with spatulated ureters.

engraftment is generally performed with the aorta and vena cava anastomosed end to side to the respective iliac vessels (Fig. 37.9). An alternative method uses an interposition graft technique involving a section of aorta and vena cava anastomosed in continuity with the corresponding iliac artery and vein (Fig. 37.10).

Results of renal transplantation using pediatric allografts

The most recent data from UNOS pertaining to the number of allografts performed and success rate are from their 1996 annual report. This indicates that of the 4997 cadaveric renal donors in the USA in 1995 9.4% of kidney donors were younger than 10 years of age, and 13.7% were between 11 and 17 years of age. Overall, pediatric donors constituted 23.9% of renal cadaveric donors. Comparing 1988 with 1995 UNOS statistics, cadaveric kidney donors aged less than age 10 years declined slightly, donors age 11–17 years increased by 15%, while overall renal donations increased by only 3%. National (UNOS) graft survival for 1988–1994 stratified by age is shown in

Figure 37.1. Patient survival is shown in Figure 37.2. Kidney graft survival show significantly poorer 1 year results using donors younger than 11 years of age (74.2%), while donor aged 11–17 years (83.7%) are comparable to optimally aged donors of 18–34 years (84.2%). Five year graft survivals show that younger donors result in durable grafts, with donors aged 10 years or younger demonstrating less risk for graft loss between 1 year and 5 years post-transplant compared with optimally aged donors (Fig. 37.1). This suggests that pediatric donors have the potential to provide superior long-term graft outcome if early graft loss due to vascular thrombosis and rejection can be minimized.

A large single-center series (1987–1997) covering 78 *en bloc* pediatric kidney transplants was reported by the University of Pittsburgh. Pediatric transplants represented 10% of their renal transplants and resulted in a 79% 43 month graft survival. These results compare favorably to UNOS data for optimally aged donors over a similar period. A review of recent single-center series revealed that urologic complications remain significant. Reviewing these series (Bretan *et al.*, 1997; Nghiem *et al.*, 1998; Ratner *et al.*, 1997) for ureteral complications demonstrated 107 recipients experiencing seven ureteral leaks, three ureteral necroses, and two ureteral obstructions. An additional bladder leak was also reported. This is considerably improved compared with previous reports (Brown *et al.*, 1988; Gruessner *et al.*, 1989; Hoyes *et al.*, 1988; Opelz, 1988; van der Vliet, 1982). Seven cases of thrombosis occurred (6.5%), including one associated with rejection (Bretan *et al.*, 1997; Nghiem *et al.*, 1998; Ratner *et al.*, 1997). This author's limit-ed *en bloc* experience (1994–1998) involving five donors less than 6 months to 6 years of age and weighing 7.5–14.5 kg resulted in no vascular thrombosis and no ureteral complications. One graft in a previously transplanted recipient with preformed antibody (99%) was lost as a result of hyperacute rejection.

Conclusion

The shortage of cadaveric organs for transplantation represents a significant health crisis. In 1995, 17 635 patients were added to the US national kidney waiting list for a total of over 31 000 patients awaiting cadaveric kidneys. Declaration of brain death for patients younger than 5 years requires longer observation periods and/or additional testing, when compared with older donors. However, the approach for requesting permission for donation and support of the brain-dead pediatric donors is similar to procedures for adult donors. Avoiding vascular and ureteral complications requires avoiding cannulation of the great vessels and preserving all collateral circulation to the ureters. Pediatric donors represent approximately 20% of all donors. While national data reveal that donors less than 11 years old have somewhat reduced 1 year graft survival, patient survival is similar to optimally aged donors and graft survival is durable. Single-center series demonstrate that even very young donors can provide outcomes equivalent to optimally aged donors.

[*Appendices appear overleaf.*]

Appendices

Appendix 1

University of New Mexico Medical Center
CHECK LIST FOR CLINICAL DIAGNOSIS OF BRAIN DEATH

Cause of Brain Death: _____

Date of Exam: _____
Time of Exam: _____

A. *Absence of Confounding Factors*:   **RESULTS**
    1. Systolic blood pressure> 90 mmHg   _____
    2. Core temperature> 32°C   _____
    3. Negative for drug intoxication or poisoning.   _____
    4. Toxicology results   _____
    5. Negative for neuromuscular blocking agents   _____

B. *Cranial Nerve Reflexes and Responses*:

    1. No spontaneous muscular movements: _____

    2. Pupils light-fixed: _____

    3. Absent corneal reflexes: _____

    4. Unresponsiveness to intensely painful

       stimuli, e.g. supraorbital pressure: _____

    5. Absent response to upper and lower

       airway stimulation, (e.g. pharyngeal and

       endotracheal suctioning):   _____

    6. Absent ocular response to head turning

       (no eye movement)

       Contraindicated if C-Spine not cleared   _____

    7. Absent ocular response to irrigation of the ears with

       100 mls. of ice water (no eye movement):   _____

    8. Apnea PaCO2> 60 mmHg

       a. PaCo2 at end of apnea test   _____

       b. PaO2 at end of apnea test   _____

       c. *See Apnea Testing procedure on reverse side*

C. *Medical Record Documentation of the above Examination*

D. *Comments*:

_____
_____
_____
_____

<u>Certification of Death</u>
Having considered the above findings, we hereby certify the death of:

_____

Physician Signature: *Printed NAME*:   *Date/Time*
I._____ , MD _____ ,MD _____

Appendix 2

Apnea Testing performed As follows:

a. **Prerequisites**
   1. Core temperature >32 °C or 94 °F.
   2. Systolic blood pressure ≥90mm Hg.
   3. ICU treatment of potentially correctable abnormalities like Diabetes Insipidus .
   4. Decreased ventilatory rate to <6 breaths / minute. After 10 minutes at that rate draw an ABG, and look for signs of respiratory effort. Is the CO2 > 60 mm/Hg? *If the patient has no respiratory effort and the CO is greater than 60 no further testing is needed.* (Items to consider: does the patient have a Hx of COPD or Asthma?)
   5. Preoxygenation with 100% oxygen.

   Option: positive fluid balance for the past several hours

b. Connect a pulse oximeter and disconnect the ventilator.

c. Place a cannula at the level of the carina and deliver 100% O2 at 8L per minute.

d. Look closely for respiratory movements (abdominal or chest excursions that produce adequate tidal volumes).

e. Measure ABG in increments ie: 3,5, and 8 minutes. Discontinue the apnea test when the PCO2 is 60 mm Hg or greater .

   Should the systolic blood pressure become < 90mm Hg or the pulse oximeter indicates significant oxygen desaturation (< 90%) and / or cardiac arrhythmia's are present; *immediately* draw an arterial blood sample and analyze arterial blood gas and immediately *connect the ventilator* thereby ending the apnea testing. Test can be repeated later when the patient is stable.

f. The apnea test result is positive if respiratory movements are absent and arterial PCO2 is 60 mm Hg (Supports the diagnosis of brain death).

g. The apnea test is negative if respiratory movements are observed. (The test does not support the clinical diagnosis of brain death).

References

Aboulgoud MS, Levy MF (1999) Principles of brain death diagnosis. In: *Organ procurement and preservation*. Klintmalm GB, Levy MF (eds) Georgetown, TX: Landes Bioscience.

Ad Hoc Committee on Brain Death, Children's Hospital, Boston (1987). Determination of brain death. *J Pediatr* **110**: 15–9.

Amante AJ, Kahan BD (1996) *En bloc* transplantation of kidneys from pediatric donors. *J Urol* **155**: 852–7.

Ashwai S, Peabody JL, Schneider S *et al.* (1990) Anencephaly: clinical determination of brain death and neuropathological studies. *Pediatr Neurol* **6**: 233–9.

Boyd GL, Phillips MG, Diethelom AG (1991) Donor management. In: *UNOS manual of organ procurement, preservations and distribution in transplantation*. Richmond, VA: UNOS.

Bretan PN, Koyle M, Singh K *et al.* (1997) Improved survival of *en bloc* renal allografts from pediatric donors. *J Urol* **157**: 1592–5.

Brown MW, Akyol AM, Bradley JA *et al.* (1988) Transplantation of cadaver kidneys from pediatric donors. *Clin. Transplant* **2**: 87–92.

Burrows L, Knight R, Polokoff E *et al.* (1996) Expanding the donor pool with the use of *en bloc* pediatric kidneys in adult recipients. *Transplant Proc* **28**: 173–4.

Gruessner RW, Matas AJ, Lloveras G *et al.* (1989) A comparison of single and double pediatric cadaver donor kidneys for transplantation. *Clin Transplant* **3**: 209.

Hayes JM, Novick A, Streem SB *et al.* (1988) The use of single pediatric cadaver kidneys for transplantation. *Transplantation* **45**: 106–10.

Lledo-Garcia E, Moncada-Iribarren F, Escribano-Patino G *et al.* (1997) Letter to Editor. Re: *En bloc* tranplantation of kidneys from pediatric donors. *J Urol* **157**: 266–7.

Medical Task Force on Anencephaly (1990) The infant with anencephaly. *N Engl J Med* **322**: 669–74.

Nghiem DD, Schlosser JD, Hsia S, Nghiem HG (1998) *En bloc* transplantation of infant kidney: ten-year experience. *J Am Coll Surg* 186.

Novitsky D, Cooper DKC, Reichart B (1987) Hemodynamic and metabolic responses to hormonal therapy in brain-dead potential organ donors. *Transplantation* **43**: 852–4.

Opelz G (1988) Influence of recipient and donors age. *Transplant Int* **1**: 95–8.

Peabody JL, Emery JR, Ashwai S (1989) Experience with anencephalic infants as prospective organ donors. *N Engl J Med*. **321**: 344–50.

Portoles J, Maranes A, Prats D *et al.* (1996) Double renal transplant from infant donors. A good alternative for adult recipients. *Transplantation* **61**: 37–40.

President's Commission for the Study of Ethical Problems in Medicine and Biomedical Research, Washington, DC (1981) Guidelines for the death. *JAMA* **246**: 2184–6.

Ratner LE, Cigarroa FG, Bender JS *et al.* (1997) Transplantation of single and paired kidneys into adult recipients. *J Am Coll Surg* **185**: 437–45.

Rosenberg JH, Alter M, Bryne T *et al.* (1995) Practice parameters for determining brain death in adults. *Neurology* **45**: 1012–4.

Roza AM, Johnson PC (1999) Optimal management for abdominal organ donation. In: Klintmalm GB, Levy MF (eds) *Organ procurement and preservation*. Georgetown, TX: Landes Bioscience.

Satterthwaiter R, Aswad S, Sunga V *et al.* (1997) Outcome of *en bloc* and single transplantation from very young cadaveric donors. *Transplantation* **63**: 1405–10.

Task Force for the Determination of Brain Death in Children (1987) Guidelines for the determination of brain death in children. *Neurology* **37**: 1077–8.

UNOS (1996) *Annual Report of the US Scientific Registry of Transplantation Recipients and the Organ Procurement and Tansplantation Network transplant data:1988–1995*. Richmond, VA: UNOS; Rockville, MD: Division of Transplantation, Bureau of Health Resources Development, US Department of Health and Human Services.

Van der Vliet JA, Cohen B, Kootstra G (1982) Transplantation of pediatric cadaver kidneys. *Transplant Proc* **14**: 74–6.

Pediatric urolithiasis

38

Michael J. Wehle and Joseph W. Segura

Introduction

Much is known and written regarding adult urolithiasis because of the widespread prevalence of adult stone disease. The prevalence of adult stone disease in the United States is up to 10/1000. The prevalence of pediatric urolithiasis is estimated to be 1/50 to 1/75 that of the adults (Polinsky *et al.*, 1987; Diamond and Menon, 1991). Pediatric urolithiasis was thought to be unique and distinct from adult urolithiasis. Although this is partly true, it has become clear that the two entities share many basic characteristics and etiologies. Technical advances, such as the advent of extracorporeal shockwave lithotripsy (ESWL) and smaller endourologic equipment, have narrowed the differences in the surgical management between pediatric and adult patients with urolithiasis. The purpose of this chapter is to review pediatric urolithiasis in its current state. Encompassed in this review is the evaluation and management of pediatric stone disease from both a medical and surgical perspective.

Epidemiology

Pediatric stone disease is unique in its epidemiologic patterns (Diamond and Menon, 1991; Drach, 1993; Kroovand, 1997). It is a relatively rare condition in the Western industrial world. In the Middle and Far East, a higher prevalence exists; in this region calculi usually occur in males and are located in the bladder (Lyrdal and Hafvander, 1988). These bladder stones commonly consist of ammonium acid urate and oxalate. The rate of recurrence for these types of stones is relatively low (Lyrdal and Hafvander, 1988; Lingeman *et al.*, 1989; Diamond and Menon, 1991; Drach, 1993; Kroovand, 1997). In the USA, pediatric urolithiasis is likely to be secondary to a metabolic disorder (Coe and Favus, 1986; Laufer and Boichis, 1989; Milliner and Murphy, 1993). Calculi in children of the USA and Europe tend to be located in the kidney as opposed to the bladder (Androulakakis *et al.*, 1982; Coe and Favus, 1986; Stapleton, 1996).

Classification

Several classifications regarding the organization of pediatric stone disease have been proposed. The schemata used by Smith seems to present the most complete and useful classification of pediatric urolithiasis (Table 38.1) (Smith and Segura, 1990).

Urinary stone presentation

In general, abdominal, flank and pelvic pain is present in 50% of children with urolithiasis. Infants often present with a picture similar to gastrointestinal colic. Infection stones or urinary tract infection (UTI) associated with stones are more commonly seen in the preschool age group. Pain and typical renal colic are more often seen in the adolescent group. Hematuria, both microscopic and macroscopic, may be present 30–90% of the time (Smith and Segura, 1990; Diamond and Menon, 1991; Kroovand, 1997). Asymptomatic microscopic hematuria in children may be secondary to hypercalciuria and may herald the development of stones in the future (Androulakakis *et al.*, 1982; Coe and Favus, 1986; Laufer and Boichis, 1989). One study demonstrated that 20% of patients with microscopic hematuria and hypercalciuria developed stones within a period of 5 years (Smith and Segura, 1990; Stapleton, 1996; Kroovand, 1997). A history of an interrupted stream or dysuria may indicate bladder or urethral stone disease. Urinary retention is often associated with urethral stones.

Table 38.1 Classification of urolithiasis in children

I.   Enzyme disorders
    Primary hyperoxaluria
      Type 1: glycolic aciduria
      Type 2: glyceric aciduria
    Xanthinuria
      1,8-Dihydroxyadeniuria
      Lesch–Nyhan syndrome (hyperuricosuria)
      Phosphoribosylpyrophosphate synthetase superactivity
    Orotic aciduria
II. Renal tubular syndromes
    Cystinuria
    Renal tubular acidosis
III. Hypercalcemic states
    Hyperparathyroidism
    Immobilization
	IV. Uric acid lithiasis
	V. Enteric urolithiasis
	VI. Idiopathic calcium oxalate urolithiasis
	    Solute excess
	      Hypercalciuria
	      Absorptive
	      Renal
	    Hyperoxaluria
	    Hyperuricosuria
	VII. Endemic bladder stone formation
	VIII. Secondary urolithiasis
	    Infection
	    Obstruction
	    Structural abnormalities
	    Urinary diversion procedures

Medical evaluation

The medical history is paramount in establishing an educated differential diagnosis and directing the physician to the final correct diagnosis. In pediatric urolithiasis, family history is very important, since pediatric stones can be associated with autosomal recessive disorders, such as cystinuria and primary hyperoxaluria (Polinsky *et al.*, 1987; Smith and Segura, 1990; Diamond and Menon, 1991; Kroovand, 1997). Other abnormalities, such as renal tubular acidosis (RTA), are often associated with urinary calculi and exhibit an autosomal dominant inherited pattern. A child with a strong family history of stone disease alerts the physician to the possibility that the patient has a more severe form of urolithiasis.

A patient's past medical history is important regarding normal daily routine such as fluid intake and dietary habits. A patient with a history of low fluid intake, dietary excesses or deficiencies can alert one to suspect certain stone types, such as those composed of calcium oxalate (Androulakakis *et al.*, 1982; Smith and Segura, 1990; Drach, 1993). A history of trauma may indicate that the patient had a period of immobilization, during which stone formation was initiated. A history of hyperthyroidism, myeloproliferative disorders, gastrointestinal disease, or chronic UTIs may be important, since these conditions can often be associated with urinary stone formation. The age of onset of stone formation is also helpful. Patients with cystinuria, primary hyperparathy-roidism, and idiopathic calcium oxalate urolithiasis usually have the onset of their stone disease in their early teens. Patients with 'infection' stones or stones associated with congenital malformation often present before the age of 5 years.

Finally, because many of the stones seen in the pediatric age group are the results of metabolic disorders, recurrence rates are relatively high. Therefore, patients with pediatric stone disease need to be evaluated thoroughly and followed carefully.

Laboratory evaluation

Laboratory evaluation for pediatric urolithiasis is straightforward. A first-morning urine analysis is helpful in many patients. The pH may indicate whether the child has a form of RTA. If bacteria are present, one should suspect infection-type stones, such as struvite. The specific gravity can also give some indication of the patient's overall fluid intake. Measurement of serum calcium, phosphorous, sodium, potassium, chloride, bicarbonate, uric acid, and creatinine levels may give insight into the type and etiology of the patient's stone disease. A 24-hour urine collection may be necessary to give a more detailed analysis of the urine chemistries. Commonly, the 24-hour urine is analysed for volume, calcium, oxalate, uric acid, citrate, cystine, sodium, phosphate, and creatinine. In reporting the data from 24-hour urine collections in children, it is impractical to use excretion rates (i.e. mg/24 hour). However, the

Table 38.2 Normal values for urine chemistries

Chemical	Normal level (mg/kg per 24 h)
Calcium	< 4.0
Oxalate	< 0.57
Uric acid	< 10.7
Citrate	> 2.0
Cystine	
Heterozygote	1.4–2.8
Homozygote	> 5.7
Magnesium	> 1.2
Phosphate	< 15.0

results must be corrected to consider the patient's size. Examples of this would include mg/g creatinine per 24 hours, mg/kg of body weight per 24 hours, and mg/1.73 m^2 per 24 hours (Smith and Segura, 1990). Normal values are shown in Table 38.2.

Enzymatic disorders

Primary hyperoxaluria

Primary hyperoxaluria is a rare, yet malignant, disorder. Genetically, primary hyperoxaluria appears to be an autosomal recessive condition. The disease is caused by two specific enzyme deficiencies. Primary hyperoxaluria is divided into two types based on these different enzymatic defects. Both enzymatic defects result in an increase in endogenous oxalate production (Smith and Segura, 1990; Danpure and Jennings, 1988; Dent, 1970; Frederick *et al.*, 1963; Smith, 1992; Wandzilak and Williams, 1990; Williams and Wandzilak, 1989). The age of onset is variable but most children present before the age of 5 years. Hyperoxaluria, urolithiasis, nephrocalcinosis, and oxalosis are the result of the oxalate excess. Deposits of calcium oxalate occur first in blood vessels and bone marrow. Death occurs usually in the early teens with a history of the disease being present for 7–8 years. The cause of death is secondary to renal failure and generalized oxalosis (extrarenal deposition of calcium oxalate).

Type I (glycolic aciduria)

Type I primary hyperoxaluria is due to a lack of alanine glyoxalate aminotransferase (AGAT) in the mitochondria of liver cells. This enzyme converts glyoxalate to glycine (Fig. 38.1). The deficiency of AGAT results in a build-up of glyoxalate which then converts to oxalate. The oxalate excess in the blood and urine results in nephrocalcinosis and oxalosis (Frederick *et al.*, 1963; Dent, 1970).

Type II: (L-glyceric aciduria)

Type II is due to deficiency in D-glyceric dehydrogenase. This condition, like type I, leads to excess oxalate production and generalized oxalosis (Dent and Stamp, 1970; Frederick *et al.*, 1963; Smith, 1992; Wandzilak and Williams, 1990; Williams and Wandzilak, 1989).

Diagnosis

Excess amounts of L-glyceric acid and glycolic acid, as well as oxalate (>100 mg/24 h) in the urine, are diagnostic of primary hyperoxaluria. Signs and symptoms of nephrocalcinosis also suggest this diagnosis (Dent and Stamp, 1970; Smith and Segura, 1990).

Treatment

Treatment should be initiated early to slow the inevitable development of nephrocalcinosis. In addition to high fluid intake, three treatment approaches are available to a patient with primary hyperoxaluria. First, pyridoxine (B$_6$) which is a coenzyme in the conversion of glyoxalate to glycine, can decrease excess oxalate formation. A dose of 1.5–3.0 mg/kg is recommended. Approximately 30% of patients with type I will respond favorably to administration of pyridoxine. Patients on high doses of B$_6$, however, may exhibit unwanted neurologic side-effects (Smith and Segura, 1990; Danpure and Jennings, 1988; Dent and Stamp, 1970; Frederick *et al.*, 1963; Smith, 1992). In addition to pyridoxine, magnesium oxide (6.5 mg/kg per day) or magnesium hydroxide (3 mg/kg per day) can be administered to form a soluble complex with oxalate, which decreases the supersaturation of oxalate in the urine. Finally, the use of oral orthophosphates (25–35 mg/kg per day) decreases both calcium and oxalate crystallization. This is in part due to an increase in urinary pyrophosphate and citrate levels, both of which act as inhibitors to calcium salt formation. The liquid form of orthophosphate (neutral sodium potassium phosphate, 28 g equaling 100 mg elemental phosphate)

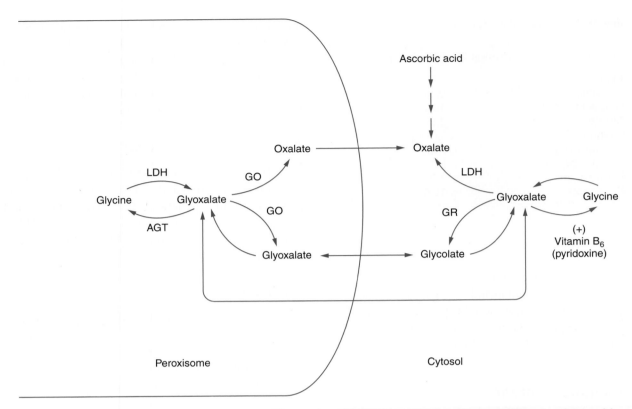

Figure 38.1 Pathway of oxalate metabolism. AGT=alanine glyoxalate aminotransferase; GO=glycolate oxidase; GR=glyoxalate reductase; LDH=lactate dehydrogenase. (From Ruml *et al.*, 1997, with permission.)

seems to be well tolerated in children. Phosphate treatment is contraindicated in patients with creatinine clearances of less than 30 ml/min. Despite these medical treatments, some patients may require a combined liver–kidney transplant for cure. An enzyme-normal, uninfected liver is necessary for the glyoxalate breakdown to glycine in preventing recurrent nephrocalcinosis in the transplanted kidney (Williams and Wandzilak, 1989; McDonald *et al.*, 1989; Watts *et al.*, 1985; Watts *et al.*, 1991).

Xanthinuria

Xanthinuria is a rare autosomal recessive disorder involving deficiency in xanthine oxidase, which is important in the degradation of purines to uric acid (Seegmiller, 1968; Wyngaarden, 1978). More commonly, xanthine stones can also be seen in patients being treated with allopurinol. Radiolucent stones can form in approximately one-third of patients with this disorder. Unlike uric acid stones, xanthine stones are unresponsive to alkalinization. This is due to the

fact that xanthine has two p*K*a values, 7.7 and 10.6. Allopurinol acts as a xanthine oxidase inhibitor, thus increasing the levels of xanthine. Medical treatment consists of prevention by instituting high fluid intake, proper allopurinol dosage and purine reduction in the diet (Seegmiller, 1968; Wyngaarden, 1978; Carpenter *et al.*, 1983; Smith and Segura, 1990).

2,8-Dihydroxyadeninuria

2,8-Dihydroxyadeninuria develops due to a deficiency of adenine phosphoribosyltransferase (APRT), which facilitates the disposal of adenines. Xanthine oxidase oxidizes adenine to 8-hydroxyadenine and 2,8-dihydroxyadenine. These substances are not soluble, and cause urinary crystallization to occur. Patients can develop stones and, infrequently, renal insufficiency. The stones characteristics resemble uric acid and xanthine stones. Allopurinol, hydration, and dietary reduction of purines are used for treatment and prevention (Gault *et al.*, 1981; Carpenter *et al.*, 1983; Smith and Segura, 1990).

Other enzymatic disorders

Hyperuricosuria in Lesch–Nyhan syndrome is caused by a deficiency in hypoxanthine guanine phosphoribosyltransferase. The overproduction of uric acid can also be due to super activity of phosphoribosylpyrophosphate (PRPP) synthetase. Both conditions are rare and will be discussed in the section devoted to uric acid stones.

Orotic aciduria

This is a very rare genetic disorder involving the abnormal metabolism of pyrimidine. Children develop an increase in urinary orotic acid resulting in urinary crystallization. Patients may present with mental and growth retardation, as well as anemia, hematuria, dysuria, and urinary obstruction secondary to stones. Treatment consists of oral uridine (100–150 mg/kg per day). Despite adequate treatment, mental deficiencies persist in these patients (Kelley and Smith, 1978; Smith and Segura, 1990).

Tubular defects

Cystinuria

Cystinuria consists of excessive urinary excretion of the amino acids cystine, ornithine, lysine, and arginine (COLA). Of these four amino acids, only cystine is relatively insoluble at ordinary urinary pH. This insolubility can lead to crystallization and cystine stone formation. The clinically important phenotypic manifestation of this disorder is cystine stone production (Dahlberg et al., 1977; Rutchik and Resnick, 1997). A nutritional deficiency does not occur, since the enzyme deficiency in the jejunum does not prevent dipeptide absorption of the essential amino acids, lysine and arginine. Furthermore, cystine is a breakdown product of another amino acid, methiamine, which can be absorbed normally. In adults, cystine stones comprise 1–2% of all urinary calculi, whereas in the pediatric population the percentage may be higher (6–8%) (Drach, 1993; Smith and Segura, 1990; Rutchik and Resnick, 1997; Burns and Finlayson, 1984). The peak age of symptomatic onset is in the late teens. A higher incidence of these stones is seen in Middle Eastern populations. Unfortunately, cystine stones are often multiple and recurrent in nature (Miliner, 1990; Singer and Sakti, 1991).

The gene responsible for cystinuria has been recently located on chromosome 2p (Pras et al., 1994). The condition is characterized by both a complete and incomplete inherited recessive genetic pattern. Three homozygote types have been identified (Rosenburg 1966; Pras et al., 1994). Type I is completely recessive and the most common. Types II and III are incompletely recessive and less severe than type I. Special oral cystine loading tests can be used to distinguish the three types (Giuglianai et al., 1987). The membrane transport defect affecting absorption of the amino acids (COLA) is present in the jejunum and proximal tubule of the kidney (Rutchik and Resnick, 1997). The inability of this proximal tubule to absorb cystine results in elevated cystine levels in the urine thats leads to supersaturation, crystallization, and stone formation. Cystinuria may also be seen in Fanconi's syndrome and in infants less than 6 months of age who have immature renal tubules.

Diagnosis

The normal cystine excretion is less than 16 mg of cystine/1.73 m^2 per 24 hours. In a normal urinary pH range, the upper limit of cystine solubility is 300 mg/l (Smith and Segura, 1990; Rutchik and Resnick, 1997). No increase in the solubility is seen until the pH reaches 7.2 or higher. Cystine stone-forming adults excrete more than 250 mg of cystine per day, whereas in children as little as 75 mg cystine/day may result in stone formation (Miliner, 1990; Rutchik and Resnick, 1997). Although rarely seen, the first-morning urine may demonstrate the pathognomonic hexagonal crystals on light microscopy (Fig. 38.2). The colorimetric sodium-nitroprusside test is a rapid and simple screening test for cystinuria. Its sensitivity for urine cystine levels can be as low as 75 mg cystine/g of creatinine. The test may present false positives in the presence of sulfa medications. Heterozygotes may also be detected with this method. Patients who have a positive nitroprusside screening test should undergo a 24-hour urine collection for ion-exchange chromatographic analysis for cystine. Radiographically, cystine stones are moderately radiopaque and homogeneous in structure without laminations or striations. The radiographic density and clarity of these stones are less than those of calcium oxalate, calcium phosphate, and most struvite stones. Cystine stones can present with a staghorn configuration (Bhatta et al., 1989).

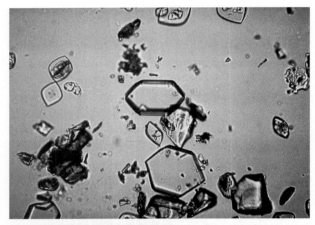

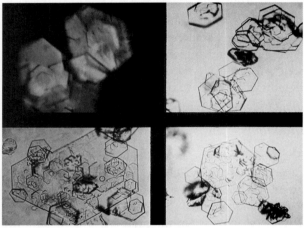

Figure 38.2 Typical cystine crystals from freshly voided urine on routine urine analysis.

Treatment

Treatment success for cystine stone disease is dependent on lowering the saturation of cystine in the patient's urine. Increased hydration, alkalinization of the urine, dietary restrictions, reducing cystine excretion, and chemolytic irrigation therapy are methods used to prevent and treat cystine stone disease (Smith and Segura, 1990; Rutchik and Resnick, 1997; Burns and Finlayson, 1984; Bhatta et al., 1989).

Dilution

Patients must maintain dilute urine to decrease cystine saturation. In a child, a urine flow of 40–50 ml/kg per 24 hours is sufficient. In order to achieve this, an almost constant intake of water is required, *including water intake during the night to prevent night-time dehydration.*

Diet

In general, it is difficult to be placed on a diet low in the amino acid methionine (the precursor to cystine) since methionine is commonly found in most proteins.

Alkalinization

The pKa of cystine is 8.3, therefore an alkaline urine will greatly enhance the solubility of cystine. A significant increase in the solubility of cystine is noted at pH 7. At pH 8, cystine increases its solubility to 1000 mg/l. A problem with alkalinizing the urine to pH 7.5 or higher is the risk of calcium phosphate precipitation and crystallization. An ideal urine pH level for cystine stone therapy is 7.0.

Reduction of cystine excretion

Methods to increase cystine solubility by complexing it to various compounds have been developed. The chemical structure of cystine, with its disulfide bonds joining two cysteine molecules, makes it amenable to reduction and chelation. Cystine binding therapy should be initiated when hydration and alkalinazation therapy are inadequate, since the cystine binders have troublesome side-effects. D-Penicillamine was the first cystine binder used in treating cystinuria (Coide et al., 1992; Halperin et al., 1981; Crawhall et al., 1963). The thiol group disassociates and forms a disulfide bond with the cystine. The compound formed is more soluble than cystine. D-Penicillamine can also directly decrease cystine excretion into the urine. Each gram of D-penicillamine can be expected to dissolve 300 mg of cystine. In attempts to dissolve cystine stones, a reduction of cystine excretion of less than 5 mg/kg 24 hours is desirable. A dose of 30 mg/kg per 24 hours of D-penicillamine in three divided doses per day may be necessary. For prevention of cystine stones, a lower dose of D-penicillamine can be used. Unfortunately, the drug is poorly tolerated and at least one-half of the patients have to discontinue its use because of adverse side-effects, including rash, proteinuria, fever, thrombocytopenia, arthralgias, and gastrointestinal distress (Rutchik and Resnick, 1997; Halperin et al., 1981; Crawhall et al., 1963).

Alphamercaptopropionyl glycine (AMPG) is structurally related to D-penicillamine with a similar cystine binding mechanism (thiol–disulfide exchange). Fewer side-effects are seen than with D-penicillamine (Rutchik and Resnick, 1997; Coide et al., 1992; Crawhall et al., 1963).

Captopril, an angiotensin-converting enzyme inhibitor, contains a thiol group and combines cystine in a fashion similar to that described earlier. Captopril's effectiveness is uncertain, but there are relatively few adverse reactions (Cohen *et al.*, 1995).

Chemolytic irrigation

Irrigation chemolytic therapy can be considered in children with persistent stone disease, when other treatments have failed. Tromethamine E and acetylcysteine have both been used to dissolve cystine stones *in vivo* and *in vitro* (Crissey and Gittes, 1979; Burns and Hamrick, 1986; Dretler, 1986; Saltman and Gittes, 1986).

Extracorporeal shockwave lithotripsy

ESWL and other related shockwave lithotripsy methods have been generally unsuccessful in cystine stone fragmentation (Leroy *et al.*, 1987; Kachel *et al.*, 1991; Abech and Andersen, 1993). The unusual crystalline properties of cystine make it difficult to fragment (Rutchik and Resnick, 1997). Rough cystine stones are composed of large, well-organized hexagonal crystals and fragment more easily than the smooth cystine stones, which have small, poorly arranged crystalline structures. Development of the holmium: yttrium-aluminum-garnet (YAG) laser has given urologists a powerful tool with which to fragment all urinary stones, including cystine calculi (Kachel *et al.*, 1991; Wu *et al.*, 1993).

Renal tubular acidosis (RTA)

The term RTA is applied to several clinical syndromes of metabolic acidosis from specific defects in renal tubular hydrogen ion secretion and urinary acidification. Three major types of RTA exist: types I, II, and IV, differentiated by the type of tubular defect present (Rohlman *et al.*, 1984; Smith, 1986; Warnock and Cogan 1989; Kinkead and Menon, 1995). It is very important to recognize RTA, since it can be associated with increased morbidity and even mortality. The recognition and correction of RTA by proper treatment can completely reverse the acidification abnormality and the destructive sequelae (Diamond and Menon, 1991; Drach, 1993; Smith and Segura, 1990; Warnock and Cogan, 1989; Kinkead *et al.*, 1991).

The function of the proximal renal tubule is to reclaim 80–90% of filtered bicarbonate. This process is facilitated by the driving force of the sodium/potassium ATPase pump located on the basolateral membrane of the tubular cell. The proximal tubule is a high-capacity, low-gradient transport system with regard to hydrogen ion secretion. Large amounts of hydrogen can be secreted, but a large hydrogen ion gradient between the blood and luminal fluid cannot be generated. Therefore, urinary pH cannot be lowered significantly. The distal nephron and collecting duct reclaim the 10–20% of bicarbonate that was not reabsorbed in the proximal tubule. The process of hydrogen ion secretion in the distal tubule differs from that in the proximal tubule. Hydrogen ion secretion occurs by means of an active hydrogen transporting pump or proton pump located in the distal nephron. This proton pump is located at the brush border of the tubule cell. A steep hydrogen ion gradient is developed between the cell and the lumen (1000:1), allowing acidification of the urine (Warnock and Cogan, 1989; Kinkead *et al.*, 1991; Kinkead and Menon, 1995).

Type I renal tubule acidosis

The functional abnormality is the inability of the distal nephron to generate and maintain a significant hydrogen ion gradient between the tubular fluid and the blood. A systemic metabolic acidosis develops with hyperchloremia, hypokalemia, and wasting of sodium, phosphorous, and calcium in the urine. An alkaline urine persists in spite of the systemic metabolic acidosis. Several mechanisms have been suggested as being responsible for the dysfunctional state that develops in the distal nephron. A backleak of hydrogen ion into the tubular cell from the lumen results in a decrease in the hydrogen ion gradient, and therefore hydrogen ion secretion is limited. Dysfunction of the proton pump in the distal nephron tubular cell will also produce type I RTA. Poor sodium reabsorption from the distal tubule can cause a voltage change from a negative to a positive charge in the tubular fluid and inhibit hydrogen ion secretion. Finally, a decrease in carbonic anhydrase in the distal collecting tubule cells results in the decreased ability to generate bicarbonate and hydrogen ion for secretion (Caruana and Buckalew, 1988; Kinkead and Menon, 1995).

Type I RTA is the most common form of RTA in children, most of these being infants. The affected infant often presents with vomiting, dehydration, weakness, and failure to thrive, resulting in ultimate growth retardation (Kossoy and Weir, 1986). Children with type I RTA may also have osteomalacia. Approximately 10% of children with RTA will exhibit nephrocalcinosis and nephrolithiasis (Brenner et al., 1982). The most common stone form is calcium phosphate and these stones are often multiple and bilateral. Stone formation is secondary to an increased urinary pH, hypercalciuria, and hypocitraturia. Hypercalciuria is a direct result of hypercalcemia resulting from bone demineralization and decreased renal production of vitamin D, both induced by systemic acidosis. The demineralization of bone results in the osteopenia that is often seen in RTA patients. Acidemia also directly inhibits both calcium and phosphate reabsorption, resulting in secondary hyperparathyroidism and worsening of urinary phosphate loss.

Citrate is a potent inhibitor of calcium crystallization and subsequent crystal growth. Severe hypocitraturia allows promotion of calcium crystallization and is probably the most important metabolic factor favoring stone formation in type I RTA. Hypokalemia is most likely to be secondary to increased aldosterone production resulting from sodium loss.

A familial form of type I RTA also exists, which appears to have an autosomal dominant inherited pattern. Acquired forms of type I RTA are associated with the following disorders: Sjögren's syndrome, Wilson's disease, lupoid hepatitis, coccidiomycosis, primary biliary cirrhosis, and jejunoileal bypass. Drugs such as amphotericin B and lithium can also cause type I RTA. Finally, spontaneous and idiopathic type I RTA can also occur (Kinkead and Menon, 1995; Kinkead et al., 1991; Osther et al., 1989; Surian et al., 1987; Van den Berg, 1987).

Diagnosis

The diagnosis of type I RTA is established when the urine remains alkaline (pH $\geq$ 5.4) despite the presence of systemic acidosis. A confirmatory second voided morning urine, after an overnight fast, should be obtained and the pH determined. If the pH is 5.4 or lower, type I RTA is not present. Care should be taken to ensure that the urine is free of bacteria, as bacteria will cause an increase in the pH. An ammonium chloride loading test (100 mg/kg per 24 h, solution 500 mg/ml) can be given. After the loading dose has been administered, the pH of urine and blood is measured, along with the serum bicarbonate level. If the urinary pH remains above 5.4 and the bicarbonate is below 20 mEq, type I RTA is confirmed (Kinkead and Menon, 1995; Smith, 1986; Osther et al., 1989; Van den Berg, 1987).

Treatment

Treatment of type I RTA consists of correction of the metabolic acidosis and electrolyte abnormalities. A sodium potassium citrate solution providing 2 mEq of base, 1 mEq of sodium, and 1 mEq of potassium per milliliter is recommended (Kinkead et al., 1991; Kinkead and Menon, 1995). Urinary citrate levels can be used to measure the adequacy of the treatment. These levels should return to normal with correction of the metabolic acidosis.

Type II (proximal) renal tubular acidosis

The primary defect in this RTA is failure of bicarbonate reabsorption in the proximal tubule. This produces hypokalemia and hyperchloremic metabolic acididosis. The kidney is able to acidify the urine appropriately and excrete the daily load of acid as distal tubule function is spared. Type II RTA is a very rare disorder seen in children. Nephrolithiasis and nephrocalcinosis are not seen in this metabolic acidosis (normal urine citrate levels). This disorder can occur in association with hypocalcemia and secondary hyperparathyroidism in children with vitamin D deficiencies. Children can present with typical features of growth retardation attributed to the metabolic acidosis (Smith, 1986; Kossoy and Weir, 1986; Kinkead and Menon, 1995).

Type IV renal tubular acidosis

This form of metabolic acidosis is seen most often in patients with chronic renal parenchymal damage. A hyperkalemic, hyperchloremic metabolic acidosis is produced. The patients are able to generate a normal acid urine response to an acid challenge. Nephrocalcinosis and nephrolithiasis are absent in type IV RTA (Kinkead and Menon, 1995).

Hypercalcemic state

Hypercalcemia is a rare cause of stone formation in children. It can be associated with several different conditions found in children, including primary hyperparathyroidism, hypervitaminosis D, sarcoidosis, milk-alkali syndrome, neoplasia, Cushing's syndrome, and hyperthyroidism (Boadus, 1989; Belezikian *et al.*, 1991; Garrick and Goldfarb, 1989; Malek and Kelalis, 1976; Parks *et al.*, 1980).

In hyperparathyroidism the level of calcium in the serum is typically high (12 mg/dl) with hypercalciuria (greater than 400 mg/24 h). Parathyroid hormone (PTH) is usually minimally elevated. If a parathyroid tumor is present, treatment should be initiated to correct this disorder before considering elective stone therapy in most instances (Malek and Kelalis, 1976; Garrick and Goldfarb, 1989; Ruml *et al.*, 1997).

Immobilization can also result in hypercalcemia with secondary stone formation. Children with severe head, orthopedic, and burn injuries seem susceptible to this disorder. Increased bone reabsorption, dehydration, and metabolic abnormalities contribute to the formation of the stones seen in the immobilized patient. Initial management includes hydration and early ambulation. Orthophosphates and calcitonin are reserved for patients in whom conservative measures are inadequate (Stewart *et al.*, 1982; Jeantet *et al.*, 1984).

Uric acid lithiasis

Uric acid is a weak acid and its solubility is determined by urinary volume, uric acid secretion, and urinary pH. Urinary pH is the principal determinant of uric acid solubility. The insolubility of uric acid in an acidic urine (pH ≤ 5.7) accounts for its crystallization and stone formation. Three sources produce uric acid: diet, *de novo* synthesis, and degradation of nucleic acids (purines). The elimination of uric acid is mainly via the kidneys, although some is eliminated through the digestive tract, hair, and nails (Gutman and Yu, 1968; Kursch and Resnick, 1984; Williams-Larson, 1990; Low and Stoller, 1997).

Uric acid stones are rare in the pediatric population (1–2%). Children with myeloproliferative disorders, hemolytic anemia, sickle cell anemia, and intestinal tract disease are most likely to exhibit uric acid stone formation. Lymphomas and leukemias in children are often treated with cytodestructive chemotherapeutic agents. Chemolytic treatment causes an increase in cell death and release of purines into the circulation, which are then metabolized to uric acid. The increased serum uric acid filtered by the kidneys results in hyperurico-suria and uric acid calculi. Patients with chronic diarrhea, dehydration, and chronically acid urine, due to intestinal loss of bicarbonate and water, will often exhibit uric acid stone formation (Low and Stoller, 1997; Pak *et al.*, 1986; Clayman and Kovoussi, 1992).

Gout

Primary gout is an autosomal dominant (with variable penetrance) inherited disease. Approximately 10–15% of patients with gout will develop uric acid stones. It is associated with hyperuricemia, hyperuricosuria, and persistent acidic urine. Uric acid overproduction and impaired renal acidification are the etiologies suspected in this disorder. The cause of urate overproduction is unclear, but is thought to be related to an increase in *de novo* purine synthesis (Yu, 1982).

Enzyme deficiencies associated with hyperuricemia

Several metabolic enzyme deficiencies are associated with the hyperuricemia and uric acid stone formation seen in children. The hyperuricemia seen in these disorders is due to PRPP (phosphoribosylpyrophosphate) substrate, which is important in the reutilization of purine synthesis (Kelley and Wyngaarden, 1978). Glucose-6-phosphatase deficiency, or type I glycogen storage disease, is a well-known disease in children. Children with type I glycogen storage disease lack glucose-6-phophatase and develop gouty arthritis with uric acid nephropathy. The lack of glucose-6-phosphatase makes PRPP substrate available, thus allowing elevated urinary uric acid levels. Hypoxanthine–guanine phosphoribosyltransferase (HGPRTase) is an enzyme responsible for the formation of hypoxanthine to inosinic acid and guanine to guanylic acid. This HGPRTase deficiency can be present in a complete form only in boys and is transmitted through a sex-linked mode of inheritance. Lesch–Nyhan syndrome is a severe form of this enzyme deficiency resulting in mental retardation, compulsive mutilating behavior, and choreoathetosis (Williams *et al.*, 1984; Smith and Segura, 1990). In addition to the above, the patients will exhibit hyperuricemia and hyperuricosuria as well as signs of gouty arthritis and uric acid stone disease. Treatment for this order consists of dietary reduction of purines, increased fluid intake, and alkalinization of the urine to pH 6.5 with potassium citrate.

Diagnosis of uric acid stones

Children with a history of chronic dehydration, previous history of stones, and acidic urine, can develop uric acid stones. Uric acid crystals in acidic urine microscopically appear similar to broken sheets of yellow glass. Uric acid stones are classically radiolucent but may appear as filling defects in the renal and ureteral collecting system on intravenous pyelograms. A computed tomographic (CT) scan can be helpful in diagnosing uric acid calculi because the density of uric acid stones is greater than 300 Hounsfield units (HU). Blood clots, sloughed papillae, and tumors usually have a density within the 20–55 HU range (Clayman and Kavoussi, 1992; Low and Stoller, 1997). Xanthine, hypoxanthine, and 2,8-dihydroadenine calculi can appear very similar to uric acid stones. It should be noted, however, that these stones are not amenable to successful dissolution by alkalinizing the urine as compared to uric acid calculi (Seegmiller, 1968; Smith and Segura, 1990).

Treatment

Uric acid stones are the only common renal stone readily amenable to dissolution therapy. Treatment is directed at increasing urine volume, alkalizing urinary pH, and decreasing the amount of urinary uric acid (Yu, 1982). Acute obstruction secondary to uric acid lithiasis may require internal or external urinary stenting. Dissolution therapy can be either systemic, with oral alkaline agents, or by direct installation of alkaline solution (Kelley and Wyngaarden, 1978; Yu, 1982; Williams *et al.*, 1984). Optimally a urinary pH of 6.5 is necessary to provoke dissolution of uric acid calculi. Caution should be taken against overalkalizing the urine, as this may cause precipitation of calcium phosphate. Alkalinization of the urine is best accomplished with potassium citrate. The use of 0.6–0.9 mEq of base/kg per 24 hours in two or three divided doses usually achieves the desired alkalinization. The urine pH can be monitored with nitrazine paper. Allopurinol, which is a xanthine oxidase inhibitor, decreases production of uric acid and can be beneficial in patients with overproduction states of uric acid. A 50% reduction in urinary excretion of uric acid can be expected with the use of allopurinol. Finally, hydration is very important to decrease the urinary concentration of uric acid. An optimal urine flow of 30–40 ml/kg per 24 hours should be encouraged.

Enteric urolithiais

Gastrointestinal disorders, most commonly inflammatory bowel disease and malabsorption syndromes, can create a favorable milieu for urinary calculi formation (Abech and Andersen, 1993; Bennett and Jepson, 1966; Dobbins, 1979; Grossman and Nugent, 1967). Water malabsorption causes decreased urine volumes, thus increasing the solute concentration and promoting supersaturation and crystallization. Chronic diarrhea can lead to loss of electrolytes such as sodium, potassium, chloride, and magnesium. Magnesium can form a complex with oxalate, thus decreasing its ability to form calcium oxalate crystals in the urine. With reduced absorption of magnesium, magnesium levels in the urine are decreased and allow oxalate to be free in the ionic form. Malabsorption of phosphate reduces the level of pyrophosphate in the urine. Pyrophosphate is known to be a strong inhibitor of calcium oxalate and calcium phosphate stone formation. The dehydration often seen in inflammatory bowel disease results in metabolic acidosis. This metabolic acidosis results in hypocitraturia and hypokalemia. Citrate is an important inhibitor in calcium oxalate stone formation. The gastrointestinal loss of citrate promotes the production of a metabolic acidosis.

In enteric hyperoxaluria, increased oxalate absorption results in an increased load of oxalate to the kidney and hyperoxaluria. Fatty acid malabsorption causes formation of calcium salts and complexes and reduces the availability of calcium within the intestinal contents. This is important because calcium often complexes with oxalate and reduces the ability of the intestine to absorb oxalate. The membranes of the intestine may also become more permeable to oxalate with high concentrations of fatty acid in the intestinal lumen.

Treatment

Treatment consists of increasing fluid intake to reduce dehydration and solute load in the urine (Bennett and Jepson, 1966; Dobbins, 1979; Grossman and Nugent, 1967) If enteric hyperoxaluria is present, attempts to decrease the oxalate in the diet may be beneficial. If urinary calcium levels are normal, the dietary calcium should be increased to approximately 20 mg/kg per day. This increased calcium load in the intestine will help to bind the oxalate and decrease oxalate absorption. If bowel malabsorption is a principal factor, then attempts to correct the diarrhea with cholestyramine may be successful. To correct the metabolic acidosis, potassium citrate in a dose of 1.5–2.0 mEq/kg per 24 hours in divided doses is most effective. Magnesium replacement can be given intramuscularly as weekly injections (15 mg magnesium/kg per week) if levels are markedly low. Uric acid urolithiasis is often seen in the setting of patients with ileostomies, who are prone to chronic dehydration and large amounts of bicarbonate loss. Treatment for these patients is outlined in the section under uric acid stones. Specifically, the urine needs to be alkalinized with potassium citrate to improve the solubility of uric acid. Allopurinol can also be given in a dose of 4 mg/kg per 24 hours to reduce uric acid excretion (Bennett and Jepson, 1966; Dobbins, 1979; Grossman and Nugent, 1967; Maratka and Nedbal, 1964).

Idiopathic calcium oxalate urolithiasis

Idiopathic calcium oxalate urolithiasis represents an entity of several urinary abnormalities that heighten the probability of calcium oxalate stone formation. The underlying metabolic reasons for these urinary abnormalities are not clearly defined. The majority of children who form calcium oxalate stones will be part of this idiopathic group, which represents the most common cause of metabolic stone formation in children (Lenmann and Gray, 1989; Pak, 1988; Churchill, 1987). An autosomal pattern of inheritance is present in some children with this disorder (Baggio *et al.*, 1986). Hypercalciuria, hyperoxaluria, hypocitraturia, and hyperuricosuria are the four urinary abnormalities that are present individually or in combination in children with idiopathic calcium oxalate urolithiasis.

Hypercalciuria

Hypercalciuria means excess excretion of calcium in the urine. A classification to explain the etiologies of hypercalciuria was devised by Pak (1979) (Table 38.3). Hypercalciuria is divided into the absorptive, of which there are three, and renal types.

Absorptive hypercalciuria

The basic abnormality in absorptive hypercalciuria is the intestinal hyperabsorption of calcium. This increase in serum concentration of calcium enhances the renal filter load and suppresses parathyroid function. Hypercalciuria is then the result of the increased filter load of serum calcium and the reduced tubular reabsorption of calcium, caused by a decrease in the parathyroid function. The serum calcium remains in the normal range in this disorder. Type I absorptive hypercalciuria is a severe form of the disease whereas type II is a milder form. A calcium loading test can distinguish between the two. Type I shows hypercalciuria on both a high and restricted calcium diet. The exact cause of the hyperabsorption of calcium is not known. Type II exhibits hypercalciuria only on a high calcium diet. In type III absorptive hypercalciuria, a renal tubular defect which allows phosphate to leak into the urine, generates an enhanced synthesis of 1,25-dihydroxy vitamin D [1,25-$(OH)_2$D]. The increased 1,25-$(OH)_2$D causes increased intestinal absorption of calcium, resulting in higher urinary calcium levels.

Renal hypercalciuria

In renal hypercalciuria the primary abnormality is thought to be an impairment in the renal tubular reabsorption of calcium. The resulting reduction in the serum calcium concentration stimulates a secondary increase in PTH. The increased

Table 38.3 Idiopathic calcium oxalate urolithiasis

With hypercalciuria	Without hypercalciuria
Absorptive hypercalciuria	Hyperoxaluria
Type I (without calcium loading)	Hyperuricosuria
Type II (with calcium loading)	Hypocitraturia
Type III (phosphate 'leak')	Inhibitor deficiency
Renal hypercalciuria	

Data from Pak (1979).

PTH stimulates renal synthesis of $1,25\text{-}(OH)_2D$. These effects increase the renal filtered load of calcium, causing significant hypercalciuria. The serum calcium remains normal, unlike the hypercalcemia seen in primary hyperparathyroidism. Some investigators believe that renal hypercalciuria may not truly exist, but may be a form of absorptive hypercalciuria.

Hyperoxaluria

Hyperoxaluria has been reported in 15–50% of patients with idiopathic calcium oxalate urolithiasis (Kahn et al., 1993; Ruml et al., 1997). The hyperoxaluria is usually caused by intestinal hyperabsorption of oxalate. Dietary restrictions therefore may play a significant role in controlling the oxalate level in the urine. Reducing dietary calcium, without reducing dietary oxalate, will cause increased absorption of oxalate, resulting in an increased urinary excretion of oxalate (Bataille, 1983; Curhan and Curhan, 1994). It would be unwise to restrict a patient's calcium intake in this instance since this would then promote oxalate intestinal aborption.

Hypocitraturia

Citrate lowers the urinary saturation of calcium salts by forming a soluble complex with calcium; thus, it is a very strong inhibitor of calcium oxalate and calcium phosphate stone formation (Churchill, 1987; Abdulahadi et al., 1993). Urine exhibiting hypocitraturia is most commonly seen with metabolic acidosis as described earlier. Hypocitraturia is present in approximately 20% of patients with idiopathic calcium oxalate urolithiasis. A diet high in acid ash (high protein diet) can also reduce the urinary excretion of citrate (Curhan and Curhan, 1994).

Hyperuricosuria

Hyperuricosuria may be the only recognizable physiologic abnormality occurring in approximately 10% of patients with idiopathic calcium oxalate urolithiasis (Pak, 1988; Churchill, 1987). Hyperuricosuria is due mainly to dietary overindulgence of purine-rich foods. Increases in uric acid production may also account for this disorder. The mechanism by which hyperuricosuria contributes to calcium oxalate stone formation is varied. It is felt that the uric acid crystals may induce a heterogeneous nuclearization of calcium oxalate. The formation of monosodium urate may act as a direct inducer of calcium oxalate stone formation. The monosodium urate may absorb certain macromolecule inhibitors, thus facilitating calcium salt formation (Burns and Finlayson, 1984).

Treatment

Treatment of idiopathic calcium oxalate urolithiasis

A proper and well thought out paradigm for treatment of patients with idiopathic calcium oxalate urolithiasis should be developed. Identifying the metabolic abnormality and specific urinary risk factors is paramount to proper treatment. Basic to all treatments in this disorder is a high fluid intake, consisting mainly of water. The fluid intake needs to be constant through a 24-hour period as any episode of dehydration may allow urinary crystallization to occur. An ideal urine output of approximately 35 ml/kg per 24 hours should be sought. Dietary restriction and manipulation should be directed towards dietary excess or deficiencies. It should be kept in mind that a balanced nutritional diet is necessary to ensure the overall health of the pediatric patient. In general, these conservative treatments should be initiated primarily to control idiopathic calcium oxalate urolithiasis. If these measures are inadequate, then more specific therapy is justified.

Treatment of hypercalciuria

Thiazide diuretics, such as hydrochlorothiazide, are excellent drugs in treating hypercalciuria (0.7 mg/kg per 24 hours in two divided doses) (Churchill, 1987; Hymes and Warshaw, 1987; Pak, 1988). A 50% reduction in urinary excretion of calcium should be observed following successful treatment. A high sodium diet will hinder the effectiveness of the thiazide treatment. In approximately 10% of the patients hypokalemia may develop, which can result in a metabolic acidosis and hypocitraturia. Potassium replacement in the form of potassium citrate is an excellent remedy (0.6–0.9 mEq/kg per 24 hours). The effect of thiazide treatment should be measured with 24-hour urine collection of calcium, sodium, citrate, and oxalate (Diamond and Menon, 1991; Drach, 1993; Smith and Segura, 1990; Ruml et al., 1997; Hymes and Warshaw, 1987).

Neutro-orthophosphate has been effective in the treatment of idiopathic calcium oxalate urolithiasis. Orthophosphate has been shown to inhibit 1,25-$(OH)_2$ D synthesis (Ruml *et al.*, 1997). This medication is indicated in patients with type III absorptive hypercalciuria. The orthophosphate decreases the saturation of calcium oxalate but can increase that of brushite. The urinary inhibitor activity is increased, probably as a result of the stimulation of renal excretion of pyrophosphate and citrate. Orthophosphate is contraindicated in nephrolithiasis complicated by UTI. Cellulose phosphate can be used to decrease absorption of calcium from the intestine in type I and II absorptive hypercalciuria. In the pediatric population, cellulose phosphate is not practical and also has the adverse effect of preventing normal bone formation (Churchill, 1987; Pak, 1988; Ruml *et al.*, 1997).

Treatment of hyperoxaluria

Hyperoxaluria in patients with idiopathic calcium oxalate stone formation is usually mild. Dietary adjustment and increased fluid intake can often be successful in decreasing the formation of calcium oxalate crystals. Neutrophosphate, however, can be used if these measures are inadequate. Potassium citrate is another alternative for the treatment of hyperoxaluria. In children, a liquid preparation seems to be the easiest to administer (polycitra-K, Willen Balkmore). The dose contains 2 mEq of base and 2 mEq of potassium per milliliter (Churchill, 1987; Pak, 1987).

Treatment of hyperuricosuria

Hyperuricosuria is often treated by limiting the amount of purines in the diet, thus decreasing uric acid formation. If dieting and hydration therapy are inadequate, then alkalinization of the urine and the use of allopurinol (as discussed earlier) can be implemented.

Treatment of hypocitraturia

Hypocitraturia can be treated with potassium citrate in divided doses as described previously. The use of the potassium citrate causes citrate levels in the urine to rise (Pak, 1987; Abdulahadi *et al.*, 1993).

Summary

Patients with idiopathic calcium oxalate urolithiasis comprise a group with heterogeneous urinary abnor-

malities. By identifying these abnormalities, successful treatment can be suited to the specific problem, thus reducing the possibility of calcium oxalate stone formation. It is essential for the physician to understand the different etiologies of these urinary abnormalities, to identify them, and to provide proper treatment. Common to all treatments is the importance of high fluid intake and elimination of dietary excesses and deficiencies. If these measures are inadequate, then the specific treatments described previously can be employed.

Idiopathic and endemic stones

At one time approximately 25% of the stones detected in children were idiopathic (Diamond and Menon, 1991; Drach, 1993; Kroovand, 1997). A more complete understanding of the metabolic etiology of urinary calculi through refined diagnostic studies has diminished the incidence of idiopathic stones. Several investigators have attempted to distinguish specific characteristics in idiopathic stone formers. An abnormally high oxalate/citrate to glycosaminoglycans ratio in idiopathic stone formers suggests a possible etiologic explanation. This imbalance in inhibitors and promoters in patients with idiopathic stone formation may represent a plausible explanation as to why stones form in these patients. Children with idiopathic stones have a tendency to present clinically at a later age and are more likely to have stones present in the ureter.

Endemic bladder stone formation in developing countries can be a major health problem in children. These calculi appear more often in males and may represent either calcium oxalate or ammonium urate stones. While the pathogenesis of endemic bladder stone disease remains uncertain, dietary factors appear to be critical. Children with a diets of a single cereal such as rice or wheat, with very little milk and animal protein, seem to have a higher urinary ammonia concentration. Children have a higher uric acid concentration in their urine than adults, until approximately the age of 10 years. This higher uric acid concentration, along with the elevated ammonia concentration, allows precipitation of ammonium urate stones (Diamond and Menon, 1991; Drach, 1993; Lyrdal and Hafvander, 1988; Pak, 1987; Baggio, 1983; Suphakaran *et al.*, 1987; Ghazali *et al.*, 1973). Several studies on endemic bladder stone formation in

Thailand demonstrate that these patients have a higher urinary oxalate, calcium, ammonia, and urate, but lower levels of urinary inhibitors, such as inorganic phosphate and pyrophosphate. These patients were shown to have diets low in animal fat and high in oxalate from eating oxalate-rich vegetables (Gault et al., 1981). Orthophosphate supplementation has decreased the amount of crystaluria found in these children. Surgery is almost always necessary for the removal of these stones and recurrence is unlikely.

Infection calculi

Infection calculi in childhood are relatively rare in the USA. One series showed the incidence to be approximately 2% of the stones seen in the pediatric population (Ghazali et al., 1973). In other countries the incidence of infection stones can be much higher (60%) (Gaches et al., 1975). Most stones associated with urinary infection are struvite and composed of magnesium ammonium phosphate ($MgNH_4PO_4$). Carbon apatite [$Ca_{10}(PO_4)_6CO_3$] is less commonly seen in association with UTIs. Struvite stones often become very large and form staghorn calculi. In order for struvite stones to form, urease-forming bacteria must be present. *Proteus mirabilis* is the most common urease-forming bacterium seen in association with infection stones. Approximately 80% of patients with struvite stones will grow *P. mirabilis* in urine cultures (Gaches et al., 1975; Kroovand, 1997). Most organisms that produce urease are in the Enterobacteriaceae family. *Escherichia coli* is often associated with urinary stones, but does not form urease. The urine culture may show mixed bacteria, rather than a single organism. *Ureaplasma urealyticum* has also been shown to be a causative organism in struvite stones however, its detection requires specialized culture techniques. Urease cleaves urea, forming ammonia, bicarbonate, and carbonate. The ammonia ion can react with water and form ammonium (NH_4^+) and a hydroxyl group (OH^-). This hydroxyl group explains why the urine is almost always alkaline when urease-producing bacteria are present. This alkalinity increases the insolubility of struvite and causes precipitation and crystallization to occur at a more rapid rate. The ammonium ion is also attracted to the glycosaminoglycan layer that coats the mucosa of the urinary tract. This attraction allows the struvite particles to become adherent to the urothelium and promotes more rapid crystallization.

When they occur, infection stones are found in children at an early age. Two-thirds of the patients in one series were under 5 years. Boys were more frequently infected than girls in a ratio of 2:1 (Gaches et al., 1975; Kroovand, 1997). Newborns, especially premature children, and children with congenital anomalies are at increased risk for infection stones. Children with foreign bodies such as stents, tubes, or catheters are also at risk for the formation of infection stones. The importance of vesicoureteral reflux (VUR) as an etiologic factor in infection stone formation is questionable. Infection stones are usually moderately radioopaque, and can be quite large, forming staghorn calculi. Most are located in either the kidney or the bladder. Treatment of infection calculi includes complete stone clearance to prevent further infection and recurrence of the stone. The overall recurrence rate may be as high as 14%. Surgical treatment of infection urinary calculi includes open procedures including partial and total nephrectomy, pyelolithotomy, extended pyelolithotomy, dismembered pyelolithotomy, anatrophic nephrolithotomy, and endourologic techniques such as percutaneous nephrolithotomy and ureteroscopy. ESWL has also been used in the treatment of infection calculi in the pediatric population (Kroovand, 1997; Drach, 1993; Smith and Segura, 1990).

Obstruction and anatomically related disorders

Urinary obstruction can increase the transient time of urine in the collecting system. This increased transient time may allow supersaturation of the solute, thereby promoting stone formation. Retrospective studies have shown an association between urinary stone disease and congenital abnormalities of the urinary tract (Ghazali et al., 1973; Gaches and Gordon, 1975; Troup et al., 1972; Bennett and Colodny, 1973). The most frequent congenital abnormality is ureteropelvic junction (UPJ) obstruction. In one series, UPJ accounted for approximately 65% of the obstructive anatomic lesions associated with urinary stones (Troup et al., 1972; Johnston and McKendrick, 1974). Lower UTIs with bladder neck obstruction, reconstructed bladders, or neuropathic bladders have been associated with bladder stones. Anatomic abnormalities seen in horseshoe kidney, polycystic kidney disease, and medullary sponge kidney have all been associated with increased stone formation. Treatment is directed towards correcting the congenital abnormality, completely removing the stone, and preventing further infection. A series from England showed a high recurrence rate in children who had stones associated with a congenital abnormality. Approximately one-third of the patients had recurrent stones, despite attempts to correct the obstruction. Patients who have persistent mild hydronephrosis or dilatation of the collecting system after surgical correction seem to be at increased risk. It is important to rule out any metabolic abnormalities in children with congenital malformation and stones, since many of these children have, in addition to their anatomic disorder, a metabolic disorder.

Surgical management

The indications for stone removal in children are similar to those in adults: a 'surgical' stone is one that is symptomatic, obstructive, or threatening to become so, or a source of infection. Although elective removal of 'non-surgical' stones is occasionally indicated, as seen in patients with metabolically active stone disease, the ready availability of considerably less invasive methods of stone management should not encourage treatment of stones that, in the past, would not have been removed surgically. Finally, it should be kept in mind that approximately 50% of stones in children may pass spontaneously (Churchill *et al.*, 1980; Kramolowsky *et al.*, 1987). Until recently, almost all stones in the pediatric age group necessitated an open surgical procedure for removal. Three developments since the mid-1980s have decreased the incidence of open surgery in most experienced practices to 1% or less:

- extracorporeal shockwave lithotripsy (ESWL)
- percutaneous lithotripsy (PL)
- ureteroscopy (US).

In this section of the chapter these new technical advances, and how they apply to the management of children with urinary calculi, will be reviewed. The indications and techniques for open stone surgery in the management of some pediatric calculi will also be presented.

Shockwave lithotripsy

Since 1984, when shockwave lithotripsy was introduced in the USA, the treatment of renal and ureteral calculi has changed dramatically. Although the literature is abundant regarding shockwave lithotripsy in adults, there are fewer data pertaining to shockwave lithotripsy in pediatric urolithiasis. However, much has been learned regarding the role that ESWL plays in the management of pediatric urolithiasis. The following is a review of current experiences and recommendations in the use of ESWL in the pediatric population. In the future, with advancements in technology and the benefit of long-term follow-up data, these current recommendations may be altered. Currently, ESWL is the treatment of choice for symptomatic or metabolically active stones located in the upper tract of children (Kramolowsky *et al.*, 1987; Bohle *et al.*, 1989; Lingeman *et al.*, 1986; Koovand *et al.*, 1987a; Lottmann and Archambaund, 1998; Longo and Netto, 1995).

Shockwaves are generated and focused by one of four systems: (1) spark-gap generated, ellipsoid focused; (2) piezoelectric generated, spherical dish focused; (3) electromagnetic generated, acoustic lens focused; and (4) explosive pellet generated, ellipsoid focused. Although spark-gap generated, ellipsoid focused systems tend to be the most powerful, this may vary depending on whether the power has been reduced by modifications to the machine or a reduction in voltage across the spark gap. The focal point, where the energy is concentrated on to the stone and any surrounding tissues, also varies considerably, from 2×11 mm in one piezoelectric machine to 2.5×8.0 cm in the most common spark-gap machine. The importance of this in children may lie not only in the anesthesic requirement but also in the amount of renal scarring that might be expected. Localization of the stone, or placing the stone in the focal point, is determined by fluoroscopy, sonography, or plain X-ray films.

In choosing ESWL as a therapeutic tool, one needs to consider not only the efficiency of the procedure, but also the risks pertaining to ESWL and the risks as they compare with alternative treatments. ESWL appears to be very effective and successful in managing most renal calculi in children (Kramolowsky *et al.*, 1987; Lingeman *et al.*, 1986; Koovand *et al.*, 1987a; Lottmann and Archambaund, 1998; Longo and Netto, 1995; Myers *et al.*, 1995). With the exception of cystine and calcium oxalate (monohydrate) stones, most stones in children can be fragmented successfully. Passage of stone debris through the ureter in children often occurs easily and the use of stents is required infrequently (Picramenos et al., 1996). Small 2 and 3 Fr stents are available for placement in patients with large stone burdens or in patients who develop obstruction secondary to stone debris. A large series (Myers et al., 1995) of 446 children treated with a second-generation shockwave lithotripter produced a renal stone-free rate of approximately 70% and an asymptomatic fragment (less than 4 mm) rate of 76%. Retreatment became necessary in 14% and ancillary procedures were required in 36%. In the same series, for ureteral stones, a stone-free rate of 91% with a retreatment rate of 3.5% and ancillary procedures in 17% was reported. Most stones in the ureter were treated without stenting and those treated without stents had a higher success rate. General anesthesia in this series was needed in 31% for the renal stones and 21% for the ureteral stones. Numerous other reports (Lingeman et al., 1986; Koovand et al., 1987a; Lottmann and Archambaund, 1998; VanHorn et al., 1995) show excellent stone-free rates in the range of 70–90% for renal stones treated with ESWL. As would be expected, large stones (> 20 mm, staghorn), those in dependent or obstructed portions of the collecting system, and calcium oxalate monohydrate stones may require a treatment strategy other than ESWL. Long-term follow-up is necessary to determine the true success or failure of shockwave lithotripsy treatment in children. Patients can continue to clear fragments for several months after treatment. In addition, Nijman et al. (1989) and Newman et al. (1989) reported retained fragment growth in 33% of patients treated with shockwave lithotripsy and frank stone recurrence in 10%. Comparisons between first- and second-generation lithotripters are difficult, since these series are fraught with multiple variables. While success rates in both generations appear similar, the retreatment rates may be higher in second-generation machines (Zanetti et al., 1993; VanHorn et al., 1995). General anesthesia is required in approximately one-third of the patients treated with the second-generation lithotripters.

Small stature or orthopedic deformities may make treatment using shockwave lithotripsy very difficult, especially with first-generation lithotripters. Modifications to the first-generation machines have, nevertheless, allowed some of these patients to undergo treatment. In the second- and third-generation machines a waterbath is not necessary and placement of the patient for effective ESWL treatment is less restricted.

In general, a lower number of total shocks and a lower voltage is used in the pediatric population compared with adult treatments, partly because of the fear of causing renal damage to the pediatric kidney. It has been demonstrated experimentally in animals that substantial kidney scars develop in the very young and that these scars are permanent (Evans et al., 1990). Animal studies have demonstrated the safety of shockwave lithotripsy to renal units, epiphyseal growth plates and nearby reproductive organs. Numerous studies have shown ESWL in children to be safe (Myers et al., 1995; Picramenos a et al., 1996; VanHorn et al., 1995; Adams et al., 1989). Lottmann et al. (1998), using pretreatment and post-treatment [99m]technetium–dimercaptosuccinic acid renal scanning, demonstrated no evidence of renal scarring in patients. In a review of the data published so far, there was no evidence of post-treatment hypertension after ESWL in the pediatric population. Mild hematuria can be seen in approximately 40% of patients treated on first-generation machines, and the incidence appears to be somewhat lower with second-generation machines (Kramolowsky et al., 1987; Myers et al., 1995; Adams et al., 1989). However, studies have demonstrated a rather high incidence of renal hematomas in adults after treatment with first-generation shockwave lithotripsy. Goel et al. (1996) demonstrated only three small hematomas in 50 children who had been treated with shockwave lithotripsy. None of these hematomas required transfusion or other treatment.

Hemoptysis has been seen in children after shockwave lithotripsy (Kramolowsky et al., 1987). Apparently, the shockwaves can transverse the lung, causing parenchymal damage. This is usually seen in children who have severe orthopedic defects that made placement in the lithotripter difficult. The use of Styrofoam to shield the lungs has been very successful in eliminating this complication (Sarica et al., 1995; Dretler and Pfister, 1984; Frick et al., 1988). Finally, sepsis can occur in patients with infection stones. Patients with infected urine should be treated with appropriate antibiotics for at least 24–48 hours before ESWL. Relative contraindications to shockwave lithotripsy in children include an uncorrected bleeding diathesis, oliguric renal failure, urinary tract obstruction distal to the calculus, and the potential inability to manage postshockwave lithotripsy ureteral obstruction by calculus fragments (Steinstrasse).

Stone composition greatly influences the effectiveness of the shockwave lithotripsy. Uric acid calculi and calcium oxalate dihydrate calculi are the most responsive to shockwave lithotripsy, whereas calcium oxalate monohydrate, struvite, and brushite are more difficult to fragment. Cystine calculi are resistant to ESWL management (Boddy *et al.*, 1987). It appears that the rough form, as described previously, may be more amenable to fragmentation than the smooth cystine stone variety. Patients with staghorn calculi are often best treated with a sandwich-type procedure, where debulking of the stone is attempted percutaneously, followed by shockwave lithotripsy and further percutaneous procedures to remove small stone fragments (Boddy *et al.*, 1987; Grasso *et al.*, 1998; Holden and Rao, 1991). Chemolysis may also play a role in these types of stone (Dretler *et al.*, 1979; Holden and Rao, 1991). It is very important, especially in struvite stones, to remove all fragments, as the recurrence rate is significant.

In summary, ESWL in children has been an effective and safe means of treatment for renal and ureteral calculi. Longer post-treatment follow-up will be necessary to access, fully, shockwave lithotripsy safety. General anesthesia is usually necessary in first-generation machines; however, second- and third-generation machines can be used with local or twilight anesthesia. Special consideration needs to be given to the location, stone type, and stone size in order to deliver optimal treatment. Not all children with upper tract stones are candidates for shockwave lithotripsy. A careful review of each patient is necessary to achieve optimal treatment results. Other procedures such as percutaneous lithotripsy, chemolytic irrigation, and ureteroscopy may be necessary in addition to shockwave lithotripsy to achieve optimal stone-free results, especially in children with a large stone burden or shockwave-resistant calculi.

Percutaneous lithotripsy

Percutaneous lithotripsy (PL) is a well-established treatment for upper tract calculi in children. Stones that are not amenable to or have failed ESWL may require PL for successful removal. Children with large stones treated with ESWL may have difficulty in passing extensive amounts of fragments. Steinstrasse has been reported in children and this condition can be a dangerous and difficult to manage (Grasso *et al.*, 1998; Fabrizio *et al.*, 1998). Ureteroscopic access to stone fragments in the pediatric ureter can be limited by the small caliber of the urethra and ureter.

Staghorn calculi are especially suited to percutaneous manipulation, either as monotherapy or in combination with ESWL (sandwich therapy) (Hulbert *et al.*, 1985; Holden and Rao, 1991; Streem, 1997). Children with severe orthopedic deformities and those with concurrent congenital abnormalities, such as UPJ obstruction and calyceal diverticula, may benefit from a PL approach (Talic, 1996; Kroovand, 1997). In addition to removing the calculi, the UPJ abnormality or calyceal diverticula may be corrected by endoscopic surgery during the surgical setting. The pediatric kidney differs from the adult kidney not only in size but also in mobility. These factors can make percutaneous access by the inexperienced radiologist or urologist difficult. Endoscopic equipment limitations call for tracts to be approximately 24 Fr in size in most cases. Trauma to the kidney from multiple tracts is a concern in the young, developing kidney. Although PL series in children are small compared with the adult experience, the successful stone-free rate appears to be comparable (Kroovand, 1997; Boddy *et al.*, 1987; Grasso *et al.*, 1998; Hulbert *et al.*, 1985; Kurzrock *et al.*, 1996). Performance of PL is almost always attempted with the patient under general anesthesia. Posterior or posteriolateral subcostal percutaneous access is achieved with fluoroscopic or ultrasonographic guidance using the Seldinger technique (Smith and Segura, 1990; Kroovand, 1997). Once the collecting system has been visualized, with either intravenous contrast material or retrograde injection of contrast, a 22 gauge needle is inserted into the upper tract collecting system. Guidewires are then placed antegrade into the ureter and bladder under fluoroscopic vision. One of the wires is used to assist dilation in establishing the nephrostomy tract. A tract of approximately 24 Fr is usually required to accommodate the rigid nephroscope. In a recent case report a smaller tract of approximately 16 Fr was established and a 15 Fr Hickman catheter peel-away type used to allow access for a 10 Fr pediatric cystoscope to identify and retrieve a solitary stone (Helal *et al.*, 1997). The rigid nephroscope is usually the instrument of choice; however, a flexible 'scope can also be used to reach stones in difficult locations, thus avoiding the possibility of multiple access tracts. Ultrasonic lithotripsy for large stones is ideal, since it tends not to make large fragments, and can evacuate the stone fragments as they are formed. Electrohydraulic lithotripsy can also be used but has a tendency to create larger fragments and can cause endothelial damage (Smith and Segura, 1990;

Kroovand, 1997; Grasso *et al.*, 1998). Cystine and calcium oxalate monohydrate stones often require use of the holmium:YAG laser to achieve successful fragmentation. The holmium:YAG laser also has the advantage of size (200 μm fiber); this allows for its use in a flexible nephroscope (Grasso *et al.*, 1998; Grasso, 1996; Shroff and Watson, 1995; Grasso *et al.*, 1995). After completion of the percutaneous calculus management, the nephrostomy tube should be positioned in the renal pelvis under uroradiographic monitoring to provide urinary drainage. A smaller catheter can also be placed down the ureter and brought out through the nephrostomy site. This tube allows access to the ureter. One or two days postoperatively, a nephrostogram and tomograms are taken to document the extent of calculus removal and fragment passage. If significant calculi remain, these can be occasionally retrieved under radiographic guidance with basketing type procedures. If this is unsuccessful, then a second endoscopic procedure is scheduled. In certain stone types, a calculytic solution can be used through a percutaneous approach to dissolve the remaining fragments (Kroovand, 1997; Smith and Segura, 1990; Dretler *et al.*, 1979). If the nephrostogram reveals no evidence of extravasation and there is no obstruction demonstrated after removal of the urethral catheter, the tube is clamped for approximately 24 hours and then removed.

Renal stone removal via percutaneous nephrolithotripsy usually requires a single session. Potential complications include blood loss requiring transfusion, loss of the kidney, sepsis, pneumothorax, hydrothorax, pulmonary edema, intestinal injury, fluid extravasation with electrolyte abnormalities, and even death (Smith and Segura, 1990; Hulbert *et al.*, 1985; Streem, 1997). Fortunately, the complication rate regarding this procedure is minimal. Several studies using radio-isotope scanning have shown no significant changes in renal function after percutaneous nephrolithotomy (Assimos and Boyce, 1985; Mor *et al.*, 1997). Anatomic scarring of the renal parenchyma also seems to be minimal. The general conclusion in the literature is that PL is an effective and safe procedure for treating certain renal stones in children.

Open surgical management of upper urinary calculi

Urinary calculi in the upper urinary tract that are symptomatic and/or metabolically active and not amenable to ESWL or PL may need open surgical management. Before undertaking any open surgical procedure, attempts to control UTIs and any medical metabolic abnormality should be undertaken. Surgical approach and management of urinary calculi are dependent on the anatomic location and the anatomic configuration of the involved urinary system; therefore, each patient's treatment must be individualized (Diamond and Menon, 1991; Kroovand, 1997; Drach, 1993; Smith and Segura, 1990).

Renal pelvic calculi

Renal pelvic calculi associated with UPJ obstruction that are not amenable to ESWL or PL can be treated successfully with open pyelolithotomy and concomitant pyeloplasty. Pyeloplasty is described in detail in other chapters of this book. Intraoperative radiographs may be helpful in avoiding retained renal stone fragments. Internal renal and ureteral tubes and stents are optional and are individualized for each case. Perirenal drains are usually used (Diamond and Menon, 1991; Kroovand, 1997; Drach, 1993; Smith and Segura, 1990).

Anatrophic nephrolithotomy is reserved for patients with large staghorn calculi and associated calyceal infundibular stenosis (Caione *et al.*, 1990; Diamond and Menon, 1991; Kroovand, 1997). The procedure is performed through a flank or anterior subcostal approach. The method is identical to that described in adults. Nephrostomies and ureteral stents are commonly utilized. Retained stone fragments can be managed with ESWL or chemolytic renal irrigation (Dretler *et al.*, 1979; Kroovand *et al.*, 1987a). When large stones are associated with UTI, their recurrence rate is quite high and patients may need long-term prophylactic antibiotics, metabolic modification, and urinary pH adjustments for prevention. The loss of renal function from anatrophic nephrolithotomy appears to be low.

Ureteral calculi

Ureteral calculi that are not amenable to ESWL and ureteroscopy require open surgical intervention. The techniques and considerations are the same as for adult ureteral open surgery.

Ureteroscopy and basket stone extraction

Basket extraction is possible in the pediatric population (Smith and Segura, 1990; Diamond and Menon,

1991; Kroovand, 1997). Basket sizes range from 2.4 to 4.5 Fr. With direct fluoroscopic visualization and an experienced surgeon, small distal ureteral stones can be removed safely with minimal morbidity. With the development of pediatric ureteral instrumentation, ureteroscopy is becoming more popular as a means of managing distal ureteral stones in children (Caione *et al.*, 1990; Hill *et al.*, 1990). Flexible ureteroscopy has even been used to remove upper ureteral and renal stones using laser technology for fragmentation. The risk of developing ureteral stricture is currently unknown. It appears from several reports that the likelihood of causing significant VUR is minimal (Hill *et al.*, 1990; Diamond and Menon, 1991; Blyth *et al.*, 1992).

Lower urinary calculi

Urethral calculi

Urethral calculi are relatively rare (Diamond and Menon, 1991; Kroovand, 1997; Drach, 1993). They usually present with the child being in urinary retention so a cystostomy is often needed. The size and location of the stone in the urethra are important factors in management. In young boys, the main concern regarding urethral stones is damage to the urethral tissues, resulting in devascularization of the mucosa and stricture. Most stones in the urethra should not be milked, as this can cause further damage to the urethra and usually is not successful. Urethral stones located in the distal urethra may be amenable to an extended meatotomy for successful removal. Endoscopic procedures are possible but extensive manipulation or trauma from instrumentation of the urethra must be avoided since strictures may form. With the holmium:YAG laser, large stones can be manipulated within the urethra and fragmented successfully (Grasso, 1996). However, open urethrotomy and removal of the stone is often the procedure of choice. If stricture is associated with stone entrapment, a first-stage urethroplasty can be performed at the time of stone removal. A complete one-stage urethroplasty is difficult, owing to the inflammation of the urethral tissue caused by the stone.

Bladder calculi

Bladder stones are more commonly seen in developing countries. Open surgical removal is usually the treatment of choice and the recurrence rate is relatively low (Diamond and Menon, 1991; Kroovand, 1997; Drach, 1993; Lyrdal and Hafvander, 1988; Smith and Segura, 1990). The etiology of the stones is described in detail elsewhere in this chapter. Bladder stones can both be seen in children with bladder outlet obstruction and metabolic stone disease. Patients who have a history of bladder augmentation, urinary diversion, or continent diversion, have a relatively high incidence of bladder or pouch calculi. This may be secondary to hypocitraturia, mucus, bacterial contamination and foreign bodies such as staples or retained sutures (Reiner *et al.*, 1979; Palmer *et al.*, 1994). For large and multiple stones, open removal is usually the treatment of choice. This procedure can be performed safely in patients who have bladder augmentations or continent urinary diversions. In the female, it is much easier to instrument the bladder with adult-sized 'scopes than in males, making endoscopic removal of bladder stones possible. In the male, because of size limitations secondary to the small urethra and fear of causing urethral stricture, endoscopic removal may be more difficult and fraught with danger. Percutaneous cystolithotomy has been described (Diamond and Menon, 1991; Kroovand, 1997; Drach, 1993). Relative contraindications to this procedure include previous lower abdominal or pelvic surgery, previous open bladder surgery, and a scarred or fibrotic bladder that cannot be distended adequately to permit percutaneous puncture. The process requires percutaneous access to the bladder while it is distended. Guidewires are placed and dilators used in a fashion similar to percutaneous nephrostomy, to establish a tract into the bladder. Instruments can then be placed through the tract for stone fragmentation and removal. A suprapubic or transurethral catheter, or both, will usually be left in place. Irrigation and chemical dissolution of residual calculus can be used, depending on the type of stone found. Fragments, particularly those lost in folds of bowel wall, can lead to recurrences following lithotripsy.

References

Abdulahadi MH, Hall PM, Streem SB (1993) Can citrate therapy prevent nephrolithiasis? *Urology* **41**: 221–5.

Abech J, Andersen JT (1993) Treatment of cystine stones: combined approach using open pyelothiotomy, percutaneous pyelolithotripsy, extracorporeal shockwave lithotripsy and chemolysis. *Scand J Urol Nephrol* **27**: 415–8.

Adams M, Newman D, Lingeman J et al. (1989) Extracorporeal shockwave lithotripsy in pediatric age population – short and long term results. *J Urol* **140**: 271–A.

Androulakakis PA, Barratt TM, Ransley PG et al. (1982) Urinary calcium in children: a 5 to 15 year followup with particular reference to recurrent and residual stones. *Br J Urol* **54**: 176–81.

Assimos DG, Boyce WH et al. (1985) Pediatric anatrophic nephrolithotomy. *J Urol* **133**: 233–8.

Baggio B et al. (1983) Juvenile renal stone disease; a study of urinary promoting and inhibiting factors. *J Urol* **130**: 1133–5.

Baggio B, Gambaro G, Marchini F et al. (1986) An inheritable anomaly of red-cell oxalate transport in 'Primary' calcium nephrolithiasis correctable with diuretics. *N Engl J Med* **314**: 599–601.

Bataille P et al. (1983) Affects of calcium restriction on renal excretion of oxalate and the probability of stones in the various pathophysiological groups with calcium stones. *J Urol* **130**: 218–21.

Belezikian JP, Silverberg SJ, Shaen E et al. (1991) Characterization, evaluation of asymptomatic primary hyperparathyroidism. *J Bone Miner Res* **2**: 121–5.

Bennett AH, Colodny AH (1973) Urinary tract calculi in children. *J Urol* **109**: 318–20.

Bennett RC, Jepson RP (1966) Uric acid stone formation following ileostomy. *Aust NZ J Surg* **36**: 153–6.

Bhatta KM, Prien EL, Dretler SP (1989) Cystine calculi – rough and smooth: a new clinical distinction. *J Urol* **142**: 937–40.

Blyth B, Eswalt DH, Duckett JW, Snyder HM (1992) Lithogenic properties of enterocystoplasty. *J Urol* **148**: 575–8.

Boadus AE (1989) Primary hyperparathyroidism. *J Urol* **141**: 725–8.

Boddy S, Kellett NJ, Fletcher MS et al. (1987) Extracorporeal shockwave lithotripsy and percutaneous nephrolithotomy in children. *J Pediatr Surg* T**21**: 223–7.

Bohle A, Knipper A, Thomas S (1989) Extracorporeal shockwave lithotripsy in pediatric patients. *Scand J Urol Nephrol* **2**: 137–43.

Brenner RJ, Spring DB, Sebastian A et al. (1982) Incidence of radiographically evident bone disease, nephrocalcinosis, and neprolithiasis in various types of renal tubular acidosis. *N Engl J Med* **307**: 217–20.

Burns JR, Finlayson B (1984) Management of the stone former. *Semin Urol Oncol* **2**: 34–9.

Burns JR, Hamrick LC Jr (1986) *In-vitro* dissolution of cystine urinary calculi. *J Urol* **136**: 850–3.

Caione P, DeGennaro M, Capozza N et al. (1990) Endoscopic manipulation of ureteral calculi in children by rigid operative ureteroscopy. *J Urol* **144**: 481–5.

Carpenter TO, Lebowitz RL, Nelson D et al. (1983) Hereditary xanthinuria presenting in infancy with nephrolithiasis. *J Pediatr* **109**: 307–10.

Caruana RJ, Buckalew VM (1988) The syndrome of distal (type I) renal tubular acidosis – clinical and laboratory findings in 58 cases. *Medicine* **57**: 84–8.

Churchill BN (1987) Medical treatment to prevent recurrent calcium urolithiasis: a guide to critical appraisal. *Miner Electrolyte Metab* **13**: 219–24.

Churchill BN, Maloney CM, Nolan R et al. (1980) Pediatric urolithiasis in the 1970s. *J Urol* **123**: 237–41.

Clayman RV, Kavoussi (1992) Endosurgical techniques for the diagnosis and treatment of non-calculus diseae of the ureter and kidney. In: Walsh PC, Retik AB, Stamey TA, Vaugh ED (eds) *Campbell's urology*. Philadelphia, PA: WB Saunders.

Coe FL, Favus MJ (1986) Disorders of stone formation. In: Brenner BM, Rector FC (eds) *The kidney*. 3rd edition. Philadelphia, PA: WB Saunders, 1403–42.

Cohen TC, Streem SB, Hall P (1995) Clinical effects of captoril on the formation and growth of cystine calculi. *J Urol* **54**: 164–6.

Coide T, Yoshioka T, Sejii Y et al. (1992) A strategy of cystine stone management. *J Urol* **147**: 112–5.

Crawhall JC, Scowen EF, Watts RW (1963) Effect of penicillamine on cystinuria. *BMJ* **1**: 588–91.

Crissey CM, Gittes RF (1979) Dissolution of cystine ureteral calculus by irrigation of tromethamine. *J Urol* **121**: 81–4.

Curhan GC, Curhan SG (1994) Dietary factors in kidney stone formation. *Compr Ther* **20**: 45–8.

Dahlberg PJ, Van den Berg CJ, Kurtz SB et al. (1977) Clinical features and management of cystinuria. *Mayo Clin Proc* **52**: 53–6.

Danpure CJ, Jennings PR (1988) Further studies on the activity and subcellular distribution of alanine:glyoxylate aminotransferase in livers of patients with primary hyperoxaluria, type I. *Clin Sci* **75**: 315–22.

Dent CE, Stamp TCB (1970) Treatment of primary hyperoxaluria. *Arch Dis Child* **45**: 735–41.

Diamond DA, Menon M (1991) Pediatric urolithiasis. *AUA Update Ser* **10**: 314–9.

Dobbins JW (1979) Oxalate and intestinal disease. *J Clin Gastroenterol* **1**: 165–9.

Drach JW (1993) Urinary lithiasis In: Walsh PC et al. (eds) *Campbell's urology*. Philadelphia, PA: WB Saunders, 2135–45.

Dretler SP (1986) Chemolysis of urinary calculi. *AUA Updade Ser* **5**: 1–7.

Dretler SP, Pfister RC (1984) Primary dissolution therapy of struvite calculi. *J Urol* **131**: 861–6.

Dretler SP, Pfister RC, Newhouse RH (1979) Renal stone dissolution via percutaneous nephrostomy. *N Engl J Med* **300**: 341–3.

Evans AP, Willis RL, Conners B et al. (1990) SW1 induces more severe renal structure and functional changes in juvenile v adult mini-pig kidney. *J Endocrinol* **4**: S58.

Fabrizio MD, Behari H, Bagley DH (1998) Ureteroscopic management of intrarenal calculi. *J Urol* **159**: 1139–43.

Frederick EW, Rabkin NT, Ritchie RH Jr, Smith LH Jr (1963) Studies on primary hyperoxaluria I. *In vivo* demonstration of a defect in a glycoxalate in metabolism. *N Engl J Med* **269**: 821–4.

Frick J, Kohle R, Kunit G (1988) Experience with extracorporeal shockwave lithotripsy in children. *Eur Urol* **14**: 181–6.

Gaches CGC, Gordon IRS *et al.* (1975) Urinary lithiasis in childhood. In the Bristol clinical area. *Br J Urol* **47**: 109–16.

Garrick R, Goldfarb S (1989) Differential diagnosis and pathophysiologic effects of hypercalcemia. *Am J Kidney Dis* **13**: 60–4.

Gault MH, Simmonds HA, Snedden W *et al.* (1981) Urolithiasis due to 1,8-dihydroxyadenine in an adult. *N Engl J Med* **305**: 1570–3.

Ghazali S, Barratt TM, Williams DL (1973) Childhood urolithiasis in Britain. *Arch Dis Child* **48**: 291–5.

Giuglianai R, Ferari I, Greene LJ (1987) Evaluation of four methods for the detection of heterozygous cystinuria. *Clin Chim Acta* **164**: 227–30.

Goel MC, Baserge NS, Babu RV *et al.* (1996) Pediatric kidney: functional outcome after extracorporal shockwave lithotripsy. *J Urol* **155**: 2044–6.

Grasso M (1996) Experience with the holmium laser as an endoscopic lithotrite. *Urology* **48**: 199–206.

Grasso M, Loisides P, Beaghler M, Bagley D (1995) A critical review of 121 extracorporeal shockwave lithotripsy failures. *J Urol* **45**: 361–71.

Grasso M, Conlin M, Bagley D (1998) Retrograde ureteropyeloscopic treatment of 2 cm. or greater upper urinary tract in minor staghorn calculi. *J Urol* **160**: 346–51.

Grossman MS, Nugent FW (1967) Urolithiasis as a complication of chronic diarrheal disease. *Am J Dig Dis* **12**: 491–7.

Gutman AB, Yu TF (1968) Uric acid nephrolithiasis. *Am J Med* **45**: 756–60.

Halperin EC, Their SO, Roseberg LE (1981) The use of D-penicillamine in cystinuria: efficacy and unreported reaction. *Yale J Biol Med* **54**: 439–41.

Helal M, Black T, Lockhart J, Figueroa TE (1997) The Hickman Peel-Away sheath: alternative for pediatric percutaneous nephrolithotomy. *J Endourol* **11**: 171–2.

Hill DE, Segura JW, Patterson DE (1990) Ureteroscopy in children. *J Urol* **144**: 481–3.

Holden D, Rao PN (1991) Management of staghorn calculus using a combination of lithotripsy, percutaneous nephrolithotomy and solution R irrigation. *Br J Urol* **67**: 13–8.

Hulbert JC, Reddy PK, Gonzalez R *et al.* (1985) Percutaneous nephrolithotomy: an alternate approach to the management of pediatric calculus disease. *Pediatrics* **76**: 610–3.

Hymes LC, Warshaw BL (1987) Thiazide diuretics for the treatment of children with idiopathic hypercalciuria and hematuria. *J Urol* **138**: 1217–20.

Jeantet A, Giachino G, Rossi P *et al.* (1984) Immobilization: the cause of resorptive hypercalciuria. *Contrib Nephrol* **37**: 31.

Johnston JH, McKendrick T (1974) Urinary calculus disease. In: Johnston JR, Goodwin WE (eds) *Reviews in Pediatric Urology*. New York: American Elsevier Publishing Company.

Kachel TA, Vijan SR, Dretler SP (1991) Endourological experience with cystine calculi in a treatment algorithm. *J Urol* **145**: 25–7.

Kahn SR, Shevock PN, Hackett RL (1993) Magnesium oxide administration and prevention of calcium oxalate nephrolithiasis. *J Urol* **149**: 413–6.

Kelley WN, Smith LH Jr (1978) Hereditary orotic aciduria. In: Stanberry JB, Wyngaarden JB, Frederickson DS (eds) *The metabolic basis of inherited disease* 4th edition. New York: McGraw-Hill, 1045–71.

Kelley WN, Wyngaarden JB (1978) The Lesch–Nyhan syndrome. In: Stanbury JB, Wyngaarden JB, Frederickson DS (eds) *The metabolic basis of inherited disease*, 4th edition. New York: McGraw-Hill, 1011–36.

Kinkead TM, Menon M (1995) Renal tubular acidosis. *AUA Update Series* **14**: 54–9.

Kinkead TM, Tan FSJ, Menon M (1991) The various forms of RTA and how to treat them. *Contemp Urol* **3**: 33–8.

Kossoy AF, Weir MR (1986) Renal tubular acidosis in infancy. *South Med J* **79**: 1256–9.

Kramolowsky EV, Willoughby BL, Loening SA (1987) Extracorporeal shockwave lithotripsy in children. *J Urol* **177**: 939–43.

Kroovand RL (1997) Pediatric urolithiasis. *Urol Clin North Am* **24**: 173–84.

Kroovand RL, Braren V, Neuman DM, Reidmiller H (1987a) ESWL use in children. *Dialog Pediatr Urol*.

Kroovand RL, Harrison LH, McCullough DL (1987b) Extracorporeal shockwave lithotripsy in children. *J Urol* **138**: 1106–10.

Kursch ED, Resnick MI (1984) Dissolution of uric acid calculi with systemic alkalinization. *J Urol* **132**: 286–90.

Kurzrock EA, Huffman JL, Hardy BE *et al.* (1996) Endoscopic treatment of pediatric urolithiasis. *J Pediatr Surg* **31**: 1413–6.

Laufer J, Boichis H (1989) Urolithiasis in children: current in medical management. *Pediatr Nephrol* **3**: 317–22.

Lenmann J Jr, Gray RW (1989) Idiopathic hypercalciuria. *J Urol* **141**: 715–8.

Leroy AJ, Segura JW, Williams HJ *et al.* (1987) Percutaneous renal calculus removal in the extracorporeal shockwave lithotripsy practice. *J Urol* **138**: 703–6.

Lingeman JE, Neuman DM, Mertz JHO *et al.* (1986) Extracorporeal shockwave lithotripsy: the Methodist Hospital of Indiana experience. *J Urol* **135**: 1134–9.

Lingeman JE, Smith LH, Woods JR *et al.* (1989) *Urinary calculi: ESWL, endourology and medical therapy*. Philadelphia PA: Lea and Febiger.

Longo JA, Netto JNR (1995) Extracorporeal shockwave lithotripsy in children. *Urology* **46**: 550–2.

Lottmann HB, Archambaund F *et al.* (1998) 99mTechnetium-dimercapto-succinic acid renal scan and evaluation of potential long term renal parenchymal damage associated with ESWL in children. *J Urol* **159**: 521–4.

Low RK, Stoller MG (1997) Uric acid-related nephrolithiasis. *Urol Clin North Am* **24**: 135–148–51.

Lyrdal F, Hafvander Y (1988) Urinary bladder stones. *Trop Doctors* **18**: 102–4.

McDonald JC, Landreanau MD, Rohr MS *et al.* (1989) Reversal by liver transplantation of the complications of primary hyperoxaluria as well as the metabolic defect. *N Engl J Med* **321**: 1100–3.

Malek RS, Kelalis PP (1976) Urologic manifestations of hyperparathyroidism in children. *J Urol* **115**: 717–21.

Maratka Z, Nedbal J (1964) Urolithias as a complication of the surgical treatment of ulcerative colitis. *Gut* **5**: 214–7.

Miliner DS (1990) Cystinuria. *Endocrinol Metab Clin North Am* **19**: 889–93.

Milliner DS, Murphy ME (1993) Urolithiasis in pediatric patients. *Mayo Clinic Proc* **68**: 241–8.

Mor Y, Elmasry YE, Kellett MJ, Duffy PG (1997) The role of percutaneous nephrolithotomy in the management of pediatric renal calculi. *J Urol* **158**: 1319–21.

Myers DA, Mobley TB, Jenkins JM *et al.* (1995) Pediatric low energy lithotripsy with Lithostar. *J Urol* **153**: 453–7.

Newman DM, Coury T, Lingeman J *et al.* (1989) Long term results of extracorporeal shockwave lithotripsy in children. *J Urol* **142**: 609–12.

Nijman RJM, Ackaert K, Scholtmeijer RJ *et al.* (1989) Longterm results of extracorporeal shockwave lithotripsy in children. *J Urol* **142**: 609–13.

Osther PJ, Hansen AB, Rohl HF (1989) Distal renal tubular acidosis and recurrent renal stone formers. *Danish Med Bull* **36**: 492–6.

Pak CYC (1979) Physiological basis for absorptive and renal hypercalciurias. *Am J Physiol* **237**: F415.

Pak CYC (1987) Citrate and renal calculi. *Miner Electrolyte Metab* **13**: 257–60.

Pak CYC (1988) Medical management in nephrolithiasis in Dallas: update 1987. *J Urol* **140**: 461–5.

Pak CYC, Sakhaee K, Fuller C (1986) Successful management of uric acid nephrolithiasis with potassium citrate. *Kidney Int* **30**: 422–5.

Palmer LS, Franco I, Reda E *et al.* (1994) Endoscopic management of bladder calculi following augmentation cystoplasty. *Neurology* **44**: 902–4.

Parks J, Coe F, Favus M (1980) Hyperparathyroidism in nephrolithiasis. *Arch Intern Med* **140**: 1479–83.

Picramenos D, Deliveliotis C *et al.* (1996) Extracorporel shockwave lithotripsy for renal stones in children. *Urol Int* **56**: 86–9.

Pohlman T, Hruski KA, Menon M (1984) Renal tubular acidosis. *J Urol* **132**: 431–7.

Polinsky MS, Kaiser BA, Baluarre HJ (1987) Urolithiasis in childhood. *Pediatr Clin North Am* **34**: 683–710.

Pras E, Arber N, Aksentijevich I *et al.* (1994) Localization of a gene causing cystinuria to chromosome 2p. *Nat Genet* **5**: 415–8.

Reiner RJ, Kroovand RL, Perlmutter AD (1979) Unusual aspects of urinary calculi in children. *J Urol* **121**: 480.

Rosenburg LE (1966) Cystinuria: gene heterogeneity and allelism. *Science* **154**: 1341–4.

Ruml LA, Pearl MS, Pak CYC (1997) Medical therapy calcium oxalate urolithiasis. *Urol Clin North Am* **24**: 117–133.

Rutchik SD, Resnick MI (1997) Cystine calculi diagnosis and management. *Urol Clin North Am* **14**: 163–71.

Saltman N, Gittes RF (1986) Chemolysis of cystine calculi. *J Urol* **136**: 846–8.

Sarica K, Kupei S, Sarica N *et al.* (1995) Longterm follow-up of renal morphology and function in children after lithotripsy. *Urol Int* **54**: 95–8.

Seegmiller JE (1968) Xanthine stone formation. *Am J Med* **45**: 789–91.

Shroff S, Watson JM (1995) Experience with ureteroscopy in children. *Br J Urol* **75**: 395–400.

Singer A, Sakti D (1990) Therapeutic dilemmas in management of cystine calculi. *Urology* **37**: 322–5.

Smith LH (1986) Renal tubular acidosis. In: *Urolithiasis update* 1986. Boston, MA: AUA Office of Education.

Smith L, Segura J (1990) Urolithiasis. In: Kelalis P, King L, Belman AB (eds). Philadelphia, PA: WB Saunders, 1327–52.

Smith LH (1992) Hyperoxaluric states. In: Coe Fl, Favus MJ (eds) *Disorders of bone and mineral metabolism*. New York: Raven Press, 707–10.

Stapleton B (1996) Clinical approach to children with urolithiasis. *Semin Nephrol* **16**: 389–97.

Stewart AF, Adler N, Byers CM *et al.* (1982) Calcium homeostasis in immobilization: an example of resorptive hypercalciuria. *N Engl J Med* **103**: 1136–9.

Streem SB (1997) Sandwich therapy. *Urol Clin North Am* **24**: 213–24.

Suphakaran VS *et al.* (1987) The effect of pumpkin seeds on oxalcrystalluria in urinary composition of children in hyperendemic areas. *Am J Clin Nutr* **45**: 115–21.

Surian M, Malberti F, Cosci P *et al.* (1987) Renal tubular acidosis and recurrent calcium Nephrolithiasis. *Contrib Nephrol* **58**: 44–8.

Talic RF (1996) Extracorporeal shockwave lithotripsy and monotherapy in renal pelvic ectopia. *Urology* **48**: 857–61.

Troup CW, Lawnicki CC *et al.* (1972) Renal calculus in children. *J Urol* **107**: 306–7.

Van den Berg CJ (1987) Renal tubular acidosis and urolithiasis. In: Rouse SN (ed) *Stone disease: diagnosis and management*. Orlando, FL: Grune & Stratton, 212–16.

VanHorn AC, Hollander JB, Kass EJ (1995) First and second lithotripsy in children: results, comparison and followup. *J Urol* **153**: 1969–71.

Wandzilak TR, Williams HE (1990) Hyperoxaluric syndromes. *Endocrinol Metab Clin North America* **19**: 851–4.

Warnock DJ, Cogan MG (1989) Renal handling of hydrogen and bicarbonate. In: Massry SG, Glasscock RJ (eds). *Textbook of Nephrology* 2nd edition. Baltimore, MD: Williams & Wilkins, 310–15.

Watts RWE, Calne RY, Williams R *et al.* (1985) Primary hyperoxaluria (type I): attempted treatment by combined hepatic and renal transplantation. *Q J Med* **57**: 697–9.

Watts RWE, Morgan SH, Danpure CJ *et al.* (1991) Combined hepatic and renal transplantation in primary hyperoxaluria (type I): clinical transport of nine cases. *Am J Med* **90**: 179–81.

Williams HE, Wandzilak TR (1989) Oxalate synthesis, transport and the hyperoxaluric syndrome. *J Urol* **241**: 742–5.

Williams JJ, Rodman JS, Peterson CM (1984) A randomized double blind study of acetohydroxamic acid in struvite nephrolithiasis. *N Engl J Med* **311**: 760–4.

Williams-Larson AW (1990) Urinary calculi associated with purine metabolism: uric acid nephrolithiasis. *Endocrinol Metab Clin North Am* **19**: 821–5.

Wu TT, Hsu TH, Chen NT *et al.* (1993) Efficiency of *in-vitro* stone fragmentation by extracorporeal electro-hydraulic and pulsed-dye laser lithotripsy. *J Endourol* **7**: 391–3.

Wyngaarden JB (1978) Heriditary xanthinuria. In: Stanbury JB, Wyngaarden JB, Frederickson DS (eds) *The metabolic basis of inherited disease*. 4th edition. New York: McGraw-Hill, 1037–44.

Yu T (1982) Urolithiasis and hyperuricemia in gout. *J Urol* **126**: 424–7.

Zanetti G, Montanari E, Guarneri A *et al.* (1993) Extracorporal shockwave lithotripsy with NPL 9000 for the treatment of urinary stone in pediatric patients. *Arch Ital DDI Urol Androl* **65**: 671–3.

Genitourinary trauma

39

Allen F. Morey and Jack W. McAninch

Introduction

Trauma accounts for almost 50% of deaths in children aged 1–14 years in the USA. Each year over 1.5 million injuries, 500 000 hospitalizations, and 20 000 deaths are sustained by children as a result of trauma (Shafermeyer, 1993). Motor vehicle accidents are the predominant cause. Pedestrian deaths are prevalent among children aged 5–9 years. Males are involved twice as frequently as females. Blacks and other minority children are at increased risk for traumatic injury and death (Centers for Disease Control, 1990).

The urinary tract is second only to the central nervous system in frequency of injury in the child, although death due to genitourinary injury is uncommon (Livne and Gonzales, 1985). While the pediatric urologist is not usually involved in the initial resuscitation of the trauma patient, his or her involvement becomes increasingly important in the management of genitourinary injuries as they become a dominant concern in the later or delayed phases of care.

Many of the principles of pediatric urologic trauma care stem from accepted principles routinely used in the care of adult patients. Although the evaluation of trauma patients has been refined, care of the pediatric trauma patient must be individualized. Caution must be exercised in the application of adult trauma management algorithms to the care of pediatric patients because of the unique anatomic and physiologic features that distinguish these two groups. This review of published data enables the formulation of a rational diagnostic approach and management plan for children with genitourinary injuries.

Renal trauma

The kidney is the most commonly injured abdominal organ, as well as the most often injured organ in the urinary system. Children appear to be more susceptible to major renal trauma than adults (Brown et al., 1998a). Several unique anatomic features have been purported to explain the greater risk of renal injury among children, such as less cushioning by perirenal fat, an underdeveloped rib cage, and less protection by muscles of the flank and abdomen. Boys suffer renal injury more often than girls (Noe and Jenkins, 1992).

Renal injury is broadly classified as blunt or penetrating. Blunt trauma is the cause of more than 90% of renal injuries in children. Blunt injuries occur secondary to motor vehicle accidents, vehicle–pedestrian accidents, sports injuries, and assault. The vast majority of blunt renal injuries are contusions and require no active therapy (Morse, 1975; Mendez, 1977; Cass et al., 1986; Hardeman et al., 1987; Mee et al., 1989; McAninch et al., 1991; Eastham et al., 1992; Miller and McAninch, 1995). Even when minor or major renal lacerations occur, they also tend to heal uneventfully with non-operative management in nearly all cases (Smith et al., 1992; Levy et al., 1993; Matthews et al., 1999). Penetrating injuries are much less common in children than in adults (Noe and Jenkins, 1992).

Pre-existing renal abnormalities such as hydronephrosis, tumors, or abnormal position predispose to injury (Miller et al., 1986). The rate of pre-existing renal anomalies in children presenting with acute renal trauma is 10% or less (Stein et al., 1994; Morey et al., 1996; Thompson-Fawcett and Kolbe, 1996). A pre-existing congenital abnormality must be suspected when seemingly trivial trauma produces signs or symptoms of renal injury. Children who have had prior renal surgery may also be at higher risk for injury from minimal trauma.

Major deceleration and flexion injuries can lead to ureteropelvic disruption, which is more common in children because of their increased flexibility and renal mobility. Ureteropelvic junction (UPJ) disruption injuries are rare and tend to occur mainly in conjunction with multisystem trauma, with most affected patients having at least three associated major injuries (Boone *et al.*, 1993; Morey *et al.*, 1996). Renal vascular damage is another rare type of injury associated with rapid deceleration. Post-traumatic thrombosis of the renal artery or its branches occurs because the media and adventitia of the renal artery are more elastic than the intima (Hass *et al.*, 1998a). An intimal tear occurs that produces turbulence, thrombosis, and occlusion with resultant complete or segmental renal ischemia (Fig. 39.1).

Evaluation

Blunt trauma

Rapid deceleration injuries such as those occurring in conjunction with a fall or high-speed motor vehicle accident should always heighten suspicion for renal injury. Most major blunt renal injuries occur in association with other major injuries of the head, chest, and abdomen. Physical findings that suggest the presence of major renal injury include abdominal mass or tenderness, flank ecchymosis or tenderness, and rib or vertebral body fractures. Retroperitoneal urinary extravasation may be associated with abdominal distension or ileus.

Since blunt renal injuries occur so often and are usually of such little consequence, efforts have been undertaken to identify children who may safely be spared radiographic imaging. For example, it is well documented that adults with microhematuria and no evidence of shock or associated abdominal injuries

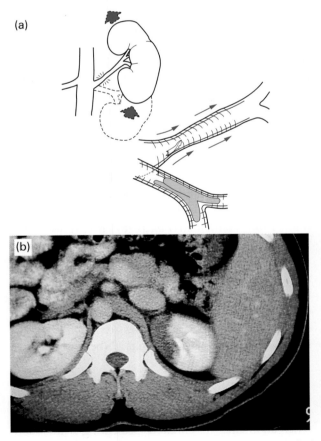

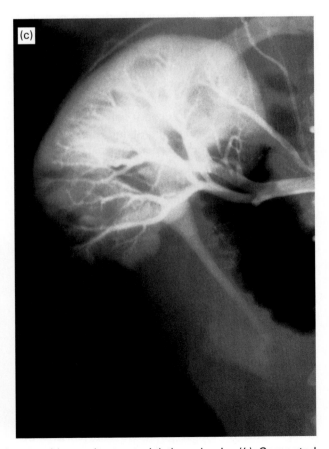

Figure 39.1 (*a*) Rapid deceleration may cause an intimal tear with resultant arterial thrombosis. (*b*) Computed tomography reveals segmental ischemia of the anterior lower pole of the right kidney after this patient fell three storys. (*c*) Arteriogram from the same patient demonstrates an absence of perfusion to the lower pole.

after blunt trauma are unlikely to have major renal injuries, and thus do not need to be studied (Cass *et al.*, 1986; Miller and McAninch, 1995). Criteria guiding the evaluation of traumatized children are less well established. Because the outpouring of catecholamines associated with major trauma can maintain a child's blood pressure in spite of a significant volume of blood loss, the absence of hypotension does not rule out significant renal injuries in children (Quinlan and Gearhart, 1990; Shafermeyer 1993; Medica and Caldamone, 1995). Further, because abnormal kidneys may be more prevalent in children and may be more susceptible to injury after minor trauma, any clinical sign suggestive of renal injury, such as ecchymosis or flank tenderness, should warrant radiographic imaging. Traditionally, therefore, all children with any degree of microhematuria after blunt trauma have been imaged acutely (Ryckman and Noseworthy, 1985; Levy *et al.*, 1993; Shafermeyer 1993; Stein *et al.*, 1994; Miller and McAninch, 1995).

In multiply injured children who are stable enough to undergo radiographic evaluation after blunt trauma, abdominal computed tomography (CT) is the study of choice. Renal CT is now used almost exclusively as the imaging study of choice for cases of suspected renal trauma, having supplanted standard excretory urography at most trauma centers (Ryckman and Noseworthy 1985; Taylor *et al.*, 1991; Morey *et al.*, 1996). CT provides superior anatomic detail regarding the depth and location of renal lacerations, the magnitude of perirenal hematomas or urinomas, and the presence of associated abdominal injuries. It also gives important information regarding the presence and location of the contralateral kidney. Several recent series have suggested that conventional intravenous pyelography (IVP) has an extremely low yield and rarely alters patient management in the setting of pediatric blunt renal trauma, especially in patients with isolated microhematuria (Lieu *et al.*, 1988; Herschorn *et al.*, 1991; Middlebrook and Schillinger, 1993; Hashmi and Klassen, 1995; Brown *et al.*, 1999).

Although hematuria is an imperfect indicator of renal injury, major blunt renal lacerations usually produce significant hematuria. Fewer than 2% of children with insignificant microhematuria [50 red blood cells/high-power field (RBC/hpf) or less] after blunt trauma have major renal injuries. Detection of significant renal injuries rises to 8% in children with significant microhematuria (>50 RBC/hpf), and 32% in those with gross hematuria after blunt trauma (Morey *et al.*, 1996). The presence of multiple major associated injuries (three or more) is associated with a higher likelihood of significant renal trauma in all groups.

Because IVP carries a small but finite risk of contrast reaction, and because the time and expense of unhelpful negative studies can be substantial, some have proposed criteria tightening the indications for imaging after blunt trauma in children. Herschorn *et al.* (1991) reported that, if only those patients with more than 20 RBC/hpf had been studied, 42% of the IVPs would have been avoided and no significant renal injury would have been missed. Likewise, Lieu *et al.* (1988) noted that 68% of IVPs would have been avoided, and no significant renal injuries missed, if only children with 50 or more RBC/hpf were imaged. Hashmi and Klassen (1995) reported that 68% of IVPs would have been avoided without missing any significant renal injuries if only those with 100 RBC/hpf or more had been imaged.

There is reason to believe that patients who are clinically suspected of having renal contusions based on history, physical examination, and urinalysis findings can safely be spared radiographic imaging. Several investigators have demonstrated that children with isolated microhematuria who were not studied radiographically did not develop complications related to renal trauma during short-term follow-up (Fleisher 1989; Morey *et al.*, 1996). Moreover, Miller and McAninch (1995) found no clinical evidence of complications relating to renal injury in 1004 adults who did not have radiographic imaging with microhematuria and no signs of shock after blunt trauma.

Instead of immediate imaging in patients suspected of having renal contusions, urinalysis should be followed closely during the recovery period. Hematuria usually clears within 72 hours after renal contusion (Fleisher 1989; Guerriero, 1991). Persistent or increasing hematuria in the follow-up period may be a useful indicator of renal injuries that warrant imaging. Follow-up urinalysis within 48 hours has revealed < 10 RBC/hpf among those without significant renal injuries, while renal laceration has been associated with > 40 RBC/hpf at 48 hours (Fleisher 1989).

Major renal injury such as UPJ disruption or segmental arterial thrombosis may occur without hematuria. However, like deep renal lacerations, both of these injuries are almost always associated with multisystem trauma that presumably would warrant abdominal imaging (Haas *et al.*, 1998a; Boone *et al.*, 1993; Morey *et al.*, 1996). In short, if forces exerted upon the child at the time of injury are sufficient to produce a major renal disruption or vascular injury, then those forces are also likely to produce multiple significant associated injuries.

The diagnosis of UPJ disruption can be difficult to make, for it may occur in the absence of a retroperitoneal hematoma (Boone *et al.*, 1993). The classic radiographic sign of UPJ disruption is non-visualization of the ureter, regardless of the imaging modality. Unfortunately, rapid-sequence helical CT scans, used commonly in contemporary urban trauma centers, may not detect urinary extravasation (Brown *et al.*, 1998b). Delayed scans are necessary to document the finding of perirenal contrast extravasation (Fig. 39.2). A post-CT plain abdominal radiograph is a helpful adjunct if further delineation of ureteral anatomy is desired.

Penetrating trauma

The extent of renal injury occurring after penetrating trauma tends to be less predictable and of greater severity than that occurring after blunt trauma. Gunshot wounds may produce extensive tissue destruction via the blast effect. Renal vascular laceration may occur as an isolated injury, without parenchymal laceration, and without producing hematuria. For this reason, it is generally accepted that any degree of microhematuria after penetrating thoracic or abdominal trauma should prompt immediate renal imaging (Miller and McAninch, 1995). Similarly, if renal injury is clinically suspected on the basis of the entrance or exit wound, renal imaging is performed.

Penetrating abdominal trauma is associated with a high incidence of associated intra-abdominal injury that may require immediate laparotomy. Abdominal CT is helpful in staging stable patients with renal stab wounds being considered for non-surgical management (Wessels *et al.*, 1997b; Armenakas *et al.*, 1999), but may be too time-consuming for use in the unstable patient with penetrating trauma. An IVP with a single bolus of 2 ml/kg of intravenous contrast given intraoperatively has been advocated to evaluate the kidneys of unstable patients selected for immediate laparotomy. Experience from San Francisco General

Hospital suggests that a single abdominal film taken at 10 min is useful in guiding renal exploration (Morey *et al.*, 1999b). Single-image IVP is particularly helpful in staging patients who have sustained multiple penetrating abdominal wounds.

Injury classification

Categorization of renal injuries according to severity helps to standardize different groups of patients, select appropriate therapy, and predict results of therapy. Categorization of injuries does not mandate operation or observation, but acts as a guide to management decision making. The American Association for the Surgery of Trauma (Moore *et al.*, 1989) has proposed a renal injury scaling system which is now used widely and has well-established prognostic value (Wessels *et al.*, 1997b; Armenakas *et al.*, 1999; Blankenship *et al.*, 1999) (Table 39.1). Injury classification is best accomplished by either abdominal CT or direct renal exploration (Karp *et al.*, 1986).

The cortical rim sign is a radiographic finding associated with acute renal arterial thrombosis, a grade 5 injury (Fig. 39.3). Recent studies suggest that this finding occurs at least 8 hours after the time of injury (Kamel and Berkowitz, 1996). The presence of a cortical rim sign warrants a non-surgical approach since renal salvage in a child is not possible after prolonged ischemia of this duration (Hass *et al.*, 1998a).

Ultrasonography has become popular in the initial evaluation of abdominal trauma because it provides a non-invasive means of detecting peritoneal fluid collections (McGahan *et al.*, 1999). In many centers, ultrasonography has replaced diagnostic peritoneal lavage as the diagnostic study of first choice when intra-abdominal fluid is suspected (Hoffmann *et al.*, 1992; Cantor and Leaming, 1998; Patrick *et al.*, 1998). However, limitations remain regarding the ability of ultrasound to evaluate suspected acute renal trauma. While ultrasound is often effective in detecting gross parenchymal disturbance associated with high-grade renal injury, McGahan *et al.* (1999) found sonography to be less reliable for detecting intermediate-grade injuries. Because it provides no information concerning renal function and is poor at defining pedicle injuries, sonography cannot at this time be recommended as a routine method of screening for acute renal injuries. Similarly, nuclear renal scans are useful in quantitating function (Wessels *et al.*,

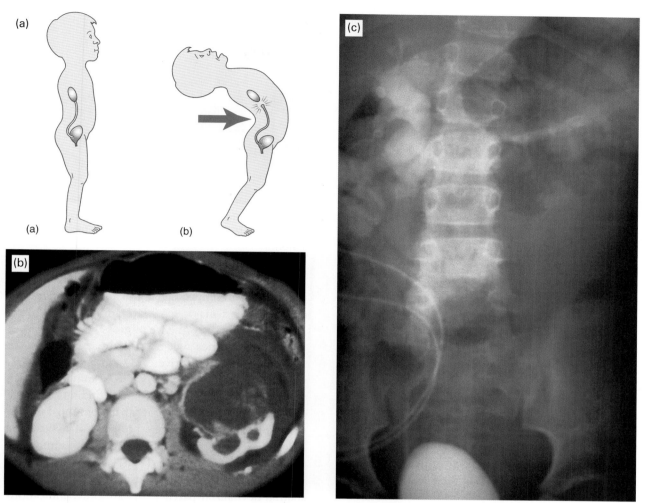

Figure 39.2 Abnormal kidneys are more susceptible than normal kidneys to injury from seemingly incidental trauma. Computed tomographic (CT) scan from a 12-year old boy struck in the flank during football practice. Urinalysis revealed an absence of hematuria. Renal imaging was performed owing to findings of abdominal distension and left flank ecchymosis and tenderness. (*a*) Mechanism of injury of ureteropelvic junction (UPJ) disruption in children. (*b*) Renal CT showing left UPJ disruption. Dilated calyces and thin parenchyma reflect chronic hydronephrosis. (*c*) Delayed plain abdominal film revealing paucity of gas in the left lower quadrant from urinoma and non-visualization of the left ureter secondary to UPJ disruption.

1997a), but do not provide the anatomic information of a CT scan. Arteriography is presently used rarely in the setting of renal trauma, although one application may be selective embolization for delayed or persistent bleeding from a renal laceration (Morey and McAninch, 1996a).

Indications for exploration

Renal exploration after trauma should be undertaken selectively, as associated life-threatening injuries often mandate that urologic intervention be efficient and systematic. In general, the goals of renal exploration are either treatment of major renal injuries, or evaluation of suspected renal injury (Nudell *et al.*, 1997). Renal imaging, while often influential, may not always be possible. Unnecessary or prolonged renal exploration must be avoided in the critically ill patient.

The decision to undertake renal exploration is based on the history (i.e. mechanism of injury) and physical, laboratory, and/or radiographic findings. Urologic management of renal injury is influenced, but not dictated by, the decision of trauma surgeons

Table 39.1 Renal injury grading scale (after Moore *et al.*, 1989).

Grade	Features
1	Contusion or non-expanding subcapsular hematoma No laceration
2	Non-expanding perirenal hematoma Cortical laceration < 1 cm deep without urinary extravasation
3	Cortical laceration > 1 cm without urinary extravasation
4	Laceration: through corticomedullary junction into collecting system, or vascular: segmental renal artery or vein injury with contained hematoma
5	Laceration: shattered kidney, or vascular: renal pedicle injury or avulsion

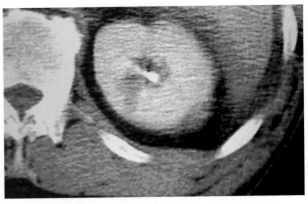

Figure 39.4 Right renal contusion with a small subcapsular hematoma (grade 1 injury): uniformly benign lesion.

to explore or observe associated abdominal injuries. If immediate laparotomy is otherwise deemed unnecessary, a non-operative urologic approach is pursued initially. If laparotomy is undertaken, indications for renal exploration include a large or pulsatile retroperitoneal hematoma or inconclusive renal imaging. Observation alone is appropriate for minor renal injuries (grade 1 and 2), which will resolve spontaneously in nearly all cases (Fig. 39.4).

Blunt trauma

In general, blunt renal injuries should be initially suspected as being minor in nature and approached according to a non-operative management algorithm

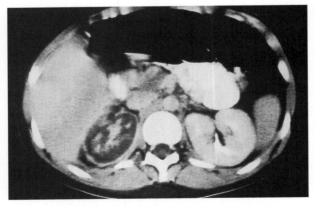

Figure 39.3 Cortical rim sign on abdominal computed tomography after traumatic thrombosis of the right kidney from blunt trauma.

unless there is compelling clinical and/or radiographic evidence that a major renal laceration exists (Morey, 1997). Even in the presence of gross hematuria, most blunt renal injuries will not require exploration. In stable patients, supportive care with bed-rest, hydration, and antibiotics is the preferred initial approach whenever possible (Fig. 39.5). The finding of a large retroperitoneal hematoma at laparotomy in a multi-trauma patient suggests the presence of a shattered kidney, an injury often best managed with immediate nephrectomy (Nash *et al.*, 1995) (Fig. 39.6). Severe renal bleeding and urinary extravasation with substantial devitalized parenchyma are other indications for immediate renal reconstruction (Fig. 39.7). Forniceal rupture is a benign entity that may occur after blunt trauma and may masquerade as a major renal injury because it produces urinary extravasation on CT scan (Borirakchanyvat *et al.*, 1995). It is important to recognize that the renal cortex remains intact in forniceal rupture and that, as a result, perirenal hematoma is absent (Fig. 39.8).

Arteriography with selective renal embolization for hemorrhage control is a reasonable alternative to laparotomy if no other indication for immediate surgery exists. Similarly, persistent urinary extravasation from an otherwise viable kidney after blunt trauma often responds to stent placement and/or percutaneous drainage (Steers *et al.*, 1985; Hass *et al.*, 1998b).

Penetrating trauma

Stab wounds of the abdomen and flank are increasingly being managed successfully non-operatively, partic-

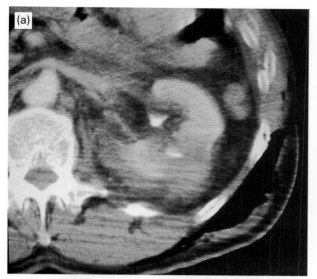

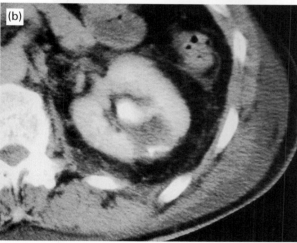

Figure 39.5 Most blunt renal injuries are amenable to non-operative therapy. (*a*) Computed tomograhic (CT) scan showing a deep (grade 4) left renal laceration which was treated non-operatively. (*b*) Follow-up CT 2 weeks later documenting excellent healing.

ularly if the entrance wound is posterior to the anterior axillary line (Armenakas *et al.*, 1999) (Fig. 39.9). CT provides precise anatomic delineation of the depth of injury, and should be used whenever possible before intervention. Superficial and peripheral renal stab wounds universally respond well to non-operative management. Renal stab wounds producing grade 3 or 4 injuries are less predictable and are associated with a higher rate of delayed complications (Wessels *et al.*, 1997b; Armenakas *et al.*, 1999) (Fig. 39.10). If CT has adequately staged the injury and the patient is otherwise stable, observation may be attempted.

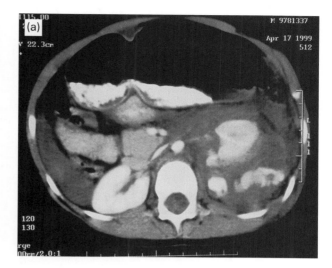

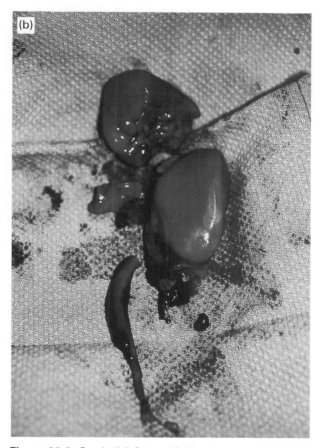

Figure 39.6 Grade 5 left renal injury in a 7-year-old girl run over by a golf cart. (*a*) Computed tomographic scan and (*b*) corresponding gross photograph of the shattered left kidney which was urgently removed in the light of life-threatening hemorrhage. (Photographs courtesy of Hunter Wessels MD.)

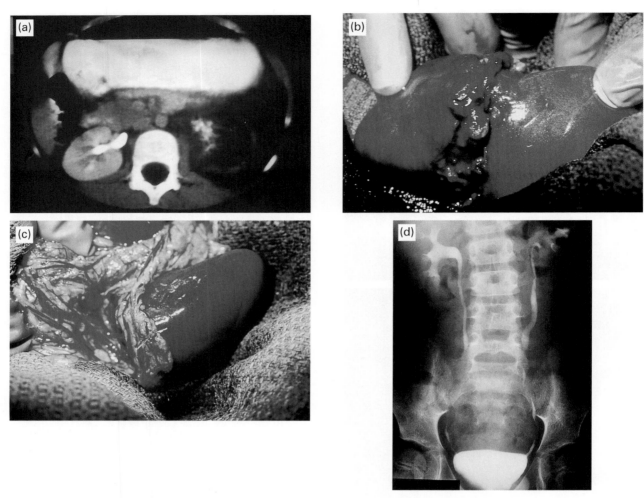

Figure 39.7 (*a*) Urinary extravasation with devitalized left renal parenchyma after blunt trauma. (*b*) Intraoperative photograph demonstrating deep central renal laceration with a non-viable lower pole (shown on the left). (*c*) Renal reconstruction performed via lower pole partial nephrectomy and omental flap. (*d*) Follow-up intravenous pyelogram revealing normally functioning left upper pole remnant.

However, if laparotomy is carried out for associated abdominal injuries, immediate reconstruction of renal stab wounds is prudent, especially if preliminary CT has not been obtained.

Abdominal or flank gunshot wounds producing hematuria should arouse a heightened suspicion for major renal destruction due to possible blast effect, even if hematuria is minimal or absent. Associated bowel or viscous injury usually warrants immediate laparotomy in gunshot victims, and the intraoperative finding of a retroperitoneal hematoma is an indication for renal exploration. Renal imaging may be obtained before exploration via an abbreviated intraoperative IVP, but resuscitation and control of associated injuries must not be delayed.

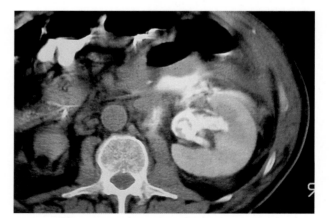

Figure 39.8 Forniceal rupture after blunt trauma in a solitary kidney. Note small contrast collection anterior to the kidney without evidence of cortical laceration or perirenal hematoma.

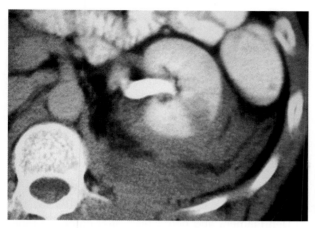

Figure 39.9 Computed tomographic scan showing a minor (grade 2) peripheral laceration of the left kidney due to a posterior stab wound with a small perirenal hematoma. This injury is amenable to observation.

Renal exploration and reconstruction

Once the decision is made to proceed to surgery, the best exposure is obtained through a midline, transabdominal incision. Repair of major visceral and vascular injuries other than those involving the kidney should first be performed, whenever possible, while the patient is resuscitated sufficiently prior to renal exploration to allow a careful reconstructive effort. If renal hemorrhage is massive and life-threatening, the kidney is approached first and other injuries secondarily.

Control of the renal vascular pedicle approached through the posterior parietal peritoneum has been associated with increased rates of renal salvage (McAninch *et al.*, 1991; Nash *et al.*, 1995). The peritoneum is incised over the aorta, just medial to the inferior mesenteric vein. The aorta is followed superiorly until the left renal vein is identified crossing it anteriorly. The left renal vein is then elevated, exposing both underlying renal arteries. Vessel loops are placed around the vessels supplying the injured kidney to facilitate occlusion, should the need arise.

Once control of the vessels has been obtained the colon is reflected medially to expose the kidney. Should a great deal of blood loss be encountered, immediate vascular control may be obtained by occlusion of the ipsilateral renal artery. Warm ischemia time should be limited to 30 min. Once the kidney has been exposed, the hematoma is swept away and the entire surface and collecting system of the kidney are inspected systematically.

Renal lacerations are débrided and oversewn with 4–0 absorbable capsular sutures. Large segmental vessels are suture ligated and the exposed collecting system is closed primarily with fine absorbable sutures. Hemostasis is facilitated by the application of absorbable collagen or gelatin sponge bolsters. Once the bleeding has been controlled, the open margins of the kidney are reapproximated and the renal capsule is closed. If polar lacerations are found to produce large areas of devitalized tissue, heminephrectomy is the best course of action. The area of reconstruction is covered by perirenal fat or a pedicle flap of omentum in order to insure against urinary leakage (McAninch *et al.*, 1991; Morey and McAninch, 1998a) (Fig. 39.11). A Penrose drain is placed in the dependent portion of the wound. Wessels and McAninch (1996) found that renal reconstruction is safe even in the presence of fecal contamination from simultaneous colon injuries.

Renal vascular injuries require prompt and efficient treatment. In the event of traumatic renal artery occlusion, arterial reconstruction may be performed via end-to-end anastomosis, autotransplantation, or various graft techniques (Noe and Jenkins, 1992). However, given the absence of any accessory blood supply to the pediatric kidney, even in the best of hands the outcome for renal arterial injuries is poor (Hass *et al.*, 1988a). Renal vein injuries may be managed by simple ligation or direct repair. Cooling of the kidney in vascular reconstruction is usually not practical in the trauma setting. In the event of

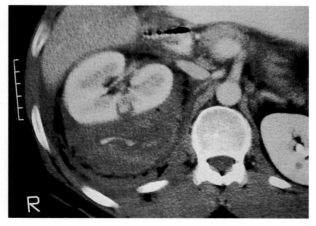

Figure 39.10 Computed tomographic scan showing a deep (grade 4) central laceration of the right kidney with a large perirenal hematoma and contrast extravasation after a stab wound. This patient required urgent renal exploration due to persistent hemorrhage.

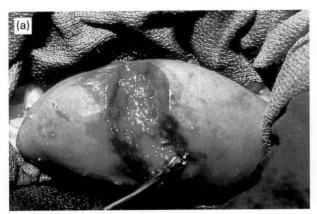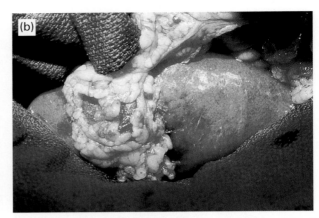

Figure 39.11 Renal reconstruction after a gunshot wound. (*a*) Débridement and hemostasis after complete renal exposure and preliminary vascular control. (*b*) The renal defect is covered by an omental flap.

penetrating injury to the renal pedicle, immediate nephrectomy is often the best solution after proving that the contralateral kidney is normal.

Nephrectomy rarely results as a complication of attempted renal reconstruction. Instead, nephrectomy is usually a life-saving maneuver undertaken in the event of irreparable renal laceration or pedicle injury, especially when combined with hemodynamic instability. Patients requiring nephrectomy after trauma are those with higher rates of hypotension and death, higher injury severity scores, and higher transfusion rates (Nash *et al.*, 1995). As an alternative to immediate nephrectomy, if the patient is hypothermic, acidotic, and coagulopathic, Coburn (1997) has recommended a damage-control approach in selected cases with initial packing of the renal fossa and subsequent pack removal, irrigation, and repair after correction of metabolic disturbances.

Complications of renal trauma

Complications of renal trauma can be early or late. Early complications include bleeding, infection, abscess, sepsis, and urinary extravasation. Delayed retroperitoneal bleeding usually occurs within several weeks of an injury or procedure and may be life-threatening. Urinary extravasation and abscess are usually best managed by percutaneous drainage. Hypertension may occur as a result of external compression (the Page kidney).

Renin-mediated hypertension is a late complication of renal trauma. But, even in the event of complete traumatic arterial occlusion, hypertension seems to be a rare event. Medical management is preferable and is usually achievable. If medical control proves difficult, surgical correction or nephrectomy is indicated.

An arteriovenous fistula should be suspected when a patient presents with the delayed onset of significant gross hematuria. Penetrating injuries account for most cases of renal vascular fistula. Percutaneous embolization is often effective for treating symptomatic arteriovencus fistulae (Noe and Jenkins, 1992), but surgical correction may be required for larger fistulae.

Although the kidney has remarkable healing properties, loss of function may occur regardless of the method of initial management. In most cases functionless renal segments remain inert and resorb, posing no threat to the patient. Wessels *et al.* (1997a) advocated nuclear renal scans as a means of documenting and tracking recovery of renal function after trauma.

Ureteral injuries

Traumatic injury to the ureter is uncommon in children. The most important injury is ureteropelvic avulsion secondary to severe flexion or deceleration injuries (Fig. 39.2). Children are felt to be more susceptible to this type of injury because of the increased flexibility of the pediatric vertebral column and the lack of protection by surrounding fat and muscle.

Evaluation

It is not uncommon for UPJ disruption to go unrecognized initially. Delayed diagnosis is often made after complications such as abscess or ileus have resulted from massive extravasation of urine (Boone *et al.*, 1993). Ureteral injury may be difficult to diagnose since hematuria and retroperitoneal hematoma are often absent. Moreover, abbreviated imaging studies often do not demonstrate contrast extravasation. Delayed IVP or CT films are usually necessary to establish the diagnosis. The radiographic hallmarks of diagnosis are a medial and periureteral pattern of contrast extravasation with non-visualization of the ipsilateral ureter (Porter *et al.*, 1998). Retrograde pyelography is an excellent test for demonstration of ureteral integrity.

Management

Surgical exploration of the ureter with direct injection of methylene blue (antegrade or retrograde) or intravenous indigo carmine is the best course of action whenever acute ureteral injury is suspected, regardless of urinary or radiographic findings (Fig. 39.12). Most cases in which the diagnosis of ureteral laceration is missed or delayed occur as a consequence of an abdominal gunshot wound (Cummings *et al.*, 1999) (Fig. 39.13). Ureteral inspection alone without dye injection may be misleading since blast injury from a gunshot wound may produce delayed necrosis, even though the ureter appears grossly intact initially. Empiric ureteral stent placement through a small cystotomy is a prudent maneuver whenever ureteral contusion is suspected.

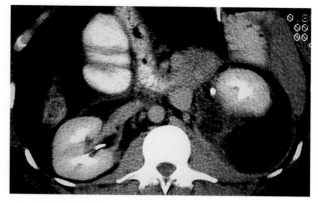

Figure 39.13 Missed ureteral injury diagnosed by the finding of urinoma on abdominal computed tomography 4 days after abdominal gunshot injury. Percutaneous drainage and nephrostomy tube placement were performed.

Penetrating injuries of the ureter are exceedingly rare in children, but the principles of management are similar to that described above. Judicious débridement and direct repair with ureteral stent placement is the preferred approach for most cases with a short defect. The goal of primary repair should be a tension-free, spatulated, watertight anastomosis (Fig. 39.14). Management of UPJ disruption is also accomplished by direct reanastomosis if the defect is short. Stent or nephrostomy tube placement is prudent if questions arise regarding tissue viability or in cases of delayed diagnosis.

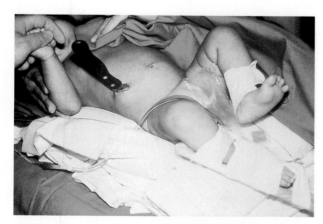

Figure 39.12 Ureteral exploration should be performed after penetrating trauma whenever injury is suspected based on an examination of the entrance and exit wounds, since urinalysis and radiographic findings may be unreliable. In this case the ureter was observed to be intact and no further urologic treatment was warranted.

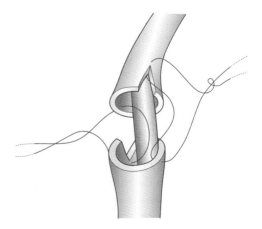

Figure 39.14 Direct repair of upper ureteral injuries is best accomplished via a spatulated, intubated, end-to-end, watertight anastomosis with fine absorbable sutures.

Injuries to the lower ureter are best repaired using a psoas hitch in conjunction with ureteroneocystostomy, with or without a Boari bladder flap. In unstable patients, delayed reconstruction may be advised after initial control by ureteral ligation and nephrostomy tube placement or exteriorization with a long single-J stent (Al-ali and Haddad 1996; Coburn, 1997). When ureteral damage is extensive, reconstruction is accomplished via transureteroureterostomy, auto-transplantation, ileal interposition or appendiceal interposition (Noe, 1992; Al-ali and Hadded, 1996; Medina *et al.*, 1999).

Bladder rupture

The bladder is a mobile organ and, hence, significant bladder trauma is a relatively rare event, accounting for only 2% of abdominal injuries requiring surgery (Morey and Carroll, 1997). Those who have bladder rupture tend to have associated injuries, the most common of which is pelvic fracture (97%). While the adult bladder derives substantial protection from the pubic symphysis, the full bladder is an abdominal organ in infants and small children and is relatively unprotected. Blunt trauma is the most common cause of bladder injury in children (Noe and Jenkins, 1992).

Intraperitoneal rupture, typically at the bladder dome, may occur secondary to severe, direct, lower abdominal blunt trauma. Because the puboprostatic ligament in the male and the pubovesical ligament in the female create a firm attachment of the inferior bladder to the posterior pubis, pelvic ring disruption may produce an extraperitoneal bladder laceration via a shearing effect. In other instances, bony fragments may directly penetrate the bladder (Noe and Jenkins 1992).

Evaluation

Conscious patients with bladder rupture due to blunt injury usually report lower abdominal pain and tenderness. Many are unable to void. Gross hematuria is nearly always present on the initial urinalysis. Bladder laceration should be suspected with any degree of hematuria after penetrating trauma to the lower abdomen, buttocks, or pelvis.

Retrograde cystography is the traditional way of establishing the diagnosis of bladder rupture. A three-film technique is employed, including a plain film, a stress cystogram (250 ml of contrast instilled for an adult), and a drainage film. Inadequate bladder distension may result in a false-negative study. In the child, bladder capacity is variable and must be estimated [(age in years + 2) × 30 ml] to enable adequate distension. Extraperitoneal laceration is confirmed by the presence of a dense, flame-shaped collection of contrast in the pelvis (Fig. 39.15). Intraperitoneal laceration is determined by the presence of contrast outlining individual loops of bowel.

Recent evidence suggests that CT scanning after adequate retrograde instillation of contrast into the bladder may be an acceptable alternative imaging

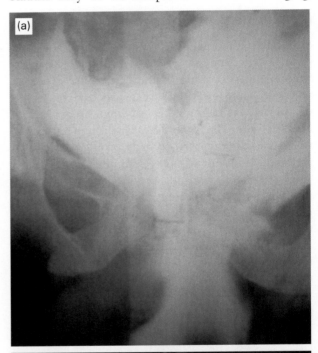

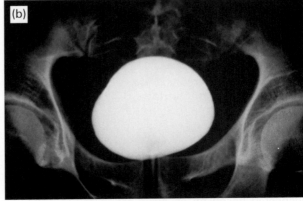

Figure 39.15 (*a*) Extraperitoneal bladder laceration after blunt trauma with extravasation into the scrotum. (*b*) Normal cystogram after 2 weeks of catheter drainage alone in the same patient.

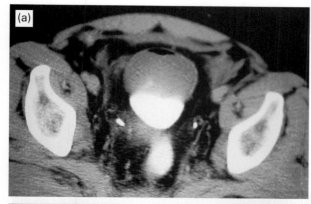

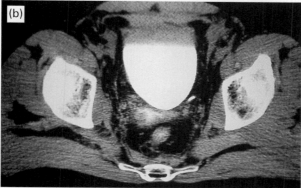

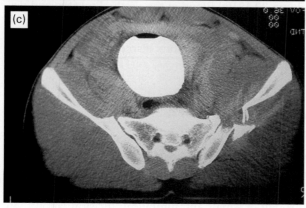

Figure 39.16 (*a*) False-negative computed tomographic (CT) cystogram due to inadequate bladder distension. (*b*) With further instillation of contrast, a small extraperitoneal laceration is identified by the pooling of contrast beneath the bladder. (*c*) Properly performed CT cystogram in a patient with a massive pelvic hematoma due to a left iliac wing fracture. No extravasation was noted.

modality for patients who require CT imaging for associated injuries (Jo *et al.*, 1996) (Fig. 39.16). Additional delayed drainage images are unnecessary during CT cystography because the retrovesicle area is well visualized. Pelvic CT relying on bladder filling

from intravenously administered contrast material, even with catheter occlusion, is an unreliable technique for evaluating bladder rupture (Hass *et al.*, 1999).

Management

Treatment of pediatric bladder rupture depends mainly on whether the rupture is extraperitoneal or intraperitoneal. Most extraperitoneal ruptures respond well to catheter drainage alone, if the catheter drains well. If clot obstruction occurs, or if laparotomy is required for associated injuries, immediate repair is prudent. Intraperitoneal rupture after trauma is best treated with prompt surgical repair. If the laceration is due to penetrating trauma, if it seems to involve the bladder neck, or if concomitant rectal or vaginal lacerations exist, urgent bladder repair is mandated (Morey *et al.*, 1999a). In all cases, the catheter should be left in place for about 2 weeks, at which time repeat cystography is performed to document complete healing. Administration of broad spectrum antibiotics appropriate to children is advisable for about 1 week during recovery.

Posterior urethral trauma

Virtually all posterior urethral injuries are associated with severe blunt trauma and the shearing and stretching effects of concomitant pelvic fracture. The posterior urethra is injured in 3–25% of male patients with pelvic fracture. Approximately 10–30% of those with posterior urethral injury will also have an associated bladder rupture (Allen, 1991). Girls may also rarely have urethral injury secondary to pelvic fracture. Usually these injuries are associated with concomitant bladder neck or vaginal injury (Fig. 39.17).

Evaluation

Blood at the urethral meatus in the patient with a pelvic fracture suggests the presence of prostatomembranous disruption. On rectal examination the prostate may be found to be elevated. Retrograde urethrography is indicated prior to attempted catheterization (Fig. 39.18). If there is no evidence of extravasation a catheter can then be safely passed into the bladder. In girls, because retrograde urethrograms are technically difficult, cystoscopy under anesthesia may be necessary for complete evaluation.

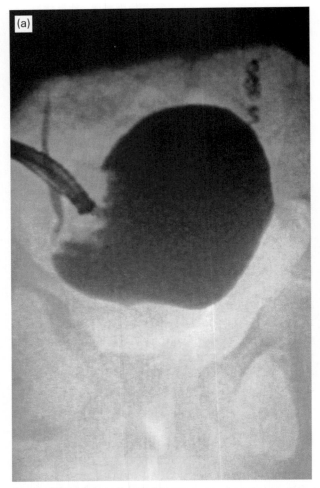

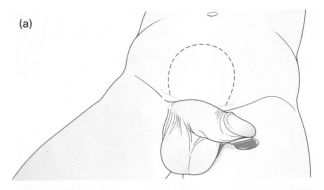

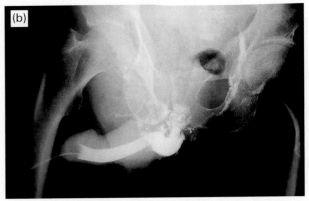

Figure 39.18 (*a*) Blood at the urethral meatus and distended bladder are the best initial signs of posterior urethral injury. (*b*) Retrograde urethrogram revealing complete posterior urethral disruption.

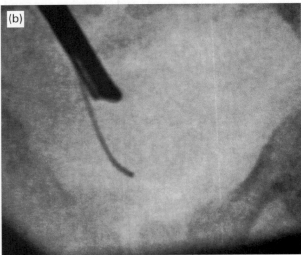

Figure 39.17 (*a*) Suprapubic cystogram in a 3-year-old girl with urethral disruption several months after pelvic fracture. (*b*) A guidewire passed through a suprapubic flexible cystoscope is passed to the level of complete posterior urethral obliteration at the site of the bone fragment.

Management

Treatment of urethral disruption remains controversial but mainly consists of either primary realignment or cystostomy with delayed urethral reconstruction. Open cystostomy tube placement through a small infraumbilical incision allows an opportunity to assess and repair any concomitant bladder laceration without disturbing the pelvic hematoma. A large-bore Foley catheter is placed in the midline at the apex of the suprapubic incision (Fig. 39.19) and withdrawn to sit at the bladder dome.

Urethral realignment may be performed either acutely or several days after injury at a time when associated injuries have stabilized. Various of realignment techniques have been reported, including magnetic sounds, Goodwin sounds, antegrade catheterization and 'cut to the light' procedures. Immediate sutured anastomosis should not be attempted. Prolonged endoscopic realignment procedures should

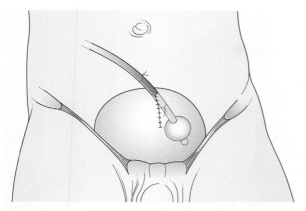

Figure 30.19 Treatment of posterior urethral disruption is best accomplished by a small suprapubic incision and placement of a large-bore Foley catheter at the apex of the lower midline incision.

be avoided in the acute setting to avoid infection of the surrounding pelvic hematoma and the risk of pelvic abscess.

Delayed reconstruction of the resultant posterior stricture should not be attempted until at least 3 months after injury. In experienced hands, prostato-membranous urethroplasty is a highly reliable procedure (Hayden and Koff, 1984; Sandler and Corriere 1989). Systematic, complete excision of fibrotic tissue from the prostatic apex until soft, pink tissues are identified is critical (Fig. 39.20). However, in small boys the membranous urethra may be difficult to approach perineally. A transpubic urethroplasty is an alternative (Waterhouse *et al.*, 1974). Kramer *et al.* (1981) reported their results with an anterior, wedge resecting transpubic repair in 12 children. Eight were completely continent on follow-up, two partially continent, and two wet. Although three patients had erectile dysfunction postopertively, this was most likely a consequence of the injury, and not the repair. None had pelvic instability after surgery. It is important to excise a portion of the pubis rather than spreading the symphysis, as the latter results in significant postoperative pain and difficult ambulation. Continence is nearly always preserved after reconstruction. Impotence tends to result not from the reconstructive procedure, but from the disruption of the vascular and nerve supply to the penis. Pelvic magnetic resonance imaging (MRI) may be a helpful adjunctive study for determining prostatic displacement prior to reconstruction (Koraitim, 1999).

Anterior urethral trauma

Trauma to the anterior urethra is rare because most of the anterior urethra is in a freely movable portion of the penis. Anterior urethral injury rarely occurs in conjunction with pelvic fracture or multisystem trauma, but is common after an isolated 'straddle' injury to the perineum. The bulbar urethra is the most commonly injured segment. This typically results from forceful compression against the underside of the pubic symphysis (Armenakas and McAninch, 1996). Patients may present years after minor perineal trauma with a symptomatic bulbar urethral stricture (Baskin and McAninch, 1993).

Evaluation

Blood at the urethral meatus should signal the possibility of urethral injury. The visible presence and extent of periurethral hematoma provides information about the status of surrounding anatomic planes. When Buck's fascia is intact, the hematoma takes on a sleeve distribution along the penile shaft. When Buck's fascia is ruptured, the hematoma extends to the scrotum and perineum (Hernandez and Morey 1999).

A retrograde urethrogram should be performed as described previously, before any attempts are made at instrumentation or catheter insertion. If contrast extravasation is absent after straddle injury, urethral contusion is diagnosed. Partial disruption is diagnosed when periurethral extravasation is noted but contrast reaches the bladder (Fig. 39.21). Following complete disruption the proximal urethra and bladder are not identified, and extravasation is massive.

Management

If extravasation as demonstrated by the urethrogram is minimal, contained by Buck's fascia, and urethral continuity is demonstrated, treatment with catheter drainage alone for about 1 week is generally successful (Corriere, 1991) However, penetrating injuries of the anterior urethra should be immediately repaired, primarily approximating the debrided edges with fine absorbable sutures over an indwelling catheter. These are often associated with genital injuries that will require concomitant reconstruction.

When complete, blunt rupture of the anterior urethra is identified, no further instrumentation of the urethra should be attempted and a suprapubic catheter is inserted for bladder drainage. Broad-spectrum

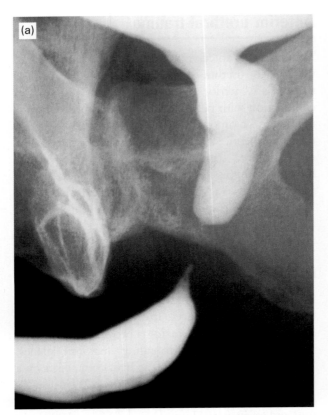

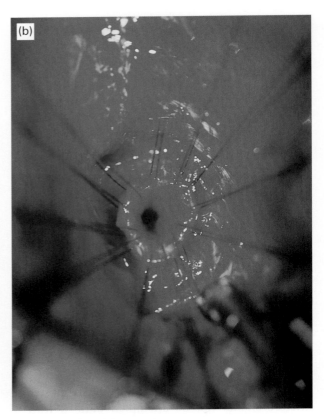

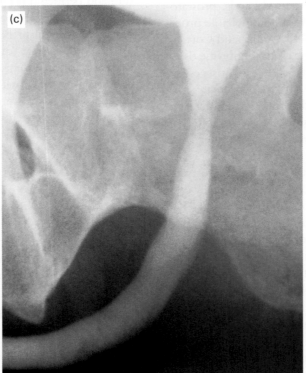

Figure 39.20 (*a*) Combined retrograde urethrogram/ cystogram demonstrating prostatomembranous disruption. (*b*) Intraoperative photograph during posterior urethral reconstruction showing complete systematic excision of fibrotic tissue from the prostatic apex. (*c*) Postoperative result revealing a widely patent urethra.

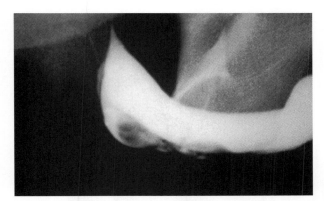

Figure 39.21 Incomplete anterior urethral injury after straddle injury, successfully treated by urethral catheterization alone.

antibiotics are instituted for 1 week, and after 2 weeks voiding cystourethrography is conducted to assess the status of the urethra. If stricture develops, delayed management may consist of either endoscopic urethrotomy or open repair, after the inflammatory process has resolved.

In general, traumatic anterior urethral strictures are short and very dense (Roehrborn and McConnell, 1994). Ideal treatment, in experienced hands, consists of complete stricture resection with end-to-end anastomosis at least 3 months after injury. Endoscopic treatments or dilations are best employed for short, flimsy strictures that are not complicated by spongiofibrosis. Urethral ultrasonography helps to determine precisely stricture length, and may be influential in the selection of reconstructive surgical technique (Morey and McAninch, 1997).

It is important to remember that periurethral erectile tissues are less developed in boys than in adults. As a result, the pediatric bulbous urethra is delicate and does not lend itself well to liberal mobilization or the support of free grafts (Morey and McAninch 1996b). Therefore, for strictures too long to be excised, penile skin flap reconstructive procedures may be preferable to those utilizing free grafts (McAninch and Morey, 1998).

Genital trauma

Testicular injuries

While scrotal trauma is common in prepubescent males, the testes, because of their mobility and size, are rarely injured. When testicular injuries occur they are

usually secondary to blunt trauma from a sports injury. Testis rupture may rarely be present in the absence of significant scrotal hematoma. Localized severe tenderness of the testis supports the diagnosis. However, a massive scrotal hematoma often obscures the testicular examination and may occur in the absence of testicular rupture. This may be a consequence of epididymal injury.

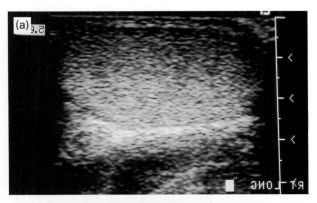

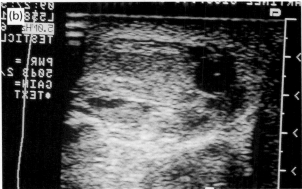

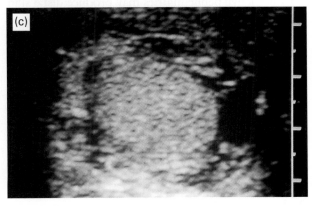

Figure 39.22 (*a*) Normal testicular ultrasound after trauma revealing homogeneous echotexture throughout the testis. (*b*) Small hypoechoic areas within the testis after blunt trauma indicative of a ruptured testis. (*c*) Hematocele surrounding a normal testis after blunt trauma.

Boys with scrotal injuries usually present acutely, because of the pain and rapid onset of dramatic swelling that such injuries often produce. Physical examination may be difficult because of exquisite tenderness. The physician must first always consider the diagnosis of testicular torsion in all boys with scrotal pain. The best way to evaluate boys with scrotal injuries is by ultrasonography. Scrotal ultrasound is rapid, non-invasive, and extremely reliable in the detection of testicular abnormalities. Normal testes have a homogeneous sonographic appearance (Fig. 39.22). If hypoechoic areas are noted within the testicular parenchyma after trauma, the diagnosis of testicular rupture must be suspected and scrotal exploration considered. Normally, testicular rupture can be treated by judicious débridement of extruded tubules with primary closure of the tunica albuginea. Most simple scrotal hematomas can be observed if the injury appears stable. Patients with large hematoceles, however, will generally recover more quickly with prompt incision and drainage (Cass and Luxenberg, 1988).

Genital skin loss

Traumatic scrotal avulsion usually occurs as a result of a rapid deceleration injury. Most scrotal defects are partial and may be successfully closed primarily in two layers with excellent results if the wound is not grossly contaminated (Fig. 39.23). Repair should be undertaken immediately since delay invites bacterial colonization of the wound (Morey and McAninch, 1999b).

Constrictive penile injuries may produce distal skin necrosis. Genital skin loss may also result from dog or human bites producing contaminated wounds that should not be closed primarily (Wolf *et al.*, 1993). For small, clean, non-circumferential penile skin defects, mobilization and closure of a local skin flap is adequate. More extensive defects may require skin grafting although penile skin regenerates, and secondary healing can be predicted to occur uneventfully. Retrograde urethrography should be performed if urethral injury is suspected.

Sexual abuse

Straddle injuries are the most common cause of genital injuries in girls (Steroff *et al.*, 1969). Unfortunately, sexual abuse is commonplace and must be suspected whenever children present to the

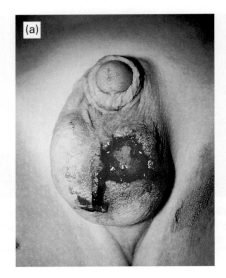

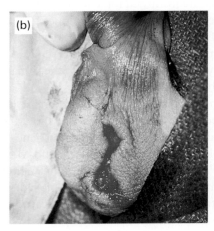

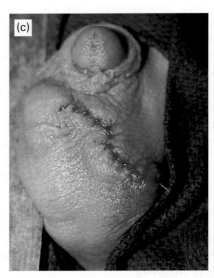

Figure 39.23 (*a*) Scrotal laceration after a deceleration injury. (*b*, *c*) Débridement and two-layer primary closure are performed using interrupted fine absorbable sutures.

emergency room with obvious signs of genital trauma that are inconsistent with the history given. Sexual abuse affects 5–20% of all children, but may be underreported because of fear or embarrassment (Finkelhor, 1994). Girls are involved two to three times as often as boys, and those at highest risk are those between the ages of 11 and 15 years (Emmert and Kohler, 1998). Tears of the vaginal, urethral, or rectal areas should prompt suspicion for abuse, and immediate reporting to the appropriate healthcare personnel experienced in the evaluation and follow-up of such children is mandatory. Examination under anesthesia may be necessary to determine the nature and extent of injuries.

Peer-group genital violence is more common in boys than girls. These injuries tend to occur around the seventh to eighth grade, in the schoolyard, and often represent some form of bullying (Finkelhor and Wolak, 1995). Men with childhood histories of genital abuse may develop disturbing urologic problems such as urogenital pain, impotence, testicular and penile injuries, genital self-mutilation, recurrent hematuria, and voiding dysfunction in adult life (McCarty *et al.*, 1996).

References

Al-ali M, Haddad LF (1996) The late treatment of 63 overlooked or complicated ureteral missile injuries: the promise of nephrostomy and role of autotransplantation. *J Urol* **156**: 1918–21.

Allen TD (1991) Editorial comment. *J Urol* **145**: 356.

Armenakas NA, McAninch JW (1996) Acute anterior urethral injuries: diagnosis and initial management. In: McAninch JW (ed.) *Traumatic and reconstructive urology*. Philadelphia, PA: WB Saunders, 543–50.

Armenakas NA, Duckett CP, McAninch JW (1999) Indications for nonoperative management of renal stab wounds. *J Urol* **161**: 768–71.

Baskin LS, McAninch JW (1993) Childhood urethral injuries: perspectives on outcome and treatment. *Br J Urol* **72**: 241–6.

Blankenship JC, Cox CE, Chauhan R, Gingrich JR (1999) Prognostic value of renal trauma grading system and importance of follow-up imaging studies for blunt renal trauma. *J Urol* **161** (Suppl): 14A.

Boone TB, Gilling PJ, Husmann DA (1993) Ureteropelvic junction disruption following blunt abdominal trauma. *J Urol* **150**: 33–6.

Borirakchanyvat S, Nash PA, McAninch JW (1995) Renal forniceal rupture following blunt abdominal trauma. *J Urol* **153** (Suppl): 315A.

Brown SL, Elder JS, Spirnak JP (1998a) Are pediatric patients more susceptible to major renal injury from blunt trauma? A comparative study. *J Urol* **161**: 138–40.

Brown SL, Hoffman DM, Spirnak JP (1998b) Limitations of routine spiral computerized tomography in the evaluation of blunt renal trauma. *J Urol* **160**: 1979–81.

Brown SL, Spirnak JP, Volsko T *et al.* (1999). Radiographic evaluation in pediatric blunt renal trauma patients with microscopic hematuria. *J Urol* **161** (Suppl): 14A.

Cantor RM, Leaming JM (1998) Evaluation and management of pediatric major trauma. *Emerg Med Clin North Am* **16**: 229–54.

Cass AS, Luxenberg M (1988) Value of early operation in blunt testicular contusion with hematocele. *J Urol* **139**: 736.

Cass AS, Luxenberg M, Gleich P *et al.* (1986) Clinical indications for radiographic evaluation of blunt renal trauma. *J Urol* **136**: 370.

Centers for Disease Control, Division of Injury Control, Center for Environmental Health and Injury Control (1990): Childhood injuries in the United States. *Am J Dis Child* **144**: 627–46.

Coburn M (1997) Damage control for urologic injuries. *Surg Clin North Am* **77**: 821–34.

Corriere JN (1991) Trauma to the lower urinary tract. In: Gillenwater JY, Grayhack JT, Howards SS, Duckett JD (eds) *Adult and pediatric urology*. 2nd edition. St Louis, MO: Mosby-Year Book, 499–521.

Cummings JM, Parra RO, Boullier JA (1999) Impact of delayed diagnosis on repair of ureteral injury. *J Urol* **161** (Suppl): 15A.

Eastham JA, Wilson TG, Ahlering TE (1992) Radiographic evaluation of adult patients with blunt renal trauma. *J Urol* **148**: 266.

Emmert C, Kohler U (1998) Data about 154 children and adolescents reporting sexual assault. *Arch Gynecol Obstet* **261**: 61–70.

Finkelhor D (1994) Abus sexuel et sante sexuelle chez l'enfant: noveaux dilemmes pour le pediatre. *Schweiz Med Wochenschr* **124**: 2320–30.

Finkelhor D, Wolak J (1995) Nonsexual assaults to the genitals in the youth population. *JAMA* **274**: 1692–7.

Fleisher G (1989) Prospective evaluation of selective criteria for imaging among children with suspected blunt renal trauma. *Pediatr Emerg Care* **5**: 8.

Guerriero WG (1991) Editorial comment. *J Urol* **146**: 277.

Haas CA, Dinchman KH, Nasrallah PF, Spirnak JP (1998a) Traumatic renal artery occlusion: a 15-year review. *J Trauma* **45**: 557–61.

Haas CA, Reigle MD, Selzman AA *et al.* (1998b) Use of ureteral stents in the management of major renal trauma with urinary extravasation: is there a role? *J Endourol* **12**: 545–9.

Haas CA, Brown SL, Spirnak JP (1999) Limitations of routine spiral computerized tomography in the evaluation of bladder trauma. *J Urol* **162**: 51–2.

Hardeman SW, Husmann DA, Chinn HKW *et al.* (1987) Blunt urinary tract trauma: identifying those patients who require radiological diagnostic studies. *J Urol* **138**: 99.

Hashmi A, Klassen T (1995) Correlation between urinalysis and intravenous pyelography in pediatric abdominal trauma. *J Emerg Med* **13**: 255.

Hayden LJ, Koff SA (1984) One-stage membranous urethroplasty in childhood. *J Urol* **132**: 311–12.

Hernandez J, Morey AF (1999) Anterior urethral injuries. *World J Urol* **17**: 96–100.

Herschorn S, Radomski S, Shoskes D *et al.* (1991) Evaluation and treatment of blunt renal trauma. *J Urol* **146**: 274–7.

Hoffmann R, Nerlich M, Muggia-Sullam M *et al.* (1992) Blunt abdominal trauma in cases of multiple trauma evaluated by ultrasonography: a prospective analysis of 291 patients. *J Trauma* **32**: 452–8.

Jo PD, Dmochowski RR, Gavant M (1996) Comparison of CT cystography and conventional cystography for detection of bladder rupture. *J Urol* **155** (Suppl); 450A.

Kamel IR, Berkowitz JF (1996) Assessment of the cortical rim sign in posttraumatic renal infarction. *J Comput Assist Tomogr* **20**: 803–6.

Karp MP, Jewett TC Jr, Kuhn JP *et al.* (1986) The impact of computed tomography scanning on the child with renal trauma. *J Pediatr Surg* **21**: 617.

Koraitim M (1999) Pelvic fracture urethral injuries: the unresolved controversy. *J Urol* **161**: 1433–41.

Kramer SA, Furlow WL, Barrett DM, Kelalis PP (1981) Transpubic urethroplasty in children. *J Urol* **126**: 767–9.

Levy JB, Baskin LS, Ewalt D *et al.* (1993) Nonoperative management of blunt pediatric major renal trauma. *Urology* **42**: 423–4.

Lieu TA, Fleisher GR, Mahboubi S *et al.* (1988) Hematuria and clinical findings as indications for intravenous pyelography in pediatric blunt renal trauma. *Pediatrics* **82**: 216.

Livne PM, Gonzales ET (1985) Genitourinary trauma in children. *Urol Clin North Am* **12**: 53.

McAninch JW, Carroll PR, Klosterman PW (1991) Renal reconstruction after injury. *J Urol* **145**: 932–7.

McAninch JW, Morey AF (1998) Penile circular fasciocutaneous skin flap in 1-stage reconstruction of complex anterior urethral strictures. *J Urol* **159**: 1209–13.

McCarty T, Roberts LW, Hendrickson K (1996) Urologic sequelae of childhood genitourinary trauma and abuse in men: principles of recognition with fifteen case illustrations. *Urology* **47**: 617–21.

McGahan JP, Richards JR, Jones CD, Gerscovich EO (1999) Use of ultrasonography in the patient with acute renal trauma. *J Ultrasound Med* **18**; 207–13.

Matthews LA, Smith EM, Spirnak JP (1997) Nonoperative treatment of major blunt renal lacerations with urinary extravasation. *J Urol* **157**: 2053–8.

Medica J, Caldamone A (1995) Pediatric renal trauma: special considerations. *Semin Urol* **13**: 74.

Medina JJ, Cummings JM, Parra RO (1999) Repair of ureteral gunshot injury with appendiceal interposition. *J Urol* **161**: 1563.

Mee SL, McAninch JW, Robinson AL *et al.* (1989) Radiographic assessment of renal trauma: a 10-year prospective study of patient selection. *J Urol* **141**: 1095.

Mendez R (1977) Renal trauma. *J Urol* **118**: 689–703.

Middlebrook PF, Schillinger JF (1993) Hematuria and intravenous pyelography in pediatric blunt renal trauma. *Can J Surg* **36**: 62.

Miller KS, McAninch JW (1995) Radiographic assessment of renal trauma: our 15-year experience. *J Urol* **154**: 352.

Miller RC, Sterioff S Jr, Drucker WR *et al.* (1986) The incidental discovery of occult abdominal tumors in children following blunt abdominal trauma. *J Trauma* **6**: 99.

Moore EE, Shackford SR, Pachter HL *et al.* (1989) Organ injury scaling: spleen, liver, and kidney. *J Trauma* **29**: 1664.

Morey AF (1997) Urologic trauma in children and priapism. In: Baskin LS, Kogan BA, Duckett JW (eds) *Handbook of pediatric urology*. Philadephia, PA: Lippincott-Raven, 51–6.

Morey AF, Carroll PR (1997) Evaluation and management of adult bladder trauma. *Contemp Urol* **9**: 13–22.

Morey AF, McAninch JW (1996a) Renal trauma: principles of evaluation and management. *Trauma Q* **13**: 79–94.

Morey AF, McAninch JW (1996b) When and how to use buccal mucosa in adult bulbar urethroplasty. *Urology* **48**: 194–8.

Morey AF, McAninch JW (1997) Role of preoperative sonourethrography in bulbar urethral reconstruction. *J Urol* **158**: 1376–9.

Morey AF, McAninch JW (1998a) Renal trauma. In: Graham SD (ed.) *Glenn's urologic surgery*, 5th edition. Philadelphia, PA: Lippincott-Raven, 599–604.

Morey AF, McAninch JW (1999b) Genital skin loss and scrotal reconstruction. In: Ehrlich RM, Alter GJ (eds) *Reconstructive and plastic surgery of the external genitalia*. Philadelphia, PA: WB Saunders, 414–22.

Morey AF, Bruce JE, McAninch JW (1996) Efficacy of radiographic imaging in pediatric blunt renal trauma. *J Urol* **156**: 2014–18.

Morey AF, Hernandez J, McAninch JW (1999a) Reconstructive surgery for trauma of the lower urinary tract. *Urol Clin North Am* **26**: 49–60.

Morey AF, McAninch JW, Tiller BK *et al.* (1999b). Single shot intraoperative excretory urography for the immediate evaluation of renal trauma. *J Urol* **161**: 1088–92.

Morse TS (1975) Renal injuries. *Pediatr Clin North Am* **22**: 379–91.

Nash PA, Bruce JE, McAninch JW (1995) Nephrectomy for traumatic renal injuries. *J Urol* **153**: 609–11.

Noe HN, Jenkins GR (1992) Genitourinary trauma. In: Kelalis P, King L, Belman AB (eds) *Clinical pediatric urology*. 3rd edition Philadelphia, PA: WB Saunders 1353–78.

Nudell D, Morey AF, McAninch JW (1997) Renal trauma – when to wait and when to operate. *Curr Opin Urol* **7**: 138–41.

Patrick DA, Bensard DD, Moore EE *et al.* (1998) Ultrasound is an effective triage tool to evaluate blunt abdominal trauma in the pediatric population. *J Trauma* **45**: 57–62.

Porter JR, Mann FA, Talner LB, Defalco AJ (1998) Computer tomographic findings in the evaluation of blunt ureteral trauma. *J Urol* **159** (Suppl): 29A.

Quinlan DM, Gearhart JP (1990) Blunt renal trauma in childhood: features indicating severe injury. *Br J Urol* **66**: 526.

Roehrborn CG, McConnell JD (1994) Analysis of factors contributing to success or failure of 1-stage urethoplasty for urethral stricture disease. *J Urol* **151**: 869–73.

Ryckman FC, Noseworthy J (1985) Multisystem trauma. *Surg Clin North Am* **65**: 1299.

Sandler CM, Corriere JN (1989) Urethrography in the diagnosis of acute urethral injuries. *Urol Clin North Am* **23**: 128.

Shafermeyer R (1993) Pediatric trauma. *Emergy Med Clin North Am* **11**: 187–205.

Smith EM, Elder JS, Spirnak JP (1992) Major blunt renal trauma in the pediatric population: is a nonoperative approach indicated? *J Urol* **148**: 691.

Steers WD, Corriere JN, Benson GS, Boileau MA (1985) The use of indwelling ureteral stents in managing ureteral injuries due to external violence. *J Trauma* **25**: 1001–3.

Stein JP, Kaji DM, Eastham J et al. (1994) Blunt renal trauma in the pediatric population: indications for radiographic evaluation. *Urology* **44**: 409.

Steroff S Jr, Izant RJ, Persky L (1969) Perineal injuries in children. *J Trauma* **9**: 56.

Taylor GA, Eichelberger MR, O'Donnell R, Bowman L (1991) Indications for computed tomography in children with blunt abdominal trauma. *Ann Surg* **213**: 212.

Thompson-Fawcett M, Kolbe A (1996) Paediatric renal trauma: caution with conservative management of major injuries. *Aust NZ J Surg* **66**: 435–40.

Waterhouse K, Abrahams JI, Caponegro P et al. (1974) The transpubic repair of membranous urethral strictures. *J Urol* **111**: 188–90.

Wessels H, McAninch JW (1996) Effect of colon injury on the management of simultaneous renal trauma. *J Urol* **155**: 1852–6.

Wessels H, Deirmenjian J, McAninch JW (1997a) Preservation of renal function after reconstruction for trauma: quantitative assessment with radionuclide scintigraphy. *J Urol* **157**: 1583.

Wessels HB, McAninch JW, Meyer A, Bruce J (1997b) Criteria for non-operative treatment of significant penetrating renal lacerations. *J Urol* **157**: 24–7.

Wolf JS Jr, Turzan CW, Cattolica EV, McAninch JW (1993) Dog bites to male genitalia: characteristics, management and comparison with human bites. *J Urol* **149**: 286.

Further reading

Al-rifael MA, Gaafar S, Abdel-Rahman M (1991) Management of posterior urethral strictures secondary to pelvic fractures in children. *J Urol* **145**: 353–6.

Dixon CM, Hricak H, McAninch JW (1992) Magnetic resonance imaging of traumatic posterior urethral defects and pelvic crush injuries. *J Urol* **148**: 1162–5.

El-abd SA (1995) Endoscopic treatment of posttraumatic urethral obliteration: experience in 396 patients. *J Urol* **153**: 67–71.

Follis HW, Koch MO, McDougal WS (1992) Immediate management of prostatomembranous urethral disruptions. *J Urol* **147**: 1259–62.

Gundogdu H, Tanyel FC, Buyukpamukcu N, Hicsonmez A (1990) Primary realignment of posterior urethral ruptures in children. *Br J Urol* **65**: 650–2.

Koraitim MM (1995) The lessons of 145 posttraumatic urethral strictures treated in 17 years. *J Urol* **153**: 63–6.

Kotkin L, Koch MO (1996) Impotence and incontinence after immediate realignment of posterior urethral trauma: result of injury or management? *J Urol* **155**: 1600–2.

McAninch JW (1989) Pubectomy in repair of membranous urethral stricture. *Urol Clin of North Am* **16**: 297–302.

McAninch JW (1981) Traumatic injuries to the urethra. *J Trauma* **21**: 291–7.

Morey AF, McAninch JW (1997) Reconstruction of posterior urethral disruption injuries: outcomes analysis in 82 patients. *J Urol* **157**: 506–10.

Mundy AR (1996) Urethroplasty for posterior urethral strictures. *Br J Urol* **78**: 243–7.

Pritchett TR, Shapiro RA, Hardy BE (1993) Surgical management of traumatic posterior urethral strictures in children. *Urology* **42**: 59–62.

Spirnak JP, Smith EM, Elder JS (1993) Posterior urethral obliteration treated by endoscopic reconstitution, internal urethrotomy, and temporary self-dilation. *J Urol* **149**: 766–8.

Waterhouse K, Laungani G, Patil U (1980) The surgical repair of membranous urethral strictures: experience with 105 consecutive cases. *J Urol* **123**: 500–5.

Wilms' tumor

40

Michael L. Ritchey

Introduction

Nephroblastoma, or Wilms' tumor, is an embryonal tumor that develops from remnants of immature kidney. It is the most common primary malignant renal tumor of childhood and typically affects children under the age of 6 years. Over the past decades the survival of children with Wilms' tumor has improved rapidly. With increasing sophistication and experience, emphasis should be on reducing the morbidity for low-risk patients and reserving more intensive treatment for selected high-risk patients for whom survival remains poor. This chapter will review the epidemiology, pathology, and recent advances in the understanding of the biology of Wilms' tumor. The current management of children with all stages of nephroblastoma will be discussed in detail.

Epidemiology

The overall annual incidence is approximately 10 cases per million children under 15 years of age, or about 500 new cases annually in the USA. Wilms' tumor accounts for 6–7% of all childhood cancers (Breslow et al., 1993). It typically affects young children (median age 3.5 years), although older children and occasionally even adults can be affected. Wilms' tumor occurs at an earlier age in children with bilateral tumors, 29.5 months for boys and 32.6 months for girls, whereas sporadic cases occur at a mean age of 3.5 years. The disease occurs nearly equally in girls and boys worldwide, but the frequency is slightly higher among girls in the USA (Breslow et al., 1994).

Children with Wilms' tumor frequently have associated congenital anomalies or recognizable syndromes. Syndromes associated with a predisposition to develop Wilms' tumor may be divided into those characterized by somatic overgrowth and those lacking this feature.

Syndromes with overgrowth include hemihypertrophy, which may occur alone or as part of the Beckwith–Wiedemann syndrome (BWS). BWS is a rare disorder consisting of developmental anomalies characterized by excess growth at the cellular, organ (macroglossia, nephromegaly, and hepatomegaly) or body segment (hemihypertrophy) levels (Beckmith, 1969; Sotelo-Avila et al., 1980). The incidence of tumor development in BWS is 10–20%, including Wilms' tumor, adrenocortical neoplasms and hepatoblastoma. The risk of Wilms' tumor development in patients with hemihypertrophy and BWS is estimated to be in the order of 4–10% (Sotelo-Avila et al., 1980; Wiedemann, 1983; Beckwith, 1996a; Debaun and Tucker, 1998). Data from the BWS registry suggest that nephromegaly is a strong risk factor for the subsequent development of Wilms' tumor (Debaun et al., 1998). The mean age at diagnosis of Wilms' tumor in hemihypertrophy patients is similar to that of the general Wilms' tumor population (Breslow et al., 1998). Other overgrowth syndromes such as the Perlman, Soto, and the Simpson–Golabi–Behmel syndromes, are also associated with the development of Wilms' tumor (Perlman et al., 1975; Neri et al., 1998).

Genitourinary anomalies (hypospadias, cryptorchidism, and renal fusion anomalies) are present in 4.5% of patients with Wilms' tumor (Breslow and Beckwith, 1982). One specific association of male pseudohermaphroditism, renal mesangial sclerosis and nephroblastoma is the Denys–Drash syndrome. (Drash et al., 1970; Coppes et al., 1993a). Genetic studies indicate that Denys–Drash syndrome is associated with mutations of the 11p13 Wilms' tumor gene (Coppes et al., 1993a). Roughly 1% of Wilms' tumor patients are diagnosed with the WAGR (Wilms' tumor, aniridia, genital anomalies, and mental retardation) syndrome (Hittner et al., 1980). Most affected individuals have a constitutional deletion on chromosome 11 and the incidence of Wilms' tumor formation is 42%.

Periodic imaging with renal ultrasonography has been recommended in children with hemihypertrophy, BWS, and aniridia. The expectation is that the tumor will then be discovered at an earlier stage. A review of such patients reported to the National Wilms' Tumor Study Group (NWTSG) found that there were more stage I tumors and small tumor diameters in patients whose tumor was detected radiographically (Green *et al.*, 1993). However, there were not enough patients in this retrospective review to determine whether early detection had an impact on patient survival. Craft *et al.* (1995) reported 13 high-risk children undergoing screening with abdominal sonogram and did not find any significant difference in stage distribution compared with children not undergoing screening. Review of most studies suggests that 3–4 months is the appropriate screening interval (Choyke *et al.*, 1999). Two recent reports have called attention to the increased incidence of non-malignant renal lesions in children with BWS (Choyke *et al.*, 1998; Borer *et al.*, 1999). In two patients, nephrectomy was performed for benign disease as a result of false-positive screening.

Biology

As an embryonal tumor of the kidney, Wilms' tumor has been studied intensely to elucidate the role of genetic alterations in tumor development. Certain groups of Wilms' tumor patients were suspected of having a germline mutation. These included children with congenital anomalies and those with a family history of Wilms' tumor. These patients and those with BWS are diagnosed at an earlier age than the average (Breslow *et al.*, 1993). It was thought that the germline mutation predisposed to both the development of multiple tumors and an earlier age of onset than the general population, as had been noted for children with retinoblastoma (Knudson and Strong, 1972).

The two-event hypothesis, or Knudson model, predicts that two genetic events are rate limiting for tumor formation (Knudson and Strong, 1972). Individuals with a genetic predisposition carry an initial lesion in their germline, either inherited from a parent or resulting from a *de novo* germline mutation. In these individuals, all body cells have already been affected by the first event. Consequently, only one new event in any one cell is required for tumor development. By contrast, in individuals who are not genetically predisposed (sporadic cases), two relatively rare independent events are required in the same cell. Subsequent genetic studies in a number of tumors have confirmed the Knudson model, demonstrating that the two postulated 'genetic hits' constitute the inactivation of both alleles of a tumor suppressor gene (Coppes *et al.*, 1994). In many cases, the first allele is inactivated by a mutation within the gene itself, while the second allele is inactivated by a gross loss of chromosomal material. The clearest example of tumorigenesis following the inactivation of both copies of a single tumor suppressor gene is the development of retinoblastoma following the inactivation of the retinoblastoma gene RB1. Unlike the genetic mechanism leading to the development of retinoblastoma, which only requires the inactivation of a single gene, the biologic pathways leading to the development of Wilms' tumor are complex and are likely to involve several genetic loci.

The identity of the first locus associated with Wilms' tumor was in patients with the WAGR syndrome. Cytogenetic studies noted a heterozygous deletion found at band 11p13 of chromosome 11. The WT1 gene was identified using cloning techniques (Call *et al.*, 1990; Gessler *et al.*, 1990; Bonetta *et al.*, 1990). This gene is expressed in the developing kidney and abnormally expressed in some Wilms' tumor specimens. WT1 mutations have been shown to occur in human DNA from sporadic Wilms' tumor, as well as the germline of patients with a genetic predisposition to cancer.

WT1 was identified as a classic tumor suppressor gene, i.e. the loss of both copies would be required for tumor development. While this is indeed the case for certain Wilms' tumors (Coppes *et al.*, 1994), it has now become clear that specific alterations in only one of the two WT1 alleles may also contribute to abnormal cell growth. WT1 appears to be a transcription factor that suppresses the expression of other genes. The normal function of WT1 is necessary for genitourinary development. Mutations at the WT1 locus, particularly in males, may confer extensive genitourinary defects, most notably hypospadias (Pelletier *et al.*, 1991; Coppes *et al.*, 1993a). The affected gonads and kidneys in patients with the Denys–Drash syndrome are heterozygous for germline mutations. The resulting phenotype is far more severe than that observed in children with a constitutional deletion of one WT1 allele (i.e. WAGR patients). This observation suggests that the altered WT1 protein in patients with the Denys–Drash syndrome is not inactivated, but rather rendered dysfunctional, resulting in a dominant-negative effect.

The majority of Wilms' tumors do not have genetic alterations at 11p13. The detection of a germline WT1 mutation reduced to homozygosity in both tumors from a bilateral Wilms' tumor patient provided molecular data indicating that inactivation of both alleles is a critical step in tumorigenesis (Huff *et al.*, 1991). Germline WT1 mutations are associated with genitourinary anomalies. No increased risk was seen in patients with nephrogenic rests, bilateral Wilms' tumor, or family history of Wilms' tumor (Diller *et al.*, 1998).

A second Wilms' tumor locus has been identified on chromosome 11p15 (Koufos *et al.*, 1989; Mannens *et al.*, 1990) and labeled WT2. Similarly to the association between WT1 at chromosome 11p13 and the WAGR syndrome, WT2 has been linked to the BWS (Koufos *et al.*, 1989; Ping *et al.*, 1989). Whether the BWS gene and WT2 are one and the same gene or two distinct but closely linked genes still needs to be elucidated. Loci at 16q (Maw *et al.*, 1992; Grundy *et al.*, 1994), 1p (Grundy *et al.*, 1994), 7p (Wilmore *et al.*, 1994), and 17p (Bardeesy *et al.*, 1994), have also been linked to the biology of Wilms' tumor. However, the latter loci do not seem to predispose to Wilms' tumor, but rather to be associated with phenotype or outcome.

Histopathology

Wilms' tumor usually compresses the adjacent normal renal parenchyma forming a pseudocapsule composed of compressed, atrophic renal tissues. Most tumors are soft and friable, with necrotic or hemorrhagic areas frequently noted. Wilms' tumor is characterized by tremendous histologic diversity. The classic triphasic pattern includes a varying proportion of three cell types: blastemal, stromal, and epithelial. The proportion of each of these components varies, with some consisting of only biphasic or even monomorphous patterns. In addition to expressing a variety of cell types found in a normal developing kidney, Wilms' tumor often contains tissues such as skeletal muscle, cartilage, and squamous epithelium. These hetero-

topic cell types probably reflect the primitive developmental potentials of metanephric blastema that are not expressed in normal nephrogenesis. Most Wilms' tumors are unicentric, but 7% are multicentric unilateral tumors. Extrarenal locations are rare and are thought to arise from displaced metanephric elements or mesonephric remnants.

One important observation was the identification of tumors with *unfavorable* histologic features that were associated with increased rates of relapse and death (Beckwith and Palmer, 1978). These unfavorable features occurred in approximately 10% of patients, but accounted for almost one-half of the tumor deaths in early NWTSG findings (Breslow *et al.*, 1985). Anaplasia, the presence of gigantic polyploid nuclei within the tumor sample, is a feature of Wilms' tumor that is clearly associated with resistance to chemotherapy. This is evidenced by the similar incidence of anaplasia in the NWTSG study (5%) and in the International Society of Pediatric Oncology (SIOP) study (5.3%) (Schmidt and Beckwith, 1995). It is rare in the first 2 years of life but the incidence increases to 13% in children aged 5 years or older (Bonadio *et al.*, 1985). The definition of focal anaplasia is based on a topographic principle and these changes may be either focal or diffuse. Focal anaplasia in this context requires that cells with anaplastic nuclear changes be confined to sharply restricted foci within the primary tumor (Faria *et al.*, 1996). Diffuse anaplasia is diagnosed when anaplasia is present in more than one portion of the tumor or if found in any extrarenal or metastatic site. When the anaplastic component is completely removed (stage I) the outcome is generally excellent (Zuppan *et al.*, 1988). This confirms the observation that anaplasia is a marker more of chemoresistance than of inherent aggressiveness of the tumor. When anaplastic changes are not present, the tumor is referred to as being of favorable histology (FH) because of the generally good outcome for these patients (Beckwith and Palmer, 1978). Clear cell sarcoma of the kidney (CCSK) and rhabdoid tumor of the kidney (RTK) were previously grouped as unfavorable histology Wilms' tumors. They are now recognized as separate malignant entities (see below).

More than one-third of kidneys resected for Wilms' tumor contain precursor lesions, known as nephrogenic rests (Beckwith *et al.*, 1990). Nephrogenic rests represent the abnormal persistence into postnatal life of embryonal cells that can produce a malignancy

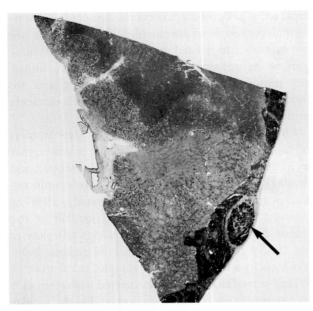

Figure 40.1 Perilobar nephrogenic rest (*arrow*) composed of blastemal cells just beneath the renal capsule (hematoxylin and eosin, × 40).

(Fig. 40.1). Two distinct categories of nephrogenic rest are currently recognized, based on the position of these lesions within the renal lobe. Perilobar nephrogenic rests (PLNR) are confined to the periphery of the renal lobe, whereas intralobar nephrogenic rests (ILNR) occur anywhere in the kidney including the renal sinus and collecting system. There are biologic differences distinguishing PLNR from ILNR (Table 40.1). The presence of multiple or diffuse nephrogenic rests will lead to the diagnosis of nephroblastomatosis. Nephrogenic rests have a varied life and most do not form Wilms' tumor. A rest can undergo maturation, sclerosis, involution, and complete disappearance. PLNR have been detected in 1% of infant kidneys on postmortem examination (Beckwith,

1998). Nephrogenic rests have also been found in 4% of multicystic dysplastic kidneys (Noe *et al.*, 1989), but only 1 in 2000 would be expected to develop a Wilms' tumor (Beckwith, 1996b). ILNR can become cystic and are indistinguishable from renal dysplasia. Hyperplastic nephrogenic rests can produce a renal mass that can be mistaken for a small Wilms' tumor. Incisional biopsy of a hyperplastic rest is of little value in distinguishing this lesion from a Wilms' tumor. Neoplastic induction of cells of a nephrogenic rest have the capability of producing Wilms' tumor and possibly other benign or malignant renal neoplasms.

Multiple rests in one kidney usually imply that nephrogenic rests are present in the other kidney (Beckwith *et al.*, 1990). Children younger than 12 months diagnosed with Wilms' tumor who also have nephrogenic rests have a markedly increased risk of developing contralateral disease. They need regular imaging surveillance to detect contralateral recurrence. Since metachronous Wilms' tumor does occur in patients previously treated with conventional chemotherapeutic regimens, one cannot assume that nephrogenic rests are always eradicated by this treatment modality.

Presentation, preoperative evaluation, and staging

The most common initial clinical manifestation of Wilms' tumor is an asymptomatic abdominal mass. Other signs and symptoms at diagnosis are abdominal pain, gross hematuria, and fever. The child may present with an acute abdomen due to rupture of the tumor with hemorrhage into the peritoneal cavity. Additional symptoms may result from compression or invasion of adjacent structures. The propensity of Wilms' tumor to grow into the renal vein and inferi-

Table 40.1 Clinical features of intralobar nephrogenic rest (ILNR) and perilobar nephrogenic rest (PLNR)

	ILNR	PLNR
Associated syndromes	WAGR Denys–Drash Genitourinary anomalies	BWS Hemihypertrophy Perlman
Median age of Wilms' tumor development	23 months	36 months
Wilms' tumor histology	Stroma predominant	Blastema, epithelial predominant

WAGR = Wilms' tumor, aniridia, genitourinary, retardation; BWS = Beckwith–Wiedemann syndrome.

or vena cava can produce atypical presentations. Varicocele, hepatomegaly due to hepatic vein obstruction, ascites, and congestive heart failure were found in fewer than 10% of patients with intracaval or atrial tumor extension in NWTS-3 (Ritchey *et al.*, 1988). Occasionally, children with Wilms' tumor will present with symptoms suggesting the production of bioactive substances by the tumor (Coppes, 1993). Hypertension is present in 25% of patients and has been attributed to elevated plasma renin levels (Voute *et al.*, 1971). During the physical examination, it is important to note signs of associated Wilms' tumor syndromes such as aniridia, hemihypertrophy, and genitourinary anomalies.

The preoperative evaluation can generally be completed in 48 hours. Emergency operation is not necessary unless there is evidence of active bleeding or tumor rupture. Laboratory evaluation should include a complete peripheral blood count, platelet count, renal function tests, liver function tests, serum calcium, and urinalysis. Elevation of the serum calcium can occur in children with congenital mesoblastic nephroma and rhabdoid tumor of the kidney. Acquired von Willebrand's disease has been found in 8% of newly diagnosed Wilms' tumor patients (Coppes *et al.*, 1993b).

The preoperative imaging evaluation of children with a solid abdominal mass has evolved over the years. All of the solid renal tumors of childhood have similar radiographic features. However, defining the exact histology is probably not as important as establishing that there is a solid renal tumor present, which will help the surgeon to plan for a major cancer operation. Children entered on NWTS-3 who had an incorrect preoperative diagnosis were found to have an increased incidence of surgical complications (Ritchey *et al.*, 1992). The majority of these patients had not undergone any preoperative imaging studies. Most importantly, imaging studies should establish the presence of a functioning contralateral kidney prior to nephrectomy.

An abdominal sonogram is obtained to demonstrate whether the mass is solid or cystic, and confirm its renal origin. Another important role of imaging is to exclude intracaval tumor extension, which occurs in 4% of Wilms' tumor patients (Fig. 40.2) (Ritchey *et al.*, 1988). Contrast-enhanced computed tomography (CT) or magnetic resonance imaging (MRI) of the abdomen is next obtained. MRI is the study of choice if extension of tumor into the inferior vena

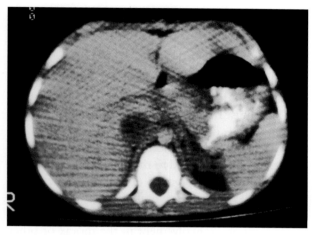

Figure 40.2 Computed tomographic scan demonstrating tumor extension into the inferior vena cava.

cava (IVC) cannot be excluded by ultrasound (Weese *et al.*, 1991).

Assessment of the contralateral kidney in Wilms' tumor patients is essential owing to the high incidence of bilaterality. Both CT and MRI are more accurate than ultrasound in identifying small lesions (nephrogenic rests or Wilms' tumor) in the opposite kidney, but a review of synchronous bilateral Wilms' tumor enrolled in NWTS-4 found that 7% of bilateral lesions were missed by preoperative imaging (Ritchey *et al.*, 1995).

There is some controversy regarding the utility of preoperative imaging for tumor staging (Cohen, 1993; D'Angio *et al.*, 1993; Ditchfield *et al.*, 1995). Accurate staging of children with Wilms' tumors is essential to define tumor extent prior to initiating treatment, as outcome is highly correlated with stage (D'Angio *et al.*, 1989). However, the current staging system used by the NWTSG relies on surgical findings and pathologic examination.

- **Stage I**: The tumor is limited to the kidney and was completely excised. The renal capsule has an intact outer surface. The tumor was not ruptured or biopsied prior to removal (fine-needle aspiration biopsies are excluded from this restriction). The vessels of the renal sinus are not involved. There is no evidence of tumor at or beyond the margins of resection.
- **Stage II**: The tumor extended beyond the kidney, but was completely excised. There may be regional extension of tumor (i.e. penetration of the renal capsule or extensive invasion of the renal sinus).

The blood vessels outside the renal parenchyma, including those of the renal sinus, may contain tumor. The tumor was biopsied (except for fine-needle aspiration), or there was spillage of tumor before or during surgery that is confined to the flank, and does not involve the peritoneal surface. There must be no evidence of tumor at or beyond the margins of resection.

■ **Stage III**: Residual non-hematogenous tumor is present, and confined to the abdomen. Any one of the following may occur. (1) Lymph nodes within the abdomen or pelvis are found to be involved by tumor (renal hilar, para-aortic or beyond). (Lymph-node involvement in the thorax or other extra-abdominal sites would be a criterion for stage IV). (2) The tumor has penetrated through the peritoneal surface. (3) Tumor implants are found on the peritoneal surface. (4) Gross or microscopic tumor remains postoperatively (e.g. tumor cells are found at the margin of surgical resection on microscopic examination). (5) The tumor is not completely resectable because of local infiltration into vital structures. (6) Tumor spill not confined to the flank occurred either before or during surgery.

■ **Stage IV**: Hematogenous metastases (lung, liver, bone, brain, etc.) or lymph-node metastases outside the abdominopelvic region are present.

■ **Stage V**: Bilateral renal involvement is present at diagnosis. An attempt should be made to stage each side according to the above criteria on the basis of the extent of disease prior to biopsy or treatment.

Staging is divided into detection of distant metastases and defining the local extent of the tumor. The local tumor burden (regional lymph-node involvement, residual disease, and diffuse tumor spillage) determines whether the child receives abdominal irradiation and also the intensity of the chemotherapy regimen. Preoperative CT can reveal evidence of regional adenopathy and suggest extrarenal tumor extension into the perirenal fat and into adjacent structures. However, prospective correlation with pathologic findings has not been done. Most children identified as having possible invasion of the liver on CT are found at the time of surgical exploration to have hepatic compression, rather than hepatic invasion (Ng *et al.*, 1991). Enlarged retroperitoneal benign lymph nodes are common in children.

Correlation between pathologic findings and lymph-node evaluation at surgical exploration in Wilms' tumor patients have found false-positive and false-negative error rates of 18 and 31%, respectively (Othersen *et al.*, 1990). It should not be expected that CT or MRI will have greater accuracy. Non-opacification of the kidney may result from tumor obstruction of the collecting system (Nakayama *et al.*, 1988), complete replacement of the renal parenchyma with neoplasm or intravascular tumor extension (Ritchey *et al.*, 1988).

Plain chest radiographs should be obtained to determine whether pulmonary metastases are present. Most centers will also use CT of the chest in the initial evaluation of children with Wilms' tumor. Additional imaging studies are helpful under specific conditions. For example, a radionuclide bone scan and X-ray skeletal survey should be obtained postoperatively on all children with CCSK (Feusner *et al.*, 1990). Brain imaging, using MRI or CT, should be obtained on all children with clear cell sarcoma or rhabdoid tumors, since both are associated with intracranial metastases (Weeks *et al.*, 1989).

Accurate staging of Wilms' tumor allows treatment results to be evaluated and enables universal comparisons of outcomes. In North America, the most widely used staging system is the one developed by the NWTSG, which is based primarily on the surgical and histopathologic findings. With the excellent survival of most patients with favorable histology Wilms' tumor, it has become increasingly difficult to find any particular histologic feature of a given tumor that will predict relapse. Several biologic factors are being investigated to predict the risk of tumor progression or relapse.

Loss of heterozygosity (LOH) for a portion of chromosome 16q and 1p has been noted in 17% and 11% of tumors, respectively (Grundy *et al.*, 1994). Patients with tumor-specific LOH for chromosome 16q had a statistically significantly poorer 2 year relapse-free and overall survival than those without LOH for chromosome 16q. This association was found to be independent of stage and histology. Loss of chromosome 1p was associated with a worse outcome, although this difference did not reach statistical significance (Grundy *et al.*, 1994).

Elevated levels of hyaluronic acid and hyaluronic acid-stimulating activity have been reported in both the urine and serum of Wilms' tumor patients (Lin *et al.*, 1995a). Following surgical removal of the tumor the levels returned to normal. Patients with persistent disease or relapse had significantly higher levels 1–6 months after surgery. Elevated urine levels of basic fibroblast growth factor have also been found in Wilms' tumor patients (Lin *et al.*, 1995b). Stage III and IV patients had significantly higher preoperative levels than did stage I and II patients. Patients with relapse or persistent disease had significantly elevated late postoperative levels compared with disease-free patients and controls. More studies are needed to define the clinical role of these markers in patients with Wilms' tumor.

Elevated plasma renin levels have been reported in Wilms' tumor patients, and following treatment there should be a reduction in plasma levels (Voute *et al.*, 1971). Recently, elevated plasma renin levels were noted in four children with relapse of Wilms' tumor (Johnston *et al.*, 1991). In all cases, the renin level had decreased after initial tumor excision and subsequently became elevated.

Surgery

The surgeon has an important role in the management of the child with Wilms' tumor. Careful removal of the tumor without rupture or spill is mandatory, as its occurrence results in an increased risk of local abdominal relapse (Shamberger *et al.*, 1999). Complete tumor resection improves patient survival. Another important surgical objective is determining tumor extent. A transperitoneal approach is preferred to allow thorough exploration of the abdominal cavity. Exploration of the contralateral kidney should be performed before nephrectomy. The colon is reflected and Gerota's fascia opened so that the kidney can be inspected on all surfaces. Any abnormalities of the kidney should be biopsied to exclude Wilms' tumor or nephrogenic rests. Lymph-node sampling is an integral step during surgery for Wilms' tumor. The presence of lymph-node metastases (stage III) has an adverse outcome on survival. Radical nephrectomy is performed, but formal lymph-node dissection is not required (Othersen *et al.*, 1990). Palpation of the renal vein and IVC should be performed to exclude intravascular tumor extension prior to vessel ligation.

One should not overlook the morbidity of surgery that can produce both acute and late complications. A recent review of NWTS-4 patients undergoing primary nephrectomy found an 11% incidence of surgical complications (Ritchey *et al.*, 1999). The most common complications were hemorrhage and small bowel obstruction. Risk factors associated with increased surgical complications include higher local tumor stage, intravascular extension, *en bloc* resection of other visceral organs, and incorrect preoperative diagnosis (Ritchey *et al.*, 1992).

Treatment and outcome

In the first half of the twentieth century, treatment consisted of surgery and radiation therapy. The development of effective systemic chemotherapy in the 1960s rapidly changed the outcome and approach to treatment of Wilms' tumor (Farber, 1966). The NWTSG was created to determine the appropriate role for each of the therapeutic modalities available. An attempt was made to stratify patients into different treatment groups based on extent of disease and histopathologic features. The goals were to allow a reduction in the intensity of therapy for most patients while maintaining overall survival. Radiation therapy, once administered routinely to all children, is now reserved for those with advanced stage disease or specific adverse prognostic features.

National Wilms' Tumor Study Group

The first two NWTSG studies, NWTS-1 (1969–1973) and NWTS-2 (1974–1978), showed that postoperative local irradiation was unnecessary for group I patients (D'Angio *et al.*, 1976; D'Angio *et al.*, 1981). The combination of vincristine (VCR) and dactinomycin (AMD) was noted to be more effective than the use of either drug alone, and the addition of doxorubicin (DOX) improved survival for higher stage patients. Important findings of NWTS-1 and-2 were identification of unfavorable histologic features and other prognostic factors that allowed refinement of the staging system, stratifying patients into high-risk and low-risk treatment groups (Farewell *et al.*, 1981). It was recognized that the presence of lymph-node metastases had an adverse outcome on survival (D'Angio *et al.*, 1976; D'Angio *et al.*, 1981). Children with lymph-node metastases, as well as those with diffuse tumor spill, were found to be at increased risk of abdominal relapse. Therefore, such patients were from then on classified as having stage III disease and given whole abdominal irradiation

(D'Angio et al., 1989). These findings were incorporated into the design of NWTS-3 to try to decrease the intensity of therapy for the majority of low-risk patients.

In NWTS-3 (1979–1986), patients with stage I, FH Wilms' tumor were treated successfully with either a 10 or 18 week regimen of VCR and AMD (D'Angio et al., 1989). This considerably decreased the amount of chemotherapy administered and the total duration of treatment. The 4 year relapse-free survival was 89% and the overall survival was 95.6%. Stage II FH patients treated with AMD and VCR without postoperative radiation therapy had an equivalent survival (4 year overall survival of 91.1%) to patients who received the same treatment plus DOX with or without radiation. This demonstrated that the cardiotoxic drug DOX is not necessary for the successful treatment of this group of patients. Radiation therapy could now be omitted for the majority of children with Wilms' tumor. For stage III FH patients, the dosage of abdominal irradiation was reduced to 10.8 Gy. This was shown to be as effective as 20 Gy in preventing abdominal relapse if DOX was added to VCR and AMD. The 4 year relapse-free survival for stage III patients was 82% in NWTS-3 and the 4 year overall survival 90.9%. Patients with stage IV FH tumors received abdominal (local) irradiation based on the local tumor stage. In addition, they all received 12 Gy to both lungs. In combination with VCR, AMD, and DOX, the 4 year relapse-free survival was 79% and the overall survival 80.9%. There was no statistically significant improvement in survival when cyclophosphamide was added to the three-drug regimen.

The goals of the fourth (1986–1994) NWTSG study were to continue improving treatment results while decreasing the cost of therapy through modification of the schedule of drug administration. Pulse-intensive chemotherapy regimens, using single doses of AMD and DOX, were compared with regimens using divided doses of the drugs. This was the first clinical pediatric cancer trial to evaluate the economic impact of two different treatment approaches. Pulse-intensive regimens used simultaneous administration of agents at less frequent intervals to decrease the number of clinic visits and hence the cost of cancer treatment. In addition, treatment durations of approximately 6 and 15 months were compared in patients with stages II–IV FH tumors. NWTS-4 demonstrated that, while the administered drug dose intensity was greater on pulse-intensive regimens, these regimens produce less hematologic toxicity than the standard regimens (Green et al., 1998a). Patients treated with pulse-intensive regimens achieved equivalent survival to those treated with standard chemotherapy regimens (Green et al., 1998b). Treatment with a 6 month duration of chemotherapy was as effective as 15 months. Overall, the 4 year survival for patients with FH Wilms' tumor now approaches 90%.

Children with anaplastic Wilms' tumors were randomized in NWTS-3 and NWTS-4 to receive VCR, AMD, DOX, or those three drugs with the addition of cyclophosphamide. The results were analysed after the tumors were reclassified using the criteria of Faria et al. (1996). There was no difference in outcome between the regimens for children with focal anaplasia who had a prognosis similar to that for FH patients (Green et al., 1994a). For stage II–IV diffuse anaplasia, the addition of cyclophosphamide to the three-drug regimen improved the 4 year relapse-free survival (27.2% vs 54.8%).

Treatment recommendations of the current intergroup study, NWTS-5, which opened in 1995, are outlined in Table 40.2. Treatment for patients with stage I or II FH, and stage I anaplastic Wilms' tumor is the same. They are to receive a pulse-intensive regimen of VCR and AMD for 18 weeks. Patients with stage III FH and stage II–III focal anaplasia are to be treated with AMD, VCR, DOX, and 10.8 Gy abdominal irradiation. Patients with stage IV FH tumors receive abdominal irradiation based on the local tumor stage and 12 Gy to both lungs. Finally, children with stage II–IV diffuse anaplasia are treated on NWTS-5 with a new chemotherapeutic regimen combining VCR, DOX, cyclophosphamide, and etoposide in an attempt to improve further the survival of this high-risk group. All of these patients will receive irradiation to the tumor bed. This is a single-arm therapeutic trial without any randomization for therapy.

Prospective collection of information regarding biologic features of Wilms' tumors is underway. A collection of banked tumor specimens is available to evaluate new prognostic factors that may be identified in the future. This study will attempt to verify the preliminary findings that loss of heterozygosity for chromosomes 16q and 1p is useful in identifying patients who are at increased risk for relapse (Grundy et al., 1994). If these molecular genetic markers are indeed

Table 40.2 Protocol for National Wilms' Tumor Study 5

	Radiotherapy	Chemotherapy
Stage I and II, favorable histology	None	Regimen EE-4A
and		
Stage I focal or diffuse anaplasia		
Stage I, favorable histology, age <2 years, tumor weight <550 g	None	Regimen EE-4A[a]
Stage III and IV, favorable histology	Yes	Regimen DD-4A
and		
Stage II, III, and IV, focal anaplasia		
Stage II–IV, diffuse anaplasia	Yes	Regimen I
and		
Stage I–IV clear cell sarcoma of the kidney		
Stage I–IV rhabdoid tumor of the kidney	Yes	Regimen RTK

[a] 1998 modification to the original protocol.
Regimen EE-4A = pulse intensive dactinomycin, vincristine (18 weeks); regimen DD-4A = pulse intensive dactinomycin, vincristine, doxorubicin (24 weeks); regimen I = dactinomycin, vincristine, doxorubicin, cyclophosphamide, and etoposide (24 weeks); regimen RTK = carboplatin, etoposide, and cyclophosphamide (24 weeks).
Stage IV/favorable histology patients are given radiation based on the local tumor stage.

found to be predictive of clinical behavior, this information will be used in subsequent clinical trials to stratify further patients for therapy.

A select group of patients under 2 years of age with stage I FH tumors weighing under 550 was selected for management with surgery alone in NWTS (Green *et al.*, 1994b). This was based on the preliminary observation of favorable outcomes on small numbers of such patients when postoperative adjuvant therapy had been omitted. A review of NWTSG patients had found excellent outcomes for such patients, albeit with postoperative chemotherapy (Green *et al.*, 1994a). This portion of the study was suspended in 1998 when the number of tumor relapses exceeded the limit allowed by the design of the study. The design of the study was that the trial would be stopped when a 2 year relapse-free survival below 95% could be excluded. It was recommended that all children with stage I tumors receive AMD and VCR. Extended follow-up of this cohort of patients continues. Observation of untreated children may yield interesting information on the role of chemotherapy in decreasing the incidence of contralateral relapse in patients with nephrogenic rests.

Preoperative therapy

International Society of Pediatric Oncology (SIOP)

The clinical protocols conducted by SIOP for treatment of Wilms' tumor have included preoperative therapy since the early 1970s. This approach usually results in tumor shrinkage, reducing the risk of intraoperative rupture or spill (Lemerle *et al.*, 1976). It is also postulated that the neoadjuvant therapy will treat micrometastases, leading to a more favorable stage distribution at the time of surgery. A greater number of patients had postchemotherapy stage I tumors. This was thought to be a significant advantage in terms of decreasing morbidity of treatment, particularly the late effects of radiotherapy. When SIOP and NWTSG began their prospective studies, all children with Wilms' tumor received postoperative radiation therapy.

The first two SIOP studies answered questions with regard to the use of prenephrectomy radiation therapy (Lemerle *et al.*, 1976). The third SIOP study, SIOP-5, showed that 4 weeks of AMD and VCR was as effective as prenephrectomy radiation therapy in avoiding surgical tumor rupture and increasing the proportion of patients with low-stage disease (Lemerle *et al.*, 1983). SIOP-6, the fourth SIOP study on Wilms' tumor, demonstrated that patients with postnephrectomy stage I disease can be treated safely with 18 weeks of AMD and VCR (Tournade *et al.*, 1993). Those with stage II, lymph-node-negative disease, however, were shown to require more intensive postnephrectomy chemotherapy, including the use of an anthracycline (Tournade *et al.*, 1993). Finally, SIOP-6 confirmed the need for a three-drug chemotherapy regimen following nephrectomy for those with more advanced stage disease, i.e. stage II lymph-node positive and stage III.

The fifth SIOP Wilms' tumor trial, SIOP-9, found no significant additional tumor shrinkage benefit after 4 weeks of preoperative AMD and VCR (Tournade *et al.*, 1994). The latest SIOP study on Wilms' tumor, SIOP 93-01, aims to determine whether postoperative therapy can be omitted in selected stage I patients and whether survival can be improved in certain high-risk patients with the use of etoposide, ifosfamide, and carboplatin (Nephroblastoma Clinical Trial and Study SIOP no. 93-01).

Preoperative treatment can produce dramatic reductions in the size of the primary tumor, thus facilitating surgical excision (Fig. 40.3). However, the staging information obtained following prenephrectomy chemotherapy does not reflect the orig-

inal tumor stage, as demonstrated by the increased frequency of intra-abdominal recurrence in non-irradiated stage II tumors (classified following 4 weeks of prenephrectomy chemotherapy) without positive lymph nodes (SIOP staging criteria) (Jereb *et al.*, 1994). Both the NWTSG and SIOP tumor staging systems are designed to stratify patients into low-risk and high-risk groups. The goal is to select out high-risk patients for more intensive therapy, while minimizing treatment and thus morbidity for low-risk patients. The NWTSG relies on surgical and pathologic staging reflecting the extent of disease at diagnosis. Although preoperative therapy may destroy the evidence of extrarenal spread of disease, e.g. lymph-node involvement or extracapsular extension, these patients have an increased risk for relapse. This raises some concern regarding the utility of postchemotherapy stage, as opposed to staging at initial surgery, to predict tumor behavior. Staging the patient after chemotherapy may inadequately define the risk of relapse (Green *et al.*, 1993b).

National Wilms' Tumor Study Group: indications for preoperative chemotherapy

The NWTSG recommends preoperative chemotherapy for some select groups of patients. These include those with bilateral involvement (Blute *et al.*, 1987; Ritchey and Coppes, 1995), tumors inoperable at surgical exploration (Ritchey *et al.*, 1994), and tumor extension into the IVC above the hepatic veins

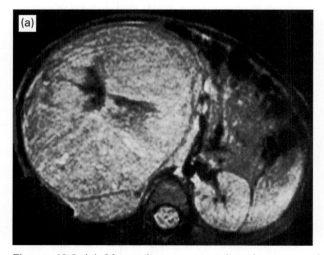 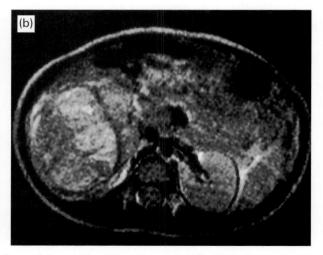

Figure 40.3 (*a*) Magnetic resonance imaging scan of a large inoperable Wilms' tumor. (*b*) After 6 weeks of chemotherapy the same tumor has dramatically decreased in size. (From Ritchey *et al.*, 1996b, Fig. 58.11, with permission from Mosby Year Book.)

(Ritchey *et al.*, 1993). The latter two conditions are associated with a markedly increased risk for surgical complications if primary nephrectomy is undertaken (Ritchey *et al.*, 1992). The rationale for preoperative chemotherapy in patients with bilateral tumors is to preserve renal parenchyma. This is important because renal failure is a significant risk in patients with bilateral disease (Ritchey *et al.*, 1996a).

Vascular extension

For vena caval involvement below the level of the hepatic veins, the caval thrombus can be removed via cavotomy, after proximal and distal vascular control is obtained. In general, the thrombus will be free floating, but if there is adherence of the thrombus to the caval wall, the thrombus can often be delivered with the passage of a Fogarty or Foley balloon catheter. If the thrombus extends above the level of the hepatic veins, preoperative chemotherapy can shrink the tumor and thrombus (Dykes *et al.*, 1991; Ritchey *et al.*, 1993), thus facilitating complete removal (Shamberger *et al.*, 2001).

Inoperable tumor

In the occasional child, the surgeon will encounter a massive tumor involving vital structures, which is not amenable to primary nephrectomy. Attempted radical resection with *en bloc* removal of surrounding organs can result in an increased risk of surgical complications (Ritchey *et al.*, 1992). The gross appearance of the tumor at the time of surgery can be misleading in interpreting tumor extent. Wilms' tumors often compress and adhere to adjacent structures without frank

invasion. If the tumor is found to be unresectable, pretreatment with chemotherapy almost always reduces the bulk of the tumor and renders it resectable (Ritchey *et al.*, 1994) (Fig. 40.3). However, treatment with preoperative chemotherapy does not result in improved survival rates, and can result in the loss of important staging information. The NWTSG recommends that patients who are determined to have unresectable tumor should be considered stage III and treated accordingly (Ritchey *et al.*, 1994). The determination of inoperability is best judged at surgical exploration. Patients who are staged by imaging studies alone are at risk for both under- and overstaging.

In general, the operative procedure can be performed within 6 weeks of initiating treatment. Serial imaging evaluation is helpful to assess response, but radiographic evidence of persistent disease can occasionally be misleading. Failure of the tumor to shrink could be due to predominance of skeletal muscle or benign elements. A second-look procedure to confirm persistent viable tumor may be necessary. Patients with progressive disease have a very poor prognosis and these patients will require treatment with a different chemotherapeutic regimen (Ritchey *et al.*, 1994).

Bilateral disease

Synchronous bilateral nephroblastoma occurs in about 5% of children, with metachronous lesions developing in only 1% (Fig. 40.4) (Blute *et al.*, 1987; Montgomery *et al.*, 1991). In the past, bilateral Wilms' tumor (BWT) patients were managed with a primary surgical approach. Consequently, many patients with synchro-

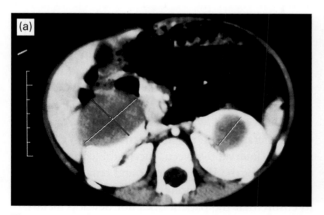
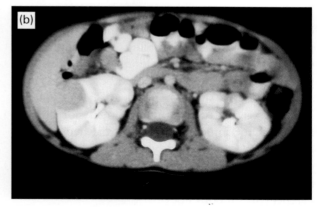

Figure 40.4 Computed tomographic scan demonstrating bilateral Wilms' tumor. (*a*) Before chemotherapy; (*b*) 6 weeks after chemotherapy, showing a marked reduction in the size of the masses.

nous BWT developed significant renal insufficiency. A review of NWTSG patients with BWT found that 9.1% with synchronous bilateral tumors and 18.8% of metachronous bilateral tumors have developed renal failure (Ritchey *et al.*, 1996a). The most common etiology for renal failure was the need for bilateral nephrectomy for persistent or recurrent tumor in the remaining kidney after initial nephrectomy.

Early experience of the NWTSG with BWT found no difference in survival between children managed with initial nephrectomy, with or without contralateral heminephrectomy, and children treated with initial biopsy alone followed by chemotherapy (Bishop *et al.*, 1977). Ten years later, Blute *et al.* (1987) reported a much larger series of 145 BWT patients enrolled in NWTS-2 and -3. Their analysis and a later update by Montgomery *et al.* (1991) confirmed the observation that patients undergoing initial biopsy followed by chemotherapy had an equivalent survival, 83% at 2 years, to patients undergoing initial surgical resection. The larger number of patients demonstrated that, as with unilateral disease, tumor stage and histology were the most important predictors of survival. Most importantly, the NWTSG investigators noted that nephrectomy could be avoided entirely in almost 50% of the group of patients undergoing initial biopsy. SIOP investigators have also reported good overall survival in patients treated with preoperative chemotherapy, with a decrease in the incidence of residual disease (Coppes *et al.*, 1989). These investigators noted that relapses have occurred as late as 4 years post-treatment and recommended long-term follow-up.

Therefore, the preferred approach for patients with BWT is initial biopsy followed by preoperative chemotherapy (Ritchey and Coppes, 1995). Bilateral biopsies should be obtained to confirm the presence of Wilms' tumor in both kidneys and define the histologic type, although sampling errors may occur. Grossly abnormal lymph nodes or other lesions suggestive of extrarenal spread should be biopsied and a surgical (local) stage assigned to both kidneys. Radical excision of the tumor should not be performed at the initial operation. Partial nephrectomy or wedge excision should be employed at the initial operation only if all tumor can be removed and there is preservation of two-thirds or more of the renal parenchyma on both sides.

After 6 weeks of chemotherapy, the patient is reassessed with an abdominal CT to determine the feasibility of resection. Experience in SIOP has shown that maximal shrinkage occurs after 4–6 weeks of chemotherapy (Tournade *et al.*, 1994). While waiting longer may not benefit a patient with unilateral tumor who will later undergo nephrectomy, that is not always the case with BWT. Even a modest further reduction in tumor size may be helpful. This is particularly true for centrally located tumors, where an additional 1 cm reduction in size may allow partial nephrectomy with sparing of the renal hilum.

However, one should not continue chemotherapy indefinitely. Some patients may not have a measurable response to preoperative chemotherapy (Zuppan *et al.*, 1991). Failure of the mass to shrink is not always due to persistent viable tumor. If serial imaging studies show no further reduction in the tumor, a second-look procedure is recommended. There may be necrosis, fibrosis, or persistence of skeletal muscle and benign elements within the original lesion. A biopsy of the kidney is necessary to confirm persistent viable tumor. At the time of the second-look procedure, partial nephrectomy or wedge excision of the tumor should be considered, but only if it will not compromise tumor resection and negative margins can be obtained.

If the tumors are not amenable to partial resections, patients with persistent viable tumor are then treated with a different chemotherapeutic regimen and/or radiotherapy. Patients who have been on AMD and VCR should then be given DOX. Those who have received all three of these drugs should receive radiation therapy (15 Gy/day × 10). The patient should be reassessed after an additional 12 weeks of chemotherapy or 4 weeks after radiation therapy to determine the feasibility of resection. If it appears that either or both of the kidneys can be salvaged, partial nephrectomies or wedge excisions of the tumors are performed. Radical nephrectomy is performed to remove the kidney with too extensive tumor involvement when only one of the two can be preserved. Bilateral nephrectomies and dialysis may rarely be required, when the tumors fail to respond to chemotherapy and radiation therapy. The recommended interval between successful completion of treatment of the Wilms' tumor and renal transplantation varies. Some advocate a waiting period of 2 years to ensure that the patient does not develop metastatic disease, while others have found that a 1-year interval is sufficient (Penn, 1979).

Partial nephrectomy in unilateral tumors

The success of renal preservation in BWT has prompted some surgeons to recommend parenchymal sparing procedures for unilateral tumors (McLorie *et al.*, 1991; Cozzi *et al.*, 1995; Moorman-Voestermans *et al.*, 1998). They cite concern about the late occurrence of renal dysfunction in children who have undergone unilateral nephrectomy. There is both clinical and experimental evidence of hyperfiltration damage of remnant nephrons after a loss of significant renal mass (McLorie *et al.*, 1991). Following treatment for unilateral Wilms' tumor, some patients may develop proteinuria and a decrease in creatinine clearance (Robitaille *et al.*, 1985; Bertolone *et al.*, 1987). However, other investigators have failed to confirm these findings (Barrera *et al.*, 1989; Bhisitkul *et al.*, 1990). A review of NWTSG patients was conducted to identify risk factors for the development of renal insufficiency (Ritchey *et al.*, 1996a). These investigators found that the incidence of renal failure in children with unilateral tumors was 0.25%. Most of those patients had the Denys–Drash syndrome and such patients have intrinsic renal disease and generally present with renal failure at diagnosis or inevitably progress to end-stage renal disease (ESRD). Therefore, the risk of developing renal failure following treatment for unilateral Wilms' tumor appears to be quite low, although continued long-term follow-up of this cohort of children for late effects of treatment is needed.

The majority of Wilms' tumors are too large for a partial nephrectomy at initial presentation. Therefore pretreatment with chemotherapy is usually necessary if renal sparing surgery is to be considered (McLorie *et al.*, 1991; Cozzi *et al.*, 1995; Moorman-Voestermans *et al.*, 1998). Staging of the patient after chemotherapy could lead to inaccuracy, as discussed above. Some authors rely on the preoperative imaging to select patients for partial nephrectomy and to stage the tumor (Bertolone *et al.*, 1987; McLorie *et al.*, 1991; Cozzi *et al.*, 1995; Moorman-Voestermans *et al.*, 1998). There are no published studies prospectively correlating staging by imaging studies and surgical/pathologic staging.

After preoperative chemotherapy, 10–15% of patients are amenable to partial nephrectomy (McLorie *et al.*, 1991; Moorman-Voestermans *et al.*, 1998). Some advocate enucleation to allow parenchymal sparing procedures for even centrally located tumors where partial nephrectomy with a rim of renal tissue would be inadvisable (Cozzi *et al.*, 1995). A recent review of patients with BWT found that the incidence of local recurrence was 7.5% following partial nephrectomy compared with 14% local recurrence after enucleation (no significant difference) (Horwitz *et al.*, 1996). Although overall survival was comparable, patients with residual disease and recurrences received added therapy to maintain this survival.

Screening of patients at an increased risk for the development of Wilms' tumor (e.g. BWS, hemihypertrophy, aniridia) will occasionally detect a small lesion, inviting the possibility of a renal sparing procedure. Others have advocated preoperative chemotherapy in all such patients to shrink the tumor and facilitate partial nephrectomy (Borer *et al.*, 1999). Data have been lacking regarding the risk for metachronous Wilms' tumor development in such patients. A recent report from the NWTSG has demonstrated an increased incidence of metachronous Wilms' tumor development in patients undergoing unilateral nephrectomy if nephrogenic rests were found in the kidney adjacent to the tumor (Coppes *et al.*, 1999). Patients with BWS, hemihypertrophy, and aniridia have an increased incidence of nephrogenic rests, or Wilms' tumor precursors, compared with patients with unilateral Wilms' tumor not associated with congenital anomalies (Beckwith, 1998). An increased risk of metachronous Wilms' tumor was found in patients with BWS (3/35 children vs 0.45 expected), hemihypertrophy (5/144 vs 1.83 expected), and aniridia (2/32 vs 0.41 expected). However, the numbers of patients were too small for reliable statistical inference.

In summary, parenchymal sparing procedures for patients with unilateral Wilms' tumor are controversial. The current recommendation of the NWTSG is to consider partial nephrectomy for patients with BWT, solitary kidney, and renal insufficiency. Patients known to have an increased incidence of nephrogenic rests (e.g. BWS, hemihypertrophy, and aniridia) are at increased risk for the development of a metachronous tumor and should be considered for parenchymal sparing procedures. The data reviewed above suggest a five-fold increase or 5% incidence of the development of metachronous Wilms' tumor in children in these high-risk categories. Does this risk justify the routine use of preoperative chemotherapy to facilitate partial nephrectomies in all patients with

BWS, hemihypertrophy, or aniridia found to have unilateral tumors? As noted in the discussion above, there is a risk for undertreatment and potentially increased risk of local recurrence. These risks must be weighed against the possible benefit of decreasing the incidence of renal failure.

Late effects of treatment

Each therapeutic modality used in the management of Wilms' tumor can result in both acute and delayed toxicities. Numerous organ systems are subject to the late sequelae of anticancer therapy. Clinicians must now become familiar with the spectrum of problems facing these children as they grow into adulthood. Long-term follow-up of treatment-related complications has been an integral role of the NWTSG. One of the major objectives of the pediatric cancer cooperative groups has been to reduce the intensity of treatment in order to prevent or lower the morbidity of multimodal therapy without reducing efficacy (Evans et al., 1991).

Children treated for Wilms' tumor are at increased risk for second malignant neoplasms (SMN). NWTSG investigators reported that 15 years after initial (Wilms' tumor) diagnosis, the cumulative incidence of a SMN is 1.6% and increasing steadily (Breslow et al., 1995). This is more than eight times the expected incidence. The risk of developing leukemia or lymphoma is greatest in the first 8 years after treatment. The risk of developing a solid tumor continues to increase over time. Most tumors occur in previously irradiated areas, but treatment for relapse and use of DOX were also associated with an increased incidence of SMNs.

Congestive heart failure is a known complication of treatment with an anthracycline (Gilladoga et al., 1976). The frequency is directly proportional to the cumulative dose of DOX received. In addition to the acute cardiotoxicity, reports are surfacing of cardiac failure up to 20 years after treatment (Steinherz et al., 1991). In a preliminary review of patients entered on NWTS-1, -2, and -3, the frequency of congestive heart failure was 1.7% among DOX-treated patients (Green et al., 1994c). The risk was increased if the patient received whole lung irradiation. In light of these findings, all children who undergo treatment with these modalities should undergo periodic reevaluation.

Damage to reproductive systems can lead to problems with hormonal dysfunction, infertility, or both. Gonadal radiation in males can result in temporary azoospermia and hypogonadism (Kinsella et al., 1989). The effect on the testis is dose related. Prepubertal germ cells also appear to be radiosensitive. In a follow-up of ten men treated for Wilms' tumor in childhood, oligospermia or azoospermia was found in eight (Shalet et al., 1978). The Leydig cells are more radioresistant than the germ cells, but higher doses can produce damage resulting in inadequate production of testosterone. This can result in delayed sexual maturation.

Chemotherapeutic agents can interfere with testicular function, particularly alkylating agents. Acute toxicity with germ-cell depletion occurs in all age groups. Some long-term studies suggested that prepubertal testes are resistant to chronic toxicity (Lentz et al., 1977). However, other studies have indicated that prepubertal testes are not protected from chemotherapy-induced damage (Aubier et al., 1989; Mustieles et al., 1995). One report found that 12 of 19 prepubertal males treated for a variety of solid tumors were sterile as a result of treatment (Aubier et al., 1989).

Female Wilms' tumor patients who received abdominal radiation have a 12% incidence of ovarian failure (Stillman et al., 1987). Of 16 women who received whole abdominal irradiation, all had evidence of ovarian failure and 75% were amenorrheic (Shalet et al., 1976). As with the testis, the effect on the ovaries is dose dependent. Chemotherapy-induced damage to the ovaries is most often associated with alkylating agents. A decrease in the number of follicles is seen in prepubertal girls treated with chemotherapy (Nicosia et al., 1985).

Several studies have addressed the risk of pregnancy in survivors after childhood cancer therapy. Women with prior abdominal radiation have the greatest potential for adverse pregnancy outcomes. In a study of patients treated for Wilms' tumor, an adverse outcome occurred in 3% among non-irradiated women compared with 30% of women who received abdominal irradiation (Li et al., 1987). Perinatal mortality rates are higher and infants are more likely to have low birth weights. The potential mutagenic effects of anticancer therapy are of concern. However, most studies have found no increase in the incidence of congenital anomalies and no cases of Wilms' tumor in the offspring of survivors (Green et al., 1982; Li et al., 1987).

Most children treated for Wilms' tumor undergo unilateral nephrectomy as part of the initial treatment. There is risk of dysfunction of the solitary, remaining kidney. Impairment of renal function may be related to irradiation, administration of nephrotoxic chemotherapeutic agents, or hyperfiltration of the remaining nephrons. Initially, compensatory hypertrophy develops in this kidney (Walker *et al.*, 1982; Levitt *et al.*, 1992). The data are conflicting regarding renal compensatory hypertrophy in patients who receive whole abdominal irradiation. Walker *et al.* (1982) found no difference in renal lengths between patients treated with chemotherapy and radiation versus chemotherapy alone. However, a later report used ultrasound to calculate renal lengths and found that patients receiving radiation had poor compensatory growth (Levitt *et al.*, 1992).

The kidney is sensitive to the effects of radiation. Radiation doses to the kidney should be limited to 12–15 Gy. Mitus *et al.* (1969) correlated functional impairment with the renal radiation dose in a review of 100 children treated for Wilms' tumor. The incidence of impaired creatinine clearance was significantly greater for children receiving greater than 12 Gy to the remaining kidney and all cases of overt renal failure occurred in patients who had received more than 23 Gy. Clinical signs of radiation nephritis may occur very acutely or begin months or years after therapy is discontinued (Mitus *et al.*, 1969). Direct radiation nephrotoxicity is the usual cause, with injury to the intrarenal vasculature.

Both experimental and clinical studies suggest that the remaining nephrons, after subtotal nephrectomy, are subject to chronic hyperfiltration which can produce renal dysfunction (Provoost *et al.*, 1991). Most experimental studies involve a loss of greater than three-quarters of the total renal mass, although one study noted abnormalities after removal of only one kidney (Provoost *et al.*, 1991). The data in humans regarding renal damage from hyperfiltration following nephrectomy are incompletely understood. Several studies have assessed long-term renal function in children following nephrectomy for Wilms' tumor (Bertolone *et al.*, 1987; Robitaille *et al.*, 1985; Barrera *et al.*, 1989; Bhisitkul *et al.*, 1990; Levitt *et al.*, 1992). The abnormalities found have included microalbuminuria, proteinuria, and a reduced glomerular filtration rate (Robitaille *et al.*, 1985; Bertolone *et al.*, 1987; Levitt *et al.*, 1992). However, other investigators have found no significant alter-ations in renal function (Barrera *et al.*, 1989; Bhisitkul *et al.*, 1990).

Investigators from the NWTSG have reported on the incidence of renal failure in 5823 children, of whom 451 had bilateral disease, registered on NWTSG trials between October, 1969 and July, 1993 (Ritchey *et al.*, 1996a). In total, 55 patients with renal failure were identified. Individuals with BWT had a much higher incidence of renal failure (Ritchey *et al.*, 1996a). In patients followed for more than 15 years, the incidence of ESRD is 16.6%, 22.3%, and 12.7% for NWTS-1, -2, and -3 patients, respectively. The most common cause of renal failure in the group of children with BWT was bilateral nephrectomy for persistent or recurrent tumor in the remaining kidney after initial nephrectomy (24/39). Treatment-related injury (radiation-induced damage or surgical complications) of the remaining kidney was the second leading cause of renal insufficiency. For patients with unilateral Wilms' tumor and an apparently normal contralateral kidney, the risk of renal failure was found to be very low (0.25%). It is noteworthy, however, that many children included with unilateral Wilms' tumor had not yet reached adulthood. They therefore remain at risk and might experience subtle renal deterioration as time goes on.

Other renal tumors of childhood

Cystic partially differentiated nephroblastoma

Cysts are common in Wilms' tumor and range in size from microscopic to several centimeters in diameter. Those tumors that are composed only of cysts with delicate septa are called cystic partially differentiated nephroblastoma. Within the septa are foci of blastema. The majority of these lesions occur in the first year of life (Joshi and Beckwith, 1989). These lesions are indistinguishable radiographically from solitary multilocular cyst described below. Surgery is curative in almost all patients, with recurrence the result of incomplete resection (Eble and Bonsib, 1998).

Multilocular cystic nephroma

Multilocular cystic nephroma, also known as solitary multilocular cyst, is an uncommon, benign renal tumor with a bimodal incidence. Fifty per cent of the multilocular cysts reported in the literature have been found in children younger than 4 years and boys predominate in a ratio of 2:1. The second peak incidence occurs in adults, and unlike the pediatric cases is usually in women (Banner *et al.*, 1981).

Cystic nephromas are commonly found incidentally on radiographic studies, but may present as an abdominal mass found on routine physical examination. All cases of multilocular cystic renal disease have been unilateral. The gross appearance of the tumor is its most distinguishing feature. The cut surfaces reveal a well-circumscribed multilocular tumor composed of cysts ranging from several millimeters to several centimeters in greatest diameter. The tumor is well encapsulated, compressing the surrounding renal parenchyma.

Multilocular cystic nephroma is a benign lesion which is cured by nephrectomy. Recurrence has occurred following incomplete excision by partial nephrectomy. If partial nephrectomy is considered, frozen section is indicated to exclude cystic, partially differentiated nephroblastoma (Joshi and Beckwith, 1989).

Congenital mesoblastic nephroma

Congenital mesoblastic nephroma (CMN) is the most common renal tumor in infants, with a mean age at diagnosis of 3.5 months (Howell *et al.*, 1982). The typical presentation is a newborn with an abdominal mass, but in recent years several cases have been recognized prenatally (Ohmichi *et al.*, 1989). Tumor induction is postulated to occur at a time when the multipotent blastema is predominantly stromagenic

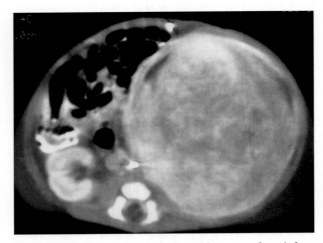

Figure 40.5 Computed tomographic scan of an infant with congenital mesoblastic nephroma.

(Tomlinson *et al.*, 1992). Imaging studies cannot reliably distinguish CMN from other renal mass lesions. Distortion of the collecting system from an intrarenal mass is noted on excretory urography. Abdominal CT shows a heterogeneous solid mass arising from the kidney (Fig. 40.5). The neoplasm is histologically distinct from Wilms' tumor. The cell population is characterized by interlacing sheets of connective cells. Recent evidence suggests a link between CMN and congenital fibrosarcoma. The cellular variant of CMN (Beckwith, 1986c; Joshi *et al.*, 1986; Gormley *et al.*, 1989) is virtually identical histologically to congenital fibrosarcoma. Molecular studies have found a similar translocation in both tumors that fuses the ETV6 (TEL) gene from 12p13 with the 15q25 neurotrophin-3 receptor gene, NTRK3 (Argani *et al.*, 1998).

Complete excision is curative for most patients with CMN (Howell *et al.*, 1982). Local recurrence has been reported in several patients with a cellular variant of CMN characterized by a high mitotic index and dense cellularity (Joshi *et al.*, 1986; Gormley *et al.*, 1989). These features are present in 25–65% of CMN specimens (Beckwith, 1986c; Anonymous, 1998). Adequacy of surgical resection and age at diagnosis appear to be more important predictors of relapse than histology (Beckwith, 1986c). The risk of recurrence is thought to be less in children under 3 months of age at diagnosis, but metastases have been reported in a few infants (Heidelberger *et al.*, 1993). Neither chemotherapy nor radiation therapy is recommended routinely (Howell *et al.*, 1982), but consideration for adjuvant treatment should be given to patients with cellular variants that are incompletely resected (Gormley *et al.*, 1989).

Clear cell sarcoma of the kidney

This tumor is also known as the bone-metastasizing renal tumor of childhood because of its predilection for these sites (Beckwith and Palmer, 1978; Marsden and Lawler, 1980). There is also an increased number of brain metastases with this entity (Green *et al.*, 1994d). CCSK accounts for 3% of renal tumors reported to the NWTS. Unlike tumors with anaplasia, even stage I CCSK lesions are associated with increased rates of relapse. Studies have demonstrated that the use of DOX is associated with a significant improvement in outcome for these children (D'Angio *et al.*, 1989). Patients with CCSK are being treated on NWTS-5 with a new chemotherapeutic regimen combining VCR, DOX, cyclophosphamide, and etoposide in an attempt to improve further the survival of this high-risk group. All of these patients will receive irradiation to the tumor bed.

Rhabdoid tumor of the kidney

Rhabdoid tumor of the kidney was first identified by NWTSG pathologists in 1978 (Beckwith and Palmer, 1978). This is a highly malignant tumor of the kidney, which accounts for 2% of renal tumors registered to the NWTSG (D'Angio *et al.*, 1989; Weeks *et al.*, 1989). This tumor is typically seen in infants and very young children, with a median age of 13 months. Rhabdoid tumor of the kidney metastasizes to the brain, which is exceedingly uncommon for Wilms' tumor. Recent studies suggest that there is a common genetic basis for central nervous system, renal, and extrarenal rhabdoid tumors (Biegel *et al.*, 1999). A deletion or mutation in the tumor suppressor gene INII on chromosome 22 predisposes to the development of this tumor. The prognosis of patients with rhabdoid tumor remains dismal with conventional chemotherapeutic regimens. In NWTS-5, children with all stages of rhabdoid tumor will be treated with carboplatin, cyclophosphamide, and etoposide. These patients will also receive abdominal irradiation.

Renal cell carcinoma

Only 5% of renal cell carcinomas occur in children (Hartman *et al.*, 1982; Broecker, 1991). These patients generally present after the age of 5 years, and it is the most common renal malignancy in the second decade of life. Survival of children with renal cell carcinoma is dependent on the ability to resect the tumor completely. Raney *et al.* (1983) found that all children with stage I lesions survived. Overall survival was about 50%. Age is also a prognostic factor, with improved survival in children younger than 11 years. These tumors do not appear responsive to chemotherapy or radiation therapy.

References

Argani P, Fritsch M, Kadkol SS, Schuster A, Beckwith JB, Perlman EJ (1998) ETV6-NTRK3 Gene fusions and trisomy 11 establish a histogenetic link between mesoblastic nephroma and congenital fibrosarcoma. *Cancer Res* **58**: 5046–8.

Aubier F, Flamant F, Brauner R *et al.* (1989) Male gonadal function after chemotherapy for solid tumors in childhood. *J Clin Oncol* **7**: 304–9.

Banner MP, Pollack HM, Chatten J, Witzleben C (1981) Multilocular renal cysts: radiologic–pathologic correlation. *Am J Roentgenol* **136**: 239–47.

Bardeesy N, Falkoff D, Petruzzi MJ *et al.* (1994) Anaplastic Wilms' tumour, a subtype displaying poor prognosis, harbours p53 gene mutations. *Nat Genet* **7**: 91–7.

Barrera M, Roy LP, Stevens M (1989) Long-term follow-up after unilateral nephrectomy and radiotherapy for Wilms tumor. *Pediatr Nephrol* **3**: 430–2.

Beckwith JB (1969) Macroglossia, omphalocele, adrenal cytomegaly, gigantism and hyperplastic visceromegaly. *Birth Defects: Original Article Series* **5**: 188–96.

Beckwith JB (1986c) Congenital mesoblastic nephroma. When should we worry? *Arch Pathol Lab Med* **110**: 98–9.

Beckwith JB (1996a) Certain conditions have an increased incidence of Wilms' tumor. *AJR Am J Roentgenol* **164**: 1294–5.

Beckwith JB (1996b) Wilms tumor in multicystic dysplastic kidneys: what is the risk? *Dialog Pediatr Urol* **19**: 3–5.

Beckwith JB (1998) Nephrogenic rests and the pathogenesis of Wilms tumor: developmental and clinical considerations. *Am J Med Genet* **79**: 268–73.

Beckwith JB, Palmer NF (1978) Histopathology and prognosis of Wilms tumor. Results from the National Wilms Tumor Study. *Cancer* **41**: 1937–48.

Beckwith JB, Kiviat NB, Bonadio JF (1990) Nephrogenic rests, nephroblastomatosis, and the pathogenesis of Wilms' tumor. *Pediatr Pathol* **10**: 1–36.

Bertolone SJ, Patel CC, Harrison HL *et al.* (1987) Long term renal function in pts. with Wilms tumor. *Proc Am Soc Clin Oncol* **6**: 265 (Abstract 1040).

Bhisitkul DM, Morgan ER, Vozar MA *et al.* (1990) Renal functional reserve in long-term survivors of unilateral Wilms tumor. *J Pediatr* **118**: 698–702.

Biegel JA, Zhou J, Rorke LB *et al.* (1999) Germ-line and acquired mutations of INII in atypical teratoid and rhabdoid tumors. *Cancer Res* **59**: 74–9.

Bishop HC, Teft M, Evans A, *et al.* (1977) Survival in bilateral Wilms' tumor – review of 30 National Wilms' Tumor Study cases. *J Pediatr Surg* **12**: 631–8.

Blute ML, Kelalis PP, Offord KP *et al.* (1987) Bilateral Wilms' tumor. *J Urol* **138**: 968–73.

Bonadio JF, Storer B, Norkool P *et al.* (1985) Anaplastic Wilms' tumor: clinical and pathological studies. *J Clin Oncol* **3**: 513–20.

Bonetta L, Kuehn SE, Huang A *et al.* (1990) Wilms tumor locus on 11p13 defined by multiple CpG island-associated transcripts. *Science* **250**: 994–7.

Borer JG, Kaefer M, Barnewolt CE *et al.* (1999) Renal findings on radiological followup of patients with Beckwith–Wiedemann syndrome. *J Urol* **161**: 235–9.

Breslow NE, Beckwith JB (1982) Epidemiological features of Wilms' tumor: results of the National Wilms' Tumor Study. *J Natl Cancer Inst* **68**: 429–36.

Breslow NB, Churchill G, Beckwith JB et al. (1985) Prognosis for Wilms' tumor patients with nonmetatastic disease at diagnosis – results of the Second National Wilms' Tumor Study. *J Clin Oncol* **3**: 521–31.

Breslow N, Beckwith JB, Ciol M, Sharples K (1988) Age distribution of Wilms tumor: report from the National Wilms Tumor Study. *Cancer Res* **48**: 1653–7.

Breslow N, Olshan A, Beckwith JB et al. (1993) Epidemiology of Wilms tumor. *Med Pediatr Oncol* **21**: 172–81.

Breslow N, Olshan A, Beckwith JB et al. (1994) Ethnic variation in the incidence, diagnosis, prognosis and follow-up of children with Wilms' Tumor. *J Natl Cancer Inst* **86**: 49–51.

Breslow NE, Takashima JR, Whitton JA et al. (1995) Second malignant meoplasms following treatment for Wilms' tumor: a report from the National Wilms' Tumor Study Group. *J Clin Oncol* **13**: 1851–9.

Broecker B (1991) Renal cell carcinoma in children. *Urology* **38**: 54–6.

Call KM, Glaser T, Ito CY et al. (1990) Isolation and characterization of a zinc finger polypeptide gene at the human chromosome 11 Wilms' tumor locus. *Cell* **60**: 509–20.

Choyke PL, Siegel MJ, Oz O et al. (1998) Nonmalignant renal disease in pediatric patients with Beckwith–Wiedemann syndrome. *AJR Am J Roentgenol* **171**: 733–7.

Choyke PL, Siegel MJ, Craft AW et al. (1999) Screening for Wilms tumor in children with Beckwith–Wiedemann syndrome or idiopathic hemihypertrophy. *Med Pediatr Oncol* **32**: 196–200.

Cohen MD (1993) Staging of Wilms' tumor. *Clin Radiol* **47**: 77–81.

Coppes MJ (1993) Serum biological markers and paraneoplastic syndromes in Wilms tumor. *Med Pediatr Oncol* **21**: 213–21.

Coppes MJ, deKraker J, vanKijken PJ et al. (1989) Bilateral Wilms' tumor: long-term survival and some epidemiological features. *J Clin Oncol* **7**: 310–15.

Coppes MJ, Huff V, Pelletier J (1993a) Denys–Drash syndrome: relating a clinical disorder to genetic alterations in the tumor suppressor gene WT1. *J Pediatr* **123**: 673–8.

Coppes MJ, Zandvoort SWH, Sparling CR et al. (1993b) Acquired von Willebrand disease in Wilms tumor patients. *J Clin Oncol* **10**: 1–7.

Coppes MJ, Haber DA, Grundy PE (1994) Genetic events in the development of Wilms' tumor. *N Engl J Med* **331**: 586–90.

Coppes MJ, Arnold M, Beckwith JB et al. (1999) Factors affecting the risk of contralateral Wilms tumor development. *Cancer* **85**: 1616–25.

Cozzi F, Schiavetti A, Bonanni M, Cozzi DA, Matrunola M, Castello MA (1996) Enucleative surgery for stage I nephroblastoma with a normal contralateral kidney. *J Urol* **156**: 1788–91.

Craft AW, Parker L, Stiller C, Cole M (1995) Screening for Wilms tumour in patients with aniridia, Beckwith syndrome, or hemihypertrophy. *Med Pediatr Oncol* **24**: 231–4.

D'Angio GJ, Evans AE, Breslow N et al. (1976) The treatment of Wilms' tumor: results of the National Wilms' tumor study. *Cancer* **38**: 633–46.

D'Angio GJ, Evans A, Breslow N et al. (1981) The treatment of Wilms' tumor: results of the Second National Wilms' Tumor Study. *Cancer* **47**: 2302–11.

D'Angio GJ, Breslow N, Beckwith JB et al. (1989) Treatment of Wilms' tumor: results of the Third National Wilms' Tumor Study. *Cancer* **64**: 349–60.

D'Angio GJ, Rosenberg H, Sharples K et al. (1993) Position paper: imaging methods for primary renal tumors of childhood: cost versus benefits. *Med Pediatr Oncol* **21**: 205–12.

Debaun MR, Tucker MA (1998) Risk of cancer during the first four years of life in children from the Beckwith–Wiedemann syndrome registry. *J Pediatr* **132**: 377–9.

Debaun MR, Siegel MJ, Choyke PL (1998) Nephromegaly in infancy and early childhood: a risk factor for Wilms tumor in Beckwith–Wiedemann syndrome. *J Pediatr* **132**: 401–4.

Diller L, Ghahremani M, Morgan J et al. (1998) Constitutional WT1 mutations in Wilms' tumor patients. *J Clin Oncol* **16**: 3634–40.

Ditchfield MR, DeCampo JF, Waters KD, Nolan TM (1995) Wilms' tumor: a rational use of preoperative imaging. *Med Pediatr Oncol* **24**: 93–6.

Drash A, Sherman F, Hartmann WH, Blizzard RM (1970) A syndrome of pseudohermaphroditism, Wilms tumor, hypertension and degenerative renal disease. *J Pediatr* **76**: 585–93.

Dykes EH, Marwaha RK, Dicks-Mireaux C et al. (1991) Risks and benefits of percutaneous biopsy and primary chemotherapy in advanced Wilms' tumour. *J Pediatr Surg* **26**: 610–12.

Eble JN, Bonsib SM (1998) Extensively cystic renal neoplasms: cystic nephroma, cystic partially differentiated nephroblastoma, multiloculuar cystic renal cell carcinoma, and cystic hamartoma of renal pelvis. *Semin Diagn Pathol* **15**: 2–20.

Evans AE, Norkool P, Evans I et al. (1991) Late effects of treatment for Wilms' tumor. A report from the National Wilms' Tumor Study Group. *Cancer* **67**: 331–6.

Farber S (1966) Chemotherapy in the treatment of leukemia and Wilms' tumor. *JAMA* **198**: 826–36.

Farewell VT, D'Angio GJ, Breslow N, Norkool P (1981) Retrospective validation of a new staging system for Wilms' tumor. *Cancer Clin Trials* **4**: 167–71.

Faria P, Beckwith JB, Mishra K et al. (1996) Focal versus diffuse anaplasia in Wilms tumor – new definitions with prognostic significance: a report from the National Wilms Tumor Study Group. *Am J Surg Pathol* **20**: 909–20.

Feusner JH, Beckwith JB, D'Angio GJ (1990) Clear cell sarcoma of the kidney: accuracy of imaging methods for detecting bone metastases. Report from the National Wilms' Tumor Study. *Med Pediatr Oncol* **18**: 225–7.

Gessler M, Poustka A, Cavenee W et al. (1990) Homozygous deletion in Wilms tumours of a zinc-finger gene identified by chromosome jumping. *Nature* **343**: 774–8.

Gilladoga AC, Manuel C, Tan CT et al. (1976) The cardiotoxicity of adriamycin and daunomycin in children. *Cancer* **37**: 1070–8.

Gormley TS, Skoog SJ, Jones RV, Maybee D (1989) Cellular congenital mesoblastic nephroma: what are the options? *J Urol* **142**: 479–83.

Graf N, Tournade MF, de Kraker J (2000) The role of preoperative chemotherapy in the management of Wilms' tumor. The SIOP studies. International Society of Pediatric Oncology. *Urol Clin North Am* **27**: 443–54.

Green DM, Fine NE, Li FP (1982) Offspring of patients treated for unilateral Wilms' tumor in childhood. *Cancer* **49**: 2285–8.

Green DM, Breslow NE, Beckwith JB, Norkool P (1993a) Screening of children with hemihypertrophy, aniridia, and Beckwith–Wiedemann syndrome in patients with Wilms' tumor: A report from the National Wilms Tumor Study. *Med Pediatr Oncol* **21**: 188–92.

Green DM, Breslow NE, D'Angio GJ (1993b) The treatment of children with unilateral Wilms tumor. *J Clin Oncol* **11**: 1009–10.

Green DM, Beckwith JB, Breslow NE et al. (1994a) Treatment of children with stages II to IV anaplastic Wilms' tumor: a report from the National Wilms' Tumor Study Group. *J Clin Oncol* **12**: 2126–31.

Green DM, Beckwith JB, Weeks DA et al. (1994b) The relationship between microsubstaging variables, tumor weight and age at diagnosis of children with stage I/favorable histology Wilms tumor. A report from the National Wilms Tumor Study. *Cancer* **74**: 1817–20.

Green DM, Breslow NE, Moksness J, D'Angio GJ (1994c) Congestive failure following initial therapy for Wilms tumor. A report from the National Wilms Tumor Study. *Pediatr Res* **35**: 161A (Abstract).

Green DM, Breslow NE, Beckwith JB et al. (1994d) The treatment of children with clear cell sarcoma of the kidney. A report from the National Wilms' Tumor Study Group. *J Clin Oncol* **12**: 2132–7.

Green DM, Breslow NE, Beckwith JB et al. (1998a) Comparison between single-dose and divided-dose administration of dactinomycin and doxorubicin for patients with Wilms' tumor: a report from the National Wilms' Tumor Study Group. *J Clin Oncol* **16**: 237–45.

Green DM, Breslow NE, Beckwith JBB et al. (1998b) Effect of duration of treatment on treatment outcomes and cost of treatment for Wilms' tumor: a report from the National Wilms Tumor Study Group. *J Clin Oncol* **16**: 3744–51.

Grundy PE, Telzerow PE, Breslow N et al. (1994) Loss of heterozygosity for chromosomes 16q and 1p in Wilms' tumors predicts an adverse outcome. *Cancer Res* **54**: 2331–3.

Hartman D, Davis C, Madewell J, Friedman A (1982) Primary malignant tumors in the second decade of life: Wilms tumor versus renal cell carcinoma. *J Urol* **127**: 888–91.

Heidelberger KP, Ritchey ML, Dauser RC et al. (1993) Congenital mesoblastic nephroma metastatic to the brain. *Cancer* **72**: 2499–502.

Hittner HM, Riccardi VM, Ferrell RE et al. (1980) Genetic heterogeneity of aniridia: negative linkage data. *Metab Pediatr Syst Ophthalmol* **4**: 179–82.

Horwitz J, Ritchey ML, Moksness J et al. (1996) Renal salvage procedures in patients with synchronous bilateral Wilms tumors: a report of the NWTSG. *J Pediatr Surg* **31**: 1020–5.

Howell CJ, Othersen HB, Kiviat NE et al. (1982) Therapy and outcome in 51 children with mesoblastic nephroma: a report of the National Wilms' Tumor Study. *J Pediatr Surg* **17**: 826–30.

Huff V, Villalba F, Riccardi VM et al. (1991) Alteration of the WT1 gene in patients with Wilms' tumor and genitourinary anomalies. *Am J Hum Genet* **49**: 44.

Jereb B, Burgers JM, Tournade MF et al. (1994) Radiotherapy in the SIOP (International Society of Pediatric Oncology) nephroblastoma studies: a review. *Med Pediatr Oncol* **22**: 221–7.

Johnston MA, Carachi R, Lindop GBM, Leckie B (1991) Inactive renin levels in recurrent nephroblastoma. *J Pediatr Surg* **26**: 613–14.

Joshi VJ, Kasznica J, Walters TR (1986) Atypical mesoblastic nephroma: pathologic characterization of a potentially aggressive variant of conventional congenital mesoblastic nephroma. *Arch Pathol Lab Med* **110**: 100–6.

Joshi VV, Beckwith JB (1989) Multilocular cyst of the kidney (cystic nephroma) and cystic, partially differentiated nephroblastoma. Terminology and criteria for diagnosis. *Cancer* **64**: 466–79.

Kinsella TJ, Trivette G, Rowland J et al. (1989) Long-term follow-up of testicular function following radiation for early-stage Hodgkin's disease. *J Clin Oncol* **7**: 718–24.

Knudson AG, Strong LC (1972) Mutation and cancer: a model for Wilms' tumor of the kidney. *J Natl Cancer Inst* **48**: 313–24.

Koufos A, Grundy P, Morgan K et al. (1989) Familial Wiedemann–Beckwith syndrome and a second Wilms tumor locus both map to 11p15.5. *Am J Hum Genet* **44**: 711–19.

Lemerle J, Voute PA, Tournade MF et al. (1976) Preoperative versus postoperative radiotherapy, single versus multiple courses of actinomycin D, in the treatment of Wilms' tumor. Preliminary results of a controlled clinical trial conducted by the International Society of Paediatric Oncology (S.I.O.P.). *Cancer* **38**: 647–54.

Lemerle J, Voute PA, Tournade MF et al. (1983) Effectiveness of preoperative chemotherapy in Wilms' tumor: results of an International Society of Paediatric Oncology (SIOP) clinical trial. *J Clin Oncol* **1**: 604–9.

Lentz RD, Berstein J, Steffens MW et al. (1977) Postpubertal evaluation of gonadal function following cyclophosphamide therapy before and during puberty. *J Pediatr* **91**: 385–94.

Levitt GA, Yeomans E, Dicks Mireaux C et al. (1992) Renal size and function after cure of Wilms tumor. *Br J Cancer* **66**: 877–82.

Li FP, Gimbrere K, Gelber RD et al. (1987) Outcome of pregnancy in survivors of Wilms tumor. *JAMA* **257**: 216–19.

Lin RY, Argent PA, Sullivan KM et al. (1995a) Urinary hyaluronic acid is a Wilms tumor marker. *J Pediatr Surg* **30**: 304–8.

Lin RY, Argenta PA, Sullivan KM, Adzick NS (1995b) Diagnostic and prognostic role of basic fibroblast growth factor in Wilms tumor patients. *Clin Cancer Res* **1**: 327–31.

McLorie GA, McKenna PH, Greenburg M *et al.* (1991) Reduction in tumor burden allowing partial nephrectomy following preoperative chemotherapy in biopsy proved Wilms' tumor. *J Urol* **146**: 509–13.

Mannens M, Devilee P, Bliek J *et al.* (1990) Loss of heterozygosity in Wilms' tumors, studied for six putative tumor suppressor regions, is limited to chromosome 11. *Cancer Res* **50**: 3279–83.

Marsden HB, Lawler W (1980) Bone metastasizing renal tumour of childhood: histopathological and clinical review of 38 cases. *Virchows Arch* **387**: 341–51.

Maw MA, Grundy PE, Millow LJ *et al.* (1992) A third Wilms' tumor locus on chromosome 16q. *Cancer Res* **52**: 3094–8.

Mitus A, Tefft M, Feller FX (1969) Long-term follow-up of renal function of 108 children who underwent nephrectomy for malignant disease. *Pediatrics* **44**: 912–21.

Montgomery BT, Kelalis PP, Blute ML *et al.* (1991) Extended follow-up of bilateral Wilms' tumor: results of the National Wilms Tumor Study. *J Urol* **146**: 514–18.

Moorman-Voestermans C, Aronson D, Staalman CR *et al.* (1998) Is partial nephrectomy appropriate treatment for unilateral Wilms' tumor? *J Pediatr Surg* **33**: 165–70.

Mustieles C, Munoz A, Alonso M *et al.* (1995) Male gonadal function after chemotherapy in survivors of childhood malignancies. *Med Pediatr Oncol* **24**: 347–51.

Nakayama DK, Ortega W, D'Angio GJ, O'Neill JA (1988) The nonopacified kidney with Wilms' tumor. *J Pediatr Surg* **23**: 152–5.

Neri G, Gurrieri F, Zanni G, Lin A (1998) Clinical and molecular aspects of the Simpson–Golabi–Behmel syndrome. *Am J Med Genet* **79**: 279–83.

Ng YY, Hall-Craggs MA, Dicks-Mireaux C *et al.* (1991) Wilms' tumour: pre- and post-chemotherapy CT appearances. *Clin Radiol* **43**: 255–9.

Nicosia SV, Matus-Ridley M, Meadows AT (1985) Gonadal effects of cancer therapy in girls. *Cancer* 1985; **55**: 2364–72.

Noe HN, Marshall JH, Edwards OP (1989) Nodular renal blastema in the multicystic kidney. *J Urol* **142**: 486–8.

Ohmichi M, Tasaka K, Sugita N *et al.* (1989) Hydramnios associated with congenital mesoblastic nephroma: a case report. *Obstet Gynecol* **74**: 469–71.

Othersen HB Jr, DeLorimer A, Hrabovsky E *et al.* (1990) Surgical evaluation of lymph node metastases in Wilms' tumor. *J Pediatr Surg* **25**: 1–2.

Pelletier J, Bruening W, Kashtan CE *et al.* (1991) Germline mutations in the Wilms' tumor suppressor gene are associated with abnormal urogenital development in Denys–Drash syndrome. *Cell* **67**: 437–47.

Penn I (1979) Renal transplantation for Wilms' tumor: report of 20 cases. *J Urol* **122**: 793–4.

Perlman M, Levin M, Wittels B (1975) Syndrome of fetal gigantism, renal hamartomas, and nephroblastomatosis with Wilms' tumor. *Cancer* **35**: 1212–17.

Ping AJ, Reeve AE, Law DJ *et al.* (1989) Genetic linkage of Beckwith–Wiedemann syndrome to 11p15. *Am J Hum Genet* **44**: 720–3.

Provoost AP, Baudoin P, DeKeijzer MH *et al.* (1991) The role of nephron loss in the progression of renal failure: experimental evidence. *Am J Kidney Dis* **17**: 27–32.

Raney RB Jr, Palmer N, Sutow WW *et al.* (1983) Renal cell carcinoma in children. *Med Pediatr Oncol* **11**: 91–8.

Ritchie ML, Coppes M (1995) The management of synchronous bilateral Wilms tumor. *Hematol Oncol Clin North Am* **9**: 1303–16.

Ritchey ML, Kelalis PP, Breslow N *et al.* (1988) Intracaval and atrial involvement with nephroblastoma: review of National Wilms' Tumor Study-3. *J Urol* **140**: 1113–18.

Ritchey ML, Kelalis PP, Breslow N *et al.* (1992) Surgical complications following nephrectomy for Wilms' tumor: a report of National Wilms' Tumor Study-3. *Surg Gynecol Obstet* **175**: 507–14.

Ritchey ML, Kelalis PP, Haase GM *et al.* (1993) Preoperative therapy for intracaval and atrial extension of Wilms' tumor. *Cancer* **71**: 4104–10.

Ritchey ML, Pringle K, Breslow N *et al.* (1994) Management and outcome of inoperable Wilms tumor. A report of National Wilms' Tumor Study. *Ann Surg* **220**: 683–90.

Ritchey ML, Green DM, Breslow NE, Norkool P (1995) Accuracy of current imaging modalities in the diagnosis of synchronous bilateral Wilms tumor. *Cancer* **75**: 600–4.

Ritchey ML, Green DM, Thomas P *et al.* (1996a) Renal failure in Wilms tumor patients: a report of the NWTSG. *Med Pediatr Oncol* **26**: 75–80.

Ritchey ML, Andrassy R, Kelalis PP *et al.* (1996b) Pediatric urologic oncology. In: Gillenwater J, Howards S, Duckett J (eds.) *Adult and pediatric urology*. Chicago, IL: Mosby Year Book, 2675–720.

Ritchey ML, Shamberger RC, Haase G *et al.* (2001) Surgical complications after nephrectomy for Wilms tumor: report from the National Wilms Tumor Study Group. *J Am Coll Surg* (in press).

Robitaille P, Mongeau JG, Lortie L *et al.* (1985) Long-term follow-up of patients who underwent nephrectomy in childhood. *Lancet* i: 1297–9.

Shamberger RC, Ritchey ML, Haase GM *et al.* (2001) Intravascular extension of Wilms tumor: report of the National Wilms Tumor Study Group. *Ann Surg* (in press).

Schmidt D, Beckwith JB (1995) Histopathology of childhood renal tumors. *Hematol Oncol Clin North Am* **9**: 1179–200.

Shalet SM, Beardwell CG, Morris-Jones PH *et al.* (1976) Ovarian failure following abdominal irradiation in childhood. *Br J Cancer* **33**: 655–8.

Shalet SM, Beardwell CG, Jacobs HS *et al.* (1978) Testicular function following irradiation of the human prepubertal testis. *Clin Endocrinol* **9**: 483–90.

Shamberger RC, Guthrie KA, Ritchey ML *et al.* (1999) Surgery-related factors and local recurrence of Wilms tumor in National Wilms Tumor Study 4. *Ann Surg* **229**: 292–7.

Sotelo-Avila C, Gonzalez-Crussi F, Fowler JW (1980) Complete and incomplete forms of Beckwith–Wiedemann syndrome: their oncogenic potential. *J Pediatr* **96**: 47–50.

Steinherz LJ, Steinherz PG, Tan CTC *et al.* (1991) Cardiac toxicity 4 to 20 years after anthracycline therapy. *JAMA* **266**: 1672–7.

Stillman RJ, Schinfeld JS, Schiff I *et al.* (1987) Ovarian failure in long term survivors of childhood malignancy. *Am J Obstet Gynecol* **139**: 62–6.

Tomlinson GE, Argyle JC, Velasco S, Nisen PD (1992) Molecular characterization of congenital mesoblastic nephroma and its distinction from Wilms tumor. *Cancer* **70**: 2358–61.

Tournade MF, Com-Nougue C, Voute PA *et al.* (1993) results of the Sixth International Society of Pediatric Oncology Wilms' Tumor Trial and Study: a risk-adapted therapeutic approach in Wilms' tumor. *J Clin Oncol* **11**: 1014–23.

Voute PA, Van Der Meer J, Staugaard-Kloosterziel W (1971) Plasma renin activity in Wilms' tumour. *Acta Endocrinol* **67**: 197–202.

Walker RD, Reid CF, Richard GA *et al.* (1982) Compensatory renal growth and function in postnephrectomized patients with Wilms tumor. *Urology* **19**: 127–30.

Weeks DA, Beckwith JB, Mierau G, Luckey DW (1989) Rhabdoid tumor of kidney. A report of 111 cases from the National Wilms' Tumor Study Pathology Center. *Am J Surg Pathol* **13**: 439–58.

Weese DL, Applebaum H, Taber P (1991) Mapping intravascular extension of Wilms' tumor with magnetic resonance imaging. *J Pediatr Surg* **26**: 64–7.

Wiedemann H (1983) Tumors and hemihypertrophy associated with the Wiedemann–Beckwith syndrome. *Eur J Pediatr* **141**: 129–41.

Wilmore HP, White GF, Howell RT *et al.* (1994) Germline and somatic abnormalities of chromosome 7 in Wilms' tumor. *Cancer Genet Cytogenet* **77**: 93–8.

Zuppan CW, Beckwith JB, Luckey DW (1988) Anaplasia in unilateral Wilms' tumor: a report from the National Wilms' Tumor Study Pathology Center. *Hum Pathol* **19**: 1199–209.

Zuppan CW, Beckwith JB, Weeks DA *et al.* (1991) The effect of preoperative therapy on the histologic features of Wilms' tumor. An analysis of cases from the Third National Wilms' Tumor Study. *Cancer* **68**: 385–94.

Rhabdomyosarcoma: prostate, bladder, vagina, and other bladder tumors

41

Paul A. Merguerian and Antoine E. Khoury

Introduction

Rhabdomyosarcoma (RMS) is the most common soft-tissue sarcoma in children under 15 years of age. It is the third most common childhood extracranial solid tumor, after neuroblastoma and Wilms' tumor, and accounts for 50% of all sarcomas and 10–15% of all solid pediatric tumors. Approximately 13–20% of these tumors arise from the genitourinary tract and another 10% from pelvic or retroperitoneal sites (Julian et al., 1995; Angell et al., 1996; Agarwal et al., 1997). Nearly one-half of these cases are diagnosed before the age of 5 years. Since its discovery by Weber in 1854, the clinical and pathologic features have been studied extensively, thus permitting the development of uniform diagnostic criteria and staging systems that are relevant prognostically (Pappo et al., 1997).

By definition, RMS is a sarcoma showing evidence of skeletal muscle differentiation. RMS can also occur in sites where skeletal muscle is not found, suggesting that this is a tumor of primitive mesenchymal skeletal muscle differentiation (Crist et al., 1995). It occurs in two large peaks of incidence: the first in the first decade and is mainly embryonal or botryoid RMS, and the second during adolescence and consists of alveolar RMS (ARMS) (Qualman et al., 1998). The histopathologic variants of RMS have different biologic courses. Embryonal RMS (ERMS) tends to occur in the head and neck and genitourinary system. The prognosis is very good, with the majority (74%) of patients surviving beyond 5 years. ARMS is often seen in the extremities and metastasizes early, with only 54% surviving beyond 5 years (Newton et al., 1995). The cure rate for patients with RMS has improved significantly, from an estimated 25% in 1970 to 70% in 1995 (Maurer et al., 1988, 1993; Crist et al., 1995). This improvement is credited to the use of increasingly effective multimodal, risk-adapted therapy, refinement in tumor grouping, and

better supportive care. Emerging information on the numerical and structural abnormalities of tumor cell chromosomes and the development of probes that can be used to identify molecular genetic lesions has led to improved diagnostic methods and have afforded new insights into the pathogenesis of this tumor. Knowledge of the genetic features of these tumors will significantly improve the ability to identify patients at lower or higher risk of treatment failure, thus paving the way for advances in risk-based therapy.

The results of cooperative group trials in the early 1970s proved the efficacy of multimodality therapy. However, the relative rarity of RMS, as well as its marked clinical and biologic heterogenicity, made the interpretation of results from small studies problematic. Thus, in 1972, three pediatric cooperative cancer study groups formed the Intergroup Rhabdomyosarcoma Study (IRS) Committee as a means of combining their patients and investigative resources. Since that time, the committee has designed, conducted and analysed four consecutive trials and is currently accruing patients for the fifth trial.

Molecular and cellular biology

Somatically acquired genetic changes underlie all forms of cancer. Until recently, the genetic characteristics for RMS were largely unknown. With improved cytogenetic techniques, the chromosomal analysis of this tumor has been found to contain both numerical and structural abnormalities (Scrable et al., 1989a, b; Pappo et al., 1993a). Recent advances in molecular and cell biology of RMS have also improved the understanding of the pathogenesis of this tumor and will aid in its diagnosis, staging, and management.

RMS appears to develop from a derangement in the final steps of myogenic differentiation. Genes of the *MyoD* family are crucial in the early differentiation of skeletal muscle precursors (Parham, 1994). These genes express DNA-binding proteins that facilitate the production of myogenic proteins such as desmin, creatine kinase, and myosin. *MyoD* expression is higher in RMS cells. This increased expression is not believed to cause tumorigenesis, but rather failure of differentiation (Parham, 1994). Failing to differentiate completely, the rhabdomyosarcoma cells continue to produce forms of actin seen only transiently in normal developing skeletal muscle cells (Schurch et al., 1994). *MyoD1* is a recently described myogenic regulatory protein that maps on chromosome 11p15.4 and is expressed during skeletal muscle development. *MyoD1* expression is a distinguishing characteristic of RMS. It is now possible, through reverse transcription polymerase chain reaction (RT-PCR) assay, to evaluate expression of *MyoD1* mRNA. This has been found to be highly sensitive and specific in detecting minimal residual disease, as well as bone marrow and peripheral blood stem cell involvement, regardless of histologic subtype (Frascella and Rosolen, 1998).

ARMS is also distinguished on the basis of structural abnormalities. Cytogenetic analysis of ARMS tumors reveal a translocation involving chromosomes 2 and 13, t(2;13)(q35-37;q14) in 70% of cases (Fig. 41.1) (Turc-Carel et al., 1986; Whang-Peng et al., 1986; Douglass et al., 1987). There have also been several reports of a t(1;13)(p36;q14) variant translocation (Whang-Peng et al., 1986; Biegel et al., 1991; Douglass et al., 1991) and single reports of cases with

other related alterations (Whang-Peng et al., 1986; Douglass et al., 1991; Sawyer et al., 1994). The t(2;13) and t(1;13) translocations have not been associated with any other tumor and appear to be specific for ARMS.

In a series of mapping experiments, the chromosome 2 locus disrupted at the t(2;13) was found to be PAX3, and translocations breakpoints were localized to the final intron of the PAX3 gene (Barr et al., 1993). This gene is a member of the paired box family and encodes a transcription factor with an N-terminal DNA binding domain containing paired box and homeobox motifs. Northern analysis of ARMS tumors with 5′ PAX3 probes demonstrated a 7.2 kb transcript that is the product of the rearranged PAX3 gene located on the derivative chromosome 13[der(13)] (Barr et al., 1993). Cloning of the corresponding cDNA revealed a fusion of PAX3 exons 5′ to the t(2;13) breakpoint with a novel sequence from the 13q14 chromosomal region. A full-length cDNA of the wild-type chromosome 13 gene was cloned and found to be a novel, widely expressed member of the fork-head transcription factor family (Galili et al., 1993; Shapiro et al., 1993a, b). This family is characterized by a conserved DNA binding motif termed the fork-head domain. Based on homology to this family, the chromosome 13 gene was named FKHR for 'fork head in rhabdomyosarcoma' (Galili et al., 1993). These combined findings indicate that the t(2;13) results in a chimeric transcript composed of 5′ PAX3 and 3′ FKHR exons (Fig. 41.1).

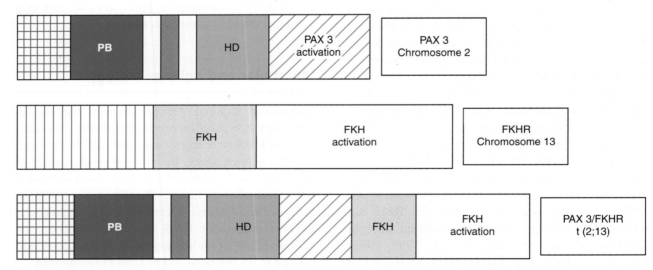

Figure 41.1 Structure of PAX3 on chromosome 2, the FKHR on chromosome 13, and the fusion product PAX-FKHR of the t(2;13) in alveolar rhabdomyosarcoma.

In summary, ARMS is characterized by a rearrangement of chromosome 2 and 13, the t(2;13) (q35;q14), in which the PAX3 gene within band 2q35 is fused with the FKHR gene within band 13q14. Both of the PAX3 DNA-binding regions (the paired box and the homeodomain) are retained in the fusion gene, whereas the carboxyl-terminal sequences are replaced by the bisected fork-head DNA-binding sequences of FKHR (Pappo et al., 1997).

In ARMS tumors with the variant t(1;13) translocation, a PAX3–FKHR fusion is not present. Southern blot and RT-PCR analyses revealed that a chromosome 1 locus encoding PAX7 (Shapiro et al., 1993b), another member of the paired box family, is rearranged and fused to FKHR in the t(1;13) conscript consisting of 5′ PAX7 and 3′ FKHR regions. This is very similar, structurally, to the 5′ PAX3–3′ FKHR transcript formed by the t(2;13) translocation (Davis et al., 1994).

Assays of expression during embryogenesis demonstrate that PAX3 and PAX7 are expressed with specific temporal and spatial patterns in early skeletal muscle progenitors, the presumed origin of ARMS, and in the developing nervous system (Goulding et al., 1991; Walther et al., 1991). In ARMS, studies indicate that the alteration of the PAX3 gene by the t(2;13) results in a gain of function. These studies are consistent with the hypothesis that the t(2;13) activates the oncogenic potential of PAX3 by dysregulating or exaggerating its normal function in the myogenic lineage. Studies indicate that the PAX3–FKHR protein affects the cellular activities of growth, differentiation, and apoptosis, and therefore may exert an oncogenic effect through multiple pathways (Bernasconi et al., 1996; Scheidler et al., 1996).

ERMS has not been associated with consistent chromosomal alterations. Molecular genetic analyses have revealed frequent allelic loss on chromosome 11 (Koufos et al., 1985). This genetic feature is specific for ERMS and is not found in ARMS (Scrable et al., 1989b). The smallest region of consistent allelic loss in ERMS cases has been localized to chromosomal region 11p15.5 (Scrable et al., 1987). Usually, the presence of a consistent region of allelic loss suggests the presence of a tumor suppressor gene that is inactivated in the associated malignancy. Studies have confirmed the presence of a tumor suppressor gene locus in the region previously demonstrated to show allelic loss in ERMS (Loh et al., 1992; Koi et al., 1993). Comparing allelic loss pattern in ERMS

tumors to the allelic status of the patients' parents has revealed that ERMS tumors preferentially maintain the paternally inherited allele and lose the maternal allele (Scrable et al., 1989a). The presence of the paternal allele suggests imprinting, the process by which individual genes from one parent are preferentially expressed over genes from the other. Even in close proximity to the genome, two genes can be oppositely imprinted, as is the case with insulin-like growth factor-2 (IGF-2) gene versus H19 and CDKN1C genes, which all map to chromosome 11p15.5. H19 gene product is an RNA molecule that is widely expressed during fetal development in association with cell differentiation but is apparently not translated into a protein product (Tycko, 1994). CDKN1C gene is expressed during development in several tissues, including skeletal muscle, and encodes a cyclin-dependent kinase inhibitor that negatively regulates cell-cycle progression by binding to and inhibiting the activity of several G1 cyclin/cyclin-dependent kinase complexes (Matsuoka et al., 1996). H19 and CDKN1C are preferentially expressed from the maternally inherited allele and IGF-2 is imprinted in the opposite direction so that the paternally inherited alleles are preferentially expressed (Tycko, 1994). Recently, another gene, GOK, has been identified at chromosome 11p15.5, which may act as a tumor-suppressor gene in RMS. It has been shown that GOK is not expressed in many RMS cell lines, which contrasts with high expression of GOK in skeletal muscle, the normal tissue of origin of RMS (Sabbioni et al., 1997). Therefore, downregulation of GOK expression may also play a role in the pathogenesis of RMS. Results of these allelic loss studies suggest that ERMS tumorigenesis frequently involves inactivation of an imprinted tumor suppressor by allelic loss of the maternal active allele and retention of the paternally inactive allele.

The combined data indicate that RMS tumorigenesis involves a variety of genetic alterations within a chromosomal region encompassing several genes. Some alterations serve to increase the number of active IGF-2 alleles, thereby resulting in overexpression of this fetal growth factor, whereas other alterations serve to mutate or inactivate expression of growth suppressive loci such as H19, CDKN1C, and GOK.

Although the PAX3/PAX7-FKHR gene fusions and allelic loss at 11p15.5 are the consistent, and possible defining, genetic alterations in ARMS and

ERMS, other alterations have also been detected. These alterations include both mutations that activate proto-oncogenes and mutations that inactivate tumor suppressor genes. These additional genetic changes indicate that ARMS and ERMS arise and evolve by a multistep process.

Studies of genomic amplification have shown differences between ARMS and ERMS. Using chromosome scanning techniques of comparative genomic hybridization there are frequent examples of whole chromosome gains in ERMS, involving chromosomes 2, 7, 8, 12, 13, 17, 18, and 19, but only one instance of amplification (Weber-Hall *et al.*, 1996). In contrast, examination of ARMS tumors reveal rare examples of chromosomal gains but evidence of amplification in almost every sample tested. Amplification of chromosomal region 12q13–15 was detected in 50% of ARMS cases which contains numerous growth-related genes including MDM2, CDK4, and GLI (Forus *et al.*, 1993; Khatib *et al.*, 1993; Meddeb *et al.*, 1996). MYCN gene amplification has been found in 10 of 40 ARMS cases and none in ERMS cases (Dias *et al.*, 1990a, b; Barr *et al.*, 1996).

Another group of proto-oncogenes that are genetically altered in RMS comprises members of the RAS gene family. Mutations of members of this family (K-RAS, N-RAS, H-RAS) have been detected in some ERMS tumors. No RAS mutations were found in ARMS tumors (Chardin *et al.*, 1985; Stratton *et al.*, 1989; Wilke *et al.*, 1993).

Of the tumor suppressor genes, alterations of the p53 gene have been most extensively studied in RMS. Using immunohistochemical assays of p53 expression that screen for tumors in which missense mutations increase the p53 protein half-life, p53 staining was detected in approximately 70% of RMS tumors (Kawai *et al.*, 1994; Wurl *et al.*, 1996). Dillert *et al.* (1995) corroborated previous findings that p53 germline mutations are seen with increased frequency in sporadic cases of RMS and that these alterations are almost uniquely seen in children younger than 3 years of age. The combined results of these studies indicate that germline and acquired p53 mutations contribute to the development of both ERMS and ARMS.

Other known tumor suppressor loci have also been investigated in RMS. A genome-wide screen of 32 RMS cases revealed several regions of allelic loss in addition to the expected 11p15 region (Visser *et al.*, 1996). In at least 25% of cases the regions showing allelic loss were 6p, 11q, 14q, 16q, and 18p. The overall frequency of allelic loss was lower in ARMS tumors than in ERMS tumors, again supporting the view that different molecular mechanisms are involved in the development of these two RMS subtypes.

In conclusion, molecular genetic studies of RMS support the premise that ARMS and ERMS represent distinct entities. These tumors are associated with specific molecular alterations, namely PAX3/PAX7-FKHR gene fusions in ARMS and 11p15.5 allelic loss in ERMS. The gene fusions in ARMS represent gain-of-function oncogenic mutations that generate potent transcriptional activators of target genes with PAX3/PAX7 binding sites. In contrast, the 11p15 allelic loss in ERMS acts on an imprinted region to inactivate expression of putative tumor suppressor loci. In addition, secondary genetic alterations of other genes occur in both ARMS and ERMS, indicating that these tumors arise in a multistep process. Both the primary and secondary events affect gene products that function in signal transduction and gene expression regulatory pathways, altering numerous key pathways in the cell, ultimately to generate the phenotypic changes of growth autonomy, abnormal differentiation, and motility (Barr, 1997).

Pathology

The significant difference in survival between ERMS and ARMS makes it imperative for the pathologist to diagnose variants of RMS accurately so that the biologic course of the disease can be predicted and appropriate therapy initiated.

In 1995, a consensus classification of RMS was published (Newton *et al.*, 1995) based on a review of a large number of tumors from IRS-II by 16 international pathologists from eight pathology groups. This produced a classification that was reproducible and could predict outcome by univariate analysis. A multivariate analysis of this new International Classification of Rhabdomyosarcoma (ICR) indicated that a survival model that included the ICR along with known prognostic factors of primary site, clinical group, and tumor size was significantly better at predicting survival than a model with only the known prognostic factors (Newton *et al.*, 1995). The ICR classification is shown in Table 41.1 along with the addition of the anaplastic variant from the Intergroup Rhabdomyosarcoma Study Group (IRS). The data

Table 41.1 International classification of rhabdomyosarcoma

Diagnosis	Histology	Incidence (%)	5-year survival (%)	Prognosis
Embryonal, botryoid	Favorable	6	95	Superior
Embryonal, spindle cell	Favorable	3	88	Superior
Embryonal NOS	Favorable	49	66	Intermediate
Alveolar, NOS or solid variant	Unfavorable	31	53	Poor
Anaplasia, diffuse	Unfavorable	2	45	Poor
Undifferentiated sarcoma	Unfavorable	3	44	Poor
Sarcoma with insufficient or inadequate tissue to make diagnosis	Unfavorable	6		Poor

NOS = not otherwise specified.

presented in this table are from ICR-related publications and IRS publications on specific RMS subtypes (Kodet *et al.*, 1993; Leuschner *et al.*, 1993; Tsokos, 1994; Newton *et al.*, 1995; Pawel *et al.*, 1997; Qualman *et al.*, 1998).

Embryonal rhabdomyosarcoma

These tumors have variable amounts of spindle and primitive round cells, which may be either tightly packed or loosely dispersed in a myxoid background (Fig. 41.2). The rhabdomyoblast, the more mature embryonal component, is characterized by bright eosinophilic cytoplasm and may appear in a variety of unusual shapes, termed 'tadpole', 'racquet', or 'strap' cells (Tsokos, 1994; Newton *et al.*, 1995). Cross-striations are seen in 50–60% of cases. These tumors are the most common genitourinary tumors. They rarely metastasize and respond well to current therapy.

Botryoid embryonal rhabdomyosarcoma

The ICR criterion for diagnosis of botryoid embryonal RMS requires demonstration of a cambium (condensed layer of rhabdomyoblasts) tumor layer underlying an intact epithelium in at least one microscopic field (Fig. 41.3). This microscopic criterion supersedes any gross demonstration of a 'grape-like' tumor mass. An extensive degree of rhabdomyoblastic differentiation can be evident both in the cambium layer and elsewhere in the tumor. The importance of diagnosing this subtype is evident given its superior prognosis with a 95% 5 year survival.

Spindle cell embryonal rhabdomyo-sarcoma

The spindle cell variant of RMS also enjoys a superior prognosis, with an 88% 5 year survival rate. It has only been recognized in the literature since 1993

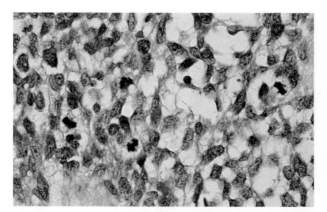

Figure 41.2 Embryonal rhabdomyosarcoma. Primitive round cells (rhabdomyoblasts) with bright eosinophilic cytoplasm are loosely dispersed in a myxoid background.

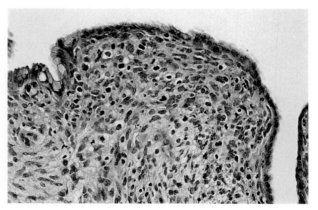

Figure 41.3 Botryoid embryonal rhabdomyosarcoma demonstrating the cambium (condensed layer of rhabdomyoblasts) tumor layer underlying an intact epithelium.

(Leuschner *et al.*, 1993). This neoplasm has a fascicular, spindled 'leiomyomatous' growth pattern which can show a marked degree of rhabdomyoblastic differentiation (Fig. 41.4). Some tumors show marked collagen deposition. This variant almost exclusively occurs in the paratesticular region, although it can rarely occur at other body sites.

Alveolar (solid) rhabdomyosarcoma

The classic cleft-like spaces lined by rhabdomyoblasts that are traditionally described (Newton *et al.*, 1995; Qualman *et al.*, 1998) for ARMS may merge with spaces filled with tumor cells that sit on thin fibrovascular septa. This latter solid variant is rarely present without the classic finding of cleft-like spaces and can be recognized with adequate tumor sampling. The key criterion is to recognize palisading of tumor cells about fibrovascular cores (Fig. 41.5). The tumor cells have a coarse chromatin pattern to their nuclei with less evident myogenesis than in ERMS (Newton *et al.*, 1995).

A review comparing IRS pathologic diagnosis with institutional diagnosis performed between 1984 and 1997 showed concordance in only 63% of cases. The high level of discordant diagnoses (37%) reflects the need for better recognition of the solid alveolar variant of this RMS subtype.

The prognosis for both the classic and solid variants is the same: both carry a poor prognosis with only a 53% 5 year survival rate. Improved concordance of review and institutional diagnosis is crucial for this malignancy, as they receive intensified therapy on current IRS protocols.

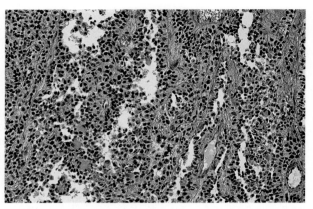

Figure 41.5 Alveolar rhabdomyosarcoma showing palisading of tumor cells with a coarse chromatin pattern about fibrovascular cores.

Anaplastic rhabdomyosarcoma

This variant also has a high rate of discordance (62%) (Qualman *et al.*, 1998). Using the IRS-I-III material, anaplastic RMS was defined using the following criteria: (1) large, lobate hyperchromatic nuclei of at least three times the size of neighboring nuclei; and (2) atypical multipolar mitotic figures (Fig. 41.6) (Kodet *et al.*, 1993; Qualman *et al.*, 1998). It is also defined further by its distribution as focal (group I), consisting of single or few anaplastic cells, or diffuse (group II), where anaplastic cells aggregate in clusters or form a continuous sheet (Kodet *et al.*, 1993; Qualman *et al.*, 1998). The occurrence of anaplasia is independent of both RMS tumor site and histopathologic subtype, although it occurs preferentially in

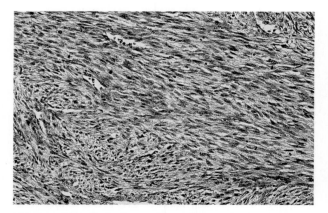

Figure 41.4 Spindle cell embryonal rhabdomyosarcoma showing the fascicular, spindled 'leiomyomatous' growth pattern with a marked degree of rhabdomyoblastic differentiation.

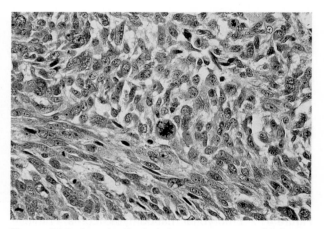

Figure 41.6 Anaplastic rhabdomyosarcoma with large, lobate hyperchromatic nuclei and atypical multipolar mitotic figures.

ERMS. The overall incidence of anaplasia in IRS-I–III was 3% (Qualman *et al.*, 1998).

Undifferentiated sarcoma

This category also has a high rate of discordance (62%) (Qualman *et al.*, 1998). This category is included in the ICR classification only because its response to therapy is similar to that of RMS (Newton *et al.*, 1995). These tumors are mainly composed of sheets of medium-packed cells with no discernible architectural structure except for delicate fibrovascular septa or a vague spindled-storiform pattern. Necrosis and inflammation are not prominent, cellularity is high with high mitotic activity [>10 mitoses per high-power field (hpf)], and the nuclei are predominantly oval with prominent chromocenters and indistinct cytoplasm (Pawel *et al.*, 1997; Qualman *et al.*, 1998). The tumors stain only with vimentin antisera (77%), if at all.

This entity is rare (3% of cases) and occurs more often in males (62%), in patients 5 years of age or older (65%), and is more common in the extremities (53%), just like ARMS (Pawel *et al.*, 1997). Five year survival with localized disease is 72% but with disseminated disease is only 44% (Qualman *et al.*, 1998).

Other diagnostic studies

Ancillary studies performed on histopathologic tissues are useful in confirming the diagnosis and in providing prognostic information on the course of the malignancy.

Immunologic studies

A comprehensive study using commercially available and experimental antibodies was undertaken in the IRS-IV study, which included 100 cases of RMS representing all subtypes (Qualman *et al.*, 1998).

The incidence of immunopositivity for the various antisera is summarized in Table 41.2. Approximately 20% of RMS cases required the use of immunohistochemistry to establish the final diagnosis (Qualman *et al.*, 1998).

Polyclonal antidesmin (P-DES) antibody was positive in all but one RMS (99%) (Fig. 41.7). Monoclonal antidesmin (M-DES) antibody was negative in many of the same tumors (38%). Antimuscle-specific actin (MSA) antibody was positive in 94% of the RMS. Antimyoglobin (MYO) antibody was positive

Table 41.2 Incidence of immunopositivity for antisera in rhabdomyosarcoma diagnostic studies

Antibody	Percentage
Polyclonal desmin	99
Monoclonal desmin	62
Muscle-specific actin	94
Alpha-smooth muscle actin	4
Myoglobin	78
Wide-spectrum keratin	7
Epithelial membrane antigen	2
S-100 protein	19
Neuron-specific enolase	6
Leukocyte common antigen	0
MIC-2	14
p53	16

in 78% and was negative mostly in the less differentiated tumors. Anti-alpha smooth muscle actin (SMA) antibody reacted positively only in a minority (4%) of ERMS (Qualman *et al.*, 1998).

The current approach at the IRS Pathology Center in cases where the diagnosis of RMS is in question is to screen the tissue with immunostaining for three antibodies: P-DES, MSA, and MIC-2; the latter helps to rule out the diagnosis of an extraosseous Ewing's sarcoma or primitive neuroectodermal tumor (Dworzak *et al.*, 1992). Approximately 14% of RMS stain positive to MIC-2 antisera but this is only a weak granular intracytoplasmic immunopositivity, while Ewing's sarcoma and primitive neuroectodermal tumors show discreet plasma membrane staining (Dworzak *et al.*, 1992). Antibodies to the various

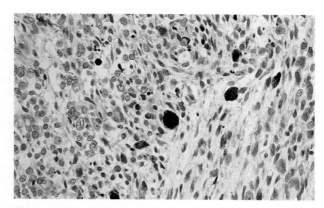

Figure 41.7 Positive polyclonal antidesmin (P-DES) antibody staining in a case of embryonal rhabdomyosarcoma.

myogenic transcription factors (Myo D1, etc.) can be tested on fresh tissue only (Triche, 1995).

Monoclonal antibody to p53 protein was also studied in pediatric RMS (Felix *et al.*, 1992). Positive immunostaining was seen in only 16% of RMS specimens (Kusafuka *et al.*, 1997; Qualman *et al.*, 1998). Conversely, immunopositivity at the grade 3–4 level (6% of RMS) was significantly associated with the occurrence of any anaplasia in ARMS and diffuse anaplasia in ERMS, independent of fusion gene status (Pascasio *et al.*, 1998). The potential linkage of p53 abnormalities with anaplasia in RMS will be further studied in the IRS-V study.

Planned future molecular studies

In IRS-V the emphasis will be on the incidence of t(1;13) and t(2;13) and their fusion genes in RMS (Qualman *et al.*, 1998). RT-PCR methodology will be employed in detecting fusion genes in frozen tissue and archival tissue (Edwards *et al.*, 1997). The t(1;13) translocation may predict a different clinical phenotype and longer event-free survival than the t(2;13) translocation (Qualman *et al.*, 1998).

Gattenloehner also demonstrated that the acetylcholine receptor gamma-subunit was strongly transcribed in 16 of 16 RMS specimens studied. They proposed that the gamma-acetylcholine receptor mRNA is a useful tumor-specific marker in RMS and in the detection of micrometastases and minimal residual disease (Gattenloehner *et al.*, 1998).

The value of ploidy analysis as a prognostic assay in RMS is uncertain, with discrepant results (Qualman *et al.*, 1998). As determined by flow cytometry, approximately two-thirds of alveolar tumors have near-tetraploid DNA content. The remaining cases are usually diploid (Shapiro *et al.*, 1991). Near-tetraploidy is almost never observed in ERMS (Pappo *et al.*, 1997). Loss of heterozygosity for closely linked foci of chromosome 11p5.5 is seen in ERMS.

Post-treatment pathologic studies

The most difficult assessment by pathologists is the prognostic significance of residual rhabdomyoblasts in post-therapeutic RMS tissue specimens. Studies support the concept that post-therapeutic cytodifferentiation occurs more frequently in botryoid or embryonal RMS (Coffin *et al.*, 1997; Heyn *et al.*, 1997). In botryoid RMS cytodifferentiation and decreased proliferation activity were associated with favorable outcome. Unchanged or increased post-therapeutic proliferation activity suggested aggressive biologic potential in embryonal or alveolar RMS. These phenomena will be further studied in IRS-V.

Staging of rhabdomyosarcoma

Both the surgically based clinical grouping system (CGS) employed in IRS I, II, and III, and the site-based TNM (tumor, node, metastases) staging system have been applied (Lawrence *et al.*, 1987a; Rodary *et al.*, 1991; Wexler and Helman, 1994).

The CGS (Table 41.3) is a surgicopathologic staging system based on whether surgical resection has been accomplished, with modifiers related to clinical and pathologic findings (Lawrence *et al.*, 1987a; Wexler and Helman, 1994).

Table 41.3 Clinical group staging for rhabdomyosarcoma

Clinical	Group	Extent of disease
I	A	Localized tumor, confined to site of origin, completely resected
I	B	Localized tumor, infiltrating beyond site of origin, completely resected
II	A	Localized tumor, gross total resection, but with microscopic residual disease
II	B	Locally extensive tumor (spread to regional lymph nodes), completely resected
II	C	Locally extensive tumor (spread to regional lymph nodes), gross total resection, but microscopic residual disease
III	A	Localized or locally extensive tumor, gross residual disease after biopsy only
III	B	Localized or locally extensive tumor, gross residual disease after major resection (> 50% debulking)
IV		Any size primary tumor, with or without regional lymph-node involvement, with distant metastases

The CGS is used to plan radiation therapy and relies on the pathologic findings, whether the tumor is confined to the primary site, whether there is presence or absence of local invasion, and whether the surgical resection is complete with tumor-free margins.

The TNM staging system (Table 41.4) takes into account tumor location, size, clinical lymph-node involvement, and the presence or absence of metastases. It is used to plan therapy and is highly predictive of outcome (Lawrence *et al.*, 1987a; Rodary *et al.*, 1991; Wexler and Helman, 1994).

According to the IRS-V protocol, representative portions of the tumor should be submitted for light microscopy or fixed for electron microscopy, placed in tissue culture medium for potential chromosome studies, and frozen and stored for molecular studies (Qualman *et al.*, 1998). When a tumor is resected, evaluation of the margins is mandatory. Recording the three-dimensional tumor size is of utmost importance, as it influences staging and outcome. The distance of the tumor from the nearest resection margins is also important for staging.

The pathologist has an important role in the proper staging and grouping of RMS, as well as its proper histopathologic classification. Accurate histologic diagnosis is important for treatment planning (Crist *et al.*, 1995).

Presentation

Bladder rhabdomyosarcoma

The mean age at presentation for patients with bladder rhabdomyosarcoma is 3.5 years. The male:female ratio is slightly greater than 2:1 (Heyn *et al.*, 1997).

The child may present with symptoms of lower urinary tract obstruction, such as strangury, urinary retention, overflow incontinence, or urinary tract infection (UTI). The most common finding is that of a large palpable lower abdominal mass. A mass can also be felt on rectal examination. The tumor may obstruct the ureters and cause hydronephrosis and impairment of renal function. Hematuria is rarely present unless the overlying bladder mucosa is disrupted by the tumor. Occasionally the child may void fragments of tumor tissue. In females, the tumor may extend out along the whole length of the urethra and protrude through the meatus (sarcoma botryoides).

Prostatic rhabdomyosarcoma

The median age of presentation for prostatic rhabdomyosarcoma is 3.5 years (Hays *et al.*, 1982). It usually presents as a solid mass rather than the botryoides form. Proximal expansion of the mass towards the bladder neck region and the trigone results in bladder outlet obstruction and possible ureteral obstruction and hydronephrosis. Posterior extension of the tumor towards the rectum produces a mass effect which may impinge on the rectum and cause constipation.

Rhabdomyosarcoma of the female genital tract

Age at presentation varies depending on the site of origin. Although the mean age of girls with vaginal tumors is less than 2 years, uterine tumors usually present during adolescence and vulvar tumors may present anywhere between 1 and 19 years of age

Table 41.4 TNM staging of genitourinary rhabdomyosarcoma

Stage	Sites	T invasiveness	T size	Regional nodes	Metastases
I	Genitourinary (non-bladder/prostate)	T_1 or T_2	a or b	N_0, N_1 or N_x	M_0
II	Bladder/prostate	T_1 or T_2	a	N_0 or N_x	M_0
	Others	T_1 or T_2	a	N_0 or N_x	M_0
III	Bladder/prostate	T_1 or T_2	a	N_1	M_0
	Others	T_1 or T_2	b	N_0, N_1, or N_x	M_0
IV	All	T_1 or T_2	a or b	N_0 or N_1	M_1

T tumor:	T_1 = confined to anatomic site of origin; T_2 = Extension.
Size:	a = < 5 cm in diameter; b = > 5 cm in diameter.
Regional nodes:	N_0 = not clinically involved; N_1 = clinically involved; N_x = clinical status unknown.
Metastases:	M_0 = no distant metastasis; M_1 = distant metastasis present.

(Hays *et al.*, 1988). Primary vaginal rhabdomyosarcoma is the most common tumor of the female genital tract in children and may present with a vaginal discharge that is foul smelling and/or bloody. The tumor may prolapse through the introitus or may be seen in the vagina (sarcoma botryoides). Although vaginal tumors may present as a palpable abdominal mass with symptoms of urethral obstruction, bladder and rectal wall infiltration are uncommon. Uterine tumors usually present as a mass and may also protrude through the cervix as a polyp. The swelling produced by vulvar tumors usually involves the labia and may be misdiagnosed as a Bartholin's gland infection (Shapiro and Strother, 1992b).

Diagnostic evaluation

The first diagnostic procedure obtained in a child who presents with an abdominal or pelvic mass and/or symptoms of urinary obstruction is an abdominal and pelvic sonogram (Fig. 41.8). This will usually show a solid tumor and will also be able to assess the status of the bladder, the postvoid residual, and the upper tracts.

The remainder of the radiographic evaluation is to determine the extent of the local and regional disease, as well as to identify metastatic foci. Computed tomographic (CT) scanning of the primary site has been the study of choice for evaluating these tumors (Fig. 41.9). Improved imaging has recently been reported

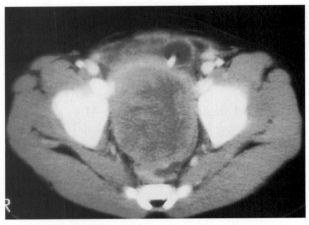

Figure 41.9 Computed tomographic scan in a 5-year-old child with embryonal group III rhabdomyosarcoma. Note that the extent of the tumor beyond the bladder is not well visualized. A catheter is seen in the bladder which is displaced anteriorly.

using magnetic resonance imaging (MRI) to delineate more clearly the local extent of the tumor. On T_2-weighted images, the extent of the tumor around the bladder and prostate can be determined. The improved contrast and spatial resolution, in addition to the sagittal and coronal views provided by the MRI, are advantageous in demonstrating the local extent of the tumor. Specifically, the expansion of the tumor distally into the urethra, proximally into the trigone and bladder wall, outside the bladder towards the pelvic floor and levators ani muscles, and posteriorly into the rectum can be determined (Figs. 41.10–41.13). MRI should be the modality of choice in evaluating the extent of the tumor in the pelvis.

Potential hematogenous and lymphatic metastatic sites need to be evaluated. This can be achieved by CT scan of the abdomen and chest or MRI, bone marrow aspiration, and bone scan.

Tissue diagnosis of RMS is confirmed by biopsy. Specimens can be obtained either by cystoscopy or needle biopsy. During endoscopic biopsy, electrocautery should be avoided as the coagulation effect may cause histologic artifacts. A cold-cup biopsy forceps or a cold-knife is preferable. An ultrasound-guided needle biopsy through the perineum or the extraperitoneal suprapubic route may also be used. Vaginal tumors are diagnosed and biopsied endoscopically, and the extent of distortion and/or infiltration of the bladder by the tumor can also be assessed by cystoscopy. Uterine tumors can be biop-

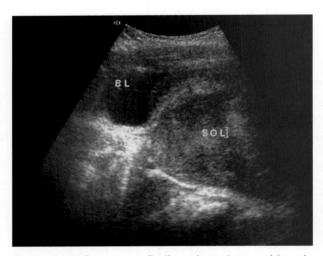

Figure 41.8 Sonogram findings in a 4-year-old male presenting with rhabdomyosarcoma. The solid tumor (SOL) is seen to be pushing the bladder anteriorly (BL).

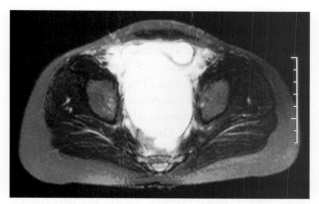

Figure 41.10 Magnetic resonance imaging scan finding in a 4-year-old male with embryonal group III rhabdomyosarcoma. On T_2-weighted images the extent of the tumor is well visualized.

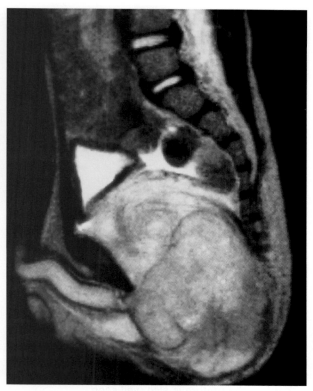

Figure 41.12 Magnetic resonance imaging scan in a 6-year-old child with embryonal group III rhabdomyosarcoma. This sagittal view on T_2-weighted image shows the extent of the tumor distally in the membranous urethra.

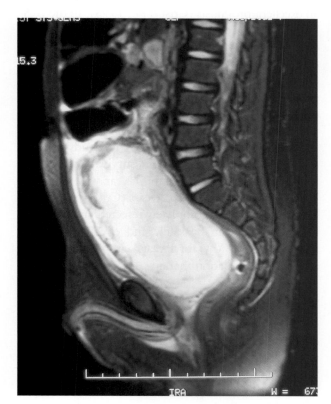

Figure 41.11 Magnetic resonance imaging scan in a 4-year-old child with embryonal group III rhabdomyosarcoma. In this sagittal view the extent of the tumor into the membranous urethra is well delineated.

sied either at the time of vaginoscopy or by performing a cervical dilation and curettage. An adequate amount of tissue is required for the pathologist to identify the histological subgroups of RMS, thus allowing correct grading and therapy. Needle biopsies that are performed to establish the diagnosis of RMS must include a sufficient number of cores.

Suprapubic catheter drainage should not be used in children who present in urinary retention, to avoid the risk of tumor spread along the suprapubic tract. A urethral Foley catheter can usually be inserted in these children. The catheter is removed once the tumor shrinks following chemotherapy and the child is able to void. Transient voiding difficulty requiring insertion of a catheter may also occur after initiation of chemotherapy, as a result of the edema that accompanies the early phases of therapy. In patients with renal impairment secondary to distal ureteral obstruction, temporary nephrostomy tube placement may be necessary to minimize the adverse effects of chemotherapy.

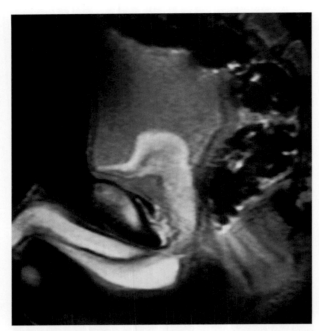

Figure 41.13 Magnetic resonance imaging scan in a 5-year-old child with embryonal group III rhabdomyosarcoma after 16 weeks of chemotherapy. The tumor is visualized extending into the bladder and its extent into the urethra is also well seen.

Treatment

The outcome of children with RMS has improved dramatically. In the early 1960s, when only local therapy such as surgery and irradiation was available, approximately one-third of patients survived (Pappo *et al.*, 1995). The only exceptions were patients with tumors in selected primary sites such as the bladder or the orbit. These patients were treated with radical surgery and the reported survival was 70% (Shapiro and Strother, 1992a, b). During the 1960s, combined chemotherapy was initiated with vincristine, dactinomycin, and cyclophosphamide (VAC), yielding promising results (Tan *et al.*, 1959; Haddy *et al.*, 1967). These early encouraging results, combined with the heterogeneity and rarity of RMS, prompted the implementation in 1972 of the first national cooperative trial.

The IRS Committee has reported the results of three consecutive trials: IRS-I (1972–1978, $n = 686$), IRS-II (1978–1984, $n = 999$), IRS-III (1984–1991, $n = 1062$) (Maurer *et al.*, 1988, 1993; Crist *et al.*, 1995). The results of the fourth consecutive trial,

IRS-IV, published in the fall of 1999, showed a similar survival to the IRS-III studies. The estimated 5 year overall survival rate steadily and significantly increased in each of the first three trials: 55% in IRS-I, 63% in IRS-II, and 71% in IRS-III.

In IRS-I treatment assignment was based on the postsurgical extent of disease, with no stratification for specific risk subgroups. The IRS-II study recognized the prognostic significance of certain risk factors (clinical group, site, and histology) and stratified patients accordingly. Patients with primary tumors in 'special pelvic' sites (bladder, prostate, vagina, uterus) received VAC chemotherapy. IRS-III further stratified patients into nine distinct risk subgroups based on extent of disease, primary tumor site, and histology.

Overview of Intergroup Rhabdomyosarcoma Study Group studies (all sites)

Clinical group I

This group consists of children whose tumors were completely resected and who were expected to have an excellent prognosis (Crist *et al.*, 1995). In the IRS-I trial, it was concluded that the 5 year overall and disease-free survival did not change with the addition of radiotherapy to VAC chemotherapy. Therefore, radiotherapy was omitted in children with clinical group I tumors (Maurer *et al.*, 1988). In this subset of patients, the IRS-II study showed that vincristine and dactinomycin chemotherapy (VA) was equivalent to VAC chemotherapy. The IRS III study showed that the 5 year progression-free survival and survival for those treated with VA for 1 year was similar to VAC for 2 years or VA for 2 years (Crist *et al.*, 1995). Thus, patients with completely resected favorable histology tumors can be safely and effectively treated with two drugs (VA) for 1 year, without the need for alkylators or radiation therapy.

Clinical group II

Children in this category usually received postoperative radiotherapy at various time points during treatment, resulting in a local control rate of 90% (Maurer *et al.*, 1988, 1993; Crist *et al.*, 1995). Based on the findings of IRS-I and IRS-II studies, VA with radiotherapy remains the therapeutic standard for children with clinical group II disease who present with a favorable histology tumor in a favorable site. IRS-III compared VA plus adriamycin and radiotherapy to VA only plus radiotherapy. Even though there seemed to be an advantage to adding adriamycin this was not statistically significant (Crist *et al.*, 1995).

Clinical group III

This is the largest group of patients enrolled in IRS-I, II, and -III (Maurer *et al.*, 1988, 1993; Crist *et al.*, 1995). In IRS-I all group III patients were randomized to receive either VAC chemotherapy and radiation, or VAC with doxorubicin (VADRC-VAC) and radiation. Addition of doxorubicin failed to improve the 5 year overall survival (Maurer *et al.*, 1988). In IRS-II, patients were randomized to receive intensified VAC or VADRC-VA therapy. Prognosis was not different between those two regimens, but the intensified treatments were superior in inducing complete responses and prolonged survival compared with IRS-I (Maurer *et al.*, 1993). In IRS-III patients were randomized to receive either pulsed VAC or VADRC-VAC-cisplatin and radiation or VADRC-VAC-cisplatin-VP-16 and radiation. At 5 years the overall survival rate was the same for all three regimens (Crist *et al.*, 1995). Several patients among these study arms received alternate induction chemotherapy with one of three drug pairs (doxorubicin–dacarbazine, dactinomycin-VP16, or dactinomycin–dacarbazine) and second-look surgery (Crist *et al.*, 1995). The outcome of these children was improved compared with that of patients who were treated in IRS-II. Preliminary data from IRS-IV showed that administration of escalating doses of cyclophosphamide was associated with significant morbidity. The overall incidence of toxic death was 7.6%. Seven of the eight deaths occurred at doses of 2.2 g/m^2. In addition, hepatic veno-occlusive disease has been recently recognized as a complication of high-dose VAC therapy in these children (Pappo *et al.*, 1997).

Clinical group IV

The 5 year survival for patients with metastatic disease continues to be poor, in spite of intensified therapy and new drug combinations. The combined agent regimens in all three IRS studies have led to 5 year overall and progression-free survival rates of below 30% (Maurer *et al.*, 1988, 1993; Crist *et al.*, 1995). IRS-IV and -V are investigating new drugs including melphalan, ifosfamide, and topotecan (Horowitz *et al.*, 1988; Houghton *et al.*, 1992;

Pappo *et al.*, 1993b). A novel treatment strategy for these patients includes immunotherapy. The National Cancer Institute research has demonstrated that by blocking the IGF-1 receptor, using the antibody alpha-IR-3, one can inhibit RMS cell proliferation (Kalebic *et al.*, 1994).

Special pelvic tumors

Early on in the IRS studies it became apparent that certain pelvic tumors (bladder, prostate, vagina, uterus) responded better to therapy than other sites. The 5 year overall survival rate in this group of patients was 74%. However, this outcome was achieved at the expense of numerous bladder extirpations for patients with genitourinary tumors, and only 23% of the patients had functional bladders 3 years after therapy (Hay, 1993). In IRS-II the treatment strategy changed to primary chemotherapy, with 4 months of VAC, followed by delayed radiation and/or surgery. This treatment approach failed to improve the bladder salvage rate, with a 3 year bladder retention rate of only 25% and a survival rate similar to IRS-I (Raney *et al.*, 1990a, b). In IRS-III, patients in clinical group III received an intensified VADRC-VAC regimen plus cisplatin to induce a complete response. Second-look surgery was recommended at 20 weeks. Alternate induction therapy with dactinomycin or dactinomycin and VP-16 was initiated for residual tumor. All patients received radiotherapy. The 3 year bladder preservation rate (60%), 5 year progression-free survival estimate (74 ± 5%) and overall survival (83 ± 4) were strikingly superior to those of IRS-I and IRS-II (Maurer *et al.*, 1988, 1993; Crist *et al.*, 1995).

The extent of surgical intervention in RMS of the bladder, vagina, and prostate remains controversial. In a series of 15 patients with tumors confined to one of these three organs, Fisch *et al.* (1995) showed that after chemotherapy, radical operative intervention with multiple biopsies at the resection margins permits complete tumor resection with excellent long-term results. This radical operative approach is in contrast to the IRS protocol. The main advantage of this treatment protocol is the elimination of radiotherapy, which is often used in conjunction with organ-sparing surgery, and has been associated with severe complications including radiation-induced cystitis and impaired growth of the pelvic bone (Agarwal *et al.*, 1997). Fichtner and Hohenfellner (1995) reported a 10% rate of radiation-induced cystitis when radiation was used alone and 30% when it was used in conjunction with chemotherapy. In a review of 11 survivors of pelvic rhabdomyosarcoma by Yeung et al. (1994), seven received radiotherapy. In all seven patients, there was markedly decreased functional bladder capacity (11–48% of mean expected value for age) and abnormal voiding patterns, although bladder compliance was not decreased and bladder emptying was almost complete in five. Four patients also had upper urinary tract dilatation and two required reconstructive bladder surgery because of severe bilateral hydronephrosis, In contrast, all four children not treated with radiation had normal bladder capacity and normal voiding patterns. They suggested that all patients treated with radiotherapy should have careful follow-up including the use of frequency–volume voiding charts.

Heyn et al. (1997) reviewed the outcome of 28 patients with group III bladder RMS. All received 20 weeks of multiagent chemotherapy and 4 weeks of radiotherapy. Of these, 13 underwent cystectomy. Cystectomy specimens demonstrated diminished tumor cells with varying degrees of maturation. They concluded that primary bladder RMS is very responsive to chemotherapy and radiotherapy, and that these tumors show further maturation following treatment, thus allowing the preservation of larger proportions of bladders with residual disease. Similarly, Lobe et al. (1996) examined the role of limited surgery in localized prostatic RMS and showed a high cure rate with relatively good bladder salvage rate. They reviewed the outcome of patients entered into the IRS-III study with prostatic RMS. In their study, all but five patients received radiotherapy. Of the 51 patients, two had group IIA tumors and were cured by primary gross excision, local radiotherapy, and vincristine and actinomycin therapy. Five had group IV metastatic disease and died despite therapy. Of 44 with group III disease, 43 underwent biopsy alone followed by chemotherapy and second-look operation. Fourteen of the 44 patients (32%) had pelvic exenteration following chemotherapy, and seven underwent prostatectomy. Fourteen of the 44 underwent laparotomy with or without biopsy and six required no further treatment after chemotherapy. They reported six relapses with a further three patients undergoing exenteration and one a prostatectomy. The cure rate in the 44 group III patients was 82% (Lobe et al., 1996).

In a recently published report on the outcome of 13 patients with lower urinary tract RMS (11 group III and two group IV), from the Hospital for Sick Children in Toronto, a strategy was proposed of intensified induction chemotherapy, followed by surgical excision and reconstruction without radiotherapy. This provided a high cure rate without the late sequelae of pelvic radiotherapy (Merguerian et al., 1998). Only two of the patients required pelvic exenteration. The survival rate in this small group of patients was 80%. Six patients received radiotherapy for residual and metastatic disease. The reliance on surgery for local control mandates that clean resection margins be achieved in this group of patients. Unfortunately, the assessment of margins on frozen sections may miss microscopic submucosal disease that is then discovered on the permanent section. In these instances, our current policy is to re-explore and excise the margins since radiotherapy in those patients in this series was associated with local recurrence. The IRS trials have not yet determined the long-term outcome of children who received radiotherapy, regarding their growth and the incidence of radiation-induced cystitis.

Unfavorable histology clinical groups I and II tumors

The poor outcome for children with clinical group I alveolar tumors was recognized in IRS-I (Maurer et al., 1988). All these children therefore received intensive VAC chemotherapy in IRS-II. This treatment modification increased the 3 year disease-free survival rate from 43% to 69% (Maurer et al., 1993). In IRS-III therapy was further intensified with the use of a VADRC-VAC-cisplatin containing regimen. The 5 year progression-free (71 ± 6%) and overall survival (80 ± 6) rates were significantly improved over those for comparable patients treated on IRS-II protocols (Crist et al., 1995).

Local therapy: results of multi-institutional trials

Although RMS is a chemosensitive tumor, the role of chemotherapy is to decrease the size of the tumor and to achieve systemic control. Surgical resection alone or in combination with irradiation is necessary for local control of the tumor. Radiotherapy has been used to eradicate residual microscopic or macroscopic tumor cells following surgery or chemotherapy. In response to the results of several trials, radiotherapy doses now vary according to the patient age, tumor site, and amount of residual tumor (Pappo *et al.*, 1997).

Intensified chemotherapy and second-look surgery have decreased the use of radiotherapy and extensive primary surgery for patients with vaginal and vulvar RMS (Andrassy *et al.*, 1995). In addition, the use of early radiotherapy, aggressive chemotherapy, and second-look surgery has dramatically decreased the use of radical surgery to treat children with genitourinary RMS (Andrassy *et al.*, 1995; Crist *et al.*, 1995).

Currently, microscopic residual disease is treated with 40 Gy of radiation to the tumor bed and a 2 cm margin. In IRS-IV, radiotherapy following complete resection of tumors with unfavorable features (large size, unfavorable site, nodal involvement) is mandated (Pappo *et al.*, 1997). Gross residual disease requires higher doses of 45–55 Gy, depending on the site and size of the tumor.

Further, to increase local control and decrease the acute and late adverse effects of radiotherapy, IRS-IV initiated a pilot protocol evaluating hyperfractionated radiotherapy in patients with unresectable or metastatic disease (Donaldson *et al.*, 1995). This study suggested that hyperfractionated radiotherapy is feasible and is associated with tolerable side-effects in children with unresected or metastatic RMS. A prospective study comparing the efficacy of hyperfractionated radiotherapy versus conventional radiotherapy is underway. Surgical approaches to the treatment of RMS have also been influenced by the multi-institutional studies. Nodal involvement is very common among patients with genitourinary tumors, therefore nodal sampling should be considered at the time of initial staging (Lawrence *et al.*, 1987b). If performed within 35 days of the primary procedure, surgical re-excision may benefit patients with microscopic positive residual tumor (Hays *et al.*, 1989; Merguerian *et al.*, 1998).

Summary

Controversy exists as to the role of radiotherapy in the treatment of group III genitourinary RMS. The IRS recommends treating most patients with group III RMS with radiotherapy. The long-term consequences of radiotherapy have not yet been fully evaluated, including pelvic growth, functional bladder capacity and the development of radiation cystitis, and erectile

dysfunction. An alternate protocol includes intense chemotherapy initially, in an attempt to decrease tumor size, followed by surgery which most often requires a continent urinary diversion with preservation of part of the bladder. Radiotherapy is reserved for those with residual disease.

IRS-III trials in patients with group III special pelvic primary tumors (bladder, prostate, vagina, uterus) clearly demonstrated that these patients benefited from the more complex therapy. The addition of doxorubicin (ADR) and cisplatin (CDDP), with or without second-look surgery, or dactinomycin (AMD) plus VP-16 to VAC, improved outcome compared with the results with VAC with or without second-look surgery in IRS-II (83% vs 72% 5-year survival rate). Of the 90 patients who achieved CR, 29% (26 of 90) were rendered tumor free by second-look surgery. They also concluded that the introduction of RT in patients with tumors at the bladder neck/trigone or prostate may have had a favorable impact on outcome. Finally, there was more than doubling of the bladder salvage rate, attributable to the more intensive therapy used in IRS-III.

Table 41.5 summarizes the treatment protocols of the IRS studies and survival data related to clinical staging.

Late effects of therapy

Because of the improved long-term survival and the use of intensified chemotherapeutic regimens, several serious and potentially life-threatening therapy-related complications have emerged. In IRS-IV the incorporation of ifosfamide into front-line therapeutic protocols for children with unresectable tumors was associated with a 14% incidence of renal toxicity. Factors contributing to that toxicity included high doses of ifosfamide (>72 g/m^2), age younger than 3 years, and pre-existing renal abnormalities such as hydronephrosis (Heyn *et al.*, 1992; Ashraf *et al.*, 1994).

Of the 109 patients with bladder and prostate tumors who were treated in IRS-I and -II, 29% developed post-therapy hematuria, 29% showed evidence of delayed pubertal development, and 10% had growth retardation (Raney *et al.*, 1993).

The occurrence of second malignant neoplasms is one of the most devastating sequelae of successful contemporary therapy. Of the 1770 patients enrolled in IRS-I and -II, 22 developed second malignant neoplasms (10 year cumulative incidence rate of

Table 41.5 Treatment protocols and outcome of children enrolled in the Intergroup Rhabdomyosarcoma Study Group Studies to date

Clinical group	IRS-I Treatment	IRS-I Survival (%)	IRS-II Treatment	IRS-II Survival (%)	IRS-III Treatment	IRS-III Survival (%)	IRS-IV Treatment	IRS-IV Survival (%)
I Favorable	VAC × 2 years	93	VAC × 2 years	85	Cyclic sequential VA × 1 year	93	VAI	84
	VAC + RT × 2 years	81	VA × 1 year	84			VIE	88
							VAC	84
II Favorable	VA + RT × 1 year	73	VA + RT × 1 year	88	VA + RT × 1 year	54	VAI + RT	
							VIE + RT	
							VAC + RT	
III Favorable	VAC + RT × 2 years	70	Pulsed VAC + RT × 1 year	79	VA + ADR + RT × 1 year	89	VAI + HF-RT	78
	—	71	Pulsed VAC ± RT ± surgery × 2 years	72	Pulsed VADRC-VAC + CDDP ± AMD + VP-16 ± RT ± surgery × 2 years	83	VIE + HF-RT	87
							VAC + HF-RT	78
I and II Unfavorable	—	57	Pulsed VAC + RT × 1 year	71	Pulsed VADRC-VAC +CDDP + RT × 1 year	80	VAI + RT	
							VIE + RT	
							VAC + RT	
IV	VAC + RT × 2 years	14	Pulsed VADRC-VAC + RT × 2 years	27	Pulsed VAC + RT × 2 years	27	VM + VAC + RT	
	VAC + ADR + RT × 2 years	26			Pulsed VADRC-VAC + CDDP + VP-16 + RT × 2 years		IE + VAC + RT	

VAC = vincristine, dactinomycin (AMD), cyclophosphamide; VA = vincristine, dactinomycin; VADRC = vincristine, dactinomycin (AMD), cyclophosphamide; CDDP = cisplatin; VAI = vincristine, dactinomycin, ifosfamide; VIE = vincristine, ifosfamide, etoposide; RT = radiation therapy; HF-RT = hyperfractionated radiotherapy; IE = ifosfamide, etoposide; VM = vincristine, melphalan.

1.7%). The most common malignancies were bone sarcomas ($n = 11$) and acute non-lymphoblastic leukemia ($n = 5$). The median time to development of these neoplasms was 7 and 4 years, respectively (Heyn *et al.*, 1993). In the IRS-III trial, acute myeloid leukemia occurred in five of the 1062 patients enrolled. All of the patients received the alkylating agent cyclophosphamide, and four received etoposide. The median time to development of acute myeloid leukemia was 39 months and median follow-up was 3.7 years (Heyn *et al.*, 1994). A large review of secondary malignancies in long-term survivors of childhood RMS was performed by Scaradavou *et al.* (1995), who reported on 130 patients with a median follow-up of 9 years. Seven patients (5.4%) developed secondary malignancies, including three with acute non-lymphoblastic leukemia and four with solid tumors. This study identified an increased risk of secondary neoplasms in patients receiving the chemotherapeutic agents carmustine and doxorubicin. They did not find radiotherapy to be a significant risk factor, in contrast to the findings from the Late Effect Study Group, which reported an increased incidence of secondary neoplasms within prior radiation fields.

Conclusion

The recent advances in understanding the biologic and genetic features of RMS, as well as the development and scheduling of new drugs, have improved the survival of these children. However, several challenges still remain. These include the refinement of risk-directed therapy based on the understanding of newly recognized, biologic, and clinical features. The use of newly developed hematopoietic growth factors will allow dose intensification, which may offer improvement in children with metastatic or recurrent disease. Finally, the recently recognized translocation-specific gene products (PAX3–FKHR and PAX-7–FKHR) in alveolar tumors may provide molecular targets for future therapies.

Other pelvic tumors

Transitional cell carcinomas

Bladder tumors rarely occur in the first two decades of life and are commonly of mesodermal origin. The largest series describe these tumors as low-grade tran-

sitional cell carcinoma and they seldom recur (Benson *et al.*, 1983; Beurton *et al.*, 1984; Madgar *et al.*, 1988; Paduano and Chiella, 1988; Khasidy *et al.*, 1990; Quillin and McAlister, 1991; Yanase *et al.*, 1991). Some of these tumors occur secondary to cyclophosphamide therapy (Samra *et al.*, 1985; Levine and Richie, 1989; Kenet *et al.*, 1995). The lesions are solitary in more than 90% of cases. Pathologic evaluation revealed 80% to be grade I tumors or papilloma, 20% grade I–II tumors and only 3% invasive through the lamina propria. Recurrence rates are low (2–5%); they are usually asymptomatic and can occur several years after the initial tumor (Paduano and Chiella, 1988; Scott *et al.*, 1989; Hoenig *et al.*, 1996).

Presenting symptoms include gross hematuria in 80% of the patients, irritative voiding symptoms or recurrent UTI in 15%, and microscopic hematuria in 5% of patients (Hoenig *et al.*, 1996).

The initial diagnosis can be made by ultrasound, which in some series was found to be 100% sensitive for identifying a bladder lesion. Intravenous pyelography and CT scans may not be able to detect small tumors. Cytologic examination is of limited value, as most of these tumors are low-grade transitional cell carcinoma (Hoenig *et al.*, 1996; Serrano-Durba *et al.*, 1999).

Cystoscopy allows definitive diagnosis, staging, and treatment of these tumors. Its role in surveillance remains ill defined, particularly because it requires general anesthesia and the risk of tumor recurrence is low. Sonography of the bladder is probably a reasonable method for periodic follow-up.

Nephrogenic adenoma of the bladder

This is a rare, benign lesion of the bladder, occurring as an epithelial response to infection or trauma. It presents as a papillary lesion resembling a low-grade, low-stage transitional cell carcinoma (Kay and Lattanzi, 1985). It most commonly occurs in adults but has also been reported in children, in whom the adenoma occurred following either surgery or localized inflammation. It is characterized histologically by the formation of tubular structures in the lamina propria resembling nephrogenic tubules (Oliva and Young, 1995). The clinical features include gross hematuria and bladder irritative symptoms secondary to inflammation. The treatment is endoscopic fulguration and long-term antimicrobial therapy (Kay and Lattanzi, 1985).

Leiomyosarcoma

Leiomyosarcomas are extremely rare in the pediatric age group (less than 2% of all soft-tissue sarcomas), and their diagnostic features and biologic behavior appear similar to those in adults. Tumor size and mitotic counts seem to be the most important features in assessing malignant potential, but absolute minimum criteria for malignancy are not well defined. Local excision usually provides adequate therapy (Weitzner, 1978; Laurenti et al., 1982; Lack, 1986; Goldschneider et al., 1990; Borzi and Frank, 1994).

Urachal adenocarcimnoma

This is a very rare tumor, accounting for only 0.17–0.34% of all bladder neoplasms. It usually occurs in adults but there have been several reported cases in children. This mucin-producing or colloid adenocarcinoma arises from the juxtavesical segment of the urachus and invades the bladder, resulting in hematuria and irritative symptoms. Surgical resection is the primary treatment. The prognosis is poor because its location predisposes to extensive local spread before detection and diagnosis (Sheldon et al., 1984; Rankin et al., 1993).

Adenocarcinoma of the exstrophied bladder

This tumor also occurs more frequently in adults than in children. It occurs in patients who have not had bladder reconstruction. The tumor rarely occurs in a reconstructed bladder (Jakobsen and Olesen, 1968; Kandzari et al., 1974; Allen, 1977; Eraklis and Folkman, 1978; Warren et al., 1980; Nielsen and Nielsen, 1983; Beynon et al., 1985; Witters and Baert-Van Damme, 1987; Krishnamsetty et al., 1988; Davillas et al., 1991).

Mesonephric adenocarcinoma of the vagina

This is a rare and highly malignant tumor that can arise at any age and approximately 30% of such tumors occur in children. Evidence that they originate from the mesonephric rests includes their tubular structure and their occurrence along the tract of the mesonephric duct or its remnants. The clinical, gross pathologic, and radiographic presentation of these vaginal mesonephric carcinomas may at times be indistinguishable from that of ERMS. The presenting symptoms are usually vaginal bleeding or discovery of a mass. Radiographic features are similar to RMS and include grape-like clusters of tumor nodules within the vagina. The treatment has been varied and includes radical surgery, radiotherapy, or both (Siegel et al., 1970).

Clear cell adenocarcinoma of the vagina or cervix

Maternal diethylstilbestrol (DES) prior to 18 weeks' gestation has been strongly implicated in the etiology of this tumor. The age of the DES-exposed patients has varied from 7 to 34 years, with the highest frequency from 14 to 22 years. The risk among the exposed is small and is in the order of 1 in 1000 (Senekjian et al., 1986; Melnick et al., 1987; Horwitz et al., 1988; Senekjian et al., 1989; Herbst and Anderson, 1990; Hanselaar et al., 1991; Hanselaar et al., 1997). The rarity of this tumor among exposed women suggests that DES is not a complete carcinogen and that some other factors are also involved in the pathogenesis of clear cell adenocarcinoma of the vagina and cervix (Melnick et al., 1987).

Cavernous hemangioma of the bladder

This hamartoma is a rare benign tumor of the bladder that usually presents with macroscopic hematuria. In about 30% of cases, the bladder tumor is associated with angiomatous lesions in other parts of the body. The diagnosis may be suspected on ultrasound examination, but it is generally made at cystoscopy. Biopsy and transurethral resection must be avoided because of the risks of hemorrhage. Laser treatment of hemangiomas has been reported and should be the initial management (Smith and Dixon, 1984). Should laser coagulation fail, partial cystectomy appears to be the most effective method of treatment (Legraverend et al., 1986).

References

Agarwal SK, Prowse OA, Merguerian PA (1997) Pediatric genitourinary tumors. *Curr Opin Oncol* **9**: 307–12.

Allen LE (1977) Adult exstrophy of the bladder with adenocarcinoma. *J Indiana State Med Assoc* **70**: 639–41.

Andrassy RJ, Hays DM, Raney RB et al. (1995) Conservative surgical management of vaginal and vulvar pediatric rhabdomyosarcoma: a report from the Intergroup Rhabdomyosarcoma Study III. *J Pediatr Surg* **30**: 1034–6; discussion 6–7.

Angell SK, Pruthi RS, Merguerian PA (1996) Pediatric genitourinary tumors. *Curr Opin Oncol* **8**: 240–6.

Ashraf MS, Brady J, Breatnach F *et al.* (1994) Ifosfamide nephrotoxicity in paediatric cancer patients. *Eur J Pediatr* **153**: 90–4.

Barr FG (1997) Molecular genetics and pathogenesis of rhabdomyosarcoma. *J Pediatr Hematol Oncol* **19**: 483–91.

Barr FG, Galili N, Holick J *et al.* (1993) Rearrangement of the PAX3 paired box gene in the paediatric solid tumour alveolar rhabdomyosarcoma. *Nat Genet* **3**: 113–17.

Barr FG, Nauta LE, Davis RJ *et al.* (1996) In vivo amplification of the PAX3–FKHR and PAX7–FKHR fusion genes in alveolar rhabdomyosarcoma. *Hum Mol Genet* **5**: 15–21.

Benson RC Jr., Tomera KM, Kelalis PP (1983) Transitional cell carcinoma of the bladder in children and adolescents. *J Urol* **130**: 54–5.

Bernasconi M, Remppis A, Fredericks WJ *et al.* (1996) Induction of apoptosis in rhabdomyosarcoma cells through down-regulation of PAX proteins. *Proc Natl Acad Sci USA* **93**: 13164–9.

Beurton D, Magnier M, Cukier J (1984) Bladder tumours in children. *Prog Clin Biol Res* 289–301.

Beynon J, Zwink R, Chow W, Sturdy DE (1985) The late presentation of adenocarcinoma in bladder exstrophy. *Br J Surg* **72**: 989.

Biegel JA, Meek RS, Parmiter AH *et al.* (1991) Chromosomal translocation t(1;13)(p36;q14) in a case of rhabdomyosarcoma. *Genes Chromosomes Cancer* **3**: 483–4.

Borzi PA, Frank JD (1994) Bladder leiomyosarcoma in a child: a 6 year follow-up. *Br J Urol* **73**: 219–20.

Chardin P, Yeramian P, Madaule P, Tavitian A (1985) N-ras gene activation in the RD human rhabdomyosarcoma cell line. *Int J Cancer* **35**: 647–52.

Coffin CM, Rulon J, Smith L *et al.* (1997) Pathologic features of rhabdomyosarcoma before and after treatment: a clinicopathologic and immunohistochemical analysis. *Mod Pathol* **10**: 1175–87.

Crist W, Gehan EA, Ragab AH *et al.* (1995) The Third Intergroup Rhabdomyosarcoma Study. *J Clin Oncol* **13**: 610–30.

Davillas N, Thanos A, Liakatas J, Davillas E (1991) Bladder exstrophy complicated by adenocarcinoma. *Br J Urol* **68**: 107.

Davis RJ, D'Cruz CM, Lovell MA *et al.* (1994) Fusion of PAX7 to FKHR by the variant t(1;13)(p36;q14) translocation in alveolar rhabdomyosarcoma. *Cancer Res* **54**: 2869–72.

Dias P, Kumar P, Marsden HB *et al.* (1990a) N-myc gene is amplified in alveolar rhabdomyosarcomas (RMS) but not in embryonal RMS. *Int J Cancer* **45**: 593–6.

Dias P, Kumar P, Marsden HB *et al.* (1990b) N- and c-myc oncogenes in childhood rhabdomyosarcoma (Letter). *J Natl Cancer Inst* **82**: 151.

Diller L, Sexsmith E, Gottlieb A *et al.* (1995) Germline p53 mutations are frequently detected in young children with rhabdomyosarcoma. *J Clin Invest* **95**: 1606–11.

Donaldson SS, Asmar L, Breneman J *et al.* (1995) Hyperfractionated radiation in children with rhabdomyosarcoma – results of an Intergroup Rhabdomyosarcoma Pilot Study. *Int J Radiat Oncol Biol Phys* **32**: 903–11.

Douglass EC, Valentine M, Etcubanas E *et al.* (1987) A specific chromosomal abnormality in rhabdomyosarcoma [published erratum appears in *Cytogenet Cell Genet* 1988; **47**: 232. *Cytogenet Cell Genet* **45**: 148–55.

Douglass EC, Rowe ST, Valentine M *et al.* (1991) Variant translocations of chromosome 13 in alveolar rhabdomyosarcoma. *Genes Chromosomes Cancer* **3**: 480–2.

Dworzak M, Stock C, Strehl S *et al.* (1992) Ewing's tumor X mouse hybrids expressing the MIC2 antigen: analyses using fluorescence CDD-banding and non-isotopic ISH. *Hum Genet* **88**: 273–8.

Edwards RH, Chatten J, Xiong QB, Barr FG (1997) Detection of gene fusions in rhabdomyosarcoma by reverse transcriptase-polymerase chain reaction assay of archival samples [published erratum appears in *Diagn Mol Pathol* 1997; **6**: 177]. *Diagn Mol Pathol* **6**: 91–7.

Eraklis AJ, Folkman MJ (1978) Adenocarcinoma at the site of ureterosigmoidostomies for exstrophy of the bladder. *J Pediatr Surg* **13**: 730–4.

Felix CA, Kappel CC, Mitsudomi T *et al.* (1992) Frequency and diversity of p53 mutations in childhood rhabdomyosarcoma. *Cancer Res* **52**: 2243–7.

Fichtner J, Hohenfellner R (1995) Damage to the urinary tract secondary to irradiation. *World J Urol* **13**: 240–2.

Fisch M, Burger R, Barthels U *et al.* (1995) Surgery in rhabdomyosarcoma of the bladder, prostate and vagina. *World J Urol* **13**: 213–18.

Forus A, Florenes VA, Maelandsmo GM *et al.* (1993) Mapping of amplification units in the q13–14 region of chromosome 12 in human sarcomas: some amplica do not include MDM2. *Cell Growth Differ* **4**: 1065–70.

Frascella E, Rosolen A (1998) Detection of the MyoD1 transcript in rhabdomyosarcoma cell lines and tumor samples by reverse transcription polymerase chain reaction. *Am J Pathol* **152**: 577–83.

Galili N, Davis RJ, Fredericks WJ *et al.* (1993) Fusion of a fork head domain gene to PAX3 in the solid tumour alveolar rhabdomyosarcoma [published erratum appears in *Nat Genet* 1994; **6**: 214]. *Nat Genet* **5**: 230–5.

Gattenloehner S, Vincent A, Leuschner I *et al.* (1998) The fetal form of the acetylcholine receptor distinguishes rhabdomyosarcomas from other childhood tumors. *Am J Pathol* **152**: 437–44.

Goldschneider KR, Forouhar FA, Altman AJ *et al.* (1990) Diagnostic pitfalls in the diagnosis of soft tissue bladder tumors in pediatric patients [published erratum appears in *Ann Clin Lab Sci* 1990; **20**: 300]. *Ann Clin Lab Sci* **20**: 22–7.

Goulding MD, Chalepakis G, Deutsch U *et al.* (1991) Pax-3, a novel murine DNA binding protein expressed during early neurogenesis. *Embo J* **10**: 1135–47.

Haddy TB, Nora AH, Sutow WW, Vietti TJ (1967) Cyclophosphamide treatment for metastatic soft tissue sarcoma. Intermittent large doses in the treatment of children. *Am J Dis Child* **114**: 301–8.

Hanselaar AG, Van Leusen ND, De Wilde PC, Vooijs GP (1991) Clear cell adenocarcinoma of the vagina and cervix. A report of the Central Netherlands Registry with emphasis on early detection and prognosis. *Cancer* **67**: 1971–8.

Hanselaar A, van Loosbroek M, Schuurbiers O *et al.* (1997) Clear cell adenocarcinoma of the vagina and cervix. An update of the central Netherlands registry showing twin age incidence peaks. *Cancer* **79**: 2229–36.

Hays DM (1993) Bladder/prostate rhabdomyosarcoma: results of the multi-institutional trials of the Intergroup Rhabdomyosarcoma Study. *Semin Surg Oncol* **9**: 520–3.

Hays DM, Raney RB Jr, Lawrence W Jr *et al.* (1982) Primary chemotherapy in the treatment of children with bladder – prostate tumors in the Intergroup Rhabdomyosarcoma Study (IRS-II). *J Pediatr Surg* **17**: 812–20.

Hays DM, Shimada H, Raney RB Jr *et al.* (1988) Clinical staging and treatment results in rhabdomyosarcoma of the female genital tract among children and adolescents. *Cancer* **61**: 1893–903.

Hays DM, Lawrence W Jr, Wharam M *et al.* (1989) Primary reexcision for patients with 'microscopic residual' tumor following initial excision of sarcomas of trunk and extremity sites. *J Pediatr Surg* **24**: 5–10.

Herbst AL, Anderson D (1990) Clear cell adenocarcinoma of the vagina and cervix secondary to intrauterine exposure to diethylstilbestrol. *Semin Surg Oncol* **6**: 343–6.

Heyn R, Raney RB Jr, Hays DM *et al.* (1992) Late effects of therapy in patients with paratesticular rhabdomyosarcoma. Intergroup Rhabdomyosarcoma Study Committee. *J Clin Oncol* **10**: 614–23.

Heyn R, Haeberlen V, Newton WA *et al.* (1993) Second malignant neoplasms in children treated for rhabdomyosarcoma. Intergroup Rhabdomyosarcoma Study Committee. *J Clin Oncol* **11**: 262–70.

Heyn R, Khan F, Ensign LG *et al.* (1994) Acute myeloid leukemia in patients treated for rhabdomyosarcoma with cyclophosphamide and low-dose etoposide on Intergroup Rhabdomyosarcoma Study III: an interim report. *Med Pediatr Oncol* **23**: 99–106.

Heyn R, Newton WA, Raney RB *et al.* (1997) Preservation of the bladder in patients with rhabdomyosarcoma. *J Clin Oncol* **15**: 69–75.

Hoenig DM, McRae S, Chen SC *et al.* (1996) Transitional cell carcinoma of the bladder in the pediatric patient. *J Urol* **156**: 203–5.

Horowitz ME, Etcubanas E, Christensen ML *et al.* (1988) Phase II testing of melphalan in children with newly diagnosed rhabdomyosarcoma: a model for anticancer drug development. *J Clin Oncol* **6**: 308–14.

Horwitz RI, Viscoli CM, Merino M *et al.* (1988) Clear cell adenocarcinoma of the vagina and cervix: incidence, undetected disease, and diethylstilbestrol. *J Clin Epidemiol* **41**: 593–7.

Houghton PJ, Cheshire PJ, Myers L *et al.* (1992) Evaluation of 9-dimethylaminomethyl-10-hydroxycamptothecin against xenografts derived from adult and childhood solid tumors. *Cancer Chemother Pharmacol* **31**: 229–39.

Jakobsen BE, Olesen S (1968) Bladder exstrophy complicated by adenocarcinoma. *Dan Med Bull* **15**: 253–6.

Julian JC, Merguerian PA, Shortliffe LM (1995) Pediatric genitourinary tumors. *Curr Opin Oncol* **7**: 265–74.

Kalebic T, Tsokos M, Helman LJ (1994) *In vivo* treatment with antibody against IGF-1 receptor suppresses growth of human rhabdomyosarcoma and down-regulates p34cdc2. *Cancer Res* **54**: 5531–4.

Kandzari SJ, Majid A, Orteza AM, Milam DF (1974) Exstrophy of urinary bladder complicated by adenocarcinoma. *Urology* **3**: 496–8.

Kawai A, Noguchi M, Beppu Y *et al.* (1994) Nuclear immunoreaction of p53 protein in soft tissue sarcomas. A possible prognostic factor. *Cancer* **73**: 2499–505.

Kay R, Lattanzi C (1985) Nephrogenic adenoma in children. *J Urol* **133**: 99–101.

Kenet G, Mandel M, Mor Y *et al.* (1995) Genetic predisposition and cyclophosphamide treatment in a girl with bladder carcinoma? *Med Pediatr Oncol* **24**: 269–70.

Khasidy LR, Khashu B, Mallett EC *et al.* (1990) Transitional cell carcinoma of bladder in children. *Urology* **35**: 142–4.

Khatib ZA, Matsushime H, Valentine M *et al.* (1993) Coamplification of the CDK4 gene with MDM2 and GLI in human sarcomas. *Cancer Res* **53**: 5535–41.

Kodet R, Newton WA Jr, Hamoudi AB *et al.* (1993) Childhood rhabdomyosarcoma with anaplastic (pleomorphic) features. A report of the Intergroup Rhabdomyosarcoma Study. *Am J Surg Pathol* **17**: 443–53.

Koi M, Johnson LA, Kalikin LM *et al.* (1993) Tumor cell growth arrest caused by subchromosomal transferable DNA fragments from chromosome 11. *Science* **260**: 361–4.

Koufos A, Hansen MF, Copeland NG *et al.* (1985) Loss of heterozygosity in three embryonal tumours suggests a common pathogenetic mechanism. *Nature* **316**: 330–4.

Krishnamsetty RM, Rao MK, Hines CR *et al.* (1988) Adenocarcinoma in exstrophy and defunctional ureterosigmoidostomy. *J Ky Med Assoc* **86**: 409–14.

Kusafuka T, Fukuzawa M, Oue T *et al.* (1997) Mutation analysis of p53 gene in childhood malignant solid tumors. *J Pediatr Surg* **32**: 1175–80.

Lack EE (1986) Leiomyosarcomas in childhood: a clinical and pathologic study of 10 cases. *Pediatr Pathol* **6**: 181–97.

Laurenti C, De Dominicis C, Dal Forno S, Bologna G (1982) Leiomyosarcoma of the bladder in a girl. *Eur Urol* **8**: 185–7.

Lawrence W Jr, Gehan EA, Hays DM *et al.* (1987a) Prognostic significance of staging factors of the UICC staging system in childhood rhabdomyosarcoma: a report from the Intergroup Rhabdomyosarcoma Study (IRS-II). *J Clin Oncol* **5**: 46–54.

Lawrence W Jr, Hays DM, Heyn R *et al.* (1987b) Lymphatic metastases with childhood rhabdomyosarcoma. A report from the Intergroup Rhabdomyosarcoma Study. *Cancer* **60**: 910–15.

Legraverend JM, Canarelli JP, Boudailliez B *et al.* (1986) Cavernous hemangioma of the bladder in children. Apropos of a case. *Ann Urol* **20**: 265–6.

Leuschner I, Newton WA Jr, Schmidt D *et al.* (1993) Spindle cell variants of embryonal rhabdomyosarcoma in the paratesticular region. A report of the Intergroup Rhabdomyosarcoma Study [published erratum appears in *Am J Surg Pathol* 1993; **17**: 858]. *Am J Surg Pathol* **17**: 221–30.

Levine LA, Richie JP (1989) Urological complications of cyclophosphamide. *J Urol* **141**: 1063–9.

Lobe TE, Wiener E, Andrassy RJ *et al.* (1996) The argument for conservative, delayed surgery in the management of prostatic rhabdomyosarcoma. *J Pediatr Surg* **31**: 1084–7.

Loh WE Jr, Scrable HJ, Livanos E *et al.* (1992) Human chromosome 11 contains two different growth suppressor genes for embryonal rhabdomyosarcoma. *Proc Natl Acad Sci USA* **89**: 1755–9.

Madgar I, Nativ O, Hanani Y, Jonas P (1988) Transitional cell carcinoma of the bladder in children under ten years of age. A case report. *Eur Urol* **14**: 216–17.

Matsuoka S, Thompson JS, Edwards MC *et al.* (1996) Imprinting of the gene encoding a human cyclin-dependent kinase inhibitor, p57KIP2, on chromosome 11p15. *Proc Natl Acad Sci USA* **93**: 3026–30.

Maurer HM, Beltangady M, Gehan EA *et al.* (1988) The Intergroup Rhabdomyosarcoma Study – I. A final report. *Cancer* **61**: 209–20.

Maurer HM, Gehan EA, Beltangady M *et al.* (1993) The Intergroup Rhabdomyosarcoma Study – II. *Cancer* **71**: 1904–22.

Meddeb M, Valent A, Danglot G *et al.* (1996) MDM2 amplification in a primary alveolar rhabdomyosarcoma displaying a t(2;13)(q35;q14). *Cytogenet Cell Genet* **73**: 325–30.

Melnick S, Cole P, Anderson D, Herbst A (1987) Rates and risks of diethylstilbestrol-related clear-cell adenocarcinoma of the vagina and cervix. An update. *N Engl J Med* **316**: 514–16.

Merguerian PA, Agarwal S, Greenberg M *et al.* (1998) Outcome analysis of rhabdomyosarcoma of the lower urinary tract. *J Urol* **160**: 1191–4; discussion 216.

Newton WA Jr, Gehan EA, Webber BL *et al.* (1995) Classification of rhabdomyosarcomas and related sarcomas. Pathologic aspects and proposal for a new classification – an Intergroup Rhabdomyosarcoma Study. *Cancer* **76**: 1073–85.

Nielsen K, Nielsen KK (1983) Adenocarcinoma in exstrophy of the bladder – the last case in Scandinavia? A case report and review of literature. *J Urol* **130**: 1180–2.

Oliva E, Young RH (1995) Nephrogenic adenoma of the urinary tract: a review of the microscopic appearance of 80 cases with emphasis on unusual features. *Mod Pathol* **8**: 722–30.

Paduano L, Chiella E (1988) Primary epithelial tumors of the bladder in children. *J Urol* **139**: 794–5.

Pappo AS, Crist WM, Kuttesch J *et al.* (1993a) Tumor-cell DNA content predicts outcome in children and adolescents with clinical group III embryonal rhabdomyosarcoma. The Intergroup Rhabdomyosarcoma Study Committee of the Children's Cancer Group and the Pediatric Oncology Group [published erratum appears in *J Clin Oncol* 1994; **12**: 440]. *J Clin Oncol* **11**: 1901–5.

Pappo AS, Etcubanas E, Santana VM *et al.* (1993b) A phase II trial of ifosfamide in previously untreated children and adolescents with unresectable rhabdomyosarcoma. *Cancer* **71**: 2119–25.

Pappo AS, Shapiro DN, Crist WM, Maurer HM (1995) Biology and therapy of pediatric rhabdomyosarcoma. *J Clin Oncol* **13**: 2123–39.

Pappo AS, Shapiro DN, Crist WM (1997) Rhabdomyosarcoma. Biology and treatment. *Pediatr Clin North Am* **44**: 953–72.

Parham DM (1994) The molecular biology of childhood rhabdomyosarcoma. *Semin Diagn Pathol* **11**: 39–46.

Pascasio J, Triche T, Sorensen P *et al.* (1998) Intergroup Rhabdomyosarcoma Study: P53 expression correlates with anaplasia in rhabdomyosarcoma. *Mod Pathol* **11**: 4p.

Pawel BR, Hamoudi AB, Asmar L *et al.* (1997) Undifferentiated sarcomas of children: pathology and clinical behavior – an Intergroup Rhabdomyosarcoma study. *Med Pediatr Oncol* **29**: 170–80.

Qualman SJ, Coffin CM, Newton WA *et al.* (1998) Current practice in pediatric pathology: Intergroup Rhabdomyosarcoma Study: update for pathologists. *Pediatr Devl Pathol* **1**: 550–61.

Quillin SP, McAlister WH (1991) Transitional cell carcinoma of the bladder in children: radiologic appearance and differential diagnosis. *Urol Radiol* **13**: 107–9.

Raney RB Jr, Crist W, Hays D *et al.* (1990a) Soft tissue sarcoma of the perineal region in childhood. A report from the Intergroup Rhabdomyosarcoma Studies I and II, 1972 through 1984. *Cancer* **65**: 2787–92.

Raney RB Jr, Gehan EA, Hays DM *et al.* (1990b) Primary chemotherapy with or without radiation therapy and/or surgery for children with localized sarcoma of the bladder, prostate, vagina, uterus, and cervix. A comparison of the results in Intergroup Rhabdomyosarcoma Studies I and II. *Cancer* **66**: 2072–81.

Raney B Jr, Heyn R, Hays DM *et al.* (1993) Sequelae of treatment in 109 patients followed for 5 to 15 years after diagnosis of sarcoma of the bladder and prostate. A report from the Intergroup Rhabdomyosarcoma Study Committee. *Cancer* **71**: 2387–94.

Rankin LF, Allen GD, Yuppa FR *et al.* (1993) Carcinoma of the urachus in an adolescent: a case report. *J Urol* **150**: 1472–3.

Rodary C, Gehan EA, Flamant F *et al.* (1991) Prognostic factors in 951 nonmetastatic rhabdomyosarcoma in children: a report from the International Rhabdomyosarcoma Workshop. *Med Pediatr Oncol* **19**: 89–95.

Sabbioni S, Barbanti-Brodano G, Croce CM, Negrini M (1997) GOK: a gene at 11p15 involved in rhabdomyosarcoma and rhabdoid tumor development. *Cancer Res* **57**: 4493–7.

Samra Y, Hertz M, Lindner A (1985) Urinary bladder tumors following cyclophosphamide therapy: a report of two cases with a review of the literature. *Med Pediatr Oncol* **13**: 86–91.

Sawyer JR, Crussi FG, Kletzel M (1994) Pericentric inversion (2)(p15q35) in an alveolar rhabdomyosarcoma. *Cancer Genet Cytogenet* **78**: 214–18.

Scaradavou A, Heller G, Sklar CA *et al.* (1995) Second malignant neoplasms in long-term survivors of childhood rhabdomyosarcoma. *Cancer* **76**: 1860–7.

Scheidler S, Fredericks WJ, Rauscher FJ III *et al.* (1996) The hybrid PAX3–FKHR fusion protein of alveolar rhabdomyosarcoma transforms fibroblasts in culture. *Proc Natl Acad Sci USA* **93**: 9805–9.

Schurch W, Bochaton-Piallat ML, Geinoz A *et al.* (1994) All histological types of primary human rhabdomyosarcoma express alpha-cardiac and not alpha-skeletal actin messenger RNA. *Am J Pathol* **144**: 836–46.

Scott AA, Stanley W, Worsham GF *et al.* (1989) Aggressive bladder carcinoma in an adolescent. Report of a case with immunohistochemical, cytogenetic, and flow cytometric characterization. *Am J Surg Pathol* **13**: 1057–63.

Scrable H, Cavenee W, Ghavimi F *et al.* (1989a) A model for embryonal rhabdomyosarcoma tumorigenesis that involves genome imprinting. *Proc Natl Acad Sci USA* **86**: 7480–4.

Scrable H, Witte D, Shimada H *et al.* (1989b) Molecular differential pathology of rhabdomyosarcoma. *Genes Chromosomes Cancer* **1**: 23–35.

Scrable HJ, Witte DP, Lampkin BC, Cavenee WK (1987) Chromosomal localization of the human rhabdomyosarcoma locus by mitotic recombination mapping. *Nature* **329**: 645–7.

Senekjian EK, Hubby M, Bell DA *et al.* (1986) Clear cell adenocarcinoma (CCA) of the vagina and cervix in association with pregnancy. *Gynecol Oncol* **24**: 207–19.

Senekjian EK, Frey K, Herbst AL (1989) Pelvic exenteration in clear cell adenocarcinoma of the vagina and cervix. *Gynecol Oncol* **34**: 413–16.

Serrano-Durba A, Dominguez-Hinarejos C, Reig-Ruiz C *et al.* (1999) Transitional cell carcinoma of the bladder in children. *Scand J Urol Nephrol* **33**: 73–6.

Shapiro DN, Parham DM, Douglass EC *et al.* (1991) Relationship of tumor-cell ploidy to histologic subtype and treatment outcome in children and adolescents with unresectable rhabdomyosarcoma [published erratum appears in *J Clin Oncol* 1991; **9**: 893]. *J Clin Oncol* **9**: 159–66.

Shapiro E, Strother D (1992a) Genitourinary rhabdomyosarcoma in childhood: current treatment alternatives and controversies in management. *Cancer Treat Res* **59**: 1–17.

Shapiro E, Strother D (1992b) Pediatric genitourinary rhabdomyosarcoma. *J Urol* **148**: 1761–8.

Shapiro DN, Sublett JE, Li B *et al.* (1993a) Fusion of PAX3 to a member of the forkhead family of transcription factors in human alveolar rhabdomyosarcoma. *Cancer Res* **53**: 5108–12.

Shapiro DN, Sublett JE, Li B *et al.* (1993b) The gene for PAX7, a member of the paired-box-containing genes, is localized on human chromosome arm 1p36. *Genomics* **17**: 767–9.

Sheldon CA, Clayman RV, Gonzalez R *et al.* (1984) Malignant urachal lesions. *J Urol* **131**: 1–8.

Siegel HA, Sagerman R, Berdon WE, Wigger HJ (1970) Mesonephric adenocarcinoma of the vagina in a 7-month-old infant simulating sarcoma botryoides. Successful control with supervoltage radiotherapy. *J Pediatr Surg* **5**: 468–70.

Smith JA, Dixon JA (1984) Neodymium-YAG laser irradiation of bladder hemangioma. *Urology* **24**: 134–6.

Stratton MR, Fisher C, Gusterson BA, Cooper CS (1989) Detection of point mutations in N-ras and K-ras genes of human embryonal rhabdomyosarcomas using oligonucleotide probes and the polymerase chain reaction. *Cancer Res* **49**: 6324–7.

Tan C, Dargeon H, Burchenal J (1959) Effect of actinomycin D in childhood cancer. *Pediatrics* **24**: 544–61.

Triche TJ (1995) Molecular biological aspects of soft tissue tumors. *Curr Top Pathol* **89**: 47–72.

Tsokos M (1994) The diagnosis and classification of childhood rhabdomyosarcoma. *Semin Diagn Pathol* **11**: 26–38.

Turc-Carel C, Lizard-Nacol S, Justrabo E *et al.* (1986) Consistent chromosomal translocation in alveolar rhabdomyosarcoma. *Cancer Genet Cytogenet* **19**: 361–2.

Tycko B (1994) Genomic imprinting: mechanism and role in human pathology. *Am J Pathol* **144**: 431–43.

Visser M, Bras J, Sijmons C *et al.* (1996) Microsatellite instability in childhood rhabdomyosarcoma is locus specific and correlates with fractional allelic loss. *Proc Natl Acad Sci USA* **93**: 9172–6.

Walther C, Guenet JL, Simon D *et al.* (1991) Pax: a murine multigene family of paired box-containing genes. *Genomics* **11**: 424–34.

Warren RB, Warner TF, Hafez GR (1980) Late development of colonic adenocarcinoma 49 years after ureterosigmoidostomy for exstrophy of the bladder. *J Urol* **124**: 550–1.

Weber-Hall S, Anderson J, McManus A *et al.* (1996) Gains, losses, and amplification of genomic material in rhabdomyosarcoma analyzed by comparative genomic hybridization. *Cancer Res* **56**: 3220–4.

Weitzner S (1978) Leiomyosarcoma of urinary bladder in children. *Urology* **12**: 450–2.

Wexler LH, Helman LJ (1994) Pediatric soft tissue sarcomas. *CA Cancer J Clin* **44**: 211–47.

Whang-Peng J, Triche TJ, Knutsen T *et al.* (1986) Cytogenetic characterization of selected small round cell tumors of childhood. *Cancer Genet Cytogenet* **21**: 185–208.

Wilke W, Maillet M, Robinson R (1993) H-ras-1 point mutations in soft tissue sarcomas. *Mod Pathol* **6**: 129–32.

Witters S, Baert-Van Damme L (1987) Bladder exstrophy complicated by adenocarcinoma. *Eur Urol* **13**: 415–16.

Wurl P, Taubert H, Bache M *et al.* (1996) Frequent occurrence of p53 mutations in rhabdomyosarcoma and leiomyosarcoma, but not in fibrosarcoma and malignant neural tumors. *Int J Cancer* **69**: 317–23.

Yanase M, Tsukamoto T, Kumamoto Y *et al.* (1991) Transitional cell carcinoma of the bladder or renal pelvis in children. *Eur Urol* **19**: 312–14.

Yeung CK, Ward HC, Ransley PG *et al.* (1994) Bladder and kidney function after cure of pelvic rhabdomyosarcoma in childhood. *Br J Cancer* **70**: 1000–3.

Testis tumors in children

42

Robert Kay

Introduction

Testicular tumors in infants and prepubertal children are very uncommon. An understanding of the biologic behavior and the treatment of these rare tumors has been confused in the past as a result of attempts at extrapolating the adult experience to infants and children. Like most diseases in pediatric urology, testicular tumors have distinct differences in the natural history and disease processes in children when compared with those of adults. Because prepubertal testis tumors are uncommon, only small series have been reported, making valid conclusions difficult to reach. In an attempt to develop a large database, the national Prepubertal Testicular Tumor Registry was established in 1980 by the Section on Urology of the American Academy of Pediatrics (Kay, 1993a). This registry continues at the time of writing and is helping to elucidate the natural history, risk factors, and optimal treatment for these rare tumors.

Nomenclature and classification

A classification system for adult testicular tumors has been based on the histologic appearance of the tumors. The establishment of this system is important because, when combined with clinical and pathologic states, clinical treatment protocols have been developed. Many different classification systems have been used for adults, including the one developed by the World Health Organization, which formalized the system and recognized the different cells of the testis. This classification functionally divided testis tumors into germ-cell and non-germ-cell tumors. Because certain carcinomas are never seen in children and the most common pediatric tumor, yolk sac tumor, is rarely seen in adults, the adult classification scheme is not entirely accurate for infants and children. Therefore, Kaplan (1984), when working initially with the Prepubertal Testicular Tumor Registry, proposed a classification of prepubertal testicular tumors. This has continued to serve as the best classification for prepubertal testicular tumors (Table 42.1).

Table 42.1 Classification of prepubertal testicular tumors

Group	Tumor type
I	Germ-cell tumors
	(a) Yolk sac
	(b) Teratoma
	(c) Teratocarcinoma
	(d) Seminoma
II	Gonadal stromal tumors
	(a) Leydig cell
	(b) Sertoli cell
	(c) Granulosa cell
	(d) Mixed
III	Gonadoblastoma
IV	Tumors of supporting tissues
	(a) Fibroma
	(b) Leiomyoma
	(c) Hemangioma
V	Lymphomas and leukemias
VI	Tumor-like lesions
	(a) Epidermoid cyst
	(b) Hyperplastic nodule secondary to congenital adrenal hyperplasia
VII	Secondary tumors
VIII	Tumors of adenexa

Table 42.2 Pathology categories for the prepubertal testicular tumor registry

Pathology	n	%
Yolk sac	243	55
Teratoma	90	21
Gonadal stromal	19	4
Sertoli cell	10	2
Leydig cell	4	1
Juvenile granulosa cell	9	2
Epidermoid cyst	13	3
Other	51	12

Incidence

Testicular tumors in childhood are exceedingly uncommon and occur with an incidence of 0.5–2.0 per 100 000 children. They rank seventh in frequency among tumors in children and account for only 1–2% of all pediatric tumors (Coppes *et al.*, 1994). Between 1980 and 1997, the Prepubertal Testicular Tumor Registry collected information on 439 tumors (Table 42.2). The registry, however, is not complete for paratesticular tumors, because the focus of the registry has been on true testicular tumors. True primary intratesticular tumors occurred in 398 patients. In this group, there were 333 germ-cell tumors (84%) and 65 non-germ-cell tumors (16%). Yolk sac tumors represented 243 (61%) of the primary testis tumors and accounted for 55% of all tumors registered.

Diagnosis

In general, a prepubertal testis tumor presents as a painless scrotal mass noticed by the parents or the physician. This may occur at any time from the newborn period throughout childhood. The mass is firm and does not transilluminate. Many of the testes may be associated with a reactive hydrocele (Fig. 42.1). In the past, the misdiagnosis of a hydrocele resulted in a 5 or 6 month delay in treatment from the time of onset of symptoms (Brosman, 1979). This is less common today with improved diagnostic acumen and scrotal sonography. A scrotal sonogram is very beneficial in detecting the characteristics of the mass, as well as examining the contralateral testis. In addition, sonography can examine the retroperitoneum to rule out metastatic disease.

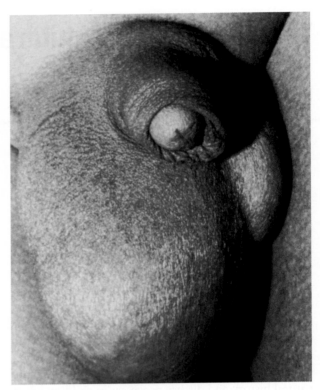

Figure 42.1 The patient is a 5-year-old prepubertal boy with a large, painless, firm scrotal mass. The testis was replaced by a leukemic infiltrate.

Alpha-1-fetoprotein (AFP) is a sensitive tumor marker for prepubertal testicular tumors, specifically yolk sac tumor. Bergstrand and Czar (1956) first described AFP in 1956 as a serum fetal protein. This protein was subsequently found to have a half-life of 5 days and is believed to represent an immature homolog of albumin (Lange *et al.*, 1982). Like other fetal proteins, such as hemoglobin F, AFP gradually disappears during development. AFP is made by the yolk sac cells and the embryo. Most yolk sac tumors have an elevation of AFP and, in general, the levels may be extremely high. It is critical, however, that the treating physician recognize that newborn infants up to the age of 6 months have elevated AFP levels (Brewer and Tanlc, 1993). Persistence of AFP after removal of a tumor in children younger than 6 months should not be mistaken for persistent disease. It is essential that physicians appreciate the expected degradation of AFP and recognize that the elevation may be the natural history of the AFP in the normal child. In addition, it has been estimated that as many as 10% of boys with yolk sac tumors do not have elevated serum AFP values (Uehling and Phillips, 1994).

The β subunit of human chorionic gonadotropin (β-hCG) is another tumor marker commonly used in adults and is produced by the syncytiotrophoblast. This level is rarely elevated in yolk sac tumors in children. Because of these excellent markers, however, preoperative AFP and β-hCG levels should always be obtained whenever a solid mass is suspected. Results need not delay surgery but will serve as a baseline for future follow-up.

Certain functional testicular tumors such as Leydig cell tumors may lead to sexual precocity or gynecomastia. Increased levels of androgen, arising from the gonadal tumor cells, create the clinical condition seen. These patients should also have baseline studies, but the presence of a mass suggests malignancy and should mandate surgery.

In general, all testicular masses should be explored for a definitive diagnosis. An inguinal incision is used to avoid contamination of the scrotum and its lymphatic drainage. The cord should be clamped with an atraumatic clamp and the scrotal contents and the intact tunica vaginalis delivered to the wound (Kay and Ross, 1998). If the sonographic finding, gross appearance and palpation do not indicate a malignant process, a biopsy or enucleation may be performed for frozen section histologic confirmation. When a malignancy is confirmed, a radical orchiectomy is performed. Postoperatively, clinical staging and management vary by tumor and are specified under the discussion of each individual tumor.

Yolk sac tumor

The most common malignant germ-cell tumor of the testis in the prepubertal male is the yolk sac tumor. Initially described by White (1910), many synonyms and eponyms have been used in the literature to describe this tumor. It is well accepted today that yolk sac tumor has become the preferred nomenclature. This tumor should not be confused with embryonal cell carcinoma of the postpubertal male, which differs both histologically and clinically.

Grossly, yolk sac tumors vary in size. They are soft tumors with rare hemorrhage and necrosis. They vary in color from pink to yellow. Microscopically, yolk sac tumors have certain characteristics that distinguish them from all other germ-cell tumors. They are composed of epithelial and mesenchymal elements. The distinctive feature is the perivascular Schiller–Duval body. This is an arrangement of cells

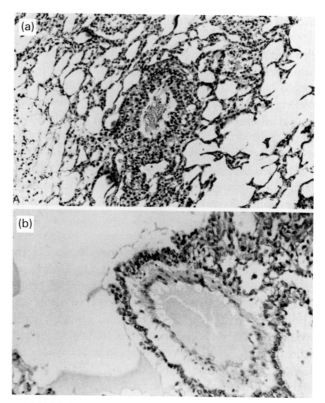

Figure 42.2 (*a*) Photomicrograph of yolk sac carcinoma demonstrating loose vacuolated network and honeycomb pattern. (*b*) Photomicrograph of perivascular Schiller–Duval body.

that form glomerulus-like structures containing AFP. These bodies are pathognomic for yolk sac tumors (Fig. 42.2).

Clinical course and treatment

Yolk sac tumors usually occur in children before 2 years of age, presenting as a scrotal mass. It is important, however, to recognize that they may occur at any age, including postpubertal adults. Evidence suggests that the prognosis is improved when children present before the age of 1 year compared with older children, particularly older than 2 years of age (Kay, 1993a). The presenting level of AFP has not been shown to be a prognostic sign, since many children present with levels as high as 20 000–30 000 units. It is of great concern, however, if the AFP levels do not return to the normal range after orchiectomy. If AFP levels do not normalize as expected, when calculated with a half-life of 5 days, metastatic disease must be suspected and further diagnosis and treatment carried out.

The management of yolk sac tumor in children has become clearer since the late 1970s. Metastatic disease and death are uncommon in children with yolk sac tumor. Metastases can occur and most commonly are spread equally via hematogenous routes to the lungs and via the lymphatic system (Grady *et al.*, 1994). It is important to recognize that this is different than the adult embryonal cell tumor, which characteristically spreads first through the lymphatic system.

The treatment of yolk sac tumor begins with a radical orchiectomy. In most patients, particularly those under 2 years of age, an orchiectomy with close postoperative surveillance and monitoring of AFP levels, chest X-ray, and a computed tomographic (CT) scan of the abdomen provide sufficient diagnostic and therapeutic treatment. The previous controversy regarding lymph node dissection, however, has been clarified over the years. Grady *et al.* (1994) reported that the number of children who would benefit from a retroperitoneal node dissection is quite limited. Furthermore, a retroperitoneal node dissection has definite complications. Intraoperative injury and late ejaculatory dysfunction may be seen in both adults and children; additionally, the incidence of bowel obstruction secondary to adhesions is higher in small children than in adults. These complications, coupled with the metastatic preference of a hematogenous spread versus a lymphatic spread, suggest that the risk of retroperitoneal lymph-node dissection outweighs the benefit. AFP serves as an excellent tumor marker, particularly when it returns to normal after initial high levels. This marker, coupled with excellent imaging techniques, allows the child to be carefully observed and accurately surveyed. Retroperitoneal lymph-node dissection in this setting, therefore, has an extremely limited role and should be reserved for persistent masses after chemotherapy. Even when present, residual masses may be comprised of only necrotic and calcified tumor (Uehling and Phillips, 1994; Terai *et al.*, 1995). Retroperitoneal lymph node dissection should definitely **not** be carried out in children with clinical stage I tumors in whom postorchiectomy AFP levels have returned to normal.

Yolk sac tumors demand close follow-up and surveillance. This includes monthly measurement of AFP levels for a minimum of 1 year. After the first year, AFP levels are obtained every 2 or 3 months. A chest X-ray should be obtained every 3 months for the first year, with alternating sonograms and CT scans to assess the retroperitoneum. These children should be followed closely for a minimum of 2 years. The Prepubertal Testicular Tumor Registry has demonstrated that no metastatic disease occurred after 14 months of follow-up (Kay, 1993b).

Chemotherapy must be used in advanced stages of yolk sac carcinoma. Despite clinical protocols from the Pediatric Oncology Group and the Children's Cancer Study Group (CCSG), meaningful information has not been obtained since metastatic disease is quite uncommon. However, the efficacy of cisplatin-

Table 42.4 POG/CCSG staging of testicular tumors

Stage	Extent of disease
I	Limited to testes
	Completely resected by high inguinal orchiectomy or transscrotal orchiectomy with no spill
	No clinical, radiographic, or histologic evidence of disease beyond the testes
	Tumor markers normal after appropriate postsurgical half-life decline; patients with normal or unknown markers at diagnosis must have a negative ipsilateral retroperitoneal node dissection to confirm stage I*
II	Transscrotal orchiectomy with gross spill of tumor
	Microscopic disease in scrotum or high in spermatic cord
	($\leq$ 5 cm from proximal end)
	Retroperitoneal lymph-node involvement ($\leq$ 2 cm)
	Increased tumor markers after appropriate half-life
III	Retroperitoneal lymph-node involvement (> 2 cm)
	No visceral or extra-abdominal involvement
IV	Distant metastases, including liver

CCSG = Children's Cancer Study Group; POG = Pediatric Oncology Group.
*Not recommended by this author.

based drugs, as in adults, has been demonstrated in children and may be considered for use in stages II, III, and IV for yolk sac carcinoma (Table 42.4). Current treatment, as recommended by the CCSG, consists of cisplatin-based chemotherapy combined with etoposide and bleomycin. At this time, treatment of advanced yolk sac tumor continues to be studied and is best treated in a national clinical protocol to gain better understanding of this rare condition.

Teratoma

Teratoma of the testis is the second most common prepubertal testis tumor in children (Grady *et al.*, 1997). Of the 333 germ-cell tumors in the registry, 90 (27%) are classified as teratomas. Teratoma has a mean age of presentation of 18 months but may be seen in the neonatal period.

Pathologically, these tumors consist of tissues representing the different germinal layers of endoderm, mesoderm, and ectoderm. They usually contain cysts and therefore may be diagnosed preoperatively by ultrasound. The optimal treatment of teratoma is surgery. Orchiectomy is curative because no metastases of teratoma in prepubertal children have ever been reported. Because these tumors are encapsulated, enucleation is both technically and clinically feasible and should be considered the treatment of choice (Fig. 42.3a, b) (Rushton and Belman, 1993). Although Manivel *et al.* (1989) demonstrated that

intratubular germ-cell neoplasia may coexist with teratomas in adults, this has not been proven in children (Rushton *et al.*, 1990). It is wise, however, to examine the normal portions of the testis attached to the specimen to ensure that no carcinoma *in situ* or coexisting pathology is present. Peripubertal and postpubertal adolescents, however, should be viewed as adults in whom teratomas may have a propensity for metastases and must be treated accordingly.

Seminoma

A germ-cell tumor seen in adults but rarely occurring in prepubertal boys is seminoma. Because seminoma is related to spermatogenesis, it has been questioned whether seminoma could truly exist in prepubertal boys. However, it has been histologically confirmed and well documented in four prepubertal children as young as 2.5 years (Navrou, 1967; Viprakasit *et al.*, 1977; Perry and Servadio, 1980; Grechi *et al.*, 1980). Most other reports of seminoma in children and adolescents did not describe the age or the presence of puberty. Postpubertal adolescents with testicular masses should be evaluated and treated as adults and therefore should not be confused with the prepubertal child. The rarity of seminoma in prepubertal children does not allow any definitive statements about treatment and therefore should default to the same therapy used in adults, with radical orchiectomy, proper staging, and radiation therapy or chemotherapy for advanced stages.

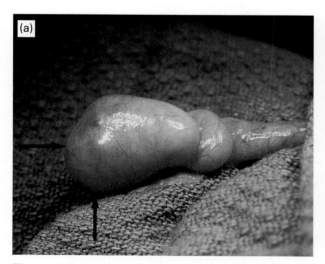 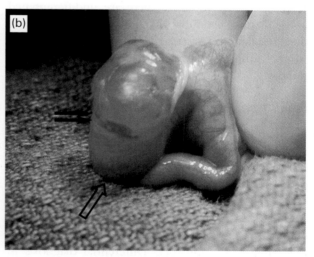

Figure 42.3 Teratoma in a 3-year-old boy: (*a*) Mass at lower pole of testis (*arrows*). (*b*) Cystic mass evident after tunica albuginea has been opened (*double arrows*). Normal remaining testicular tissue (*open arrows*). Tumor was enucleated.

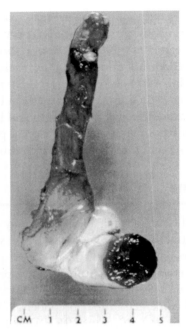

Figure 42.4 Gross pathologic specimen following radical orchiectomy for testicular tumor in a prepubertal male demonstrating a spherical, round mass; subsequently the mass proved histologically to be a Leydig cell tumor.

Gonadal stromal tumors

The most common non-germ-cell testicular tumors in children are tumors that arise from the stroma and are collectively referred to as gonadal stromal tumors. These include tumors arising from Leydig cells or Sertoli cells. In addition, there are undifferentiated gonadal stromal tumors that cannot be classified. In the Prepubertal Testicular Tumor Registry, gonadal stromal tumors represent about 9% of testicular tumors.

Leydig cell tumors

Leydig cell tumors or interstitial cell tumors are fascinating tumors in children because of their functional capability. They produce high levels of androgen and patients usually present with precocious puberty (Fig. 42.4). These children usually present between the ages of 5 and 10 years, and signs of virilization including pubic hair, increased penile size, and acne clinically suggest the disorder. Differential diagnosis in this clinical setting must include all causes of precocious puberty, including congenital adrenal hyperpla-

sia (CAH), adrenocortical carcinoma, and isosexual precocious puberty. In addition, children who have known congenital adrenal hyperplasia and testicular tumors need to be considered as showing a testicular tumor of the adrenogenital syndrome, which is discussed later in this chapter. In most cases, however, the presence of a scrotal mass with precocious puberty suggests Leydig cell tumor, the presence of which should be confirmed by ultrasound and subsequently by surgical removal.

Preoperatively, children with Leydig cell tumors should be evaluated with an endocrinologic evaluation including serum testosterone levels, follicle-stimulating hormone (FSH) levels, luteinizing hormone (LH) levels, and bone age. A sonogram of the scrotum should be obtained. If a mass is confirmed in the presence of an elevated serum testosterone, as well as low or normal FSH and LH levels, the presumed diagnosis is a Leydig cell tumor.

No metastases have been reported in children with Leydig cell tumors, and orchiectomy is curative treatment for this disease. Because these tumors are encapsulated and benign in children, some authors have suggested enucleation (Urban *et al.*, 1978).

Sertoli cell tumors

Sertoli cell tumors represent the next most common gonadal stromal tumors that can be well defined. These tumors are generally benign. However, metastatic disease has been described in at least four prepubescent boys (Kolon and Hochman, 1997). In general, orchiectomy is curative.

Sertoli cell tumors also have unusual variations. They may be associated with certain disorders, such as Peutz–Jeghers syndrome, and may produce hormonal abnormalities leading to feminization (Young *et al.*, 1995; Hertl *et al.*, 1998). Children with Peutz–Jeghers syndrome may also develop bilateral tumors, usually with the unique histologic finding of a large-cell, calcifying Sertoli tumor (Niewenhuis *et al.*, 1994; Dreyer *et al.*, 1994; Dudiak *et al.*, 1994; White *et al.*, 1997; Chang *et al.*, 1998). This unusual variant must be noted because of its association with other abnormalities (Noszian *et al.*, 1995). Carney *et al.* (1985) first described these unusual syndromes, associated with cardiac myxomas and endocrine hyperactivity. Carney's complex describes patients who have an autosomal dominant condition with macular pigmented mucocutaneous changes similar in nature and location to those seen with Peutz–Jeghers syndrome. These tumors are often multicentric and bilateral and usually affect the very young child. It is important for the pediatric urologist to recognize these syndromes, so that other pathology may be located and accurate counseling given.

Other gonadal stromal tumors may not be classified histologically. Some patients in the Prepubertal Testicular Tumor Registry had malignant undifferentiated gonadal stromal tumors, including one child who died despite multimodal therapy (Rosvoll and Woodard, 1968). In general, gonadal stromal tumors are benign but unusual variances may be observed and must be managed carefully.

Juvenile granulosa cell tumor

Juvenile granulosa cell tumor of the testis is very rare but usually occurs in the infant (Uehling *et al.*, 1987). Crump (1983) first described this tumor, in a 30-week-old fetus. The majority of cases described have been found in newborns, with all the remaining cases (except one) diagnosed in the first year of life. Several of these cases have been described in patients with abnormal external genitalia and karyotypic abnormalities (Young *et al.*, 1985).

Juvenile granulosa cell tumor presents as an asymptomatic mass without any endocrine manifestations and normal tumor markers. Differential diagnosis of a testicular lesion in the newborn should include cystic testicular dysplasia, teratoma, epidermoid cyst, cystic lymphangioma, testicular torsion, yolk sac tumor, and neuroblastoma. Levy *et al.* (1994) reviewed neonatal testis tumors and of 22 tumors found, six were yolk sac tumor, six were gonadal stromal tumors, and six were classified as juvenile granulosa cell tumors. Orchiectomy is curative and no further treatment is necessary (Chan *et al.*, 1997).

Gonadoblastoma

Gonadoblastoma is a rare tumor in children that occurs in intersex patients with abnormal gonads (Scully, 1970). This tumor is found most commonly in either phenotypic females or children with ambiguous genitalia who have genetic karyotypes with a Y chromosome. Eighty per cent of these children are phenotypic females with intra-abdominal testes, similar to that seen in the testicular feminization (complete androgen insensitivity) syndrome. The remaining patients with gonadoblastoma have other diseases of intersexuality. In most cases the gonads are either streak or cryptorchid.

Gonadoblastoma is a neoplasm containing a mixture of germ cells and stromal cells. The tumor may be

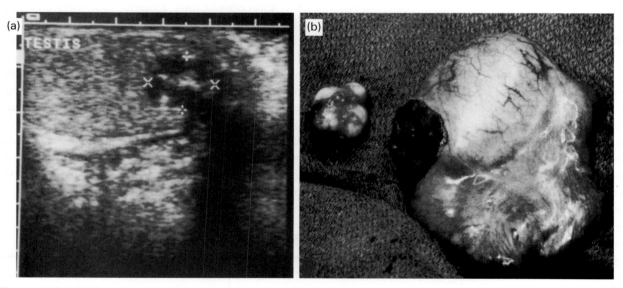

Figure 42.5 (*a*) Ultrasonogram demonstrates a complex mass in the lower pole of the right testis. (*b*) Gross specimen of a mass following enucleation of the lobulated encapsulated mass subsequently proved to be an epidermoid inclusion cyst.

bilateral. It occurs more commonly after puberty but may rarely be seen in the prepubertal child. Gonadoblastoma is usually benign and orchiectomy is curative treatment. In cases in which germ cells become malignant, the tumor resembles a dysgerminoma, which is similar to a seminoma in an adult male.

Epidermoid cysts

Epidermoid cysts are rare, benign tumors in prepubertal children (Gilbaugh et al., 1967; Price, 1969). Because they are intratesticular, it may be difficult to make the correct preoperative diagnosis and completely distinguish this tumor from a teratoma. However, ultrasonography may demonstrate a complex heterogeneous mass, which should suggest the possibility of an epidermoid cyst (Fig. 42.5). Histologically these tumors consist of squamous-lined cysts with keratinized debris. They are distinct from teratomas in that epidermoid cysts do not have all layers of the germinal epithelium. They are benign and cured by orchiectomy or enucleation (Ross et al., 1993). If enucleation is performed, histologic examination of the normal attached tubules is done to rule out carcinoma *in situ* in other locations, as indicated by Manivel et al. (1989). It should be noted that carcinoma *in situ* has not been seen concomitantly in these tumors in prepubertal children but has been associated with the disease in postpubertal males.

Tumors of the adrenogenital syndrome

An unusual clinical setting of testicular masses occurring in patients with CAH has been described (Rutgers et al., 1988; Srikanth et al., 1992; Oberman et al., 1993). Rutgers et al. (1988) initially reviewed the literature and identified 40 patients with adrenogenital syndrome and testicular lesions. Most patients were adults but in the pediatric patients it was discovered, either at autopsy or on testicular biopsy, that most of the masses were bilateral, consisting of nodules composed of Leydig cell hyperplasia. These tumors must be distinguished from Leydig cell tumors that are neoplastic. In hyperplastic nodules, growth is seen when stimulating hormonal levels are elevated and not controlled.

New, conservative treatments for these patients have been described. Surgical enucleation can be performed successfully, preserving most of the testes (Walker et al., 1997). Conversely, medical treatment has also been shown to be effective, obviating the need for surgery (Rich et al., 1998). Corticosteroid therapy has led to a decrease in the size of the tumors in many of the patients. If the tumor has not decreased in size but is not growing, these patients may be followed and no surgery is indicated. It is important that testicular tumors of the adrenogenital syndrome be recognized and distinguished from Leydig cell tumors so that unnecessary orchiectomies do not take place.

Secondary tumors of the testes

Secondary tumors in the prepubertal testes are most commonly seen in patients with lymphoma and leukemia. Four per cent of patients with lymphoma and 11–25% of patients with leukemia have testicular involvement (Oakhill et al., 1980; Klein et al., 1984). Leukemic infiltrates occur in the prepubertal testes both during and after therapy. Wilms' tumor and neuroblastoma have also been reported to metastasize to the testis.

The testes represent an interesting location for leukemia because they appear to be a sanctuary for tumor cells. It has been postulated that the blood–testes barrier, like the blood–brain barrier, prevents chemotherapy from reaching the testes. Therefore, the testes should have a higher rate of involvement than other organs, and there is some evidence to confirm this phenomenon. In a series by Oakhill et al. (1980), 60% of patients with acute lymphoblastic leukemia who developed testicular leukemia had no other evidence of tumor. When patients with leukemia develop testicular masses, either during therapy or after therapy, a biopsy is performed for confirmation. The patients are then treated with gonadal radiation and intensive chemotherapy, with consideration given to alternative treatment such as bone marrow transplantation.

Testicular microlithiasis

Testicular microlithiasis is a rare condition that may be associated with an increased prevalence of testicular tumors. It has been reported to be as common as 1 in every 600 boys but increases to 1 in 15 for boys with cryptorchidism (McEnitt *et al.*, 1995). Men with the condition are often infertile or subfertile. Although the etiology of microlithiasis is unclear, it has been shown to be associated with carcinoma *in situ*, as well as other tumors including seminoma and embryonal cell tumors, and in children with teratomas and yolk sac tumor (Horwitz and Abiri, 1997). Testicular microlithiasis has recently been reported in association with yolk sac tumor in a child who was discovered on routine follow-up for his testicular microlithiasis (McEnitt *et al.*, 1995). Follow-up of boys identified with microlithiasis is probably important but how often and by what means has not been established.

Paratesticular rhabdomyosarcoma

Paratesticular rhabdomyosarcoma must be considered in any child with a scrotal mass. It represents 12% of all childhood scrotal tumors (Wiener *et al.*, 1994). In general, rhabdomyosarcomas account for 5–10% of all childhood tumors and are the fourth most common tumor seen in children. Of rhabdomyosarcomas, paratesticular tumors account for only 7%. Rhabdomyosarcoma most commonly occurs in the head and neck, followed by the genitourinary system, the extremities, the trunk, and the retroperitoneum.

Presentation of paratesticular rhabdomyosarcoma has a mean age of approximately 10 years, but age varies with clinical group. It may be seen at any age, including adult, with older children usually having the worst prognosis, because they have a higher stage at presentation. This suggests that the age of the child may be a favorable prognostic sign, with older children presenting with more extensive and metastatic disease.

The Intergroup Rhabdomyosarcoma Study (IRS) demonstrated that there were two types of histologic pattern: those with a favorable outcome and those with an unfavorable outcome (see Chapter 41). Favorable histology included subtypes that have been classified as embryonal, embryonal–botryoid, pleomorphic, mixed, undifferentiated, and extraosseus Ewing's sarcoma. Unfavorable histology was attributed to any tumor with an alveolar pattern. Of the patients in the IRS with paratesticular rhabdomyosarcoma, 97% were known to have an embryonal histologic subtype. This is significantly different from the overall IRS data in which embryonal histology constituted only 53% of all rhabdomyosarcomas.

Clinically, rhabdomyosarcoma in the scrotum presents as a painless mass. Ultrasonography may detect the solid mass as arising from the paratesticular structures and may be able to differentiate it from the normal testis. Tumor markers, such as AFP and β-hCG levels, should be obtained before surgical removal, to ensure that the testicular mass is not a yolk sac tumor.

The treatment of rhabdomyosarcoma begins with clinical and pathologic staging. A high, inguinal, radical orchiectomy must be performed. If a needle biopsy or previous scrotal approach has violated the scrotum, the conservative and standard approach is to perform a hemiscrotectomy. The necessity for routine hemiscrotectomy in this setting is being reviewed and is currently evolving. A hemiscrotectomy may also be required for recurrent local disease, palpable masses, contamination, or positive margins (Rogers *et al.*, 1995).

After surgical and pathologic confirmation, the patient should undergo staging. This includes a CT scan of the chest and abdomen and a bone scan. Controversy continues regarding surgical examination of the retroperitoneum and its lymph nodes. Raney *et al.* (1987). The IRS demonstrated that 41% of patients had abnormal retroperitoneal lymph-node dissection, justifying the need to examine these nodes. However, the IRS-II group showed that this decreased to approximately 26%. Overall, retroperitoneal node involvement in the IRS-III for paratesticular rhabdomyosarcoma was 31%. The IRS-III recommended a limited unilateral retroperitoneal lymph-node dissection to accurately stage the disease. The controversy over retroperitoneal lymph-node dissection has continued and remains an issue in other national studies.

In a series from Italy and other countries, it was demonstrated that current adjuvant chemotherapy regimens can control subclinical microscopic disease and retroperitoneal lymph-node dissection is not necessary (Gamba *et al.*, 1994; Ferrari *et al.*, 1998). The current IRS-IV protocol recommends thin-cut CT scans but no retroperitoneal lymph-node biopsy or sampling for clinical stage I patients. In addition, IRS-IV recommends adjuvant actinomycin D and vincristine for stage I, group I patients. For advanced disease, accurate staging and adherence to protocol are essential.

The results of treatment for paratesticular rhabdomyosarcoma in the IRS-III are excellent, with an 84% 5 year survival. This compares with a 5 year survival rate of 73% for all patients in IRS-III, regardless of primary site. These favorable results are consistent with the characteristics of paratesticular rhabdomyosarcoma including early diagnosis, predominance for embryonal histology (93%) and a 27% proportion of the more favorable spindle-cell variant histology (Leuschner *et al.*, 1993).

The overall prognosis for patients with paratesticular rhabdomyosarcoma is excellent. With such a relatively rare tumor, it is important to enroll these patients in a national clinical protocol, both for better understanding of the tumor and for optimal treatment plans.

References

Bergstrand CG, Czar B (1956) Demonstration of a new protein fraction in serum from human fetus. *Scand J Clin Invest* **8**: 174.

Brewer JA, Tank ES (1993) Yolk sac tumors and alpha-fetoprotein in first year of life. *Urology* **42**: 79.

Brosman SA (1979) Testicular tumors in prepubertal children. *Urology* **13**: 581.

Carney JA, Gordon H, Carpenter PC *et al.* (1985) The complex myxomas, spotty pigmentation and endocrine overactivity. *Medicine* **64**: 270–83.

Chan YF, Restall P, Kimble R (1997) Juvenile granulosa cell tumor of the testis: report of 2 cases in newborns. *J Pediatr Surg* **32**: 752–3.

Chang B, Borer JG, Tan PE, Diamond DA (1998) Large-cell calcifying Sertoli cell tumor of the testis: case report and review of the literature. *Urology* 520–2.

Coppes M, Rackley R, Kay R (1994) Primary testicular and paratesticular tumors of childhood. *Med Pediatr Oncol* **22**: 329–40.

Crump WD (1983) Juvenile granulosa cell tumor of the fetal testis. *J Urol* **129**: 1057–8.

Dreyer L, Jacyk WK, du Plessis DJ (1994) Bilateral large-cell calcifying Sertoli cell tumor of the testes with Peutz–Jeghers syndrome. *Pediatr Dermatol* **11**: 335–7.

Dudiak CM, Vade A, Isaac RM (1994) Sonographic demonstration of bilateral large-cell calcifying Sertoli cell tumors of the testes. *J Ultrasound Med* **13**: 232–5.

Ferrari A, Casanova M, Massimino M *et al.* (1998) The management of paratesticular rhabdomyosarcoma: a single institutional experience with 44 consecutive children. *J Urol* **159**: 1031–4.

Gamba PG, Cecchetto G, Katende M *et al.* (1994) Paratesticular rhabdomyosarcoma (RMS) and paraaortic lymphadenectomy. *Eur J Pediatr Surg* **4**: 158–60.

Gilbaugh JH Jr, Kelalis PP, Dockerty MB (1967) Epidermoid cysts of the testis. *J Urol* **97**: 876.

Grady J, Ross JH, Kay R (1994) Patterns of metastatic spread in prepubertal yolk sac tumor of the testis. *J Urol* **153**: 1259–61.

Grady R, Ross JH, Kay R (1997) Epidemiologic features of teratomas of the testis in a prepubertal population. *J Urol* **158**: 1191–92.

Grechi G, Zampi GC, Selli C *et al.* (1980) Polyorchidism and seminoma in a child. *J Urol* **123**: 291.

Hertl MC, Wiebel J, Schafer H *et al.* (1998) Feminizing Sertoli cell tumors associated with Peutz–Jeghers syndrome: an increasingly recognized cause of prepubertal gynecomastia. *Plast Reconstruct Surg* **102**: 1151–57.

Horwitz MB, Abiri MM (1997) US case of the day. Benign cystic teratoma and testicular microlithiasis. *Radiographics* **17**: 793–6.

Kaplan GW (1984) Prepubertal testicular tumors. *World J Urol* **2**: 238.

Kay R (1993a) Prepubertal Testicular Tumor Registry. *J Urol* **150**: 671–4.

Kay R (1993b) Prepubertal testicular tumor registry. In: Klein E, Kay R (eds) *Urologic clinics of North America*. Philadelphia, PA: WB Saunders, 1–5.

Kay R, Ross JH (1998) Testis tumors. In: King L (ed) *Urologic surgery in infants and children*. Philadelphia, PA: WB Saunders, 255–61.

Klein E, Kay R, Norris D (1984) The incidence and detection of testicular leukemia in children. *Cleve Clin Q* **51**: 502–4.

Kolon TF, Hochman HI (1997) Malignant Sertoli cell tumor in a prepubescent boy. *J Urol* **158**: 608–9.

Lange PH, Vogelzang NJ, Goldman A *et al.* (1982) Marker half-life analysis as a prognostic tool in testicular cancer. *J Urol* **182**: 708.

Leuschner I, Newton WA Jr, Schmidt D *et al.* (1993) Spindle cell variants of embryonal rhabdomyosarcoma in the paratesticular region. A report of the Intergroup Rhabdomyosarcoma Study. *Am J Surg Pathol* **17**: 221–30.

Levy D, Kay R, Elder J (1994) Neonatal testis tumors: a review of the prepubertal testis tumor registry. *J Urol* **151**: 715–17.

Manivel JC, Reinberg Y, Nifans GA (1989) Intratubular germ cell neoplasia in testicular teratomas and epidermoid cysts. *Cancer* **64**: 175.

Mavrou C (1967) Hypothyroidism and seminoma in association with Down's syndrome. *J Pediatr* **70**: 810.

McEniff N, Doherty F, Katz J *et al.* (1995) Yolk sac tumor of the testis discovered on a routine annual sonogram in a boy with testicular microlithiasis. *AJR Am J Roentgenol* **164**: 971–2.

Niewenhuis JC, Wolf MC, Kass EJ (1994) Bilateral asynchronous Sertoli cell tumor in a boy with Peutz–Jeghers syndrome. *J Urol* **152**: 1246–8.

Noszian IM, Balon R, Eitelberger FG, Schmid N (1995) Bilateral testicular large-cell calcifying Sertoli cell tumor and recurrent cardiac myxoma in a patient with Carney's complex. *Pediat Radiol* **25** (Suppl): S236–7.

Oakhill A, Mainwaring D, Hill FGH *et al.* (1980) Management of leukemic infiltration of the testis. *Arch Dis Child* **55**: 564.

Oberman AS, Flatau E, Luboshitzky R (1993) Bilateral testicular adrenal rests in a patient with 11-hydroxylase deficient congenital adrenal hyperplasia. *J Urol* **149**: 350–2.

Perry C, Servadio C (1980) Seminoma in children. *J Urol* **124**: 932.

Price EB (1969) Epidermoid cysts of the testis: a clinical and pathologic analysis of 69 cases from the Testicular Tumor Registry. *J Urol* **102**: 708.

Raney RB, Tefft M, Lawrence WJ *et al.* (1987) Paratesticular sarcoma in children and adolescence. *Cancer* **60**: 2337.

Rich MA, Keating MA, Levin HS, Kay R (1998) Tumors of the adrenogenital syndrome: an aggressive conservative approach. *J Urol* **160**: 1838–41.

Rogers DA, Rao BN, Meyer WH *et al.* (1995) Indications for hemiscrotectomy in the management of genitourinary tumors in children. *J Pediatr Surg* **30**: 1437–9.

Ross JH, Kay R, Elder J (1993) Testis sparing surgery for pediatric epidermoid cysts in the testis. *J Urol* **149**: 353–6.

Rosvoll RV, Woodard JR (1968) Malignant Sertoli cell tumor of the testis. *Cancer* **22**: 8.

Rushton HG, Belman AB (1993) Testis-sparing surgery for benign lesions of the prepubertal testis. In: Klein E, Kay R (eds) *Urologic clinics of North America*. Philadelphia, PA: WB Saunders, 27–37.

Rushton HG, Belman AB, Sesterhenn I *et al.* (1990) Testicular sparing surgery for prepubertal teratoma of the testis: a clinical and pathological study. *J Urol* **144**: 726.

Rutgers JL, Young RH, Scully RE (1988) The testicular 'tumor' of the adrenogenital syndrome. *Am J Surg Pathol* **12**: 503.

Scully RE (1970) Gonadoblastoma: a review of 74 cases. *Cancer* **25**: 1340.

Srikanth MS, West BR, Ishitani M *et al.* (1992) Benign testicular tumors in children with congenital adrenal hyperplasia. *J Pediatr Surg* **27**: 639–41.

Terai A, Ishitoya S, Hashimura T *et al.* (1995) A case of metastatic yolk sac tumor of testis in a child. *Int J Urol* **2**: 135–8.

Uehling DT, Phillips E (1994) Residual retroperitoneal mass following chemotherapy for infantile yolk sac tumor. *J Urol* **152**: 185–6.

Uehling DT, Smith JE, Logan R, Hafez GR (1987) Newborn granulosa cell of the testis. *J Urol* **138**: 385.

Urban MD, Lee PA, Plotnick LP, Migeon CJ (1978) The diagnosis of Leydig cell tumors in children. *Am J Dis Child* **132**: 494.

Viprakasit D, Navaroo E., Guarin VK *et al.* (1977) Seminoma in children. *Urology* **9**: 568.

Walker BR, Skoog SJ, Winslow BH *et al.* (1997) Testis sparing surgery for steroid unresponsive testicular tumors of the adrenogenital syndrome. *J Urol* **157**: 1460–3.

White CP (1910) A case of carcinoma myxomatodes of the testis in infancy. *J Pathol* **14**: 522.

White MD, Loughlin MW, Kallakury BV *et al.* (1997) Bilateral large-cell calcifying Sertoli cell tumor of the testis in a 7-year old boy. *J Urol* **158**: 1547–8.

Wiener ES, Lawrence W, Hays D *et al.* (1994) Retroperitoneal node biopsy in paratesticular rhabdomyosarcoma. *J Pediatr Surg* **29**: 171–7.

Young RH, Lawrence WD, Scully RE (1985) Juvenile granulosa cell tumor – another neoplasm associated with chromosomes and ambiguous genitalia. A report of 3 cases. *Am J Surg Pathol* **9**: 737.

Young S, Gooneratne S, Straus FH II *et al.* (1995) Feminizing Sertoli cell tumors in boys with Peutz–Jeghers syndrome. *Am J Surg Pathol* **19**: 50–8.

Tumors of the retroperitoneum

43

Gordon A. McLorie and Darius J. Bägli

Introduction

Retroperitoneal tumors of non-renal origin are relatively uncommon in children. The most significant are neuroblastoma, sacrococcygeal teratoma, the rare childhood pheochromocytoma and adrenal carcinoma. This chapter will focus on these four tumor types, with primary emphasis on the first two. The listing given in Table 43.1 of non-renal retroperitoneal tumors is included for completeness.

Neuroblastoma

Neuroblastoma accounts for 8–10% of all childhood cancers. Following the original description by Virchow in 1864, it has continued to capture the imagination and interest of pediatricians, surgeons, and scientists. Historic landmarks in the biology of neuroblastoma include the understanding of the relationship of this childhood malignancy to the secretion

Table 43.1 Non-renal retroperitoneal tumors

Benign	Malignant
Lymphangioma	Neuroblastoma
Neurofibroma	Pheochromocytoma
Ganglioneuroma	Sacrococcygeal teratoma
Lipoma	Non-genitourinary pelvic
Sacrococcygeal	rhabdomyosarcoma
teratoma	Lymphoma
	Liposarcoma
	Fibrosarcoma
	Leiomyosacoma
	Malignant fibrous
	histiocytoma
	Secondary tumors

of neuroactive substances in 1957, followed by the ability to establish a biochemical diagnosis based on the urinary secretion of catecholamines. Cushing described its transition in biologic activity from a malignant tumor to one of a benign nature while Beckwith and Perin (1963) noted that clusters of neuroblastic nodules resembling neuroblastoma *in situ* were an incidental finding in the adrenal glands in children dying of other diseases. These clues provided the initial impetus that led to the recognition of the now well-known phenomenon of spontaneous regression of some neuroblastomas. Newer advances in molecular research have provided significant further insight into the biology of neuroblastoma. Furthermore, the paradigms described for neuroblastoma have acted as a template for diagnostic staging and applications of molecular and genetic insights to clinical therapies of other childhood malignancies. Fingerprinting the tumor's molecular characteristics (beyond MYCN proto-oncogene expression) has allowed stratification of children with neuroblastoma into distinctive clinical subsets. These stratification and staging methodologies provide better applications of therapeutic options and appropriate balancing of therapies that are more aggressive to children with poor prognostic disease. They also allow us to pursue a goal of less aggressive therapies to be used for those children in whom better prognosis can be defined (Castleberry, 1997).

Recent insights have unfolded as a result of neonatal screening programs in Japan and Canada. In these programs, the secretion of urinary vanillylmandelic acid (VMA) in the newborn has been used as a method of neuroblastoma detection. However, early detection has reduced neither the occurrence nor improved the prognosis of those children who are discovered to have higher grade tumors in later infancy and childhood. This has led to the thesis that the tumors detected during neonatal screening programs are those that have a natural propensity for spontaneous resolution (Woods *et al.*, 1996, 1997). The results suggest that mass screening for neuroblastoma, while feasible, is unlikely to alter the course of those patients destined to succumb to the disease.

Clinical and biological features

Neuroblastoma ranks as the most common extracranial solid malignancy of childhood (Gurney *et al.*, 1997) and early infancy. The incidence may be increasing slightly (Gurney *et al.*, 1997; Kenney *et al.*, 1998). In children presenting with neuroblastoma, 65% will occur in the retroperitoneum, of which 40% will originate in the adrenal gland (Bonovarus *et al.*, 1986).

Few, if any, environmental risk factors have been identified for neuroblastoma. Recently, maternal vaginal infections, their treatment, and prenatal maternal hormone use have been weakly suggested to increase the risk of neuroblastoma in offspring (Michalek *et al.*, 1996). Pesticide exposure has been suggested as being associated with an increased risk of carcinogenesis in children compared with adults; the risk included but was not specific for neuroblastoma (Zahm and Ward, 1998).

While newer molecular modalities are helping to refine prognostic groupings and treatment assignment, the overwhelming variables distinguishing high-from low-risk groups continue to be age at diagnosis, tumor stage, and histologic grade (Saito *et al.*, 1997). Diagnosis before 12 months of age is more clinically favorable than later diagnosis.

Any predisposition for neuroblastoma appears to follow an autosomal dominant pattern, as elucidated by the two-hit hypothesis of Knudson and Strong (1972). Also described for Wilms' tumor and pheochromocytoma, inherited forms of neuroblastoma may occur in patients who harbor a mutation in a gene that pre-existed in a parental germ line (preconception or germinal mutation). A subsequent spontaneous mutation of the other copy of the same gene (a somatic mutation) in a cell of the appropriate background (neural crest cell) leads to malignant transformation of that cell. This has led to estimates that over one-fifth of all neuroblastoma may be of the inherited variety (Knudson and Strong, 1972). The occurrence of non-familial neuroblastoma must therefore await these two critical mutations or 'hits' as two independent spontaneous events. This explains the reduced likelihood (incidence) of non-familial or sporadic disease. With one of two mutations possibly present in all cells of a given child with a strong family history of neuroblastoma, it is easy to see why earlier incidence, bilaterality and multifocality, and higher recurrence rates are the norm in those with familial disease. Exceptions to the two-hit hypothesis have been reported (familial neuroblastoma in older children), suggesting that other genetic mechanisms may also underlie familial disease (Ichimiya *et al.*, 1999). While several reports exist of neuroblastoma being found in children with a chromosomal abnormality, few chromosomal predispositions have been definitively associated with neuroblastoma. Abnormal rearrangements have been described involving chromosomes 1 and 17 (see below). Deletions involving 1p36 have implicated this region as containing a neuroblastoma tumor suppressor gene, and gains in the 17q region have been associated with poor prognosis (Caron, 1995; Caron *et al.*, 1996; Lastowska *et al.*, 1997a,b; Plantaz *et al.*, 1997; Ichimiya *et al.*, 1999). Finally, loss of heterozygosity (LOH), a molecular phenotype characterized by the loss of the subtle differences that normally exist between the two allelic (parental) copies of any gene signifying that one of the copies is missing, has been identified as a more general phenomenon in neuroblastoma. Subjects with LOH are, therefore, homozygous instead of heterozygous for that particular chromosomal region. When a disease becomes evident in association with LOH in particular regions of a chromosome, this implies that the missing region of that chromosome encodes a gene or genes responsible for suppressing that disease, i.e. tumor suppressor genes. Although LOH does not identify the missing gene itself, LOH in neuroblastoma has been reported present in a number of chromosomes, including 1p, 11q and 14q, 2q, 9p and 18q (Takita *et al.*, 1997).

Clinical manifestations: primary, metastatic, and paraneoplastic features

The presenting signs and symptoms are variable and may reflect the effects of the tumor, the presence of metastatic disease, or the results of tumor hormone production. As mentioned earlier, prenatal screening may also identify neuroblastoma. Infants may present with an abdominal mass that is often huge. A unique feature of neuroblastoma in children is the potential for widespread liver metastatic disease that may signify stage 4S disease (Fig. 43.1).

Children with stage 4S have a potential survival rate of up to 90%, in spite of metastases to either liver, skin, or bone marrow, but not to cortical bone. Subcutaneous nodules are another manifestation of this early presentation (Peled *et al.*, 1992). In some patients tumors regress spontaneously. Alternatively, metastases may regress following excision of the primary tumor (Evans *et al.*, 1976; Brodeur *et al.*, 1984). In children older than 1 year of age the size of the abdominal mass is variable and may not be the presenting symptom. Malaise and/or pain reflecting the presence of metastatic disease is the presenting complaint in up to 60%. Anemia (from bone marrow involvement in 50% of patients) is also a common presenting sign. The new or sudden onset of constipation or urinary retention may herald the well-known propensity of neuroblastoma to invade the spinal cord. In addition, transient pain attributable to bony metastases may mimic rheumatoid arthritis. Lung or brain metastases are common sites of relapse and late-stage disease.

Paraneoplastic syndromes occur in fewer than 5% of neuroblastoma patients. Intractable diarrhea may result from the secretion of vasoactive intestinal peptide (VIP) (Mendelsohn *et al.*, 1976). However,

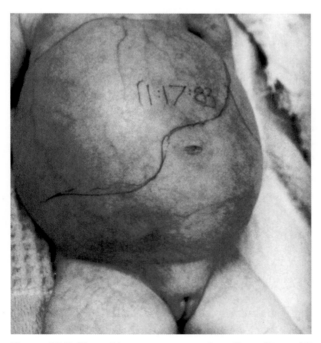

Figure 43.1 Neuroblastoma metastatic to liver. Stage 4S neuroblastoma underwent spontaneous regression. (From Snyder *et al.*, with permission.)

this symptom, mimicking malabsorption syndrome, is more often associated with the better differentiated ganglioneuroma or intermediately differentiated ganglioneuroblastoma. Resolution follows removal of the tumor. Another unusual symptom is cerebellar ataxia and opsomyoclonus (dancing feet, dancing eyes; myoclonic encephalopathy of infants). This syndrome is of unknown pathogenesis and is more often associated with thoracic tumors (Bonovarus *et al.*, 1986). While symptoms of catecholamine excess (palpitations, tachycardia, hypertension) are rare in neuroblastoma, they can occur from excess circulating tumor-derived norepinephrine. However, norepinephrine is less potent than its metabolite, epinephrine, in inducing these symptoms. These symptoms are more commonly found in patients with pheochromocytoma. The responsible enzyme is phenylethanolamine *N*-methyl transferase (PNMT), which plays a role in the conversion of norepinephrine to epinephrine.

Gross, histologic, molecular pathology, and markers

Neuroblastomas arise from cells of neural crest origin, which ultimately form the sympathetic nervous systems (sympathogonia). The sites of origin may be found at any location in the sympathetic nervous system with over one-half occurring in the neonatal abdominal cavity, and up to two-thirds from the adrenal gland. The remainder occur in the sympathetic ganglia and, more rarely, in the organ of Zuckerhandel. The spectrum of biologic behavior or potential of these tumors is broad. Malignant neuroblastomas comprise the majority. Ganglioneuroblastoma and ganglioneuroma represent progressively more benign forms of the tumor, reflecting more indolent clinical manifestations, better prognoses, as well as distinct morphology and biochemical profiles.

The histopathologic features that define the malignant potential are unique. Homer–Wright pseudorosettes, the diagnostic histologic presence of eosinophilic neutrophils surrounded by neuroblasts, occur in only one-half of cases (Black, 1997). The presence of associated neuropils (pigmented neuritic processes) is pathognomonic for neuroblastoma. The other type of cell is the Schwann cell, which may be recruited into the tumor and comprises the Schwannian stroma which makes up the mesenchymal component of the tumor. The degree of histologic differentiation is classified according to a variety of schemes but the most popular is that developed by Shimada, which has recently been revised by Joshi (Table 43.2), and a combination of the two is the basis of planned prospective trials (Shimada *et al.*, 1984; Joshi *et al.*, 1992).

Molecular pathology

Molecular understanding of neuroblastoma has identified several newer features of the disease that may aid in all aspects of its management, including diagnosis, natural history, prognostic stratification, and treatment selection. These include analyses of nuclear and chromosomal material, and neuronal phenotyping through assessment of various neuron-associated growth factors. While karyotyping has identified specific chromosomal abnormalities (see below), analysis of DNA ploidy has also revealed significant information. Paradoxically, neuroblastomas of the

Table 43.2 Histopathologic classifications of Shimada and Joshi

Prognosis	Histopathologic features/age
Favorable	
Shimada	Stroma rich, all ages, no nodular pattern
	Stroma poor, age 1.5–5 years, differentiated, MKI < 100
	Stroma poor, age < 1.5 years, MKI < 200
Joshi	Grade 1, all ages; grade 2, < 1 year
Unfavorable:	
Shimada	Stroma rich, all ages, nodular pattern
	Stroma poor, age > 5 years
	Stroma poor, age 1.5–5 years, undifferentiated
	Stroma poor, age 1.5–5 years, differentiated, MKI > 100
	Stroma poor, age < 1.5 years, MKI > 200
Joshi	Grade 2, age > 1 years; grade 3, all ages

Grade 1 = low mitotic rate (< 10 mitotic figures per 10 high power fields) and calcification present; grade 2 = either low mitotic rate or calcification present; grade 3 = neither low mitotic rate nor calcification present.
MKI = mitosis–karyorrhexis index (number of mitoses and karyorrhexis per 5000 cells).
Adapted from Brodeur and Castleberry (1997) with permission.

hyperdiploid variety are more likely to respond favorably to chemotherapy. Diploid or near-diploid tumors are associated with higher stage disease (including unresectable tumors), poorer prognosis, a lower response to chemotherapy, and recurrence or progression (Morris *et al.*, 1995; Bowman *et al.*, 1997; Cheung *et al.*, 1997; Katzenstein *et al.*, 1998).

The most widely reported genetic marker for neuroblastoma has been amplification of the MYCN (or N-myc) proto-oncogene (Brodeur *et al.*, 1984; Seeger *et al.*, 1985). The association between MYCN amplification and high-grade (Shimada *et al.*, 1995), advanced stage disease at presentation, rapid progression, and overall poor prognosis is well established. Recently, an etiologic relationship between MYCN and neuroblastoma has been demonstrated by two complementary studies. Chan and co-workers from the Hospital For Sick Children in Toronto reported that elevations in MYCN protein expression in neuroblastoma tissues is independently associated with poor prognosis in high-stage disease (III, IV, IVS) even in the absence of MYCN gene amplification (Chan *et al.*, 1997). Furthermore, MYCN protein levels were prognostic, independent of the most significant variables of age or stage (Chan *et al.*, 1997), thus strongly supporting the concept that MYCN expression is directly involved in the cellular events of neuroblastoma progression. Conversely, in the subgroup of patients who did well with normal MYCN gene expression, MYCN protein levels were undetectable (Chan *et al.*, 1997). In a related animal study, the targeted overexpression of the MYCN gene in neuroectodermal cells led to the development of neuroblastoma in MYCN transgenic mice (Weiss *et al.*, 1997). MYCN tumorigenesis is further augmented in the absence of the recognized tumor suppressor genes NF1 or RB1 (Weiss *et al.*, 1997). This demonstrates that MYCN's transforming effect can be influenced by other genes, consistent with the emerging concept of multistep processes in malignant transformation. MYCN gene amplification is present in approximately 40% of patients with advanced stage III or IV disease (compared with < 10% in low-stage patients) and its absence augurs a slower disease progression in these patients.

As mentioned above, deletions of chromosome 1 and gains in chromosome 17 have been shown to carry strong prognostic information in advanced neuroblastoma. A landmark report from a collaborative group in Europe has shown a very powerful association between gains in chromosome 17q and adverse neuroblastoma outcome. The study is important because of its large numbers, the availability of all clinical and genetic data variables for 85% of the patients in the cohort, and the close coordination between a team of basic and clinical researchers. In total, 313 children from six European centers were studied. Often, but not exclusively, the gain of 17q was linked to the loss of 1p. Most significantly, in univariate and multivariate analyses, 17q gain was independently predictive of poor outcome (30.6% 5 year survival with 17q gain vs 86% 5 year survival without 17q gain) (Bown et al., 1999).

A longstanding notion in tumorigenesis states that transformation (neoplasia) is the result of aberrant differentiation pathways leading away from the normal cell phenotype. As a result, neuroblastoma may represent an aberration of normal neuronal development. As such, several neuronal differentiation markers have been investigated in this disease, including chromogranin A, neuropeptide Y, and receptors for neurotropins such as nerve growth factor. Neuropeptide Y is detectable in abundance in the serum of neuroblastoma patients and may be useful in following tumor burden both before and after therapy (Kogner et al., 1993). In tumor tissue, it reaches its highest levels in poorly differentiated neuroblastoma, compared with ganglioneuroblastoma or ganglioneuroma (Kogner et al., 1993). Conversely, chomogranin A derivatives may become useful markers of more favorably differentiated tumors (Kogner et al., 1995).

Acting through various receptors, neurotropic factors are, by definition, involved in the differentiation of neural tissues. One family of neurotropin receptors, the tyrosine kinase receptors TRK-A, TRK-B, and TRK-C, is showing promise in understanding neuroblastoma biology. It appears that TRK-A gene expression is associated with favorable outcome, yielding its highest expression in more well-differentiated tumors (Brodeur et al., 1997; Combaret et al., 1997). Furthermore, TRK-A levels are inversely correlated with MYCN gene expression (Brodeur et al., 1997). Expression of TRK-C and shortened forms of TRK-B also portend better outcome (Brodeur et al., 1997). Together, these observations have also led to speculation that functioning, intact neurotropin/TRK receptor pathways in these tumors may be further linked to their propensity to mature (differentiate) into ganglioneuromas, or regress through a cell-death pathway (from a presumed eventual unavailability of factor for the receptor, or receptor malfunction). However, as our knowledge of the role of these pathways evolves, it is becoming clear that they carry potential as powerful markers of disease, or even as molecular therapeutic targets to manipulate neuroblastomas to assume differentiation or regression pathways.

Drawing on the foregoing discussion, neuroblastomas may be stratified into specific prognostic subgroups based on the genetic interplay represented by MYCN expression, LOH, DNA ploidy, and neurotropin receptor expression. Combined with age and stage, three genetic neuroblastoma profiles can be determined with differing survival rates (Table 43.3).

Diagnosis, staging, and treatment

The diagnosis of neuroblastoma is confirmed by histologic sampling of tumor tissue or bone marrow. Standard light and electron microscopic evaluation may be followed by immunohistochemical identification of tissue of neuronal origin. The vast majority of the tumors secrete catecholamines synthesized from the amino acid tyrosine in the sequence: dopa, dopamine [both excreted as homovanillic acid

Table 43.3 Genetic neuroblastoma profiles

Feature	Type 1	Type 2	Type 3
MYCN amplification	None	None	Present
DNA ploidy	Hyperdiploid	Near-diploid	Near-tetraploid
LOH	Rare	25–50%	Present
Neurotropin gene expression	High	Low/absent (except TRK-B, high)	
Age	1 year	>1 year	
Stage	1, 2, 4S	3, 4	
3 year survival	95%	25–50%	< 5%

LOH = loss of heterozygosity; TRK = tyrosine kinase receptor.
Adapted from Brodeur (1998) with permission.

(HVA)], and finally norepinephrine. In contrast to pheochromocytomas, neuroblastomas lack the ability to convert norepinephrine to epinephrine. Norepinephrine and epinephrine are both excreted as vanillyl-mandelic acid (VMA).

Imaging techniques

Traditionally, the presentation of an abdominal neuroblastoma has been either by the discovery of an abdominal mass on physical examination, or the result of investigations to explain symptoms related to either metastatic disease or the neurendocrine manifestations of the tumor. Abdominal ultrasonography will detect a great percentage of those tumors that occur in the abdominal cavity. Occasionally they are found as an incidental finding in the course of pursuing an otherwise unrelated symptom. With increased sonographic screening this has now become a more common cause for presentation of these tumors (Graham and McHenry, 1998). In the authors'recent experience at a large children's hospital there have been two instances in the past year when children who were being followed in the course of an investigation for antenatal hydronephrosis had neuroblastomas that become apparent and had not been present on prior examinations (Fig. 43.2a–c).

Diagnostic imaging techniques are evolving and improving with great rapidity, and there is no consensus as to which method is best. The choices include ultrasonography, computed tomography (CT), and magnetic resonance imaging (MRI). The availability and the non-invasive nature of ultrasonography endorse this technology as the choice for the initial screening test. The time required for both CT and MRI makes their selection for young children more critical. Either of these techniques may be used to delineate and define the extent of the disease. Availability may be the most critical determinant of which should be used. CT imaging currently seems to be the most widely available modality. (Figs. 43.2, 43.3).

In seeking metastatic disease a chest radiograph is a useful initial step. Radioisotope bone scanning using technetium-99m-methylene diphosphonate is more accurate than a standard X-ray skeletal survey for the detection of bony metastases (Fig. 43.4).

Prognostic markers

Both clinical and biochemical markers have evolved that are helpful in the management of neuroblastoma. The best recognized are the traditional clinical para-

meters of age at diagnosis and tumor stage. Patients diagnosed at 1 year of age appear to show consistently better survival outcomes than older children, even in the presence of advanced disease at presentation. Survival also stratifies dramatically with respect to disease stage, with 75–90% 5 year survival for stage 1, 2, and 4S patients, compared with 10–30% 2 year survival for stage 3–4 disease.

Various biochemical and cell associated parameters have also been assessed for their prognostic ability in the management of neuroblastoma. Serum ferritin is elevated during periods of rapid tumor growth and/or large tumor burden. Whether this reflects a growth requirement for ferritin by the tumor or is a product of neuroblastoma cell metabolism is unknown. Ferritin levels appear to discriminate between stage 4 and stage 4S disease (Hann et al., 1981). Lactate dehydrogenase (LDH) is elaborated non-specifically in several tumor types including neuroblastoma, where it may reflect rapid tumor cell turnover and (Sakakibara et al., 1999) tumor burden. Neuron-specific enolase is a cytoplasmic enzyme found in cells of neural (Massaron et al., 1998) origin. Neuroblastoma prognosis appears worse if elevated levels are detected in serum, although this marker is not specific to neuroblastoma (Massaron et al., 1998). Serum and tissue ganglioside GD2 is a glycosphingolipid shed by neuroblastoma tumor cells. It may reflect tumor burden, and decreasing levels may be seen as a positive response to successful reduction of tumor load. The presence of GD2 on the cell surface has attracted interest in targeting this molecule using immunotherapy strategies (Cheung IY et al., 1998; Cheung NK et al., 1998; Klingebiel et al., 1998). Finally, matrix metalloproteinases (MMPs) are cellular enzymes required to break down the extracellular matrix and facilitate cell movement through the matrix during the metastatic process. Very recently, tumor cell expression of a membrane-associated MMP was found to correlate with advanced stage and poor outcome in neuroblastoma (Sakakibara et al., 1999).

Staging

A disease with such diverse manifestations as neuroblastoma in childhood needs a comprehensive staging system to allow precise diagnostic criteria and a method for categorizing and quantifying disease. Such a staging system then acts as a template upon which diagnostic criteria can be applied to various subgroups of disease, and permits definition of out-

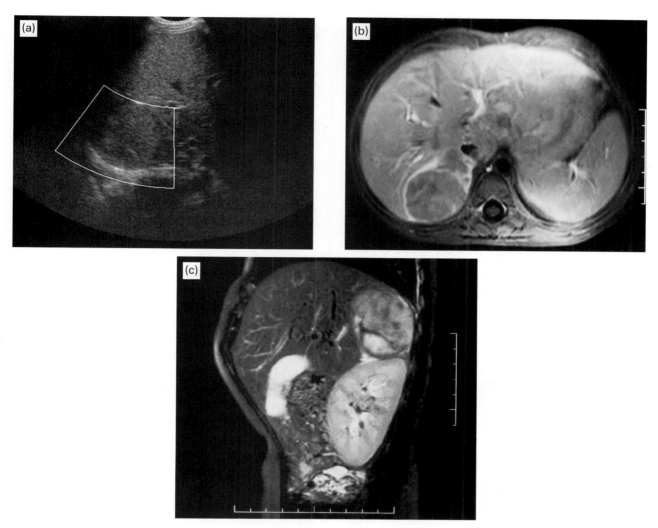

Figure 43.2 (*a*) Ultrasound image discovered in a 1-year-old child as 'incidentaloma' in the course of investigating contralateral antenataly diagnosed hydronephrosis. Prior sonogram 6 months. earlier with good views of the same area showed no evidence of mass lesion. (*b,c*) Transverse and sagittal magnetic resonance images of the same lesion, showing relationships in the retroperitoneum.

come measures that will allow collaboration between centers in implementing and assessing clinical trials. An international working group published the outcome of its deliberations in 1988 (Brodeur *et al.*, 1988). The staging system recommended is known as the International Neuroblastoma Staging System (INSS) and the response criteria are referred to as the International Neuroblastoma Response Criteria (INRC). This staging system has now replaced previous systems by Evans, originally established by the Pediatric Oncology Group (POG). Table 43.4 outlines the three staging systems, thus facilitating some comparison of previously published data.

Treatment

Therapy of neuroblastoma requires close coordination of medical, surgical, and radiation oncologists and clearly represents a prime example of multimodal cancer therapy. Surgical intervention plays a dual role. At the time of diagnosis, open or laparoscopic approaches may be necessary to obtain adequate and thorough samples for histologic and molecular diagnosis and marker analysis. Needle biopsy materials are most often inadequate for these purposes. For selected tumors, primary surgical excision may be possible, particularly for small, locally confined cases. In this

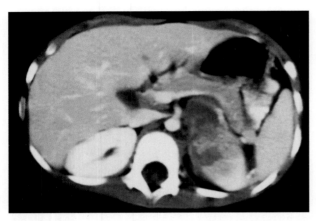

Figure 43.3 Transverse computed tomographic scan of retroperitoneal recurrence of a previously excised stage 3 neuroblastoma.

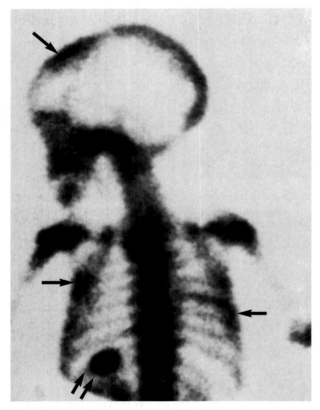

Figure 43.4 Posterior view of thorax and skull. Increased uptake is seen in skull-upper thoracic spine and left and right ribs (*arrows*) as a result of metastatic neuroblastoma. The decreased uptake at T12 is an unusual manifestation of metastatic tumor. The right suprarenal uptake of tracer is within the primary tumor (*double arrow*).

regard, laparoscopic surgery may be considered and has been used successfully for small tumors identified by screening (Nakajima *et al.*, 1997). Given that infant screening detects tumors that are generally biologically favorable, laparoscopic surgery may be a safe modality on oncologic grounds. Open surgical dissection is also employed to both assess response to therapy and excise residual disease after initial courses of chemotherapy have been completed. Recent reports have suggested a higher incidence of nephrectomy in children with neuroblastoma who were treated with primary surgical intervention (Cañete *et al.*, 1998; Shamberger *et al.*, 1998).

Chemotherapy is a major component of the treatment of neuroblastoma. Both single-agent and synergistic multiagent drug regimens are used, combining cell-cycle-specific and cell-cycle-independent drugs to achieve the maximum ratio of therapeutic benefit to toxicity. Ionizing radiation has a role in neuroblastoma treatment as the tumor is radiosensitive. It is most useful in achieving local control on the one hand, and palliation of disease uncontrollable by other modalities on the other. As a primary modality, however, radiotherapy is limited by the extensive metastatic proclivity of many neuroblastomas. The agent methyliodobenzylguanidine (MIBG), used in the localization of neuroblastomas and pheochromocytomas, has been studied for its ability to bind to neuroblastoma tumors systemically and carry with it radioligands such as iodine-131 that are toxic to the tumor cells (Klingebiel *et al.*, 1998; Mastrangelo *et al.*, 1998; Matthay *et al.*, 1998). This approach has also been used as a surgical adjunct to guide tumor tissue resection using the gamma camera intraoperatively once the tumor is radiolabeled by preoperative injection of [131I]MIBG (Heij *et al.*, 1977).

Given the aggressive nature of advanced and higher staged disease, efforts continue to attempt improved disease control in this subset of patients while refining therapy to limit toxicity in lower stage and more favorable disease.

Treatment strategy

The ability to stratify patients into distinctly risk-related groups, by application of the varied but highly accurate histologic and molecular diagnostic and staging methodologies, has permitted the much more judicious and specific use of the therapeutic regimens.

Table 43.4 Neuroblastoma Staging System

Evans and D'Angio	POG	INSS
Stage I Tumor confined to the organ or structure of origin	*Stage A* Complete gross resection of primary tumor, with or without microscopic residual. Intracavitary lymph nodes, not adhered to and removed with primary (nodes adhered to or with tumor resection may be positive for tumor without upstaging patient to stage C), histologically free of tumor. If primary in the abdomen or pelvis, liver histologically free of tumor	*Stage I* Localized tumor with complete gross excision without microscopic residual disease; representative ipsilateral lymph nodes negative for tumor microscopically (nodes attached to and removed with the primary tumor may be positive)
Stage II Tumor extending in continuity beyond the organ or structure of origin but not crossing the midline. Regional lymph nodes on the ipsilateral side may be involved		*Stage 2A* Localized tumor with incomplete gross excision; representative ipsilateral non-adherent lymph nodes negative for tumor microscopically
Stage III Tumor extending in continuity beyond the midline. Regional lymph nodes may be involved bilaterally	*Stage B* Grossly unresected primary tumor. Nodes and liver same as stage A	*Stage 2B* Localized tumor with or without complete gross excision, with ipsilateral non-adherent lymph nodes positive for tumor. Enlarged contralateral lymph nodes must be negative microscopically.
Stage IV Remote disease involving the skeleton, bone marrow, soft tissue, distant lymph-node groups, etc. (see stage IV-S)	*Stage C* Complete or incomplete resection of primary. Intracavitary nodes not adhered to primary histologically positive for tumor. Liver as in stage A	*Stage 3* Unresectable unilateral tumor infiltrating across the midline, with or without regional lymph-node involvement; or localized unilateral tumor with contralateral regional lymph-node involvement; or midline tumor with bilateral extension by infiltration (unresectable) or by lymph-node involvement.
State IV-S Patients who would otherwise be stage I or II, but who have remote disease confined to liver, skin, or bone marrow (without radiographic evidence of bone metastases on complete skeletal survey)	*Stage D* Any dissemination of disease beyond intracavitary nodes (i.e. extracavitary nodes, liver, skin, bone marrow, bone)	
	Stage DS Infants <1 year of age with Stage IV-S disease (see Evans and D'Angio)	*Stage 4* Any primary tumor with dissemination to distant lymph nodes, bone, bone marrow, liver, skin, and/or other organs (except as defined for stage 4S)
		Stage 4S Localized primary tumor as defined for stage 1, 2A, or 2B with dissemination limited to skin, liver, and/or bone marrow (limited to infants <1 year of age)

POG = Pediatric Oncology Group; INSS = International Neuroblastoma Staging System.
From Halperin *et al*. (1994).

Stage 1 and 2 tumors (low risk) are treatable by primary surgical resection alone, with no need for initial chemotherapy or radiotherapy. A prognosis of up to 89% survival has been reported in this group of patients (Nitschke *et al.*, 1991; Castleberry, 1997; Matthay *et al.*, 1998). Stage 4S tumors will undergo spontaneous remission and are thus considered low risk. However, if symptoms are present related to severe hepatic metastatic disease or respiratory compromise, they may benefit from chemotherapy or radiation therapy in small doses.

Stage 3 tumors (intermediate risk) still have an excellent overall survival rate of up to 89% (Nitschke *et al.*, 1991) but chemotherapy is advised following primary surgical excision. Second-look surgery may also be appropriate after chemotherapy. The goal of therapy in this group is to reserve more intense therapy for those children with biologically unfavorable tumors.

Patients with stage 4 disease (high risk) have derived minimal benefits from even the most intensive regimens. Multiagent chemotherapy remains the standard primary treatment strategy for these patients. There have been isolated applications of ablative chemotherapy and bone marrow transplantation and these intensive therapeutic approaches are currently being explored in multicenter trials. The overall prognosis in this group of children remains very low (15–35% survival) (Stram *et al.*, 1996).

Ganglioneuroma

A more histologically benign counterpart of neuroblastoma is the ganglioneuroma. Ganglioneuroblastoma is an intermediate malignant classification between ganglioneuroma and neuroblastoma, and for treatment purposes is regarded with neuroblastoma. Ganglioneuromas are most often seen in older children and present as abdominal masses. It is intriguing to hypothesize that late development of a more benign variant may represent a 'second hit', but these tumors do not exhibit an 'explosive' form of metastatic behavior (Moschovi *et al.*, 1997). Nonetheless, by virtue of their inexorable growth and distortion of adjacent tissues they can have a very morbid clinical course. Such a case is illustrated in Figure 43.5a–c, in which both gastrointestinal and genitourinary tissues are grossly displaced. The urologic system, in particular, may exhibit such profound destruction that urinary diversion may be deemed necessary. The figures illustrate the results of MRI, which can

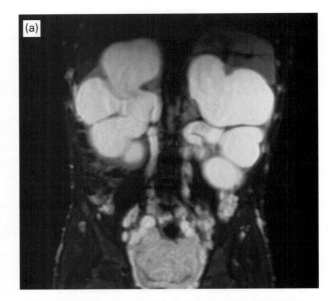

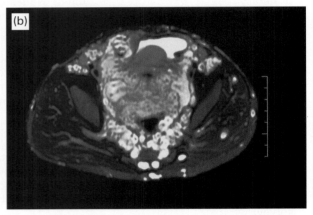

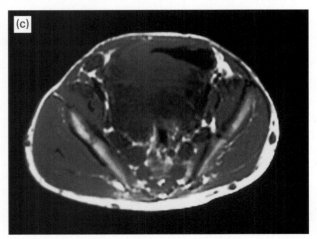

Figure 43.5 (*a*) Magnetic resonance scan of patient with a ganglioneuroma, showing obstruction of the ureters. (*b*) Primary neuronal masses displacing the bladder anteriorly and the rectum posteriorly. (*c*) T_2-weighted image of the same pelvic area as in (*b*), showing the different appearance of neural tissues.

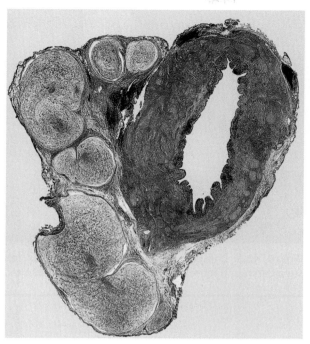

Figure 43.6 Pathologic section of area of excised ureter, with ureter encased in, but not invaded by tumor tissue.

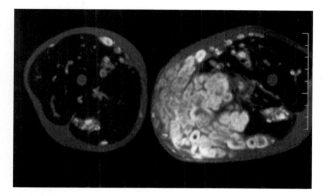

Figure 43.7 Extension of ganglioneuroma down the sheath of the sacral nerve.

provide eloquent detail of the soft-tissue involvement by these tumors, while there is no evidence of direct histologic invasion of the compressed tissues (Fig. 43.6).

The correlation of the MRI features with latent malignant potential in these tumors has recently been documented by Ichikawa *et al.* (1996). They were able to show that punctate calcification on the CT scan and low or intermediate attenuation are common in ganglioneuromas. The MR images are mainly of low intensity on T_1-weighted images (T_1WI) and of high intensity on T_2-weighted images (T_2WI). Dynamic MR studies show a lack of early involvement but gradually increasing enhancement. The authors concluded that the absence of these features, judged 'typical' for ganglioneuroma, should suggest a potential for a more malignant course. The slow-growing nature of ganglioneuromas may also have a devastating effect on vascular and neurologic function by virtue of its compressive effects on adjacent structures. Figure 43.7 demonstrates extension along the sacral nerve prior to the appearance of clinical degeneration. This and other cases have demonstrated the potential for clinical morbidity that may be associated with ganglioneuroma despite its non-metastatic nature. To prevent these localized effects, incomplete surgical resection may be justified in the absence of effective chemotherapy or radiotherapy.

Pheochromocytoma

Clinical features and presentation

Pediatric pheochromocytoma is an extremely uncommon primary tumor of the adrenal medulla, although it is the most common hyperfunctioning form of this tissue in children. Over a period of 5 years at the Hospital for Sick Children in Toronto, of 30 patients presenting with a primary adrenal tumor, only one, a 16-year-old girl, had a pheochromocytoma. The tumors arise in the autonomic system, with 90% originating in the adrenal gland. Catecholamine production is the norm and is the basis for both the clinical manifestations and laboratory diagnosis. Pediatric pheochromocytomas can be seen in association with a variety of diseases including neurofibromatosis, von Hippel–Lindau disease, Sturge–Webber syndrome, and multiple endocrine neoplasia (MEN-2). Those associated with MEN-2 are more likely to occur later in life and are more likely to be bilateral.

Imaging, biochemical features, and new prognostic markers

The diagnosis of pheochromocytoma in childhood is suggested by the rare coexistence of hypertension and abdominal mass detectable on sonographic evaluation. Non-palpable pheochromocytoma causing secondary hypertension in children is exceedingly rare. The diagnosis is confirmed by means of either serum or urine confirmation of hypersecretion of catecholamines.

As stated previously, the principal catecholamine that produces the classic characteristic symptoms of flushing, palpitations, hypertension (vasoconstriction), and anxiety in patients with pheochromocytoma is epinephrine. Epinephrine is a metabolite of its precursor, norepinephrine. The latter is a less potent mediator of the clinical constellation seen in pheochromocytoma. However, compared with neuroblastoma, both catecholamines are more commonly produced by pheochromocytomas. Pheochromocytomas, particularly those of adrenal origin, produce the enzyme PNMT, which converts norepinephrine to epinephrine. As such, the norepinephrine to epinephrine ratio has been used to distinguish pheochromocytomas of adrenal from those of extra-adrenal origin.

With respect to diagnostic imaging, the initial methodology in suspected cases is ultrasonography (Fig. 43.8). Thereafter, either CT or MRI can be employed to confirm the diagnosis of an adrenal or a para-adrenal mass (Fig. 43.9). Serologic or creatinine-specific measures of catecholamine excretion in the urine are then undertaken. The most specific diag-

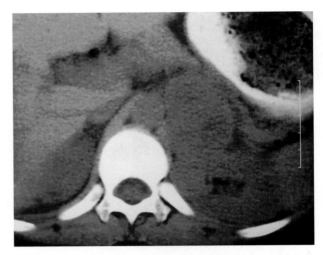

Figure 43.9 Computed tomographic image of left suprarenal pheochromocytoma, as seen in ultrasound in Figure 43.8.

nostic imaging methodology is radionucleotide scanning using [131I]MIBG scintigraphy (Fig. 43.10). With this approach, the sensitivity is greater than 90% (Dunnick et al., 1996). [131I]MIBG scanning is particularly valuable in the localization of tumors located outside the adrenal gland (Francis and Korobkin, 1996; Nielsen et al., 1996).

One of the persisting challenges in pheochromocytoma management remains the inability to define precisely whether a given tumor is benign or malignant. The current gold standard criterion for

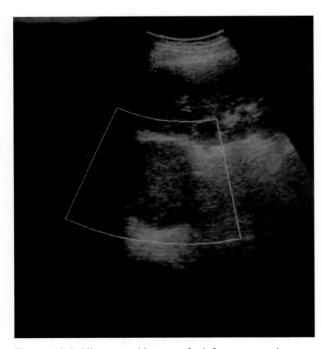

Figure 43.8 Ultrasound image of a left suprarenal tumor in a 16-year-old child presenting with hypertension.

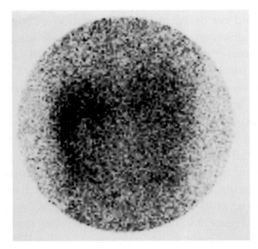

Figure 43.10 MIBG abdominal scan, with uptake of radionuclide in the left suprarenal area, in a 16-year-old with pheochromocytoma.

malignancy remains the appearance of metastases. As a predictor of malignancy, this is analogous to predicting that automobile brakes are defective based on the occurrence of a collision. Clearly, more accurate markers for determining malignancy of pheochromocytoma are needed. Recent studies have identified biologic features of pheochromocytomas that may hold promise in determining the metastatic proclivity of the tumor. For example, telomeres are comprised of repeated nucleotide sequences on the ends of chromosomes. During normal cell aging, they progressively shorten during successive normal cell replications. In normal cells, this shortening is thought to be associated with waning activity of the enzyme that produces the telomeres. Recent retrospective molecular analysis of pheochromocytoma tumors known to be benign or malignant reveals that telomerase, the RNA polymerase enzyme responsible for the production of telomeres, shows increased activity exclusively in tumors known to be malignant (Kinoshita *et al.*, 1998; Kubota *et al.*, 1998). Similarly, antibody-based approaches that detect proliferating cells are being used increasingly to describe the malignant phenotype in tumors. One such antibody, MIP-1, selectively recognizes cells engaged in the cell cycle (i.e. scheduled to undergo mitosis, but not necessarily in the process of mitosis). Its predictability was explored in a survey of pheochromocytomas in which malignancy was confirmed by the existence of metastases. A positive MIB-1 labeling index (defined as >3% of tumor cells staining positive for MIB-1 versus the total number of cells counted) showed a specificity of 100% (benign tumors stained negative) and sensitivity of 50% (half of the malignant tumors stained positive) (Clarke *et al.*, 1998). Although sensitivity was poor, the ability to define benign disease accurately in this manner would be clinically reassuring.

Therapy

The historic importance of pheochromocytomas with respect to surgery is not the technical nature of their excision but the associated anesthetic risks. These relate to the potential for drastic changes in the excretion of catecholamines upon manipulation and subsequent removal of the tumor. The challenges revolve around stabilization of blood pressure intraoperatively and the prevention of potential cardiovascular collapse at the time of tumor removal or ligation of the veins delivering catecholamines to the systemic circulation. In infants, particularly in the preoperative state, these risks pose a great concern. In view of the high specificity and reduced invasiveness of modern serologic and radionuclide diagnostic methodologies, risk factors are reduced. Prevention of problems when pheochromocytoma is considered the rule. As in adults, the mainstay of preoperative therapy includes blockade of α-adrenergic receptors (phenoxybenzamine) accompanied by adequate systemic volume repletion once the vasoconstrictive and volume-contracted state has been overcome. Cardiac β-blockade (propranolol) in every case to prevent reflex tachyarrythmias remains controversial but should at least be considered in selected cases. Clearly, preoperative pharmacologic management of affected children should be undertaken in collaboration with the pediatric endocrinologist and anesthesiologist. If adequate blockade and volume replacement are achieved preoperatively, manipulation of the tumor is usually not accompanied by large variations in blood pressure and large additional volume requirements are usually not found necessary upon tumor removal.

Open surgical excision by the flank or posterior lumbotomy approach has been the classic means of treatment. However, Rutherford *et al.* (1995) have published an excellent review of the laparoscopic experience of excision of these tumors. They noted that patients treated laparoscopically have a significant reduction in recovery time as well as a low complication rate. It may well be that this will become the most widely accepted method of surgical excision.

Sacrococcygeal teratoma

Sacrococcygeal teratoma (SCT) is the most common neoplasm in the newborn, and one of the first tumors successfully excised surgically (Wolley, 1986). Virchow coined the term 'teratoma', referring to a coccygeal growth with diverse anatomic characteristics. The tumors originate from all three embryologic tissues: ectoderm, mesoderm, and endoderm. Although they have provoked great interest because of their occurrence early in life and their dramatic appearance at birth, they have achieved even more current interest because of the facility and frequency with which they can be diagnosed by antenatal ultrasonography (Altran *et al.*, 1974; Ein *et al.*, 1985).

The appearance and character of the tumors are highly variable since they may be internal or external. SCTs have no known etiology. They are usually benign, but may undergo malignant degeneration.

Pathology

A teratoma is a neoplasm composed of multiple tissues that are foreign to the area in which it arises. Teratomas are grouped into those benign lesions with mature tissue (70%), those having malignant anaplastic elements (20%), and a third, embryonic group (10%), that may contain histologically immature-appearing benign tissue that does not progress to mature organ formation (Mahour *et al.*, 1975). This latter group carries a generally favorable prognosis following total excision. In the benign varieties, elements such as skin, teeth, central nervous system (CNS) tissue, cartilage, bone, and respiratory and alimentary mucosa may be seen.

Infants diagnosed with SCT at greater than 1 year of age as well as older children are more likely to have malignant elements. To detect these elements, the pathologist must undertake an extensive search through all of the varied elements within the tumor. The term 'yolk sac' or endodermal sinus tumor is the name appropriately used for the malignant elements in such tumors. These tissues represent a separate element of the teratomatous cell line. Elevated serum levels of α-fetoprotein may be seen in these cases.

Clinical features and presentation

The traditional mode of presentation of these tumors has been discovery at birth. In most developed countries where antenatal sonography is now either mandatory or prevalent, they are discovered by antenatal sonography. A recent review (Holterman *et al.*, 1998) of antenatally diagnosed SCTs demonstrated a high incidence of *in utero* mortality (19%) coupled with a perinatal mortality of 14%. The incidence of premature labor in this series was 50%. Thus, although the pathology of SCT is often benign, the overall outcome is associated with considerable morbidity and mortality. Those clinical features in the antenatal state that correlated with a poorer prognosis included polyhydramnios (an early sign of fetal distress and predictor of placental megaly-hydrops fetalis), tumor hypervascularity, or the presence of a solid tumor (a risk factor for both malignancy and vascular steal syndrome), large tumor size at delivery (>10 cm

in its greatest dimension), and a fast rate of tumor growth relative to cranial growth.

A solid tumor is the most ominous predictor of poor outcome. A fetus with a solid tumor has a mortality rate of 66% compared with a mortality of 11% for cystic or mixed tumors. Thus, mothers carrying a fetal diagnosis of SCT at the time of clinical obstetric presentation are definitely at risk for prenatal and perinatal complications. The presence of polyhydramnios appears to be a relative predictor or warning sign of premature labor.

There is a 5–25% association with other congenital anomalies in infants with benign SCT. Seventy-five per cent of the infants are female, harboring primarily benign tumors (Ein *et al.*, 1991). The sex distribution is more evenly distributed between males and females in those whose tumors develop malignant degeneration.

Classification

The classification of SCT was proposed in 1974 by Altman and includes: type 1, totally external; type 2, primarily external with internal component; type 3, almost completely internal; and type 4, totally internal (Altman *et al.*, 1973) (Fig. 43.11).

Today, since most SCTs may well be diagnosed in the antenatal state following obstetric ultrasonography, an improved prognosis may be anticipated following delivery by cesarean section. The latter is advised as an initial attempt to decrease perinatal mortality and morbidity. The major early cause for morbidity relates to tumor rupture, for which cesarean section is the best prophylaxis. In Altman's classification, large tumors were defined as being greater than 10 cm and these appear to be associated with greater morbidity.

When not diagnosed prior to birth, external tumors are found at delivery. Internal tumors may present as an abdominal mass with the diagnosis of SCT noted by neonatal ultrasonography. Some authors (Rauch, 1979) propose that all newborns should have a rectal examination to exclude internal SCT, but acknowledge that the rarity of the tumor would result in positive identification in only 1 out of 400 000 babies.

Laboratory

Tumors that undergo malignant degeneration may produce α-fetoprotein and/or β-human chorionic gonadotropin (β-hCG). These proteins are indicators of malignant degeneration in the dermal sinus or choriocarcinomatous components of the tumor (Wolley, 1986; Tsuchida *et al.*, 1989).

Imaging

Imaging studies for complete assessment include CT and MRI. Radiographic detection of calcification does not distinguish between benign and malignant tumors (Figs. 43.12, 43.13).

Treatment

With the increasing availability of antenatal diagnosis the question of antenatal intervention has had a logical appeal. Other forms of intrauterine therapy, such as intrauterine transfusion and decompression of a dilated urinary tract, have been successful as early as 16 weeks gestational age. However, large or completely external SCTs have not yet been uniformly successfully approached surgically (Ikeda *et al.*, 1990; Flake, 1993). It has been speculated that ligating the blood supply to the tumor prenatally may be effective in decreasing its size and/or controlling the hyperdynamic state in the perinatal period (Robertson *et al.*, 1995; Angel *et al.*, 1998). In spite of the attractive apparent potential for intrauterine treatment, no success has been seen in antenatal treatment or antenatal surgical excision.

Postnatal therapy of SCT is primarily surgical. Devascularization of the tumor may be of benefit; however, this is best applied as the first intraoperative

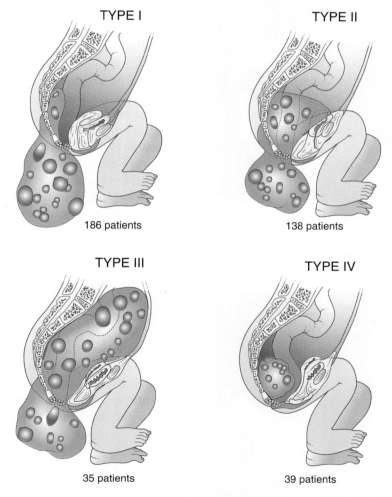

TYPE I

186 patients

TYPE II

138 patients

TYPE III

35 patients

TYPE IV

39 patients

Figure 43.11 Classification of sacrococcygeal teratomas. Type 1: tumors are predominantly external (sacrococcygeal) with only a minimal presacral component. Type 2: tumors present externally but with a significant intrapelvic extension. Type 3: tumors are apparent externally but the predominant mass is pelvic and extends into the abdomen. Type 4: tumors are presacral with no external presentation. (Adapted from Altman *et al.*, 1973.)

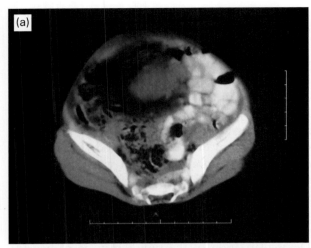

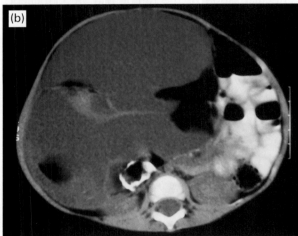

Figure 43.12 Computed tomographic images of cystic teratoma in a 6-month-old child, arising from the pelvis (*a*) and filling the abdomen (*b*).

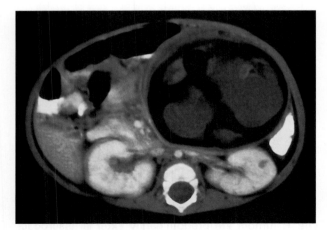

Figure 43.13 Computed tomographic image of a more solid teratoma filling the central abdomen in a 6-month-old child.

component of surgical removal (Robertson *et al.*, 1995; Angel *et al.*, 1998). Complete surgical excision should be the rule, with *en bloc* removal of the involved portion of the coccyx.

The two clinical groups of presentation include those that appear early in the neonatal period with large, benign tumors, and those that appear later (>1 year of age), which are often smaller, fixed, and malignant. In the first group, total removal is the rule and is best achieved by a midline sacral or chevron incision. The coccyx should be removed in the process of excising the tumor. With the retroperitoneal extension of the teratoma, urinary, internal genital, and gastrointestinal organs may be displaced. They can usually be dissected free, with minimal injury to the viscera, and good access to the vascular supply of the tumor is usually afforded by this retroperitoneal approach. However, in more extensive cases, anterior abdominal exploration may be warranted. A generous surgical exposure to obtain control of the presacral vessels is recommended. Avulsion of the vessels is a hazard to be avoided. In some rare instances, SCT may involve the dura or extend to the spine. This potential extension can be defined by meticulous preoperative imaging (Gross *et al.*, 1951; Donnellan and Sivenson, 1968; Ashcraft and Holder, 1974). An inadvertent entry into the dura may result in a cerebrospinal fluid leak, which is associated with a higher morbidity. Modern imaging techniques, particularly MRI, will allow a much more achievable definition of these potential extensions to the CNS.

The second group of patient presentation is represented by those children in whom tumors present at an age beyond 1 year. These tumors are generally symptomatic, fixed, and firm. Diagnosis is established by ultrasound and/or physical examination and confirmed by CT or MRI. These tumors are often of a malignant variety and serum α-fetoprotein is a sensitive marker. The appropriate surgical approach is initially directed at biopsy, followed by either multiagent chemotherapy or radiotherapy, in an attempt to decrease the size of the tumor, followed by surgical removal.

Results of therapy

There are only rare reports of success in therapy in the antenatal stage (Flake, 1993). In postnatal excisions, those undertaken in infancy for both external and internal SCT are remarkably successful in achieving complete removal of tumors with relatively little long-term morbidity (Shanbhogue *et al.*, 1990). Incontinence is rare (Ein *et al.*, 1980). However, in those cases where high sacrococcygeal extension is present necessitating transabdominopelvic excision, long-term fecal soiling and incontinence may be more prevalent. These sequelae may be related to more direct injury of skeletal muscular components or to some more occult neurogenic impairment of the viscera (Bass *et al.*, 1991). These sequelae may also be seen in the newborns after the excision of large, benign tumors.

Malignant SCT is rare in children under 6 months of age but, beyond that, the incidence rises sharply (Hickey and Layton, 1954). Malignant tumors may invade adjacent tissues or may recur in up to 40% of cases. During the 1990s, chemotherapeutic regimes have added considerably to the improved outcomes (Shanbhogue *et al.*, 1989; Bilik *et al.*, 1993).

Long-term follow-up

A recent evaluation of long-term follow-up in children with SCT showed that mature teratomas may have a recurrence rate of up to 11%. Further treatment with surgical excision and combined chemotherapy resulted in an 85% cure rate (Göbel *et al.*, 1998). On long-term follow-up, a 3% recurrence rate was noted for immature teratomas. They were detected by a rising α-fetoprotein level 6 months after the initial procedure. These responded well to local excision. Endodermal sinus tumors detected and treated initially with surgical excisions represented only 9% of the tumors presenting at birth, whereas they represented 27% of the patients presenting at an older age. With long-term follow-up, 89% are still alive in spite of the higher recurrence rate.

Adrenal carcinoma

Adrenal carcinoma represents fewer than 0.0001% of neoplastic tumors in children. The most common presentation is abnormal virilization, occurring in two-thirds (Hayles *et al.*, 1996). Symptoms consistent with Cushing's syndrome account for most of the remainder. Individual case reports have reported occasional aldosterone-secreting tumors. Given the widespread availability of ultrasound imaging technology, the most common presentation may now be that of an incidental finding on an abdominal ultrasound.

Adrenocortical tumors may also be a component of more global genetic malformations. These include children with congenital adrenal hyperplasia, multiple endocrine syndromes (MEN 1), and Beckwith–Wiedemann syndrome.

Clinical presentation

Virilizing adrenal tumors

Of the functioning adrenal cortical tumors, virilizing forms account for two-thirds, usually occurring in children older than 2 years. The tumors produce dehydroepiandrosterone (DHA), a weak androgen but one that is converted to delta-4-androstenedione and testosterone, which are more potent virilizing hormones. Boys with such tumors present with signs of precocious puberty. Girls respond with an increase in clitoral size, similar to that seen with congenital adrenal hyperplasia (Fig. 43.14). Pubic and axillary hair may be seen in children of either gender.

Alternate causes of premature virilization in boys include interstitial cell tumors of the testis or as a delayed manifestation of congenital adrenal hyperplasia. Clinical evaluation may give some clues

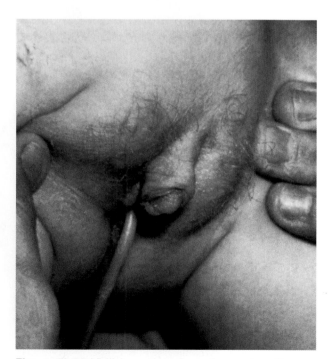

Figure 43.14 Virilizing adrenal carcinoma in a 5-year-old girl. Note clitoral hypertrophy and pubic hair. There is no posterior labial fusion, as would be seen in congenital adrenal hyperplasia.

towards distinguishing the underlying etiology. Unilateral or asymmetric testicular enlargement suggests a Leydig cell tumor. In patients with centrally stimulated precocious puberty, testicular enlargement is bilateral. With virilizing adrenal tumors, the testes are usually small.

The differential diagnosis in female children includes ovarian arrhenoblastoma and other rare tumors of the adrenal cortex.

Cushing's syndrome

Approximately one-third of children with adrenocortical tumors have the stigmata of Cushing's syndrome. Carcinoma may be responsible in up to one-half, with the others having bilateral adrenal hyperplasia. A benign adenoma may rarely be seen. The clinical appearance is in response to the excessive production of cortisol. This leads to protein catabolism, increased gluconeogenesis, and the typical

obesity associated with cortisol excess. The moon facies and truncal obesity (Fig. 43.15) of Cushing's disease are generally obvious when they are present in infants.

The differential diagnosis in patients exhibiting excess adrenocortical activity includes adrenal adenomas and iatrogenic administration of steroids. This latter iatrogenic excess is commonly seen in children receiving transplanted organs.

Feminizing adrenal tumors

Feminizing adrenal tumors are rare. They occur more frequently in males and in these cases the more commonly seen primary gynecomastia must be excluded.

Diagnostic evaluation

The critical diagnostic feature is the biochemical demonstration of adrenal hyperfunction. Urinary

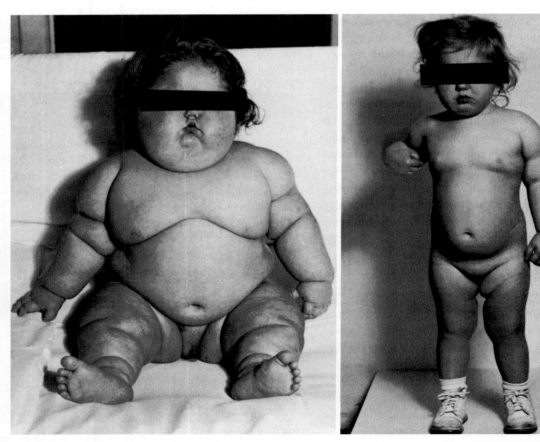

Figure 43.15 (Left) Striking features of cortisol excess in a 17-month-old girl with adrenocortical carcinoma. In addition, pubic hair and mild enlargement of the clitoris were present. (Right) At 10 months after removal of the adrenocortical carcinoma, there was complete regression of the signs of Cushing's syndrome.

steroids typically show a markedly elevated 17-ketosteroid level. The free cortisol, DHA, and 17-hydroxysteroid levels may also be elevated (Lipsett and Weson, 1962). Radioimmune assays of serum hormonal levels usually show elevation of DHA, delta-4-androstenedione, testosterone and cortisol (Suez *et al.*, 1971; Cahen *et al.*, 1978). Serum estrogen levels are elevated in the rare feminizing cases (Axelrod *et al.*, 1968). Occassionally, an elevated serum aldosterone level can be demonstrated in cases of adrenocortical carcinoma (Jackson *et al.*, 1958).

In Cushing's syndrome caused by adrenocortical carcinoma, the plasma cortisol level and urinary corticosteroids are markedly elevated above the levels typically seen with adrenal hyperplasia or an adrenal adenoma. A significant elevation in 17-ketosteroids, pregnanetriol, and estrogens may suggest carcinoma. The adrenocorticotropic hormone (ACTH) stimulation test produces no change in adrenocortical carcinomas, whereas these with adrenal hyperplasia show an exaggerated normal response. In exogenous obesity, which occasionally may enter the differential diagnosis, the ACTH test result is normal. When benign adenomas are present, the ACTH test exhibits a subnormal response. Metyrapone blocks 11-hydroxylation in the adrenal cortex and leads to a fall in cortisol level with an increase in endogenous ACTH. Thus, a test with metyrapone produces results similar to those produced by the ACTH test. The diurnal variation usually seen in normal cortisol levels is absent with both tumors and adrenal hyperplasia. Dexamethasone blocks ACTH release in normal patients. The dexamethasone suppression test is useful to separate adrenal hyperplasia from tumors in that a large dose (8 mg) typically suppresses hyperplasia but not a tumor (Liddle, 1963; Linn *et al.*, 1967) (Table 43.5).

Modern diagnostic imaging has led to the greatest advances over the past decade. (See section on imaging techniques under *Neuroblastoma*.) In addition to the ultrasound findings, MRI scanning has led to tremendous advances in the ability to distinguish adrenal carcinoma from benign adenomas (Schwartz *et al.*, 1997; McGrath *et al.*, 1998).

Treatment

Treatment of adrenal cortical carcinoma is surgical. In children, open surgical removal may be accomplished by large, transverse abdominal incisions or, in some instances, by extended flank incisions. Laparoscopic removal is now widely used in adults but the current lack of small instrumentation limits its use in children (Godellas and Prinz, 1998). The advances in imaging allow more limited surgical approaches than may have been previously encountered. Tumor diameter of more than 5 cm is a reasonable predictor of malignancy, whereas small adenomas may be approached in a more limited manner. Preoperative care must recognize the need for corticosteroid replacement in cases where corticoid excess is anticipated.

The prognosis for adrenal carcinoma is poor. Surgery is the primary motive therapy and chemotherapy has not been effective in controlling widespread disease.

Table 43.5 Test results with various adrenocortical lesions

| Condition | Plasma cortisols | | Dexamethasone test[a] | | Metyrapone test response | Plasma ACTH |
	Concentration	Diurnal rhythm	Low-dose suppression	High-dose suppression		
Normal	Normal	Yes	Yes	Yes	Yes	Normal
Cushing's disease	High	No	No	Yes	Yes	Increases
Tumor	High	No	No	No	No	Decrease
Non-ACTH-dependent hyperplasia	High	No	No	No	No	Decrease
Ectopic ACTH syndrome	High	No	No	No	No	Increase

[a] Low dose = 0.22 mg/10 kg for 2 days; high dose = 0.84 mg/10 kg for 3 days.
ACTH = adrenocorticotropic hormone.

Lymphangiomas

Lymphangiomas are benign tumors comprised of a mass of anastomosing lymphatic channels. These are rare and most commonly affect the extremities. Most are congenital and may not become evident until a few years of age. When in the retroperitoneum they are found by the evaluation of abdominal pain, which may be caused by the onset of spontaneous hemorrhage into the mass. However, they may extend through the inguinal canal and present with the misdiagnosis of hernia. Diagnosis is made on CT, at which time the low-density characteristic of lymphatic tissue is noted.

Surgical excision of the majority of the wall of the tumor is ideal, but may not be technically possible without causing significant damage to adjacent organs. Large cysts may be drained into the peritoneal cavity.

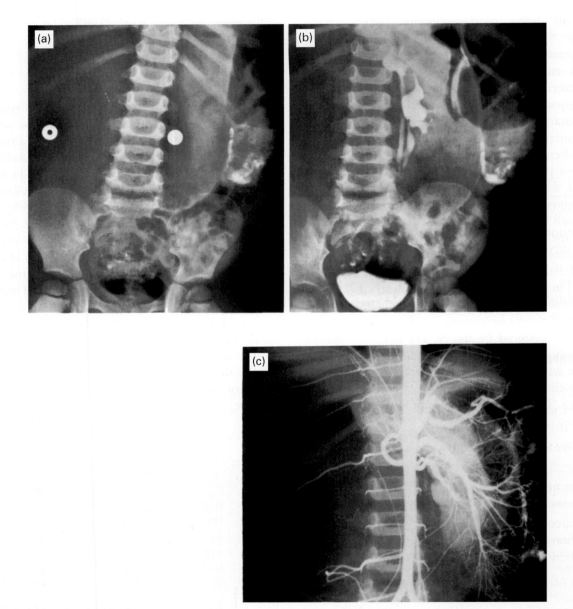

Figure 43.16 Retroperitoneal lipoma. (*a*) Abdominal film (KUB) demonstrating a retroperitoneal mass obliterating the right psoas shadow and displacing the bowel to the left. (*b*) Excretory urogram showing the right kidney and ureter displaced across the midline to the left. Note the absence of hydronephrosis. (*c*) Aortogram shows displacement of the right renal artery. The right kidney is now superior to the left kidney. The absence of neovascularity suggests the benign nature of the tumor.

Neurofibroma

Patients with neurofibromatosis (von Recklinghausen's disease) may present with abdominal neurofibromas similar to but as a more benign variant of ganglioneuromas. As outlined in the previous section on benign ganglioneuromas, partial excision may be an appropriate surgical treatment.

Lipoma

Retroperitoneal lipomas are usually benign, presenting as an abdominal mass in infants and young children (Fig. 43.16). CT defines the characteristically low-density lesions. These are generally benign and well encapsulated. Local excision is the treatment of choice.

Other malignant retroperitoneal tumors

Hodgkin's and non-Hodgkin's lymphomas may involve intra-abdominal viscera including the urinary and gastrointestinal tracts. Lateral deviation of the ureters is the most common genitourinary feature; however, ureteral obstruction may be the primary presenting symptom. Ureteral catheterization may become necessary in advance of chemotherapy.

Liposarcoma

Liposarcoma is rare in children, being seen more often in the teenage years leading into young adulthood. If it is identified early, surgical excision may result in complete cure.

Fibrosarcoma

Fibrosarcoma may be difficult to distinguish from neurofibroma. These lesions also occur primarily in the extremities, although retroperitoneal sites may be seen.

References

Altman RP, Randolph JG, Lilly JR (1973) Sacrococcygeal teratoma: American Academy of Pediatrics surgical section survey. *J Pediatr Surg* **9**: 389.

Altran R, Randolph JG, JRL, Lilly JR (1974) Sacroccygeal teratoma: American Academy of Pediatrics Surgical Section Surgery – 1973. *J Pediatr Surg* **9**: 389–98.

Angel CA, Murillo C, Mayhew J (1998) Experience with vascular control before excision of giant, highly vascular sacrococcygeal teratomas in neonates. *J Pediatr Surg* **33**: 1840–2.

Ashcraft KW, Holder TN (1974) Hereditary presacral teratoma. *J Pediatr Surg* **9**: 691–7.

Axelrod LR, Goldzieher JW, Woodhead DM (1968) Steroid biosynthesis in feminizing adrenal carcinomas. *J Clin Endocrinol Metab* **29**: 1481.

Bass J, Luks F, Yazbeck S (1991) Long-term follow-up of sacrococcygeal teratomas with emphasis on anorectal function. *Pediatr Surg Int.* **6**: 119–21.

Beckwith JB, Perrin EV (1963) *In situ* neuroblastoma: a contribution to the natural history of neural crest tumors. *Am J Pathol* **43**: 1089.

Bilik R, Shandling B, Pope M *et al.* (1993) Malignant benign neonatal sacrococcygeal teratoma. *J Pediatr Surg* **28**: 1158–60.

Black C (1997) Neuroblastoma. *Semin Pediatr Surg* **6**: 2–10.

Bonovarus A, Kirks DR, Grossman H (1986) Imaging of neuroblastoma: an overview. *Pediatr Radiol* **16**: 89–106.

Bowman LC, Castleberry RP, Cantor A *et al.* (1997) Genetic staging of unresectable or metastatic neuroblastoma in infants: a Pediatric Oncology Group study. *J Natl Cancer Inst* **89**: 373–80.

Bown N, Cotterill BA, Lastowska M *et al.* (1999) Gain of chromosome arm 17q and adverse outcome in patients with neuroblastoma. *N Engl J Med* **340**: 1954–61.

Brodeur G (1998) Clinical and biological aspects of neuroblastoma, In: Vogelstein B, Kinzler K W (eds) *The genetic basis of human cancer*. New York: McGraw-Hill.

Brodeur GM, Barrett A, Berthold F *et al.* (1998) International criteria for diagnosis, staging, and response to treatment in patients with neuroblastoma. *J Clin Oncol* **6**: 1874.

Brodeur GM, Castleberry RP (1997) Neuroblastoma. In Pizzo PA, Poplack DG (eds): *Principles and Practice of Pediatric Oncology*. Philadelphia, PA: JB Lippincott, 7712;

Brodeur GM, Nakagawara A, Yamashiro DJ *et al.* (1997) Expression of TrkA, TrkB and TrkC in human neuroblastomas. *J Neuro-Oncol* **31**: 49–55.

Brodeur GM, Seeger RC, Schwab M *et al.* (1984) Amplification of n-myc in untreated human neuroblastomas correlates with advanced stage of disease. *Science* **224**: 1121.

Cañete A, Jovani C, Lopez A *et al.* (1998) Surgical treatment for neuroblastoma: complications during 15 years' experience. *J Pediatr Surg* **33**: 1526–30.

Cahen LA, Villee DB, Powers ML *et al.* (1978) A virilizing adrenocortical tumor in a female infant: *in vivo* and *in vitro* biochemical characteristics. *J Clin Endocrinol Metab* **47**: 300.

Caron H, van Sluis P, de Kraker J *et al.* (1996) Allelic loss of chromosome 1p as a predictor of unfavorable outcome in patients with neuroblastoma. *N Engl J Med* **334**: 225–30.

Caron H. (1995) Allelic loss of chromosome 1 and additional chromosome 17 material are both unfavourable prognostic markers in neuroblastoma. *Med Pediatr Oncol* **24**: 215–21.

Castleberry RP (1997) Neuroblastoma. *Eur J Cancer* **33**: 1430–7; discussion 1437–8.

Chan HS, Gallie BL, DeBoer G et al. (1997) MYCN protein expression as a predictor of neuroblastoma prognosis. *Clin Cancer Res* **3**: 1699–706.

Cheung IY, Barber D, Cheung NK (1998) Detection of microscopic neuroblastoma in marrow by histology, immunocytology, and reverse transcription-PCR of multiple molecular markers. *Clin Cancer Res* **4**: 2801–5.

Cheung NK, Kushner BH, Cheung IY et al. (1998) Anti-G(D2) antibody treatment of minimal residual stage 4 neuroblastoma diagnosed at more than 1 year of age. *J Clin Oncol* **16**: 3053–60.

Cheung NK, Kushner BH, LaQuaglia MP et al. (1997) Survival from non-stage 4 neuroblastoma without cytotoxic therapy: an analysis of clinical and biological markers. *Eur J Cancer* **33**: 2117–20.

Clarke MR, Weyant RJ, Watson CG, Carty SE (1998) Prognostic markers in pheochromocytoma. *Hum Pathol* **29**: 522–6.

Combaret V, Gross N, Lasset C et al. (1997) Clinical relevance of TRKA expression on neuroblastoma: comparison with N-MYC amplification and CD44 expression. *Br J Cancer* **75**: 1151–5.

Donnellan WA, Swenson O (1968) Benign and malignant sacrococcygeal teratoma. *Surgery* **64**: 834–46.

Dunnick NR, Korobkin M, Francis I (1996) Adrenal radiology: distinguishing benign from malignant adrenal masses. *AJR Am J Roentgenol* **167**: 861–7.

Ein LH, Adeyemi AD, Mancer K (1980) Benign sacrococcygeal teratomas in infants and children. A 25 year review. *Ann Surg* **191**: 382–4.

Ein SH, Adeyemi SD, Mancer K (1991) Benign sacrococcygeal teratomas in infants and children: a 25 year review. *Ann. Surg* 382–4.

Ein SH, Mancer K, Adeyemi SD (1985) Malignant sacrococcygeal teratoma – endodermal sinus, yolk sac tumours – in infants and children: a 32 year review. *J Pediatr Surg* **20**: 473–7.

Evans AE, Albo V, D'Angio GJ et al. (1976) Factors influencing survival of children with non-metastatic neuroblastoma. *Cancer* **38**: 661.

Flake AW (1993) Fetal sacrococcygeal teratoma. *Semin Pediatr Surg* **2**: 113–20.

Francis IR, Korobkin M (1996) Pheochromocytoma. *Radiol Clin North Am* **34**: 1101–12.

Göbel U, Calaminus G, Engert J et al. (1998) Teratomas in infancy and childhood. *Med Pediatr Oncol* **31**: 8–15.

Godellas CV, Prinz RA (1998) Surgical approach to adrenal neoplasms: laparoscopic versus open adrenalectomy. *Surg Oncol Clin North Am* **7**: 807–17.

Graham KJ, McHenry CR (1998) The adrenal incidentaloma. *Surg Oncol Clin North Am* **7**: 749–62.

Gross RE, Clatworthy HWJ, Meeker IAJ (1951) Sacrococcygeal teratoma in infants and children: a report of 40 cases. *Surg Gynecol Obstet* **92**: 341–54.

Gurney JG, Ross JA, Wall DA et al. (1997) Infant cancer in the U.S.: histology-specific incidence and trends, 1973 to 1992. *J Pediatr Hematol Oncol* **19**: 428–32.

Halperin EC, Constine LC, Tarbell NJ, et al. (1994) Neuroblastoma. In: *Pediatric Radiation Oncology*. 2nd edition, Halperin EC (ed.). New York: Raven Press, 182–3.

Hann HW, Evans AE, Cohen IJ, Leitmeyer JE (1981) Biologic differences between neuroblastoma stages IV-S and IV. Measurement of serum ferritin and E-rosette inhibition in 30 children. *N Engl J Med* **305**: 425–9.

Hayles AB, Hanh HB, Sprague RG et al. (1996) Hormone-secreting tumors of the adrenal cortex in children. *Am J Med* **41**: 581.

Heij HA, Rutgers EJ, de Kraker J, Vos A (1997) Intraoperative search for neuroblastoma by MIBG and radioguided surgery with the gamma detector. *Med Pediatr Oncol* **28**: 171–4.

Hickey RC, Layton JM (1954) Sacrococcygeal teratoma. *Cancer* **7**: 1031–43.

Holterman A-X, Filiatrault D, Lallier M, Youssef S (1998) The natural history of sacrococcygeal teratomas diagnosed through routine obstetric sonogram: a single institution experience. *J Pediatr Surg* **33**: 899–903.

Ichikawa T, Ohtomo K, Araki T et al. (1996) Ganglioneuroma: computed tomography and magnetic resonance features. *Br J Radiol* **69**: 114–21.

Ichimiya S, Nimura Y, Kageyama H et al. (1999) p73 at chromosome 1p36.3 is lost in advanced stage neuroblastoma but its mutation is infrequent. *Oncogene* **18**: 1061–6.

Ikeda H, Okumura H, Nagashima K et al. (1990) The management of prenatally diagnosed sacrococcygeal teratoma. *Pediatr Surg Int* **5**: 192–4.

Jackson WPU, Zilberg B, Lewis B, McKenzie D (1958) Cushing's syndrome in childhood: report of case of adrenocortical carcinoma with excessive aldosterone production. *BMJ* **ii**: 130.

Joshi V, Cantor A, Altshuler G et al. (1992) Age-linked prognostic categorization base on a new histologic grading of neuroblastoma. *Cancer* **69**: 2197.

Katzenstein HM, Bowman LC, Brodeur GM et al. (1998) Prognostic significance of age, MYCN oncogene amplification, tumor cell ploidy, and histology in 110 infants with stage D(S) neuroblastoma: the pediatric oncology group experience – a pediatric oncology group study. *J Clin Oncol* **16**: 2007–17.

Kenney LB, Miller BA, Ries LA et al. (1998) Increased incidence of cancer in infants in the U.S.: 1980–1990. *Cancer* **82**: 1396–400.

Kinoshita H, Ogawa O, Mishina M et al. (1998) Telomerase activity in adrenal cortical tumors and pheochromocytomas with reference to clinicopathologic features. *Urol Res* **26**: 29–32.

Klingebiel T, Bader P, Bares R et al. (1998) Treatment of neuroblastoma stage 4 with 131I-meta-iodo-benzylguanidine, high-dose chemotherapy and immunotherapy. A pilot study. *Eur J Cancer* **34**: 1398–402.

Knudson AGJ, Strong LC. (1972) Neuroblastoma and pheochromocytoma. *Am J Hum Genet* **24**: 514.

Kogner P, Björk O, Theodorsson E (1993) Neuropeptide Y in neuroblastoma: increased concentration in metastasis, release during surgery, and characterization of plasma and tumor extracts. *Med Pediatr Oncol* **21**: 317–22.

Kogner P, Bjellerup P, Svensson T, Theodorsson E (1995) Pancreastatin immunoreactivity in favourable childhood neuroblastoma and ganglioneuroma. *Eur J Cancer* 31A: 557–60.

Kubota Y, Nakada T, Sasagawa I *et al.* (1998) Elevated levels of telomerase activity in malignant pheochromocytoma. *Cancer* **82**: 176–9.

Lastowska M, Cotterill S, Pearson AD *et al.* (1997a) Gain of chromosome arm 17q predicts unfavourable outcome in neuroblastoma patients. U.K. Children's Cancer Study Group and the U.K. Cancer Cytogenetics Group. *Eur J Cancer* **33**: 1627–33.

Lastowska M, Roberts P, Pearson AD *et al.* (1997b) Promiscuous translocations of chromosome arm 17q in human neuroblastomas. *Genes Chrom Cancer* **19**: 143–9.

Liddle GW (1963) Tests of pituitary-adrenal suppressibility in the diagnosis of Cushing's syndrome. *Arch Intern Med* **111**: 471.

Linn JE Jr, Boudoin B, Farmer TA, Meador CK (1967). Observations and comments on failure of dexamethasone suppression. *N Engl J Med* **277**: 403.

Lipsett MB, Weson H (1962) Adrenocortical cancer: steroid biosynthesis and metabolism evaluated by urinary metabolites. *J Clin Endocrinol* **22**: 906.

Mahour HG, Wooley MM, Trivedi SN, Landing BH (1975) Sacrococcygeal teratoma. *J Pediatr Surg* **10**: 183–8.

Massaron S, Seregni E, Luksch R *et al.* (1998) Neuron-specific enolase evaluation in patients with neuroblastoma. *Tumour Biol* **19**: 261–8.

Mastrangelo R, Tornesello A, Mastrangelo S (1998) Role of 131I-metaiodobenzylguanidine in the treatment of neuroblastoma. *Med Pediatr Oncol* **31**: 22–6.

Matthay KK, DeSantes K, Hasegawa B *et al.* (1998) Phase I dose escalation of 131I-metaiodobenzylguanidine with autologous bone marrow support in refractory neuroblastoma. *J Clin Oncol* **16**: 229–36.

McGrath PC, Sloan DA, Schwartz RW, Kenady DE (1998) Advances in the diagnosis and therapy of adrenal tumors. *Curr Opin Oncol* **10**: 52–7.

Mendelsohn G, Eggleston JC, Olson JL *et al.* (1976) Vasoactive intestinal polypeptide and its relationship to ganglion cell differentiation in neuroblastoma. *Cancer* **37**: 846.

Michalek AM, Buck GM, Nasca PC *et al.* (1996) Gravid health status, medication use, and risk of neuroblastoma. *Am J Epidemiol* **143**: 996–1001.

Morris JA, Shcochat SJ, Smith EI *et al.* (1995) Biological variables in thoracic neuroblastoma: a Pediatric Oncology Group study. *J Pediatr Surg* **30**: 296–302; discussion 302–3.

Moschovi M, Arvanitis D, Hadjigeorgi C *et al.* (1997) Lat malignant transformation of dormant ganglioneuroma. *Med Pediatr Oncol* **28**: 377–81.

Nakajima K, Fukuzawa M, Fukui Y *et al.* (1997) Laparoscopic resection of mass-screened adrenal neuroblastoma in an 8-month-old infant. *Surg Laparosc Endosc* **7**: 498–500.

Nielsen NR, Nielsen BV, Rehling M (1996) Location of adrenal medullary pheochromocytoma by I-123 metaiodobenzylguanidine SPECT. *Clin Nucl Med* **21**: 695–9.

Nitschke R, Smith EI, Altshuler G *et al.* (1991) Treatment of grossly unresectable localized neuroblastoma: a Pediatric Oncology Group study. *J Clin Oncol* **9**: 1181.

Peled N, Baby NP, deNanossy Q (1992) The computed tomographic appearance of subcutaneous nodules occurring in neuroblastoma. *Can Assoc Radiol J* **43**: 491–442.

Plantaz D, Mohapatra G, Matthay KK *et al.* (1997) Gain of chromosome 17 is the most frequent abnormality detected in neuroblastoma by comparative genomic hybridization. *Am J Pathol* **150**: 81–9.

Rauch MM (1979) Sacrococcygeal teratoma. In: Rauch MMWK, Benson CD *et al.* (eds) *Pediatric surgery*. Chicago, IL: Year Book.

Robertson FM, Crombleholme TM, Frantz IDR *et al.* (1995) Devascularization and staged resection of giant sacrococcygeal teratoma in the premature infant. *J Pediatr Surg* **30**: 309–11.

Rutherford JC, Gordon RD, Stowasser M *et al.* (1995) Laparoscopic adrenalectomy for adrenal tumours causing hypertension and for 'incidentalomas' of the adrenal on computerized tomography scanning. *Clin Exp Pharmacol Physiol* **22**: 490–2.

Saito T, Tsunematsu Y, Saeki M *et al.* (1997) Trends of survival in neuroblastoma and independent risk factors for survival at a single institution. *Med Pediatr Oncol* **29**: 197–205.

Sakakibara M, Koizumi S, Saikawa Y *et al.* (1999) Membrane-type matrix metalloproteinase-1 expression and activation of gelatinase A as prognostic markers in advanced pediatric neuroblastoma. *Cancer* **85**: 231–9.

Schwartz LH, Panicek DM, Doyle MV *et al.* (1997) Comparison of two algorithms and their associated charges when evaluating adrenal masses in patients with malignancies. *AJR Am J Roentgenol* **168**: 1575–8.

Seeger RC, Wada R, Brodeur GM *et al.* (1985) Association of multiple copies of the N-myc oncogene with rapid progression of neuroblastomas. *N Engl J Med* **313**: 1111.

Shamberger RC, Smith EI, Joshi VV *et al.* (1998) The risk of nephrectomy during local control in abdominal neuroblastoma. *J Pediatr Surg* **33**: 161–4.

Shanbhogue LKR, Bianchi A, Doig CM, Gough DCS (1990) Management of benign sacrococcygeal teratoma: Reducing mortality and morbidity. *Pediatr Surg* **5**: 41–4.

Shanbhogue LKR, Gough DCS, Jones PM (1989) Malignant sacrococcygeal teratoma: improved survival with chemotherapy. *Pediatr Surg Int* **4**: 202–4.

Shimada H, Chatten J, Newton WA *et al.* (1984) Histopathologic prognostic factors in neuroblastic tumors. *J Natl Cancer Inst* **73**: 405–16.

Shimada H, Stram DO, Chatten J *et al.* (1995) Identification of subsets of neuroblastomas by combined histopathologic and N-myc analysis. *J Natl Cancer Inst* **87**: 1470–6.

Snyder HM, D'Angio GJ, Evans AE *et al.* (1986) Paediatric oncology. In: Walsh PC, Girres RF, Perlmutter AD, Raney RB (eds) *Campbell's urology*, 5th edn. Philadelphia, PA: W.B. Saunders, p. 2269.

Stram DO, Matthay KK, O'Leary M *et al.* (1996) Consolidation chemoradiotherapy and autologous bone marrow transplantation versus continued chemotherapy for metastatic neuroblastoma: a report of two concurrent Children's Cancer Group studies. *J Clin Oncol* **14**: 2417–26.

Suez JM, Lorans B, Morera AM *et al.* (1971) Studies of androgens and their precursors in adrenocortical virilizing carcinomas. *J Clin Endocrinol Metab* **32**: 462.

Takita J, Hayashi Y, Yokota J (1997) Loss of heterozygosity in neuroblastomas – an overview. *Eur J Cancer* **33**: 1971–3.

Tsuchida Y, Kaneko M, Fukui M *et al.* (1989) Three different types of alpha-fetoprotein in the diagnosis of malignant solid tumors: use of a sensitive lectin-affinity immunoelectrophoresis. *J Pediatr Surg* **24**: 350–5.

Weiss WA, Aldape K, Mohapatra G *et al.* (1997) Targeted expression of MYCN causes neuroblastoma in transgenic mice. *Embo J* **16**: 2985–95.

Wolley MM (1986) Teratoma. In: Welch KJ, Randolph JG, Revich MM *et al.* (eds) *Pediatric surgery.* 14th edition. Chicago, IL: Year Book, 265–76.

Woods WG, Tuchman M, Robison LL *et al.* (1996) A population-based study of the usefulness of screening for neuroblastoma. *Lancet* **348**: 1682–7.

Woods WG, Tuchman M, Robison LL *et al.* (1997) Screening for neuroblastoma is ineffective in reducing the incidence of unfavourable advanced stage disease in older children. *Eur J Cancer* **33**: 2106–12.

Zahm SH, Ward MH (1998) Pesticides and childhood cancer. *Environ Health Perspect* **106** (Suppl 3): 893–908.

Index

Page numbers in *italics* indicate illustrations; page numbers in **bold** indicate tables.